THE UNFAVORABLE RESULT IN PLASTIC SURGERY

AVOIDANCE AND TREATMENT

THIRD EDITION

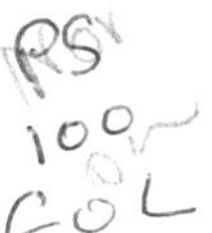

THE UNFAVORABLE RESULT IN PLASTIC SURGERY

AVOIDANCE AND TREATMENT

THIRD EDITION

ROBERT M. GOLDWYN, MD

Clinical Professor of Surgery
Harvard Medical School
Beth Israel Deaconess Medical Center
Boston, Massachusetts

MIMIS N. COHEN, MD

Professor and Chief of Plastic Surgery
University of Illinois at Chicago, and
Cook County Hospital
Chicago, Illinois

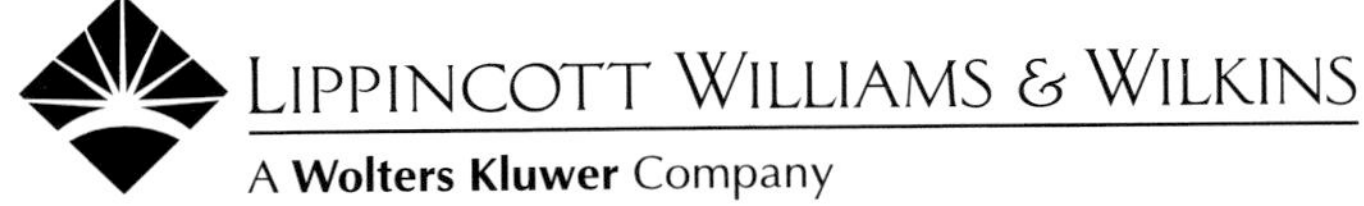
LIPPINCOTT WILLIAMS & WILKINS
A **Wolters Kluwer** Company
Philadelphia • Baltimore • New York • London
Buenos Aires • Hong Kong • Sydney • Tokyo

Acquisitions Editor: Beth Barry
Developmental Editor: Joanne Bersin/Delois Patterson
Production Editor: Tony DeGeorge
Manufacturing Manager: Benjamin Rivera
Cover Designer: Mark Lerner
Compositor: Maryland Composition
Printer: Maple Press

530 Walnut Street
Philadelphia, PA 19106 USA
LWW.com

Printed in the USA

Library of Congress Cataloging-in-Publication Data

The unfavorable result in plastic surgery : avoidance and treatment / edited by Robert M. Goldwyn, and Mimis N. Cohen.—3rd ed.
p. cm.
Includes bibliographical references and index.
ISBN 0-7817-1819-8
1. Surgery, Plastic—Complications. I. Goldwyn, Robert M. II. Cohen, Mimis.

RD118.7 .U54 2001
617.9′5—dc21

2001023445

Care has been taken to confirm the accuracy of the information presented and to describe generally accepted practices. However, the authors, editors, and publisher are not responsible for errors or omissions or for any consequences from application of the information in this book and make no warranty, expressed or implied, with respect to the currency, completeness, or accuracy of the contents of the publication. Application of this information in a particular situation remains the professional responsibility of the practitioner.

The authors, editors, and publisher have exerted every effort to ensure that drug selection and dosage set forth in this text are in accordance with current recommendations and practice at the time of publication. However, in view of ongoing research, changes in government regulations, and the constant flow of information relating to drug therapy and drug reactions, the reader is urged to check the package insert for each drug for any change in indications and dosage and for added warnings and precautions. This is particularly important when the recommended agent is a new or infrequently employed drug.

Some drugs and medical devices presented in this publication have Food and Drug Administration (FDA) clearance for limited use in restricted research settings. It is the responsibility of the health care provider to ascertain the FDA status of each drug or device planned for use in their clinical practice.

10 9 8 7 6 5 4 3 2 1

To our wives, Tatyana and Andrea

CONTENTS

SECTION IV: SKIN AND ADNEXA 269

SECTION V: HEAD AND NECK 301

SECTION VI: TRUNK 619

SECTION VII: HAND 691

CONTRIBUTING AUTHORS

Bruce M. Achauer, MD, FACS Professor of Surgery, Department of Plastic Surgery, University of California, Irvine Medical Center, Orange, California

William P. Adams, Jr., MD Assistant Professor, Department of Plastic Surgery, University of Texas Southwestern Medical Center at Dallas; Chief, Department of Plastic Surgery, Parkland Health and Hospital Systems, Dallas, Texas

Adrien Aiache, MD, FACS Attending Plastic Surgeon, Cedars-Sinai Medical Center, Beverly Hills, California

Gilbert Aiach, MD Private Practice, Paris, France

Tina S. Alster, MD Clinical Associate Professor, Department of Medicine, Georgetown University Hospital; and Director, Washington Institute of Dermatologic Laser Surgery, Washington, DC

David B. Apfelberg, MD Assistant Clinical Professor, Plastic Surgery, Stanford University Medical Center; Director, Atherton Plastic Surgery Center, Atherton, California

Louis C. Argenta, MD, FACS Professor and Chair of Plastic and Reconstructive Surgery, Wake Forest University School of Medicine, Medical Center Boulevard, Winston-Salem, North Carolina

Eric Arnaud, MD Consultant, Craniofacial Unit Hospital Necker, Paris, France

Phillip G. Arnold, MD Chair, Department of Plastic Surgery, Mayo Clinic, Rochester, Minnesota

Hirotaka Asato, MD Department of Plastic and Reconstructive Surgery, Graduate School of Medicine, University of Tokyo, Tokyo, Japan

Thomas J. Baker, MD, FACS Instructor, Department of Plastic Surgery, University of Miami School of Medicine, Miami, Florida; Department of Plastic Surgery, Mercy Hospital, Miami, Florida

Tracy M. Baker, MD Instructor in Plastic Surgery, Department of Plastic Surgery, University of Miami School of Medicine, Miami, Florida; Department of Plastic Surgery, Mercy Hospital, Miami Florida

Michael S. Beckenstein, MD Faculty, Plastic Surgery, St. Vincent's Hospital, Birmingham, Alabama

Teresa Benacquista, MD Assistant Professor, Department of Plastic Surgery (Microsurgery), Montefiore Medical Center, Bronx, New York

Prosper Benhaim, MD Assistant Professor, Departments of Surgery and Orthopaedic Surgery, University of California, Los Angeles, Los Angeles, California

Kristin Boehm, MD Division of Plastic Surgery, University of Utah Medical Center, Salt Lake City, Utah

J. Brian Boyd, MD, FACS Professor, Department of Surgery, Ohio State University, Columbus, Ohio; Chairman, Department of Plastic Surgery, Cleveland Clinic Hospital, Fort Lauderdale, Florida

Burton D. Brent, MD Private Practice, Woodside, California

Gregory M. Buncke, MD Assistant Clinical Professor, Division of Plastic Surgery, University of California at San Francisco; Co-director Microsurgery Service, Microsurgical Replantation and Transplantation, Davies Medical Center, San Francisco, California

Harry J. Buncke, MD, FACS Clinical Professor, Department of Surgery, Division of Plastic Surgery, University of California at San Francisco; Co-Director, Microsurgical Replantation and Transplantation, Davies Medical Center, San Francisco, California

Rudolf F. Buntic, MD Attending Surgeon, Microsurgical Replantation and Transplantation Department, Davies Medical Center, San Francisco, California

Patricia E. Burrows, MD Professor, Department of Radiology, Harvard Medical School; Director, Interventional Radiology, Department of Radiology, Children's Hospital, Boston, Massachusetts

Paul J. Carniol, MD, FACS Clinical Associate Professor, Department of Surgery, University of Medicine and Dentistry of New Jersey, Murray Hill, New Jersey

Lloyd N. Carlsen, MD, CM, FRCS(C), FACS Assistant Clinical Professor, Department of Surgery, McMaster University, Hamilton, Ontario, Canada; Division of Plastic Surgery, Scarborough Hospital, General Division, Scarborough, Ontario, Canada

Mack L. Cheney, MD, FACS Associate Professor, Department of Otolaryngology, Harvard Medical School, Boston, Massachusetts; Director Of Facial Plastic and Reconstructive Surgery, Department Of Otolaryngology, Massachusetts Eye and Ear Infirmary Boston, Massachusetts

David T. W. Chiu, MD, FACS Thomas S. Zimmer Professor of Clinical Surgery, Division of Plastic Surgery, Columbia-Presbyterian Medical Center, New York, New York

Thomas P. Cimino, Jr., JD Partner, Vedder, Price Law Firm, Chicago, Illinois

Mark A. Codner, MD Clinical Assistant Professor, Plastic Surgery, Emory University, Atlanta, Georgia; Paces Plastic Surgery, Atlanta, Georgia

I. Kelman Cohen, MD, PhD (Hon) Professor, Department of Surgery, Division of Plastic and Reconstructive Surgery, Medical College of Virginia, Richmond, Virginia

Meir Cohen, MD, MPS Instructor in Plastic Surgery, Department of Surgery, Sackler Faculty of Medicine, Tel-Aviv, Israel; Attending Surgeon, Department of Plastic Surgery, Schneider Childrens' Medical Center of Israel, Petach Tikva, Israel

Mimis N. Cohen, MD, FACS Professor and Chief, Divisions of Plastic Surgery, University of Illinois at Chicago, and Cook County Hospital, Chicago, Illinois

Steven R. Cohen, MD Center for Craniofacial Disorders, Scottish Rite Children's Medical Center, Atlanta, Georgia

John Joseph Coleman III, MD James E. Bennett Professor of Plastic Surgery, Department of Surgery, Indiana University School of Medicine; Chief, Division of Plastic Surgery, Indiana University, Medical Center, Indianapolis, Indiana

Mark B. Constantian, MD, FACS Adjunct Assistant Professor of Surgery, Dartmouth Medical School, Hanover, New Hampshire

Joseph Daw, MD Assistant Professor, Craniofacial Center, Division of Plastic Surgery, University of Illinois at Chicago, Illinois

Charles R. Day, MD Paces Plastic Surgery, Atlanta, Georgia

Rafael de la Plaza, MD Former Associate, Professor, Centro de Quemados Y Cirugia Plastica Cruz Roja, Universidad Complutense; Director, Plastic and Aesthetic Surgery Unit, La Luz Hospital, Madrid, Spain

Jorge I. de la Torre, MD Assistant Professor, Division of Plastic Surgery, University of Alabama at Birmingham, Birmingham, Alabama

Rosa L. Dell'Oca, MD Stanford University Medical Division of Hand Surgery, Palo Alto, California

A. Lee Dellon, MD Professor of Plastic Surgery and Neurosurgery, Johns Hopkins University, Baltimore, Maryland

Craig R. Dufresne, MD Clinical Professor, Department of Plastic Surgery, Georgetown University; Chief, Section of Plastic Surgery, INOVA Fairfax Hospital, Falls Church, Virginia

L. Franklyn Elliott, MD, FACS Atlanta Plastic Surgery, Atlanta, Georgia

Gregory R. D. Evans, MD, FACS Professor and Chief, Division of Plastic Surgery, The University of California, Irvine, College of Medicine and Health System, Orange, California

Afshin Farzadmehr, MD Department of Surgery, University of California, Irvine, California; Resident, Division of Dermatology, King/Drew Medical Center, University of California Los Angeles, School of Medicine, Los Angeles, California

Alvaro A. Figueroa, DDS, MS Co-director, Rush Craniofacial Center, Presbyterian-St. Luke's Medical Center, Chicago, Illinois

Jack Fisher, MD Associate Clinical Professor, Department of Plastic Surgery, Vanderbilt University; Chief, Department Of Plastic Surgery, Baptist Hospital, Nashville, Tennessee

R. Jobe Fix, MD Professor, Department of Surgery, The University of Alabama at Birmingham, Birmingham, Alabama

Peter B. Fodor, MD, FACS Associate Clinical Professor, Department of Plastic Surgery, University of California at Los Angeles; and Chief, Department of Plastic Surgey, Century City Hospital, Los Angeles, California

Elizabeth Fox, MD Miami, Florida

David W. Furnas, MD, FACS Clinical Professor of Surgery (Plastic), Division of Plastic Surgery, University of California, Irvine, Orange, California

Laurence J. Garey, MD Division of Neuroscience, Imperial College School of Medicine, Charing Cross Hospital, London, United Kingdom

Paul M. Glat, MD Assistant Professor, Department of Surgery, Medical College of Pennsylvania, Philadelphia, Pennsylvania; Chief, Division of Plastic Surgery, Saint Christopher's Hospital for Children, Philadelphia, Pennsylvania

Robert M. Goldwyn, MD Clinical Professor of Surgery, Harvard Medical School, Beth Israel Deaconess Medical Center, Boston, Massachusetts

Mark H. Gonzalez, MD Chief, Hand Service, Department of Surgery, Division of Orthopaedic Surgery, Cook County Hospital, Chicago, Illinois

Mark Gorney, MD, FACS Medical Director, The Doctors' Company, Napa, California

William P. Graham III, MD Professor of Surgery and Anatomy, Department Of Surgery, Division of Plastic Surgery, Pennsylvania State University and M.S. Hershey Medical Center, Hershey, Pennsylvania

Mark S. Granick, MD, FACS Professor of Surgery, Medical College of Pennsylvania—Hahnemann University; Chief, Division of Plastic Surgery, Medical College of Pennyslvania Hospital and Hannemann Hospital, Philadelphia, Pennsylvania

James C. Grotting, MD Clinical Professor, Department of Plastic Surgery, University of Alabama at Birmingham; and Grotting, Core, Wolfley, and Clinton Plastic Surgery Clinic, Birmingham, Alabama

Ronald P. Gruber, MD, FACS Clinical Assistant Professor, Department of Plastic and Reconstructive Surgery, Stanford University, Stanford, California; Department of Surgery, Hawthorne and Webster, Oakland, California

José Guerrerosantos, MD, FACS Chairman and Professor, Division of Plastic Surgery, University of Guadalajara; Chairman and Director, The Valisco Plastic Surgery Institute, Guadalajara, Jalisco, Mexico

Karsten K. H. Gundlach, MD, DDS, MSD Professor, Department of Maxillofacial and Facial Plastic Surgery, Rostock University; Chairman, Department of Maxillofacial and Facial Plastic Surgery, University Hospital Rostock, Rostock, Germany

Abhay Gupta, MD, FRCSC Fellow, Department of Plastic Surgery, University of Texas MD Anderson Cancer Center, Houston, Texas

Bahman Guyuron, MD, FACS Clinical Professor of Plastic Surgery, Department of Plastic Surgery, Case Western Reserve University, Cleveland, Ohio

Mutaz B. Habal, MD, FRCSC, FACS Director, Tampa Bay Craniofacial Center, Research Professor, University of Southern Florida, Tampa, Florida; Adjunct Professor of Material Sciences, University of Florida; President of the Medical Staff, St. Joseph Health Center; Surgeon, University Community Hospital, Tampa, Florida

Geoffrey G. Hallock, MD, FACS Consultant, Division of Plastic Surgery, Lehigh Valley Hospital, Allentown, Pennsylvania

Kiyonori Harii, MD Professor, Department of Plastic and Reconstructive Surgery, Graduate School of Medicine, University of Tokyo; Chair, Department of Plastic and Reconstructive Surgery, University of Tokyo, Tokyo, Japan

Vincent Rodney Hentz, MD Professor, Department of Surgery, Stanford University, Palo Alto, California; Chief, Division of Hand Surgery, Stanford, California

Saul Hoffman, MD Clinical Professor of Surgery, Mount Sinai School of Medicine, New York , New York

Michael S. Hohlastos, BS Department of Plastic and Reconstructive Surgery, Rush-Presbyterian-St. Luke's Medical Center, Chicago, Illinois

Larry Hollier, Jr., MD Assistant Professor, Department of Plastic Surgery, Baylor College of Medicine, Houston, Texas

Nicholas Iliff, MD Associate Professor, Department of Ophthalmology and Plastic Surgery, John Hopkins University School of Medicine, Baltimore, Maryland

Yves-Gerard Illouz, MD Chief, Department of Aesthetic Surgery, Saint Louis Hospital, Paris, France

Ian T. Jackson, MD, DSc (Hon), FACS, FRCS, FRACS (Hon) Director Institute for Craniofacial and Reconstructive Surgery, Southfield, Michigan; Chief, Division of Plastic Surgery, Providence Hospital, Southfield, Michigan

Jonathan S. Jacobs, DMD, MD, FACS Associate Professor of Clinical Plastic Surgery, Department of Surgery, Eastern Virginia Medical School, Norfolk, Virginia; Chairman, Surgical Executive Committee, Sentara Leigh Hospital, Sentara Hospitals—Norfolk, Norfolk, Virginia

Vivek Jain, MCh (Ortho) Clinical Fellow of Plastic and Reconstructive Surgery, Chang Gung Memorial Hospital, Taipei, Taiwan

Aldona Jedrysiak, MD Resident, Division of Plastic Surgery, Baylor College of Medicine, Houston, Texas

Craig H. Johnson, MD Assistant Professor, Mayo Medical School, Rochester, Minnesota; Consultant, Division of Plastic Surgery, Mayo Clinic, Rochester, Minnesota

Neil Ford Jones, MD, FRCS Professor, Division of Plastic and Reconstructive Surgery; and Department of Orthopedic Surgery, University of California Los Angeles,

Los Angeles, California; Chief of Hand Surgery, University of California Los Angeles Medical Center, Los Angeles, California

Jennifer C. Kim, MD Department of Otology and Laryngology, Massachusetts Eye and Ear Infirmary, Boston, Massachusetts

Gabriel Kind, MD Assistant Clinical Professor, Department of Surgery, Division of Plastic Surgery, University of California, San Francisco, San Francisco, California; Assistant Director of Fellowship and Research, Hand and Microsurgery Fellowship, The Buncke Clinic at the Davies Campus of California Pacific Medical Center, San Francisco, California

Stanley Klatsky, MD Associate Professor, Department of Plastic Surgery, Johns Hopkins University, Baltimore, Maryland

Michael Klebuc, MD Texas Children's Hospital, Houston, Texas

Stephen S. Kroll, MD (deceased) Formerly Professor of Plastic Surgery, University of Texas MD Anderson Cancer Center, Houston, Texas

Amy Lai, MD Clinical Instructor, Department of Otology and Laryngology, Massachusetts Eye and Ear Infirmary, Boston, Massachusetts; Department of Surgery, Winchester Hospital, Winchester, Massachusetts

W. Thomas Lawrence, MPH, MD Professor, Section of Plastic Surgery, University of Kansas Medical School, Kansas City, Kansas; Chief of Plastic Surgery, Section of Plastic Surgery, Kansas University Medical Center, Kansas City, Kansas

William C. Lineaweaver, MD, FACS Professor, Department of Surgery, Department of Physiology, University of Mississippi Medical Center, Jackson, Mississippi

J. William Little, MD Director Emeritus and Clinical Professor of Plastic Surgery, Division of Plastic Surgery, Georgetown University School of Medicine, Washington, DC; Chief of Plastic Surgery, Medstar—Georgetown Center for Ambulatory Surgery, Washington, DC

Ted E. Lockwood, MD, FACS Associate Clinical Professor, Department of Surgery, Division of Plastic Surgery, University of Kansas Medical School, Kansas City, Kansas

Donald R. Mackay, MD Associate Professor, Department of Surgery and Pediatrics, Pennsylvania State University, Hershey, Pennsylvania; Chief, Division of Plastic Surgery, Milton Hershey Medical Center, Hershey, Pennsylvania

Susan E. Mackinnon, MD, FACS Shoenberg Professor and Chief, Division of Plastic and Reconstructive Surgery, Washington University School of Medicine, Saint Louis, Missouri; Plastic Surgeon-in-Chief, Department of Surgery, Barnes—Jewish Hospital, Saint Louis, Missouri

Gaston-François Maillard, MD Associate Professor, Department of Plastic Surgery, Lausanne University, Lausanne, Switzerland

Ernest K. Manders, MD Professor, Department of Surgery, University of Pittsburgh Medical Center, Pittsburgh, Pennsylvania

Paul N. Manson, MD, FACS Professor, Department of Surgery, The Johns Hopkins Hospital, Baltimore, Maryland

Daniel Marchac, MD Associate Professor, College Medicine, Hopitaux de Paris, Paris, France; Director Craniofacial Unit, Hospital Necker Enfants Malade, Paris, France

Jeffrey L. Marsh, MD Professor, Division of Plastic Surgery, Washington University School of Medicine, St. Louis, Missouri; Director, Pediatric Plastic Surgery, St. Louis Children's Hospital, St. Louis, Missouri

Jeannette Martello, MD, JD Private Practice, Plastic and Hand Surgery, Pasadena, California; Medical Consultant, Enforcement Program Probation Unit, Medical Board of California

Joseph G. McCarthy, MD Lawrence D. Bell Professor of Plastic Surgery, Director, Institute of Reconstructive Plastic Surgery, New York University Medical Center, New York, New York

Peter McKinney, MD, FACS Professor of Plastic Surgery, Department of Plastic Surgery, Northwestern University Medical School, Chicago, Illinois; Professor of Plastic Surgery, Department of Plastic Surgery Rush Medical College, Chicago, Illinois

Blair M. Mehling, MD Department of Plastic Surgery, University of Texas MD Anderson Cancer Center, Houston, Texas

Frederick J. Menick, MD Private Practice, Saint Joseph's Hospital, Tuscon, Arizona

Berkan Mersa, MD Department of Surgery, Eastern Virginia Medical School, Norfolk, Virginia

Fernando Molina, MD Hospital Angeles del Pedregal, Mexico City, Mexico

John B. Mulliken, MD, FACS Associate Professor of Surgery, Harvard Medical School, Boston, Massachusetts; Director, Craniofacial Center, Co-director,

Vascular Anomalies Center, The Children's Hospital, Boston, Massachusetts

Satoru Nagata, MD Director, Department of Reconstructive Plastic Surgery, Chiba Tokushukai Hospital, Funabashi, Chiba, Japan

Foad Nahai, MD, FACS Clinical Professor, Division of Plastic Surgery, Emory University, Atlanta, Georgia; Paces Plastic Surgery, Atlanta, Georgia

David T. Netscher, MD Professor, Division of Plastic Surgery, Baylor College of Medicine, Houston, Texas; Chief, Plastic Surgery Section, Veterans Affairs Medical Center, Houston, Texas

R. Barrett Noone, MD, FACS Clinical Professor of Surgery, Department of Surgery, University of Pennsylvania, Philadelphia, Pennsylvania; Chief, Division of Plastic Surgery, Main Line Hospitals, Bryn Mawr Hospital, Bryn Mawr, Pennsylvania

Fernando Ortiz Monasterio, MD Professor Emeritus, School of Medicine, Universidad Nacional Autónoma de México; Professor of Plastic Surgery, Department of Plastic & Reconstructive Surgery, Hospital General "Manuel Gea Gonzalez," Mexico City, Mexico

Douglas K. Ousterhout, MD, DDS Clinical Professor, Division of Plastic Surgery, University of California, San Francisco, California; Davies Medical Center, California Pacific Medical Center San Francisco, California

Stephen Pap, MD Plastic Surgeon, Department of Surgery, University of Massachusetts Medical School, Worcester, Massachusetts; Department of Surgery, Division of Plastic Surgery, University of Massachusetts Memorial Health Care, Worcester, Massachusetts

Jennifer Parker Porter, MD Assistant Professor, Bobby R. Alford Department of Otolaryngology and Communicative Sciences, Baylor College of Medicine, Houston, Texas; Department of Otolaryngology, The Methodist Hospital, Houston, Texas

John A. Persing, MD Professor, Chief, Department of Plastic Surgery, Yale University School of Medicine, New Haven, Connecticut; Chief, Plastic Surgery, Yale-New Haven Hospital, New Haven, Connecticut

Linda G. Phillips, MD, FACS Professor, Department of Surgery, University of Texas Medical Branch, Galveston, Texas; Chief, Division of Plastic Surgery University of Texas Medical Branch, Galveston, Texas

Ivo Pitanguy, MD, FACS, FICS Head Professor, Department of Plastic Surgery, Pontifical Catholic University of Rio de Janeiro, and the Carlos Chagas Institute of Post-Graduate, Medical Studies; Chief, 38th Infirmary, Santa Casa General Hospital, Rio de Janeiro, Brazil

John W. Polley, MD Department of Plastic and Reconstructive Surgery, Rush-Presbyterian-St. Luke's Medical Center, Chicago, Illinois

Jeffrey C. Posnick, DMD, MD, FRCS(C), FACS Clinical Professor, Plastic Surgery, Otolaryngology, Oral and Maxillofacial Surgery and Pediatrics, Georgetown University, Washington, DC; Director, Posnick Center for Facial Plastic Surgery, Chevy Chase, Maryland

Jason N. Pozner, MD Jupiter, Florida

Julian J. Pribaz, MD Associate Professor, Department of Plastic Surgery, Harvard Medical School, Boston, Massachusetts; Plastic Surgeon, Brigham and Women's Hospital, Boston, Massachusetts

Oscar M. Ramirez, MD Plastic and Aesthetic Surgery Center of Maryland, Timonium, Maryland

Neal R. Reisman, MD, JD Associate Clinical Professor of Plastic Surgery, Department of Plastic Surgery, Baylor College of Medicine, Houston, Texas; Associate Chief, Department of Plastic Surgery, St. Luke's Episcopal Hospital, Houston, Texas

Dominique Renier, MD Director of Neurosurgery, Craniofacial Unit, Service Neruochirurgie, Hôpital Necker Enfants Malades, Paris, France

Thomas L. Roberts III, MD, FACS Carolina Plastic Surgery, Spartanburg, South Carolina

Rod J. Rohrich, MD, FACS Professor and Chairman, Department of Plastic Surgery, University of Texas Southwestern Medical Center; Chief, Department of Plastic Surgery, Zale Lipshy University Hospital, Dallas, Texas

Elliott H. Rose, MD Associate Clinical Professor, Division of Plastic Surgery, Mount Sinai Medical Center; Director, The Aesthetic Surgery Center, New York, New York

Harvey M. Rosen, MD, DMD Clinical Associate Professor, Department of Surgery, University of Pennsylvania, Philadelphia, Pennsylvania; Chief, Division of Plastic Surgery, Pennsylvania Hospital Philadelphia, Pennsylvania

Gary J. Rosenberg, MD, FACS Florida Aesthetic Surgery Center, Delray Beach, Florida

J. Peter Rubin, MD Chief Resident in Plastic Surgery, Harvard University, Boston, Massachusetts

Ramon L. Ruiz, DMD, MD Clinical Fellow, Pediatric Craniofacial and Maxillofacial Surgery, Posnick Center for Facial Plastic Surgery, Chevy Chase, Maryland; and Instructor, Oral and Maxillofacial Surgery, University of North Carolina, Chapel Hill, North Carolina

A. Michael Sadove, MD Professor of Plastic Surgery, Indiana University School of Medicine, Indianapolis, Indiana

Roger E. Salisbury, MD Burn Unit – Macy Pavilion, New York Medical College and Westchester Medical Center, Valhalla, New York

Renato Saltz, MD, FACS Department of Surgery, University of Utah Medical Center, Salt Lake City, Utah

Kenneth E. Salyer, MD, FACS, FAAP Founding Director, International Craniofacial Institute, Medical City Dallas Hospital, Dallas, Texas

David B. Sarwer, PhD Departments of Psychiatry and Surgery, and Division of Plastic Surgery, University of Pennsylvania School of Medicine; and The Edwin and Fanny Gray Center for Human Appearance, Philadelphia, Pennsylvania

Robert R. Schenck, MD Hand Surgery Ltd., Chicago, Illinois

Jatin P. Shah, MD, FACS, FRCS (Hon) Professor of Surgery, Weill Medical College of Cornell University, New York, New York; Chief, Head and Neck Service, Chair in Head and Neck Oncology, Memorial Sloan-Kettering Cancer Center, New York, New York

Saleh M. Shenaq, MD, FACS Professor and Chief, Division of Plastic Surgery, Baylor College of Medicine, Houston, Texas; Chief, Plastic Surgery Service, The Methodist Hospital, Houston, Texas

Sumner A. Slavin, MD Associate Clinical Professor of Surgery, Beth Israel-Deaconess Hospital, Brookline, Massachusetts

Bonnie E. Smith, PhD, CCC-SLP Associate Professor—Speech Pathology, Department of Otolaryngology—Head and Neck Surgery, Department of Surgery, University of Illinois at Chicago, Chicago, Illinois; Director, Division of Speech Pathology, University of Illinois Hospital, Chicago, Illinois

Scott L. Spear, MD, FACS Professor, Department of Surgery, Georgetown University, Washington, DC; Chief, Division of Plastic Surgery, Georgetown University Hospital, Washington, DC

Melvin Spira, MD Baylor College of Medicine, Houston, Texas

Samuel Stal, MD, FACS Associate Professor, Department of Plastic Surgery, Baylor College of Medicine, Houston, Texas; Chief, Department of Plastic Surgery, Texas Children's Hospital, Houston, Texas

Thomas R. Stevenson, MD Professor and Chief, Division of Plastic Surgery, University of California, Davis, Sacramento, California

Berish Strauch, MD Professor and Chairman, Plastic Surgery, Albert Einstein College of Medicine, Bronx, New York; Professor and Chairman, Plastic Surgery, Montefiore Medical Center, Bronx, New York

James M. Stuzin, MD, FACS Plastic Surgery Associates, P.A., Miami, Florida

Walter G. Sullivan, MD, JD, FAAP, FCLM Private Practice, Nevada Plastic Surgery, Las Vegas, Nevada

John B. Tebbetts, MD, FACS Inamed Corporation, Dallas, Texas

Edward O. Terino, MD Medical Director, Plastic Surgery Institute of Southern California, Thousand Oaks, California; Los Robles Medical Center, Thousand Oaks, California

Julia K. Terzis, MD, PhD, FCRS(C) Professor, Department of Surgery, Division of Plastic and Reconstructive Surgery, Eastern Virginia Medical School, Norfolk, Virginia; Senior Staff Surgeon, Department of Plastic Surgery, Sentara Norfolk General Hospital, Norfolk, Virginia

Seth R. Thaller, MD Professor and Chief, Division of Plastic Surgery, University of Miami School of Medicine, Miami, Florida; Chief and Professor, Division of Plastic Surgery, Jackson Memorial Hospital, Miami, Florida

J. Kevin Thompson, PhD Department of Psychology, University of South Florida, Tampa, Florida

Dean M. Toriumi, MD, FACS Department of Otolaryngology-HNS, Chicago, Illinois

Walter P. Unger, MD University of Toronto, Toronto, Ontario, Canada

Joseph Upton, MD Associate Clinical Professor, Department of Surgery, Harvard Medical School, Boston, Massachusetts; Director, Division of Plastic Surgery, Beth Israel Deaconess Medical Center, Boston, Massachusetts

Victoria M. Vanderkam, RN, BS, CPSN Clinical Nurse III, Division of Plastic Surgery, University of California Irvine Medical Center, Orange, California

Henry C. Vasconez, MD, FACS Professor, Department of Surgery, University of Kentucky, Lexington, Kentucky; Chief, Division of Plastic Surgery, University of Kentucky Medical Center, Lexington, Kentucky

Luis O. Vásconez, MD Professor and Chief, Division of Plastic Surgery, University of Alabama at Birmingham, Birmingham, Alabama

James E. Vogel, MD Division of Plastic Surgery, The Johns Hopkins School of Medicine, Baltimore, Maryland

Fun-Chan Wei, MD, FACS Professor of Plastic and Reconstructive Surgery, Chang Gung Memorial Hospital, Taipei, Taiwan

Jeffrey Weinzweig, MD Clinical Instructor, Division of Plastic Surgery, University of Pennsylvania Medical Center, Philadelphia, Pennsylvania

Norman Weinzweig, MD Associate Professor of Plastic Surgery and Orthopedic Surgery, Divisions of Plastic Surgery and Orthopedic Surgery, University of Illinois at Chicago and Cook County Hospital, Chicago, Illinois

Bradon J. Wilhelmi, MD Division of Plastic Surgery, Southern Illinois University School of Medicine, Springfield, Illinois

H. Bruce Williams, MD, FRCSC Professor of Surgery, McGill University; Surgeon-in-Chief Department of Surgery, Montreal Children's Hospital, Montreal, Quebec, Canada

Richard Williams III, JD Partner, Vedder, Price Law Firm, Chicago, Illinois

S. Anthony Wolfe, MD Division of Plastic Surgery, University of Miami School of Medicine, Miami Children's Hospital, Miami, Florida

Michael J. Yaremchuk, MD Clinical Professor, Department of Surgery, Harvard Medical School, Boston, Massachusetts; Chief, Craniofacial Surgery, Department of Plastic and Reconstructive Surgery, Massachusetts General Hospital, Boston, Massachusetts

Elvin G. Zook, MD Chairman, Division of Plastic Surgery, Southern Illinois University School of Medicine, Springfield, Illinois

Ronald M. Zuker, MD, FRCSC, FACS, FAAP Professor, Department of Surgery, University of Toronto, Toronto, Ontario, Canada; Head, Division of Plastic Surgery, Department of Surgery, The Hospital for Sick Children, Toronto, Ontario, Canada

PREFACE

This third edition comes 28 years after the first and 16 years after the second. During those intervals, significant advances occurred in plastic surgery and in all medical disciplines. We now can do more for patients. Yet inevitably, unfavorable results, minor and major, still occur. This edition, like its predecessors, concerns these unpleasant realities.

When I was gathering material about complications for the first edition, I reported my own and enlisted others to do the same. A few senior plastic surgeons advised me to desist because they feared the medicolegal repercussions for our specialty and the personal consequences for myself if my name were to be forever linked to bad outcomes. Fortunately, perhaps miraculously, these predictions have proven false. In fact, attorneys for defendants have used this information to demonstrate to juries that a complication for which their client has been charged with negligence has been well described. Patients still come to me despite a reputation built partially on failed procedures, luckily not all mine.

By custom, this preface should have been written by both editors, Mimis Cohen and myself. As the (considerably) senior editor, I prevailed on him to let me author it because I wanted to praise and thank him for his constant enthusiasm, his prodigious work, and his sage counsel. If I had not enlisted him—and if he had not graciously agreed—this third edition would likely not have appeared. In this endeavor, as in my entire professional life, I have been blessed and am truly grateful.

We both appreciate more than we can express the labors of the contributing authors and discussants whose book this really is. We also want to thank the highly skilled professionals at Lippincott Williams & Wilkins who helped make this book possible, including Beth Barry, Joanne Bersin, Tony DeGeorge, Penny Bice, and Allison Risko.

Robert M. Goldwyn, MD

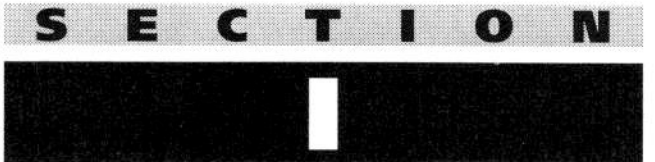

SECTION I

INTRODUCTION

1

WHY WE FAIL

ROBERT M. GOLDWYN

Men are men, they needs must err.
Euripides, *Hippolytus*

The ancients were right: to err is human. No patient and no surgeon can live a full life without being the victim or perpetrator of an error. This fact does not condone mistakes but recognizes their reality. The genesis of human fallibility has been variously ascribed to Original Sin, divine retribution, arrested evolution, astral mismatch, capricious fate, simple chance, malintent, and poor judgment. Whatever the cause or causes, the effect can be the same: despair and defeat.

Following a failure, most of us seek an explanation. Paré's philosophy, "I dress and God heals," may be valid for many medical situations but not all. Should God be blamed for a poorly designed flap? We tend to externalize responsibility: to look heavenward is easier than to look inward.

Oscar Wilde, however, recognized a basic truth: "There is a luxury in self-reproach. When we blame ourselves we feel that no one else has a right to blame us."

The title of this chapter, "Why We Fail," was chosen with care. Originally I called it "Why Things Go Wrong," but that would imply that an unfavorable result occurs because we are helpless victims of circumstances. Responsibility for actions is the cornerstone of Judeo-Christian religion. The burden on the individual is unrelenting. In our Western culture, whose development has been intimately related to science, it is unacceptable to say only that "something happened." We are compelled to probe why it occurred, although the explanation may not be obvious. For example, if on a wintry day someone falls, the easy answer might be that it was due to the ice. Indeed, that may be true, but the real cause might have been that the person was in poor health or was not wearing proper shoes or was rushing because he had risen too late from poor planning or laziness.

The purpose of this book is not just to name specific complications and unfavorable results. The reader should become aware of the more subtle conditions and factors that predispose to failure. These situations constitute what might be called the matrix of mistakes. The surgeon, like any other erring human being, in order to improve, must not only recognize and correct the mistake but, if possible, identify its cause and avoid it in the future. Admittedly, to be able to do this requires the talents of a Sherlock Holmes and a Sigmund Freud. Only by taking an unswerving look at ourselves during the course of treating patients can we find the critical points where errors commonly arise.

PREOPERATIVE

Incomplete Initial History and Hasty Physical Examination

The initial consultation can be either the moment of truth or the moment of deception. The most common cause of selecting the wrong patient, making the wrong diagnosis, or recommending the wrong treatment is not spending enough time with that patient. The assembly-line approach in the office invites disaster.

Hazards are inherent in different stages of our professional life. Success, for example, does not always make for continued success. On the contrary, it may confer defeat because of false security. When one begins a practice, one tries to establish a name. Later, the name by itself may come to represent the skills and care that the doctor once had but consciously or unconsciously no longer exercises. The doctor becomes sloppy, and the patient is the victim. The traps and trappings of a flourishing practice replace sound judgment and hard work. The surgeon may hire someone to take the history and even to talk to the patient about what to expect from the procedure and how to pay for it. The doctor may do the physical examination but in a superficial manner. Trying to operate on more patients may transform a physician into a policeman directing the medical traffic in the office. Under these circumstances, it is not hard to imagine how an error might occur.

No matter how well we plan our day, there frequently is not enough time for an adequate history and physical ex-

R. M. Goldwyn: Division of Plastic Surgery, Beth Israel Deaconess Medical Center, Harvard Medical School, Boston, Massachusetts

amination. It is better to inform the patient of that fact and to invite him or her back, at no charge, for proper evaluation. Most patients will appreciate honesty and thoroughness and will not mind the inconvenience of having to make another appointment. Just as the major cause of automobile accidents is driving at excessive speed for existing conditions, so the major cause of error in a physician's office is seeing too many patients too hastily. Some physicians truly believe that it is their duty to help as many patients as possible. Others, less nobly motivated, realize that more patients mean greater income. High aspirations and income are not in themselves objectionable, but too often the patient becomes the casualty. Perhaps for most physicians, seeing an excessive number of patients results not from design but from inadvertence, the inevitable outcome of the "fit her in somewhere" philosophy. The surgeon and his or her staff over the years gradually have become stretched beyond their capacity.

That most plastic surgeons do aesthetic surgery may predispose them to regard their procedures as just skin deep. Because cosmetic patients usually are in good health, the surgeon may not believe that a thorough physical examination is crucial, the assumption being that, whatever the procedure, the patient will come through unscathed except for local scarring. The surgeon may not inquire about systemic illnesses, past operations and emotional reactions to them, drug sensitivities, smoking history, and so forth. Furthermore, because the patient for aesthetic surgery has a focus, the nose or breast, the surgeon may limit his or her attention to one segment of the patient. In fact, it would be considered odd and inappropriate if the plastic surgeon did a pelvic examination on a 40-year-old woman desiring a facelift. However, in viewing the patient narrowly, the plastic surgeon may forget that he or she is a physician with the duty to think of that individual globally and not only regionally. The patient may reinforce the plastic surgeon's superficial approach because he or she does not want to believe that a rhinoplasty, for example, is a real operation with true hazards.

Operating for the Wrong Reasons

The decision to operate should be made for medical or surgical reasons with regard to the patient and not for the surgeon's ambition, convenience, pride, or fiscal needs. If we think that we cannot improve a situation, we should leave it alone. If we believe that we cannot give a patient the result he or she expects, either consciously or unconsciously (1,2), we should not undertake that operation. Selecting the proper patient and giving him or her the proper operation are the ultimate objectives of the initial consultation (3). As plastic surgeons, we justifiably place great reliance on technique, but a well-executed procedure does not necessarily produce a happy patient. This is particularly so in aesthetic surgery, where factors psychological may predominate over those anatomical.

Types of patients who should raise our antennae as well as our threshold for operating are those who write an excessively long letter to arrange the initial consultation, therein revealing their obsessive and perhaps neurotic nature; those who are rude or pushy, who want to be treated as an exception, and who have a high titer of self-entitlement; those who are unkempt or dirty and therefore may be severely disturbed and need a psychiatrist rather than a plastic surgeon; those who praise you excessively and denigrate your colleagues; those who give a false history or are indecisive or vague about what they wish to have done; those who have a minimal deformity but maximal concern; those who refuse to conform to your usual regimen, in such matters as undressing or being photographed; those who have shopped for the "right" plastic surgeon and have come to you as the fourth or fifth on the list; those who are the compulsive seekers and bearers of multiple operations—masochists on the make; those who acquiesce to have an operation in order to please someone else, a disinterested husband, or an overbearing parent; those who are paranoid or visibly depressed; those who are in psychotherapy without having obtained the approval of their therapist, without your having communicated with their therapist, and without your having obtained the approval of their therapist; the older male patient who seeks a rhinoplasty in order to resolve sexual inadequacy; the "special" patient who is so important socially that he or she does not want to be bound by the usual conventions of medical care; and, finally, the patient whom you dislike (4).

The reality is that we vary in our intuition. However, in reviewing my own experience and in speaking to many plastic surgeons who had dissatisfied patients, I have found that we too often disregarded our presentiments. When we have more than an inkling that a patient for elective surgery will be too difficult emotionally for us to manage, it is better to say no at the initial consultation than to invite the patient back for additional appraisals and bend over backward, literally contorting our judgment, to give him or her another opportunity for an operation that should not be done, at least not by us. Sometimes a member of our staff will voice uneasiness about a patient because of an incident that should alert us to potential disaster. Ignoring this information may cause considerable regret later.

Not Seeking a Consultation

With objectivity, we should periodically assess our own abilities. If a procedure requires a skill that we do not possess, we should be prompt to refer or at least to consult. Plastic surgeons have criticized other surgeons for venturing beyond their competence. We should not do the same. The era of the omnificent plastic surgeon has ended. The patient is gravely endangered, as is the surgeon, by the undertaking of an unfamiliar procedure. Today, there are enough plastic surgeons with a sufficient variety of skills to make referral not only possible but mandatory. Because most plastic and reconstructive surgery is elective, there is opportunity to guide the patient to the right physician.

Sometimes a surgeon builds a reputation in a particular area, such as maxillofacial surgery, but, in truth, with time, he or she seldom performs those procedures. The surgeon may be unwilling to relinquish them and to admit to having a practice that is more "aesthetic" than "traumatic." He or she still likes to retain the self-image of a young prowler of the emergency room and a "real doctor." For old time's sake, he may do an operation that preserves his image, he thinks, but it soon harms his reputation and, more importantly, injures the patient. For many plastic surgeons, there is an inevitable shift in what they do over the years. In my own career, I did a considerable amount of hand surgery when I was first in practice, but this work decreased as other procedures came to predominate. I recall my discomfort when I first made the hard decision of referring a patient who needed a tendon graft to someone who was doing this operation every week rather than, in my instance, about once every 2 months. A good rule is that a surgeon and patient should feel comfortable with one another; whenever this rule is transgressed, error and rancor are more likely to result. I have yet to meet a patient who has not respected a physician more for having admitted his or her limitations. Pretending prowess where none exists is wrong medically, ethically, and legally.

A Poorly Informed Patient

If a patient and his or her family do not understand the when, why, or what of a procedure, trouble is on the way—not only from the medicolegal standpoint but from the total therapeutic aspect. A patient may actively dislike an objectively good result if he or she did not comprehend the pain, time, and cost involved, as well as the nature of the scars and the limitations of the procedure. Sometimes the patient does not know what the surgeon has in mind because the surgeon does not really know. He or she has not taken the time to plan the treatment properly. In aesthetic surgery, the fact that a patient has prepaid and has signed an informed consent does not necessarily mean that he or she has completely understood and, more importantly, remembered what the doctor has said. But even under the best of circumstances, when the patient is intelligent and the surgeon painstaking in his or her explanation, verbally, in writing, and perhaps even with the aid of audiovisual materials, the recall by the patient is modest. What chance does a patient or surgeon have under less than ideal circumstances, if the information is too scanty and too rapidly presented?

Finances

Many a surgeon and his or her patient have foundered on these rough shoals. Certainly medicine involves more than finances, but when misunderstandings occur in this realm, the relationship between the patient and the surgeon is doomed. The payment of a bill by a patient who is unhappy or dissatisfied is the common impetus for him or her to seek an attorney. This does not necessarily mean that patients who sue for malpractice are only those who have been stressed or distressed by a bill. However, paying someone for services whose quality is doubtful, either subjectively or objectively, is disturbing, at the very least. As mentioned before, it is imperative that before any procedure is undertaken, the financial aspects must be clearly stated, understood, and remembered by the patient and the surgeon. Prepayment for the surgery of appearance, of course, has solved many but not all of these problems. Prepayment has the additional advantage of having the patient indicate a commitment. If he or she has conflict about the operation, it is likely to come to the fore at the time of writing a check. Should the surgeon detect vacillation, instead of getting angry, he or she should welcome this opportunity for learning that a patient is not a good candidate for the procedure and should tell the patient to wait until he or she is more certain. I never charge a patient for an operation that I have not done because the patient canceled. I do not want to coerce someone unwilling to submit to surgery.

INTRAOPERATIVE

A Poorly Planned or Poorly Performed Operation

Although it is true that bad preoperative and postoperative management can destroy a good operation, only infrequently can a bad operation be transformed into a good one by bedside attentions. This is true particularly in plastic and reconstructive surgery, where results depend directly although not totally upon technique.

When the surgeon performs the procedure in the operating room, it should not be for the first time. It should have been done in the mind's eye before, perhaps in the office but certainly in the 12 hours or so before the operation, if the case is elective. The design of the flap, the type of immobilization, the availability of blood and proper equipment—such considerations should not be left to happenstance. The ability to *ad lib* may lend a virtuoso quality to surgical performance, but it should never replace tactical thinking. It is surprising and distressing to note how many surgeons start thinking about the case when they take up the knife.

No operation is truly minor. Someone once said that a "minor operation" is what happens to someone else. Every surgeon and patient should be wary of the "simple case." We all can recall with anguish and embarrassment the sin of underestimating, of enduring awake a surgical "nightmare." How apt the Russian proverb: "More drown in the puddles than in the sea."

Subtle factors may ruin a good result. For example, a surgeon may be stimulated to try something that he or she ordinarily would not do in order to impress a new resident or a visiting surgeon. Another surgeon may not give a particular operation his or her full effort because he or she is battling the clock—another case, a meeting, patients in the office, a dinner party at home. The fourth operation on a surgeon's schedule should be done with the same high standards as the first. If the patient is in satisfactory condition, no procedure should be terminated until it has been executed as well as possible. Boredom, fatigue, or the press of a schedule should not compromise judgment or quality. A result that looks just fair at operation generally will look worse in the office. If that final glance discloses a remediable fault, we should not be reluctant to heed our assessment. A few more minutes can make a startling difference. Time spent then is more worthwhile than excuses and explanations later. Stitches are not sacred: they can and should be removed and replaced until the desired result is achieved. Michelangelo wisely commented: "Trivials make perfection but perfection is not trivial."

A good surgeon is not necessarily someone whose hands move fast but someone whose brain keeps ahead of the next step in the procedure. He or she does not repeat unnecessarily. When I was a resident and rotated onto the anesthesia service, it soon became apparent to me from the other end of the table how easy it was to distinguish the excellent surgeons from those who were only good or fair. The distinction was not based on digital dexterity but on planning and judgment. The best do not waste time. Although an operation should not be a tense affair, it certainly is not a social event. Those who unnecessarily prolong a procedure are usually the surgeons who have the smallest practices and want to savor each minute or, to be exact, each hour of the session.

Like any professional, the surgeon who is committed to doing an excellent job must concentrate and avoid distractions that can result in disaster. We must remember that in any operation the patient might die or get a suboptimal outcome.

We surgeons must be attentive to many things and not just to what we are doing. We must be alert to possible breaks in asepsis; we must check all solutions before using them; we must be sure that the patient has been properly placed on the operating table with all bony prominences padded; we must check that alternating pneumatic boots on the legs, if used, are functioning even before the patient is given anesthesia; we must communicate with the anesthesiologist about vital signs. If we have a cavalier approach to our duties, those around us will adopt a similar attitude. Patients trust the surgeons to whom they have committed themselves. That responsibility deserves our best. What makes M*A*S*H a successful television production will not do the same for the surgeon's performance and the patient's outcome.

Although the surgeon is in charge and must oversee the activities of many, he or she should do this without becoming a martinet. Making everyone around you uncomfortable and fearful produces an environment inimical to success. Those who are there to aid you and the patient should not be afraid to speak or to advise when they see something that could be improved.

POSTOPERATIVE

Concluding the Case with the Operation

In reality, the operation is not over until the patient is discharged from the surgeon's care. The hit-and-run technique has no place in surgery. The patient and his or her problems should not fade from the surgeon's consciousness as soon as the dressing is applied.

Careful observations, detailed orders, and clear instructions are critical, especially with the ascendancy of ambulatory surgery. If a patient is admitted, we should be fully aware of the hospital course and should not abrogate our responsibility to residents. One should know, for example, about unusual pain or vomiting or some other important incident or complaint. We should be fully aware of the patient's medications, as well as blood pressure, pulse, and temperature. Our standards should not go down with the setting sun. If a dressing or splint warrants removal, it should be done as quickly at night as during the day. The "wait for the morning" attitude may be effective for growing crocuses but not for managing patients.

In our follow-up, we should take an active part and not assign accountability to others in the office. We should know how a wound is healing, and we should be available to listen to a patient's fears and anxieties. We should not create an atmosphere that intimidates a patient into silence. If a postoperative situation presents problems beyond our usual ken, we should be quick to utilize consultants before the patient asks or a tragedy occurs—not just to keep ourselves "clean" medicolegally but, more importantly, to ensure the patient receives the best treatment. One head, even that of a surgeon, is not always better than two.

We must fight the tendency to become fair-weather doctors, attentive and helpful when all goes well but distant and punitive when a complication develops. A patient who has to bear an unwanted result usually feels isolated and angry, and often guilty. Such a patient should be encouraged to express his or her sentiments without fear of reprisal. Unconsciously, the patient might think of his or her complication as divine retribution for the self-indulgence of an elective procedure, especially a cosmetic one, which friends and family considered unnecessary. The physician's responsibility is to guide the patient through this difficult period with genuine sympathy. This is certainly not the occasion for rancor and desultory care (see Chapter 2).

The Follow-up that Isn't

The surgeon who fails to continue to observe his or her patient long enough will lose a valuable chance to learn. In contrast, the surgeon who believes in extended observation will behold many things, sometimes wondrous, occasionally painful, always instructive. A year later, the revised scar that initially looked so disappointing will have improved miraculously. This being a hard world, the reverse also is true. The rhinoplasty that appeared "just perfect" at 6 months may end with many imperfections. It is always tempting to quit while ahead—discharge the facelift patient, for example, after a few months, when he or she is feeling rejuvenated and grateful. If we truly wish to improve our techniques and to learn our patients' reactions to their operations, however, we should follow them for longer than several weeks and, in many instances, such as after augmentation mammaplasty, for many years. During this period, we must be genuinely committed to objective evaluation and resist the temptation to fit the facts to an old thinking mold. There is a difference between 20 years of experiences and 20 years of 1-year experience. Spare us the fate of the Bourbons, about whom Talleyrand observed: "They have learned nothing and forgotten nothing."

The Iron Man (Woman) Delusion

"Neither snow, nor rain, nor heat, nor gloom of night. . . ." This delusion can now become the property of women also. No surgeon—no human being—is invincible. Recall what happened to Caesar, Cleopatra, and Napoleon.

An operation is a series of interdigitating sequential acts, whose quality depends on the soma and psyche of the surgeon as well as of the patient. The overworked, overstressed surgeon does himself or herself little good and may do the patient considerable harm. It seems logical for us to try to keep fit physically and emotionally for our daily performance. Certainly, any athlete knows this. We are not infinitely distensible. Although we should not shirk our tasks, we must take time to replenish ourselves. Periodic vacations as well as a day chasing a white ball over green acreage are helpful. Whatever it takes to lower our peripheral resistance and to raise our inner glow should be done from time to time. A professional life is a marathon, not a sprint.

Chance

No surgeon, even the most careful, skillful, and knowledgeable, can control every variable in the treatment of the patient. Pertinent is the passage from Ecclesiastes: ". . . time and chance happeneth to them all." From that perspective, it is remarkable that most outcomes are good and most patients are satisfied. However, the unusual and unexpected can occur. A patient in the hospital may not receive the right medication or may develop a sensitivity to it or, following a recent rhinoplasty, injure the nose. The scenarios are infinite. Although the surgeon is not responsible for these capricious turns of fate, he or she must deal with them appropriately and with equanimity.

CONCLUSION

The recognition of certain prime ingredients in failure should make us less willing to accept an unfavorable result as an event related only to the patient or emanating only from the heavens. In many instances, although not all, its genesis lies at the surgeon's doorstep; his or her treatment style, which is, after all, integral to his or her lifestyle. Although we cannot always assume total responsibility for an unwanted outcome, we must not delude ourselves into thinking that we had no part in the occurrence of any complication. No matter how attentive we are, fallibility unpredictability marks the human condition, and mistakes will occur. Of this sad reality, Hippocrates observed:

> Mistakes, no less than benefits, witness to the existence of the art, for what benefited did so because correctly administered, and what harmed did so because incorrectly administered. Now, where correctness and incorrectness each have a defined limit, surely there must be an art. For absence of art I take to be absence of correctness and of incorrectness, but where both are present art can not be absent.
>
> *The Art, V* (W.H.S. Jones, translator)

We are not self-correcting computers. Our capacity to learn is present but not always used. An error, although painful and unwanted, nevertheless presents a unique opportunity for self-betterment.

REFERENCES

1. Dunofsky M. Psychological characteristics of women who undergo single and multiple cosmetic surgeries. *Ann Plast Surg* 1997;39:223–228.
2. Wengle H-P. The psychology of cosmetic surgery: old problems in patient selection seen in a new way—part II. *Ann Plast Surg* 1986;16:487–493.
3. Goldwyn RM. *The patient and the plastic surgeon,* 2nd ed. Boston: Little, Brown and Company, 1991.
4. Wengle H-P. The psychology of cosmetic surgery: a critical overview of the literature 1960–1982—part I. *Ann Plast Surg* 1986;16:435–442.

2

THE DISSATISFIED PATIENT

ROBERT M. GOLDWYN

The dissatisfied patient is an unfortunate, stressful reality that can be avoided only by retiring from practice. Because this is an impractical alternative for most of us who wish to take care of patients and must make a living, there are more practical and fulfilling ways to manage the patient who is unhappy after our surgical efforts. Although infrequent, the patient who is not satisfied has an enormous negative emotional impact. No picture of the surgical landscape would be complete without showing somewhere the patient whose expectations we were unable to meet (1).

BACKGROUND

As physicians, we seek to help others and to obtain their approbation. It is terribly distressing to have to deal with a person whom we not only have failed to help, but possibly have made worse; who, instead of being grateful, is hostile; and who, instead of applauding our motives and talents, openly accuses us of greed and incompetence and may actually seek legal redress.

A plastic surgical residency, like most other educational experiences in our culture, does not usually equip us to manage the unpleasant side of our métier. As residents, we took care of the grief of somebody else's efforts, and even when it was our own patient, when we were chief residents, we had the glimmer of hope that the rotation would soon be over and we might even be leaving town to begin our practice. But now, as professionals, we all are in a position so well described by Harry Truman as "The buck stops here."

Today's plastic surgeon frequently is in an urban area, usually unknown to the patient before the initial consultation, has only brief contact with the patient, and projects an image of wealth. Statistically, most plastic surgeons are at the upper end of the socioeconomic ladder, and the media ceaselessly seeks and finds plastic surgeons who delight in displaying their wealth as well as their talents.

R. M. Goldwyn: Division of Plastic Surgery, Beth Israel Deaconess Medical Center, Harvard Medical School, Boston, Massachusetts

The average patient seeking aesthetic surgery comes with the belief that perfection is just around the corner. Again, members of our own specialty, coupled with the media, have reinforced this false reality. Although it is true that most patients will be satisfied and that the surgical results will be exemplary, this obviously is not true for every patient and every outcome.

THE PATIENT

As mentioned, some patients arrive with inflated expectations and unrealistic beliefs of the prowess of the plastic surgeon. However, many come distrustful of medicine in general and of any doctor in particular. A few patients are openly hostile and have the attitude "show me what you can do." Unlike 35 years ago, when I first began practice, patients today pointedly ask about your training, experience, capability, and even previous malpractice suits. The last information is available, at least in my state, Massachusetts, from the Board of Registration in Medicine and on computer.

Many patients have been referred by primary physicians whose incomes are generally less than those of plastic surgeons, especially those doing a preponderance of aesthetic operations. If something does go wrong, the family physician may not be the most understanding or helpful because of his or her resentment about the disparity in the financial rewards.

WHY IS THE PATIENT DISSATISFIED?

The first task of the surgeon is to know why the patient is unhappy. Usually the patient will remove all ambiguity by a strong, unequivocal statement of complaint, but if this is not forthcoming, one should be alert to veiled discontent—a sullenness, an irritability, or some form of passive-aggressive behavior, such as the patient not keeping appointments or not paying the bill if, unwisely, we had not established the ground rules prior to the operation. In some way, it seems easier to let the patient leave the office, and we feel relief because he or she did not verbalize the unpleasantness that we would have to confront. Sooner or later, however, the seamy side will appear and must be faced. We must not become so unreceptive that the patient's resentment reaches the proportions of a lethal abscess. Before this occurs, a helpful comment might be, "You don't seem too happy today. What is troubling you?"

Some patients seem more unhappy than they prove to be. Unless they have told you what bothers them, sometimes after having been asked, they may respond more positively than you had thought possible. This becomes a good foundation on which to build the ensuing discussion and management.

For many patients, dissatisfaction disappears with reassurance that circumstances justify. For example, someone who is concerned about swelling 2 weeks after eyelidplasty can be told that the swelling will subside as healing progresses over the next several weeks or months. A patient may worry about the bulkiness of a recently turned flap. Here, too, reassurance about the progressive flattening will be comforting, particularly because it is true. It should be an axiom that one never reassures a patient if reality dictates otherwise.

Occasionally, postoperative unhappiness centers on the minimal or the nonexistent. In this situation, it is important to probe into "why this now?" Is the person depressed and guilty about having an elective operation about something else? Has there been a recent loss, such as a divorce or death? I remember a 35-year-old married woman who had a very good result following a rhinoplasty and chin implant but seemed depressed a few weeks later. She then told me her girlfriend next door had "kept away" and finally confessed to my patient that she feared rejection because she thought that my patient, now better looking, would need her less. Occasionally the culprit in postoperative depression of a mild sort is the family physician, who may have said to the patient soon after a facelift, "You went through all this to look like that?" This unkind and destructive remark may have been prompted by the patient's not consulting him or her about the surgery or proceeding without advice or, as mentioned, the practitioner's or internist's resentment of what he or she considers an excessive fee for something that is not life threatening.

Several patients have told me following aesthetic surgery that female friends rejected them because they believe that the patient is now a threat to them because their spouse might find them more attractive.

Another situation, with an unusual twist: Is the spouse a lover who may have enjoyed the personal dominance that resulted from the mate's feelings of inferiority about her disliked feature? Because the patient is now rid of it, the partner may become less secure about the leverage he or she formerly possessed. For example, following a breast reconstruction, a patient left her husband who was having affairs because he thought that, with her deformity, she would be lucky to have him and would never object to his other activities. One cannot save a marriage through plastic surgery, and sometimes the procedure may prompt a divorce.

The patient who complains legitimately about an undesirable result, for example, infection, asymmetry, or bad scarring, deserves prompt attention of the right sort. To detail the spectrum of complications is beyond the present task and is not our purpose here. The point is that if the patient's dissatisfaction has an objective basis, it, like any reality, merits respect and empathy. Someone who had aesthetic surgery, for example, frequently sought it against the advice of family, friends, and other physicians and may have paid a large fee. When something goes wrong, he or she may feel foolish, ashamed, guilty, and, not unexpectedly, angry. The patient may believe that this complication is divine recompense for vanity that led him or her to risking his or her health for something "frivolous" that now has become a distinct liability.

MISMANAGING THE DISSATISFIED PATIENT

The following quotations from my patients emphasize the points I wish to make.

> He (another plastic surgeon), always tries to minimize the problem. He hasn't really been honest with me. I don't want to go back to him even though he said he would do it over for nothing. I don't trust him. Suppose he makes a mistake again. But if I go to someone else, it will cost a lot of money and I can't afford it. I already paid him $8,000 and for what (facelift)?

> I am bringing my wife here to see you for a second opinion. It would have helped if Dr. — had suggested it. He never would. His ego could fill a ballroom.

> He expects me to like him after all I have been through. He is lucky that I won't sue him and I really might. I have trouble enough seeing him for this hole in my face (concavity after liposuction). He avoids me like the plague. Maybe an attorney can get to him.

> He was there for the money but he is not there for me now. All I get to talk to is his nurse (secretary). He really doesn't give a damn.

> If I really thought this would have happened, I wouldn't have had it done.

> Every time I see her, she tries to talk me into thinking that it (noticeable ectropion) will go away with time. It has already been 10 months. She won't admit that she goofed. I can't get a word in edgewise with her.

> I thought that with your reputation, this wouldn't have happened.

> My boyfriend hasn't come near me since the operation. I really can't blame him. This big hole (skin loss after abdominoplasty) would disgust me, too.

Today's patients generally are well informed, often have sought more than one consultation, and, even though they have been informed about the possibility of a complication, have not been prepared emotionally to accept it. We all know that loved ones will die, but few among us can accept that reality with equanimity, especially if death is sudden and consciously unanticipated.

A complication is even harder to accept if the patient went to a surgeon with a well-known reputation. Yet, we know that no matter who the surgeon is or how long he or she has been in practice, things can go wrong; the mighty also fail and fall.

AVOIDING THE REALITY

As surgeons, especially because most of our results are favorable, we instinctively turn away from the adverse outcome, but the sooner we accept it, the better we can manage it. I remember being in a colleague's office when a patient complained of asymmetry of her nipples following breast reduction. The problem was obvious to me, but the other plastic surgeon tried to convince the patient that she was wrong. In my opinion, he compounded the injury by insulting her intelligence. Most patients and most of their friends or family are capable of judging a scar that is thick (hypertrophic or keloid) or a tip that is bulbous. Trying to fast-talk the patient out of a problem may succeed for a few hours, but ultimately it will fail. It will make the patient angrier and less willing to follow advice. If there is anything that can drive a patient to another plastic surgeon or to an attorney, it is distorting reality.

BLAMING THE PATIENT OR BECOMING ANGRY AT THE PATIENT

To accuse the patient of producing an unfavorable result usually is unjustified. Although it is true that some patients, by not following directions, e.g., smoking after a breast reduction, can produce an adverse result, usually it is the surgeon or the circumstances of the operation that bring about the unfavorable result. If that is so, why take the low road and accuse the patient of causing it? The duet of patient and physician then becomes a duel. It is much better to recognize the reality and to work together to correct it.

Not uncommonly, surgeons become angry at patients when something goes wrong. Although that is understandable as an expression of the surgeon's frustration, it is unacceptable professional behavior.

A plastic surgeon whom I knew very well used to accuse her patients of "poor eating habits and nutrition" whenever a wound healed unsatisfactorily. One patient, whom I saw in consultation, was incensed by this kind of treatment. She happened to be an Olympic skier with nothing wrong in her diet.

When a patient is angry and the surgeon retaliates in kind, both regress together. The patient becomes angrier because he or she becomes more fearful to be in the presence and hands of a surgeon who has lost control. At the moment when the patient is looking to the surgeon for guidance and maturity, it is devastating to have the healer decompensate. This makes a difficult situation worse.

On a few occasions, I have said to a patient, "I know that you are angry and I also would be if I were in your position. However, it is important that we work together. I need your support, also, to get through this and I can assure you that I will be there for you."

BEING DISTANT OR UNAVAILABLE

One should not erect a barrier between you and the patient; one should make oneself available at all times. The unfavorable result may actually be an opportunity to deepen the relationship and sometimes can be converted from a potentially miserable disaster into a satisfying experience. It is interesting that, over the years, several patients who developed postoperative problems and were managed with a modicum of decency actually became enthusiastic supporters and subsequently referred other patients. Everyone in the office should be instructed that the patient with an unfavorable result has direct and immediate access. I give patients my home telephone number to make her or him more secure. This actually results in fewer telephone calls. If one becomes hard to reach, the easy-to-reach attorney will be on the scene. But, medicolegal considerations aside, it is not fair that one should make oneself scarce after one has contracted to do a job, even if it has not turned out as either the surgeon or the patient expected. We certainly would resent this attitude if, for example, a carpenter came to our home, performed a task, did not produce the outcome we expected, and then would not respond to our telephone calls.

Many years ago, a colleague referred a patient from the West Coast who was going to school in Boston and on whom he had operated but the rotation flap became necrotic in the lower leg. The patient required debridement and subsequent skin grafting. During the course of her hospitalization, the doctor was in town for a meeting but failed to see the patient in the hospital. The patient, as well as her family, knew that he was in town, and although they forgave him for the complication, they never excused his running away and his lacking the decency to see the patient in follow-up. I was not surprised to learn that a court battle ensued.

FAILING TO STRUCTURE A TREATMENT PLAN

No patient, especially a dissatisfied one, should be left swinging in the breeze. No matter what the situation, it is always possible to structure a plan even if one cannot give specifics.

For example, in a patient whose flap has become necrotic, one can say: "I want to see you in the office at least twice a week so that I can get rid of the dead tissue. How large the wound becomes will determine whether or not a skin graft will be necessary. I wish I could tell you that precisely now, but I cannot. However, I assure you that you will know everything that I am thinking at the time of your visit."

It is not necessary to be precise, but one should to offer the security that any patient, especially one in distress, craves. How wrong it would be to tell the same patient: "I am really not sure what will happen. I guess I should see you frequently. We can set up some schedule over the next 2 or 3 weeks. You might need a skin graft, but you might not. I will let you know when I think that it is necessary, but for now, my secretaries will be in touch with you and keep in touch with us."

FAILING TO CONSULT

Another aspect of managing the dissatisfied patient is proper use of a consultant. Most patients want to remain with the original physician, but it can comfort the patient, as well as the surgeon, to get another opinion, especially if it is warranted. You should sense when a patient wishes a consultation, and you should not make the patient jump hurdles to obtain one; however, the patient should not feel tossed off or shunted, but directed to the other physician. I usually dictate a letter in the patient's presence stating what the problem is and that I would like his or her advice, which can be discussed freely with the patient.

Occasionally, you may sense that the patient does not feel that he or she should pay for "your mistake." I would hope that we would consent to see patients for colleagues at no charge to maintain a delicate balance between the unhappy individual and the hard-pressed physician. If you, as the referring physician, believe that a patient should be charged for the consultation, you should so inform the surgeon and offer to pay for it yourself. Most of us, I am sure, would not allow a colleague to do so, but this practice has precedence and does not imply that you are guilty of any wrongdoing. If the patient chooses to continue his or her care under another doctor, either the consultant or someone else, do not make the patient feel guilty. In similar situations, I have made sure that I knew when the patient was going into the hospital and have even called the patient in the hospital or at home afterward. The patient realizes that you are truly interested in his or her well-being, and the doctor who has cared for the patient also will welcome your support and not feel that he or she has lost a professional friend.

Many patients have told me that when they suggested to the doctor a "second opinion," the response was hostile. A recent patient who had loss of skin behind the ear following a facelift recalled that the surgeon said that he never wanted to see the patient back if he went to someone else. That behavior is puerile and irrational, because the patient was a reasonable individual, justifiably concerned about her face. Fortunately, time and dressing changes resulted in a satisfactory outcome.

The patient may require a consultation with a psychiatrist or a psychotherapist if he or she becomes depressed and seems unable to handle the stress. It is better to suggest this sooner than later. Sometimes it is difficult to get the patient to agree. In this situation, the family physician may be helpful.

IGNORING PAIN

Some patients reveal their unhappiness by complaining of pain long beyond the time that would seem appropriate. People vary greatly in their pain tolerance, and it is impossible to know how much pain another person is having or should have. Chronic pain after an aesthetic operation usually signifies a depressed and displeased patient. The busy plastic surgeon, if not vigilant, may prescribe a tranquilizer in order to have the patient stop bothering him or her. Which medication to select is obviously in the province of an expert such as a psychiatrist or pain specialist.

Those patients who have puzzling persistent pain after reconstruction, requiring analgesics and allegedly preventing their return to work, should make one suspect malingering for secondary gain emotionally and financially. Depression also is a possibility, and here again one should make an effort to enlist a therapist in order to determine the dynamics of the behavior and to offer an effective treatment.

NEGLECTING THE SUPPORT SYSTEM

The patient, like most human beings in difficulty, needs support. I find it helpful to involve the close and relevant members of the family and friends, even showing some of them how to change dressings if there has been breakdown of the wound. The referring doctor should be informed in order to enlist his or her help.

Most of us like to hide an embarrassing situation. Although that is instinctual, it is unwise. That something has gone wrong with an operation mirrors life: bad things happen.

If the surgeon has a secretive way of dealing with a problem, the patient will sense the shame of it and will become even more unwilling to deal with the reality. Guilt increases, as does anxiety.

INCREASING THE FINANCIAL BURDEN

In considering the management of an unfavorable result, the financial aspects are important. For patients who had reconstructive surgery, the cost of treating a complication usually is borne by insurance. Not so when things go wrong after a cosmetic operation. He or she must pay the bill. A great advantage for the patient is the surgeon who has his or her own operating room so that the patient need not be charged for its use. Not all plastic surgeons have such a facility and depend on the hospital. I stipulate in my consent form that the patient undergoing cosmetic surgery is responsible not only for the expense of that operation, but also for those associated with any complication that will involve the hospital. Although I would not charge a patient for revision after an aesthetic procedure, I cannot assume the additional expenses of the hospital. Perhaps it is a cliche to state that every situation must be evaluated according to each patient's surgeon. On occasion, we may sense that another financial stress for an individual would be unfair and inappropriate. Some attorneys advise billing a patient for any work to relieve a complication because not doing so would imply guilt. Others say that if we do not charge the patient and note in the record that we are not doing so in order to lighten his or her financial load, this is an acceptable alternative in a trying situation and, rather than implying guilt, it denotes compassion, something a jury might readily understand. This is a sticky wicket, so before writing out a check to a patient, it would be wise to consult with a representative of a malpractice insurance company.

One colleague had a patient whose umbilicus was off center following abdominoplasty. He charged her for its relocation. The patient did not mind paying for the hospital but was irate that the surgeon made additional money from a mistake that he made. Again, we would not tolerate that kind of behavior from a carpenter, plumber, or painter. They are professionals, too, whom we would allow to make mistakes but expect them to rectify the errors without added cost.

It is perhaps too simple to say that we should treat the patient, satisfied or dissatisfied, as we ourselves would want to be treated. In so doing, Emerson's words should be comforting: "Bad times . . . are occasions a good learner would not miss."

WHEN THE DISSATISFIED PATIENT IS SOMEBODY ELSE'S

The consultant who sees a patient with an unfavorable result arising from the work of another surgeon is in a singular position to do considerable good or irrevocable harm. Although in this situation, as in any other medical circumstance, the first obligation is the patient, one also can help or try to help the other doctor.

The first step is to obtain as objective a history as possible. Exclamations of disbelief at the patient's story or the other surgeon's behavior should be assiduously avoided. Usually the patient who is angry and distraught gives too brief a history because he or she wishes something done immediately to correct the undesirable result. Since the operation, the patient has relived the unfortunate surgical events thousands of times and may be impatient with you, the consultant, for laboriously trying to gather the sequence; however, securing a full account is crucial.

I always inform the patient that I wish to get in touch with the other doctor in order to improve his or her care. If the patient does not allow this, I am reluctant to continue treatment. It is illegal to communicate with another doctor without the patient's permission—by phone or innuendo at a chance meeting in the corridor or in the dining room of the hospital.

Following are typical statements from patients whom I have seen in consultation.

> I went to him because he was supposedly tops in his field. How could he have done this?
>
> He never told me this could happen. I was in and out of his office 1-2-3.

In reply to the first statement, I usually am able to say, because it is true, that I have had the same kind of problem or that this is not an unheard of difficulty. To the second statement with its implication that the patient was not properly informed, it is certainly better to say nothing and to hear the other side of the story.

As part of the history, it is advisable to ask the patient about his or her general health, and professional and family life, as one would do if that person had come to you initially. What are his or her relations with spouse, parents, employer? Is the patient now abnormally depressed? How has he or she reacted to previous operations?

When a patient expresses anger at another physician, it certainly is unwise to join in the chorus. Far better to say to the patient, "I can understand that you are angry. I am sure Dr. — is upset also. No good doctor wants to have an unhappy patient. I can tell you that I wish all my patients had wonderful results, but that is not true. Perhaps he is seeing one of my patients as I am seeing you now."

The physical examination usually is less of a problem than the history, because the examination is more objective. The patient is almost eager to show the scars that "shouldn't be there," the breasts that "don't match," the nose that "looks awful," the tendon graft that "doesn't work." For the consultant, the pitfall is being so absorbed in the local problem that he or she neglects the patient in totality. A consultant might fail to notice, for example, how scars have healed from past operations; or he or she might not detect systemic disease, such as a malfunctioning thyroid. During the examination, it is best, once again, to avoid comments or articulate or not, such as a low whistle, a stare of surprise, or an "Oh my" head shake. The patient will be alert to any sign of how bad the consultant feels the problem is or how badly he or she thinks the other surgeon performed.

The patient should be asked to return to the consulting

room for a proper discussion with both of you seated. Most likely the patient feels the other doctor is not spending enough time with him or her and would not want another opinion on the fly no matter how impressive the consultant's credentials.

Now comes the most difficult part of the consultation, literally, "the moment of truth." My experience has been that it is best to give the patient as honest an appraisal of his or her problem as is possible, but to do so with warmth and empathy and to avoid any pejorative statements. One can begin simply, "Mrs. —, as you know, you have had a breast reduction and your problem is that the scars are more noticeable than you want. It is true, also, as you said, that the breasts are not symmetric. I am sure that for both you and Dr. —, this has been very distressing because you both know that he would have wanted the best for you." Having structured the problem, one can proceed to the treatment, which, for the patient, is the most important derivative of the consultation. "Now, Mrs. —, we would all agree that we have to decide what to do. Looking backward is not productive and can be very upsetting." Although at times a consultant should defer his or her opinion because the other surgeon has requested it, it generally is wise to give a candid but not condemning evaluation when the patient is seen. Patients fear conspiracy among doctors; they believe that physicians will protect the worst actions of the most incompetent to maintain the solidarity of our guild. Unfortunately, in some instances, this is not mere paranoia.

A practical matter must soon be resolved. Who now is responsible for the patient's future care? Sometimes the patient will settle the matter by refusing to return to the former doctor. Frequently the other surgeon who arranged the consultation will continue to care for the patient.

I do not believe that it is wise medically or correct ethically to force patients to return to a doctor whom they no longer trust or like, even though their attitude might be unjustly founded. The plastic surgeon who consults, as we all do, must be willing to assume responsibility for difficult situations, as we routinely do for the patient coming to us from surgeons not in our specialty. The fear of being unpopular and avoiding a lawsuit should not lead us to avoid aiding the patient. As a practical matter, the patient whom we have seen as a second or third surgeon and refuse to treat is more likely to seek redress by going to an attorney.

At some point in the consultation, the truth should be reiterated: that in surgery, as in all of life, perfection is the aim but rarely the attainment. We must emphasize again that we also have results that are not excellent and patients who are dissatisfied. In indicating the limitations of our own talents, we must at the same time not make the patient feel that he or she has been so deformed as to be beyond help. This is a most delicate balance to achieve. Occasionally, it happens that nothing further can be done from a surgical point of view, but one should be able to continue to see the patient and to support him or her during this difficult period. This is not the time to be cool or distant or insensitive.

The consultant should be sufficiently mature not to use the patient's misery to denigrate a colleague and to plump his or her own ego. The golden rule is eminently pertinent here. Because all who operate are bound to have failures, rejoicing secretly in someone else's professional misfortune is immature and short sighted. Beware the boomerang!

A consultant who is able to help a patient in trouble also helps a family and a colleague. Few situations in medicine demand greater sense and sensibility but yield more satisfaction.

REFERENCE

1. Goldwyn RM. *The patient and the plastic surgeon,* 2nd ed. New York: Little, Brown and Company, 1991.

3

PSYCHOLOGICAL CONSIDERATIONS IN COSMETIC SURGERY

DAVID B. SARWER

Psychological investigations of cosmetic surgery patients have a long history dating back to the 1940s (1,2). Over the last 60 years, these studies have contributed greatly to our understanding of the relevant psychological issues of cosmetic surgery patients. In addition, they have helped us begin to understand the psychological effects of a surgical change of physical appearance. These studies primarily were designed to address two fundamental questions: (i) Do cosmetic surgery patients share a common psychological profile?; and (ii) Do cosmetic surgery patients experience positive psychological changes postoperatively? Studies designed to address the first question have sought to uncover the psychological motivations of persons who seek cosmetic surgery. These investigations also had a more practical objective—to identify patients with psychological conditions that may be treated more appropriately by psychotherapy than cosmetic surgery. Investigations that focused on the second question have attempted to confirm an intuitive assumption of cosmetic surgery—that a surgical change in appearance leads to psychological benefit. Furthermore, these studies sought to identify psychological factors that are related to a poor psychological outcome and, therefore, contraindicate cosmetic surgery.

Understanding the relevant psychological issues of cosmetic surgery patients is critical on at least two levels. First, appropriate patient selection and screening is vital to the survival of the individual surgeon. A patient whose psychological status is not appropriately assessed and addressed can be, at a minimum, a headache to the surgeon, nurse, and office staff. At worst, this patient may bring legal action, threaten, or actually commit violence against the surgeon and/or staff. Understanding the psychological issues of patients also is important to the survival of the profession of plastic surgery as a whole. In an era of increased competition for cosmetic surgery patients by non-plastic surgery physician groups, it behooves the profession to understand the relevant psychological issues of persons who seek cosmetic surgery. With such information, surgeons can honestly and accurately inform patients about the effects of surgery on self-esteem, quality of life, and body image. This information is critical to ensure both the credibility and legitimacy of the profession both now and in the future.

This chapter is organized in three sections. The first section reviews the existing psychological literature on cosmetic surgery. The second section discusses more recent advances in the relevant psychological issues in cosmetic surgery, focusing on issues of physical appearance and body image. Finally, the third section provides guidelines for patient screening and selection.

PSYCHOLOGICAL INVESTIGATIONS IN COSMETIC SURGERY

As noted, studies of the psychological status of cosmetic surgery patients primarily were designed to address two fundamental questions: (i) Do cosmetic surgery patients share a common psychological profile?; and (ii) Do cosmetic surgery patients experience positive psychological changes postoperatively? Studies addressing this first question have attempted to identify patients with psychological difficulties—to prevent the unfavorable result before it occurs. The hope for these investigations is that they would yield a reliable and valid tool that surgeons could use to screen out inappropriate patients. Studies focusing on the second issue have attempted to address a fundamental question of physicians regardless of their discipline—do patients benefit from a given treatment? As the "treatment" of cosmetic surgery is considered, the question becomes: Do patients experience psychological benefits following cosmetic surgery?

These two questions also allow for an organization of the research into two categories. The first question addresses the preoperative psychological status of cosmetic surgery pa-

D. B. Sarwer: Departments of Psychiatry and Surgery, and Division of Plastic Surgery, University of Pennsylvania School of Medicine; and The Edwin and Fannie Gray Hall Center for Human Appearance, Philadelphia, Pennsylvania

tients. The second question addresses the potential postoperative changes in psychological status following cosmetic surgery. In addition, these studies can be organized by the type of research method utilized: clinical assessments, which have primarily relied on patient interviews, as compared to psychometric assessments, which have used paper-and-pencil measures of psychological status. By using this organizational framework, it becomes easier to determine if these investigations have addressed the questions they set out to study.

PREOPERATIVE STUDIES OF COSMETIC SURGERY PATIENTS

Clinical Assessments

Clinical assessments of patients typically have relied on similar methodology. These studies most frequently involved patients being interviewed by psychologists or psychiatrists working in collaboration with plastic surgeons. The interviews typically consisted of question-and-answer sessions that focused on symptoms of psychopathology. Clinical interview investigations have, almost uniformly, found high rates of psychopathology in patients. In several studies, approximately 70% of patients who sought a variety of cosmetic procedures were diagnosed with a psychiatric disturbance (3–13). Patients in these studies have been described as experiencing increased psychiatric symptoms of depression, anxiety, guilt, and low self-esteem (3,4,10,12,13). In two investigations of breast augmentation patients, for example, 55% of prospective patients were described as being "in need of therapy" and 70% in another study as "deviating from the normal picture." A more recent investigation of breast augmentation patients found greater use of alcohol and oral contraceptives, as well as a greater number of sexual partners, in patients as compared with controls, potentially suggesting greater psychological difficulties in breast augmentation candidates (14).

Although consistent in their findings, these investigations have several methodologic shortcomings that raise questions about their validity. Many of these studies were conducted in the 1960s and early 1970s by psychiatrists working from a psychodynamic or Freudian perspective, the dominant school of psychiatric thought of the time. From this perspective, appearance-related concerns typically were interpreted as symbolic displacements of intrapsychic conflicts. For example, a 16-year-old girl with a large nose who sought rhinoplasty might have had her desire for surgery interpreted by a psychiatrist as a strategy to remove unwanted characteristics of her father's personality from her own. In contrast, a more straightforward and equally plausible interpretation might have been that the patient had an appropriate concern about an overly prominent facial feature and not an unconscious personality conflict with her father. Thus, the high levels of psychopathology reported in these studies may have reflected the biases of the primarily psychoanalytically trained psychiatrists (1,2). Unfortunately, this categorization of cosmetic surgery patients moved into both the professional and popular cultures without the support of valid and reliable evidence and, to some extent, still exists in the present day.

More contemporary studies have additional methodologic problems. In most studies, the nature of the clinical interview was not described, and control or comparison groups were not used. Furthermore, studies typically did not use widely accepted diagnostic criteria, such as those found in the *Diagnostic and Statistical Manual of Mental Disorders,* fourth edition (DSM-IV) (15). As a result of these methodologic problems, it is not clear if these studies accurately represent the degree of psychological disturbance in these patients.

A more recent interview investigation of cosmetic surgery patients that used the *Diagnostic and Statistical Manual of Mental Disorders,* revised third edition (DSM-IIII-R) (16) diagnostic criteria reported that 19.5% had a major psychiatric disorder (predominantly mood and anxiety disorders) and 70% a personality disorder (predominantly narcissistic and borderline personality disorders) (17). Although this study improved on earlier investigations by using widely accepted diagnostic criteria, the use of an unspecified clinical interview and the absence of interrater reliability of diagnoses could account for the extremely high prevalence of personality disorder diagnoses in this sample (1,2).

Psychometric Assessments

In contrast to the interview-based investigations, studies that used valid and reliable psychometric tests generally reported less psychological disturbance. Studies of patients who sought rhinoplasty, rhytidectomy, and breast augmentation, and who were assessed by standardized measures, found relatively few symptoms of psychopathology (18–22). In contrast, two studies found only mild symptoms of depression and anxiety in patients preoperatively (23,24).

Although the psychometric studies present a more favorable picture than the interview-based investigations, the former studies also have limitations. Several failed to use control or comparisons groups. Investigations that compared patients to normative samples frequently failed to describe the demographic characteristics of the two groups. As a result, the prevalence of psychopathology in women seeking cosmetic surgery, as compared to that of women not seeking surgery, is unknown.

In summary, preoperative investigations of cosmetic surgery patients have produced contradictory results. Clinical interview investigations reported high rates of psychopathology, whereas studies that used standardized psychometric tests found far less disturbance. Methodologic concerns with both sets of studies limit the conclusions that can be drawn. Therefore, the typical psychological presentation of cosmetic surgery patients cannot be asserted reliably, thereby making it difficult to determine which, if any, psychiatric diagnoses serve as contraindications to cosmetic surgery.

POSTOPERATIVE STUDIES OF COSMETIC SURGERY PATIENTS

Postoperative investigations of cosmetic surgery patients have focused on two issues: patient satisfaction and changes in psychological status. Studies of patient satisfaction following cosmetic surgery have, with few exceptions, been largely anecdotal. They consist primarily of surgeons' reports of their patients' satisfaction. These reports suggest that the vast majority of patients report satisfaction with their outcome (3,25–29). In several studies of breast augmentation patients, however, 10% to 30% of women reported some degree of dissatisfaction postoperatively, typically associated with some postoperative complication (25–27,29–32).

Other studies have focused on psychological changes following cosmetic surgery. As with the preoperative investigations, these studies can be classified as clinical and psychometric assessments.

Clinical Assessments

The majority of postoperative interview investigations reported that women experience psychological benefits from cosmetic surgery (5–8,10,11,33). Two studies reported some negative consequences (4,9), and two other studies noted no change or mixed results (13,34). In several studies, improvements in self-esteem and body image were reported by a majority of patients postoperatively (7,13,21,25–27, 29,31,35,36). These studies, which are similar to the preoperative interview investigations, also have significant methodologic shortcomings. The interviews typically were not standardized, and the criteria for judging outcome were not clearly articulated. Most of the studies were retrospective and frequently did not include preoperative assessments or control groups. Furthermore, several studies had high attrition. These significant methodologic concerns limit the confidence that can be placed in the claims that women experience psychological benefit from cosmetic surgery (1,2,37,38).

Psychometric Assessments

Of studies that used standardized tests to assess psychological outcome in other cosmetic surgery groups, two showed favorable changes (20,27), three observed no greater change than that found in comparison groups (22,24,39), and two described an increase in depressive symptoms (19,40). Similar to the interview studies, the psychometric investigations also had methodologic shortcomings; therefore, it is difficult to confidently draw conclusions from these studies.

A recent study, however, suggests that cosmetic surgery patients experience psychological benefit following cosmetic surgery. Rankin and colleagues (41) asked 105 patients seeking a variety of cosmetic procedures to complete measures of depressive symptoms, quality of life, social support, and coping preoperatively and at 1 and 6 months postoperatively. Patients reported significant improvements in depression and quality of life 6 months postoperatively as compared to preoperative levels. This investigation improved on previous studies by its use of a prospective design and valid and reliable psychometric measures. Replication of these findings in studies that include a nonsurgical control group are needed in order to conclude confidently that cosmetic surgery leads to improvements in depression and quality of life.

Clinical experience also has suggested the potential role of two additional variables—the patients' motivation for surgery and the patients' gender—as predictors of psychological outcome. Anecdotally, patients who are externally motivated and are having surgery to please others (rather than to please themselves) as well as male patients have been considered greater risks for a poor psychological outcome. The role of patient motivation as a predictor of outcome has yet to be investigated, in part because it is hard to quantify motivations. A recent investigation of male patients identified few differences in body image concerns as compared to female patients (42). Postoperative outcome has yet to be studied in men.

In summary, postoperative investigations, like the preoperative studies, have shown mixed results. Most studies suggested that the majority of cosmetic surgery patients are satisfied with their postoperative result. Several studies suggested that patients may experience psychological benefits postoperatively; however, methodologic concerns with many of these studies limit the confidence that can be placed in their results.

SUMMARY OF THE RESEARCH

Attempts at drawing firm conclusions from the psychological research in cosmetic surgery is difficult at best. Overall, the findings are contradictory. Preoperative interview-based investigations suggested that patients are highly psychopathological, whereas studies that used valid and reliable paper-and-pencil measures found little psychopathology. These latter studies are perhaps more consistent with the experiences of surgeons in the present day—that the majority of patients do not present with significant psychopathology. However, given that not every individual who is dissatisfied with his or her appearance seeks cosmetic surgery, my colleagues and I have suggested that there must be some personality characteristic(s), although not necessarily a psychopathological one(s), that differentiates those who seek cosmetic surgery from those who do not (1,2).

The postoperative findings are just as limiting. Although the vast majority of patients report satisfaction with their postoperative outcome, it is unclear whether or not this satisfaction is related to psychological change. Studies that specifically looked at psychological changes following surgery have, for the most part, suffered from many of the same methodologic flaws as the preoperative studies. Thus, at this time it may be premature to state that cosmetic surgery leads to psychological benefit in a majority of patients (1,2).

Perhaps the most appropriate conclusion at this time is that the existing research has failed to answer the main questions that prompted the work. Perhaps with the exception of the patient who is actively psychotic (and patients who suffer from body dysmorphic disorder [BDD], as discussed later), there do not appear to be any psychological conditions that are absolute contraindications to surgery. Presently, there are only limited data suggesting that patients benefit psychologically from cosmetic surgery. Given the disappointing findings of this psychopathology-based approach, my colleagues and I have proposed a new avenue for psychological study with cosmetic surgery patients that focuses on body image (1,2).

BODY IMAGE AND COSMETIC SURGERY

Research over the past 25 years has consistently demonstrated the importance of physical appearance in daily life. Persons who are considered physically attractive, as compared to those less attractive, are consistently judged more positively across a variety of personality traits (43). Not only are attractive people seen more positively by others, they also are thought to receive preferential social treatment in virtually every social situation, including education, employment, medical care, legal proceedings, and romantic encounters (44). Whether or not we like to admit it, in our culture, appearance matters. Not surprisingly, this emphasis on physical appearance is thought to influence the increasing demand for cosmetic surgery, although this topic has received far less attention in the cosmetic surgery literature than studies of psychopathology.

The most distinguishing characteristic of cosmetic surgery patients may be their thoughts and feelings about their appearance. Cosmetic surgery patients may be more dissatisfied with their appearance that other individuals, or they may obtain larger portions of their self-esteem from their appearance. Alternatively, they may be highly motivated individuals who, when dissatisfied with an aspect of their lives, take action to fix it. Regardless, their interest in cosmetic surgery suggests an increased interest and focus on their physical appearance.

The psychological construct of body image specifically addresses issues of appearance and appearance-related concerns. Dissatisfaction with body image is pervasive in the United States (45) and is thought to motivate the pursuit of cosmetic surgery (1,2,36). One consistent finding of the preoperative studies of cosmetic surgery patients is that women who seek cosmetic surgery have reported increased dissatisfaction with body image (12,18,21,46,47). Body image dissatisfaction also may differentiate persons who seek cosmetic surgery from those who do not. Furthermore, Pruzinsky (37,38) has suggested that cosmetic surgery is body image surgery—that by modifying the body surgically, psychological improvement can occur.

Body image has been defined in numerous ways. Perhaps one of the most parsimonious and useful definitions is that of Cash and Pruzinsky (48), who defined body image as perceptions, thoughts, and feelings about the body and bodily experiences. This definition captures both the multidimensional nature (i.e., thoughts, feelings, and behaviors), as well as the external/objective and internal/subjective elements of body image (48). From the tenets of this definition, my colleagues and I have proposed a model of the relationship between body image and cosmetic surgery (2). The model considers both physical and psychological influences on the development of body image. It expands on this knowledge by specifically discussing how thoughts and feelings about appearance may influence the decision to seek cosmetic surgery.

Theoretical Relationship Between Body Image and Cosmetic Surgery

We theorized that there are several factors that may influence body image and the decision to seek cosmetic surgery (1,2). The first is the physical reality of one's appearance, which, we believe, lays the foundation for an individual's body image. As noted earlier, physical appearance is a potent determinant of person perception (43). Furthermore, there is increasing evidence of genetic and physiologic influences in perceptions of beauty. Relevant psychological influences of the model include perceptual, developmental, and sociocultural factors (1,2). Perceptual influences account for an individual's ability to accurately determine the physical features of a given body part. Patients frequently will report to their surgeon that a body part is different in size, shape, or appearance from the objective reality of the feature. Developmental influences consider the contribution of childhood and adolescent experiences to the adult body image. This influential factor accounts for the negative experiences of teasing about a specific appearance feature that many patients report during their initial consultation. Finally, sociocultural influences account for the interaction of the mass media and cultural ideals of appearance (which frequently portray unrealistic, exaggerated, or unattainable images of beauty that have been digitally enhanced and airbrushed to perfection), with the tendency for individuals to compare themselves to others. Perceptual, developmental, and sociocultural factors are thought to influence an individual's attitudes toward the body (1,2).

We theorized that attitudes toward the body have at least two dimensions (2). The first consists of a valence, defined as the degree of importance of body image to one's self-esteem. Persons with a high body image valence, in contrast to those with a low valence, are thought to derive much of their self-esteem from their body image. In addition, body image has a value (i.e., positive or negative). Presently, body image dissatisfaction is thought to be at its all-time high in the United States (45). It is difficult, however, to determine the point at which an individual's perceptions, attitudes, and behaviors regarding his or her body image become problematic. Therefore, we hypothesized that body image dissatisfaction falls on a continuum (1,2). Such dissatisfaction may range from a dislike of a specific appearance feature to psychopathologic dissatisfaction, in which thoughts about appearance distress and preoccupy the individual, and behavior is negatively influenced by these concerns (1,2). This more extreme dissatisfaction may be a symptom of clinically significant psychopathology that contraindicates cosmetic surgery.

We believe that it is the interaction between body image valence and body image value that influences the decision to pursue cosmetic surgery. Persons with a low body image valence and little body image dissatisfaction are unlikely to seek cosmetic surgery. In contrast, persons with a high body image valence, for whom body image is an important part of self-esteem, and who have a heightened degree of dissatisfaction with a specific feature may comprise the majority of cosmetic surgery patients.

Empirical Studies of Body Image in Cosmetic Surgery Patients

As noted earlier, several investigations suggested that cosmetic surgery patients report increased body image dissatisfaction. However, many of these investigations failed to use valid and reliable measures to assess body image concerns. It is only recently through a series of empirical investigations that the degree of body image dissatisfaction in cosmetic surgery patients has been established.

Our initial study in this area examined body image dissatisfaction in prospective cosmetic surgery patients (49). Prior to their initial consultation, 100 women who were seeking a variety of procedures completed a general measure of body image, as well as a measure of the degree of dissatisfaction with the specific feature for which they were seeking surgery. Results were compared to those of the normative samples for each of the measures. Prospective cosmetic surgery patients did not report a greater investment or increased dissatisfaction with their overall body image as compared to the normative values; however, they reported heightened dissatisfaction with the specific body feature for which they were pursuing surgery. Similar results subsequently were found in an investigation of male cosmetic surgery patients, as well as a study of women who sought rhytidectomy and blepharoplasty (42,46). Together, these results substantiated that cosmetic surgery patients had heightened dissatisfaction with the specific body feature considered for surgery, rather than more global dissatisfaction with the entire body.

Three recent studies of breast augmentation patients found similar results (50–52). In the first investigation, body image dissatisfaction in prospective breast augmentation and breast reduction patients was assessed (52). As expected breast augmentation patients reported less dissatisfaction with their breasts than did breast reduction patients, although both groups reported greater dissatisfaction than did other cosmetic surgery patients. Breast reduction patients reported greater dissatisfaction with their overall body image, part of which can be understood as a function of their increased body weight. Reduction patients also reported greater dissatisfaction with their breasts, marked by increased dysphoria and maladaptive behavioral change, including embarrassment about their breasts in public and social settings and avoidance of physical activity. More than 50% of both groups, however, reported significant behavioral change in response to negative feelings about their breasts. This included avoidance of being seen undressed by others, checking the appearance of their breasts, and camouflaging the appearance of their breasts with clothing or special bras. Results of this investigation also found that, in the year before surgery, 37% of reduction patients and 27% of breast augmentation patients reported a significant life change (i.e., change of employment, change in residence, separation, or divorce); 27% of reduction and 20% of augmentation patients reported increased anxiety and depression; and 6% of reduction and 10% of augmentation patients reported seeing a mental health professional. These results suggest that not only do women who seek cosmetic breast surgery experience increased breast dissatisfaction, but a substantial minority experience significant dysphoria that may warrant further psychological assessment or treatment (52).

In the second investigation, women who sought breast augmentation were compared to an age-matched sample of small-breasted women who were not seeking augmentation (50). Breast augmentation patients reported significantly greater dissatisfaction with their breasts, as well as greater discomfort in social situations, than did non-surgery seekers. However, the two groups did not differ on self-esteem. The third study also compared women who sought breast augmentation to physically similar women who were not seeking surgery on body image as well as self-esteem, quality of life, and appearance-related teasing (51). As with the previous study, augmentation patients reported greater body image and breast dissatisfaction. Although the two groups did not differ on self-esteem and quality of life, augmentation patients reported increased appearance-related teasing as well as increased use of psychotherapy, suggesting that these women may be experiencing a more general dysphoria as a result of their breast dissatisfaction.

Therefore, it appears that women who seek cosmetic surgery report greater body image dissatisfaction than women not seeking surgery. Early investigations, which did not use appropriate control groups, suggested that these differences were limited to the concerns with the feature considered for surgery. Studies of breast augmentation patients using physically similar women as controls, however, appear to suggest that not only do these women have increased dissatisfaction with their breasts, but they also have greater investment in their appearance, greater overall dissatisfaction, and greater concerns about their bodies in social situations. Furthermore, these women appear to use psychotherapy more frequently. Thus, it appears that body image dissatisfaction may be related to a more general dysphoria.

Body Image Dissatisfaction and Cosmetic Surgery: How Much is Too Much?

Results of these more recent studies raise the question of how much body image dissatisfaction is too much for cosmetic surgery. Extreme body image dissatisfaction is a central component of BDD, which is defined as a preoccupation with an imagined or slight defect in appearance that leads to significant impairment in functioning (15). Persons with BDD are often so preoccupied with a feature(s) of their appearance that they will examine, check, or alter their appearance repeatedly. These behaviors often prevent these individuals from attending school, holding a job, or maintaining romantic and social relationships. Although any body area may be the focus of concern for persons with BDD, the most commonly affected areas are the skin, hair, and nose (53–55).

BDD has many distinctive features that distinguish it from more normative appearance concerns. Many persons engage in repetitive behaviors to examine or improve the defect. Others may engage in avoidance behaviors, such as not looking at mirrors or refusing to leave the house. These behaviors may range in severity, but typically involve one or more hours a day (53).

The following case example illustrates many of the symptoms of BDD.

> Terry was a 42-year-old woman who presented for plastic surgery seeking laser resurfacing of her perioral area. She was married, had two children of high-school age, and was employed as a teacher. She was an attractive woman who arrived at her consultation well groomed. For the past several years, she had become concerned about several wrinkle lines between her upper lip and nose. When she was asked to show the surgeon the specific areas of concern, she scrutinized her mouth with a hand-held mirror for several minutes from different angles. She reported that she wore a great deal of makeup on a daily basis to camouflage these wrinkles, often reapplying the makeup several times in the morning until it was "just right." This activity frequently made her late for the start of school, which, over time, forced her to obtain permission from her principal to arrive late each morning. She also indicated that she would not let her students or other teachers get close to her right side, where she believed the wrinkles were most visible. Over time, she stopped socializing with the other teachers at school and stopped leaving her house on the evenings and weekends. She reported that she feared that others would think less of her if they saw her wrinkles. Following the consultation (the surgeon elected not to perform the surgery and referred her for a psychological consultation) she called the surgeon's office on three separate occasions to ask extremely detailed questions about the surgeon's impression of her appearance.

The prevalence of BDD in the general population is thought to be approximately 2% (53). A recent study found that 7% of female cosmetic surgery patients met diagnostic criteria for BDD (49). However, it often may be difficult to make this diagnosis in plastic surgery patients (49,56). Cosmetic surgery patients frequently present with relatively slight defects in appearance, presumably consistent with the first criteria of the diagnosis of BDD. Such slight defects, however, frequently are judged as observable and correctable by the plastic surgeon. As a result, judgment of a defect as "slight" becomes highly subjective in these patients. We have suggested that the degree of emotional distress and behavioral impairment, rather that the nature of the physical defect, may be more accurate indicators of body dysmorphic symptoms in plastic surgery populations (49,56).

The typical presentation of BDD patients for cosmetic surgery is relatively unknown. Pruzinsky (37,38) suggested that patients previously classified in the cosmetic surgery literature as "minimal deformity" patients may, in fact, have BDD. However, the "insatiable" patient who returns for multiple revisions without satisfaction also may be a candidate for the diagnosis. Preliminary clinical reports found that persons with BDD typically do not benefit from cosmetic surgery (54,55), either remaining focused on the presenting defect postoperatively or becoming focused on a different appearance feature. These results suggest that BDD may contraindicate cosmetic surgery (56); however, this has yet to be empirically studied.

Body Image Changes Following Cosmetic Surgery

The question remains, however, does body image improve following cosmetic surgery? Anecdotal clinical reports suggested that patients report improved feelings about their appearance postoperatively. Preliminary empirical data suggest that, 6 months after surgery, cosmetic surgery patients reported a significant reduction in the degree of dissatisfaction with the body feature surgically altered (57). However, they reported no significant changes in their investment or degree of satisfaction with their overall body image. Therefore, it appears that cosmetic surgery had a positive effect on feelings about a specific feature, but not global body image. Additional studies are needed to confirm improvements in body image following surgery and to investigate the stability of these changes over longer periods of time.

Reconstructive Surgery Patients

Reconstructive surgery patients, whether presenting with a congenital deformity, traumatic injury, or following oncologic treatment, also may experience a variety of psychological issues. Many studies have documented the psychological difficulties of children and adolescents with disfigured appearances. As a whole, these studies suggested that these children are at increased risk for psychological problems as a result of their appearance. A recent investigation from our group suggested that young adults born with craniofacial disfigurement, as compared to nonfacially disfigured adults, experience greater dissatisfaction with appearance and lower self-esteem and quality of life in early adulthood (58). In another investigation of adults seeking reconstructive procedures, 16% of patients (all scar revision patients) reported a level of distress and preoccupation with their appearance consistent with the diagnosis of BDD (59).

These preliminary investigations suggest that reconstructive surgery patients also may be experiencing psychological difficulties related to their appearance that warrant mental health care. Although additional research is needed to understand more fully the psychological issues for these patients, plastic surgeons should be aware that these individuals may be experiencing significant psychological difficulties, which may include extreme body image dissatisfaction, depression, social anxiety, or, in the case of victims of trauma, posttraumatic stress disorder. Given the plastic surgeon's role in the physical treatment of these conditions, surgeons also are in an optimal position to identify psychological difficulties and provide appropriate psychotherapeutic referrals.

PATIENT SCREENING AND SELECTION

Psychological screening of cosmetic surgery patients is critical for at least two reasons. First, such screening can help assess if patients' postoperative expectations are realistic. Second, this screening is vital to identify patients who have psychiatric conditions that may contraindicate cosmetic surgery. Thorough assessment of prospective patients can help identify patients who, at a minimum, may become a management problem to the surgeon and office staff, or who may threaten or follow through with threats of legal action or violence postoperatively.

Psychological screening of patients should focus on several areas: motivations and expectations; psychiatric status and history; and body image concerns (including BDD). In addition, the patient's behavior in the office should be observed carefully. Providing patients with referrals to mental health professionals when needed is an important part of patient selection.

Motivations and Expectations

It is important to determine the patients' motivations for surgery. Several researchers have attempted to categorize motivations for surgery as internal (undergoing the surgery to improve one's self-esteem) or external (undergoing the surgery for some secondary gain, such as obtaining a promotion or starting a new romantic relationship) (9,19). To assess the nature of patients' motivations, it may be useful to ask: "How come you are interested in surgery now?" This question may help determine if the patient is having the surgery for himself or herself and modest improvements in appearance, or if he or she having the surgery for others. Although a clear distinction between an internal and external motivation may be difficult, internally motivated patients are thought to be more likely to meet their goals for surgery (5).

Pruzinsky (38) categorized postoperative expectations as surgical, psychological, and social. Surgical expectations address the specific concerns about physical appearance (discussed later). Psychological expectations include the potential improvements in body image, self-esteem, and quality of life that may occur postoperatively. Social expectations address the potential social benefits of cosmetic surgery. Many persons interested in cosmetic surgery believe they will become more attractive to current or potential romantic partners following surgery. Although plastic surgery can enhance physical appearance, it may not improve the quality of romantic relationships. Thus, prospective patients should be aware that an improvement in appearance probably will not result in a change in the social responses of others. To assess postoperative expectations, it may be useful to inquire: "How do you anticipate your life will be different following the surgery?" Patients who are internally motivated and have realistic expectations may be most likely to be satisfied with the postoperative result.

Psychiatric Status and History

An important step in determining the psychological appropriateness of patients is collecting a psychiatric history. This information should be collected routinely as part of the history and physical examination. Patients should be asked about present and past psychiatric diagnoses, as well as any ongoing treatment. Patients with a history of psychopathology who are not currently under psychiatric care should be questioned closely about the potential need for psychiatric care. These patients may warrant a psychiatric consultation preoperatively to determine their current psychological status. Patients currently under psychiatric care should be asked if their mental health professional is aware of their interest in surgery. These professionals should be contacted by the surgeon to confirm that cosmetic surgery is appropriate for the patient at this time. Patients who have not mentioned their interest in cosmetic surgery to their mental health provider, or who refuse to allow the surgeon to contact him or her, should be viewed with caution. These patients warrant a psychiatric consultation. Patients with a psychiatric history who are dissatisfied with the postoperative result may use their psychiatric history as part of their legal action against the surgeon, arguing that their psychiatric condition prevented them from fully understanding the procedure and its potential outcomes. Therefore, it is critical that surgeons are aware of the psychiatric status of each of their patients.

Body Image and Body Dysmorphic Disorder

Assessment of body image concerns is a central component of the initial consultation with a cosmetic surgery patient. One useful way to begin to assess body image concerns is to ask, "What is it that you dislike about your appearance?" Patients should be able to articulate specific concerns about their appearance (i.e., "I dislike this bump on my nose.") Their physical concerns should be visible with little effort. Previous studies found no relationship between degree of physical deformity and degree of emotional distress in cosmetic surgery patients (5,23,60). Patients who are markedly distressed about slight defects that are not readily visible may be suffering from BDD.

The degree of dissatisfaction also should be thoroughly assessed. Ask: "When does the feature bother you the greatest amount?" "Do you ever 'camouflage' or hide the feature from others?" "Do you ever wish you could think about your appearance less?" "Do your feelings about your appearance keep you from doing certain activities?" These questions can indicate the degree of distress and impairment a person may be experiencing. Practitioners also may wish to familiarize themselves with the Body Dysmorphic Disorder Examination (61) in order to more thoroughly assess patients who show signs of BDD.

Office Behavior

Patients' behavior during their office visits should be observed closely. A 30- to 45-minute consultation is a brief period of time to learn about patients' psychiatric status. In addition, prospective patients are on their best behavior during the preoperative consultation and often will expend a great deal of effort to present as "appropriate" for surgery. Therefore, every bit of information either obtained during the consultation or observed during interactions with the nursing or office staff should be used in making a determination of appropriateness for surgery. Nonsurgical personnel frequently see different aspects of patients' behavior during other interactions in the office. These individuals may gather valuable insight into patients' psychological functioning that may alert the surgeon to a potential psychological problem. Patients who have difficulty following the office routine warrant further attention. Patients who frequently cancel appointments, ask for appointments outside of office hours, or do not wish to talk to anyone other than the surgeon should be reconsidered for surgery. Patients who raise concerns should, at a minimum, be seen for a second preoperative consultation. If concerns persist, these patients should be referred to a psychologist or psychiatrist for evaluation.

Mental Health Referrals

If the surgeon or staff have concerns about the psychological status of prospective patients, a referral to a psychologist or psychiatrist for an evaluation should be made. Given the relationship between body image dissatisfaction, BDD, and cosmetic surgery, a psychologist or psychiatrist with interest or expertise in body image may be the ideal consultant. These mental health professionals often work with other forms of psychopathology with a body image component, such as eating disorders. Professionals who work in areas of health psychology or behavioral medicine also may have some expertise in body image. Regardless of the expertise of the consultant, it is important that the surgeon communicate to the consultant the specific nature of the referral question. A well-qualified mental health professional with a good understanding of body image dissatisfaction and BDD can be a valuable asset to a cosmetic surgery practice.

Patients often will react to mental health referrals with anger and denial and frequently will refuse to accept the referral. Patients who refuse to see the consultant probably are not good candidates for surgery. Unfortunately, many of these patients eventually will find a surgeon who will operate on them, thereby not receiving the mental health care they need. Nevertheless, it is important that the surgeon treat the referral to the psychologist or psychiatrist like any other referral to a medical professional. This frequently will help destigmatize the mental health professional to the patient and make the referral more acceptable to them. It is important to communicate to the patient the reason for the consultation. It may be useful to say: "Undergoing cosmetic surgery is an important decision. You are considering making changes to your appearance that are more or less permanent. Cosmetic surgery often leads to changes in how you feel about your appearance—some that may be positive and others that may be less positive. I think it is important that we both are 100% sure that surgery is right for you at this time. Therefore, I would like you to see a psychologist (psychiatrist) who often works with us to help us decide if this is the right time for surgery." Such a statement underscores the importance of the consultation to the patient in a nonthreatening away and hopefully prevents the patient from responding with anger or hostility.

Plastic surgeons also may need to refer patients to a mental health professional postoperatively. This typically occurs in one of the scenarios—the cosmetic surgery patient is dissatisfied with successful surgery, the reconstructive patient is having difficulty coping with some residual deformity postoperatively, or the cosmetic or reconstructive patient is experiencing an exacerbation of psychopathology that was not detected preoperatively. Patients in each of these examples warrant further assessment and often psychotherapeutic care.

CONCLUSIONS

The psychological issues of cosmetic surgery patients have been of great interest to plastic surgeons since the origination of the specialty. Early studies in this area set out to identify those persons thought to benefit from surgery as well as those who might be psychologically inappropriate for surgery. Methodologic problems with this research, however, have left these questions largely unanswered. Within the last decade, body image has taken a central role in the study of cosmetic surgery patients. Body image dissatisfaction is thought to motivate persons to seek surgery, and body image appears to improve postoperatively. In addition, there appears to be an increased incidence of profound body image dissatisfaction, as characterized by BDD, among cosmetic surgery patients. Unfortunately, these individuals do not appear to benefit from cosmetic surgery. Given the increased incidence of BDD, coupled with the increasing popularity of cosmetic surgery in general, patient screening and selection has become increasingly important. Assessment of current psychological functioning, with specific attention to extreme body image dissatisfaction and BDD, is a critical element in determining patient appropriateness. Careful screening and selection of patients can increase the likelihood that those who have surgery meet their expectations and that those who do not receive the most appropriate care.

REFERENCES

1. Sarwer DB, Pertschuk MJ, Wadden TA, et al. Psychological investigations of cosmetic surgery patients: a look back and a look ahead. *Plast Reconstr Surg* 1998;101:1136–1142.
2. Sarwer DB, Wadden TA, Pertschuk MJ, et al. The psychology of cosmetic surgery: a review and reconceptualization. *Clin Psychol Rev* 1998;18:1–22.
3. Beale S, Lisper H, Palm B. A psychological study of patients seeking augmentation mammaplasty. *Br J Psychiatry* 1980;136: 133–138.
4. Edgerton MT, Jacobson WE, Meyer E. Surgical-psychiatric study of patients seeking plastic (cosmetic) surgery: ninety-eight consecutive patients with minimal deformity. *Br J Plast Surg* 1960;13:136–145.
5. Edgerton MT, Langman MW, Pruzinsky T. Plastic surgery and psychotherapy in the treatment of 100 psychologically disturbed patients. *Plast Reconstr Surg* 1991;88:594–608.
6. Edgerton MT, McClary AR. Augmentation mammaplasty: psychiatric implications and surgical indications. *Plast Reconstr Surg* 1958;21:279–305.
7. Edgerton MT, Meyer E, Jacobson WE. Augmentation mammaplasty: II. Further surgical and psychiatric evaluation. *Plast Reconstr Surg* 1961;27:279–303.
8. Marcus P. Psychological aspects of cosmetic rhinoplasty. *Br J Plast Surg* 1984;37:313–318.
9. Meyer E, Jacobson WE, Edgerton MT, et al. Motivational patterns in patients seeking elective plastic surgery. *Psyc Med* 1960;22:193–202.
10. Ohlsen L, Ponten B, Hambert G. Augmentation mammaplasty: a surgical and psychiatric evaluation of the results. *Ann Plast Surg* 1978;2:42–52.
11. Robin AA, Copas JB, Jack AB, et al. Reshaping the psyche: the concurrent improvement in appearance and mental state after rhinoplasty. *Br J Psychiatry* 1988;152:539–543.
12. Schlebusch L, Levin A. A psychological profile of women selected for augmentation mammaplasty. *South Afr Med J* 1983;64: 481–483.
13. Sihm F, Jagd M, Pers M. Psychological assessment before and after augmentation mammaplasty. *Scand J Plast Reconstr Surg* 1978;12:295–298.
14. Cook LS, Daling JR, Voigt LF, et al. Characteristics of women with and without breast augmentation. *JAMA* 1997;277: 1612–1617.
15. American Psychiatric Association. *Diagnostic and statistical manual of mental disorders,* 4th ed. Washington, DC: American Psychiatric Press, 1994.
16. American Psychiatric Association. *Diagnostic and statistical manual of mental disorders,* 3rd ed rev. Washington, DC: American Psychiatric Press, 1987.
17. Napoleon A. The presentation of personalities in plastic surgery. *Ann Plast Surg* 1993;31:193–208.
18. Baker JL, Kolin IS, Bartlett ES. Psychosexual dynamics of patients undergoing mammary augmentation. *Plast Reconstr Surg* 1974;53:652–659.
19. Goin MK, Burgoyne RW, Goin JM, et al. A prospective psychological study of 50 female face-lift patients. *Plast Reconstr Surg* 1980;65:436–442.
20. Goin MK, Rees TD. A prospective study of patients' psychological reactions to rhinoplasty. *Ann Plast Surg* 1991;27:210–215.
21. Shipley RH, O'Donnell JM, Bader KF. Personality characteristics of women seeking breast augmentation. *Plast Reconstr Surg* 1977;60:369–376.
22. Wright MR, Wright WK. A psychological study of patients undergoing cosmetic surgery. *Arch Otolaryngol* 1975;101:145–151.
23. Hay GG. Psychiatric aspects of cosmetic nasal operations. *Br J Psychiatry* 1970;116:85–97.
24. Hollyman JA, Lacey JH, Whitfield PJ, et al. Surgery for the psyche: a longitudinal study of women undergoing reduction mammoplasty. *Br J Plast Surg* 1986;39:222–224.
25. Hetter GP. Improved patient satisfaction with augmentation mammoplasty: the transaxillary subpectoral approach. *Aesthetic Plast Surg* 1991;15:123–127.
26. Park AJ, Chetty U, Watson ACH. Patient satisfaction following insertion of silicone breast implants. *Br J Plast Surg* 1996; 49:515–518.
27. Schlebusch L, Marht I. Long-term psychological sequelae of augmentation mammaplasty. *South Afr Med J* 1993;83:267–271.
28. Wells KE, Cruse CW, Baker JL, et al. The health status of women

following cosmetic surgery. *Plast Reconstr Surg* 1994;93: 907–912.
29. Young VL, Nemecek JR, Nemecek DA. The efficacy of breast augmentation: breast size increase, patient satisfaction, and psychological effects. *Plast Reconstr Surg* 1994;94:958–969.
30. Handel N, Wellisch D, Silverstein MJ, et al. Knowledge, concern, and satisfaction among augmentation mammaplasty patients. *Ann Plast Surg* 1993;30:13–20.
31. Kilmann PR, Sattler JI, Taylor J. The impact of augmentation mammaplasty: a follow-up study. *Plast Reconstr Surg* 1987; 80:374–378.
32. Placheff-Wiemer M, Concannon MJ, Conn VS, et al. The impact of the media on women with breast implants. *Plast Reconstr Surg* 1993;92:779–785.
33. Goin MK, Goin JM, Gianini MH. The psychic consequences of a reduction mammaplasty. *Plast Reconstr Surg* 1977;59:530–534.
34. Hay GG, Heather BB. Changes in psychometric test results following cosmetic nasal operations. *Br J Psychiatry* 1973;122: 89–90.
35. Kaslow F, Becker H. Breast augmentation: psychological and plastic surgery considerations. *Psychotherapy* 1992;29:467–473.
36. Schouten JW. Selves in transition: symbolic consumption in personal rites of passage and identity reconstruction. *J Consum Res* 1991;17:412–425.
37. Pruzinsky T. Psychological factors in cosmetic plastic surgery: recent developments in patient care. *Plast Surg Nurs* 1993;13: 64–71.
38. Pruzinsky T. The psychology of plastic surgery: advances in evaluating body image, quality of life, and psychopathology. In: Habal MB, Lineaweaver WC, Parsons RW, et al., eds. *Advances in plastic and reconstructive surgery,* vol. 12. Philadelphia: Mosby 1996:153–170.
39. Slator R, Harris DL. Are rhinoplasty patients potentially mad? *Br J Plast Surg* 1992;45:307–310.
40. Meyer L, Ringberg A. Augmentation mammaplasty—psychiatric and psychosocial characteristics and outcome in a group of Swedish women. *Scand J Plast Reconstr Surg* 1987;21:199–208.
41. Rankin M, Borah GL, Perry AW, et al. Quality-of-life outcomes after cosmetic surgery. *Plast Reconstr Surg* 1998;102:2139–2145.
42. Pertschuk MJ, Sarwer DB, Wadden TA, et al. Body image dissatisfaction in male cosmetic surgery patients. *Aesthetic Plast Surg* 1998;22:20–24.
43. Alley TR. *Social and applied aspects of perceiving faces.* Hillsdale, NJ: Lawrence Erlbaum, 1988.
44. Hatfield E, Sprecher S. *Mirror, mirror . . . The importance of looks in everyday life.* Albany, NY: SUNY Press, 1986.
45. Garner DM. The 1997 body image survey results. *Psyc Today* 1997;31:30–87.
46. Sarwer DB, Whitaker LA, Wadden TA, et al. Body image dissatisfaction in women seeking rhytidectomy or blepharoplasty. *Aesthetic Surg J* 1997;17:230–234.
47. Schlebusch L. Negative bodily experience and prevalence of depression in patients who request augmentation mammoplasty. *South Afr Med J* 1989;75:323–326.
48. Cash TF, Pruzinsky T. *Body images: development, deviance, and change.* New York: Guilford, 1990.
49. Sarwer DB, Wadden TA, Pertschuk MJ, et al. Body image dissatisfaction and body dysmorphic disorder in 100 cosmetic surgery patients. *Plast Reconstr Surg* 1998;101:1644–1649.
50. Nordmann JE. Body image and self-esteem in women seeking breast augmentation. (Unpublished doctoral dissertation).
51. Sarwer DB. An investigation of the psychological characteristics of cosmetic breast augmentation patients. (Unpublished data).
52. Sarwer DB, Bartlett SP, Bucky LP, et al. Bigger is not always better: body image dissatisfaction in breast reduction and breast augmentation patients. *Plast Reconstr Surg* 1998;101: 1956–1961.
53. Phillips KA. *The broken mirror: understanding and treating body dysmorphic disorder.* New York: Oxford University Press, 1996.
54. Phillips KA, Diaz SF. Gender differences in body dysmorphic disorder. *J Nerv Ment Dis* 1997;185:570–577.
55. Phillips KA, McElroy SL, Keck PE, et al. Body dysmorphic disorder: 30 cases of imagined ugliness. *Am J Psyc* 1993;150: 302–308.
56. Sarwer DB. The "obsessive" cosmetic surgery patient: a consideration of body image dissatisfaction and body dysmorphic disorder. *Plast Surg Nurs* 1997;17:193–209.
57. Sarwer DB, Wadden TA, Pertschuk MJ, et al. Changes in body image following cosmetic surgery. Paper presented at the Nineteenth Annual Meeting of the Society of Behavioral Medicine, New Orleans, LA, March 25–28, 1998.
58. Sarwer DB, Bartlett SP, Whitaker LA, et al. Adult psychological functioning of individuals born with craniofacial anomalies. *Plast Reconstr Surg* 1999;103:412–418.
59. Sarwer DB, Whitaker LA, Pertschuk MJ, et al. Body image concerns of reconstructive surgery patients: an underrecognized problem. *Ann Plast Surg* 1998;40:404–407.
60. Boone OR, Wexler MR, Kaplan De-Nour A. Rhinoplasty patients' critical self-evaluations of their noses. *Plast Reconstr Surg* 1996;98:436–439.
61. Rosen JC, Reiter J. Development of the body dysmorphic disorder examination. *Behav Res Ther* 1996;34:755–766.

SUGGESTED READING

Sarwer DB, Pertschuk MJ, Wadden TA, et al. Psychological investigations of cosmetic surgery patients: a look back and a look ahead. *Plast Reconstr Surg* 1998;101:1136–1142.

Sarwer DB, Wadden TA, Pertschuk MJ, et al. Body image dissatisfaction and body dysmorphic disorder in 100 cosmetic surgery patients. *Plast Reconstr Surg* 1998;101:1644–1649.

Phillips KA. *The broken mirror: understanding and treating body dysmorphic disorder.* New York: Oxford University Press, 1996.

Discussion

PSYCHOLOGICAL CONSIDERATIONS IN COSMETIC SURGERY

J. KEVIN THOMPSON

In Chapter 3, David Sarwer not only provides a compelling yet succinct analysis of the methods and findings for the past 50 years, but he also offers a template for theorizing and investigating the topic for the next 50 years. Importantly, he and his colleagues have already begun the enterprise, having completed several studies that provide an exposition of his model, which is largely based on the integration of the concept of body image into the examination of psychological factors and cosmetic surgery.

His overview of past methodological shortcomings needs only the briefest mention herein, but includes such critical design recommendations as (a) inclusion of control and/or comparison groups, (b) greater specificity of clinical interview components, (c) detailing of demographic characteristics, (d) assessment of preoperative levels of disturbance, (e) standardization of interview methods, (f) consideration of patient's motivation and gender as moderating factors, and (g) utilization of prospective designs. His cautionary conclusion that "it is premature to conclude that cosmetic surgery produces psychological benefits" is an apt summary of the available data, as well as a strong comment on the need for future research.

By conceptualizing cosmetic surgery as "body image surgery," Sarwer and other researchers have connected two relatively disparate fields of research—body image and cosmetic surgery—which, unfortunately, have proceeded somewhat independently of one another. For virtually the entire 20th century, researchers have been interested in the internal representation of one's appearance (1,2). In the past decade, researchers have explored the connection between objective and subjective aspects of appearance (i.e., quantifiable "attractiveness" level and the internal view [body image]) and found that the overlap is quite small (3,4). In addition, a plethora of assessment measures has emerged, providing the researcher and clinician an assortment of reliable and valid questionnaires for the collection of body image disturbance ratings (5). Finally, it is apparent that surgery need not be the only solution for body image enhancement. Several well-controlled studies have demonstrated that cognitive-behavioral strategies can improve appearance satisfaction levels (6,7).

Thus, the time is quite right for an integration of the extant database on body image into the research designs of cosmetic surgery, which is what Sarwer and colleagues have proposed and accomplished in their recent work. They have done a stellar job of selecting widely used and psychometrically valid measures in their research, and we would do well to follow their lead in designing our own investigations. Thus far, I have focused primarily on the issue of research; however, Sarwer also details critical issues related to patient selection and screening. It is in this area that I would consider suggesting a few additional considerations by the cosmetic surgeon.

Sarwer provides a list of questions to guide the initial evaluation of patients for surgery, including those that might reveal body dysmorphic symptoms. He also notes the importance of evaluating patient motivation for surgery and expectations regarding the outcome. He encourages a second preoperative consultation when concerns regarding appropriateness for surgery are apparent, followed by a consultation with a psychologist or psychiatrist versed in the body dysmorphic disorder literature and trained in its assessment. My own addition to his recommendations might be seen as extreme. I believe that surgeons might consider the potential utility of adding a consultant who takes part in the evaluation of virtually any patient considering cosmetic surgery.

My reasoning for this is twofold. First, I am not sure it reasonable to expect a surgeon to actually develop, without extensive training, proficiency in assessing body dysmorphic disorder, especially (and this is an issue upon which I agree with Sarwer) if the Body Dysmorphic Disorder Examination (4,7) is used as a screening measure for debatable cases. Related to this concern is the need for other potential assessment materials, such as questionnaire data, to augment clinical interview. A consultant with expertise in the body image arena would be able to select appropriate measures,

J. K. Thompson: Department of Psychology, University of South Florida, Tampa, Florida

for diverse patient samples, with a focus on the reliability and validity of various methods.

Second, I think that surgeons should consider the adjunctive, or primary, use of psychological treatment procedures (4,6) for those cases that are either inappropriate for surgery or might benefit from additional psychological work postoperatively. Mild cases of body dissatisfaction, with surgical contraindications, might readily respond to tried and tested directive cognitive-behavioral techniques. Patients with unmet expectations postoperatively also might benefit from this type of intervention.

In sum, Sarwer has provided us with an extremely important review of the problems with past research, along with an outline for future investigation and clinical practice. My own, certainly debatable, proposition is that surgeons strongly consider the use of a trained consultant in the area of body image assessment and treatment.

REFERENCES

1. Fisher S. *Development and structure of the body image.* Hillsdale, NJ: Lawrence Erlbaum, 1986.
2. Thompson JK. *Body image disturbance: assessment and treatment.* Elmsford, NY: Pergamon Press, 1990.
3. Cash TF, Pruzinsky T. *Body images: development, deviance, and change.* New York: Guilford, 1990.
4. Thompson JK, Heinberg LJ, Altabe M, et al. *Exacting beauty: theory, assessment and treatment of body image disturbance.* Washington, DC: American Psychological Association, 1999.
5. Thompson JK. *Body image, eating disorders, and obesity: an integrative guide for assessment and treatment.* Washington, DC: American Psychological Association, 1996.
6. Cash TF. *What do you see when you look in the mirror?* New York: Bantam, 1995.
7. Rosen JC. Body dysmorphic disorder: assessment and treatment. In: Thompson JK, ed. *Body image, eating disorders and obesity: an integrative guide for assessment and treatment.* Washington, DC: American Psychological Association, 1996:149–170.

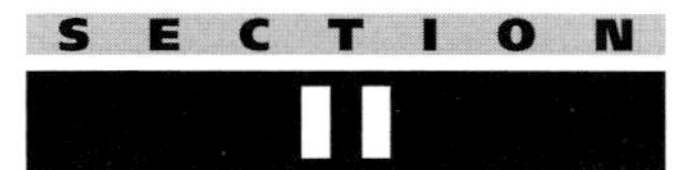

LEGAL ISSUES

4

INFORMED CONSENT, RECORD KEEPING, AND DOCUMENTATION

WALTER G. SULLIVAN

INFORMED CONSENT

A lawsuit based solely on an alleged lack of informed consent is quite rare. More commonly, an informed consent claim is added to the main complaint of medical negligence. In the context of plastic surgery cases, the unfavorable result frequently is the basis of the suit. Whether or not supported by the facts, the patient alleges that had she been informed about the possibility of this unfavorable result, she never would have consented to the procedure. This is used as yet another bargaining chip by the plaintiff's attorney in ongoing negotiations. Thus, obtaining and documenting the informed consent becomes a valuable exercise for the plastic surgeon.

Background

Historically, failure to obtain permission before a medical procedure was considered the tort of battery (1). Battery is an unlawful (i.e., without permission) touching that need not be harmful to be actionable against the physician. Today, battery is rarely the basis of a lawsuit against a surgeon. Although a procedure done without consent is an unlawful touching and no harmful result needs to be proved, the monetary value of damages may be quite small. In addition, battery is an intentional tort (i.e., the result of an intentional act rather than a negligent act) and will not be covered by the physician's malpractice insurance. This makes the case less attractive to a plaintiff's attorney, because a surgeon is more likely to settle a case if the settlement is paid from the insurance company's money rather than his own. Consequently, the claim will be filed as a medical negligence case rather than a battery action to bring it within the insurance policy's coverage. This approach is widely accepted by the courts, because failure to obtain consent before a procedure is considered a breach of the standard of care and, consequently, is an act of medical malpractice. Surprisingly, it was not until 1957 that the term "informed consent" was first used by a court (2). Following the 1960s, legal theories of patient autonomy expanded, and the patient became a partner in the doctor–patient relationship entitled to an adequate understanding of contemplated treatment plans. Physicians have a legal and ethical obligation to obtain an informed consent from their patients before treatment. The duty to obtain consent before treatment is rooted, first, in the long recognized principle of English common law that no free man may be touched without his permission. Second, a right of privacy and individual autonomy that gives an individual sovereignty over his own body has been elucidated by the United States Supreme Court as flowing from the Bill of Rights and the 14th Amendment.

W. G. Sullivan: Nevada Plastic Surgery, Las Vegas, Nevada

Elements Required in an Informed Consent

It is easy to enumerate the kinds of information that are required to be disclosed to the patient, but it is a much more complicated task to list the details of what must be disclosed. In some cases, it will depend on the state in which the surgeon practices. In other cases, it will depend on the individual nature of the particular patient. These complicating factors will be discussed later in the chapter. In general, five types of information are required, and additional information may be required stemming from the physician's role as a fiduciary. The standard five types of information required are as follows.

Diagnosis

This is rarely an important issue in the context of plastic surgery, and it is rarely litigated.

Nature and Purpose of the Proposed Treatment

A detailed description of the procedure is not required, and, although it may be good practice, there is no case law requiring the discussion of the likelihood of success (3).

Availability of Alternative Treatments

This is an extensively litigated area. The patient must be informed about any medically acceptable alternative treatment that could be used under the circumstances. This includes procedures that the informing physician could not, in fact, perform, and the patient would have to see another physician for the alternative treatment. However, it is not necessary to inform the patient about procedures that neither the informing physician nor another specialist would recommend (4).

Risks, Complications, and Consequences

This is clearly the "mother lode" of informed consent litigation in plastic surgery. More frequently than is justified by the facts: there is an unfavorable result, a suit for malpractice is filed, and an informed consent claim is added claiming that the patient never would have had the procedure if she had be informed of the possibility of that unfavorable result. A risk or complication is something that might happen as a result of the procedure, e.g., a postoperative hematoma occurs after a facelift. A consequence is something that either normally occurs after a procedure, e.g., a joint will not move after an arthrodesis, or is something that results from the occurrence of a complication, e.g., skin loss following a postfacelift hematoma.

Courts do not require that every risk be disclosed to a patient. Extremely unlikely risks generally are not required to be disclosed, but this is subject to exceptions in some states. Case law indicates that risks that are "commonly known" need not be discussed (5), but, in our present medicolegal milieu, reliance on this by the physician is not recommended to avoid being second guessed later. Finally, although rarely mentioned in talks and in the literature directed at physicians, what you legally need to disclose to a patient is dependent on the informed consent standard adopted in your particular state, which will be addressed shortly.

Result if No Treatment

A physician is under the legal duty to inform the patient about any unfavorable results that may occur without treatment. For example, a biopsy of a suspicious lesion may be indicated, but the patient refuses. The patient must be informed that the result of not having a biopsy may be a delay in diagnosis of a malignancy increasing the extent of later treatment or raising the probability of mortality (6).

The Physician as Fiduciary

The physician–patient relationship imposes on the physician the highest standard of duty imposed by law, that of the fiduciary. A fiduciary is one who undertakes to act in the interest of another person while subordinating the fiduciary's personal interests to that of the other person (7). This has led a court to find that a physician had a duty to disclose his alcoholism to a patient (8) and another to find a duty to disclose a physician's human immunodeficiency virus (HIV)-positive status (9). Although not strictly an issue of informed consent, physicians are obligated to disclose a failure of treatment or the happening of a maloccurrence during a procedure (e.g., "the nerve was accidentally cut and I repaired it") (10).

State Variations in Duty to Disclose

There are two standards used to judge the adequacy of an informed consent: the physician-based standard* and the patient-based standard.** Some states use a hybrid rule.† Although the number of physician-based states (at 22) outnumber the patient-based states (20 plus DC), a majority of the hybrid states are more patient oriented than physician oriented, effectively making the patient-based standard the majority rule in the United States.

Initially, courts allowed the medical profession to set the standards for informed consent. What was required was what the doctors in the community thought was necessary. This evolved into the physician-based standard. Within the past few decades, some states have, instead, adopted a rule that requires disclosure of what the patient would consider material to his decision. This is the patient-based standard.

Physician-based Standard

A plastic surgeon in a physician-based standard state needs to inform the patient what the reasonable plastic surgeon would tell the patient under the same or similar circumstances (14). This standard is basically the same as that used for medical malpractice, where the question is whether the physician violated the standard of care as determined by the physician's specialty group. Such a standard can only be determined by an expert witness who can testify to the standards of the specialty. In an informed consent case in a physician-based standard state, the prevailing standard of informed consent in that specialty must be testified to by an expert witness.

Patient-based Standard

In a patient-based standard state, the plastic surgeon must give the patient all the information "material" to the deci-

* Physician-based standard states: AL, AZ, AR, DE, ID, IN, IL, KS, ME, MI, MO, MT, NE, NV, NH, NY, NC, SC, TN, VT, VA, WY (11).
** Patient-based standard states: AK, CA, CT, DC, GA, IA, LA, MD, MA, MN, MS, NJ, NM, OH, OK, PA, RI, SD, WA, WV, WI (12).
† CO, FL, HI, KY, ND, OR, TX, UT (13).

sion that the patient must make. Rather than inform the patient about what plastic surgeons think the patient should know, the information given must be what the patient needs to know to make a decision. What the patient needs to know is what a patient would find important (i.e., material) in making the decision.

Complicating matters is whether you need to tell that patient what that particular patient needs to know (subjective standard), or is it adequate to tell the patient what the reasonable and prudent patient would want to know under the same or similar circumstances (objective standard). In the groundbreaking case that first elucidated the patient-based standard (15), the court applied the "objective" patient-based standard. By far, the objective standard is the most commonly adopted standard in the states using the patient-based approach. However, even using the objective approach, where you must make the patient aware of risks that the theoretical reasonable patient would want to know, the courts still insist that a physician take into account any special fears, values, or sensibilities of his particular patient.

The disadvantage for the physician-defendant in a patient-based standard state is that the plaintiff-patient need not have an expert witness testify that the physician should have told him about a particular risk before surgery. Because the standard is what the reasonable patient-layman would want to know, the jury can simply put itself in the reasonable patient's position and decide for itself if the members of the jury would have wanted to be informed. From the plaintiff attorney's point of view, this is much better position to be in, because, almost regardless of the weakness of his case, he is not dependent on finding an expert and the judge will most likely allow the case to go to the jury to let the jury decide the issue. Juries, unfortunately, do not always decide rationally.

Causation Test

Even if the patient can convince the jury that she should have been told, the case is not over. The patient also must prove causation. First, she must show that the procedure done actually caused her injury, and that the physician should have known that this injury could occur following the procedure. This usually is straightforward, but a expert medical witness usually is necessary. Second, she must show that had she been informed of the risk, she would not have had the procedure. For example, a patient has a complete facial nerve palsy after a deep-plane facelift. She contends that had she known that a nerve injury was possible, she would not have had the procedure. This is possible. Another patient has a squamous cell carcinoma and develops a postoperative infection. He contends that he would have never had his cancer removed had he been told that he could develop a wound infection. This is not believable. In the latter case, the causality test fails because there is no cause-and-effect relationship between not being told about the complication and having the procedure in the first place. The jury needs to decide if the patient would have had the procedure had he been told. States then use yet another objective or subjective standard. The great majority of states use the objective decision causality test. They ask if the reasonable and prudent would have not had the procedure had they been told about the risk in question. In a minority of states, the subjective decision causality test is used, and the jury tries to decide if this particular patient would have had the procedure or not.

Hybrid Rule States

These states have generally modified either the physician-based or patient-based rules by statute (16). Texas, for example, created a Medical Disclosure Panel to prescribe what needed to be disclosed for particular procedures of their choosing. However, the courts found that this statute had the effect of replacing the physician-based standard with the patient-based standard for any procedures that the panel did not address (17). In Florida, the disclosure must meet the physician-based standard and be sufficient for a reasonable person to have a general understanding of the procedure, medically acceptable alternatives, and substantial risks inherent in the procedure (18). Some states (e.g., CA, ME, MA, MN) have statutes covering specific situations, e.g., what must be disclosed in the treatment of breast cancer.

When an Informed Consent is not Required

There are a number of situations when an informed consent is not required.

Waiver

A competent patient may waive an informed consent. Patients have the right to refuse disclosures otherwise required for an informed consent and may not be forced to hear them. A waiver must be voluntarily given without duress, and the patient must be aware that he has the right to hear the information. It is suggested that a physician give the patient enough information so that it is clear what types of information the patient is waiving the disclosure of. Physicians are urged to document the patient's waiver.

Emergency Treatment

When prompt treatment is needed and the patient is incapable of giving an informed consent, courts generally will allow consent by proxy from the patient's nearest relation who is available. If no such proxy is available or known, the courts presume that the patient would want such emergency care if he were able to consent absent evidence to the contrary (e.g., "Living Will"). However, states differ on how serious the emergency need be to allow the physician a free hand. Certainly, the physician may proceed if necessary to preserve life and limb. If consent is refused by the next of kin, the physician is put in a difficult situation. If time is available, emergency permission from the court may be obtained. Hospital legal departments usually are very helpful in such situations. If there is no time, the surgeon is put in a difficult position. If treatment is refused by a spouse and the surgeon does not proceed and the patient loses a limb, legally he should be on strong ground, but allegations of inadequately informing the relative may come up later. In this situation where a relative refuses needed treatment, it is advisable to get another party involved to stress the importance of action. If the surgeon goes ahead with treatment despite a relative's objection and in the absence of court permission, the surgeon opens himself up not only to a failure to obtain an informed consent (medical malpractice), but also to a battery charge if permitted by the jurisdiction. Battery, an intentional tort, probably will be excluded from coverage by his malpractice policy and his personal assets will be at risk. This gives the plaintiff a very strong bargaining position.

Therapeutic Privilege

A physician may abstain from a complete disclosure to the patient when, in the physician's sound judgment, the disclosure itself poses a significant risk of harming the patient. For example, a physician decided that a seriously ill patient with hypertension and a suspected thoracic aortic aneurysm should not be told the risks of thoracic aortography. The patient developed paralysis after the aortogram and contended that had he been told of the risk he would not have consented. The court held for the doctor on the basis of therapeutic privilege (19). Such situations should be rare in plastic surgery, and, although not required by law, it has been suggested by courts that the surgeon disclose the risks to a spouse or other close relation even though this may be a breach of confidentiality. Documentation of the reasons for the physician's action should be noted in the patient's record. In addition, a second concurring opinion by an uninvolved physician would be helpful should legal complications later occur. Fear that the patient will not have the procedure if informed of the risk is not a situation where the therapeutic privilege will apply. The constitutional right to refuse treatment even where strongly indicated is the basis of the right to receive an informed consent.

Patient's Prior Knowledge

Where the physician is aware that the patient has adequate prior knowledge, it is not necessary to inform the patient again. Also, courts have repeatedly stated that it is not necessary to inform patients about matters within common knowledge or about risks that are very remote. However, even if the risk is remote, if it involves death, paralysis, loss of sexual or reproductive function, or other very serious unfavorable result, it might be required. Thus, it is safer practice to mention it.

Implied Consent

A patient's conduct may legally imply consent. For example, a patient who poses for preoperative photographs in the office without objection has given implied consent to be photographed.

Special Patient Categories

Minors

By statute, adulthood begins at age 18 years in most states (19 years in AL, NE, WY; 21 years in MS and MO) (20). Although it is commonly believed that only the parent's consent is needed to treat an adolescent minor, this is not generally correct. Many states have passed statutes that allow minors varying from age 14 to 16 years to consent to any form of medical treatment. In addition, many states have adopted the "mature minor" rule, which does not specify an age, but rather allows minors who understand and appreciate the consequences of the proposed treatment to give consent (16). This has a great deal of relevance to plastic surgery. A 16-year-old rhinoplasty patient must herself give an informed consent to the procedure. Generally, the more unnecessary the procedure (e.g., cosmetic), the more important is the minor's consent. Interestingly, there has not been a recorded case in the last 30 years in which a parent has recovered damages from a physician for appropriate treatment for which consent had not been given by the parent but was given by the minor patient who was over the age of 15 years (21). In the situation where the failure to treat would result in serious injury, the physician may petition the court for permission to treat in the absence of parental or minor consent.

When parents are separated or divorced, the parent with legal custody or actual possession of the child can give consent. Where the child is with the noncustodial parent and needs treatment for an injury, the noncustodial parent may give consent.

In the emergency setting, courts are very willing to let the physician proceed with treatment when a parent cannot be reached for consent, even in the absence of a serious injury. Courts do not want children in pain or frightened for prolonged periods while waiting for their parents to be found.

Incompetent Patients

When the patient has been legally adjudicated as incompetent, consent is obtained from the individual designated as guardian by the court. Usually, however, the circumstances are not that convenient. If a patient does not give consent to a needed procedure because he does not appear to be mentally competent to understand the seriousness of the situation, there is no easy answer for the surgeon. The law presumes that an adult is competent unless adjudicated otherwise. Short of petitioning the court for a guardian to be appointed, surgeons should try to enlist the support of the patient's family, ask for a second medical opinion, and discuss the situation with the hospital attorney.

When the Procedure Exceeds the Consent

The Extension Doctrine

The extension doctrine allows the surgeon to extend the scope of the procedure when unforeseen circumstances arise that make it advisable to do so. This doctrine does not allow a surgeon carte blanche. If the extension was foreseeable and the patient was not informed about its possibility, then the doctrine does not apply. Similarly, it will not apply in situations where the extension is not so urgent that it can be postponed until the patient can give consent. For example, during an authorized oophorectomy, a surgeon removed a suspicious mole from a patient's thigh without consent. The court held against the surgeon, since there was no necessity to proceed without first getting the patient's consent (22). In another case, a surgeon harvested tensor fascia lata without consent to use in an authorized hand procedure. The court found that surgeon was unjustified (23). The additional procedure was a foreseeable possibility of which the patient could have been informed.

Unauthorized Surgeon

A substitute surgeon may not be used without the patient's consent. In an emergency, necessary treatment may be instituted by an unauthorized physician.

Documentation

Contrary to common belief, a consent need not be in writing. What a written consent may provide, however, is documentation that the informed consent actually took place. This frequently becomes an issue in litigation following an unfavorable result. Strictly speaking, a verbal disclosure meeting the legal requirements followed by a verbal assent by the patient is all that is required. However, the surgeon, for his own protection, should record in the patient's medical record that an informed consent was given by the patient. Listing the risks discussed also may be helpful.

Another approach is to have a written consent to assure that the legal requirements are fulfilled. A very complete written consent signed by the patient is not a complete defense. Plaintiffs may contend that they were not given enough time to read it, that they did not understand it, and that they had no opportunity to ask questions, in short, that they did not know what they were doing. There is no foolproof way of preventing an informed consent claim, but some states, bowing to tort reform, have helped to make a defense easier if certain conditions are met. At least 12 states* make a signed consent form presumptively valid (25). The list of required disclosures is generally short. Plastic surgeons practicing in these states should consider taking advantage of their states' laws and use a written consent. I have found the information and consent forms available from the American Society of Plastic Surgeons, Inc., to be very helpful. Others have found them too detailed to the point of being speculative. For example, is it really necessary to disclose to a patient that they may get toxic-shock syndrome following an augmentation mammoplasty?

Courts have generally looked unfavorably at "blanket" consent forms that give the surgeon virtually unlimited discretion in performing the procedure. Courts will strike down consents that include waivers of prospective liability as void against public policy. Such waivers to sue physicians for future possible malpractice are never valid.

MEDICAL RECORDS

Physicians have a legal and ethical obligation to maintain adequate medical records. The importance of the patient's medical record in our litigious society cannot be overstated. Remarkably, medical evidence is thought to be involved in three-fourths of all civil cases and about one-fourth of criminal cases brought to trial (26). The medical record is vital in the communication of medical information among physicians and other health care entities. It allows continuity of care when the patient changes physicians, allowing future medical professionals to evaluate the patient with the benefit of knowing what came before. More narrowly, the medical record allows the physician to document clearly the progress of the patient's treatment. This will be of major importance should a legal dispute arise in the future.

Medical records should be accurate and timely. A note should reflect each patient visit. Although very difficult to be consistently carried out in practice, notations should be made for every patient contact, including telephone calls. The patient's noncompliance with treatment plans and failure to return for office visits should be documented. Patient's complaints and dissatisfactions should be noted. When dealing with pediatric patients, it is the parent or guardian who will determine compliance with treatment, and discussions with them should be noted. Documentation of informed consents should be reflected in the chart. The record should be legible. Inadequate medical records could be the basis of the court finding a violation of the standard of care. There are state and federal statutes that mandate that medical records be retained for a specific number of years, usually 5 to 15 years, and longer for children (27). If a patient decides to see another physician, a copy of the medical record should be sent to the new physician. In plastic surgery, copies of the patient's photographs are particularly useful to the new surgeon. If a surgeon moves or retires from practice, his records still need to be retained, at least for the statutorily mandated time. Ideally, the records could be transferred to the surgeon taking over the practice. Otherwise, there still needs to be some way for the patients to gain access to them.

Alteration of Medical Records

Errors in medical records are frequent and usually involve a spelling or transcription error. However, an error as simple as

* FL, GA, ID, IA, LA, ME, NV, NC, OH, TX, UT, WA (24).

transcribing "there is evidence of necrosis" when what was dictated was "there is no evidence of necrosis" could make a great deal of difference in a malpractice suit for a delay in the treatment of a complication. In addition, simple but costly errors, such as that just described, are difficult to pick up without carefully reading the record. Mistakes should be corrected as soon as possible. The proper way to correct a medical record is to put a simple line through the improper entry, so that it still can be read. Then, the appropriate entry should be placed nearby, with the date of the correction added followed by the corrector's initials, which in most cases would be the physician who dictated the note. If it is not obvious from the context why the change needed to be made, then the reason should be noted. Never try to erase or obliterate an error. Never substitute an entirely new note for the old one with the intention of making the evidence of the error disappear. When the worst happens and your own words, whether an erroneous entry or not, will damn you in a malpractice case, never, never, never attempt to cover it up. You must always assume that the opposing party already has a copy of the record and would love to find an altered record on discovery. If this occurs, the case is over. You lose. However, that may be the least of your troubles. In some states, it is a criminal offense to falsify a medical record to conceal negligence or a criminal act (28). The physician would be looking at the possible loss of his medical license and a term in the penitentiary. Physicians should know that the science of documentation examination has advanced to such a point that it is very difficult to successfully falsify a medical record. Plaintiff attorneys use such experts for any suspicious entry, because the effects of finding such an alteration mean a virtually guaranteed win. As an example, did you know that the ink used in pens is labeled for the year in which it manufactured? Try explaining a 1997 entry with 1999 ink! The greatest temptation to alter a record is when the physician is really blameless and the entry was an honest mistake. Never attempt to alter the record in any way except the correct way. In this situation, discuss this with your attorney before making a change in a case that is or will be involved in litigation.

Confidentiality

Flowing from the fiduciary physician–patient relationship is the duty to preserve the patient's privacy and keep his medical records confidential. Legally, the physical medical record belongs to the physician, but the information contained within belongs to the patient. State laws vary, but the patient largely has a right to a copy of his records. Exceptions usually exist for psychiatric records. Unless there is a statute providing an exception, the physician may not release the patient's medical records without the patient's permission. The medical record cannot be released, even by request from the patient's attorney or insurance company, without the patient's consent. A good office policy is not to allow any medical record to leave the office without it being checked by the physician. Filing errors occur, and it is possible to send someone else's note or laboratory result that was misfiled into another patient's chart. Before sending out the copy of the record, the presence of the patient's consent can be verified. Such permission should be in writing.

All information about the patient is confidential. It is the patient's privilege to waive, and, with rare legal exception, the physician may not reveal information about the patient without permission. For example, in one case where a plastic surgeon used a patient's preoperative and postoperative photographs in a presentation at a department store and on television without permission, the court found that this was a violation of the patient's right to confidentiality (29). Breach of confidentiality can lead to a lawsuit on multiple grounds, e.g., breach of privacy, breach of confidentiality, breach of fiduciary duty, breach of loyalty, breach of contract, negligence, infliction of emotional distress, as well as liability for violation of privacy statutes (30). By statute, the patient usually waives his right to confidentiality when he puts his health in question in litigation, e.g., a malpractice action.

REFERENCES

1. *Schloendorff v. Society of New York Hospital,* 211 N.Y. 125, 105 N.E. 92 (1914).
2. *Salgo v. Leland Stanford Jr. Univ. Bd. of Trustees,* 154 Cal. App. 2d 560, 317 P.2d 170 (1957).
3. Rosoff AJ. Consent to medical treatment. In: MacDonald MG, Kaufman RM, Capron AM, et al., eds. *Treatise on health care law.* New York: Matthew Bender & Co., 1998:17–17.
4. *Vandi v. Permanente Medical Group,* 7 Cal. App. 4th 1064, 9 Cal. Rptr. 2d 463 (1992).
5. *Cobbs v. Grant,* 8 Cal. 3d 229, 104 Cal. Rptr. 505, 502 P.2d 1 (1972).
6. *Truman v. Thomas,* 27 Cal. 3d 285, 165 Cal. Rptr. 308, 611 P.2d 902 (1980).
7. Scott AW. *The Fiduciary Principle.* 37 Cal. L. Rev. 539 (1949).
8. *Hidding v. Williams,* 578 So. 2d 1192 (La. Ct. App. 1991).
9. Rosoff AJ. Consent to medical treatment. In: MacDonald MG, Kaufman RM, Capron AM, et al., eds. *Treatise on health care law.* New York: Matthew Bender & Co., 1998:17–18.2.
10. LeBlang T, King J. *Tort Liability for Nondisclosure: The Physician's Legal Obligation to Disclose Patient Illness and Injury.* 89 Dick. L. Rev. (1984): 1.
11. Rosoff AJ. Consent to medical treatment. In: MacDonald MG, Kaufman RM, Capron AM, et al., eds. *Treatise on health care law.* New York: Matthew Bender & Co., 1998:17A-1.
12. Rosoff AJ. Consent to medical treatment. In: MacDonald MG, Kaufman RM, Capron AM, et al., eds. *Treatise on health care law.* New York: Matthew Bender & Co., 1998.
13. Rosoff AJ. Consent to medical treatment. In: MacDonald MG, Kaufman RM, Capron AM, et al., eds. *Treatise on health care law.* New York: Matthew Bender & Co., 1998.
14. *Natanson v. Kline,* 186 Kan. 393, 350 P.2d 1093 (1960).
15. *Canterbury v. Spence,* 464 F. 2d 772 (D.C. Cir. 1972).
16. Nev. Rev. Stat. 129.030(2) (1986).
17. Rosoff AJ. Consent to medical treatment. In: MacDonald MG, Kaufman RM, Capron AM, et al., eds. *Treatise on health care law.* New York: Matthew Bender & Co., 1998:17–34.
18. Rosoff AJ. Consent to medical treatment. In: MacDonald MG, Kaufman RM, Capron AM, et al., eds. *Treatise on health care law.* New York: Matthew Bender & Co., 1998:17A-5.
19. *Nishi v. Hartwell,* 473 P.2d 116 (Haw. 1970).

20. Rosoff AJ. Consent to medical treatment. In: MacDonald MG, Kaufman RM, Capron AM, et al., eds. *Treatise on health care law.* New York: Matthew Bender & Co., 1998:17–18.3.
21. Holder AR. Special categories of consent: minors and handicapped newborns. In: MacDonald, p. 19-7.
22. *Lloyd v. Kull,* 329 F. 2d 168 (7th Cir. 1974).
23. *Millard v. Nagle,* 402 Pa. Super. 376, 587 A. 2d 10 (1991).
24. Rosoff AJ. Consent to medical treatment. In: MacDonald MG, Kaufman RM, Capron AM, et al., eds. *Treatise on health care law.* New York: Matthew Bender & Co., 1998:17–84
25. Rosoff AJ. Consent to medical treatment. In: MacDonald MG, Kaufman RM, Capron AM, et al., eds. *Treatise on health care law.* New York: Matthew Bender & Co., 1998.
26. Hirsh HL. Medical records. In: Sanbar SS, Gibofsky A, Firestone MH, et al., eds. *Legal medicine,* 4th ed. St. Louis: Mosby, 1998:280
27. DeWitt RE, Harton AE, Hoffman WE Jr, et al. Patient information and confidentiality. In: MacDonald MG, Kaufman RM, Capron AM, et al., eds. *Treatise on health care law.* New York: Matthew Bender & Co., 1998:16–20.
28. Mich. Stat. Ann. 14.624(1) (Callaghan 1976).
29. *Vassiliades v. Garfinckel's,* 492 A. 2d 580 (D.C. 1985).
30. *Doe v. Roe,* 93 Misc. 2d 201, 400 N.Y.S. 2d 668 (Sup. Ct. 1977).

Discussion

INFORMED CONSENT, RECORD KEEPING, AND DOCUMENTATION

NEAL R. REISMAN

Dr. Sullivan has nicely summarized the law and protections every plastic surgeon should know about informed consent, the medical record, and documentation. The key elements presented are the foundation of our protections. One key element is that the patient should be adequately informed about treatment and care. Although states may vary as to the legal standard, physicians have a duty to portray some level of possible risks to the patient in an understandable fashion. It is this balance between detailed information provided and patient understanding that creates the documentation dilemma.

It is unrealistic and prohibitive to document the entire physician–patient interaction. It may be advisable to create as favorable and educational an experience as possible. This involves altering the "old" adage that a patient remembers 50% of what is explained. In fact, it is now thought that learning styles of the listener account for what is retained and explain what is not. One can create such a positive learning environment and consultation experience by understanding and using leaning styles. Patients usually learn through three basic methods: visual, auditory, and kinesthetic. The plastic surgical office should create an informed consent process that captures all three styles. The visual learner requires some visual aids, often schematic diagrams or photographs to fully grasp what is presented. Diagrams or similar aids in addition to brochures will allow this patient to understand and retain the information. One must be careful not to create a warranty by representing the photographic result to be this patient's result. This can be easily prevented by not making additional representations, promises, or unrealistic statements. The auditory patient learner requires a detailed verbal description of the process. Although photographs and brochures may be used, this patient's retention will be far greater if someone on the plastic surgical team explains and answers all questions, thereby creating the informed consent process. The kinesthetic patient learner requires some degree of personalized association and relationship to fully grasp what is being presented. This usually involves a personal anecdotal story the patient can understand. An example would be a story of a moderate-to-severe sunburn at the beach being compared to a laser resurfacing. The patient, having experienced a sunburn, will now be able to better understand a possible effect from laser treatments. It is difficult to find anecdotal stories or experiences without a full knowledge of each patient's past. It would be advisable to create and use a number of similar experiences to draw from, permitting the kinesthetic patient to understand what is being presented.

This process may appear difficult and cumbersome, but in fact most physicians already function in this manner. A complete informed consent process should include varied aspects of what is proposed and continue until the patient is given suitable information to make an informed choice. The more complete the process, the happier the patient and possibly the more appropriate the expectations will be. An ex-

N. R. Reisman: Department of Plastic Surgery, Baylor College of Medicine; and Department of Plastic Surgery, St. Luke's Episcopal Hospital, Houston, Texas.

ample of a recommended patient informed consent process for laser resurfacing would include a detailed interactive description of the operative and perioperative process (auditory), photographs or visual aids such as brochures demonstrating risks and skin changes (visual), and a discussion to the patient of remembering when they may have had a sunburn and even some blisters on their face allowing them to personally experience what is being presented (kinesthetic).

These recommendations assume the plastic surgeon has the communication skills to complete this process, but many surgeons may not; therefore, the practice should use a team formed of physician, nurse, and other assistants trained to fulfill the patient's needs. The products used for the process then would become part of the medical record. This would include brochures, anecdotal examples for different procedures, and any diagrams, photographs, and explained information. This fulfills the informed consent process requirements while also fulfilling the documentation and medical record-keeping requirements.

Dr. Sullivan importantly emphasizes the confidential component of the medical record. This is another key element that imposes increased demands on patient information, thereby increasing risks for the practitioner to release what is required while the patient may be concerned about the office gossip. An increasing trend is the self-insured company. There is often a company employee assigned to represent the insurance needs of the employees. Although this employee, like the surgeon, has a fiduciary responsibility to confidentiality, not infrequently, "gossip" spreads around the office about "other" procedures the employee undergoes. This "mouthy" indiscreet employee now oversees the company's self-insured insurance claims. There may be a reason why the patient will not permit a release of information on a cosmetic procedure when performed in conjunction with a reimbursable procedure. The plastic surgical office should be aware of the patient's rights to confidentiality despite managed care or legal interactions. The marketing plan of the practice also should be aware of these rights and never display a patient photograph without explicit written permission. The medicolegal managed care environment now contains not only informed consent issues, but also fraud and confidentiality issues. The plastic surgical practice should be cautious and steadfast about maintaining an ethical patient interaction. The zeal by which some surgeons seek patients raises ethical and legal questions about misrepresentations and warranty issues if a legal challenge occurs. As Dr. Sullivan notes, the plaintiff's attorney will use all available allegations to place pressure on the defendant plastic surgeon and the insurance carrier. The plastic surgeon may not have practiced negligently or committed malpractice, but these other "activities" may force a trial and a verdict against the doctor.

This entire arena of the plastic surgical practice is an important one, as it has such potential for negative exposure. The plastic surgery practice should develop methods to address all of the points raised and consistently provide the suitable informed consent process for the patient with adequate documentation while preserving the integrity of the medical record. There can be a balance that is not overly burdensome and actually quite functional. Many trial attorneys believe that if a good educational experience and warm relationship ensues between physician, practice, and patient, there is less of a likelihood of being sued.

Another and most important area of legal awareness arises when treating the unhappy patient treated by another plastic surgeon. The plastic surgeon now assuming care must be extremely aware of confidentiality issues as well as what often is perceived as prior negligence by the past treater. There is a strong belief that many lawsuits begin by the patient listening to "innocent" comments made by the current care provider about the care of the previous surgeon. Comments such as "Who did that to you?" or "What happened . . . I've never seen that before!" create a higher degree of suspicion and often precipitate a visit to the plaintiff attorney. It is certainly advised not to comment, because no matter the level of sophistication of the current surgeon, he or she was not there at the prior surgery or office experience and certainly did not see the patient before this point in time. One can never exactly reproduce those experiences after the fact. If a complication has occurred and the current surgeon is asked for a second opinion, the surgeon should seek permission to inquire about the prior care and discuss the facts with the prior treater. If this request is denied, the surgeon should proceed carefully, caring for the patient as he or she now presents and not commenting about why the complication occurred or questioning prior care. Of course, there should be good documentation of exactly what is observed and absolutely refraining from comment about the prior treater in the medical record .

This entire area is challenging for the surgeon. Ethical behavior must be adhered to, and although there may be a desire to comment that " . . . this is the fifth such complication from Dr. PriorMD I've seen this month," do not make that statement, even to other surgeons. There is a question, relative to the state one practices, whether there is a duty to report actual substandard practices to the State Board of Medical Examiners. That is a confidential reporting as compared to what may be a slanderous comment if made to other surgeons. The best activity is to think what you would like said to the patient and others if you were the surgeon others were discussing. Think about what is recorded in the medical record. Be factual and assume nothing. The prior treating surgeon may have a completely different record and experience with the patient than what the patient relates to you.

In summary, Dr. Sullivan has covered many of the important protective areas of a plastic surgical practice. I have tried to balance the practice enhancement pressures with a reasonable approach to patient care and documentation. One should be alert as to additional areas of concern arising from marketing efforts and increased patient demands as well as patients often seeking care from many plastic surgeons. In my opinion, if a plastic surgeon actually practices what is proscribed, rather than being cumbersome, there may be increased patient acceptance with positive economic results, as well as more sleep-filled nights.

SUGGESTED READING

Medicolegal Issues

Peimer C, ed. *Surgery of the hand and upper extremity,* vol. 1. New York: McGraw-Hill, 1996.

Liability Issues with Ultrasonic-assisted Lipoplasty

Rohrich R, ed. *Ultrasonic assisted liposuction.* 1998.
Plastic surgery office boutique—practice enhancement or risk? *APSA NETWORK Newsletter.*
Unavailable doctor syndrome. *APSA NETWORK Newsletter.*
The Plastic Surgery Office—How Risky? A.P.S.A., Dallas, TX, 1996.
Harassment in the workplace. *APSA NETWORK Newsletter.*
ASPRS—Risk Management Symposium, Moderator, Speaker, Seattle, WA, 1996.
Office personality. *APSA NETWORK Newsletter.*
Medico-Legal Risks of Health Care Reform—Areas of the Law. ASPRS, Practice Development Session, San Francisco, CA, 1997.
Medico-Legal Risk and the Plastic Surgery Nurse. American Society of Plastic & Reconstructive Surgical Nurses, San Francisco, CA, 1997.
Surviving a deposition. ASPRS Instructional Course.
Avoiding New Areas of Risk in Plastic Surgery. Spring Institute, ASPRS, Phoenix, AZ, 1998.
The Risk Free Office—At What Cost. SPSSCS, Annual Meeting Presentation, Los Angeles, CA, 1998.
Risk for the Plastic Surgical Office. APSA National Meeting Speaker Presentation, Boston, MA, 1998.

5

MEDICAL MALPRACTICE AND PLASTIC SURGERY: THE CARRIER'S POINT OF VIEW

MARK GORNEY

A plastic and reconstructive surgeon practicing in the United States in the last three decades of the 20th century may find it virtually impossible to end his or her career unblemished by a claim of malpractice. Social and economic circumstances combined with the explosive growth of a plaintiffs' bar specializing in medical malpractice have made it imperative that anyone entering the specialty be at least conversant with the basic principles of risk management and claims prevention. In a moment of exasperation, Associate Justice Antonin Scalia of the United States Supreme Court is reported to have said, "It is virtually impossible to underestimate the ability of the plaintiffs' bar to keep expanding the envelope of judicial restraint beyond anyone's imagination!" This cogent observation underscores the fact that most claims against plastic surgeons involve elective surgery, a situation in which the treating surgeon, in contrast to other physicians, is making well patients temporarily "unwell" to make them better. Clearly, the psychodynamics that underlie any malpractice claim against a plastic surgeon are quite different than a claim involving a patient who was unwell initially.

That said, it also is true that well over half the malpractice claims are preventable. Most are based on failures of communication and patient selection criteria, rather than on technical faults. Patient selection is the ultimate inexact science. It is a melange of surgical judgment, gut feelings, personality interactions, the surgeon's ego strength and, increasingly, the substitution of surgical judgment (or common sense) for economic considerations. Accurate and clear communication, on the other hand, is the *sine qua non* of building the all-important doctor–patient relationship. Unfortunately, the ability to communicate well comes with one's genes, or it may be learned at mother's knee. It is not something that can be readily learned in adulthood. Regardless of technical ability, anyone who appears cold, arrogant, or insensitive is far more likely to be sued than someone who relates to others at a much more "human" level.

M. Gorney: The Doctors' Company, Napa, California

THUMBNAIL SKETCH OF LEGAL PRINCIPLES APPLICABLE TO PLASTIC SURGERY

Standard of Care

Malpractice is defined as "treatment which is contrary to accepted medical standards and which produces injurious results in the patient." Most medical malpractice actions are based on laws governing negligence. The law recognizes that medicine is an inexact art and that there can be no absolute liability. Thus, the cause of action is usually the "failure of defendant/physician to exercise that reasonable degree of skill, learning, care and treatment ordinarily possessed by others of the same profession in the community." In the past, the term "community" was accepted as a geographic reference. Now, based on the supposition that doctors everywhere keep up with the latest developments in their fields, "community" is generally interpreted as "specialty community." "Standards of care" are now those of the entire specialty without regard to geographic location.

Warranty

The law holds that by merely engaging to render treatment, a physician warrants that he or she has the learning skill and competence of the average member of his or her specialty and will apply that learning skill with ordinary and reasonable care. This warranty of due care is legally implied: it need not be mentioned specifically by the physician or the patient. However, the warranty is for service, not for cure. Thus, the surgeon should never imply that the operation will be a success, the results will be favorable, or that he or she will never commit a medical error. Remember: there is a warranty for service, not for cure.

Informed Consent

When attempting to define the yardstick of disclosure, the courts divide medical and surgical procedures into two categories:

1. Common procedures that incur minor or very remote serious risk (including death or serious bodily harm), e.g., the administration of antibiotics
2. Procedures involving serious risks for which the doctor has an "affirmative duty to disclose the potential of death or serious harm and explain, in detail, the complications that might occur."

Affirmative duty means that the physician is obligated to disclose risks on his own, without waiting for the patient to ask. The courts have held that it is the patient, not the physician, who has the prerogative of determining in which direction his or her best interests lie. Thus, the physician is obliged to discuss therapeutic alternatives and their particular hazards.

How much explanation is appropriate, and in what detail, is required to achieve a balance between the surgeon's feeling about his or her patient and the legal requirements? It simply is not possible to tell patients everything that could happen without scaring them out of their surgery. Rather, the law states that patients must be told of probable known dangers and the percentage of that probability. The rest may be disclosed in general terms, and patients also may be reminded of the statistical possibility of being in an automobile accident that very same day.

Obviously, the most common complications should be volunteered frankly and openly, and their probability, based on the surgeon's experience, also should be discussed. Finally, any or all of this information is completely wasted unless it is documented in the patient's record. For purposes of subsequent legal inquiries, if it is not written down, it simply did not happen.

Elements of Documentation

When treatment is urgent and the condition is serious, it is inappropriate to engage in an orgy of open-ended disclosure with hair-raising details that might tend to magnify existing anxiety. Nevertheless, it is important that the patient, or at least the immediate family, understand the risks and consequences of the proposed treatment. In general, there are six elements that comprise true complete disclosure:

1. Diagnosis, or possible diagnosis
2. Description of treatment and its purposes
3. Inherent risks and possible complications
4. Probability of outcome
5. Alternative treatments, if available, and
6. Consequences of refusing treatment.

Therapeutic Alliance

The ritual of obtaining informed consent need not be a dry, impersonal, or bothersome proceeding. The process can actually establish between doctor and patient what might be called a "therapeutic alliance." This will not only solidify the rapport between physician and patient so essential to avoiding postoperative acrimony, but, more importantly, will involve the patient in the decision-making process. In this way, whatever the outcome of the treatment, the patient, whose natural reaction is always to blame the surgeon, is psychologically obligated to share some of the responsibility of whatever the outcome might be. It certainly will tend to reduce the tendency to point fingers.

PSYCHOLOGICAL AND PSYCHIATRIC ASPECTS OF ELECTIVE SURGERY

The growing popularity of aesthetic surgery makes it imperative to establish clear criteria of patient selection. Without these criteria, there will be an inevitable parallel increase in patient dissatisfaction and litigation.

Who, then, is the "ideal" candidate for aesthetic surgery? There is no such person, but the surgeon certainly should note any personality factors that will enhance or detract from the physical improvements sought.

There are basically two categories for acceptance or rejection of a patient seeking elective aesthetic surgery. The first is anatomical unsuitability. The second is emotional or psychological inadequacy. Because the latter is by far the more important, the surgeon must differentiate between healthy and unhealthy reasons for seeking aesthetic improvement.

Strength of motivation is critical. It has a startlingly close relationship with patient satisfaction. Furthermore, a strongly motivated patient will have less pain, a better postoperative course, and a significantly higher index of satisfaction, regardless of result.

It is possible to establish some nearly objective criteria of patient selection and liability potential. Figure 5-1 depicts the patient's objective deformity (as judged by the surgeon) on the horizontal axis versus the patient's degree of concern with that deformity on the vertical axis. Two opposite extremes emerge:

1. The patient with major deformity but minimal concern (lower right-hand corner)
2. The patient with minor visible deformity but extreme concern (upper left-hand corner).

The latter extreme is by far the poorest candidate. Although one seldom sees patients with major deformity and minimal concern, most of the patients that come to the plastic surgeon's office fit somewhere on a diagonal between the contralateral corners. The closer the patient comes to the upper left-hand corner, the more likely is an unfavorably perceived outcome followed by a visit to the attorney. Because a patient may seek consultation but postpone the decision on actually having the surgery done, it is a good idea to chart one's impression of such a patient's eligibility

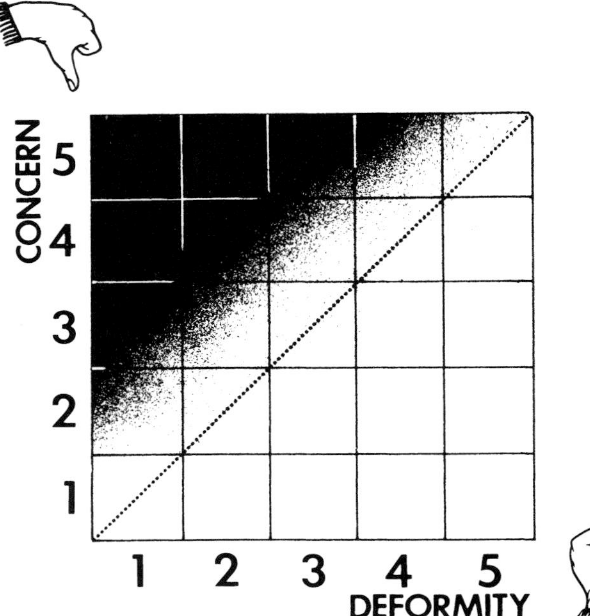

FIGURE 5-1. The patient's objective deformity (as judged by the surgeon) on the horizontal axis versus the patient's degree of concern with that deformity on the vertical axis.

for the procedure as a reminder against the day when the patient may decide to go ahead with surgery. If the patient is anywhere near the upper left-hand corner, it is strongly recommended that he or she be referred elsewhere.

Communication

The common denominator in all litigation in plastic surgery is poor communication. Underlying all dissatisfaction is a breakdown in the rapport between patient and surgeon. This vital relationship often is shattered by the surgeon's arrogance, hostility, coldness (real or imagined), or the perception that "he or she didn't care." There are only two ways to avoid such a debacle: (i) make sure that the patient has no reason to feel that way, or (ii) avoid a patient who is going to feel that way no matter what is done.

Although the doctor's skill, reputation, and other intangible factors contribute to a patient's sense of confidence, rapport between patient and doctor must be based on forthright and accurate communication. Faulty communications often lead to this inevitable vicious cycle: disappointment, anger, or frustration on the part of the patient; reactive hostility, defensiveness, and arrogance from the doctor; and deepening patient anger. The culmination is a visit to the attorney by the angry, unhappy patient.

The art of listening, as well as that of verbal and nonverbal expression, merits serious attention in the effort to reduce malpractice claims.

One of the most common patient complaints involves physicians' use of complex terminology or medical jargon. Words should be chosen that do not produce anxiety. Whereas "excise" might be misunderstood, "cutting it out" sounds painful. "Removing it" is better.

Various studies show that the average patient retains 35% of what he or she was told. Thus, it does no harm to repeat, in summary form, the essential points at the end of the consultation or examination, which strongly reinforces what has been said. The anxiety inherent in an office visit often causes patients to forget important questions or information. They should be encouraged to write down their questions and bring the list on the next visit.

Starting with the first handshake, nonverbal communication establishes and maintains patient confidence. It becomes absolutely critical if things go wrong.

Physicians should not permit their own emotions or frustrations to be seen by the patient. The patient's anxiety often magnifies the physician's body language.

"Who Did That To You"?

Another common catalyst in the chemistry of malpractice suits is the inadvertent or deliberate critical comment by a health professional concerning another colleague's actions. Experienced defense attorneys estimate that 25% of all claims may be triggered by such an event. It is not necessary to actually say anything critical. "Body language" (frowning, sighing, raising eyebrows, emphatic "hmphs," or looking down and shaking of head) constitutes eloquent comments to a patient who already is concerned. A surgeon acting as a consultant physician, particularly in second opinion situations, should make every effort to avoid communicating by word or action any criticism of colleagues. Anyone who was not there during the initial treatment is in no position to know what really happened and should make that clear to the patient.

The need to maintain a nonjudgmental stance is a caution that applies particularly to office staff. A casual innocent remark by an empathetic aide preparing a patient for examination can be all it takes to trigger a claim. Surgeons should brief their staff to refrain from such comments.

If the treatment or procedure was egregiously wrong or truly harmful, the physician has a clear responsibility to disclose the truth. In most situations, the questions are not so sharply defined. The consultant surgeon should carefully avoid coming to a conclusion without knowing all the facts. Obviously, a thorough review of prior medical records is mandatory. A direct call to the first physician can provide important insight into the situation. Remember that the patient may either inadvertently or deliberately omit significant information, or may distort facts out of hostility or resentment.

Anger: A Root Cause of Malpractice Claims

Patients feel a sense of bewilderment and anxiety when elective surgery does not go smoothly. The borderline between anxiety and anger is tenuous, and the conversion factor is uncertainty—fear of the unknown. A patient frightened by a postoperative complication or uncertain about the future may surmise: "If it is the doctor's fault, the responsibility is the doctor's to correct."

The patient's perceptions may clash with the physician's anxieties, insecurities, and wounded pride. The patient blames the physician, who in turn becomes defensive. At this critical and delicate juncture, the physician's natural reaction can set in motion or prevent a natural chain reaction. The physician must put aside feelings of disappointment, anxiety, defensiveness, and hostility and understand that he or she is probably dealing with a frightened patient who is using anger to gain "control" of the situation. Subsequent negative developments can be avoided by whatever understanding, support, or encouragement seems appropriate to the situation.

The patient's perception that the physician understands the uncertainty and will join with him or her to help conquer it may determine whether the patient will seek legal counsel. When faced with someone who is upset or angry, it is best to remain silent and let that person talk about the problem. The physician should only respond with noncommittal comments until the emotionally charged patient has calmed down. The technique of attentive silence often defuses angry people. Once the angry speaker has finished expressing his or her dissatisfaction, it is best to calmly ask the speaker to reiterate part of the message, even though it was fully understood already. The request for additional information or explanation reinforces in the speaker's mind the importance attached to the message.

One of the worst errors in dealing with angry or dissatisfied patients is to try to avoid them. It is necessary to participate actively in the process rather than avoid the issue. Avoidance will never make the problem go away; on the contrary, it is guaranteed to quickly aggravate the situation.

The Med-Mal Hit Parade

Every medical malpractice insurance carrier who covers plastic and reconstructive surgeons knows that the majority of their claims stem from the elective/aesthetic surgery component of the insureds' surgeon's practice. Following is an analysis of the loss experience of approximately 700 plastic and reconstructive surgeons over a period of 20 years. It constitutes a reliable picture of the genesis of most claims against plastic surgeons. Surprisingly, although the frequency and severity of such claims have risen out of proportion to the increasing numbers of practicing surgeons, the genesis of the claims has remained constant. Medical liability carriers continue to see the same generic problems in elective aesthetic surgery claims: poor documentation with missing or poor quality preoperative photographs, inadequate informed consent, poor patient selection criteria, and substandard postoperative results. All but the last are entirely avoidable.

Let us look at specific procedures. Clearly, the constant loss leader in all categories is surgery of the breast. It should be evident from the breast implant crisis that augmentation mammoplasty stands in a category all its own.

Setting aside the dubious merit of the systemic disease claims, now proven invalid by both extensive scientific and legal criteria, we see capsular contracture as the most common complaint. It is disturbing to the carrier to hear this problem labeled as a "complication." It is *not* a complication: it is an inherent risk of the procedure, in the same sense that crashing is an inherent risk of flying. People who board planes are aware of this, yet they consciously board the aircraft anyway. The main difference between these two situations is that women contemplating augmentation do not know, and are often not told fully and truthfully, the percentage possibility of contracture. Every aesthetic surgeon should have on hand a sample of his or her preferred prosthesis, which when squeezed can simulate the feel of capsular contracture. If this also were noted in the record, it would dramatically decrease the number of claims based on improper disclosure.

Were it not for the silicone hysteria, reduction mammoplasty would surely be the leading cause of claims against plastic surgeons. The primary causes of these claims are (i) unexpectedly ugly scars; (ii) too much or too little removed; (iii) partial loss, distortion, or misplacement of nipples; (iv) dissatisfaction with the resulting shape; and (v) necessity of revision and attendant costs. The primary complaint is back and shoulder pain. When the pain is relieved, the dissatisfaction quotient is considerably less.

Not surprisingly, the third most common complication involves nasal surgery. In this procedure, arguably the most difficult and unpredictable, surgeons have often had to face unhappiness with (i) disappointing results, (ii) airway obstruction, (iii) visible irregularities or scars, (iv) asymmetry, and (v) "emotional distress."

In no other operation is the gulf between expectations and results more likely to be wider than in nasal surgery. In no other procedure is the emotional investment (the dangerous, invisible bulk of the iceberg below the surface) so likely to emerge even when, in the eyes of the surgeon, the result is good. In no other procedure is it so critically important to select the right candidate for emotional stability as well as physical characteristics. Most experienced rhinoplastic surgeons can identify the "SIMON" as the most troublesome patient of all. This is a patient who is Single, Immature, Male, Overexpectant, Narcissistic. Typically this is an individual between the ages of 17 and 40 years, usually unmarried, with a grossly exaggerated fixation on a genetic or familial nasal characteristic that may or may not even be evident to the surgeon. This patient generally belongs in the upper left-hand corner of Fig. 1-1.

Next on the list of most claims against plastic surgeons is blepharoplasty. The pitfalls in this area are (i) ectropion or scleral show with exposure keratitis ("I look starey"); (ii) visible scars; (iii) real or alleged impairment of vision; and (iv) "change of expression" (whatever that means). It is surprising to review these cases and find that, more often than not, excision of skin was performed without compensating for gravity, i.e., patient supine, or excess skin measured without having the patient look up or open the mouth. In the rare but devastating postoperative blindness cases, we find universally that the typical expanding hematoma was not identified and immediately relieved. Another common denominator is a sudden increase in blood pressure in the head (sudden exertion, sneezing, bending over, or constipated bowel efforts, etc.) at the peak of the reactive hyperemia after reabsorption of the local anesthetic. It is strongly recommended that all blepharoplasty cases be kept under observation for at least 3 hours since the last injection with epinephrine containing local anesthesia. These patients also should be given written instructions emphasizing the importance of no exertion or bending over for at least the next 12 hours.

Rhytidectomy claims follow, involving (i) visible or hypertrophic scars; (ii) sloughs or wound disruptions (most often in heavy smokers); (iii) facial nerve damage; (iv) inadequate result from insufficient or excessive tightening; (v) persistent pain or numbness; and (vi) cost and time for secondary revision. Again, we find that the common denominator in these cases is a crisis of expectations based on inadequate disclosure. It is imperative to discuss the risks and limitations of this operation in clear language and to document that discussion. It should be understood that the effect of heavy smoking on healing is now well known to the plaintiffs' bar. Accepting a patient who smokes automatically exposes the surgeon to greater risk.

Suction-assisted lipectomy is now the most requested aesthetic operation in the United States. Regrettably, it is perceived as a procedure that can be done by virtually any physician without any formal surgical training. It is a rapidly growing leading cause of medical malpractice claims against a variety of specialists. The most common allegations are (i) waviness, lumpiness, or asymmetric irregularities; (ii) disappointment with the degree of changes achieved; (iii) persistent numbness and pain; and (iv) cost of revision.

It should be noted that, in the last 5 years, there have been somewhere over 100 documented fatal outcomes directly related to large-volume liposuction. By common consensus, "large volume" is defined as any aspiration over 5,000 mL. The profound physiologic and fluid balance changes in such procedures are not unlike that of a significant burn injury. Insurers are finding it increasingly difficult to defend such cases if they were done on an outpatient basis instead of a full hospital setting. Aside from the morbidity or fatal outcome associated from fluid overload, the most common causes for serious complications in lipoplasty are (i) pulmonary embolism, (ii) abdominal perforation with subsequent complications, and (iii) anesthetic problems, including lidocaine overdose. With the addition of ultrasonic energy, one may only speculate on the nature of new, undefined problems that may be encountered in the future.

As with any developing technology, the laser-based resurfacing techniques so popular today among various specialties are beginning to produce their share of problems similar to the problems seen with traditional peeling and dermabrasion: (i) excessive depth, with or without attendant infection resulting in hypotrophic scarring; and (ii) permanent pigmentary changes. These claims result from either improper patient selection or just plain overly enthusiastic treatment.

An unfortunate trend is developing among aesthetic surgeons that involves combining several procedures at one sitting. Whereas this approach is appropriate in two small- or medium-length procedures, it is doubtful (and certainly difficult to defend) when several major procedures are combined in one long surgery in an office facility without full life-support capability. Several such cases have triggered settlements in the seven-figure range. It is highly preferable to plan on staggered treatment sessions rather than overdoing at one sitting.

The last and most increasingly disturbing trend is the rising number of claims in which it is clear that economic considerations were put ahead of sound surgical judgment: the patient did not really need that procedure; it was the wrong patient on whom to perform that operation; the surgeon was inexperienced, but went ahead anyway; the result was at best mediocre, but the bill was turned over to a collection agency; and so on.

Of all the crosses a beleaguered medical liability risk manager has to bear, the heaviest is best illustrated by Fig. 5-2, which needs no caption. It is entirely natural to assume a reactively defensive posture when our best laid plans go awry. Unfortunately, there also is a tendency among plastic and reconstructive surgeons to assume a certain air of invincibility. Humility and diffidence can hardly be described as

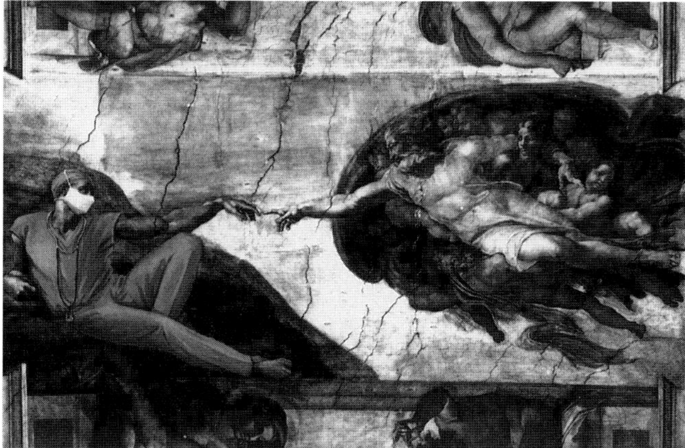

FIGURE 5-2. The most difficult and intractable problem facing the medical liability risk manager is shown in this self-explanatory illustration.

generic to the specialty. Defensiveness breeds avoidance, which is readily interpreted as arrogance. Under those circumstances, any hint of arrogance will surely encourage a visit to the attorney's office.

What triggers a claim is not as much what the doctor did or failed to do, but how he or she behaved after it happened. Regardless of the underlying cause, all medical malpractice claims have in common surprise, disappointment, and anger, followed by a breakdown in communications. In summary, the reader is gently reminded, again, that a warm body and a valid credit card alone are poor indications for elective plastic surgery. Regardless of economic circumstances, the only absolutes in claims prevention are surgical competence and intelligent patient selection.

6

MEDICAL MALPRACTICE AND PLASTIC SURGERY: A TRIAL LAWYER'S PERSPECTIVE

THOMAS P. CIMINO, JR.
RICHARD L. WILLIAMS III

A young man scans your advertising materials as he contemplates cosmetic surgery. Later, he walks into your office seeking your assistance in improving his physical appearance. After conducting an examination and assessment of his condition, you inform him that several surgical options are available. He selects one option over the others and you schedule the surgery. At this point, what do you know about this particular individual? Does this man hope that the outcome of the surgery will change his life for the better and cure all of his social ills? If his hopes are unfulfilled, will he blame you and file a lawsuit alleging that you committed medical malpractice?

In protecting yourself against medical malpractice claims, it is important to first understand the basic legal principles surrounding medical malpractice litigation. What is medical malpractice? In general, medical malpractice occurs when a physician fails to meet the minimum standard of care then prevailing in that physician's area of specialty. In most cases, a plaintiff will need to resort to the testimony of a paid expert to support his or her claim.

The number of medical malpractice claims filed has increased dramatically since the early 1980s. This increase has had a number of adverse consequences. Medical malpractice insurance premiums have risen almost as dramatically as jury verdicts. Additionally, medical costs have been driven up by the need to practice "defensive medicine" as a precaution against being sued. Moreover, a cottage industry of testifying experts has developed. The use of "forensic experts" has resulted in an increase of opinion testimony unsupported by valid scientific methodology and unrestrained by peer-reviewed research. Some courts and commentators have referred to such opinion testimony as "junk science." Fortunately, the United States Supreme Court has recently put into place procedures whereby trial courts can limit and, in some cases, exclude questionable or unreliable expert testimony.

This chapter explores medical malpractice litigation from the perspective of the plastic surgeon. The legal process involved in such litigation is explained and common defenses are examined. Additionally, suggestions are offered on how the practitioner can avoid costly and embarrassing malpractice litigation.

MEDICAL MALPRACTICE CLAIMS

Often, the first indication a surgeon has that a suit is about to be filed is a request by a patient for his or her medical records. This is because a plaintiff's lawyer usually will want and need to review these records before instituting litigation. The attorney also may need to discuss the records with an expert before suit is filed. As a general rule, patients have a legal right to obtain copies of their medical records (1). Moreover, if there is a chance to salvage your relationship with the patient, stonewalling a request for records almost always will eliminate that chance. Accordingly, although it is unpleasant to contemplate the possibility of a lawsuit, a request by a patient for his or her records should be promptly acknowledged. Should you suspect, however, that a malpractice claim is behind a request for medical records, it would be wise to consult an attorney before responding to the request.

If litigation is initiated, it will begin with the filing of a complaint at law. The complaint contains the plaintiff's allegations of wrongdoing and his or her prayer for damages. Once filed, the complaint must be served upon the physician. In most states, a defendant served with a complaint only has a certain number of days to respond (usually between 20 and 30 days from the service of the complaint). Failure to respond to a complaint can result in a judgment being entered against the defendant, ending the defendant's right to defend the case. Moreover, most medical malprac-

T.P. Cimino, Jr., and R.L. Williams III: Vedder, Price Law Firm, Chicago, Illinois

tice insurance policies require prompt notice to the insurer of any claims made against the physician. Failure to properly notify an insurer can result in the insurer refusing to defend and indemnify the defendant. Accordingly, should you be served with a complaint or should you otherwise learn that a claim is about to be filed against you, promptly notify your insurance company and contact your attorney. In addition to generally protecting your interests, your attorney can advise you as to the strength and legal sufficiency of the plaintiff's claim.

Importantly, once you seek legal advice from an attorney, you and the attorney enter an attorney–client relationship. That relationship imposes certain obligations on the attorney in his or her representation of you. Specifically, all information you convey to your attorney must be kept in the highest confidence. This duty of confidentiality enables your attorney to learn of all facts concerning your case, while giving you the security of knowing that your disclosures will be kept private. Full disclosure to your attorney is key because if harmful facts exist and your attorney is unaware of them, he or she will not be prepared to rebut those facts. This will weaken your defense to the plaintiff's claim.

After the lawsuit is commenced, your attorney will need to file a response to the complaint. This response is known as an answer. Your answer to the complaint is simply a reply to the allegations made in the plaintiff's lawsuit. Your attorney will need to consult with you and review records regarding the treatment of the plaintiff in order to accurately prepare an answer to the complaint.

Your attorney also may file formal legal defenses to the claims made against you. You can assist your attorney in his or her decision regarding what legal defenses to assert by providing your attorney with as much information as possible regarding your treatment of the plaintiff. For example, your files may contain documentation showing that you fully and properly informed your patient of the risks involved in the surgical procedure at issue. This information may allow your attorney to request that the court dismiss the plaintiff's claim.

After the filing of your answer, both sides of the litigation will engage in discovery. As the name implies, discovery is a process by which each side learns the facts of the case. This process is significant because it allows the attorneys to assess the validity of the lawsuit and to become familiar with the strengths and weaknesses of the entire case. Discovery can be written, in the form of requests for documents or written questions, called interrogatories, which you and your attorney must answer under oath. It also can involve live testimony, in the form of a deposition. A deposition is a discovery tool that allows parties to a lawsuit to take sworn testimony from witnesses. In addition to providing facts about the case, this testimony can be used later at trial to impeach the witness.

After completing the discovery phase of the litigation, your attorney will likely attempt to resolve the litigation. Your attorney may attempt to convince the court that even if the facts alleged by the plaintiff are true, there is no legal basis on which the court may hold the physician liable. This argument is presented via a motion for summary judgment. Assuming that it is well founded, a summary judgment motion can be helpful. This step often is warranted because even if the motion is denied, it will force the plaintiff to come forward with evidence to support his or her case. This will further educate your attorney as to the plaintiff's theory. Your attorney also may engage in settlement negotiations. If settlement negotiations fail, the case will be set for trial.

In preparing for a trial, your attorney will need to procure an expert witness, most likely another plastic or reconstructive surgeon, to testify that you provided treatment that was reasonable and proper under the circumstances. Because you practice in this area of medicine, you may be able to assist your attorney in finding a competent physician to testify on your behalf.

At trial, the court imposes upon the plaintiff the burden to prove that the defendant-physician was negligent. To demonstrate a physician's negligence, the plaintiff must prove

1. the existence of a duty of care,
2. a breach of that duty of care,
3. a causal connection between the breach of the duty of care and the patient's alleged injuries, and
4. damages as a result of the physician's breach of care (2).

If all four elements are proven, the jury can find the physician guilty of negligence.

Duty of Care to the Patient

In general, a physician owes a duty of care to a patient whenever a physician–patient relationship exists. Such a relationship is created when the physician examines a patient, reviews medical records, charges a fee, orders a patient's release, schedules postoperative care, or supervises the care given to a patient by another physician (3). Issues in this area typically focus on the particular facts surrounding a physician's involvement in treating the patient. As a general guideline, the more affirmative steps the physician takes in providing care to the patient, the more probable it is that a court will determine that a physician–patient relationship exists.

With plastic surgeons, many physician–patient relationships arise as the result of a referral for consultation. That the plastic surgeon is brought onto a case merely to consult does not negate the existence of a physician–patient relationship. Accordingly, care must be given in all cases to ensure that the *patient* understands the limits of the relationship and the plastic surgeon's role—particularly where the patient is being treated by a number of physicians from different specialty areas.

Breach of the Duty of Care

Once a duty to a patient is established, a physician is required to exercise the reasonable degree of skill, knowledge, and care as is used by others in his or her area of specialty. Most courts require specialists to abide by national standards, which typically are higher and more objective than local, community standards. Holding plastic surgeons to a national standard is considerably easier in this era of modern technology, given that computers, e-mail, the Internet, and other media allow for the instantaneous transfer of information from nearly anywhere in the country (4).

A deviation from the applicable standard is a breach of the duty of care. However, an allegation that the surgery or procedure did not turn out as expected is not sufficient to demonstrate a breach of the duty of care. Rather, in most cases, expert testimony from another physician will be required because of the complexity of the issues that surround medical diagnosis and treatment (5). This expert must be qualified to testify as to the standard of care in the field of plastic surgery. The expert need not, however, be a board certified plastic surgeon. Rather, he or she only needs to demonstrate expertise in the treatment or surgical procedure at issue (6). The expert testimony must establish that the physician did not conform to the degree of care required and that the failure to use the requisite degree of care resulted in the injury alleged.

Causation

A plaintiff in a medical malpractice case is required to establish that his or her injury was proximately caused by the surgeon's breach of care. "Proximate cause" refers to the legal cause of the injury. Proximate cause exists when the injury is the natural or probable result of an act or omission by the surgeon and where a reasonable surgeon ought to have foreseen the injuries (7).

Proximate cause cannot be established by speculation. Instead, courts apply a reasonable certainty test, which requires a foreseeable connection between the alleged breach of duty and injury. This often requires an inquiry into the recognized complications from a surgical procedure. Expert testimony usually is required to establish this element.

Damages

Finally, in order to establish a malpractice claim, a plaintiff must prove damages. There are several different types of damages that may be compensable. For example, a patient may receive damages for pain and suffering. These are *noneconomic damages,* which the jury or trial judge finds reasonable to compensate the patient for having to endure the injury. Such damages include amounts for alleged disfigurement (8). In the past, the amount of this award was completely up to the trial judge or jury. This led to many multimillion dollar judgments against physicians in medical malpractice cases. As discussed later, many states recently have attempted to place a cap on noneconomic damages as part of their tort reform efforts.

Additionally, a plaintiff may be entitled to *special damages,* which are the actual damages incurred by the plaintiff as a result of the negligence. The damages that most commonly fall into this category are lost wages or earnings, medical expenses for future medical treatment, or subsequent surgery costs. In many cases, the amount of special damages owed to the plaintiff is significantly less than the noneconomic damages sought or received by the plaintiff.

A physician also may be exposed to *punitive damages.* Punitive damages allow the jury or judge to punish the defendant for conduct that grossly deviates from the standard of care. Some states place a cap on the amount of punitive damages; other states do not allow any punitive damages against health care providers. The particular statute in your state will be key in determining your exposure to a medical malpractice action.

INFORMED CONSENT

Courts uniformly require physicians to disclose all material information to their patients regarding the contemplated medical procedure. The definition of material information includes all inherent risks associated with the treatment. It is a well-recognized principle of law that a patient must consent and agree to treatment. Informed consent is important because a patient has a right to reject any treatment that poses unwanted risks. Additionally, if a patient agrees to undergo only certain treatments or procedures, the surgeon cannot exceed the scope of the agreement and perform other procedures or render additional treatment (9).

A patient may bring a medical malpractice action against the physician on a theory of lack of informed consent. To prove a malpractice claim under this theory, the plaintiff must show that a reasonably prudent physician would have disclosed the risks and alternatives to the plaintiff or that a reasonable plaintiff would not have consented to the procedure had he or she been properly informed of the risks and alternatives. Although the informed consent theory is not as common as a negligence claim, courts have held physicians liable for failing to adequately disclose to the patient the risks involved from surgical procedures (10).

Usually, a plaintiff will be required to produce expert testimony to show that a reasonable plastic surgeon would have disclosed the risks or alternatives under similar circumstances and that a reasonable person in the plaintiff's shoes would not have consented to the surgical procedure had he or she been properly advised. If a plaintiff fails to offer expert testimony to support his or her claim of lack of informed consent, a court can dismiss the action. For example, in a New Jersey state court case, the trial court dismissed the patient's medical malpractice action against a physician, which was based on a lack of informed consent (11). The court reasoned that because the plaintiff failed to produce an expert to testify that the risk of injury incurred by the plaintiff was recognized within the medical community, the plaintiff could not prove his cause of action.

Closely related to lack of informed consent is a claim for breach of contract. Such claims can arise when a surgeon "guarantees" a result. This is particularly applicable to plastic surgeons who advertise using "before and after" photos or other techniques that expressly, or by way of implication, promise a better appearance following surgery. The breach of contract claim centers on whether an objective and reasonable patient could understand the physician's claim of future condition to be a guaranty or a warranty. This is usually a question of fact, which means that it must be decided by the jury.

In guarding against claims for lack of informed consent or breach of contract, it is important to properly communicate with your patient and to fully document all discussions. When meeting with the patient to discuss a course of treatment, a plastic surgeon should pay special attention to the patient's understanding of the risks and disclose to the patient any and all well-accepted complications attendant to the surgery or treatment. Care must also be given to avoid potentially misleading advertisements upon which a plaintiff might rely to claim that the plastic surgeon guaranteed a certain result or physical appearance.

RES IPSA LOQUITUR

In some cases, a bad result will occur where there is no direct evidence that shows that a breach of the duty of care occurred. Courts allow claims in such cases under the theory of *res ipsa loquitur. Res ipsa loquitur* is a Latin term meaning "the thing speaks for itself" (12). The doctrine usually is reserved for those cases in which the patient sustains an injury during surgery, but where there is no evidence as to how the injury occurred. Under the judicial doctrine of *res ipsa loquitur,* courts sometimes allow the jury to infer negligence merely by a showing that the plaintiff had no culpability for his or her injury, that the physician was in control of the patient or the surgical equipment at the time of the injury, and that the injury is not one that normally occurs in the absence of a breach of the standard of care (13). The last point is critical because, in many cases, the claimed injury is a recognized complication from the procedure, even when no negligence occurs.

Because of the need to show that the injury is not one that occurs in the absence of negligence, courts usually require expert testimony to make out a *res ipsa* claim. In one case, however, the court allowed the jury to infer negligence under a *res ipsa* theory in the absence of expert testimony. In that case, the surgeon applied alcohol to the patient and then used an electric cautery to perform a medical procedure. As a result, the patient suffered burns. There was, however, no evidence as to how the burns occurred. The court ruled that, even in the absence of expert testimony, it could find that such a burn would not have occurred without negligence. Therefore, the court allowed the use of *res ipsa loquitur* and the jury found negligence (14).

ROLE OF EXPERTS IN PROVING MEDICAL MALPRACTICE

The use of experts to provide testimony, opinions, and information to the jury has increased exponentially since the mid-1970s. This is especially true in medical malpractice litigation. Experts testify as to the standard of care, whether the methods and procedures used by the physician met the standard of care and, if not, whether that failure caused the plaintiff's injuries. In today's legal climate, it is all but impossible to litigate a medical malpractice case without extensive expert testimony. This trend is not limited, however, to medical malpractice litigation. One survey found that 44% of judges and lawyers had to deal with scientific evidence and expert testimony in over 30% of their cases (15). Although there has been an increase in the use of scientific evidence in the courtroom, there also has been an increase in the amount of unverified and unsupported expert testimony.

A New Standard: *Daubert v. Merrell Dow Pharmaceuticals, Inc.*

In the face of increased attempts by plaintiff's lawyers to expand the use of expert testimony, the United States Supreme Court in *Daubert v. Merrell Dow Pharmaceuticals, Inc.* adopted a new standard governing the admissibility of expert opinions (16). Under the previous standard, enunciated by the Court in 1923 in a case known as *Frye v. United States,* an expert's testimony was admissible only insofar as it was based on a technique "that was generally accepted" in the scientific community (17). Now, under the new standard enunciated in *Daubert,* an expert's testimony is admissible only so long as the process or technique used by the expert in formulating the opinion is "reliable."

Daubert expanded the discretion of trial courts to evaluate the reliability and relevance of contested evidence by concluding that the "general acceptance" test for the admissibility of scientific evidence enunciated in *Frye* had been superseded by the adoption of Rule 702 of the Federal Rules of Evidence. Rule 702 explicitly requires that the scientific expert's testimony "assist the trier of fact to understand or determine a fact in issue." *Daubert* concluded that this "helpfulness" standard "requires a valid scientific connection to the pertinent inquiry as a pre-condition to admissibility" (18).

The Supreme Court in *Daubert* emphasized that trial courts must maintain a "gatekeeping responsibility" to ensure that admitted scientific testimony is both relevant and reliable. As they perform this "gatekeeping" task, trial courts are instructed to engage in a two-prong analysis. First, the court must determine whether the proffered expert testimony consists of "scientific knowledge," which is essentially a reliability inquiry. Second, even if the "scientific knowledge" prong is satisfied, the court must inquire further to ascertain whether the proposed testimony is relevant and whether it will "assist the trier of fact."

The Supreme Court has interpreted the first prong of the admissibility test, the "scientific knowledge" requirement of Rule 702, as "establish[ing] a standard of evidentiary reliability" or "trustworthiness." The Court held that "evidentiary reliability" means, in effect, "scientific validity." To be scientifically valid, an expert's opinion must be "ground[ed] in the methods and procedures of science" and "supported by appropriate validation." Conjecture, hypothesis, "subjective belief, or unsupported speculation" are impermissible grounds on which to base an expert opinion. In short, *Daubert* commands that, in court, the science must do the speaking, not merely the scientist.

Several factors may affect the validity, or reliability, of a particular expert opinion, but the *Daubert* Court noted four in particular. They are as follows:

1. Whether the theory or technique used by the expert can be, and has been, tested;
2. Whether the theory or technique has been subjected to peer review and publication;
3. The known or potential rate of error of the method used; and
4. The degree of the method's or conclusion's acceptance within the relevant scientific community.

With the second prong of the admissibility test, the Supreme Court gave trial courts a more familiar role to play. This second prong focuses on the relevance of the proffered opinion to an issue in the case and on the "fit" of the proposed testimony and evidence to the facts of the case. Under this prong, not only must the opinion be scientifically valid, or reliable, but it also must advance the trier of fact's understanding of a material issue in the case.

The distinction between "scientific validity" and "fit" is not always clear, and at times the inquiries may overlap. For instance, there may be a case where an expert relies on published and widely accepted, tested theories in forming her opinion, and her ultimate conclusion is clearly relevant to an issue in the case, but if those published studies and theories purport to prove XYZ, and from them the expert concludes ABC, it may be that the expert's reasoning process itself is not scientifically valid. Courts generally disallow testimony or evidence when there is no "fit" between the tested theories relied upon and the ultimate conclusion reached.

The *Daubert* Court indicated that the inquiry as to whether a particular scientific technique or method is reliable is a flexible one. The Court rejected "general acceptance" as a necessary precondition to the admissibility of scientific evidence under the Federal Rules of Evidence. It stated, however, that the Rules of Evidence assigned to the trial court the task of ensuring that an expert's testimony both rests on a reliable foundation and is relevant to the task at hand. Pertinent evidence based on scientifically valid principles generally will satisfy those demands.

Daubert's Application to Claims Against Plastic Surgeons

Generally speaking, the *Daubert* test is a strong tool to use in defending a malpractice claim; however, it is not a panacea. Although *Daubert* allows a defendant-surgeon to exclude unsupported opinions proffered by a plaintiff's expert, it does not mean that an expert automatically will be excluded just because he or she is not a board-certified plastic surgeon. For example, in one case, a *dermatologist* was allowed to testify as to the standard of care required of a plastic surgeon even though he never personally used the product involved in the patient's lip augmentation and was not a board-certified surgeon (19). The court deemed the witness qualified because he demonstrated that he had knowledge, experience, and education with regard to the surgical procedure.

Notwithstanding the case cited, most courts now scrutinize all experts, and they do not readily deem any physician an expert. For instance, an internist, who admitted that he did not have expertise in the surgical procedure at issue and that he was unfamiliar with the standards of practice used by surgeons, was held by the court to be unqualified to act as an expert for the plaintiff and to testify as to the standard of care required of a surgeon (20).

In attempting to set out some guidelines, at least one court has held that the qualifications required of an expert to testify in a medical malpractice action against a plastic surgeon are whether the expert (i) is licensed to practice medicine; (ii) is certified by the American Board of Plastic and Reconstructive Surgery; (iii) has practiced as a plastic surgeon; (iv) is on staff with a hospital; (v) has any affiliations with societies or academic research groups; and (vi) has any practical experience in performing the particular type of operation (21).

Silicone Breast Implant Litigation and *Daubert's* Role in Defending Such Claims

Although it does not fall into the category of "medical malpractice," the product liability litigation brought against silicone breast implant manufacturers demonstrates the practical use of the *Daubert* doctrine. After years of tumultuous debate over the safety of silicone breast implants, courts are beginning to reject the scientific evidence used by the plaintiffs' expert witnesses. For example, the United States District Court of Oregon recently applied *Daubert* to exclude the plaintiffs' experts (22). In that litigation, the plaintiffs claimed that silicone breast implants caused a host of autoimmune and connective tissue diseases. These claims brought four areas of science into play: epidemiology, rheumatology, immunology/toxicology, and polymer chemistry. To determine the scientific validity of the plaintiffs' claims, the court appointed an independent panel of advisors. The judge and panel subjected the plaintiffs' experts and their theories to questioning on the issues of medical causation, the scientific reliability and general acceptance of tests and studies relied upon by the experts, and the methodology and scientific reasoning underlying the experts' opinions.

After this hearing, the court determined that the plaintiffs' scientific assertions did not hold up under *Daubert.* Specifically, the court's scrutiny exposed the fact that many of the plaintiffs' theories were untested, not generally accepted in the scientific community, and lacked a scientific basis. Moreover, the court noted that the plaintiffs' theories failed to prove a causal connection between the silicone from the breast implants and the alleged diseases contracted by the plaintiffs.

Many of the arguments used to attack the plaintiffs' experts in the silicone breast implant litigation can be used to challenge a plaintiff's expert in a medical malpractice case. The most important teaching of the breast implant litigation is that, when confronted with an expert, the science and methodology supporting the proffered opinion must be valid before the opinion is admissible in court.

TORT REFORM EFFORTS

Another way states have attempted to stem the tide of rising personal injury verdicts is to enact tort reform legislation. These reforms were passed not only because of the attention paid to inconsistent results from the courtroom, especially when dealing with scientific evidence, but also because of the significant rise in insurance premiums. The emerging problems with skyrocketing health care costs fueled by personal injury and medical malpractice litigation also drove this effort. Nearly all states now have enacted some type of legislation to reform or modify the ability of plaintiffs to recover in personal injury cases (Table 6-1) (23).

One measure commonly adopted was to ban or place a limit on the amount of noneconomic or punitive damages a plaintiff can recover. States enacting such limits have placed caps on such damages ranging from $100,000 to $500,000.

TABLE 6-1. NUMBER OF STATES RECENTLY ENACTING MEASURES OF TORT REFORM

Year	No. of states (reference no.)
1995	19 (24)
1996 and 1997	22 (25)

Additionally, some states have taken steps to try to limit frivolous malpractice litigation. For example, Illinois requires a plaintiff, as a prerequisite to filing a malpractice claim against a physician, to provide the court with an affidavit of an expert, stating that the expert has reviewed the facts and medical records and is prepared to testify that there is a meritorious basis for the claim (26). The plaintiff's failure to comply with this requirement can result in immediate dismissal of the plaintiff's lawsuit. Therefore, the defendant-physician should contest the sufficiency of the affidavit if it appears that the plaintiff's expert failed to inspect the records or to otherwise adequately support his opinion.

Some states also have lowered or capped the fees a plaintiff's attorney can recover based on a contingent fee arrangement. A contingent fee arrangement is one in which the plaintiff's attorney receives a percentage of the award or settlement. Under such legislation, an attorney normally accustomed to taking a fee in the amount of one-third of any settlement or jury verdict may have to accept a case for less than the standard fee. In some instances, some statutes impose a 25% fee as the maximum an attorney can charge in a contingency fee case (27). The theory is that if an attorney cannot earn as much money in a particular claim, there will be less litigation.

Although tort reform efforts have been passed by state legislatures, they are subject to review by the courts of each state. Across the country, many state courts have limited or overturned tort reform as an unconstitutional infringement on one's opportunity to recover for injuries. In fact, the high courts in 24 states have delivered 61 different decisions rejecting, in whole or in part, laws that attempted to cap damages or erect hurdles to discourage tort suits (28). The darkened states in Fig. 6-1 are the states in which tort reform legislation has been limited or overturned by the courts.

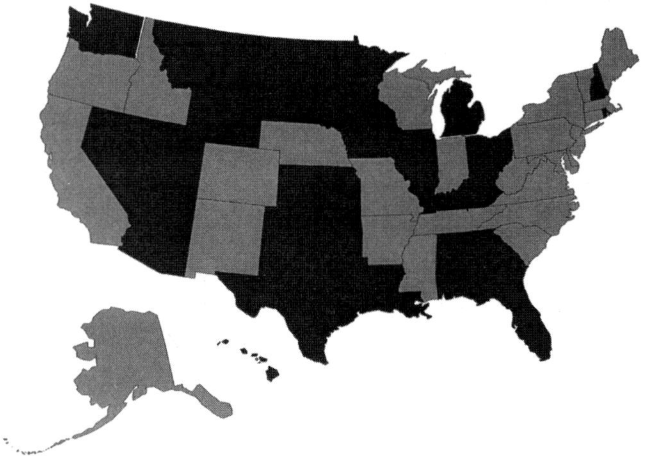

FIGURE 6-1. Tort reform legislation in the United States. The darkened areas represent states in which tort reform legislation has been limited or overturned by the courts.

In addition, tort reform has been heavily criticized by members of the plaintiff's bar. They argue that caps on noneconomic damages are inconsistent with the principle or fundamental goal of tort law—to fully compensate an injured plaintiff for his or her injuries. Other criticisms are that caps on damages remove the jury from making the decision as to who is wrong and as to what the award should be. Clearly, the debate over the constitutionality of tort reform and its merits will continue to rage.

DEFENSES TO MALPRACTICE CLAIMS

In general, a plastic surgeon can defend a medical malpractice claim in a number of different ways. Typically, defense counsel will contest whether a physician–patient relationship existed, whether the surgeon breached the standard of care required, or whether the surgeon's acts or omissions caused the injuries alleged by the plaintiff. A failure of the plaintiff to prove any of these elements will result in a verdict for the physician, so it is important to contest each element vigorously.

When confronted with a lack of informed consent claim or a claim for breach of contract, a successful defense can be mounted by producing documents to show that the patient received adequate and proper disclosure and that no guaranties or promises were made as to the result of the surgery. In order to guard against such claims, a plastic surgeon should document all steps taken to inform the patient about the inherent risks and alternatives.

In addition to defending a malpractice claim on its merits, there are statutes in place in most states that limit the time in which a malpractice claim may be brought. The defenses—the statute of limitations and statute of repose—are in place to guard against stale claims and to provide some time limit beyond which claims may not be asserted.

A statute of limitations bars a claim from being brought after a certain time period. The purpose of a statute of limitations is to keep claims fresh. Courts and legislatures are concerned that, after a certain number of years, the validity of testimony and evidence will diminish as witnesses' memories fade. Typically, the time period starts when the patient knows, or should reasonably know, that he or she has sustained an injury and that the injury may have been caused by another's act. In many states, the statute of limitations for medical malpractice claims is 2 years after the alleged negligent act or omission.

Like statutes of limitation, statutes of repose seek to impose finality by limiting the time in which medical malpractice claims can be brought. Unlike statutes of limitation, however, they do not depend on the plaintiff's knowledge of the existence of a cause of action. To the contrary, under a statute of repose, a plaintiff's cause of action ceases to exist once the requisite time limit has passed. Many statutes of repose for medical malpractice are between 8 and 10 years, running from the date of the alleged negligent act or omission.

Most states toll the running of the statute of limitations if the plaintiff is a minor. When this occurs, the statute of limitations begins to run as soon as the plaintiff reaches majority. Many states also toll the running of the statute of repose when the plaintiff is a minor. In most of these states, however, the plaintiff does not obtain the benefit of the entire statute of repose (e.g., 8 years) upon reaching majority. Rather, the time period is shortened to a time that often is equivalent to the statute of limitations (e.g., 2 years).

AVOIDING MEDICAL MALPRACTICE CLAIMS

Clearly, medical malpractice litigation is burdensome, time consuming and costly. Also, it can injure one's professional reputation. Thus, it is imperative for a plastic surgeon to attempt to avoid such claims. The best way to protect yourself is to do high-quality work and to insist that those persons under your direction, such as medical residents and nurses, also maintain high standards in their practice. By being diligent in your practice, you can avoid most situations that would allow someone to question your decisions or cause of treatment. Apart from simply being the best surgeon you can be, the following are some additional suggestions for avoiding malpractice litigation.

Develop a Good Rapport with Patients

Patients generally are loyal to their physician if they believe that their doctor is pulling for them. Developing a good rapport is more than just performing good work. It also requires you to show concern for your patient's well-being and to take steps above and beyond what is required according to your fee arrangement. A good "bedside manner" or a phone call after surgery to see how the patient is doing will go a long way to building a relationship between you and your patient. Oftentimes, even if there is some question as to the treatment provided, a patient will not bring a claim against his or her physician out of loyalty, respect, and the knowledge that the surgeon cared and tried his or her very best.

Do Not Create Unrealistic Expectations Through Your Advertising

Many patients seeking cosmetic changes want to become beautiful, sexy, or handsome. In many cases, an aesthetically improved image may be created. However, it is best to deal, on a patient-by-patient basis, with the realities and risks associated with the surgery. By not creating unrealistic expectations, there is a better chance that the patient will be more reasonable in dealing with the outcome.

One way to lower expectations is to limit advertising that uses "before and after" or comparison photographs, diagrams, or videos. Although such advertisements may prove effective in garnering patients, they also may cause patients to assume that their surgery will result in an equally sensational result, even if it is not a physical possibility. Patients also may point to such advertisements in claiming that an implied guarantee was created. If before and after or comparison advertisements are used, care should be given to explaining to the patient that results vary from patient to patient and that the surgeon cannot guarantee a result. The patient should acknowledge this discussion in writing and should agree that he or she has not relied on any advertisements in deciding to go forward with the surgery.

Be Sensitive to Patients with Unrealistic Expectations

Plastic surgeons may encounter individuals who have psychological problems that they seek to remedy through physical changes. Emotional problems cannot be cured by performing cosmetic surgery. Sometimes, it may be best to avoid an individual who seeks more than just a physical change. Additionally, you may run into a patient who has a track record of not only filing lawsuits, but in particular filing lawsuits against physicians. The practitioner should attempt to identify these patients and should pay particular attention to detail when documenting disclosures to, or discussions with, the patients.

Keep Accurate and Complete Documentation

As a general rule, all discussions with a patient should be memorialized in writing in the patient's medical records. In addition to documenting patient interviews, medical procedures, and preoperative and postoperative visits, medical records should include details of phone conversations with the patient. Such records can prove vital to defending or avoiding a medical malpractice claim.

Assume, for example, that, shortly after completing a breast reduction procedure, you are contacted by telephone by your patient. The patient asks whether she can go swimming. You caution her that, because of the risk of infection, under no circumstances should she swim before a date certain. If your patient ignores your advice and suffers a severe infection, how will you prove that you properly advised her? Remember that, in front of the jury, it will be your word against hers.

By making a note contemporaneous with your telephone conversation, you can establish your cautionary instructions to the plaintiff. This likely would be enough to convince a jury that no malpractice occurred. More importantly, however, you may avoid a claim altogether if the plaintiff's attorney believes that the note so weakens the case that he or she decides never to bring it.

Keep Apprised of New Developments

Developments in medical technology and surgery occur quickly. As someone in your field seeking to deliver the best medical care to your patient, it is important to keep up to speed on the latest developments. Failure to do so not only can injure your patient, it also can make you look foolish in front of a jury when asked why you did not use an improved technique. Nothing could be more embarrassing than to have someone from your field testify that you failed to use a recently developed treatment or method that could have provided an improved result in your patient's surgery. Accordingly, you should make it a regular practice to read articles, attend seminars and conferences, and use sources such as the Internet to keep your practice on the cutting edge.

Follow Up with Your Patients

Patients may have questions or may elect to have future surgeries to correct problems that were not fixed in the first surgery. By following up with the patients, you not only work in developing patient rapport, you also discover ways to treat the patient before serious problems arise. Simple things can make the difference. Follow-up, follow-up, follow-up.

Use and Fully Explain Consent Forms

When a patient comes to you and elects to have cosmetic surgery, surgeons often request that he or she fill out a consent form. Although this can serve as evidence of that person's consent, it will be a much stronger piece of evidence if you explain to the patient what is in the consent form and document the discussion in your records. In this way, a patient knows to what he or she is consenting, and the surgeon will have an opportunity to answer questions about that consent.

When in Doubt, Seek Legal Advice

Many doctors who have been entangled in medical malpractice litigation dislike the legal system and avoid it at all costs. Do not let your dislike for the legal system stand in your way of seeking legal advice. Trial attorneys, like physicians, can provide advice that will lessen the risk involved, before a problem occurs. More importantly, you will need to develop a relationship with your attorney so that you can trust him or her with important details and important aspects of your medical practice. Lawyers are under a duty to keep confidential all information disclosed to them. By developing a relationship with and trust in your attorney, you will be able to obtain the advice you need without worrying that the information provided in connection with obtaining the advice will be disclosed to competitors or patients.

Refer Out Cases That Are Beyond Your Capabilities

Oftentimes, professionals enjoy taking on tasks that are challenging. However, know where to draw the line between a case that is challenging and one that is beyond the realm of your capabilities. By referring out to a more highly trained specialist in a particular area, you are able to avoid causing injury to a patient and becoming entangled in medical malpractice.

Become Involved in Your State and National Medical Societies

Many states have passed various tort reform measures. These reforms are due, in no small part, to the efforts of medical associations. Nevertheless, over 60 of these measures have been struck down. Accordingly, medical associations are left with the task of advocating the reenactment of meaningful tort reform. Your support and assistance in that effort can protect your practice from frivolous and costly litigation.

These suggestions are only some ways to avoid malpractice claims. They are, by no means, the only measures you can take to protect yourself. Moreover, the unfortunate fact is that there is no set of guidelines one can use that will guarantee that you will not be the subject of a malpractice lawsuit. Physicians, like lawyers, accountants, engineers, and all other professionals who hold themselves out as providers of advice or specialized services, are vulnerable to such claims. All one can do is be diligent and attempt to provide high-quality health care to all patients.

REFERENCES

1. See, e.g., *Cannell v. Medical & Surgical Clinic,* 21 Ill. App. 3d 383, 315 N.E.2d 278 (1974) (discussing duty of hospital or clinic to disclose a patient's medical records upon request).
2. Lynn JSR. *Connecticut Medical Malpractice,* 12 Bridgeport L. Rev. 381, 383 (1992) (discussing the basic elements of a negligence claim).
3. Kerns C, Gerner CJ, Ryan C (Sedgwick, Detert, Moran & Arnold). *Health Care Liability Deskbook,* Medical Malpractice Liability, § 1:2 (3rd Ed. 1997).
4. See *McMillan v. Durrant,* 312 S.C. 200, 439 S.E. 2d 829 (1993), cited in Kerns, Gerner, Ryan, supra note 3.
5. Adams MB, Dopf GW. *Trial Practice in a Medical Malpractice Case: A Defense Perspective,* 109 Practising Law Institute (1992).
6. Adams MB, Dopf GW. Supra note 5, at 359; see also *Nunley v. Kloehn,* 888 F. Supp. 1483, 1488 (E.D. Wis. 1995) (ruling all that is required is that the expert have experience in the field; therefore, the expert can belong to another medical field, such as dermatology or internal medicine, if she has experience with the particular treatment or procedure used in the case).
7. St. Julian RD. *Malpractice, Illinois Jurisprudence: Personal Injury & Torts,* 29:15, 29:24 (1994); see also *Malpractice AM, Jur. 7 Proof of Facts* 479.
8. Annotation, *Cost of Future Cosmetic Plastic Surgery as Element of Damages,* 88 A.L.R.3d 117 (1978).
9. Rigney DE, *Annotation, Medical Malpractice in Connection with Breast Augmentation, Reduction or Reconstruction,* 28 A.L.R. 5th 497 (1995).
10. Rigney DE. Supra note 9, discussing *Korman v. Mallin,* 858 P. 2d 1145 (Ala. 1993); see also 28 A.L.R. 5th 845.
11. See *Febus v. Barot, M.D.,* 260 N.J. Super. 322, 616 A.2d 933 (1992).
12. *Black's Law Dictionary,* 1305 (6th Ed. 1990).
13. See *Magner v. Beth Israel Hospital,* 120 N.J. Super 529, 295 A.2d 363, cited in Holder AR, *Plastic Surgeon's Liability in Cosmetic Surgery Cases, AM. Jur. 22 Proof of Facts* 721.
14. Holder AR. Supra note 13, at 728-729.
15. National Center for State Courts Reports, vol. 7, no. 8 (Aug. 1980).
16. 509 U.S. 579 (1993).
17. See *Frye v. United States,* 293 F. 579 (D.C. Cir. 1923).
18. *Daubert,* 590 U.S. at 591-92.
19. See *Nunley v. Kloehn,* 888 F. Supp. 1483 (E.D. Wis. 1995).
20. See Adams MB, Dopf GW. Supra note 5, 121-22.
21. *Ditto v. McCurdy,* 947 P.2d 961 (HI App. 1997).
22. *Hall v. Baxter Healthcare Corp., et al.,* 947 F. Supp. 1387 (D. Ct. Or. 1996).
23. Pace KA. *Recalibrating the Scales of Justice Through National Punitive Damages Reform, American Univ. Law Review,* June 1997. According to one commentator, 46 states have enacted some form of tort reform legislation.
24. Schwartz VE, Behrens MA. *Stamping Out Tort Reform, 147 New Jersey Law Journal* 897 (1997).
25. Thompson M. *Letting the Air Out of Tort Reform: After Making Inroads in State Legislatures, Proponents of Restrictions on Tort Suits Now Are Fighting in the Courts to Protect Their Gains, 83 A.B.A. Journal* 64 (May 1997).
26. 735 ILCS 5/2-622; see *Estate of Cassara by Cassara v. State of Illinois,* 853 F. Supp. 273.
27. Schneyer T. *Legal-Process Constraints on the Regulation of Lawyers' Contingent Fee Contracts,* 47 Depaul L. Rev. 371 (1998) (discussing contingency fee rate structures).
28. Finzen BA, Haley BJ. Shaw KA. *Illinois High Court Latest to Nix Tort Reform Law, National Law Journal,* Feb. 16, 1998.

Discussion

MEDICAL MALPRACTICE AND PLASTIC SURGERY: A TRIAL LAWYER'S PERSPECTIVE

JEANNETTE MARTELLO

As a medical consultant for the Medical Board of California and an independent reviewer of medical malpractice cases for the past 16 years, I have had the opportunity to review several medical malpractice cases. The practicing attorney who wrote this chapter discussed several good points that must be stressed. Other additional new points should be brought to light.

FIRST SIGN

Unfortunately, the interface between medicine and the law is not found in the medical school curriculum. Therefore, physicians oftentimes are rudely awakened and must become educated on such medical legal matters when they are first served with subpoena papers.

If you receive a request from a patient for medical records, immediately notify your malpractice insurance carrier and notify your attorney. If you do not do so promptly, your insurance company may not defend the malpractice allegations. Oftentimes, it is helpful to have a separate attorney from the one who is assigned to you by the malpractice insurance company. Discuss with and educate your attorney with respect to the details of the case. Do not worry about confidentiality, because once the attorney–client relationship is established, it can only be waived by you, the defendant-physician.

ELEMENTS OF A MEDICAL MALPRACTICE CLAIM

The burden of proof lies with the plaintiff-patient to prove a case of medical malpractice. The defendant is the physician or other entity who is defending himself against the allegations of medical malpractice.

J. Martello: Plastic and Hand Surgery, Pasadena, California; and Medical Consultant, Enforcement Program Probation Unit, Medical Board of California

The tort of negligence is defined as "conduct which falls below the standard established by law for the protection of others against unreasonable risk of harm" (1).

In order for this tort of negligence to exist, four legal elements must be proven:

1. The physician must have owed a duty of care to the patient.
2. The standard of care must have been violated by the physician.
3. This violation of the standard of care must have proximately caused . . .
4. An injury or loss that occurred for which the patient can be compensated.

Point 1: Duty of Care

Once a physician–patient relationship is established, the physician owes a duty to the patient. For example, a physician who undertakes to render medical care to a patient creates a professional relationship with the patient. In fact, it is important to note that a physician can undertake to treat a patient without ever setting eyes on the patient! If a patient discusses a medical problem with a physician over the telephone and the physician offers medical advice, the physician has undertaken to treat the patient. If an intermediary such as a nurse is involved, a physician can be found to have rendered medical care without ever knowing or seeing the patient!

Beware of the cases involving patient transfers. Oftentimes, we are called as consultants on trauma cases and asked to accept traumatized patients in transfer from another hospital or from another service. Make sure that the patient is stable and has no other underlying potentially life- or limb-threatening problems before accepting the patient in transfer.

Affirmative acts of rendering medical care as well as omissions can be defined as medical care and therefore subject to the duty owed the patient.

This duty of care is owed and cannot be broken unless it is terminated in one of three different ways:

1. Via mutual agreement
2. Via the patient's request
3. Via the physician's request. This notice must be reasonable advance notice. The definition of reasonable depends on the patient's medical condition. The notice must be given far enough in advance for the patient to be able to obtain effective medical management elsewhere. Notice should be performed in writing via a registered letter with a return receipt requested.

If the patient–physician relationship is not terminated via one of these aforementioned ways, the physician may be found guilty of patient abandonment.

DOCTRINE OF VICARIOUS LIABILITY

A physician may be held legally responsible for the negligent acts of others via the legal doctrine of vicarious liability. Direct negligence on the part of the physician need not be proven. Negligence will be imputed to the defendant-physician as the result of another's' actions or omissions.

Via this doctrine, a defendant-physician can be held liable for the acts or omissions of others, such as interns, residents, nurses, hospital or office employees, or other ancillary staff. In legal terms, these third parties are considered "borrowed servants." That is, "[A] servant directed or permitted by his master to perform services for another may become the servant of such other in performing the services" (2). In order for this "vicarious liability" or "borrowed servant" doctrine to apply, a few requirements must be met:

1. A relationship must exist between the defendant-physician and the person or "servant" who actually committed the negligent act.
2. The "servant" who committed negligence must have been acting within the scope of the relationship.
3. The "servant" must have been negligent.
4. The defendant-physician must have possessed the requisite degree of control over the "servant."
5. The "servant" must have been acting within the scope of his relationship with the defendant-physician.

Note that a defendant-physician may be found vicariously liable for the negligent acts of another physician who is a partner, especially if the negligent act was committed within the scope of the partnership.

Additionally, the defendant-physician may be found liable for the acts of a substitute surgeon if the defendant-physician did not notify the patient that a substitute surgeon was going to be performing the operation. Note that a defendant-physician may be held responsible for the negligent acts of an anesthesiologist if the defendant-physician had control or the right to control the anesthesiologist.

RES IPSA LOQUITUR ("THE THING SPEAKS FOR ITSELF")

Usually, negligence is proven via direct evidence. Negligence also can be proven via circumstantial evidence. This doctrine is rarely utilized. In order for it to be proven, three elements must be proven:

1. An event resulted that does not ordinarily occur in the absence of negligence.
2. A person or instrument was under the exclusive control or management of the defendant.
3. The event that occurred and caused injury to the plaintiff was not the result of contributory negligence or a voluntary act on the part of the plaintiff-patient.

Classic examples include those of retained sponges or instruments; and burns or trauma to parts of a patient's body that were not in the immediate operative field and those of pressure sore formation. In these cases, expert testimony often is not needed.

Point 2: The Standard of Care Must Have Been Violated by the Physician

A physician must adhere to an applicable standard of care. This standard of care is defined as the care that would be rendered by a reasonable physician under like or similar circumstances. The standard of care is evaluated in light of the state of medical knowledge and skill available at the time of the allegedly negligent conduct.

This standard of care is delineated by medical expert testimony. In general, the medical expert must be in the same specialty as the defendant. In some instances, the courts have allowed physicians in other specialties to testify as medical experts so long as the alleged negligence involves matters within the knowledge of every physician (3). Therefore, although you may be a board-certified plastic surgeon, a non–board-certified physician may be the medical expert for the plaintiff's case.

In general, physicians are held to a more objective, national standard of care; therefore, an expert can be acquired from across the nation.

Point 3: This Violation of the Standard of Care Must Have Proximately Caused . . .

The plaintiff must prove that the injury or loss that resulted would not have occurred "but for" the negligent conduct of the defendant-physician. Alternatively, the plaintiff must show that the defendant-physician's negligent conduct was a "substantial factor" in bringing about and "more likely than not" caused the patient's injury or loss.

Point 4: A Loss or Injury Must Have Occurred for Which the Patient Can Be Compensated

This requirement is in order for the plaintiff-patient to be "made whole" because "but for" the defendant-physician's "negligence," the patient would have been a "whole person." Even if the tort of negligence is proven, if compensable damages are not present, a judgment in favor of the plaintiff will not be awarded (4).

Classically, the largest damages have been awarded for noneconomic damages, such as "pain and suffering," although many states now have placed caps on these damages ranging from $250,000 to $500,000.

Actual damages can be awarded for lost wages or earnings; medical expenses actually incurred; and future medical treatment (including rehabilitation) or subsequent surgery costs.

Punitive damages can be awarded for the punishment of the defendant for gross deviations from the standard of care. These damages rarely are awarded in medical malpractice cases.

PRETRIAL DISCOVERY

It is essential that you become intimately involved with your own medical malpractice case. In most cases, it is important for you to obtain your own counsel (independent of the insurance company). This is so that you can ensure that a case will not be settled without your consent, as well as to ensure that you have an objective legal advocate who does not have a potential conflict of interest with your insurance company.

Make sure that you educate your attorney and assist him or her with the preparation of the interrogatories as well as in the acquisition and preparation of the defense expert witness.

The most important part of pretrial discovery, though, remains the deposition. In fact, according to Melvin Belli, the world-famous plaintiff medical malpractice attorney, a deposition is a "good way to win without going to court" (5). Make sure that you thoroughly prepare, and are well-coached by your attorney, for your deposition. Your deposition will be taken under oath and can literally impact both your career and personal life. Your deposition testimony can be used against you and read during your trial in order to impeach your credibility.

INFORMED CONSENT

In the last 5 years, most medical liability carriers have experienced a significant increase in the claims that allege a failure to obtain a proper informed consent before treatment. A breach in the standard of care of rendering an informed consent will be determined by testimony from expert witnesses and ultimately decided on by a judge or jury. Even if the standard of care with respect to informed consent is met, if compensable damages do not result, there will not be an award to the plaintiff-patient.

Note that an informed consent is not simply a form that has to be filled out and signed. Rather, an informed consent is an ongoing process between the physician and the patient. No one but the physician can give the patient an informed consent. An informed consent is not obtained by simply writing or calling in an order to "obtain an informed consent for a breast augmentation" (for example). Ancillary staff and hospital or office personnel can simply supplement an informed consent. If supplemental materials, such as pamphlets, brochures, or videos, are given to or viewed by the patient, make sure that your medical record refers to them.

An informed consent must be rendered to a patient who has no mind-altering medication in his or her system. Informed consents obtained in the preoperative holding room are to be frowned upon unless an emergency procedure is about to be performed. In one malpractice case, the cosmetic surgery patient stated that she was asked to sign the consent form in the operating room itself!

In most states, physicians have an "affirmative duty" to disclose such information. That is, as a physician, you must volunteer the information and not simply wait for questions from the patient. Patients need to be provided with sufficient information with regard to risks, benefits, and treatment alternatives, including nontreatment. Patients are to be given all information about risks that are relevant to a meaningful decision-making process.

Most states follow the "prudent patient" test. That is, the judge will inform the jury that there is no liability on the doctor's part if a prudent person in the patient's position would have accepted the treatment had he or she been adequately informed of all significant and relevant risks.

BREACH OF CONTRACT

Beware of the appearance of guaranteeing a result to a patient. Before and after computer imaging systems (especially when the actual hard-copy photograph is given to the patient) can come back to haunt a surgeon. Avoid misleading advertisements that may appear to guarantee a specific postoperative result.

In general, a medical malpractice case can be proven only when the tort of negligence is proven. When a guarantee or warranty is thought to exist, then the arena of contract law is entered. In negligence cases, the statute of limitations for filing a case varies from 1 to 2 years. That is, the plaintiff-patient has 1 to 2 years to file the case. In breach of contract cases (with respect to guarantees and warranties), the statute of limitations is much longer (between 5 and 7 years), and the burden of proof in proving the case is lower for the plaintiff-patient.

PRODUCT LIABILITY

As previously mentioned, in order for a case of medical malpractice to be proven, the tort of negligence (and its legal requirements) must be met. In the case of product liability, though, strict liability (not negligence) is all that is needed. For example, if a patient buys skin care from your office and this skin care is found to cause damage to the patient, you will be found liable because you provided the skin care to the patient. This is a reason why it is a good idea for you to personally see the patient before selling him or her the skin care products. Do not forget that the fact that your aesthetician employee saw the patient will not protect you, because you are still liable through the vicarious liability/borrowed servant doctrines. Even if the aesthetician is an independent contractor, you may be found liable through the principles of Agency Law. That is, the aesthetician may be perceived by the patient as an agent of your practice or office.

REFERENCES

1. Restatement (Second) of Torts, secs. 282–3 (1965).
2. Restatement (Second) of Agency, sec. 227 (1958).
3. Furrow BR, Greaney TL, et al. *Health law.* Hornbook Series. St. Paul, MN: West Publishing Co., 1995.
4. *Morse v. Moretti,* 403 F2d 564 CADC (1968).
5. Belli M, Carlova J. *For your malpractice defense.* Oradell, NJ: Medical Economics Books, 1986:39–140, 142.

SUGGESTED READING

For further information regarding medical legal issues in plastic surgery and the avoidance of medical malpractice claims, refer to the January 1999 issue of the *Clinics in Plastic Surgery, An International Quarterly,* edited by Dr. Mark Gorney and myself. Additionally, Dr. Robert Goldwyn's book, *The Patient and the Plastic Surgeon* is well worth reading.

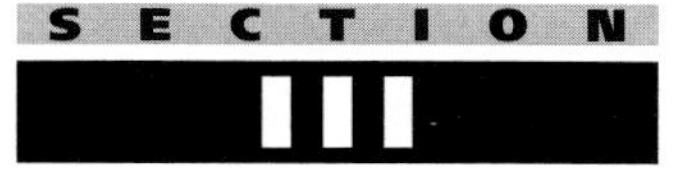

GENERAL PROBLEMS

7

SCARS AND SCAR REVISIONS

DAVID W. FURNAS
AFSHIN FARZADMEHR

"I thought plastic surgery didn't leave any scars!" "I know you are so much better at surgery than that last doctor—I can hardly see the scar you left on my eyelid and the other surgeon left a great big scar on my shoulder!" "I know I get keloids—see this keloid on my arm!" (The patient points to a thin, pale, linear scar.) Every plastic surgeon has heard such statements many times. Of course, any wound that penetrates the dermis causes some degree of scar. The scar may be virtually invisible or, at the other extreme, it can cause gross deformity and impairment of function, or the patient may be correct; it may indeed be "a keloid." Although many problems with scars are preordained, the surgeon usually can exert influence over the final outcome. If the surgeon has the opportunity to close the original wound, then meticulous attention to surgical details and postoperative wound care most often will yield a scar that needs no revision. When the patient's presenting problem is an unsatisfactory scar, the surgeon's first step is to obtain an accurate diagnosis and to determine the prognosis for improvement. Watchful waiting is often the treatment of choice. Application of pressure, massage, and other conservative steps sometimes are indicated during the waiting period. At other times, early or late surgical intervention is needed to obtain the most favorable result.

WOUND HEALING AND SCARS

The Healing Wound

Scar formation begins when wound healing reaches the collagen phase. Proliferation of fibroblasts, with synthesis and polymerization of collagen, gives increasing strength during the first weeks after injury. As rapid turnover of the collagen molecules proceeds, the cross linkages regroup the molecules in a more compact, stronger configuration. The scar contracts, diminishes in bulk, and increases in strength. The early, immature scar is hard, red, and raised due to the bulk of proliferating fibroblasts and unmodeled collagen, and the blush of dense capillaries. As wound maturity progresses, the fibroblasts and capillaries recede, the collagen continues to remodel, and, over a period of 6 to 12 months (or more), the scar becomes flat, soft, usually pale, and diminished in size (Fig. 7-1A,B) (1).

D. W. Furnas: Division of Plastic Surgery, University of California, Irvine, Orange, California

A. Farzadmehr: Department of Surgery, University of California, Irvine Medical Center, Orange, California; Division of Dermatology, Los Angeles County–King/Drew Medical Center, University of California Los Angeles, School of Medicine, Los Angeles, California

Scar Contraction and Contractures

Contraction of a scar is a normal stage in maturation, and it occurs in three dimensions. The margins of an open wound will inexorably creep together until the wound is closed, unless exceptionally unfavorable conditions prevail. Contraction also occurs in a vertical direction, so that deep wounds tend to be indented and adherent to underlying structures. Awaiting the completion of wound contraction is sometimes a definitive surgical strategy for wound closure, but contraction of a wound also can lead to disabling contractures if the wound is over the flexor surface of a joint or involves a mobile feature, such as the eyelid.

Collagen, Capillaries, and Pigmentation

Scar tissue contains no elastin, and the collagen bundles are oriented along stress lines rather than in the random weave seen in dermis. For these reasons, scar tissue lacks elasticity. Scar tissue also lacks hair, sweat glands, and sebaceous glands, making it dry and dense. If scar tissue impinges on hair follicles or cutaneous glands, chronic cysts and sinuses can result. The epidermal layer of a scar is not anchored by rete ridges and is stripped off more easily than normal epidermis. Even though the immature scar is pink from abundant capillaries, the mature scar has a paucity of capillaries. Repeat injury to mature scar tissue is slow to heal because of this diminished blood supply. This problem is magnified if the perfusion of the anatomical area is diminished. Scar tissue typically lacks normal pigmentation. Although mature scars usually are pale (Figs. 7-1B and 7-2D), they can be dark in patients with pigmented skin (see Fig. 7-4A). Particularly in burns, a mixture of both hypopigmentation and hyperpigmentation may be seen (Fig. 7-3A).

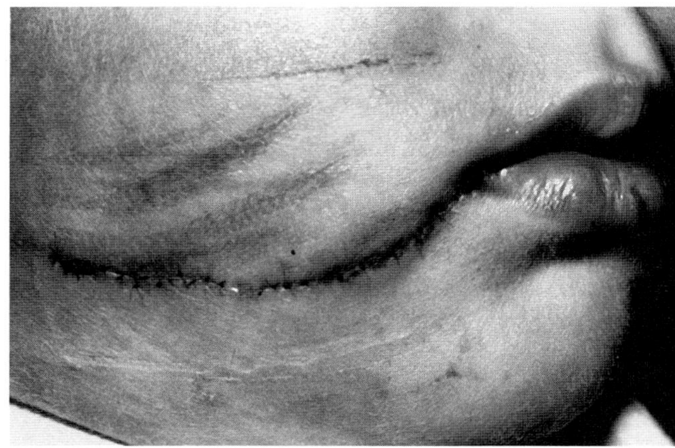

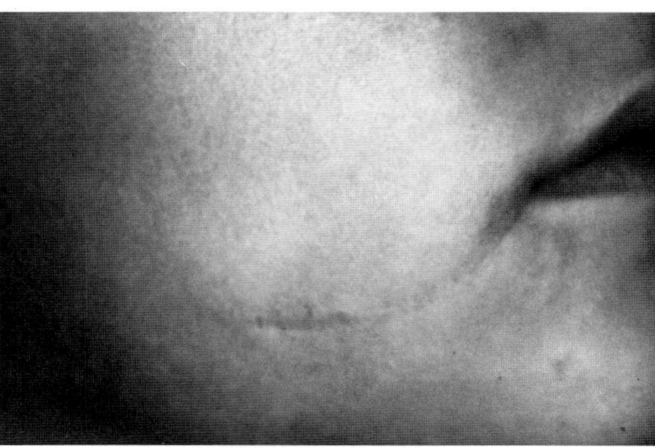

FIGURE 7-1. Closure of cheek wound that crossed crease lines. **A:** Laceration across the skin crease lines from barbed wire in 3-year-old boy. The wound was closed meticulously under magnification. **B:** Four years postoperatively, the scar has spread slightly and is still reddish in the central area where it crosses the skin creases at 90°, but it is inconspicuous elsewhere. If the reddish capillary blush persists, it can be removed with a 585-nm laser.

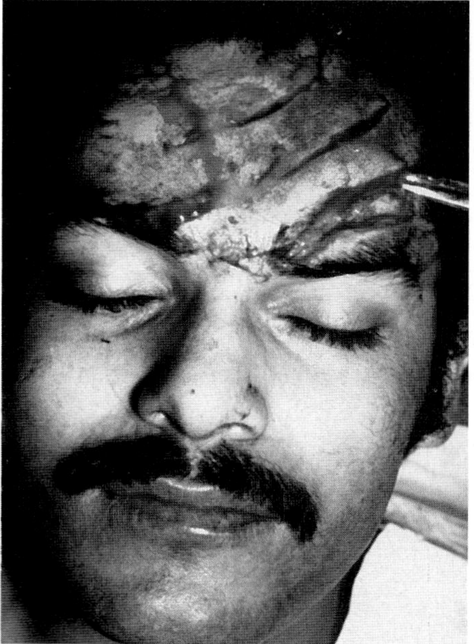

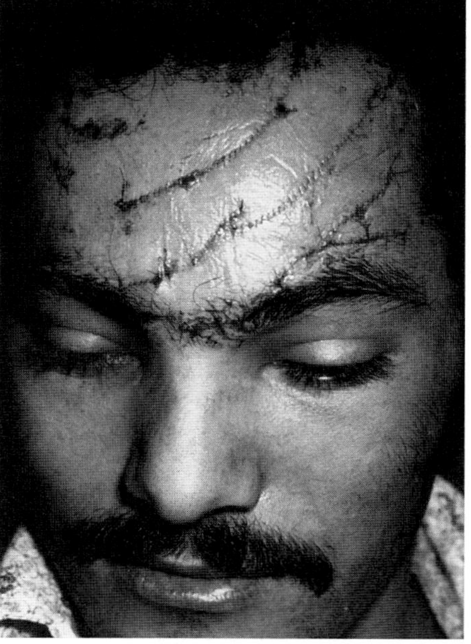

FIGURE 7-2. Application of pressure to immature wound. **A:** Slicing beveled lacerations from a windshield. Such wounds tend to heal with a protruding center in a "trap-door" or "pincushion" effect. **B:** Wounds trimmed and closed under magnification. *(Continued)*

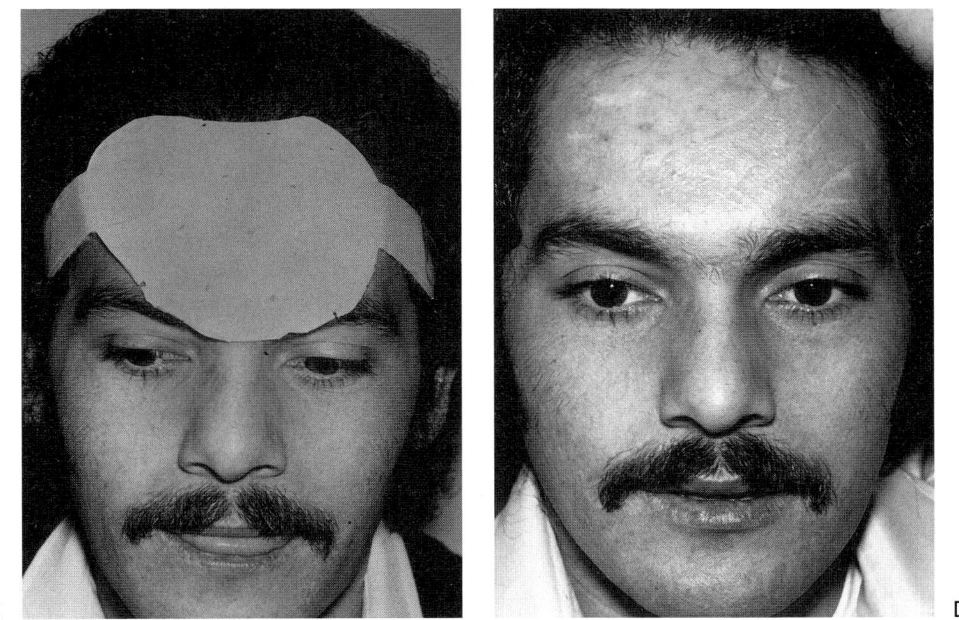

FIGURE 7-2. (*Continued*) **C:** The maturing wounds are compressed with a silicone gel sheet under a thermoplastic splint. **D:** One year postoperatively, the scars are soft and flat. The pallor of the mature scars is accentuated by the natural pigmentation of the patient's normal skin.

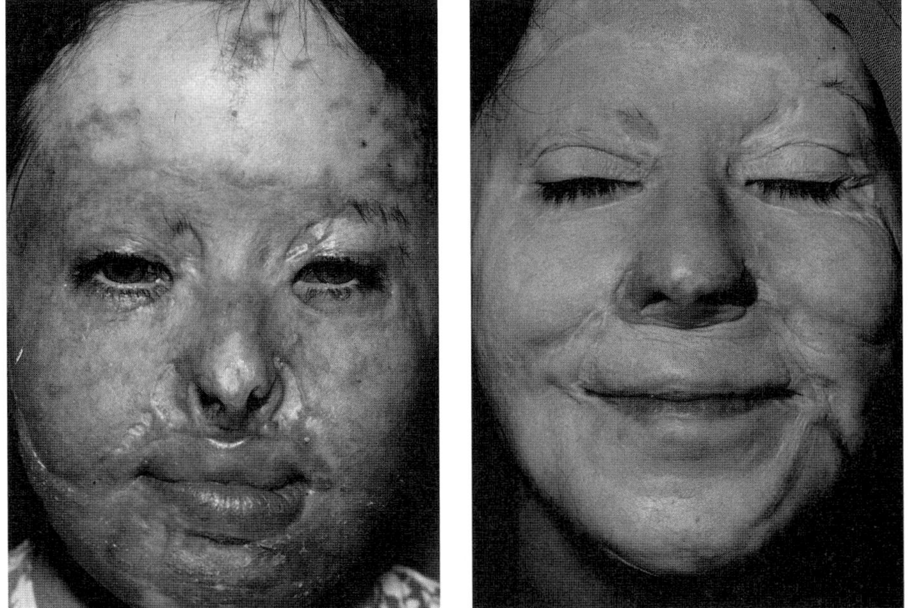

FIGURE 7-3. Severe facial burn scars—revision by skin grafts and flaps. **A:** Tight, irregular scars of lower cheeks and mandibular margin, ectropion of mouth and eyelids, and loss of nasal alae from automobile explosion and fire. **B:** Replacement of facial scars and thin contracted skin grafts with large full-thickness skin grafts from lower abdomen to the cheeks. Correction of ectropion of eyelids with split-skin grafts. Construction of nasal alae with composite skin grafts from ear lobes. Small local flaps were used at strategic points.

Predisposition to Problem Scars

As a general rule, patients with more pigmented skin are prone to hypertrophic scars or keloids (see Fig. 7-4A). Young children tend to develop a more florid hypertrophy of immature scars.

BIOMECHANICS AND ANATOMY OF SCARS

Crease Lines and Langer's Lines

Crease lines* cross the skin at right angles to the long axis of muscle contraction, as observed in living patients. Langer's lines are cleavage lines observed in cadavers that, in Langer's original illustrations, are parallel to the crease lines in some areas and not so in other areas. Gibson (3), who studied the biomechanics of skin, and who also translated Langer's papers, felt that crease lines and Langer's lines were not necessarily different systems. The inconsistencies in comparing Langer's drawings with drawings and photos of other authors may represent variation among the subjects. On the human face, the crease lines are perpendicular to the long axis of the muscles of facial expression. In the limbs, they run parallel to the axis of joints, which also is perpendicular to the long axis of the muscles in the limbs. The skin creases augment the skin area of flexor surfaces and provide for extensibility in functional movements. The furrowed line formed by the crease traces the axis of minimum extensibility. According to Gibson's review, Langer's cleavage lines plot the direction of minimal extensibility of the skin of cadavers. Langer made multiple perforations in the skin with a round awl. The circular punctures deformed into elliptical defects because of the directional extensibility of the skin. Langer connected the long axes of multiple ellipses to plot cleavage lines. Gibson observed that the direction of minimum extensibility varies from area to area, from individual to individual, and from infancy to old age. Scars aligned with the crease lines favor an aesthetic outcome, whereas scars that cross crease lines or are in areas of high skin tension where crease lines intersect (shoulders, sternum) have a poorer prognosis for satisfactory aesthetics.

Skin Tension and Age

Skin tension decreases with age, as noted by Gibson. Facial wounds in young children, therefore, have a greater tendency to hypertrophy; conversely, surgical scars in the elderly patient often are virtually invisible.

GEOMETRY OF SCARS

Convexities and Concavities

Scars that cross concavities or recesses, such as the medial canthal hollow, postauricular groove, alar groove, or flexor side of joints, tend to form bowstrings, bridal bands, or webs (see Fig. 7-7). Even a scar that is outside of the medial canthal hollow may contract unfavorably, transmitting a web to the intact but thin and extensible skin of the hollow. Scars that cross convexities have a tendency to spread, and they may be vulnerable to wounds from minor trauma. A linear scar across the convexity of the nose may cause a groove as it contracts and indents the thicker, softer sebaceous nasal skin.

Trap Doors and Bevels

A scar, caused by an oblique, semicircular "trap-door" laceration, tends to cause bulging of the skin enclosed in the semicircle. As the maturing semicircle contracts, the skin may bulge with a "pincushion" effect. Revision of such scars should be staged, excising only a segment of the arc each time. A scar from a beveled cut will tend to heap up in a ridge as healing proceeds and contraction causes bulging of the superficial, thinner side of the bevel. Conservative management in the postinjury period may prevent a permanent bulge. Oblique through-and-through lacerations of the vermillion of the lip have a special propensity to bulging of the wedge-shaped side as the wound matures. The mature bulge may require individualized trimming for an optimum result.

Depressed Scars and Step-off Scars

A scar that causes mobile skin to adhere to immobile deep structures, such as seen after a tracheotomy, results in fixation and indentation of the scarred skin. After freeing the underlying attachments, superficial muscle and fascia are interposed between the superficial and deep portions of the scar. Where wound edges have been opposed inaccurately or where the sutured edges have shifted from their original position, a stair-step or step-off scar may result. Revision is by realignment.

Anatomical Mismatch

If a laceration of the vermillion margin is closed inaccurately, a jog in the margin will be evident. If a shaved hairline or eyebrow has not been carefully matched, the discrepancy will be obvious as the hair grows. A small single Z-plasty, with the misplaced vermillion or brow forming one triangle and normal skin forming the other triangle, will correct the mismatch when the flaps are transposed.

AESTHETICS AND PSYCHOLOGY OF SCARS

Aesthetic Considerations

Scars range through an entire aesthetic spectrum, from an inconspicuous white dot to a grotesque deformity. The capability of a plastic surgeon to improve on the appearance of a scar also has a spectrum. Furthermore, the surgeon can never predict with complete reliability where on this spectrum his results will lie, or even how many operations will be needed to

---

* A number of words and phrases are, in essence, synonyms for Gibson's "crease lines," such as *relaxed skin tension lines* (RSTLs) *of Borges, Kraisal's lines, cleavage lines, wrinkle lines,* and more (2).

gain an optimum result. Whether the concern is with scars from proposed surgery or scars from past injury or surgery, a clear understanding between the surgeon and the patient about the subject of aesthetics of the scar in question is mandatory. This communication is one of the most important features in avoiding an unfavorable result. The patient must understand that scar removal can never eradicate a scar but can only minimize it. The surgeon must accurately convey to the patient his prediction of the natural history, chronology, and ultimate outcome of the scar to the best of his ability, and the patient must learn of potential complications, and uncertainties, and how they should be put in perspective.

Psychological Considerations

The surgeon must become knowledgeable about the patient, the patient's strong points, and the patient's vulnerabilities. He must earn the patient's confidence and friendship. Such preparation will lead to the best surgical decisions, the most satisfactory outcome, and the most favorable relationship and cooperation in the event of a complication. The surgeon must be prepared to say "No, I don't recommend trying to improve the appearance of your scar with surgery," in a firm but tactful and supportive manner, or "Yes, I think we have a good chance of gaining worthwhile improvement of your scar," in a positive and attentive manner. Or the surgeon might say, "I'm not enthusiastic about our prospects of gaining the improvement you deserve, but I think we have a reasonable chance of making *some* improvement, and it is unlikely that our effort will prove meddlesome—I'm going to put the decision in your hands as to whether you want to try for these small gains at a minimal risk of making the scar worse." It is the surgeon's task to determine whether the patient truly comprehends this dialogue and to communicate further with the patient, family, and previous physicians if there is doubt.

Unfavorable Psychological Factors

Freud described a patient who fixated on a barely perceptible scar from electrocautery of a tiny nasal pore (4). Inconspicuous as the blemish was, it was a disabling focal point to this seriously disturbed patient, which masked layers of psychopathology that were to become the material for Freud's landmark publication. The surgeon must get to know his patient well enough to detect not only misperceptions due to ignorance and normal anxiety, but also to detect misperceptions from distortions of reality.

TOPOGRAPHICAL ANATOMY AND SCARS

Favorable Anatomical Sites

Sites most favorable for inconspicuous scars are those where the blood supply is abundant and the skin is extensible. The face and neck, particularly the eyelids, the flexor surface of the hands, and the genitals are favorable areas.

Unfavorable Sites

Unfavorable sites are those where the skin is under greatest tension, as mentioned earlier (deltoid, presternal), where blood supply is least abundant (pretibial), where the area is vulnerable to chronic trauma (lower limbs), and other sites for which the cause of vulnerability is not obvious.

Aesthetic Units

The more distinct convexities and concavities of the face can be viewed as separate aesthetic units. Scars that pass from one distinct aesthetic unit to another, such as cheek—nose or cheek—lip, tend to be conspicuous. They cross crease lines, cast shadows, and disrupt aesthetic units. Scars that cross the mandibular margin to the cheek are perpendicular to the skin creases but, as they pass upward on the cheek, they are parallel; the mandibular segment often becomes wide and conspicuous. The cheek portion usually will fade. Longitudinal scars that cross the flexor creases of the wrist will tend to hypertrophy, whereas any distal extension into the palm that parallels the thenar eminence will heal invisibly.

Hidden Scars

Scars at the junction of anatomical features such as the alar base, eyebrow, hairline, and subciliary margin, or scars out of sight within the nostril, mouth, scalp, or suprapubic area, are inconspicuous and rarely need extra surgical attention. These sites are chosen for elective incisions. (A patient with the bad fortune of sustaining a laceration may have the good fortune that the wound site is favorable.)

UNFAVORABLE SCARS

Predisposition of Patient to Unfavorable Scarring

Some patients have a tendency to form unfavorable scars, even at favorable sites. An association between the density of melanin pigmentation of skin and severe scar hypertrophy or keloids has been observed. Whereas a Millard lip repair, properly performed, provides a symmetrical, even Cupid's bow, the scar contracts in some patients, raising one peak of Cupid's bow. With time, the scar usually returns to its normal level as maturation and softening take place, but not always. A later secondary rotation-advancement procedure usually solves the problem permanently. Two exceptions in our experience have been a Korean child whose secondary rotation scar showed florid hypertrophy and contracted even worse than the first. A third rotation, done several years later, showed neither hypertrophy nor contraction, and resulted in an excellent aesthetic repair—a demonstration of different wound responses at different ages. Another cleft lip patient who had an excellent, aesthetic lip repair went through a teenage growth spurt in which he grew 10 inches in 1 year. The cleft scar developed a marked relative contracture during the same period, and rerotation was needed. A similar phenomenon may be noted after successful correction of scars of the flexor surface of the hand and fingers in a child. In the teenage growth spurt, the patient loses extension of the fingers as the normal tissues outgrow the scarred flexor surface, and surgical corrections must be repeated.

Contractures

The normal healing process of contraction is a benign process in most small wounds on most parts of the body. However, contraction of a severe wound on a flexor surface, or involving mobile facial features, leads to pathologic contracture formation. The edges of a contracting wound creep closer together and bring any moveable anatomical parts along with them. Facial features are distorted, and joints lose their range of motion as scars contract. In children, contracting scar tissue can collapse pliant limbs into crippled appendages and contort the growing skeleton into grotesque configurations. Untreated burns with extensive surface damage are the most notorious cause of such severe contractures.

Unstable Scars

The paucity of vascularity in scar tissue was noted earlier. Optimum healing requires optimum blood supply. Therefore, if injury occurs within a previously scarred site, healing is slow and may be of poor quality. Also, wound closure in some patients with underlying systemic or local disease will be of inferior quality. Repeated chronic stress or injury of vulnerable wounds will cause a chronic, unstable, scar in which a repeating cycle of healed wound—open wound—healed wound is seen. Common sites are weight-bearing surfaces, areas of poor circulation (lower limbs), flexor areas with webbed, contracted scars (which are stretched beyond their limitations) (see Fig. 7-8), or in unpadded convexities such as the knee or elbow. If arterial supply is diminished or if venous stasis or lymphedema is present, the instability is worsened. An unstable scar is prone to repeated injury and chronic ulceration. If ulceration persists for many years (usually 2 to 3 decades), metaplasia and finally squamous cell carcinoma (Marjolin's ulcer) may occur.

Hypertrophic Scars

Sometimes early fibroblastic proliferation is pronounced, giving a hypertrophic scar. Marked hypertrophy is seen, particularly in the young, growing child whose skin is under more tension than a mature adult. Also, some sites of the body that have pronounced, multidirectional skin tension (deltoid area, upper chest) tend to form hypertrophic scars. Some patients have a constitutional proclivity toward scar hypertrophy, such as that seen with keloids. A deep, partial thickness burn in a child is notorious for causing hypertrophic scars, and sometimes scar maturation does not occur for 4 or 5 years (long after it seems it will never mature).

Keloids

Occasionally a massive overgrowth of scar tissue invades the normal surrounding skin and creates unsightly gnarled protuberances, or keloids. Keloids have a great propensity for recurrence when excised. They are particularly common over the sternum, deltoid area, and earlobes, although any part of the body can be affected (Fig. 7-4A,B). A true keloid represents one of the most difficult problems to treat in the field of plastic surgery.

Collagen Defects

Defects in collagen synthesis, such as in Ehlers-Danlos syndrome (Fig. 7-5A,B), scurvy, protein deficiency, or corticosteroid treatment can interfere with the healing process and cause abnormal scar formation. Radiation changes cause diminished blood supply and instability of scar tissue.

Pain and Paresthesias

Nerve regeneration in the area of a scar causes itching and other paresthesias in the early maturation process. Some hypertrophic scars cause intense itching for a prolonged period as regeneration progresses. Painful scars often are the result of tiny neuromas that are trapped in scar tissue. The pain usually is transient. An explanation of the process to the patient usually is sufficient therapy.

Foreign Bodies and Traumatic Tattoos

Foreign bodies increase scarring. Dirt or explosive particles cause traumatic tattooing of scar tissue (Fig. 7-6A,B). The tattoos usually are blue-black in color due to the Tyndall effect. Painstaking removal of pigmented particles under magnification prevents permanent tattooing. Established tattoos can be removed with a Q-switched YAG laser.

Suture Marks

Heavy sutures, tight sutures, large bites, and sutures that are left in place for a long time cause suture marks. These range from light, punctate indentations to heavy, unsightly "railroad track" scars. Epidermis may grow into the suture tracts if sutures are left in place too long, causing sinuses and cysts.

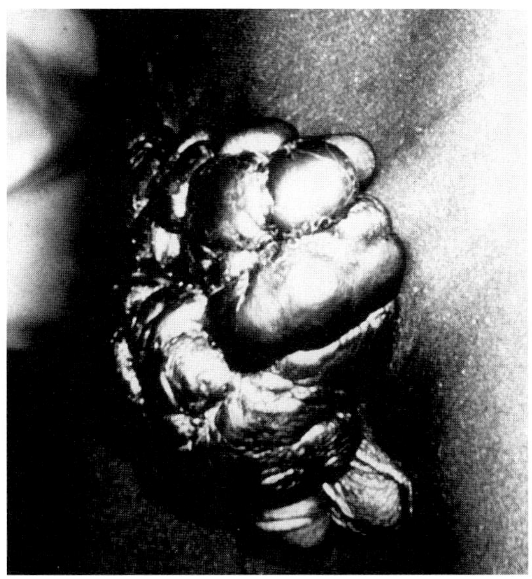

A

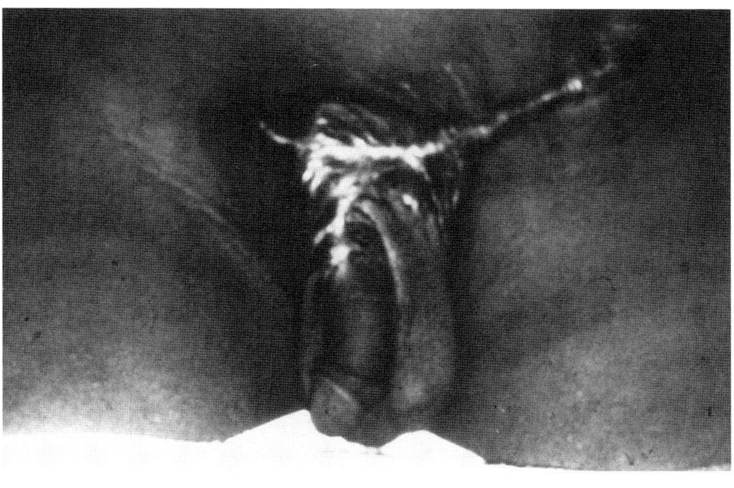

B

FIGURE 7-4. Recurrent keloid of inguinal region—radiation treatment. **A:** Recurrent keloid at site of incision for inguinal hernia repair. Keloid recurred and enlarged after excision and triamcinolone injections. **B:** Result after reexcision, with delivery of 1,200 rads of radiation and subsequent triamcinolone injections.

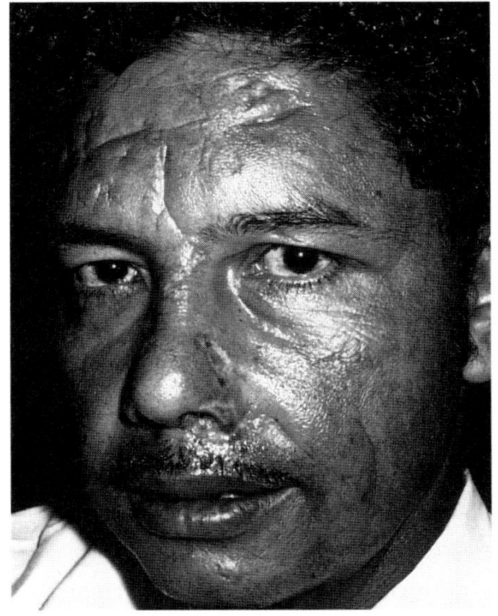

A

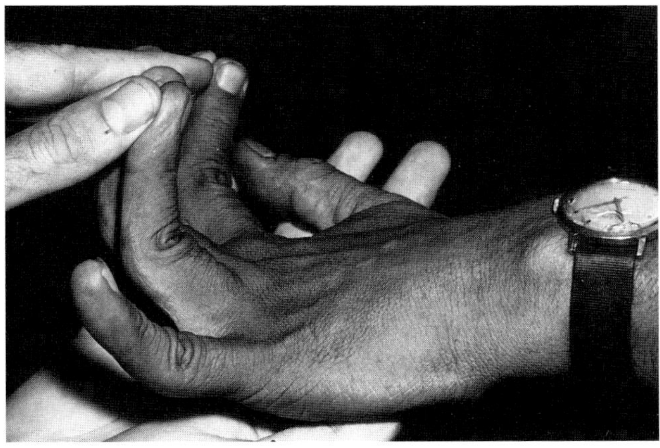

B

FIGURE 7-5. Ehlers-Danlos syndrome. **A:** Unexpected spreading and indentation of carefully repaired facial wounds led to identification of this patient's Ehlers-Danlos syndrome. **B:** Hyperextensibility of fingers in the same patient.

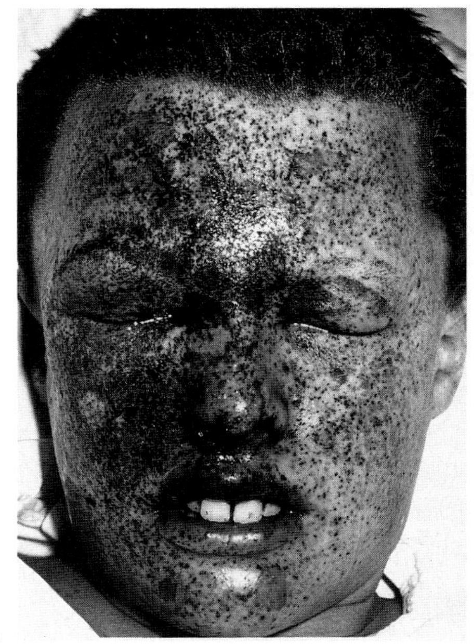
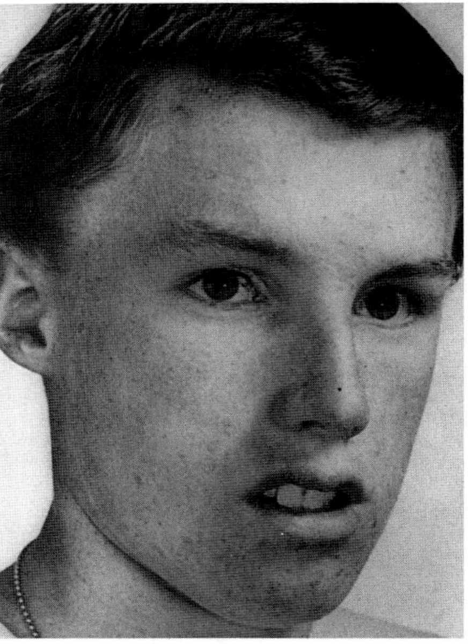

A B

FIGURE 7-6. Prevention of traumatic tattoos. **A:** Traumatic tattoos from a firecracker explosion. Operating room search for embedded particles of pigment was carried out under microscope, and particles were removed (particles were not removed from sclerae). **B:** Postoperatively, skin is essentially free of traumatic tattoos, but the sclerae show blue-black specks where pigmented particles remained.

Infections

Wound infections, acne, hidradenitis, chronic folliculitis, and draining osteomyelitis are all infectious processes that exacerbate scarring. They must be controlled to gain a satisfactory outcome. A site of chronic infection persisting 10 or 20 years can result in the development of squamous cell carcinoma (see section on Unstable Scars).

SURGICAL TREATMENT

Diagnosis and Planning

Accurate wound diagnosis is essential in planning the surgical treatment of a scar. The surgeon must determine what he can do better than was done before. If the original scar was complicated by the result of an infection, foreign body, or unskilled wound repair, surgical revision may be in order, and the surgeon must select the plan most likely to deliver a favorable result. Major skin losses usually cannot be corrected by simple techniques. Once the scar has been removed, the defect may expand dramatically, requiring a skin graft or pedicle for repair (Fig. 7-3A–B).

Simple Scar Revision

On the face, our usual technique for scar revision is to excise the offending scar, mobilize the neighboring skin, and then build the wound up in layers with adsorbable synthetic sutures. Continuous over-and-over sutures of very fine (6-0 or 7-0) monofilament polypropylene provide surface sutures (Fig. 7-2B). Interrupted sutures are added as needed. Interrupted sutures alone can be used (Fig. 7-1B). Small horizontal mattress sutures are used if they are essential for wound eversion. Sutures can be removed from well-supported wounds of the face in 4 to 6 days because of the excellent blood supply, thus avoiding suture marks. In small children and infants, continuous subcuticular pullout sutures are preferred in small wounds of the face because of ease of removal. However, we close the surface of a delicate complex wound, such as a cleft lip in an infant, with continuous 7-0 monofilament polypropylene suture. EMLA (eutectic mixture of local anesthetics) cream, a well-placed infant restraint, and high-power loupes provide for pain-free removal of the sutures. We feel that the convenience of fast absorbing catgut in such wounds is outweighed by the compromise in the quality of wound closure. Elsewhere on the body, particularly on the limbs and trunk, healing is less rapid and early suture removal presents the risk of the wound opening from minimal trauma. Intradermal surface sutures are used in these wounds to avoid the need for early suture removal. Small inaccuracies in the intradermal closure can be corrected with a few tiny interrupted monofilament finishing sutures that are removed early. The ends of the subcuticular suture are secured with tape inasmuch as knots tend to erode the skin. Adsorbable suture material that is knotted and left to dissolve in a subcuticular position tends to leave lumps or irregularities. In revising an indented scar, the base of the scar is left in place. The scar is deepithelialized and adjacent skin is advanced over it, giving fullness to the closure (5). Scars that tend to spread (chest, back, limbs) are sutured in several layers with long-acting adsorbable sutures. Wound support may be provided by tape strips during the months of wound maturation. If small lesions are to be removed from the back, deltoid area, sternum, or upper chest, it may be better to remove the lesion with as small a margin of normal tissue as possible and then simply allow the defect to heal-in by epithelialization. The scar is likely to be the smallest and least conspicuous obtainable. Octylcyanoacrylate cement currently shows promise for sutureless closure of the surface layer of revised scars (6).

Shaving and Dermabrasion

Small, heaped-up epithelial protrusions from flap-like lacerations or stair-step deformities can be corrected by simply shaving off the protruding portion with a scalpel blade or by the use of a dermabrader. Superficial cutaneous irregularities frequently are improved by shaving or dermabrasion. However, significant improvement in the scar tissue itself rarely is achieved with these techniques.

Skin Grafts and Major Flaps

If the overall area of scarring is extensive both in length and width, a skin graft or a flap most likely will be needed to give a sufficient release (Fig. 7-3A–B). (The choice of procedures is beyond the scope of this chapter.)

Dermal Overgrafting

Thin fragile scars with little padding, such as on the malleolar area in older people, sometimes can be improved by dermal overgrafting. The surface is freshened with a dermabrader or knife, and a skin graft is placed on the raw surface. After intervals of several weeks, this maneuver may be repeated, further augmenting the thickness of the dermis.

Z-plasties

Z-plasties occasionally are useful in breaking up and realigning forces in linear surface scars, or in repositioning displaced anatomical structures. Diagrams of Z-plasties most often show two isosceles triangular flaps on a flat plane in which the three limbs are equal, laid out in the figure of a "Z" or a reverse "Z". Beyond these two figures, the surgeon has numerous choices to exercise (7). Wider angles provide more lengthening on the long axis but more tension on the short axis. Asymmetrical angles may deal with the local topography better. Some asymmetry of the limbs can be accommodated by gathering a closure line. Z-plasties are exceptionally useful in redistributing the skin where web deformities are present (Fig. 7-7). The Z-plasty gives its most dramatic result when the scar is a simple cord-like bridle contracture with healthy skin surfaces on either side. If the surfaces meet at a sufficient angle, the Z-plasty releases the web by a simple interchange of surfaces of an imaginary tetrahedron.

Serial Z-plasties

The serial Z-plasty and the W-plasty (2) rearrange the tension in linear scars that traverse the crease lines of the face.

A

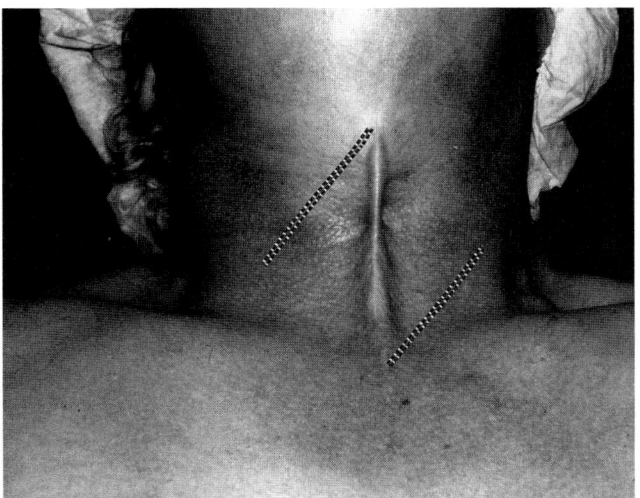

B

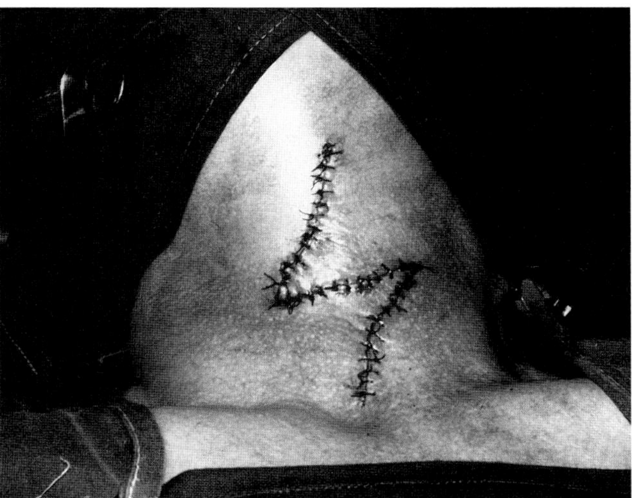

FIGURE 7-7. Two-plane Z-plasty for webbed scar of neck. **A:** Webbing due to contraction of vertical scar of flexion area of neck. The web is composed of two distinct planes of skin. *Broken lines* show proposed z-plasty incisions. **B:** The pair of triangular flaps is transposed, obliterating the web.

However, a simple scar revision, meticulously performed, which is supported with tape strips for 6 months postoperatively, often will give the best result. A serial Z-plasty has the disadvantages of an unnatural shape (Fig. 7-8A,B), small elevations and depressions (standing and lying cones of Limberg), and a total linear distance longer than the original scar. Z-plasties do not lend themselves to easy revision, and the limbs that run at the greatest angle to the crease lines tend to spread. W-plasties elongate the wound less and show fewer protrusions, but normal skin must be discarded; the appearance is unnatural and alternate limbs generally spread more than intervening limbs. Random geometric patterns (interlocking triangles, squares, and semicircles instead of *W*s or *Z*s) are another means of breaking up straight-line scars. Advantages and drawbacks are similar to Z-plasties and W-plasties. On the face in particular, these procedures usually should be held in reserve, until simple scar revision has been given ample trial.

In the case of a linear circumferential scar contracture on a limb or a finger, a circumferential serial Z-plasty often is the treatment of choice. If vascular compromise appears to be a risk, the Z-plasty can be staged.

Zigzag Incisions

For access to the flexor surface of the fingers, Bruner (8) and Littler (9) advocate zigzag incisions that cross no major transverse creases. These provide clear access to the complex structures beneath without danger of a flexor scar contracture. Munro and Fearson (10) recommend zigzag scalp incisions for craniofacial exposure, because the closure line is less obvious than the hairless pale stripe left by a straight bicoronal incision. The authors have seen a groove in the skull of a growing child caused by the force of contraction of a straight-line bicoronal incision. If a zigzag bicoronal incision is not a surgeon's preference, ample sine-shaped curves should be incorporated into bicoronal incisions in infants and young children.

Filling Defects

Buried grafts of dermis or fascia may be of help to build up an indented scar. Recent improvements in injection of autologous fat for contouring show some promise. Bovine collagen serves as a very temporary filling substance.

NONSURGICAL METHODS OF PREVENTING AND TREATING SCARS

Splinting the Scar with Tape

Immature collagen is influenced by external pressure and stresses. Supporting a scar with tape strips to overcome the tension of the surrounding skin is helpful in minimizing the spreading of the scar over time. The tape also exerts some direct pressure on the scar.

Application of Direct Pressure to the Scar

A contoured thermoplastic splint with a sheet of silicone gel for the wound interface, held in position with pressure by elastic bands, can effectively diminish hypertrophic scarring (Fig. 7-2A–B). This technique is most effective if an underlying bony surface is present to facilitate the compression (e.g., forehead). At other sites, elastic garments can provide pressure; silicone gel patches can be placed beneath the garment at strategic points. Silicone gel held in place with tape alone probably provides some benefit.

A
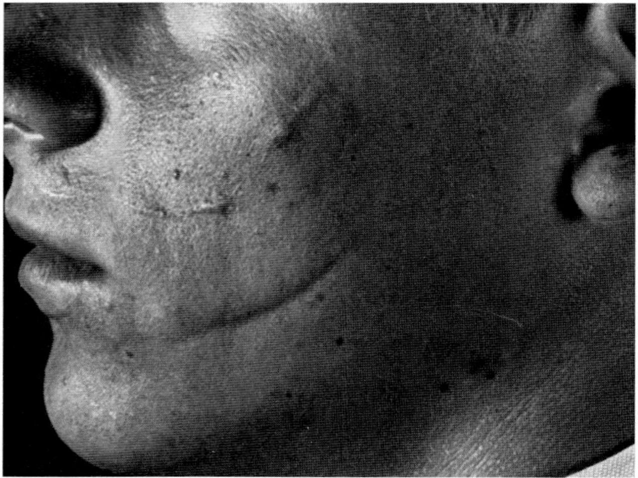

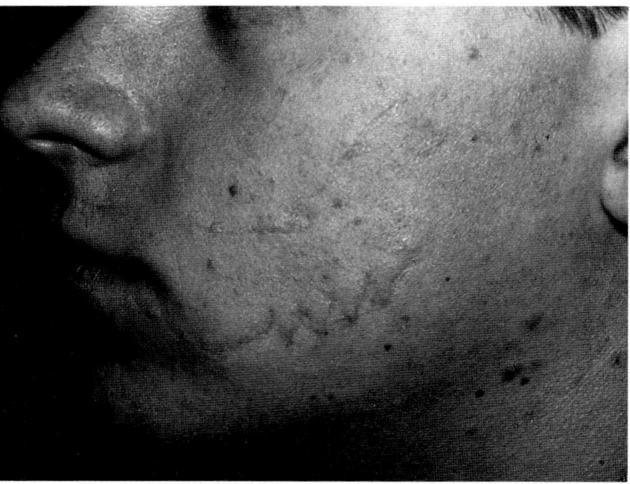
B

FIGURE 7-8. Serial Z-plasty for straight-line scar. **A:** Indented, wide scar on a single plane surface from a laceration that traversed skin creases of the face. **B:** Serial Z-plasty designed to break up and reorient the straight line of the scar. The Z-plasty will be less conspicuous with maturation. Nonetheless, it is a less than an ideal solution for the problem.

Dynamic and Serial Splinting

For scar contractures that exert force on a mobile part of the skeleton, such as those seen in a burn of the hand or neck, splinting is a valuable adjunct. Dynamic splints applied with graded force can be effective in overcoming the tension of a contracting wound and preventing contractures. The keys to splinting are early application, while wound collagen is in a malleable state, and careful follow-up with adjustments and serial replacement as needed.

Corticosteroids

The injection of triamcinolone or betamethasone into hard, raised, red immature scars can accelerate maturation and diminish hypertrophy. These agents may have the side effect of skin atrophy, which may or may not be temporary. Topical application of cortisone cream or cortisone impregnated tape strips is of some limited value.

Massage

Firm frequent massage of wounds may be recommended, but we warn against massaging downward on the upper eyelid for fear of stretching the levator aponeurosis. Patients often ask about topical vitamin E. Our reply is that it is of unproved value, but that it is a satisfactory lubricant for massaging scars.

Collagen-affecting Agents

The use of penicillamine, betaminopropylnitrile (BAPN), and colchicine to diminish keloids or severe scarring have proved useful in limited trials. They are a potent combination with potentially serious side effects. We have seen in consultation a teenage boy with an extremely severe keloid of the upper lip and nose that was refractory to repeated excision, skin grafts, and steroid injections. He was treated elsewhere with penicillamine, colchicine, and low-dose radiation with satisfactory results.

X-ray

Keloids that are persistent after several efforts at conventional treatment can be treated by excision, careful closure with intradermal sutures, and low-dose x-rays of 1,000 to 1,200 roentgens. In those very few patients in whom we have requested radiologic collaboration, the results have been consistently satisfactory. This good record may be a reflection of the small size of our series, because keloids are known to recur after radiation.

FUTURE ADVANCES IN PREVENTION AND TREATMENT OF UNSATISFACTORY SCARS

Several areas of research show promise for improved means of dealing with scarring. Some are being tried clinically. The use of growth factors and other agents for acceleration and improvement of the quality of wound healing appears to be beneficial (5,11). Current investigations of the mechanisms of cellular biology of basic wound healing are revealing new information, some of which will provide for improved clinical results (12). Inasmuch as wounds of the intrauterine fetus show scarless healing, it is hoped that efforts to gain understanding of this phenomenon will improve the surgeon's ability to avoid unsatisfactory scars in children and adults (13,14).

REFERENCES

1. Porras-Reyes BH, Mustoe T. Wound healing. In Cohen M, ed. *Mastery of plastic and reconstructive surgery.* Boston: Little, Brown and Company, 1994:3–13.
2. Borges AF. *Elective incisions and scar revision.* Boston: Little, Brown and Company, 1973.
3. Gibson T. Physical properties of skin. In McCarthy JG, ed. *Plastic surgery, vol. 1.* Philadelphia: WB Saunders, 1990:207–220.
4. Buckley P. Fifty years after Freud: Dora, the rat man, and the wolfman. *Am J Psychiatry* 1989;146:1394–1403.
5. Steed DL. Modifying the wound healing response with exogenous growth factors. *Clin Plast Surg* 1998;25:397–404.
6. Quinn J, Wells G, Sutcliffe T, et al. A randomized trial comparing octylcyanoacrylate tissue adhesive and sutures in the management of lacerations. *JAMA* 1997;277:1527–1530.
7. Furnas DW, Fischer GW. The Z-plasty: biomechanics and mathematics. *Br J Plast Surg* 1971;24:144–160.
8. Bruner JM. Incisions for plastic and reconstructive (nonseptic) surgery of the hand. *Br J Plast Surg* 1951;4:48–55.
9. Littler JW. Digital extensor-flexor system, vol. 6. In Converse JM, ed. *Reconstructive plastic surgery,* 2nd ed. Philadelphia: WB Saunders, 1977:3203.
10. Munro IR, Fearon JA. The coronal incision revisited. *Plast Reconstr Surg* 1994;93:185–187.
11. Hunt TK, LaVan FB. Enhancement of wound healing by growth factors. *N Engl J Med* 1989;321:111–112.
12. Hardesty RA. What's new in plastic surgery. *J Am Coll Surg* 1998;186:212–218.
13. Longaker MT. The biology of fetal wound healing: a review. *Plast Reconstr Surg* 1991;87:788–798.
14. Mackool RJ, Gittes GK, Longaker MT. Scarless healing of the fetal wound. *Clin Plast Surg* 1998;25:357–363.

SUGGESTED READING

Rudolph R. Wide spread scars, hypertrophic scars, and keloids. *Clin Plast Surg* 1987;14:253–260.

Discussion

SCARS AND SCAR REVISIONS

I. KELMAN COHEN

These comments are based on the outline of the text to provide the reader with a simple way to follow my comments on the chapter.

INTRODUCTION

Many surgeons and some other health professionals are able to close a wound as well as any board-certified plastic surgeon. Therefore, one must be very careful not to place blame of the appearance of a scar on the primary health care provider unless there are obvious telltale signs of neglect, such as suture marks. Moreover, closure of many wounds under emergency conditions cannot obtain maximal aesthetic results. The doctrine of "save all parts" and "never do today what you can honorably put off until tomorrow" holds in the emergency closure of some wounds, especially those of the face. This is not true in distally based flaps, especially in the elderly, where leaving this tissue often leads to necrosis of the flap. Often, the tissue should be excised and a skin graft applied for the best chance at a favorable result.

One need not have a wound through the dermis to result in unsightly scarring. Once the basement membrane of the epidermis has been violated, an inflammatory reaction is triggered and severe scarring may occur. There are no clear data that pressure, massage, or taping has anything to do with the ultimate appearance of the scar. However, use of these measures by patients gives them something to do and lets them feel a participatory role in the healing process. Use of silicone sheeting, silicone gels, or other preparations, which claim to improve scar appearance, have no solid basis for use.

WOUND HEALING AND SCARS

Healing begins long before the "collagen phase" but is initiated immediately when wounding occurs. We have noted increased collagen synthesis within 10 hours of wounding, during which time coagulation occurs and growth factors are released (1). It is quite clear that alterations in these early phases may improve the appearance and strength of the scar. Data are accumulating to demonstrate that it is more than collagen remodeling that determines the structure of scar. Several other matrix proteins besides collagen, such as fibronectin, and the complex carbohydrates, which make up the glucosaminoglycans (hyaluronic acid being one), are important in the healing and final structure of the scar. Moreover, it is not only the synthesis and deposition of collagen and other matrix proteins that account of the quality of the scar, but also the structure that is laid down. This has been learned from fetal healing where there is no inflammation and matrix is totally normal (2–9)—there is no scar!

The authors give the impression that all scars contract. This is not true. Many linear closures do not contract at all. Somehow, those linear wounds that cross tension creases tend to contract, but this must not be confused with other linear closures. "Proliferating fibroblasts" do not cause the bulk of tissue visible in the early skin wound after closure, as claimed by the authors. The bulk of the raised scar is derived from the excessive matrix deposited in the early healing stages. Most of this is collagen. It recedes because collagenases and other proteolytic enzymes remodel the matrix and the inflammatory responses recedes.

SCAR CONTRACTION AND CONTRACTURE

Contraction is an active process. Contracture is a deformity, which results from the active process in contraction. To state that all healing tissues contract demonstrates a misunderstanding of the data on this phenomenon. The most compelling data to date present strong evidence that inflammation in the healing process produces cytokines, such as transforming growth factor-β, that transform the fibroblast into a specialized cell termed the "myofibroblast," which has smooth muscle actin within the cytoplasm. These transformed cells are capable of exerting their muscular force to bring the edges of the wound together and hence contract. These same cells appear involved in such processes

I. K. Cohen: Department of Surgery, Medical College of Virginia, Richmond, Virginia

and Dupuytren's contracture and firm breasts, which have capsular contraction around breast prosthesis. Although pharmacologic intervention surely will be available in the future, the problem of excessive contraction, which leads to contracture, remains serious and unsolved.

SKIN TENSION AND AGE

There are no clear data to support the authors' conclusion that children form hypertrophic scar with greater frequency than do adults or the elderly because there is more tension in children's skin. Clearly, during the fetal period where there is tremendous growth and tension on skin, incisions heal without any clinical or histologic evidence of scar and without any inflammatory response. In infancy, scars are visible but rarely hypertrophic. From age 6 months until after puberty, all scars tend to go through a more prolonged hypertrophic phase than in adults or the elderly. This is because of the inflammatory response and the products thereof and has nothing to do with skin tension! With time, most of the hypertrophic scares in young people resolve spontaneously.

TRAP DOORS AND BEVELS

The authors state that trap-door scar forms a pincushion effect because of scar contraction. This is conjecture. There also is evidence suggesting that the trap-door shape of the scar is formed because there is little lymphatic outlet. Therefore, edema within the pincushion is the etiology of the problem. Thence, total excision of the trap-door deformity may be far superior to multiple Z-plasties, which themselves can be a tell-tale deformity. The bulging of the lip after injury is the result of scar accumulation, which seems quite particular to the lip. Moreover, lip muscle hypertrophies after injury.

UNFAVORABLE PSYCHOLOGICAL FACTORS

The authors did not mention the psychiatric diagnosis of dysmorphogenesis. These patients have an insatiable dislike for their appearance and, regardless of what surgical procedure may be done to correct deformities, they will never be satisfied. In general, they are resistant to psychiatric intervention. Promising results have been obtained by neurologic ablation procedures.

UNFAVORABLE SITES

Although tension will lead to the formation of wide scars, it does not result in keloid or hypertrophic scar. With keloid, this rationale presented by the authors does not apply. For example, the earlobe, which is a favorite site for keloid development, is vascular and tension free!

UNFAVORABLE SCARS

The bottom line with the statement that "some patients have a tendency to form unfavorable scars, even at favorable sites" is that the problem is genetic. Unfortunately, we have not reached the point of sophistication in our molecular genetic techniques where we can predict which patients are destined to develop unfavorable scars. Family history can be of some limited predictive value.

CONTRACTURES

The authors might have presented more material on the etiology of contracture and possible methods to avoid these deformities. Clearly, burn contractures occur when there is a significant loss of skin and the normal biologic process of contraction occurs, resulting in contracture deformity. This can be avoided at times by splinting and early grafting to replace the lost skin. However, this often is inadequate because of the severity of the inflammatory process that coincides with the burn injury. Products of inflammation stimulate the production of myofibroblasts, resulting in further contracture. Without splinting, the skin graft placed in the defect wrinkles up and the original contracture recurs. Nothing happens to the graft! It is the underlying connective tissue matrix that contracts. Correction of contractures often can be best accomplished by bringing in new healthy tissue as a free tissue transfer or pedicled flap. These tissues are free of the inflammatory cells found in the base of the turn wound and, therefore, are resistant to further contraction.

UNSTABLE SCARS

Remember that a scar never attains the tensile strength of normal skin. The collagen bundles are not well organized, and there is no elasticity to the scar tissue. One must not excise all scar to close a wound. Surgically closed scar heals with acceptable tensile strength in most instances. Remember that malnutrition, bacteria, pain, and certain drugs (such as corticosteroid and immunosuppressive agents), as well as immunosuppressive diseases, all can lead to wound healing problems and unstable scar. You will recall that 2 centuries ago, British sailors on long sea voyages were found to have scars many years old that fell apart during the voyage. It was found that ingestion of fresh lime juice (which contains ascorbic acid) prevented the wound breakdown—hence, the British sailors became known as "limeys," a name that has stuck to this very day.

KELOIDS

The authors did not mention informed consent. If you are going to excise a keloid, you had better make careful note in your permission that recurrence occurs commonly and have the patient sign it. There have been many malpractice claims over this issue. There is no cure for keloids. Although we know a great deal about the biology of the lesions, the "magic bullet" for treatment has not been found. In the beginning of the 21st century, perhaps the best we have to offer is excision (if the lesion is bulky) followed by the use of triamcinolone 40 mg/mL and never exceeding 2 cc every 6 to 8 weeks. Doses in children should be less. Patients who follow this regimen often can be saved from having massive recurrence and, at times, are even cured. Always remember that there are some keloid patients who should not have their keloids removed. If the goal is to stop burning and itching, antihistamines, intralesional triamcinolone, and occasional use of topical clobetasol propionate (Temovate) can be used. All steroids must be used with caution because of skin thinning, fat atrophy, and depigmentation.

COLLAGEN DEFECTS

Many of us have been plagued by problems of collagen defects. They can be very insidious. For example, I have seen unhappy patients following breast ptosis correction or reduction mammoplasty with recurrent sagging of the breast, with recurrence even after revision. Clearly, these few cases, which were done by competent plastic surgeons, are due to genetically controlled defects in collagen metabolism. Many of the collagen defects we see from keloid to wound dehiscence are genetic and not the fault of the surgeon. It is frustrating that actual molecular tools are available to make these diagnoses, but few facilities have been established to look at this problem. Moreover, once a defect in collagen metabolism has been detected, we do not know how to correct the defect.

One cannot leave the subject of collagen defects without mention of the "factitious wound." Perhaps because of my particular interest in scars and healing, I either see, or diagnose by phone, 10 to 15 factitious wounds per year. Anyone interested in this problem should read the excellent review by Brenman and Serafin (10).

INFECTIONS

A few basic principles must be remembered. Open wounds with more than 1×10^5 bacteria from a wound biopsy culture are clear evidence that the wound should not be closed until the bacterial count is lowered (11). Topical antibiotics are most suitable to obtain this goal. Antibiotics are unnecessary in most clean surgical cases, unless there are factors that increase the risk of infection. If used in normal clean surgical cases, antibiotics should only be used in the perioperative period and started before surgery. If acute wounds are left open for secondary closure because of the increased risk of infection, closure may be attempted when the wound "looks good" or after obtaining quantitative bacteriology. Acute wounds with more than 1×10^5 bacteria per gram of tissue should not be closed until the counts have been lowered by use of systemic or topical antibiotics and aggressive dressing changes.

Systemic antibiotics are incapable of reaching the chronic wound; hence, these wounds should be treated with appropriate topical antibiotics unless systemic symptoms occur.

SURGICAL TREATMENT

For simple scar revision, there is no incontrovertible evidence that multiple layers of closure will combat the inexorable tension of a closure, which is against tension lines. Scars across the knee or perpendicular to the closure may be closed with several layers and even splinted, but they still will recur as wide scars. If you perform a revision on such a scar, you will find that the suture material may be intact and in the center of the deep planes of the wide scar. Simply, tension leads to tissue remodeling and the scar widens around the intact suture. Sutures and splinting are useless for control of scar width.

The authors mention skin eversion. Eversion allows final healing with a flat scar. If an inverted scar is the long-term result of closure, it will be a much more noticeable scar. This is because angled light passing over an inverted scar causes a shadow, which is noted by the observer. Every plastic surgeon knows that if one takes a photo of a patient with severe scarring, it will virtually disappear if the photo is obtained with overexposure. It is the same effect, as overexposure removes shadows.

Z-plasties were covered thoroughly by the authors. Perhaps Z-plasties and W-plasties are the most overdone exercises in all of scar revision surgery. They must be used very conservatively to lengthen a contracted scar or to direct the majority of a scar back into lines of relaxation. In 28 years of practice, I have seen more deformity than improvement from procedures.

NONSURGICAL METHODS OF PREVENTING SCARS

Scars mature with time. The data that pressure enhances healing of burn scar are reasonable. There are no data that a piece of silicone sheeting placed on a primary closed wound is any better than simple inexpensive tape placed on the wound. It amazes me that surgeons and the public alike are attracted to this placebo therapy.

The authors' suggestion that corticosteroid injection will "accelerate maturation and diminish hypertrophy" of scars must be taken with caution. These agents may result in skin atrophy and depigmentation. The patient must be warned of these complications before these agents are used.

REFERENCES

1. Clore JN, Cohen IK, Diegelmann RF. Quantitation of collagen types I and III during wound healing in rat skin. *Proc Soc Exp Biol Med* 1979;161:337–340.
2. Krummel TM, Nelson JM, Diegelmann RF, et al. Fetal response to injury in the rabbit. *J Pediatr Surg* 1987;22:640–644.
3. Krummel TM, Michna BA, Thomas BL, et al. Transforming growth factor beta (TGF-β) induces fibrosis in a fetal wound model. *J Pediatr Surg* 1988;23:647–652.
4. DePalma RL, Krummel TM, Durham LA, et al. Characterization and quantitation of wound matrix in the fetal rabbit. *Matrix* 1989;9:224–231.
5. Mast BA, Flood LC, Haynes JH, et al. Hyaluronic acid is a major component of the matrix of fetal rabbit skin wounds: implications for healing by regeneration. *Matrix* 1991;11:63–68.
6. Mast BA, Flood LC, Haynes JH, et al. Hyaluronic acid is a major component of the matrix of fetal rabbit skin wounds: implications for healing by regeneration. *Matrix* 1991;11:63–68.
7. Mast BA, Diegelmann RF, Krummel TM, et al. Fetal wound healing: a review of scarless tissue repair. *Surg Gynecol Obstet* 1992;174:441–451.
8. Frantz FW, Diegelmann RF, Mast BA, et al. Biology of fetal wound healing: collagen biosynthesis during dermal repair. *J Pediatr Surg* 1992;27:945–949.
9. Mast BA, Frantz FW, Haynes JH, et al. Ultrastructural comparison of fetal wounds and skin: mammalian healing by regeneration. *Wound Repair Regen* 1997;5:243–248.
10. Brenman S, Serafin D. Factitious problems in wound healing. In: Cohen IK, Diegelmann RF, Yager DR, et al., eds. *Wound care and wound healing.* In: Schwartz SI, ed. *Principles of surgery,* 7th ed. New York: McGraw Hill Book Co., 1998.
11. Robson MC, Stenberg BD, Heggers JP. Wound healing alterations caused by infection. *Clin Plast Surg* 1990;17:485–492.

8

SURGICAL INFECTIONS

BRADON J. WILHELMI
LINDA G. PHILLIPS

For centuries, our knowledge of infectious diseases rested on theories, which only recently have been replaced by the discoveries of science and the advances of technology. Until the development of bacteriology in the mid-19th century, the comprehension of infection in Western civilization was based on theoretical doctrines, and few preventative and therapeutic approaches had any validity. Finally, near the end of the 20th century, scientific investigation augmented the understanding of infectious diseases by identifying hundreds of microorganisms and producing a diverse spectrum of antimicrobial agents for use in prophylactic and therapeutic regimens. In treating surgical infections, plastic surgeons encounter two types of problems: those occurring in our own wounds and those referred to us.

EPIDEMIOLOGY

Accounting for a quarter of nosocomial infections, wound infections remain a major source of postoperative morbidity (1–3). With the trend for performing operations in the outpatient setting, many wound infections are first recognized in the outpatient clinic or the patient's home (3). Thus, the frequency by diagnosis and report of this complication has declined (Table 8-1). The rate of wound infection varies with surgeon, hospital, procedure, and patient. In 1961, one of the earliest comprehensive studies demonstrated an overall postoperative wound infection rate of 7.4% (2). Data collected from studies in the last two decades identified additional contributors to decreasing rates of wound infection, including the appropriate institution of prophylactic antibiotics and the identification of high-risk patients and procedures (3–6). Overall, this decline in wound infection rates has resulted in decreases in the duration of hospital stays and overall cost of care for surgical patients (3) (Table 8-1).

Bradon J. Wilhelmi: Division of Plastic Surgery, Southern Illinois University School of Medicine, Springfield, Illinois
Linda G. Phillips: Department of Surgery, Division of Plastic Surgery, University of Texas Medical Branch, Galveston, Texas

SURGICAL WOUND CLASSIFICATION

To examine the indication for and use of prophylactic antibiotics appropriately, surgical wounds are classified as clean, clean-contaminated, contaminated, or dirty wounds. Clean wounds include uninfected wounds free of inflammation. These wounds do not involve the respiratory, alimentary, or genitourinary tracts. Clean wounds occur under ideal circumstances (i.e., in the operating room) and may be primarily closed. Clean-contaminated wounds include those occurring in the respiratory, alimentary, and genitourinary tracts without unusual contamination. Contaminated wounds comprise fresh traumatic wounds, nonpurulent inflamed wounds, and surgical wounds exposed to contaminant because of a break in sterile technique or spillage of gastrointestinal contents. Dirty wounds include old traumatic wounds, wounds containing foreign bodies or devitalized tissue, and wounds contaminated by perforated viscera (7) (Table 8-2). The wound infection rates reported for the various classes of wounds are as follows: 1% to 5% for clean, 3% to 10% for clean-contaminated, 10% to 20% for contaminated, and 30% to 40% for dirty wounds (7–10) (Table 8-2).

PROPHYLACTIC ANTIBIOTICS

Preoperative antibiotic prophylaxis can reduce the incidence of wound infection in selected cases. For clean, uncomplicated surgical wounds, antibiotics have no effect on the incidence of postoperative infection (11–15). The use of prophylactic antibiotics is indicated for clean-contaminated and contaminated wounds, as reduced infection rates for these wounds have been reported (7,11,16–19). The treatment of dirty wounds requires a full course of antibiotic therapy (7).

Certain patients with clean wounds may benefit from prophylaxis, such as patients with impaired host defenses, patients with increased bacterial colonization of various anatomic sites, and those undergoing procedures in which

TABLE 8-1. EPIDEMIOLOGY

Study	Reported rate (%)	Comments
National Academy of Sciences, 1964	7.4	2.5-year five-hospital survey 15,613 operations
Cruse, 1981	4.7	10-year single-hospital study 69,939 operations
Haley, 1985	2.8	1-year nationwide survey 18,271,858 operations
Olson and Lee, 1990	2.5	10-year single-hospital study 40,915 operations

Trend for decreased wound infection rate.

infections are potentially devastating, including insertion of prostheses (14,20–23).

To be at an appropriate concentration at the operative site, a prophylactic antibiotic must be administered before any incision is made or possible inoculation performed—preferably at least 1 hour before the procedure is begun (17–19,24–27). Postoperatively, continuing to administer an antibiotic for more than 48 hours provides no advantage. In fact, most investigators recommend a 24-hour course of treatment for prophylaxis (19,28). A full 7- to 10-day course is indicated when definite evidence of a wound infection is found (3,7) (Table 8-2). The antibiotic must be effective against possible pathogens among resident flora in a given institution, and selection is guided by the location of a procedure.

RISK FACTORS

Other factors, in addition to the administration of prophylactic antibiotics, proven to influence the development of postoperative wound infection include preoperative hospital stay, preoperative cleansing, shaving techniques, operative length, remote infections, and impaired host defenses (Table 8-3). Other factors implicated but not proven to cause postoperative wound infection include preoperative scrub technique, surgical glove damage, barrier materials, and laminar flow air systems in the operating room.

A direct correlation has been noted between the length of preoperative hospitalization and the development of postoperative wound infection. Cruse and Ford (9) reported that an overall infection rate of 1.1% for a 1-day preoperative stay doubles with each preoperative week of stay. Northey (29) observed that patients undergo colonization with infective bacteria within 2 weeks of hospitalization, often with resistant, hospital-acquired organisms. Most patients undergoing elective operations today are admitted the morning of surgery instead of earlier; this arrangement greatly decreases colonization with hospital bacteria and thus risk for infection. Accordingly, patients admitted for other medical problems should not undergo elective procedures during the same stay to decrease the risk for postoperative wound infection (9,29).

Early reports supported preoperative showering with chlorhexidine to decrease the incidence of postoperative infection (9). However, one large multihospital study of 5,536 clean operative procedures demonstrated no advantage to preoperative shower with chlorhexidine detergent over detergent alone, thus disproving the role for preoperative chlorhexidine shower (30).

Razor shaving one day before surgery is associated with higher wound infection rates because bacteria have time to

TABLE 8-2. CLASSIFICATION OF SURGICAL WOUNDS

Wound	Example	Infection rate (%)	Antibiotics
Clean	Noncontaminated skin, elective procedure, closed primarily	1–5	Not indicated
Clean-contaminated	Contaminated areas, such as oral cavity, respiratory tract, axilla, or perineum	3–10	24-h course
Contaminated	Traumatic wounds; major breaks aseptic technique; acute, nonpurulent inflamed cysts	10–20	24-h course
Dirty	Grossly contaminated or infected, foreign bodies or devitalized tissue	30–40	7–10 d

TABLE 8-3. RISK FACTORS FOR WOUND INFECTIONS

Preoperative hospital stay
Shaving technique
Long operation
Remote infection
Immune compromise
Ischemia

proliferate in skin cuts (9). Seropian and Reynolds demonstrated a lower wound infection rate with hair removal by depilatory agent (0.6%) versus razor preparation the day before surgery (5.6%). Because many surgeons prefer to operate in a hairless field, an additional alternative of immediate preoperative hair clipping was studied and found acceptable, with a low 1.7% infection rate (31). All these studies indicate that shaving the night before the operation increases the potential for bacterial proliferation in injured skin. Therefore, if hair removal is desired, it appears prudent to remove hair in the immediate preoperative period with either a clipper or a razor (3).

Another risk factor for wound infection includes length of operation, as infection rates almost double with each hour of surgery (9). Shapiro et al. (32) reported that a longer hysterectomy procedure is associated with a decreased effect of antibiotic prophylaxis in preventing wound infection. Another study of postoperative wound infections, in 676 children, demonstrated an increased risk with procedures lasting longer than 1 hour (33). Even the plastic surgery literature confirms the operative length to be a risk factor (8). This increased wound infection rate for longer procedures relates to the pharmacokinetics of prophylactic antibiotics and the increased bacterial contamination that occurs during prolonged, complex procedures (32).

An active remote infection at the time of an elective operation increases the risk for postoperative wound infections (34,35). The most common locations for these remote infections include the urinary tract, skin, and respiratory tract (34,35). Treatment of skin infections with prophylactic antibiotics on the night before surgery did not reduce the risk for wound infections (35). However, the administration of prophylactic antibiotics 24 hours before surgery did significantly reduce the incidence of infection to the same level as that of patients without remote infection (25,35) (Table 8-3).

Another risk factor for postoperative wound infection includes impairment of host resistance, associated with systemic conditions of obesity, diabetes, uremia, old age, advanced malignancy, immunosuppression, and immunodeficiency disorders. When patients with these problems are treated, special precautions should be taken to prevent wound infection complications, including correction or control of underlying diseases, whenever possible.

No convincing evidence has been found to prove that other potential risk factors correlate with postoperative rates of wound infection, including preoperative scrub technique, surgical glove damage, and barrier materials (e.g., caps, masks, shoe covers).

DIAGNOSIS

Infection is defined as the product of the entrance, growth, metabolic activities, and pathophysiologic effects of microorganisms in the tissues of a patient (8,36). The normal biologic state of humans is not germ-free. Both transient and permanent flora reside on all skin and mucosal surfaces, all with the potential to cause infection. The absence of infection represents an equilibrium between the factors of host resistance and the actions of bacteria (37). Clinical infection may result once this equilibrium is upset, by either an increase in bacterial inoculum or an impairment in the host defense system (38).

Because they often deal with contaminated wounds and demand high-quality results, plastic and reconstructive surgeons appreciate the importance of detecting any upset of bacterial balance and the need to reset the equilibrium. The diagnosis of a wound bacterial imbalance is initially made on the basis of the history and clinical examination. However, a significant advance in the prevention and treatment of surgical infections was the discovery that the mere presence of organisms in a wound is less important than the level of bacterial growth (39). Experimental and clinical data have demonstrated that bacterial levels in excess of 1,000,000 organisms per gram of tissue are necessary to cause wound infection (37,40). Only β-hemolytic streptococci appear capable of causing infection at levels below 100,000 organisms per gram of tissue (41).

Microorganisms can be recovered in the majority of instances, provided the specimen is properly collected and transported to the laboratory. Generally, the favorite device for collecting a specimen, the cotton swab, provides an insufficient amount of material for culture. Furthermore, samples of specimen are not readily released from a standard cotton swab. Moreover, cotton contains substances injurious to some microorganisms. Accordingly, commercially available porous plastic cotton substitutes were developed to improve the utility of swabs by releasing the entire specimen and protecting against desiccation. However, as swabs sample only the bacteria on the wound surface, they are no substitute for quantitative tissue cultures. Furthermore, studies have demonstrated a lower predictive value of culture from swabs in comparison with culture from tissue specimens (42–45).

The technique of tissue collection for quantitative culture involves obtaining 1 cm^3 of tissue sharply with a scalpel or core biopsy device after the wound has been cleansed and debrided (39,46). Because the number of microorganisms diminishes with the duration of infection, the more chronic the infection, the larger the portion of a lesion that should be obtained (39,47). Also, multiple specimens should be recovered from larger wounds (37,47). The specimen is aseptically weighed, decontaminated, homogenized, serially diluted, and inoculated onto blood agar and into thioglycolate broth. These cultures must be incubated for 24 hours at 37°C before colonies are counted (38,46,47) (Fig. 8-1).

A modification of this procedure, termed *rapid slide analysis,* can be used to apply quantitative bacteriology in acute settings (46,47) (Fig. 8-1). This modification requires that 0.02 mL of undiluted homogenate be transferred to a clean glass microscope slide and spread over an area less than 15 mm in diameter. The slide is dried for 15 minutes in an oven at 75°C and prepared with Gram's stain. On microscopic examination of all fields of the slide, the presence of a single organism correlates with a bacterial load of at least 10^6 organisms (38,47–49). If β-hemolytic streptococci are present, the rapid slide technique may yield a false-negative result. Fewer organisms of this species can cause invasive infection; it is more virulent because of the enzymes it elaborates.

In addition to the diagnosis of wound infections, quantitative bacteriology of wound biopsy specimens has proved useful in the management of acute and chronic wounds by delayed closure, skin grafting, or flap reconstruction (49–53). Robson and Heggers (49) showed that the presence of fewer than 10^6 organisms is critical to the successful delayed primary closure of a wound. Liedburg et al. (51) demonstrated in rabbits that skin grafts fail in beds inoculated with more than 10^5 organisms. Additionally, U.S. Army Surgical Research Unit studies showed that sepsis in burn wounds requires more than 10^5 organisms per gram of tissue (54,55). Breidenbach and Trager (42) reported the value of preoperative quantitative cultures to predict infection following free-flap reconstruction of extremity wounds (42). Thus, most of the data implicate a critical bacterial load of more than 10^5 organisms.

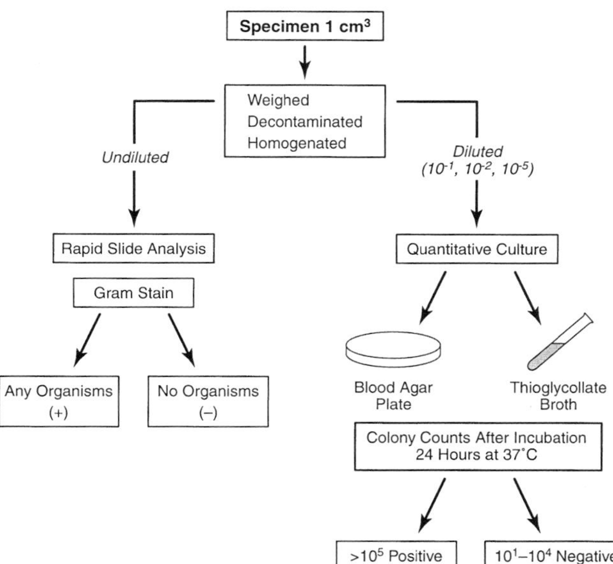

FIGURE 8-1. Diagnosis. The technique of obtaining a quantitative culture involves removing 1 cm^3 of tissue sharply or with a core biopsy instrument after the wound has been cleansed. The specimen is aseptically weighed, decontaminated, homogenized, serially diluted, and inoculated onto blood agar and into thioglycolate broth. The cultures must be incubated for 24 hours at 37°C before colonies are counted.

NORMAL SKIN FLORA

Because the skin is an unfavorable medium for the growth of most microbes, relatively few species of microorganisms consistently comprise the normal resident cutaneous flora, although many can be found transiently on the skin surface (56,57). Several factors limit the normal flora to only a few microbes, including an intact stratum corneum, a low pH, and the host immune system. An intact stratum corneum impedes the attachment and entry of most microorganisms. Most microbes do not adhere well to cutaneous surfaces, so they cannot thrive or reproduce on the skin for sustained periods. The dryness of an intact stratum corneum also discourages the growth of many microorganisms, such as gram-negative bacilli and *Candida* species, which require moisture to thrive. The low pH (5.5) of the skin, a consequence of the production of acid by the normal flora from lipids and sebum, produces an unfavorable environment for most organisms. Lastly, the host's immune system plays a role in the prevention of microbial survival and reproduction, via cell-mediated mechanisms and the secretion of antibodies, immunoglobulins A and G, which are present in sweat (57).

Furthermore, the composition of microorganisms varies depending on body location. More prevalent in moist areas, aerobes populate intertriginous zones and web spaces with a density of $10^7/cm_2$, versus a density of $10^2/cm^2$ in dry skin. Although the sweat glands and ducts are sterile, anaerobes populate the deepest portions of hair follicles and sebaceous glands. In fact, anaerobes reach concentrations of 10^4 to $10^6/cm^2$ in areas with abundant sebaceous glands, whereas they are sparse in other cutaneous locations (58).

Of the gram-positive cocci, *Staphylococcus epidermidis* is the most predominant, comprising more than half of resident staphylococci. *S. epidermidis* colonizes the upper body. Although *Staphylococcus aureus* usually does not colonize the skin, it may be found in intertriginous areas and intranasally in up to 20% of normal people (57,59). *Staphylococcus saprophyticus* is a common cause of urinary tract infections. Other *Staphylococcus* species populating the skin include *S. hominis, S. haemolyticus, S. capitis, S. warneri, S. cohnii,* and *S. simulans.* The anaerobe *Peptococcus asaccharolyticus* comprises the normal flora in 20% of the population, concentrating on the forehead and intertriginous zones, areas with abundant sebaceous glands.

Not of the normal skin flora, group B streptococci colonize mucous membranes and may exist transiently in perioral skin. Also, group A streptococci, which have been shown to die quickly on normal intact skin, rarely colonize the skin (63). For the cutaneous pathogen *Streptococcus pyogenes* (group A streptococci) to cause infection, disruption of the stratum corneum is required (59). In some normal hosts, *S. pyogenes* may survive a few days, but infection develops in most of them shortly thereafter (57,59,60).

Another major component of the normal skin flora, the gram-positive bacillus, and *Corynebacterium* (diphtheroids/lactobacilli) are lipophilic and thrive in areas rich in lipids. They concentrate in moist, intertriginous areas (57,58).

ANTIBIOTICS AND COMMON WOUND PATHOGENS

Among the postoperative wound pathogens, *S. aureus* causes many wound infections, although the incidence of gram-negative infections continues to rise (15). The reported incidence of anaerobic wound infections probably underestimates their actual frequency because of the difficulty of cultivating anaerobes in the laboratory and the failure of clinicians to obtain appropriate culture specimens.

The incubation period for *S. aureus* infections is 4 to 6 days. These infections tend to be localized, with initial erythema, edema, pain, and eventual abscess formation. The pus is usually thick, creamy, white or yellow, and odorless. Spread to lymph nodes is unusual, but bacteremia is common. Fever and leukocytosis may be present. Furthermore, exotoxin release in *S. aureus* infections can lead to toxic shock syndrome, characterized by fever, rash, desquamation, involvement of three or more organ systems, and hypotension (56,61,62). Although treatment by opening the infected portion of the wound usually suffices, antibiotic therapy may be necessary when the infection is not well localized. A penicillinase-resistant penicillin or cephalosporin provides reliable *S. aureus* coverage (15,38,63).

The number of wound infections caused by *S. epidermidis,* which is a normal component of the skin flora, is increasing. The presence of this organism in wounds containing a foreign body (prostheses) is a reason for concern. A penicillinase-resistant penicillin or cephalosporin is required for adequate coverage of this organism, as strains resistant to penicillin are becoming increasingly common. If the infection involves a wound that contains a prosthesis, successful treatment may require removal of the prosthetic device (15,57).

Wound infections caused by gram-negative bacilli are increasing in frequency, although they are more common after general surgery procedures as a result of contamination with enteric contents. Because the incubation period is 7 to 14 days, many patients are at home when the infection becomes evident. Infections caused by gram-negative organisms are associated with less erythema, edema, and pain than are staphylococcal infections. Instead of local inflammation, systemic signs, including fever or tachycardia, develop. Aminoglycosides and third-generation cephalosporins provide consistent gram-negative coverage, and quinolones are an acceptable alternative when oral administration is desired (15).

Infections with group A streptococci can run a fulminant course after initial presentation as diffuse cellulitis, lymphangiitis, or lymphadenopathy. The cellulitis is characterized by an area of rapidly advancing erythema with a raised, delineated border. Large, blood-filled blebs may form around the primary focus of infection, with the potential for local breakdown and progression to gangrene or necrotizing fasciitis if untreated. The characteristic exudate is thin and watery. Streptococcal wound infections appear within 1 to 3 days of inoculation. Chills, fever, tachycardia, sweats, prostration, and other signs of toxemia are common. Streptococcal cellulitis usually responds to high doses of parenteral penicillin. However, aggressive debridement may be required to treat infections progressing to gangrene or tissue necrosis.

Infections caused by enterococci, *S. faecalis,* or other group D streptococci are less invasive than those caused by group A streptococci. Enterococcal infections are usually mixed, with enteric gram-negative organisms present. Thus, enterococcal infections should be treated with ampicillin and an aminoglycoside.

INFECTIONS IN PATIENTS UNDERGOING PLASTIC SURGERY

Depending on the circumstances of wounding and the wound location, certain organisms have the potential to cause infection (Table 8-4). Not always obvious, the decision to administer prophylactic antibiotics requires that the risk factors for infection (i.e., dirty wound or devastating consequence to infection) be considered. A published poll taken among 1,718 practicing plastic surgeons demonstrated trends toward antibiotic prophylaxis for certain procedures (50).

The treatment of maxillofacial injuries, including facial fractures and lacerations, incurs a moderate risk for infection because the placement of hardware within dirty wounds is often required. In the treatment of open facial fractures, studies have demonstrated lower infection rates in groups treated with prophylactic antibiotics (64,65). In cases of closed facial trauma, in which the skin or mucosa has not been broken, prophylactic antibiotics do not appear to be indicated (66). Accordingly, this factor appears to be the major determinant for the use of prophylactic antibiotics among the plastic surgeons surveyed (50). Fractures within dirty skin wounds require prophylaxis for *S. aureus* and other cutaneous flora (66). Fractures communicating with the oral mucosa require prophylaxis for streptococci

TABLE 8-4. PROPHYLAXIS FOR PLASTIC SURGERY

Procedure	Circumstances	Organisms	Antibiotic
Maxillofacial	Dirty laceration	Streptococcus, anaerobes	Penicillin
	Open fracture	Staphylococcus	Nafcillin
Head and neck	Oropharynx	Streptococcus, GNR Anaerobes	Broad-spectrum
Facial aesthetic	Blepharoplasty		None
	Rhinoplasty		None
	Rhytidectomy		None
	Laser	Herpesvirus	Acyclovir/valacyclovir
Congenital	Cleft lip/palate		None
deformity	Ear reconstruction	Staphylococcus	Nafcillin
Breast		Staphylococcus	First-generation cephalosporin
Body contouring	Liposuction		None
	Abdominoplasty		First-generation cephalosporin
Pressure sores		GNR, anaerobes GPC	Broad-spectrum

GNR, gram-negative rod; GPC, gram-positive cocci.

and the anaerobes *Peptostreptococcus* and *Clostridium,* which are common organisms of the oral flora (67). Overall, in the treatment of open fractures, infection rates were lowest when cephalothin was the antibiotic given for prophylaxis (65). We commonly use penicillin and nafcillin for streptococcal, anaerobic, and staphylococcal coverage. In addition to treatment with antibiotics, infected, exposed hardware may require removal, especially if within radiated tissue (68–70).

In surgery for head and neck cancer, violation of the oropharynx appears to be a major risk factor for infection (66). Studies have demonstrated that infection rates are lower with the administration of antibiotic prophylaxis to patients undergoing tumor resection that violates the oropharynx (64,71). Antibiotic prophylaxis for procedures in which the oropharynx is not entered, including parotidectomy, thyroidectomy, and radical neck dissection, appears to be of no benefit (64,66,71). Furthermore, Krizek et al. (50) found that the plastic surgeons in the survey followed this trend. Antibiotics selected for prophylaxis or treatment in this patient population should provide coverage for *S. aureus, Streptococcus, Peptostreptococcus,* and gram-negative organisms (66).

Cases of cellulitis have been reported following aesthetic surgery of the face, but they are rare (< 1%) (72–75). As previously discussed, antibiotic prophylaxis is not indicated for clean procedures. Furthermore, no studies are available to support antibiotic prophylaxis for facelifts, blepharoplasties, or other clean cases. Because rhinoplasty may involve contamination with organisms from the nasal mucosa, antibiotic prophylaxis for this procedure has been studied. A prospective, blinded study of rhinoplasty procedures demonstrated no increased risk for infection without prophylactic antibiotics (76). Teichgraeber et al. (75) identified antecedent sinus infection and turbinate surgery as risk factors for infection. Rarely, *S. aureus* toxic shock syndrome following nasal surgery has been described as potentially related to intranasal packing (62,77,78). Overall, most plastic surgeons forego the use of prophylactic antibiotics for routine facial aesthetic procedures (50). However, when alloplast is inserted, prophylactic antibiotics are given by most plastic surgeons to avoid potentially devastating sequelae of infection (50,79). No studies exist to support this practice. Like ultraviolet light, laser may activate dormant herpes simplex virus. Devastating cases of herpes infection following laser resurfacing have been reported; therefore, prophylaxis with 400 mg of oral acyclovir three times daily or 500 mg of valacyclovir twice daily preoperatively and until postoperative reepithelialization is complete is justified (72,80). Herpes infections after laser may require intravenous antiviral therapy until a Tzanck smear confirms the diagnosis.

Infections rarely complicate plastic surgical procedures to correct congenital anomalies (81). Accordingly, most plastic surgeons abstain from antibiotic prophylaxis for cleft lip and palate repairs (50). A prospective, randomized, double-blinded study demonstrated no increased risk when cleft lip and palate repairs were performed without antibiotic prophylaxis (82). However, when performing ear reconstructions, most plastic surgeons administer prophylactic antibiotics, whether their support construct is formed of cartilage (58%) or alloplast (76%) (50). Studies to support this practice demonstrated statistically higher rates of wound infection for auricular procedures than for procedures involving the rest of the face (83,84).

Infections following breast operations occur relatively frequently (1% to 20% of cases) because breast tissue has its own endogenous flora (11,82,85–87). As a consequence of communication with external skin through lactiferous ducts, deep breast tissue contains a flora similar to that of normal breast skin (88). The organisms most frequently cultured from breast tissue include coagulase-negative *Staphylococcus* (53%), *Propionibacterium acnes* (30%), and diphtheroids/lactobacilli (9%) (88). Coagulase-negative staphylococci have been implicated in periprosthetic contracture formation following augmentation mammoplasty (89,90). Shah et al. (91) confirmed this finding with an animal model study, in which thicker capsules formed around implants infected with *S. epidermidis.* Although antibiotic prophylaxis decreased the number of bacteria isolated from pockets created for implants, it did not significantly affect the rate and severity of contracture formation in a randomized, double-blinded study by Gylbert et al. (92), despite an earlier report by Burkhardt et al. (93). The use of prophylactic antibiotics statistically decreased wound infections in a study of breast procedures, including reduction mammoplasty, augmentation mammoplasty, and breast reconstruction (82). Antibiotic prophylaxis was found to prevent 38% of predicted infections in a prospective, randomized, multicenter study of 2,587 cases of reduction mammoplasties, lumpectomies, and mastectomies (94). Among the survey of plastic surgeons by Krizek et al. (50), the frequency of prophylactic antibacterial use for various breast operations was as follows: reductions (44%), flap reconstruction (53%), augmentation (59%), and reconstruction with implants (63%). The offending organism chiefly isolated from breast infections is *S. aureus* (79,90,95,96). A first-generation cephalosporin is the prophylactic antibiotic of choice for the aforementioned breast procedures. Although mycobacterial and fungal infections following breast procedures have been described, routine prophylaxis for these organisms is unnecessary (97–99). In addition to the administration of antibiotics, the removal of exposed infected breast expanders and implants is generally required, although cases of implant salvage have been reported (79,90,100–104). Prosthesis removal is devastating to the patient and complicates future breast reconstruction by causing shrinkage of the breast envelope. Therefore, many surgeons attempt and successfully salvage some breast implants. The salvage technique is less successful in poorly vascularized tissue, such as in breasts reconstructed without adequate muscle flap coverage or breasts in which the incision was placed in the dependent portion rather than the periareolar area (79,90).

Infection following body contouring with suction lipectomy is uncommon (< 1%) (105–109), and few plastic surgeons routinely use antibiotic prophylaxis for liposuction procedures according to the survey of Krizek et al. (50). Specific indications for antibiotic prophylaxis in liposuction include older patients, aspiration of more than 2 L of fat, and a procedure combined with dermolipectomy (105,110). After suction lipectomy procedures, postoperative infections have been effectively treated with ciprofloxacin, which has excellent penetration and concentrates in adipose tissue (110). The rate of wound infection complicating abdominoplasty has been reported to be as high as 7.3% in a survey of 958 plastic surgeons by Grazer and Goldwyn (111). Antibiotic prophylaxis may have a role in this procedure. In the survey of Krizek et al. (50), only 43% of plastic surgeons administered antibiotic prophylaxis for abdominoplasty procedures (50). When abdominoplasty is performed with other abdominal or pelvic procedures, it seems obvious that the risk for infection would be increased and that antibiotic prophylaxis would be warranted (112). In performing panniculectomy on the obese patient, several authors recommend prophylactic antibiotics in addition to bowel preparation in the event of an unappreciated ventral hernia (113).

The initial management of pressure sores and other chronic wounds involves obtaining quantitative cultures to identify and quantify the bacteria present. Studies have demonstrated the delayed healing of pressure sores in tissue with a bacterial density of more than 10^5/g (114), and have also shown that quantitative cultures predict wound infection complications of flap reconstructions; quantitative cultures may indicate the optimal timing for wound reconstruction (42,115). Topical antimicrobials can be used to decrease the local bacterial count in preparation for reconstruction. Debridement of devitalized tissue may be necessary to control infection, improve healing, or prepare for reconstruction. Infections of pressure sores are usually polymicrobial. Gram-negative and anaerobic organisms are frequently isolated from pressure sores, given their location and topography (116–119). After determination of the offending organisms by qualitative and quantitative cultures, specific antibiotic therapy can be selected (Table 8-4).

In general, the partial loss of plastic surgical flap reconstructions may be caused by infection or may result in infection (52,120). In these circumstances, the application of topical antimicrobials has been shown to improve flap survival (121). In an animal model, McGrath (121) demonstrated a longer survival of questionable flaps after the application of silver sulfadiazine or vehicle cream.

INFECTIONS REQUIRING PLASTIC SURGERY

Plastic surgical closure techniques are required to place soft tissue over infected areas of the sternum in cases of osteomyelitis and over infected, exposed prostheses. Although it had been previously described by Stark in 1946 (122), Mathes et al. (123,124) popularized the reconstruction of infected wounds with muscle flaps to improve blood flow and thus the delivery of oxygen, immune factors, and systemic antibiotics. In an animal model study, Mathes and colleagues (123) demonstrated increased oxygen tension in the distal portion of muscle flaps in comparison with random flaps. Demonstrating the relevance of this finding, they noted better survival of muscle flaps than of random flaps covering wounds inoculated with *S. aureus* (10^7 organisms). Applying the knowledge gained from this study, they successfully reconstructed 11 chronic osteomyelitis wounds with muscle flaps (123). In another animal model study,

Chang and Mathes (125) observed greater bacterial inhibition and elimination of bacterial growth under musculocutaneous flaps than under random flaps. Using a similar study design, Calderon et al. (126) demonstrated the superiority of the muscle flap to the fasciocutaneous flap in reconstructing infected wounds. Furthermore, an animal study by Murphy et al. (115) confirmed the superiority of the muscle flap to the random flap for reconstructing wounds with minimal and moderate bacterial contamination (10^4 and 10^5 organisms, respectively), but flap failure with 10^6 organisms. Clinically, Mathes reported stable wound coverage for 93% of infected wounds reconstructed with muscle flaps in 54 patients with osteomyelitis, pressure sores, soft tissue wounds, or osteoradionecrosis (124). Thus, because it has been shown to survive bacterial challenge and also inhibit and eliminate bacteria, the muscle flap has become the preferred flap for infected wounds. Other reported applications of the muscle flap in the reconstruction of wound infections include median sternotomy wounds, exposed prosthetic joints, vascular prostheses, and abdominal mesh (42,127–134).

CONCLUSION

In summary, approaches to the prevention and treatment of wound infections have evolved such that indications for the use of prophylactic antibiotics and the selection of appropriate antibiotics are now based on the classification of surgical wounds and established risk factors. In the diagnosis of a wound infection, quantitative bacteriology most accurately identifies the offending organisms and the appropriateness of debridement or reconstruction (Fig. 8-2). Finally, in addition to incision and debridement, operative procedures have been described that potentiate the host's ability to resist or overcome infection by bringing well-vascularized tissue to the infected area.

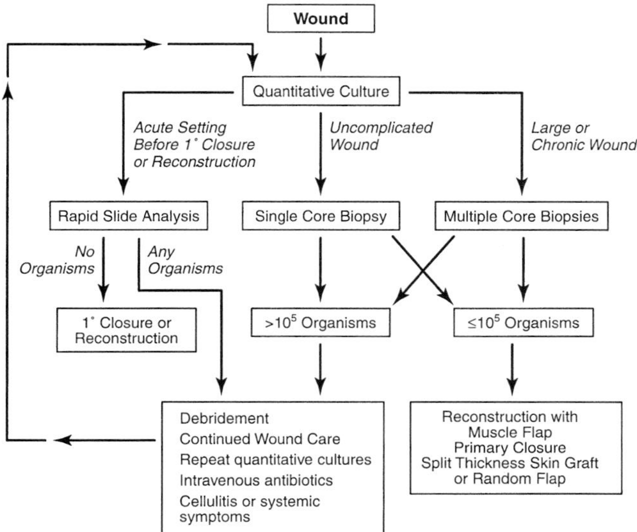

FIGURE 8-2. Algorithm for the evaluation of a suspect wound.

REFERENCES

1. Haley RW, Culver DH, White JW, et al. The nationwide nosocomial infection rate: a new need for vital statistics. *Am J Epidemiol* 1985;121:159–167.
2. Nichols RL. Postoperative wound infection. *N Engl J Med* 1982;307:1701–1702.
3. Nichols RL. Surgical wound infection. *Am J Med* 1991; 91(Suppl 3B):54–64.
4. National Academy of Sciences, National Research Council. Postoperative wound infections: the influence of ultraviolet irradiation of the operating room and of various other factors. *Ann Surg* 1964;160(Suppl 2):1.
5. Green JW, Wenzel RP. Postoperative wound infection: a controlled study of the increased duration of hospital stay and direct cost of hospitalization. *Ann Surg* 1977;185:264–268.
6. Haley RW, Quade D, Freeman HE, et al. The SENIC project. Study on the efficacy of nosocomial infection control (SENIC Project). Summary of study design. *Am J Epidemiol* 1980; 111:472–485.
7. Sebben JE. Prophylactic antibiotics in cutaneous surgery. *Dermatol Surg Oncol* 1985;11:901–906.
8. Andenaes K, Amland PF, Lingaas E, et al. A prospective, randomized surveillance study of postoperative wound infections after plastic surgery: a study of incidence and surveillance methods. *Plast Reconstr Surg* 1995;96:948–956.
9. Cruse PJE, Ford R. A five-year prospective study of 23,649 surgical wounds. *Arch Surg* 1973;107:206–210.
10. Garner JS. CDC guidelines for the prevention and control of nosocomial infections: guideline for prevention of surgical wound infections. *Am J Infect Control* 1986;14:71–82.
11. Becker GD. Chemoprophylaxis for surgery of the head and neck. *Ann Otol Rhinol Laryngol* 1981;90:8–12.
12. DiPiro JT, Bowden TA Jr, Hooks VH 3rd. Prophylactic parenteral cephalosporins in surgery. Are the newer agents better? *JAMA* 1984;252:3277–3279.
13. DiPiro JT, Cheung RPF, Bowden TA Jr, et al. Single dose systemic antibiotic prophylaxis of surgical wound infections. *Am J Surg* 1986;152:552–559.
14. Lewis RT. Antibiotic prophylaxis in surgery. *Can J Surg* 1981;24:561–566.
15. Simmons RL. Wound infection: review of diagnosis and treatment. *Infect Control* 1982;3:44–51.
16. Polk HC Jr, Lopez-Mayor JF. Postoperative wound infection: a prospective study of determinant factors and prevention. *Surgery* 1969;66:97–103.
17. Stone HH, Hester TR Jr. Incisional and peritoneal infection after emergency celiotomy. *Ann Surg* 1973;177:669–678.
18. Stone HH, Hooper CA, Kolb LD, et al. Antibiotic prophylaxis in gastric, biliary, and colonic surgery. *Ann Surg* 1976; 184:443–452.
19. Stone HH, Haney BB, Kolb LD. Prophylactic and preventive antibiotic therapy: timing, duration, and economics. *Ann Surg* 1979;189:691–699.
20. Boyd RJ, Burke JF, Colton T. A double blind clinical trial of prophylactic antibiotics in hip fractures. *J Bone Joint Surg Am* 1973;55:1251–1258.
21. Charnley J. Postoperative infection after total hip replacement

with special reference to air contamination in the operating room. *Clin Orthop* 1972;87:167–187.
22. Levine AS, Siegel SE, Schreiber AD, et al. Protected environment and prophylactic antibiotics: a prospective controlled study of their utility in the therapy of acute leukemia. *N Engl J Med* 1973;288:477–483.
23. Pavel A, Smith RL, Ballard A, et al. Prophylactic antibiotics in clean orthopedic surgery. *J Bone Joint Surg Am* 1974;56: 777–782.
24. Alexander JW, Sykes NS, Mitchell MM, et al. Concentration of selected intravenously administered antibiotics in experimental surgical wounds. *J Trauma* 1973;13:423–434.
25. Burke JF. The effective period of preventive antibiotic action in experimental incisions and dermal lesions. *Surgery* 1961;50: 161–168.
26. Classen DCN, Scott Evans R, Pestonik SL, et al. The timing of prophylactic administration of antibiotics and the risk of surgical wound infection. *N Engl J Med* 1992;326:281–286.
27. Rodeheaver G, Marsh D, Edgerton MT, et al. Proteolytic enzymes as adjuncts to antimicrobial prophylaxis of contaminated wounds. *Am J Surg* 1975;129:537–544.
28. Mendelson J, Portnoy J, DeSaint Victory JE, et al. Effect of single and multidose cephradine prophylaxis on infectious morbidity of vaginal hysterectomy. *Obstet Gynecol Surg* 1979; 53:31–35.
29. Northey D. Microbial surveillance in a surgical intensive care unit. *Surg Gynecol Obstet* 1974;139:321–326.
30. Rotter ML, Larsen SO, Cooke EM, et al. A comparison of the effects of preoperative whole-body bathing with detergent alone and with detergent containing chlorhexidine gluconate on the frequency of wound infections after clean surgery. *J Hosp Infect* 1988;11:310–320.
30a. Seropian R, Reynolds BM. Wound infections after preoperative depilatory versus razor preparation. *Am J Surg* 1971;121: 251–254.
31. Balthazar ER, Colt J, Nichols RL. Preoperative hair removal: a random, prospective study. *South Med J* 1982;75:799–801.
32. Shapiro M, Munoz A, Tager IB, et al. Risk factors for infection at the operative site after abdominal or vaginal hysterectomy. *N Engl J Med* 1982;307:1661–1666.
33. Bhattacharyya N, Kosloske AM. Postoperative wound infection in surgical patients: a study of 676 infants and children. *J Pediatr Surg* 1990;25:125–129.
34. Edwards LD. The epidemiology of 2056 remote site infections and 1966 surgical wound infections occurring in 1865 patients: a four-year study of 40,923 operations at Rush-Presbyterian-St.Luke's Hospital, Chicago. *Ann Surg* 1976;184:758–766.
35. Valentine RJ, Weigelt JA, Dryer D, et al. Effect of remote infections on clean wound infection rates. *Am J Infect Control* 1986;14:64–67.
36. Committee on Control of Surgical Infections of the Committee on Pre- and Post-operative Care of the American College of Surgeons. *Manual on control of infection in surgical patients.* Philadelphia: JB Lippincott, 1976.
37. Robson MC, Krizek TJ, Heggers JP. Biology of surgical infections. *Curr Probl Surg* 1973; Mar ;1–62.
38. Robson MC. Infection in the surgical patient: an imbalance in the normal equilibrium. *Clin Plast Surg* 1979;6:493–503.
39. Robson MC. Equilibrium between bacteria and the host. In: Heggers JP, Robson MC, eds. *Quantitative bacteriology: its role in the armamentarium of the surgeon.* Boca Raton, FL: CRC Press, 1991:1–8.
40. Elak SD. Experimental staphylococcal infections in the skin of man. *Ann N Y Acad Sci* 1956;65:85–90.
41. Robson MC, Heggers JP. Surgical infections. II. The beta-hemolytic streptococcus. *J Surg Res* 1969;9:289–292.
42. Breidenbach WC, Trager S. Quantitative culture technique and infection in complex wounds of the extremities closed with free flaps. *Plast Reconstr Surg* 1995;95:860–865.
43. Mackowiak PA, Jones SR, Smith JW. Diagnostic value of sinus tract cultures in chronic osteomyelitis. *JAMA* 1978;239: 2772–2775.
44. Merrit K. Factors increasing the risk of infection in patients with open fractures. *J Trauma* 1988;28:823–827.
45. Moore TJ, Mauney C, Barron J. The use of quantitative bacterial counts in open fractures. *Clin Orthop* 1989;248:227–230.
46. Isenberg HD. Clinical microbiology. In: Gorbach SL, Bartlett JG, Blacklow NR, eds. *Infectious diseases,* 2nd ed. Philadelphia: WB Saunders, 1998;123–144.
47. Cooney WP, Fitzgerald RH, Dobyns JH, et al. Quantitative wound cultures in upper extremity trauma. *J Trauma* 1982;22: 112–117.
48. Phillips LG, Heggers JP, Robson MC. History of quantitative bacteriology in qualitative bacteriology. In: Heggers JP, Robson MC, eds. *Quantitative bacteriology: its role in the armamentarium of the surgeon.* Boca Raton, FL: CRC Press, 1991:9–14.
49. Robson MC, Heggers JP. Bacterial quantification of open wounds. *Mil Med* 1969;134:19–24.
50. Krizek TJ, Gottlieb LJ, Koss N, et al. The use of prophylactic antibacterials in plastic surgery: a 1980's update. *Plast Reconstr Surg* 1985;76:953–963.
51. Liedburg NCF, Reiss E, Artz CP. The effect of bacteria on the take of split-thickness skin grafts in rabbits. *Ann Surg* 1944; 120:268.
52. Phillips LG, Mann R, Heggers JP, et al. *In vivo* ovine flap model to evaluate surgical infection and tissue necrosis. *J Surg Res* 1994;56:1–4.
53. Strain B. Quantitative bacteriology: tissues and aspirates. In: Isenberg HD, ed. *Clinical microbiology procedures handbook.* Washington, DC: American Society for Microbiology, 1992:1.16a.1–1.16a.4.
54. Lindberg RB, Moncrief JA, Switzer WE, et al. The successful control of burn wound sepsis. *J Trauma* 1965;5:601.
55. Teplitz C, Davis D, Mason AD, et al. *Pseudomonas* burn wound sepsis. I. Pathogenesis of experimental burn wound sepsis. *J Surg Res* 1964;4:200.
56. Leyden JJ, McGinly KJ, Nordstrom KM, et al. Skin microflora. *J Invest Dermatol* 1987;88:65s–72s.
57. Roth RR, James WD. Microbiology of the skin: resident flora ecology, infection. *J Am Acad Dermatol* 1989;20:367–390.
58. Leach RD, Eykyn SJ, Phillips I, et al. Anaerobic axillary abscess. *Br Med J* 1979;2:5–7.
59. Leyden JJ, Stewart R, Kligman AM. Experimental infections with group A streptococci in humans. *J Invest Dermatol* 1980;75:196–201.
60. Bernard P, Dedane C, Mounier M. Streptococcal cause of erysipelas and cellulitis in adults. *Arch Dermatol* 1989;125: 779–782.
61. Gosain AK, Larson DL. Toxic shock syndrome following latissimus dorsi musculocutaneous flap breast reconstruction. *Ann Plast Surg* 1992;29:571–575.
62. Tobin G, Shaw RC, Goodpasture HC. Toxic shock syndrome following breast and nasal surgery. *Plast Reconstr Surg* 1997;80:111–113.
63. Sheagren JN. *Staphylococcus aureus*: the persistent pathogen. *N Engl J Med* 1984;310:1368–1373.
64. Eschelman LT. Prophylactic antibiotics in otolaryngologic surgery: a double blinded study. *Trans Am Acad Ophthalmol Otolaryngol* 1971;75:387–394.
65. Patzakis MJ, Harvey JP Jr, Ivler D. The role of antibiotics and the management of open fractures. *J Bone Joint Surg Am* 1974;56A:532–541.

66. Herzon FS. The prophylactic use of antibiotics in head and neck surgery. *Otolaryngol Clin North Am* 1976;9:781–787.
67. Wagner JD, Morris DM. Odontogenic infections. In: Fry DE, ed. *Surgical infections.* Boston: Little, Brown and Company 1995:487–494.
68. Boyd JB, Mulholland RS. Fixation of the vascularized bone graft in mandibular reconstruction. *Plast Reconstr Surg* 1993;91: 274–282.
69. Cohen M, Schultz RC. Mandibular reconstruction. *Clin Plast Surg* 1985;12:411–422.
70. Davidson J, Birt BD, Gruss J. A-O plate mandibular reconstruction: a complication critique. *J Otolaryngol* 1991;20: 104–107.
71. Dor P, Klastersky J. Prophylactic antibiotics and oral and pharyngeal surgery for cancer: a double-blinded study. *Laryngoscope* 1973;83:1992–1998.
72. Baker TJ. Facial laser resurfacing. Panel discussion, American Society of Plastic Reconstructive Surgery meeting, Dallas, 1996.
73. LeRoy JL Jr, Rees TD, Nolan WB III. Infections requiring hospital readmission following facelift surgery: incidence, treatment and sequelae. *Plast Reconstr Surg* 1994;93:533–536.
74. Morgan SC. Orbital cellulitis and blindness following a blepharoplasty. *Plast Reconstr Surg* 1979;64:823–826.
75. Teichgraiber JF, Wiley WB, Parks DH. Nasal surgery complications. *Plast Reconstr Surg* 1990;85:527–531.
76. Donaldson JA, Snyder IS. Prophylactic chemotherapy in nasal surgery. *Laryngoscope* 1966;76:1201.
77. Hull HF, Mann JM, Sands CJ. The toxic shock syndrome related to nasal packing. *Arch Otolaryngol* 1983;109:624–626.
78. Thomas SW, Baird IM, Frazier RD. Toxic shock syndrome following submucous resection and rhinoplasty. *JAMA* 1982; 247:2402–2403.
79. Wilkinson TS. Complications in aesthetic malar augmentation. *Plast Reconst Surg* 1983;71:643–647.
80. Rapaport MJ, Kamer F. Exacerbation of facial herpes simplex after phenolic face peels. *J Dermatol Surg* 1984;10:57–58.
81. Whitaker LA, Munro IR, Salyer KE, et al. Combined report of problems and complications in 793 craniofacial operations. *Plast Reconstr Surg* 1979:64:198–203.
82. Amland PR, Andenaes K, Samdal F, et al. A prospective, double-blind, placebo-controlled trial of a single dose of azithromycin on postoperative wound infections in plastic surgery. *Plast Reconstr Surg* 1995;96:1378–1383.
83. Sylaidis P, Wood S, Murray DS. Postoperative infection following clean facial surgery. *Ann Plast Surg* 1997;39:342–346.
84. Tabet JC, Johnson JT. Wound infection in head and neck surgery: prophylaxis, etiology and management. *J Otol* 1990;19:197–200.
85. Gibney J. The long-term results of tissue expansion for breast reconstruction. *Clin Plast Surg* 1987;14:509–518.
86. Maxwell GP, Falcone PA. Eighty-four consecutive breast reconstructions using a textured silicone tissue expander. *Plast Reconstr Surg* 1992;89:1022–1034.
87. Radovan C. Breast reconstruction after mastectomy using the temporary expander. *Plast Reconstr Surg* 1982;69:195–208.
88. Thornton JW, Argenta LC, McClatchey KD, et al. Studies of endogenous flora of the human breast. *Ann Plast Surg* 1988;20:39–42.
89. Blue AI. *Staphylococcus epidermidis* and infection following augmentation mammaplasty. *Plast Reconstr Surg* 1985;76:969.
90. Courtiss EH, Goldwyn RM, Anastasi GW. The fate of breast implants with infections around them. *Plast Reconstr Surg* 1979;63:812–816.
91. Shah Z, Lehman JA, Tan J. Does infection play a role in breast capsular contracture. *Plast Reconstr Surg* 1981;68:34–38.
92. Gylbert L, Asplund O, Berggren A, et al. Preoperative antibiotics and capsular contracture in augmentation mammaplasty. *Plast Reconstr Surg* 1990;86:260–267.
93. Burkhardt BR, Fried M, Schnur PL, et al. Capsules, infection, and intraluminal antibiotics. *Plast Reconstr Surg* 1981;68:45–47.
94. Platt R, Zucker JR, Zaleznik DF, et al. Perioperative antibiotic prophylaxis and wound infection following breast surgery. *J Antimicrob Chemother* 1993;31(Suppl B):43–48.
95. Broadbent TR, Woolf RM. Augmentation mammaplasty. *Plast Reconstr Surg* 1967;40:517–523.
96. DeCholnoky T. Augmentation mammoplasty: survey of complications in 10,941 patients by 265 surgeons. *Plast Reconstr Surg* 1970;45:573–577.
97. Clegg HW, Bertagnoll P, Hightower AW, et al. Mammaplasty-associated mycobacterial infection: a survey of plastic surgeons. *Plast Reconstr Surg* 1983;72:165–169.
98. Toranto IR, Malow JB. Atypical mycobacteria periprosthetic infections. *Plast Reconstr Surg* 1980;66:226–228.
99. Truppman ES, Ellenby JD, Schwartz BM. Fungi in and around implants after augmentation mammaplasty. *Plast Reconstr Surg* 1979;64:804–806.
100. Johnson HA. Silastic breast implants: coping with the complications. *Plast Reconstr Surg* 1969;44:588–591.
101. Perras C. The prevention and treatment of infections following breast implants. *Plast Reconstr Surg* 1965;35:649–656.
102. Rempel JH. Treatment of an exposed breast implant by muscle flap and by fascia graft. *Ann Plast Surg* 1978;1:229–232.
103. Snyder GB. Treatment of an exposed breast implant by reimplantation behind the posterior wall of the capsule. *Plast Reconstr Surg* 1975;56:97–98.
104. Weber J, Hentz RV. Salvage of the exposed breast implant. *Ann Plast Surg* 1986;16:106–110.
105. Cohen S. Lipolysis: pitfalls and problems in a series of 1,246 procedures. *Aesthetic Plast Surg* 1985;9:207–214.
106. Dillerud E. Suction lipoplasty: a report on complications, undesired results, and patient satisfaction based on 3511 procedures. *Plast Reconstr Surg* 1991;88:239–249.
107. Gargan TJ, Courtiss EH. The risks of suction lipectomy. *Clin Plast Surg* 1984;11:457–463.
108. Pitman GH, Teimourian B. Suction lipectomy: complications and results by survey. *Plast Reconstr Surg* 1985;76:65–72.
109. Teimourian B, Adham MN, Gulin S, et al. Suction lipectomy—a review of 200 patients over a six-year period and a study of the technique in cadavers. *Ann Plast Surg* 1983;11:93–98.
110. Lockwood T. Lower body lift with superficial fascial system suspension. *Plast Reconstr Surg* 1993;92:1112–1125.
111. Grazer FM, Goldwyn RM. Abdominoplasty assessed by survey, with emphasis on complications. *Plast Reconstr Surg* 1977;59: 513–517.
112. Perry AW. Abdominoplasty combined with total hysterectomy. *Ann Plast Surg* 1986;16:121–122.
113. Matory WE, O'Sullivan J, Fudem G, et al. Abdominal surgery in patients with severe morbid obesity. *Plast Reconstr Surg* 1994;94:976–987.
114. Bendy RH, Nuccio PA, Wolfe E, et al. Relationship of quantitative wound bacterial counts to healing of decubiti: effect of topical gentamicin. *Antimicrob Agents Chemother* 1965;4:147.
115. Murphy RC, Robson MC, Heggers JP, et al. The effect of microbial contamination on musculocutaneous and random flaps. *J Surg Res* 1986;41:71–80.
116. Bryan CS, Dew CE, Reynolds KL. Bacteremia associated with decubitus ulcers. *Arch Intern Med* 1983;143:2093–2095.
117. Galpin JE, Chow AW, Bayer AS, et al. Sepsis associated with decubitus ulcers. *Am J Med* 1976;61:346–350.
118. Reuler JB, Cooney TG. The pressure sore: pathophysiology and principles of management. *Ann Intern Med* 1981;94:661–666.

119. Sapico FL, Ginunas VJ, Thornhill-Joynes M, et al. Quantitative microbiology of pressure sores in different stages of healing. *Diagn Microbiol Infect Dis* 1986;5:31–38.
120. Mann R, Phillips LG, Heggers JP, et al. The effect of venous obstruction in infected pedicled flap. *Arch Surg* 1990;125: 1177–1180.
121. McGrath MH. How topical dressings salvage "questionable" flaps: experimental study. *Plast Reconstr Surg* 1981;67:653–659.
122. Stark WJ. The use of pedicled muscle flaps in the surgical treatment of chronic osteomyelitis resulting from compound fractures. *J Bone Joint Surg* 1946;28:343.
123. Mathes SJ, Alpert BS, Chang N. Use of the muscle flap in chronic osteomyelitis: experimental and clinical correlation. *Plast Reconstr Surg* 1982;69:815–828.
124. Mathes SJ, Feng LJ, Hunt TK. Coverage of the infected wound. *Ann Surg* 1983;198:420–429.
125. Chang N, Mathes SJ. Comparison of the effect of bacterial inoculation in musculocutaneous and random-pattern flaps. *Plast Reconstr Surg* 1982;70:1–9.
126. Calderon W, Chang N, Mathes SJ. Comparison of the effect of bacterial inoculation in musculocutaneous and fasciocutaneous flaps. *Plast Reconstr Surg* 1986;77:785–792.
127. Arnold PG, Witzke DJ. Management of failed total hip arthroplasty with muscle flaps. *Ann Plast Surg* 1983;11:474–478.
128. Irons GB. Rectus abdominis muscle flaps for closure of osteomyelitis hip defects. *Ann Plast Surg* 1983;11:469–473.
129. Luce EA, Gottlieb SE, Romm S. Total abdominal wall reconstruction. *Arch Surg* 1983;118:1446–1448.
130. Mixter RC, Turnipseed WD, Smith DJ, et al. Rotational muscle flaps: a new technique for covering infected vascular grafts. *J Vasc Surg* 1989;9:472–478.
131. Nahai F, Rand RP, Hester R, et al. Primary treatment of the infected sternotomy wound with muscle flaps: a review of 211 consecutive cases. *Plast Reconstr Surg* 1989;84:434–441.
132. Pairolero PC, Arnold PG. Thoracic wall defects: surgical management of 205 consecutive patients. *Mayo Clin Proc* 1986;61: 557–563.
133. Pearl SN, Dibbell DG. Reconstruction after median sternotomy infection. *Surg Gynecol Obstet* 1984;159:47–52.
134. Voegele LD, Metcalf MM, Prioleau WH, et al. Median sternotomy infection: management and reconstruction. *Am Surg* 1985;51:645–647.

SUGGESTED READING

Baker DC. Complications of cervicofacial rhytidectomy. *Clin Plast Surg* 1983;10:543–562.

Darouiche RO, Landon GC, Klima M, et al. Osteomyelitis associated with pressure sores. *Arch Intern Med* 1994;154:753–758.

Mckinney P, Cook JQ. A critical evaluation of 200 rhinoplasties. *Ann Plast Surg* 1981;7:357–361.

Padovan IF, Jugo SB. The complications of rhinoplasty. *Ear Nose Throat J* 1991;70:454–456.

Schimpff SC, Greene WH, Young VM, et al. Infection prevention in acute nonlymphocytic leukemia. Laminar flow room reverse isolation with oral nonabsorbable antibiotic prophylaxis. *Ann Intern Med* 1975;82:351–358.

Strong MS. Wound infection in otolaryngologic surgery and the inexpediency of antibiotic prophylaxis. *Laryngoscope* 1961; 73:165.

Sugarman B, Hawes S, Musher DM, et al. Osteomyelitis beneath pressure sores. *Arch Intern Med* 1983;143:683–688.

Wangensteen OH, Wangensteen SD, Kinger CF. Some pre-Listerian and post-Listerian antiseptic wound practices and the emergence of asepsis. *Surg Gynecol Obstet* 1973;137:677.

Discussion

SURGICAL INFECTIONS

WILLIAM C. LINEAWEAVER

Drs. Wilhelmi and Phillips summarize the biology of surgical infections and illustrate several areas of the diagnosis and treatment of infections in patients undergoing plastic surgery. The significance of their chapter is best appreciated, however, by combining its content with the broadest definition of reconstructive plastic surgery practice.

A thoroughly trained plastic surgeon is, ideally, a postgraduate surgeon who has additional skills in graft and flap execution, hand surgery, microsurgery (with its applications to flap surgery, replantation, and nerve reconstruction), and numerous other techniques applicable to the restoration of form and function throughout the body. Therefore, the general surgeon may usefully define his or her role in the treatment of surgical infection as " . . . eradication of bacterial invaders and other inflammatory stimuli, and

W. C. Lineaweaver: Department of Surgery, Department of Physiology, University of Mississippi Medical Center, Jackson, Mississippi

TABLE 8D-1. REGIONS OF SURGICAL INFECTION TREATED FROM 1992 THROUGH 1995

Body region	Cases	Percentage of total cases
Head and neck	14	9.5
Trunk and pelvis	58	39.5
Upper extremity	32	21.8
Lower extremity	43	29.3

From Lineaweaver W, Hui K, Yim K, et al. The role of the plastic surgeon in the management of surgical infection. *Plast Reconstr Surg* 1999; 103: 1553–1560, with permission.

dissipation of the host mediator response to such stimuli" (1). The plastic surgeon may also claim this role in the treatment of infection in most regions of the body. In addition, the plastic surgeon may move from the eradication of infection to optimal repair and reconstruction of the damage caused by disease and treatment.

This broad scope of practice allows the plastic surgeon to play a potentially eminent role in the management of surgical infection. The role can be manifested in such ways as the provision of chronic wound management services and comprehensive operative approaches, and the organization of a comprehensive network for the treatment of surgical infections.

Chronic wounds can be managed in a hospice-like approach that accepts a wound as an entity causing attendant discomforts that can be minimized (2,3). The plastic surgeon can contribute critical perspective on the use of wound agents, equipment (including beds and wheelchairs), and adjuncts (e.g., hyperbaric oxygen and hydrotherapy). The plastic surgeon can subject all these elements to rational standards based on the biology summarized by Wilhelmi and Phillips and provide a framework for the selection of therapies and evaluation of their efficacy.

The plastic surgeon can demonstrate in his or her practice a comprehensive approach to the eradication of surgical infection and repair and reconstruction in which timing and techniques are specifically tailored to each problem. Descriptions of the treatment of lower extremity osteomyelitis illustrate the efficacy of wide debridement and prompt flap coverage in curing this disease (4,5). This approach can be generalized by the plastic surgeon, who can confidently undertake thorough debridement and apply reconstructive strategies throughout the body (6). Recently, my colleagues and I published a review of surgical infections treated within our plastic surgery practice (7). In 3 years, we treated 147 infections, with 92% resolution of these lesions. Our practice in fact addressed infections in all body regions (Table 8D-1). Our aggressive approach to these infections included 131 ablative and 126 reconstructive procedures, ranging from primary closures to microsurgical flaps (Table 8D-2). We also found that we were in an optimal position to coordinate specialized surgical procedures (including major vessel reconstruction, craniotomy, and skeletal fixation), discharge planning, and follow-up.

This experience led us to hypothesize a surgical infection service, an entity that could be a very sophisticated expression of the plastic surgeon's ability to deal with surgical infections comprehensively. The utility of such a service seemed justified by the complicated and often urgent nature of these problems, the volume of cases elicited by the informal availability of an interested referral point, and the observation that, in 1998–1999, a review of Diagnostic Related Groups (DRGs) in our department showed that infections and complicated wounds formed a cluster that outnumbered any other single DRG (based on Medicare records). Infection and complicated wound DRGs, however, were not

TABLE 8D-2. PROCEDURES PERFORMED IN 147 CASES OF SURGICAL INFECTION: 1992–1995

	Head/ neck	Trunk/ pelvis	Upper extremity	Lower extremity	Total
Ablative procedures					
Incision, drainage	0	9	24	7	40
Debridement	3	30	12	36	81
Sequestrectomy	0	2	1	1	4
Amputation	0	0	3	3	6
Reconstructive procedures					
Primary closure	2	1	0	2	5
Delayed primary closure	0	1	5	12	18
Split-thickness skin graft	0	3	2	10	15
Full-thickness skin graft	0	0	1	1	2
Local flaps	1	7	1	2	11
Fasciocutaneous flaps	2	13	0	2	17
Muscle flaps	1	19	0	6	26
Microsurgical flaps	12	3	2	11	28
Flap revision	3	1	0	0	4

From Lineaweaver W, Hui K, Yim K, et al. The role of the plastic surgeon in the management of surgical infection. *Plast Reconstr Surg* 1999; 103: 1553–1560, with permission.

TABLE 8D-3. OUTLINE FOR A SURGICAL INFECTION SERVICE

I. Personnel
  A. Plastic surgeon
  B. Infectious disease specialist
  C. Ancillary staff (e.g., wound care nurse)
II. Consultant network
  A. Orthopedist
  B. General surgeon
  C. Neurosurgeon
  D. Otorhinolaryngologist
  E. Gynecologist
  F. Urologist
III. Inpatient services
  A. Medically and surgically evaluate consults and emergencies
  B. Coordinate specialist examinations and recommendations
  C. Coordinate team and sequential procedures
  D. Oversee antibiotic management
IV. Clinic services
  A. Coordinate post-discharge clinical management
  B. Coordinate radiologic and scan follow-ups
  C. Oversee antibiotic administration and monitoring
  D. Evaluate for further surgical therapy
  E. Compile data for analyses
  F. Evaluate new patients and initiate their management plans

handled in any coordinated way. On the basis of complexity, urgency, and volume, therefore, an organized approach to this group of patients seems justified.

How could such a service be organized? One scheme is outlined in Table 8D-3. Ideally, the service should include an inpatient team that would respond to emergency cases and hospitalized patients. This team would consist of an infectious disease specialist and a plastic surgeon, who could make initial determinations of medical and surgical elements in each case, proceed to surgery as necessary, and assemble further consultations and teams from an established network of consultants (including general surgeons, orthopedists, neurosurgeons, and otorhinolaryngologists). An outpatient clinic could likewise be organized with an infectious disease specialist and a plastic surgeon. This clinic could coordinate follow-up for discharged patients, including antibiotic administration and monitoring, radiology and scan follow-ups, and ongoing reconstructive surgery. New patients could also be seen in the clinic as outpatients, and the treatment of cases would be coordinated according to the same principles as those applied to inpatients.

This service could provide aggressive, focused care for a large population of patients who now are treated in a disjointed and improvised fashion or sometimes not treated at all. Outcomes and costs could also be analyzed much more thoroughly in such a framework.

Combining a thorough cognitive basis for the understanding of surgical infection with the clinical skills of plastic surgeons and imaginative frameworks for managing patients could define a whole new area of activity for reconstructive plastic surgeons, one that could improve the care of unfavorable results in many surgical domains.

REFERENCES

1. Dougherty SH. Principles of surgical treatment. In: Howard RJ, Simmons RL, eds. *Surgical infectious disease,* 3rd ed. Norwalk: Appleton & Lange, 1995:617.
2. Granick MS, Solomon MP, Wind S, et al. Wound management and wound care. *Adv Plast Reconstr Surg* 1996;12:99–118.
3. Granick M, McGowan E, Long CD. Outcome assessment of an in-hospital cross-function wound care team. *Plast Reconstr Surg* 1998;101:1243–1248.
4. Anthony J, Mathes S, Alpert B. The muscle flap in the treatment of chronic lower extremity osteomyelitis: results in patients over five years after treatment. *Plast Reconstr Surg* 1991;88:311–315.
5. Gayle L, Lineaweaver W, Oliva A, et al. Treatment of chronic osteomyelitis of the lower extremities with debridement and microvascular muscle transfer. *Clin Plast Surg* 1992;19:895–908.
6. Lineaweaver W, Follansbee S, Valauri F. Antibiotics and the management of infected wounds. In: Buncke HJ, ed. *Microsurgery.* Philadelphia : Lea & Febiger, 1991:743–747.
7. Lineaweaver W, Hui K, Yim K, et al. The role of the plastic surgeon in the management of surgical infection. *Plast Reconstr Surg* 1999;103:1553–1560.

9

SOFT TISSUE COVERAGE

ELVIN G. ZOOK

The coverage of vital structures with soft tissue and the restoration of body form are the basic goals of plastic surgery. Plastic surgery was born during World War I when a small number of surgeons trained in various fields attempted to replace soft tissue lost in wounds or burns sustained in combat.

First attempts were many times clumsy and poorly planned (basically because of lack of knowledge), and plastic surgeons, much like children who fall while learning to walk, frequently were unsuccessful in their efforts. Fortunately for us, our predecessors picked themselves up and tried again. Slowly and laboriously over the years, plastic surgeons learned which techniques almost always worked, sometimes worked, or never worked. They were also forced to deal with the concept and the fact that certain techniques seemed to be successful only in the hands of certain individuals. These practitioners were willing to share their secrets and knowledge with others, and their techniques came into widespread use. I remember that as a resident in the 1960s, the main topic that took up our time in conferences and discussions was how to delay flaps so that more tissue could be included reliably in a tissue transfer. The measure of progress is that I can count on one hand the number of flaps that I have delayed during the past 20 years.

Unfortunately, even though vastly improved techniques and knowledge have been disseminated throughout the field of plastic surgery, poor judgment and lack of planning are still with us. The majority of soft tissue complications are a consequence of these two factors. A statement attributed to Louis Vasconez, "The portion of a flap that dies is the portion necessary to make the operation a success," is all too frequently true. The classic example of poor planning is designing a flap that is too short to reach the distal portion of the defect and then adding a little stretch to close the hole. This frequently ends in disaster because the tension causes tip ischemia and flap necrosis.

Other frequent mistakes are designing a flap with the donor site scars not aligned in the direction of the skin tension lines to achieve the best cosmetic appearance. Tissue that is not optimal is chosen to close a defect because of a lack of judgment or a desire for expediency. In all but a few instances, it is wiser to cover an open wound with moist saline dressings, allografts, homografts, or autografts and perform a well-planned, considered closure after a few days rather than embark on a hastily conceived closure (Fig. 9-1). It has been shown by many authors that the complication rates for wounds closed within a few days after trauma are essentially no higher than the rates for wounds closed immediately.

Essentially two types of soft tissue coverage are available in our armamentarium.

SKIN GRAFTS

The major problems encountered in skin grafting are lack of durability and suboptimal appearance. There are many reasons to use a skin graft. One is to provide temporary coverage; allograft or homograft is used and then removed and replaced with autogenous tissue. This coverage keeps the wound moist and decreases the growth of bacteria.

The advantages of split-thickness skin grafts are well-known. They include less need to place the graft onto a well-vascularized bed and relatively uncontaminated wound and, in some cases, contraction. The disadvantages are lack of durability, appearance of the surface of the graft, depression of the surface, and contraction of the grafted wound. The advantages of a full-thickness skin graft are a better color and texture match and less contraction of the grafted wound. The disadvantages are the need to place the graft onto a well-vascularized and relatively uncontaminated wound.

These facts can be used to the surgeon's advantage in the care of a wound. If one is faced with an avulsion injury that cannot be closed primarily or only partially closed primarily, a split-thickness skin graft may suffice to heal the wound, and contraction will make the wound smaller. At a secondary procedure, the skin graft can be excised and the wound closed with a longitudinal scar (Fig. 9-2). This is

E. G. Zook: Division of Plastic Surgery, Southern Illinois University School of Medicine, Springfield, Illinois

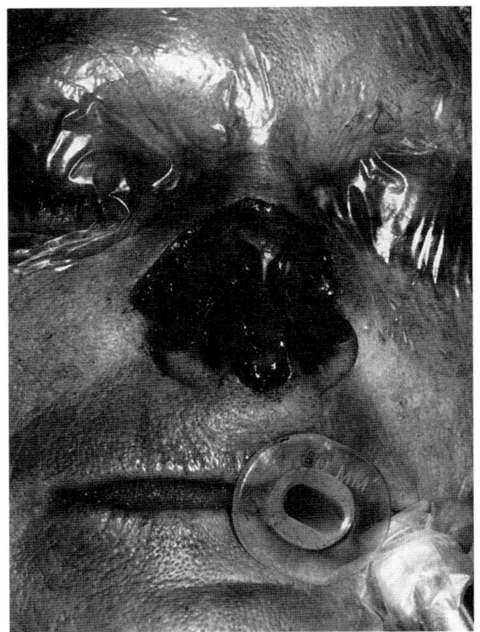

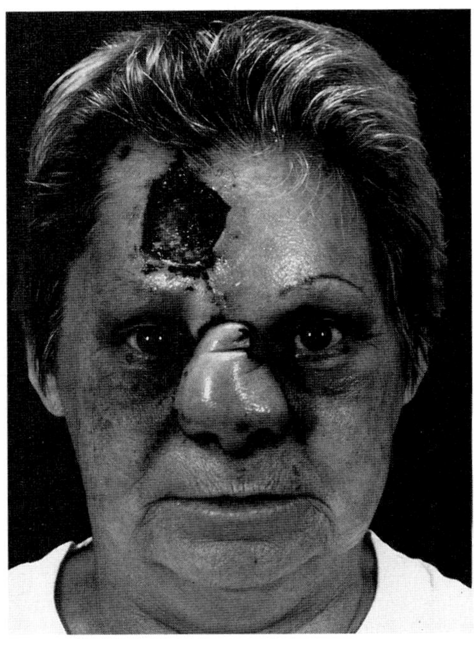

A B

FIGURE 9-1. A: A Mohs' technique rhinectomy presenting for emergency closure. **B:** A hastily planned and executed forehead flap with a large defect. With more planning, this might have been obviated by the use of tissue expander or other techniques.

much better than rotating a flap, with the resultant added scarring of the donor area. When a split-thickness skin graft is chosen for temporary closure, one need not be concerned about color match because the skin graft eventually is removed. The surgeon must consider the donor site and how it will be hidden. A common site for the harvest of a split-thickness skin graft is the anterior midthigh. Although this is the quickest and simplest donor site, a visible scar is left on almost every patient. The donor site scar is particularly unfavorable in female patients or persons who like to wear

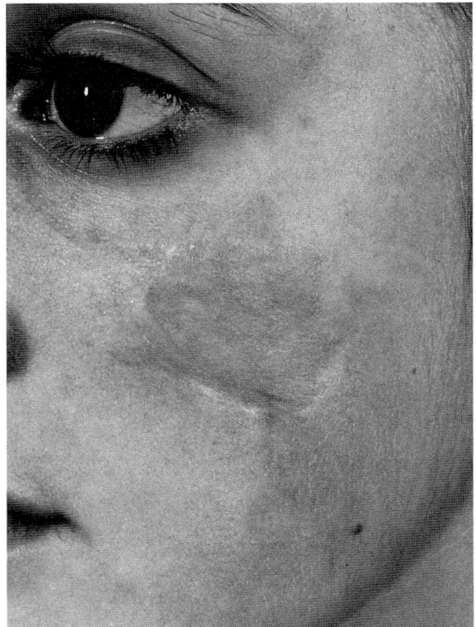

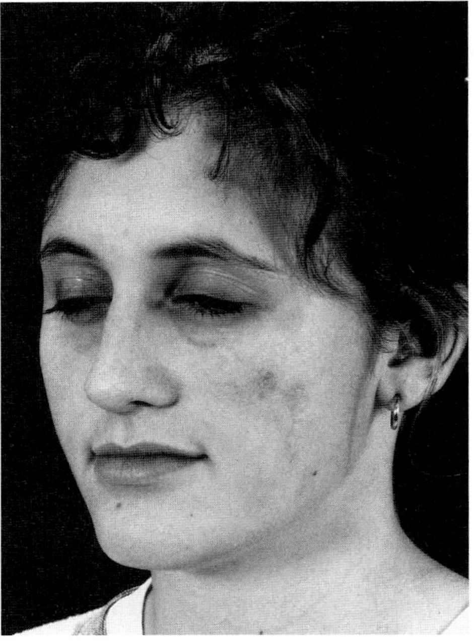

A B

FIGURE 9-2. A: A young woman with avulsion of a portion of the cheek and lacerations resulting from a dog bite. A retroauricular full-thickness skin graft was placed initially. **B:** Fractional excision of the skin graft has left a straight scar on the cheek.

shorts (Fig. 9-3). A skin graft is best taken from areas concealed by a bathing suit, shorts, or panties. These areas may be somewhat more difficult to harvest, and the week to 10 days of healing may be more difficult, but in the long run the scar will form in a less conspicuous area.

A split-thickness skin graft is frequently meshed to allow egress of body fluids through the graft, particularly in an area where contamination, serum oozing, or bleeding may be present. If the graft is going to be excised later, meshing is of no consequence. However, if the graft is going to stay in place, mesh scars will remain scattered over the graft (Fig. 9-3). If one meshes a skin graft, the longitudinal lines of the mesh cut should be parallel to the skin tension lines present on the recipient site before the injury to give the best cosmetic result. We frequently see burn patients with meshed skin grafts on the back of the hand; these are cosmetically unfavorable because the scars do not run transversely in the skin lines.

If a full-thickness skin graft is used for permanent coverage, it should be taken from an area with a color similar to that of the recipient site. Full-thickness grafts are commonly used on the face, and the ideal donor site, depending on the amount of skin needed, is the hairless skin in front of the ear or behind the ear or the skin of the supraclavicular area. These are known as *blush areas* and provide the best color match. Small pieces for full-thickness grafts, up to 1.5 cm in women and 1 cm in men, can be harvested from in front of the ear. Care must be taken not to include beard in the full-thickness graft if it is to be applied to the nose or a hairless recipient site because the hair may grow. Pulling the beard of a male patient back against the ear for closure may create a shaving problem in a heavily bearded man. A large piece of full-thickness skin graft can be taken from the hairless area of the scalp behind the ear and the posterior aspect of the ear. If the perichondrium and periosteum are left intact, a split-thickness skin graft can be placed over the donor site when a large piece of full-thickness graft is needed. If one is covering a large area on the face with retroauricular skin, only one chance at success is possible, and therefore the bed must be ideal, hemostasis complete, and immobilization successful. Shearing of a full-thickness graft from the recipient bed is, along with hematoma, the most frequent cause of graft loss. In an area of facial mobility, it is frequently better to use moderate or soft foam as a tie-over stent, which will allow more facial motion, than a less mobile stent, such as wet cotton.

Caution should be taken when harvesting full-thickness skin grafts from the neck of female patients above the clavicle. If they wear clothing that reveals the area, they will frequently find the scar unacceptable. Remember when you take a piece of skin and close that you will be closing under tension and that the scar may spread significantly. It is wise before undertaking a full-thickness skin graft to discuss with the patient which donor site will be most acceptable.

The depression left by a skin graft is often considered an unfavorable result by the patient (Fig. 9-3). Correction of this problem may require excision and primary closure, excision and flap rotation, or elevation and grafting beneath the depression to elevate it. The latter procedure is difficult with a split-thickness graft but may be more successful with a full-thickness graft. Unfortunately, the injection of various filling agents at present has provided early but little long-term elevation. Injections of bovine collagen, fat, and other material are all too frequently resorbed over a period of months and improve the appearance very little.

Excision and Reclosure

Scars should not be revised for at least 6 months or until maturation has occurred unless an obvious malalignment of the scar is noted.

Excision and reclosure of a scar narrow the scar by 25%

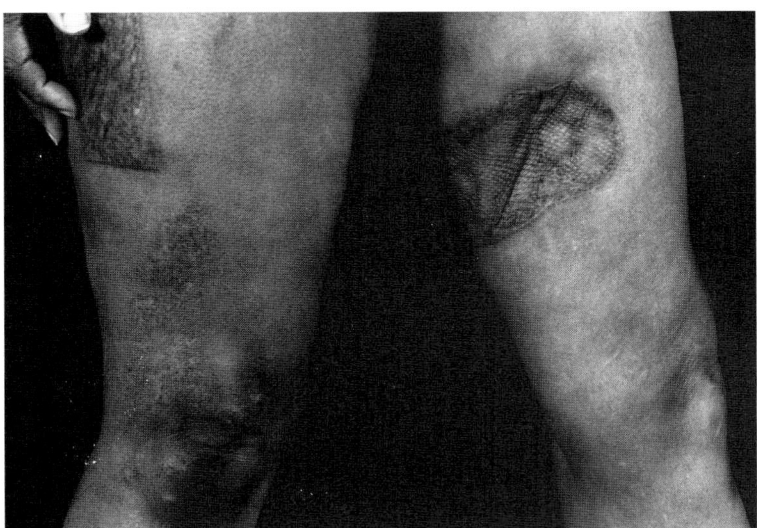

FIGURE 9-3. Note the appearance of a donor site on the right thigh near the hand, which will always be visible when the subject wears shorts or a bathing suit. Also note the depression of the left thigh where a meshed skin graft has left a typical irregular appearance.

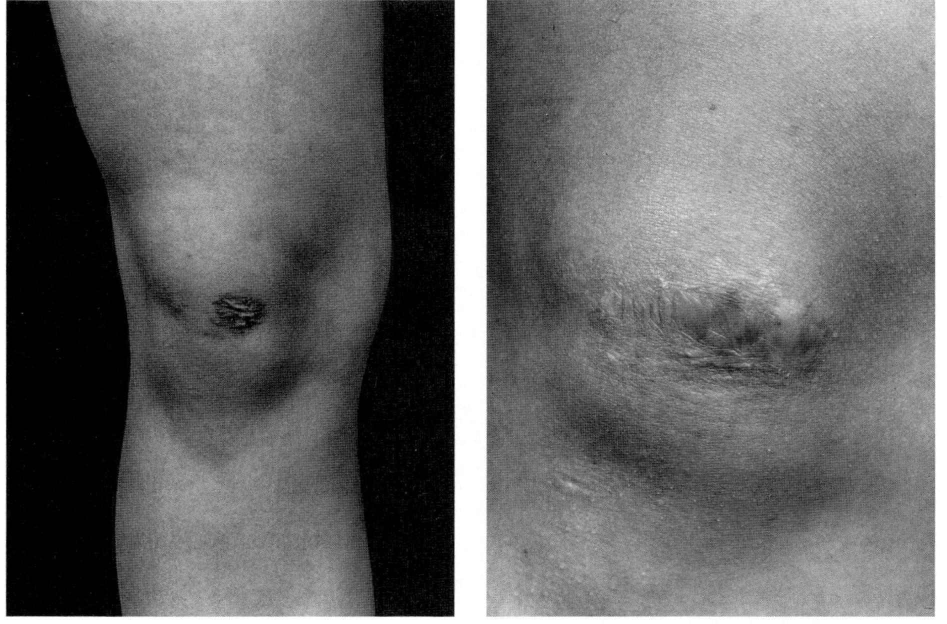

FIGURE 9-4. **A:** Full-thickness loss over the knee allowed to heal secondarily with a wide scar and puckering. **B:** The scar is narrowed after revision but is still significant because of constant stretching of the skin over the extensor surface.

to 75% (average of 50%). The improvement is less with scars over the knee (Fig. 9-4), elbow, and back because of powerful stretching forces on the scar during joint motion. Excision will also remove tattooing from the scar that was not removed at the time of primary closure (Fig. 9-5). Serial excision, if it can be performed in two procedures, has advantages over tissue expansion (Fig. 9-6), although tissue expansion has its place (Fig. 9-7).

Excision of a depressed scar is best accomplished by reepithelializing only the scar and leaving the deep portion of the scar in place. The adjacent soft tissue is mobilized and approximated over the deeper scar, which acts a platform and

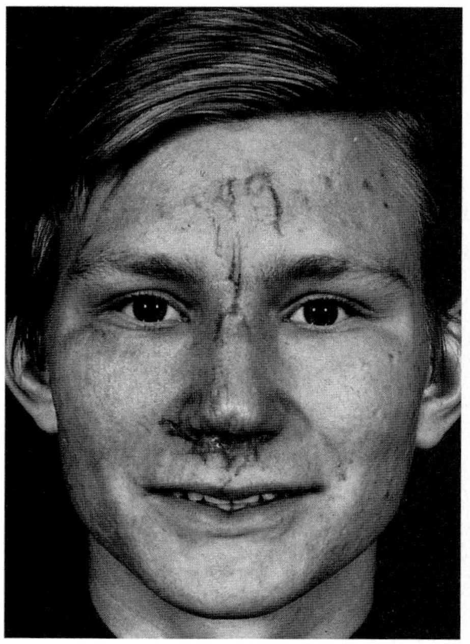

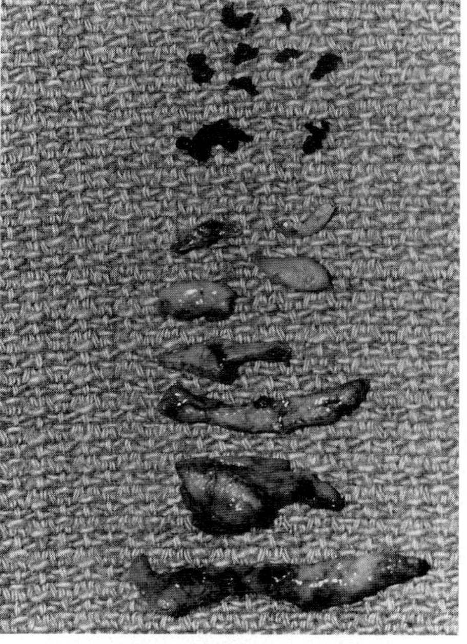

FIGURE 9-5. **A:** Multiple pigmented scars resulting from failure to remove carbon particles from the wound at the initial procedure. **B:** The carbon-bearing fragments of scar removed surgically at a secondary procedure. *(Continued)*

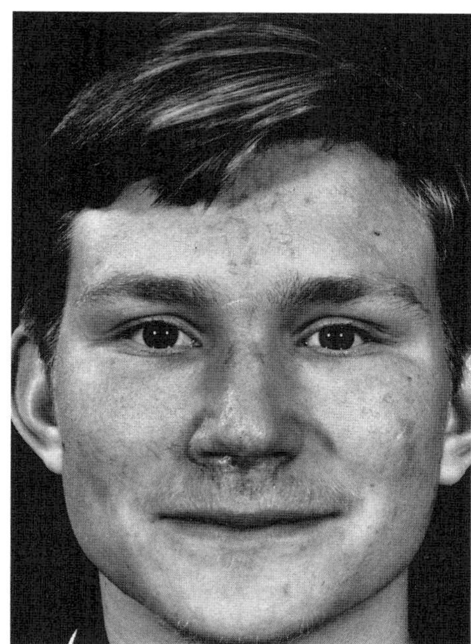

C

FIGURE 9-5. *(Continued)* **C:** The patient with most of the pigment removed.

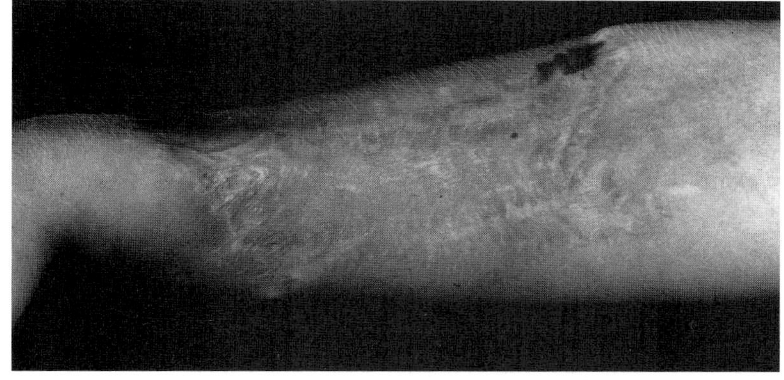

A

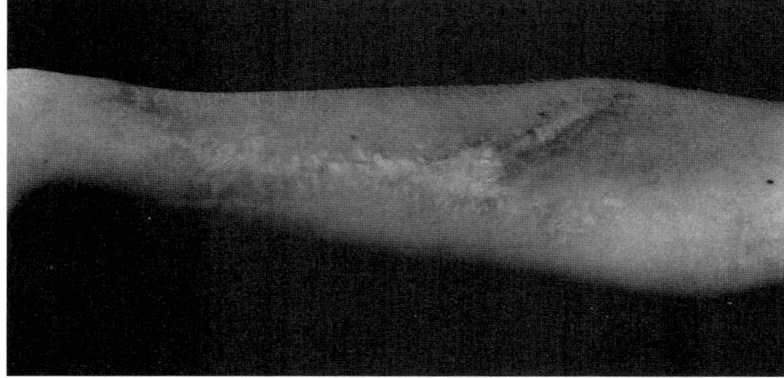

B

FIGURE 9-6. A: A patient with wide scar of the forearm, which was fractionally excised in two settings without the use of tissue expanders. **B:** The resultant scar.

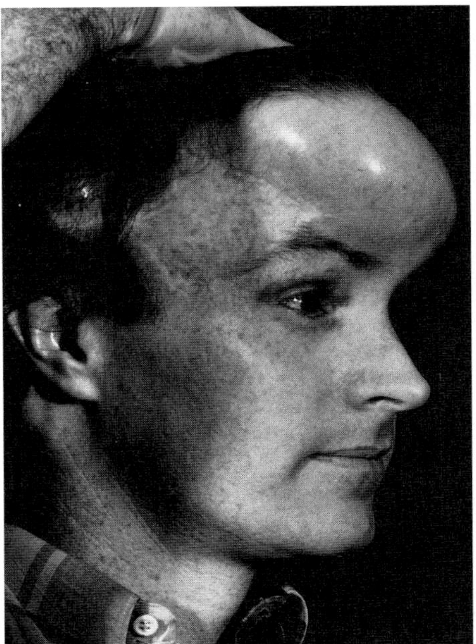

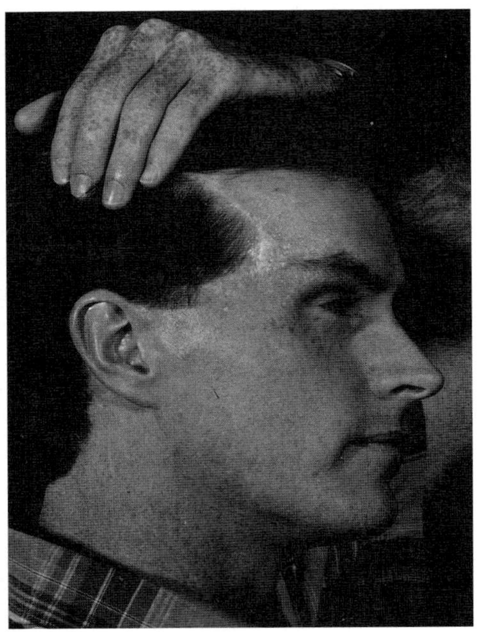

FIGURE 9-7. **A:** The anterior lateral hairline and a portion of the forehead has been replaced by a skin graft. Tissue expanders are placed over the forehead and the scalp. **B:** After tissue expansion, the hairline is replaced into its normal position.

improves the depression. When suture marks are present, it is usually better not to include them in the scar excision because the wider excision increases the wound closure tension and widening of the scar after revision (1) (Fig. 9-8).

Lacerations of the lip frequently cause redundancy of the vermilion border because of the flaplike nature of many of these injuries and enlargement of the mucous glands. Mucous glands seen beneath the mucosa at the time of the primary repair should be removed to prevent enlargement. Revision of bulging lip scars should be conservative. A second revision is much easier and more likely to be successful than taking off too much soft tissue at the first procedure and leaving a depression that is very difficult to correct (Fig. 9-9).

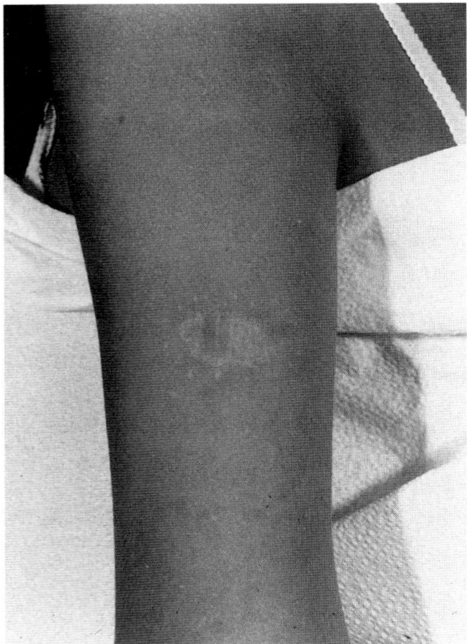

FIGURE 9-8. Closure of the wound under tension leaves stitch marks. Removal of suture marks causes even more tension and a wider scar. Suture marks are usually best left in place.

Exposure of wet mucosa during smiling is a complication of lip laceration repair (Fig. 9-10). It is best treated by transverse excision at the junction of the wet and dry mucosa of the volume of tissue necessary to remove the protruding vermilion.

FLAPS

In general, flaps are tissue composites. They provide improved contour and padding and allow the placement of other grafts, such as tendon, nerve, and bone, beneath them. The old adage, "Rob Peter to pay Paul," particularly applies to the use of flaps. Flap creation requires a decision by the surgeon and the patient as to whether Peter can afford to pay Paul. In this way, a result that will be a draw or a loss to both can be avoided.

The most common flaps used on the face and scalp are relatively small ones that close limited defects. V-Y advancement flaps, random flaps, or rotation flaps are most common. Planning is necessary to place as many donor site clo-

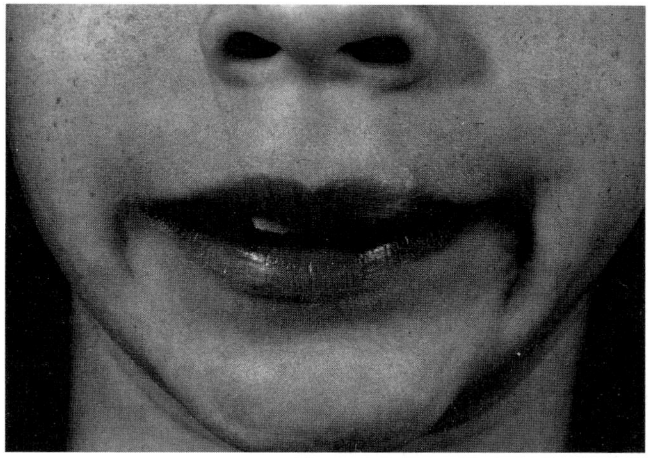
A

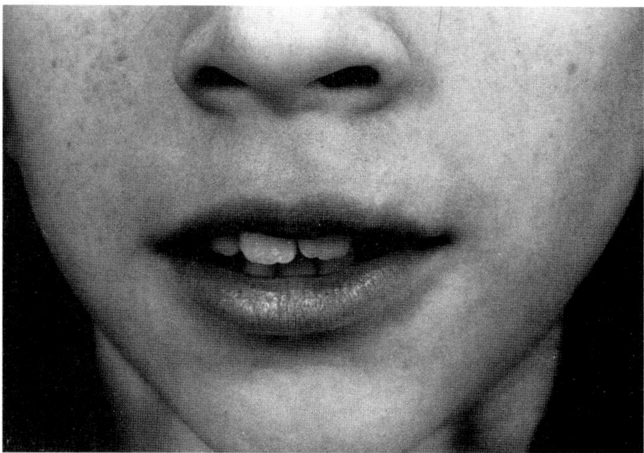
B

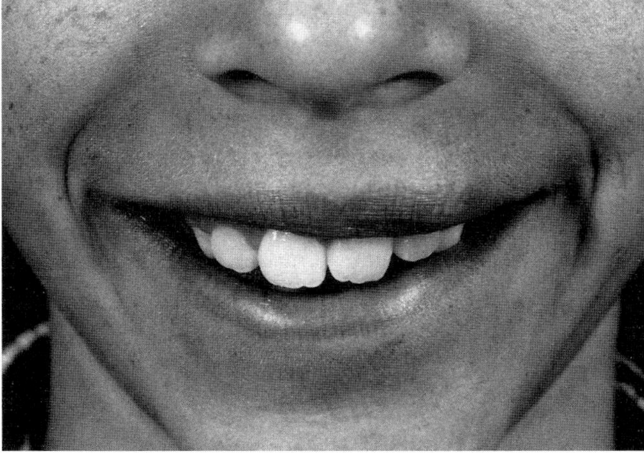
C

FIGURE 9-9. A: A patient after laceration of the lip. Thickening has resulted from mucous gland hypertrophy and biscuiting of the scar. **B:** A transverse bilenticular configuration of mucous membrane is removed at the wet–dry junction and hypertrophic mucous glands are removed. **C:** The patient's smile shows much improvement.

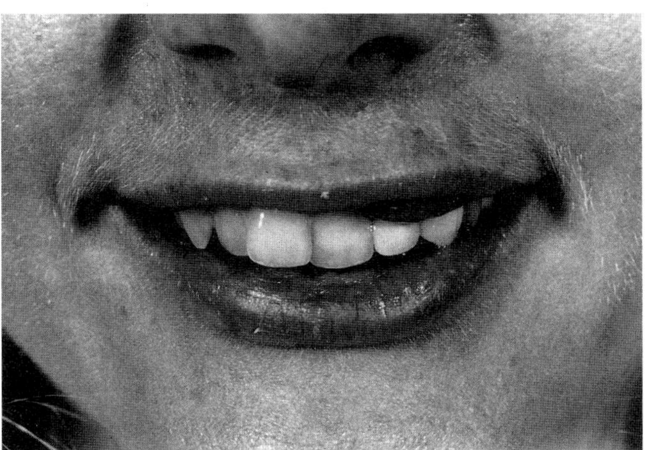
A

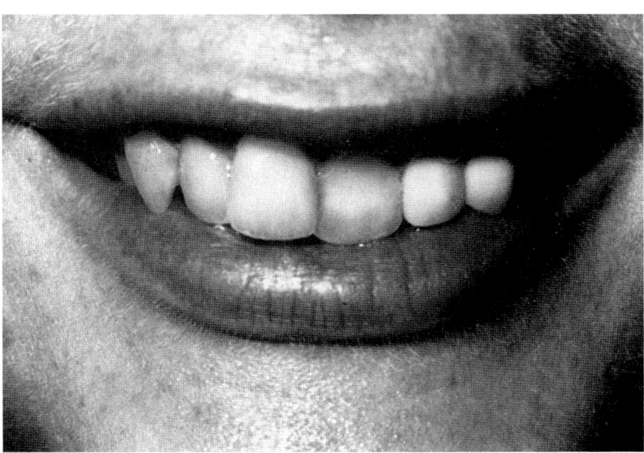
B

FIGURE 9-10. A: Redundant mucous membrane following laceration of the lip hangs down like a curtain when the patient smiles. **B:** A transverse bilenticular configuration removed at the wet–dry junction eliminates the redundant apron.

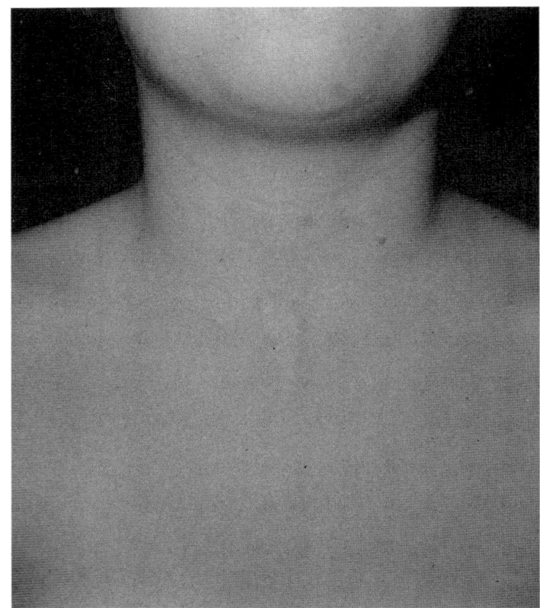

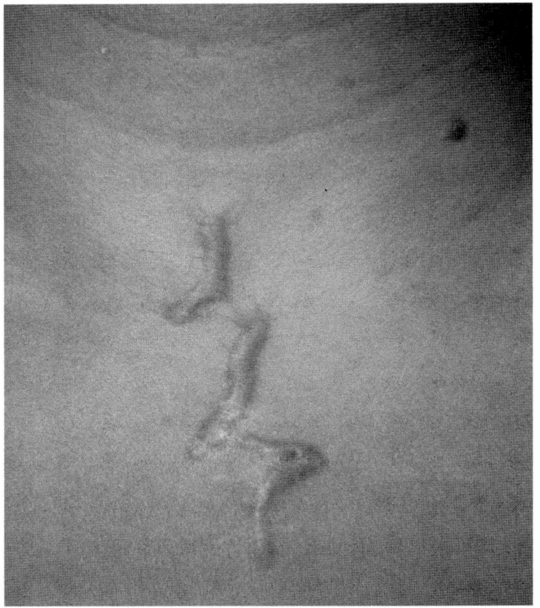

A B

FIGURE 9-11. A: A vertical tracheostomy scar. **B:** An attempt to break up the vertical scar has improved the transverse arms but has left multiple diagonal hypertrophic scars and a much worse appearance than before the revision.

sure scars or scars in the direction of skin lines or skin folds as possible (Fig. 9-10). Unfortunately, once these flaps are designed and closed off from normal skin tension lines and folds, it is extremely difficult to reposition the scars (Fig. 9-11). The running W-plasty and Z-plasty may improve them, but it is almost impossible to place them back in the lines of tension. As a rule, random flaps with more than a one-to-one dimension are tenuous and should be avoided if possible.

Z-Plasty

The Z-plasty (2) is designed to move the longitudinal component of a scar to reestablish normal skin tension or wrin-

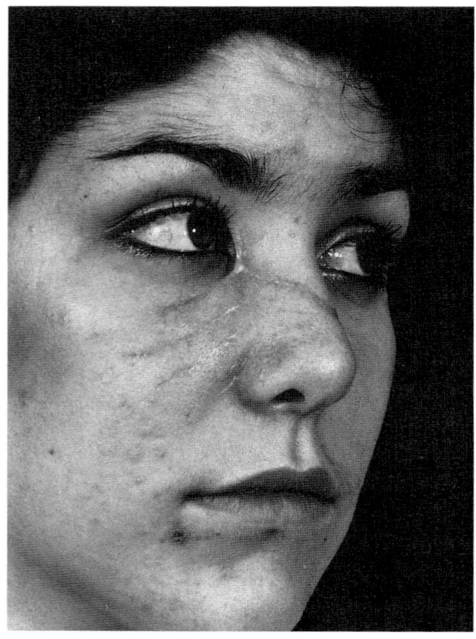

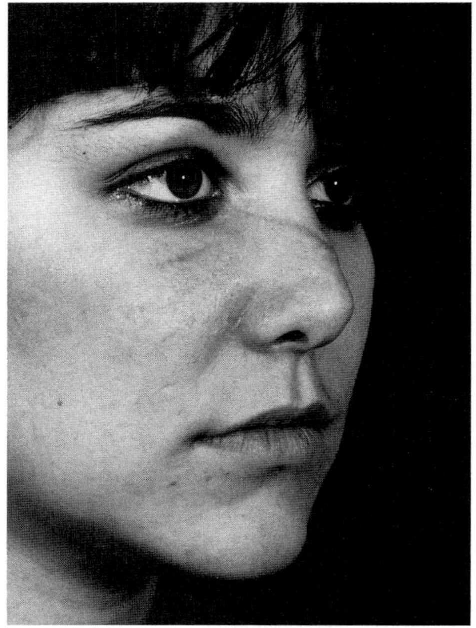

A B

FIGURE 9-12. A: A laceration of the medial canthal area causes a scar band resembling an epicanthal fold. **B:** Z-plasty reorientation of the scar relieves the epicanthal fold.

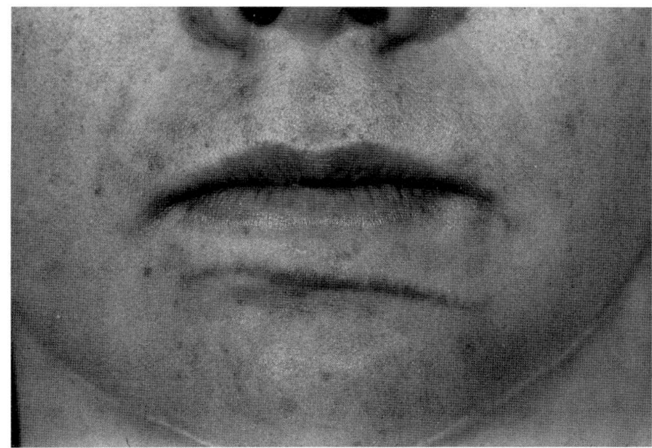

A

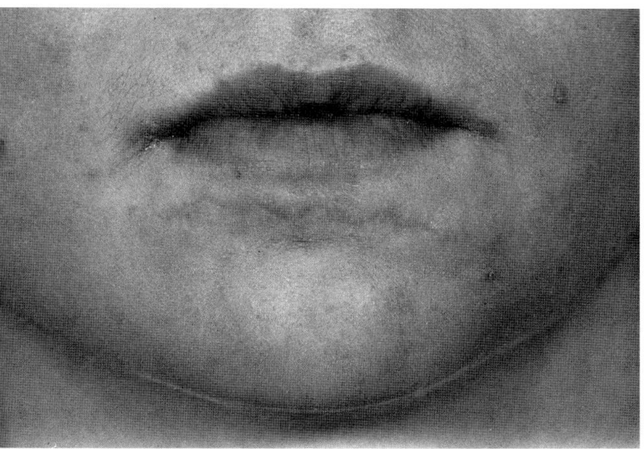

B

FIGURE 9-13. **A:** A transverse scar of the chin–lip junction is noticeable with lip motion. **B:** A running W-plasty relieves the stringlike effect and hides the scar.

kle lines and relieve tension (Fig. 9-12). On the face, it is better to use several small Z-plasties than one large Z-plasty. I have seen a 1-in vertical scar of the forehead turned into a 3-in scar of the forehead in a Z-pattern, which was far less cosmetically acceptable than the 1-in vertical scar that antedated the operation. Z-plasties should be well planned because once they are cut it is extremely difficult to correct them.

W-Plasty

The running W-plasty (3) has the advantages of breaking up a longitudinal scar so that it is less noticeable. In addition, it relieves tension so that the "string" effect when the ends of the scar are pulled is avoided (Fig. 9-13). It is best used over flat areas where skin tension lines are not distinct. The disadvantage is that some normal tissue on each side of the scar is discarded. Therefore, the surgeon must judge whether the tension on the surrounding skin will allow some normal tissue to be discarded.

The saw-toothed final appearance of the running W-plasty may be improved with dermabrasion or laser application at a later date. Minimal makeup will also help cover the sawtooth scar (Fig. 9-14). At times, all the aforementioned entities are necessary to achieve optimal soft tissue coverage and appearance (Fig. 9-15).

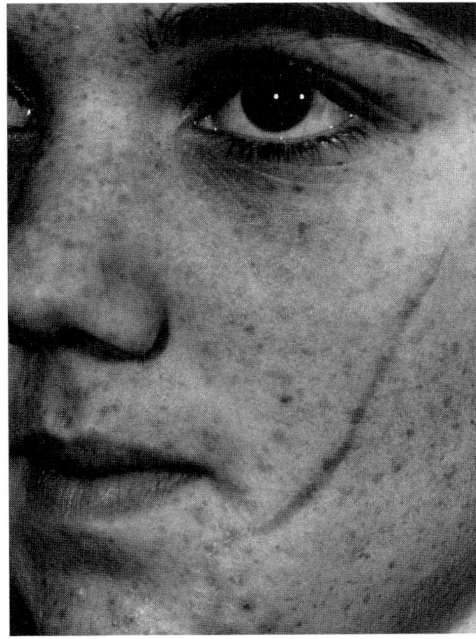

A

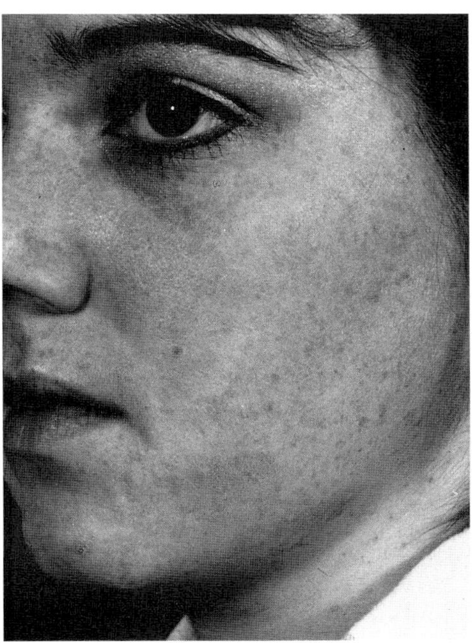

B

FIGURE 9-14. **A:** A diagonal scar across the cheek causes a stringlike effect and depression of the scar with motion. **B:** A running W-plasty and sanding results in a greatly improved scar that can be covered with a touch of makeup.

The rotation flap must be designed so that like skin is rotated if possible. Using nasal skin on the nose rather than rotating a flap from the cheek gives a better cosmetic result. Also, it is obvious that rotating a scalp flap to close a defect of the forehead is acceptable only as a last-ditch effort to close a wound.

Forehead Flap

The forehead flap is commonly used to reconstruct the nose and in most cases gives an excellent result. The forehead flap can be problematic in the patient with a low hairline, in whom the length of the flap needed to cover the distal nose or be folded inside includes scalp hair. One should consider hair removal in the portion of the flap and scalp needed before transfer. Others have advocated a saber-shaped flap below the hairline extending laterally on the forehead (Fig. 9-16). In my experience, this often results in an unacceptable forehead scar along with permanent elevation of the brow. It is important to remember that in most middle-aged people, a 2- to 3-cm-wide flap can be removed from the midline of the forehead with primary closure, but in most older persons, particularly if they are thin, a wider flap can frequently be removed with an excellent midline scar. However, in the younger person, much less tissue can be removed without the use of tissue expansion, delay of flap, or other techniques to allow primary closure. The concept of aesthetic units on nose is correct, but the amount of tissue available must be considered. If one ala can be replaced with a forehead flap and the donor site closed primarily with little scarring, the overall result will frequently be better than if the normal skin on the opposite ala is removed and a larger forehead flap is used to cover the entire tip aesthetic unit, creating a much less acceptable forehead scar (Fig. 9-17). Again, one must consider whether Peter can afford to pay Paul. It is important in reconstruction of the nose that there be support for the soft tissue moved for coverage. This may involve placement of cartilage graft under the forehead flap before its rotation onto the nasal area. This is a good time to perform a delay of the forehead flap because it will improve

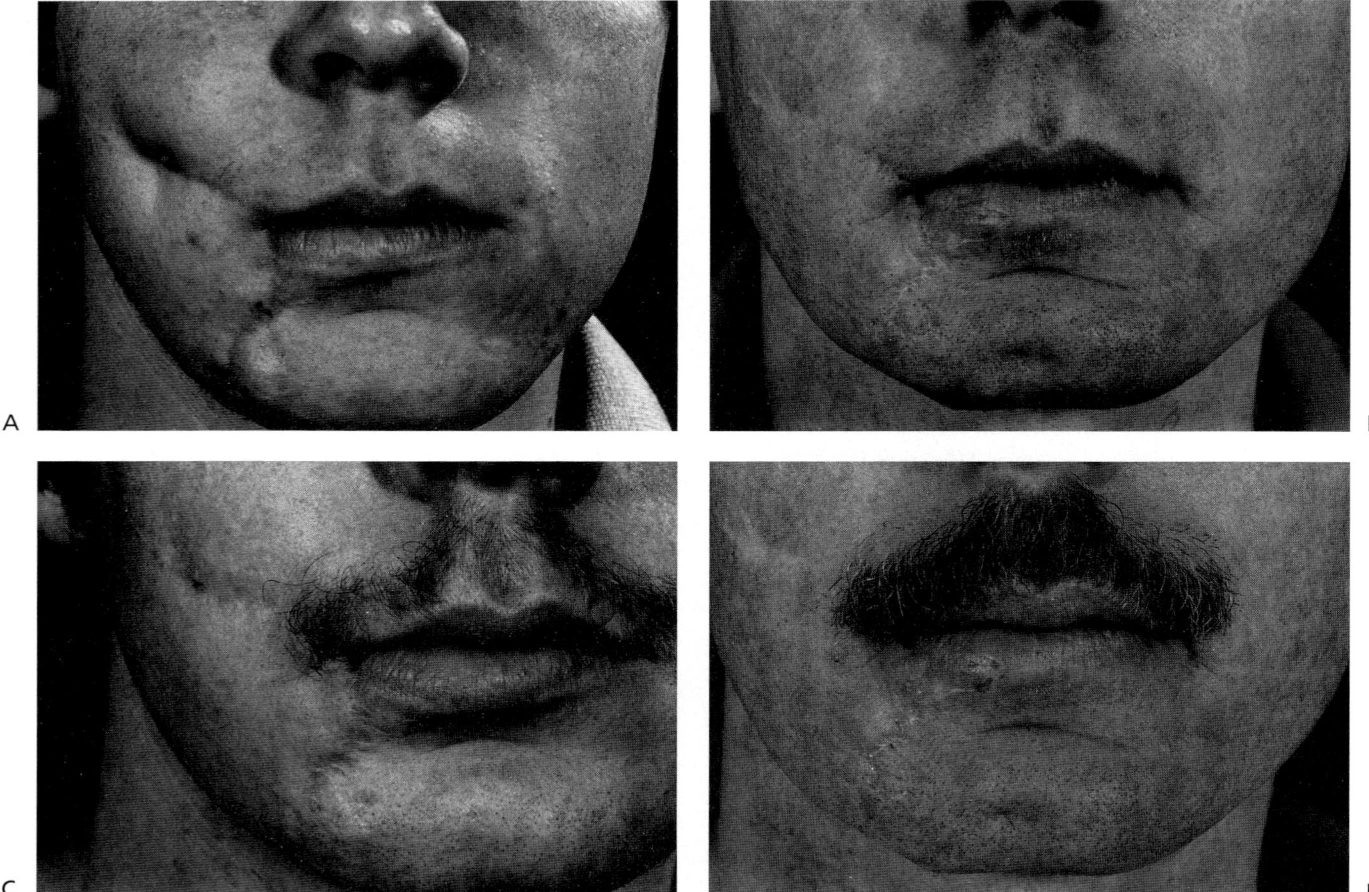

FIGURE 9-15. A: A young man with a depressed scar of the right cheek, pulling of the right lower lip, and an irregular, depressed scar of the chin. **B:** Running W-plasties were performed to revise the scar of the cheek and chin and Z-plasties to release the pull on the lower lip. **C:** A few years later, the appearance of the scar is improved. **D:** With growth of a mustache, the scar appearance is even better.

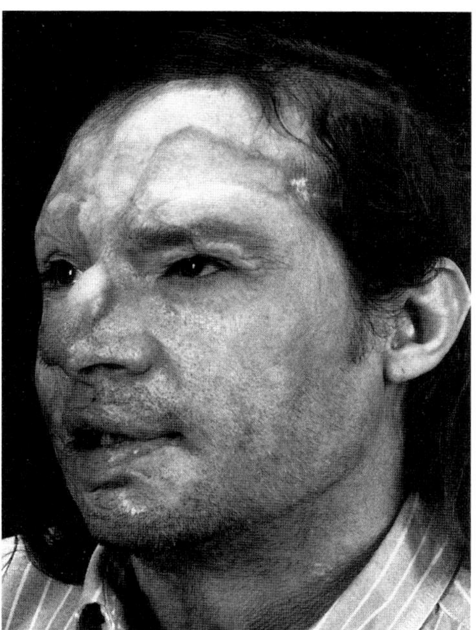

FIGURE 9-16. A saber-shaped forehead flap is used in a burn patient to resurface the nose. An unsightly scar of the forehead results, and hair is transferred onto the tip of the nose.

the blood supply, cause less scarring, and allow more tissue to be moved.

The use of Moh's technique may not allow for proper planning, and the final result may be compromised (Fig. 9-1).

When embarking on the closure of a soft tissue defect, the surgeon must have more than one plan. The surgeon must consider what to do if the flap or graft fails. A plan to "bail out" must be considered beforehand. If a procedure will give a satisfactory result but fails and a backup option is available that will also give a satisfactory result, it may be better to use it rather than a more risky procedure to achieve the best cosmetic result. If the flap or tissue procedure fails and no backup has been planned, the result is likely to be significantly more unfavorable.

Large Flaps

Since the advent of microsurgery, the plastic surgeon has been able to transfer large volumes of tissue from one area to another. Because of the urgent need for tissue that is supplied by a single vessel or small number of vessels, the myocutaneous flap, which does not have to be detached, has become a frequent tool of the plastic surgeon. In the past, moving enough tissue to fill and cover a defect adequately was problematic. With the use of myocutaneous and free flaps, sometimes the problem is transferring too much tissue (Fig. 9-18). If a myocutaneous flap has too much volume, it is advisable to wait for muscle atrophy to develop secondary to lack of insertion. If adequate atrophy of the muscle to provide acceptable flap contour is not achieved, surgical division of the nerve supply to the flap may cause additional muscle atrophy. If the volume of the flap is a consequence of excess fat, elevation of the flap with visual defatting or liposuction will decrease the flap volume. There is some indication that ultrasonically assisted liposuction is more effective for defatting a flap than regular liposuction. The placement of the donor site scar must always be considered

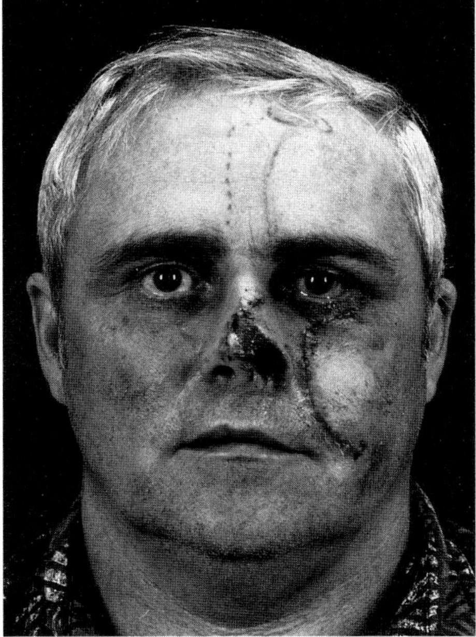

A

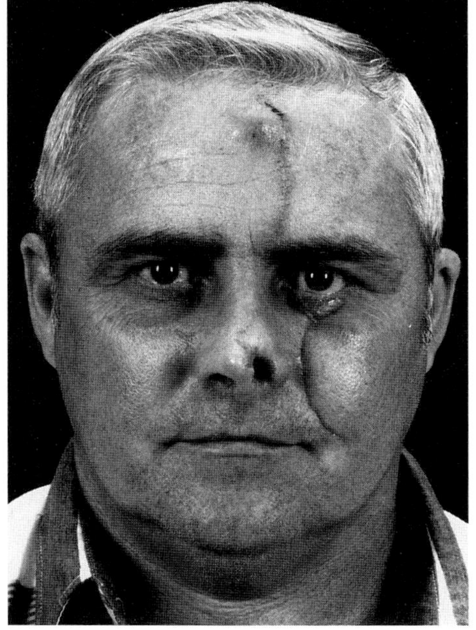

B

FIGURE 9-17. A: Amputation of one ala and the tip of the nose covered with autograft. A midline forehead flap with a fragment of conchal cartilage is planned for nasal reconstruction. **B:** The forehead flap has been delayed and the cartilage implanted. *(Continued)*

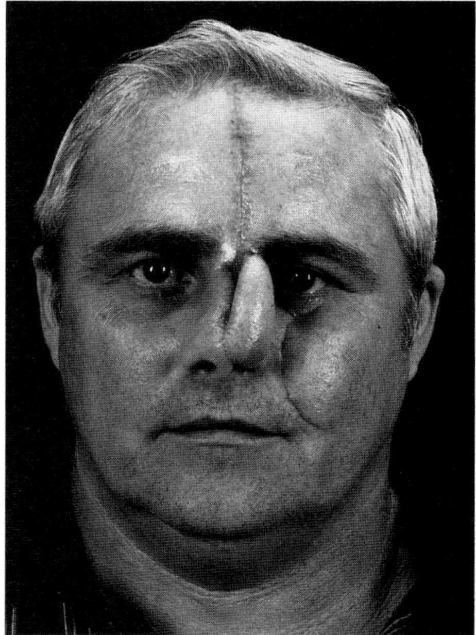

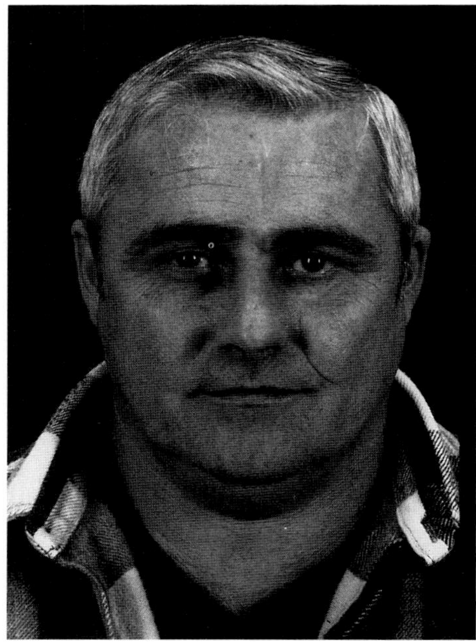

C D

FIGURE 9-17. *(Continued)* **C:** A midline scar results, and the flap is turned down to replace one ala rather than reconstructing the entire tip and discarding much normal tissue. **D:** Completed nasal reconstruction shows an excellent texture and color match without use of a much larger flap to reconstruct the entire cosmetic unit of the nasal tip.

preoperatively, with input from the patient, to achieve the greatest overall satisfaction. The plastic surgeon needs to be especially careful not to make the flap too bulky if muscle covered with a skin graft is being used. It is significantly more difficult to resect muscle secondarily to thin a flap without disturbing the blood supply than it is to remove fat.

An unstable skin graft that is abraded and breaks down can be a significant problem. This may be corrected by resecting the unstable area with further rotation or advancement of the flap, or by removing the epidermis from the unstable area and performing one or a series of skin grafts to allow added layers of dermis to increase the durability.

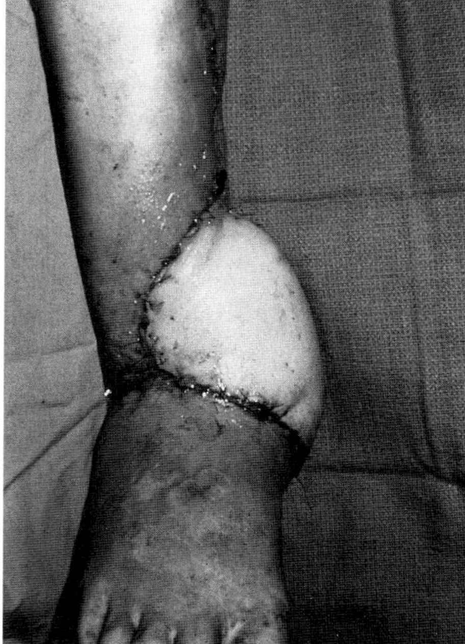

FIGURE 9-18. A flap that is too thick bulges. It is not only unsightly but also functionally less than ideal.

REFERENCES

1. Borges AF. Suture removal and stitch marks. In: *Elective incisions and scar revision.* Boston: Little, Brown and Company, 1973:83.
2. Borges AF. Z-plastic scar revision. In: *Elective incisions and scar revision.* Boston: Little, Brown and Company, 1973:155–177.
3. Borges AF. W-plastic scar revision. In: Elective incisions and scar revision. Boston: Little, Brown and Company, 1973:177–197.

Discussion

SOFT TISSUE COVERAGE

W. THOMAS LAWRENCE

As suggested by Dr. Zook, soft tissue coverage is the basic goal of plastic surgery, and a discussion of the advances in the coverage of soft tissue defects mirrors the history of plastic surgery. He has highlighted many of the factors that can lead to unfavorable results with skin grafts and flaps, and has also discussed options for revising unattractive or dysfunctional scars. Unfavorable results can ultimately be related to imperfect application of the basic principles of wound and tissue management in most cases.

Inappropriate application of the principles regarding the timing of wound closure is one cause of unfavorable results in soft tissue coverage. *Wounds should not be closed if hemostasis is incomplete, if the wound contains nonviable tissue, or if the bacterial count is excessive.* Most commonly, bleeding can be controlled, although hemostasis can occasionally be difficult to achieve in extensive injuries or in patients with coagulopathies. In such cases, the incidence of complications can be limited by packing the wound and carrying out delayed wound closure. Despite surgeons' best efforts, postoperative hematomas occasionally occur. Minor hematomas often resorb secondarily, and slightly larger hematomas can often be aspirated after they liquefy in 1 to 2 weeks. Significant hematomas require drainage to prevent secondary problems of infection or imperfect healing.

Tissue viability is sometimes difficult to assess. Questions regarding the vascularity of surgically or traumatically elevated flaps are not uncommon. A variety of methods exist for the assessment of flap and tissue viability (1–8), although many of them require special equipment. When such equipment is unavailable, one must rely on careful physical examination or fluorescein injections followed by tissue evaluation under a Wood's lamp (1,2) to decide where debridement is required. Delaying definitive wound closure until the flap has defined itself is sometimes the best option.

It is often difficult to assess whether the bacterial count in a wound is excessive. Closing wounds with bacterial counts greater than 10^5/g of tissue generally leads to infection (9,10). β-Hemolytic streptococci are the only bacteria that can produce infections at lower concentrations (11). Quantitative bacteriology allows the most definitive assessment of bacterial counts in a wound (12). Delaying wound closure until bacterial control has been accomplished minimizes the incidence of infectious complications (13). If quantitative bacteriology is not available, bacterial counts can be reasonably accurately surmised by assessing factors such as how long the wound has been open and untreated and the mechanism of injury. Older wounds are much more likely to harbor excessively high bacterial counts (14). Judgment needs to be applied in assessing how long a wound can remain open and still be safely closed. Wounds in immunocompromised patients and wounds in areas of vascular compromise should not be closed if they have been open for even 4 to 6 hours, whereas wounds on the face can be closed even if they have been open for 12 hours or possibly longer. Some mechanisms of injury, such as the human bite, are known to be excessively contaminated with bacteria from their inception and should generally not be closed (15). Contaminated wounds can be transformed into clean wounds by excisional debridement.

Wounds can also become infected through the transmission of bacteria from some other body site. Wound closure should generally be postponed until the patient is free of infection.

In chronic wounds, evidence of active wound contraction or epithelialization is suggestive of limited bacterial

W. T. Lawrence: Section of Plastic Surgery, University of Kansas Medical School and Medical Center, Kansas City, Kansas

contamination. One must ensure that adequate debridement is carried out before such chronic wounds are closed, however. Wound chronicity in such cases can often result from a nidus of bacterially contaminated, nonviable tissue. A common example is the development of a chronic wound in a lower extremity secondary to devascularization of a bone segment after a severe fracture. The devascularized bone must be adequately debrided before wound closure to avoid secondary wound infections and wound breakdown. Significant experience is often required to assess accurately and reliably when debridement is adequate.

Once the decision has been made that a wound is "tidy" and can be closed, the next decision concerns what method of closure to use. *The spectrum of closure options that exists is often referred to as the* reconstructive ladder (Table 9D-1). *In general, the simplest method of closure that can produce the desired aesthetic and functional results is preferred. The basic Halstedian surgical principles of gentle handling of tissues and avoidance of excessive tension are key to avoiding unfavorable results with any method of wound closure.*

Precision in operative technique is critical whenever soft tissue defects are closed. Greater levels of surgical precision are required for more complex wound closures. When flaps are elevated or extensive debridement is carried out, one must be intimately familiar with the anatomic area in which one is working to avoid inadvertent technical errors created by straying from the correct surgical plane. When anastomoses are performed, as in transfers of free tissue, stitches must be precisely placed to preserve flap blood flow and viability. Postoperatively, wounds must be protected to limit problems that can result from excessive tension or pressure on a flap pedicle. Careful examination allows early diagnosis of complications such as hematomas or vascular thromboses when they do occur. The early diagnosis and treatment of such problems maximize the opportunities for salvage of the wound closure.

The simplest of wound closure options is direct wound approximation. This is the method of choice for incisional wounds or wounds that involve limited tissue deficits. For direct wound approximation to be successful, it must be accomplished with limited tension.

If direct wound closure is not a possibility, the next option to be considered on the reconstructive ladder is the skin graft. Dr. Zook has nicely outlined the pros and cons of skin graft closures and has pointed out ways to optimize results. *For a skin graft to be successful, the wound must have a blood supply adequate to revascularize the grafted tissue.* Wounds with relatively avascular structures at their bases, such as bone denuded of periosteum, tendon denuded of peritenon, nerve denuded of perineurium, and cartilage denuded of perichondrium, should not be grafted. Other factors that can lead to graft loss in noninfected wounds with adequate hemostasis are seroma collection under the graft and movement of the graft on the wound bed. Adequate wound immobilization and utilization of a compressive dressing to hold the graft on the wound can minimize the incidence of these complications.

TABLE 9D-1. RECONSTRUCTIVE LADDER

Direct wound approximation
Skin graft
Local flap
Distant flap

When direct wound approximation and grafting are not feasible, flaps are required for wound closure. *A flap of adequate size must be chosen to allow wound closure with well-vascularized tissue that is not subjected to excessive tension.* Local flaps are generally simpler to perform and are preferred when available. As suggested by Dr. Zook, flap complications that are not technical most commonly result from choosing a flap of inadequate size to fill the wound in question. In such cases, the surgeon often extends the flap to a point where its length outstrips its blood supply; the result is tip loss. Alternatively, a not-quite-adequate flap may be stretched and closed under tension; tissue ischemia and wound breakdown are the consequences. Either of these problems can lead to the fulfillment of Vasconez' law. As described by Dr. Zook, Vasconez' law states that *"the portion of a flap that dies is the portion necessary to make an operation a success."* The utility of local flaps can be increased by tissue expansion, which lengthens flaps so that they can successfully close wounds they would not be able to close in an unexpanded state.

If local flaps are not available to allow closure of a wound with well-vascularized tissue approximated under limited tension, a distant flap should be utilized. Like local flaps, distant flaps must be designed such that the tissue transferred is well vascularized and adequate tissue is provided to allow for tension-free wound closure. With free-tissue transfers, it is also critical that the recipient vessels be adequate to provide a reliable blood supply to the flap. In anatomic areas that have been subjected to significant trauma in the past, utilizing a recipient vessel outside the traumatized area can minimize complications. Significant judgment is required to assess the adequacy of recipient vessels accurately in such patients.

If all the above-mentioned principles are adhered to, soft tissue coverage of wounds can be successfully accomplished in the vast majority of cases. As plastic surgeons, however, our goal in wound closure is not simply closing the wound but also restoring both form and function in as anatomic a manner as possible. Dr. Frank McDowell commented on the rapidly expanding repertoire of flaps available for wound closure as follows: *"In many instances there can no longer be any doubt that a larger log of tissue can be transported more quickly to more difficult places with more certainty by these recently developed techniques. What we need to see now are a few harpsichords, rather than so many logs—recognizable, new, artistic, and fully acceptable noses, cheeks, chins, necks, legs, and arms rather than indistinguishable globs and blobs of transported tissue in those areas"* (16). Optimal reconstruction involves the creation of "harpsichords," not logs. The basic principles that allow reconstruction of defects in this manner were outlined by Millard (17), who stated, *"Know the ideal beautiful normal. Diagnose what is present, what is diseased, destroyed, displaced or distorted, and what is in excess. Then, guided by the normal in your mind's eye, utilize what you have to make what you want—and when possible, go for even better than what might have been."* Results can be less than ideal if inadequate attention is paid to the anatomic form that is being restored. The magnificent nasal reconstructive work of Gary Burget highlights how precise attention to the restoration of as exact an anatomic form as possible can change a possibly acceptable result to a magnificent one (18). Maximizing result quality may necessitate actually enlarging the wound to correspond to an "aesthetic unit."

Optimal reconstruction may involve the utilization of a more complex reconstructive modality than would minimally be required. For example, wounds on the nasal tip can often be closed with a skin graft. Although wound closure can be accomplished, skin grafts, even from the head and neck area, do not provide a good match for the thicker skin of the nasal tip. Flap closure of these wounds can often provide a more natural-appearing reconstructive result in terms of color and texture.

Another wound for which a more complex solution than that minimally required would be preferred is the wound involving the loss of multiple types and/or layers of tissue. Mandibular defects that involve bone, oral lining, and skin could often be grafted, although the aesthetic and functional result would be abysmal. Optimizing the repair of such complex defects requires assessment of what tissues are missing and restoring all those tissues to the best degree possible. For complex mandibular defects involving bone, oral lining, and skin, free osteocutaneous flaps that restore all missing layers independently often produce the best results.

The degree of improvement created by the wound closure method chosen must be balanced against the severity of the defect created in closing the wound. As suggested by Gilles and Millard (19) and echoed by Zook, *"Borrow from Peter to pay Paul only when Peter can afford it."* Donor sites for grafts should be carefully chosen to ensure that they are as inconspicuous as possible, and Dr. Zook has suggested ways of accomplishing this. When flaps are utilized, they must be designed such that the additional scars created are not in prominent areas. Flaps that leave donor scars that do not reside in natural skin creases are less desirable. The feelings and lifestyle of the patient must also be considered in assessing the severity of disfigurement produced by a donor site scar. For example, a donor scar on the back created by the utilization of a latissimus dorsi myocutaneous flap may be unimportant to some patients but very distasteful for a woman who enjoys wearing dresses, tops, or swimwear that expose significant portions of her back.

Unfavorable results in soft tissue coverage can generally be traced to violations of one or more of the basic plastic surgery principles highlighted in this discussion. The violations may be errors in judgment regarding the timing of wound closure or the method chosen for the closure of a particular type of wound. Furthermore, errors in surgical technique can cause additional damage to the wounded tissue or to the flap or graft being used for wound closure. Alternatively, although wound closure may be successfully accomplished, inadequate attention to the anatomic nature of the original defect or the significance of the secondary donor defect created for wound closure may make the reconstructive result unfavorable. Strict attention to these principles is the best way to minimize the incidence of unfavorable results in soft tissue coverage. It has been stated, *"Good judgment is a result of experience and experience is a result of bad judgment."* Although this statement is accurate, the correct application of basic principles often allows one to make good decisions before suffering through the results of bad ones.

REFERENCES

1. Myers MB. Prediction of skin sloughs at the time of operation with the use of fluorescein dye. *Surgery* 1962;51:158–162.
2. McCraw JB, Myers B, Shanklin KD. The value of fluorescein in predicting the survival of arterialized flaps. *Plast Reconstr Surg* 1977;60:710–719.
3. Silverman DG, Norton KJ, Brousseau D.A. Serial fluorometric documentation of fluorescein dye delivery. *Surgery* 1985;97: 185–193.
4. Kerrigan CL, Daniel RK. Monitoring acute skin-flap failure. *Plast Reconstr Surg* 1983;71:519–524.
5. Tsur H, Orenstein A, Mazkereth R. The use of transcutaneous oxygen pressure measurement in flap surgery. *Ann Plast Surg* 1982;8:510–516.
6. Thorne FL, Georgiade NG, Wheeler WF, et al. Photoplethysmography as an aid in determining the viability of pedicle flaps. *Plast Reconstr Surg* 1969;44:297–284.
7. Svensson H, Svedman P, Holmberg J, et al. Detecting arterial and venous obstruction in flaps. *Ann Plast Surg* 1985;14:20–23.
8. Banis JC, Schwartz KS, Acland RD. Electromagnetic Flowmetry—an experimental method for continuous blood flow measurement using a new island flap model. *Plast Reconstr Surg* 1980;66:534–544.
9. Teplitz C, Davis D, Mason AD, et al. *Pseudomonas* burn wound sepsis I. Pathogenesis of experimental burn wound sepsis. *J Surg Res* 1964;5:200–216.
10. Shuck JM, Moncrief JA. The management of burns I. General considerations and the sulfamylon method. *Curr Probl Surg* 1969;Feb:3–52.
11. Robson MC, Heggers JP. Surgical infection II. The beta-hemolytic streptococcus. *J Surg Res* 1969;9:289–292.
12. Heggers JP, Robson MC, Ristroph JD. A rapid method of performing quantitative wound cultures. *Mil Med* 1969;134: 666–667.
13. Robson MC, Heggers JP. Delayed wound closure based on bacterial counts. *J Surg Oncol* 1970;2:379–383.

14. Robson MC, Duke WF, Krizek TJ. Rapid bacterial screening in the treatment of civilian wounds. *J Surg Res* 1973;14:426–430.
15. Peebles C, Bowick JA, Scott FA. Wounds of the hand contaminated by human or animal saliva. *J Trauma* 1980;20:383–389.
16. McDowell F. Logs vs. harpsichords, blobby flaps vs. finished results. *Plast Reconstr Surg* 1979;64:249.
17. Millard DR Jr. *Principalization of plastic surgery.* Boston: Little, Brown and Company, 1986.
18. Burget GC. Aesthetic restoration of the nose. *Clin Plast Surg* 1985;12:463–480.
19. Gillies H, Millard DR. *The principles and art of plastic surgery.* Boston: Little, Brown and Company, 1957:51.

10

AUTOGENOUS TISSUE TRANSFER: FAT, DERMIS, CARTILAGE, FASCIA

ROD J. ROHRICH
WILLIAM P. ADAMS, JR.

The restoration of structure and function with the use of similar tissue remains the challenge of the plastic surgeon. The optimal reconstruction of a given defect requires the application of one or more options on the reconstructive ladder, including healing by primary repair and the use of nonvascularized grafts, pedicled flaps, and composite free-tissue transfer. Alloplastic implants and materials have become increasingly popular; however, these products have specific limitations.

This chapter reviews some of the specific components of autogenous tissue reconstruction, including grafts of nonvascularized fat, dermis, cartilage, and fascia. These options may be extremely useful in primary or secondary reconstruction and often are utilized with other techniques to fine tune and optimize results. In general, nonvascularized grafts are indicated for mild to moderate defects with adequate donor bed vascularity (1). Each component is addressed separately, and we consider the fate of autogenous grafts and review the techniques and settings that optimize results.

NONVASCULARIZED FAT GRAFTS

Free-fat grafting from one part of the body to another has intrigued and challenged surgeons for more than a century. The history of autogenous fat grafting has been reviewed by Billings and May (2) in detail. In 1893, Nueber (3) reconstructed soft tissue depressions with small fat grafts, but was less successful with larger defects (> 2 cm) and larger grafts. He concluded that grafts larger than "an almond" yielded poor results.

In the early 1900s, Lexer (4) reported excellent results with free autogenous fat grafting; however, he acknowledged that up to two-thirds of the original graft would be resorbed. Furthermore, Lexer noted that the degree of fat shrinkage was related to graft trauma during the transplantation procedure. As a result of his observations, the concept of bulk fat grafting was conceived to minimize fat cell trauma during transfer and overcorrect to compensate for inevitable resorption.

Peer (5) reported on the biology and fate of free autologous fat grafts. He noted that by the fourth day, blood flow was reestablished in the smaller graft blood vessels, and he attributed the recovery of circulation to revascularization between the smaller recipient bed blood vessels and the graft. The majority of degenerative adipocytes were noted in the periphery and were most likely traumatized during the transplantation process. Up until the fourth month, the graft underwent further cellular decay and evenly distributed cyst formation. Neutrophils, lymphocytes, plasma cells, and macrophages infiltrated and scavenged the cellular debris. It was the appearance of the large, lipid-filled macrophages that led early investigators to believe, erroneously, that these were new fat cells replacing dead cells (host replacement theory). A richly vascularized connective tissue capsule surrounded the fat graft.

From the fourth month to a year, grafts were characterized by a progressive recovery to normal adipose tissue. The cyst and macrophages disappeared, the fat took on a normal adipose morphology, and the connective tissue capsule became thinner. Peer estimated that approximately 45% of the original mass was resorbed. He demonstrated that multiple smaller grafts were resorbed more quickly than one large graft of equal volume because the smaller grafts had a larger ratio of traumatized surface area to volume. (This concept was subsequently found to be inaccurate.) Ultimately, the connective tissue capsule thinned yet persisted and was observed surrounding a 13-year-old fat graft. These mature grafts were dynamic, like other adipose tissue in the body, as evidenced by Peer's observation of one patient who experienced weight gain with a corresponding increase in graft volume.

In the 1980s, Ellenbogen (6) advocated the use of 4- to 6-mm autologous "pearl" fat grafts to maximize viability. He also advocated treatment of the grafts with vitamin E and insulin, a technique that has not been widely used in

R. J. Rohrich and W. P. Adams, Jr.: Department of Plastic Surgery, University of Texas Southwestern Medical Center, Dallas, Texas

clinical practice, although it is supported by some laboratory data (7). Overall, the use of free autologous fat grafts is controversial. The results are variable and often surgeon- and situation-dependent (2).

The explosive growth of suction-assisted lipoplasty for body contouring in the past two decades reestablished the need for an efficient and predictable fat-grafting procedure, and refinements in lipoinjection have provided promising early results. The fat harvested via liposuction loses its organized tissue character and is amenable to syringe injection (8), like the "pearl" fat graft premise established by Ellenbogen. It is hypothesized that individual adipocytes during lipoinjection fall within the oxygen diffusion range required to maintain cell viability until neovascularization occurs. Nevertheless, early lipoinjection trials resulted in resorption rates of at least 30% to 50% (9–13). Cyst formation was not seen in lipoinjection, as it was in bulk fat grafts.

The high initial resorption rates were attributed to the traumatic handling of fat during harvesting and injection. Nguyen et al. (14) noted that lipoaspiration at one atmosphere (atm) damaged 90% of adipocytes, whereas syringe aspiration damaged only 5%. Several reports have recommended half the normal suction pressure to minimize adipocyte trauma during the lipoinjection harvest (9,12,13). Even with reduced suction, adipocytes are fragile and still traumatized, and the harvest may be performed with large-bore needles (9,11,12,15) or, preferably, specialized cannulas that are now available (9,16–18). The use of a superwet injection (infiltrate-to-aspirate ratio of 1:1) before harvesting is recommended to minimize blood and serum in the aspirate.

Asken (11,12) recommend that harvest sites be areas resistant to volume changes during fluctuations in body weight, such as the trochanteric and hip regions. Niechajev and Sevcuk (9) also recommend use of the trochanteric region because of its low vascularity, which minimizes the amount of blood in the aspirate. Our preference is to use the deep fat compartment of the lower abdomen or other areas of typical deep fat, including the anterior hips and lateral thigh regions, which may be more amenable to harvest during certain procedures because of positioning.

Aspirate purification, including the removal of tumescent fluid, blood, serum, destroyed fat cells, and oil, remains controversial. Guerrerosantos (18), Ersek et al. (16), and Niechajev and Sevcuk (9) recommend rinsing the fat in saline solution to remove contaminants and fibrin. Carraway and Mellow (15) recommend gravity sedimentation, whereas Asken (11) and Coleman (17) use mild centrifugation. Coleman (17) discourages rinsing the aspirate because he considers it to comprise small packets of organized tissue; he feels that rinsing disrupts the organization and further traumatizes the fat. Insulin was previously thought to inhibit lipolysis; however, no conclusive evidence exists, and the aspirate has not routinely been treated with insulin.

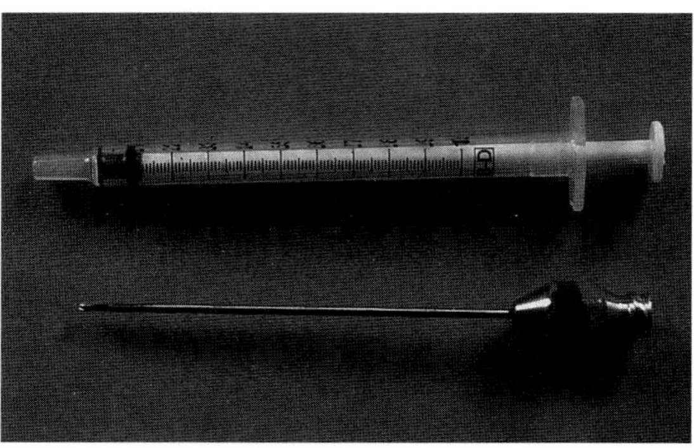

FIGURE 10-1. Blunt 3-mm cannula with 1-mL syringe to minimize adipocyte damage.

Blunt cannulas with 1-mL syringes are favored for the injection phase to minimize host site damage (Fig. 10-1); however, lipoinjection has also been described with the use of large-bore needles. Isolated small quantities of fat must be surrounded by host tissue to ensure adequate early diffusion and nutrition before revascularization occurs. Coleman (17) recommends minimal positive pressure during injection. The cannula should be inserted entirely in prograde fashion, with the injection performed during cannula withdrawal. The fat is placed in isolated tunnels stacked on top of one another until the anticipated volume is reached (hence the name *liposculpture*). Primary overcorrection in anticipation of resorption has been practiced; however, Coleman (17,19) does not provide for any graft resorption but does overcorrect slightly to compensate for resorption of impurities in the aspirate.

Most consider lipoinjection to be a safe technique; however, fat embolism and central nervous system damage have been reported (20–22). Extreme care should be taken in the glabella region because branches of the ophthalmic artery connect with the vasculature of this region. Intravascular injection may occur even when retrograde techniques are used.

Key Points

1. Free autologous fat grafts may be used for small defects; however, they must be placed in a well-vascularized bed, and expected resorption rates approach 50%.
2. Refinements in lipoinjection have made this the preferred technique in treating small contour deformities with autologous fat.
3. Fat graft harvesting is a critical step to avoid individual fat cell trauma and subsequent fat cell resorption. Key steps include the following:
   a. Inject area with superwet technique for blood-free fat aspiration.
   b. Use minimal aspiration pressure (manual) in small 5- to 100-mL syringes.

TABLE 10-1. UNIVERSITY OF TEXAS SOUTHWESTERN SUPERWET SOLUTION

1-L lactated Ringer's solution
30-mL 1% lidocaine
1-mL 1:1000 epinephrine

c. Use large-bore 14F to 16F blunt cannulas.
d. Centrifuge and decant (do not strain fat).
e. Inject small 0.1-mL aliquots slowly during withdrawal of a blunt 14F to 16F cannula. Use a 1-mL tuberculin syringe.

4. Our preferred technique for fat harvest includes injection of the abdominal or lateral thigh donor site with the superwet technique (Table 10-1).
5. In our experience, we routinely see 35% to 40% volume resorption over time, with maintenance volume at approximately 1 year (Fig. 10-2).

DERMAL-FAT GRAFT

Dermal-fat grafts are a useful adjunct in plastic surgery, and their application has paralleled the studies of fat grafting previously reviewed. This section reviews the pertinent science of dermal-fat grafts and describes their recommended clinical uses.

Bames (23) recognized the importance of early fat revascularization in viability and suggested the use of a dermal-fat graft to enhance the revascularization process. Peer (5,24) also favored dermal-fat grafts over fat grafts; however, unlike Bames, he felt that the improved long-term viability was secondary to the dermal protection of the graft from trauma. The volume loss seen in dermal-fat grafts ranges from 10% to 50% (23,24); however, the inclusion of dermis enhances the relative graft volume permissible. Large dermal-fat grafts (> 3 cm) take almost as well as moderately small fat grafts (24).

The exact mechanism of dermal enhancement has not been fully elucidated; however, Watson (25) reported capillary bed enhancement in addition to undefined vasoactive effects provided by the inclusion of dermis. He recommended placing the dermis side against the most vascular tissue available and clinically described fat-fascial-dermal grafts of up to 250 g that showed no significant long-term shrinkage in a series of patients.

Sawhney et al. (26) examined the fate of small dermal-fat grafts in a porcine model. They concluded that the grafts are vascularized from their dermal surface, but that this vascularization does not affect the eventual replacement of fat by fibrous tissue. Interestingly, by 8 weeks, they noted a 33% decrease in net graft volume, and 90% to 100% of the fat had been replaced by fibrous tissue. The volume of the dermal component remained constant over time and in the skin appendages except that sweat glands and ducts degenerated. Other investigators have reported similar replacement of fat by fibrous tissues in dermal-fat grafts (27). Of note, other studies (5,6), most notably Peer's, do not demonstrate

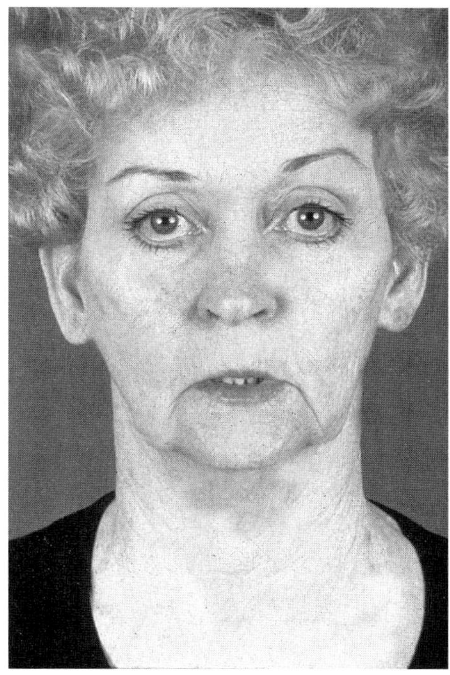
A

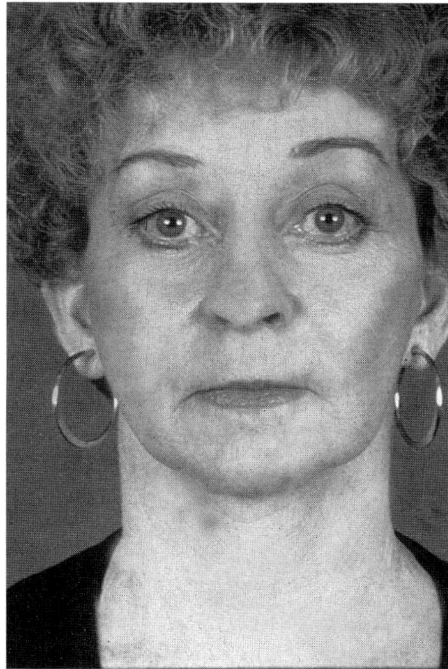
B

FIGURE 10-2. A: Preoperative. **B:** Postoperative 1.5 years after autologous fat injection (centrifuged) into nasolabial folds (2-mL per side, 1.5-mL per side into each marionette line, and 2-mL per side into each malar region).

fibrous replacement, as evidenced by the investigator's biopsy of a 13-year-old fat graft demonstrating normal adipose tissue enclosed by a connective tissue capsule.

Key Points

1. Dermal-fat grafts are based on many of the principles applied in standard fat grafting.
2. The addition of dermis introduces a large capillary manifold over the fat component and also may protect the adipocytes from trauma.
3. The addition of dermis allows a graft with a larger volume to be used.
4. Resorption is inevitable and unpredictable, ranging from 10% to 50% in dermal-fat grafts, especially in larger contour deformities.
5. Our preferred technique is to use dermal-fat grafts for larger contour deformities (> 3 cm in width and > 1 cm in depth) that may not be amenable to lipoinjection (Fig. 10-3A).
6. Anticipate 30% to 40% long-term volume reduction in the graft; therefore, overcorrect initially by 30% to 40% (Fig. 10-3B).
7. Strict adherence to atraumatic technique is essential for graft harvest and recipient bed preparation, including meticulous hemostasis to maximize bed vascularity.
8. Placement with the dermis deep is particularly useful in the face. It optimizes long-term surface contour and results in a lesser degree of palpable surface fibrosis.
9. Our preference is to limit graft thickness to less than 1.5 cm, as advocated by other centers (9), and to immobilize the graft strictly with fine sutures and splints when possible for 5 to 7 days.

DERMIS-ONLY GRAFTS

Grafts of dermis alone have also been advocated for contour deformities, particularly of the nose. Thin single or multilayer dermal-only grafts have been use with good long-term results (28). In our experience, use of the dermis alone as an onlay for the nasal dorsum has been somewhat disappointing at 2 to 3 years. A dermal graft inlay to correct dorsal irregularities has been more successful. We have also had a favorable experience with a cellular dermal homograft for nasal dorsal augmentation and comoflaging of dorsal irregularities particularly in secondary rhinoplasty.

CARTILAGE GRAFTS

Autogenous cartilage grafts have withstood the test of time, yielding excellent results in reconstructive plastic surgery. Numerous authors have obtained extensive experience in the use of rib, auricular, or septal cartilage grafts with excellent long-term results, low resorption rates, and minimal complications (29–32).

The fact that the cartilage graft is immunologically privileged results in its clinical longevity. The metabolic rate of

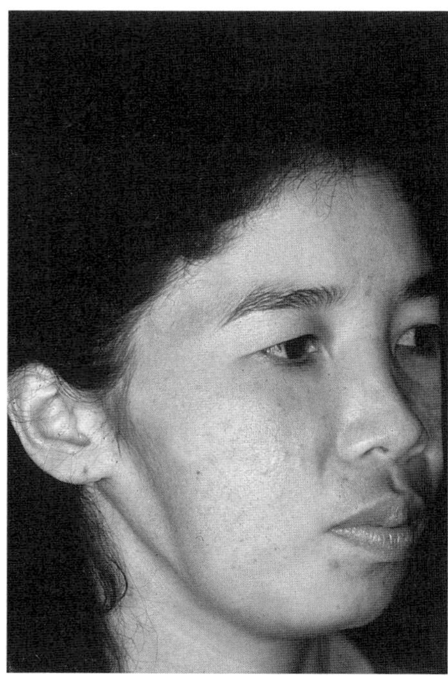
A

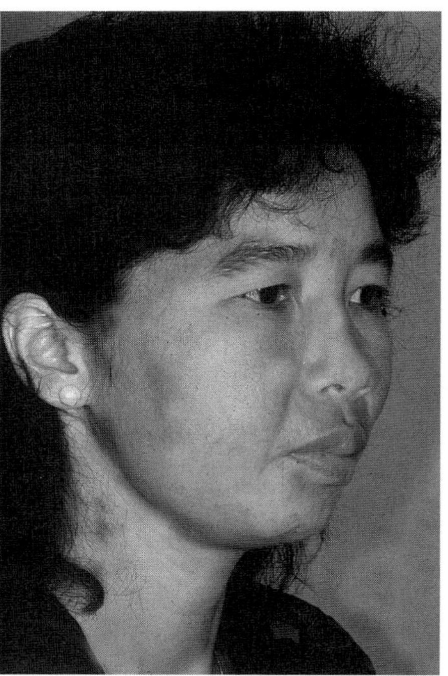
B

FIGURE 10-3. A: Preoperative congenital soft tissue hypoplasia. **B:** One and one-half years following 4 x 5-cm dermal-fat graft placed with 50% overcorrection (initially) and reasonable contour.

cartilage is a fraction of that in other human tissues, owing to its small cell population and relatively low vascularity. Chondrocytes, or cartilage cells, are relatively isolated from their surroundings by a medium consisting primarily of chondroitin sulfate, a mucopolysaccaride, and elastin and collagen, which make up the cartilaginous matrix. Because of this unique matrix, immunologic stimulation is minimal and resorption rates are very low. In fact, it has been shown that cartilage grafts actually grow (29,33). The key to successful and functioning cartilage grafts is the chondrocyte, and so nonviable cartilage grafts, such as those that have been irradiated, can be expected to yield less-than-optimal results and show significantly higher resorption rates. Cartilage grafts should be placed in well-vascularized pockets. When cartilage, particularly rib cartilage, is carved, a balanced cross section should be constructed to minimize warping (34). The warping characteristics of irradiated cartilage have been shown not to be significantly different from those of nonirradiated cartilage (35). Unlike many other autogenous grafts, cartilage does not undergo metaplastic changes after implantation; thus, it is ideal for many reconstructive procedures in plastic surgery.

With the advent of more precise methods of nasal analysis and an increase in iatrogenically induced nasal deformities, the number of augmentation rhinoplasties, rather than the traditional reduction rhinoplasties, has increased, so that suitable donor sites that provide consistent and effective autogenous supportive tissue are needed. We prefer to use autogenous tissue, especially in the nose, and do not feel that alloplasts are indicated.

Septal cartilage remains the cartilage of choice in that it is available in the same operative field and is easily contoured for dorsal augmentation, columellar struts, or tip grafts as needed (36). It does not have the convolutions found in other cartilage, such as ear cartilage. However, especially in a secondary rhinoplasty, it is sometimes lacking or insufficient for nasal reconstruction.

Ear cartilage provides a large volume of cartilage, but because of its flaccidity and convolutions, it is best used when these characteristics are desired, especially in reconstructing the lower lateral cartilages. Rib cartilage is used when a large volume or length is required, as in a dorsal augmentation, but warping problems can develop, as will be discussed.

The remainder of this chapter describes our technique in harvesting cartilage grafts, specifically septum, ear, and rib cartilage grafts, which we feel are excellent autogenous sources for use in primary and secondary rhinoplasty.

Septal Cartilage

Septal cartilage is our primary choice for all grafts in rhinoplasty. It is an excellent source of straight cartilage with versatile capabilities in primary and secondary rhinoplasty. It is easily harvested and available within the operative field, and minimal donor morbidity is another advantage.

Technique

When harvesting septal cartilage for use in a graft, we prefer to use a hemitransfixion or Killian incision to minimize the loss of tip projection. At least 2 mm of tip projection is lost with an extended full transfixion incision, particularly when it is carried well down over the anterior nasal spine. Septal harvesting also can be performed through an open approach, through a marginal and transcolumellar incision, by separating the medial crura and upper lateral cartilages from the septum.

Next, carry the dissection subperichondrially on one side of the septum over the caudal edge of the septal cartilage down to the anterior nasal spine. Using a sharp Cottle elevator, elevate the soft tissues away from the anterior nasal spine (Fig. 10-4).

To facilitate the dissection, use a long Vienna speculum with the tips on either side of the spine to provide soft tissue retraction. Use a dental amalgam packer to begin the skeletonization at the caudal edge of the septal cartilage and create bilateral subperichondrial flaps. The skeletonized cartilage usually has a distinct grayish-bluish appearance.

If it does not, you need to go deeper to be sure that your location is subperichondrial, but be careful not to penetrate the cartilage. Using the elevator, expose the entire quadrilateral cartilage bilaterally from the vomer to the dorsum and continue subperiosteally over the perpendicular plane of the ethmoid. Continue the subperiosteal dissection in continuity inferiorly and posteriorly over the posterior vomer. With care, it is possible to elevate the periosteal con-

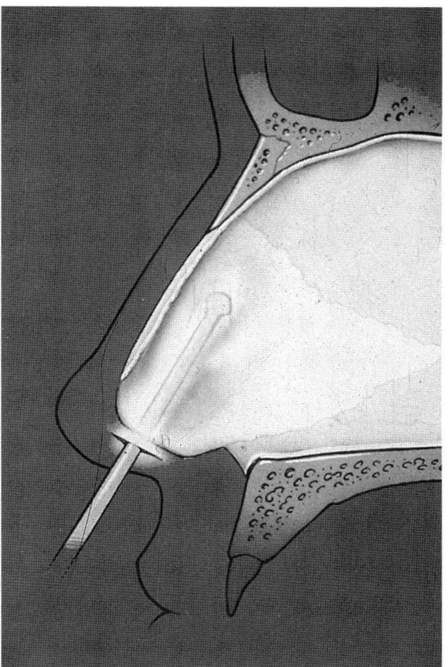

FIGURE 10-4. Submucoperichondrial dissection with Cottle elevator.

nections between these two bones without perforating the lining. Using your Cottle elevator, carefully dissect sharply along the vomerine-cartilaginous junction in a posterior to anterior direction.

Next, progressively remove submucosally small horizontal wedges of cartilage spurs just superior to the vomer to exposing the bony crest along the vomer and premaxilla and allow sharp elevation of the periosteum and perichondrium in continuity. In this way, the premaxilla and vomer are isolated to allow manipulation by either resection or osteotomies without injury to the lining. The dissection is completed to allow submucous resection of the quadrilateral cartilage for use as a graft.

Next, with a No. 15 blade, a full-thickness cut is made 10 mm behind the caudal septum. Angled septal scissors are used to disarticulate the cartilage from its junction with the ethmoid plate, with at least a 10-mm intact dorsal cartilaginous strut left in place (Fig. 10-5). The detached piece of cartilage is removed with a long, straight hemostat. Once the septal cartilage graft and bone have been separated from the perpendicular plate, the periosteum can be elevated and the deviated portions of the ethmoid and vomer bone removed. In this way, any bony interferences that might prevent the cartilage from moving into the midline are removed. With each blade of the speculum protecting the lining on either side of the perpendicular plate of the ethmoid or vomer, deviated portions can be removed with a rongeur. Unless an intrinsic deformity of the septal cartilage or its attachment to the anterior nasal spine is present, the septum should come into the midline. Silastic nasal splints (Xomed) are sutured and stabilized in place anteriorly with 3-0 nylon. No nasal packing is done.

Ear Cartilage

The auricle can provide a large amount of cartilage for rhinoplasty; however, it is flaccid and convoluted. It is reserved as a backup to septal cartilage for specific needs. Ear cartilage is good for reconstructing lower lateral cartilage components and tip grafts, and if properly contoured, it can also serve as a dorsal onlay graft.

Technique

Two methods are available, with the choice dependent on how the ear cartilage graft is to be used. If one needs a graft for lower lateral cartilage or tip only, then an anterior approach is preferred (Fig. 10-6). The incision is made 3 mm inside the conchal bowl for camouflage and to preserve the rim of the conchal bowl. The conchal bowl skin is hyperinflated with 3 mL of 1% lidocaine with epinephrine to ease the dissection plane.

The initial incision is made with a No. 15 blade and a sharp scissor is used to dissect the conchal bowl skin off the perichondrium (Fig. 10-7). Next, a full-thickness cartilage cut is made 3 mm inside the conchal bowl through the posterior perichondrium, and scissors are used to dissect the posterior perichondrium off the postauricular skin. The ear graft harvest is completed by removing the desired ear cartilage with a No. 15 blade (Fig. 10-8). Hemostasis is obtained

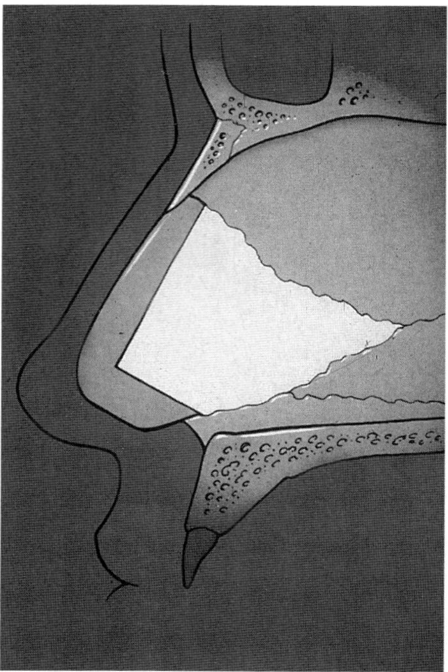

FIGURE 10-5. Retain mm dorsal and caudal septal strut.

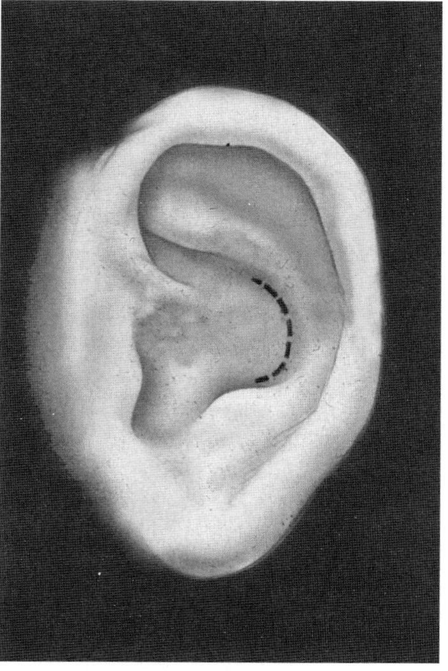

FIGURE 10-6. Incision placed 3 mm inside conchal bowl.

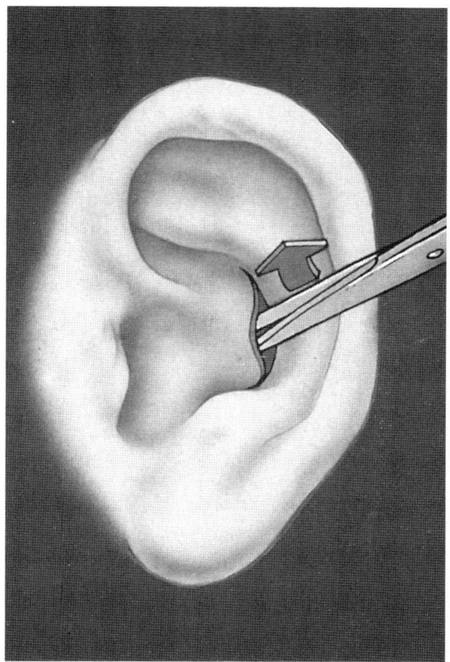

FIGURE 10-7. Anterior dissection.

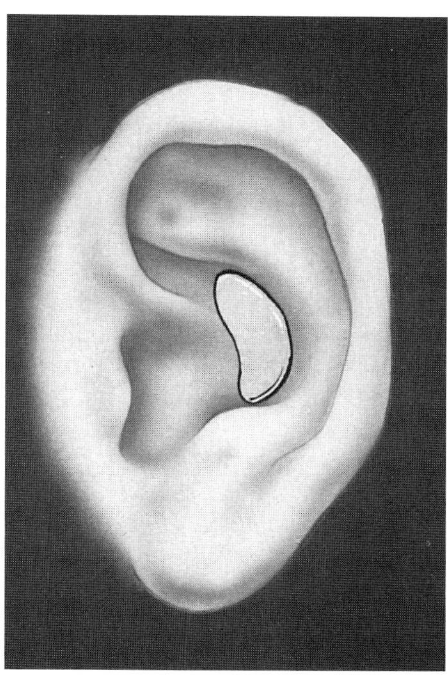

FIGURE 10-8. Conchal bowl harvest sparing vertical height.

and closure accomplished with 5-0 chromic. A through-and-through full-thickness 4-0 chromic suture is run over the length of the dissection to prevent hematoma formation and obviate the need for a bolster.

If one requires a longer piece that may be more malleable, a postauricular incision is used. The postauricular skin is again hyperinflated with 3 mL of 1% lidocaine and epinephrine, and a 3-cm postauricular incision is made through skin only. The entire posterior subcutaneous soft tissue and perichondrium are preserved and harvested as a unit with the postauricular conchal bowl. Again, 3 mm of the conchal bowl rim is preserved to maintain the integrity of the ear. Next, the skin is dissected to the postauricular groove. A No. 15 blade is used to create a full-thickness cut 3 mm behind the conchal bowl, and the anterior dissection is completed with a sharp scissor. The ear graft resection is completed with another full-thickness incision through the inner conchal bowl, with care taken not to perforate the skin of the anterior conchal bowl. Hemostasis is obtained and the closure performed with 5-0 chromic. A cotton/Xeroform tie-on bolster is applied, as previously described.

Rib Cartilage

Rib cartilage is excellent when support is a primary consideration. Rib cartilage has no blood vessels and receives its nourishment via tissue fluid diffusion. This property allows the cartilage autograft to adjust to almost any environment because the chondrocytes survive as living cells that maintain their surrounding matrix. Once transferred as a free graft, autogenous cartilage undergoes no metaplastic changes. Hyaline matrix remains hyaline; thus, rib cartilage remains firm upon being transferred. Autogenous rib cartilage is unaffected by functional stress and can be contoured into any desired shape, retaining both form and bulk if basic surgical principles are followed.

Rib cartilage grafts have been used to provide nasal support and to correct major saddle nose deformities. The grafts must be fashioned to comply with Gibson's principles of balanced cross-sectional carving (Fig. 10-9). Stresses built within rib cartilage, like those within septal cartilage, necessitate careful sculpting to prevent undesirable warping.

Costal cartilage autografts survive satisfactorily, do not require contact with the nasal bony framework (a requirement of bone grafts), and are specifically indicated when such contact cannot be established (37).

Technique

The optimal site for harvesting rib cartilage is the lower chest wall, specifically the anterior medial synchondrosis of rib cartilages 7, 8, and 9 (Figs. 10-10 and 10-11). The lower ribs are marked on the chest wall after palpation of the appropriate rib to be harvested.

A 2-cm incision is made anteriorly and laterally, depending on the type of cartilage (usually from rib 8) to be harvested (Fig. 10-7). The chest wall skin is very mobile, so that one can expose and harvest a large amount of cartilage through a small, 2-cm incision with good lighting and retraction. The ease of accessibility allows for ample harvest-

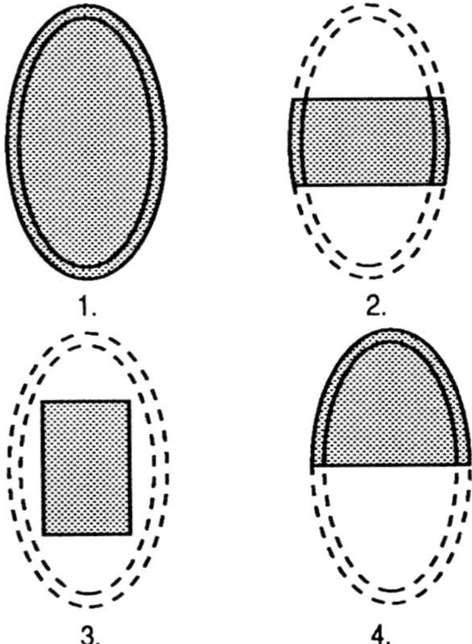

FIGURE 10-9. Gibson principles of balanced cross-sectional carving.

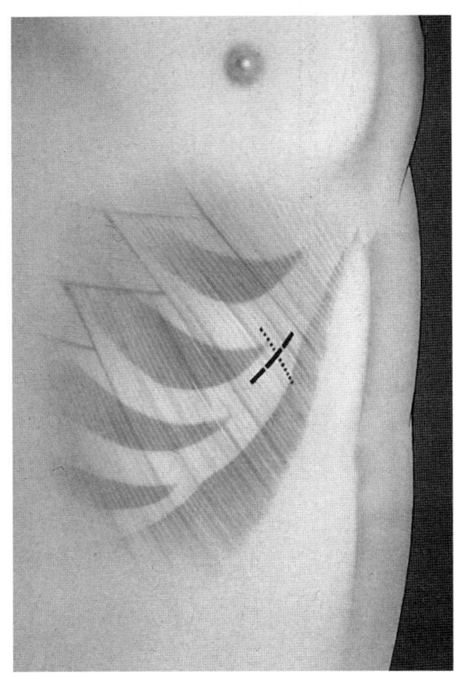

FIGURE 10-10. Optimal incision for rib harvest—2 cm over ribs 7, 8, and 9.

ing of cartilage (Fig. 10-8). The perichondrium is dissected out meticulously with a dental elevator and a Joseph elevator used alternately. Care is taken to prevent a pneumothorax. The desired amount of cartilage is then taken.

After meticulous hemostasis has been obtained and the cartilage enucleated, the perichondrium is closed it has been determined that no pneumothorax is present. Usually, no drain is placed. Closure of the wound in layers with deep suture is followed by subcenticular skin closure. Steri-strips are applied. Injection of 0.25% Marcaine into the area around the site and an intercostal area above and below the incision site provides prolonged postoperative analgesia and prevents chest wall splinting and subsequent atelectasis.

It is prudent to harvest a slightly larger amount of rib cartilage than is needed. One must keep in mind the principles of Gibson and Davies (34) that rib cartilage must be carved

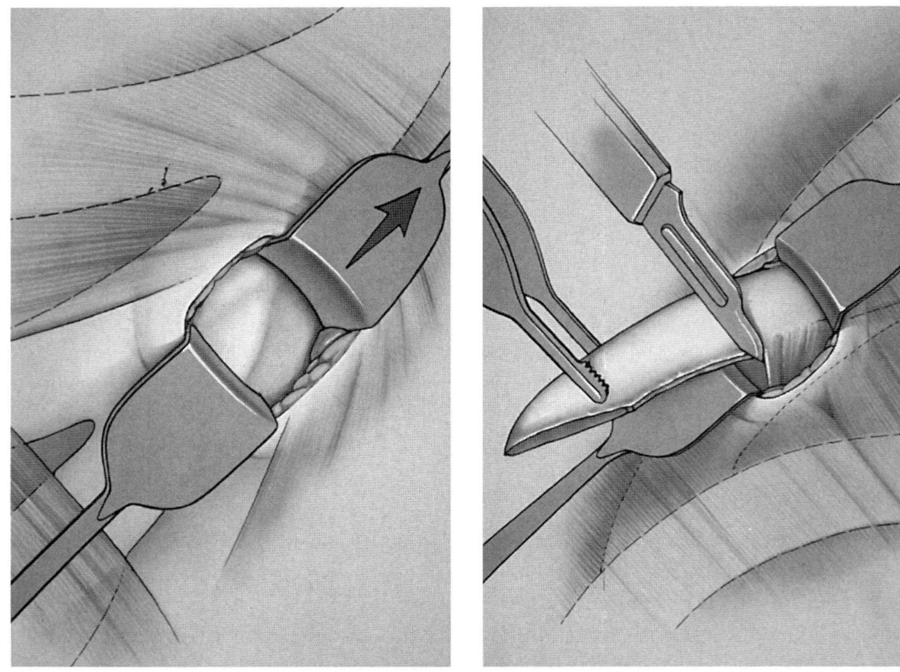

FIGURE 10-11. Rib harvest. Subperichondrial exposure of rib **(A)** and meticulous removal of rib **(B)**.

to remove equal amounts from both sides (balanced cross section) to prevent warping and bending.

End slices of rib cartilage have a tendency to curl and can be used for lower lateral alar replacement of selective onlay grafts. Rib cartilage grafts harvested in this way are ideal for maxillary augmentation, dorsal onlay grafting, tip grafting, and columellar strut. All these cartilage grafts are appropriately contoured and suture-stabilized in place. This is usually done in an open approach to rhinoplasty.

The ninth rib alone is often ideal because it offers a long, relatively straight segment of bone and cartilage and is wrapped in perichondrium, so that warping is minimized and survival enhanced. It is harvested in a similar fashion.

Key points

1. We have presented three specific techniques to obtain ample cartilage for rhinoplasty or other reconstructive procedures, specifically when a large amount of autogenous support tissue is required.
2. Autogenous cartilage grafts can be used with minimal resorption and good long-term success.

FASCIAL GRAFTS

Since the early 1900s, fascial grafts have been recognized as a useful adjunct in reconstructive surgery. We will limit our discussion of fascial grafts to critical data and common uses.

Fascial grafts are unique, particularly in comparison with fat grafts, in that they retain their underlying structure once grafted. Peer (38) performed an extensive examination of fascial grafts and demonstrated microscopically that cells present in long-standing fascial grafts are the same cells that were originally grafted. Furthermore, fascial grafts do not elicit the inflammatory responses or encapsulation typically seen with fat grafting (38,39). Many favorable outcomes with the use of fascial grafts for facial and nasal reconstructive procedures have been reported (39,40). The primary donor sites for fascial grafts include the tensor fasciae latae and the deep temporal fascia. Miller (39) examined temporalis fascial grafts for facial and nasal contour augmentation. He found temporalis fascia to be a better donor site than the tensor fasciae latae, providing ease of harvesting under local anesthesia, maintenance of a single operative field, minimal postoperative discomfort, and a hidden donor site scar within hair-bearing tissue. Furthermore, biopsy specimens taken from these grafts at 3 to 4 months demonstrated no inflammatory response or encapsulation. He found that the grafts maintained the "characteristic sheen of fascia." He did note compaction of the collagen, fibers, and fibrous tissue, consistent with previous reports (38). This compaction is felt to occur during the first 4 to 6 weeks and may result in up to a 20% shrinkage of the graft volume. For this reason, slight overcorrection should be obtained when fascial grafts are used to treat small contour deformities.

Guerrerosantos (41) has shown good results with cartilage grafts wrapped or covered by fascia grafts in secondary rhinoplasty. Of note, partial fascia resorption was seen in approximately 10% of these cases; however, this occurred in secondary and tertiary rhinoplasties, where scarring was extensive and vascularization of the graft bed less than optimal. A similarly positive experience with the use of temporalis fascial grafts in open secondary rhinoplasty, especially in thin-skinned patients, has been reported (40).

The use of tensor fasciae latae or temporalis fascial grafts as a facial sling in the treatment of facial paralysis has been advocated. Because of its excellent tensile strength, long-term viability, and lack of an associated inflammatory response, this graft is optimal for facial sling procedures. Furthermore, because encapsulation is absent, the fascia is easily identified during reoperative surgery, so that secondary corrections through readvancement are possible.

Key Points

1. Fascial grafts are an excellent adjunct in the treatment of small contour deformities of the face and nose and in facial sling procedures.
2. Donor site morbidity is less with use of the temporalis fascia.
3. Data support good viability of fascial grafts without any inflammatory response or encapsulation; however, the fascia does undergo compaction, which can result in volume shrinkage of up to 20%.

CONCLUSIONS

Free grafts of autogenous fat, dermis, cartilage, and fascia are a useful adjunct to the plastic surgeon. They can be used to optimize results in primary operations or to correct deformities in secondary procedures. Ideally, plastic surgeons should be familiar with all these techniques, including the indications and optimal circumstances for each method.

ACKNOWLEDGMENT

We acknowledge the excellent assistance of Frank Saporito, second year medical student, University of Texas Southwestern Medical School, in the preparation of this article.

REFERENCES

1. Mordick TG, Larossa D, Whitaker L. Soft-tissue reconstruction of the face: a comparison of dermal-fat grafting and vascularized tissue transfer. *Ann Plast Surg* 1992;29:390–396.

2. Billings E, May JW. Historical review and present status of free fat graft autotransplantation in plastic and reconstructive surgery. *Plast Reconstr Surg* 1989;83:368–381.
3. Neuber G. Asepsis und kunstliche Blutleere. *Verh Dtsch Ges Chir f (Berl)* 1910;22:159.
4. Lexer E. Fatty tissue transplantation. In: *Die Transplantationen,* part 1. Stuttgart: Ferdinand Enke, 1919:265,273, 282–302, 311, 543.
5. Peer MA. Loss of weight and volume in human fat grafts. *Plast Reconstr Surg* 1950;5:217–230.
6. Ellenbogen R. Free autogenous pearl grafts in the face: a preliminary report of a rediscovered technique. *Ann Plast Surg* 1986;16:179–193.
7. Adams WP Jr, Trott S, Robinson JB Jr. Personal communication, 1998.
8. Illouz YG. The fat cell "graft": a new technique to fill depressions [Letter]. *Plast Reconstr Surg* 1986;78:122–123.
9. Niechajev I, Sevcuk O. Long-term results of fat transplantation: clinical and histological studies. *Plast Reconstr Surg* 1994;94:496–506.
10. Pinski KS, Roenigk HH. Autologous fat transplantation: long-term follow-up. *J Dermatol Surg Oncol* 1992;18:179–184.
11. Asken S. Microliposuction and autologous fat transplantation for aesthetic enhancement of the aging face. *J Dermatol Surg Oncol* 1990;16:965–972.
12. Asken S. Facial liposuction and microlipoinjection. *J Dermatol Surg Oncol* 1988;14:297–305.
13. Chajchir A, Benzaquen I. Fat-grafting injection for soft-tissue augmentation. *Plast Reconstr Surg* 1989;84:921–934.
14. Nguyen A, Pasyk KA, Bouvier TN, et al. Comparative study of survival of autologous adipose tissue taken and transplanted by different techniques. *Plast Reconstr Surg* 1990;85:378–386.
15. Carraway JH, Mellow CG. Syringe aspiration and fat concentration: a simple technique for autologous fat injection. *Ann Plast Surg* 1990;24:293–296.
16. Ersek RA, Chang P, Salisbury MA. Lipo layering of autologous fat: an improved technique with promising results. *Plast Reconstr Surg* 1998;101:820–826.
17. Coleman SR. Facial recontouring with lipostructure. *Clin Plast Surg* 1997;24:347–367.
18. Guerrerosantos J. Autologous fat grafting for body contouring. *Clin Plast Surg* 1996;23:619–631.
19. Coleman SR. Long-term survival of fat transplants: controlled demonstrations. *Aesthetic Plast Surg* 1995;19:421–425.
20. Feinendegen DL, Baumgartner RW, Vuadens P, et al. Autologous fat injection for soft tissue augmentation in the face: a safe procedure? *Aesthetic Plast Surg* 1998;22:163–167.
21. Lee DH, Yang HN, Kim JC et al. Sudden unilateral visual loss and brain infarction after autologous fat injection into nasolabial groove. *Br J Ophthalmol* 1996;80:1026–1027.
22. Teimourian B. Blindness following fat injections [Letter]. *Plast Reconstr Surg* 1988;82:361.
23. Bames HO. Augmentation mammoplasty by lipo-transplant. *Plast Reconstr Surg* 1953;11:404–413.
24. Peer MA. The neglected free fat graft. *Plast Reconstr Surg* 1956;18:233–250.
25. Watson MA. Some observations on free fat grafts: with reference to their use in mammoplasty. *Br J Plast Surg* 1959;12:263–274.
26. Sawhney CP, Banerjee TN, Chakravarti RN. Behaviour of dermal fat transplants. *Br J Plast Surg* 1969;22:169–176.
27. Mackay DR, Manders EK, Saggers GC, et al. The fate of dermal and dermal-fat grafts. *Ann Plast Surg* 1993;131:42–46.
28. Reich J. The application of dermis grafts in deformities of the nose. *Plast Reconstr Surg* 1983;71:772–781.
29. Stoll DA, Furnas DW. The growth of cartilage transplants in baby rabbits. *Plast Reconstr Surg* 1970;45:356–359.
30. Tanzer RC. Microtia: a long-term follow-up of 44 reconstructed auricles. *Plast Reconstr Surg* 1978;61:161–166.
31. Brebt B. Total auricular reconstruction with sculpted costal cartilage. In: Brent B, ed. *The artistry of reconstructive surgery.* St. Louis: Mosby, 1987:113–127.
32. Sheen JH. *Aesthetic rhinoplasty,* 2nd ed. St. Louis: Mosby, 1987.
33. Dupertuis SM. Actual growth of young cartilage transplants in rabbits. *Arch Surg* 1941:43:32.
34. Gibson T, Davies WB. The distortion of autologous cartilage grafts: its cause and prevention. *Br J Plast Surg* 1958;10:257.
35. Adams WP Jr, Gunter JP, Rohrich RJ, et al. The role of irradiation in rib cartilage warping: a controlled comparison and clinical implications. *Plast Reconstr Surg* 1999;103:265–270.
36. Peer LA. Cartilage grafting. *Br J Plast Surg* 1955;7:250.
37. Chase S, Herndon C. The fate of autogenous and homogenous bone grafts: a historical review. *J Bone Joint Surg* 1955;37A:809.
38. Peer L. *Transplantation of tissues.* Baltimore: Williams & Wilkins, 1955.
39. Miller T. Temporalis fascia grafts for facial and nasal contour augmentation. *Plast Reconstr Surg* 1988;81:524–533.
40. Baker TM, Courtis EH. Temporalis fascia grafts in open secondary rhinoplasty. *Plast Reconstr Surg* 1994;93:802–810.
41. Guerrerosantos J. Temporoparietal free fascia grafts to the nose. *Plast Reconstr Surg* 1985;76:328–332.

Discussion

AUTOGENOUS TISSUE TRANSFER: FAT, DERMIS, CARTILAGE, FASCIA

JOSE GUERREROSANTOS

I read this chapter on autologous tissue transfer with great interest. Autologous grafts remain within the focus of my plastic surgical activities because, at the present time, no substitute for autologous material is widely accepted as ideal. Drs. Rohrich and Adams present an excellent review of some of the more common uses of autologous grafts. Many data have been collected and reported. The chapter raises some important issues, which I would like to address.

A plastic surgeon who undertakes to perform body contour augmentation or modification accurately plans each individual case and considers every anatomic zone. Whenever I apply new material to a specific anatomic region with thin-layered soft tissues, such as the nose and ears, I personally prefer to use autologous grafts and refuse to use implants. I use the latter only when they are to be introduced into anatomic areas of thick-layered soft tissue in which they will be totally covered, such as the chin and the malar and mammary regions. Implant extrusions are very frequent on the nose and ears during the early postoperative period, and sometimes even several months or years after the surgery.

I present my comments on the use of autologous grafts as described by Rohrich and Adams, keeping in mind the fact that nonvascularized grafts are indicated for mild or moderate defects with adequate bed vascularity.

FAT GRAFTS

Fat transplantation can be divided into two historical stages: the first before the introduction of liposuction, when big or small pieces of fat were grafted, and the second after the introduction of liposuction and lipoinjection.

I personally agree with the four principles on which this type of transplant is based, as follows: (a) To guarantee the long-term survival of a fat transplant, as stated by Nueber in 1983 (1), long before the liposuction era, the fat tissue has to be applied in small pieces or, at present, injected as thin rolls to maintain the viability of the grafted tissue by means of good vascularity and blood flow and thus good cell nourishment. (b) Therefore, the grafted material must be placed or injected into a well-vascularized anatomic area. (c) Trauma must be reduced to a minimum during harvesting and preparation of the fat to be transplanted (2). (d) The tissue transplant must be homogeneous (3). Any impurities, such as local anesthetic, oil, and blood, must be removed, and the exact amount to be applied must be determined. Following these principles guaranteed predictable fat transplant results, so that overcorrections were unnecessary. Through late December 1999, we saw at the Jalisco Institute for Reconstructive Plastic Surgery and the Guerrerosantos Clinic a total of 2,428 patients who underwent fat transplants, of whom 1,936 had facial, palate, and pharyngeal contour augmentation. These statistics helped us ensure that well-harvested, well-prepared, and appropriately positioned fat transplants would last for a long time.

Some technical recommendations follow: (a) We perform fat harvesting with manual maneuvers and use No. 14 needles and 10-mL syringes. We avoid using the suction machine because we feel that the fat cells may be subjected to trauma: (b) Fat tissue can be washed with saline solution for cleansing (3). (c) Before injecting fat, we draw back on the syringe to prevent the intraarterial or intravenous injection of a bolus of fat, which can result in a fat embolism. (d) We strongly recommend injecting the fat during horizontal maneuvers on the face to avoid injuries to the branches of the facial nerve, facial arteries and veins, and parotid duct. (e) Spreading and molding of the fat to obtain an adequate contour is accomplished by kneading and rolling the skin, as one would do when modeling clay with digital pressure. (f) After the injection, the area is massaged gently to help disperse the fat. (g) Care must be taken that the deposition is accurate. (h) Overcorrections should be avoided. (i) The simplicity of this method permits repetition of the procedure if desired. (j) I recommend waiting 6 months if additional volume is necessary.

Some authors have advocated the use of certain substances presumptively to promote fat transplant integration under better conditions. Such substances include insulin and vitamin E. Some authors also advocate utilizing emerging approaches to the tissue engineering of fat, which are complex and quite expensive procedures (4–7). In my

J. Guerrerosantos: Division of Plastic Surgery, University of Guadalajara; and The Valisco Plastic Surgery Institute, Guadalajara, Jalisco, Mexico

opinion, fat transplantation is a very simple, inexpensive, and safe surgical procedure, and the great majority of patients have an unlimited source of fat tissue available for transfer to other areas of the body. I think tissue engineering of fat should be utilized only in patients who are extremely thin, in whom the harvesting of fat grafts is extremely difficult; it should not be used in routine cases.

The following case illustrates long-term survival of a fat transplant.

Sequelae of Facial Paralysis

Fat autografting is an extremely good alternative for the aesthetic improvement of faces with sequelae of facial paralysis. In paralyzed faces, when a striated muscle fiber loses its motor innervation, profound changes occur, with a progressive decrease in fiber size from 50% to 80%. Augmenting facial contour to thicken soft tissues, especially the muscles, is mandatory, and placement of fat grafts is one solution. A patient presented for consultation at the age of 25 years with sequelae of facial palsy after having suffered an acute episode of Bell's paralysis 5 years previously (Fig. 10D-1A). The entire left side of the face was compromised, and all facial expressions were drawn toward the right side. Considerable atrophy marked the left half of the face. After a meticulous study of this case, we designed a facial rehabilitation plan with suspension dermal flaps for the left side of the face, plus a segmental rhytidoplasty and lipoinjection. To reduce muscle traction on the

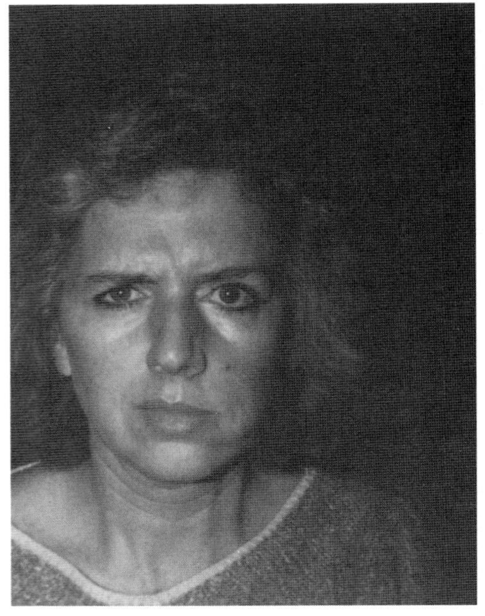

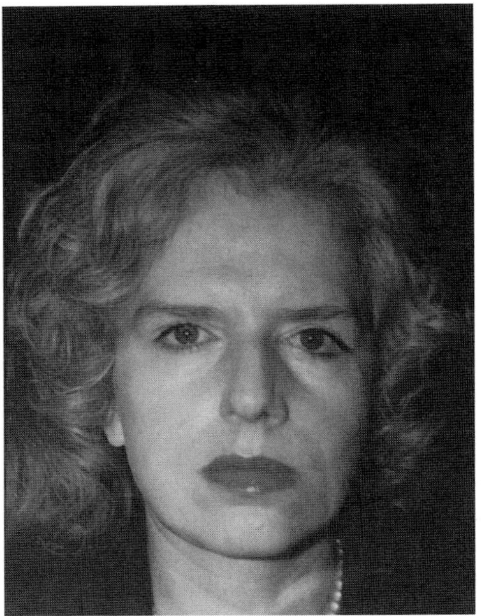

FIGURE 10D-1. A 25-year-old female patient with sequelae of facial palsy and considerable atrophy of the left half of the face. **A:** Preoperative condition. **B,C:** Patient 6 years after initial treatment. *(continued)*

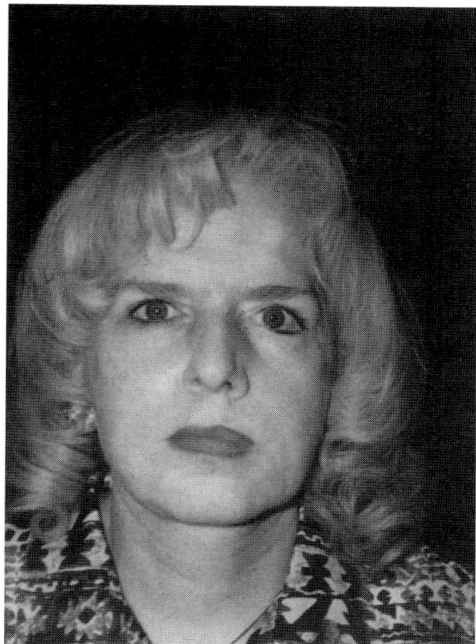

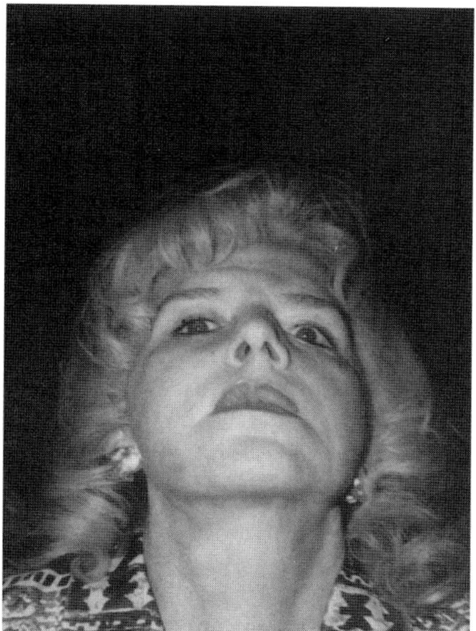

FIGURE 10D-1. *Continued* **D,E:** Patient 12 years after first lipoinjection session and 4 years after second lipoinjection session.

right side, we planned myotomies of the quadratus labii superioris, zygomaticus, and quadratus labii inferioris muscles through an incision on the melolabial sulcus. The complete surgical procedure was planned to achieve an improvement in facial symmetry. The right muscular traction was largely relieved by the myotomies, and the applied lipoinjection enhanced the facial contour, considering the previous soft tissue atrophy on the left facial side. On the left side of the face, 8 mL of fat was injected on the cheek, and 3 mL on the upper lip and melolabial sulcus. On the right side of the face, 2 mL was placed on the buccal fat pad compartment, 1 mL on the melolabial sulcus, and 1 mL on the upper lip. After 6 years of follow-up, we could observe a persistently augmented facial contour after long-term survival of the injected fat tissue (Fig. 10D-1B,C). Eight years after the initial lipoinjection session, a second fat infiltration was performed to apply 2 mL on the left cheek, 1 mL on the left side of the upper lip, and 2 mL on the right cheek. Follow-up 4 years after the second lipoinjection session showed a good contour of her face (12 years after the initiation of treatment) (Fig. 10D-1-D,E).

DERMAL-FAT GRAFTS

In my surgical practice, I successfully use dermal-fat grafts to correct facial depressions. Zarem (8) pointed out some years ago that integration failure with this type of graft is a consequence of the use of thick dermal-fat grafts by most surgeons to achieve an aesthetic contour correction of facial depressions. As a result, the center of the graft, because of poor nourishment, becomes fibrotic. The loss of fat tissue is aesthetically detrimental, and therefore he recommended that dermal-fat grafts have a maximum thickness of 3 mm. Ever since then, we have used dermal-fat grafts no thicker than those described by Zarem, and we have had very good results correcting facial depressions that were sequelae of Parry-Romberg's disease and craniofacial microsomia. Especially in Parry-Romberg's disease, in which tissue nourishment is usually poor, we use them in conjunction with a galeal pedicle flap, which improves vascularity in the affected area and produces the best possible aesthetic result. If the depression is very deep, we employ bone and cartilage grafts, and as a routine procedure, we include lipoinjection of the deep soft tissues and galeal flap. With this technique, we have not yet observed any fibrosis nor any net reduction in graft volume. I prefer placing the grafts with the dermis facing up in direct contact with the galeal flap, which then receives excellent nourishment and yields a smooth surface. This is not the case if the fat of the graft is facing the skin.

DERMAL GRAFTS

I learned from Reich (9,10) how to use dermal grafts for nasal reconstruction, and I consider this to be a useful procedure. However, I now use fascia as nasal filling. I occasionally still use dermal micrografts (11) to fill up other soft tissue depressions.

CARTILAGE GRAFTS

Rohrich and Adams have done a magnificent job of reviewing the use of cartilage grafts, and I can hardly add anything else, so I will just point out my technical preferences regarding this superb autologous material. For aesthetic rhinoplasty, to enhance the shape and projection of the nasal tip, I prefer using a combined septal, alar, and concha cartilage graft. Septal cartilage is my first choice in combination with alar cartilage if the quantity is sufficient for the procedure, but if not, I then harvest cartilage from the auricular concha and use a procedure and scheme very similar to those of Gruber and Grover (12). I approach both alar areas and the nasal tip through an open-tip rhinoplasty without skin columella incision technique (13). I use costal cartilage grafts for larger nasal and paranasal reconstructions, congenital anomalies, and sequelae of trauma, and also for complex nasal reconstructions after partial or total amputations resulting from cancer ablation. It is often mentioned that in aesthetic corrections of the nasal dorsum, thin cartilage grafts shrink or lose alignment, especially if a graft harvested from the concha is applied. To prevent this, I recommend

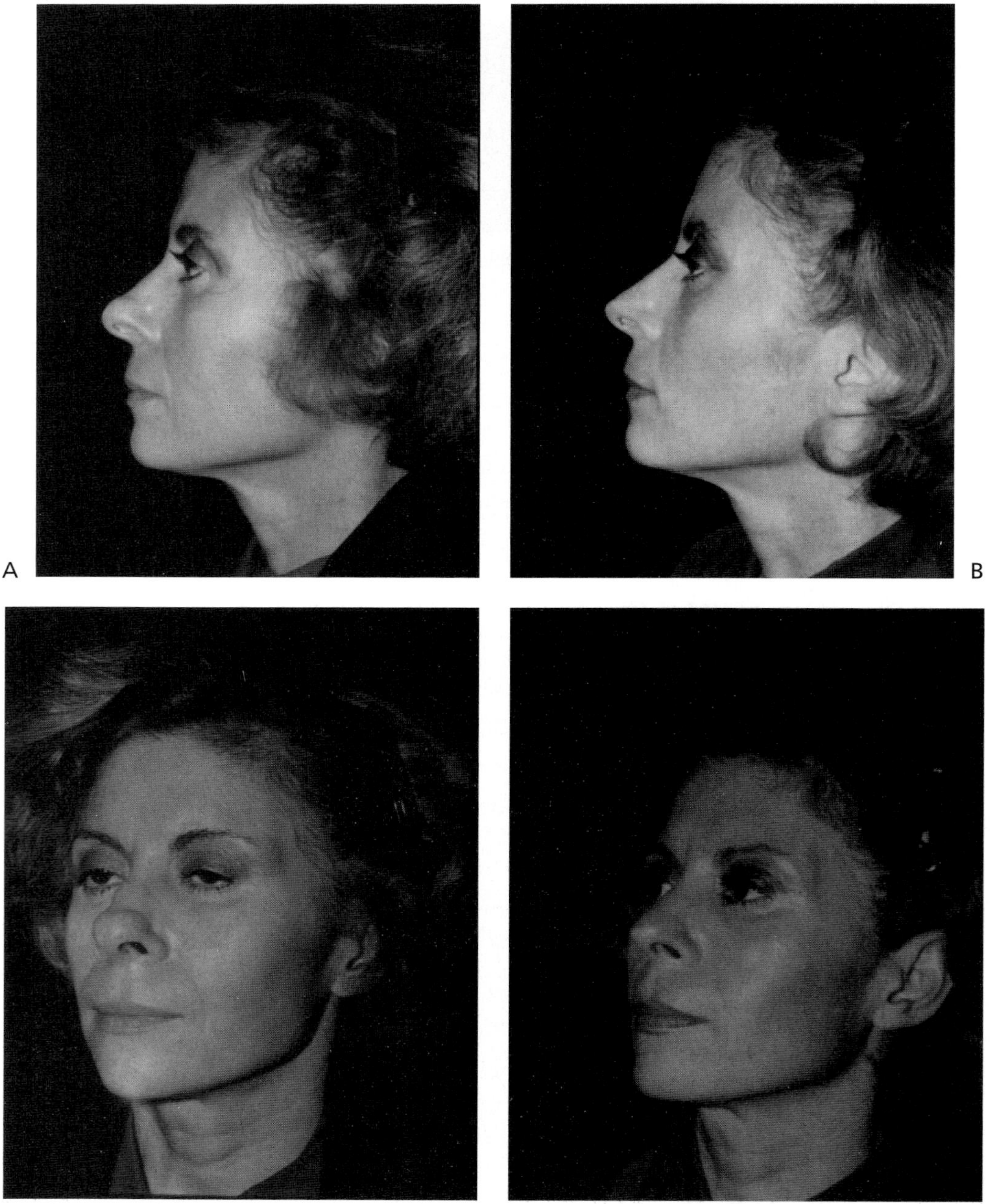

FIGURE 10D-2. Female patient with remarkable bulbous nasal tip resulting from thick and convex alar crura and thin skin. **A,C:** Preoperative condition. **B,D:** Result 2 years after rhinoplasty with cartilage and fascia graft on the tip.

making a straight, tight, and deep nasal dorsum pocket with the use of very narrow instruments, then making short cuttings on the carved cartilage graft, and continuing to wrap it up completely with fascia (14). With this technique, the grafts remain intact without shrinkage or deviation. In another group of patients, after preparing the nasal dorsum as previously explained, we prepared several small pieces of cartilage, which are then wrapped up with fascia and likewise introduced as a combined graft in the nasal dorsum. Excellent aesthetic results can be achieved with this technique, and the grafts are barely visible or palpable.

FASCIAL GRAFT

In 1979, I began to use fascial grafts for nasal reconstruction and presented my first reports in 1984 (14). Then came Miller (15), Baker and Courtiss (16), and Sheen (17), who outlined their experiences with the use of fascial grafts in nasal aesthetic surgery. In his book, Sheen (17) discusses his experience using superficial temporal fascia with disappointing results within 18 months of follow-up. It is important at this point to mention that in my early series 20 years ago, I used superficial temporal fascia in some instances, and

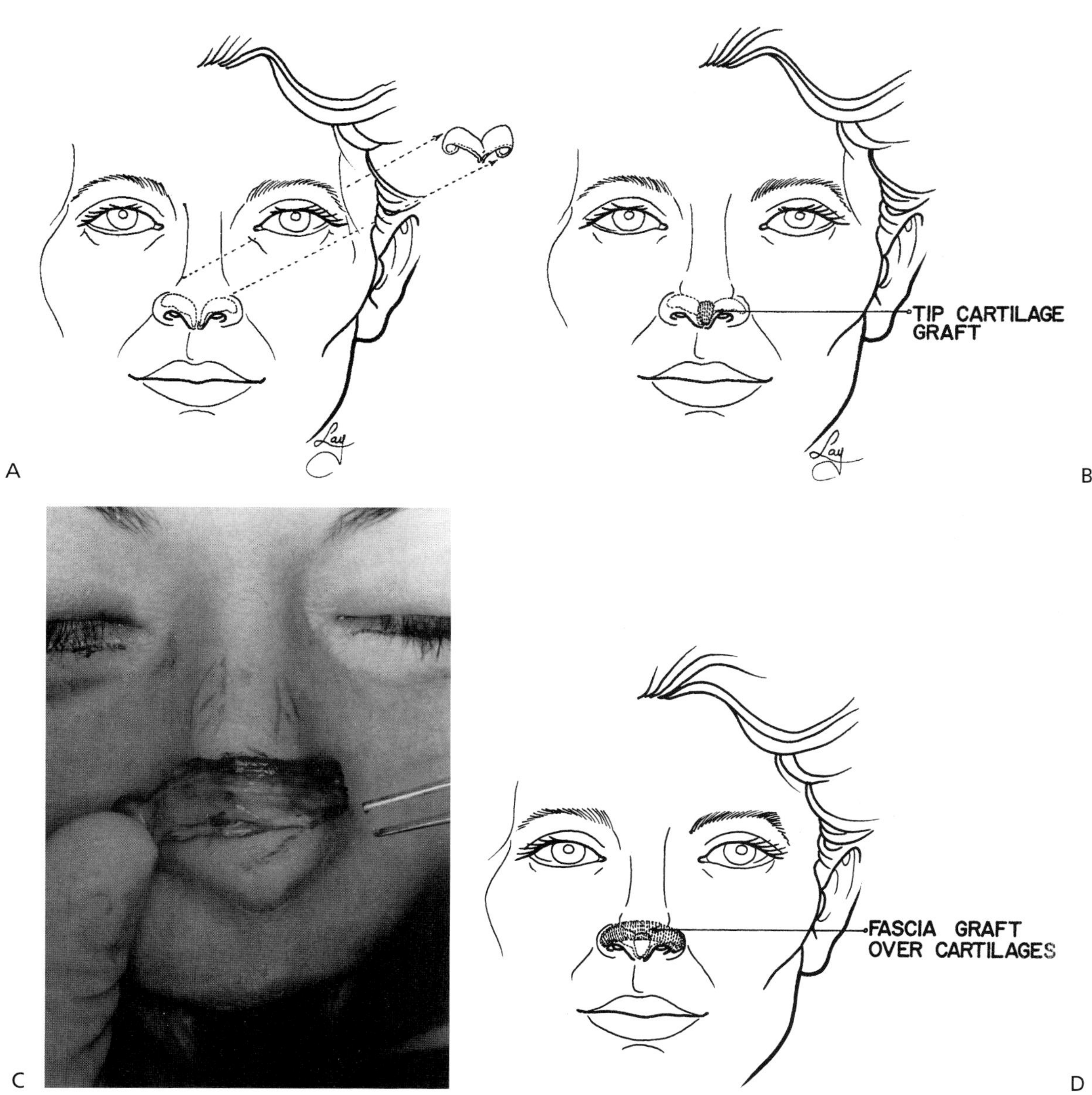

FIGURE 10D-3. Drawings of the surgical procedure utilized for the patient in Fig. 2. **A:** Excision of the excess cephalic lateral crura. **B:** Placement of tip cartilage graft at dome. **C:** Fascial graft before insertion. **D:** Dome, lateral crura, and tip cartilage graft covered by fascia.

in others deep temporal fascia. I should make it very clear, for surgeons who want to wrap fascia over cartilage or bone grafts or just use it for nasal augmentation, that the superficial temporal fascia is always resorbed, whereas deep temporal fascia grafts remain intact indefinitely, as demonstrated by Peer (2) and also by us in our large experience. We have patients at 8, 10, and 15 years of follow-up with excellent permanent integration of fascia. Therefore, with the use of deep temporal fascia, we believe that it is mandatory for the surgeon to identify deep fascia for graft harvests.

I have had the opportunity to treat several hundred of patients with fascial grafts. In cases with sequelae of eyelid palsy or leprosy, I have used fascial slings for reconstruction. In cases with grade 3 palpebral ptosis, I have used them with frontalis muscle adhesion. I have employed them on the nose in several ways: (a) As a single fascial graft for nasal dorsum augmentation, initially with the fascia rolls technique, but lately by creating the receiving pocket on the nasal dorsum and then introducing the fascial strip without curling until the desired augmentation is achieved. (b) Wrapping up cartilage strips with fascia for dorsum augmentation, using from one to four cartilage strips depending on the volume required. (c) Also in dorsum augmentation, using cartilage pieces wrapped up in fascia. (d) Conchal cartilage micropieces covered up with fascia are a great option for augmentation of the paranasal area. I have also used fascia to reduce the nasolabial sulcus, and for labial contour augmentation.

I agree absolutely with Rohrich and Adams that fascial grafts are an excellent adjunct for facial augmentation. To illustrate the advantage of using a fascial graft in patients with thin nasal skin undergoing rhinoplasty, a demonstrative case is included.

A female patient had an extremely bulbous nasal tip (Fig. 10D-2A,C) resulting from large, bulky, excessively thick, and convex alar cartilages, with minimal skin thickness and proportional overprojection. Because of her thin skin, she required precise alar sculpturing with excision of a large portion of the cephalic lateral crura (Fig. 10D-3A), a tip graft (Fig. 10D-3B), and an overlying fascial graft (Fig. 10D-3C,D). The advantage of the fascial graft was to camouflage the cartilage borders of both alar crura and the tip graft. Two years later, the patient had a nice aesthetic result (Fig. 10D-2B,D).

REFERENCES

1. Neuber GA. Fettransplantation. *Chir Kongr Verhandl Deutsch Gesellsch Chir* 1983;22:66.
2. Peer LA. *Transplantation of tissues,* vol 2. Baltimore: Williams & Wilkins, 1955:195–230.
3. Lewis CM. Personal communication, 1984.
4. Eppley BL, Sadove AM. A physicochemical approach to improving free fat grafts survival: preliminary observations. *Aesthetic Plast Surg* 1991;15:215–218.
5. Eppley BL, Sidner RA, Platis JM, et al. Bioactivation of free-fat transfer: a potential new approach to improving graft survival. *Plast Reconstr Surg* 1992;90:1022–1030.
6. Har-Shai Y, Lindenbaum ES, Gamliel-Lazarovich A, et al. An integrated approach for increasing the survival of autologous fat grafts in the treatment of contour defects. *Plast Reconstr Surg* 1999;104:945–954.
7. Katz AJ, Llull R, Hedrick MH, et al. Emerging approaches to the tissue engineering of fat. *Clin Plast Surg* 1999;26:587–603.
8. Zarem HM. Personal communication, 1982.
9. Reich J. Personal communication, 1989.
10. Reich J. The application of dermis graft in deformities of the nose. *Plast Reconstr Surg* 1983;71:772–782.
11. Hinderer UT. Personal communication, 1989.
12. Gruber RP, Grover S. The anatomic tip graft for nasal augmentation. *Plast Reconstr Surg* 1999;103:1744–1753.
13. Guerrerosantos J. Open rhinoplasty without skin-columella incision. *Plast Reconstr Surg* 1990;85:955–960.
14. Guerrerosantos J. Temporoparietal free fascia grafts in rhinoplasty. *Plast Reconstr Surg* 1984;74:465–475.
15. Miller TA. Temporalis fascial grafts. *Plast Reconstr Surg* 1980;65:236–237.
16. Baker TM, Courtiss EH. Temporalis fascia graft in open secondary rhinoplasty. *Plast Reconstr Surg* 1994;93:802–810.
17. Sheen JH. Superficial temporal fascia graft. In: Sheen JH, Sheen A, eds. *Aesthetic rhinoplasty.* St. Louis: Mosby, 1987: 407–417.

SUGGESTED READING

Bircoll M, Novack BH. Autologous fat transplantation employing liposuction techniques. *Ann Plast Surg* 1987;18:32–329.

Guerrerosantos J. Recontouring of the middle third of the face with onlay cartilage plus free fascia graft. *Ann Plast Surg* 1987;18: 409–420.

Guerrerosantos J. Facial grafts in augmentation rhinoplasty. In: Stark RB, ed. *Plastic surgery of the head and neck.* New York: Churchill Livingstone, 1987: 712.

Guerrerosantos J, González MA, López Luque J. Further experience with free temporoparietal fascia grafts in rhinoplasty. *Plast Surg Forum* 1989;12:210.

Guerrerosantos J. Nose and paranasal augmentation: autogenous fascia and cartilage. *Clin Plast Surg* 1991;18:65–86.

Moscona R, Ullman Y, Har-Shai Y, et al. Free-fat injections for the correction of hemifacial atrophy. *Plast Reconstr Surg* 1989;84: 501–507.

11

BONE GRAFTS

MUTAZ B. HABAL

In the past, surgeons considered only the survival of a bone graft to measure the outcome of their procedure and evaluate the final result. Failure of the bone graft to survive was an unfavorable result, interpreted as a technical failure of bone graft surgery. Today, we know more about the pathophysiologic processes involved in bone graft healing and assume that surgeons who perform surgical procedures have mastered the technical aspects of bone graft surgery. We are therefore left to analyze the physiologic processes that affect the survival of a transplanted bone graft. Failure to maintain volume is considered failure to achieve the desired outcome, and survival alone is no longer an indicator of the success or failure of a procedure, or of a favorable or unfavorable result. The result is now equated with the real-time final volume of the transplanted bone graft. Therefore, pharmacologic, mechanical, and genetic manipulation by gene transfer are used to improve the final outcome.

It is imperative in a discussion of the unfavorable result in bone graft surgery to start with an account of the processes underlying bone repair and bone healing. The biologic factors involved in bone healing and repair are similar to the biologic and histopathologic mechanisms involved in bone graft repair. Healing of a bone graft eventually leads to incorporation of the graft and remodeling as the graft blends in with adjacent bone structures. The process of bone repair will shed some light on the scientific information that is being presented. A bone graft is living material and remains as such throughout the life of the receipt site. Sometimes, a bone graft must be removed for various reasons, particularly cancer recurrence. The histologic study of such grafts provides valuable information on reparative processes and presents a good opportunity to study the biologic and mechanical factors involved in the healing and repair of bone grafts and a favorable or unfavorable outcome.

Bone graft surgery is an integral part of the practice of modern plastic surgery. Every plastic surgeon should be adept in the harvesting, application, and fixation of bone grafts. These are the major skills required of a bone graft surgeon. By the turn of the 20th century, surgeons had noted the value of bone grafting in clinical situations, so they directed their attention to the technical aspects of harvesting and applying bone for discontinuity defects. The craniofacial skeleton was studied most closely. The skull was the first part of the human body to be treated and repaired with bone grafts. The earliest repairs were posttraumatic in nature (1). Other parts of the skeleton were then treated with bone grafts—initially for traumatic injury, then defects left by cancer resection, birth defects, and lastly cosmetic problems. Different sets of indications and contraindications exist for each of those categories (2). For the purposes of the discussion in this chapter, an unfavorable result in bone graft surgery is basically a failure of the bone graft to develop as planned by the surgical team. Failure can be attributed to various etiologic factors that may lead to an unfavorable outcome.

HISTORICAL BACKGROUND

Dr. Fred Albee is considered among the few surgeons in the modern era who directed attention to the importance of autologous bone grafts in the total rehabilitation of the patient with skeletal defects. He popularized his techniques during two decades, working in both New York and Florida, where he had to convert a new hotel to a hospital to accommodate all his patients (3). However, more than 100 years before Albee's era, surgeons were attempting to graft bone from different donors and species to acquired skull defects. They attributed bone graft failure in these situations to infection of the application site. Not until the development of modern immunology in the last 30 years did we become more familiar with the rejection phenomenon, on a cellular level for allografts and on a humoral level for xenografts. Thus, a major controversy was removed as we focused on autografts and their applications in the skeletal system (Fig. 11-1). At present, an autograft is considered the ideal bone graft to use in the craniofacial skeleton, and every other material used is compared with the autogenous bone graft. A free bone graft is a bone graft that does not have a vascular pedicle. Survival of the graft depends on the degree and efficiency of the vascularization it can acquire to ensure its permanent survival and incorporation (4).

M. B. Habal: Tampa Bay Craniofacial Center; Department of Material Sciences, University of Florida; and Department of Surgery, University Community Hospital, Tampa, Florida

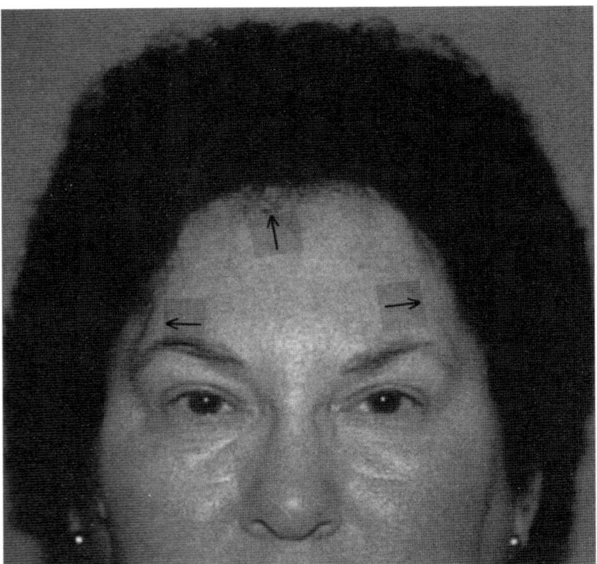

FIGURE 11-1. Patient who had a cranial bone graft fixed to the skull with metallic plates. The contour was adequate, but extrusion of the plates developed, and they had to be removed 5 years after reconstruction.

BONE GRAFT HEALING

The healing of bone grafts depends on two factors. The first is the ability of the bone graft to undergo vascularization. Blood vessels may form in canaliculi already present and connect to the vascular network. This process is more prevalent in dense cortical bone. Alternatively, blood vessels create their own channels, a process referred to as *neovascularization.* Neovascularization is more prevalent in cancellous bone or in bone graft that is structureless, such as slurry or particulate bone (Fig. 11-2). The first process is slow and certain; the second process is fast and unlimited. Both processes depend on the physical structures of the recipient bed and on the hormonal and local environmental milieu in which the bone graft is applied. Abundant vascularity in the craniofacial skeleton is the reason for unlimited success in grafting, whereas the sluggish system of vessels in the lower extremities is the reason for limited success. The second factor is the cellular component of the graft (4), which is still a controversial and uncertain issue. However, it is believed that new pluripotent cells and stem cells arrive at the bone graft site via the circulation and undergo transformation into bone-forming cells, osteoblasts and osteocytes, to maintain the volume of the bone graft and ensure survival (5). Multiple other elements play a role in graft healing, such as the bone matrix, cytokines, hormones, and generated nutrients (6). Cytokines play a major role in bone graft healing. However, they must be generated *de novo* in the wound by cellular elements and cannot be added to the bone graft to produce a "jump start" (7). To date, no definable system can enhance or accelerate the natural processes of bone graft incorporation. For a favorable outcome, natural processes must be allowed to take their course without alteration. Then, adhering to technique and following principles become imperative in achieving a favorable outcome. The denser the bone, the slower are vascularization, healing, incorporation, and eventual adaptation. The structure of dense bone is better able to withstand mechanical forces. The less dense the bone, the faster are vascularization, incorporation, and adaptation. Volume retention is also better. Because mechanical forces are less well tolerated, external augmentations may be necessary (4).

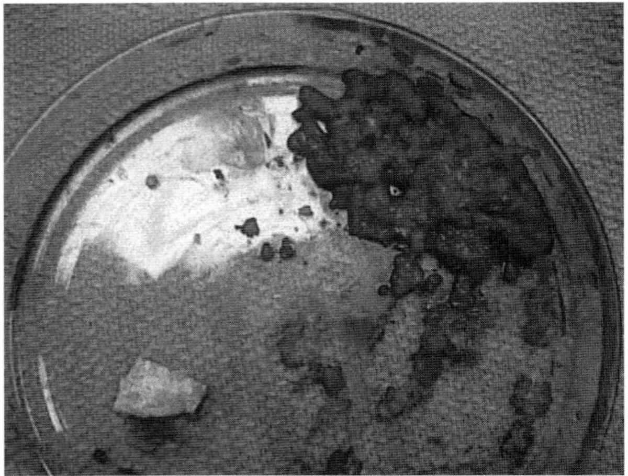

FIGURE 11-2. Corticocancellous bone graft. This bone does not have any mechanical structure and is best used to support or fill a static defect.

ANATOMIC SITES FOR BONE GRAFTS

The main anatomic site for a successful bone graft is the bony skeleton. The site chosen depends on the familiarity of the surgeon with the harvesting process from various sites and the associated morbidity. The harvesting sites are not diseased; therefore, it is imperative to preserve them to achieve a successful clinical outcome. It is important to stress that the harvesting of a bone graft and its healing are not site-dependent. To heal, the bone graft must be autogenous, able to undergo vascularization, and totally covered by soft tissue to avoid extrusion and infection. Multiple surveys have shown that at present, autologous bone grafts are used about 95% of the time (Fig. 11-3). Still in limited use are bone allografts and, even less frequently, bone xenografts (8). The use of allografts is recommended for certain aspects of ablative surgery (9). The lack of enthusiasm for allografts is related to our understanding of the immunologic mechanism of rejection (10). Bone can be harvested from any site on the human skeleton. However,

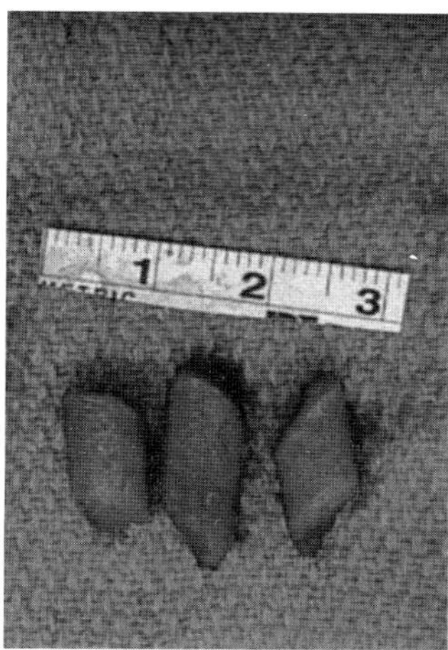

FIGURE 11-3. Bicortical autologous bone graft from the hip removed by a semipercutaneous incision.

today the most popular sites include the skull, maxilla, ribs, ilium, and tibial plateau (Fig. 11-4). The techniques for harvesting are conventional and have not changed much since first described (11). Morbidity is the main reason for research into the development of bone substitutes, and the impetus for the development of new forms in surgical research (12). It is important to understand repair by regeneration before unfavorable outcomes in the use of bone grafts are outlined (13). Bone grafts eventually must be replaced by the regeneration of new bone as the old graft acts as a strut for new bone (14).

In the following sections, unfavorable outcomes are divided into two categories—major and minor, or serious and not serious. These categories are related to the outcome of bone grafts. Serious, unfavorable outcomes may result in the loss of a bone graft, whereas nonserious, unfavorable outcomes are related to donor site morbidity and therefore have a minimal effect on the outcome of a bone graft (Fig. 11-5).

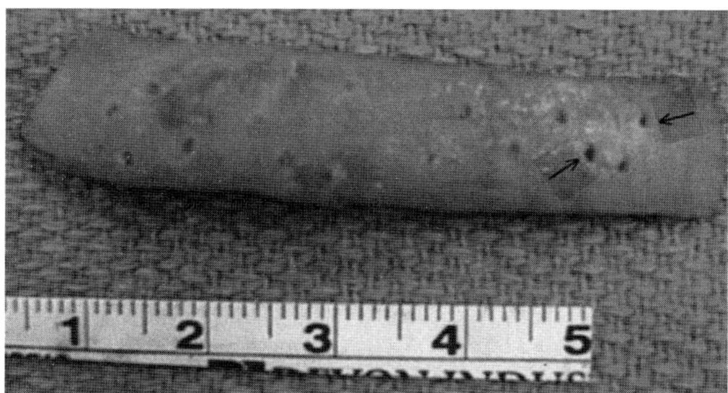

FIGURE 11-4. Rib bone graft. Note the fenestrations to enhance vascularization of the graft for a faster incorporation.

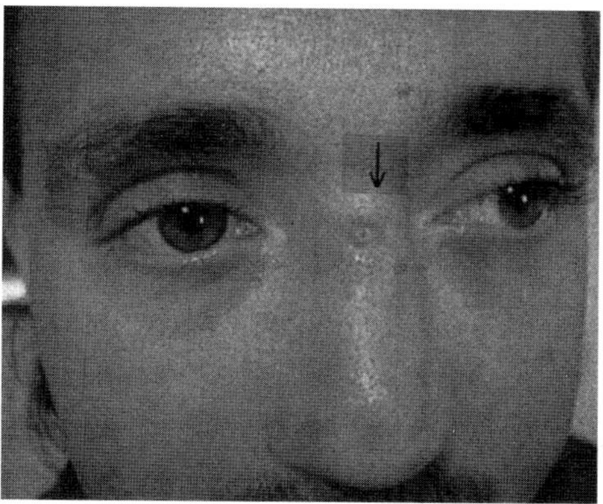

FIGURE 11-5. A nose 7 years after reconstruction with a bone graft. The skin breakdown was caused by the fixation screw.

MAJOR UNFAVORABLE OUTCOMES

Unfavorable outcomes take numerous forms, which are listed in Table 11-1. They may be intrinsic, inherent to the bone graft itself, or extrinsic, related to the site where the bone graft is embedded. The first unfavorable outcome, which is frequently seen, is incorrect placement of a bone graft, which results in a major distortion of the area to be reconstructed (Fig. 11-5). The bone graft in these situations may have to be removed, or the patient may have to undergo a second operation to correct the unfavorable result. The most common cause of this problem is lack of familiarity on the part of the treating surgeon with the intricacies of bone grafting. Another cause may be inadequate contouring of a bone graft to fit the defect. Sometimes, excessive enthusiasm about a procedure can result in such an outcome. An example of the latter is the use of cranial bone grafts. Certain defects do not lend themselves to bone grafting, and the biologic nature of these grafts is such that they cannot be contoured. Unfavorable outcomes decrease with time as the improved skill and clinical judgment of surgeons is coupled with a reduced enthusiasm for a new and less effective procedure.

A second unfavorable outcome is extrusion of a bone graft. The most common cause of such an outcome is re-

TABLE 11-1. UNFAVORABLE RESULTS IN AUTOLOGOUS BONE GRAFTS SURGERY

	Cranial	Rib	Hip	Tibia
Poor fit	±	±	–	–
Mismatch	+/–	+	±	–
Mechanical	+++	+	+	+
Resorption	+	+	+	–
Incorporation	+	+	+	+
Rejection	–	–	–	–
Extrusion	–	±		±
Infection	±	±	±	±
Donor morbidity	+	+	++	+++

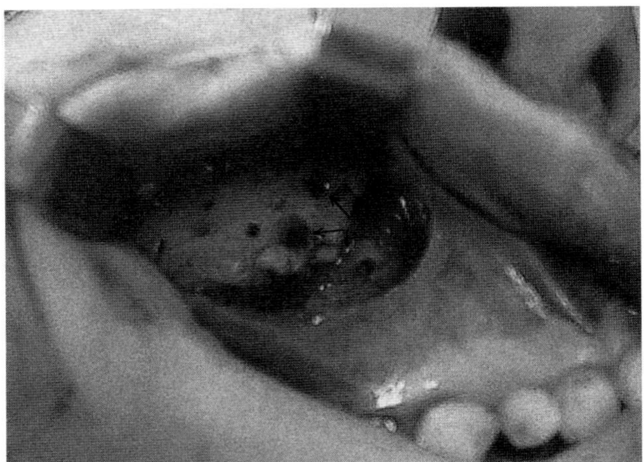

FIGURE 11-6. Bone graft to the maxilla in a youngster. The bone graft was fixed with absorbable screws.

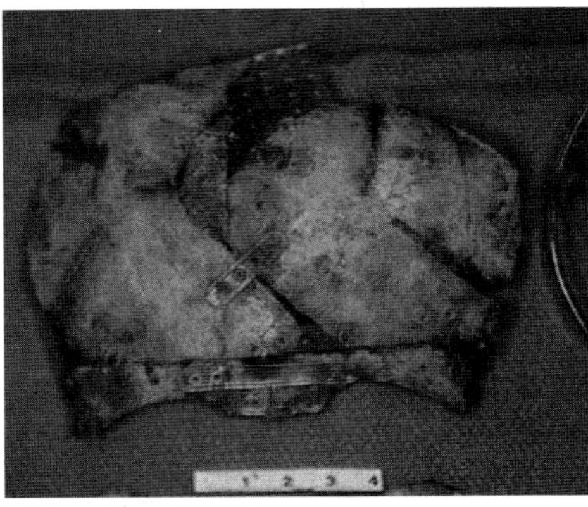

FIGURE 11-7. Cranial bone removed for reshaping. It will be returned to that location and will undergo the same processes as an orthotopic bone graft.

lated to a discrepancy between the defect to be corrected with the bone graft and the size of the bone graft to be used. The problem with a free bone graft is that once it is exposed to the external environment outside the body, it is doomed to failure unless it is salvaged very quickly. Salvage includes the restoration of coverage with soft tissue or a reduction in the size of the bone graft. These problems lead to an unfavorable outcome, particularly if the whole graft has to be removed. However, careful management of the problem may lead to an acceptable result and salvage, so that the unfavorable eventual outcome can be avoided.

Another bone graft problem that may lead to an unfavorable outcome is migration of the bone to a different site. This problem is related to a lack of familiarity of the treating surgeon with bone fixation. Today, there is not a hospital in the world without a rigid fixation apparatus (Fig. 11-6). With the use of stainless steel fixation for the bone graft, the chance for migration is less and the possibility for total healing by regeneration is greater because partial mobility is allowed. Mobility is related to healing by regeneration. To heal well, a bone graft must be completely immobilized (Fig. 11-7). Any micromotion will result in loss of volume, delayed healing, and an eventual unfavorable outcome. To avoid this major unfavorable outcome, good immobilization must be arranged, even if the patient requires a second operation. A mobile bone graft, particularly in an area of dynamic mobility, will be doomed to an unfavorable outcome, manifested as a major loss of volume. Hematoma formation around the grafted site will result in excessive scarring, extrusion, or infection. All these problems will lead to partial or total loss of the graft and an unfavorable outcome. Any observed hematoma formation is an indication to evacuate the blood clots immediately and look for persistent bleeding, so that it can be stopped. This last measure obviates an unfavorable outcome. Infection is another factor that may lead to the eventual loss of a bone graft and an unfavorable outcome. Any factor that can cause an eventual infection, such as extrusion or hematoma formation, can affect the viability of a bone graft.

It is necessary to institute special measures to combat these problems. The free graft is washed with a dilute solution of antibacterial agents. Our preference is 50,000 U of bacitracin in 500 mL of saline solution. The same solution allows us to irrigate the recipient bed well. Both these measures eradicate infection. The patient receiving a bone graft receives a large dose of a long-acting systemic antibiotic to ensure a reduction in any hematogenous cause of infection. Other problems that may lead to infection are treated before an infection takes hold in a bone graft. All these measures prevent an unfavorable outcome.

The last aspect we need to address is poor "take" or poor healing of the bone graft. This event is related to the biologic system, degree of healing power, recipient bed where the bone graft has been placed, and external environmental factors, such as radiation administered to the patient (Fig. 11-8). This phenomenon is age-related. Bone grafts heal and regenerate much more readily in a child than in an older person, particularly in regions of the facial and cranial skeleton. In neonates and children up to the age of 6 years, the dura is more osteogenic than in an older patient. For comparison and an understanding of the favorable outcome, the age of the patient is of utmost importance. The nature of the bone graft is also of extreme importance in regard to final outcome. An orthotopic bone graft, one returned to its original biologic site, has a better outcome than a bone graft from a different donor site (Fig. 11-8). A heterotopic bone graft one taken from one donor site and placed in another site (Fig. 11-6). Heterotopic grafts have an unfavorable outcome more often than grafts placed in their original site after contouring or transplantation, even though both grafts are immunologically the same (15). These are local factors that may lead to an unfavorable outcome in bone grafting.

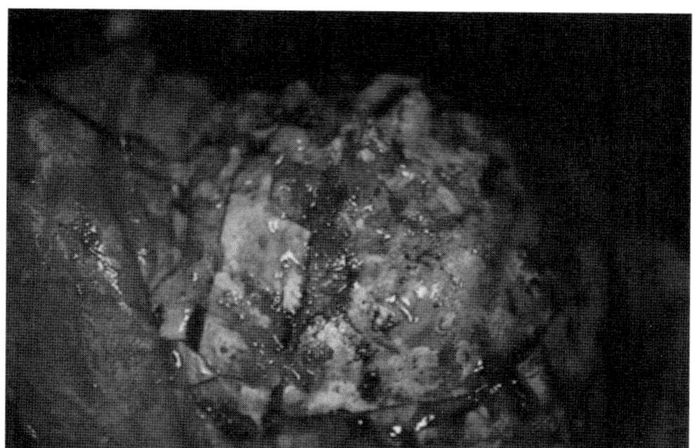

FIGURE 11-8. Example of an orthotopic bone graft. The bone is fixed with absorbable screws to prevent any mobility during healing.

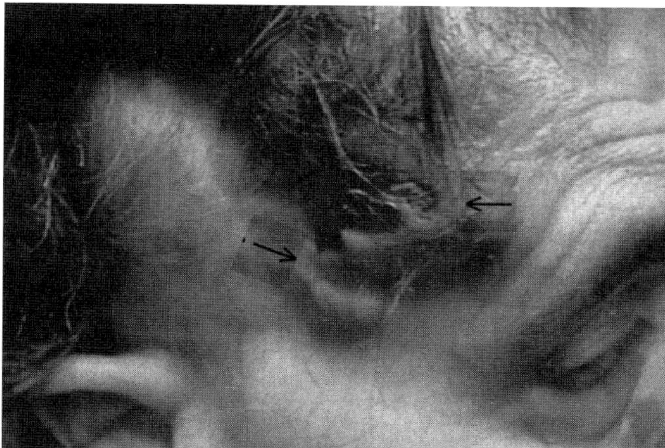

FIGURE 11-9. An unfavorable result in a bone graft placed 5 years previously in a patient treated with a heavy dose of radiation.

Other factors that may contribute to the unfavorable outcome of a bone graft are systemic or general. The most common of these is apparent when a bone graft is applied in irradiated tissue, mostly as part of the treatment for malignant disease. The chance for graft survival in these circumstances is usually guarded because irradiated tissue is not capable of regeneration, as are nonirradiated recipient sites. Certain measures can be instituted at such bone graft sites to obviate an unfavorable outcome. One is the use of vascularized, nonirradiated tissues in operated sites and the use of hyperbaric oxygen. Other supportive measures can also be applied successfully (Fig. 11-9).

In addition to the factors noted above is a second category of unfavorable outcomes in bone graft surgery—bone graft failure. If bone graft failure is total, there is no evidence of the graft in the applied site except for local scarring. Total bone graft failure is the most unfavorable outcome seen (Fig. 11-10). Failure can also be subtotal. In this situation, part of the bone graft survives, but most is lost because of any of the etiologic factors previously discussed, such as infection or hematoma formation. Exposure of part of the bone graft may lead to loss. If the graft can be salvaged, then the loss is subtotal. If it cannot, the whole bone graft is lost. In this case, the surgeon should attempt to reoperate provided that the factors that contributed to the loss of the bone graft can be alleviated (Fig. 11-11). The volume of the bone

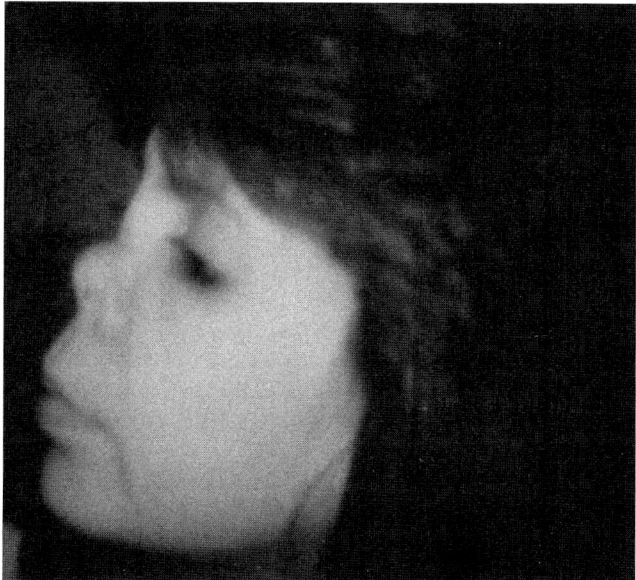

A

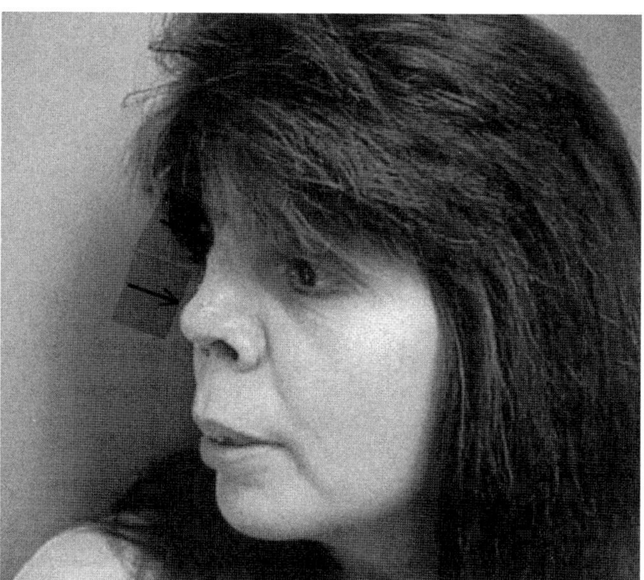

B

FIGURE 11-10. A: A patient with significant deformity resulting from multiple cosmetic procedures to the nose. **B:** Correction of the deformity with a bone graft.

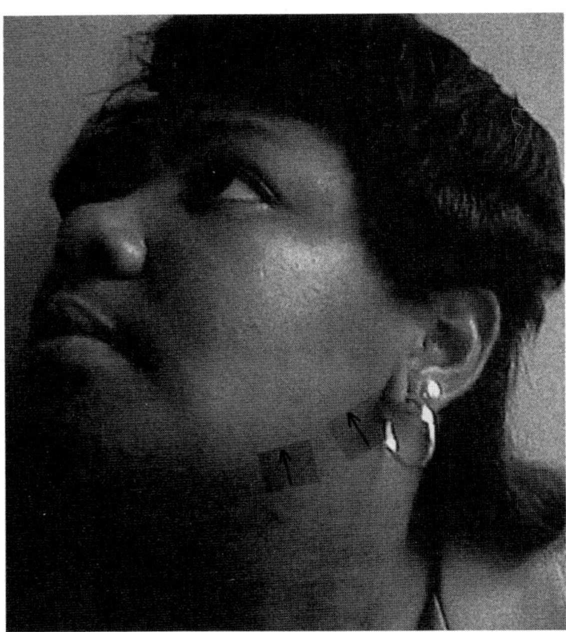

FIGURE 11-11. Left side of the mandible reconstructed with a bone graft after tumor resection. Note normal contour. Interdental osseointegrated implants placed one year after grafting.

graft may be lost subtotally because of the biologic nature of the bone graft healing process, even if contributing factors are absent (16). This last phenomenon is time-oriented. Therefore, bone graft survival, patient outcome, and any unfavorable result should be analyzed in the clinical setting at least 18 months after the implantation of a bone graft in the desired site.

An evaluation is performed for both onlay grafts and for grafts placed in a discontinuity defect in the facial and cranial skeleton. Graft survival is a function of graft vascularity. The faster grafts undergo vascularization, the greater are resorption and volume control and the less desirable the outcome that can be achieved. A graft in direct contact with an active muscle retains less volume in the long term (17). This phenomenon is related to fixation of the bone graft when it is applied (18) and is important in overall survival of the bone graft. A free-floating bone graft in a dynamic zone of the face in constant motion will fail because constant motion leads to volume loss secondary to demineralization and lack of vascularization. This phenomenon is important in maintaining a living bone graft, particularly over a period of time, and was well noted at the experimental level as a correlate to the clinical situation (19). Long-term maintenance is an important factor in graft viability that is assessed by noninvasive methodology the simplest of which is the use of radiography (20). As a bone graft heals and becomes incorporated, the recipient site passes through different phases toward a favorable outcome (21). Failure of any of these phases will result in an unfavorable outcome and contribute to loss of the graft. To activate bone incorporation, particularly in the patient who had been treated with extensive radiation for cancer, hyperbaric oxygen is an important modality to consider (22). Osteoinductive factors can be applied in bone grafting as a composite for enhancement of healing purposes (23).

DONOR SITE MORBIDITY

A discussion of unfavorable results in bone graft surgery would not be complete without mentioning the factors that are a driving force behind the development of bone substitutes to obviate the need for bone-grafting procedures. The best substance to use for a discontinuity defect or a contour defect that requires a bone graft is autogenous bone. The removal of such bone should be associated with minimal morbidity and no mortality. However, any bone removal is associated with some form of morbidity that should be taken into consideration and avoided at the desired anatomic site. As discussed previously, the architectural status of a bone graft and its healing are related to its density, not to its embryonic origin. Attention to the donor site morbidity is an integral part of a consideration of unfavorable results in bone graft surgery. Bone substitutes are discussed together with bone grafts whether they are inductive (23), conductive (12), the enhanced type (24), or just demineralized bone component (25).

Bone harvesting requires that the surgeon be well acquainted with the surgical anatomy of the donor region so that unfavorable results can be minimized. Certain problems are common to all harvest sites, such as bleeding and infection. The accumulation of blood in the donor site may be a primary factor in contaminating a region and lead to the development of infection in a site previously free from disease. Pain is another factor to be considered and is sometimes the only unfavorable result noted. In addition to these general problems, others specific to each donor site must be considered.

The maxilla and mandible are used in certain situations as donor sites for bone grafts. The indications for use of the maxilla are limited; when the maxilla is used as a donor site, soft tissue can herniate into the sinuses and cause infection, particularly in a patient with chronic sinus problems (26). This form of bone graft is used primarily to repair an orbital floor defect (27). The bone graft from that region is thin and pliable and lends itself well to the orbital floor. Maxillary bone grafts are also applied in the maxillofacial region.

The cranial bones as a harvesting site became popular in the last decade (28). Specific unfavorable results studied closely were those of neuralgic complications during the harvest. Bone grafting in this situation is mainly an *in situ* harvest without inclusion of the full thickness of cranial bone as part of the bone flap; even this in a way constitutes

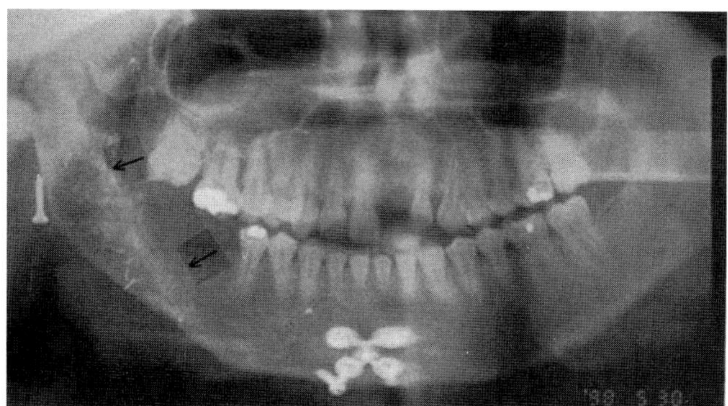

FIGURE 11-12. Right side of the mandible reconstructed with a bicortical hip graft. Note incorporation of the graft into the original mandibular bone.

a bone graft. Such a bone flap is nonetheless an orthotopic bone graft and follows the natural rules of bone graft take and healing (Fig. 11-12). The number of neurologic unfavorable outcomes has been minimal in relation to the number of bone grafts removed from the skull (28). Another unfavorable outcome is irregularity of the skull surface, which now is corrected by preventing soft tissue from filling the defect created by harvesting of cranial bone (Fig. 11-13). Controlled bone regeneration is achieved by presenting soft tissue from herniation into donor site. Bone harvesting from this area should not be performed without adequate training because of the danger involved in entering the cranial fossa. Persons trained in brain surgery limit their practice to the brain. They are not usually familiar with the harvest techniques involved in bone grafting, particularly the *in situ* methodology of splitting the outer table of the skull. The failure of a bone flap to heal in a patient undergoing a major craniofacial procedure is related primarily to infection at the recipient site; as noted previously, this represents an orthotopic bone graft.

Use of the rib cage as a donor site is associated with the fewest unfavorable outcomes in bone graft surgery. Rib bone has a thin cortical and a central cancellous component, so that vascularization is rapid and maintenance of volume is not very good. However, the bone structure provides for good stability (Fig. 11-14). A specific unfavorable outcome relates to violation of the pleural cavity and the development of pneumothorax. Careful coordination with the anesthesiologist will obviate the need for a chest tube and prolonged hospitalization. The use of positive-pressure ventilation will prevent the lung from collapsing when the pleural cavity in entered inadvertently. Other unfavorable outcomes may also include pain in the region. Tension pneumothorax has been noted in the past, but today, with the use of positive-pressure ventilation for most surgical procedures, this unfavorable outcome is rare.

The iliac bone continues to be the most common site for bicortical, monocortical, and cancellous bone graft harvest. A specific unfavorable outcome here is pain, which has been reported even 2 years after the surgical procedure. Pain affects the site where the dissection was performed and the distribution of the cutaneous nerve if it is injured (29). Other unfavorable outcomes include herniation of the abdominal contents, which must be corrected (30). Besides

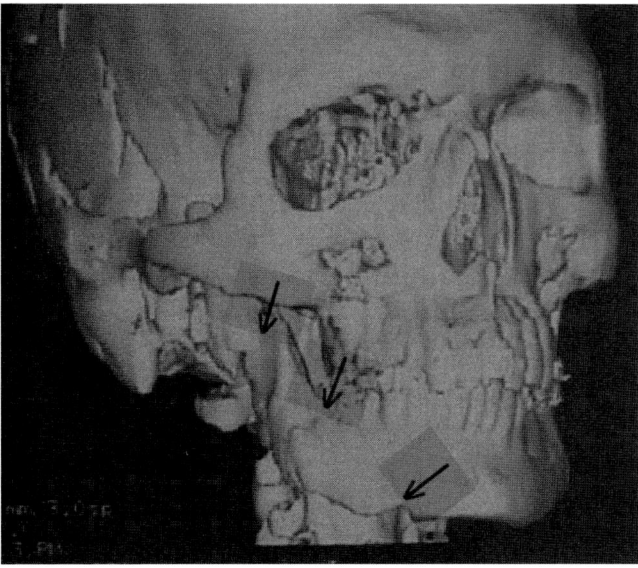

FIGURE 11-13. Bone graft placed after the patient underwent radiation to the mandible for malignant disease.

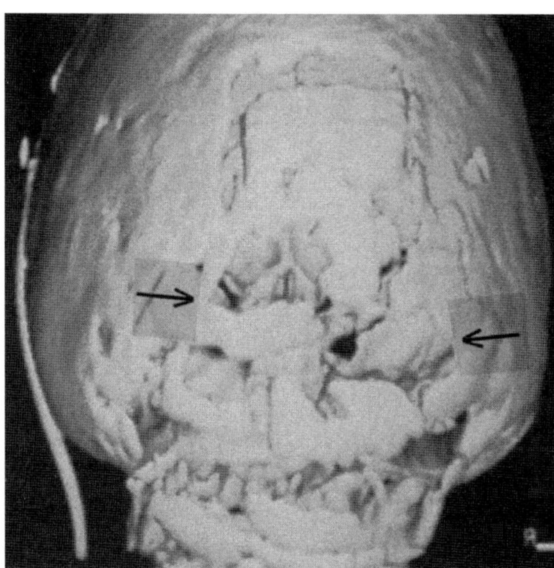

FIGURE 11-14. Cortical cranial bone in the occipital region as part of the treatment of an encephalocele.

abdominal herniation, vascular injuries and fracture of the iliac wing can occur and produce an unfavorable result, with a functional derangement (31). All these problems require a second operation for correction. The iliac bone should be reconstructed after all large iliac bone grafts have been harvested to obviate problems with instability and discomfort after surgery (32).

In all the studies already noted, one common finding eventually interfered with the outcome and precipitated an unfavorable result—hematoma formation. Hematomas can be avoided by limiting bone exposure to the harvested components and providing good hemostasis in the open area (33). We found in our experience that the use of hemostatic agents, such as microfibrillar collagen (Avatine), can obviate this problem completely. We have not noticed any abdominal herniation in our patients, who are followed closely during the postoperative period. These observations have been made in more than 1,000 iliac bone grafts performed by one surgeon (34). Paying attention to the skin incision and staying away from the anterior iliac spine to avoid injury to the lateral femoral cutaneous nerve prevents neurologic problems (35).

If we look at all the series reviewing bone graft harvesting, we find that hematoma formation, even if minor, is the most common unfavorable result at any site. Some surgeons tend to drain the donor site after any bone graft surgery. However, we prefer to utilize hemostatic agents in the wound. We have not had to drain hematoma from any donor site.

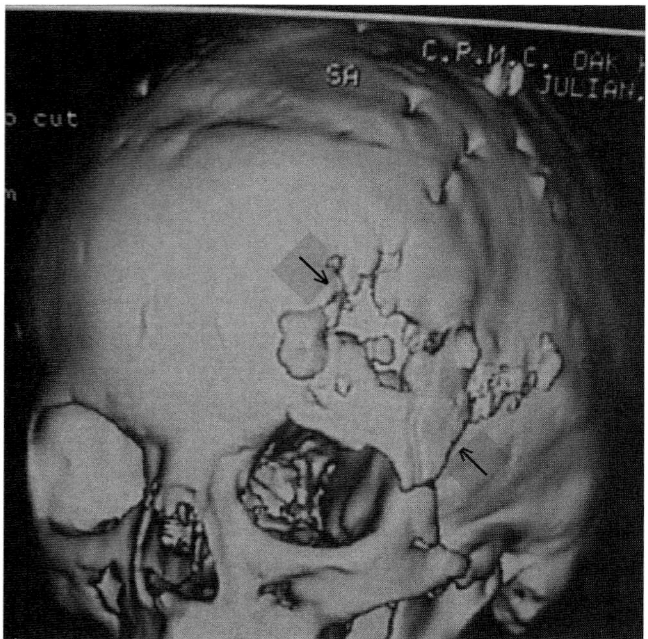

FIGURE 11-15. Cranioorbital reconstruction in a patient with a congenital anomaly. Note the well-healed bone incorporated in the left orbit.

The last donor site to be considered is the tibia and fibula (36). This site was very popular few years back. However, surgeons today, for obvious reasons, rarely use the tibial bone graft because disability far outweighs benefits. For that reason, it should be utilized only in special circumstances in nonambulatory patients (37). The bone harvested is cancellous and undergoes faster vascularization, healing, and incorporation. The main utility for such a bone graft is as filler for a discontinuity defect in the craniofacial skeleton. The bone surgeon should be familiar with this method in case it should be needed (Fig. 11-15).

CONCLUSION

In summary, unfavorable results in bone graft surgery can be divided into two main categories. The first is related to bone graft survival in the newly designed site. The second is related to donor site morbidity, which exacerbates any unfavorable result of bone graft surgery. A bone graft may be totally or partially lost. Volume loss is related to underlying biologic mechanisms that affect survival and also to the presence of local tissue problems—inadequate soft tissue to cover the exposed bone graft, infection, and hematoma formation. Hematoma formation appears to lead to an unfavorable outcome in both categories. Avoidance of those problems with good hemostasis and attention to the soft tissue at both the donor and recipient sites is key to ensuring a favorable outcome. The gradual loss of the bone graft is part of the process of incorporation, vascularization, and remodeling of the bone graft. To deal with this last problem, overcorrection is performed to allow for the effect of soft tissue elastic recoil. Extra bone in the graft allows for uncontrolled resorption and loss of volume. Overcompensation avoids an unfavorable result, and extra in the bone graft will produce a much more favorable result. Early loss is the result of exposure and ensuing infection in the recipient site.

An unfavorable result in bone graft surgery is a salvageable situation. Two important points are to be considered. The first is that problems must be recognized early, so that corrective measures can be applied. The second is that in such circumstances, procrastination can lead to an unfavorable outcome that cannot be corrected surgically or medically, so that the bone graft is eventually lost (Fig. 11-16).

Bone graft surgery is an art in regard to application and a science in regard to acquiring an understanding of healing and the processes of incorporation, remodeling, and eventual survival that result in a favorable outcome. Failure to deal with any of the problems that interrupt these processes will lead to an unfavorable result.

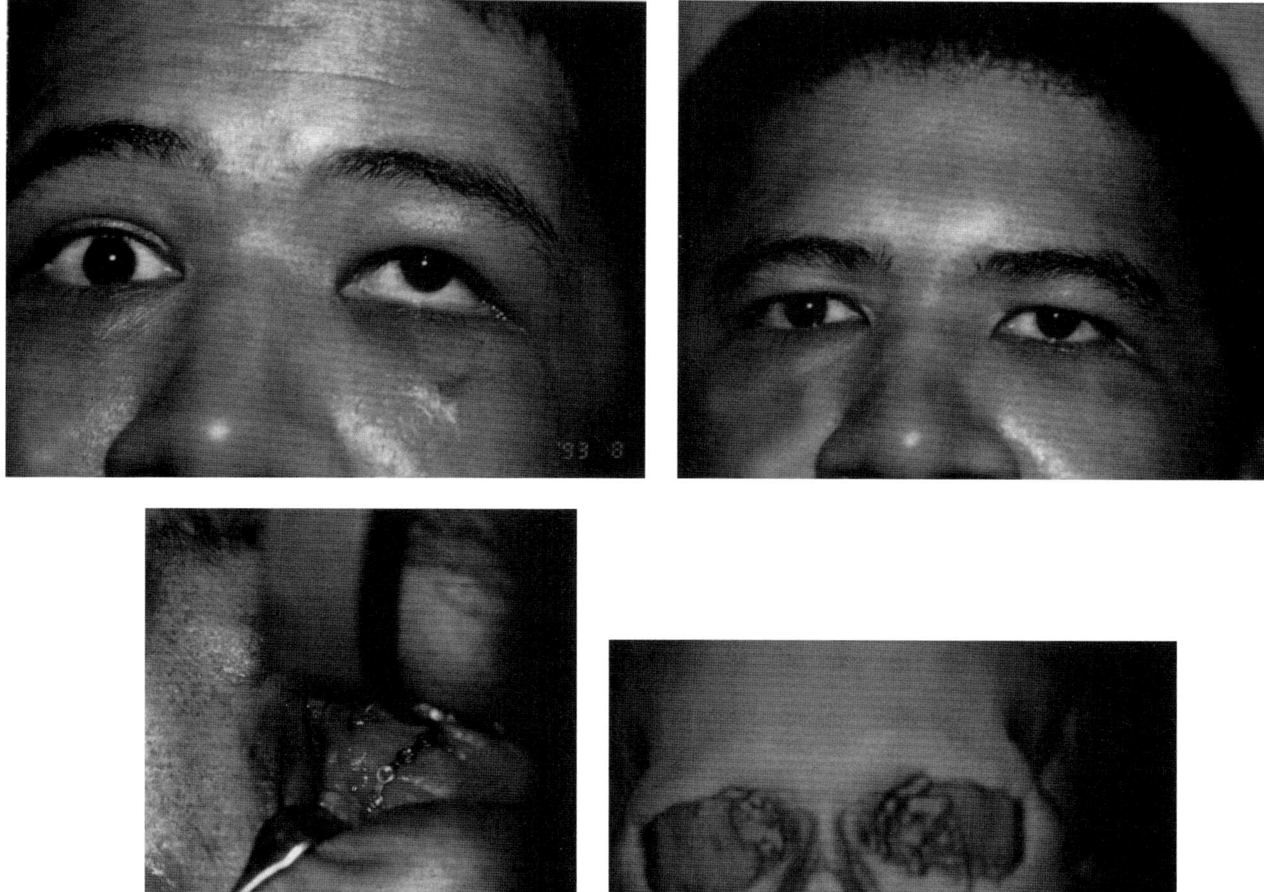

FIGURE 11-16. Patient with an orbital fracture treated with a bone graft. **A:** Patient has severe residual diplopia. **B:** The bone graft and the fixation apparatus were removed and reshaped to give the patient balanced vision. Intraoperative photo **(C)** and three-dimensional computed tomogram **(D)** demonstrate the problem.

REFERENCES

1. Sanan A, Hains SJ. Repairing holes in the head: a history of cranioplasty. *Neurosurgery* 1997;40:588–603.
2. Habal MB. Bone repair by regeneration. *Clin Plast Surg* 1996;23:93–101.
3. Albee FA. *Bone grafts surgery.* Philadelphia: WB Saunders, 1915.
4. Habal MB, Reddi HA. *Bone grafts and bone substitutes.* Philadelphia: WB Saunders, 1992.
5. Ozaki W, Buchman SR. Volume maintenance of onlay bone grafts in the craniofacial skeleton: microarchitecture vs. embryonic origin. *Plast Reconstr Surg* 1998;102:291–299.
6. Sumner DR, Turner TM, Purchio AF, et al. Enhancement of bone ingrowth by transforming growth factor beta. *J Bone Joint Surg Am* 1995;77:1135–1147.
7. Luster AD. Chemokines—chemotactic cytokines that mediate inflammation. *N Engl J Med* 1998;338:436–444.
8. Iwamoto Y, Sugioka Y, Chuman H, et al. Nationwide survey of bone grafting performed from 1980 through 1989 in Japan. *Clin Orthop* 1997;335:292–297.
9. Lewandrowski KU, Tomford WW, Scomacker KT, et al. Improved osteoinduction of cortical bone allografts: a study of the effects of laser perforation and partial demineralization. *J Orthop Res* 1997;15:748–756.
10. Hofmann GO, Falk C, Wangermann T. Immunological transformation in the recipient of allografted human bone. *Arch Orthop Trauma Surg* 1997;116:143–150.
11. Habal MB. Advances in bone repair surgery: induction, distraction, and just bone grafting. *Adv Plast Reconstr Surg* 1996;13:47–66.

12. Costantino PD, Friedman CD. Synthetic bone grafts substitutes. *Otolaryngol Clin North Am* 1994;27:1037–1047.
13. Dado DV, Izquierdo R. Absorption of onlay bone grafts in immature rabbits: membranous vs. enchondral bone and bone struts versus paste. *Ann Plast Surg* 1989;23:39–48.
14. Alonso N, Machado AO, Jorgetti V, et al. Cranial vs. iliac onlay bone grafts in the facial skeleton: a macroscopic and histomorphometric study. *J Craniomaxillofac Surg* 1995;6:113—118.
15. Ermis I, Pool M. The effects of soft tissue coverage on bone grafts resorption in the craniofacial region. *Br J Plast Surg* 1992;45:26–29.
16. Philips JH, Rahn BA. Fixation effects on membranous enchondral onlay bone graft revascularization and bone deposition. *Plast Reconstr Surg* 1990;85:891–897.
17. Chen NT, Glowacki J, Bucky LP, et al. The role of revascularization and resorption on endurance of craniofacial onlay bone grafts in the rabbit. *Plast Reconstruct Surg* 1994;93:714–722.
18. Block MS, Kent JN, Kallukaran FU, et al. Bone maintenance 5 to 10 years after sinus grafting. *J Oral Maxillofac Surg* 1998;56:706–714.
19. Pogrel MA, Podlesh S, Anthony JP, et al. A comparison of vascularized and non-vascularized bone grafts for reconstruction of mandibular continuity defects. *J Oral Maxillofac Surg* 1997;55:1200–1206.
20. Nigro N, Grace D. Radiographic evaluation of bone grafts. *J Foot Ankle Surg* 1996;36:378–385.
21. Stevenson S, Emery SE, Goldberg VM. Factors affecting bone grafts incorporation. *Clin Orthop* 1996;324:66–74.
22. Ashmalla HL, Thom SR, Goldwein JW. Hyperbaric oxygen therapy for the treatment of radiation-induced sequelae in children. *Cancer* 1996;77:2407–2412.
23. Boden SD, Schimandle JH, Hutton WC, et al. *In vivo* evaluation of resorbable osteoinductive composites as a graft substitute for lumber spinal fusion. *J Spinal Disord* 1997;10:1–11.
24. Constanz BR, Ison IC, Fulmer MT, et al. Skeletal repair by *in situ* formation of the mineral phase of bone. *Science* 1995;267:1796–1799.
25. Ehrnberg A, De Pablos J, Martinez LG, et al. Comparison of demineralized allegoric bone matrix grafting, the Urist procedure, and Ilizarov procedure in large diaphysial defects in sheep. *J Orthop Res* 1993;11:438–447.
26. Pasetti P. Bone harvesting from the oral cavity. *Int J Dent Symp* 1994;2:46–51.
27. Lee HH, Alcaraz N, Reino A, et al. Reconstruction of orbital floor fractures with maxillary bone. *Arch Otolaryngol Head Neck Surg* 1998;124:56–59.
28. Kline RM, Wolfe SA. Complications associated with the harvesting of cranial bone grafts. *Plast Reconstr Surg* 1995;95:5–13.
29. Cheney ML, Gliklich RE. The use of calvarial bone in nasal reconstruction. *Arch Otolaryngol Head Neck Surg* 1995;121: 643–648.
30. Goulet JA, Senunas LE, DeSilva GL, et al. Autogenous iliac crest bone graft. Complications and functional assessment. *Clin Orthop* 1997;339:76–81.
31. Arrington ED, Smith WJ, Chambers HG, Bucknell AL, et al. Complications of iliac crests bone graft harvesting. *Clin Orthop* 1996;329:300–309.
32. Banwart JC, Asher MA, Hassanein RS. Iliac crest bone graft harvest donor site morbidity: a statistical evaluation. *Spine* 1995;20:1055–1060.
33. Wippermann BW, Schratt HE, Steeg S, et al. Complications of spongiosa harvesting of the ilial crest: a retrospective analysis of 1,191 patients. *Chirurg* 1997;68:1286–1291.
34. Weikel AM, Habal MB. Meralgia paresthetica: a complication of iliac bone procurement. *Plast Reconstr Surg* 1977;60:572–579.
35. Aszmann OC, Dellon ES, Dellon AL. Anatomical course of the lateral femoral cutaneous nerve and its susceptibility to compression and injury. *Plast Reconstr Surg* 1997;100:600–604.
36. Vail TP, Urbaniak JR. Donor site morbidity with the use of vascularized autogenous fibular graft. *J Bone Joint Surg Am* 1996;78:204–211.
37. Saltrick KR, Caron M, Grossman J. Utilization of autogenous corticocancellous bone graft from the distal tibia for reconstructive surgery of the foot and ankle. *J Foot Ankle Surg* 1996;35:406–412.

Discussion

BONE GRAFTS

CRAIG R. DUFRESNE

Throughout the centuries, surgeons have sought to correct craniofacial skeletal deformities and tissue loss safely and predictably with autografts, allografts, and xenografts. Historically, the most successfully attempts at reconstruction have been with the use of autogenous tissues. These autografts, whether nonvascularized or vascularized, still remain the "gold standard" in craniofacial skeletal reconstruction. Dr. Habal, with his extensive experience in craniofacial surgery has thoroughly reviewed the unfavorable outcomes that can occur in bone graft surgery, even in the most experienced hands.

C. R. Dufresne: Department of Plastic Surgery, Georgetown University, Washington D.C.; and Section of Plastic Surgery, INOVA Fairfax Hospital Center, Fairfax, Virginia

Bone is a complex, dynamic tissue that is capable of marked adaptive responses to local, physical, and environmental influences during growth and throughout life. Bone remodeling occurs constantly; structural changes may result from variations in nutrition, vascular support, local bone stresses, and endocrine factors. It is often difficult to control all these variables during the planning and execution of complex reconstructions (3,4).

Autogenous bone grafts are, by definition, segments of bone transplanted from one anatomic location of the skeleton to another within the same person. The three most common sites of nonvascularized donor bone are the calvarium, rib, and iliac crest. Less common harvest sites are the tibia and radial bone. Vascularized donor bone sites include the fibula, scapular spine, iliac crest, radial bone, rib, and calvarium (3).

Calvarial bone has become an increasingly popular source of donor grafts for congenital, traumatic, or surgically created defects of the craniofacial skeleton. The outer table of the nondominant parietal bone is the most common harvest site. The cranium is easily accessed if the planned surgical approach requires a coronal incision, as in most cases of craniofacial surgery. Alternatively, when a coronal approach is not indicated, an incision can be made in the hair-bearing scalp over the right or left parietal bones. With either incision, the periosteum is reflected over the parietal bone. The graft may be harvested as a full-thickness or partial-thickness graft. If a partial-thickness graft is planned, the desired size and shape of the graft are then scored to the level of the diploë on the parietal calvarium with a rotating burr. The diploë layer can be recognized by bone bleeding within the newly scored troughs. A curved osteotome and mallet are then used to separate the outer-table (partial-thickness) graft from the inner calvarial table. The dissection plane is the diploë. Penetration of the inner table must be avoided to prevent dural laceration or brain injury. When the outer-table graft is properly obtained, morbidity at the calvarial donor site is minimal. After graft removal, the edges of bone at the donor site can be smoothed with a shaping burr to prevent bony irregularities.

If a full-thickness graft is planned, a craniotomy is performed. The cranial bone flap can be split into its inner and outer tables with a sagittal saw and osteotomes. The inner table can be used as a partial-thickness calvarial bone graft. The outer table is returned to the donor site to prevent contour deformities. These procedures produce blocks of cortical bone that can be contoured for specific defects anywhere in the craniofacial skeleton.

The inner- and outer-table bone grafts are quite rigid and can be placed in areas that require strong structural support. Because of their rigidity, these bone grafts are not malleable. They must be contoured with a shaping burr to achieve the necessary dimensions to repair a specific craniofacial defect. Some frequent uses of calvarial grafts in the craniofacial skeleton are cranial vault reconstruction, placement of cantilever dorsal nasal bone grafts, repair of bone comminution and bone gaps in facial trauma, orbital reconstruction, and onlay augmentation of the maxilla, zygoma, and mandible (Fig. 11D-1). Cranial bone can also be harvested in forms other than the inner- or outer-table blocks. Thin calvarial bone strips can be obtained by leaving the periosteum intact over an area of calvarium and harvesting a thin layer of the external table with a sharp osteotome. The resulting thin, pliable bone segments have been used to reconstruct inner orbital defects (13).

Calvarial bone "paste" can be produced by using a neurosurgical perforating burr to create partial-thickness cranial burr holes to the level of the diploë. This procedure produces bone shavings that can be used to smooth the contour between bone flaps or defects or for other purposes, such as obliteration of the frontal sinus.

The rib is another common bone graft donor site for craniofacial applications. Ribs can be harvested through an inframammary incision on the anterior chest wall. The incision should be carried through the periosteum overlying the donor rib. The fifth or sixth rib is the most common harvest site. The rib is usually dissected in a subperiosteal fashion. If required, osteochondral cartilage can be harvested with the rib graft by extending the dissection medially. If this cartilage is not needed, the rib graft can be sectioned at the costochondral junction and at a lateral posterior site that is determined by the length of bone required. During rib dissection, care should be taken to avoid injury to the parietal pleura (which results in a pneumothorax). Entry into the pleural space can be evaluated by direct observation or a fluid seal test.

Depending on the application, rib grafts can be used as whole or split grafts. Split rib grafts are produced by sectioning the rib longitudinally into two cortical halves with an osteotome. Splitting the rib effectively doubles the amount of donor graft. Split rib grafts are malleable and easily amenable to shaping with a Tessier rib-contouring forceps. Because they are easily contoured, split rib grafts are highly desirable for orbital reconstruction in particular.

The costochondral rib graft is also used for nasal reconstruction. Rib grafts can be used whole, shaped with rotating burr, for dorsal nasal reconstruction as cantilever grafts. The cartilage portion is contoured and placed within the nasal dome, camouflaged beneath the medial crura of the lower lateral cartilages. The bony portion of the graft is then shaped for the nasal dorsum. Some problems can occur when rib grafts are used for nasal reconstruction in young patients. These can warp with time if a cartilaginous portion of the graft is included in the reconstruction (13) (Fig. 11D-2).

Rib grafts have also been used extensively for reconstruction in the midface and mandibular areas to correct deformities secondary to trauma, congenital anomalies, and surgically created defects (tumor resection). Costochondral rib grafts are used to reconstruct the mandibular condyle after severe trauma. The cartilage portion of the graft can be

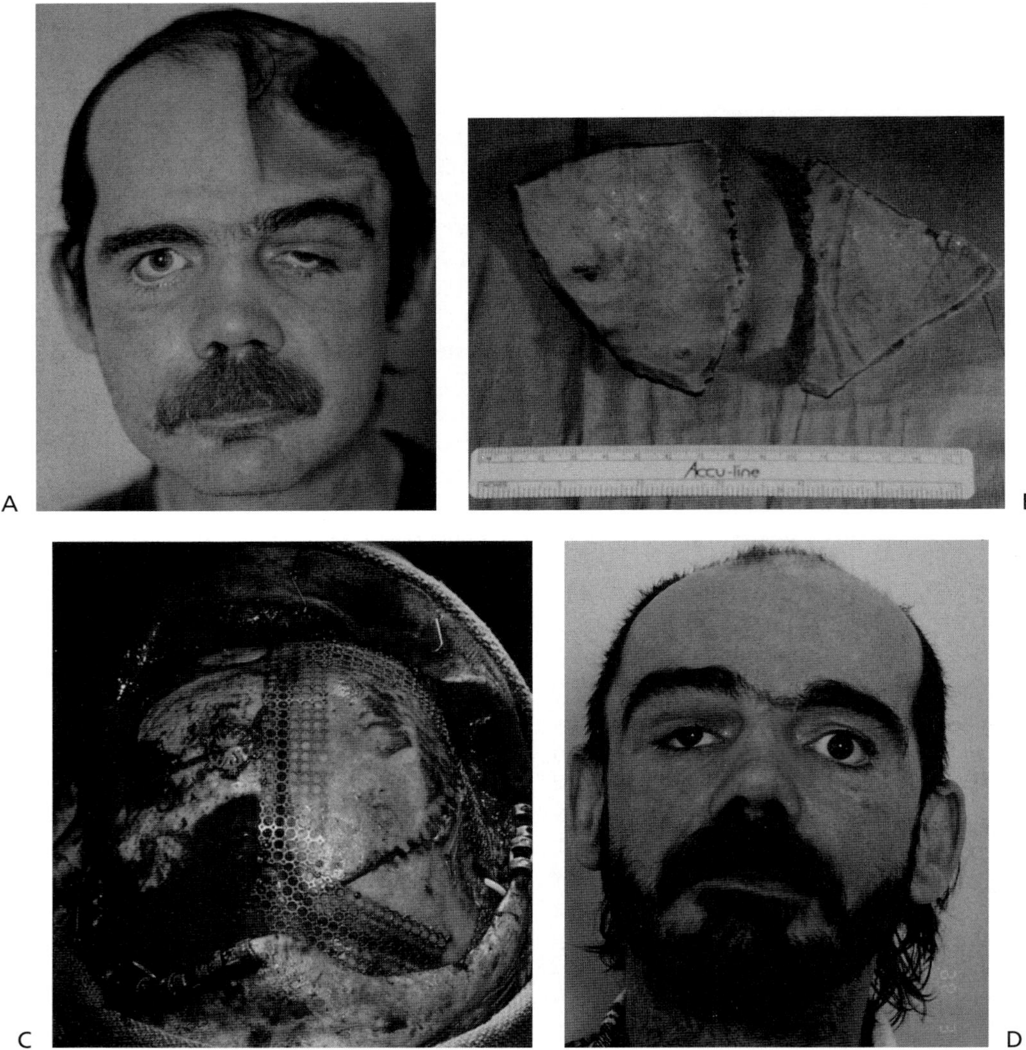

FIGURE 11D-1. A: This 42-year-old man sustained a crushing blow to the head that resulted in extensive cranial bone fragmentation and brain injury with a significant deformity. **B:** Full-thickness calvarial grafts were split to reconstruct the donor and recipient sites. **C:** Final reconstruction with split calvarial grafts secured by rigid fixation. **D:** The final result 4 months after surgery.

shaped to fit the glenoid fossa of the temporomandibular joint. Like calvarial grafts, rib grafts can be used as onlay or interpositional grafts in the zygoma, maxilla, and mandible. One problem noted with the use of costochondral rib grafts is a tendency to overgrow or hypertrophy (Fig. 11D-3). In extreme cases, mandibular set-back procedures have been required to correct the anomaly.

In the past, the iliac crest has been a popular bone graft donor site. It can be harvested in cortical block form or as particulate cancellous marrow. Iliac crest cortical bone can be obtained through an incision just below the iliac tuberosity. The incision is carried down to the periosteum overlying the anterior iliac crest. The anterior muscle is then stripped subperiosteally and reflected to expose the anterior iliac bone. Care must be taken to avoid injury to the lateral femoral cutaneous nerve, which results in numbness or paresthesias in the lateral aspect of the thigh. Anterior cortical block bone segments can be removed from the center of the iliac wing by careful osteotome sectioning. The hip also provides a plentiful source of cancellous bone. This is easily harvested with a curette after removal of the cortical bone graft. If only cancellous bone is required, the outer, cortical block can be hinged medially or inferiorly and replaced into position after the cancellous bone has been harvested.

The most popular use of iliac bone grafts has been mandibular reconstruction. Small, limited defects of the mandible can be packed with cancellous bone after initial rigid stabilization. Cancellous bone has also been used to fill alveolar gaps in cleft surgery. Like cranial grafts, iliac cortical grafts are strong and rigid. Therefore, limited, full-thick-

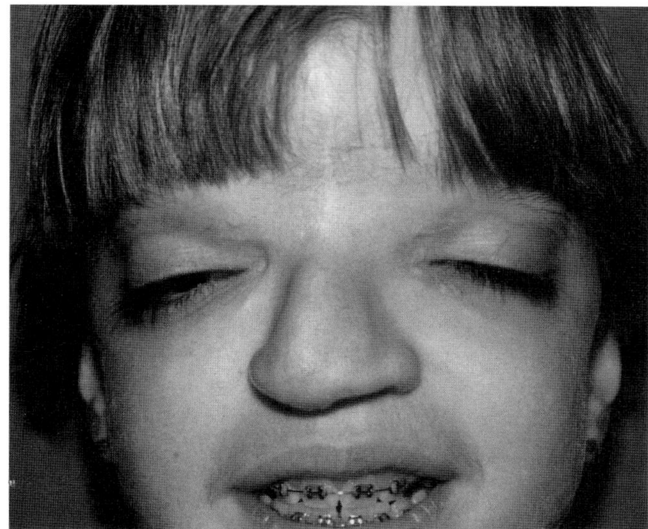

FIGURE 11D-2. A girl was born with a congenital midline teratoma. She required resection of the large midline mass and immediate reconstruction of the cranium. The hypoplastic nasal dorsum was reconstructed with a costochondral graft. After 10 years, it appeared to grow and deviate to the right, reflecting the inherent growth pattern of the thoracic rib.

ness, segmental mandible defects (< 5 cm in length) can be reliably repaired with rigidly fixed iliac cortical grafts. Postoperative morbidity at the iliac donor site is manifested as local discomfort and difficult initial ambulation. The degree of morbidity is most likely related to the amount of bone graft harvested (10).

Certain caveats have evolved for the proper handling of autografts: (a) Harvested bone should be wrapped in a blood-soaked sponge to maintain bone cell viability. (b) Before transplantation, harvested bone should not remain exposed to air longer than 30 minutes to preserve bone cell viability and prevent bone dessication; (c) Antibiotic solutions and physiologic saline solution (after prolonged exposure) can be toxic to bone cells within the graft. (d) Temperatures in excess of 42°C will kill cells. (e) Any dead space around the graft at the time of placement should be avoided. (f) Graft survival can be improved if the graft is implanted into a bed that is already actively producing new vessels and new bone. Adherence to these guidelines allows a graft of better quality to be harvested that heals more readily (10,13).

The recipient site of implantation of a bone graft influences the stimulus for repair. Certain areas of the craniofacial skeleton in particular are resorptive (i.e., undergo periosteum-induced resorption of bone), whereas other areas are depository (i.e., undergo periosteal deposition of bone). This is why multiple bone grafts are often required in certain syndromes (i.e., bone grafts to the malar area in Treacher Collins syndrome) and not in others. The influence of graft orientation is also important—that is, the position of the cancellous and periosteal surfaces relative to the soft tissue envelope on the onlay bone grafts. Bone grafts with their periosteal surface in contact with soft tissues and their cancellous surface in contact with host bone lose less volume than do grafts with their cancellous surface in contact with soft tissue (5,15).

Transferring bone tissue with its vascular supply allows healing to proceed much more reliably and rapidly. In the craniofacial area, certain flaps can be designed from local tissue that result in minimal long-term resorption of the transferred tissue. Lower facial or mandibular reconstruction can be carried out with other local osteomyocutaneous flaps (e.g., trapezius and scapular flaps) or with free-tissue transfers from distant locations (e.g., free fibular flap). Several advantages unique to vascularized free flaps should be kept in mind when a reconstruction is being planned. Transfers of vascularized tissue should be considered in the following situations: (a) Segmental defects larger than 6 cm are present in stress-bearing sites; (b) the recipient bed is compromised (i.e., scarred, infected, or irradiated); (c) rapid healing of a graft rather than slower healing is needed, as in the case of a graft healing with creeping substitution; (d) growth of the segment is important, as in a young child (1,2).

Early concepts of bone graft healing theorized that transplanted bone graft did not survive, eventually became necrotic, and was gradually resorbed and replaced by new living bone. This process was referred to as *creeping substitution.* Some believed that the process of new bone formation with transplanted bone grafts originated in the periosteum, whereas others postulated that surface bone cells on the transplanted autograft survived and aided in forming new living bone within the graft, a process referred to as *osteogenesis.* Many studies have shown that periosteal preservation significantly enhances new bone formation in both cortical and trabecular bone (17). Preservation of the periosteum also favorably influences graft revascularization and graft integrity. This is important during harvesting and the reconstruction phase. It is also known that periosteum is actively osteogenic in youth and becomes less so in adulthood. This is an important factor to be considered when reconstructions are performed in patients of various ages (14).

In a comparison of cancellous bone grafts with cortical bone grafts, several points are important to consider when a decision must be made regarding which graft to use. Cancellous grafts are initially mechanically weak but revascularize more rapidly and more completely than cortical bone grafts. In cortical bone grafts, mechanical weakness (to 60% of normal strength) develops between from 1-1/2 and 6 months after grafting, and the internal porosity of the graft increases because of resorption. Mechanical factors play a dominant role in the long-term function of cells within a graft. Bone grafts subjected to net compressive forces in the physiologic range generally become hypertrophic, whereas grafts not subjected to deforming force or a net tensile force are generally replaced with nonosseous tissue (5).

As our understanding of bone healing increases, new

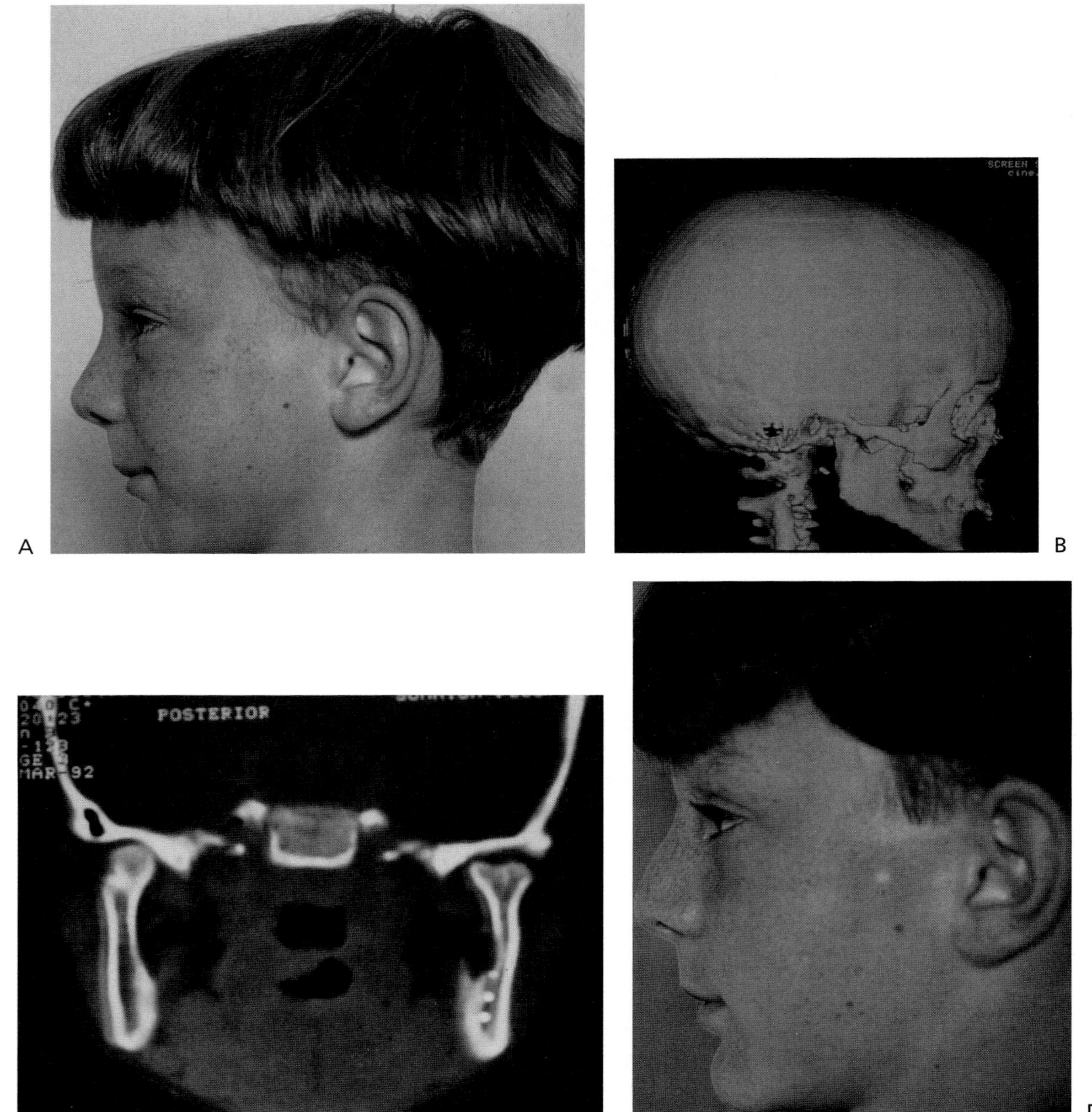

FIGURE 11D-3. A: A 6-year-old boy involved in a car accident sustained panfacial and bilateral condylar fractures. Note lateral facial appearance with foreshortening in the lower region. **B:** Three-dimensional computed tomogram demonstrates loss of the condyle and subsequent loss of lower facial height. **C:** Radiograph demonstrates bilateral costochondral grafts in place, with hypertrophy of the left cartilaginous portion beyond the glenoid fossa. **D:** Lateral photograph demonstrates the protruding portion of the graft around the glenoid fossa.

technologic advances are improving outcomes and reducing complications and unfavorable results. One such advance has been the use of rigid fixation. The beneficial effects on bone graft survival can be explained in three ways: (a) Bone graft immobilization favors more rapid vascularization; (b) compression of the bone graft to the recipient site expands the area of contact between the bone graft and its recipient bed, thereby facilitating creeping substitution and minimizing the resorptive phase; and (c) earlier consolidation of the bone graft in its bed allows an earlier onset of the appositional phase of healing and more efficient ingrowth of osteogenic cells (15,16,17). Clinically, analysis of the results of rigid fixation techniques has led to the following conclusions: (a) Rigid skeletal fixation of bone grafts produces better bone graft volume survival than does wire fixation of grafts; (b) membranous bone grafts are associated with better graft volume survival than are endochondral bone grafts; (c) membranous bone grafts demonstrate greater bone graft volume survival and greater bone graft weight survival; (d) inlay bone grafts demonstrate greater weight and volume survival than do onlay bone grafts; and (e) bone grafts fixed with rigid techniques are incorporated by bony union, whereas bone grafts fixed with wire techniques are incorporated with fibrous union (7–9,11,15).

In summary, many conditions and variables affect the ultimate outcome of bone grafts. The surgeon who optimizes favorable factors will avoid the unfavorable outcome in bone graft surgery.

REFERENCES

1. Cutting CB, McCarthy JG, Knize DM. Repair and grafting of bone. In: McCarthy JG, ed. *Plastic surgery,* vol 1. Philadelphia: WB Saunders, 1990:583–629.
2. Cutting CB, McCarthy JG. Comparison of residual osseous mass between vascularized and nonvascularized onlay bone transfers. *Plast Reconstr Surg* 1983;72:672–675.
3. Leipziger LS, Dufresne CR. Autogenous and allogenic materials. In: Dufresne CR, Carson BS, Zinreich SJ, eds. Complex craniofacial problems. New York: Churchill Livingstone, 1992: 489–494.
4. Gross TP, Jinnah RH, Clarke HJ, et al. The biology of bone grafting. *Orthopedics* 1991;14:563–568.
5. Zins JE, Whitaker LA. Membranous versus endochondral bone: implications for craniofacial reconstruction. *Plast Reconstr Surg* 1983;72:778–785.
6. Bartlett SP, Whitaker LA. Growth and survival of vascularized and nonvascularized membranous bone: an experimental study. *Plast Reconstr Surg* 1989;84:783–788.
7. DeLacure MD. Physiology of bone healing and bone grafts. *Otolaryngol Clin North Am* 1994;27:859–874.
8. Romana MC, Masquelet AC. Vascularized periosteum associated with cancellous bone graft: an experimental study. *Plast Reconstr Surg* 1990;85:587–592.
9. Manson PN. Facial bone healing and bone grafts. A review of clinical physiology. *Clin Plast Surg* 1994;21:331–348.
10. Sullivan WG, Szwajkun PR. Revascularization of cranial versus iliac crest bone grafts in the rat. *Plast Reconstr Surg* 1991;87: 1105–1109.
11. Phillips JH, Rahn BA. Fixation effects on membranous and endochondral onlay bone-graft resorption. *Plast Reconstr Surg* 1988;82:872–877.
12. Prolo DJ, Oklund SA. The use of bone grafts and alloplastic materials in cranioplasty. *Clin Orthop* 1991;268:270–278.
13. Enlow DH. *The handbook of facial growth,* 2nd ed. Philadelphia: WB Saunders, 1990;75–126.
14. Ermis I, Poole M. The effects of soft tissue coverage on bone graft resorption in the craniofacial region. *Br J Plast Surg* 1992;45: 26–29.
15. Fisher J, Wood MB. Experimental comparison of bone vascularization by musculocutaneous and cutaneous flaps. *Plast Reconstr Surg* 1987;79:81.
16. Han CS, Wood MB, Bishop AT, et al. Vascularized bone transfer. *J Bone Joint Surg Am* 1992;74:1441–1449.
17. Weiland AJ, Moore JR, Daniel RK. Vascularized bone autografts. Experience with 41 cases. *Clin Orthop* 1983;174:87.

SUGGESTED READING

de Boer HH, Wood MB. Bone changes in the vascularized fibular graft. *J Bone Joint Surg Br* 1989;71:374–378.

Dufresne CR, Cutting CB, Valauri F, et al. Reconstruction of mandibular and floor of mouth defects using the trapezius myocutaneous and osteomyocutaneous flaps. *Plast Reconstr Surg* 1987;79:687–696.

Kusiak JF, Zins JE, Whitaker LA. The early revascularization of membranous bone. *Plast Reconstr Surg* 1985;76:510–516.

Thompson N, Casson JA. Experimental onlay bone grafts to the jaws. A preliminary study in dogs. *Plast Reconstr Surg* 1970;46:341–349.

12

NERVE GRAFTS

SUSAN E. MACKINNON

Unlike many other tissues, the peripheral nerve is relatively intolerant to a surgical injury. A "surgical mishap" is immediately obvious to both surgeon and patient and may cause an unfavorable result that lasts for a very long, if not indefinite, period of time. An injury to a cutaneous nerve during a ganglion removal or to a small portion of the median nerve during an open carpal tunnel release is not "outside the standard of care," but it may irreparably alter the patient's life. Similarly, seemingly inconsequential digital nerve injuries that progress to a painful neuroma and a chronic pain syndrome can render patients and their families more functionally disabled than a painless limb amputation. The sensory and motor impairment associated with peripheral nerve injuries can be profound, but it is the painful sequelae of peripheral nerve injuries that are the most disturbing and difficult to treat. There appears to be little to no room for error in peripheral nerve surgery. Fortunately, certain techniques can be used to avoid an unfavorable result, and others have proved useful in the treatment of such complications when they occur. This chapter addresses the peripheral nerve procedures most commonly performed by plastic surgeons, including nerve repair and grafting, neuroma surgery, carpal tunnel release, and ulnar nerve transposition. Methods to minimize the complications associated with these procedures and suggestions on how to treat complications are reviewed.

NERVE RECONSTRUCTION

Timing

The most critical factor to ensure a favorable result following a nerve injury is to intervene with electrodiagnostic studies or surgery at the appropriate time (Figs. 12-1 and 12-2). I am frequently presented with clinical scenarios in which the surgeon is technically competent to perform a given procedure but is uncertain about when to proceed with either electrodiagnostic studies or surgery. A young woman who had been scheduled for a nerve graft for a complete facial palsy following removal of an acoustic neuroma sought a second opinion. At 2 months following the tumor surgery, the suggestion of a nasolabial fold was noted. An electromyographic study at 3 months showed evidence of motor unit potentials, and at 6 months, normal facial movement was recovered. Surgery "done too early" on this patient would have been unnecessary and would have resulted in a less favorable result than that achieved by spontaneous recovery. By contrast, patients with lower extremity nerve injuries or proximal upper extremity nerve injuries are typically referred "too late," a situation that also reduces the likelihood of an excellent result. Thus, key to preventing an unfavorable result following nerve injury is an understanding of the timing of nerve reconstruction. The appropriate timing of nerve reconstruction depends on a very clear understanding of the classification of nerve injury.

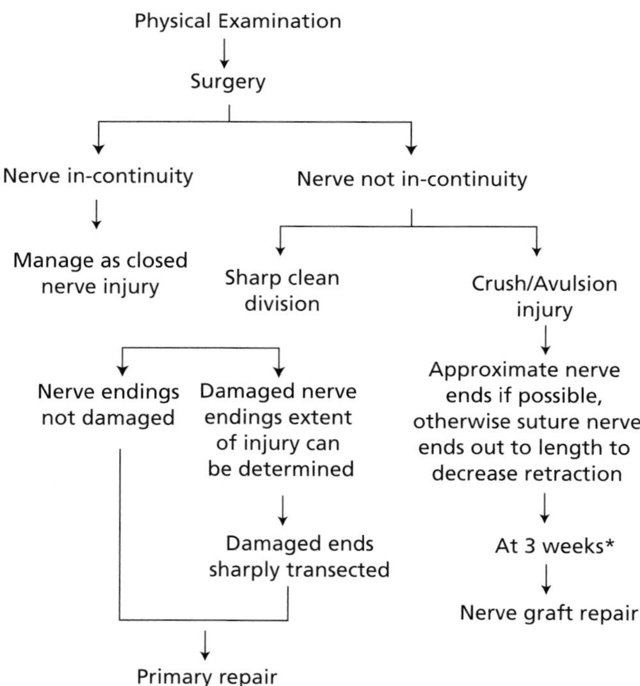

FIGURE 12-1. Open nerve injury algorithm.

S. E. Mackinnon: Division of Plastic Surgery and Reconstructive Surgery, Washington University School of Medicine; and Department of Surgery, Boones-Jewish Hospital, St. Louis, Missouri

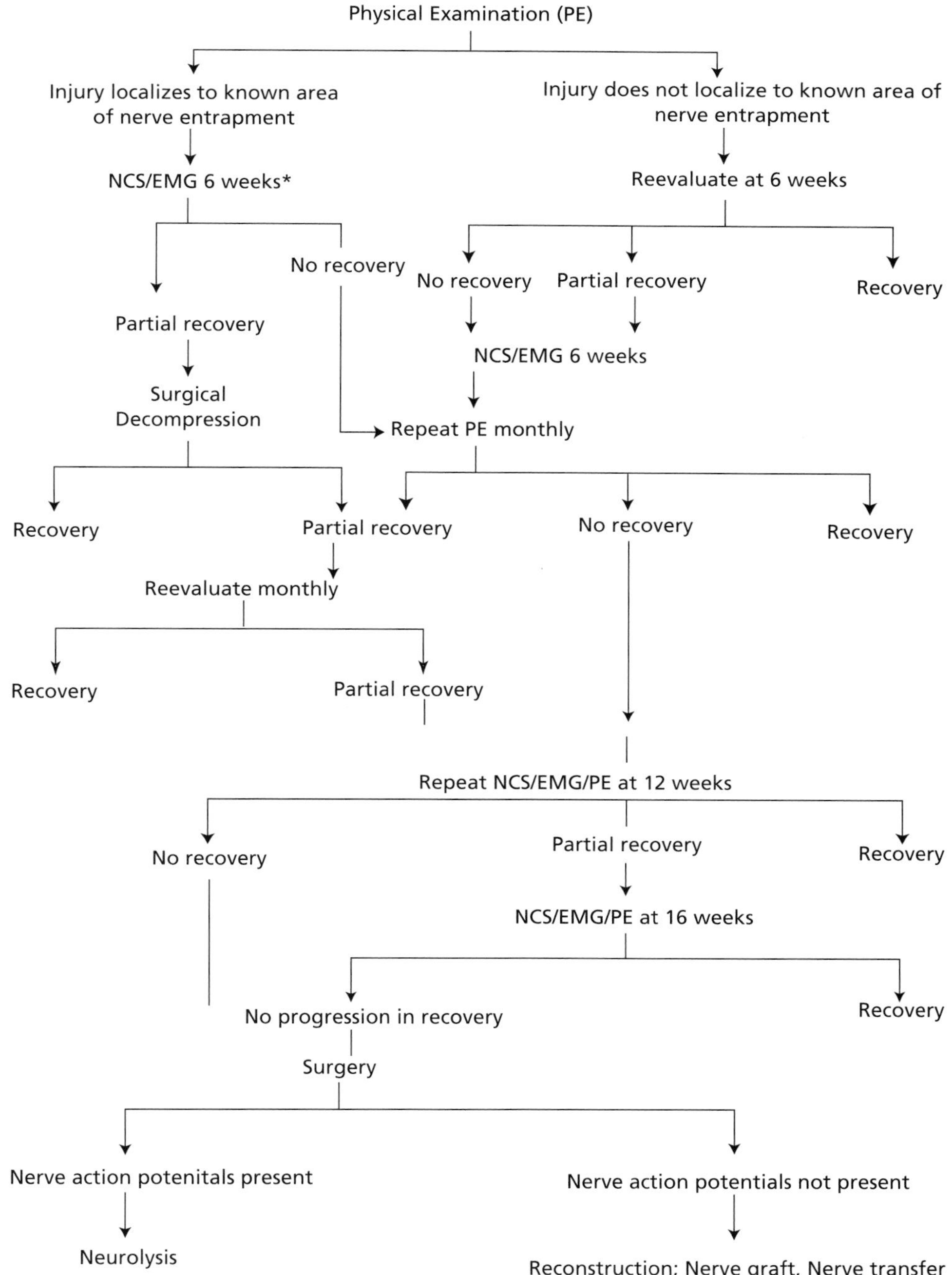

FIGURE 12-2. Closed nerve injury algorithm.

Classification of Nerve Injury

Sir Herbert Seddon in 1943 described three types of nerve injury: neurapraxia, axonotmesis, and neurotmesis. Sir Sydney Sunderland in 1951 presented a second classification describing five degrees of nerve injury. He expanded Seddon's classification to include a third-degree injury that involved some scarring within the endoneurium, and a fourth-degree injury that involved such extensive scarring within the nerve that no regeneration could occur across the injury. The author has popularized a combination injury that includes various injury patterns (i.e., sixth-degree injury) (Table 12-1 and Fig. 12-3).

TABLE 12-1. RELATIONSHIP OF INJURY TO RECOVERY

Degree of Injury	Tinel's Sign Present Disability Progresses	Recovery Pattern	Rate of Recovery	Surgical Procedure
1. Neurapraxia	–/–	Complete	Fast, days to 12 weeks	None
2. Axonotmesis	+/+	Complete	Slow (1 inch per month)	None
3.	+/+	Great variation[a]	Slow (1 inch per month)	None or neurolysis
4. Neuroma in continuity	+/–	None	No recovery	Nerve repair or graft
5. Neurotmesis or nerve	–/–	None	No repair	Nerve repair or graft
6. Mixed injury varies with each fascicle, depending on the combination of injury patterns as noted above.				

[a] Recovery is at least as good as with a nerve repair but can vary from excellent to poor, depending on the degree of endoneurial scarring and the amount of sensory or motor axonal misdirection that is possible within the injured fascicle.
From Mackinnon SE, Dellon AL. *Surgery of the peripheral nerve*. New York: Thieme Medical Publishers, 1988, with permission.

First-degree Injury (Neurapraxia)

Neurapraxia involves a conduction block along a localized length of a peripheral nerve. Without any disruption of the axon, the axon nevertheless does not regenerate. Thus, no Tinel's sign is present. At most, histologic evaluation demonstrates an area of segmental demyelination (Table 12-1). It may take up to 12 weeks for remyelination to occur and neurologic function to recover. Thus, the timing for recovery may vary from days to 12 weeks. The nature of the mechanism of injury coupled with the lack of a Tinel's sign is useful in determining a first-degree injury. Electrodiagnostic studies will show no conduction across the area of injury but normal conduction distal to the area of injury. This electric finding is unique for a neurapraxia, or first-degree injury.

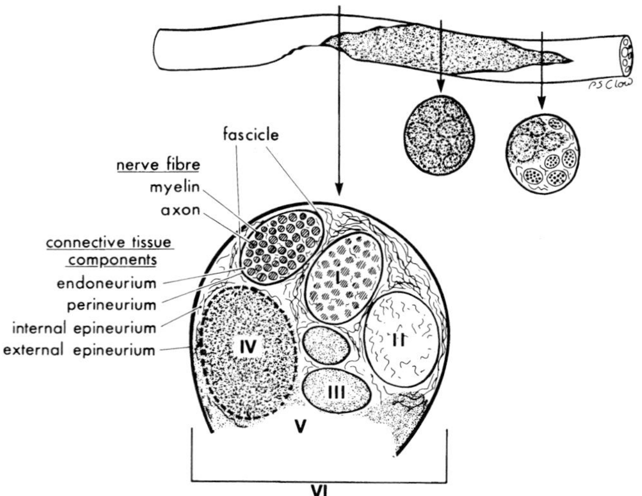

FIGURE 12-3. In this "mixed" (sixth-degree) injury, elements of Sunderland's five degrees of injury are noted. At 1 o'clock, a normal fascicle is seen. *I,* a fascicle demonstrating a first-degree injury (i.e., neurapraxia with segmental demyelination). *II,* a fascicle demonstrating a second-degree Sunderland injury (i.e., axonotmesis, in which the endoneurium is normal and the perineurium is preserved). *III,* a fascicle demonstrating a third-degree injury (i.e., scarring is present within the endoneurium but the perineurium is preserved). *IV,* a fascicle with a fourth-degree injury (i.e., the nerve is in continuity, but only with scar tissue). *V,* fifth-degree injury (i.e., neurotmesis, in which the nerve has been divided). The surgeon must separate the fourth- and fifth-degree injury patterns, which require reconstruction, from normal fascicles and fascicles demonstrating first-, second-, and third-degree injuries. These latter patterns of injury require at most a neurolysis. The drawing demonstrates the fact that an injury can change along the longitudinal axis of the nerve. (From Mackinnon SE, Dellon AL. *Surgery of the peripheral nerve.* New York: Thieme Medical Publishers, 1988, with permission.)

Second-degree Injury (Axonotmesis)

An axonotmetic injury with axonal damage results in axonal degeneration distal to the site of nerve injury. For recovery from this type of injury to occur, regeneration of the axon is required. Thus, a Tinel's sign will be present at the level of the nerve injury, and with regeneration, the Tinel's sign will be seen to advance distal to the nerve injury, progressing at a rate of approximately a millimeter a day or an inch a month. For examination, the surgeon should begin tapping well distal to the area of nerve injury and percuss proximally along the course of the nerve to elicit the level of the most distal Tinel's sign. A stronger Tinel's sign is usually present at the level of the nerve injury for many months. Functional recovery following a second-degree injury should be complete unless the injury is so far proximal to the target end-organs that a prolonged period of denervation negatively affects the ultimate result.

Third-degree Injury

In the "finer print" of Seddon's original description of nerve injuries, he did in fact describe a third-degree injury. However, it was Sunderland who highlighted the description of this type of injury. In a third-degree injury, a varying amount of scar tissue is present within the endoneurium. The axons regenerate at the classic rate, but the amount of recovery is less than with a second-degree injury. The amount of recovery in a third-degree injury is more variable and less predictable than in the other injuries, depending on the amount of scar tissue within the nerve and on whether or not the nerve involved comprises purely motor or sensory fascicles or has a mixed fascicular pattern. With mixed-nerve

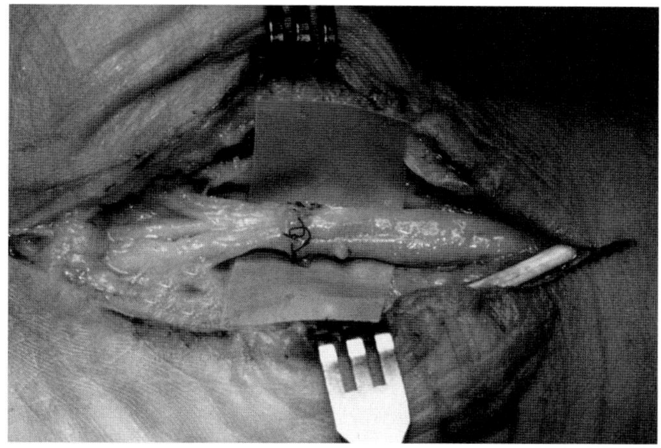

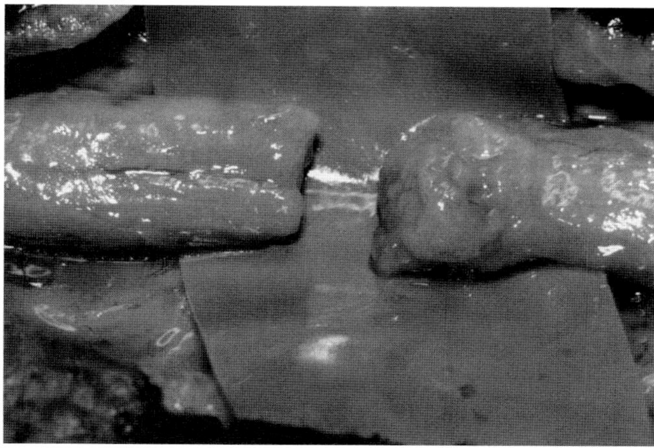

FIGURE 12-4. After an open carpal tunnel release, this patient had no median nerve function. The history from the referring surgeon stated that the nerve "was found" in two pieces and repaired. **A:** Exploration of the surgical site demonstrates a poor attempt at nerve repair. **B:** When the large sutures were removed, a completely divided median nerve was seen. (From Cartotto RC, McCabe S, Mackinnon SE. Two devastating complications of carpal tunnel surgery. *Ann Plast Surg* 1992;28:472–474, with permission.)

injuries, the opportunity for mismatching of appropriate sensory and motor regenerating fibers, which results in a poorer functional result, is greater. Thus, in a second- and third-degree injury, recovery can vary from almost complete to very poor, depending on the nature of the fascicular pattern and the degree of endoneurial scarring within the nerve. A third-degree injury is the common "medicolegal" injury. With a first- or second-degree injury, recovery is complete and any deficit is transient. With a fourth- or fifth-degree injury to a major nerve in a primary surgical procedure, no recovery occurs and there is little room for debate regarding negligence (Figs. 4 and 5). However, with a third-degree injury, despite the fact that this is recognized as an unavoidable injury, the recovery is not perfect, and there is opportunity for "discussion in the medicolegal arena."

Fourth-degree Injury

With a fourth-degree injury, the nerve is in continuity but with complete scarring, such that no regeneration occurs across the area of injury. A Tinel's sign is present at the level of the injury but does not advance. Electrodiagnostic studies show no evidence of reinnervation.

Fifth-degree Injury

A fifth-degree injury involves a complete transection of the involved nerve. The clinical and electric findings are similar to those in a fourth-degree injury. A Tinel's sign is present at the level of the injury but does not advance, and no electric evidence of reinnervation is noted.

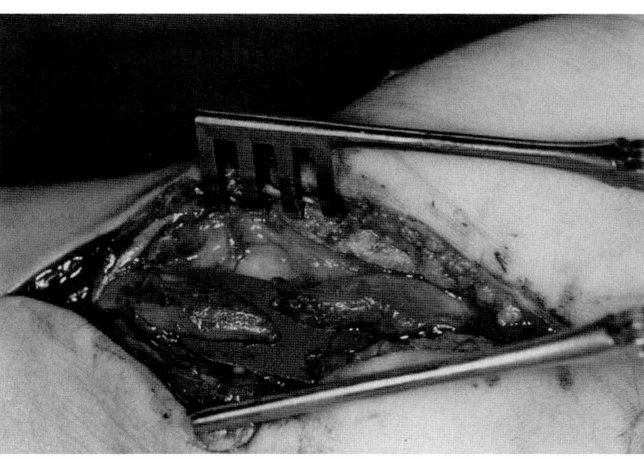

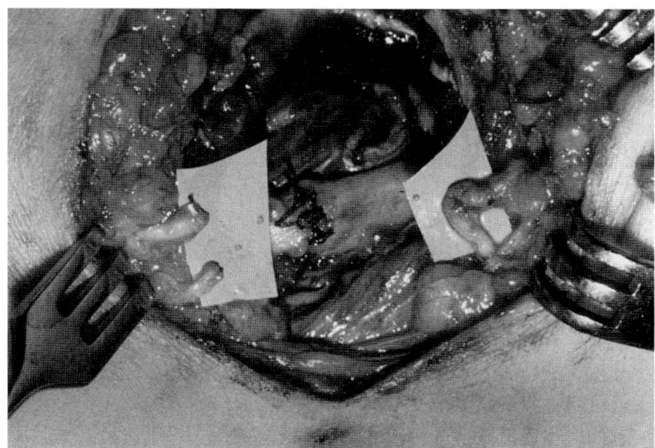

FIGURE 12-5. A: During an endoscopic carpal tunnel release, the median nerve was divided in an oblique fashion. **B:** This ulnar nerve was inadvertently divided and repaired with very large silk sutures. The overlying branches of the medial antebrachial cutaneous nerve were not treated because such treatment would likely have added insult to injury and caused painful neuromas to form.

Sixth-degree Injury

As has already been described, a sixth-degree injury, which is a combination of various degrees of nerve injuries in which some fascicles demonstrate recoverable injuries and others nonrecoverable injuries (fourth- and fifth-degree injuries). Within this type of injury, some fascicles may be entirely normal. Similarly, along the longitudinal extent of the nerve injury, the injury pattern may vary. The sixth-degree injury is the most challenging to repair surgically. During the procedure, the surgeon must identify the fourth- and fifth-degree injury patterns and reconstruct them, and at the same time not downgrade the functioning normal fascicles or those fascicles that are capable of recovery (first-, second-, and third-degree injuries).

The timing of surgical intervention is depends directly on the type of nerve injury. Injuries with the possibility of recovery (first-, second-, and third-degree injuries) are managed conservatively unless they localize to a known area of nerve entrapment. In these cases, if recovery fails to occur or is incomplete, or if regeneration does not progress past the known area of nerve entrapment, then a release of the nerve at this level should be considered. Frequently, a Tinel's sign will be present at the known area of entrapment (e.g., carpal tunnel, cubital tunnel, fibular head, arcade of Frohse). With these recoverable injuries, it is not particularly urgent to perform the release, and it is usually appropriate to wait a few weeks to see whether regeneration is forthcoming before the release is considered. An exception would be a dense neurologic deficit in the situation of an acute hematoma or compartment syndrome.

Once the surgeon is convinced that nerve regeneration and recovery are not forthcoming (i.e., a fourth- or fifth-degree injury is present), then surgical intervention is indicated. With mixed-degree injuries, the surgeon may be aware very early on that a component of the injury is a fourth- or fifth-degree injury and that surgical intervention will be required. However, the timing of surgical intervention depends on whether or not a potential for recovery is present in other components of the nerve injury. In this situation, the surgeon will "wait out" the component of injury that may be recoverable, delaying surgery on the fourth- or fifth-degree component of the nerve injury until it is clear that other elements of the nerve injury are more favorable. For example, a patient might present with clear evidence of avulsion of a portion of the brachial plexus, which certainly would not recover spontaneously. Other elements of the plexus that were not avulsed might in fact have a potential for recovery. Thus, surgery could be indicated immediately for the avulsion component of the injury but would be delayed until the potential for recovery (first-, second-, and third-degree injuries) could be determined in the remainder of the plexus. Similarly, with a gunshot wound to a major nerve, immediate exploration of the wound might identify a physical disruption in some component of the nerve that would likely require a nerve graft procedure, whereas the other elements of the nerve might be in continuity. Thus, the initial surgery would involve "approximation"* of the portion of the nerve that was not in continuity. Because of the mechanism of injury, definitive reconstruction for the injured part of the nerve would likely require a nerve graft, and this surgery would be delayed until the remaining in-continuity portion of the nerve had been established as either a recoverable (first-, second-, or third-degree) injury or a nonrecoverable (fourth-degree) injury that also required surgical reconstruction. Frequently, in sixth-degree injuries, a portion of the nerve obviously requires a definitive nerve graft but another portion of the nerve appears likely to go on to recovery. *Definitive surgery should be delayed until the potential for the remainder of the nerve to recover has been ascertained.* In general, by 3 months, either clinical or electric evidence of recovery will allow a surgeon to determine whether or not a closed nerve injury is a third- or fourth-degree injury (i.e., will or will not require surgical intervention).

NERVE REPAIR

The unfavorable result of a nerve repair is a lack of motor or sensory recovery, the development of neuropathic pain, or both (1–4). Poor functional recovery is usually associated with increased painful sequelae as the nerve fibers that otherwise would provide neurologic recovery are blocked at the level of the nerve repair; this process results in neuroma formation and pain. If the longitudinal extent of injury is underestimated and the nerve repair is performed within the zone of neurologic injury, regenerating nerve fibers will be blocked by scar tissue, and a satisfactory result will not be obtained. Similarly, a technically outstanding nerve repair performed without tension and outside the zone of injury can facilitate excellent axonal regeneration with no functional recovery if the motor and sensory fascicles are misaligned. The following central tenets are important in predicting a favorable result following a nerve repair:

1. A neurologic deficit including subjective sensory loss associated with an open injury requires surgical exploration as soon as the clinical and surgical conditions permit.
2. Microsurgical technique with appropriate magnification, instrumentation, and suture material should be used.
3. The proximal and distal extent of the nerve injury must be carefully assessed so that the damaged nerve is resected or the nerve repair will not heal with scar tissue.
4. A nerve repair must be tension-free.
5. When a tension-free nerve repair is not possible, an interposition interfascicular nerve graft should be used.

* Because gunshot injuries have a great potential for recovery, they are treated as closed injuries (Fig. 12-2). Initial exploration, as noted above, would be performed only in a case with another indication for immediate surgery, such as vascular compromise.

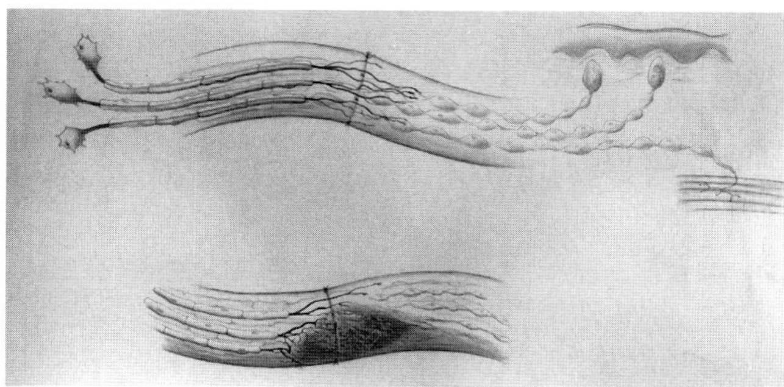

FIGURE 12-6. The top drawing demonstrates the ideal nerve repair, coapting healthy proximal and distal nerve. The bottom drawing emphasizes that if the nerve repair is performed between damaged proximal and distal nerve, then nerve regeneration will be inhibited, even when perfect microsurgical technique has been used. (From Mackinnon SE. Upper extremity nerve injuries: primary repair and reconstruction. In: Cohen ML, ed. *Mastery of plastic and reconstructive surgery.* Boston: Little, Brown and Company, 1994:1598–1624, with permission.)

6. Extreme postural positioning of an extremity to facilitate an end-to-end repair should be avoided. Both a nerve repair and a nerve graft must be carried out without tension at the repair site(s).
7. An epineural repair should be performed unless the intraneural topography dictates a group fascicular repair (e.g., ulnar nerve in the forearm and wrist). Early protected mobilization of the nerve repair or graft will minimize scar adhesion.
8. In the case of an injury requiring a very proximal repair or a very long nerve graft, a distal nerve transfer should be considered.
9. Postoperative motor and sensory reeducation with desensitization will maximize the surgical result and minimize painful sequelae.

The importance of fine microneurosurgical techniques and microsuture must be emphasized (5). In the failed primary repairs that I have treated, operative reports usually describe excellent surgical techniques. Accordingly, fine microsutures are noted at the time of reoperation, but a large amount of scar tissue is seen at the nerve repair site. Once the scar tissue has been excised, only a short gap separates the proximal and distal healthy fascicular patterns. This suggests that underestimating the longitudinal extent of a nerve injury is a key reason for failure of functional recovery following nerve repair (Fig. 12-6).

ELECTRODIAGNOSTIC STUDIES

Electrodiagnostic studies are very useful in determining the appropriate timing for surgical intervention; operating too early can downgrade an otherwise recoverable injury, and operating too late can preclude an excellent motor result. Thus, electrodiagnostic studies are extremely useful in determining the degree and management of a given nerve injury. A few points should be emphasized. The myelin influences conduction velocity and distal latency. By contrast, the function of the axon is reflected in the amplitude of the resulting response. A neurapraxia with demyelination will be associated with a decrease in conduction velocity across the lesion. Any injury involving the axon will be associated with a decrease in amplitude. False-positive results are easily generated in electrodiagnostic testing. For example, a decrease in temperature of 1°C will decrease the conduction velocity by approximately 5% and the distal latency by up to 0.2 to 0.3 msec. Similarly, on needle electromyography, a reduction in temperature will increase the polyphasic units and duration of waveforms and give the impression of a neurogenic injury. A neurapraxia will resolve with remyelination over a period of days to 3 months. With injuries to the axon, it may be possible to stimulate regions distal to the injury even up to 7–10 days after the injury. However, after this time, the ability to stimulate and record a response distal to the injury is lost. A week after a complete axonal injury, the response to motor and sensory nerve stimulation is lost. However, fibrillations are not seen until approximately 3 weeks after the injury. If the muscle is completely denervated and is not reinnervated, the fibrillations generally dissipate within a year. However, in partially denervated muscles, fibrillations may be seen for years following injury. Reinnervation in cases of partial denervation begins with collateral axonal sprouting from any remaining viable axons as they send small sprouts to the denervated muscle fibers. This results in a long duration and polyphasic units of the remaining motor units, but most of these motor units retain a normal amplitude. These changes are generally first seen 4 to 6 weeks following axonal injury. The motor units are a sign of reinnervation, and the presence of a large amplitude suggests collateral sprouting. Short-duration, low-voltage, immature polyphasic units are evidence of axonal regrowth and reinnervation, not of collateral sprouting. They can generally be recorded approximately 2 months before any clinical evidence of muscle reinnervation is noted. As the reinnervation process continues and more muscle fibers are reinnervated, the motor units over a period of months to years increase in size, and as the amplitude increases, the number of polyphasic units decreases. Fibrillations dissipate as the muscle is reinnervated, and ultimately, as the reinnervation process is completed, motor units larger than 5 mV and frequently 8 to 12 mV are noted. Polyphasic units dissipate and fibrillations resolve as the motor units are reorganized. Thus, in general, electrodiagnostic studies are initially performed approximately 6 weeks after a closed injury, and at that time, the examiner should be able to detect evidence of reinnervation if the injury pattern has allowed collateral sprouting. Before 6 weeks, absence of fibrillations distal to the level of injury will distinguish a neurapraxia from second-, third-, fourth-, and fifth-degree injuries. However, electric studies before 6 weeks do not distinguish "recoverable" (second- and third-degree) injuries from "nonrecoverable" (fourth- and fifth-degree) injuries. Thus, the author generally recommends obtaining electrodiagnostic studies at 6 to 8 weeks, when signs of reinnervation (motor unit potentials and nascent units) will distinguish second- and third-degree injuries from fourth- and fifth-degree injuries. With a closed injury, if no evidence of reinnervation is noted after 3 months, then surgical intervention is indicated (Fig. 12-2). During surgery, intraoperative electrodiagnostic testing is performed to confirm the preoperative findings.

PATIENT SELECTION

Patients with a sensory or motor neurologic deficit and electrodiagnostic studies supporting such functional loss are in general excellent candidates for surgical intervention. By contrast, patients with sensory and motor complaints but normal electrodiagnostic findings and patients with pain as their predominant complaint, even those with abnormal electrodiagnostic findings, are frequently not surgical candidates. When pain is a significant component of the clinical presentation, the utmost care must be taken in the patient selection. *The nuances of surgical technique are important for successful management, but equally if not more important is the selection of appropriate patients for surgical intervention.* We have modified a pain evaluation scale during the last decade to help identify patients with significant a psychological overlay (6) (Fig. 12-7). Even with the most outstanding surgical technique, inattention to the psychological aspects of peripheral nerve pain precludes a successful surgical outcome. Our pain evaluation questionnaire (Appendix 12-1) includes demographic data (age, sex, occupation); a list of 19 pain descriptors; body diagrams; five visual analogue scales; and 22 multiple choice questions. The 10-cm visual analogue scales are used to measure pain level, stress levels at home and at work, and stress coping levels at home and at work. For pain and stress levels, a higher rating indicates more pain and stress. For coping levels, higher ratings indicate a better ability to cope with stress. The multiple choice questions address pain and difficulty in performing work tasks; current work status; pain intensity; depression; illness behaviors; physical, emotional, and sexual abuse histories; and current pain medications. A questionnaire score between 0 and 60 is assigned on the basis of the patient's responses to the multiple choice questions. A questionnaire score above 23 indicates a higher likelihood of functional overlay in pain perception. The pain descriptors circled from the given list are counted, and the use of more than four adjectives suggests a tendency to exaggerate pain response. A drawing on the body diagram outside the anatomic area suggested by the nerve injury also suggests functional overlay problems. If a patient's score is positive in all three of these areas (adjectives, body diagram, questionnaire), then a psychiatric referral is recommended and surgery is not performed. If the patient's score is positive on two of these measurements, then surgery may be performed, but only after an appropriate psychological/psychiatric evaluation has been completed.

NEUROMAS

Painful neuromas are one of the most challenging problems to manage (7,8). The clinical diagnosis of a neuroma is made when significant pain is associated with the scar and sensibility is altered in the distribution of the involved nerve. More than 200 recommendations have been made for the management of neuroma formation. An understanding of the pathophysiology of the painful neuroma is critical in the clinical management of these problems. The microenvironment of a sensory nerve significantly influences its regeneration. If a sensory nerve is placed in an innervated muscle, regeneration will be inhibited. By contrast, if it is placed underneath denervated skin and scar, regeneration is encouraged. The neuroma itself is sensitive to mechanical stimulation, so that excision of the mature neuroma is recommended. Several general points can be made with respect to the surgical management of this problem:

1. Patient selection is key to the successful management of this problem.
2. Careful preoperative identification of the nerve(s) or fascicles involved in the neuroma formation is important. Preoperative anesthetic nerve blocks are useful in identifying the various nerves which may innervate the neuroma.
3. Restoration of the continuity of the peripheral nervous system is an appropriate first line of surgical management, with use of either a nerve repair or a nerve graft. If this fails, then proximal transposition is indicated, but the proximal transposition must relocate the new neuroma into an area that is not mechanically sensitive and is well away from the overlying skin and scar.
4. In general, surgery to manage neuromas involves excision of the established neuroma and proximal transposition of the involved nerve(s) away from any area of mechanical stimulation and well away from any scar or denervated skin.
5. Preoperative blockade with an antisympathetic medication such as bretylium and careful postoperative pain management with an antineuropathic medication such as gabapentin (Neurontin) are important aspects of intraoperative and overall management.
6. A peripheral nerve stimulator can be considered as a good salvage operation for pain control in a carefully selected patient (9) (Fig. 12-8).

the slightly more distal brachialis branches allows more powerful elbow flexion. As we become more familiar with the internal topography of the peripheral nerve and can carry out nerve grafts or nerve transfers to target specific motor and sensory fascicles, our results should improve dramatically. This chapter does not permit a detailed description of the nuances of the internal topography of all the peripheral nerves, and the reader is referred to other sources (1,4,5,11). Certainly, the most common cause of a failed nerve graft is inappropriate sensory and motor identification and nerve reconstruction, provided that otherwise appropriate microneurosurgical technique has been used.

Donor Grafts

The sural nerve remains the traditional donor nerve graft. However, several other expendable nerves can be utilized in reconstruction. The anterior branch of the medial antebrachial cutaneous nerve is an excellent donor graft. If only the anterior branch of the medial antebrachial cutaneous nerve is used, then the sensory loss is in the anterior surface of the forearm, not around the elbow and on the ulnar border of the forearm. If necessary, both anterior and posterior branches of the medial antebrachial cutaneous nerve can be used. The lateral antebrachial cutaneous nerve is identified adjacent to the cephalic vein in the proximal forearm. The sensory loss is minimal given the overlap of sensory distribution with the radial sensory nerve. We have recently used the terminal branch of the median nerve, which innervates the pronator quadratus. Use of the distal portion of the anterior interosseous nerve results in no motor or sensory functional loss. When a completely injured median nerve is reconstructed, use of the ulnar or medial portion of the median nerve innervating the third web space can be considered. Thus, the patient is not subjected to a new donor nerve sensory loss. Similarly, in a complete ulnar nerve loss, the dorsocutaneous branch of the ulnar nerve can be used as nerve graft material to reconstruct the main ulnar nerve.

NERVE TRANSFERS

Nerve transfers have traditionally been used within the brachial plexus for avulsion injuries. In the last 8 years, I have used nerve transfers whenever possible as an alternative to long nerve grafts. The transfer of a more distal nerve to the injured nerve eliminates the need for a long nerve graft. In most cases, a direct end-to-end repair of the transferred nerve to the recipient nerve is possible. Intraoperative electric stimulation will identify expendable, normal, pure motor nerves that can be used in the transfer. When more than one nerve is available for transfer, the use of a nerve that innervates a muscle whose action is synergistic with that of the target muscle is appropriate. Retraining of the reinnervated muscle is most easily achieved when nerves from muscles with synergistic action are used in the nerve transfer. The medial pectoral nerve is extremely useful in reinnervating

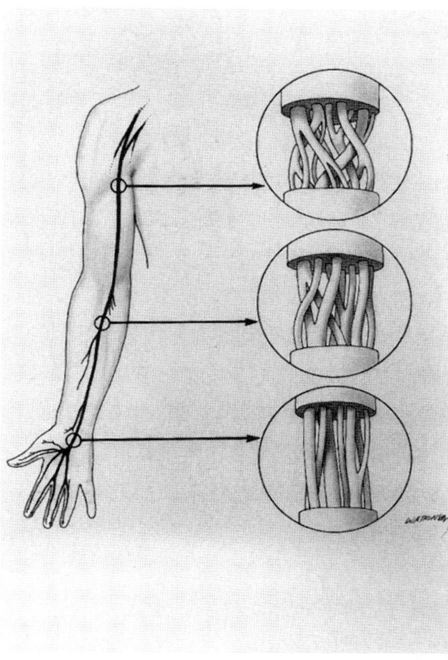

FIGURE 12-11. Although considerable plexus formation is noted between fascicles in the proximal portion of the extremity, this pattern changes considerably in the distal portion, where little plexus formation is found. (From Mackinnon SE, Dellon AL. *Surgery of the peripheral nerve.* New York: Thieme Medical Publishers, 1988:6, with permission.)

within the brachial plexus for both shoulder and elbow function. A thoracodorsal nerve transferred to the musculocutaneous nerve also provides excellent recovery of elbow flexion. With high ulnar nerve injuries, the distal portion of the anterior interosseous nerve, which innervates the pronator quadratus, can be transferred to the deep motor branch of the ulnar nerve (11) (Fig. 12-12). With high median nerve injuries, transfer of the ulnar nerve to the fourth web space over to the radial digital nerve to the index finger and the ulnar digital nerve to the thumb will rapidly provide important sensibility in the thumb and index finger. In patients who lack pronation because of brachial plexus neuritis, a redundant portion of the ulnar nerve (branches to the flexor carpi ulnaris) can be repaired directly to the nonfunctioning pronator teres branch. In patients with a functioning flexor digitorum superficialis muscle, the nerve to the superficialis muscle has been transferred to the nerve to the denervated pronator muscle with successful reinnervation of the pronator teres muscle.

Nerve transfers have become our treatment of choice for proximal injuries and have dramatically altered our expectations for functional recovery following nerve injury (12).

CARPAL TUNNEL RELEASE

Carpal tunnel surgery is generally performed well and yields excellent results. Because of the increased incidence of repetitive work-related disorders of the upper extremity, the sur-

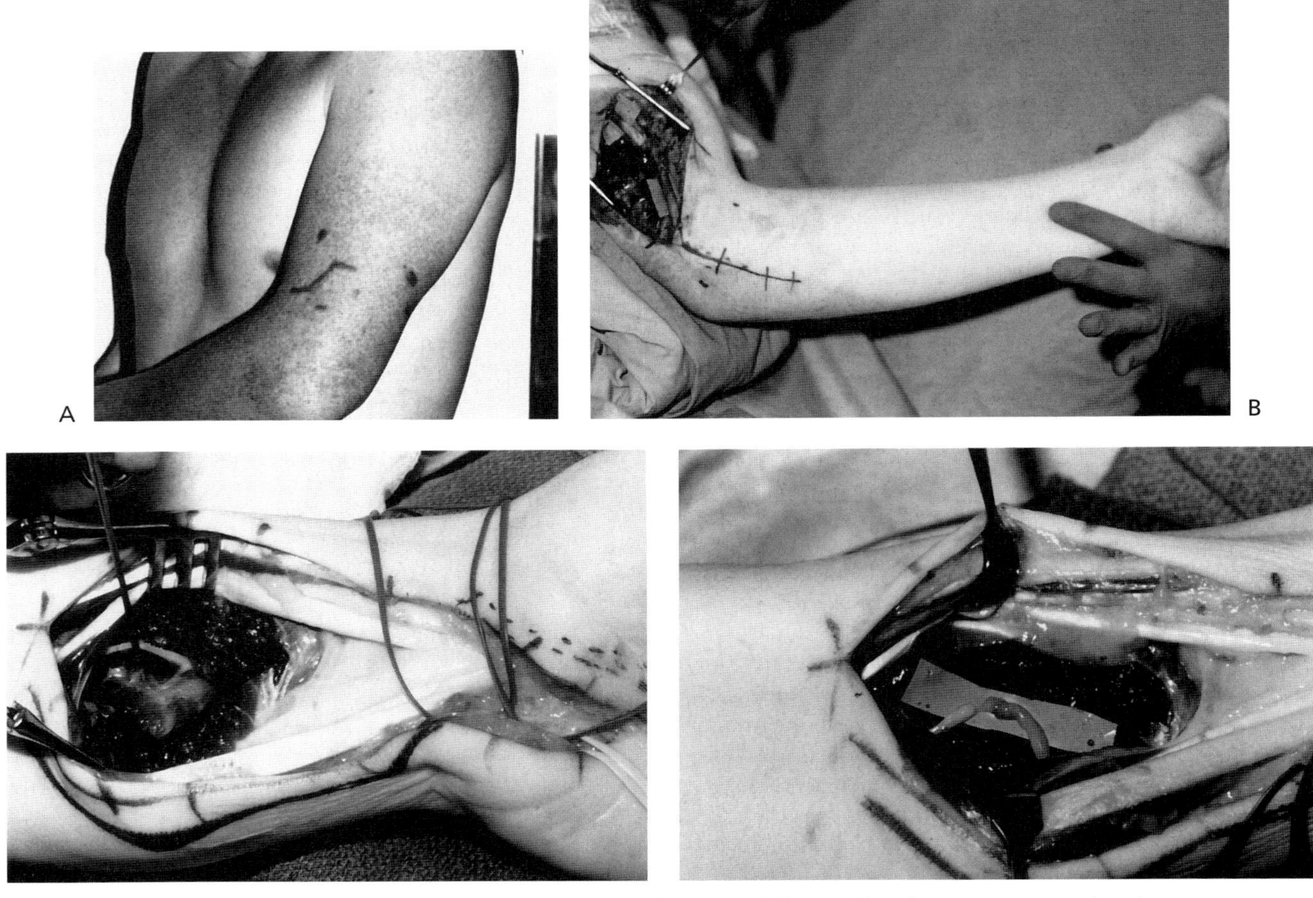

FIGURE 12-12. A: This patient had a proximal ulnar nerve injury. **B:** The ulnar nerve was explored and repaired proximally. **C:** The terminal branch of the anterior interosseous nerve innervating the pronator quadratus is identified and followed into the midportion of the pronator quadratus. The sensory and motor fascicular groups of the ulnar nerve are identified in the hand. **D:** A direct repair between the anterior interosseous nerve and the motor branch of the ulnar will provide satisfactory, although not entirely normal, reinnervation of the intrinsic muscles in the hand. (From Mackinnon SE, Novak CB. Nerve transfers: new options for reconstruction following nerve injury. *Hand Clin* 1999, with permission.)

geon should be very careful to examine the patient for more proximal levels of nerve compression. A body diagram drawing that demonstrates sensory disturbance and especially pain beyond the area of the median nerve distribution in the hand should alert the surgeon to other, associated problems, such as median nerve compression in the proximal forearm, ulnar nerve compression at the elbow, thoracic outlet syndrome, or muscle strain. An "unfavorable" result following a complete carpal tunnel decompression with failure to relieve symptoms is usually the consequence of failure to diagnose associated problems. Symptoms will clearly not be relieved with a second operation, and the possibility of nerve injury increases with repeated surgery. I have recently presented our protocol for the evaluation and management of patients with complains of upper extremity nerve compression (6,13). If time is taken to perform a complete examination of the upper extremity, including an evaluation of the neck and shoulder in patients presenting with carpal tunnel syndrome, patients will not be led to expect that their symptoms will be relieved by a carpal tunnel release when other, associated problems are present.

Because of the variation in branching patterns of the median nerve, especially in the distal portion of the carpal tunnel, iatrogenic nerve injuries involving a portion of the median nerve do occur, especially to the fascicles to the third web space. With the national increase in obesity, such injuries are becoming more common as the "simple carpal tunnel release" becomes more difficult. The use of loupe magnification and tourniquet control can assist in ensuring a good result. With more than half of all Americans ages 20 to 74 now overweight, the use of forearm tourniquets to perform carpal tunnel releases will decrease the incidence of venous tourniquet problems in larger arms. Also, less anesthetic is needed, so that tourniquet time is shorter. Special care and attention must be taken at the most distal and most proximal levels of the release. When releasing the distal antebrachial fascia, I position myself at the end of the operating table to be able to visualize the fascia clearly. If there is any concern, I extend the incision proximally rather than compromise visualization of the antebrachial fascia and median nerve.

An incision placed well medial to the thenar crease in line with the fourth ray decreases the chance of injury to the palmar cutaneous branch of the median nerve. This incision is also positioned between the median and ulnar nerves, so that any scarring is well away from the nerves (14). The fact that pillar pain is not seen with this approach may be related to a decreased incidence of injury to the small cutaneous nerves. To minimize the occurrence of postoperative reflex sympathetic dystrophy, chronic regional pain syndrome, or painful sequelae, I include 1.5 mg of bretylium per kilogram of body weight in the intravenous regional anesthesia.

Postoperative management is key to a good result following carpal tunnel release. The dressing is removed 2 days after surgery. Range of movement is encouraged, and the patient is told to wear a wrist-neutral splint at night for 3 weeks and during the day for comfort as necessary. If the patient has bilateral symptoms, an excellent result from the first surgery should be obtained before a second surgery is undertaken on the contralateral arm, especially in worker's compensation cases. The simultaneous release of both carpal tunnels is contraindicated because of the associated limitation of activity in both arms and hands.

A common iatrogenic nerve injury in carpal tunnel release is to the palmar cutaneous branch of the median nerve. This is treated effectively by exploration of the median nerve well proximal to the wrist. The palmar cutaneous branch from the main median nerve is identified and neurolysis performed such that it can be turned back proximally to lie in the muscle interface between the superficial and deep digital flexors in the mid-forearm. The second most common iatrogenic nerve injury is to the ulnar side of the median nerve. This area of injury to the median nerve can be excised and grafted. However, if the patient has significant pain, does not want a nerve graft, and will agree to numbness in the third web space versus pain in this area, then the fascicles innervating the third web space can be transposed proximally to lie in the muscle interface between the deep and superficial flexor muscle mass. The ulnar side of the median nerve, which innervates the third web space, can be separated from the main portion of the median nerve for a long distance. If a nerve graft is needed to repair a damaged portion of the median nerve, then upper extremity nerve grafts are usually superior to sural nerve grafts because they cause less morbidity. Use of the anterior branch of the medial antebrachial cutaneous nerve creates a cosmetically acceptable donor scar that is hidden in the medial aspect of the arm. Use of the lateral antebrachial cutaneous nerve causes little donor deficit because of significant overlap with the radial sensory nerve. More recently, I have used the terminal portion of the anterior interosseous nerve, which innervates the pronator quadratus, as a short nerve graft that causes no donor sensory or motor functional deficit. Offering patients the opportunity to choose between these various nerve grafts gives them some sense of control in decision making, which is especially important in patients with an iatrogenic nerve injury.

The technique of surgical management of problems relating to carpal tunnel surgery has been extensively discussed and reviewed (15).

CUBITAL TUNNEL SYNDROME

In comparison with carpal tunnel syndrome, the surgical results of cubital tunnel syndrome are generally less satisfactory. The fact that five or six operations are recommended for the management of cubital tunnel syndrome reflects the lack of consensus among surgeons regarding the superiority of any one particular procedure. Unfortunately, a common unfavorable result following cubital tunnel surgery is severe pain and dysfunction. The avoidance of this problem is relatively straightforward. The surgeon should learn a technique that is tried and true. This is not a procedure that the surgeon can learn from a textbook. Successful results depend on good surgical technique. A novice surgeon should learn a technique for the management of cubital tunnel syndrome from a more experienced surgeon who performs a large number of cubital tunnel surgeries with good results. For surgeons who have not yet found a procedure that reliably gives excellent results, I recommend a modification of the anterior submuscular transposition (16). I have performed this procedure for 18 years on approximately 50 patients per year. (In a study of subjective patient outcome following this surgical procedure, with a mean follow-up of 37 months, 77% of patients reported that they were better and 13% said they were no different.) Key points in the technique involve careful identification and protection of the medial antebrachial cutaneous nerve, removal of the medial intermuscular septum, creation of fascial flaps that are closed above the transposed ulnar nerve in a lengthened position so as not to compress the ulnar nerve, and removal of all the tendinous bands within the origin of the flexor pronator muscle, where they can compress the ulnar nerve in its newly transposed position. Attention must be directed to any distal fascial bands that might compress the ulnar nerve as it is moved from its normal position in the flexor carpi ulnaris muscle up to its new anterior position in the transposed location. These thin but strong distal fascial bands will compress the ulnar nerve at the distal transposition site.

A technically perfect surgical procedure can be compromised by mismanagement in the postoperative period. The suction drain is removed on the first postoperative day, and on the second or third postoperative day, all the dressings are removed. Range of movement is encouraged at this time. Early postoperative movement is imperative for a favorable result. By 3 weeks, full range of movement should be achieved. For the first 3 weeks, the patient wears a sling at night and during the day for comfort. At 4 weeks, strengthening exercises are started. For those surgeons interested in learning this procedure, a video is available through the American Society for Surgery of the Hand.

The most common and most disturbing complication of surgical treatment for cubital tunnel syndrome is injury to the medial antebrachial cutaneous nerve. This nerve usually crosses the incision approximately 1 inch distal to the medial epicondyle, and a more proximal, smaller branch is noted approximately 2 inches proximal to the medial epicondyle. The surgeon may need to mobilize the medial antebrachial cutaneous nerve to elevate the soft tissue flaps above the pronator muscle origin. Dissection of the soft tissue flap above the flexor pronator muscle origin should be performed at the level of the muscle fascia, with reflection of all the soft tissue superiorly. Because the medial antebrachial cutaneous nerve runs in the soft tissue, this practice will ensure that the nerve is not injured as it is being elevated in the subcutaneous flap. If the nerve is injured, neurolysis should be performed proximally. The distal end is then cauterized with microbipolar cautery and turned back proximally to lie well away from the overlying skin and scar. Alternatively, it can be dropped to lie below the flexor pronator muscle origin well away from the skin and scar and in a muscle environment. It is well recognized that the medial intermuscular septum can kink the ulnar nerve when the nerve is transposed anteriorly. It is less recognized that the fascia between and within the flexor carpi ulnaris muscle can compress the ulnar nerve at its most distal location once the nerve has been moved anteriorly. The surgeon should check and recheck both proximally and distally to ensure that no structures are kinking the ulnar nerve once it is transposed anteriorly. The surgeon should be able to run a finger along the course of the ulnar nerve and not feel any tight bands compressing the nerve. In the vast majority of the failed submuscular transpositions that I have seen, the tendinous bands within the flexor pronator muscle origin have not been removed, and these bands then significantly compress the ulnar nerve. It is appropriate to emphasize again that early postoperative movement, so that scarring does not tether the ulnar nerve, is key to successful treatment.

Patients who have had an unfavorable result following an ulnar nerve transposition are candidates for revisionary surgery with the technique described before. When other surgically failed transpositions are redone, special attention should be directed to the medial antebrachial cutaneous nerve. If there is any question preoperatively of medial antebrachial cutaneous nerve injury, the involved branch should be transferred back into the triceps muscle or into the soft tissue of the upper arm, well away from the overlying skin and scar. Occasionally, it is easier to identify the medial antebrachial cutaneous nerve proximally adjacent to the basilic vein and then follow the nerve distally. The posterior branch of the medial antebrachial cutaneous nerve is frequently injured, and the anterior branch is usually not injured. If a portion of either branch is involved, then the entire branch should be treated with proximal transposition. Previous failed decompression and subcutaneous transposition are fairly simply managed by neurolysis and elevation of the ulnar nerve, creation of the fascial flaps, and performance of the procedure noted previously. Previously failed intermuscular or submuscular cases are more difficult. The surgeon will have to find the ulnar nerve proximally and distally and then work back and forth through the previous surgical site. Tendinous bands compressing the nerve must be removed. Occasionally, the surgeon will be able to leave some of the soft muscle that was previously transposed above the nerve intact, but all the tendinous bands must be removed. Postoperative management includes the use of bupivacaine anesthesia in the incision and a bupivacaine anesthetic pain pump. Early movement is as important in the repeated ulnar nerve operation, as it is in the primary ulnar transposition.

If the revisionary surgery fails, then the patient should be evaluated as a potential candidate for a peripheral nerve stimulator. To qualify for a nerve stimulator, the patient should respond positively to an anesthetic block of the ulnar nerve and should "pass" a Minnesota Multiphasic Personality Inventory or other psychological type of evaluation. The vast majority (80%) of patients who are carefully selected for peripheral nerve stimulators respond positively and obtain significant pain relief.

CONCLUSION

Unfortunately, unfavorable results following peripheral nerve surgery do occur. Similarly, iatrogenic nerve injuries following unrelated surgeries occur with some frequency. In the event of an iatrogenic nerve injury, it is recommended that the responsible surgeon acknowledge and apologize for this incidence as soon as it is recognized. Complications relating to the peripheral nerve can be well within standard of care but are still extremely painful, if not disabling, for the patient. When explaining standard of care complications to patients, I draw a box and label that procedure *A*. I explain to the patient that in my opinion their complication is or is not acceptable for that given procedure (i.e., I mark the complication as an *X* either within or outside the procedure box). Because these complications can be painful or neurologically disabling and still be within standard of care, it is up to the surgeon to help the patient understand their particular complication. For example, an injury to the sural nerve during removal of a tumor or an ankle procedure is not outside the standard of care. A phrenic or long thoracic nerve palsy in a

TABLE 12-2. NERVE INJURY RECOVERY

Degree of Nerve Injury	Recovery	Rate of Recovery	Surgery
1. Neurapraxia	Complete	Fast, days to 12 weeks	None
2. Axonotmesis	Complete	Slow (1 inch per month)	None
3.	Incomplete	Slow (1 inch per month)	None or neurolysis
4.	No recovery		Nerve repair or graft
5. Neurotmesis	No recovery		Nerve repair or graft
6. Mixed injury	Recovery and reconstruction vary depending on the combination of injury patterns as noted above.		

From Mackinnon SE, Dellon AL. *Surgery of the peripheral nerve*. New York: Thieme Medical Publishers, 1988, with permission.

brachial plexus/first rib resection is a known complication and not outside the standard of care, given the very small size of these nerves. However, these injuries cause the patient significant pain and dysfunction and may require a second surgical procedure for correction. By contrast, an injury to the accessory nerve during removal of a lymph node in a primary surgery without previous surgical scar or radiation is outside the standard of care. It is difficult if not impossible for patients to understand that a neurologic problem does not imply surgical negligence. Much time and emotion can be saved if the surgeon explains nerve injury and regeneration to the patient.

If a given surgeon has had an unfavorable result following peripheral nerve surgery, it is appropriate to seek the advice of another surgeon who can be objective in analyzing the complication. This surgeon may be a more appropriate person to address the issue of whether the injury is within the standard of care. If secondary surgery is necessary, referral to an independent surgeon with expertise in managing nerve problems is recommended.

Finally, because of the time required for nerves to recover, especially when problems occur proximally in the extremity, it is necessary for the surgeon to explain the pathophysiology of nerve injury and regeneration to the patient. A simplified chart of nerve injuries and recovery will assist patients in understanding their complicated nerve problems. I show Table 12-2, which is a simplified version of Table 12-1, to my patients. Patients helped to understand the cause of an unfavorable result and the constructive plan for its resolution are better able to tolerate the complication. Such understanding enables patients and surgeons to work together to achieve a successful, favorable outcome.

APPENDIX 12-1.

Pain Questionnaire.

ID:________________________________ Date:______________________

SSN:____/___/______ DOB: ___/___/___ Age:________ Sex: Male___ Female____

Diagnosis:____ Hand Dom: Right___ Left___

1. Pain is difficult to describe. Circle the words that best describe your symptoms:

Burning	Throbbing	Aching	Stabbing	Tingling	Dull
Twisting	Cramping	Cutting	Shooting	Numbing	Vague
Stinging	Squeezing	Pulling	Smarting	Pressure	Coldness
Indescribable	Other:________________________________				

2. Mark your average level of pain in the last month?

____

No Pain Most Severe Pain

3. Where is your pain? (Draw on diagram)

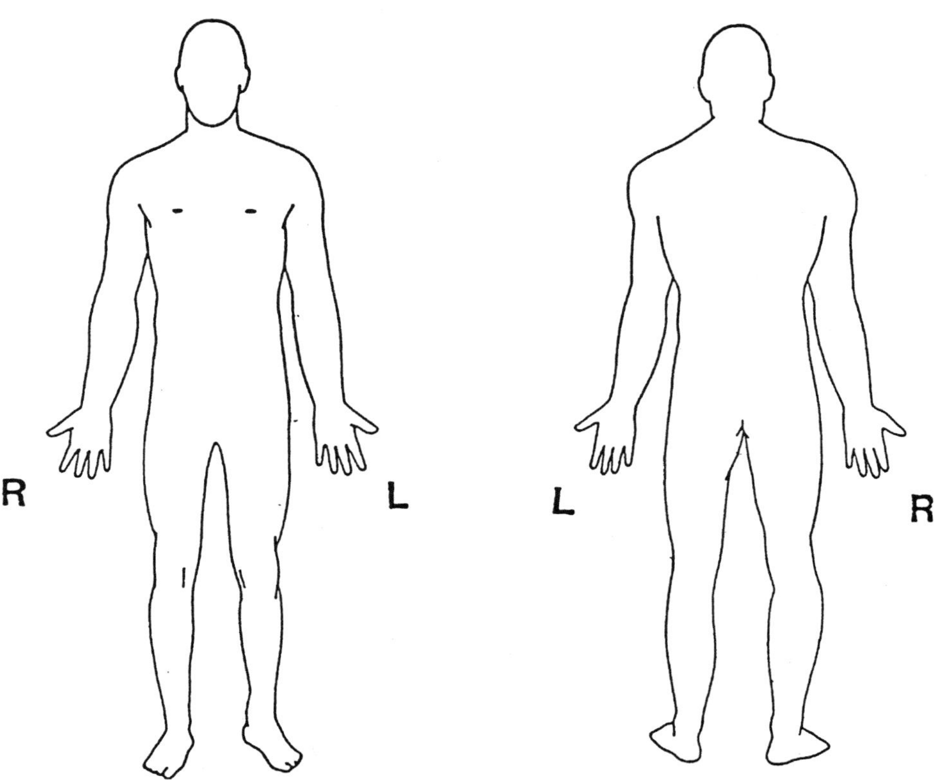

ID:______________________

4. Mark your average level of stress in the last month?

at home ____________________________________
0 10

at work ____________________________________
0 10

5. How well are you able to cope with that stress?

at home ____________________________________
Very Well Not at all

at work ____________________________________
Very Well Not at all

6. Does movement have any effect on your pain?
   a. The pain is always worsened by use or movement
   b. The pain is usually worsened by use and movement
   c. The pain is not altered by use and movement

7. Does weather have any effect on your pain?
   a. The pain is usually worse with damp or cold weather.
   b. The pain is occasionally worse with damp or cold weather.
   c. Damp or cold weather have no effect on the pain.

8. If you are retired, a student or homemaker, proceed to Question 8B.

8A. Are you still working?
   a. Works every day at the same pre-pain job.
   b. Works every day but the job is not the same as the pre-pain job with reduced responsibility or physical activity
   c. Works occasionally.
   d. Not presently working.

8B. Are you able to do your household chores?
   a. Does same level of household activities without discomfort.
   b. Does same level of household chores with discomfort.
   c. Does a reduced amount of household chores.
   d. Most household chores are now performed by others.

ID:__________________________

9. Do you ever have trouble falling asleep or awaken from sleep?
   a. No - Proceed to Question 10 **b.** Yes - Proceed to 9A & 9B

9A. How often do you have trouble falling asleep?
   a. Trouble falling asleep every night due to pain
   b. Trouble falling asleep due to pain most nights of the week
   c. Occasionally having difficulty falling asleep due to pain
   d. No trouble falling asleep due to pain
   e. Trouble falling asleep which is not related to pain

9B. How often do you awaken from sleep?
   a. Awakened by pain every night
   b. Awakened from sleep by pain more than 3 times per week
   c. Not usually awakened from sleep by pain
   d. Restless sleep or early morning awakening with or without being able to return to sleep, both unrelated to pain

10. Has your pain affected your intimate personal relationships?
   a. No **b.** Yes

11. Are you involved in any legal action regarding your physical complaint?
   a. No **b.** Yes

12. Is this a Workers' Compensation case?
   a. No **b.** Yes

13. Have you ever thought of suicide?
   a. No **b.** Yes **c.** Previous suicide attempts

14. Are you presently receiving psychiatric treatment?
   a. No **b.** Yes **c.** Previous psychiatric treatment

15. Are you a victim of emotional abuse?
   a. No **b.** Yes **c.** No comment

16. Are you a victim of physical abuse?
   a. No **b.** Yes **c.** No comment

17. Are you a victim of sexual abuse?
   a. No **b.** Yes **c.** No comment

18. Are you presently a victim of abuse?
   a. No **b.** Yes **c.** No comment

ID:________________________

19. How many surgical procedures have you had in order to try to eliminate the cause of your pain?
   a. None or one
   b. Two surgical procedures
   c. Three or four surgical procedures
   d. Greater than four surgical procedures

20. How did the pain that you are now experiencing occur?
   a. Sudden onset with accident or definable event
   b. Slow progressive onset
   c. Slow progressive onset with acute exacerbation without an accident or definable event
   d. A sudden onset without an accident or definable event

21. What medications have you used in the past month?
   a. No medications
   b. List medications:____

   ____

   ____

22. If you had three wishes for anything in the world, what would you wish for?

   1. ____

   2. ____

   3. ____

Name: ______________________ Date: ______________

RIGHT

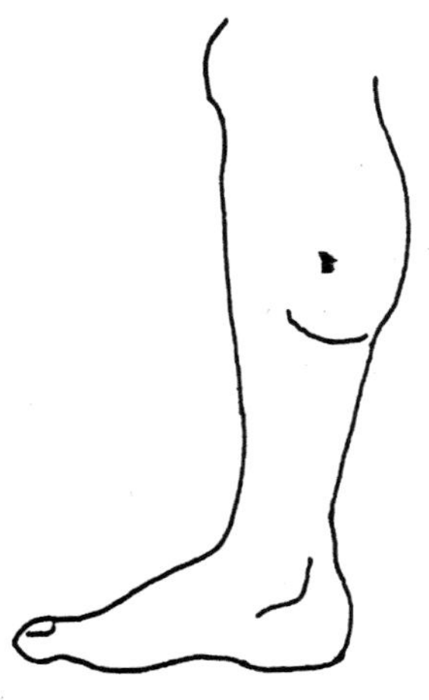
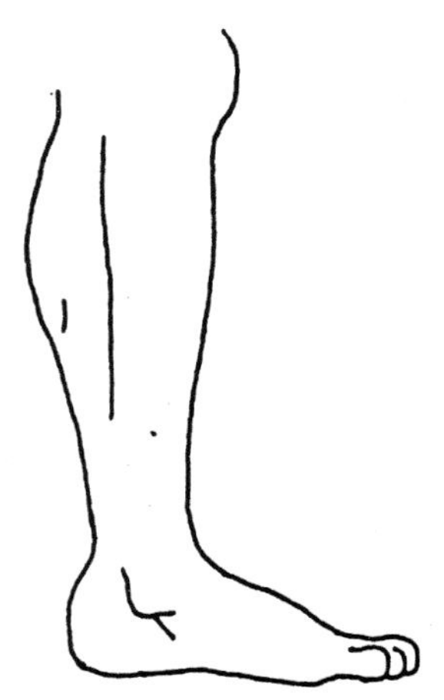
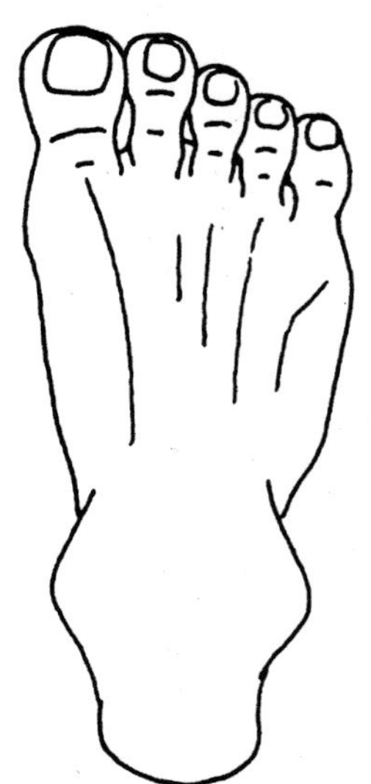
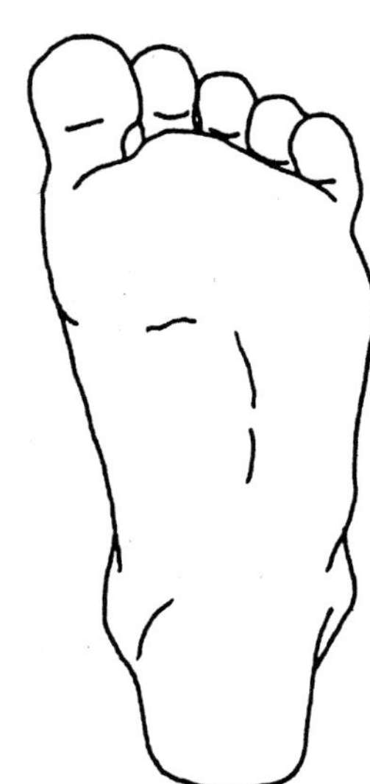

LEFT

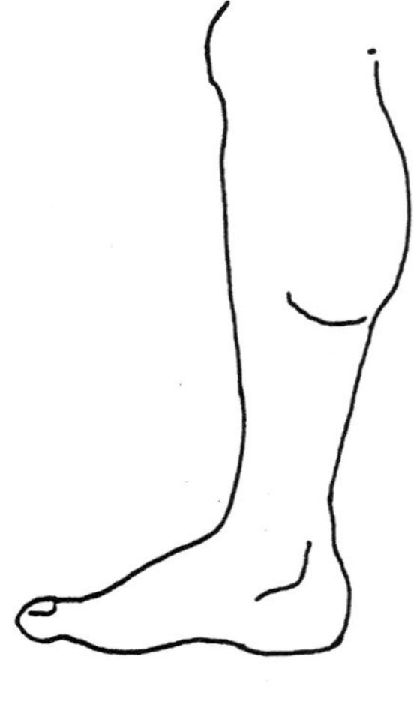
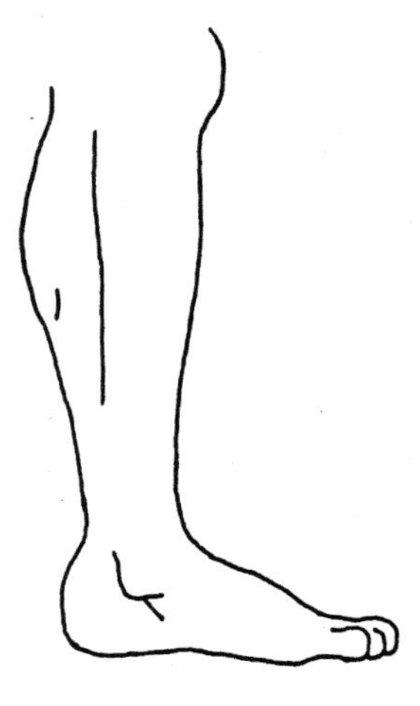
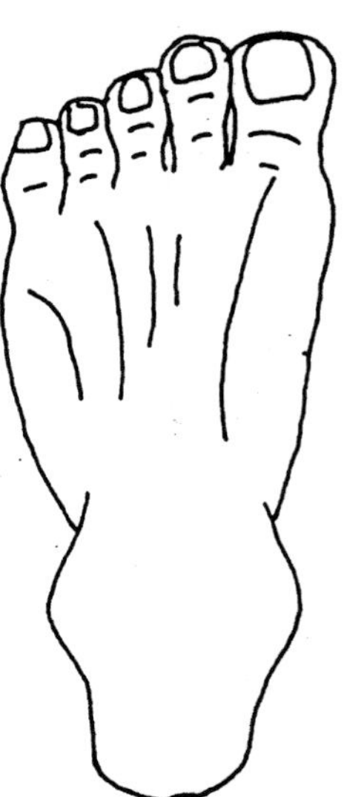
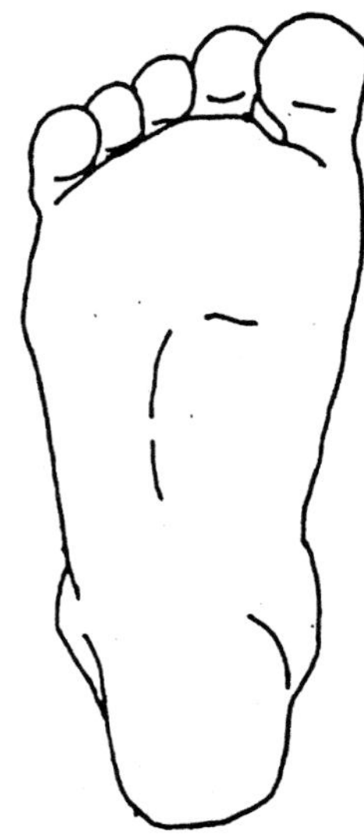

Name: ______________________________ Date: ______________

Dominant Hand: Right ___ Left ___

Right

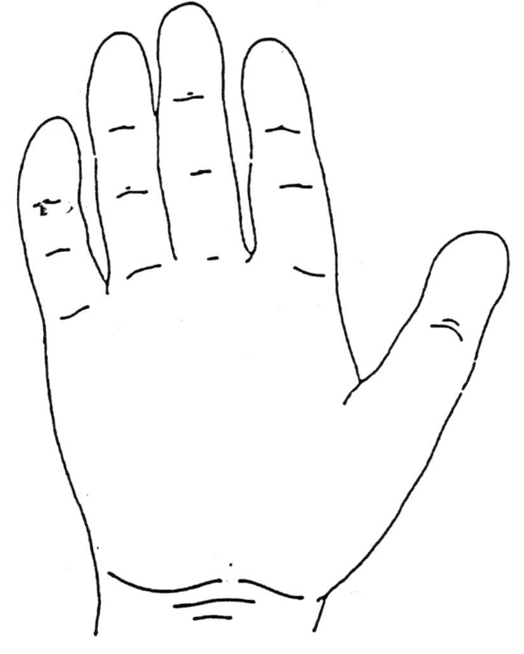

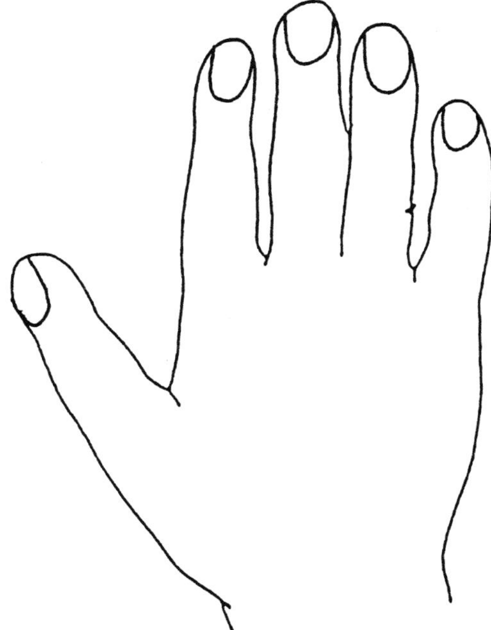

Left

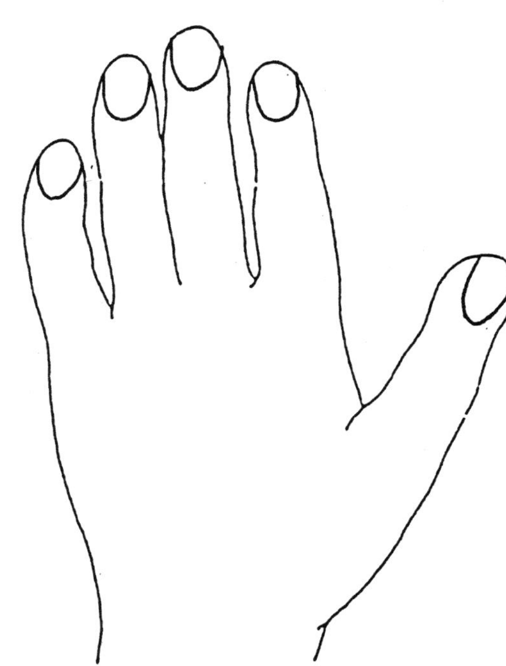

REFERENCES

1. Brandt KE, Mackinnon SE. Microsurgical repair of peripheral nerves and nerve grafts. In: Aston SJ, Beasley RW, Thorne C, eds. *Grabb & Smith's plastic surgery.* Philadelphia: Lippincott–Raven Publishers, 1997;5:79–90.
2. Mackinnon SE. Peripheral nerve injuries. In: Light T, ed. *Hand surgery update.* Englewood, CA: American Society for Surgery of the Hand, 1999:199–210.
3. Watchmaker G, Mackinnon SE. Nerve repair and reconstruction. In: Peimer CA, ed. *Surgery of the hand and upper extremity.* New York: McGraw-Hill, 1996:1251–1276.
4. Watchmaker GP, Mackinnon SE. Advances in peripheral nerve repair. *Clin Plast Surg* 1997;24:63–73.
5. Mackinnon SE. Techniques of nerve repair. In: Tindall GT, Cooper PR, Barrow DL, eds. *The practice of neurosurgery.* Baltimore: Williams & Wilkins, 1996:2879–2908.
6. Mackinnon SE, Novak CB. Evaluation of the patient with thoracic outlet syndrome. *Chest Surg Clin North Am* 1999;9:725–746.
7. Mackinnon SE. Evaluation and treatment in painful neuroma. In: Weiland A, ed. *Techniques in hand and upper extremity surgery.* Philadelphia: Lippincott–Raven Publishers, 1997:1–19.
8. Mackinnon SE. Neuromas. In: Gould JS, ed. *Foot and ankle clinics: nerve problems of the foot and ankle.* Philadelphia: WB Saunders, 1998;3:385–404.
9. Novak CB, Mackinnon SE. Outcome following implant of peripheral nerve stimulator in patients with chronic nerve pain. *Plast Reconstr Surg* 1999;105:1967–1985, 2806.
10. Mackinnon SE. Surgical approach to the radial nerve. In: Weiland A, ed. *Techniques in hand and upper extremity surgery.* Philadelphia: Lippincott–Raven Publishers, 1999;3:87–98.
11. Mackinnon SE. Evaluation of nerve gaps: upper and lower extremities. In: Omer GE, Spinner M, Van Beek AL, eds. *Management of peripheral nerve problems.* Philadelphia: WB Saunders, 1998:328–339.
12. Mackinnon SE, Novak CB. Nerve transfers: new options for reconstruction following nerve injury. *Hand Clin* 1999;15: 643–666.
13. Mackinnon SE. Thoracic outlet syndrome: a current overview. *Chest Surg Clin North Am* 1999;9:701–712.
14. Watchmaker GP, Weber D, Mackinnon SE. Avoidance of transection of the palmar cutaneous branch of the median nerve in carpal tunnel release. *J Hand Surg* 1996;21A:644–650.
15. Mackinnon SE, Tung T. Management of nerve lesions after open or endoscopic carpal tunnel release. In: Luchetti R, ed. *Carpal tunnel syndrome.* Rome: Verduci Editore, 2001 *(in press).*
16. Mackinnon SE. Submuscular transposition of the ulnar nerve at the elbow. In: Rengachary SS, Wilkins RH, eds. *Neurosurgical operative atlas.* Park Ridge, IL: American Association of Neurological Surgeons, 1995:225–233.

Discussion

NERVE GRAFTS

DAVID T. W. CHIU

Dr. Susan Mackinnon has presented a voluminous chapter in which she addresses the methods used to minimize the complications associated with nerve repair and grafting, neuroma surgery, carpal tunnel release, and ulnar nerve transposition. She also reviews the approaches suggested to treat such complications. In general, the author's objectives have been met with glowing success. However, I believe that certain areas of particular interest invite further discussion.

ON "TIMING"

As a prelude to nerve reconstruction, the importance of timely electrodiagnostic studies and the proper timing of surgery has been stressed. An illustrative case of a complex facial nerve palsy following an acoustic neuroma extirpation is cited. This is a very common scenario. What makes this example interesting is that the surgeon who removed acoustic neuroma was very proud of the fact that the facial nerve (CN VII) was well preserved intraoperatively. The key in this case is a thorough history and examination. The likelihood of CN VII not having been destroyed and the incompleteness of the CN VII palsy should be revealed in the history; the reemergence of the nasolabial fold ought to provide the lucky consultant with a hint to withhold the scalpel. The electrodiagnostic study was simply confirmatory, as any test should be. I believe this case example indicates that diagnostic acumen is the most important "good" beginning of a potentially long journey. Diagnostic acumen derives from detailed history taking and careful examination. Once the diagnosis is correctly made, the decision regarding when to

D. T. W. Chiu: Division of Plastic Surgery, Columbia-Presbyterian Medical Center, New York, New York

intervene or, more importantly, whether to intervene at all becomes elementary.

ON "CLASSIFICATION"

The author elaborates on and correlates the classification of Sir Herbert Seddon with that of Sir Sydney Sunderland, as well as her own additions to the latter.

Sir Sydney Sunderland's classification is based on the nature and extent of the damage to the intrinsic anatomy of the nerve trunk. The five degrees of injury so designated were intended to indicate increasing severity of injury, ranging from functional blockage of a structurally intact axon (first-degree injury) to complete severance of the entire nerve trunk (fifth-degree injury). As explained with insight by Sir Sydney Sunderland, depending on the nature of the offending mechanism, the severity of the injury inflicted can vary either across or along the length of the nerve trunk; as a consequence, mixed lesions are produced, with the first four degrees of injury occurring in various combinations (1). The sixth degree added by the author is convenient in that a box is provided to be checked when the existence of mixed injuries is suspected. However, it is mathematically incomplete. After all, for four variables, eleven possible combinations are given. The provision of only one box will very likely drive a mathematically inclined purist insane. My recommendation is to keep it simple.

ON "NERVE REPAIR"

The author enumerates nine points on nerve repair that certainly represent the valuable opinion of an expert in this area. I believe that one caveat should be offered regarding the first point: "A neurologic deficit including subjective sensory loss associated with an open injury requires surgical exploration as soon as the clinical and surgical conditions permit." I suggest that the following qualifications be added: (a) if the area of penetration or laceration corresponds to the course of the nerve or nerves in which a motor or sensory function deficit has been detected after the injury, and (b) if no well-intentioned emergency doctor in the referring facility has administered local anesthesia to ease the patient's pain.

In addition, regarding the fifth point, I would like to add that when a tension-free nerve repair is not possible, a bridge graft should be used. For nerve gaps larger than 3 cm, a critical sensory nerve of varying size or an interposition autogenous nerve graft should be used. However, for nonessential sensory nerves with gaps smaller than 3 cm, an autogenous venous nerve conduit should be considered (2).

Epineural repair has the advantage of simplicity, particularly when the vasa nervorum are clearly recognizable; however, it carries the disadvantage of uncertain fascicular alignment. Perineural repair, on the contrary, offers precise fascicular alignment, but it is handicapped by the unavoidably excessive trauma that results from the manipulation of individual fascicles and the introduction of foreign bodies, namely sutures. A happy medium is the technique of perineural repair in which the epiperineural suturing technique is utilized. For the median nerve at the wrist level, I too favor perineural repair, but with the epi-perineural suturing technique. For the common digital nerve, perineural repair is more strategic (3).

ON "ELECTRODIAGNOSTIC STUDIES"

The author (a) emphasizes the value of electrodiagnostic studies in determining the timing for surgical intervention, (b) touches upon the physiologic basis for electrodiagnostic studies, (c) cautions about the technical sensitivity of the test, and (d) chalks up several strategic time points for electrodiagnostic testing.

Electrodiagnosis, since the first publication of Hodes et al. in 1948 (4), in which they described altered nerve conduction in human diseases and the slowing of nerve conduction velocity in regenerating nerves, has been useful in (a) localizing the site of a nerve lesion, (b) measuring the severity of an injury, and (c) gauging the progress of recovery. Electrodiagnosis is in fact an extension of the clinical examination of the neuromuscular system. As useful as it is as a diagnostic tool, numerous biologic as well as technical variables deserve attention, notably the following: (a) limb temperature, (b) age of the patient, (c) height of the patient, (d) proximity to the spine, and (e) interexaminer variability.

Dr. Mackinnon has mentioned the effect of temperature. Dengs (5) reported that skin temperature of the limb below 30°C reduces nerve conduction velocity, increases the amplitude of the action potential, and enhances neuromuscular transmission. Moreover, fibrillation may not be detectable in a cool limb. Age is another interesting variable and probably reflects age-related myelination. In children of 5 years old or younger, the nerve conduction velocity is about one-third to one-half that of older children or adults. On the other side of the spectrum, sensory nerve action potentials decline with age. Over the age of 65, the sural nerve sensory potential may not be recordable in normal subjects (6).

The conduction velocity of the proximal portion of a nerve is difficult to measure. Special techniques, such as the f response, has been developed to estimate the proximal nerve conduction. The f response, first recorded from a muscle of the foot, registers a late response evoked by peripheral stimulation; it propagates antidromically to activate the anterior horn cell. The lower motor neurons discharge and generate a secondary action potential, which then traverses orthodromically down the path of the axon (7). The body height of the subject has been found to be a variable in nerve conduction velocity. In the sural, tibial, and peroneal nerves, conduction velocity is inversely correlated with height (8). Ultimately, however, one should recognize the significant interexaminer variability in the measurement of nerve action potentials (e.g., sensory action potential and compound motor action potential) (9,10). Nerve conduction velocity is less affected by interexaminer variability and is a better parameter to use for longitudinal study.

Caution should be used in ordering an electrodiagnostic study. One must screen patients who are receiving anticoagulants. Proper precautions must be taken and preparations made before testing. In choosing a facility for electrodiagnostic study, the referring physician must be assured of a facility's compliance with sterile technique because needle puncture is required to obtain an electromyographic recording.

ON "NEUROMAS"

I am in complete agreement with the author's view that painful neuromas are one of the most challenging problems to manage. This problem indeed taxes and tests the treating physician's diagnostic acumen, patience, tenacity, and surgical skill.

The author has offered six pointers that in general are very helpful guidelines. However, accurate diagnosis, rather than patient selection, is the key to success. Diagnosis involves the determination first of whether a painful neuroma is present, and second of whether the neuroma is fed by one or multiple sensory nerves. To address the first question, the examining physician can, during the initial evaluation, (a) identify the point of maximal discomfort by examination or (b) inject the focal point of pain with local anesthetics. If the injection test is successful in relieving all the symptoms, then the diagnosis is confirmed. If there is reason to suspect multiple nerve involvement, then one can perform a selective nerve block in a separate setting. Another technique that I have been using for more than a decade is positive identification of the neuroma preoperatively. Before the patient is anesthetized, the target point is injected with a mixture of lidocaine and methylene blue. Again, complete resolution of the neuroma pain is used as proof that the target is color-coded. For deep-seated and small neuromas, such as those of the anterior and lateral femoral system, this technique has proved extremely helpful.

In regard to patient evaluation, Dr. Mackinnon described a clinical test that is helpful to identify which nerve or which portion of a nerve is involved in the neuroma formation. A positive response is a Tinel-like sign proximal to the neuroma. I have encountered such findings in neuromas involving the superficial radial nerve and the dorsal branch of the ulnar nerve but have found them to be inconsistent. I agree with Dr. Mackinnon that such a positive percussion sign most likely represents regeneration of injured nerve fibers in an orthodromic progression. I therefore do not expect such findings to be constant or consistent.

ON "NERVE GRAFTING"

Dr. Mackinnon presents a strong argument for the concept of prioritization and selective reinnervation. When the number of usable proximal motor fibers is limited, the strategic move is to channel these fibers to the motor nerve of the muscle performing the most desirable function. Ideally, the transfer is between synergistic motor nerve fibers.

The intraoperative sensory and motor identification regimen that is advocated by Dr. MacKinnon is a very sound approach. However, in most instances, particularly in the distal regions of the peripheral nerves, the internal fascicular topography is so specific that it is easily recognized by the experienced examiner when confined by strategic distal dissection. An accurate matching of the motor and sensory fascicles is readily obtained without elaborate intraoperative nerve stimulation and enzyme staining.

As for donor nerve grafts, the distal sural nerve, medial and lateral antebrachial nerves, and the anterior interosseous nerve are all very useful donor nerves indeed, particularly the sural nerve. Other donor nerves can come from an amputated and unsalvageable limb or digit. For small nerve gaps (< 3 cm) in a noncritical sensory nerve, application of an autogenous vein graft as a conduit is recommended. This technique has been in use for two decades and has been highly effective (2).

ON "CARPAL TUNNEL RELEASE"

I subscribe to Dr. Mackinnon's opinion that the most common cause of failure in symptom relief following carpal tunnel release is misdiagnosis. The other likely cause is technical failure.

As clearly stated by Dr. MacKinnon, if time is taken to perform a complete history and examination of the upper extremity, including the neck, an accurate assessment should be ascertained. In addition, an electrodiagnostic study, which I routinely obtain as a confirmatory test and as objective documentation of the severity of involvement, serves well as a safeguard. Concomitant pathology, such as cervical radiculopathy, can easily be discerned (11). The most disturbing untoward results arising from carpal tunnel release are iatrogenic injuries. After his comprehensive review, Kessler (12) came to the conclusion that the basic factor in complications is an inappropriate incision. I believe that the most important surgical prerequisite for this essentially simple operation is good visualization. If the surgeon cuts only with full visual command of the surgical field, agile control of the instrument, and a clear recognition of the structure under the sharp edge of the instrument, then damage to the median nerve is highly unlikely. Nothing is perfectly safe because anatomic anomalies are always possible; fortunately, however, these are rare. As to the question, "What is the best approach?" the choices are numerous: endoscopic technique (palm and wrist), open technique full palmar approach, and limited palmar approach. The advice I would offer is to use the approach that affords you the greatest comfort and skill, so that the transverse carpal ligament can be fully transected without injury to the median nerve, superficial arch, palmar cutaneous nerve, or transverse branch of the palmar cutaneous nerve. *Additional advice: When you need to gain proficiency, practice on cadavers, not on patients.*

I endorse Dr. Mackinnon's open approach, although, with the aid of a lighted Alfricht retractor, I routinely use the limited palmar open approach—that is, a longitudinal incision along the radial border of the ring finger that extends from the midpalmar level proximally to about 1.5 cm from the distal palmar flexor crease of the wrist joint. The incision is designed to avoid injury to the palmar cutaneous nerve and the transverse branch (13).

ON "CUBITAL TUNNEL SYNDROME"

The ulnar nerve descends toward the elbow from behind the epicondyle of the humerus. It then emerges from the submuscular plane and traverses the postcondylar groove under fascia covering the subcutaneous plane. It enters the forearm through an opening and a short passage bound by the tendinous arcade—the arcuate ligament, olecranon, epicondyle, and medial collateral ligament of the elbow joint. This opening and short passage, known as *cubital tunnel* (14), were recognized as a potential site of compression long ago by Farquhar Buzzard (15) and later by Osborne (16–20). Osborne further recognized that the arcuate ligament is slack during elbow extension and tightened during elbow flexion. The arcuate ligament is a tendinous ligament bridging the humerus and the ulnar origin of the flexor carpi ulnaris. Intrinsic hypertrophy of this ligament, often associated with proximal conjoining of the two heads of the flexor carpi ulnaris, predisposes the ulnar nerve to compression.

Sunderland (1) categorized cubital tunnel syndrome into three subgroups, as follows:

1. *Primary cubital tunnel compression.* This is caused by narrowing of the cubital tunnel during flexion of the elbow in the absence of bone and joint disease and external trauma.
2. *Secondary cubital tunnel compression.* This is caused by local disease that increases the diameter of the nerve (e.g., leprosy), decreases the space of the cubital tunnel (e.g., outpouching of the medial collateral ligament, seen in rheumatoid arthritis with follicular synovitis of the elbow joint), serious valgus deformity of the elbow, bony spur (e.g., in osteoarthritis), benign soft tissue tumor, or hematoma.
3. *Multifactorial cubital tunnel compression.* This is caused by a chronic underlying pathologic condition or systemic illness, such as alcoholism or stroke, in which the patient tends to flex the elbow for a prolonged period over an unyielding surface. Debilitated, ill-nourished, bedridden patients are most prone to this type of lesion (20).

The key to successful management and a reduction in untoward results is, again, accurate determination of the cause of ulnar nerve compression. This is accomplished by thoughtful history taking, thorough and systematic examination, and the use of electrodiagnostic studies and imaging.

Regarding the treatment of primary cubital tunnel syndrome and most of the multifactorial types, simple decompression is adequate, as demonstrated in the series presented by Nathan et al. (21), in which good relief was maintained in 79% of 131 patients with an average follow-up of 4.3 years.

Regarding secondary cubital tunnel syndrome, transposition of the ulnar nerve, either submuscularly or subcutaneously, can be considered. Based on her experience, Dr. Mackinnon has provided numerous expert suggestions for performing such submuscular transpositions. A word of caution: It is essential to recognize the potential hazard of devascularization of the ulnar nerve (22).

Dr. Mackinnon concludes her chapter with some pearls of wisdom. She advises one never to hesitate to seek advice from colleagues whenever one is in doubt. Physicians should work together as a team to give patients the best of care. We should indeed increase our endeavors in public education. A knowledgeable patient is often more appreciative of the physician's devotion and perseverance, and is more confident on the way to recovery.

REFERENCES

1. Sunderland S. A classification of peripheral nerve injuries producing loss of function. *Brain* 1951;74:491.
2. Chiu DTW, Strauch B. A prospective clinical evaluation of autogenous vein graft used as a nerve conduit for distal sensory deficit of 3 cm or less. *Plast Reconstr Surg* 1990;86:928–934.
3. Chiu DTW. Management of nerve injury, including tendon transfer. In: Jurkiewich MJ, Kriezek J, eds. *Principles of plastic surgery,* vol 1. St. Louis: Mosby, 1990:727–760.
4. Hodes R, Larrabee MC, German W. The human electromyogram in response to nerve stimulation and the conduction velocity of motor axons. *Arch Neurol Psychiatry* 1948;60:240–365.
5. Dengs EH. The influence of temperature in clinical neurophysiology. *Muscle Nerve* 1991;14:795–811.
6. Hyllienmark L, Ludvigsson J, Brismar T. Normal values of nerve conduction in children and adolescents. *Electroencephalogr Clin Neurophysiol* 1995;97:208–214.
7. Fisher MA. H reflexes and F waves: physiology and clinical indications. *Muscle Nerve* 1992;15:1223–1233.

8. Rivner MH, Swift TR, Crout BO, et al. Toward more rational nerve conduction interpretations: the effect of height. *Muscle Nerve* 1990;13:232–239.
9. Chandry V, Cornblath DR, Mellits ED, et al. Inter- and intra-examiner reliability of nerve conduction measurements in normal subjects. *Ann Neurol* 1991;30:841–843.
10. Chandry V, Corse AM, Freiner ML, et al. Inter- and intra-examiner reliability of nerve conduction measurements in patients with diabetic neuropathy. *Neurology* 1994;44:1459–1462.
11. Upton ARM, McComas AJ. The double crush in nerve entrapment syndrome. *Lancet* 1973;3:359–361.
12. Kessler FB. Complications of the management of carpal tunnel syndrome. *Hand Clin* 1986;2:401–406.
13. Abouzhar MK, Chiu DTW. Carpal tunnel release using limited direct vision. *Plast Reconstr Surg* 1995;1:152–155.
14. Feindel W, Straford J. The role of the cubital tunnel in tardy ulnar. *Malig Can J Surg* 1958;1:287–300.
15. Farquhar Buzzard E. Some varieties of traumatic and toxic ulnar neuritis. *Lancet* 1922;1:317.
16. Osborne GV. The surgical treatment of tardy ulnar neuritis. *J Bone Joint Surg Br* 1957;39:782.
17. Osborne GV. Spontaneous ulnar nerve paresis. *Br J Med* 1958;1:218.
18. Osborne GV. Ulnar neuritis. *Postgrad Med J* 1959;35:392.
19. Osborne GV. Compression neuritis of the ulnar nerve at the elbow. *Hand* 1970;2:10–13.
20. Wadsworth JG, Williams JR. Cubital tunnel external compression syndrome. *Br J Med* 1973;1:662.
21. Nathan PA, Kenistin RC, Meadows KD. Outcome study of ulnar compression in the elbow treated with simple compression and an early program of physical therapy. *J Hand Surg* 1995;20B:628–637.
22. Messina A, Messina JC. Transposition of the ulnar nerve and its vascular bundle for the entrapment syndrome at the elbow. *J Hand Surg* 1995;20B:638–651.

13

BIOMATERIALS (EXCLUDING BREAST IMPLANTS AND EXPANDERS)

J. PETER RUBIN
MICHAEL J. YAREMCHUK

Alloplastic implants are widely used in craniofacial surgery. We review several of the most commonly used implants: acrylic for cranioplasty, metal plates and screws for rigid fixation, and implants for reconstruction of the orbital floor. Complications are varied and can be related to the physical characteristics of the device, the quality of the tissues in which it is implanted, and surgical technique. Common complications and their management are discussed.

ACRYLIC CRANIOPLASTY

Acrylic is an implantable material that is used across many specialties. It is easy to mold, has a high tensile strength, and elicits a minimal reaction from the surrounding tissue. The implant is formed by mixing powdered polymer with a hardening agent (liquid monomer). Potential problems with this material intraoperatively include systemic toxicity from free monomer and tissue damage from the heat of the curing process. In the postoperative period, infection and exposure of the device are the primary concerns. Other postoperative problems include implant displacement and hematoma formation. Migration of the device can be avoided with screw or wire fixation to the underlying bone, and the incidence of hematomas can be reduced through careful surgical technique.

Acrylics such as methylmethacrylate have been associated with acute systemic toxicity in the operating room. During the insertion of hip prostheses with freshly mixed methylmethacrylate into the femur, patients have suffered acute hypotension that has sometimes progressed to cardiovascular collapse and death (1–3). The free monomer form of methylmethacrylate has been shown experimentally to have direct vasodilator effects. Presumably, the monomer leaches out of the cement and into the exposed medullary vasculature before the compound is fully cured (4). The large volume of methylmethacrylate used to cement a hip prosthesis, combined with a large intramedullary surface area, likely provides the best setting for this type of reaction. Recognition of the potential vasoactive effects of acrylic monomer by anesthesiologists has allowed for preemptive management in the operating room and a subsequent decrease in hemodynamic events. No episodes of cardiovascular depression have been reported with the use of methylmethacrylate in craniofacial surgery. However, a single case of an allergic response during cranioplasty, manifested as acute bronchospasm, has been reported (5). In general, the risk for systemic toxicity resulting from the use of acrylic cement for craniofacial applications should be considered very low.

Another potential danger associated with acrylics is local tissue necrosis caused by the high heat produced during the exothermic curing reaction. Clinical data from Manson et al. (6) demonstrate that continuous irrigation with iced saline solution results in temperature rises of less than 3°C. Stelnicki and Ousterhout (7) developed an *in vitro* model to quantify the effects of saline solution irrigation on acrylic curing temperature with varying implant thickness. In their study, unirrigated implants produced exothermic reactions lasting an average of 6 minutes and reaching peak temperatures between 177°F (3-mm implant) and 222°F (12-mm implant). The duration of the peak temperatures averaged 21 seconds. With saline solution irrigation, the peak temperature on the underside of 6-mm implants reached only 125°F for less than 15 seconds. At an implant thickness of 7 mm, temperature on the underside of the acrylic plate became more difficult to control. At an implant thickness of 10 mm or more, saline solution irrigation failed entirely to reduce the temperature on the underside of the implant. Stelnicki and Ousterhout concluded that *in situ* polymerization of acrylic implants with saline solution irrigation is safe if the implant is 6 mm or less in thickness. We recommend copious saline solution irrigation of all implants during *in situ* curing.

The infection rate for acrylic cranioplasty is 2.2%, averaged from several large clinical series (6,8–12) comprising 1,094 patients. As was recognized during wartime experience

J. P. Rubin: Department of Plastic Surgery, Harvard University, Boston, Massachusetts
M. J. Yaremchuk: Department of Surgery, Harvard Medical School; and Department of Plastic and Reconstructive Surgery, Massachusetts General Hospital, Boston, Massachusetts

(13,14), a history of previous infection can dramatically increase the risk for infection. Manson et al. (6) found the timing of cranial reconstruction to be more important than the material used in cases with a history of infection. Regardless of whether bone or alloplast is used, waiting at least 1 year after resolution of the initial infectious process reduces the risk for infection after cranioplasty. Additional factors that increase the risk for infection after cranioplasty are communication between the reconstructive plate and the nasal and frontal sinus cavities, and residual ethmoidal or frontal sinus inflammatory disease. We advocate treating all sinus disease before cranioplasty and eradicating any communication between the sinus cavities and the site of reconstruction. If an alloplastic cranial implant becomes infected or exposed, removal of the implant is always indicated. With any smooth-surfaced alloplastic implant, infection of the surrounding pocket will not resolve while the foreign body is in place. After removal of the implant and resolution of the infection, another alloplastic implant can be used if soft tissue coverage is adequate. It is paramount that the tissues overlying the implant are of good quality and not placed under tension. Additionally, the implant pocket should be remote from the incision. Failure to follow these principles can increase the likelihood of implant exposure or fistula formation (Fig. 13-1). In general, we will attempt a second (but not a third) alloplastic cranioplasty after appropriate treatment of the infection. The rate of infection after redo acrylic cranioplasty is not well defined in the literature, but we have not observed it to be much higher than the rate after primary procedures so long as conditions have been optimized.

Clinical Case No. 1.

A 45-year-old woman underwent excision of a brain tumor through a frontal craniotomy. The craniotomy flap was subsequently removed secondary to infection. She then received a course of radiation as adjuvant therapy for the brain tumor. When she presented for reconstruction, the following factors were considered: (a) previous infection in the operative field, (b) radiated tissues, and (c) a prior coronal incision that would lie over the reconstruction. When alloplastic material is used to treat a complication, it is paramount to consider variables that may contribute to further complications after another procedure. Because of the previous infection, reconstruction was delayed until 1 year after removal of the craniotomy flap. A composite graft was used; acrylic was placed on the patient's forehead to provide precise contour, and split-rib grafts were used above the hairline in the radiated tissues and beneath the craniotomy scars (Fig. 13-2).

Recently, a hydroxyapatite cement (BoneSource, Leibinger, Dallas, Texas) has become commercially available for craniofacial applications. It is manufactured in powder form and mixed with either water or sodium phosphate at the operating table to form a moldable paste. It is indicated for the repair of bony defects and bony augmentation (Fig. 13-3). Although bony ingrowth does occur (15), this material should not be used for stress-bearing applications.

METAL PLATES FOR CRANIOFACIAL SURGERY

Metal plate and screw fixation has been adapted to the craniofacial skeleton for more than 25 years. Plate fixation allows for the precise three-dimensional reconstruction of facial bones and early return to function. Use of this beneficial technology does, however, come with potential complications. Artifact from the implants on imaging studies may interfere with surveillance after cancer surgery. The materials used to manufacture the plates may be potentially toxic to the patient. Plates and screws can become infected, exposed,

A
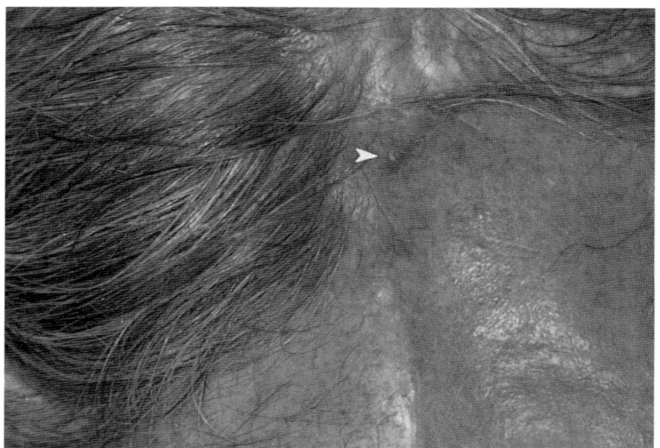

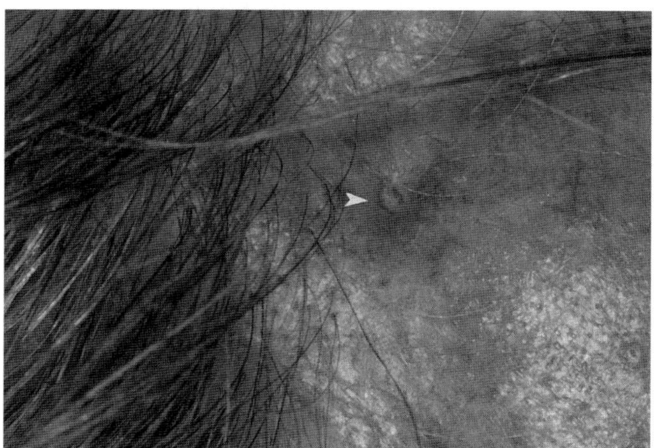
B

FIGURE 13-1. A: Acrylic implant in the temporal region with chronic draining sinus along incision at superior pole. The incision should not overlie an alloplastic implant; its placement should be remote from the pocket. **B:** Close-up view of sinus tract.

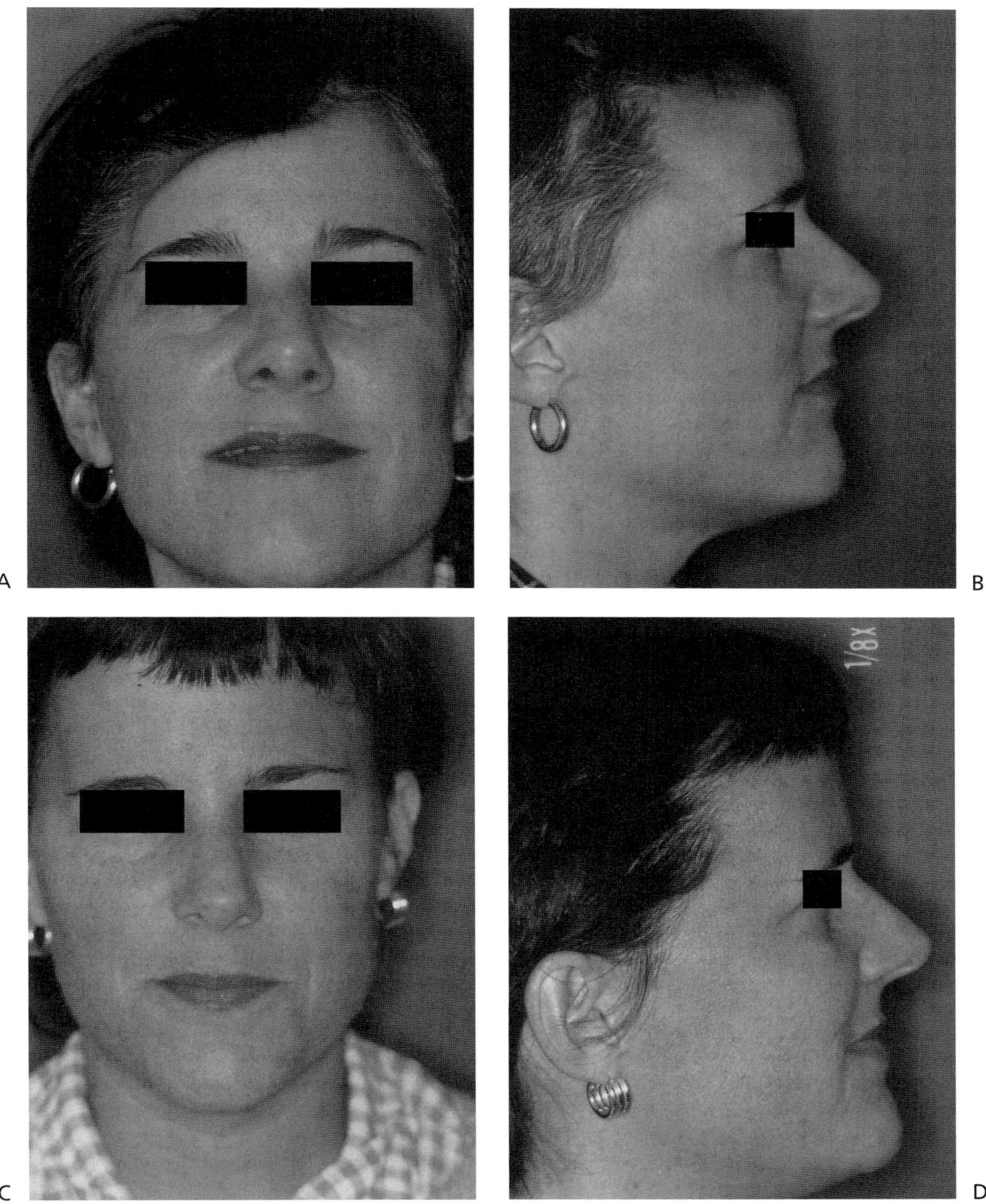

FIGURE 13-2. Patient after removal of infected craniotomy flap **(A,B)** and after reconstruction with acrylic and split-rib composite graft **(C,D)**.

or loosened from the bones to which they are anchored. Plates may also cause pain, become prominent under thin soft tissue cover, or be associated with local intolerance to cold. Additionally, the use of metal plates and screws on the facial skeleton of a child warrants consideration of growth restriction and plate translocation. Overall, these devices are well tolerated and have significant clinical advantages over closed reduction techniques and wire fixation. We do not recommend routine hardware removal; rather, we favor removal of plates and screws only for documented complications.

Artifact on Imaging Studies

Commercially available fixation plates are made from stainless steel, cobalt–chromium alloy (Vitallium), or titanium (either pure or as an alloy with aluminum and vanadium). Artifact on imaging studies caused by hardware can reduce

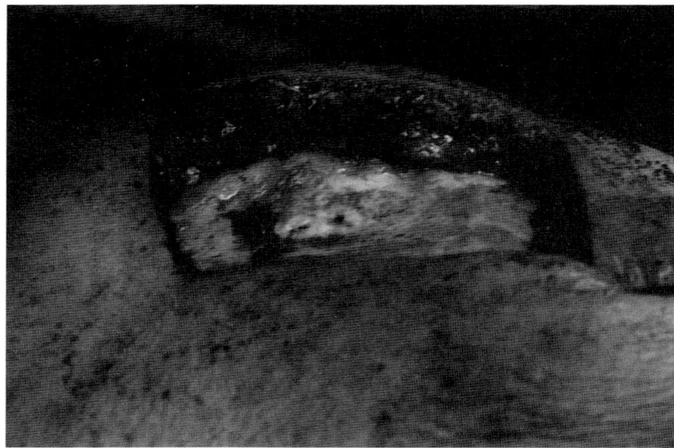

A

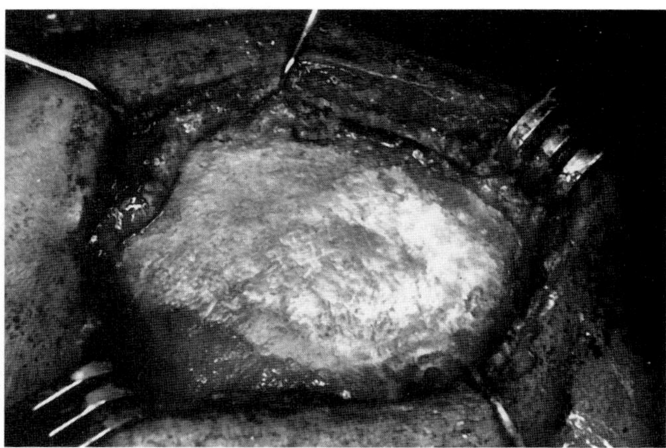

B

FIGURE 13-3. A: Intraoperative view of untreated depressed anterior wall frontal sinus fracture. The sinus was obliterated with hydroxyapatite cement, and the frontal contour was restored. **B:** Intraoperative view after reconstruction.

the ability to assess soft tissue changes in the vicinity of the fixation device and may necessitate plate removal if tumor surveillance is impeded. The artifact caused by titanium hardware on magnetic resonance imaging is substantially less than that caused by stainless steel or cobalt–chromium (16), so that better assessment of the surrounding tissue is possible (Fig. 13-4). A similar reduction in artifact with titanium in comparison with stainless steel is seen on computed tomography (17).

Toxicity of Metal Implants

Corrosion of metal implants leads to the release of metal ions, raising questions about the risk of systemic toxicity from these degradation products. In humans, an accumulation of metal has been found adjacent to maxillofacial fixation plates (18,19) and in a submandibular lymph node after mandibular plating (20). The corrosion process can result in a local fibroblastic tissue reaction (21,22), which has been implicated in implant failure in maxillofacial plates (23) and also long-bone fixation devices (24). Using transmission electron microscopy, Kim et al. (25) examined biopsy specimens of soft tissue overlying titanium miniplates that were taken from 14 patients with craniofacial implants during elective plate removal (mean of 7.1 months after implantation). Dense particles were seen within the connective tissue of all specimens. Additionally, random bone biopsy specimens taken from two patients showed the same particles in the bone matrix. Postmortem studies of patients with stainless steel and cobalt–chromium long-bone implants demonstrated elevated levels of these metals in local and distant lymph nodes, bone marrow, liver, and spleen (26). Although the local and systemic spread of metal ions has been documented in humans, no adverse effects have

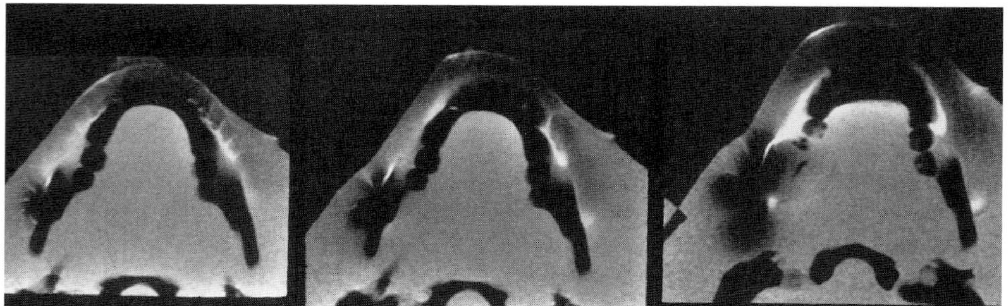

FIGURE 13-4. Representative views of magnetic resonance imaging artifacts produced by mandibular reconstruction plates. **Left to right:** Axial views of titanium, Vitallium, and stainless steel mandibular reconstruction plates. The mandibular reconstruction plate and corresponding artifacts can be seen along the external margin of the mandible, most prominently on the left side of the image along the ramus of the mandible. Dimensions of the pictured artifacts along the rami are 24 x 13 mm, 37 x 20 mm, and 61 x 32 mm for titanium, Vitallium, and stainless steel reconstruction plates, respectively. Note the significant artifact produced by stainless steel plates. (Reprinted from Fiala TGS, Paige KT, Davis TL, et al. Comparison of artifact from craniomaxillofacial internal fixation devices: magnetic resonance imaging. *Plast Reconstr Surg* 1994;93:725, with permission.)

been associated with these findings. It is estimated that 88,200 hip replacements were performed in 1975 (27), and that 11 million people currently carry implanted metallic fixation devices (28). With this large number of implants in place and a 25-year latency period passed, one might expect sequelae from implant corrosion to have developed by this time. Currently, no data are available to suggest that the risk for toxicity from metal implants exceeds the risks associated with hardware removal.

Metal Plates: Scope of Common Complications in Published Series

Data from published clinical series concerning the complication rates of metal fixation devices were tabulated, and weighted averages by sample size were calculated for different complications in various applications (Table 13-1). Complications relating closely to surgical technique, such as early hematoma and nerve injury, were not included. Additionally, elective removal of plates in asymptomatic patients was not counted as a complication. Certain complications arising by a similar process were grouped together for simplicity; these include infection/fistula and exposure/extrusion. When reporting on complication rates in this review, we sometimes refer to a study as having no implant-related complications. This does not indicate that the series was free of all complications, but that no complications were reported that were attributed directly to the implant itself.

A large experience with metal plates for mandibular fractures is reflected in the literature. Twelve studies (29–40), comprising data from 1,368 patients, show the average incidence of infection to be 6.7%. Infection can lead to screw loosening and osteomyelitis and is an indication for plate removal. Exposure of plates occurred in 1.3% of cases and is a relative indication for plate removal. In the absence of gross infection, an exposed intraoral plate may be left in place provided the site can be kept clean and irrigated and the hardware is not loose. Once bony union occurs, the plate can be removed electively (37). If the fixation is not completely rigid or there is any question of evolving infection, the plate must be removed. Surgical options following plate removal include placement of a new plate in a clean field, provided another surgical approach is available, or use of an external fixator.

Plates used to fix mandible fractures are placed under load, and as a consequence, a small incidence of plate fracture (< 0.5%) and hardware loosening is reported (< 0.5%). The robust surrounding soft tissue makes prominence an uncommon complication of mandible plating. Chronic pain is reported in 1% of cases and necessitates plate removal if it does not resolve after bone healing. Less commonly, placement of screws into or very close to a root canal can lead to necrosis of the tooth pulp (41). In these studies, 5.3% of patients underwent hardware removal for complications related to the plate and screws.

Studies assessing outcomes of plating for all facial fracture sites (not just the mandible) demonstrate a slightly different spectrum of complications. Five studies, comprising 880 patients, examined the use of metal plates and screws for various facial fractures (42–46). The average incidence of infection was 6.6%, with 2% of the implants becoming exposed. The thin soft tissue over the upper facial skeleton led to complaints of prominence in 0.9% of patients. Chronic pain at the site of the plate was reported in 1.3% of cases. Plate removal after bony union is therapeutic for these symptoms. Hardware loosening and plate fracture were rare when facial bones other than the mandible were plated. Overall, 10.1% of plates were removed for hardware-related complications.

As might be expected, a slightly lower incidence of infection (3.9%) was seen with plates used for elective (not trauma-related) craniofacial procedures (42,47–49). In this

TABLE 13-1. COMPLICATION RATES FOR METAL FIXATION DEVICES IN FACIAL SURGERY

	Type of Fixation Device and Application				
	Plates for Various Facial Fractures	Plates for Mandible Fractures	Plates for Elective Procedures	Plates for Mandible Reconstruction	Overall
Number of studies reviewed	5	12	4	11	32
Total number of patients	880	1,368	280	343	2,871
Average complication rates (%)					
Infection	6.6	6.7	3.9	14.3	7.1
Exposure/extrusion	2.0	1.3	< 0.5	14.9	3.1
Plate fracture	0	< 0.5	0	0.9	< 0.5
Prominence	0.9	0	2.1	0	0.5
Pain	1.3	1.0	3.9	0	1.3
Hardware loosening	0	< 0.5	0	2.6	< 0.5
Implants removed for IRC	10.1	5.3	10.0	19.5	8.9

IRC, implant-related complications.
Modified from Rubin JP, Yaremchuk MJ. Complications and toxicities of implantable biomaterials used in facial reconstructive and aesthetic surgery. *Plast Reconstr Surg* 1997; 100:1336, with permission.

patient population, however, complaints of prominence and pain at the plate sites were higher, at 2.1% and 3.9% respectively. Plates were removed from 10.0% of these patients.

The highest complication rates with metal plates were observed in cases of mandibular reconstruction after tumor resection, in which plates were applied in patients undergoing chemotherapy and radiation treatment (50–60). Infection rates and plate exposure were 14.3% and 14.9%, respectively. With the loss of normal skeletal architecture, bridging plates are used to stabilize the remaining mandibular segments. When used as a sole support structure (e.g., without interposing bone graft), these plates are particularly prone to failure. The higher load requirements on these plates make both hardware fracture (0.9%) and hardware loosening (2.6%) more likely. Patients in these studies, many followed for an average of 24 months, required plate removal in 19.5% of cases. Clinical experience indicates that plates alone used to bridge mandibular defects inevitably fail.

Clinical Case No. 2.

A 46-year-old man was treated for a carcinoma with a resection that included excision of the right hemimandible. A metal reconstruction plate was used to span the defect in the mandible. Postoperative radiation therapy was administered. The patient presented to follow-up with erosion of the metal plate through the skin (Fig. 13-5). This complication was treated with removal of the metal plate and application of an external fixation device. After the infection was controlled, a bone graft was placed in the defect and a vascularized flap was used for soft tissue cover. This case highlights the point that metal plates cannot be used as the permanent sole support in place of a mandibular defect.

Intracranial Plate Translocation

The use of miniplates for pediatric craniofacial use has yielded an interesting complication; hardware placed on the

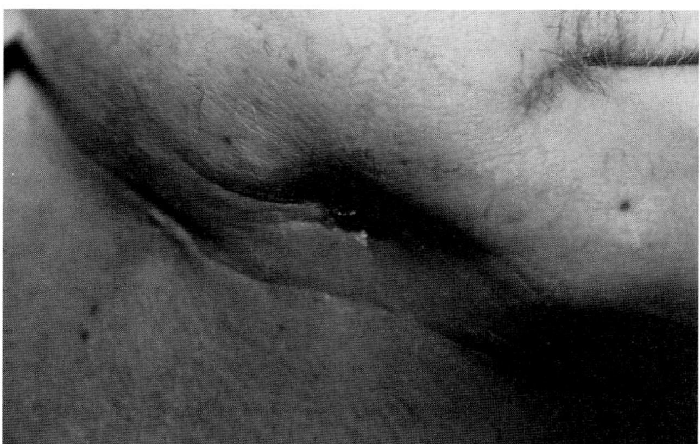

FIGURE 13-5. Patient with mandibular bridging plate extruding through the skin laterally.

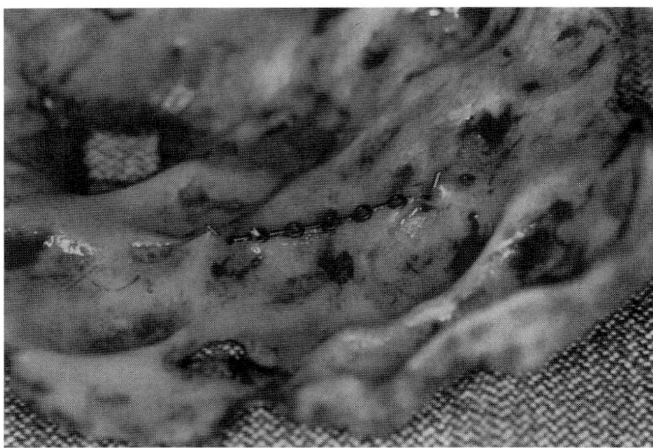

FIGURE 13-6. Inner table of calvarial flap during secondary reconstruction in a child. A metal plate that was placed on the outer table during the initial procedure has translocated to an intracranial position.

outer table of the skull can migrate through the cranial bone and rest directly against the dura (Fig. 13-6). This "intracranial plate translocation" has been described by Pappay et al. (61), who noted that plates originally placed on the outer table of the skull were found on the inner table in 7 of 20 children during reoperation for a second cranial remodeling procedure. The mean age at first operation was 6.8 months (range, 7 days to 13 months), and the average interval between first and second operation was 33 months (range, 12 months to 48 months). No screws were found to have pierced through the dura in this study, although adherence of the hardware led to a dural tear in one patient during removal of the plates and screws. None of the patients with translocated plates had a perioperative history of meningitis, seizure disorder, or other new neurologic symptoms. Goldberg et al. (62) used computed tomography to assess plate translocation in 27 patients who had undergone cranial vault reconstruction at a mean age of 11.5 months (range, 6 months to 36 months). The average follow-up time was 25 months (range, 12 months to 48 months). Of 227 microplates studied, 32 (14.1%) were found between the inner and outer tables (17 plates) or beneath the inner table (15 plates). Using regression analysis, the authors of this study found four factors that were statistically related to plate translocation in this patient population: placement of plates in the temporal region, younger patient age at operation, presence of syndromic craniosynostosis, and use of longer plates (average of 10 holes, 40 mm). No symptoms relating to plate translocation, such as seizure disorder or brain dysfunction, could be found in this patient population. To assess the experience with plate translocation encountered by a number of surgeons, Persing et al. (63) polled 67 members of the International Craniofacial Surgery Society. More than half of the surgeons polled

(51%) reported seeing hardware intracranially in 10% or fewer of reoperative cases. A small number of surgeons (9%) reported intracranial translocation in 76% to 100% of their reoperative cases. Penetration of the dura by screws or wires occurred in 4% or fewer of reoperated cases, as reported by 95% of respondents. No recognized brain injuries or intracranial hemorrhages were reported as a consequence of metal fixation devices.

It has been postulated that as the skull grows, endocranial bone is resorbed beneath the plate and ectocranial bone is laid down over it. The very substance into which the plate is anchored disappears, and the hardware drifts toward the dura. Experimentally, microplates with screws and wires used to fixate supraorbital osteotomies in 6-week-old Yucatan minipigs migrated toward the dura at a mean monthly rate of 0.9 mm. By 6 months, evidence of hardware was no longer present on the surface of the skull. Fluorescent bone labeling indicated that the hardware migrated inward at the same rate at which bone was deposited above it. Although some hardware moved to rest directly on the dura, no dural penetration was found (64). Honig et al. (65) showed that plate translocation still occurs in a pig model if the plate is placed over the periosteum, although at an initially slower rate than that of plates secured directly to bone. The rate of translocation would be expected to be slower in humans, in whom the calvarium has reached 50% of adult size at birth and 90% of adult size by age 5 to 7 years (66).

The primary concern with translocation is whether the underlying brain tissue is adversely affected. Yu et al. (67) used microplates to fixate fronto-orbital advancements in 3-week-old Yorkshire pigs. When sacrificed at 6 months, the animals demonstrated complete translocation of 28% of plates and partial translocation of the remainder. All plates stayed above the leptomeninges. However, gross indentations were noted in the dura and underlying cortex caused by the translocated screws projecting into the cranial cavity. No subdural hemorrhage, cerebritis, gliosis, or hypoxic changes were found, but mild focal histologic changes resulting from compression by the hardware were seen. If dural perforation were to occur, data from a rabbit study in which common microfixation hardware was placed directly against the brain suggest that a chronic inflammatory response would ensue (68).

In addition to being associated with plate translocation, experimental evidence suggests that rigid fixation of the immature craniofacial skeleton has the potential to restrict growth. Yaremchuk et al. (69) performed left frontal and supraorbital osteotomies on infant rhesus monkeys (Fig. 13-7). The bone flaps were then fixed with either interfragmentary wires, standard microplate fixation, or "extensive" fixation, which involved the use of longer plates purposely crossing coronal and sagittal sutures (Fig. 13-8). Multiple cephalometric measurements at a mean age of 16.7 months (past the completion of 95% of cranial growth) demonstrated subtle but definite growth restriction that was proportional to the complexity of fixation (Fig. 13-9). Extrapolation of these findings to humans rests on the concept that the rhesus monkey is suitable for craniofacial growth experiments. The orbitozygomatic anatomy of the rhesus monkey is similar to that of humans. In addition, the pattern of development of the facial skeleton is similar in the rhesus monkey and in humans. Despite these attributes, the model is still somewhat limited because the rhesus monkey brain has attained 75% of its adult weight at birth, whereas the human brain does not reach that proportional stage of growth until approximately age 3.

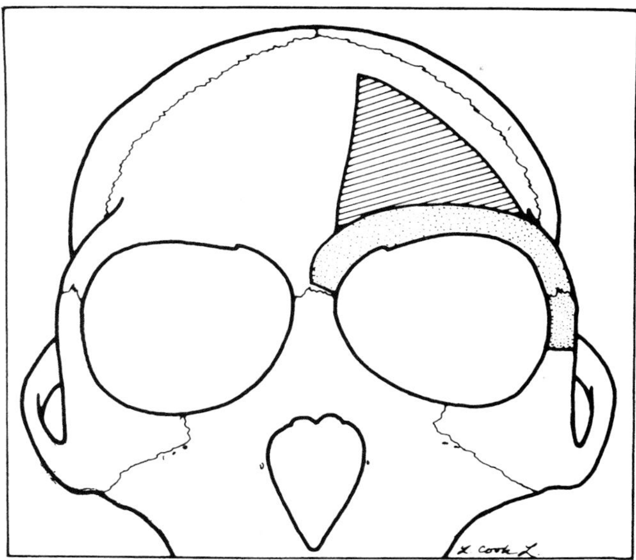

FIGURE 13-7. Osteotomy design. *Hatching* indicates area of frontal osteotomy; *stippling* indicates supraorbital rim osteotomy. (Reprinted from Yaremchuk MJ, Fiala TGS, Barker F, et al. The effects of rigid fixation on craniofacial growth of rhesus monkeys. *Plast Reconstr Surg* 1994;93:1, with permission.)

The available clinical and experimental data indicate that plate translocation can be expected to occur in some children after cranial procedures. The risk for dural penetration appears to be small. Despite the documented occurrence of hardware translocation, the significance is unclear. To date, no brain injury or adverse reactions to translocated plates have been reported; however, long-term data are not yet available. Routine removal of plates in children has not been advocated because reoperation, especially with plates embedded in bone, can cause injury to a patient who may not currently be at great risk. Because of the potential for intracranial translocation of metallic plates, their use is very selective in pediatric and particularly infant craniofacial surgery.

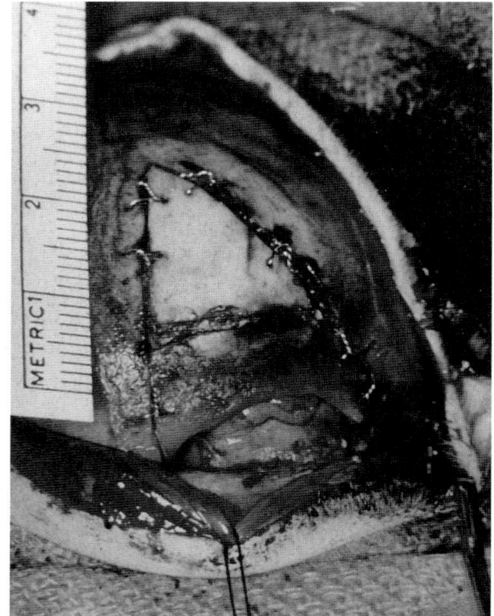

A

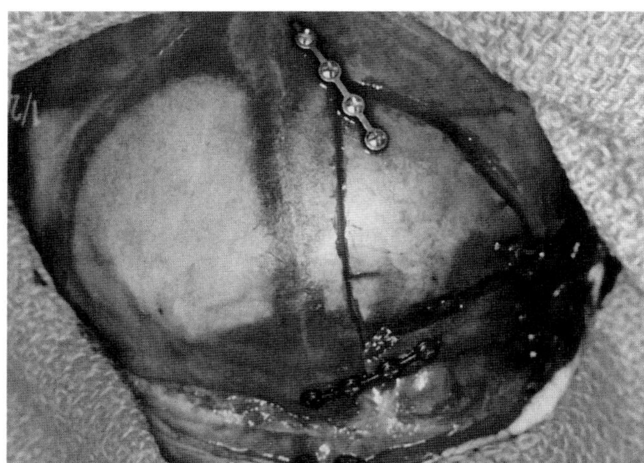
B

C

FIGURE 13-8. Representative postreduction intraoperative photographs taken from above showing the three types of fixation utilized in this primate study. **A:** Wire fixation. **B:** Microplate fixation. **C:** Extensive microplate fixation. (Reprinted from Yaremchuk MJ, Fiala TGS, Barker F, et al. The effects of rigid fixation on craniofacial growth of rhesus monkeys. *Plast Reconstr Surg* 1994;93:1, with permission.)

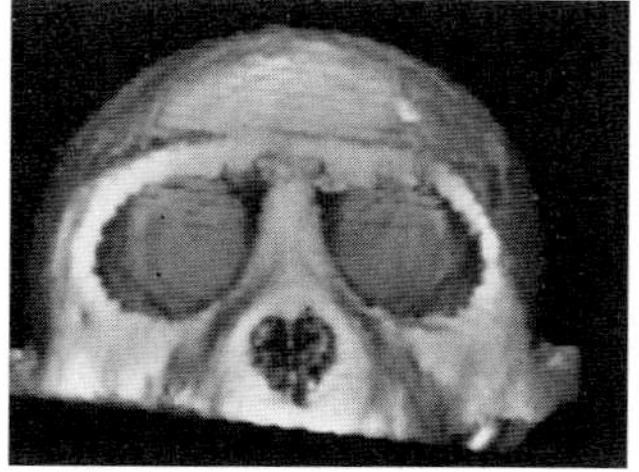

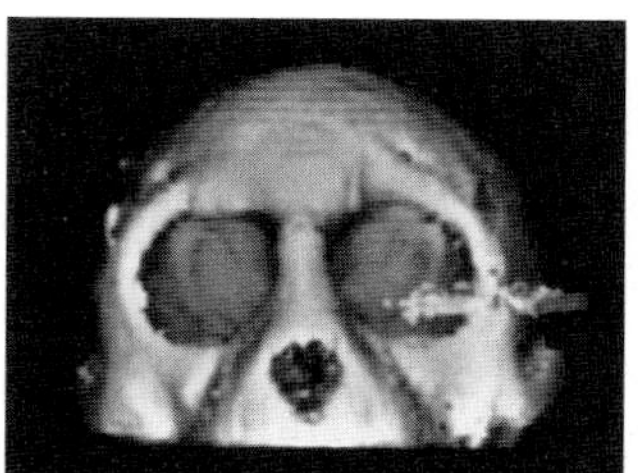

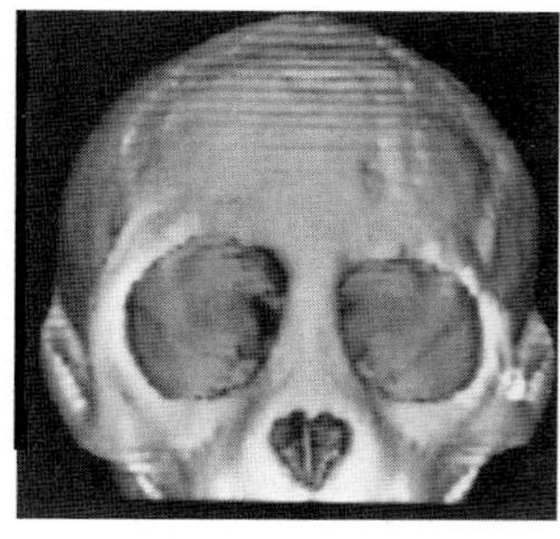

FIGURE 13-9. Representative late postoperative frontal three-dimensional computed tomographic images of rhesus skulls. **Left to right:** Wire fixation, microplate fixation (artifact is the result of a screw that was not removed before imaging), and extensive microplate fixation. (Reprinted from Yaremchuk MJ, Fiala TGS, Barker F, et al. The effects of rigid fixation on craniofacial growth of rhesus monkeys. *Plast Reconstr Surg* 1994;93:1, with permission.)

Resorbable Plates As a Solution to Intracranial Translocation

The use of resorbable plates and screws in craniofacial surgery is a fairly new development and could be especially beneficial in infant patients, in whom intracranial plate translocation is known to occur. Early studies of the use of polymer plates in adults revealed significant problems resulting from prolonged biodegradation. Gerlach (70) used poly-L-lactide (PLLA) plates and screws to repair zygomatic fractures in 15 patients. Although all fractures and wounds healed uneventfully, the plates were still palpable through the skin after 2 years. At 30 months, a noninfectious inflammatory reaction developed at the operative site in two patients. PLLA could be aspirated from the area of inflammation. Bos et al. (71) used PLLA plates and screws in 10 patients with zygomatic fractures. Long-term follow-up, reported by Bergsma et al. (72,73), showed that all patients experienced acceptable wound and fracture healing. However, a sterile foreign body reaction developed at the repair site in all patients in this series at approximately 3 years postoperatively. Fragments of PLLA were found during wound exploration as long as 5.7 years after the initial repair.

Plates manufactured from polylactic acid and polyglycolic acid copolymers may represent a significant advance toward practical resorbable plating systems. Eppley et al. (74) reported the use of 912 copolymer plates (LactoSorb, Walter Lorenz Surgical, Jacksonville) in 100 children undergoing correction of calvarial defects. The young age of the patients (range, 6 to 12 months; average, 8.9 months) allowed for the use of plates with a thickness of only 0.5 mm. The plates were secured with metal screws because polymeric screws of that small size could not be produced. With 85% of patients followed for at least 1 year, no inflammatory or foreign body reactions were noted. No occurrences of plate infections, bony collapse, or hardware loosening were reported. Four patients returned to the operating room between 9 and 18 months after the initial procedure for either bony recontouring or removal of prominent screws. Inspection of 22 plated sites revealed no evidence of residual polymer. This study suggests that small plates which are absorbed completely within 1 year may provide adequate structural support for the rapidly growing pediatric craniofacial skeleton, and that their use may prevent the sequelae of metallic plates. It must be noted, however, that these plates were not placed under a load.

ALLOPLASTIC ORBITAL FLOOR RECONSTRUCTION

Autogenous bone graft remains the gold standard for orbital floor reconstruction. However, unpredictable resorption of the bone graft and donor site morbidity have led clinicians to experiment with a variety of alloplastic materials. The fact that orbital floor implants do not affect facial contour minimizes the requirements for a precise profile and consistency of the device. Indeed, almost every available material has been used in this application.

A review of the literature on orbital floor repair becomes a tutorial on biomaterials. We have reviewed clinical series and extracted data on complication rates. As in the review of cranial skeleton fixation studies, weighted averages based on sample size have been calculated for different complications (75). Overall, the reported complication rates of orbital implants are low—a 2.1% incidence of infection and a 1.6% rate of extrusion in 1,481 patients. When individual devices are examined, the rate of complications can vary and often correlates with the physical qualities of the material (Tables 13-2 and 13-3). It must be recognized that it is difficult to attribute complications solely to the implant material itself. The overlap between surgical technique, host response, and

TABLE 13-2. COMPLICATION RATES FOR ORBITAL IMPLANTS

	Implant Material				
	PTFE	Silicone	Porous Polyethylene	Dense Polyethylene	Proplast
Number of studies reviewed	4	7	2	3	2
Total number of patients	437	519	52	78	22
Average complication rate (%)					
Infection	0.9	4.6	1.9	2.6	0
Exposure/extrusion	< 0.5	3.1	0	0	0
Displacement	0	0	0	0	0
Persistent edema	0	< 0.5	0	3.9	0
Prominence	0	< 0.5	1.9	0	0
Pain	0	1.4	0	0	0
Inflammatory reaction	0	0	1.9	0	0
Implants removed for IRC	1.1	9.3	1.9	1.3	0

IRC, implant-related complications; PTFE, polytetrafluoroethylene.
Modified from Rubin JP, Yaremchuk MJ. Complications and toxicities of implantable biomaterials used in facial reconstructive and aesthetic surgery. *Plast Reconstr Surg* 1997;100:1336, with permission.

TABLE 13-3. COMPLICATION RATES FOR ORBITAL IMPLANTS

	Implant Material					
	Nylon Plate	Surgical Mesh	Resorbable Devices	Metal Plates	Methylmethacrylate	Overall
Number of studies reviewed	2	2	2	4	1	29
Total number of patients	58	69	48	92	106	1,481
Average complication rate (%)						
Infection	0	0	0	4.4	0	2.1
Exposure/extrusion	12.1	0	0	0	0	1.6
Displacement	0	0	0	0	0.9	< 0.5
Persistent edema	0	0	0	0	0	< 0.5
Prominence	0	0	0	0	0	< 0.5
Pain	3.5	0	0	0	0	0.6
Inflammatory reaction	0	0	8.3	0	0	< 0.5
Implants removed for IRC	12.1	0	0	3.3	0.9	4.5

IRC, implant-related complications.
Modified from Rubin JP, Yaremchuk MJ. Complications and toxicities of implantable biomaterials used in facial reconstructive and aesthetic surgery. *Plast Reconstr Surg* 1997;100:1336, with permission.

potential toxicity of the implant is considerable. For example, widely differing perioperative antibiotic regimens combined with varying attention to aseptic technique can influence infection rates for a given material and site.

One of the more common materials used in this application is polysiloxane (silicone). Probably the most familiar implant material, silicone can be manufactured with consistencies ranging from liquid to hard solid. The manufacturing process plays an important role in the purity and integrity of silicone. The natural host response to this smooth-surfaced material is fibrous encapsulation or, if the soft tissue cover is thin or under tension, extrusion of the implant. When silicone was implanted in the orbital floor, infection was seen in 4.6% of 519 patients. The smooth surface and somewhat rigid structure of silicone devices contributed to extrusion in 3.1% of cases. Pain was encountered with silicone implants in 1.4% of cases. Ultimately, 9.3% of these devices were removed in the studies reviewed.

Silicone also comes in a room temperature vulcanized (RTV) form. In contradistinction to the standard heat temperature vulcanized (HTV) form, RTV silicone is mixed with a hardening agent and custom-molded by the surgeon either before implantation or *in situ*. RTV silicone has been used for volume augmentation in the anophthalmic socket. The elastomer is mixed with a curing agent, injected into the desired tissue plane, and allowed to harden *in situ*. Success with this technique has proved to be highly operator-dependent, and data from these studies have not been tabulated with those for the other orbital implant materials. Occasional shifting of the polymer as it hardens leads to displacement rates as high as 44%.

Nylon is the general name used to describe a group of polymerized amides (polyamides). A smooth-surfaced nylon plate is produced with trade names such as Suprafoil (S. Jackson, Alexandria, Virginia). Like silicone, the smooth surface of nylon encourages either encapsulation or extrusion. Nylon plates are extremely rigid and have sharp edges. When combined with a smooth surface, these characteristics led to extrusion in 12.1% of 58 patients (Fig. 13-10). Chronic pain was noted in 3.5% of patients, which may have been a manifestation of shifting of the implant against the surrounding tissue.

Polyethylene has a simple carbon chain structure and serves as the reference standard for an inert substance in assays of tissue reaction to biomaterials. Like silicone, it can be produced in a variety of consistencies, from grease to hard solid. Early clinical use involved a dense, smooth-surfaced form of polyethylene. Infection was seen in 2.6% of patients and persistent edema in 3.9%. Currently available implants are constructed from a porous form of polyethylene such as Medpor (Porex, Fairburn, Georgia). The porous structure allows the ingrowth of both soft tissue and bone, which makes the implant resistant to extrusion and difficult to remove during reoperation. Experimental data suggest that the growth of tissue into the porous device can decrease the risk for infection. In studies comprising 52 patients, the infection rate was noted to be 1.9%. Proplast (formerly by Vitek, Houston, Texas) is another porous material composed of polytetrafluoroethylene combined with either carbon fibers (Proplast I) or aluminum oxide (Proplast II). Proplast is no longer manufactured in the United States because inflammatory reactions were elicited by implant fragments when the device was used as an interposition graft in the temporomandibular joint. However, complication rates were very favorable in the small number of patients who received Proplast orbital floor implants.

Polytetrafluoroethylene is best recognized as Gore-Tex (W. L. Gore, Flagstaff, Arizona). This material is produced in pliable sheets that can be easily cut and shaped. Small interstices allow for some tissue ingrowth. The characteristics of this material have contributed to low rates of infection (0.9%) and extrusion (< 0.5%) in studies comprising 437 patients.

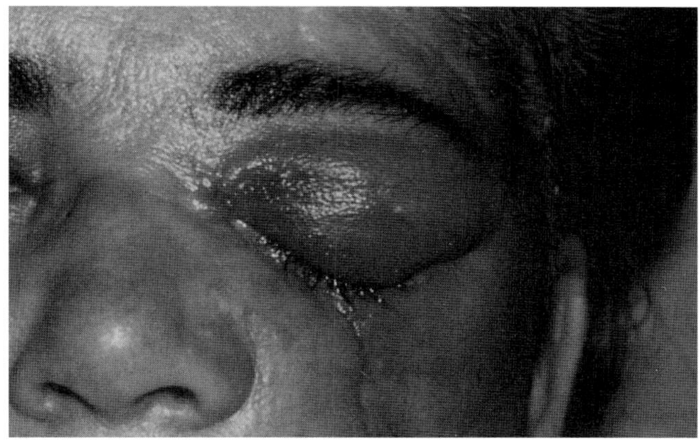
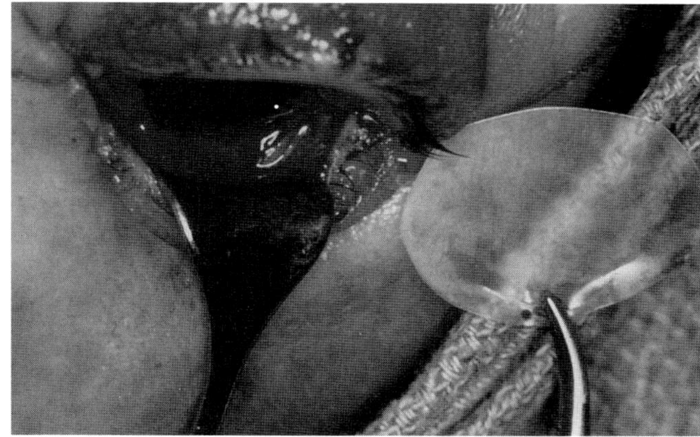

FIGURE 13-10. A: Patient with infected orbital floor implant. **B:** Intraoperative photograph of implant being removed. The rigid structure and sharp edges of this nylon plate implant may contribute to failure rates that are higher than average.

Acrylic implants, such as methylmethacrylate, have also been placed in the orbital floor. The dense, smooth-surfaced material was prone to displacement in 106 patients. Polypropylene, the material used in the manufacture of nonabsorbable sutures, is used to construct surgical mesh. Growth of fibrous tissue through the mesh secures it firmly in place. This material was very well tolerated in the orbital floor in 69 patients. Metal plates, when used in the orbital floor, were prone to become infected in 4.4% of cases. These devices are traditionally secured to adjacent bone with screws to prevent extrusion. In published studies describing the use of resorbable polymer plates for orbital floor repair, devices were used that were produced before refinements were made in the polymer composition. Consequently, an 8.3% incidence of sterile inflammatory reactions was observed.

There are many reports in the literature of late complications with orbital implants, especially with silicone, polytetrafluoroethylene, and nylon plate. These have been noted to occur as late as 21 years after placement and include the following: infection, extrusion, migration with hematoma formation, migration with obstruction of the lacrimal duct, erosion into the maxillary sinus, and lower eyelid deformity.

Without exception, infected orbital floor implants must be removed. Antibiotics alone are not adequate with a foreign body in place. After complete resolution of the infection, the safest approach is to employ autogenous bone graft for the secondary reconstruction.

CONCLUSION

Currently used implantable materials, including acrylic, polyethylene, and metal alloys, are well tolerated in most craniofacial applications. The greatest postoperative concerns are for infection and exposure/extrusion of the device. Meticulous surgical technique cannot be overemphasized when alloplastic implants are used. Moreover, soft tissue coverage above the implant must be adequate and not under tension. If an alloplastic implant becomes infected, removal is mandatory because the infection cannot resolve with the foreign body in place. After the infection is cleared, it is reasonable to consider a second alloplastic reconstruction, but the safest approach is to use autogenous materials. The decision to remove or revise an implant secondary to other complications, such as displacement or pain, should be individualized for each patient.

Rigid fixation in the growing craniofacial skeleton carries the potential for plate translocation and growth restriction. For this reason, its use in the infant skeleton should be highly individualized according to the severity of the deformity and the need for stability. Further refinement of resorbable fixation methods may obviate the need for permanent skeletal fixation devices.

REFERENCES

1. Kepes ER, Underwood PS, Becsey L. Intraoperative death associated with acrylic bone cement: report of two cases. *JAMA* 1972;222:576–577.
2. Milne I. Hazards of acrylic bone cement: a report of 2 cases. *Anaesthesia* 1973;28:538–543.
3. Monteny E, Oleffe J, Donkerwolke M. Methylmethacrylate hypersensitivity in a patient with cemented endoprosthesis. *Acta Orthop Scand* 1978;49:554–556.
4. Peebles D, Ellis R, Stride S, et al. Cardiovascular effects of methylmethacrylate cement. *Br Med J* 1972;1:349–349.51.
5. Wong HY, Vidovich MI. Acute bronchospasm associated with polymethylmethacrylate cement. *Anesthesiology* 1997;87:696–698.
6. Manson PN, Crawley WA, Hoopes JE. Frontal cranioplasty: risk factors and choice of cranial vault reconstructive material. *Plast Reconstr Surg* 1986;77:888–900.
7. Stelnicki EJ, Ousterhout DK. Prevention of thermal tissue injury induced by the application of polymethylmethacrylate to the calvarium. *J Craniofac Surg* 1996;7:192–195.

8. Hammon W, Kempe L. Methyl methacrylate cranioplasty: 13 years' experience with 417 patients. *Acta Neurochir* 1971;25:69–77.
9. Cabanella ME, Coventry MB, MacCarty CS, et al. The fate of patients with methyl methacrylate cranioplasty. *J Bone Joint Surg Am* 1972;54:278–281.
10. Rish B, Dillon J, Meirowsky A, et al. Cranioplasty: a review of 1030 cases of penetrating head injury. *Neurosurgery* 1979;4: 381–385.
11. Malis LI. Titanium mesh and acrylic cranioplasty. *Neurosurgery* 1989;25:351–355.
12. Vaandrager JM, van Mullem PJ, de Wijn JR. Craniofacial contouring and porous acrylic cement. *Ann Plast Surg* 1988;21: 583–593.
13. Woolf J, Walker A. Cranioplasty. *Int J Surg* 1945;81:1–9.
14. White J. Late complications following cranioplasty with alloplastic plates. *Ann Surg* 1948;128:743–755.
15. Stelnicki E, Ousterhout D. Hydroxyapatite paste (BoneSource) used as an onlay implant for supraorbital and malar augmentation. *J Craniofac Surg* 1997;8:367–372.
16. Fiala TGS, Paige KT, Davis TL, et al. Comparison of artifact from craniomaxillofacial internal fixation devices: magnetic resonance imaging. *Plast Reconstr Surg* 1994;93:725–731.
17. Saxe AW, Doppman JL, Brennan MF. Use of titanium surgical clips to avoid artifacts seen on computed tomography. *Arch Surg* 1982;117:978–979.
18. Schliephake H, Lehmann H, Kunz U, et al. Ultrastructural findings in soft tissues adjacent to titanium plates used in jaw fracture treatment. *Int J Oral Maxillofac Surg* 1993;22:20–25.
19. Rosenberg A, Gratz KW, Sailer HF. Should titanium miniplates be removed after bone healing is complete? *Int J Oral Maxillofac Surg* 1993;22:185–188.
20. Onodera K, Ooya K, Kawamura H. Titanium lymph node pigmentation in the reconstruction plate system of a mandibular bone defect. *Oral Surg Oral Med Oral Pathol* 1993;75:495–497.
21. Swann M. Malignant soft-tissue tumour at the site of a total hip replacement. *J Bone Joint Surg Br* 1984;66:629–631.
22. Thomas KA, Cook SD, Harding AF, et al. Tissue reaction to implant corrosion in 38 internal fixation devices. *Orthopedics* 1988;11:441–451.
23. Byrne JE, Lovasko JH, Laskin DM. Corrosion of metal fracture fixation appliances. *J Oral Surg* 1973;31:639–645.
24. Cohen J, Wulff J. Clinical failure caused by corrosion of a Vitallium plate. *J Bone Joint Surg Am* 1972;54:617–628.
25. Kim YK, Yeo HH, Lim SC. Tissue response to titanium plates: a transmitted electron microscopic study [see Comments]. *J Oral Maxillofac Surg* 1997;55:322–326.
26. Case CP, Langkamer VG, James C, et al. Widespread dissemination of metal debris from implants. *J Bone Joint Surg Br* 1994;76:701–712.
27. Hori R, Lewis J, Zimmerman J, et al. The number of total joint replacements in the United States. *Clin Orthop* 1978;132:46–52.
28. Praemer A, Furner S, Rice D. *Musculoskeletal conditions in the United States.* Rosemont, IL: American Academy of Orthopedic Surgeons, 1992.
29. Chu L, Gussack GS, Muller T. A treatment protocol for mandible fractures. *J Trauma* 1994;36:48–52.
30. Hoffman WY, Barton RM, Price M, et al. Rigid internal fixation vs. traditional techniques for the treatment of mandible fractures. *J Trauma* 1990;30:1032–1035.
31. Morgan CE, Hicks JN, Eby TL, et al. Repair of mandibular fractures: plating vs. traditional techniques. *Otolaryngol Head Neck Surg* 1992;106:245–249.
32. Nakamura S, Takenoshita Y, Oka M. Complications of miniplate osteosynthesis for mandibular fractures. *J Oral Maxillofac Surg* 1994;52:233–238.
33. Smith BR, Johnson JV. Rigid fixation of comminuted mandibular fractures. *J Oral Maxillofac Surg* 1993;51:1320–1326.
34. Stone IE, Dodson TB, Bays RA. Risk factors for infection following operative treatment of mandibular fractures: a multivariate analysis. *Plast Reconstr Surg* 1993;91:64–68.
35. Tuovinen V, Norholt SE, Sindet-Pedersen S, et al. A retrospective analysis of 279 patients with isolated mandibular fractures treated with titanium miniplates. *J Oral Maxillofac Surg* 1994;52:931–935.
36. Valentino J, Levy FE, Marentette LJ. Intraoral monocortical miniplating of mandible fractures. *Arch Otolaryngol Head Neck Surg* 1994;120:605–612.
37. Zachariades N, Papademetriou I. Complications of treatment of mandibular fractures with compression plates. *Oral Surg Oral Med Oral Pathol Oral Radiol Endod* 1995;79:150–153.
38. Souyris F, Lamarche J, Mirfakhrai A. Treatment of mandibular fractures by intraoral placement of bone plates. *J Oral Surg* 1980;38:33–35.
39. Strezlow V, Strezlow A. Osteosynthesis of mandibular fractures in the angle region. *Arch Otolaryngol* 1983;109:403–406.
40. Champy M, Lodde J, Schmitt J, et al. Mandibular osteosynthesis by miniature screwed plates via a buccal approach. *J Maxillofac Surg* 1978;6:14–21.
41. Chandler NP, Cathro PR. Endodontic sequelae of miniplate bone fixation. *Oral Surg Oral Med Oral Pathol Oral Radiol Endod* 1996;81:467–471.
42. Brown JS, Trotter M, Cliffe J, et al. The fate of miniplates in facial trauma and orthognathic surgery: a retrospective study. *Br J Oral Maxillofac Surg* 1989;27:308–315.
43. Francel TJ, Birely BC, Ringelman PR, et al. The fate of plates and screws after facial fracture reconstruction. *Plast Reconstr Surg* 1992;90:568–573.
44. Ikemura K, Hidaka H, Etoh T, et al. Osteosynthesis in facial bone fractures using miniplates: clinical and experimental studies. *J Oral Maxillofac Surg* 1988;46:10–14.
45. Klotch DW, Gilliland R. Internal fixation vs. conventional therapy in midface fractures. *J Trauma* 1987;27:1136–1145.
46. Zachariades N, Papademetriou I, Rallis G. Complications associated with rigid internal fixation of facial bone fractures. *J Oral Maxillofac Surg* 1993;51:275–278.
47. Schmidt BL, Perrott DH, Mahan D, et al. The removal of plates and screws after Le Fort I osteotomy. *J Oral Maxillofac Surg* 1998;56:184–188.
48. Rosen HM. Miniplate fixation of Le Fort I osteotomies. *Plast Reconstr Surg* 1986;78:748–754.
49. Smith SC, Pelofsky S. Adaptation of rigid fixation to cranial flap replacement. *Neurosurgery* 1991;29:417–418.
50. Davidson J, Birt BD, Gruss J. A-O plate mandibular reconstruction: a complication critique. *J Otolaryngol* 1991;20:104–107.
51. del Hoyo JA, Sanroman JF, Bueno PR, et al. Primary mandibular reconstruction with bridging plates. *J Craniomaxillofac Surg* 1994;22:43–48.
52. Disher MJ, Esclamado RM, Sullivan MJ. Indications for the AO plate with a myocutaneous flap instead of revascularized tissue transfer for mandibular reconstruction. *Laryngoscope* 1993;103: 1264–1268.
53. Klotch DW, Prein J. Mandibular reconstruction using AO plates. *Am J Surg* 1987;154:384–388.
54. Koch WM, Yoo GH, Goodstein ML, et al. Advantages of mandibular reconstruction with the titanium hollow screw osseointegrating reconstruction plate (THORP). *Laryngoscope* 1994;104:545–552.
55. Kim MR, Donoff RB. Critical analysis of mandibular reconstruction using AO reconstruction plates. *J Oral Maxillofac Surg* 1992;50:1152–1157.

56. Lindqvist C, Soderholm AL, Laine P, et al. Rigid reconstruction plates for immediate reconstruction following mandibular resection for malignant tumors. *J Oral Maxillofac Surg* 1992;50: 1158–1163.
57. McCann KJ, Irish JC, Gullane PJ, et al. Complications associated with rigid fixation of mandibulotomies. *J Otolaryngol* 1994; 23:210–215.
58. Papazian MR, Castillo MH, Campbell JH, et al. Analysis of reconstruction for anterior mandibular defects using AO plates. *J Oral Maxillofac Surg* 1991;49:1055–1059.
59. Schusterman MA, Reece GP, Kroll SS, et al. Use of the AO plate for immediate mandibular reconstruction in cancer patients. *Plast Reconstr Surg* 1991;88:588–593.
60. Shah JP, Kumaraswamy SV, Kulkarni V. Comparative evaluation of fixation methods after mandibulotomy for oropharyngeal tumors. *Am J Surg* 1993;166:431–434.
61. Pappay F, Hardy S, Morales L, et al. "False" migration of rigid fixation appliances in pediatric craniofacial surgery. *J Craniofac Surg* 1995;6:309–313.
62. Goldberg D, Bartlett S, Yu J, et al. Critical review of microfixation in pediatric craniofacial surgery. *J Craniofac Surg* 1995;6: 301–306.
63. Persing JA, Posnick J, Magge S, et al. Cranial plate and screw fixation in infancy: an assessment of risk. *J Craniofac Surg* 1996; 7:267–270.
64. Stelnicki EJ, Hoffman W. Intracranial migration of microplates versus wires in neonatal pigs after frontal advancement. *J Craniofac Surg* 1998;9:60–64.
65. Honig JF, Merten HA, Luhr HG. Passive and active intracranial translocation of osteosynthesis plates in adolescent minipigs [see Comments]. *J Craniofac Surg* 1995;6:292–298; discussion 299–300.
66. Enlow D. Facial growth. In: Dyson J, ed. *Facial growth.* Philadelphia: WB Saunders, 1990:173–192.
67. Yu J, Bartlett S, Goldberg D, et al. An experimental study of the effects of craniofacial growth on the long-term positional stability of microfixation. *J Craniofac Surg* 1996;7:64–68.
68. Mofid M, Thompson R, Pardo C, et al. Biocompatibility of fixation materials in the brain. *Plast Reconstr Surg* 1997;100:14–20.
69. Yaremchuk M, Fiala T, Barker F, et al. The effects of rigid fixation of the craniofacial growth of. rhesus monkeys *Plast Reconstr Surg* 1994;93:1–10.
70. Gerlach KL. *In vivo* and clinical evaluations of poly(L-lactide) plates and screws for use in maxillofacial traumatology. *Clin Mat* 1993;13:21–28.
71. Bos RRM, Boering G, Rozema FR, et al. Resorbable poly(L-lactide) plates and screws for the fixation of zygomatic fractures. *J Oral Maxillofac Surg* 1987;45:751–753.
72. Bergsma J, Rozema F, Bos R, et al. Foreign body reactions to resorbable poly(L-lactide) bone plates and screws used for fixation of unstable zygomatic fractures. *J Oral Maxillofac Surg* 1993; 51:666–670.
73. Bergsma JE, de Bruijn WC, Rozema FR, et al. Late degradation tissue response to poly(L-lactide) bone plates and screws. *Biomaterials* 1995;16:25–31.
74. Eppley B, Sadove A, Havlik R. Resorbable plate fixation in pediatric craniofacial surgery. *Plast Reconstr Surg* 1997;100:1–7.
75. Rubin JP, Yaremchuk MJ. Complications and toxicities of implantable biomaterials used in facial reconstructive and aesthetic surgery: a comprehensive review of the literature. *Plast Reconstr Surg* 1997;100:1336–1353.

Discussion

BIOMATERIALS (EXCLUDING BREAST IMPLANTS AND EXPANDERS)

DOUGLAS K. OUSTERHOUT

Biomaterials are an important part of the plastic surgeon's armamentarium in both aesthetic and reconstructive surgery. Not everything can be accomplished by osteotomies or augmentation with autogenous materials; for example, cheek augmentation is best handled, at this time, with prosthetic materials because bone grafts undergo significant, irregular, and uncontrolled resorption no matter what their origin (cranium, iliac crest, rib). The chapter by Drs. Rubin and Yaremchuk briefly reviews some of the common facial implant materials and the problems associated with their use. Implants have the potential to save a tremendous amount of surgical time. Filling in a cranial defect in an adult patient with methylmethacrylate may require only a fraction of the time needed to obtain a bone graft, adapt it to the appropriate contour, and stabilize it. However, problems can occur; prosthetic materials, like mostly everything else, are not perfect.

The choice of implant material may be the most important factor in avoiding complications. For example, in

D. K. Ousterhout: Division of Plastic Surgery, University of California, San Francisco; and Davies Medical Center, California Pacific Medical Center, San Francisco, California

cranioplasties, methylmethacrylate is stable in position and time. I have patients who have undergone a forehead cranioplasty in which methylmethacrylate was used whose implants have remained in position for more than 25 years without a single problem (Fig. 13D-1). On the other hand, micromovements generally develop in prefabricated silicone implants to the skull after some period of time (a few years). These movements cause a significant accumulation of fluid, which eventually ruptures through the skin and causes implant exposure and infection, so that removal of the implant becomes necessary. I have been told that all the custom-made silicone forehead cranioplasty implants placed by the Stanford University plastic surgery staff and residents (of whom I am one) between 1968 and 1982 became exposed through such a mechanism, and that all had to be removed (1).

Methylmethacrylate has in my experience been a superb material for augmenting the calvarium. Since 1973, I have used it to develop a normal forehead contour and brows (with appropriate orbital protection from above) in all my craniofacial patients who required augmentation. They have all been placed after skull growth was complete or nearly so (primarily in the early teenage years) (2). The results are as good as if the surgeon was a sculptor. I have used it in more than 300 cases without a single infection or loss of an implant with one exception. In 1985, I completed such an augmentation on a teenager with Apert syndrome. In 1991, he was badly injured when his head was struck by the outside of an automobile windshield while he was crossing a highway. Computed tomography did not show any fracture and the skin was intact, but 8 months later, pus began to drain from his left temple. He returned to San Francisco, where the implant was removed through the old coronal incision by splitting the implant down the middle with a burr. A fracture was identified on the anterior wall of the right frontal sinus, obviously the area of bacterial contamination to the implant. The fracture was treated with a thin piece of split calvarial bone graft overlying the bony cleft of the fracture. Eighteen months later, the same implant (resterilized) was recemented to the now complete forehead, like all my prefabricated implants, with a thin mix of methylmethacrylate (2). The patient has now gone another 6 years without a recurrent infection. I suspect that the implant saved his life in the automobile accident.

When I place small implants on the skull, I do not use a screw or wire, as suggested by the authors for fixation. Rather, I place two converging holes in the outer table of the cranial bone (Fig. 13D-2). If an infection occurs and the implant has to be removed, the implant can be cut down the middle and the halves removed laterally without difficulty (2). This avoids the tedious process of burring methylmethacrylate away until the retaining devices, such as screws and wires, can be found and removed. It saves a tremendous amount of time. It also saves some expense.

I do not think that methylmethacrylate should ever be used in association with an exposed sinus. It will automatically and immediately become contaminated and will certainly fail. On the other hand, I do not know when a patient is necessarily free of sinus inflammatory disease. I have entered many sinuses in asymptomatic patients and found dis-

A 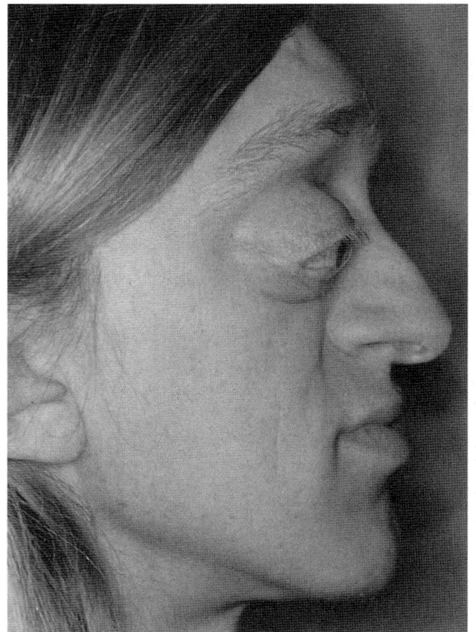

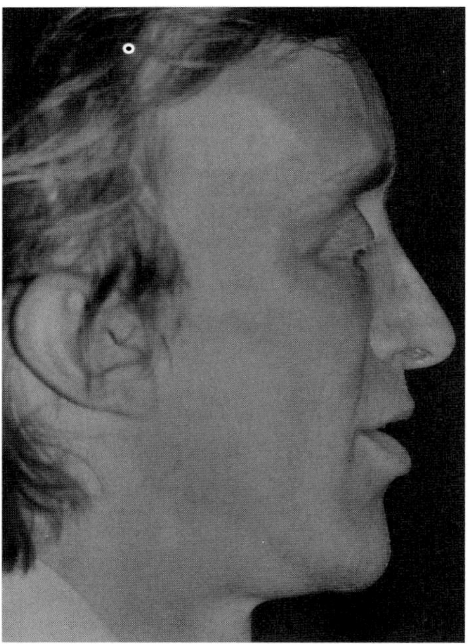 B

FIGURE 13D-1. A: Patient with Crouzon syndrome before surgery. **B:** Patient 2 years after Le Fort III operation, sliding genioplasty, rhinoplasty, and methylmethacrylate cranioplasty. This patient continues to do well 25 years after surgery.

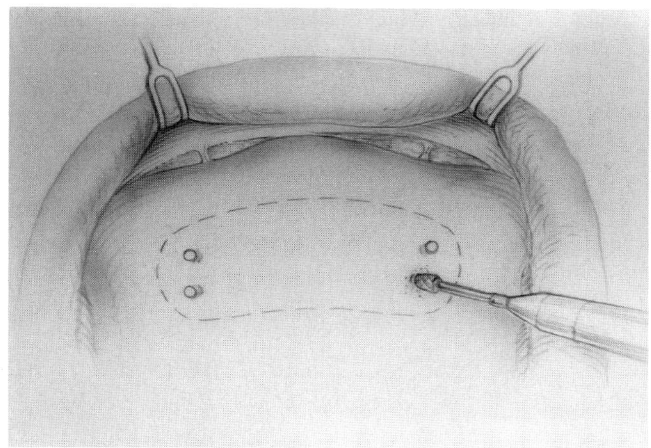

FIGURE 13D-2. Placement of two to four converging holes in the outer table of cranial bone nicely holds a methylmethacrylate cranioplasty, even when it is quite large.

ease not previously suspected or noticed by history or in radiographs. I suspect that at least some of my surgery patients who have received methylmethacrylate onlay implants have had sinus problems, but, as stated before, such problems have never caused an implant to become infected, so that removal was required. In deference to the authors, I do not feel the patients need to be free of sinus disease so long as the bone is intact.

The authors have presented a brief paragraph on the use of hydroxyapatite cement in which they state, "It is indicated for the repair of bony defects and bony augmentation." To the best of my knowledge, it has never proved successful for long-term augmentation (longer than a year) (3). Why should it work better than bony augmentation, which does not work for long-term augmentation? I have used the material in several children to fill bony defects. Computed tomography in two of them showed at least calcification (questionable ossification) within a few months. Interestingly, a few months later (6 and 8 months after surgery), the bony defect had returned. A great deal more needs to be known about this expensive material before its use can be recommended in reconstruction, and particularly augmentation, in craniomaxillofacial surgery.

The authors discuss Medpor. Personally, I have found it to be a very useful implant material for augmentation of the angle of the mandible and the cheek. I have not used it in the temporal fossa, as I prefer methylmethacrylate in this area. However, its use in the nose, at least in my hands, has rarely been successful. I reported on the use of Medpor in the nostril area in 1995 (4). It was not successful in a single case on a long-term basis. Even after several months of being nicely contained within the mucosa, it eventually erodes through the mucosa and has to be removed. I have not found it possible for skin or mucosa to grow over its surface, as has been reported (5).

The authors do not discuss hydroxyapatite granules (Interpore Cross International, Irvine, California), which I have found to be very useful for filling in bony defects (e.g., at the step-off between the proximal and distal pieces of a sliding genioplasty to prevent a deep groove in the sublabial crease and around the piriform margin, particularly in children with cleft lip, in which one side is depressed in comparison with the other). It does present a problem in dependent areas (e.g., at the inferior border of the mandible, where it occasionally seems to drift and then solidify to become a hard, protruding mass that has to be reapproached and recontoured). However, I have never seen it become infected, even with exposure. Hydroxyapatite granules around the piriform margin are resistant to infection and stable, whereas silicone implants want to move and are not resistant to bacterial contamination. Prefabricated silicone or Medpor implants are desirable for cheek implants, whereas methylmethacrylate would be difficult to form and hydroxyapatite granules would be difficult to position and stabilize.

The authors nicely discuss the use of metal plates and screws in craniofacial surgery. This has been one of the great advances of the past 30 years in cranial and maxillofacial surgery. However, the use of plates and screws in infant craniofacial surgery, as the authors explain, is not without significant problems. The translocation of plates may develop in a future that we have not yet seen. Will there ever be a problem in a football player when he is hit hard on the head? We obviously hope not, but time will tell. Our craniofacial team at the University of California, San Francisco, has not used internal plate fixation in infant craniofacial surgery. We have found wire fixation to be quicker and more useful in the final positioning and stabilization of bony pieces. Additionally, although it is not addressed by these authors, the cost of plates and screws in a child's skull can be extreme, certainly a major consideration in today's price-cutting market.

CONCLUSION

Implants have been and will remain for a long time an important adjunct in reconstructive and aesthetic surgery, particularly in the craniofacial region. Perhaps someone someday will develop a soft tissue filler that works, lasts, and is safe. New materials must be evaluated in regard to their general and specific desirability. They must also be evaluated for their biodegradability, stability as an implant within tissues, toxicity, carcinogenicity, potential for migration, effects on bone and soft tissues, and potential to cause problems in diagnostic studies (e.g., magnetism in magnetic resonance imaging). Implants have their specific uses, and no one material is ideal for all situations and free of complications, especially when the choice has been unwise.

REFERENCES

1. Vistnes L. Personal communication, 1987.
2. Ousterhout DK. Prosthetic forehead augmentation. In: Ousterhout DK, ed. *Aesthetic contouring of the craniofacial skeleton.* Boston: Little, Brown and Company, 1991:199–220.
3. Stelnicki E, Ousterhout DK. Hydroxyapatite paste (BoneSource) used as an onlay implant for supraorbital and malar augmentation, *J Craniofac Surg* 1997;8:367–372.
4. Ousterhout DK. Medpor nasal implants. Panel No. 4: The role of alloplastic materials in facial surgery. ASPRS/EF/ASMS Meeting, Montreal, Canada, October 9, 1995.
5. Wellisz T. Reconstruction of the burned external ear using a Medpor porous polyethylene pivoting helix framework. *Plast Reconstr Surg* 1993;91:811–818.

14

MICROSURGERY

TERESA BENACQUISTA
BERISH STRAUCH

Microsurgery is both exciting and exacting, allowing the surgeon to apply the techniques of free-tissue transfer and replantation within the full gamut of reconstructive surgery.

Microvascular free-tissue transfer has enhanced the ability of the plastic surgeon more accurately to reconstruct defects with similar tissue, so that better functional and aesthetic results are obtained. However, in no other area of plastic surgery is an unfavorable outcome more devastating than in microsurgery. An unfavorable outcome usually means a free-flap failure. In most microsurgical procedures, few other options are available for a good reconstruction, and in many cases, the other options have been tried and have failed; a free flap is the only possible way to salvage the situation. In the case of replants, the only alternative after a failure is amputation of that part. To minimize the possibility of an unfavorable result in microsurgery, one must plan carefully preoperatively, carry out a technically flawless procedure, monitor the flap and patient postoperatively, and be prepared to return to the operating room as soon as a problem is detected.

PREOPERATIVE PLANNING

The key to trying to prevent problems in microsurgery is thorough preoperative planning. The first decision to be made is whether a free flap is indicated, or whether the reconstruction can be carried out with simpler techniques. In the management of an open wound, the steps of the reconstructive ladder are followed: from primary closure, to split-thickness skin grafts, to local flaps, to free flaps. Indications for using free flaps are specific for various sites on the body. Large wounds with exposed vital structures, hardware, or denuded bone are indications for free flaps, if sufficient local tissue is not available or the local tissue is otherwise unsuitable (traumatized).

In reconstruction following ablation, the indications for free flaps are also specific to the defect and to the patient. For example, in breast reconstruction after a mastectomy, a free flap (e.g., free transverse rectus abdominis myocutaneous [TRAM] flap, perforator flap, or free gluteus flap) or a pedicle flap (e.g., pedicle TRAM or latissimus dorsi) may be chosen. Patient selection is based on such factors as weight, medical conditions, smoking status, previous surgeries, and the patient's wishes (1). These same criteria must be taken into account in all reconstructive cases, including trauma cases.

Once the choice for a microsurgical transfer has been made, multiple decisions follow. The recipient site dictates many of these decisions.

The timing of reconstruction is determined by the condition of the recipient site. In the case of lower extremity trauma, for example, the timing of coverage is quite a significant factor in determining successful outcome. Adequately debrided wounds, covered in the first few days after trauma, are more likely to heal successfully than those covered in the so-called subacute phase. Frequent debridement during a period of a few weeks may be required to prepare the wound for a free flap adequately (2). In postablative surgery, immediate reconstructions usually yield better functional and aesthetic results than delayed reconstructions. This is especially true in the head and neck, where postablative scar contractures and irradiation work together to make delayed reconstructions more difficult and the results less than optimal. However, in other areas, immediate reconstruction may not always be possible, either from a medical viewpoint or because of the patient's wishes.

Once the timing has been determined, the best donor site must then be chosen. Again, the requirements of the recipient site are the primary determinants of the donor site. The recipient site must first be categorized as to location on the body, size, three-dimensional shape, depth, types of tissue required, and functional needs. Sometimes, one needs only to fill in a hole with vascularized tissue (e.g., open tibial-fibular fractures in a lower extremity). At other times, one must reconstruct a complex head and neck defect, including intraoral lining, bone, and skin. Even reinnervation may be required. In these instances, flap design becomes critical. When a hole with depth is filled in, a free muscle flap covered with a split-thickness skin graft is usually the

T. Benacquista and B. Strauch: Department of Plastic and Reconstructive Surgery, Albert Einstein College of Medicine and Montefiore Medical Center, Bronx, New York

best choice. Depending on the size of the defect, a number of different muscle donor sites are fairly easy to harvest and provide adequate pedicle sizes and lengths. The workhorses are the rectus abdominis (pedicle—deep inferior epigastric vessels) and the latissimus dorsi (thoracodorsal vessels). Smaller muscles include the serratus (based on the serratus branch of the thoracodorsal) and the gracilis (gracilis branch). The latissimus dorsi, serratus, and gracilis muscles can all be innervated based on their respective nerves in the pedicle.

The donor site choices for complex head and neck reconstructions are numerous and have been described in detail in the literature. As examples, common donor sites for jaw reconstructions include the fibular osteocutaneous flap, iliac crest with internal oblique muscle, and scapular bone with skin. Free-flap breast reconstruction options include the free TRAM flap, the deep inferior epigastric artery perforator (DIEAP) flap, gluteal free flap, gluteal perforator flap, and lateral thigh flap. Each of these flaps has specific advantages and disadvantages.

Choosing among the different donor sites available for a certain recipient area may be difficult. Donor site morbidity should be taken into account. In the case of jaw reconstruction, a fibula free flap may produce less morbidity than an iliac crest in terms of pain at the donor site and postoperative patient mobility (3).

The donor flap pedicle size and pedicle length are also important in determining which of the available options is chosen. Usually, a longer and larger-caliber pedicle is preferable because it makes the technical aspects of the case easier. For this reason, flaps such as the free TRAM flap are more popular than the gluteus free flap for breast reconstruction. It is also the reason why the groin flap, with its very small-caliber vessel, the superficial circumflex femoral artery, has lost favor to other skin flaps, such as the scapular flap, based on the larger-caliber subscapular artery (4).

The recipient vessels must also be addressed. If these vessels are very small in caliber, then the smaller-caliber pedicle flaps may be more advantageous. Of course, the vessel diameter may not be known preoperatively, unless an angiogram has been obtained or the recipient site is first dissected before a definitive donor site is chosen intraoperatively. If an end-to-side anastomosis is going to be performed, then matching the recipient and donor vessel sizes is not as critical.

Angiography

Preoperative angiograms of recipient sites are advantageous in some cases and critical in others. In cases of upper and lower extremity trauma, they are mandatory. In cases of reconstruction of the lower extremities in vascular patients, they are critical, but if the vascular surgeon is performing a bypass and the flap is being taken off the bypass, then the angiogram is not mandatory for the plastic surgeon, although it may be useful for the vascular surgeon.

Preoperative angiograms of donor sites are indicated in certain cases, the most common being the fibula free flap. A report of one series (5) recommends the routine use of preoperative angiography in planned fibula harvest, whereas more recent articles recommend it only in cases of abnormal preoperative vascular examination findings (6). An angiogram may also be indicated for a radial forearm flap if the Allen's test result is abnormal.

VEIN GRAFTS

In many cases, it can be determined preoperatively that vein grafts will be needed. In cases of lower extremity trauma, if an angiogram indicates that a significant zone of injury exists, vein grafts will be required to anastomose the flap away from this zone. Vein grafts may also be used electively in head and neck microsurgery for scalp and jaw reconstructions, to take advantage of large-caliber inflow from the carotid system. A temporary arteriovenous fistula is created and divided when the surgeon is ready to perform the arterial and venous anastomoses.

The use of vein grafts intraoperatively emergently, either because the pedicle does not reach the inflow vessel or because thrombosis has developed from a primary anastomosis, is associated with a higher rate of complications and unfavorable outcomes. The overall use of vein grafts is associated with a higher rate of free-flap failure; this is not a consequence of the vein grafts themselves but of the fact that they are used in high-risk cases, especially trauma cases.

In addition to all the factors mentioned above, ease of harvest and the patient positioning required to harvest the flap are critical deciding factors. Once again, the free TRAM flap wins over the gluteus flap for breast reconstruction, according to the mentioned criteria.

A special word is required about patient positioning. Any time the patient needs to be repositioned during surgery to harvest a flap, the operating time is lengthened (because of the actual time it takes to change the patient's position, which ordinarily must be done more than once); furthermore, ablation and flap harvesting cannot be carried out simultaneously. Thus, many hours can be added to an already lengthy procedure. Therefore, flaps that do not require patient repositioning should always be considered first.

Finally, when a donor site is chosen, the microsurgeon's expertise is also a factor. One must develop a certain facility with a number of different flaps, but not necessarily with every flap ever described. Most defects can be adequately reconstructed by choosing from a limited number of free-flap donor sites. Many times, the surgeon's preference is the deciding factor, when all else is equal.

INTRAOPERATIVE PLANNING

The intraoperative conduct of a microsurgical procedure basically determines the outcome of the case. A technically smooth procedure, although it does not guarantee a favorable outcome, usually results in success. However, a procedure fraught with technical problems increases the chances of an unsuccessful transfer.

The development of a consistent routine ensures the smooth conduct of a microsurgery case. One of the best ways to accomplish this is to have a particular microsurgery team in which all the members are familiar with the procedures, equipment, and setup, so that each case can proceed efficiently without any waste of time or effort. Many steps are required in each microsurgical case, and each one can cause a great deal of delay or problems if not carried out properly. It is best always to proceed with the steps in the same order and manner, so that no step is inadvertently missed or repeated. This also allows the surgical team to anticipate the next step.

Most of the time, it has been determined preoperatively which donor site and which recipient vessels will be used. Thus, the patient is placed in a position that will allow for recipient site preparation and donor flap harvesting simultaneously. This is not always possible, and in some cases, the patient must be repositioned during the procedure. The easiest position, of course, is the supine position, to which many donor sites are amenable (e.g., TRAM, rectus, gracilis, radial forearm, fibula). However, if a latissimus dorsi muscle, serratus muscle, or scapular flap is to be used, then the patient's back must be accessible.

A common procedure is a latissimus dorsi muscle transfer to an open leg wound. If the posterior tibial artery is chosen as the recipient vessel, then a contralateral latissimus dorsi muscle is best. The patient is placed in a modified lateral decubitus position, which allows access to the medial aspect of the leg and back simultaneously. If the anterior tibial artery is to be the recipient vessel, then an ipsilateral latissimus dorsi muscle is harvested.

From a technical standpoint, consistent and meticulous dissection is imperative. In no other area of plastic surgery is the correlation between tissue handling and unfavorable outcome so direct. The slightest injury to a flap pedicle or recipient vessel can cause intimal damage and subsequent thrombosis of the anastomosis. Maintaining meticulous hemostasis allows for an easier dissection because it prevents tissue staining.

The recipient vessels should always be dissected out and prepared before the donor pedicle is clamped to allow for the shortest ischemia time and to determine inflow and outflow status. Although this seems quite a simple concept, these steps are not always carried out by the microsurgeon; the result is a longer ischemia time or even failure if adequate inflow or outflow cannot be established once the donor flap has been transferred.

Recognizing what constitutes adequate outflow or inflow requires experience. Determining adequate inflow is easier than determining adequate outflow. A soft, pulsatile artery with good forward bleeding is not difficult to recognize. In cases of vascular disease with calcified vessels, it is more difficult to decide where the best take-off is or whether the artery is adequate at all. Preoperative angiograms are helpful in these situations. Determining the adequacy of venous outflow can be even more difficult. Preoperative duplexes of the venous system of the legs may be helpful in some cases (e.g., in severe crush injuries, in a patient with a history of venous stasis, or in a very edematous extremity). Testing venous outflow during the procedure with an injection of heparinized saline solution is surgeon- and equipment-dependent and should be performed in a consistent manner each time.

Before flap transfer, the patient's hemodynamic condition and pulmonary status should be ascertained by the anesthesiologist, and if it is not optimal, it should be corrected. If the procedure has to be delayed during ischemia time to correct any hemodynamic problems, irreversible changes can occur, especially if the flap is a muscle with less reserve than a skin or bone flap.

In jaw reconstructions with a fibular free flap, the fibula is shaped into a neomandible by performing the osteotomies and placing the plates while the fibula is still attached to its vascular supply on the leg; this decreases ischemia time. Placing the patient in intermaxillary fixation and using templates that are prepared from a one-to-one computed tomogram and a cephalogram are the most accurate ways of shaping the fibula into a neomandible that accurately matches the patient's preoperative contour.

The resected jaw specimen itself can also be used as the template, but this is unwieldy and may not be as accurate, especially if the specimen is distorted by a large tumor.

Transfer of the fibula neomandible is usually accomplished by first plating the bone to the native mandible, with the patient in intermaxillary fixation, before the flap is revascularized. This can be a rapid procedure if the shape and size of the neomandible are accurate; if not, then adjustments will increase ischemia time.

The anastomosis should also be performed in a consistent and meticulous fashion. Many different techniques are used, and each can be successful if expertly performed. Many surgeons prefer to perform the venous anastomosis first, whereas others perform the arterial first but do not release the clamps. Whether two veins are necessary is also not clear, and successful results can be obtained with only one vein. The use of running versus interrupted sutures does not affect outcome. Size discrepancies of up to 2:1 between the recipient and donor vessels can be overcome with judicious stitch placement, or an end-to-side anastomosis can be performed. The use of an operating microscope is not always necessary during microsurgery, and excellent results are obtained by some surgeons using only loupe magnification.

In-setting the flap also requires planning. Thoughtful preoperative flap design will eliminate many of the problems that can develop at this stage of the procedure (7). The length of the pedicle required should be carefully measured before transfer. Adequate soft tissue coverage of the pedicle must be available, either from local tissue or from the flap itself. The latissimus muscle is a good flap in this respect, in that its tendon can be used to cover the pedicle. A parascapular flap also can cover its own pedicle by if the flap is extended superiorly. No tension should be placed on the anastomosis during flap in-setting, and the liberal use of split-thickness skin grafts can be very helpful in avoiding tension. The careful placement of drains is also important, and it is best to place the drains away from the vessels beneath the flap. Suturing the drain in place under the flap with a rapidly absorbable suture can prevent migration of the drain and prevent later problems.

TREATMENT OF TECHNICAL MISHAPS

No matter how meticulous and consistent the care or how much preoperative planning, some procedure will always not go as planned. The surgeon must be prepared to correct the problem or have a backup solution. In trauma cases, if the recipient vessels are inadequate or in an area of injury, then the dissection must be carried out either more proximally, away from the area of injury, or further distally, so that retrograde flow can be obtained. If dissection proceeds a considerable distance from the defect, then vein grafts will be required. One must always be prepared for vein grafting in microsurgery. In cases without trauma, if the chosen recipient vessels are inadequate, other vessels in the vicinity can be dissected out.

It is very rare for the donor pedicle to be of inadequate caliber and length. But if this does occur, then harvesting another flap may be required. If an injury has occurred to the pedicle, then vein grafting should be considered immediately. If a technically flawless anastomosis has been carried out without tension and inflow and outflow vessels are adequate but thrombosis occurs during the procedure, then spasm must be ruled out. Lidocaine (2%) or papaverine will help to alleviate early spasm, but it may not be useful in established spasm. The use of these two antispasmodic agents during vessel dissection can help prevent spasm. Dissecting off the adventitial layer of the vessel can also alleviate spasm. If thrombosis occurs, the anastomosis must be opened, checked for any suture mishap or intimal injury, and repeated. Hemodynamic and coagulation factors must also be considered.

A long ischemia time can lead to irreversible changes within a flap or replanted part and prevent reperfusion during the subsequent reestablishment of circulation. This is called the *no-reflow phenomenon,* in which the anastomosis is patent but perfusion is absent in the flap. Although not yet in clinical application, some enhanced ischemic tissue survival has been shown in animal models with high-energy phosphates (e.g., adenosine), superoxide dismutase (an oxygen free radical scavenger), urokinase (a thrombolytic agent), and dexamethasone, alone or in combination (8,9).

At the completion of the procedure, dressings, if used, are kept light and are loosely wrapped so as not to place any compression on the flap pedicle. A window should be left for flap monitoring. The pedicle should be marked if postoperative monitoring by Doppler is to be carried out. For the first few days, it may be advisable to prevent excessive movement that could result in injury to the pedicle. Immobilization of the extremities can be carried out with external fixators, as splints may compress the flap.

POSTOPERATIVE CARE

During the postoperative period after a free flap has been created, the patient and flap are closely monitored. The patient can be put into an intensive care unit, a step-down unit, or a specifically designed flap-monitoring unit. It is best if experienced personnel render the care and monitor the flap.

First, the patient is monitored for organ function, especially from a hemodynamic and pulmonary standpoint, because adequate hydration and oxygenation are imperative for flap survival. Besides the determination of routine vital signs, urine output, and laboratory values, the placement of central venous pressure and arterial lines may be required, the better to assess volume status. Rarely is a Swan-Ganz catheter needed, except when a patient has cardiac disease.

Close monitoring of the flap itself is imperative if salvage is to be attempted in the event of a pedicle thrombosis. The majority of thromboses occur within the first 3 days postoperatively, with most occurring in the first 24 hours after surgery. Arterial thromboses are more frequent earlier in this period, and venous thromboses are more frequent later in the postoperative period. Most series agree that venous obstructions occur more often than arterial obstructions. Therefore, careful monitoring of the flap on an hourly basis is warranted for the first 3 days, and then less frequent monitoring until about 7 days postoperatively (10).

Monitoring

The ideal monitoring technique should cause no injury to the patient or the flap, should reliably and accurately provide a rapid response to circulatory changes in the flap, and should be usable with all types of flaps, buried or not. Although different methods are available to monitor a free flap, no single method is infallible, and so different techniques are used in different clinical cases; sometimes, a combination of monitoring techniques is used.

Physical examination is still quite reliable if carried out by experienced personnel. It does require that the flap not be buried. Even when other methods of monitoring are employed, the physical examination of a free flap is always necessary because mechanical problems can cause false readings with some of the monitoring techniques. Also, one must look for problems developing in the flap, such as hematoma formation or excessive swelling or bleeding, all of which can eventually cause pedicle problems if left unchecked.

Skin flaps lend themselves most readily to monitoring by physical examination. The color, capillary refill, and warmth of skin flaps are easily assessed. A muscle flap can be examined for color, turgor, and warmth, but more experience is required. Pinprick of skin and muscle flaps is sometimes helpful to clarify vascularity when a change in the physical examination findings has occurred. Temperature probes are also helpful in monitoring skin flaps and replants, but they are less reliable in monitoring muscle flaps, even when they are implanted.

For digital replants, the most reliable method is to use a pulse oximeter; this is a continuous monitoring technique and is very accurate, and the results can easily be compared with findings in a control digit.

More technical and expensive monitoring techniques are also available, including laser Doppler flowmetry. An advantage is that this is a noninvasive, objective, continuous, and instantaneous monitoring device that is very accurate in determining tissue perfusion. Most important, abnormal flow measurements precede the manifestation of clinical signs. Its main disadvantage is the sensitivity of the instrument to patient movement, and large variations in blood flow baselines between individual patients make it difficult to establish "normal" flow values. However, the pattern or trend of blood flow into a free flap can be used as a basis for monitoring, and this device is in wide use.

The limitation of the monitoring techniques previously described is the requirement for an accessible, exposed portion of the free flap. For buried flaps and intraoral flaps, these devices either may not be accurate or may not be usable at all. A conventional Doppler signal can be used in buried as well as in exposed flaps if flow through the pedicle of a free flap is monitored. This is best done in a portion of the flap that is far from the recipient site; otherwise, the transmitted signal from recipient bed vessels can be misinterpreted as flow through the pedicle. Many flaps lend themselves to this type of monitoring, especially the free fibula flap used in mandibular reconstruction, which is often buried if no skin paddle is present. The Doppler signal should be monitored well away from the carotid vessels. The main disadvantage is that this is not a continuous monitoring system, and misleading results can be produced by surrounding vasculature.

An implantable, 20-mHz ultrasonic Doppler device is an effective and direct means of monitoring blood flow through microvascular anastomoses. It can be used in both buried and exposed flaps. The probes can be placed on either the artery or the vein of the free-flap pedicle. When the device is placed on the artery, arterial disturbances are promptly detected; however, venous problems are not easily determined. If the probe is placed on the vein, venous obstruction is instantaneously identifiable, and arterial occlusion is also detected within minutes of its occurrence. One disadvantage is that experienced personnel are needed to interpret the sound signals. Other disadvantages include the invasive nature of the device, the possibility of probe failure, and interference from other electronic machinery (11).

Tissue oxygen measurement is another minimally invasive method of monitoring. Implantation of a microcatheter Po_2 sensor into the flap allows measurement of tissue Po_2 by direct contact of the probe with the flap tissue. If arterial obstruction occurs in the free flap, the Po_2 drops slowly. Absolute values for Po_2 are not used; rather, again, the trend is used. Dislodgement of the catheter can cause errors (12).

Other methods of monitoring include color flow ultrasonography and tissue pH monitoring. The advantage of the latter is that pH values are consistent in all flaps, regardless of tissue type or location.

If any indication that pedicle thrombosis is occurring is noted, then emergent reexploration is undertaken. Thrombosis develops in about 5% to 10% of free flaps and requires reexploration; the rate of thrombosis is highest in the lower extremity and lowest in the head and neck. At exploration, the pedicle is inspected first. A determination is made as to whether the problem is arterial or venous. One must also determine whether the anastomotic problem is intrinsic (primary) or extrinsic (secondary).

Extrinsic problems include compression from a hematoma or an in-setting that is too tight, or twisting of the pedicle. In some instances, a secondary anastomotic problem can be relieved only by correction of an underlying problem. However, if it has been present long enough to have caused thrombosis of the vessels, the anastomosis must be opened and explored, as it must be when a primary anastomotic thrombosis is suspected. If the problem stems from either an inflow or outflow obstruction of the recipient vessels, then this must be relieved if possible, or different recipient vessels must be used. Sometimes, the use of vein grafts is required if other vessels are not readily available in the field. Repeated in-setting after exploration often requires the liberal use of split-thickness skin grafting to decrease tension, as marked edema is usually present secondary to vascular insult.

The salvage rate of free flaps at exploration varies in different series from 35% to 100% and is most commonly found to be about 70%. Salvage rates are higher when the time from thrombotic occurrence to exploration is shorter, so that the overall ischemic time is limited. The rate is higher also when the thrombosis occurs within the first 3 days after surgery, perhaps because the flap is more closely monitored during this time (13).

Many postoperative systemic therapeutic agents are used as possible means for improving anastomotic patency, although randomized clinical trials are not available to prove their efficacy. However, most do appear to improve patency in laboratory studies. Aspirin, dipyridamole, dextran, and prostacyclin analogues primarily affect platelet aggregation, and heparin and streptokinase primarily affect fibrin clot. Prophylactically, dextran and aspirin are used most commonly. Heparin and streptokinase are used more often when a thrombosis has occurred or the flap has been reexplored. Aspirin can be started preoperatively, but its use will increase the possibility of hematoma formation. Dextran can cause some serious complications, such as anaphylaxis, pulmonary edema, or fluid overload.

Leeches still have a role in the postoperative care of a failing free flap. In some cases of venous congestion that do not resolve despite reexploration of the venous outflow, the use of leeches for a period of 5 to 7 days can sometimes salvage the flap.

Although infrequently (2% to 10% of cases), a free flap occasionally fails and cannot be salvaged. If the flap cannot be successfully revascularized at the initial transfer in the operating room (despite all previously mentioned maneuvers) and it must be discarded, the next step depends on the type of clinical case. In many cases, especially if the upper or lower extremities are involved, the wound can be left open. Dressing changes are made, and wound coverage is addressed on another day when the microsurgical team is no longer tired. Sometimes, a biologic dressing or split-thickness skin graft can be placed in some lower extremity wounds to keep them from desiccating while a new plan is formulated. In many cases of head and neck reconstruction, if a free-flap failure occurs on the table, closure of the wound can be accomplished with the use of local or regional flaps, such as a temporalis flap, pectoralis flap, latissimus dorsi pedicled flap, or deltopectoral flap. Although none of these flaps provides the versatility of a free flap or good bone stock for jaw reconstruction, they all can provide stable wound closure at a difficult moment.

In the case of breast reconstruction, if a flap fails on the table, a tissue expander can be placed provided preoperative consent has been obtained from the patient. However, most flaps do not fail on the table; rather, as discussed previously, they fail within the first 72 hours after surgery. Many of these can be salvaged at reexploration, but a percentage cannot.

In some instances, delaying the debridement of failing flaps can be helpful in avoiding another flap. In some noncritical wounds, if the flap has survived for a sufficiently long period of time (perhaps between 12 and 72 hours), local revascularization of the deep portion of the flap (Crane principle) may occur. Thus, at debridement, enough granulation tissue may be present at the base of these wounds to allow coverage with a split-thickness skin graft. This technique works best in the management of wounds in which bones are exposed, but it is not applicable in wounds in which flap coverage is critical, such as wounds with exposed orthopedic hardware (14).

A certain percentage of flap failures are slow and demonstrate that free-flap failure is not necessarily an all-or-nothing phenomenon. Weinzweig and Gonzales (15) reported that 62.5% of their free-flap losses demonstrated this phenomenon. They hypothesized that secondary thrombosis of the vascular pedicle initiates a slow, progressive form of free-flap failure, so that neovascularization occurs and flap death is limited. They also recommend delayed and conservative debridement of these dying free flaps. In their series, most of the wound closures were accomplished by split-thickness skin grafts. Figures 14-1A–D demonstrate a parascapular free flap that became congested on postoperative day 7 and survived, except for minimal loss in its central portion, which left a scar.

Of lower extremities with failed flaps, one series showed that a large number went on to amputation (22%). In the remaining 78% of cases, the extremities were salvaged with split-thickness skin grafts, local flaps, or a second free flap. Long-term wound problems plagued 35% of the patients with salvaged extremities (16).

However, many wounds or reconstructions do require another flap. Sometimes, a local or regional flap can be used, although if this option was rejected before the free flap was created, it may not be a possibility after a failed flap either.

A second free flap may be required to accomplish the reconstructive goals. In the decision to perform another free flap, all the same judgments that the surgeon made before the first flap must be repeated, but this time with even greater care because the stakes are higher.

The surgeon may do a more thorough hematologic screening, looking for a hypercoagulable state. The flap that is chosen may need to be larger (e.g., latissimus dorsi or rectus abdominis vs. gracilis), with larger-caliber vessels. A repeated arteriogram may be required in the upper or lower extremity after a free-flap thrombosis has occurred to rule out propagation of clot into the main vessels. One may be more liberal with the use of vein grafts in a second attempt, especially if the cause of failure is suspected to be intimal injury in the recipient vessels.

Fearon and colleagues (17) showed that a second attempt at a free-tissue transfer can be quite successful in a number of different clinical cases (six of seven second attempts in their series were successful). Therefore, one should not hesitate to create a second free flap if this is the indicated procedure. Figures 14-2A–E show a patient who had a failed latissimus dorsi/serratus muscle combination for a squamous cell carcinoma of the head. A second free-flap procedure in which a TRAM flap was used was subsequently successful.

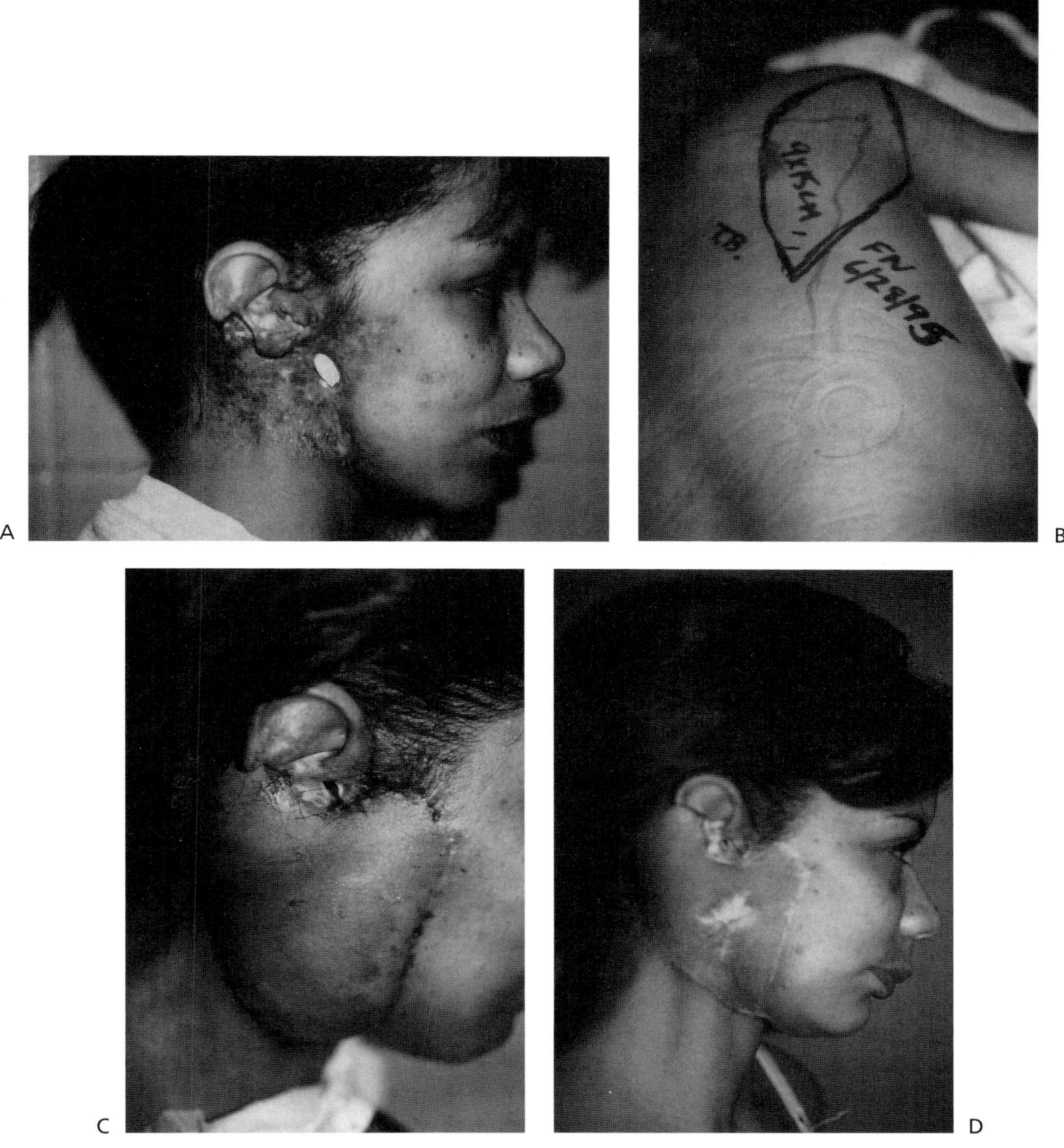

FIGURE 14-1. A: Young woman with osteoradionecrosis of the right mandible, partial destruction of the ear, and skin breakdown of the right side of the neck and right cheek. **B:** Right parascapular free flap. **C:** Venous congestion of the parascapular free flap on postoperative day 7. **D:** Long-term follow-up of the parascapular free flap shows a central scar.

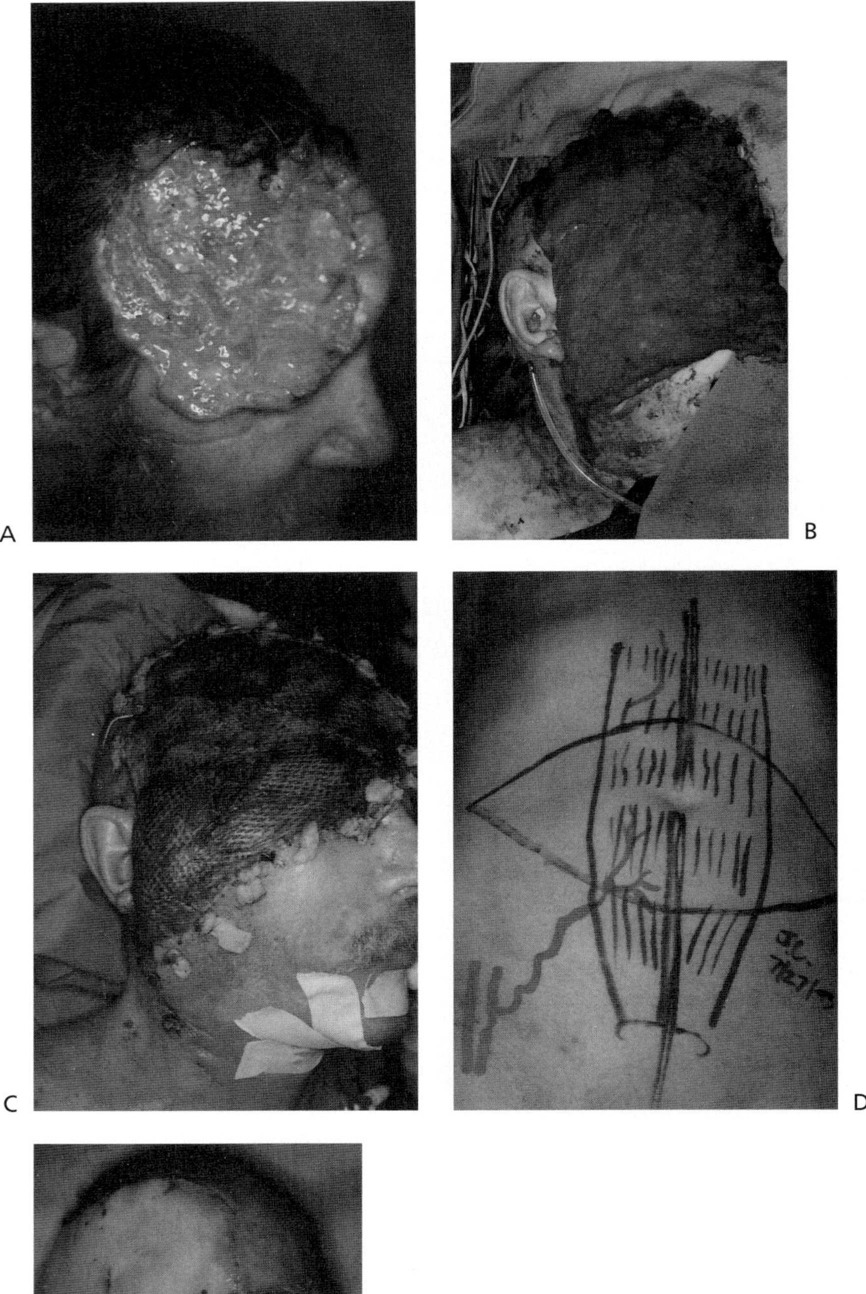

FIGURE 14-2. A: Veteran with massive squamous cell carcinoma of the scalp invading the dura mater and right globe. **B:** Intraoperative photograph of the revascularized latissimus dorsi/serratus free flap used for reconstruction. **C:** Failed flap at postoperative day 6. **D:** Second free-tissue transfer with use of a TRAM (transverse rectus abdominis myocutaneous) flap. **E:** Healing TRAM flap after second free-tissue transfer.

CONCLUSION

Very high success rates of free-tissue transfers are reported in most large series, with percentages ranging between 90% and 98%. To achieve these excellent results, good clinical judgment, experience, and technical expertise are necessary. The surgeon must prepare a thoughtful preoperative plan and backup plan. The procedure should be carried out expediently and with reasonable ischemia times. Postoperatively, the patient and the flap should be monitored by experienced personnel. Vascular obstructions in the flap pedicles, if caught early, can be frequently corrected on flap reexploration, and many failing flaps can be salvaged.

Once a flap failure has occurred, all the same rules apply, and even greater clinical judgment and experience are needed at this time to achieve a successful outcome.

REFERENCES

1. Grotting JC, Urist M, Maddex WA, et al. Conventional TRAM flap versus free microsurgical TRAM flap for immediate reconstruction. *Plast Reconstr Surg* 1989;83:842.
2. Attinger C. Soft tissue coverage for lower extremity trauma [Review]. *Orthop Clin North Am* 1995;26:295.
3. Anthony JP, Rawnsley JD, Benhaim P, et al. Donor leg morbidity and function after fibula free flap mandible reconstruction. *Plast Reconstr Surg* 1995;96:146.
4. Kroll SS, Shusterman MA, Reece GP, et al. Choice of flap and incidence of free flap success. *Plast Reconstr Surg* 1996;98:459.
5. Young DM. The need for preoperative leg angiography in fibula free flaps. *J Reconstr Microsurg* 1994;10:283.
6. Disa JJ, Cordeiro PG. The current role of preoperative arteriography in free fibula flaps. *Plast Reconstr Surg* 1998;102:1083.
7. Khouri RK. Avoiding free flap failure. *Clin Plast Surg* 1992;19:773.
8. Ablove RH, Moy OJ, Peimer CA, et al. Effect of high energy phosphates and free radical scavengers on replant survival in an ischemic model. *Microsurgery* 1996;17:481.
9. Shah DK, Zhang WX, Forman DL, et al. Combination therapy for salvaging a failing, experimental skin flap. *J Reconstr Microsurg* 1996;12:365.
10. Kroll SS, Shusterman MA, Reece GP, et al. Timing of pedicle thrombosis and flap loss after free tissue transfer. *Plast Reconstr Surg* 1996;98:1230.
11. Swartz WM, Izquierdo R, Miller MJ. Implantable venous Doppler microvascular monitoring: laboratory investigation and clinical results. *Plast Reconstr Surg* 1994;93:152.
12. Wechselberger G, Rumer A, Schoeller T, et al. Free flap monitoring with tissue-oxygen measurement. *J Reconstr Microsurg* 1997;13:125.
13. Hidalgo DA, Jones CS. The role of emergent exploration in free tissue transfer: a review of 150 consecutive cases. *Plast Reconstr Surg* 1990;86:492.
14. Wheatley MJ, Meltzer TR. The management of unsalvageable free flaps. *J Reconstr Microsurg* 1996;12:227.
15. Weinzweig N, Gonzales M. Free tissue failure is not an all-or-none phenomenon. *Plast Reconstr Surg* 1995;96:648.
16. Benacquista T, Kasabian AK, Karp NS. The fate of lower extremities with failed free flaps. *Plast Reconstr Surg* 1996;98:834.
17. Fearon JA, Cuddros CL, Way JW. Flap failure after microvascular free tissue transfer: the fate of a second attempt. *Plast Reconstr Surg* 1990;86:746.

SUGGESTED READING

Khouri RK, Cooley BC, Kunselman AR, et al. A prospective study of microvascular free flap surgery and outcome. *Plast Reconstr Surg* 1998;102:711.

Place MJ, Witt P, Hendricks D. Cutaneous blood flow patterns in free flaps determined by laser Doppler flowmetry. *J Reconstr Microsurg* 1996;12:355.

Strauch B, Yu HL, Chen ZW, et al. *Atlas of microvascular surgery: anatomy and operative approaches*. New York: Thieme Medical Publishers, 1999.

Discussion

MICROSURGERY

JULIAN J. PRIBAZ

The authors of this chapter are experienced microsurgeons, and they have carefully and thoroughly reviewed their methods of managing patients undergoing microsurgical procedures to ensure a good outcome. As microsurgeons, we learn from one another, experiences in the operating room, presentations at meetings, and articles in journals (1). Generally speaking, we all share the same general philosophy regarding how patients should be managed, so this commentary will to a large extent echo many of the sentiments that have already been expressed. However, I do hope to emphasize some additional aspects of patient management and provide a slightly different perspective for the readers.

I should begin by stressing that microsurgery is not a *separate specialty,* but rather a *technique* that has greatly expanded the repertoire of reconstructive surgeons. Although free-tissue transfer was practiced before the 1973 report of Daniel and Taylor of a free groin flap (2), it was this event that sparked interest and really heralded the advent of the microsurgical era. Initially, few free flaps were available, and the major interest was in obtaining flap survival. A revolution followed whereby a return to basic anatomical studies eventually led to the development of multiple available flaps for transfer, which led to many refinements in microsurgical reconstruction.

In the early days, if the microanastomosis remained patent and the flap survived, a procedure was heralded as a success. However, if clots formed in the vessels, the flap failed totally. As experience was gained, the success rate of free-tissue transfers increased, so that most centers now report a success rate of 95% or higher (3–5). Thus, if flap viability is the only parameter of a successful outcome, then unfavorable outcomes are rare.

However, we should now expand our definition of success or failure to include not only whether flaps remain viable, but also whether reconstructive goals are met and defects are satisfactorily and optimally reconstructed. In free-tissue transfer, one has to borrow from "Peter" to pay "Paul," so there is always a donor site. It is important to consider whether donor site complications and morbidity have been prevented or reduced, as they can be the reason for an unhappy patient. Furthermore, other complications that are the result of a lengthy operation or of drugs and medications administered (which may be necessary for a successful microanastomosis) must be considered. Finally, it is important to consider whether patients are generally happy with the outcome of their procedures, whether their expectations have been met, and whether they have been led to have unrealistic expectations. All the above factors, not just the technical aspects of microsurgery, must be considered before we can judge that a result has been favorable or unfavorable.

INITIAL CONSULTATION

The initial consultation is critical, and it is at this time that all the groundwork must be done. As the authors correctly point out, the appropriate indications for a free-tissue transfer should be present, and other, simpler options for the reconstruction should have been considered and discussed with the patient. A clear reconstructive goal needs to be established initially. A very thorough history must be taken and an examination performed at the initial consultation. In addition, the flaps available and the relative merits, advantages, and disadvantages of each one with respect to achieving the reconstructive goal should be considered in great detail and discussed with the patient.

As the authors point out, the timing of the reconstruction is also important. Any oncologic reconstruction is typically performed acutely at the same session as the extirpative surgery. In traumatic cases, however, the microvascular reconstruction is usually delayed, although authors such as Godina have clearly shown the benefit of acute reconstruction in trauma of the lower extremity versus the higher complication rates when reconstruction is performed subacutely (6).

As much information as possible should be obtained from the patient about general medical conditions, medications, and smoking history, as all these factors may affect the type of reconstruction that is chosen and the eventual outcome.

Clear goals of reconstruction need to be presented and understood, and for complex problems, it is best to see the patient on more than one occasion together with the patient's family so that all questions can be answered and a

J. J. Pribaz: Department of Plastic Surgery, Harvard Medical School; and Department of Plastic Surgery, Brigham and Women's Hospital, Boston, Massachusettes

clear picture presented to the patient. It is important to stress that all reconstructive efforts are very much a compromise, and that it may not be possible to restore the patient to total normality because the tissues to be used in the reconstruction are not the same as those that have been removed in the tumor extirpation or lost in the injury. Both functional and aesthetic aspects need to be addressed, stressed, and understood so that the result can be more appropriately gauged not only by the physician, but also by the patient and the patient's family. In this way, a misunderstanding of the outcome can be avoided.

This author believes that is very difficult to obtain completely informed consent in complex reconstructions. It is very difficult for lay persons to comprehend fully the nature of their problem and the technical aspects of a reconstructive procedure that is being recommended by the surgeon. Herein lies a major difficulty, for even a result judged as excellent by the treating surgeon may be viewed a dismal failure by the patient if the patient's expectations are not realistic.

OPERATION

As emphasized by Benacquista and Strauch, when the patient eventually does come into the operating room for the surgical procedure, it is important that the surgeons, anesthesiologists, and nursing staff work as a "team" to prepare the patient for a lengthy operation. It may take 1 hour of preparation before the procedure can commence. All the lines, monitors, and medications are administered. Also, the staff must attend to all the important parameters, such as room temperature, careful positioning, and protection of all the pressure areas and other vital areas to avoid inadvertent complications and errors of omission that are not related to the microsurgery. If such complications do occur, they will become the problem of the reconstructive surgeon, even if the surgeon was not directly responsible, because it is the surgeon who will continue to follow the patient postoperatively.

The surgeon will already have formulated a general reconstructive plan and backup plan well before the operation, but once the patient is fully prepared for surgery, it is wise to spend additional time planning and designing the flap that will be used for reconstruction. This process begins with making a very accurate anatomical diagnosis of the defect requiring reconstruction; the surgeon must not only consider the presenting defect but also appreciate that the defect will enlarge with debridement, recipient vessel dissection, and other extirpative measures. The more time spent in diagnosing the exact defect, the better. The use of templates and intraoperative models can be especially helpful in cases of complex defects in the head and neck by providing an accurate assessment of what is missing and, therefore, what is required (7).

Once an accurate picture has been obtained, then the various donor sites are reconsidered. Generally, the donor site has been selected preoperatively, but sometimes unpredictable changes resulting from surgical intervention on the recipient side necessitate a change of plan, and the reconstructive surgeon must always have a backup plan for each type of reconstruction.

Microvascular free-tissue transfer is a lengthy operation, and I wholeheartedly agree with the authors that it is best to avoid moving an anesthetized patient intraoperatively because it adds significantly to operating time and potential complications. This fact should be taken into account when a flap is selected, and positional changes should be avoided if at all possible.

A careful analysis of the problem to be corrected includes dissecting the recipient vessels and analyzing the relationship of these to the defect, so that a flap with a pedicle of appropriate length can be selected. If it is recognized that the pedicle length will not be adequate, an alternative flap may be selected, or a vein graft or arteriovenous loop can be planned electively so that no scrambling will take place at the time of anastomosis and flap detachment if it is discovered that the pedicle is not long enough. If this is done prospectively, the operation usually can proceed expeditiously. Well into a case, a tired and unprepared surgeon may attempt to suture the microanastomosis under tension, significantly increasing the chances of major complications. Another situation that commonly arises in microsurgery is that during flap dissection, anatomical variations are discovered that require a modification of the initial plan. The Boy Scout motto, "Be prepared," is an excellent *vade mecum* for the microsurgeon.

Although this discussion deals with microsurgery, the reconstructive surgeon prefers to anastomose larger vessels rather than very small vessels, and again, it is appropriate to select flaps with larger pedicles to minimize the chances of vascular complications. Many maneuvers to ensure a large anastomotic site, including simple techniques such as cutting vessels obliquely or utilizing a T-junction, can facilitate the microsurgical procedures.

The microsurgeon should be comfortably positioned and have good magnification while performing vascular repairs. With an experienced surgeon, the microvascular anastomosis is the easiest part of the operation, whereas the actual analysis and design of the flap are crucial in that they allow the best aesthetic and functional result for the patient (8,9).

Careful handling of the vessel to minimize spasm and the need to avoid twisting (especially with vein grafts) or compressing the pedicle with tight dressings are well discussed by the authors. This last point is indeed very important, and microsurgeons typically remain in the operating room until all the dressings are in place, even though they may be exhausted, because it is well-known that a poorly applied dressing can compromise the entire procedure if it interferes with blood flow to the flap.

A multitude of different rituals and medications have

been used by microsurgeons over the years, many of which are quite empirical and without scientific merit. In a multicenter study by Khouri et al. (10), many of these were shown not to affect vessel patency or the success rate. In fact, certain medications have been shown to be associated with a higher complication rate (e.g., the routine use of systemic heparin). In recent years, many surgeons have simplified and modified the adjunctive regimes that they use without any change in their overall success rates.

Attention to detail at every phase of the operative procedure is imperative in avoiding an unfavorable result. This can be difficult, especially during prolonged operations, as the operating team becomes fatigued.

POSTOPERATIVE CARE

I concur with the authors that postoperative monitoring is crucial, especially during the first 12 to 24 hours. It is within this period that most anastomotic complications become manifest. Various sophisticated methods of flap monitoring have been described and are outlined in the text; however, in busy microsurgical centers, the general shift has been away from complex, expensive monitoring devices to simpler means of assessing flap viability, such as frequent clinical examination, Doppler ultrasonography, and perhaps temperature probe monitoring. A prompt return to the operating room if there is any doubt about the integrity of the anastomosis is mandatory for flap salvage.

Although flap failure is a devastating complication, it is relatively rare in the hands of an experienced microsurgeon. Success rates in excess of 95% are the norm among experienced microsurgeons. Total flap failure is obviously a major complication but is relatively rare. Unfavorable results of a reconstruction may be a consequence of any of the factors that have been mentioned. Thus, a consideration of all aspects of the reconstruction and prolonged surgery and the means to reduce complications is even more important than the actual execution of the microanastomosis in avoiding an unfavorable outcome.

REFERENCES

1. Khouri RK. Avoiding free flap failure. *Clin Plast Surg* 1992;19:773–781.
2. Daniel RK, Taylor CI. Distant transfer of an island flap by microvascular anastomoses. A clinical technique. *Plast Reconstr Surg* 1973;52:111–117.
3. Parry SW, Toth BA, Elliot LF. Microvascular free tissue transfer in children. *Plast Reconstr Surg* 1985;81:838–840.
4. Schusterman MA, Miller MJ, Reece CP, et al. A single center's experience with 308 free flaps for head and neck cancer defects. *Plast Reconstr Surg* 1994;93:472–478.
5. Shestak KC, Jones NF. Microsurgical free tissue transfer in the elderly patient. *Plast Reconstr Surg* 1991;88:259–263.
6. Godina M. Early microsurgical reconstruction of complex trauma of the extremities. *Plast Reconstr Surg* 1986;78:285–292.
7. Pribaz JJ, Morris D, Mulliken JB. Three-dimensional free flap reconstruction of complex facial defects using intraoperative modeling. *Plast Reconstr Surg* 1994;93:285–293.
8. Acland RD. *Microsurgery—a practice manual.* St. Louis: Mosby, 1980.
9. O'Brien BM, Morrison WA. *Reconstructive microsurgery.* New York: Churchill Livingstone, 1987.
10. Khouri RK, Cooley BC, Kunselman AR, et al. A prospective study of microvascular free-flap surgery and outcome. *Plast Reconstr Surg* 1998;102:711–721.

15

CRANIOFACIAL SURGERY

IAN T. JACKSON

Craniofacial techniques are now applied to the management of craniofacial deformities, acute trauma and its residual deformities, and tumors of the skull base. Whatever the primary reason for surgery, the significant complications and the treatment they require are basically similar.

WOUND PROBLEMS

Placement of the coronal incision has changed significantly. The neurosurgical fraternity favored an incision at or just within the frontal hairline. The former, with ultracareful suturing, can produce a good scar, but the latter never does. The scar is seen through the hair, and worse still, the hair on either side of the scar may fall in different directions and make the scar line even more noticeable. In men who become bald, the scar may cause significant deformity and embarrassment. It cannot be corrected satisfactorily.

Management

Change to a pre-hairline scar with careful deep and subcuticular suturing and overlap of the upper edge over hair-bearing dermis in the hope that hair will grow through the scar. The result is often good.

The coronal incision used in the past by some plastic surgeons and neurosurgeons was pre-auricular to pre-auricular. This could spread and become obvious in the temporal area, especially in male patients.

Convert to large W-plasty closure. After scar excision, close in layers deep with nonabsorbable sutures or staples. The ideal coronal incision should end in a *postauricular* position, which places the scar much further posteriorly but still allows adequate frontal exposure. The scar is well hidden in both male and female patients. It can be designed as a large W-plasty incision if desired; whether or not this is done, the need for revision is uncommon. Use a Colorado needle to incise the scalp.

I. T. Jackson: Institute for Craniofacial and Reconstructive Surgery; and Division of Plastic Surgery, Providence Hospital, Southfield, Michigan

WOUND INFECTION

Wound infection is rare in craniofacial cases and may be associated with hematoma.

Management

Allow to settle with dressings and antibiotics as indicated. Drain any infected hematoma. It may be necessary to raise the flap once more for good exposure. This is absolutely indicated if an underlying cause (e.g., devascularized bone) is present. The procedure is described in the section on scalp necrosis with underlying nonvascular bone.

Prophylaxis

Make sure the drains are placed through the posterior scalp on either side of the sagittal midline and are taken into the temporal region, where the hematoma most frequently occurs. Dressings should be well padded and firm.

SCALP NECROSIS

Scalp necrosis, which is rare, is usually associated with multiple scarring of the scalp, previous radiation, or closure under tension.

Management

Allow to demarcate; excise and, if the bed is suitable, skin graft. If not, raise a *large* scalp rotation flap and, if necessary, graft the resulting secondary defect.

SCALP NECROSIS WITH UNDERLYING NONVASCULAR BONE

This situation occurs when a craniofacial procedure has been performed and devascularized bone lies deep to the totally devascularized scalp.

Management

Treat conservatively if the patient is well; the skin and outer table may sequestrate with the development of granulation tissue. Skin graft as soon as possible. Frequently, a full-thickness removal of all necrotic tissue is necessary. Cover is established with a local flap and skin grafting of the secondary defect. The latter need not be immediate—the base should be prepared until the skin graft take is certain.

The long-term solution in this situation is tissue expansion, scalp reconstruction, and cranial reconstruction with split-skull or split-rib grafts. Should this not be possible, the area can be camouflaged with a wig.

POSTOPERATIVE CHRONIC DISCHARGING SINUS

A chronic discharging sinus indicates dead bone, an infected implant, or infection around hardware—plates, screws, or wires. The clinical diagnosis is confirmed by sinus probe and roentgenography.

Management

Remove the focus of infection, preferably by a remote approach (e.g., coronal flap for upper face, upper buccal sulcus for the maxilla up to the infraorbital rim and zygoma).

MIDLINE SWELLING EXTENDING INTO UPPER LIDS

This is usually caused by a localized infectious process. It may be related to devascularized bone, an infection in the ethmoid sinuses, or an infected hematoma. The swelling can be significant if alloplastic material has been inserted at the original procedure. Aspiration will determine the nature of the effusion, and computed tomography (CT) will reveal the cause.

Management

If the fluid obtained is sterile and CT shows no abnormalities, delay with close observation and antibiotics is acceptable. If the culture is positive for organisms and the patient is well, even with an intracranial collection, a similar "wait and see" course can be adopted. If the patient does not recover normally and fluid reaccumulates clinically and on scan, then both the intracranial and extracranial area should be reexplored. Any loose bone or alloplastic material should be removed. More importantly, the anterior skull base should be examined, and if a connection is found between the intracranial and extracranial area, it should be repaired. This is discussed in greater detail later, but briefly, the defect should be closed with vascularized local or distant tissue. Secure closure is essential.

Whatever the cause, it should be ascertained that the brain can expand completely and that no residual extradural defect is present. Closure is in the routine fashion with temporal drains. It is not advisable to place drains centrally for fear of reestablishing an intracranial nasal connection.

If the situation does not resolve satisfactorily, an intracranial nasopharyngeal connection should be suspected.

RESIDUAL INTRACRANIAL NASOPHARYNGEAL CONNECTION

A residual intracranial nasopharyngeal connection may occur with an anterior fossa procedure, whether performed for exploration in acute trauma, reconstruction of a posttraumatic or congenital deformity, or resection of a skull base tumor.

The patient may be unwell after surgery, with fever, frontal inflammation, and puffy periorbital inflammation that fails to resolve after 4 to 5 days. The latter is the most significant feature in this scenario and may be the only indication that something is significantly wrong, especially in cases with fever.

In certain patients, everything settles well, but a skin defect develops later in relation to the osteotomy in the frontal, glabellar, or medial canthal areas. CT will reveal retruded frontal lobes and a resulting defect behind the frontal bone, although this is not always the case. Should this condition persist undiagnosed or if the patient delays presentation, the frontal bone will be gradually lost. The craniotomy flap must have contact with the periosteum and the dura to ensure adequate vascularity and survival.

Management

This can be an urgent situation, but in most cases, it is not an emergency. The coronal flap is raised, and the frontal bone flap is removed. If exploration is performed early in the postoperative phase, some purulence and a small dead space may be noted. The anterior cranial fossa floor is explored to determine the size and position of the defect, which is usually small and centrally located in the cribriform area. If a local flap has not been used previously, the galeal frontalis myofascial periosteal flap is ideal in such a case (1) (Fig. 15-1). The flap is raised based inferiorly from the center of the coronal flap, and the dimensions should be at least two to three times those of the defect. The flap is then folded down to cover the defect with wide overlapping of the surrounding bone. It is stabilized with sutures through drill holes in the bone surrounding the defect. Another useful method of stabilizing the flap to use the fibrin glue compound Tisseal (Baxter Healthcare, Glendale, California). When a galeal

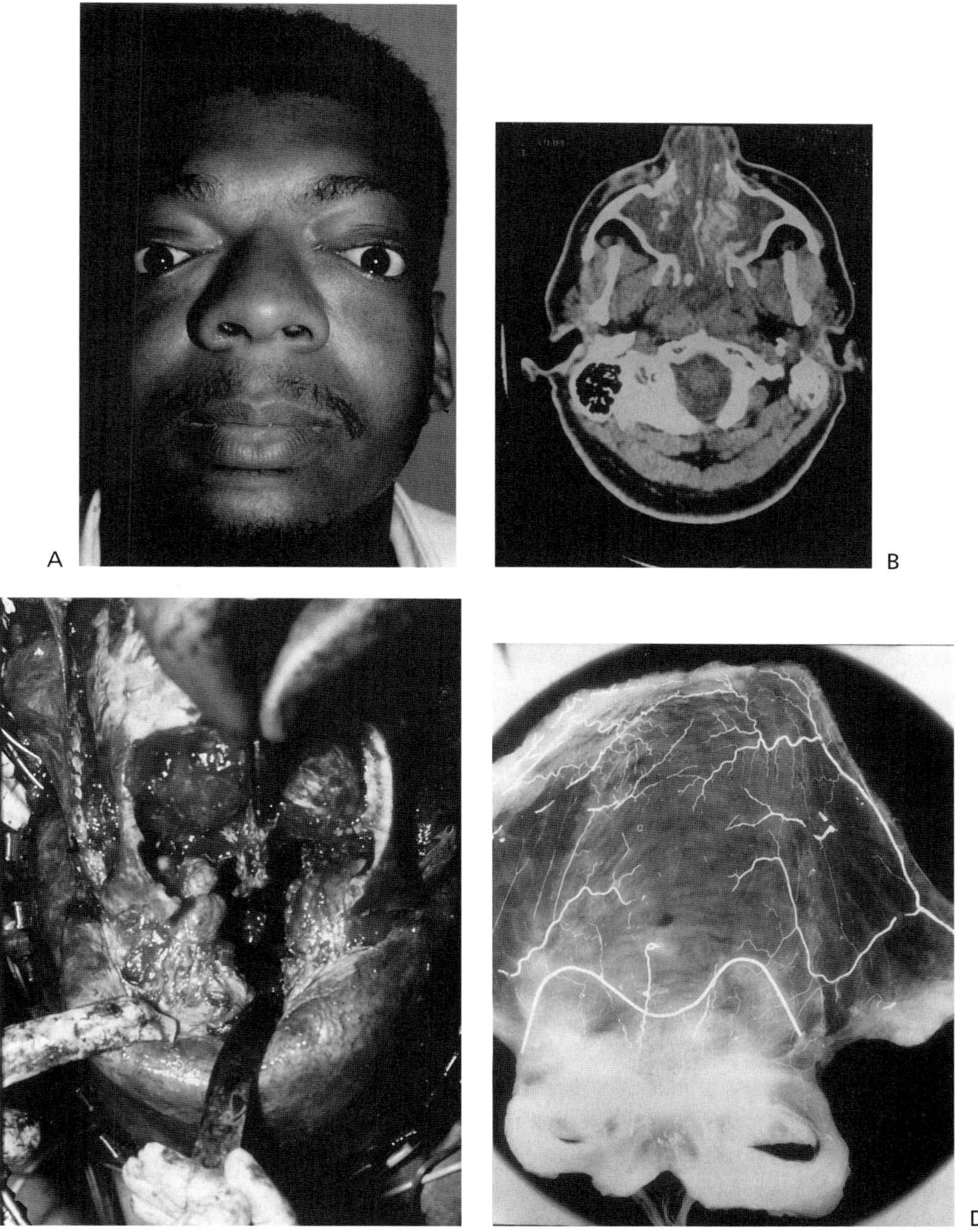

FIGURE 15-1. Use of the galeal frontalis myofascial flap. **A:** Massive involvement of all craniofacial sinuses with aggressive polyps. Right frontal bone, right dura, and right frontal lobe are invaded. **B:** Axial computed tomography shows extensive involvement of sinuses and parasinus areas with polyps. **C:** A connection is formed between the anterior cranial fossa and the nasopharynx through the floor of the anterior cranial fossa after radical polyp removal. **D:** Blood supply of the isolated galeal frontalis myofascial flap is somewhat scanty beyond its lower third. *(continued)*

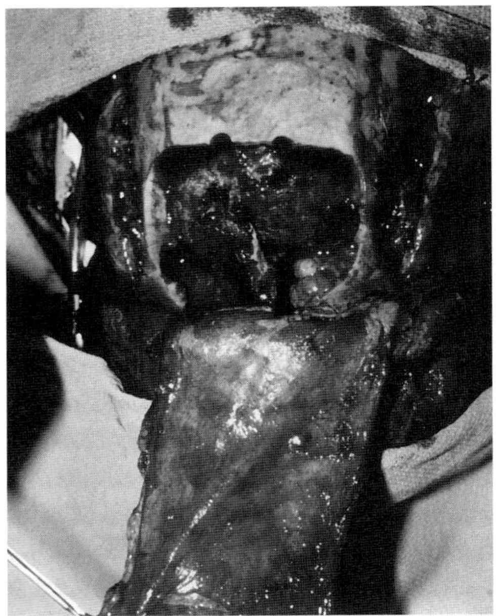

E

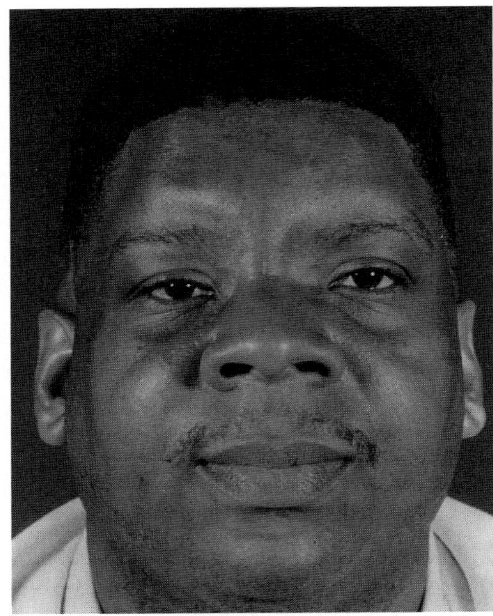

F

FIGURE 15-1. *Continued* **E:** Elevated galeal frontalis myofascial flap will be used to cover the floor of the anterior cranial fossa. **F:** End result 5 years after surgery.

frontalis flap is not available, a temporal galeal flap can be used; this is based laterally and can extend beyond the cribriform plate to the other side.

It is mandatory that any foreign material used in the primary repair be removed. Also, copious irrigation is performed during the surgery with saline solution with or without antibiotic.

In cases in which the diagnosis is delayed, profuse granulation tissue will be found around the osteotomies and around any frontal bone erosion, and it also fills the dead space anterior the frontal lobe. Meticulous debridement of the granulation tissue will expose the defect into the nasopharynx. Copious irrigation is employed to cleanse the area of any loose and avascular material. Because these cases are often referred from other institutions, foreign material (e.g., methylmethacrylate) may have been used. This must be removed completely.

It is essential to place vascularized tissue into the extradural defect. The only two choices are omentum or a free-muscle transfer. The reason for this is that the brain probably will not be able to expand because of prolonged inflammation with resultant dural thickening; thus, the dead space must be filled completely. Local flaps do not have sufficient volume. The omentum was used in the past before muscle flaps were identified. The results were excellent because the omentum provides a long vascular pedicle that reaches the neck without difficulty. In addition, the vessels are large, and a large amount of pliable soft tissue is available to fill the defect (2). However, an intraabdominal intervention is required, which can cause problems (e.g., peritonitis, abscess, adhesions).

The rectus abdominis, serratus, and latissimus dorsi free-muscle flaps have proved very satisfactory (3–6); our own preference and that of many others is the rectus abdominis flap (Fig. 15-2). A skin paddle is included if indicated, as when a significant skin defect is present. The vessels can be conveniently anastomosed to the temporal, facial, or neck vessels, but occasionally, in the latter, vein grafts are necessary. Flaps such as the radial forearm flap have no place in this situation; these skin flaps have insufficient bulk to fill the defect, and the initial problem may well recur.

It is important to pack the flap down into the defect in the skull base. If it can be fixed with sutures in that area, so much the better, because this allows a complete seal to be achieved. Tisseal can again be used in this situation.

If the bone is healthy and can be replaced without compressing the muscle flap, it is carefully placed in position and fixed with plates and screws. Care must be taken not to compress the vascular pedicle in any way. If this occurs, the bone flap is sacrificed, as it is if infection is present around the bone. This is not always the case; judgment is required.

Drains are inserted and the coronal flap is replaced and stapled into position. In five cases treated in this way, which represent approximately 1% of our skull base tumor cases, and in two craniofacial deformity cases, which represent an incidence considerably less than 1%, the postoperative progress was uneventful. When the bone was replaced at a later date, no problems were encountered. Initially, split rib was used, but now we use split cranial bone.

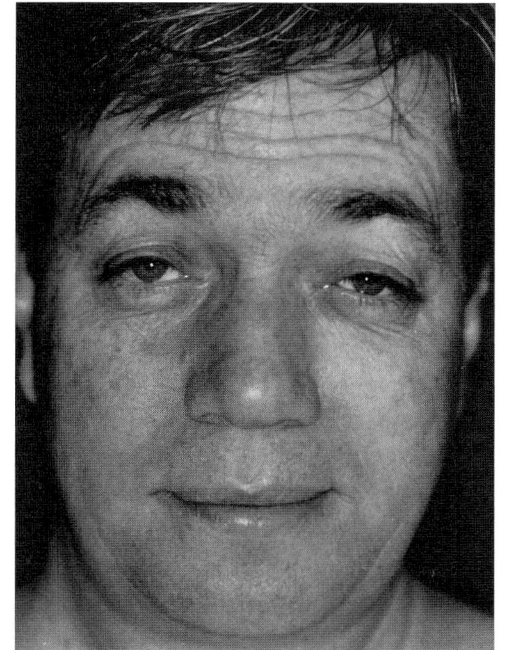
A

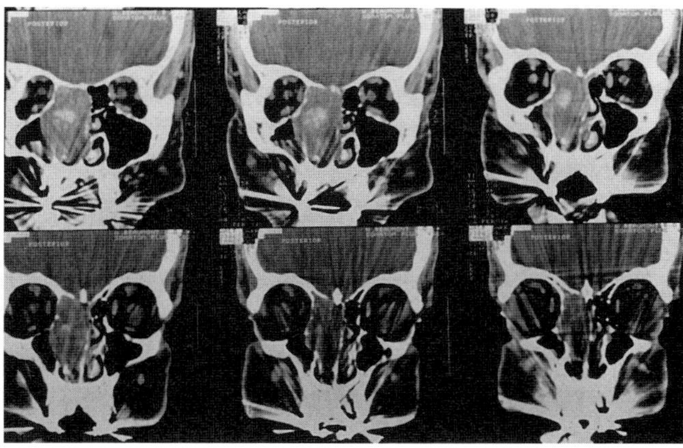
B

C

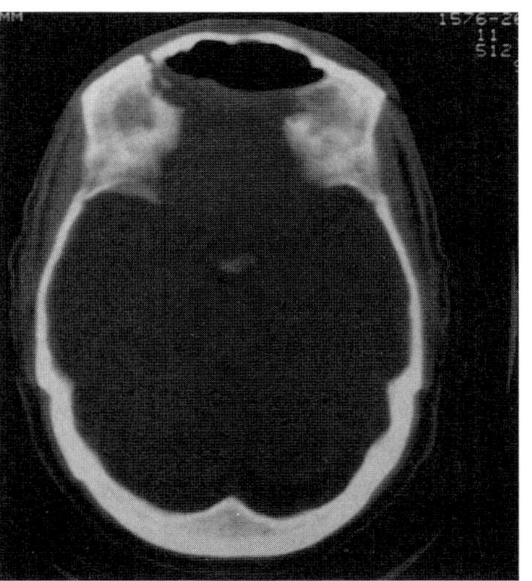
D

FIGURE 15-2. Use of free-tissue transfer in an infection of the anterior cranial fossa. **A:** A 46-year-old man with an esthesioneuroblastoma of the anterior cranial fossa and nasal cavity. **B:** Appearance of the lesion on coronal computed tomogram with and without contrast. **C:** Exposed frontal bone after surgery. **D:** Axial computed tomogram showing typical appearance of the "dead space" behind the frontal bone flap. *(continued)*

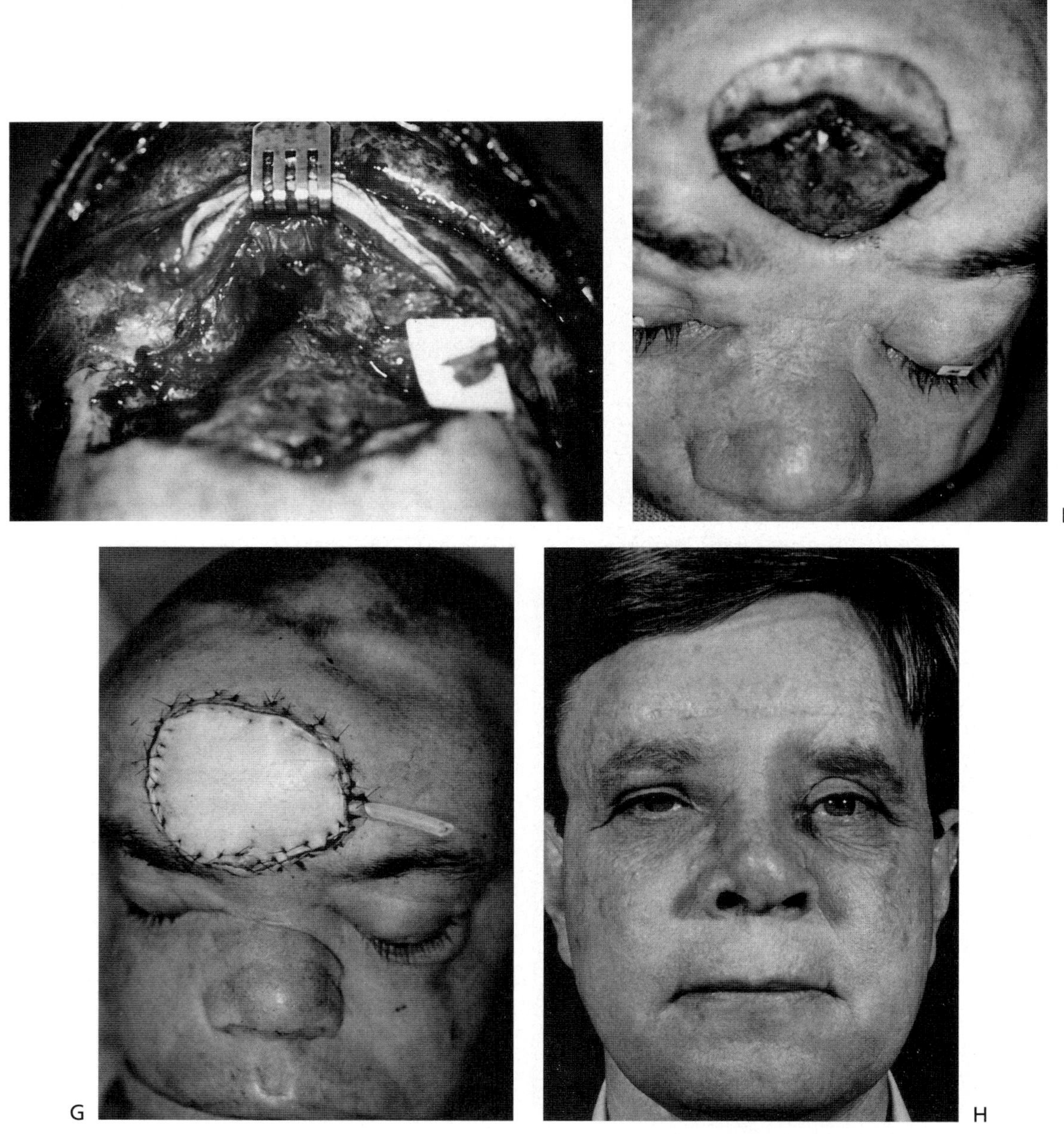

FIGURE 15-2. *(Continued)* **E:** At reexploration, the cause of the infection and the dead space, a connection between the anterior cranial fossa and the nose, can be seen. **F:** Frontal skin defect following debridement. **G:** Skin defect and anterior cranial fossa filled with a rectus myocutaneous free flap. **H:** Final appearance after two-stage resection of the rectus flap cutaneous paddle. Patient is alive and doing well 6 years after surgery.

In the single case in which a skin paddle had to be incorporated in the flap, the latter was removed totally in two later serial excisions.

FRONTAL BONE IRREGULARITIES

Irregularity of the skull is not uncommon after craniofacial procedures, and this is aesthetically significant in the frontotemporal areas. In other regions, the deformity is covered by the hair-bearing scalp; it should be remembered, however, when the need for reconstruction is being considered, that some male patients will eventually become bald.

Management

In the past, methylmethacrylate was the material of choice to effect a satisfactory reconstruction, and it is still used by many surgeons. To obtain good adhesion of the methylmethacrylate, small screws are placed into the bone with one-third to one-half of each screw left exposed, depending on the thickness of the methylmethacrylate to be applied. Any full-thickness defect is padded with multiple layers of Surgicel. The screws allow the material to be fixed securely, and the Surgicel helps to protect the dura from the exothermic reaction that is generated as the acrylic hardens. Once the reconstruction is solid, it is contoured and irrigated profusely, and the scalp is closed and drained. Antibiotic cover is maintained for 10 days (7).

An alternative is to use BoneSource (Howmedica Leibinger, Dallas, Texas) or Norian CRS (Synthes Maxillofacial, Monument, Colorado) (Fig. 15-3). When mixed with a sodium phosphate buffer solution (BoneSource) or a combination of calcium phosphate powder and sodium phosphate solution (Norian CRS), these substances become like putty and can be applied and molded to reconstruct the defect (8–10). The setting time depends on the volume of sodium phosphate added. Experimentally at 1 year, new bone replaces 77% of the hydroxyapatite cement. The material can be exposed to open

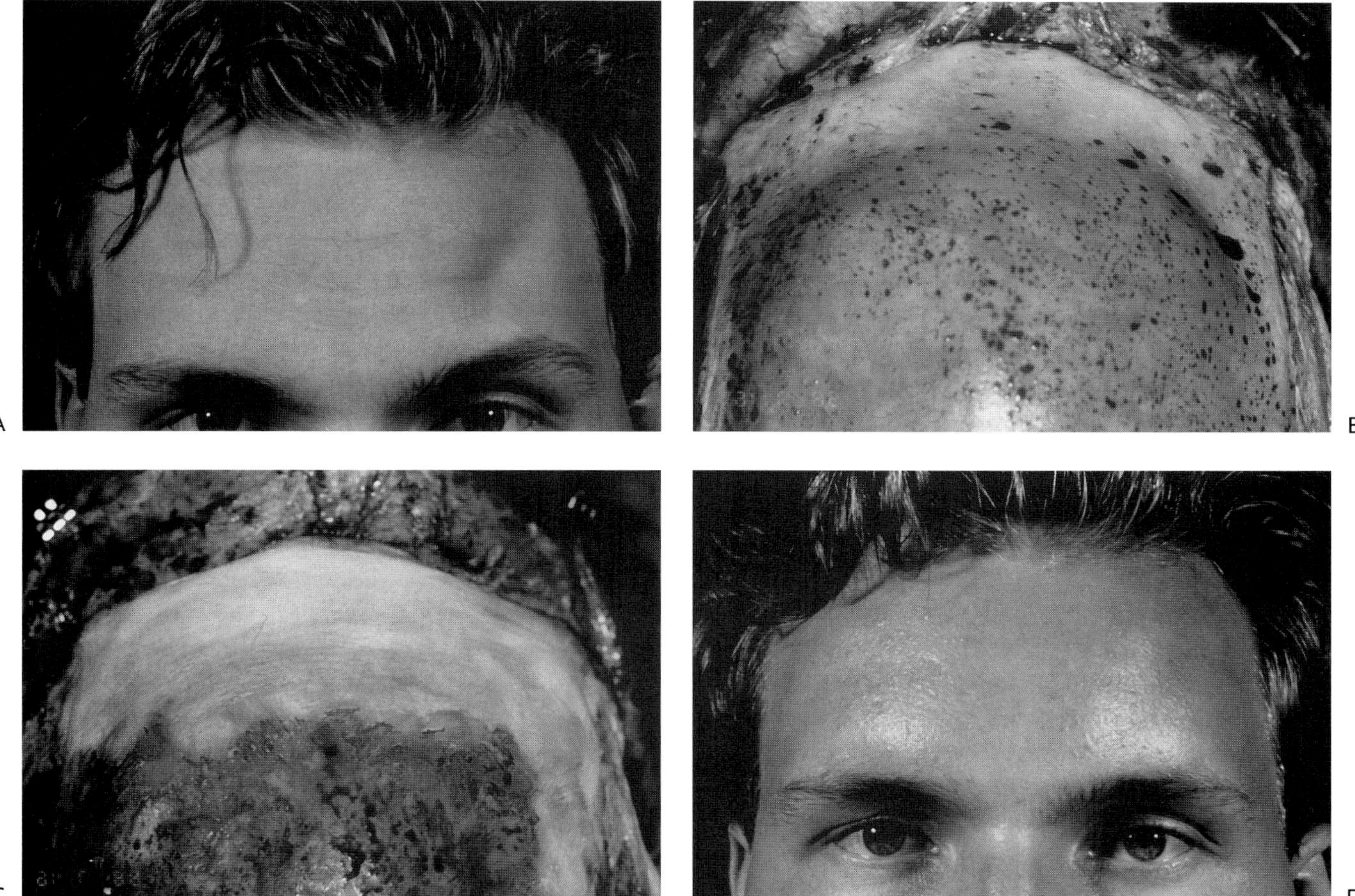

FIGURE 15-3. The use of hydroxyapatite cement (BoneSource) to reconstruct skull defects. **A:** Concavity of the left frontal area—no obvious cause. **B:** Frontal area exposed by a coronal flap shows some degree of bilateral deformity. The left side is worse than the right. **C:** BoneSource applied. **D:** The result after 6 months.

sinuses, and provided the brain is covered (e.g., with layers of moist Surgicel), the full thickness of the skull can be reconstructed satisfactorily.

CRANIAL BONE DEFECTS

Cranial bone defects may occur following surgical correction of a deformity, loss of bone resulting from infection, or cranial bone harvest. They are corrected if they are of concern to the patient (e.g., a soft spot or irregularity), or to both surgeon and patient (e.g., if they are large).

Management

Small defects can be reconstructed with Surgicel, BoneSource, or methylmethacrylate, as described previously. Moderately large defects are best replaced with split-skull grafts. The cranium can be taken as a full-thickness harvest and split with a thin osteotome. In this way, both defect and donor site are reconstructed. The bone is stabilized with titanium or resorbable polylactate plates and screws (Bionx Implants, Lampere, Finland); the latter can be contoured without heating (11). In children, defects are usually closed with fragments of bone not required in the original reconstruction; if necessary, these are augmented with bone dust obtained with the craniotome. Surgicel is placed over the defect, the graft is placed in position, and a further layer of Surgicel is placed on top. This process usually, but not always, provides a satisfactory reconstruction. On occasion, hydroxyapatite granules are used to provide bulk.

HARVEST OF SKULL BONE GRAFTS

It is also possible to harvest split-bone grafts *in situ,* but care and experience are required, especially in female patients. This procedure is not advocated for children before adolescence.

First, one uses an instrument (e.g., a periosteal elevator; the same one should always be used) to tap the skull. Depending on the pitch of the tone, the thickness of the skull can be determined. This sound allows the surgeon to decide whether to take an *in situ* full- or partial-thickness graft.

The graft design is outlined with a lead pencil, and a contouring burr is used to penetrate the outer table. Laterally, the contouring burr reduces the outer table down to the diploë. The outer table is now like an island, and a thin, sharp curved or straight osteotome is placed between the tables; the surgeon gently taps and moves around the bony island to remove the outer table safely. This must be done carefully to prevent a full-thickness penetration with damage to the dura and brain.

Frontal defects in children require harvest of a full-thickness bone graft, which is usually taken from the temporal area. The neurosurgeon uses burr holes and a protected drill to harvest the bone. For the plastic surgeon, it is safer to use the contouring burr and gradually remove bone to expose the dura all around. As the skull becomes thinner, the dural vessels can be seen; these are just under the inner table. The inner table is cut through slowly; the dura is moderately resistant to the drill. The graft should be completely freed all around because during elevation, retained bony spicules could tear the dura. At this point, the graft is separated from the dura by means of a fine periosteal elevator. It is gradually loosened and removed. The resulting defect is reconstructed, as previously mentioned, with fragments of leftover bone.

ALTERNATIVES FOR CRANIAL RECONSTRUCTION

This is an area of considerable interest at this moment. In the past, molded solid titanium sheeting was used, and it is still used in some centers. The manufacture of such a replacement is expensive. The same can be said for premade polypropylene (Medpor, Porex Surgical, College Park, Georgia) or hydroxyapatite reconstructions. Titanium mesh is an alternative and can be very satisfactory.

BoneSource and Norian CRS can also be used. Initially, a metal mesh or polylactate/polyglycolide mesh is used to cover the defect, and the bone replacement material is spread on top of this.

CONTOUR DEFORMITIES

These can result from deficiencies or from excess tissue (e.g., excess or displaced bone). Alternatively, plates and screws can be made more obvious by slight surrounding resorption of bone.

Management

Through local incisions on the scalp or a coronal incision for the frontal area, the irregularities are exposed. The excess bone or, in situations in which a plate is the cause of the problem and removal is difficult, the plate is contoured until the desired surface contour of metal and skull is obtained. If possible, plates and screws are removed and contouring proceeds accordingly. The use of resorbable plates and screws eliminates much of the need for contouring.

TEMPORAL HOLLOWING

After application of the coronal flap approach to the craniofacial region, an obvious concave deformity of the temporal region can develop, unilaterally or bilaterally. In most cases, this undoubtedly occurs because of failure to reposition the temporalis adequately at the end of the original procedure. The muscle should be securely positioned by placing many drill holes in the lateral orbital rim and in the temporal crest; in this way, the muscle can be stabilized in its correct position with nonabsorbable sutures.

Management

The coronal flap is again lifted and the temporalis is exposed down to the zygomatic arch. The galea is elevated in continuity with the temporalis, and the latter is mobilized completely. The contracture lies in the layer of scar tissue on the posterior surface of the muscle, and this is expanded by making vertical and horizontal incisions, preferably confined to the scar tissue. Once the correct dimensions of the muscle are obtained, it is fixed in position as described for the initial closure. Should this procedure fail to correct the contour deformity, methylmethacrylate or hydroxyapatite cement can be placed deep to the muscle and modified as necessary to achieve the correct temporal contours. Bone grafts placed in this situation tend to be resorbed, possibly because of overlying temporalis activity. The muscle is positioned as described previously.

ORBITAL AND EYE COMPLICATIONS: MALPOSITION OF THE ORBIT OR PORTIONS THEREOF

Malposition of the orbit is most frequently caused by incorrectly repositioned type IV orbitozygomatic fractures. The result is an expanded orbit with displacement of the globe inferiorly and laterally; enophthalmos also develops. The zygoma rotates posterolaterally, so that the lateral orbital wall, zygoma, and lateral portion of the inferior rim are displaced posteriorly. Similar clinical pictures with different eye positions are associated with isolated floor and medial wall displacement. The enophthalmos is usually secondary to the displacement of orbital fat as a result of periorbital defects rather than to a true loss of fat. Diplopia is usually an accompanying feature in this situation, resulting from either malposition of the globe or malfunction of the extraocular muscles, or a combination of both.

Management

Clinical assessment of the orbital rim and malar and eye position requires standard and preferably three-dimensional CT to confirm and enhance the clinical impression. The three-dimensional CT should be interactive to allow total assessment of the problem and accurate comparison with the unaffected side, and it should have the capacity to perform mock surgery to aid the surgeon in deciding on the correct procedure. In our institution, the Analyze system (Mayo Medical Foundation, Biomedical Engineering, Rochester, Minnesota) is used because it fulfills these requirements (12–14) (Fig. 15-4).

If an isolated floor displacement, which is rare, is the cause, this can be approached transconjunctivally through the inferior fornix, through a blepharoplasty approach, or through a cheek incision over the infraorbital rim. The periosteum of the floor is elevated with the contents, and the floor is reconstructed with a cranial bone graft or an alloplastic material firm enough to maintain the eye and its contents in the correct position. Medpor is such a material, as is polypropylene polylactate. The error most frequently seen in this situation is failure to extend the dissection far enough posteriorly. The extent of dissection should preferably be determined by three-dimensional CT measurements; if these are not available, it is wise to dissect carefully after a distance of 4.5 cm. Medial and lateral wall displacement is approached by a coronal incision; again, the contents are freed and the medial wall reconstructed, as for the floor. Cranial bone is preferred, but alloplastic material can be used. The medial canthus is replaced in its correct position (see section on medical canthus displacement). Lateral wall displacement can be isolated, but most frequently, the whole malar complex is involved (Fig. 15-5). There may be a rotational element to the displacement, which can be fully analyzed by the three-dimensional CT system. In this case, the displaced segment is approached through a coronal incision, and the orbital soft tissue is dissected from the displaced bone. The latter is then mobilized by manipulation or osteotomy and correctly positioned and stabilized with plates and screws. Any resulting defect in the lateral orbital wall or floor is reconstructed with cranial bone, and any residual enophthalmos is corrected by placing a bone graft or alloplastic material deep in the posterior orbit to advance the eye.

LATERAL CANTHAL DISPLACEMENT

This may be the result of a canthus that is too anterior or too inferior, or a combination of both. It is important to verify that the lateral orbital rim is in the correct position.

Management

A horizontal incision is made at the lateral canthal area, and the canthus is dissected out with sharp pointed scissors and disinserted. With toothed forceps, it is repositioned, usually by a combination of superior and lateral movement, until the canthal appearance is correct in relation to the contralateral, normal side. Its position in relation to the rim is noted, and the periosteum of the lateral wall is elevated. Two drill holes are made in the rim, and wire is placed through the canthus and double-looped. The ends are

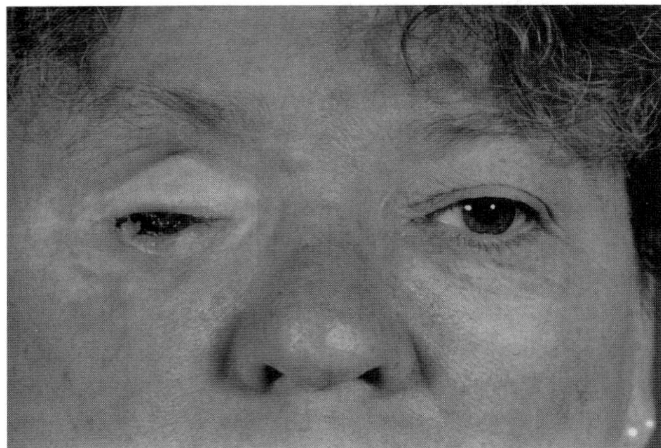

A

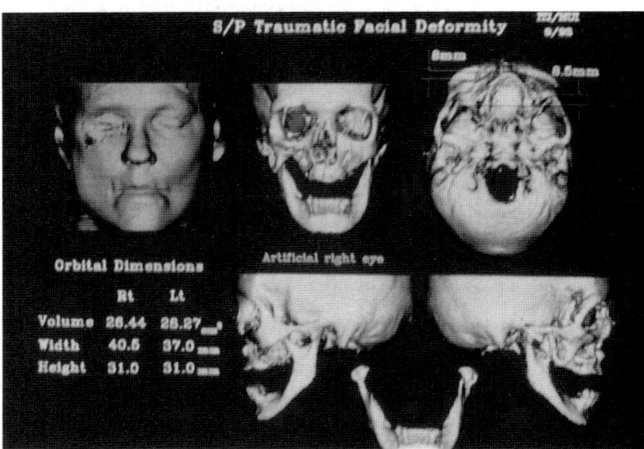

B

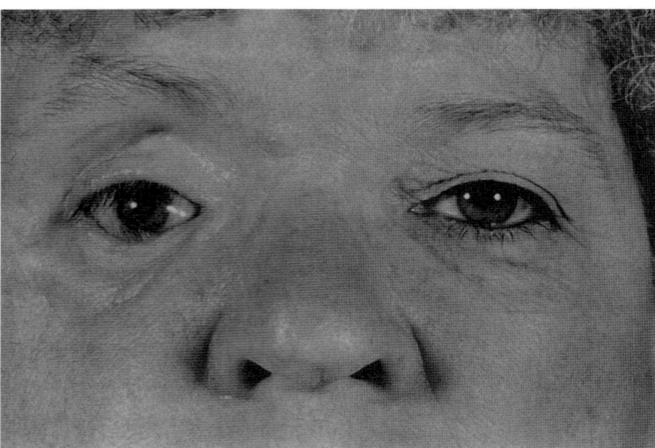

C

FIGURE 15-4. Management of orbital malposition with use of the Analyze system. **A:** Posttraumatic orbital deformity—displacement and fat atrophy with loss of eye. **B:** Three-dimensional computed tomography with use of the Analyze program. The malpositioned orbit with its altered dimensions can be clearly seen. **C:** The result following exploration by means of a coronal flap and expansion and repositioning of the orbit with the appropriate osteotomies. The prosthesis is in a good position, but the lower lid still must be corrected.

brought out through the rim holes, and the wire is tightened on the lateral aspect of the rim. The most common error is to fix the wire too far anteriorly.

MEDIAL CANTHAL DISPLACEMENT

This is commonly seen after old trauma correction, hypertelorism correction, or asymmetrical conditions, such a facial clefts. An epiphora may be associated if the lacrimal drainage system has been damaged (15).

Management

By clinical examination and CT, interactive three-dimensional if possible, it can be determined whether the displacement is secondary to ligament displacement alone, incorrect positioning of the medial orbital wall, or excess bone on the medial orbital wall, and whether it is symmetrical or asymmetrical.

A Y-shaped incision is made at the medial canthus. The single limb extends from the canthus to the nose, and the other two limbs extend onto the upper and lower lids. Through this incision, the whole medial canthal and nasal area can be dissected out to allow accurate identification of the lacrimal drainage system. The subperiosteal dissection and the incision and/or excision of scar tissue is continued until the canthus can be placed in its correct position effortlessly. When this achieved, the position on the medial orbital wall is marked, and a hole is drilled of sufficient size to take the canthus.

Under the medial end of the contralateral eyebrow, an incision is made down through the periosteum. A subperiosteal dissection is carried out to expose the underlying bone. With a wire-passing drill, two holes are made through the bone and down to the hole on the medial wall of the contralateral orbit. A No. 2-0 gauge stout wire cut to a sharp point is securely looped through the medial canthal ligament. Using a reversed straight needle with an eye or a syringe needle, inserted from the opposite side, the wire is brought from the hole in the medial orbital wall and out through one of the holes in the contralateral glabellar area. The other end of the wire is brought through the other drill hole using the same technique. The wire can now be tightened without concern because of the thick bone in this area. In this way, the medial canthus is brought into its correct anatomical position. This is a totally stable situation (Fig. 15-6).

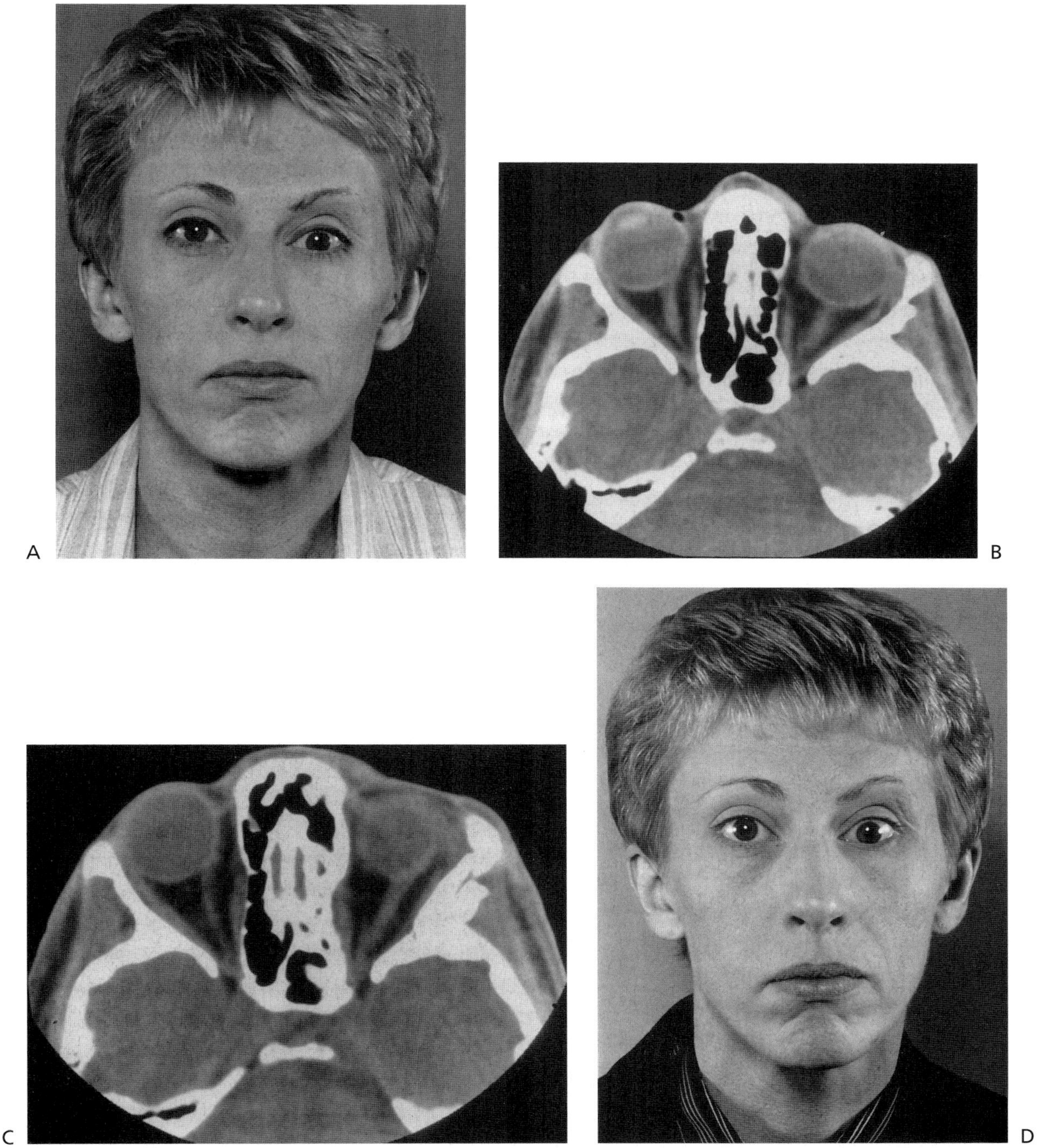

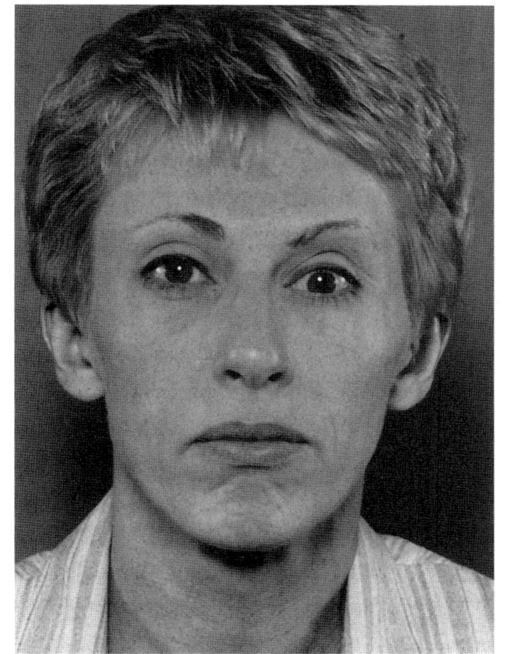

A

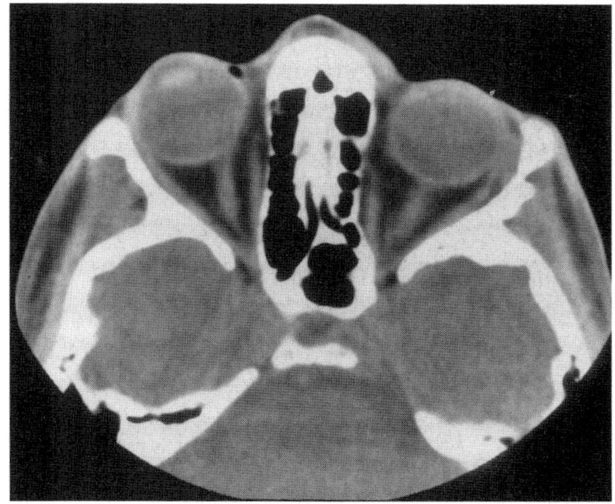

B

C

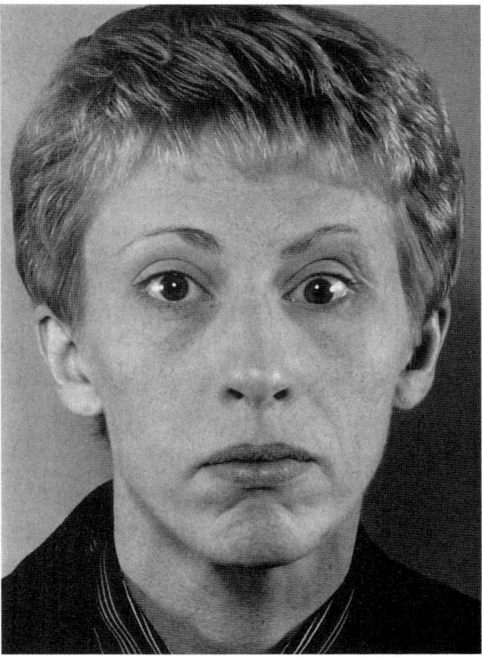

D

FIGURE 15-5. Management of enophthalmos resulting from lateral wall displacement. **A:** Left posttraumatic enophthalmos together with inferior displacement of the globe. **B:** Axial computed tomography shows enlargement of the left orbit resulting from displacement of the lateral orbital wall. **C:** Reconstruction of the orbit by advancement osteotomy of the lateral orbital wall and reduction of the orbit by means of the cranial bone graft on the inner aspect of the lateral orbital wall. **D:** After the eye position improves, further surgery will be performed on the upper eyelid.

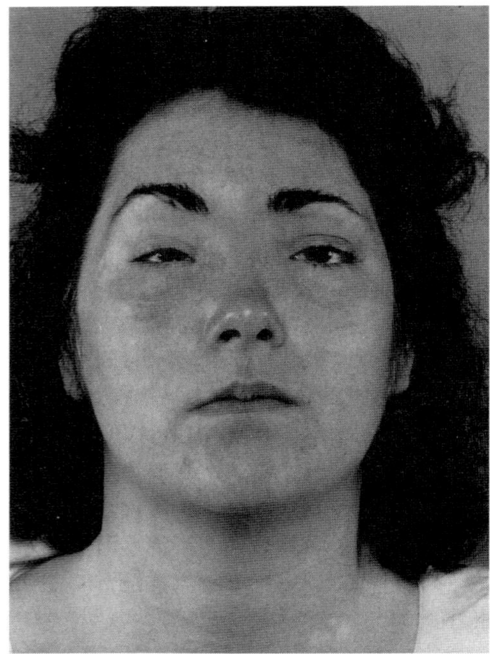

A

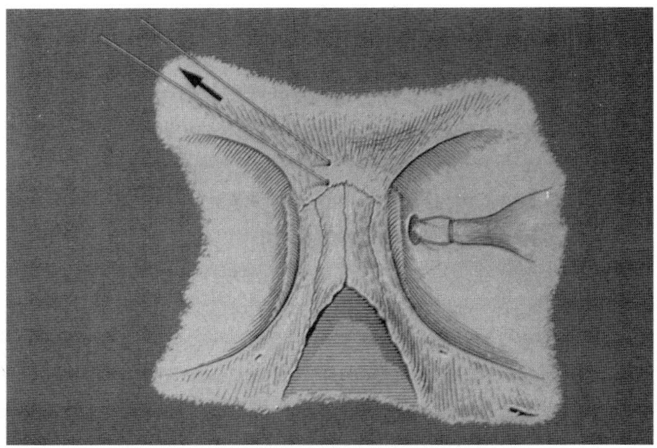

D

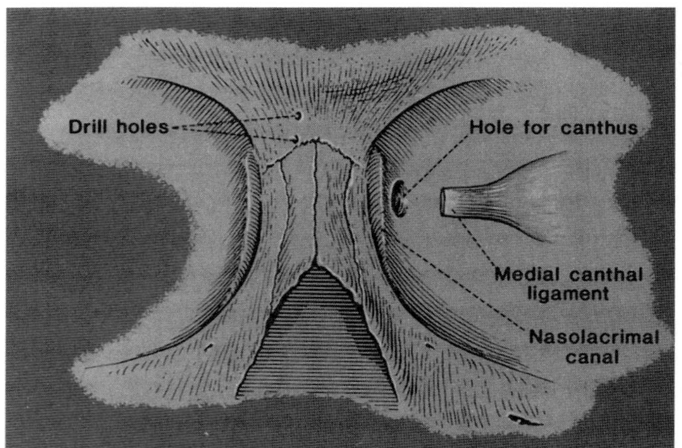

B

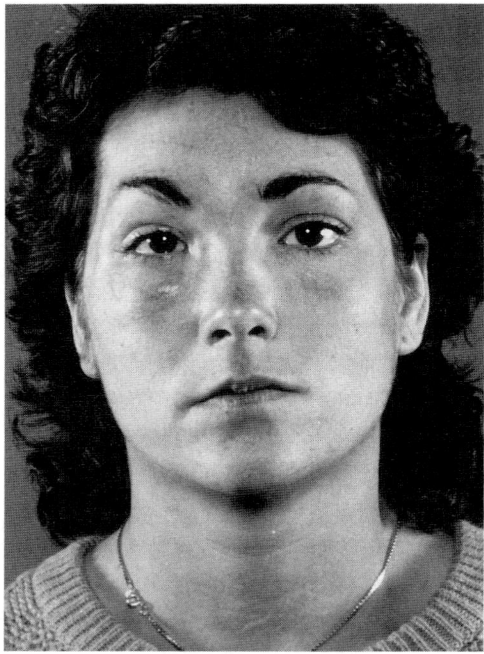

E

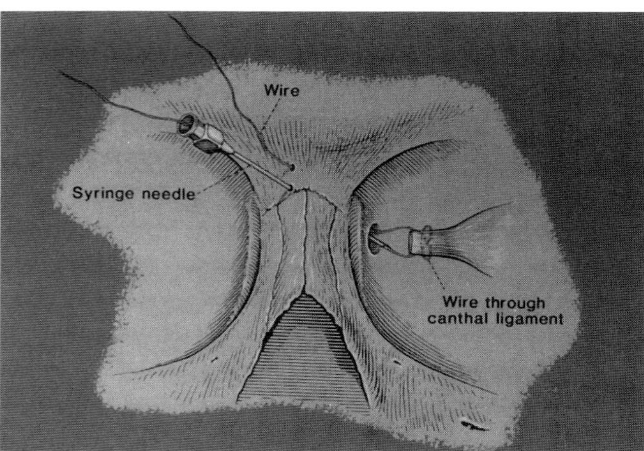

C

FIGURE 15-6. Management of posttraumatic right enophthalmos and bilateral medial canthal displacement. **A:** Preoperative appearance. Note ptosis of the right upper eyelid. **B:** The insertion area of the medial canthal ligament is shown, and also the point for its stabilization on the contralateral glabellar area. **C:** Wire looped through the medial canthal ligament. The wire is brought into the secure fixation area with the use of a syringe needle of appropriate size. **D:** The two ends of the wire have been passed through and will be tightened to bring the canthus into its correct position. **E:** Postoperative result. A further small correction of the right medial canthus will be necessary.

MAXILLA

Cheek Irregularities

These are usually caused by plates or screws following bone resorption, especially in cases requiring augmentation of the cheek bones (e.g., Treacher Collins syndrome). The bone is resorbed and the screws become obvious and, of course, palpable.

Management

If a further craniofacial exposure is being performed, the area can be exposed and the screws removed under reasonable vision. If a coronal exposure is not contemplated, an alternate approach is through the upper buccal sulcus. The screw heads are exposed and reduced to the level of the bone graft with a contouring burr. This procedure requires considerable forceful retraction, and the patient should be warned of postoperative swelling, tenderness, and possible bruising.

Maxillary Hypoplasia

This is not a complication but it may become noticeable when the maxilla is advanced and the dental occlusion is ideal but paranasal hypoplasia is present. The patient may or may not be aware of the situation, which can also develop after trauma, in association with unilateral or bilateral clefts, or in Binder's syndrome.

Management

Maxillary hypoplasia can be corrected with bone grafts, but a donor site must be used (e.g., skull, lip), which is usually the last thing the patient wants. The simplest method is to make upper buccal sulcus incisions bilaterally, elevate the periosteum, and place hydroxyapatite granules into the subperiosteal defect. Because the granules come in a narrow-diameter tube, the entry incision in the buccal sulcus can be very small, and enough granules can be inserted to establish normal facial contours. The process is aided by extensive massage over the area. Closure of the buccal sulcus incisions should be accurate. The technique provides a stable augmentation, and complications are few. In more than 100 cases, aspiration of a seroma was required in one, and granules came through the wound in a few, but the problem resolved within a few days. The technique is really valuable for this particular condition. Hydroxyapatite granules can also be used to correct any maxillary bony asymmetries that are present and that can be reached from an upper buccal sulcus incision. The technique can be used in the mandible or any other area where augmentation is required.

Maxillary Relapse

After advancement of the maxilla in, for example, Crouzon or Apert syndrome, a slight relapse may develop.

Management

If maxillary relapse is spotted early, the teeth can be put back into intermaxillary fixation, which should be maintained for 1 month. In some cases, it will be necessary to administer general anesthesia to manipulate the maxilla into a satisfactory position. The interdental splint is inserted and intermaxillary fixation applied and maintained for 1 month. If a class III maloclusion becomes estblished, Lefort I advancement may be indicated.

OTHER PROBLEMS ARISING IN THE POSTOPERATIVE PERIOD

Continuing Cerebrospinal Fluid Leak

This problem usually presents as a clear or blood-stained fluid that does not clot and tests positive for glucose. Often, an inexperienced surgeon will suspect nasal secretions, which can be significant after these procedures, to be a cerebrospinal fluid leak.

Management

The patient should be sedated, laid flat, and given broad-spectrum antibiotics. The problem usually then resolves. Should the leak continue, it is necessary to perform an intracranial exploration, with repair of the dural defect responsible for the leak. The repair is performed with fascia lata, stored fascia, or more recently AlloDerm (LifeCell Corporation, The Woodlands, Texas).

Failure to Regain Consciousness

Management

If this occurs, the neurosurgeon should be consulted. A CT investigation is organized. The most likely cause is an intracranial bleed, which will be explored by the neurosurgeon. If no evidence of an intracranial lesion is found, brain edema may be the cause, and high doses of steroids are given intravenously. Close observation is continued, with CT performed as necessary.

In cases of respiratory compromise, a tracheostomy is performed.

Blindness

A sudden onset of blindness is difficult to diagnose. Changes in the pupil reaction may be sluggish or absent.

MANAGEMENT

Megadoses of steroids should be given and the CT findings examined. If no evidence of optic nerve compression is found, which would require a surgical solution, the megadose steroids are continued. These may or may not be successful, but little else can be done in this situation.

Needless to say, an ophthalmologic consultation should be obtained as soon as possible. If any mechanical compression of the optic nerve (e.g., a bone spicule) is present, an immediate craniotomy and release of the causative agent should be performed.

Meningitis

This is an extremely rare situation. Occasionally, signs of meningism are noted, but these resolve within a few days or less.

Management

When frank meningitis is diagnosed with signs of meningism (raised temperature, stiffness), CT and lumbar puncture are performed, and the fluid is sent for culture. In the meantime, an antibiotic with a suitable spectrum that is capable of reaching the meningeal area is prescribed. With diagnosis and early treatment, most patients do well.

Complications of Plates and Screws

The complications of plates and screws most commonly encountered are surface irregularities, loosening, and localized infection. Hardware invading the skull and ending up within the cranium, or becoming embedded in the dura or, worse still, the brain, has been described. The latter situation may be, at least in theory, associated with focal symptoms.

Many patients are aware of surface deformities following plate application but find this acceptable so long as they are asymptomatic or hidden. Pain can be a complaint and is difficult to explain; it is assumed to be a host reaction to the metal.

Loosening is extremely unusual. It occurs in children, in whom the bone is thin, or in persons with abnormal bone (e.g., after irradiation or when portions of fibrous dysplastic bone are used *de novo* or after autoclaving).

Surface irregularities are noted most frequently on the forehead, cheek bone, infraorbital rim, and nasal areas. These have decreased since the use of low-profile plates and screws, especially of the micro variety.

Invasion of the skull by plates and screws is certainly possible. Before they were used, wire was employed and could later be found in the dura. The questions are, Is this a frequent occurrence? Does it cause any problems? The author has rarely seen this problem despite having performed a very large number of craniofacial procedures for congenital deformities, trauma, and tumors during a period of 30 years, and certainly has never encountered symptoms of any kind.

Management

As stated earlier, if pain, contour problems, loosening, or infection is present, the hardware should be removed through a coronal or buccal sulcus approach. Occasionally, a transconjunctival approach through the lower fornix can be the simplest way to reach an inferior orbital rim screw or plate. Occasionally, a localized screw may be approached through a stab incision. In the case of infection, all granulation tissue should be removed and the area copiously irrigated; drainage should be considered if appropriate.

Occasionally, it may be wiser to contour a plate or screw, such as when removal would cause a defect that in turn would result in a contour irregularity. Contouring would be done only if the hardware was stable.

Because of contour concerns (e.g., placing plates on the frontal areas, particularly in young children), a new technique was adopted in this situation 20 years ago. In frontal osteotomies or in cases requiring barrel staving, the plates were applied on the *inner* surface of the skull. No complications of this technique have been reported, nor have any problems been noted in cases requiring reexploration for further reconstructions. Certainly, no plates have moved through the skull to present on the external surface!

All these problems have been obviated by the use of resorbable plates and screws. These are made with calcium polymers of polylactic and polyglycolic acids and are particularly useful in children. In addition, they do not interfere with magnetic resonance imaging or CT. This material retains its maximal strength for 3 to 4 months and is resorbed completely in 9 to 15 months. The polymers have different characteristics. Polylactic acid is resorbed slowly and can be found from 6 to 7 years after its placement. Polyglycolic acid, on the other hand, is rapidly resorbed, and at the end of a month after implantation, it has lost its strength.

Self-reinforced poly-L-lactide (SR-PLLA) plates and screws compare well with metal. The reinforcement is provided by sintering parallel polymeric fibers into the matrix of the polylactide material. This increases all the mechanical properties of the implant. Furthermore, it is possible to bend the plates without heating and to reuse a plate that is unsuitable in a particular case. For all these reasons, SR-PLLA plates and screws are our fixation system of choice. They have been used extensively in the skull, upper face, and maxilla of children and adults.

With the strength, convenience, and resorptive features of this material, the use of metal plates and screws, especially in children, is rarely indicated.

CONCLUSION

What has been learned during a long experience in craniofacial surgery is that effective measures can be taken to prevent the significant problems seen in the past. Ground rules have been established and applied in any procedure that extends beyond the anterior skull base and results in a nasopharyngeal–intracranial connection. The connection must be sealed, preferably with local vascularized tissue (e.g., galeal frontalis myofascial periosteal flap). Otherwise, the brain will not expand and dead space will result. All dural defects should be repaired directly if possible; otherwise, a fascial patch should be used rather than artificial material.

Undoubtedly, the most important requirement in craniofacial surgery is cooperation between surgeons in different specialties—neurosurgery, plastic surgery, maxillofacial surgery, and surgery of the ear, nose, and throat. The surgeons, in turn, must cooperate with the anesthesiologist. Without such cooperation and without a good surgical nursing team, these major cases can be hazardous. With experience, harmony, and good cooperation, the results are rewarding and complications are few.

REFERENCES

1. Jackson IT, Adham MN, Marsh WR. Use of the galeal frontalis myofascial flap in craniofacial surgery. *Plast Reconstr Surg* 1986;77:905–910.
2. Fisher J, Jackson IT. Microvascular surgery as an adjunct to craniomaxillofacial reconstruction. *Br J Plast Surg* 1989;42:146–154.
3. Jones NF, Schramm VL, Sekhar LN. Reconstruction of the cranial base following turnover resection. *Br J Plast Surg* 1987;40:155–162.
4. Jones NF, Sekhar LN, Schramm VL. Free rectus abdominis muscle flap in reconstruction of the middle and posterior cranial base. *Plast Reconstr Surg* 1986;78:471–479.
5. Jones NF. The contribution of microsurgical reconstruction to craniofacial surgery. *World J Surg* 1989;13:454–464.
6. Neligan PC, Mulholland S, Irish J, et al. Flap selection in cranial base reconstruction. *Plast Reconstr Surg* 1995;98:1159–1168.
7. Smith AW, Jackson IT, Yousefi J. The use of screw fixation of methyl methacrylate to reconstruct large craniofacial contour defects. *Eur J Plast Surg* 1999;99:17–21.
8. Costantino PD, Friedman CD, Jones K, et al. Hydroxyapatite cement I. Basic chemistry and histologic properties. *Arch Otolaryngol Head Neck Surg* 1991;117:379–384.
9. Friedman CD, Costantino PD, Jones K, et al. Hydroxyapatite cement II. Obliteration and reconstruction of the cat frontal sinus. *Arch Otolaryngol Head Neck Surg* 1991;117:385–389.
10. Jackson IT, Yavuzer R. Hydroxyapatite cement: an alternative for craniofacial skeletal contour refinements. *Br J Plast Surg* 2000;53:24–29.
11. Peltoniemi HH, Tualmo RM, Toivonen T, et al. Intraosseous plating: a new method for biodegradable osteofixation in craniofacial surgery. *J Craniofac Surg* 1998;9:247.
12. Bite U, Jackson IT, Forbes GS, et al. Orbital volume measurements in enophthalmos using three-dimensional CT imaging. *Plast Reconstr Surg* 1985;75:502–507.
13. Forbes G, Gehring DG, Gorman CA, et al. Volume measurements of normal orbital structures by computed tomographic analysis. *AJNR Am J Neuroradiol* 1985;6:419–424.
14. Schuknecht B, Carls F, Valavanis A, et al. CT assessment of orbital volume in late post-traumatic enophthalmos. *Neuroradiology* 1996;38:470–475.
15. Jackson IT. Resection of tumors involving the anterior and middle cranial fossa. In: Barclay TL, Kernahan DA. *Operative surgery—plastic surgery,* 4th ed. Boston: Butterworth-Heinemann, 1986:572–598.

Discussion

CRANIOFACIAL SURGERY

KENNETH E. SALYER

Craniofacial surgery has provided new methods for the reconstruction of deformities. The avoidance of complications depends on more than the expertise of the surgeon. It requires a dedicated, experienced team. When craniofacial surgery is attempted by persons without expertise, the results can be devastating. Ian Jackson's chapter outlines very nicely many of the possible complications associated with craniofacial surgery. As the subspecialty of plastic surgery has matured, a new spectrum of complications has evolved that the pediatric neurosurgeon, who is an integral part of the surgical team, may be called on to treat. Meningitis, ma-

K. E. Salyer: International Craniofacial Institute, Dallas, Texas

jor intracranial infections, cranial or facial bone loss, increased intracranial pressure, blindness, cerebrospinal fluid leak, major blood loss, and even death are all potential devastating sequelae of this challenging form of surgery.

Achieving excellence in craniofacial surgery often means pushing the envelope to its limits with the use of wide planes of dissection associated with extensive intracranial and facial exposure. Today, total cranial vault remodeling or complete separation of the facial and cranial skeleton by osteotomies is performed in one operation. Improved technology and surgical technique provided by a dedicated team and an experienced surgeon make all the difference in reducing complications and achieving excellent results.

In 1976, I performed my first four monobloc advancement operations of the face. Three of those four cases became infected. The infections developed because a dead space was created in the frontonasal region, a new problem not encountered before. Learning how to deal with dead space and how to prevent this complication is indicative of new problems created by craniofacial surgery. Advancement in this new subspecialty has taken us into unknown territory; assessment and further modification of techniques are often required, in addition to judgment about the timing of procedures. Thus, the prevention of potential complications depends on experience, judgment, and technical expertise.

An important factor often contributing to complications is inexperience of the surgeon. Today, craniofacial surgery is frequently performed by many surgeons. Fifty percent of the craniofacial patients presenting at our center today have undergone surgery elsewhere with unsatisfactory or unfavorable results. Many of these cases have been attempted by surgeons who should never have performed such surgery. The unfavorable results include poor contour, major irregularities, destruction of features, and major bone loss.

Tessier initially stated that craniofacial surgery should be performed only in centers that have extensive experience. Thirty years later, I would echo that plea. A minimum number of intracranial craniofacial cases should be performed per year to facilitate competence and, it is hoped, reduce complications. That number has been placed at about 20 intracranial cases per year. We know today that when craniofacial surgery is performed on a regular basis by a well-organized team, complications are minimal. However, complications occur even in the hands of the most experienced teams.

WOUND PROBLEMS

Secondary complications of scarring from the coronal incision have been markedly reduced since a zigzag incision or W-plasty has been used instead of a straight line. The placement of the scar is in the hair, and no hair is shaved. Many in the neurosurgical "fraternity" continue to shave heads in the belief that shaving prevents infection. In our center, we have shown that this is not the case; we do not shave the patient's head for any elective craniofacial or pediatric neurosurgical procedure. The old neurosurgical axiom or premise that the head must be entirely shaved is passé, so long as the hair is washed adequately preoperatively and an appropriate preparation is used. Shaving is not necessary; furthermore, not shaving the head spares the patient a significant amount of embarrassment as the hair grows out over a period of months.

Spreading of the scar can be a problem; I believe that placing deep sutures, such as Monocryl or Vicryl (Ethicon), in the galeal subcutaneous layer prevents spreading of the scar. Because the removal of sutures in children is disadvantageous, we tried using catgut in the dermal scalp. However, we found more scarring and areas of alopecia than when staples were used. Staples, in association with deeper sutures to prevent spreading, give us the best results with minimal scarring. I do not agree that postauricular extension of the incision is an ideal placement, as it does not allow full exposure of the face. A properly placed preauricular incision leaves minimal evidence of scarring and provides better access to the midface.

WOUND INFECTION

Any persistent swelling in and around the orbital region, either unilaterally, at the midline, or bilaterally, is an indication of a potential postoperative infection. In congenital cases requiring surgery on a nondiseased ethmoid, I have never seen an infection result from removal of the ethmoid sinus. Postoperative infection is most frequently evidenced in the frontal sinus and, very occasionally, the maxillary sinus following an osteotomy across the sinus. I agree that aspiration of the effusion and computed tomography (CT) usually reveal the cause. Persistent air found in the frontal region is a negative finding and suggestive of a connection with the nasal pharynx or an infectious process. The aspirate should be Gram's-stained and antibiotics initiated. One may, then, initiate a wait-and-see course, as outlined by Dr. Jackson. If the patient is not recovering on antibiotics and fluid continues to accumulate clinically, then exploration, which most likely will include intracranial exploration, is required. At the time of exploration for frontal bone infection, the decision must always be made regarding how much frontal bone has to be removed. All necrotic bone must be removed, but when the surgeon reaches an area that is vascularized, that portion can be preserved. Debridement is important, but not total debridement and total removal of all the frontal bone. We have frequently been able to salvage a significant amount of bone. A number of suction drains are inserted intraoperatively. During the postoperative period, continuous dilute Betadine, antibiotic solution, or saline solution is run through one catheter and suctioned through others. This continuous lavage, over a period of days, has resulted in improved wound healing and eliminated the need for total cranial bone removal. Taking the patient back to the operating room every 2 to 3 days to undergo repeated exploration and careful debridement is also a good technique to add to the use of drains for irrigation.

Dead Space in the Frontal Region

The primary cause of infection in the frontal area is the residual dead space resulting from frontal bone advancement. Dead space after frontal bone advancement is not a problem in infants and children up to 5 to 6 years of age because of rapid dura expansion. However, in the older child and adult, expansion does not occur as rapidly and the persistence of dead space contributes to the development of infection in the region of the frontal sinus. Dead space plus a nasopharyngeal connection will result in a frontal bone infection. Where there has been a persistent connection from the nose to the intracranial cavity, it must be sealed off and the dead space filled. Only in very rare occasions in children have we found it necessary to use a vascularized tissue flap. One can take the advanced bone, if necessary, where an infection is present and simply set the bone back onto the dura, removing the dead space and allowing healing and correction of the wound once the necrotic tissue has been removed. Skull-based surgery for cancer lends itself to this problem in the adult patient where it is frequently necessary to use a vascularized flap. Postoperatively, drains are not used in craniofacial surgery today as they are not necessary in the initial surgery. However, the use of drains in the postoperative period after an infection is present is important as a basic premise of wound care.

RESIDUAL INTRACRANIAL NASOPHARYNGEAL CONNECTION

One of the ways to prevent a residual intracranial nasopharyngeal connection is to use a galeal frontalis myofascial periosteal flap, as described, at the time of the procedure. We frequently use fibrin tissue adhesive to seal the anterior cranial base or floor, applying it over any potential areas of dural leak.

FRONTAL BONE IRREGULARITIES

I agree that irregularity of the skull is common after craniofacial procedures and that it is aesthetically significant in the frontal temporal regions and other areas where it shows on the face.

Management

The use of methylmethacrylate as a reconstruction material in craniofacial surgery, either primarily or secondarily, is not recommended. Neurosurgeons have used it successfully, and it is their method of choice; however, this has been in cases in which the cranial vault was sealed from the facial region. In numerous cases in craniofacial surgery, communication between the face and the cranium creates an increased risk for the development of infection. Long-term follow-up of the use of methylmethacrylate in craniofacial surgery has demonstrated cases in which removal of the implant was required. Methylmethacrylate should not be used in a growing child. If one is absolutely sure that the cranial region is isolated from the frontonasal region or the nose, performing primary or secondary surgery in an adult with the use of methylmethacrylate may be a satisfactory technique.

The Growing Child

No alloplastic materials should be used in the head or face of a growing child. The use of methylmethacrylate, hydroxyapatite, titanium plates and screws, or any other foreign body is strongly contraindicated. The cranial vault and facial bones undergo remodeling, and alloplastic material does not undergo the same remodeling and acts as a foreign body that can migrate or remain stationary while the rest of the craniofacial skeleton grows and remodels. As a result, plates and screws can penetrate the dura. Other materials may produce contour defects or deformity during growth and cause an unfavorable result. Having performed secondary surgery on a large number of children in whom alloplastic materials were utilized, I feel that this practice is contraindicated in children. However, after growth is complete, I believe these materials may be used by a surgeon with appropriate experience provided precautions are taken. More recently, in the growing child, BoneSource (Leibinger) and Norian CRS (Synthes) have been used. "Experimentally at 1 year new bone replaces 77% of the hydroxyapatite cement" (1). It has been my clinical experience with these children that cement is not replaced with bone. Little or no evidence has been found in the patients I have seen or followed that cement is replaced by bone. In an evaluation of Norian CRS in the last year, we have used it in 16 cases with four infections. The material may be tolerated for a few months, then subsequently an area of breakdown develops that may lead to infection. We can no longer recommend the use of this material in craniofacial surgery. Irregularities of the craniofacial skeleton in children should be reconstructed with autogenous tissue or, if this is not available, demineralized bone, which is osteoinductive (Fig. 15D-1).

CRANIAL BONE DEFECTS: DEMINERALIZED BONE

Many children presenting as secondary cases have major cranial defects. Securing autogenous bone to reconstruct these defects is a major problem. When no cranial bone remains

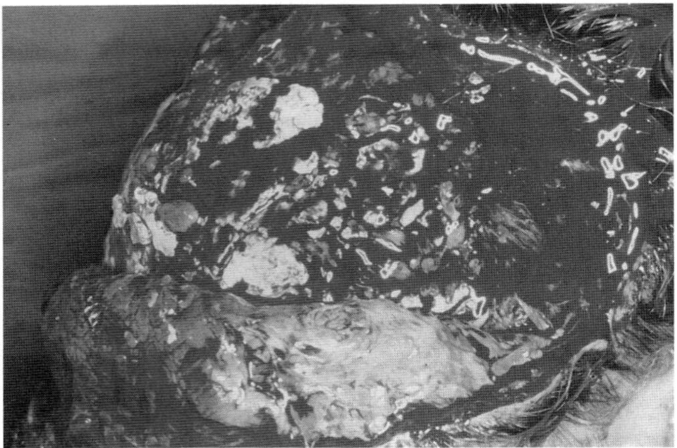

FIGURE 15D-1. Intraoperative view using a coronal incision showing complications of hydroxyapatite paste. After Norian CRS (Synthes Maxillofacial) was implanted in this 17-year-old patient for contour irregularities, areas of breakdown developed with infection and tissue reaction. Exploration was required to remove the hydroxyapatite paste.

to be harvested, our first choice is osteoinductive demineralized bone. The rib and iliac crest are harvested for special cases. We have used demineralized bone for the past 10 years, with an experience of more than 1,600 separate implants in various forms (2–4). The use of demineralized bone is beneficial in patients requiring reconstruction of the cranial vault, including children with an absent frontal bone as a consequence of previous infection or a loss of major sections of bone in the cranial vault. Our infection rate with the use of demineralized bone is 2.3%. Our overall infection rate has been 1.9% in more than 5,000 skeletal craniomaxillofacial cases. We frequently save and use the bone dust to cover all the burr holes. When enough bone dust is not available, demineralized bone paste is added. We have had excellent long-term results with this approach. Resorption, which has been a major complaint with demineralized bone, has not been a problem when material supplied by the Pacific Coast Tissue Bank of Los Angeles was used. Again, we would not use hydroxyapatite granules to cover defects in children. I have never used hydroxyapatite granules for small craniofacial defects. Marchac (5), who has had extensive experience in the use of hydroxyapatite granules, found that in the long term it produces irregularities and has therefore stopped using this material (5).

TEMPORAL DEFORMITIES

The main reason for temporal hollowing after use of the coronal approach in the craniofacial region is devascularization, with resulting atrophy of the temporalis muscle. I agree that it is important to reposition the muscle; however, even when it has been repositioned carefully, temporal hollowing may occur. The temporalis muscle should be elevated only when necessary and as little as necessary for any given procedure. For example, exposure of the entire lateral orbit and zygoma and face can be obtained while the temporalis muscle is left intact. For the Le Fort III operation or major hypertelorism correction, it is necessary to release the temporal, orbital, and frontal attachments of the temporalis muscle to gain exposure to perform the procedure. It is in these cases that muscle atrophy may occur.

In the secondary correction, an implant below the temporalis muscle works well if it is of the correct shape. I prefer demineralized bone, although I have used blocks of hydroxyapatite in the past. I find that demineralized bone can be contoured much more easily than hydroxyapatite or methylmethacrylate; it is also osteoinductive and corrects this deformity very nicely. I do agree that cranial bone grafts placed in this position tend to be resorbed. The key to temporalis atrophy is prevention by limiting the initial dissection when possible.

ORBITAL AND EYE COMPLICATIONS: MALPOSITION OF THE ORBIT OR PORTIONS THEREOF

The single most frequent secondary posttraumatic deformity seen at the International Craniofacial Institute is incorrect positioning of the orbital zygomatic fracture. Dr. Jackson's description is entirely appropriate, and I agree with it.

Management

Three-dimensional CT is very useful in all craniofacial deformities. A newer technique that is useful in planning and improving results is a three-dimensional stereolithographic model that is accurate to within 1 mm. The three-dimensional model or template is sterilized and used in the operating room to design the reconstruction with greater accuracy. It offers several advantages.

Preoperative and intraoperative evaluation and planning of the reconstructive procedure, especially in complex craniofacial malformations, are greatly facilitated with this tactile model. An accurate surgical simulation can be achieved by cutting, drilling, and sawing the model, which saves operative time and eliminates any unforeseen "surprises" during actual performance of the reconstruction. The model acts as an effective tool and a visual aid in preparing the patient for surgery and also serves as a reference for case discussions with colleagues and related specialists. Implant customization and prior bending of fixation devices have been particularly easy with the use of these models in a variety of situations, such as augmentations, reconstructions, and especially distraction osteogenesis. The model is sterilized and used in the operative field.

The Analyze system referred to by the author is a specialized unit developed at the Mayo Clinic. I do not believe it is currently used by many centers except those introduced to it at the Mayo Clinic. I would think that if the system had merits, others would use it. I have not found any computer interactive system to date that has offered any long-term advantage in improving results or simplifying surgery. In the future, I am sure, it will be a useful three-dimensional computer model for perioperative simulation and surgical planning. We have evaluated a number of computer programs for simulated surgery and not found any that are useful to date. The deformity is three-dimensional, and the computer does not indicate the exact movement and volume that are necessary to correct the deformity.

In this deformity, if the affected eye is positioned like the opposite, normal eye, the enophthalmos will likely relapse or recur because of scar contracture. Soft tissue scarring in addition to bone deformity contributes to the problem. This is one of the most difficult deformities to correct, particularly the diplopia in both the primary and secondary fields of vision. Many patients must undergo repeated procedures in expert hands for optimal results to be achieved. Again, in secondary correction of these cases, we use osteotomies with overcorrection of the enophthalmos and release of the contracted scarred periorbital tissue. We also decrease the orbital volume in comparison with the normal side. I prefer demineralized bone in the posterior orbit to advance the eye and overcorrect it. The grafts must be placed behind the equator of the eye. It is necessary to reconstruct all four orbital walls and rims correctly if they are involved. Frequently, a C-shaped osteotomy of the superior, lateral, and inferior orbital rims and portion of the adjacent wall is adequate.

LATERAL CANTHAL DISPLACEMENT

Frequently, not only is the canthus in the wrong position, but the bony lateral orbit is abnormal. It is very difficult to achieve a perfect aesthetic contour in a congenital or acquired deformity with marked displacement and abnormal shape. This may contribute to the abnormal displacement of the lateral canthus. The technique described here is the one I use; however, it is very important in cases with severely contracted soft tissue to overcorrect the lateral canthus because the pull of the soft tissues will be tremendous. The periosteal attachment along the lower orbital rim must be totally released and mobilized to get the lateral canthus to stay in its proper position postoperatively and prevent the sclera from showing. It may even be necessary to perform a subperiosteal dissection and lift over the entire maxilla and zygoma. Also, it is important to place the canthus within the bony orbit and make certain that the bony orbit is of the right size and shape and in the right position. This requires a three-dimensional reconstruction, which is not often easy to achieve with or without an intraoperative model in hand.

MEDIAL CANTHAL DISPLACEMENT

In addition to postsurgical medial canthal displacement, a secondary epicanthal fold is frequently seen following the correction of posttraumatic or congenital hypertelorism or other orbital asymmetries. The displacement of the medial canthus and epicanthal fold correction may or may not be a result of underlying bony abnormality; they may also be a consequence of soft tissue excess in this region that is inadequately accounted for following bony correction.

Management

The associated epiphora that may occur with a damaged nasal lacrimal drainage system can be prevented at the time of primary hypertelorism correction by totally unroofing the nasolacrimal system to prevent subsequent bony or surgical injury with bone translocation. If CT shows that the abnormality is caused only by ligament displacement, then this is corrected with an appropriate soft tissue procedure. If it is caused by bony abnormality, then the bony interorbital distance must be appropriately corrected and any obstructing bone removed. Frequently in hypertelorism correction, if the medial inferior orbital rim has been moved medially and left intact, the translocation of the medial canthal tendon and orbit is obstructed. A portion of this must be removed or contoured out to allow proper positioning of the medial canthal tendon. The incision for access to the medial canthus described by del Fuente (6), a form of Z-plasty that converts and allows proper correction of the epicanthal fold with minimal medial canthal scarring, is excellent. The old approach of Mustardé of correcting the epicanthal fold causes considerable medial canthal scarring. Also, following hypertelorism correction, a frequent cause for persistent deformity is the surgeon's failure to reduce the distance between the supraorbital medial rims in the glabellar region, which remains too wide. When this occurs, an hourglass deformity with an abnormally shaped orbit is seen, in which the interorbital distance remains too wide at the upper portion of the orbit. Proper removal of the bony orbit is important, in addition to reshaping, translocation, and positioning of the medial canthus, following correction of a congenital deformity. Many different techniques can be used for transnasal wiring or correction of the medial canthal positioning. Becoming adept at one that consistently works is important. Many surgeons never master a technique that gives consistently good medial canthal contour and positioning.

MAXILLARY HYPOPLASIA

In the deformed maxilla, if the planning of the new position of the maxilla is based on the dental occlusal level, then paranasal or malar deficiency may persist. Correction of the deformity should produce a balanced projection of the entire skeletal face. How this is achieved is the choice of the surgeon. Experience, planning, and careful differential adjustment of the skeletal and soft tissue facial structures are required. Artistic reconstruction of the skeletal segments is important in craniofacial deformity correction. A restoration of the skeletal volume, projection and aesthetic contour, balance and harmony, and attractiveness of the face can be achieved.

Management

Correcting the paranasal and malar deficiency, with or without maxillary advancement, has been most easily accomplished with the use of demineralized bone when cranial bone is not readily available or the patient wants off-the-shelf material to be used rather than a donor site. Demineralized bone is readily accepted by the patient, is osteoinductive, and has given a consistently good result. Hydroxyapatite granules may migrate or produce irregularities. Hydroxyapatite is not a good choice for contour reconstruction in any area in which the underlying irregularity may be seen.

MAXILLARY RELAPSE

After advancement of the maxilla in cases of major congenital craniofacial deformity, such as Crouzon or Apert syndrome or cleft cases, relapse may occur.

Management

We have treated this problem mostly with the use of a face mask, such as that developed by Delaire (7), during the postoperative period to eliminate the need for intermaxillary fixation. Intermaxillary fixation is best applied at the time of surgery. It eliminates edema in the temporomandibular joint and other tissues, which can alter the occlusion. Another technique to prevent relapse in the Le Fort III procedure is to apply an internal rigid fixation plate from the base of the skull around to the front of the maxilla. That, combined with an occlusal wafer and postoperative elastics and/or face mask, prevents and resolves relapse in most patients.

DISTRACTION

The other advancement in craniofacial surgery that has improved results in the correction of major deformities and prevents relapse is distraction osteogenesis (8,9). It not only prevents relapse of the maxilla but can eliminate dead space in the frontal cranial region with the accompanying risk for infection. The Le Fort III or monobloc osteotomy is performed and then gradually distracted over time to eliminate the dead space. To date, no internal midface distraction device is available that allows good, three-dimensional positioning of the maxilla. This will be accomplished in the future. In the interim, it is necessary to use external devices (10). Distraction also allows soft tissue to expand and prevents additional relapse. This is a new and exciting chapter in the field of craniofacial surgery.

OTHER PROBLEMS ARISING IN THE POSTOPERATIVE PERIOD

Continuing Cerebrospinal Fluid Leak

Occasionally, patients who have undergone craniofacial surgery present with a continuous cerebrospinal fluid leak. Our incidence to date, with very careful dissection and the use of multiple techniques, is less than 1% in a large series of patients. This low incidence can be attributed to the pediatric neurosurgeons, who perform meticulous dural closures and prevent tears.

Management

Any patient with a cerebrospinal fluid leak is admitted to the hospital and may require placement of a spinal drain to lower the intracranial pressure. Decreasing the pressure frequently allows the dura to seal. In the early 1970s, we used spinal fluid drainage routinely postoperatively but found it unnecessary. It is still a very good technique for decompressing potential or actual cerebrospinal fluid leaks. If the leak persists, then intracranial exploration is important. Preoperative radionuclide CT can help identify the possible site of a leak. Again, prevention at the time of surgery is key. In high-risk defects, we have found fibrin tissue adhesive useful. Fibrin tissue sealant has proved very effective when water-tight closure is difficult to achieve. We have no experience with fascia lata or AlloDerm. Our team uses adjacent temporal fascia, which works well when a graft is needed.

Tracheostomy

Management

We would not perform a tracheostomy early on if the patient were slow to awaken, as described by Dr. Jackson. Observation with CT is always of benefit for these patients. Tracheostomy is rarely, if ever, performed on craniofacial patients today at our center. In the 1970s and early 1980s, tracheostomy was almost a routine procedure. Advances in anesthesia, the use of hypotensive anesthesia, good airway control, and good postoperative pediatric intensive care have allowed us to eliminate tracheostomy. The temporary placement of an endotracheal tube provides an efficient, safe method for interim care until the patient regains consciousness and control.

Blindness

Blindness has been reported in the literature in association with craniofacial surgery. This is a rare but ever-present concern when this type of surgery is performed. The surgeon must continuously be aware of the optic nerve and globe while performing osteotomies in and around the orbit and in the intracranial region.

Management

Decreased vision or sudden blindness is an emergency, and CT should be performed immediately. Compression of the optic nerve, an intraorbital hematoma, or compression of the eye by a bony fragment dictates immediate exploration. Large doses of steroids are indicated to decrease swelling.

Meningitis

This is an extremely rare situation in controlled craniofacial surgery. However, it may occur, and if so, appropriate diagnosis and treatment are mandatory.

Management

All craniofacial cases are treated perioperatively with broad-spectrum antibiotics. That, plus the prevention of postoperative cerebrospinal fluid leaks by meticulous intraoperative closure of all holes, prevents leakage and lowers the incidence of meningitis. If signs and symptoms of meningitis develop, then a spinal fluid tap, cultures, and appropriate treatment are indicated.

Complications of Plates And Screws

In the growing child, the craniofacial skeleton is remodeling and ever changing, laying down new bone during growth. As this occurs, any type of foreign body, whether plates and screws or other material, is basically translocated or moves with new bone apposition. Remodeling of bone around the nonbiologic material results in translocation. At the International Craniofacial Institute, we have observed plates and screws on or in the dura. In a large series of cases recently assayed by Persing (11), to his knowledge, no case with significant symptoms or with perforation of the dura as a result of hardware translocation has been reported. Resorbable plates and screws offer an improvement. The problem with resorbable plates and screws is that, to date, their resorption rate of 6 to 18 months is too long. I have observed persistence of this material 6 to 12 months later. Regarding the new "technique" of 20 years ago in which the plates are placed on the inside of the frontal bone or bandeau, I recently returned to a case in which I had performed the surgery and placed the resorbable plate on the inside of the frontal bone. Six months later, indentations from the screw heads and the plates were evident on the dura. Placing plates and screws on the internal surface of the frontal bone is potentially hazardous.

CONCLUSION

Major advances have been made in craniofacial surgery during the last 30 years. The key to reducing complications is to prevent them. The key to preventing complications is to have surgery performed by experienced surgeons and dedicated multidisciplinary, coordinated teams. Better results can be obtained in any field of surgery when the surgery is performed on a regular basis. Craniofacial surgery is complex and associated with major potential hazards and complications. I am aware of complications, including death, that have occurred during surgery performed by both inexperienced and experienced surgeons. Complications can occur with any surgeon but can be reduced or nearly eliminated by an experienced, dedicated team and surgeon. At our center in the past 13 years, we have performed more than 5,000 craniofacial operations, with two deaths, two known cases of meningitis, a 1.9% infection rate, and a less than 1% incidence of dural leaks. The average hospital stay for intracranial procedures has been 4.2 days. These results can be found only in dedicated centers, and craniofacial surgery, which is complex, should be performed only in such centers.

REFERENCES

1. Costantino PD, Friedman CD, Jones K, et al. Experimental hydroxyapatite cement cranioplasty. *Plast Reconstr Surg* 1992;90: 174–185.
2. Salyer KE, Gendler E, Squier C. Long-term outcome of extensive skull reconstruction using demineralized perforated bone in Siamese twins joined at the skull vertex. *Plast Reconstr Surg* 1997;99:1721–1726.
3. Salyer KE, Gendler E, Menendez JL, et al: Demineralized perforated bone implants in craniofacial surgery. *J Craniofac Surg* 1992;3:55–62.
4. Salyer KE, Bardach J, Squier C, et al. Cranioplasty in the growing canine skull using demineralized perforated bone. *Plast Reconstr Surg* 1995;96:770–779.
5. Marchac D. Personal communication, 1997.
6. Del Fuente AC. Surgical treatment of the epicanthal fold. *Plast Reconstr Surg* 1984;73:566–570.
7. Delaire J. Confection du masque orthopédique. *Rev Stomatol* 1971;72:579–584.
8. McCarthy JG, Schreiber J, Karp N, et al. Lengthening the human mandible by gradual distraction. *Plast Reconstr Surg* 1992;89:1–8.
9. Corcoran J, Hubli EH, Salyer KE. Distraction osteogenesis of costochondral neomandibles: a clinical experience. *Plast Reconstr Surg* 1997;100:311–315.
10. Polley JW, Figueroa AA. Management of severe maxillary deficiency in childhood and adolescence through distraction osteogenesis with an external, adjustable, rigid distraction device. *J Craniofac Surg* 1997;8:181–185.
11. Persing J. Personal communication, 1998.

16

DISTRACTION OSTEOGENESIS

LARRY H. HOLLIER
JOSEPH G. McCARTHY

The technique of distraction osteogenesis was popularized by Ilizarov, a Russian surgeon who began his practice during the years after World War II in Siberia, where he encountered a large population of veterans with lower extremity malunions and nonunions. In the design of his external fixator, the primary goal was to provide sufficient stability to allow the fractures to heal. The discovery that bone was generated in the gap as a result of slow distraction of the device was serendipitous, but recognition of the therapeutic potential led Ilizarov to make this the focus of his life's work.

Distraction was first applied to the craniofacial skeleton by Snyder, who resected a portion of the dog mandible, compressed the bone ends, and distracted the resected site (1). The first clinical cases were performed by McCarthy et al. (2) in a series of children with congenital mandibular deficiencies. Since their report in 1990, distraction osteogenesis has had a profound effect on the field of craniofacial surgery. It has been used on virtually every anatomic component of the craniofacial complex, including the mandible, condyle, zygoma, maxilla, midface, and cranial vault (3–8).

One of the most attractive aspects of distraction osteogenesis as a surgical technique is its relative simplicity and low morbidity rate. Traditional techniques of craniofacial surgery have typically required complex osteotomies, autogenous bone grafts, and rigid internal fixation to achieve skeletal repositioning. Because of the prolonged operative time and the extensive surgical exposure required, blood transfusions are not uncommon. Distraction techniques have, however, simplified surgical treatment. The process of distraction creates bone at the site of the osteotomy that is histologically indistinguishable from the surrounding bone (9). No supplemental bone grafts are necessary (10). Furthermore, because distraction does not require intraoperative repositioning and internal stabilization of the skeletal elements, it generally takes less time than conventional operations and does not require transfusions (10). The length of hospitalization has also been significantly reduced.

Another advantage of distraction has been the relative infrequency of significant skeletal relapse (10). With standard craniofacial techniques, the bone segments are quickly advanced intraoperatively against a restrictive soft tissue envelope. The recoil of the overlying soft tissues can lead to relapse of the surgically positioned bone. Relapse has become less frequent with the advent of rigid internal fixation but is occasionally still problematic, particularly in orthognathic procedures, in which relapse of even a few millimeters can lead to occlusal problems (11). With distraction, the overlying soft tissues, including skin, fat, and muscle, are *gradually* lengthened, a situation analogous to that of tissue expansion. In essence, a new soft tissue envelope is created, and the tendency to relapse is reduced (12).

Despite these advantages, distraction osteogenesis, like any surgical procedure, is not entirely free of complications. This is particularly true of distraction of the endochondral bones of the lower extremity, in which the overall rate of complications has been relatively high in most series (13), especially when minor infections associated with the pin sites of the external fixators are included. In craniofacial distraction, however, the reported complication rates have been much lower (10,12,14). One possible explanation is the increased vascularity of the head and neck region relative to the extremities. The dimensions of the craniofacial bones are smaller. Additionally, the amount of distraction necessary in cases involving an extremity is generally greater, and a longer treatment time is required (15). This alone would be expected to increase the associated complications. However, a distinct set of complications remains associated with craniofacial distraction, of which the surgeon must be aware.

NERVE INJURY

In distraction of the middle and upper craniofacial skeleton, the risk to nerves is really only that associated with the standard incisions and exposure techniques utilized in craniofacial surgery. The nerve at greatest risk is the frontal branch of the facial nerve, particularly during reflection of the coronal flap for exposure of the zygomatic arch and midface. To prevent damage to the nerve as much as possible, one must incise the superficial layer of the deep temporal fascia at the level of the supraorbital rim and continue the dissection on the surface of the temporal fat pad (16). The technique of

L. H. Hollier and J. G. McCarthy: Institute of Reconstructive Plastic Surgery, New York University Medical Center, New York, New York

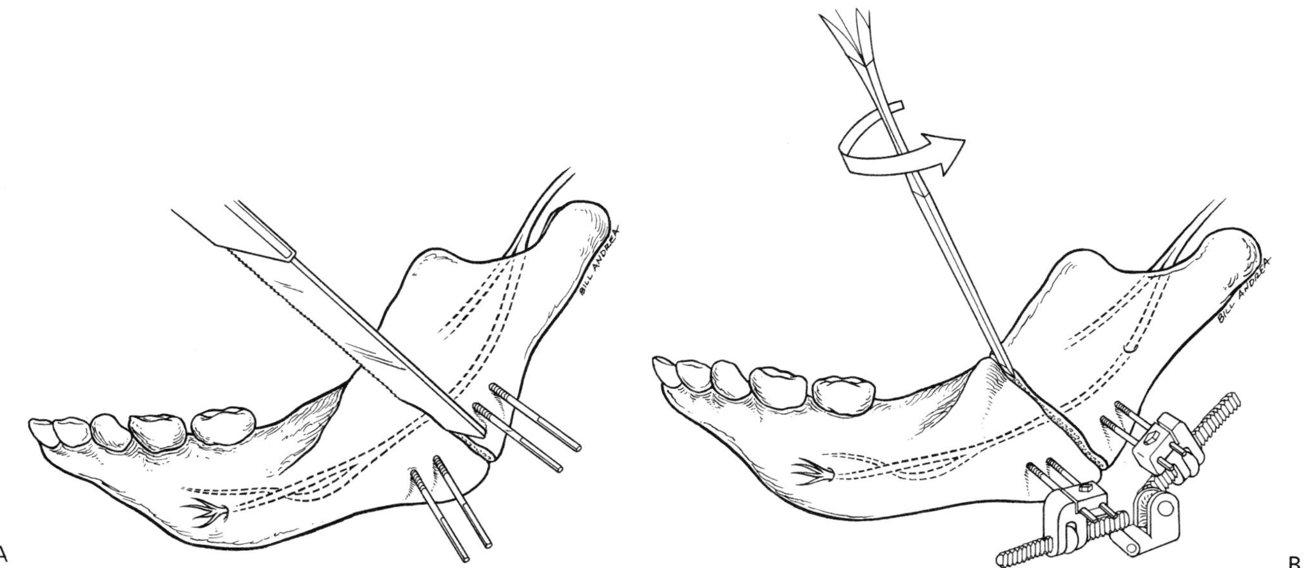

FIGURE 16-1. A: To preserve the integrity of the inferior alveolar nerve, the inferior border and buccal cortex of the mandible should be sectioned with a reciprocating saw. **B:** Next, the lingual cortex is disrupted by inserting an osteotome and twisting. In this way, the osteotomy is completed and the nerve is not subjected to any risk.

distraction thus adds no additional risk of injury to this nerve.

In mandibular distraction, two nerves may potentially be damaged—the inferior alveolar and the facial nerves. The inferior alveolar nerve is at greatest risk and can be injured in several ways. The first is at the site of the mandibular osteotomy. A linear osteotomy, which is not used in orthognathic surgical cases, is used in mandibular distraction, most frequently in the region of the angle. To prevent damage to the nerve, the osteotomy is usually left incomplete; initially, a corticotomy of the buccal cortex and the superior and inferior mandibular borders is performed. To complete the osteotomy, an osteotome is inserted into the site of the buccal corticotomy and rotated to disrupt the lingual cortex (10) (Fig. 16-1). To ensure a complete osteotomy, one must visualize complete separation of the segments with this maneuver. Molina and Ortiz Monasterio (14) have advocated leaving the lingual cortex intact. This technical modification derives from their effort to ensure preservation of the inferior alveolar nerve. With this technique, once distraction is initiated, the lingual cortex is fractured by the force of the distraction device, and the process then proceeds as though a complete osteotomy has been performed. The importance of preserving the lingual cortex and continuity of the medullary bone in mandibular distraction has never been demonstrated.

With the use of either of the above techniques no cases of permanent inferior alveolar nerve injury have been reported, but formal two-point discrimination studies have not been performed. Even transient numbness of the lip has been only rarely reported (17). It should be remembered that in the condition most frequently treated by mandibular distraction, craniofacial microsomia, the nerve may be absent or, if present, may not be normally positioned within the substance of the mandible. In these situations, it would not be placed at risk by the osteotomy. This may account, in part, for the low reported incidence of nerve injury. However, because of the straightforward nature of the osteotomy, the nerve is undoubtedly placed at less risk than when the sagittal split technique is used (18).

Another theoretical mechanism by which the inferior alveolar nerve can be damaged is the distraction process itself. With the initiation of distraction, the nerve is obviously lengthened along with the bone and overlying soft tissues. Excessive stretch can injure nerves, as has been reported in distraction of the extremity (13,19). In one study, electrodiagnostic evidence of deep peroneal nerve injury was found in six of six patients studied after tibial distraction (19). After mandibular distraction, examination of the inferior alveolar nerve in animal studies has demonstrated histologic changes consisting of axonal damage and demyelination (20,21). However, nerve function, as assessed by jaw jerk voltages, was normal in all animals in which it was tested (20). Clinically, this has not been shown to be a problem in mandibular distraction. Only transient numbness in the distribution of the inferior alveolar nerve has been reported (17). No permanent injuries have been reported.

The facial nerve branches may also be at risk in mandibular distraction procedures, particularly those in which an external incision is utilized (22). This applies to all the standard external or percutaneous approaches, but because the mandibular osteotomy is most frequently performed in the region of the angle, a Risdon (submandibular) incision is most commonly used. This incision places the marginal mandibular branch within the field of dissection. Care must be taken to avoid this type of nerve injury as the mandible is exposed. One method of doing this is to identify the facial vessels overlying the mandibular border after the platysma is incised (16). The vessels are ligated inferiorly, divided, and rotated cephalad. As the marginal branch crosses these vessels superficially, the latter maneuver should elevate the nerve superiorly, away from the field of dissection.

Even without an external incision, the facial nerve branches may still be damaged by the external device used for the distraction. The pins of the distractors are placed percutaneously after a 2- to 3-mm incision has been made in the skin, and small scissors are used to spread the soft tissues down to the level of the mandible (10). The pins and distractor are positioned, and the mandibular osteotomy is made through an intraoral incision. With the use of this technique, the branches of the facial nerve can be avoided. However, once distraction is begun, separation of the pins may place traction on the nerve, which results in facial muscle weakness or paralysis. The marginal branch is most likely to be at risk when the distractor is placed in the most common orientation, with an oblique vector in the region of the angle of the mandible. As the vector is oriented in a more vertical direction, traction is more likely to be placed on the branches of the facial nerve that run cephalad—the buccal, zygomatic, and even frontal branches. Any paresis resulting from this mechanism should be temporary, resolving after deactivation of the distraction device.

INFECTION

Infections secondary to craniofacial distraction procedures are uncommon. However, in any discussion of this subject, a distinction should be made between superficial and deep infections. An infection resulting from a distraction procedure that required reoperation and drainage has been reported only once in the literature (23). Serious infections have generally not been a problem with craniofacial distraction. The reason for this is likely related to the blood flow in the region of distraction. It has been shown experimentally that blood flow at the distraction site peaks at seven times the level before distraction, and an almost 300% increase is noted throughout the period of bone remodeling (24). This increase would certainly be expected to improve the resistance of the operative site to infection.

It should also be noted that, in comparison with standard craniofacial procedures, in which bone grafts and internal fixation hardware are used, distraction procedures leave no indwelling foreign body to act as a potential nidus for infection. Although during the distraction either an internal device or pins in the bone affix an external distractor, at the conclusion of the consolidation phase of distraction, the only addition to the distraction site should be bone that is essentially indistinguishable from the surrounding, unoperated bone (9).

In the report of Molina and Ortiz Monasterio (14) of 106 patients undergoing mandibular distraction with an external device, no serious infections occurred. Three cases of inflammation around pin sites were controlled with oral antibiotics. Smaller series of craniofacial distraction report somewhat higher rates of pin tract inflammation, but again without involvement of the deep soft tissues or bone (10,17,25).

It is debatable whether local inflammation around the pin sites of a distraction device should even be considered a complication. One might argue that this is to be expected when a foreign body is left protruding from the skin for a period of 3 months or longer. Indeed, in lower extremity distraction, the rate of pin site inflammation is even higher than in craniofacial cases (13,24); in one series, 95% of 100 cases experienced this problem, but without deeper bony involvement (24).

In the event of a pin site infection, patients should be placed on oral antibiotics to cover *Staphylococcus* organisms (usually a first-generation cephalosporin). The device should be examined to ensure its stability within the bone. It is also advisable to obtain radiographs to examine the pin–bone interface. Any extension of the infection to this level may manifest as osteolysis around the pin, a significant finding that mandates removal of the involved pins. Ideally, the patient should be returned to the operating room and another set of pins placed distal to the involved pin site. Another device should be adjusted, then placed for stabilization before removal of the first device and the infected pins. In follow-up, radiographs should be obtained periodically to check for resolution of the bone involvement.

SCARRING

Scarring resulting from craniofacial distraction procedures has been a primary criticism since the introduction of the technique for the treatment of mandibular deformities. When external distraction hardware is used, with either a cutaneous or an intraoral incision, pins must be placed into the bone transcutaneously. With subsequent distraction, a short scar is created at each pin site along the vector of the distraction. Some have argued that this scar is problematic in the majority of cases (26). However, the rates of scar revision in series of mandibular distraction have been low (none to 3%) (2,14,17), and it has been our experience that the majority of parents and patients are not displeased by the scar (Fig. 16-2). Two technical modifications have been suggested in an effort to minimize the scar that is produced (14,22). The first is to place the scar as low as possible by elevating the skin from below the mandibular border cephalad before the pins are placed (Fig. 16-3A). In this way, the

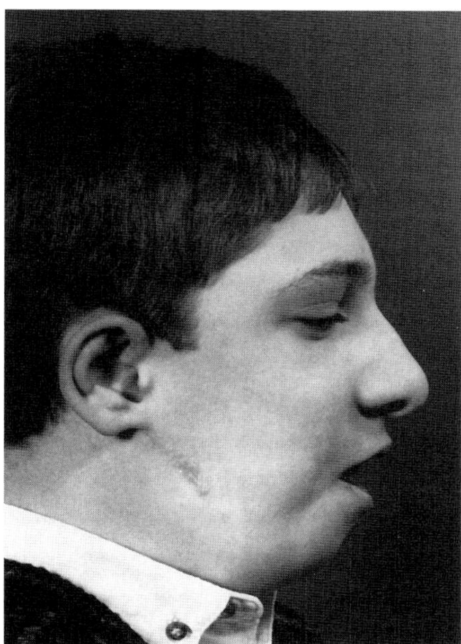

FIGURE 16-2. Mature but poorly placed facial scar resulting from bilateral mandibular distraction.

scar is moved from the face to the neck, where it is less noticeable. Additionally, after placement of the first set of pins, it is helpful to pinch the skin up against them before the second set of pins is placed (Fig. 16-3B). This results in an excess of tissue between the pins that are to be distracted apart. Consequently, migration of the pins through the skin is reduced, with a resulting shorter scar.

The issue of scarring has been the primary impetus behind the development of internal distraction hardware. Although the scar is often very acceptable, no scar is better than even a "good" scar. Mandibular distraction devices have been developed that allow for placement and activation through an intraoral route (26–28). Many devices for midface distraction are also internal, placed through a coronal incision and activated via a percutaneous screw (3,25,29). The drawback of the mandibular devices is the limited amount of bone available. In cases of extreme hypoplasia, placement and adequate stabilization of the device in the proper orientation become extremely difficult or even impossible. External devices have the advantage of requiring minimal bone stock (approximately 20 mm for mandibular distraction) and, as such, are applicable in even the most severe cases.

PREMATURE CONSOLIDATION AND FIBROUS UNION

Premature consolidation and fibrous union are uncommon complications. Consolidation of the regenerate during the process of distraction prevents further lengthening. The only mechanism by which this can be corrected is a reoperation with a secondary osteotomy and liberation of the frag-

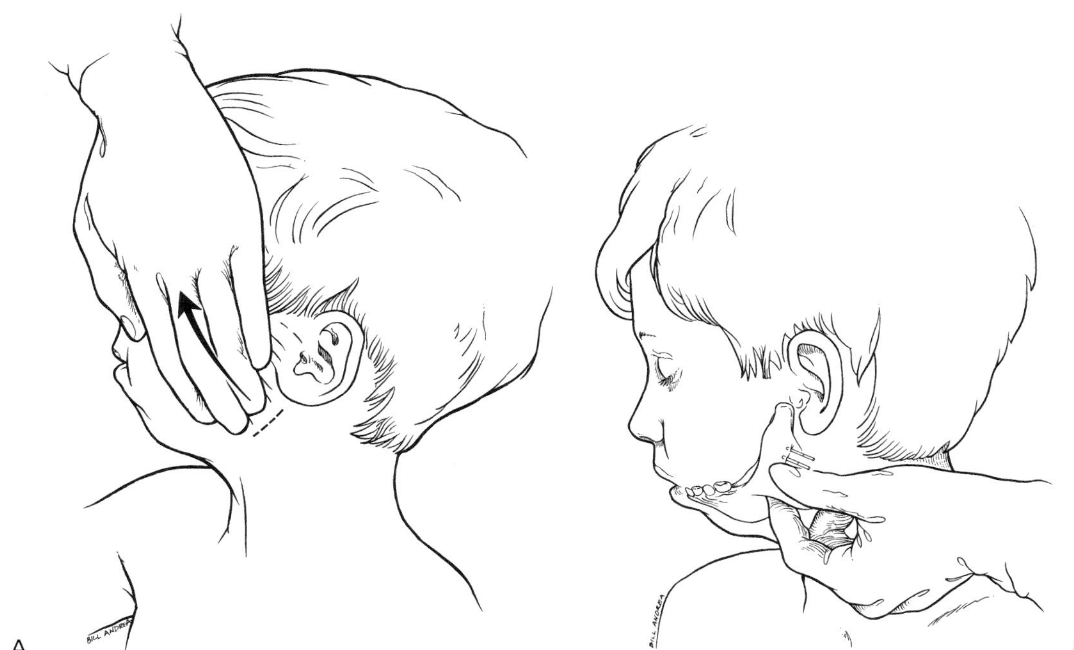

FIGURE 16-3. Technical modifications to reduce the scar resulting from mandibular distraction. **A:** The cheek skin should be elevated from below the inferior border of the mandible before the percutaneous pins are placed. This allows the scar to fall below the mandible on the neck after the pins are removed. **B:** Before the second set of pins is placed, the skin should be pinched to create an excess between the two pin sites. Consequently, the resultant scars will not be as long.

ments. If the bone segments are in an acceptable position, it should be possible to resume distraction postoperatively and take advantage of the regenerate already formed.

The main cause of premature consolidation is distraction at a rate that is too slow to maintain the central, nonossified portion of the regenerate. As has been described by Karp and associates (21), the distraction zone can be divided into four areas. A central fibrous zone consists of organized collagen. Adjacent to this on either side are three zones in various stages of bone formation. Continued distraction depends on maintenance of the fibrous central zone. Generally, the bone ends are moved apart 1 mm/24 h. Ilizarov determined this rate as optimal after extensive experimental and clinical experience (30). In most cases of endochondral and membranous bone distraction, this rate seems to be ideal and only rarely leads to consolidation before the cessation of distraction (25,31). When it does, several explanations are possible. It is possible that the device movement is not being fully transferred to the bone, so that distraction occurs at a rate of less than 1 mm/d. This situation may result from a technical error in the placement of the device or from failure of the device itself. In the case of external devices, we have found that placing the device on the pins farther from the bone interface results in a less efficient transfer of the distraction forces to the bone (i.e., a rate of distraction that is slower than intended) (unpublished data). One should always place external distractors as close as possible to the skin without actually impinging on it. This practice should ensure the maximum possible efficiency of transfer of distraction forces.

Another potential cause of premature consolidation is distraction along secondary vectors. Recently developed distraction devices allow movement of the bone ends in three planes (32); in other words, in addition to distracting bone in an anteroposterior direction, one can also distract along the vertical and horizontal axes. In cases of mandibular distraction, this has been shown to help in the closure of anterior open bites and in increasing the bigonial distance (33). However, angulation of the distractor to accomplish these secondary movements can move the bone segments closer together at a cortical surface, actually compressing the regenerate (33). Compression rather than continuous distraction will lead to consolidation. As such, it is imperative to continue or even accelerate the rate of linear distraction during secondary distraction movements to ensure that the net movement of the bone ends is always apart, with maintenance of a nonossified central zone to the regenerate. Distraction at a rate of 1.5 to 2 mm/d may be required in patients less than 3 years of age.

The problem of fibrous union in craniofacial distraction is rare (17). Two basic mechanisms may lead to this complication—motion at the distraction site and an overly rapid distraction rate. The most likely reason for motion in the distraction gap is a technical error in fixation of the distractor to the bone. The construct of bone and distractor should be absolutely rigid, whether external or internal devices are used. Any motion of the distractor after fixation is unacceptable and mandates repeated fixation.

A less common explanation for fibrous union in cases of mandibular distraction is ankylosis of the proximal skeletal segment in the region of the glenoid fossa. This is most likely to occur when a preexisting ankylosis is released at the same time that the distraction procedure is performed. The forces of mastication are then transferred to the distraction zone, which functions as a pseudarthrosis to allow mandibular excursion. The only reported case of fibrous union in craniofacial distraction occurred through such a mechanism (17). In any case in which a temporomandibular joint ankylosis is released at the time of a mandibular distraction, the patient should be instructed in a routine of vigorous jaw-opening exercises. As described by McCormick et al. (33a), the articulating surface of the proximal bone segment becomes covered with connective tissue that functions remarkably well as a neocondyle, so long as it is allowed to remodel by repeated motion after it has contacted the glenoid fossa. This is a form of transport distraction, in which bone is distracted into a region from which bone has been resected.

Fibrous union may also be caused when the rate of distraction is too rapid. This leads to a distraction zone that is too wide to allow for ossification of the regenerate (9). Although no firm clinical evidence is available regarding the maximal or even the optimal rate of distraction in the craniofacial skeleton, Ilizarov clearly established that a rate of 1 mm/d is optimal in the endochondral bones of the lower extremity (30). Rates in excess of 1 mm/d can lead to increasing problems with fibrous union. In experimental studies, distraction of the dog mandible at the rate of 3 mm/d has been shown to result in fibrous union (unpublished data). Generally, the distraction rate should be maintained at 1 mm/d. An exception to this would be a distraction in a child under 4 years of age and a distraction during which movements in the vertical or horizontal planes are to be carried out simultaneously with sagittal distraction. If these movements result in a net compression of the bone ends, the rate of distraction in the anteroposterior direction should be accelerated to prevent premature consolidation.

Fibrous union will be manifested as a failure of radiographic consolidation of the regenerate despite a post-distraction stabilization period of 8 to 12 weeks. If this occurs, the patient should be returned to the operating room and the tissue in the distraction gap resected. The bone edges should also be resected to the point at which bleeding bone is visualized. Following this, the distraction device may be used to compress rather than distract the bone segments. After an interval of 5 to 7 days, distraction may be resumed.

MALOCCLUSION

In most cases of craniofacial distraction involving the jaws, the endpoint of treatment is not the status of the occlusion but rather the position of the bone (or jaw) being distracted. This principle is particularly true for the younger patient. Orthodontic treatment and subsequent growth can compensate for most occlusal discrepancies resulting from the distraction process in the child.

The most common occlusal change seen with unilateral mandibular distraction is a posterior open bite on the distracted side (2,14). In our pediatric experience, this generally requires nothing more than the insertion and serial reduction of a bite plate to promote descent of the posterior maxillary dentoalveolusure. Indeed, in children less than 4 years of age, the open bite often closes spontaneously without the need for any type of orthodontic appliance intervention (34). In their series of 106 patients, Molina and Ortiz Monasterio found the need for treatment to be related to the severity of the original mandibular deformity (14). Patients with the most severe hypoplasia (Pruzansky IIB) required bite plates in addition to dynamic orthodontic appliances to correct the posterior open bite. However, no further surgical intervention was necessary.

Other authors have reported more significant difficulties with occlusal problems after distraction. Pensler and colleagues (35) reported that unacceptable occlusal relationships developed in six of nine patients in their series of mandibular distractions. For this problem, the authors report that in a secondary procedure, " . . . the mandible was reduced by digital manipulation of the regenerate into the optimal occlusion and stabilized in the new position." Other, similar reports of occlusal problems requiring device modification during treatment or significant post-distraction intervention for correction have been published (29,36). Such cases must bring into question the vector chosen for the distraction. Distraction of the midface or mandible should never be performed along a vector such that an occlusal relationship will result that cannot be corrected orthodontically. When unidirectional devices are used, one is committed to the vector established when the device is applied to the bone. Therefore, the direction of distraction must be planned preoperatively. However, with multidirectional devices, the vector may be adjusted during the distraction process, although a clear preoperative plan is still essential (33). Some authors have proposed mathematical formulas based on measurements taken from cephalometric radiographs and three-dimensional computed tomography (37). However, in cases of mandibular distraction, the severity of ramal hypoplasia is usually the best indicator (14,38). As the ramus becomes increasingly hypoplastic, the vector should be set in a more *vertical* orientation (Fig. 16-4A). This allows the distraction process to reestablish the posterior facial height on the affected side by creating a bone segment that more closely resembles the contralateral normal ramus. With time, the muscles of mastication act to produce a counterclockwise rotation of the mandible, which results in sagittal advancement of the chin point and restoration of a gonial angle. In cases in which the ramus is normally proportioned and the primary problem is retropositioning of the pogonion, a *horizontal* vector is most appropriate (Fig. 16-4B). This allows maximal sagittal advancement of the mandible. In the majority of patients, an increase in both ramal height and sagittal advancement are needed. In these situations, an *oblique* vector between the straight vertical and horizontal is most likely to achieve the desired result (Fig. 16-4C).

This discussion of occlusion applies primarily to pediatric craniofacial distraction. In adults, the occlusion is most

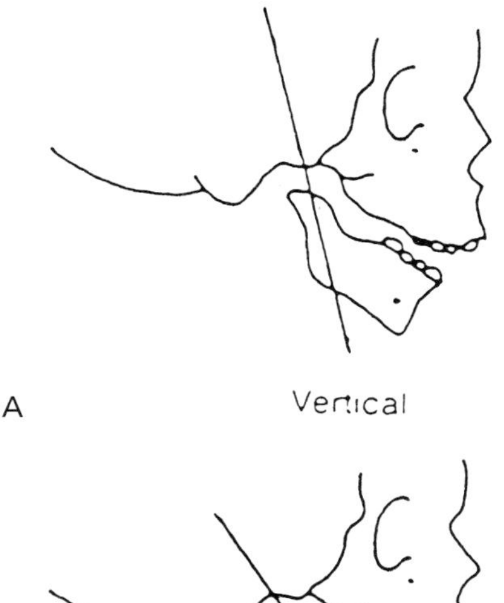

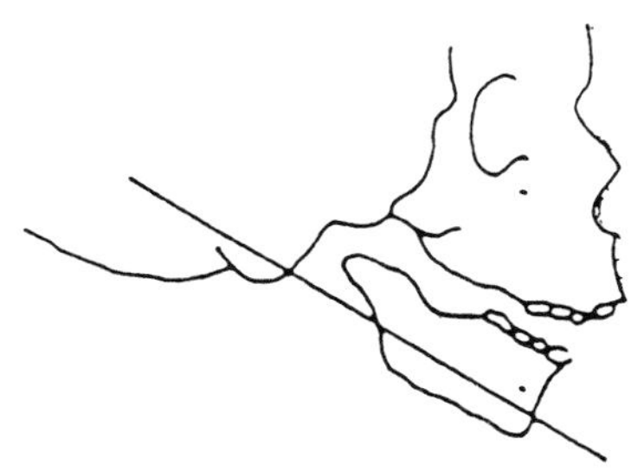

FIGURE 16-4. The vector of distraction depends on the mandibular deformity. **A:** With an extremely hypoplastic ramus, a vertical orientation ensures the restitution of ramal height. **B:** With inadequate projection of the pogonion, the horizontal vector achieves maximal advancement, particularly in bilateral cases. **C:** In situations in which the ramus height and chin point projection are both inadequate, an oblique vector is most appropriate.

frequently well adapted to the existing maxillary or mandibular deformities, and changes in the occlusion are not easily corrected by orthodontic therapy. Ortiz Monasterio et al. (12) have proposed simultaneous mandibular and maxillary distraction in this group of patients. In seven adult patients with craniofacial microsomia and a stable functional occlusal relationship, mandibular distraction devices were applied, after which a mandibular corticotomy and an incomplete Le Fort I osteotomy were performed. The pterygomaxillary suture on the unaffected side was left intact to serve as a fulcrum for the distraction. On the fifth postoperative day, the patients were placed in maxillomandibular fixation and distraction was initiated. In all patients, the occlusal plane was leveled and the occlusal relationships were preserved. It is mandatory to control for the occlusion in an adult patient undergoing distraction; failure to do so is likely to result in an occlusal relationship that can be corrected only by secondary orthognathic surgery. Recently, with the use of tooth-borne distractors, distraction has even been used to treat orthodontic problems such as dental crowding (34).

DEVICE FAILURE

The hardware used for distraction in the craniofacial skeleton is currently undergoing a period of development and modification. The focus of development has been to produce smaller devices capable of distracting in multiple planes. Ultimately, the goal would be to have a miniature internal device capable of distracting bone according to a preprogrammed position. Technology is currently far from able to achieve this goal, and device failure has been reported in many series of distraction cases (17,25,26,39).

The causes of device failure can be divided into several categories. One is failure of the gear mechanism in the distractor (39). In the case of external devices, dried blood within the mechanism can cause it to lock, so that further distraction is prevented. It is important to instruct the families of patients to clean the device daily with hydrogen peroxide, particularly during the first postoperative week. It is easiest and most effective simply to pour the peroxide on the device. This helps to remove blood or drainage that has already dried within the gearing. With internal distractors, failure of the external connector that is turned to distract the device is possible. This has been seen in intraoral devices in which a flexible rod is utilized to minimize intraoral irritation (26,27). The connector must be sufficiently strong to transfer the force necessary to distract the bone segments.

Another potential problem with distraction devices is difficulty in achieving rigid fixation to the bone, particularly in cases of midface distraction. When internal devices are used, fixation is best accomplished on the temporoparietal skull and the malar eminence. In children, especially those with syndromic conditions, the zygoma may not provide adequate bone for rigid stabilization of the device. This is particularly true when the midface is distracted against a restrictive soft tissue envelope. Chin and Toth measured the force necessary to advance the Le Fort III segment in children with midface hypoplasia (25). Advancement beyond 10 mm was found to require between 7 and 9 kg of force. If bone is felt to be insufficient, an external device should be used.

In the event of device failure, the only option is to replace the distractor. When an internal device has been used, the patient must be returned to the operating room. With external distractors, the replacement can usually be performed in the office. If possible, one should make an effort to affix the replacement device to the bone pins before the malfunctioning device is removed. This ensures maintenance of the position of the bone segments. If this is not possible, removal of the failed device may result in the ends of the bone assuming a different orientation with respect to one another, and the end result of the distraction will be affected.

CONCLUSION

Distraction osteogenesis has revolutionized the field of craniofacial surgery. Although Ilizarov experienced a great deal of success in lower extremity distraction, there can be no question that the craniofacial skeleton, with its smaller osseous dimensions and abundant vascular supply of the surrounding soft tissues, is more amenable to the technique. It is perhaps the first surgical procedure to enable the body to regenerate its own missing or damaged tissue, and it does so with minimal associated morbidity and without the need for bone grafts or blood transfusions required in earlier techniques. Those complications that are associated with distraction are infrequent and can often be avoided by careful attention to preoperative planning and surgical detail.

REFERENCES

1. Snyder CC, Levine GA, Swanson HM, et al. Mandibular lengthening by gradual distraction. Preliminary report. *Plast Reconstr Surg* 1973;51:506–508.
2. McCarthy JG, Schreiber J, Karp N, et al. Lengthening the human mandible by gradual distraction. *Plast Reconstr Surg* 1992;89:1–8.
3. Cohen SR, Burstein FD, Stewart MB, et al. Maxillary-midface distraction in children with cleft lip and palate: a preliminary report. *Plast Reconstr Surg* 1997;99:1421–1428.
4. Grayson BH, McCormick S, Santiago P, et al. Vector of device placement and trajectory of mandibular distraction. *J Craniofac Surg* 1997;8:473–480.
5. McCormick SU. Reconstruction of the mandibular condyle using transport distraction osteogenesis. *J Craniofac Surg* 1997;8:48–52.
6. Polley JW, Figueroa AA. Management of severe maxillary deficiency in childhood and adolescence through distraction osteogenesis with an external, rigid distraction device. *J Craniofac Surg* 1997;8:181–185.

7. Polley JW, Figueroa AA, Charbel FT, et al. Monobloc craniomaxillofacial distraction osteogenesis in a newborn with severe craniofacial synostosis: a preliminary report. *J Craniofac Surg* 1995;6:421–423.
8. Remmler D, McCoy FJ, O'Neil D, et al. Osseous expansion of the cranial vault by craniostasis. *Plast Reconstr Surg* 1992;89:787–797.
9. Karp NS, McCarthy JG, Schreiber JS, et al. Membranous bone lengthening: a serial histologic study. *Ann Plast Surg* 1992;29:2–7.
10. McCarthy JG. The role of distraction osteogenesis in the reconstruction of the mandible in unilateral craniofacial microsomia. *Clin Plast Surg* 1994;21:625–631.
11. McCarthy JG, Kawamoto HK, Grayson BH, et al. Surgery of the jaws. In: McCarthy JG, ed. *Plastic surgery.* Philadelphia: WB Saunders, 1990:1188–1374.
12. Ortiz Monasterio F, Molina F, Andrade L, et al. Simultaneous mandibular and maxillary distraction in hemifacial microsomia in adults: avoiding occlusal disasters. *Plast Reconstr Surg* 1997;100:852–861.
13. Tjernstrom B, Olerud S, Rehnberg L. Limb lengthening by callus distraction. Complications in 53 cases operated 1980–1991. *Acta Orthop Scand* 1994;65:447–455.
14. Molina F, Ortiz Monasterio F. Mandibular elongation and remodeling by distraction: a farewell to major osteotomies. *Plast Reconstr Surg* 1995;96:825–840.
15. Mafulli N, Lombari C, Matarazzo L, et al. A review of 240 patients undergoing distraction osteogenesis for congenital posttraumatic or post-infective lower limb length discrepancy. *J Am Coll Surg* 1996;182:394–402.
16. Glat PM, Staffenberg DA, Karp NS, et al. Multidimensional distraction osteogenesis: the canine zygoma. *Plast Reconstr Surg* 1994;94:753–758.
17. Diner PA, Kollar EM, Martinez H, et al. Intraoral distraction for mandibular lengthening: a technical innovation. *J Craniomaxillofac Surg* 1996;24:92–95.
18. Trauner R, Obwegeser H. Surgical correction of mandibular prognathism and retrogenia with consideration of genioplasty. *Oral Surg* 1957;10:677.
19. Young NL, Davis RJ, Bell DF, et al. Electromyographic and nerve conduction changes after tibial lengthening by the Ilizarov method. *J Pediatr Orthop* 1993;13:473–477.
20. Block MS, Daire J, Stover J, et al. Changes in the inferior alveolar nerve following mandibular lengthening in the dog using distraction osteogenesis. *J Oral Maxillofac Surg* 1993;51:652–660.
21. Karp NS, Thorne CH, McCarthy JG, et al. Bone lengthening in the craniofacial skeleton. *Ann Plast Surg* 1990;24:231–237.
22. McCarthy JG. Mandibular distraction. In: McCarthy JG, ed. Distraction of the craniofacial skeleton. New York: Springer-Verlag New York 1998.
23. Cohen SR, Rutrick RE, Burstein FD. Distraction osteogenesis of the human craniofacial skeleton: initial experience with new distraction system. *J Craniofac Surg* 1995;6:368–374.
24. Aronson J. Experimental and clinical experience with distraction osteogenesis. *Cleft Palate Craniofac J* 1994;31:473–481.
25. Chin M, Toth BA. Le Fort III advancement with gradual distraction using internal devices. *Plast Reconstr Surg* 1997;100:819–830.
26. Diner PA, Kollar E, Martinez H, et al. Submerged intraoral device for mandibular lengthening. *J Craniomaxillofac Surg* 1997;25:116–123.
27. Ellis E, Zide M. Transfacial approaches to the mandible. In: Ellis E, Zide M, eds. *Surgical approaches to the facial skeleton.* Baltimore: Williams & Wilkins, 1995:123–138.
28. McCarthy JG, Staffenberg DA, Wood RJ, et al. Introduction of an intraoral bone-lengthening device. *Plast Reconstr Surg* 1995;96:978–981.
29. Corcoran J, Hubli EH, Salyer KE. Distraction osteogenesis of costochondral neomandibles: a clinical experience. *Plast Reconstr Surg* 1997;100:311–315.
30. Ilizarov GA. The principles of the Ilizarov method. *Bull Hosp Joint Dis Orthop Inst* 1988;48:1–11.
31. Aldegheri R, Renzi-Brivio L, Agostini S. The callotasis method of limb lengthening. *Clin Orthop* 1989;241:137–141.
32. McCarthy JG, Williams JK, Grayson BH, et al. Controlled multiplanar distraction of the mandible: device development and clinical studies *(submitted).*
33. Williams JK, Rowe NM, Mackool R, et al. Controlled multiplanar distraction of the mandible: laboratory studies of anteroposterior and vertical movements *(submitted).*
33a. McCormick SU, McCarthy JG, Grayson BH, et al. Effect of mandibular distraction on the temporomandibular joint: part II, clinical study. *J Craniofac Surg* 1995;6:364–367.
34. Hollier LH, Kim J, McCarthy JG, et al. Mandibular growth after distraction in children less than 48 months of age *(submitted).*
35. Pensler JM, Goldberg DP, Lindell B, et al. Skeletal distraction of the hypoplastic mandible. *Ann Plast Surg* 1995;34:130–136.
36. Rachmiel A, Levy M, Laufer D. Lengthening of the mandible by distraction osteogenesis: report of cases. *J Oral Maxillofac Surg* 1995;53:838–846.
37. Losken HW, Patterson GT, Lazarou SA, et al. Planning mandibular distraction: preliminary report. *Cleft Palate Craniofac J* 1995;32:71–76.
38. Guerrero CA, Bell WH, Contasti GI, et al. Mandibular widening by intraoral distraction osteogenesis. *Br J Oral Maxillofac Surg* 1997;35:383–392.
39. Weil TS, VanSickels JE, Payne CJ. Distraction osteogenesis for correction of transverse mandibular deficiency: a preliminary report. *J Oral Maxillofac Surg* 1997;55:953–960.

SUGGESTED READING

Chin M, Toth BA. Distraction osteogenesis in maxillofacial surgery using internal devices: review of five cases. *J Oral Maxillofac Surg* 1996;54:45–53.

McCormick SU, McCarthy JG, Grayson BH, et al. Effect of mandibular distraction on the temporomandibular joint: part 1, canine study. *J Craniofac Surg* 1995;6:358–363.

Discussion

DISTRACTION OSTEOGENESIS

FERNANDO MOLINA

Distraction osteogenesis, which simplifies the treatment for congenital mandibular hypoplasia, is becoming a very popular technique. It is a relatively minor surgical procedure that preserves the vascular supply and nerve function of the mandible. Distraction osteogenesis produces excellent aesthetic and functional results and restores facial symmetry; it horizontalizes the chin and buccal commissure in unilateral cases, and elongates the ramus and mandibular body with good projection of the chin in bilateral cases (1–5).

Drs. Hollier and McCarthy have thoroughly and carefully reviewed all the possible complications of mandibular distraction, including nerve injury, infection, skin scarring, problems related to bone healing, and occlusal changes. The various devices in use are also analyzed.

Since performing the initial case in our clinical series of distraction osteogenesis, we have observed that the most critical factor in obtaining good results with long-term stability is planning the proper distraction vector on the cephalogram, and then achieving the same vector in the operating room. Other surgical teams from different countries have made the same observation.

In our opinion, distraction osteogenesis in the craniofacial skeleton involves two important goals: first, to induce the formation of new bone to correct bone hypoplasia, and second, to reconstruct the normal anatomy of the mandible as closely as possible with the new bone.

If these goals are accomplished, the occlusal changes produced by the distraction procedure will be minimal and amenable to correction with standard orthodontic procedures (4), and the function of the temporomandibular joint will be improved because of the beneficial effects of distraction on the condyle. In addition, facial symmetry will be restored to provide a more cosmetically pleasing appearance.

It does not make sense to produce a large amount of new bone in a hypoplastic mandible if the elongation process does not roughly resemble normal mandibular growth. It also does not make sense to elongate the mandible of a patient with hemifacial microsomia grade 2A by using a horizontal distraction vector. The mandibular horizontalization resulting from the new bone formation will cause a loosening of the angle, with a complete change of the position of the condyle and its relationship to the glenoid fossa. Erroneous bone elongation will cause a major malocclusion and result in unacceptable facial symmetry. In every patient with hemifacial microsomia grade 2A, the most critical point is the reconstruction of the ascending ramus in addition to the mandibular angle.

In our experience of 265 patients with hemifacial microsomia treated with mandibular distraction during the last 9 years, we have found that three different distraction vectors can be used: the oblique, the semioblique, and the vertical. And for the group of patients with micrognathia (56 patients), we have used bidirectional devices to achieve two simultaneous vectors of distraction: a vertical vector for the ascending ramus, and a horizontal one for the mandibular body.

In 90% of cases, with correct use of the different types of vectors and with individualization according to each bone deformity, we can obtain excellent aesthetic and functional results.

However, in a few cases, it is necessary to change the distraction vector during a procedure. The purpose of such vector changes is to obtain simultaneous bone elongation and remodeling and a roughly normal final anatomy of the mandible in comparison with the contralateral side. To exemplify this situation, I present the case of a 5-year-old girl who had hemifacial microsomia grade 2B with severe hypoplasia of the angle and ascending ramus and a very rudimentary condyle (Fig. 16D-1. The surgical plan was to use distraction osteogenesis to reconstruct the angle and ascending ramus, with simultaneous repositioning of the condyle to create a better relationship with the glenoid fossa. After performing a corticotomy extending from the retromolar triangle toward the gonion and inserting a unidirectional flexible device, we used an oblique vector to recreate the angle, elongating it by 18 mm (Fig. 16D-2). Then, with the use of local anesthesia, we inserted a third pin to create a vertical distraction vector. After elongating it by 24 mm, we rebuilt the ascending ramus (Fig. 16D-3). At the end of the distraction period, we observed radiographically that a complete and anatomical reconstruction of the mandible had been achieved. New bone formation was observed in the angle and ascending ramus, which were very similar to those of the con-

F. Molina: Hospital Angeles del Pedregal, Mexico City, Mexico

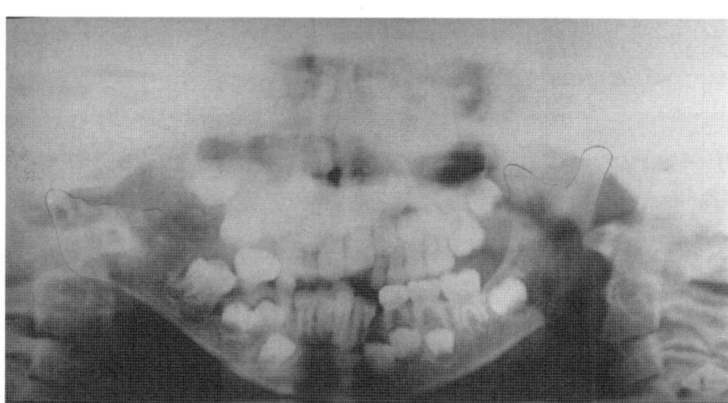
A

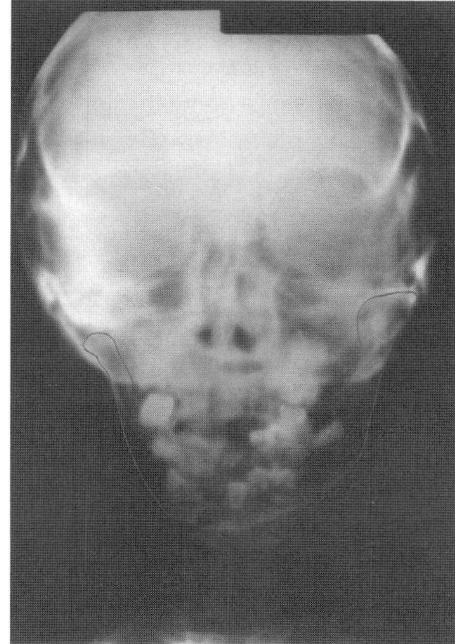
B

FIGURE 16D-1. A: Preoperative Panorex showing severe hypoplasia of the angle and ascending ramus (grade 2B). The condyle is very rudimentary, with dislocation of the glenoid fossa. **B:** Preoperative posteroanterior cephalogram showing right mandibular hypoplasia. The bone hypoplasia involves the mandibular angle and ascending ramus. The bigonial distance is decreased because of absence of the angle in the affected side. Note the lateral displacement of the condyle.

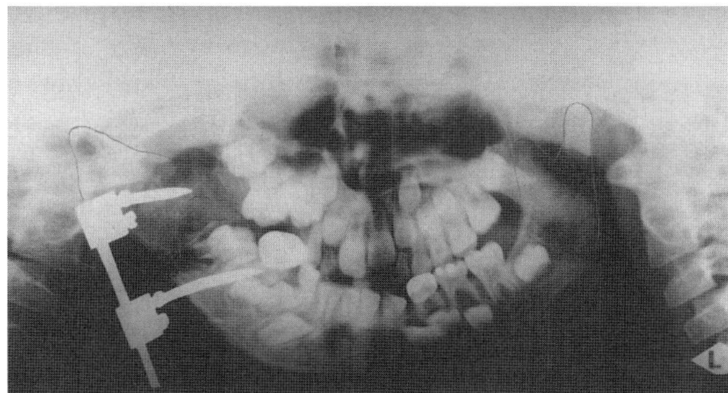
A

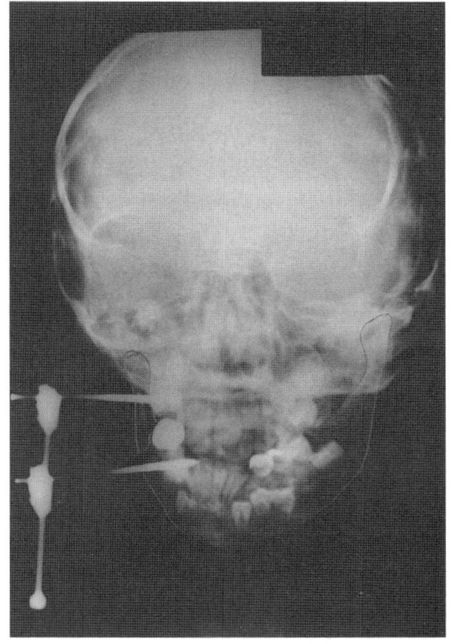
B

FIGURE 16D-2. A: Panorex showing the bone elongation (18 mm) produced by use of the oblique vector. A large amount of new bone is found at the site of the mandibular angle. Also note that the area of new bone formation is between the inferior point of the angle and the ascending ramus. The mandibular body dimension has been preserved. **B:** In this view, it is possible to observe the initial remodeling effect of the corticotomy plus the use of a flexible device. The angle has been enlarged, and the condyle has been medialized.

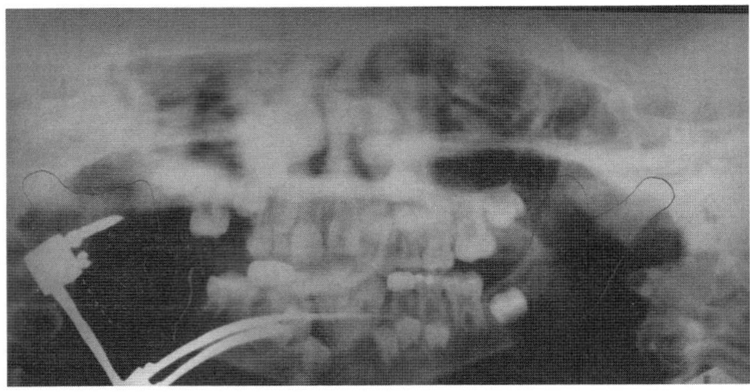

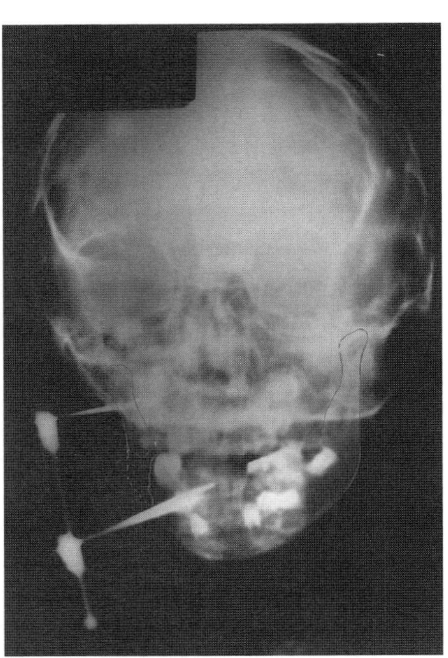

FIGURE 16D-3. A: After changing the oblique vector into a vertical one and at the end of the distraction period, we found a complete elongation and remodeling of the mandible. A new mandibular angle and a new dimension of the ascending ramus have been created. Note the presence of a third pin in the mandible. **B:** With use of the vertical vector, 28 mm of new bone has been added to the ascending ramus. The size and shape of the condyle have been increased, so that it is now very similar to the contralateral condyle in regard to position and relationship with the fossa. The bigonial distance has been increased considerably. All these changes allow better function and have provided good aesthetic results.

tralateral side. The bigonial distance was enlarged by remodeling of the new angle. The new ascending ramus closely resembled the normal one in both length and width. It was very interesting to observe the initial position of the condyle and then how it had shifted after the distraction procedure to a more medial position, which improved its shape and size and provided a better relationship to the fossa.

Undoubtedly, distraction osteogenesis has revolutionized the treatment of mandibular deformities. This technique is associated with minimal morbidity and a very low rate of complications. Because of the abundant vascular supply in the craniofacial skeleton, the most frequent complications of distraction that arise in orthopedic surgery are infrequent in cases involving the mandible, and very often they can be avoided by careful attention to preoperative planning and surgical details.

REFERENCES

1. McCarthy JG, Schreiber J, Karp N, et al. Lengthening the human mandible by gradual distraction. *Plast Reconstr Surg* 1992;89:1–8.
2. Molina F, Ortiz Monasterio F. Extended indications for mandibular distraction: unilateral, bilateral and bidirectional. *International Craniofacial Congress* 1993;5:79.
3. Molina F. Mandibular distraction in hemifacial microsomia: technique and results in 56 patients. Cambridge: The Craniofacial Society of Great Britain, 1994.
4. Molina F, Ortiz Monasterio F. Mandibular elongation and remodelling by distraction: a farewell to major osteotomies. *Plast Reconstr Surg* 1995;96:825–840.
5. Molina F, Ortiz Monasterio F, Aguilar M de la P, et al. Maxillary distraction: aesthetic and functional benefits in cleft lip-palate and prognathic patients during mixed dentition. *Plast Reconstr Surg.* 1998 101:951–963.

17

TISSUE EXPANSION

LOUIS C. ARGENTA

Tissue expansion is an aesthetic refinement in reconstructive plastic surgery. Because of the significant investment of time and effort, in addition to the anticipated positive aesthetic outcome, complications and results that are less than favorable are particular disappointments to both patients and physicians. Because tissue expansion involves both surgical and mechanical skill, a significant "learning curve" is required. In the 1970s and 1980s, complication rates of 30% to 50% were not unusually reported (1–4). As prostheses have become more sophisticated, indications for the technique have been refined and patients have been more properly selected. In the 1990s, complication rates have been more uniformly in the 5% to 6% range. Thus, the prediction of Fenton (5) that "tissue expansion will not realize its full potential until the complication rate is consistently below 10%" has been realized. Today, tissue expansion is practiced successfully throughout the world, with acceptable complication rates and often dramatic results.

Generic complications of tissue expansion have classically been categorized as major or minor. Major complications are those that interfere with the intended outcome of the procedure and result in abandonment of the procedure. More frequently encountered minor complications are those that do not affect the final outcome of the procedure, but that require time-consuming and costly treatment. The vast majority of tissue expansion complications are minor, and with some experience they can be overcome so as not to result in termination of the procedure. Major complications include failure of the implant with deflation, extrusion of the expander, major infection of the prosthesis, significant tissue ischemia, and necrosis of the overlying tissue. Minor complications include leaking of the inflation reservoir, reservoir rotation, pain, intermittent ischemia of the overlying tissue, and inadequate tissue expansion.

L.C. Argenta: Department of Plastic and Reconstructive Surgery, Wake Forest University School of Medicine, Winston-Salem, North Carolina

GENERAL SUGGESTIONS FOR AVOIDING COMPLICATIONS

Complications are better avoided than treated. Careful preoperative planning to accomplish a rapid, safe, and effective expansion is critical. Tissue expansion is a refinement used in conjunction with existing, accepted flap techniques. The quality of donor tissues needs to be assessed carefully preoperatively. The more traumatized, scarred, and compromised the donor tissue is preoperatively, the higher the risk for complications during and after tissue expansion. Although the process of tissue expansion does act as a delay and increases the vascularity of tissue, tissue that has been previously compromised will ultimately compromise the final results.

Flaps should be planned so that the ultimate transposition, rotation, or free flap will come to rest with its suture lines in safe, aesthetically pleasing areas. This is particularly important in tissue expansion of the scalp and face. The ultimate aesthetic result is determined not only by the quality of transposed tissue, but also by how it is incorporated into the recipient area. The number of tissue expanders to be placed is also critical in preoperative planning. Although a single large expander may suffice in many cases on the trunk, defects on the face, scalp, and extremities may require multiple expanders so that excessive individual volume placement is not necessary. The use of multiple small expanders allows the recruitment of viable, aesthetically normal tissue from more than one adjacent area. Expansion with multiple small expanders is usually accomplished in a shorter period of time with a lower rate of complications. Complications associated with one of multiple implants can often be tolerated, and the procedure can be carried to completion rather than aborted.

The incision for placement of the prosthesis should be considered carefully. Small incisions distant from the flap border minimize wound dehiscence and implant exposure. However, the placement of such incisions must be carefully planned so that excessive scarring and compromise of later flaps do not occur. The incision should be large enough to allow visualization of the pocket created for placement of the expander. Although balloon inflation devices are available that can create pockets blindly, the author prefers direct visualization of the pocket so that careful hemostasis and a uniformly thick plane of overlying tissue can be guaranteed.

The pocket for the main prosthesis can be dissected subcutaneously, submuscularly, or subfascially. The vast majority of tissue expanders are placed subcutaneously. This allows rapid expansion and the advancement or rotation of large skin flaps unencumbered by vascular and fascial pedicles. When a permanent prosthesis is to be placed in the expanded space, the expansion of overlying muscle, such as the pectoralis in breast reconstruction, minimizes contamination of the prosthesis and usually leads to more aesthetically pleasing long-term results. Likewise, known myocutaneous flaps can be expanded submuscularly to create a larger surface area allowing extremely large flaps to be transferred. The incorporation of fascia over the prosthesis requires that greater force be applied to expand the prosthesis but probably creates a safer flap because an additional layer is provided to minimize exposure. Initially, we placed expanders under the platysma muscle for facial reconstruction, but we have abandoned the practice because incorporating this muscle does result in some later compromise of rotation.

Some surgeons prefer placing the inflation reservoir external to the skin to avoid the discomfort of percutaneous injection (6). We prefer a system that is completely incorporated within the patient. This minimizes the risk for bacterial contamination and capsular inflammation, which usually occur around the prosthesis when an external port is used. External ports should never be used when alloplastic materials are to be implanted. In our experience, completely buried ports require less care than external ports and are tolerated by the vast majority of patients without difficulty. A eutectic mixture of lidocaine 2.5% and prilocaine 2.5%, EMLA®, or an ice pack applied to the tissue over the inflation reservoir usually make percutaneous injection painless.

The pocket dissected for the prosthesis should be sufficiently large to accommodate the prosthesis without any risk of encroachment on the suture line. Implants should be at least 3 cm from the closest incision because they tend to migrate with collection of serum in the early postoperative period.

Drains are almost never used with expanders. Hemostasis should be meticulously obtained at the time of surgery. Filling expanders intraoperatively to take up dead space results in a significant reduction in hematoma and seroma formation around the implant.

The risk for infection is greatest in the perioperative period. Intraoperative antibiotics are administered intravenously before the prosthesis is placed. Cephalosporins are usually given because most perioperative infections are caused by gram-positive organisms. Routine gram-negative coverage is not necessary unless the operation is to be performed in an area where gram-negative infection is anticipated, such as the perineum. The use of irrigating solutions containing antibiotics or Betadine also helps minimize the risk for infection. We prefer 50,000 U of bacitracin per liter of saline solution or 20 mL of Betadine per liter of saline solution for irrigation.

Postoperatively, inflation is carried out at weekly intervals, usually beginning a week after insertion of the prosthesis. Frequent small inflations are safer and better tolerated by the patient. Particularly in children, weekly or biweekly small inflations are better tolerated than larger, less frequent inflations. The amount of saline solution infused depends on comfort of the patient and integrity of the overlying tissue. If the overlying tissue blanches and does not regain its normal color within 5 minutes, saline solution should be removed from the expander. Pain may occur with initial inflations, particularly in the scalp and forehead (7,8). Oral analgesics given before inflation are helpful and may be required for several hours. Intraluminal analgesics are rarely indicated.

CONTRAINDICATIONS TO TISSUE EXPANSION

Absolute contraindications for placement of an expansion prosthesis are few. First, an expander should not be placed adjacent to obvious or even suspected malignancy. Recurrence of the malignancy in the periprosthetic space results in widespread dissemination of the neoplasm, which makes extirpation difficult and sometimes impossible. Second, a prosthesis should not be placed in an area of known infection. Because a foreign body is being placed in the wound, the odds of successfully controlling the infection with antibiotics or any other means is minimal. Distant infections, such as pneumonia and urinary sepsis, are relative contraindications because contamination of the implant can occur secondary to bacteriemia.

The number of relative contraindications to the placement of expansion prostheses is larger. Poorly vascularized tissue secondary to local factors or systemic disease predisposes to a higher rate of complications. Active chemotherapy results in a higher but usually tolerable risk for complications. Adjuvant chemotherapy following mastectomy is common, and successful reconstruction of the breast by tissue expansion can be accomplished during active chemotherapy. The use of tissue expansion during chemotherapy with "potent" chemotherapeutic agents, such as Adriamycin, cisplatin, and similar drugs, carries a higher rate of complications.

Tissue that has been previously irradiated can be very difficult to expand successfully. The risk for extrusion and complication is significantly higher in tissue exposed either preoperatively or postoperatively to radiation. Furthermore, long-term sequelae, such as fibrosis or capsular contracture, may compromise the final aesthetic result.

Psychological problems have often been advanced as a relative contraindication to tissue expansion. However, studies have demonstrated that with preoperative explanation to the patient and proper support of the patient during expansion, tissue expansion can be well tolerated.

Tolerance to tissue expansion varies considerably in different areas of the body. In general, areas covered with soft, thick tissue, such as the breast, trunk, back, upper leg, upper arm, and scalp, tolerate expansion with little difficulty. The face and forearm tolerate judicious expansion well. Tissue expansion is more difficult in the lower extremity, particularly below the knee, when previous soft tissue trauma has occurred. Difficulty is frequently the result of compromised lymphatics and venous channels that result in stasis and infection later in the course of expansion. Isolated injuries to the lower extremity when massive tissue trauma has not occurred, however, can be treated without difficulty. The hands and feet generally should not be expanded because expansion causes extreme pain.

MANAGEMENT OF SPECIFIC COMPLICATIONS

Implant Failure

Implant failure with subsequent deflation occurs much less frequently today than previously. Prostheses have been highly refined so that the vast majority can tolerate two to three times their recommended inflation volume without rupturing. Most deflations occur in the immediate perioperative period and are probably iatrogenic. Protheses are often compromised during wound closure, so that an immediate or delayed leakage occurs. The handling of any silicone protheses with instruments should be religiously avoided. Hemostat and forceps "bite" marks are frequently the site of later implant leakage. Disruption in the tubing at the point of the in-line connector is also frequent. Once the proper length of tubing has been determined, the tubing can be shortened to an appropriate length and the in-line connector secured with a permanent suture. Excessive force on the knot of the suture, however, may result in failure of the silicone later, and this should be avoided. When the inflation tube is placed across a joint, additional tubing must be allowed to remain so that in-line sutures are not disrupted during active motion.

Deflation occurring several weeks after placement is usually the result of trauma. Excessive force placed on the prosthesis during play, work, or acts of violence can cause implants to rupture. This is particularly true when the implant volume is approaching capacity. Leakage from the inflation reservoir is not uncommon. Puncture by needles larger than 23 gauge result in leakage over time. Lacerations of the valve by needles placed at an oblique angle or through the valve result in failure of sealing. Occasionally, puncture of the implant itself can occur when reservoirs are incorporated into the prosthesis. We have found that the use of magnetic port detectors can be quite deceiving, particularly in implants placed submuscularly.

Defective implants can be avoided by testing all implants before placement. Some authors have advocated placing methylene blue in the implant, but we feel that saline solution is more than adequate (9).

If deflation occurs early in the process of expansion, before adequate amounts of tissue can be generated, the prosthesis must be replaced at a second procedure. If deflation occurs late in the course of expansion, the surgeon must decide whether it is best to use the generated tissue to achieve the desired result, whether the flap should be advanced partially and reexpanded later, or whether a new prosthesis should be placed. Unless adequate amounts of tissue are available to accomplish an optimal result, it has been our experience that the prosthesis is better replaced. Partial advancements are possible if the implant has not been exposed, but the resulting scar is usually such that the second expansion is considerably more difficult.

Perioperative Hematoma and Seroma

Hematomas are usually the result of inadequate hemostasis at the time of surgery. Delayed rupture of vessels and disturbances of coagulation are rarely the cause (10). Direct visualization of the pocket is critical. Drains should not be used in the hope of avoiding a hematoma. Intraoperative placement of saline solution into the expander helps to minimize dead space and is very effective in reducing oozing from capillary beds.

Seromas not infrequently form around a prosthesis, particularly following immediate breast reconstruction, or in areas that have previously been traumatized or irradiated. The risk for infection of seromas, particularly when drains are used, must always been borne in mind. Patients in whom seromas develop should be aggressively treated with antibiotics. It has been suggested that external ports help drain seromas, but in our experience, seromas usually become infected and fibrotic when external ports are used.

Infection

Placement of any foreign material in the body always creates a risk for infection. Strict sterile technique at the time of implant placement is critical. Short, clean operations during which tissues are handled carefully minimize the risk. Perioperative infection is more common when expanders are placed following a long procedure, such as a major orthopedic reconstruction, modified radical mastectomy, or an operation during which other prosthetic materials are placed. Perioperative antibiotics routinely administered, but not intraluminal antibiotics, have in our experience been helpful (11).

The tissue overlying an expander usually becomes indurated during expansion. Excessive warmth, excessive pain, general prolonged malaise, or *peau d'orange* should alert the surgeon that subclinical infection is occurring.

Infection also occurs when inflation reservoirs are contaminated during injection. Absolute adherence to sterile technique is critical. Preparation of the valve area with Betadine and the use of sterile gloves are recommended.

If infection occurs early after the placement of tissue expanders, some authors have advocated attempts at salvage. This can be successful if the infection is well localized and minimal. Removal of the expander, copious irrigation with local antibiotics or Betadine, sterilization of the expander by repeated autoclaving, and replacement of the expander with a closed suction drain can occasionally salvage an infected prosthesis. If any symptoms of an aggressive infection, such as generalized inflammation, fever, chills, or a general feeling of malaise, are present, then the implant is best removed. The wound is copiously irrigated after removal of the prosthesis and then loosely closed with a suction drain.

If an infection occurs late in the course of expansion, the vast majority of procedures can be salvaged if enough tissue has been generated. After removal of the prosthesis, the wound is copiously irrigated and debridement of any compromised tissue performed. The flap is then rotated or advanced and sutured in place with monofilament suture. Closed suction drains are used until all seroma has subsided. In no case should a permanent prosthesis be placed when an expander prosthesis has been infected. Although such a permanent prosthesis may not become infected immediately, late complications almost always occur.

In general, 4 to 6 months should pass before a second attempt is made at expansion. At the time of the second operation, one frequently will find a remnant of the capsule and occasionally some fluid within it. This fluid should be Gram's-stained and cultured for bacteria before a new prosthesis is placed.

Exposure of the Implant

Any portion of the expansion device can become exposed during the process of tissue expansion. Exposure of the valve and tubing is less deleterious than exposure of the implant itself. Exposures most often occur with disruption of the suture line, traumatic injury to overlying tissue during placement of the prosthesis, virulent infection, or excessively rapid and forceful tissue expansion. Nonetheless, exposures do occur for which no good explanation can be found.

Care must be taken to locate valves in an area where excessive pressure will not be applied. When a valve is placed over firm tissue, such as the mastoid, skull, or ribs, prolonged and relatively painless pressure will result in compromise of the overlying tissue and exposure (Fig. 17-1). Exposure of the valve does not doom the procedure. Frequently, exteriorization of the valve is all that is necessary. If the valve is exteriorized several weeks after implantation, the prosthesis is usually sufficiently encapsulated so that contamination of the main prosthesis does not occur. The use of topical ointments, such as Silvadene or bacitracin, at the point of skin exit is helpful to minimize infection of an exteriorized port.

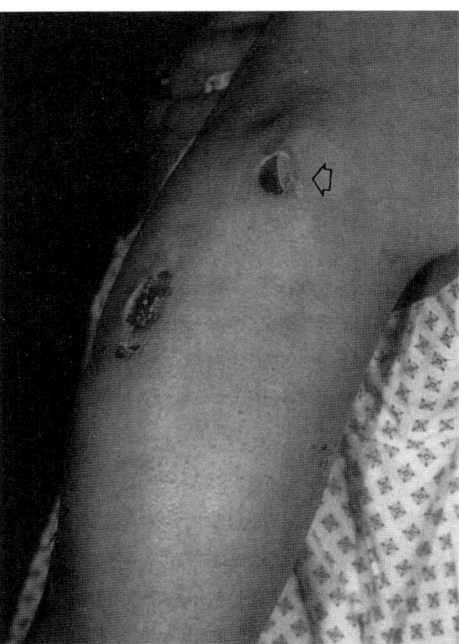

FIGURE 17-1. Extrusion of a valve in the upper arm over the humerus. A valve has rotated onto its side, and the lead edge is formed by the undersurface of the valve. This valve would have been better situated more medially on the forearm.

Tubing usually becomes exposed when it is excessive and a kink occurs. Provided that the portion of the tube immediately adjacent to the prostheses is not exposed, the balloon portion of the expander usually does not become contaminated. Topical treatment with antibiotic creams such as Silvadene is helpful in controlling such implant exposure (Fig. 17-2). Exposure of both the reservoir and tubing occurs most frequently in the head and neck area.

Exposure of the inflation implant itself presents a significant problem. Most exposures occur in the suture line when an incision is made in what is to be the advancing edge of the flap (Fig. 17-3). To minimize this risk, the surgeon should dissect a pocket adequate to allow the prosthesis to be placed 3 to 5 cm away from the incision. The incision should be closed with multiple layers of absorbable monofilament deep suture and permanent monofilament skin suture.

The use of a prosthesis that does not have a reinforced backing and the use of multiple small expanders rather than a single large prosthesis will help minimize the risk for exposure of the implant. Placing some fluid in the implant at the time of surgery also affords the surgeon the opportunity to manipulate the expander and work out folds before the wound is closed.

Impending exposure of an implant, manifested by thinness and blueness of overlying tissue, should be addressed immediately. Massaging the prosthesis to work out kinks will occasionally help. The application of Steri-Strip or tape directly over the thin, questionable area will help to prevent excessive tension.

If a prosthesis becomes exposed early in the course of tissue expansion, it is by definition infected. If a technical

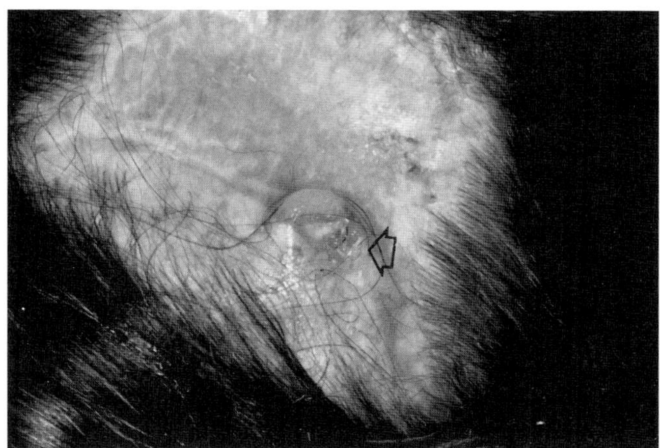

FIGURE 17-2. Exposure of the fill tube in an area of previous scar in the scalp. The valve should ideally be situated where the fill tube will not be adjacent to or under compromised tissue. This exposure was treated with topical antibiotics, and the expansion continued.

source for the extrusion can be determined, such as a broken suture, the implant can occasionally be autoclaved again, the pocket irrigated, and the procedure salvaged. However, if the extrusion is the result of compromise of tissues in the suture line or in the overlying tissue, the procedure is probably best aborted and reattempted at a later date.

If the extrusion occurs late in the course of tissue expansion, the vast majority of reconstructions can still be accomplished. If an adequate amount of tissue has been generated, the prosthesis is removed and the reconstructive flap turned. Drains are placed beneath this flap because the flap is contaminated. Flaps closed under such conditions are usually less than optimal, and excessive scar can be anticipated. Revision of scars is usually necessary, but the reconstructive procedure can usually be salvaged.

Ischemia and Necrosis of Overlying Tissue

The loss of tissue during the process of tissue expansion is relatively uncommon. It occurs most frequently when the tissue to be expanded has already been compromised by systemic disease, radiation injury, or previous trauma. Excessive thinning of the overlying skin resulting from irregular dissection may result in ischemia that progresses to necrosis with increasing expansion. Circulatory compromise of expanded tissue is most common in the lower extremity and forearm, in burns, and in young children (12–14).

Excessively aggressive tissue expansion may result in ischemia and loss of tissue. The use of multiple small inflations to the point of discomfort but not pain helps minimize this problem. Overly aggressive expansion can compromise overlying tissue such that the final aesthetic result is less than optimal, even if necrosis does not occur. The loss of hair follicles and other adnexal structures will compromise the quality of the tissue to be expanded.

Necrosis can also occur during the second stage, when flaps are rotated or expanded grafts are placed. If flaps are excessively thin, expansion has been inadequate for the defect to be covered, or if too much capsule and the adjacent vasculature are divided during the rotation–advancement phase, ischemia and necrosis can occur (Fig. 17-4).

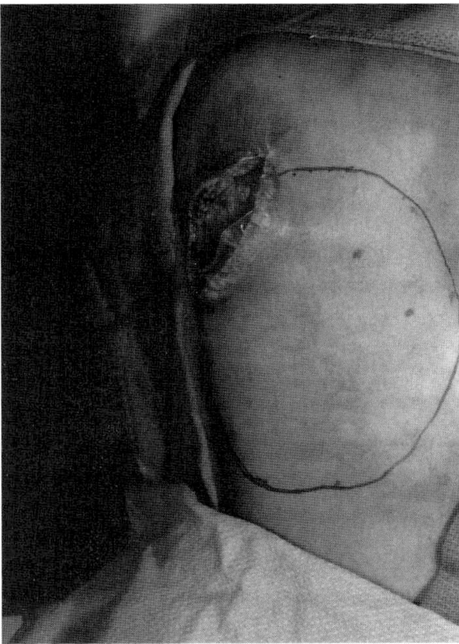

FIGURE 17-3. Implant exposure through the original placement and incision in the axilla. This incision was in scar in an area subject to tension. A single prosthesis was placed partially around the incision while the patient was sleeping. The flap was rotated into the axilla without difficulty despite the exposure.

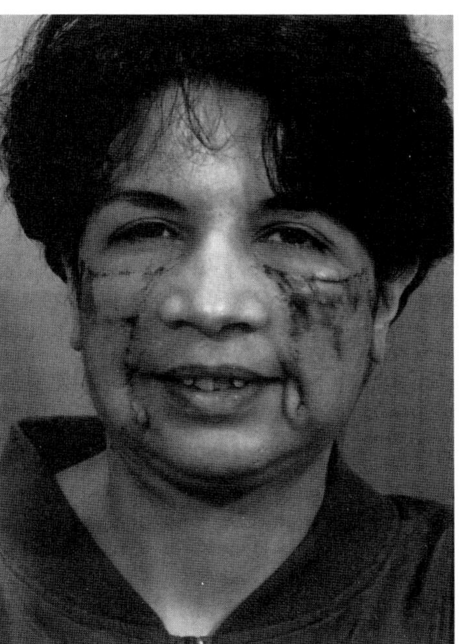

FIGURE 17-4. Ischemia of bilateral cheek rotation flaps used to replace radiation damaged tissue. The patient recovered with minimal scarring that did not require revision. The dog ears at the labial angles were revised secondarily.

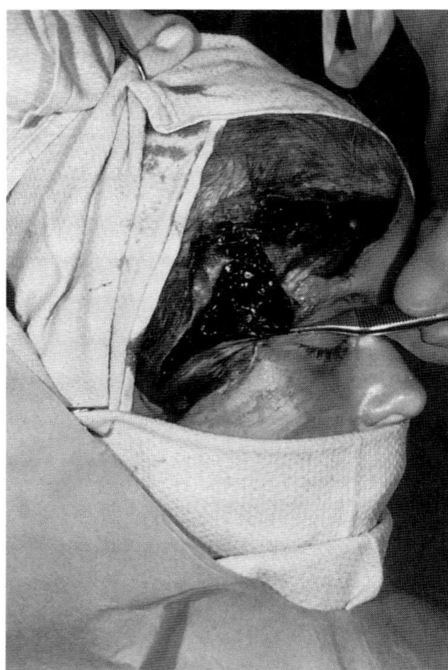

FIGURE 17-5. Loss of an expanded full-thickness flap placed over the forehead and lateral face of a child who underwent excision of a giant hairy nevus. Hematoma under the graft resulted in total loss. A second graft was harvested from the original donor site in the supraclavicular area and was used to replace the necrotic graft successfully.

When tissue becomes compromised during tissue expansion, it is best to deflate the implant partially and allow the tissue to attempt to recover. If ischemia occurs immediately following flap rotation, removal of some sutures to minimize tension on the flap may be helpful. A large scar will result, but scar revision is usually much easier to accomplish than a repeated expansion.

Necrosis and loss of expanded full-thickness grafts usually result from hematoma, infection, or poor adherence of the graft (Fig. 17-5). Such grafts should be removed expeditiously and regrafted. A second expanded full-thickness graft can usually be harvested from the original source if adequate expansion was accomplished.

SITE-SPECIFIC UNTOWARD RESULTS

Reconstruction of the Scalp

Tissue expansion has been extensively used in reconstruction of the scalp because it is the only reconstructive procedure that allows hair follicles to be redistributed to produce an aesthetically pleasing result. Tissue expansion redistributes hair follicles by distracting them from one another so that they are more evenly distributed. Distraction by a factor of two (i.e., doubling the surface area of the hair-bearing scalp) is usually tolerated without its becoming noticeable. Expansion beyond this point or excessive expansion of localized areas causes obvious hair thinness that may compromise the final result. The entire scalp should be considered as a donor area for scalp expansion. Distraction of hair follicles over a large area produces an aesthetically more pleasing result than does excessive expansion of an isolated area. For this reason, multiple tissue expanders are usually recommended. Scalp defects requiring very extensive expansion and hair redistribution (e.g., some burns) will result in thinning of hair. In such cases, patients can be advised to lighten their hair color to minimize the appearance of thinning hair.

The regrowth of hair in expanded flaps is directly proportional to the blood supply of the flaps. Flaps that are excessively ischemic result in relative or even total alopecia of that segment. Whenever possible, flaps should be designed so that the expanded flap incorporates one of the major vessels of the scalp. Careful preoperative planning makes it possible to incorporate a major vessel in almost any flap on the scalp.

Scarring in the scalp may be obvious after tissue expansion, particularly in dark-haired persons and in blacks. When tissue expansion is carried out in infants, it can be universally anticipated that some scar widening will occur with growth and that some revision will be necessary later in life (Fig. 17-6). The secondary correction of scars is facilitated by multiple Z-plasties, particularly in black children. Relative alopecia at the margins of a scar will make it more conspicuous. The excessive use of electrocautery during flap rotation is discouraged because it causes some loss of hair follicles.

Extensive tension on flaps also results in hair loss and scarring. Whenever possible, the expanded scalp flap should be rotated or advanced and various positioning attempted with staples. The area of alopecia or abnormal tissue is excised after various alternatives have been assessed to ensure adequacy and maximal use of tissue.

The establishment of a relatively normal hairline is paramount in achieving a final aesthetic result. In general, the establishment of an anterior hairline is more important than the establishment of a temporal hair cover. With adequate styling, hair can be combed to conceal most temporal alopecia. Secondary expansion of the scalp to create more tissue laterally is better undertaken as a later procedure after the anterior hairline has been established. Lateral scalp margins should be naturally curvilinear rather than straight.

It should also be remembered that the scalp and forehead are basically the same tissue and that relative increases or decreases of 20% in the amount of forehead visible are usually not perceptible to the lay viewer. Therefore, expansion of the forehead and its redistribution to previous hair-bearing areas may sometimes be necessary in very extensive deformities. It is critical that the brows be maintained in a symmetrical position during forehead and scalp reconstructions.

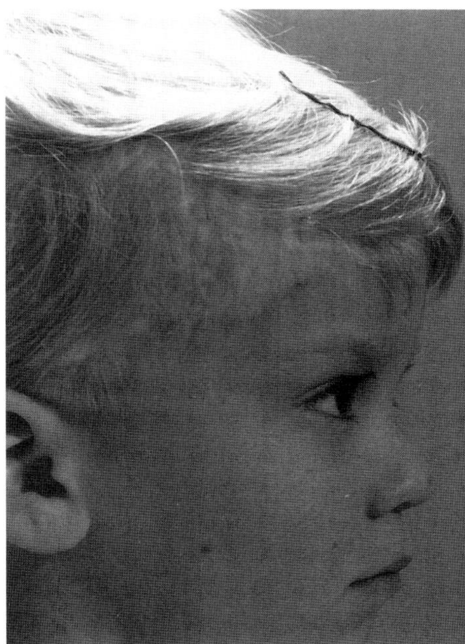

FIGURE 17-6. This child required three sessions of tissue expansion in infancy to remove more than half of his scalp because of a giant hairy nevus. As the skull grew, the scalp margins became more obvious. Secondary reconstruction is best delayed as long as possible.

Secondary correction of the brow position may occasionally be necessary.

Scalp expansion is usually delayed until 2 years of age, when the skull is more ossified and pressure deformation minimized. Almost all pressure deformities of the skull correct spontaneously once the prosthesis is removed and are clinically well tolerated.

Reconstruction of the Face

The use of tissue expansion in reconstruction of the face requires considerable expertise and planning. The ultimate aim is to reconstruct abnormal areas of the face with other facial tissue that matches in color, consistency, and hair-bearing quality. Surgery should be planned ideally to reconstruct entire facial aesthetic units, with suture lines lying in the margins of aesthetic units. The surgeon must also keep in mind the potential hair-bearing properties of the face, so that reconstructions performed in infancy will have proper aesthetic qualities later in life.

The forehead is best reconstructed by expanding and moving tissue transversely from either side. Attempts at moving tissue in the vertical direction result in irregularities and malposition of the brow or hairline and rarely succeed except in minor deformities. Moving tissue laterally on the forehead requires integrity of the anterior branch of the temporal artery because the supratrochlear and supraorbital arteries are usually divided. Patients should be warned that sensation in the forehead will be significantly impaired after such procedures.

In large losses of the nose, the forehead can be expanded and rotated inferiorly for reconstruction. Expanders should encompass the entire forehead so that the donor site can be primarily closed. It is critical that the infrastructure of the nose be reconstructed, or the expanded flap will contract and become distorted. Cantilevered cranial bone grafts are required to reconstruct the dorsum, and conchal cartilage grafts to reconstruct the alae. The expanded flap is then draped over these structures to create an aesthetic and functional nose.

The lateral face and neck are similar in color, texture, and hair-bearing quality. Classically, the neck is expanded and rotated as a large flap to reconstruct the aesthetic unit of the cheek. Suture lines should rest along the nasolabial fold and infraorbital area (Fig. 17-4). The tension and mass of such tissue predispose to ectropion of the lower lid, and therefore this flap must be secured in position both medially and laterally to the orbit with buried permanent sutures. In addition, the flap should be constructed so that it extends lateral and superior to the lateral canthus, as described by Mustardé. Incorporating the overlying platsyma increases the vascularity of the neck flap but compromises its rotation.

The periorbital and perioral regions, and occasionally the forehead, can be reconstructed with full-thickness skin grafts from the neck. The area immediately above the clavicles and below the hair-bearing tissue of the neck matches the periocular and perioral areas extremely well. It is transferred as an expanded or nonexpanded full-thickness graft to accomplish reconstructions within aesthetic units. Donor defects are closed primarily in a transverse direction.

These are ideal aims, and many times the compression of local tissue by disease and trauma makes it impossible to achieve an optimal situation. The surgeon must then decide when and how to compromise to achieve the best possible result. Sometimes, the expansion procedure must be abandoned and a prefabricated flap or a distant free flap used.

Expansion in the Trunk

Massive quantities of tissue are available for expansion in the trunk and back areas. Tissues in these areas are usually thick, and adipose tissue is adequate for expansion with large prostheses to be carried out quickly with relatively low risk. The placement of prostheses below muscle allows the expansion of myocutaneous flaps with large adjacent skin paddles that can be moved either as a classic myocutaneous flap or as a free flap.

In general, expansion and movement of tissue in a radial fashion are more easily accomplished than is the movement of tissue in an axial pattern. Although the scars resulting from an axial pattern of expansion and flap movement are usually aesthetically better, considerably more expansion is required, and the movement of tissue is considerably more difficult.

Planning is necessary to avoid displacing the nipple–areolar complex to an asymmetrical position in both male and female patients, particularly infants. Expanded flaps should be mobilized so that suture lines do not come to rest axially in the axilla, as later contracture is frequently seen.

Expansion in the areas of the back and buttocks requires considerable cooperation by the patient to avoid excessive pressure and extrusion. Even the most cooperative patient may encounter some difficulty secondary to pressure and positioning at night. For this reason, the use of multiple expanders, which can be expanded relatively rapidly to minimize the filling phase, makes it easier to achieve a final reasonable result. The use of extremely large prostheses, even in the back and anterior trunk, may result in considerable gravitational deformation and thinning of flaps inferiorly.

Breast Reconstruction

Following its introduction by Radovan and modifications by others later, tissue expansion became the method of choice for most surgeons performing breast reconstruction between 1980 and 1995. Refinements in autologous tissue transfer and controversy regarding silicone prostheses have made physicians look more carefully at the complications and less-than-optimal aesthetic results associated with the use of prostheses. Subsequent refinements in technique have been useful in minimizing complications and improving aesthetic results.

Tissue expansion in breast reconstruction is unique. Tissue must be developed to form a breast mound, and a significant degree of softness and resistance to later deformation are required. Radovan initially expanded in the subcutaneous space above the muscles. Although his results were at the time significant, later deformation and capsular contracture plus exposure have made this technique obsolete. Even with the use of polyurethane or other textured prostheses, very few surgeons continue to expand in the prepectoral space. Modifications in which the expansion prosthesis is placed beneath the pectoralis and other chest wall muscles have significantly improved aesthetic results and decreased complication rates (15).

Contoured protheses with integrated valves, and textured prostheses that appear to cause less capsular contracture and minimize migration of the implant during expansion, have been significant advances and are recommended. Prostheses with various geometrical shapes that more adequately mimic the shape of the normal breast produce better results than the older, round prostheses. Reconstruction of the breast can be performed either simultaneously with the mastectomy in selected cases or at a later date following recovery from the initial mastectomy.

Immediate Breast Reconstruction

With recent advances in preoperative evaluation, it is relatively easy to select those patients who will benefit from immediate breast reconstruction with tissue expanders at the time of mastectomy. Minimal periareolar, inframammary, or axillary incisions to treat localized neoplasms greatly facilitate the use of expanders at the time of mastectomy. Patients with localized disease and a moderate-size breast who are not expected to undergo radiation therapy are ideal patients for reconstruction with this technique. Implants with a base size equal to or slightly greater than the base size of the opposite breast, rather than the volume size, are selected. Excessive inflation of prostheses is well tolerated and can usually be accomplished to correct most volume asymmetries. A prosthesis should be placed in the subpectoral space to isolate it from the mastectomy and axillary dissection plane. The inframammary fold should be preserved if possible at the time of mastectomy so that better definition and symmetry with the opposite side can be obtained. Transposition of the serratus anterior, anterior rectus, pectoralis minor, or latissimus dorsi muscle may be necessary to augment the pectoralis and create an entirely separate submuscular plane. The inflation valve is usually allowed to egress through the muscle and is placed in a subcutaneous space either in the axilla or below the inframammary fold. The accumulation of lymphatic fluid in the mastectomy and axillary dissection site significantly predisposes the prosthesis to infection (16) (Fig. 17-7). The drainage of the subpectoral and the prepectoral space by separate closed suction drains minimizes the risk for excess lymphatic collection and infection.

Migration of the prosthesis, particularly after immediate breast reconstruction, is a problem that may lead to an asymmetrical breast reconstruction. It can be minimized by the use of textured expanders. Closure of the implant completely within a subpectoral muscle space is also helpful. The lateral margin of the submuscular closure is frequently tenuous and is the most frequent site of extrusion of the prosthesis laterally into the axillary space.

Careful attention to flap thickness during the mastectomy is necessary to preserve the vascular integrity of the

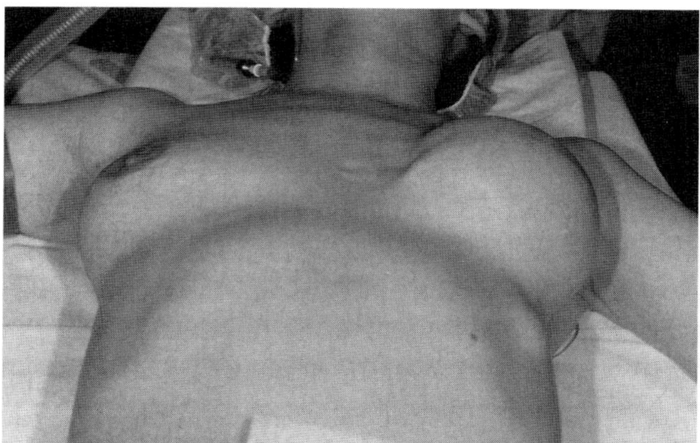

FIGURE. 17-7. Massive collection of lymph following immediate breast reconstruction. Although this patient did not become infected, a significant number of such cases do become compromised.

flap. Only enough fluid to eliminate dead space is placed in the prosthesis at the time of the initial mastectomy. Excess tension should not be placed on the overlying flaps because necrosis can quickly develop. Usually, 10 days are allowed to pass before inflation of the prosthesis is begun. Leaving the drain in the submuscular space during the first one or two inflations helps to force serum from this space.

Because implants tend to migrate superiorly, particularly during the course of expansion, the prosthesis is usually placed at or slightly lower than the inframammary fold of the opposite side. Placing the implant too low to compensate for a ptotic breast on the opposite side may make it difficult for the patient to wear a brassiere later because of discrepancies in the inframammary fold.

Inflation should be carried out weekly or biweekly with smaller volumes. In our experience, tissue expands more rapidly in immediate reconstruction than in delayed reconstruction. The prosthesis is usually overinflated by 500 to 600 mL for a period of 4 months to create later ptosis. The effect of overinflation on later capsular contracture continues to be debated (17). The capsule formed in this period, however, is helpful in tissue rearrangements at the time of permanent implant placement. High-profile implants with volumes that match that of the opposite side are used. Modern saline implants still do not produce results comparable with those attained with the old gel implants.

At the time of permanent implant placement, maneuvers such as the Ryan abdominal advancement can be helpful to reconstruct the inframammary fold. Permanent sutures are almost always required in these cases.

Capsular contracture and distortion of the breast remain the major problems following breast reconstruction with tissue expanders. Most breasts reconstructed by this technique do not have the projection and ptosis that are achieved with autologous tissue transfer. With adequate explanation to the patient, a breast reconstructed in this way is usually an acceptable alternative that is well tolerated.

Secondary Breast Reconstruction

Most mastectomy patients undergo reconstruction at a later, second procedure following the initial mastectomy. Ideally, one should wait 2 to 3 months after mastectomy for delayed reconstruction. Although tissue may be more scarred and more resistant to expansion during secondary reconstruction, the process offers several advantages. The flaps on the chest wall have usually recovered from surgery, and the maintenance of separate prepectoral and retropectoral pockets is less important than in immediate reconstruction. Usually, the upper medial two-thirds of the prosthesis is covered with pectoral muscle, and the inferior lateral aspect of the expander remains in the subcutaneous space. Except in a very few patients, expansion can be carried out rapidly and safely. Seroma collection in delayed reconstruction is significantly less than in immediate reconstruction.

Positioning of the expander is important in obtaining symmetry with the opposite side. If the opposite breast is large and ptotic, the inframammary fold on the reconstructed side can be lowered to create the illusion of better symmetry. Placing the implant too low, however, makes it difficult later for the patient to wear a brassiere. It is helpful to overexpand and leave the expander in place for 4 to 6 months following maximal expansion when reconstructing a ptotic breast.

As in immediate breast reconstructions, capsular contracture and deformation of the breast remain the major problems in delayed reconstructions.

Extrusion of breast implants almost always occurs through previous incisions. Layered closure of muscle and subcutaneous spaces with large, absorbable sutures is recommended. The formation of striae on the breast may be noted during expansion. This is usually a complication of excessively rapid expansion but can occur in young patients for unknown reasons.

REFERENCES

1. Antonyshyn O, Gruss JS, Mackinnon SE, et al. Complications of soft tissue expansion. *Br J Plast Surg* 1988;41:239–250.
2. Austad ED. Contraindications and complications in tissue-expansion. *Fac Plast Surg* 1988;5:379–382.
3. Manders EK, Schenden MJ, Furrey JA, et al. Soft tissue expansion: concept and complications. *Plast Reconstr Surg* 1984; 74:493–507.
4. Neale HW, High RM, Billmire DA, et al. Complications of controlled tissue expansion in the pediatric burn patient. *Plast Reconstr Surg* 1988;82:840–845.
5. Fenton O. Complications of soft-tissue expansion. *Br J Plast Surg* 1988;41:49–50.
6. Jackson JT, Sharpe DT, Polley J, et al. Use of external reservoirs in tissue expansion. *Plast Reconstr Surg* 1987;80:266–271.
7. Cohen IK, Roberts C. Lidocaine to relieve pain with tissue expansion of the breast. *Plast Reconstr Surg* 1987;79:489.
8. Cole RP, Gault DT, Mayou BJ, et al. Pain and forehead expansion. *Br J Plast Surg* 1991;44:41–43.
9. Goldstein RD, Schuster SH. Methylene blue, a simple adjunct to aid in soft tissue expansion. *Plast Reconstr Surg* 1986;77:452.
10. Ashall G, Quaba A. A hemorrhagic hazard of tissue expansion. *Plast Reconstr Surg* 1987;79:627–630.
11. Nordstrom REA. Antibiotics in the tissue expander to decrease the rate of infection [Letter]. *Plast Reconstr Surg* 1988;81: 137–138.
12. Argenta LC. Controlled tissue expander. *Br J Plast Surg* 1984;37:520–529.
13. Donelan MB Jr. Complications of controlled tissue expansion in the pediatric burn patient. *Plast Reconstr Surg* 1988;82:846–848.
14. Elias DL, Baird WL, Zubowicz VN. Applications and complications of tissue expansion in pediatric patients. *J Pediatr Surg* 1991;226:15–21.
15. Dickson MG, Sharpe DT. The complications of tissue expansion in breast reconstruction: a review of 75 cases. *Br J Plast Surg* 1987;40:629–635.
16. Armstrong RW, Berkowitz RL, Bolding F. Infection following breast reconstruction. *Ann Plast Surg* 1989;23:284–288.
17. Holmes JD. Capsular contracture after breast reconstruction with tissue expansion. *Br J Plast Surg* 1989;42:591–594.

Discussion

TISSUE EXPANSION

ERNEST K. MANDERS

Dr. Argenta's chapter is a thorough primer on soft tissue expansion, in which he clearly outlines the principles underlying the safe and effective use of this technique. Of the advice given, the admonition that planning is the essence of success is of paramount importance. Careful planning ensures better results through the development of an expanded flap of optimal geometry. A well-planned surgery in which scars are carefully positioned not to be obvious at the conclusion of the reconstructive program will result in a superior aesthetic appearance.

PSYCHOLOGICAL ASPECTS

The proper psychological preparation of the patient should be given special emphasis. It may be said that most patients undergoing soft tissue expansion are in a hurry. The surgeon must deal with this fact on an up-front basis. Patients must be told that the surgeon is sympathetic but that impatience works against a successful result, and that one cannot plan to make an advancement on a given date so many weeks or months after the insertion of expanders. The expansion process must continue until measurement shows that an adequate flap has been created to allow a successful reconstruction. During the course of expansion, especially when expanders become more difficult to conceal, the surgeon must be sensitive to the patient's feelings and help the patient cope with the change in appearance. A case may be made that the psychological aspects of tissue expansion are the most neglected part of the experience from the patient's point of view.

INCISIONS

Incisions can be made close to or distant from the edge of a defect. Always, in the placement of incisions, the question of where the final scars will lie should be considered. The technique should be directed at imposing a minimal scar burden on the patient. Very often, this is best accomplished by incising within the defect if it is a congenital nevus, or at the edge of the defect if it is an area of skin graft to be replaced. Then the scar of the initial placement incision will be eliminated at the time of tissue advancement. Although I have tried placing expanders through remote incisions, I have generally abandoned this technique in favor of the quicker, easier, more direct approach through an incision at the edge of the defect. It should be emphasized that this is safe provided one makes certain to create a pocket to accommodate the expander that is large enough so that the edge of the device will lie well away from the line of closure.

VALVE PLACEMENT

The placement of the filling port is a matter of some importance. Valves may be integrated into the envelope of the expander or attached to it by a tube. In the head and neck area and in breast reconstruction, integrated valves have a place and may significantly simplify surgery (1). It is a nuisance to make a separate pocket for the expander port and then retrieve it when it is embedded in a fibrous capsule. Under general anesthesia, this is less difficult, but if one is operating under local anesthesia, it is most assuredly a great inconvenience for both patient and surgeon.

An alternative to placing the valve in a remote position is to place it on top of the expander. One should place it near the *edge* of the expander, where it will typically ride atop a cushion of saline solution and be very well tolerated. It is best not to place the port over the exact center of the dome of the expander because the tension on the skin is greatest at this point, and so is the dermal thinning that occurs. Also, more pressure is placed on the skin when the patient rests on the expander dome with the port on top. By observing these precautions, one can use this means of port placement successfully in many cases. This approach has shortened significantly the time required for expander insertion and retrieval. The valve is readily palpable, and families can safely perform expansion at home even with the expander port placed above the envelope.

E. K. Manders: Department of Surgery, University of Pittsburgh Medical Center, Pittsburgh, Pennsylvania

USE OF LOCAL ANESTHESIA

At the time of placement, local anesthesia may be the technique of choice for keeping the patient comfortable during surgery. This is another advantage of tissue expansion; when the expanders are placed in a subcutaneous plane, or in a subgaleal plane in the case of the scalp, the patient can be kept comfortable very successfully with local anesthesia with or without sedation. In the case of children, a general anesthesia will be needed, but many adults appreciate undergoing surgery with a minimum of recovery from anesthesia.

DRAINS

In reading Dr. Argenta's description of how he uses drains, it occurs to me that I may be overly zealous in my use of drains. Obviously, like most surgeons, I do not drain the pockets created for breast augmentation. One can ask, If the expander pocket is not significantly different, should it be drained?

In some situations, it may be advantageous to drain—for example, when large expander pockets are created over the scalp, particularly around the forehead. A drain may decrease facial swelling, especially of the eyelids. Also, when expanders are placed in the lower extremity, the tendency for seroma formation is greater. Therefore, drains may be helpful when expanders are placed in the lower extremity.

INFLATION

The process of inflation is crucial to success. We frequently employ home expansion carried out by parents, other members of the family, neighbors, or on occasion even the patient (Fig. 17D-1). We instruct patients and their families to inject until the first sensation of tightness is experienced. We know that this sensation corresponds to a pressure that is below or just at the level of capillary pressure; in minutes, the pressure recedes because the investing capsule relaxes, and the patient is comfortable. High pressures are to be avoided. Also, if one is expanding over muscle, one must be particularly careful because if the muscle is rendered ischemic, it will swell and cause an unremitting severe pain. Should such pain occur, the proper treatment is simple removal of a small volume of fluid to make the expander soft and restore circulation to the underlying ischemic muscle.

In the case of children or persons who cannot communicate, or in the case of areas that are relatively insensate, one can use a 23-gauge scalp vein needle as a manometer. If one simply stretches the tubing in the air above the needle as it stands in the filling port, one has a manometer that corresponds approximately to pressure of 20 mm Hg. This is a simple test. If the fluid runs out over the top of the needle when the syringe is detached from the tubing, then the pressure is greater than 20 mm Hg. If the meniscus falls in the tubing, then the pressure is less. This test can add safety to the process of expansion and give confidence to those who are new to it.

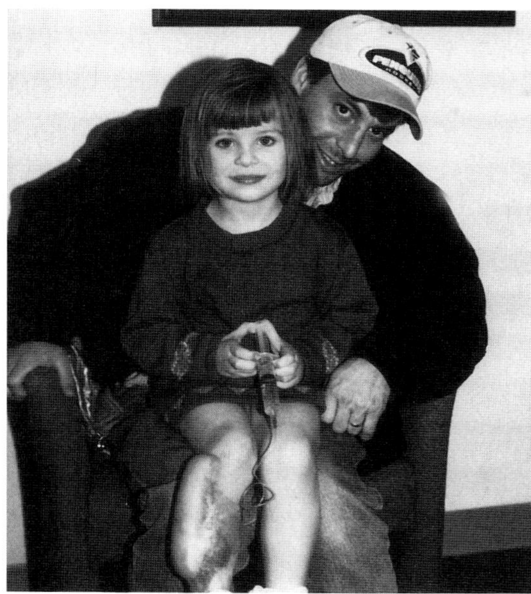

FIGURE 17D-1. A child can administer her own injection with parental supervision.

CONTRAINDICATIONS

Contraindications are mentioned, including inadequate vascularity, as occurs in areas of excessive scarring or previous radiation therapy. Open sores are another contraindication. They can lead to contamination of the skin with a lawn of bacteria. It has been our practice to treat superficial wounds until they are healed or to cover them with allograft so that they are effectively closed. This makes the process of tissue expander placement much safer.

One must also be aware of foreign bodies, which can confound the placement of expanders. Wires used to reconstruct the cranium after open fractures may be a source of contamination from associated granulation tissue and puncture from sharp wire ends.

Irradiation does alter the elasticity of tissue, but it seems that if a patient has received 5,000 rads or less to the pectoral area, then soft tissue expansion can probably be used successfully in a subsequent breast reconstruction. The chances of success are increasingly diminished as the total dose of radiation therapy increases.

Many patients are self-conscious about their appearance, and this problem should be addressed. It is unfortunate that a major impediment to the use of soft tissue expansion for the treatment of undesired male pattern baldness is self-consciousness of the male patient. In 4 months' time, if he were routinely confident, he could be completely converted from hippocratic baldness with a fringe around the top to a complete cover of natural hair. Unfortunately, even hats are often not enough camouflage for sensitive men. Nevertheless, with proper encouragement, it should be possible to help patients cope so that the benefits of expansion can be enjoyed by all. It is important to note that virtually all expanders can be hidden except for those placed around the midface. As our experience has grown, we find that expansion in the central face is indicated less and less often, and therefore today virtually all expanders can be hidden by the use of scarves, shawls, hats, and bulky garments.

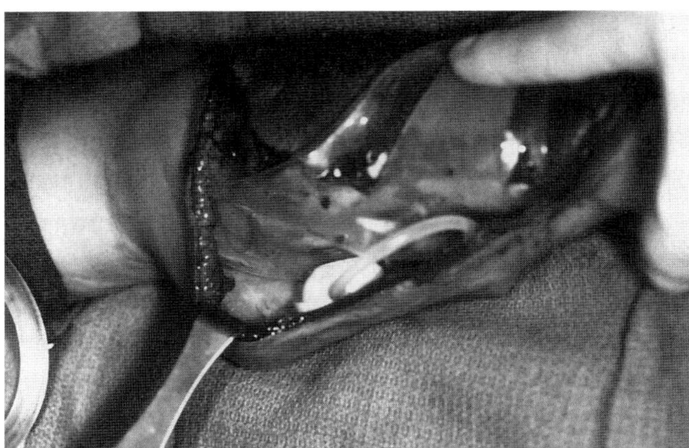

FIGURE 17D-2. The injection port became displaced and inverted after a seroma distended this expander pocket located in the lower leg.

COMPLICATIONS

The management of complications should include strategies to deal with several problems (2,3). Implant failure is one of the chief problems. Needle holes are the usual culprit. Puncture can be caused at the time of implantation by the injudicious placement of a suture for wound closure, at the time of filling if the envelope is punctured, or more rarely at the time of searching for the filling port if the fill tube itself is punctured. The fill tube cannot seal itself, and a puncture inevitably results in a slow leak.

Another rare complication leading to implant failure is a fibrin plug within the injection port or the fill port tubing. We have seen this after evacuating all the air from an expander. The result was a negative pressure within the device. Serum entered through the needle hole and a serum clot formed within the fill port and tubing. We demonstrated that when the device is removed, an injection of urokinase, as is used to open central venous fluid lines, can open the expander. Should it be difficult to inject an expander immediately after placement and before successful fluid administration, the surgeon might try to inject urokinase to open the tube in case a fibrin clot is present.

At one time, we routinely injected air into soft tissue expanders and immersed them in a basin of saline solution to check for leaks before implantation. We no longer do this. We have never seen a defective soft tissue expander delivered from its protective wrapping to the surgeon. The defects have always been caused by surgical misadventures.

Occasionally, the surgeon may be concerned that a rupture or puncture of the expander has been caused inadvertently during placement. If this should be a concern, the injection of saline solution with or without methylene blue will usually reveal the leak.

Deflation can be a significant problem if a large hole has developed. Two sources of envelope failure with rapid deflation are an opening at the site of entry of the remote fill port tubing, and an opening at the site where the envelope is bonded to a rigid base. Deflation can also be caused by so-called fold flaw deformities, in which a small fold has been mechanically stressed back and forth so that the material becomes fatigued and the envelope cracks. If a leak occurs, sometimes it is possible to continue the expansion with more frequent injection of saline solution. At other times, it is best to move to the operating room and either carry out the advancement with the tissue available or replace the expander by substituting a new device to complete the job.

Seromas can be a problem if proper drainage has not been instituted. We have seen soft tissue expanders with integrated valves turn upside down in seroma-filled cavities in the lower extremity. The only good way to detect such malposition is with ultrasonography or radiography. In our experience, we have not been able to turn an expander with an integrated port successfully so that the valve can be entered again. We have also seen a seroma cause rotation of a remote valve placed on top of an expander at the edge of the expander pocket (Fig. 17D-2).

Infection

The biggest problem today is infection. Occasionally, one sees a redness in the skin without any detection of purulent fluid in the pocket during aspiration over the expander port. We have seen several such cases through the years, and they have resolved after treatment with antibiotics. If cloudy fluid is noted in the pocket containing the injection port, however, then the expander must be removed and the pocket drained. If no significant tissue-phase infection is present, it may be possible to carry out the advancement, as described by Dr. Argenta. Also as noted, if the expansion is intended to create a pocket for a subsequent breast implant, this goal cannot be accomplished in the face of bacteriologic contamination.

Periprosthetic infections probably occur in most cases when bacteria are introduced at the time of expander placement. However, it is important to note that in the case of children, the hematogenous route is not unknown. Most recently, we have seen periprosthetic infection develop fol-

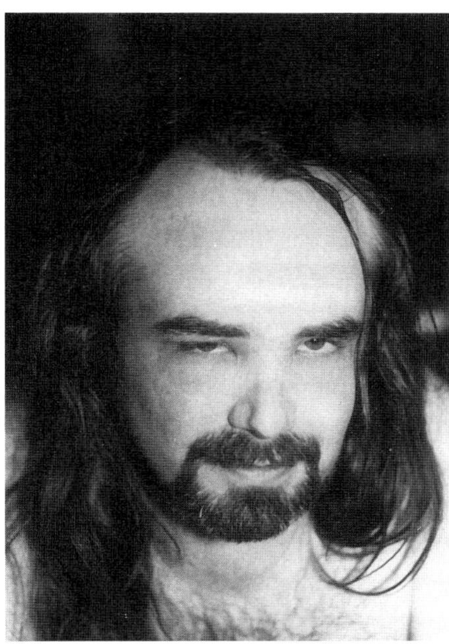

FIGURE 17D-3. Temple and upper eyelid swelling signal the presence of a late postoperative infection around scalp expanders placed for the treatment of male pattern alopecia.

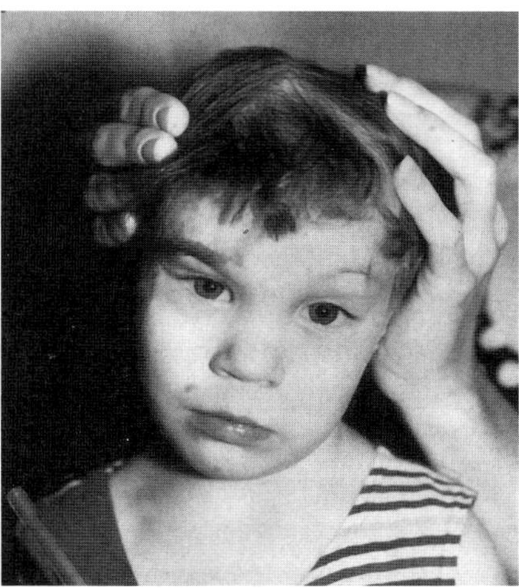

FIGURE 17D-4. This postoperative bony ridge, which formed at the edge of the expander cavity, eventually receded without treatment.

lowing middle ear infection (4). Also, it is important to note that exposure of the expander at any point may lead to periprosthetic infection.

One can recognize infection from the signs of tenderness and swelling, and by the aspiration of cloudy fluid above the expander dome. If the infection occurs around an expander in the head and neck, swelling is often present in the face. In particular, in the case of a scalp expander infection in the frontal area, the eyelids are often swollen, a sign that something is amiss. Early after surgery, one expects some eyelid edema with a forehead or frontal expander. However, if this sign appears several weeks into expansion, it is very probably the herald of infection (Fig. 17D-3).

Exposure

Exposure is a complication that the surgeon should avoid by carefully choosing an expander that lies relatively flat within a large pocket. The other factor that is so important in avoiding this complication is a careful, deliberate, slow filling. Often, exposure is the result of overzealous inflation by the patient, the physician, or both of them. Thin spots can often be recognized, as described by Dr. Argenta, as blue or opalescent gray areas. When one palpates the area, the skin feels distinctly thin. Before a problem develops, one can transilluminate the expander in a dark room. When this is done, the thin areas of impending exposure appear as bright points of light. This is another way to identify a sharp envelope fold that may lead to exposure.

In our experience at present, most exposures result from infection. At one time, exposures were the result of placing an overly large expander in a pocket that was too small. Occasionally, the exposure resulted from the use of an expander with a stiff backer. A stiff backer on the curve of a child's calvarium or on a child's extremity at times lifted the corner of the expander off the underlying muscle, so that the corner eventually pushed itself through the skin to produce a dreaded exposure (Fig. 17D-4). Stiff backers over curved surfaces should be avoided.

The process of advancement requires careful consideration. In the first place, one should always plan for advancement by measuring across the dome of the expander. One then measures by sight the base width of the expander dome. By subtracting the base width from the arc measured with a tape lying over the expander from edge to edge at the base, one gets an idea of the increase in arc of the expanded flap. One can then measure the width of the defect to see if the increase in flap arc length equals or exceeds the width of the defect.

That said, it is still necessary during surgery to release the flap and carry out a trial before the lesion to be removed is entirely eliminated. It is very discouraging to resect an area of skin graft or nevus and then carry out an advancement only to find that one is short of tissue. A trial advancement and marking the farthest reach of the leading edge will prevent this sort of dilemma.

Capsule

Lastly, one must always consider how to deal with the capsule. At times, mobility and advancement will be increased if one scores or partially cuts the capsule. One should be conservative. The capsule does confer a greater blood supply to the expanded flap (1). If the expansion has been designed well, it should not be necessary to remove or extensively excise it at the base and mobilize it. However, it will frequently be necessary to incise the capsule at the edge of the flaps so that the tissue advances more easily and lies flatter afterwards.

REGIONAL CONCERNS

Scalp

In dealing with scalp advancements, it is always wise to try to avoid *T*-shaped closures at the hairline (2–7). These scars widen, and the perpendicular intersection of the closure and the hairline results in an area of alopecia that is a nuisance and usually requires correction.

One should counsel patients regarding hair loss. Very often during expansion, the scalp rubs on the pillow or bed, and hair loss may ensue. Some induction of the telogen phase of the hair follicle cycle may occur during expansion, so that hair seen in the shower causes the patient some concern. An effluvium commonly follows surgery, and the patient needs to be reassured during this time that given some 6 weeks to 3 months of time, hair growth will resume and the hair density will be much improved.

At the time of surgery, it is very important to have patients shower or otherwise bathe to keep the areas of surgery clean. We shampoo patients' hair on the operating table after surgery and have them shampoo themselves the day after surgery. If efforts are not made to keep the scalp clean, crusts of serum and clot form that often result in the loss of hair when the coagulum itself is removed.

Changes in the cranial contour have been noted by all surgeons performing scalp expansion (Fig. 17D-4). These changes almost always correct themselves with no intervention on the surgeon's part. It is not necessary to address the edges of a bathtub deformity. It is not necessary to address bony ridges. Given time, these invariably become flat, and the symmetrical curves of the skull are restored.

Forehead

The forehead still poses significant obstacles to easy aesthetic reconstruction. With time, I have personally grown more conservative, recognizing that it is difficult to expand the forehead with the intent of moving the expansion a large distance from one side to the other. In the past, some expansions were marched across the forehead by carrying out long incisions at the hairline and above the eyebrow. This led to unwanted scars and diminished cutaneous sensibility. A carefully applied partial-thickness skin graft still has its place, especially on the lateral forehead (Fig. 17D-5). It may make it possible to avoid incisions centrally and over the contralateral eyebrow and lead to an aesthetically superior result.

Nasal Reconstruction

For nasal reconstruction, fashioning a stable skeleton for the new nose is absolutely essential, as Dr. Argenta points out. We have moved from using bone to utilizing cartilage. The most difficult area to manage is the columellar strut, which must be invested by the expanded flap or other tissues (2,8). Often, tissues in the area of the nasal spine are inadequate. The surgeon who is contemplating a reconstruction of the anterior maxillary alveolus, or who sees that soft tissue is inadequate in the area of the nasal spine, should consider a first procedure to move adequate tissue into the area before placing the strut and covering it for a total nasal reconstruction.

Neck

Although neck skin does indeed resemble facial skin, it is exceedingly difficult to elevate the skin of the neck up across the line of the mandible onto the cheek. An optical illusion is created here in that when one carries out an expansion on the underside of the chin, one has filled a concavity. One has not actually made more skin, but has rather moved the concavity underlying the mandible outward to form a convexity with what is essentially almost the same amount of skin. This results in difficult advancements that have caused great unhappiness on many occasions. A better strategy to expand soft tissues for the reconstruction of large cheek defects was developed by Dr. Robert Spence (9). He has taught us the value of supraclavicular expansion to create large flaps for neck and facial reconstruction with great success.

Central Face

Few reasons are left to expand in the central face. This process is difficult in that it often produces a fat atrophy that leads to contour irregularities. We now know that one can perform reverse facelift serial advancements and remove even large defects.

Trunk

Expansion on the trunk, both front and back, can be somewhat difficult if one does not pay attention to careful placement of the injection port. Truncal expanders tend to migrate downward, and therefore remote ports should always be placed on or above the expander. If it is placed below, the expander envelope may actually descend over the injection port and make continued filling impossible (Fig. 17D-5).

One should also be very careful to place the expander fill port at a depth where it can be easily palpated and filled. If the patient has a fairly thick subcutaneous fatty layer, care must be taken to place the valve superficially enough that it can be easily injected.

Breast Reconstruction

Breast reconstruction has been significantly improved by the use of soft tissue expansion (10–13). Perhaps three of ev-

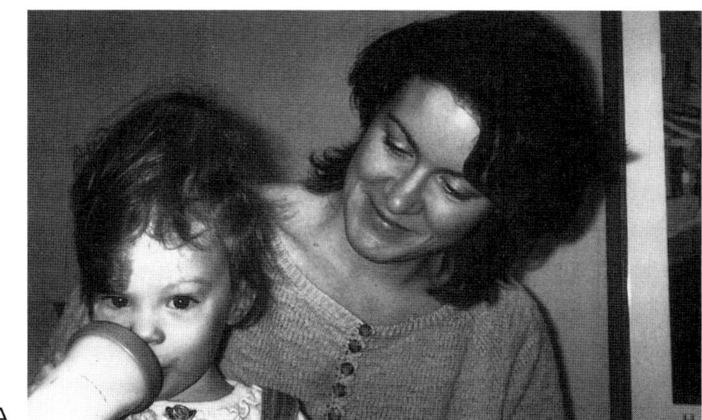

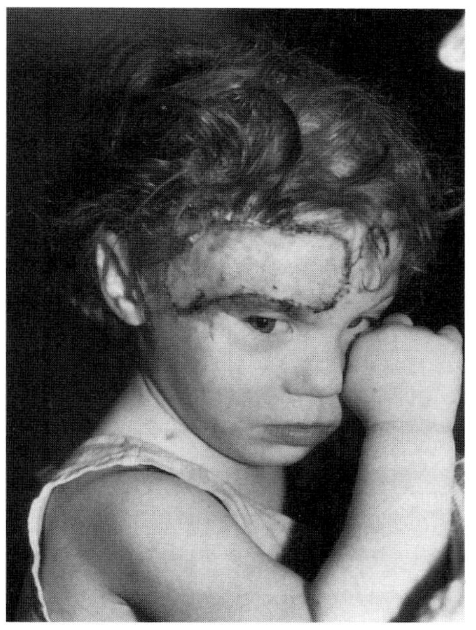

A B

FIGURE 17D-5. A: Scalp expansion is under way for replacement of a right frontal congenital melanocytic nevus. The right forehead will be skin-grafted. **B:** Early after excision of the forehead nevus and application of a split-thickness skin graft from the left parietal scalp..

ery four breast reconstructions were accomplished through the use of tissue expansion before the silicone gel breast implant scare. Fearing the legal consequences of using silicone gel implants, plastic surgeons and their patients moved toward an increasing use of autogenous tissue reconstruction. With the debunking of the spurious legal claims, the use of tissue expansion is now on the rise again, and tissue expansions will probably constitute two-thirds to three-fourths of reconstructions in this cost-conscious era.

The technique can be very predictable if one measures the degree of expansion (14). The surgeon can predict the patient's appearance if the dimensions of the skin envelope on the unoperated side are measured. Selecting a point on the clavicle and measuring across the breast to the inframammary fold and noting the distance will allow the surgeon to determine the shortage of tissue by making a comparable measurement on the operated side. As the expansion is carried out, the surgeon should repeat this measurement to determine progress in the regeneration of the appropriate skin envelope. When the full dimension has been reached, the surgeon should remove fluid from the expanded side until the breast volume is like that of the unoperated breast. At this point, the skin dimension should be measured again. It is common to find a contraction of the skin envelope of as much as 1 to even 4 cm when the tension in the expander is reduced. This tells the surgeon that if a prosthesis filled with saline solution is placed within the pocket, the dimensions will be smaller and the breast less ptotic than desired.

The solution is to restore the fluid to the expander and to continue to expand for another 1, 2, 3, or 4 cm as needed to obtain the full dimensions of the breast envelope for an ideal expansion. This is a simple engineering approach that will yield a predictable result when the final prosthesis is put in place.

CONCLUSION

Tissue expansion is elegant in its simplicity. This apparent simplicity should not beguile the operator into thinking that the steps are absolutely obvious and without some subtlety. As in any endeavor, experience leads to ever better results, and the neophyte will certainly find this to be the case in tissue expansion.

Tissue expansion has many values. Chief among them is that it allows for the reconstruction of defects with adjacent tissues resembling those that were lost. Tissue expansion is particularly valuable when special adnexal features, such as hair, need to be restored in a uniform pattern. Scalp reconstruction through expansion has led to extraordinarily satisfying results.

Soft tissue expansion takes time, but it is a safe and reliable means of reconstruction that is very rarely attended by tissue loss. Even in the event of infection or extrusion, tissue is not normally lost; the greatest cost is delay.

The technique is highly rewarding for patient and physician alike. With careful planning, attention to details, and regular continued emotional support for the patient, tissue expansion can be a most rewarding reconstructive adventure.

REFERENCES

1. Mottaleb M, Wong RKM, Manders EK, et al. Tissue expansion. In: Riley WB, ed. *Instructional courses,* vol 1. St. Louis: Mosby, 1988:277–304.
2. Manders EK, Schenden MJ, Furrey JA, et al. Soft tissue expansion: concepts and complications. *Plast Reconstr Surg* 1984;74:493–507.
3. Manders EK, Da Paula P. Repeated tissue expansions. In: Grotting JC, ed. *Reoperative aesthetic and reconstructive plastic surgery.* St. Louis: Quality Medical Publishing, 1995:137–153.
4. Mason AC, Davison SP, Manders EK. Tissue expander infections in children: look beyond the expander pocket. *Ann Plast Surg* 1999;43:539–541.
5. Antonyshyn O, Gruss JS, Zucker R, et al. Tissue expansion in head and neck reconstruction. *Plast Reconstr Surg* 1988;82:58–64.
6. Argenta LC. Controlled tissue expansion in facial reconstruction. In: Baker SR, Swanson NA, eds. *Local flaps in facial reconstruction.* St. Louis: Mosby, 1995: 517–544.
7. Manders, EK, Graham WP III, Schenden MJ, et al. Scalp expansion to eliminate large scalp defects. *Ann Plast Surg* 1984;12:305–312.
8. Manders EK, Carlton JM, Wong RKM. Soft tissue expansion in the head and neck. In: Paparella, Shumrick, eds. *Otolaryngology,* vol 4. Philadelphia: WB Saunders, 1990:2871–2881.
9. Spence RJ. Experiences with novel uses of tissue expanders in burn reconstruction of the face and neck. *Ann Plast Surg* 1992;28:453–464.
10. Radovan C. Breast reconstruction after mastectomy using the temporary expander. *Plast Reconstr Surg* 1982;69:195–201.
11. Argenta LC, Austad ED. Principles and techniques of tissue expansion. In: McCarthy JG, ed. *Plastic surgery.* Philadelphia: WB Saunders, 1990:475–507.
12. Sasaki GH. Tissue expansion. In: Jurkiewicz MJ, Krizek TJ, Mathes SJ, et al., eds. *Plastic surgery: principles and practice.* St. Louis: Mosby, 1990:1609–1634.
13. Maxwell GP. Breast reconstruction following mastectomy and surgical management of the patient with high-risk breast disease. In: Smith JW, Aston SJ, eds. *Grabb and Smith's plastic surgery,* 4th ed. Boston: Little, Brown and Company, 1991:1203–1247.
14. Manders EK, Furrey JA. The evolution of soft tissue expansion for the reconstruction of the breast. In: Bohmert HH, Leis HP, Jackson IT, eds. *Breast cancer: conservative and reconstructive surgery.* New York: Thieme Medical Publishers, 1989:238–242.

18

LASERS

DAVID B. APFELBERG
TINA S. ALSTER

Complications of laser surgery can be understood best by reviewing the evolution of laser technology over the past 3 decades. Lasers initially were designed to operate in a continuous-wave (CW) mode, which produced a continuous beam of radiation that subsequently was absorbed by a target chromophore. Although particular skin structures could be targeted using these early lasers, their use was limited because the energy emitted not only altered the target, but also spread by heat conduction into adjacent normal tissue. The nonselective thermal damage produced in adjacent tissue resulted in significant side effects and complications, namely, scarring and hypopigmentation.

The safety and efficacy that we have come to expect from modern lasers can be attributed to the ground-breaking work of Anderson and Parrish (1) in the early 1980s. Their theory of selective photothermolysis set the rules for specific tissue destruction through manipulation of the type of laser energy produced and the manner in which it was delivered. Thus, a specific chromophore or target can be selectively destroyed with minimal collateral thermal tissue damage when the laser wavelength matches that absorbed by the chromophore and when the target is exposed to the laser energy for an interval less than its thermal relaxation time (the time it takes after laser impact for the target to cool by 50%).

Lasers designed upon the theory of selective photothermolysis are more specific and have a lower risk profile in terms of scarring yet have their own unique side effect profiles. Depending upon the wavelength and pulse durations delivered, pigmentary changes, epidermal cell injury, textural changes, as well as crusting and tissue splatter potentially can occur. It is important to remember that even the safest of lasers can cause injury if used incorrectly. Repetitive or overlapping pulses, excessive energy or power settings, and improper patient selection potentially can result in a high rate of morbidity with the use of any medical laser. The following provides an overview of the complications encountered with currently available laser systems.

D.B. Apfelberg: Atherton Plastic Surgery Center, Atherton, California, and Department of Plastic Surgery, Stanford University Medical Center, Stanford, California
T.S. Alster: Washington Institute of Dermatologic and Laser Surgery; and Departments of Medicine, Georgetown University Hospital, Washington, DC

LASER SKIN RESURFACING

Background

The use of lasers for resurfacing skin is now a well-accepted modality for the treatment of rhytides, photoaging, and atrophic acne scars. Many series have been published documenting the improvement that can be obtained in regional and full-face treatments with various carbon dioxide (CO_2) lasers (2–16). In many practices, this technique has replaced the more traditional chemical peel and dermabrasion as a procedure of choice. Laser resurfacing offers precise micron-level control with excellent visualization and involves the progressive removal of thin layers of tissue in a controlled manner, with minimal heat damage to the surrounding skin structures. Photovaporization of the epidermis and a variable amount of the dermis can be achieved by varying the fluence and number of passes applied to the skin. The CO_2 laser has been used to resurface the skin for many years, and recent refinements in pulsing or scanning techniques have allowed it to be used safely with few side effects. Newer lasers, such as the erbium:yttrium aluminum garnet (YAG) laser, offer other benefits (17–26).

Carbon Dioxide Lasers

CW CO_2 lasers have been used since the 1960s for photovaporization of a variety of superficial skin lesions. Because the 10,600-nm wavelength of the CO_2 laser is absorbed principally by water, this laser has a high affinity to skin, which is composed of 90% water. The high water absorption coefficient results in absorption of 90% of the laser light within a 20- to 30-μm layer of tissue. Taking into account the principles of selective photothermolysis (1), not only must the laser wavelength be specific for the target, but in the case of resurfacing, sufficient energy needs to be delivered in a brief time period in order to effect tissue vaporization without char formation (or overheating residual dermal tissue). Thus, CO_2 laser energy density needs to exceed 5 J/cm^2 in less than 1 ms in order to ablate 20 to 30 μm of tissue with minimal residual thermal damage (27).

Two different CO_2 laser technologies can be used to achieve this goal. The first applies high-energy, short pulses (e.g., Coherent Ultrapulse), and the second involves a continuous-mode system with a computerized scanner (e.g., Sharplan/ESC SilkTouch or FeatherTouch). The microprocessor-controlled scanner that accompanies the latter laser systems provides rapid movement of a focused laser beam across the skin, such that the radiation dwell time on any given point of tissue is less than 1 ms. Scanning sizes can be varied between 3 and 16 mm in diameter, and fluences between 5 and 16 J/cm^2 can be delivered with this system. Although several other skin resurfacing lasers now are available for resurfacing (e.g., Luxar Novapulse, Tissue Technologies TruPulse), the aforementioned systems typify well the range of lasers.

Erbium:Yttrium Aluminum Garnet Lasers

The erbium:YAG laser, which emits light at 2,940 nm, is absorbed approximately 10 to 12 times more by water-containing tissue than is the CO_2 laser. In addition, its brief pulse duration (250 to 350 μs) ablates tissue more efficiently, producing inconsequential amounts of residual thermal damage in the dermis. The ablation threshold of tissue (1.25 to 1.6 J/cm^2) is easily exceeded by erbium laser irradiation, resulting in immediate and forceful epidermal photovaporization. Because the ratio of energy used for ablation versus tissue heating is very high, 10 to 40 μm of tissue is ablated and only a narrow rim (5 to 20 μm) of residual thermal damage remains. Thus, approximately 2 to 3 μm/J/cm^2 is ablated with each erbium laser pass. Faster reepithelialization rates and shorter erythema durations are observed after erbium:YAG laser irradiation compared to CO_2 laser vaporization on a pass per pass basis. As additional erbium passes are made (and deeper dermal penetration is effected), pinpoint bleeding occurs due to the inability of the erbium laser to produce sufficient heat to coagulate small blood vessels.

Side Effects and Complications

As the depth of laser ablation increases in an attempt to efface more rhytides and scars, the patient may be at greater risk for the development of side effects or complications. Increased postoperative pain, prolonged erythema, and delayed wound healing have been associated with increased number of laser passes. The incidence of side effects and complications associated with laser resurfacing has been reported by several authors (28–34). Apfelberg (35) summarized the results of the laser task force survey of the members of the American Society of Aesthetic Plastic Surgery and members of the American Society of Plastic and Reconstructive Surgery concerning laser resurfacing. Responses to a questionnaire by 885 laser surgeons were analyzed and a detailed report on routine patient preparation, postoperative management, and complications of laser resurfacing was provided.

Typical Sequelae of Laser Resurfacing

All patients experience postlaser resurfacing erythema for a variable period of time (average 8 to 12 weeks). The erythema may vary in intensity, ranging from pale pink to fiery red. Gradual fading of erythema occurs over the first 2 to 3 months. Alster and West (36) reported decreased postoperative erythema intensity with the daily use of topical vitamin C beginning 2 to 5 weeks after resurfacing. Some surgeons advocate intermittent use of a topical steroid cream to decrease erythema related to irritation. At approximately 2 to 4 weeks, many patients experience pruritus, which can be additionally relieved by cool compress application and iced facial misting.

During the first couple of postoperative months, many patients also develop milia as a normal part of the wound healing response. The patient should be reassured that the milia typically disappear spontaneously; however, creams containing retinoic acid and/or manual extraction can be used to facilitate the process. Due to the blockage of pilosebaceous glands by occlusive dressings and/or petrolatum-based ointments, the patient also may experience an acne flare-up. This can occur at any time (typically 2 to 6 weeks postoperatively) and, in addition to the cessation of occlusive skin preparations, may require treatment with topical or systemic antibiotics and/or topical retinoic and azelaic acid.

The line of demarcation (Fig. 18-1) that is apparent between the laser-treated skin and normal skin normally will disappear within a few months after surgery. Camouflage makeup and reassurance typically are all that are necessary when patients are adequately prepared for its inevitable development. In an attempt to soften the line, some surgeons feather the edges of the treatment areas using decreased laser energy or by defocusing the laser beam by aiming it tangentially (rather than perpendicularly). Others peel with trichloroacetic acid to blend adjacent nonlased skin with the lased skin.

Patients who are tanned or who have excessive solar dyspigmentation of adjacent skin may complain about the abnormally pale appearance of their skin after the procedure. Reassurance regarding its normalcy and/or the use of a topical self-tanner typically suffice to treat the problem. After reepithelialization of skin that had been severely dyspigmented, long-standing, previously unnoticed telangiectasias or mild rosacea may become clinically apparent. These unwanted blood vessels can be treated effectively with a vascular-specific laser (see later). Synechia, or adherence of reepithelializing wound edges, may produce abnormal creases in

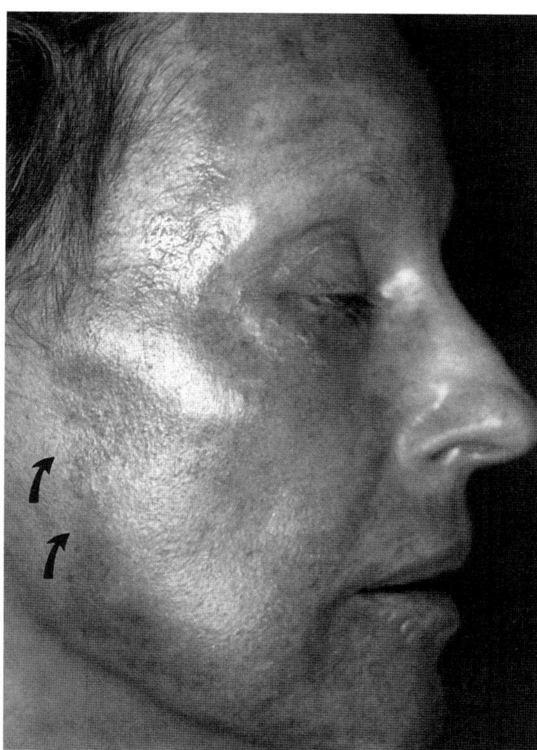

FIGURE 18-1. Patient 12 weeks after laser resurfacing demonstrating a line of demarcation *(arrows)* between the laser treated skin of the central facial area and the nonlasered skin at the periphery in the preauricular area.

the skin. These can be separated manually with lubrication of denuded skin to prevent readhesion (Fig. 18-2).

Approximately 8% to 12% of patients will experience either persistence or recurrence of rhytides. Several months after the procedure, when healing is complete, it is possible to perform "touchup" laser treatment in selected areas that have not had the expected degree of improvement with the anticipation that more satisfactory results will be effected.

Complications of Laser Resurfacing

Fortunately, true complications of laser resurfacing are rare. Postoperative bacterial or viral infections, left untreated, potentially could lead to sepsis and/or scarring. Herpes simplex viral infections often are heralded by a tingly or burning sensation, accompanied by punctate erosions and/or vesicles. Patients who are suspected of having a herpetic infection should have a Tzanck stain for detection of multinucleated giant cells and/or a viral culture of a skin swab and be started immediately on high (zoster) doses of antiviral agents (e.g., acyclovir [Zovirax], famciclovir [Famvir], valacyclovir [Valtrex]) (37). Bacterial infections also are possible, most commonly *Staphylococcus* and *Pseudomonas*. If an infection is suspected, bacterial cultures should be obtained and the patient given appropriate systemic antibiotics. Topical antibiotics, such as bacitracin and neomycin, commonly have produced allergic contact dermatitis and should be avoided after laser resurfacing. Fungal (e.g., *Candida*) infections also are possible (Fig. 18-3). A potassium hydroxide microscopic examination of pustules should be conducted. If pseudohyphae are seen, topical and/or oral antifungal agents (e.g., fluconazole) should be prescribed. The routine prophylactic use of antibiotics has been debated among laser surgeons, with just over 50% of laser surgeons routinely placing their patients on a 5- to 10-day course of antibiotics and antiviral agents.

Hypertrophic or keloid scarring has been seen after laser resurfacing, presumably due to cutaneous infection and/or overaggressive laser treatment (e.g., overlapping laser scans, multiple laser passes). Additionally, the use of isotretinoin (Accutane) within 1 year prior to laser skin resurfacing may diminish pilosebaceous gland activity, thereby creating a delay in the reepithelialization process and an impairment in wound healing with subsequent hypertrophic scar formation. A proactive approach to detect the possibility of hypertrophic scarring should be advocated, including palpation and inspection of skin at regular intervals postoperatively to assess for induration, variegation in erythema, and symptoms suggestive of hypertrophic scar formation. Topical fluorinated corticosteroids, intralesional steroid injections, topical silicone gel sheeting, or Cordran tape should be instituted. Some laser surgeons advise the use of intralesional 5-fluorouracil or verapamil (2.5 mg/mL), whereas others recommend pulsed dye laser irradiation. Alster and Nanni (38) reported significant improvement of laser-induced burn scars after an average of three pulsed dye laser treatments at 6- to 8-week intervals.

CO_2 laser resurfacing of the neck generally is not recommended by most laser surgeons because the neck skin is thinner and contains fewer pilosebaceous glands than does facial skin for reepithelialization (Fig. 18-4). Fitzpatrick and Goldman (39) reported on ten patients who had CO_2 laser resurfacing on the neck; three patients developed hypertrophic scar bands and four others demonstrated unacceptable hypopigmentation. However, other investigators successfully treated the neck without adverse sequelae, using less aggressive laser parameters (40,41).

Hyperpigmentation resulting after laser treatment may be a difficult problem for the patient, but fortunately it always is temporary (Fig. 18-5). It may result from inadvertent sun exposure on freshly lased skin; however, most cases are simply due to the natural presence of pigment in the skin. Thus, hyperpigmentation is seen more commonly in patients with dark skin tones. Hyperpigmentation diminishes with time, but it may last several months. It may be cleared more rapidly with the use of bleaching agents such as hydroquinone, kojic acid, or a combination treatment of 0.1% tretinoin topical (Retin-A) cream, 5% hydroquinone, and steroid (Kligman's formula) (42). The use of bleaching agents before the laser resurfacing procedure does not ap-

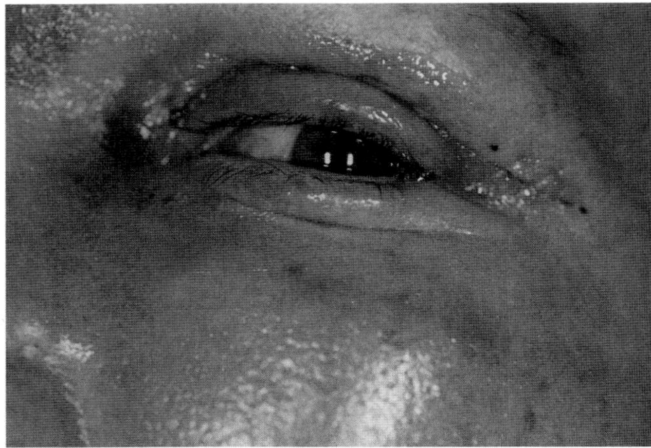

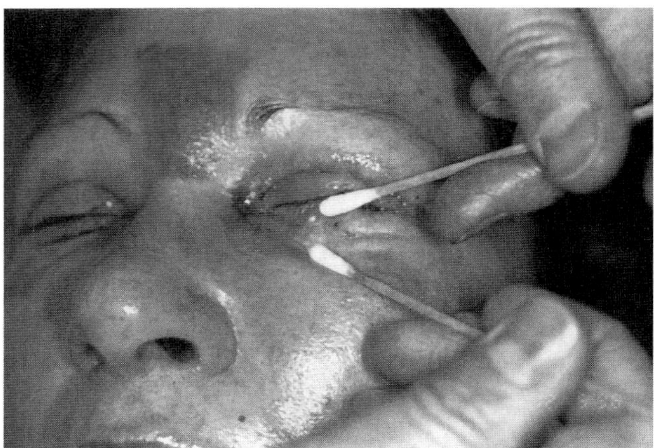

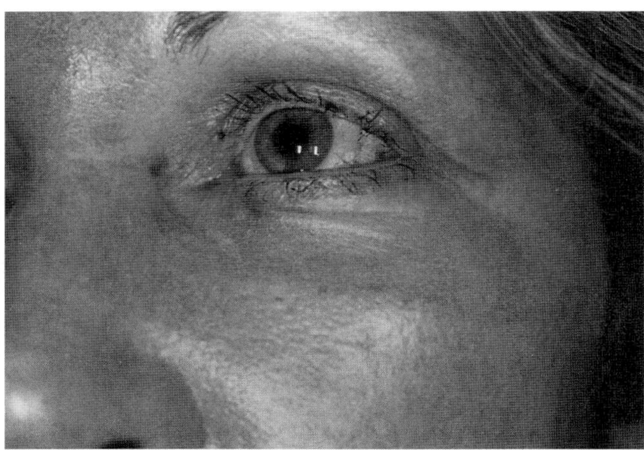

FIGURE 18-2. **A:** Synechia or abnormal infolding of the skin of the eyelid 2 weeks after laser resurfacing. **B:** Demonstration of manual release of adhesed skin edges. **C:** Final result is smooth nonindented skin.

pear to reduce the risk or resolution of postoperative hyperpigmentation (43). In a study of 100 patients randomly assigned to three pretreatment groups, West and Alster (44) did not find significant differences in the rate of postoperative hyperpigmentation in nontreated controls compared to patients using combined retinoic acid/hydroquinone or glycolic acid cream.

In contrast to hyperpigmentation, postoperative hypopigmentation appears to be permanent. It may result from resurfacing that has produced a deep dermal injury or could simply be related to unmasking of fibrosis from previous treatment (e.g., dermabrasion, phenol peel). Camouflage makeup continues to be the best treatment option for hypopigmentation.

Patients who have undergone laser resurfacing are sensitive to various topical agents and cosmetics. It is not unusual

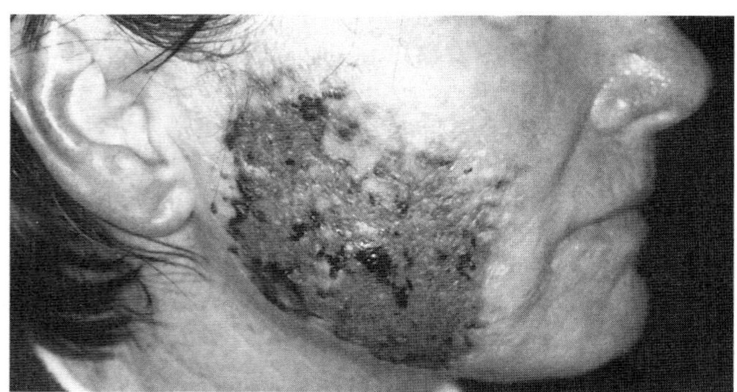

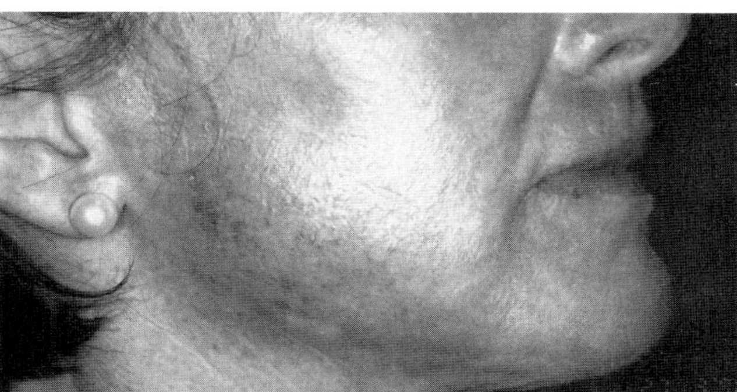

FIGURE 18-3. **A:** Laser wound 4 days after full-face resurfacing with obvious infection in the cheek area with positive cultures of *Candida* and *Staphlococcus.* **B:** Satisfactory resolution of infection and wound healing without scarring after aggressive systemic and topical antibiotic therapy.

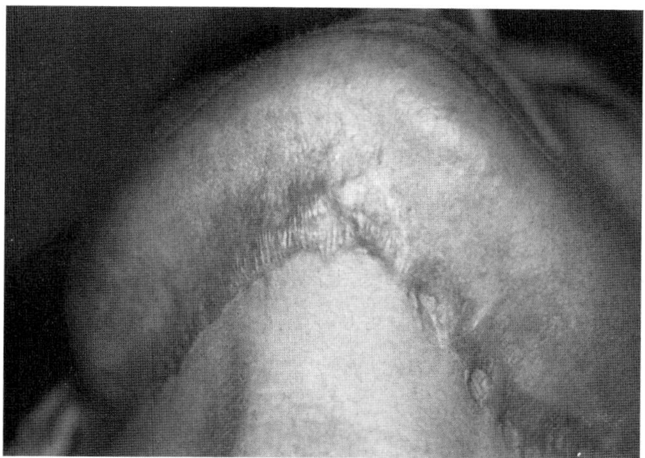

FIGURE 18-4. Hypertrophic scar of the neck.

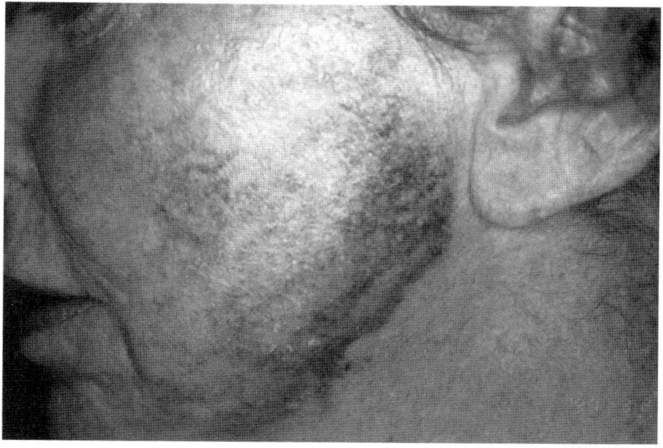

FIGURE 18-6. Hypersensitivity reaction of cheek 4 weeks after laser resurfacing resulting from exposure to fabric softener.

for a patient to report that a particular cosmetic that previously had not caused a problem produced a skin reaction postoperatively. Lased skin is more sensitive to many agents, and contact or allergic dermatitis is seen in 10% to 15% of patients. In particular, topical antibiotics, such as bacitracin or neomycin, have been known to cause extreme allergic reactions that require the use of systemic steroids (e.g., methylprednisolone [Medrol] dose pack). Sensitivity reactions also have been reported to fabric softeners, astringents, and aloe-containing products (Fig. 18-6).

Tooth enamel injury has occurred when an unprotected tooth was lased inadvertently. The enamel may be fractured by the initial impact of the laser or by subsequent heat production. The judicious use of nonreflective metal mouth guards or placement of moist gauze over the teeth will prevent enamel injury. Similarly, the eyes must be protected from inadvertent exposure to laser light. Because corneal injuries have occurred as a direct result of laser irradiation, routine use of scleral eye shields or a Jaeger plate is advocated in all cases involving periorbital resurfacing.

Patients who had laser resurfacing of the lower eyelids may develop a scleral show or a temporary or permanent ectropion. Most cases of ectropion will resolve spontaneously with time and application of gentle massage and lubrication. Patients who are having lower eyelid resurfacing should be evaluated carefully for tarsal adequacy (Fig. 18-7). Any patient who is observed to have inadequate tarsal integrity should have a tarsal tightening procedure prior to, or in conjunction with, resurfacing of the lower eyelid.

LASER FACIAL COSMETIC SURGERY

Using a fine beam of focused laser light, a surgeon is able to make a hemostatic incision because the laser can cut while simultaneously coagulating feeding blood vessels. Thus, it

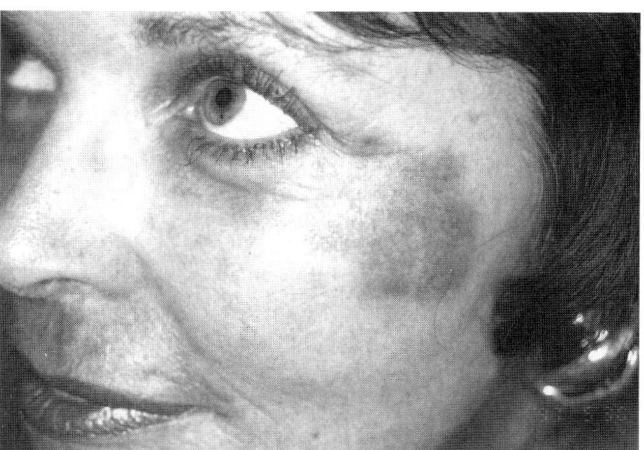

A

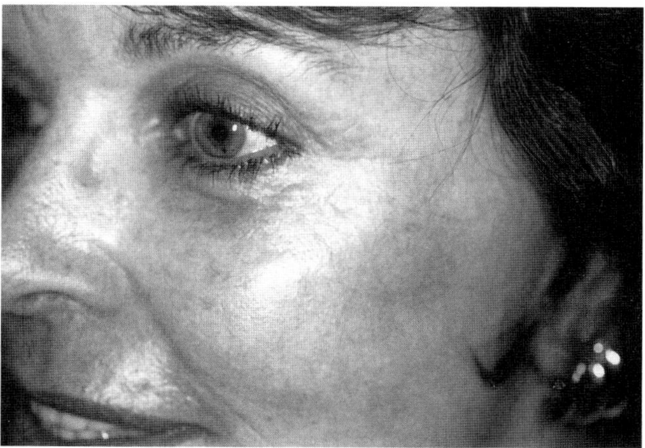

B

FIGURE 18-5. A: Hyperpigmentation of the malar/lateral canthal area resulting from sun exposure 6 weeks after periorbital laser resurfacing. **B:** Satisfactory fading 3 weeks after use of combination 5% hydroquinone, 0.1% tretinoin topical cream, and steroid (Kligman's formula).

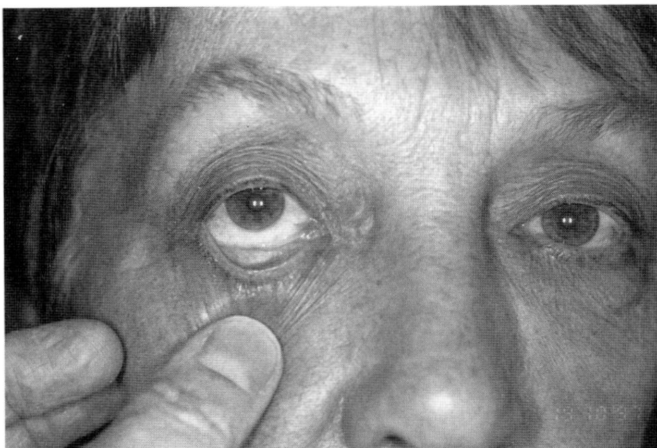
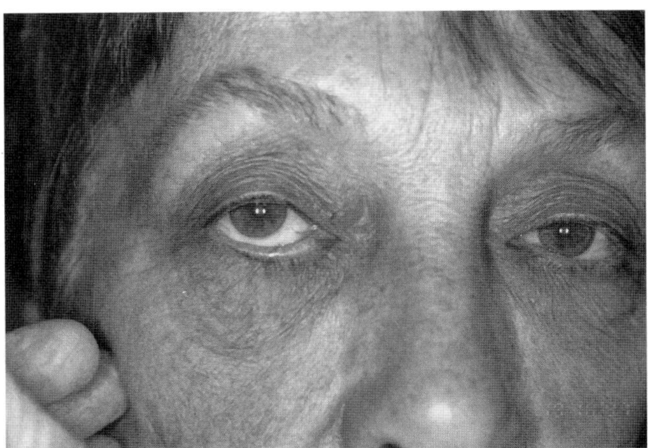

A B

FIGURE 18-7. A: "Snap" or lid distraction test demonstrating laxity of tarsus of lower lid. **B:** Upon release, the eyelid is slow in recovery and still presents with a lowered position and significant scleral show.

seemed natural to apply the laser beam to cosmetic surgery where precision and hemostasis also is very important. There is growing evidence in reports from many authors that sequelae such as pain, bruising, and swelling could be reduced markedly by the use of lasers. The YAG laser is the most hemostatic laser with the greatest ability to coagulate small blood vessels. The YAG laser energy may be transmitted through fiber optics to scalpels equipped with special sapphire tips so that the laser may be used as "light knife". Apfelberg (45) reported on a series of facelifts and blepharoplasties performed with the YAG laser and demonstrated a 30% reduction in postoperative bruising and swelling compared to conventional laser surgery. Kulick and Apfelberg (46), Kulick (47), and Keller (48,49) used the frequency-doubled KTP (potassium titanyl phosphate)-YAG laser with contact fibers in the same manner. Apfelberg (50), Keller and Cray (51), Keller (52), Morrow and Morrow (53), and Lent and David (54) also demonstrated excellent results using the CO_2 laser for facelift and eyelid surgery. Many authors have demonstrated the beneficial effects of the CO_2 laser in blepharoplasty (55–59). The laser is used in a focused mode, with a 0.2-mm spot size and either 4 to 5 W of continuous beam or 15 to 25 mJ in the ultrapulse range. Lower blepharoplasty is accomplished using the transconjunctival approach and often combined with laser resurfacing of the lower eyelid. Several authors demonstrated the benefit of the CO_2 laser in conjunction with endoscopic forehead lift use.

There is a continuing controversy about the safety of using the laser to resurface skin flaps that have been elevated during facelift, forehead lift, or blepharoplasty surgery. Numerous authors demonstrated the safety of resurfacing the forehead after an endoscopic forehead lift (60–62). There is an excellent blood supply to the forehead secondary to the depth of the dissection, which normally is in the subperiosteal plane. Similarly, resurfacing the lower eyelid skin flap after a transconjunctival blepharoplasty is done frequently without complications or problems. Studies have shown that resurfacing undermined facelift flaps is hazardous and may lead to flap injury and subsequent necrosis. Guyuron et al. (63) reported a clinical and animal study of flaps that were elevated and then subsequently laser resurfaced. In Yucatan minipigs, the mean healing time for skin treated with laser alone was 12.05 days. In comparison, the healing time for the laser-treated area subsequent to flap elevation averaged 17.95 days, and two flaps failed to heal completely in 24 days. The authors also reported their clinical experience with patients who suffered delayed healing in the undermined area of the lateral cheek flap with subsequent reepithelialization showing marked surface telangiectasia and textural change. The authors recommended against laser resurfacing over an undermined facelift flap. In contrast, Mayl and Felder (64) reported successful resurfacing of undermined face flaps using lower (80% of normal) laser energy densities and termed the process "laser blend resurfacing."

Complications of Laser Blepharoplasty

Complications that arise from laser blepharoplasty procedures may occur in the intraoperative or postoperative period (65,66). Intraoperative complications include those arising from violation of laser safety standards, inappropriate use of the laser, and loss of anatomic orientation within the eyelid. Standards of laser safety must be strictly observed for the patient's protection during the procedure. Use of the laser beam shortly after the application of a flammable skin solvent, such as alcohol, acetone, or ether, should be discouraged because of the possibility of ignition with subsequent thermal burn. Similarly, the use of oxygen, which is delivered close to the eyes and may be combustible, should be carefully limited. The use of wet towels to protect the skin around the eyes will prevent accidental laser burning of adjacent skin. The patient's globe and cornea must be protected against inadvertent damage by a laser beam. Scleral shields of a nonreflective metal design have been shown to be totally protective (Fig. 18-8) (67). Alternatively, a protective "Baker-David" clamp, which consists of a large metal plate that is placed between the upper eyelid and the globe and fixed in position by a toothed clamp, will protect the upper eyelid during blepharoplasty surgery. A "Jaeger" plate of either dull finished metal or plastic may be placed against the cornea behind the lower eyelid for protection. If a laser beam strikes the cornea directly, visual injury or even blindness can result.

The laser beam should be used in a focused mode (at the focal length of the laser) to produce clean cutting of the skin with the least thermal injury. Defocusing the laser beam creates increasing amounts of peripheral thermal damage and can lead to poor wound healing, dehiscence, and excessive scar formation. The laser beam must be applied carefully only to the area of surgery, and care must be taken to avoid inadvertent injury to eyelashes, which could result in permanent injury to the lash follicle and loss of hair. In the upper eyelid, the orbital septum, which must be divided in order to remove the orbital fat pads, is very close to the levator aponeurosis. If the orbital septum is divided too deeply, the risk of dividing the levator aponeurosis is increased, which would result in eyelid ptosis. Deeper laser penetration would actually penetrate the eyelid and cause possible corneal injury. For safety, because the levator muscle aponeurosis is separated at the greatest distance from the orbital septum at the level of the superior orbital rim, the septum should be opened just below this rim. The lacrimal gland is very close to the lateral edge of the central fat pad and should not be disturbed or laser irradiated or a dry eye condition may result.

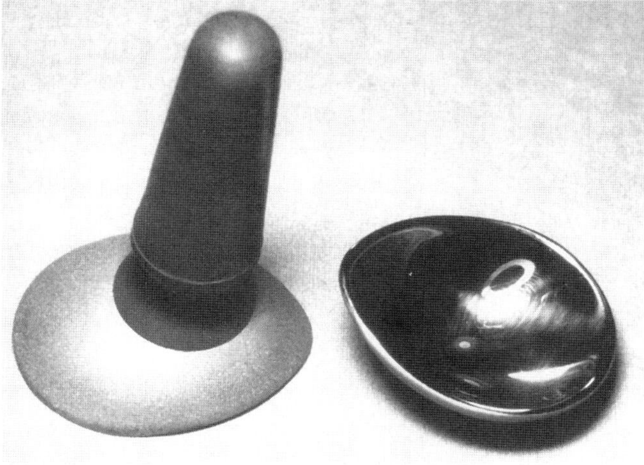

FIGURE 18-8. Demonstration of metal scleral shield eye protectors and suction cup used for their removal.

Transconjunctival lower blepharoplasty surgery is associated with several risks. The transconjunctival approach to lower eyelid surgery penetrates the lower eyelid retractors but does not divide the orbital septum, a structure that can cause significant scarring and postoperative ectropion. The surgeon must be careful not to orient the incision too far anteriorly, which not only could penetrate the septum but could cause a full-thickness injury directly through the lower eyelid onto the skin, resulting in an external scar (Figs. 18-9 and 18-10). When removing the nasal and the central fat pads, the inferior oblique muscle is encountered between these structures, and care must be taken not to divide or burn this muscle, which would result in a loss of eyelid mobility and diplopia.

Other possible complications from laser blepharoplasty include unacceptable scarring, which may be a result of defocusing the laser, thus producing larger zones of thermal damage in the adjacent skin as well as wound dehiscence. Chemosis or excessive conjunctival edema may occur more frequently with laser transconjunctival lower blepharoplasty (Fig. 18-11). Fortunately, this situation is short lived, limiting itself to 2 to 5 days. Treatment includes frequent use of lubricating or cortisone eyedrops, and either eyelid suspension with a temporary suture or occasionally temporary suture tarsorrhaphy. Temporary dry eye syndrome sometimes occurs after laser blepharoplasty.

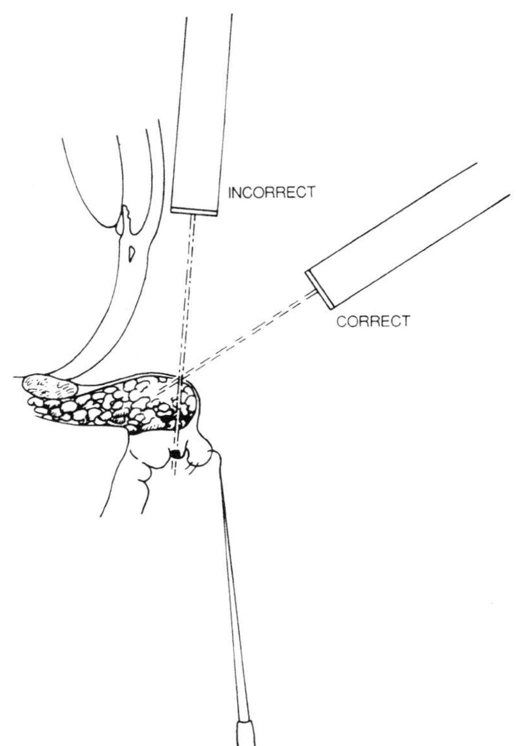

FIGURE 18-9. Diagram of correct versus incorrect orientation of laser beam. Incorrect angle will result in full-thickness penetration of the lower lid.

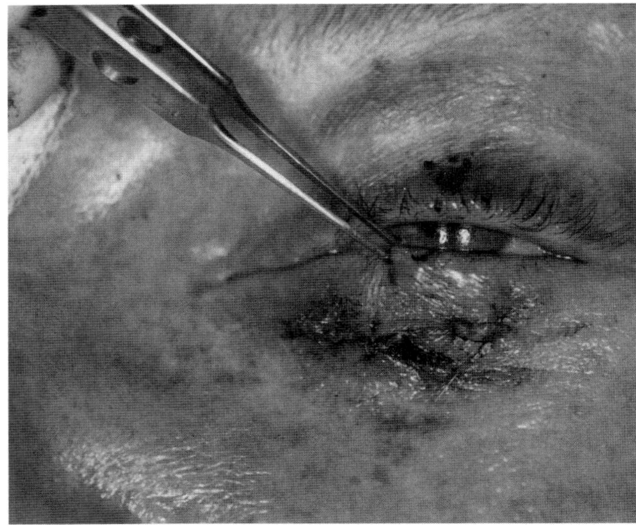

A

FIGURE 18-10. A: Full-thickness penetration and laceration of the lower eyelid resulting from improper orientation of the laser beam in a transconjunctival lower blepharoplasty. B: Result 8 weeks after eyelid laceration repair. C: Final satisfactory result 16 weeks after eyelid injury and repair.

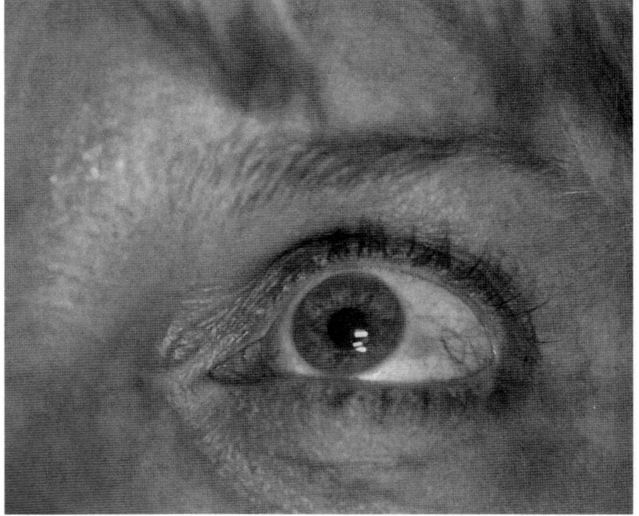

B

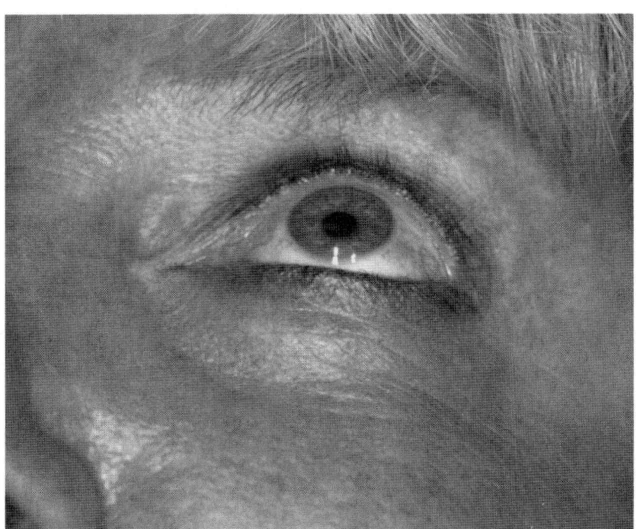

C

A report of the joint laser task force study of the American Society for Aesthetic Plastic Surgery and the American Society of Plastic and Reconstructive Surgeons provided a summary of these complications (35).

VASCULAR-SPECIFIC LASERS

Argon Lasers

Argon lasers were the first types of CW lasers in widespread clinical use for the treatment of vascular lesions such as port-wine stains and hemangiomas (68,69). The CW argon laser emits blue-green light at 488 to 514 nm and effectively targets oxyhemoglobin, but it also is absorbed by epidermal melanin. As a CW system, the argon laser produces radial tissue damage through heat dissipation, with tissue exposure times in excess of the thermal relaxation time of cutaneous blood vessels (70,71). Significant hypertrophic scarring of port-wine stains, particularly within the pediatric population and in the perinasal and perioral/lip regions, has been shown to develop within 3 to 6 weeks after argon laser treatment in as many as 38% of patients (71–73). In addition to the usual treatment for such scars (including intralesional and topical corticosteroids, silicone gel application, and surgical revision), it has been shown that pulsed dye laser treatment (see later) can significantly improve the scars' erythema, texture, pliability, bulk, and symptoms (e.g., pruritus). CW argon laser treatment also may produce permanent pigmentary changes, manifested typically as hypopigmentation (Fig. 18-12), for which little can be done (71–76). Isolated reports of pyogenic granulomas and cutaneous lupus erythematosus have occurred after argon laser irradiation (77,78). Because of the high risk of untoward sequelae except in the most experienced laser surgeons'

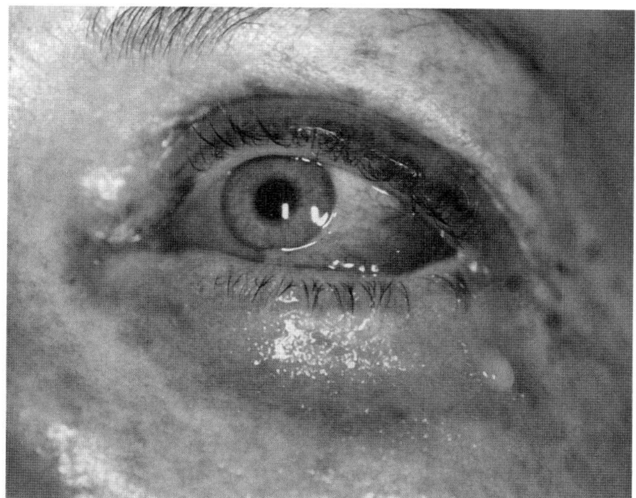

FIGURE 18-11. Chemosis or excess conjunctival edema after laser transconjunctival lower blepharoplasty.

hands, current use of CW argon lasers is limited to the treatment of facial telangiectasias.

In contrast to its CW counterpart, the argon-pumped tunable dye laser generates yellow light at wavelengths ranging from 577 to 595 nm in a quasi-continuous (quasi-CW) mode through the use of a mechanical shutter that effectively delivers laser pulses as short as 20 ms. Theoretically, the shuttered "pulses" produce less thermal damage in normal surrounding tissue, thereby limiting side effects to erythema, vesiculation, transient pigmentary alteration, and linear crusting, rather than to hypertrophic scarring (79,80). Because of the temporary nature of the side effects seen, no specific treatment generally is needed, except to observe for and promptly intervene with antibiotic therapy or local wound care if secondary bacterial infection or prolonged healing is suspected. Treatment sessions tend to be lengthy and results are highly operator dependent because blood vessels need to be manually traced; however, a computer scanner may be used to shorten treatment time.

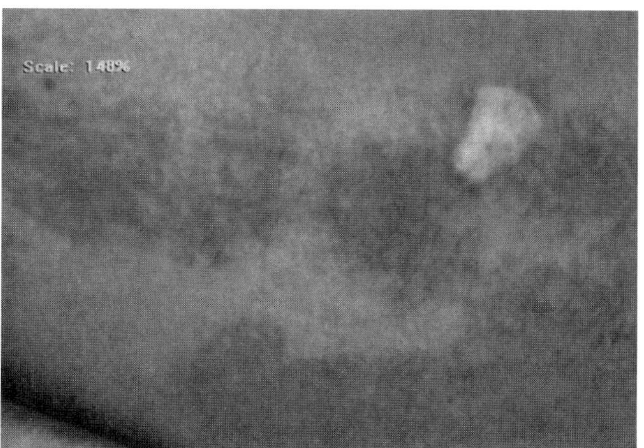

FIGURE 18-12. Hypopigmented scar in a continuous-wave argon laser test spot for port-wine stain removal.

Potassium Titanyl Phosphate Lasers

KTP lasers emit light at 532 nm and can be used to treat a variety of vascular and pigmented lesions (81,82). As with the argon-pumped tunable dye laser, the KTP laser handpiece is used in a quasi-continuous mode at varying repetition rates to individually trace blood vessels, or a scanner can be used to facilitate treatment. Side effects generally are limited to linear crusting of skin overlying treated blood vessels, transient pigmentary changes, and mild fibrosis that spontaneously improve without any specific intervention (81–83). Although posttreatment purpura does not occur as with the use of the pulsed dye laser (see later), the 532-nm pigment-specific wavelength potentially can increase the risk of postoperative hypopigmentation, especially when treating darkly pigmented skin. Thus, its use is not recommended in patients with tans or in those with naturally darker skin tones.

Krypton/Copper Vapor/Copper Bromide Lasers

Each of these laser systems emits light at two different wavelengths: yellow light (568 to 578 nm) to treat vascular lesions and green light (511, 520 to 530 nm) to treat pigmented lesions. They are operated in a quasi-CW mode and, similar to other lasers that require the operator to trace a particular target, they demand technical expertise and produce variable clinical results (84–89). Side effects include immediate postoperative erythema that lasts several hours, soft tissue edema, and punctate scabbing along treated vessels (84,87,88). Ten to fifteen percent of patients may develop postinflammatory hyperpigmentation that generally resolves within 6 to 8 weeks. Hypopigmentation has been reported in up to 47% of patients (86,89). Local anesthesia usually is not required during treatment; however, 28% of patients report mild pain and 18% complain of severe pain during facial telangiectasia treatment (86). Hypertrophic scarring and transient skin atrophy have been reported in up to 20% patients (87).

Flashlamp-pumped Pulsed Dye Lasers

The flashlamp-pumped pulsed dye laser (FPDL) was designed specifically for the treatment of cutaneous vascular lesions, bearing in mind the principles of selective photothermolysis. With its ability to target blood vessels with minimal risk of collateral thermal injury and subsequent scar formation, it is the safest vascular laser available today. It uses a high-powered flashlamp and rhodamine dye to produce a pulse of yellow light at 585 nm that can selectively

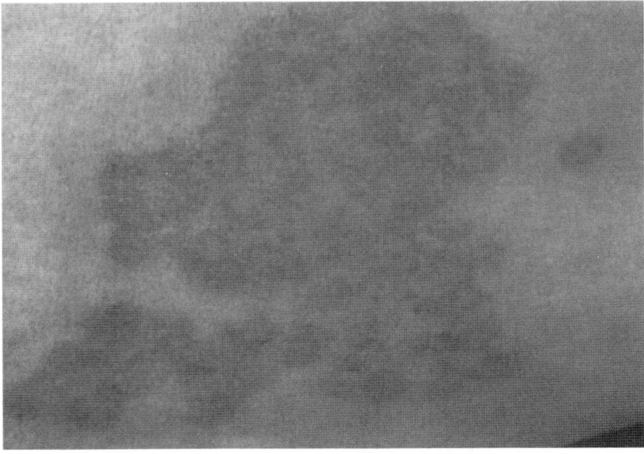

FIGURE 18-13. Immediate purpura and reactive hyperemia after 585-nm pulsed dye laser irradiation.

target blood vessels in vascular lesions, as well as in hypertrophic scars, striae, and verrucae (38,90–100). In a study of 500 patients treated with the FPDL for a variety of vascular conditions, there were no reported cases of hypertrophic scarring and the incidence of atrophic scarring was less than 0.1% (101). Isolated cases of hypertrophic and keloid scar development after FPDL treatment of vascular lesions have been seen in patients concomitantly taking isotretinoin or with application of excessive energy densities and/or pulse overlapping (94,102). Therefore, caution is advised with this or any other laser system when treating patient taking retinoids. Other mild and transient side effects that generally do not require intervention include edema and mild scaling that may persist up to 1 week.

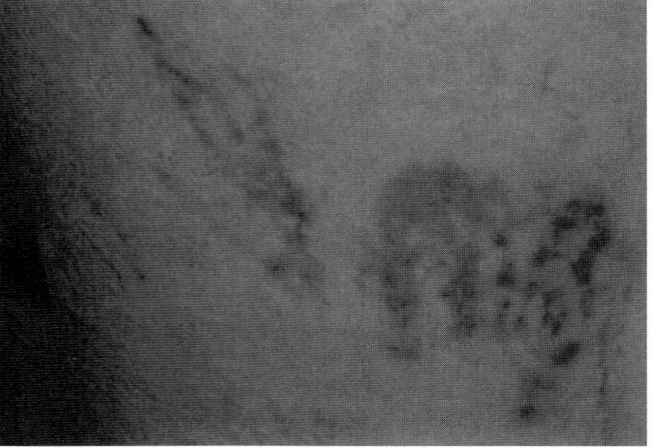

FIGURE 18-14. Hyperpigmentation of leg veins after vascular-specific laser irradiation. (This can be seen with pulsed dye, potassium titanyl phosphate, long-pulsed green, and red light laser systems.)

Immediate posttreatment purpura is a universal occurrence and typically lasts 7 to 14 days (Fig. 18-13). Transient pigmentary changes, such as hyperpigmentation, may occur in up to 85% of patients (Fig. 18-14), and hypopigmentation lasting 3 to 6 months develops in 2.2% to 26% of patients (79,92–94,101). Mild-to-moderate discomfort (similar to that of a rubber band snap) during pulsed dye laser treatment of facial telangiectasias has been reported in 35% to 85% of patients, but it does not require more than a topical or local anesthetic in the majority of patients (79,80,103). Because the treatment of warts involves the delivery of multiple overlapping pulses of high fluences, local infiltration of lidocaine often is essential to achieve adequate treatment (100). As many as 50% of patients being treated for warts experience pain that lasts several hours (100).

PIGMENT AND TATTOO-SPECIFIC LASERS

Q-switched Ruby Lasers

The ruby laser, with a wavelength of 694 nm, is used for the treatment of epidermal and dermal pigment. This laser operates in a quality-switched (QS) mode that produces high-energy light in nanosecond pulses. An ultrashort tissue dwell time is ideal for treating melanocytic lesions and dermal pigments and minimizes the risk of unwanted collateral thermal damage. However, during ruby laser treatment, side effects include tissue splatter, punctate bleeding, edema, pruritus, vesiculation, and purpura (104–107). Like all of the QS pigment-specific lasers, the ruby laser produces an immediate ash white epidermal tissue response on impact. Because normal epidermal melanin also may absorb ruby light, transient hypopigmentation may be seen in 25% to 50% of patients (Fig. 18-15). Postinflammatory hyperpigmentation, hair whitening, and hair loss also have been observed in areas treated with ruby laser (106–111). Crust formation commonly develops locally after treatment, and epidermal atrophy has been reported to occur in as many as 50% of patients after ruby irradiation. However, permanent textural changes, such as scarring, occur in less than 5% of patients overall (105–107,109,110,112,113).

Immediate and irreversible pigment darkening of cosmetic tattoos (particularly white, pink, and flesh-colored inks) has been reported to occur after ruby laser irradiation, presumably due to chemical reduction of the iron-containing tattoo pigment from ferric oxide to the ferrous oxide form (114). Although continued ruby laser treatment eventually may clear the darkened pigment, results are not predictable, and additional procedures, such as surgical excision or CO_2 laser resurfacing, may be needed to effectively eliminate it (115). Type IV cutaneous allergic reactions to laser tattoo removal also have been reported. It is hypothesized that laser treatment liberates intracellular pigment into the extracellular space, where it becomes antigenic. Both gener-

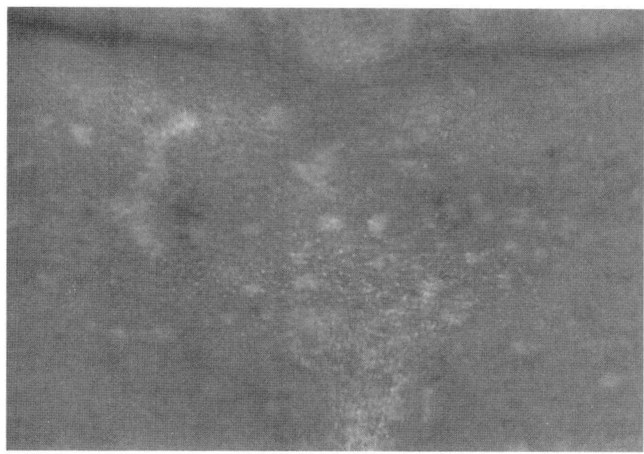

FIGURE 18-15. Hypopigmentation and fibrosis on the anterior chest after the use of excessive laser fluences for solar lentigines. (This can occur with any of the pigment or tattoo-specific lasers.)

alized and localized urticarial, pruritic, and eczematous reactions may develop (116) and can be treated with oral or mid-potency topical corticosteroids and oral antihistamines. Rarely, a granulomatous allergic reaction can occur with subsequent hypertrophic scar formation (Fig. 18-16). Intralesional steroid injections or occlusion/pressure therapy can be used to reduce the bulky nature of such lesions without further worsening of the inciting allergic reaction.

Q-switched Alexandrite Lasers

Like the ruby laser, the alexandrite laser also operates by a QS mechanism and emits red light (755 nm) to effectively treat a variety of pigmented lesions and tattoos (117–121).

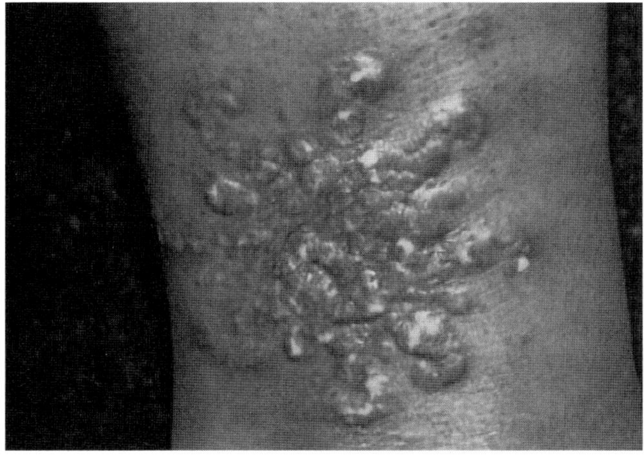

FIGURE 18-16. Hypertrophic scarring and pigmentary alteration due to a granulomatous allergic reaction (to red ink) in a quality-switched laser-treated multicolored professional tattoo.

Hypopigmentation and hyperpigmentation have been reported after treatment with the alexandrite laser (117,118). Up to 50% of patients being treated for tattoos may experience postoperative hypopigmentation for 3 to 6 months (117,120). Skin lightening tends to occur more commonly in darker skin types and is related to the total number of laser treatments, with an average of seven treatments necessary to induce significant hypopigmentation (117). Punctate bleeding and tissue splatter may occur with the alexandrite laser, especially at high fluences, but is generally less common than splatter with neodymium (Nd):YAG laser treatment (117,118,120). Older faded tattoos tend to show a milder tissue response in terms of bleeding and epidermal erosions. However, when tattoos (especially those of the distal lower extremity) are treated with the alexandrite or any of the other QS laser systems, hemorrhagic bullae may form. Young and densely pigmented tattoos require a fluence of 7.5 J/cm^2 to induce bleeding, whereas older, faded tattoos require fluences of up to 9.0 J/cm^2 (120). Rarely, scarring and tissue fibrosis may occur with the alexandrite laser as a result of poor wound management (117). Immediate irreversible pigment darkening of cosmetic, white, flesh-tone, and pink tattoos may occur with any of the QS systems used for tattoo removal, including the alexandrite laser (Fig. 18-17) (114).

Q-switched Neodymium:Yttrium Aluminum Garnet Lasers

The Nd:YAG laser emits a wavelength of 1,064 nm with a pulse duration of 10 ns. It has been used to effectively treat primarily dermal pigment such as blue and black tattoos, melanocytic nevi, and nevi of Ota and Ito (122,123).

An immediate ash white tissue response occurs at laser treatment sites with a subsequent wheal-and-flare reaction (122). Other significant side effects of Nd:YAG laser treatment include tissue splatter and bleeding, textural changes, hypopigmentation, and hyperpigmentation (122–128). Textural changes may occur in up to 8% of patients, but generally they are transient and only evident when patients are examined earlier than 4 weeks after treatment

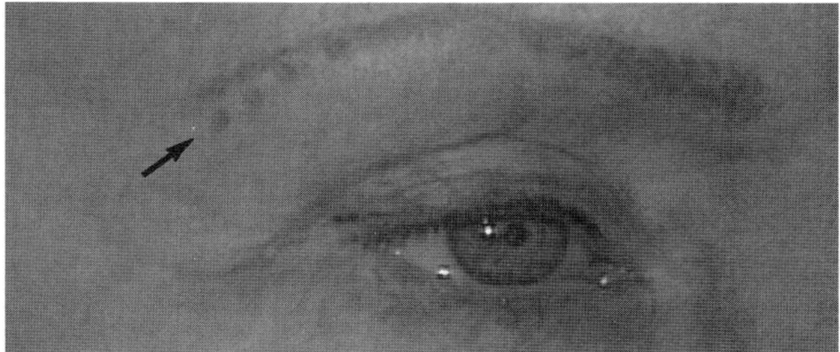

FIGURE 18-17. Tattoo ink darkening in quality-switched laser-treated cosmetic eyebrow tattoo that contained iron or titanium oxide pigment.

(122,125,126). Hypopigmentation also may develop after several treatments (123).

Generalized cutaneous allergic reactions to tattoo laser removal have been reported with this laser as well as with the ruby laser (126). As described with the QS systems, immediate and irreversible ink darkening of white, flesh-tone, and pink cosmetic tattoos may occur with QS Nd:YAG treatment (114).

Frequency-doubled Q-switched Neodymium:Yttrium Aluminum Garnet Lasers

The frequency-doubled Nd:YAG laser is used for the treatment of epidermal pigment as well as red and yellow tattoos (105,125,127). By passing 1,064-nm Nd:YAG light through a potassium diphosphate crystal, the frequency is doubled, producing a 532-nm wavelength. The resultant green light targets epidermal pigment due to its marked absorption by melanin (105,127).

Complications experienced with this laser include transient erythema, which may persist for up to 6 weeks and appears to be fluence dependent, purpura for up to 1 week, pigmentary alteration, textural changes, and blistering (105,126). There have been no reports of permanent scarring. Postinflammatory hyperpigmentation occurs in up to 8% of patients and occurs more often in darker skin types (105,126). Pinpoint bleeding occurs at higher fluences (4 to 5 J/cm^2) (125,126). Pain and postoperative bleeding have been reported to be greater with the Nd:YAG than with the ruby laser (125). A mild burning sensation during treatment is expected with a sunburn feeling that may persist for 1 to 2 days after treatment (126).

510-nm Pulsed Dye Lasers

The pigmented lesion dye laser (PLDL) produces a wavelength of 510 nm and a pulse duration of 300 ns, which targets epidermal melanin. This green light laser has a much greater affinity for melanin than for oxyhemoglobin, making it an ideal laser to treat benign epidermal pigmented lesions with minimal risk of dermal injury and scarring (129–133).

Complications such as transient hyperpigmentation occurs in approximately 15% to 33% of patients, with complete resolution by 2 to 6 months (129,130,132,133). Avoidance of sun exposure is advocated after treatment and topical lightening agents (e.g., hydroquinone) may be used to facilitate fading. Hypopigmentation occasionally occurs and usually resolves quickly; however, it has been reported to last 6 months after PLDL treatment of a *café-au-lait* macule (129). There have been no reports of scarring, atrophy, or textural changes.

A mild snapping pain and an ash-white appearance of laser-treated skin occurs during treatment (129,133), after which time purpura may be observed in up to 60% of patients (131). No residual tissue effects have been noted as a result of the purpura formation, which spontaneously resolves within 1 to 2 weeks.

Immediate and irreversible pigment darkening of cosmetic tattoos, particularly those inks colored white, pink, and flesh tone, has been noted to occur with PLDL treatment. This darkening is believed to be due to the reduction of iron in tattoo pigment from ferric oxide to the ferrous oxide upon laser impact (114).

LASER-ASSISTED HAIR REMOVAL

There currently are several lasers and light sources available and marketed for the treatment of unwanted or excessive hair. Those with wavelengths in the red and infrared portion of the electromagnetic spectrum (e.g., ruby, alexandrite, diode, Nd:YAG) are used most often for hair removal because they effectively target melanin in the hair follicle and potentially can penetrate to the appropriate depth of the dermis (134–145), In order to target the follicle, these lasers rely either on endogenous melanin within the follicular epithelium and hair shaft or on the placement of an exogenous carbon solution that can be targeted in the hair follicle.

Although the goal of laser-assisted hair removal is permanent follicular damage, there also is a risk of epidermal injury during the hair removal process. Any melanin-containing structure, such as a melanocyte, keratinocyte, or nevus, also may sustain thermal injury when irradiated by red and infrared light (146). Although hair shafts often are darker in color than the surrounding skin, partial absorption of applied laser energy may occur by epidermal chromophores. Methods to protect the epidermis during laser-assisted hair removal have included contact cooling laser tips, cryogen sprays, and topical application of cooling gels. Epidermal cooling thus serves to reduce the amount of superficial thermal damage sustained upon laser impact.

Despite all efforts to protect the epidermis from damage, photoepilation may result in clinically significant adverse reactions. Nanni and Alster (147) performed a retrospective chart review of 900 consecutive laser-assisted hair removal treatments in 156 patients treated with either a QS Nd:YAG (Thermolase SoftLight), long-pulsed ruby (Palomar EpiLaser), or long-pulsed alexandrite (Cynosure LPIR) laser (147). Perifollicular edema and posttreatment erythema were the most common side effects observed within all laser groups and usually resolved spontaneously within 1 to 4 hours after treatment. Mild and transient treatment pain occurred in up to 87% of patients treated with any laser system, with the need for topical or local anesthesia in fewer than 1% of patients. (The use of a cooling mechanism greatly reduces the need for anesthetic use.)

In general, the QS Nd:YG laser system results in the fewest side effects; however, it is less effective in providing long-term hair reduction (142,147). Folliculitis has been reported to occur in 35% of patients (when pretreatment wax epilation was used during the process) (147). Because of the low energies used in the process, pigmentary alteration is rarely seen.

Long-pulsed ruby, alexandrite, and diode laser systems theoretically can produce more side effects due to their pigment-specific wavelengths and higher energy densities used to effect long-lasting hair removal. Side effects are influenced by skin type, body location, seasonal variations, and patient history of recent sun exposure. The extremities tend to suffer the most side effects, and sun-protected areas such as the axillary and inguinal regions suffer the least. Blistering and/or fine epidermal crusting (Fig. 18-18) as well as hypopigmentation and purpura are experienced more commonly in darker skin tones (phototypes III and higher) or in tanned skin (147). Average duration of postinflammatory hyperpigmentation is 2 months, whereas hypopigmentation can persist for several months.

Whereas long-term adverse sequelae and scarring typically are not observed with the use of any of the hair removal systems, the side effects of laser-assisted hair removal are not always trivial, particularly if left untreated. The most important factors affecting negative outcomes from laser-assisted hair removal relate to melanin and/or melanocyte activation (e.g., dark skin type, tanned skin, chronically sun-exposed body areas such as the forearms and face) and to the use of excessively high energy densities. Even when proper patient selection and treatment parameters are followed, laser-assisted hair removal may result in unwanted cutaneous side effects. Thus, the process should be given the same respect typically shown to other laser procedures. Fortunately, the majority of photoepilation side effects are mild and transient and, when proper postoperative care is administered, permanent complications may be easily avoided.

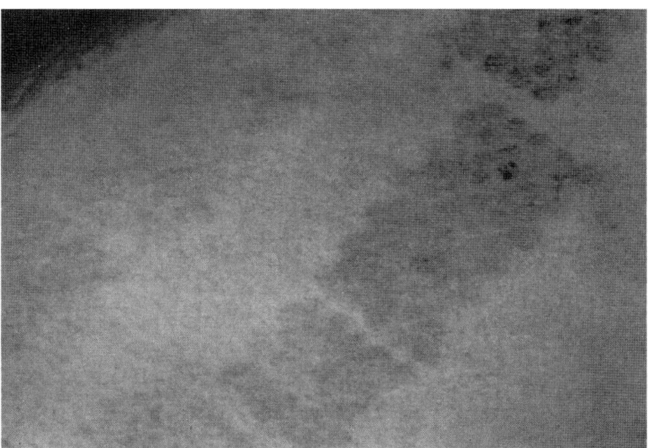

FIGURE 18-18. Crusting seen after laser-assisted hair removal procedure. This occurs more commonly in patients who are tan or in those with naturally darker skin phototypes.

SUMMARY

CW lasers, the first medical lasers to be used, continue to be effective, but they are extremely operator dependent and potentially can result in significant risks, including scarring. In 1983, the theory of selective photothermolysis was introduced, which enabled physician-scientists to design lasers that were highly selective and safer to operate. These newer lasers are capable of affecting a specific target tissue while minimizing the risk of scarring and pigmentary changes. They accomplish this task by producing a wavelength and pulse duration that is best absorbed by a specific target. However, not all modern lasers use this theory and, therefore, may operate in either a CW, quasi-CW, pulsed, or QS mode. CW lasers are least selective and tend to produce unwanted tissue damage and scarring through heat dissipation. Quasi-CW lasers attempt to limit unwanted thermal damage by producing a series of brief laser pulses or by the chopping of a CW beam; however, they still may pose a higher risk of nonspecific tissue damage and thermal injury. The pulsed and QS systems adhere most closely to the principles of selective photothermolysis and result in the most selective destruction with the lowest risk of scarring and unwanted thermal diffusion. Of course, any laser system potentially can result in scarring and tissue damage; therefore, adequate operator education and skill are essential when using surgical lasers. Side effects and complications that occur as a consequence of laser treatment can be significantly influenced and improved upon if diagnosed and treated early.

REFERENCES

1. Anderson RR, Parrish JA. Selective photothermolysis: precise microsurgery by selective absorption of pulsed radiation. *Science* 1983;220:524–527.
2. Apfelberg DB. UltraPulse carbon dioxide laser resurfacing and facial cosmetic surgery. *Can J Plast Surg* 1995;3:133–136.
3. Apfelberg DB. The UltraPulse carbon dioxide laser with computer pattern generator automatic scanner for facial cosmetic surgery and resurfacing. *Ann Plast Surg* 1996;36:522–530.
4. Apfelberg DB. Adjunctive considerations for laser resurfacing. *Op Tech Otolaryngol Head Neck Surg* 1997;8:35–30.
5. Apfelberg DB. A critical appraisal of high-energy pulsed carbon dioxide laser facial resurfacing for acne scars. *Ann Plast Surg* 1997;38:95–101.
6. Apfelberg DB. UltraPulse carbon dioxide laser with CPG scanner for full face resurfacing for rhytids, photo-aging, and acne scars. *Plast Reconstr Surg* 1997;99:1817–1826.
7. Apfelberg DB. Perioperative considerations in laser resurfacing. *Int J Aesthetic Restor Surg* 1997;5:21–28.
8. Weinstein C, Alster TS. Skin resurfacing with high-energy, pulsed carbon dioxide lasers. In: Alster TS, Apfelberg DB, eds. *Cosmetic laser surgery.* New York: Wiley-Liss, 1996:9–27.

9. Chernoff WG, Schoenrock LD, Cramer H, et al. Cutaneous laser resurfacing. *Aesthetic Restor Surg* 1995;3:57–68.
10. Fitzpatrick RE, Goldman MP, Satur NM, et al. Pulsed carbon dioxide laser resurfacing of photo-aged facial skin. *Arch Dermatol* 1996;132:395–402.
11. Lowe NJ, Lask G, Griffin ME. Laser skin resurfacing. *Dermatol Surg* 1995;21:1017–1019.
12. Waldorf HA, Kauvar ANB, Geronemus RG. Skin resurfacing of fine to deep rhytides using a char free carbon dioxide laser in 47 patients. *Dermatol Surg* 1995;21:940–946.
13. Alster TS, West TB. Resurfacing of atrophic acne scars with a high-energy pulsed CO_2 laser. *Dermatol Surg* 1996;22: 151–155.
14. Bernstein LJ, Kauvar ANB, Grossman MC, et al. The short and long term side effects of carbon dioxide laser resurfacing. *Dermatol Surg* 1997;23:519–525.
15. Alster TS. Comparison of two high-energy pulsed carbon dioxide lasers in the treatment of peri-orbital rhytides. *Dermatol Surg* 1996;22:541–545.
16. Alster TS, Garg S. Treatment of facial rhytides with the UltraPulse high energy carbon dioxide laser. *Plast Reconstr Surg* 1996;98:791–794.
17. Goldberg DJ, Meine J. Photo-aged neck skin: treatment with the Er:YAG laser. *Dermatol Surg* 1998;24:619–621.
18. Teikemeir G, Goldberg DJ. Skin resurfacing with Er:YAG laser. *Dermatol Surg* 1997;23:685–687.
19. Hohenleutner U, Hohenleutner S, Baumier W, et al. Fast and effective skin ablation with an Er:YAG laser: determination of ablation rates and thermal damage zones. *Lasers Surg Med* 1997;20:242–247.
20. McDaniel DH, Ash K, Lord J, et al. The Er:YAG laser: a review and preliminary report on resurfacing of the face, neck, and hands. *Aesthetic Surg* 1997;17:157–164.
21. Perez MI, Bank DA, Silvers D. Skin resurfacing with the Er:YAG laser. *Dermatol Surg* 1998;24:653–659.
22. Manaloto RMP, Alster TS. Erbium:YAG laser resurfacing for refractory melasma. *Dermatol Surg* 1999;25:121.
23. Ross EV, Anderson RR. The erbium laser in skin resurfacing. In: Alster TS, Apfelberg DB, eds. *Cosmetic laser surgery,* 2nd ed. New York: John Wiley & Sons, 1998:57–84.
24. Bass LS. Er:YAG laser skin resurfacing: preliminary clinical evaluation. *Ann Plast Surg* 1998;40:328–335.
25. Weinstein C. Computerized scanning Er:YAG laser for skin resurfacing. *Dermatol Surg* 1998;24:83–91.
26. Alster TS. Clinical and histologic evaluation of six erbium:YAG lasers for cutaneous resurfacing. *Lasers Surg Med* 1999;24: 87–92.
27. Green HA, Domankevitz Y, Nishioka NS. Pulsed carbon dioxide laser ablation of burned skin: in vitro and in vivo analysis. *Lasers Surg Med* 1990;10:476–484.
28. Roberts TL, Lettieri JT, Ellis LB. CO_2 laser resurfacing: recognizing and minimizing complications. *Aesthetic Surg Q* 1996;143–148.
29. Apfelberg DB. Side effects, sequelae, and complications of carbon dioxide laser resurfacing. *Aesthetic Surg J* 1997;365–372.
30. Alster TS, Nanni CA. Complications of cutaneous laser surgery. In: Biesman B, ed. *Carbon dioxide lasers in facial aesthetic and reconstructive surgery.* Baltimore: Williams & Wilkins, 1998.
31. Nanni CA, Alster TS. Complications of carbon dioxide laser resurfacing: an evaluation of 500 patients. *Dermatol Surg* 1998;24:315–325.
32. Nanni CA. Postoperative management and complications of carbon dioxide laser resurfacing. In: Alster TS, Apfelberg DB, eds. *Cosmetic laser surgery,* 2nd ed. New York: John Wiley & Sons, 1998:37–56.
33. Fulton JE. Complications of laser resurfacing: methods of prevention and management. *Dermatol Surg* 1998;24:91–101.
34. Sriprachya-Anunt S, Fitzpatrick RE, Goldman MP, et al. Infections complicating laser resurfacing for photo-aged skin. *Dermatol Surg* 1997;23:527–536.
35. Apfelberg DB. Summary of the 1997 ASAPS/ASPRS laser task force survey on laser resurfacing and laser blepharoplasty. *Plast Reconstr Surg* 1998;101:511–518.
36. Alster TS, West TB. Effect of topical vitamin C on postoperative carbon dioxide laser resurfacing erythema. *Dermatol Surg* 1998;24:331–334.
37. Alster TS, Nanni CA. Famciclovir prophylaxis for herpes simplex virus reactivation after cutaneous laser resurfacing. *Dermatol Surg* 1999;25(Mar):242–246.
38. Alster TS, Nanni CA. Pulsed dye laser treatment of hypertrophic burn scars. *Plast Reconstr Surg* 1998;102:2190–2195.
39. Fitzpatrick RE, Goldman MP. Resurfacing of photodamage of the neck using the UltraPulse CO_2 laser. *Lasers Surg Med* 1997;20[Suppl 9]:33.
40. Rosenberg G. Full face and neck laser skin resurfacing. *Plast Reconstr Surg* 1997;100:1846–1854.
41. Fanous N, Prinja N, Sawat M. Laser resurfacing of the neck: a review of 48 cases. *Aesthetic Plast Surg* 1998;22:73–179.
42. Kligman AM, Willis I. A new formula for depigmenting human skin. *Arch Dermatol* 1975;111:40–48.
43. Horton S, Alster TS. Preoperative and postoperative considerations for carbon dioxide laser resurfacing. *Cutis* 1999;64: 399–406.
44. West TB, Alster TS. Effect of pretreatment on the incidence of hyperpigmentation following cutaneous CO_2 laser resurfacing. *Dermatol Surg* 1999;25:15–17.
45. Apfelberg DB. YAG laser meloplasty and blepharoplasty. *Aesthetic Plast Surg* 1995;19:231–236.
46. Kulick MI, Apfelberg DB. Aesthetic laser surgery. In: Kulick MI, ed. *Lasers in aesthetic surgery.* New York: Springer, 1998:88–143.
47. Kulick MI. Evaluation of the KTP laser in aesthetic facial surgery. *Aesthetic Plast Surg* 1996;20:53–57.
48. Keller GS. KTP laser rhytidectomy. *Facial Plast Surg Clin North Am* 1993;1:153–162.
49. Keller GS. Use of the KTP laser in cosmetic surgery. *Am J Cosmetic Surg* 1992;9:177–180.
50. Apfelberg DB. Laser-assisted blepharoplasty and meloplasty. In: Alster TS, Apfelberg DB, eds. *Cosmetic laser surgery.* New York: John Wiley & Sons, 1996:29–40.
51. Keller GS, Cray JC. Laser assisted surgery of the aging face. *Facial Plast Surg Clin North Am* 1995;3:319–341.
52. Keller GS. Suprafibromuscular and endoscopic rhytidectomy with the high-output carbon dioxide laser and flexible waveguide. In: Alster TS, Apfelberg DB, eds. *Cosmetic laser surgery.* New York: John Wiley & Sons, 1996:43–54.
53. Morrow DM, Morrow LB. Carbon dioxide laser-assisted lower facelift: a preliminary report. *Am J Cosmetic Surg* 1993; 9:159–168.
54. Lent WM, David LM. Laser-assisted rhytidectomy: a preliminary report. *Dermatol Surg* 1995;21:1039–1041.
55. Baker SS, Muenzler WS, Small RG, et al. Carbon dioxide laser blepharoplasty. *Ophthalmology* 1984;91:238–244.
56. David LM, Sanders G. CO_2 laser blepharoplasty: a comparison to cold steel and electrocautery. *J Dermatol Surg Oncol* 1987;13:110–114.
57. Beeson WM, Kabaker S, Keller GS. Carbon dioxide laser blepharoplasty: a comparison to electrosurgery. *Int J Aesthetic Restor Surg* 1994;2:33–36.
58. Mittelman MD, Apfelberg DB. Carbon dioxide laser blepharoplasty—advantages and disadvantages. *Ann Plast Surg* 1990; 24:1–6.

59. Morrow DM, Morrow LB. CO_2 laser blepharoplasty. *J Dermatol Surg Oncol* 1992;18:307–313.
60. Weinstein C. Carbon dioxide laser resurfacing combined with endoscopic forehead lift, laser blepharoplasty, and transblepharoplasty corrugator muscle resection. *Dermatol Surg* 1998; 24:63–69.
61. Roberts TL, Ellis LB. In pursuit of optimal rejuvenation of the forehead: endoscopic browlift with simultaneous carbon dioxide laser resurfacing. *Plast Reconstr Surg* 1998;101:1075–1084.
62. Ramirez OM, Pozner JN. Laser resurfacing as an adjunct to endoforehead lift, endofacelift and biplanar facelift. *Ann Plast Surg* 1997;38:315–321.
63. Guyuron B, Michelow B, Schmelzer R, et al. Delayed healing of rhytidectomy flap resurfaced with CO_2 laser. *Plast Reconstr Surg* 1998;101:816–819.
64. Mayl N, Felder DS. CO_2 laser resurfacing over facial flaps. *Plastic Reconstr Surg* 1998;102:1768–1769.
65. Trelles MA, Baker SS, Ting J, et al. Carbon dioxide laser transconjunctival lower lid blepharoplasty complications. *Ann Plast Surg* 1996;37:465–468.
66. Biesman BS. Complications of laser-assisted blepharoplasty. In: Alster TS, Apfelberg DB, eds. *Cosmetic laser surgery,* 2nd ed. New York: John Wiley & Sons, 1998:41–154.
67. Ries WR, Clymer MA, Reinisch L. Laser safety features of eye shields. *Lasers Surg Med* 1996;18:309–315.
68. Brauner G, Schliftman A, Cosman B. Evaluation of argon laser surgery in children under 13 years of age. *Plast Reconstr Surg* 1991;87:37–43.
69. Apfelberg DB, Maser MR, Lash H. Argon laser treatment of cutaneous vascular abnormalities. *Ann Plast Surg* 1978;1:14–18.
70. Scheibner A, Wheeland RG. Use of the argon-pumped tunable dye laser for port-wine stains in children. *J Dermatol Surg Oncol* 1991;17:735–739.
71. Dixon J, Huether S, Rotering RH. Hypertrophic scarring in argon laser treatment of portwine stains. *Plast Reconstr Surg* 1984;73:771–780.
72. Cosman B. Experience in the argon laser therapy of port-wine stains. *Plast Reconstr Surg* 1980;65:119–129.
73. Noe JM, Barsky SH, Geer DE, et al. Port wine stains and the response to argon laser therapy: successful treatment and the predictive role of color, age, and biopsy. *Plast Reconstr Surg* 1980;65:130–136.
74. Dolsky RL. Argon laser skin surgery. *Surg Clin North Am* 1984;64:861–870.
75. Craig RDP, Purser JM, Lessells AM, et al. Argon laser therapy for cutaneous lesions. *Br J Plast Surg* 1985;38:148–155.
76. Apfelberg DB, Maser MR, Lash H. Extended clinical use of the argon laser for cutaneous lesions. *Arch Dermatol* 1979; 115;719–721.
77. De Rooij MJ, Nuemann HA. Granuloma telangiectaticum after argon laser therapy of a spider nevus. *Dermatol Surg* 1995; 21:356–357.
78. Wolf JT, Weinberg JM, Elenitsas R, et al. Cutaneous lupus erythematosus following laser-induced thermal injury. *Arch Dermatol* 1997;133:392–393.
79. Boska P, Martinho E, Goodman MM. Comparison of the argon tunable dye laser with the flashlamp pulsed dye laser in the treatment of facial telangiectasia. *Dermatol Surg Oncol* 1994; 20:749–753.
80. Ross M, Watcher MA, Goodman MM. Comparison of the flashlamp pulsed dye laser with the argon tunable dye laser with robotized handpiece for facial telangiectasia. *Lasers Surg Med* 1993;13:374–378.
81. Apfelberg DB, Bailin P, Rosenberg H. Preliminary investigation of KTP/532 laser light in the treatment of hemangiomas and tattoos. *Lasers Surg Med* 1986;6:38–42.
82. Silver BE, Livshots YL. Preliminary experience with the KTP/532 nm laser in the treatment of facial telangiectasia. *Cosmetic Dermatol* 1996;9:61–64.
83. West TB, Alster TS. Comparison of the 590 nm long-pulse (1. 5 ms) and KTP (532 nm) lasers in the treatment of facial and leg telangiectasias. *Dermatol Surg* 1998;24:221–226.
84. Key M J, Waner M. Selective destruction of facial telangiectasia using a copper vapor laser. *Arch Otolaryngol Head Neck Surg* 1992;118:509–513.
85. McCoy S, Hanna M, Anderson P, et al. An evaluation of the copper-bromide laser for treating telangiectasia. *Dermatol Surg* 1996;22:551–557.
86. Thibault PK. Copper vapor laser and microsclerotherapy of facial telangiectases. A patient questionnaire. *J Dermatol Surg Oncol* 1994;20:48–54.
87. Pickering JW, Walker PHB, Halewyn CN. Copper vapour laser treatment of port-wine stains and other vascular malformations. *Br J Plast Surg* 1990;43:272–282.
88. Waner M, Dinehart SM, Wilson MB, et al. A comparison of copper vapor and flashlamp pumped dye lasers in the treatment of facial telangiectasia 1993 *J Dermatol Surg Oncol* 1993; 19:992–998.
89. Dinehart SM, Waner M, Flock S. The copper vapor laser for the treatment of cutaneous vascular and pigmented lesions. *J Dermatol Surg Oncol* 1993;19:370–375.
90. Morelli JG, Tan OT, Garden J, et al. Tunable dye laser (577 nm) treatment of port wine stains. *Lasers Surg Med* 1986; 6:94–99.
91. Tan OT, Sherwood K, Gilchrest BA. Treatment of children with port-wine stains using the flashlamp-pulsed tunable dye laser. *N Engl J Med* 1989;320:416–421.
92. Alster TS, Wilson F. Treatment of port-wine stains with the flashlamp-pumped pulsed dye laser: extended clinical experience in children and adults. *Ann Plast Surg* 1994;32:478–484.
93. Lowe NJ, Behr KL, Fitzpatrick R, et al. Flashlamp pumped dye laser for rosacea-associated telangiectasia and erythema. *J Dermatol Surg Oncol* 1991;17:522–525.
94. Renfro L, Geronemus RG. Anatomical differences of port-wine stains in response to treatment with the pulsed dye laser. *Arch Dermatol* 1993;129:182–188.
95. Geronemus RG. Poikiloderma of Civatte. *Arch Dermatol* 1990;26:547–548.
96. Alster TS. Improvement of erythematous and hypertrophic scars by the 585 nm pulsed dye laser. *Ann Plast Surg* 1994; 32:186–190.
97. Alster TS, Williams CM. Treatment of keloid sternotomy scars with 585 nm flashlamp-pumped pulsed-dye laser. *Lancet* 1995;345:1198–1200.
98. Alster TS. Laser treatment of hypertrophic scars. *Facial Plast Surg* 1996;4:267–274.
99. Tan OT, Hurwitz RM, Stafford TJ. Pulsed dye laser treatment of recalcitrant verrucae: a preliminary report. *Lasers Surg Med* 1993;13:127–137.
100. Kauvar ANB, McDaniel DH, Geronemus RG. Pulsed dye laser treatment of warts. *Arch Fam Med* 1995;4:1035–1040.
101. Levine VJ, Geronemus RG. Adverse effects associated with the 577- and 585-nanometer pulsed dye laser in the treatment of cutaneous vascular lesions: a study of 500 patients. *J Am Acad Dermatol* 1995;32:613–617.
102. Bernstein LJ, Geronemus RG. Keloid formation with the 585-nm pulsed dye laser during isotretinoin treatment. *Arch Dermatol* 1997;133:111–112.
103. Alster TS. Laser treatment of vascular lesions. In: Alster TS, ed. *Manual of cutaneous laser techniques.* Philadelphia: Lippincott-Raven Publishers, 1997:24–44.
104. Goldman L, Hornby P, Meyer R. Radiation from a Q-switched

ruby laser. *J Invest Dermatol* 1965;44:69–71.
105. Kilmer S, Anderson R. Clinical use of the Q-switched ruby and the Q-switched Nd:YAG (1064 nm and 532 nm) lasers for treatment of tattoos. *J Dermatol Surg Oncol* 1993;19:330–338 .
106. Lowe N, Luftman D, Sawcer D. Q-switched ruby laser: further observations on treatment of professional tattoos. *J Dermatol Surg Oncol* 1994;20:307–311.
107. Scheibner A, Kenny G, White W, et al. A superior method of tattoo removal using the Q-switched ruby laser. *J Dermatol Surg Oncol* 1990;16:1092–1096.
108. Achauer B, Nelson J, Vander Kam V, et al. Treatment of traumatic tattoos by Q-switched ruby laser. *Plast Reconstr Surg* 1994;93:318–323.
109. Reid WH, Miller ID, Murphy MJ, et al. Q-switched ruby laser treatment of tattoos: a 9-year experience. *Br J Plast Surg* 1990;43:663–669.
110. Taylor CR, Gange W, Dover J, et al. Treatment of tattoos by Q-switched ruby laser: a dose response study. *Arch Dermatol* 1990;126:893–899.
111. Taylor CR, Anderson R. Treatment of benign pigmented epidermal lesions by Q-switched ruby laser. *Pharmacol Ther* 1993;32:908–912 .
112. Levins PC, Anderson R. Q-switched ruby laser for the treatment of pigmented lesions and tattoos. *Clin Dermatol* 1995; 13:75–79.
113. Levins PC, Gravelink JM, Anderson RR. Q-switched ruby laser treatment of tattoos. *Lasers Surg Med* 1991;11[Suppl 13]:255.
114. Anderson RR, Geronemus R, Kilmer SL, et al. Cosmetic tattoo ink darkening: a complication of Q-switched and pulsed-laser treatment. *Arch Dermatol* 1993;129:1010–1014.
115. Alster TS. Laser treatment of tattoos. In: Alster TS, ed. *Manual of cutaneous laser techniques.* Philadelphia: Lippincott-Raven Publishers, 1997:63–80.
116. Ashinoff R, Levine VJ, Soter NA. Allergic reactions to tattoo pigment after laser treatment. *Dermatol Surg* 1995;21:291–294.
117. Fitzpatrick RE, Goldman MP. Tattoo removal using the alexandrite laser. *Arch Dermatol* 1994;130:1508–1514.
118. Alster TS. Q-switched alexandrite laser treatment (755 nm) of professional and amateur tattoos. *J Am Acad Dermatol* 1995; 33:69–73.
119. Alster TS. Successful elimination of traumatic tattoos by the Q-switched alexandrite (755 nm) laser. *Ann Plast Surg* 1995; 34:542–545.
120. Stafford T J, Lizek R, Tan O T. Role of the alexandrite laser for removal of tattoos. *Lasers Surg Med* 1995;17:32–38.
121. Alster TS, Williams CM. Treatment of nevus of Ota by the Q-switched alexandrite laser. *Dermatol Surg* 1995;21:592–596.
122. Kilmer S, Lee M, Grevelink J, et al. The Q-switched Nd:YAG laser effectively treats tattoos. *Arch Dermatol* 1993;129: 971–978.
123. Goldman MP. Fitzpatrick RE. *Cutaneous laser surgery: the art and science of selective photothermolysis.* St. Louis: Mosby, 1994:168–173.
124. Grevelink JM, Casparian JM, Gonzalez E, et al. Undesirable effects associated with treatment of tattoos and pigmented lesions with the Q-switched lasers at 1064 nm and 694 nm—the MGH experience. *Lasers Surg Med* 1993;13[Suppl 5]:53.
125. Levine VJ, Geronemus RG. Tattoo removal with the Q-switched ruby laser and the Q-switched Nd:YAG laser: a comparative study. *Cutis* 1995;55:291–296.
126. Tse Y, Levine V, McClain S, et al. The removal of cutaneous pigmented lesions with the Q-switched neodymium:yttrium-aluminum-garnet laser: a comparative study. *J Dermatol Surg Oncol* 1994;20:795–800.
127. Kilmer S, Wheeland R, Goldberg D, et al. Treatment of epidermal pigmented lesions with the frequency-doubled Q-switched Nd:YAG laser. *Arch Dermatol* 1994;130:1515–1519.
128. Anderson RR, Dover JS. Selective photothermolysis of cutaneous pigmentation by Q-switched Nd:YAG laser pulses at 1064, 532, and 355 nm. *J Invest Dermatol* 1989;93:28–32.
129. Alster TS. Complete elimination of large cafe-au-lait birthmarks by the 510-nm pulsed dye laser. *Plast Reconstr Surg* 1995; 96:1660–1664.
130. Alster TS, Williams CM. Cafe-au-lait macule in type V skin: successful treatment with a 510 nm pulsed dye laser. *J Am Acad Dermatol* 1995;33:1042–1043.
131. Fitzpatrick RE, Goldman MP, Ruiz-Esparza J. Laser treatment of benign pigmented epidermal lesions using a 300 nsecond pulse and 510 nm wavelength. *J Dermatol Surg Oncol* 1993;19:341–347.
132. Scheepers JH, Quaba AA. Clinical experience with the PLDL-1 (pigmented lesion dye laser) in the treatment of pigmented birthmarks: a preliminary report. *Br J Plast Surg* 1993;46: 247–251.
133. Grekin RC, Shelton RM, Geisse JK, et al. 510-nm pigmented lesion dye laser. Its characteristics and clinical uses. *J Dermatol Surg Oncol* 1993;19:380–387.
134. Nanni CA, Alster TS. A practical review of laser-assisted hair removal using the Q-switched Nd:YAG, long-pulsed ruby, and long-pulsed alexandrite lasers. *Dermatol Surg* 1998;24: 1399–1405.
135. Chernoff WG. Selective photothermolysis for hair removal. *Int J Aesthetic Restor Surg* 1997;5:50–54.
136. Grossman MC, Dierickx C, Farinelli W, et al. Damage to hair follicles by normal-mode ruby pulses. *J Am Acad Dermatol* 1996;35:889–894.
137. Lask G, Elman M, Slatkine M, et al. Laser-assisted hair removal by selective photothermolysis: preliminary results. *Dermatol Surg* 1997;23:737–739.
138. Nanni CA, Alster TS. Long-pulsed alexandrite laser-assisted hair removal at 5, 10, and 20 millisecond pulse durations. *Lasers Surg Med* 1999;24:332–337.
139. Finkel B, Eliezri YD, Waldman A, et al. Pulsed alexandrite laser technology for noninvasive hair removal. *J Clin Laser Med Surg* 1997;15:225–229.
140. Gold MH, Bell MW, Foster TD, et al. Long-term epilation using the EpiLight broad band, intense pulsed light hair removal system. *Dermatol Surg* 1997;23:909–913.
141. Goldberg DJ, Littler CM, Wheeland RG. Topical suspension-assisted Q-switched Nd:YAG laser hair removal. *Dermatol Surg* 1997;23:741–745.
142. Nanni CA, Alster TS. Optimizing treatment parameters for hair removal using a topical carbon-based solution and 1064-nm Q-switched neodymium:YAG laser energy. *Arch Dermatol* 1997;133:1546–1549.
143. Littler CM. Laser hair removal in a patient with hypertrichosis lanuginosa congenita. *Dermatol Surg* 1997;23:705–707.
144. Wheeland RG. Laser-assisted hair removal. *Dermatol Clin* 1997;15:469–477.
145. Dierickx CC, Grossman MC, Farinelli WS, et al. Permanent hair removal by normal-mode ruby laser. *Arch Dermatol* 1998;134:837–842.
146. Nanni CA, Alster TS. Treatment of Becker's nevus using a 694-nm long-pulsed ruby laser. *Dermatol Surg* 1998;24: 1032–1034.
147. Nanni CA, Alster TS. Laser-assisted hair removal: side effects of Q-switched Nd:YAG, long-pulsed ruby and alexandrite lasers. *J Am Acad Dermatol* 1999;41:165–171.

Discussion

LASERS

GARY J. ROSENBERG

Dr. Apfelberg and Dr. Alster have written an excellent chapter that will be useful to all laser surgeons. The discussion of physiology and laser choices is complete. There is very little that I can add to this well-written chapter.

The authors describe the two different carbon dioxide (CO_2) laser technologies. It is important to note that the first they describe as high energy with short pulses (Coherent Ultrapulse) is a collimated laser. The second is a fixed focal point laser (Sharplan/ESC SilkTouch or FeatherTouch). Herein lies the difference between the two lasers; that is, the collimated laser when used at density 5 or 6 automatically provides the 10% to 15% overlap that is precisely within the realm of the standard gaussian curve. The fixed focal point laser has hard shoulders, therefore resulting in more user error (1).

The discussion of the erbium:yttrium aluminum garnet (YAG) laser is short and does not address what we know clinically. That is, that the erbium:YAG laser does not achieve the same results as the CO_2 laser. There is less skin shrinkage and tightening, and unless one is willing to make excessively numerous passes, the erbium will be restricted to the superficial dermis. In order to see the most beneficial effects of laser resurfacing, the deep dermis should be involved to provide transdermal neocollagenesis as well as deep dermal neoelastogenesis. Neoelastogenesis only occurs in the deep reticular dermis (2).

Although the authors point out ways to diminish postoperative erythema and refer to this as an undesirable effect of laser resurfacing, I have found quite the opposite to be true. Although I treat my patients with hydrocortisone 1% b.i.d. to suppress itching, I find that that the longer the erythema lasts, the better the result. Therefore, I stress this to my patients and educate them to the desirability of erythema lasting 4 to 6 weeks.

The authors recommend against CO_2 laser resurfacing of the neck. They state that the neck skin is thinner and contains fewer pilosebaceous glands. I do not find that the number of pilosebaceous glands is relevant. Compare the neck skin histologically to that of the temples, forehead, and upper eyelids and take note that these areas heal very nicely. The histology of all these areas was well worked out by Gonzales-Ulloa et al. (3) in 1954. I first reported laser resurfacing of the neck in 1994. I have not had scarring of the neck in many hundreds of patients. The key is diligent and frequent postoperative care (4). Long-term follow-up of these patients will be published by the time of this printing (5).

The authors recommend that if the patient has experienced persistence or recurrence of rhytides, it would be possible to perform a touchup laser treatment several months later. I have found that the optimal time to do a touchup is 6 to 12 weeks later, which is when neocollagenesis and neoelastogenesis are initiated. The timing may be of importance and warrants further investigation. However, the superior results of touchup at 6 to 12 weeks compared to 6 months or later are most evident.

I prefer an open technique for postoperative care of laser resurfacing patients. I have found that by using the open technique, the incidence of infection is much lower than with the closed technique. This was confirmed by Sriprachya-onunt et al. (6). Also, with the open technique, patients are very involved and see the improvement daily. If done properly, postoperative pain is nonexistent or negligible. After initiating the open technique in my practice in 1995, I have found that my complication rate has dropped significantly.

I also always use preoperative antibiotics and antiviral medications. At this time, the antiviral of choice is valcyclovir (Valtrex) 500 mg p.o. t.i.d. The tissue availability is high and the lack of hepatic toxicity makes this a particularly attractive medication. Valcyclovir should be used until reepithelialization is complete. Cephalexin (Keflex) or azithromycin (Zithromax) is initiated 24 hours preoperatively and continued for 7 days postoperatively.

Each patient attends a preoperative visit with the office nurse. A thorough review of the postoperative care instructions first is given verbally and then reviewed a second time in writing. It is impressed upon the patient that he or she will have very little discomfort or pain if the instructions are

G. J. Rosenberg: Florida Aesthetic Surgery Center, Delray Beach, Florida

followed properly. It is also impressed upon the patient that, during the period of postoperative edema and exudate (7 days), he or she will not want to have any visitors.

Over the first 24 hours, the patient applies cool saline compresses with gauze to the face, followed by petrolatum (Vaseline), which acts as an occlusive dressing. After 24 hours, the patient washes his or her face in the morning with baby shampoo and water and applies Vaseline. Then, throughout the day, the patient applies alternating compresses of diluted hydrogen peroxide (mixed 50/50 with water and aluminum acetate [Domeboro] solution, one packet mixed in 16 oz of water). Each compress is followed by an application of petrolatum. Before going to bed, the patient washes his or her face again with baby shampoo and water and applies petrolatum. This is continued for 7 days or until reepithelialization occurs.

Once reepithelialization is complete, hydrocortisone 1% is applied twice a day. Moisturizers are used throughout the remainder of the day, as needed. The patient will use an no. 45 sunblock of titanium oxide. Direct sun exposure is avoided for 1 month.

Hyperpigmentation also is treated successfully using microdermabrasion. Patients can expect three to six treatments over a 3-week period, with almost total resolution in most cases. However, those cases that persist are well treated with the management suggested by Apfelberg and Alster. When it occurs, hypopigmentation can be blended in by judicious laser resurfacing. Areas of demarcation can be camouflaged by gradual diminution of the fluence.

Another point regarding laser cosmetic surgery is the authors' reference to the successful resurfacing of undermined facial flaps. As we have gained more long-term experience with CO_2 laser resurfacing, new applications have been explored. The authors discuss the concomitant use of full-face CO_2 laser resurfacing with face and necklift. This should not be attempted until the surgeon has gained proficiency in both techniques and understands that this is applicable in selected cases only. Long-term follow-up of these patients will be published by the time of this printing (5,7).

The discussion of vascular-specific lasers, pigment and tattoo-specific lasers, and hair removal lasers is complete. There is now a new generation of lasers that allows all of these applications to be included in one machine. The convenience as well as the facility of multimode lasers is apparent.

The reader is strongly encouraged to follow the advice of Drs. Apfelberg and Alster. In addition to being pioneers in the field of cosmetic laser surgery, their combined experience speaks for itself.

REFERENCES

1. Rosenberg GJ. A comparative study of the Coherent Ultrapulse and Sharplan Silk-touch CO_2 laser system for skin resurfacing. Presented at the Annual Meeting of the American Society of Plastic and Reconstructive Surgeons, Dallas, Texas, November 1996.
2. Rosenberg GJ, Brito MA, Aportella R, et al. Long-term histologic effects of the CO_2 laser. *Plast Reconstr Surg* 1999;104:2239.
3. Gonzalez-Ulloa M, Castillo A, Stevens E, et al. Preliminary study of the total restoration of the facial skin. *Plast Reconstr Surg* 1954;13:151.
4. Rosenberg GJ. Full face and neck laser skin resurfacing. *Plast Reconstr Surg* 1997;100:1846.
5. Rosenberg GJ. Combination of CO_2 laser resurfacing and incisional cosmetic facial surgery. *Clin Plast Surg* 2001 *(in press).*
6. Sriprachya-onunt S, Fitzpatrick RE, Goldman MP, et al. Infections complicating CO_2 laser resurfacing. *Dermatol Surg* 1997;23:527.
7. Rosenberg GJ. Face and necklift with full face CO_2 laser skin resurfacing: is it safe? Presented at the Annual Meeting of the American Society of Aesthetic Plastic Surgery, Los Angeles, California, 1998.

19

ENDOSCOPY

RENATO SALTZ
KRISTIN BOEHM

Endoscopic surgery has become a popular procedure among surgical specialties. Surgeons around the world have taken advantage of this technique to obtain acceptable results with smaller scars and reduced morbidity. Specifically, the technique involves the introduction of a rigid tube that transmits the image to a video screen. After an optical cavity is developed, the endoscope reflects the light, and an image is created by the camera chip and transmitted to a video monitor. Through additional incisions, different instruments can be introduced to allow the surgeon to perform the operative procedure. The surgeon's hands perform the maneuvers with indirect feedback from a two-dimensional video screen.

Because of the separation of hand/eye coordination, additional training often is required to become proficient in endoscopic surgery. Although plastic surgery has been somewhat slow in adopting endoscopic techniques, the past 7 years show plastic and reconstructive surgeons taking this technology to new dimensions. In endoscopic plastic surgery, it is essential that the surgeon develop the necessary skill through training. For younger surgeons trained in laparoscopy during their general surgery years, endoscopy is a natural continuation of their previously acquired skills. Older surgeons have found that the learning is not difficult and can be accomplished fairly rapidly through hands-on courses, particularly those that include the use of cadavers. In contrast to general surgery laparoscopy, most of the plastic surgery endoscopic procedures are not performed in natural body cavities, thus necessitating the creation of a space between soft tissues and bone, or between soft tissue and soft tissue before introduction of the endoscope. Consequently, a variety of sophisticated instruments unique to endoscopic plastic surgery have been developed and are critical for accomplishing satisfactory results. Understanding the basics of endoscopy, becoming familiar with the equipment. and developing the necessary skills to perform the procedures will save the practitioner time and frustration, shorten the learning curve, and hopefully minimize the complications. The different applications of endoscopy in plastic surgery encompass both the aesthetic and reconstructive fields. Concomitant with the advancement of endoscopic techniques in these two important areas, however, has been the development of associated complications. The following review details specific complications associated with various endoscopic plastic surgery procedures, in an effort to elucidate certain pitfalls and help better prepare the endoscopic plastic surgeon.

ENDOSCOPIC BROWLIFT/FOREHEAD

The coronal browlift uses a large incision to effect eyebrow elevation. Because of the lengthy incision, scarring, alopecia, scalp dysesthesias, and overelevation of the medial eyebrow are potential problems with this traditional technique. The endoscopic browlift, with its more limited incisions and minimal scarring, has gained acceptance and popularity since its introduction by Core et al. (1) in 1992. Swift et al. (2) validated the procedure with their evaluation of 50 endoscopic brows. They found an overall increase in brow height coupled with significant improvement in frontalis furrows when preoperative and postoperative photographs were analyzed (2).

Despite its obvious advantages, the endoscopic browlift is not without its occasional complications. Data from the Endoscopy in Plastic Surgery: A Consensus Multidisciplinary Symposium at the University of Alabama in July 1994 indicated a 3.4% major complication rate, including six hematomas, one transcutaneous electrical burn, and four frontal branch paralyses (3). More recently, Saltz et al. (4) reviewed 800 cases of endoscopic browlift with a 6-year follow-up. The complications observed were all related to technique and appeared to have declined as the authors became more proficient with the technique (Table 19-1). Swift et al. (2) reported no injuries to the frontal branch of the facial nerve in

R. Saltz and K. Boehm: Department of Surgery, University of Utah Medical Center, Salt Lake City, Utah

TABLE 19-1. COMPLICATIONS IN 800 ENDOSCOPIC BROWLIFTS

Complication	No. of Patients (%)
Forehead numbness (<3 wk)	462 (58%)
Temporal alopecia	33 (4%)
Need for revision	7 (<1%)

the 50 brows they examined. That same series demonstrated that alopecia occurred in 25% of patients, although the areas were small and at screw fixation sites (2). Daniel and Tirkantis (5) reported a 15% transitory alopecia around the screws. The alopecia is believed to be caused in part by pressure necrosis of the hair follicles during the endoscopic procedure, or by local scalp ischemia during the screw fixation. The Swift group has now changed to the use of nonabsorbable suture fixation of the galea to tunnels drilled into the outer table of the calvarium, with reportedly decreased incidence of spot alopecia. Other alternatives include absorbable screws, suture fixations, tissue glues, and external dressings (Figs. 19-1 through 19-3).

Injury to the supratrochlear and supraorbital nerves with resultant paraesthesias represents another potential complication of this procedure. Lorenc et al. (6) reported neurosensory preservation in ten consecutive patients undergoing endoscopic complication. Isse (7) found 1 month of postoperative numbness in two of 61 patients. Knize (8) has offered suggestions to preserve the deeper division of the supraorbital nerve by adequate scalp incision placement. A subperiosteal dissection plane retains the vascular subgaleal fascia plane within the forehead flap, which serves to maximize flap blood supply. These steps will avoid injury to the deep branch of the supraorbital nerve, which runs superficial to the periosteum and within the galea.

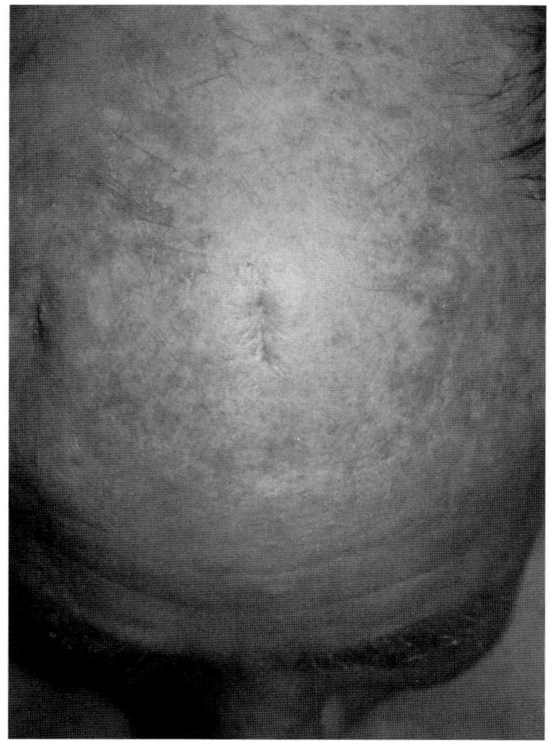

FIGURE 19-2. Wound infection with buried screw fixation, requiring removal of foreign body.

Slade and Cohen (9) described a case of bradycardia followed by a junctional escape rhythm believed to have been elicited by the oculocardiac reflex during endoscopic forehead lift surgery. Initiation of this reflex likely resulted from direct traction on the supraorbital nerve. Surgeons in a po-

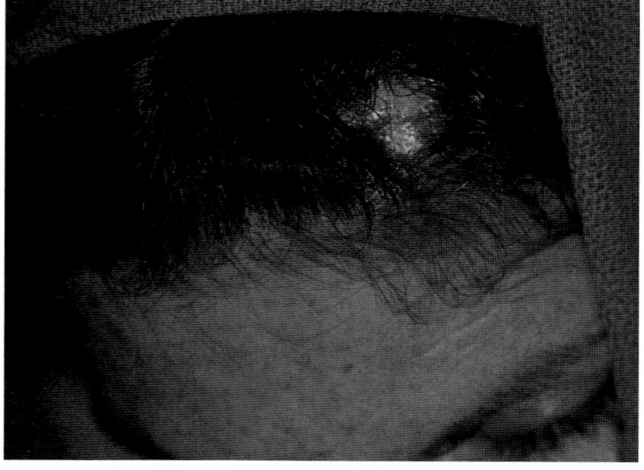

A

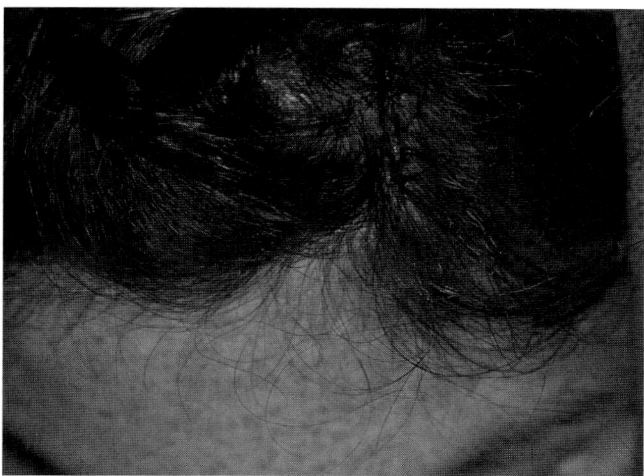

B

FIGURE 19-1. A: Area of alopecia after screw and staple fixation. **B:** Revision with primary closure under local anesthesia.

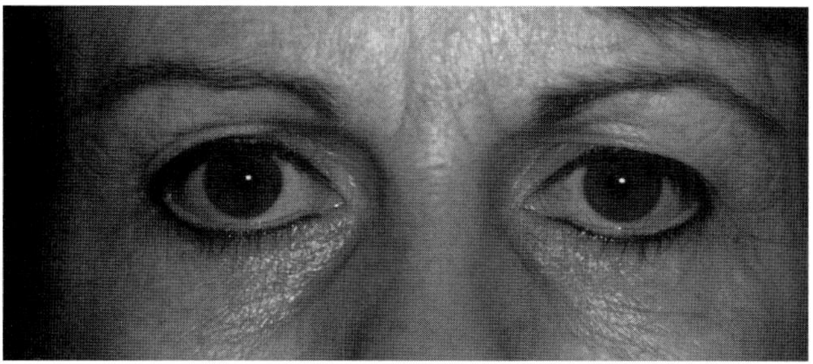
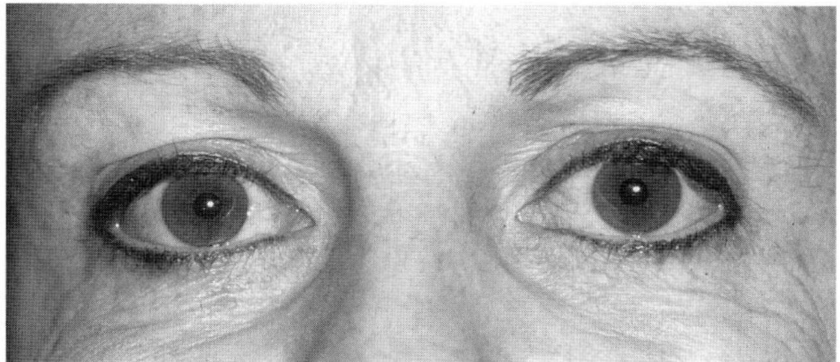

FIGURE 19-3. A: Preoperative endoscopic brow lift. **B:** Medial brow elevation and glabella widening due to release of central periosteum. Complication avoided by keeping a central "periosteal window" intact.

sition to induce this phenomenon should be prepared to promptly recognize the problem and treat it.

MASTOPEXY/BREAST REDUCTION

Endoscopic versions of these procedures were first performed in 1992. Once again, the surgery group at Porto Alegre reported a series of 56 patients who underwent this technique (10). Incisions are placed in the inconspicuous submammary sulcus, through which a retromammary pocket is created between the breast tissue and pectoralis tissue using a tomoscope and laparoscopic scissors connected to electrocautery. A video arthroscopic shaver is used to aspirate and resect tissue. By resecting only the base of the breast cone, function and sensation are preserved. Transcutaneous endoscopically assisted sutures reposition the mammary gland and fashion it to the pectoralis fascia. Their only complication was hematoma when no drains were used. The maintenance of the mastopexy depends on good skin elasticity for retraction; thus, the endoscopic procedure is most effective in young patients who do not have significant excess skin. Once again, the success of this technique lies in using it when properly indicated.

ENDOSCOPIC BREAST AUGMENTATION

Ho (11) reported the first series of endoscopic transaxillary subpectoral breast augmentation in 1993. In his initial series of 13 patients, his only complication was an intraoperative hematoma that was evacuated at the end of the procedure. In 1995, the Emory Group reported their first 50 cases of endoscopic breast augmentation (12). Their reported complications were transient nipple paresthesia and transient inner arm hyperesthesia. There is no greater instance of capsule contracture when compared to traditional subpectoral saline implant breast augmentation. Other complications related to endoscopic transaxillary breast augmentation include transcutaneous burns in the inframammary region secondary to cautery dissections in that area, and breast asymmetries.

ENDOSCOPIC ABDOMINOPLASTY

The ability to treat abdominal wall deformities without a large visible scar and frequent dog-ears represents an improvement to the currently practiced standard. Faria-Correa and his group (10) from Porto Alegre, Brazil, introduced video endoscopic techniques to abdominoplasty procedures in 1991. The technique involves two incisions, one umbilical and one suprapubic, through which a subcutaneous tomoscope is introduced to allow visualization of the subcutaneous dissection while preserving perforating vessels and nerves in an attempt to reduce occurrence of seroma, hematoma, and hypoesthesia. The rectus abdominis muscles then are plicated under endoscopic guidance, and liposuction is performed to shave fat from the underside of the undermined area. There is not an extensive skin resection. In their series of 54 cases, 12 developed seroma that was treated by serial aspiration. Recent efforts to preserve as many perforators as possible apparently have reduced seroma formation rate. More recently, the Emory Clinic published results of 32 women who underwent endoscopic abdominoplasty (13). Complications occurred in five of the 32 patients. Two developed infection, two developed seroma, and one had partial fascial dehiscence. Of note, none experienced intraabdominal perforation, deep vein thrombosis, or loss due to tissue ischemia.

It should be noted that dissecting in the cephalad direction can prove technically challenging and potentially limits candidates for this procedure to those with lower abdominal deformities only. Failure to successfully plicate the upper abdominal fascia may produce a relative upper abdominal

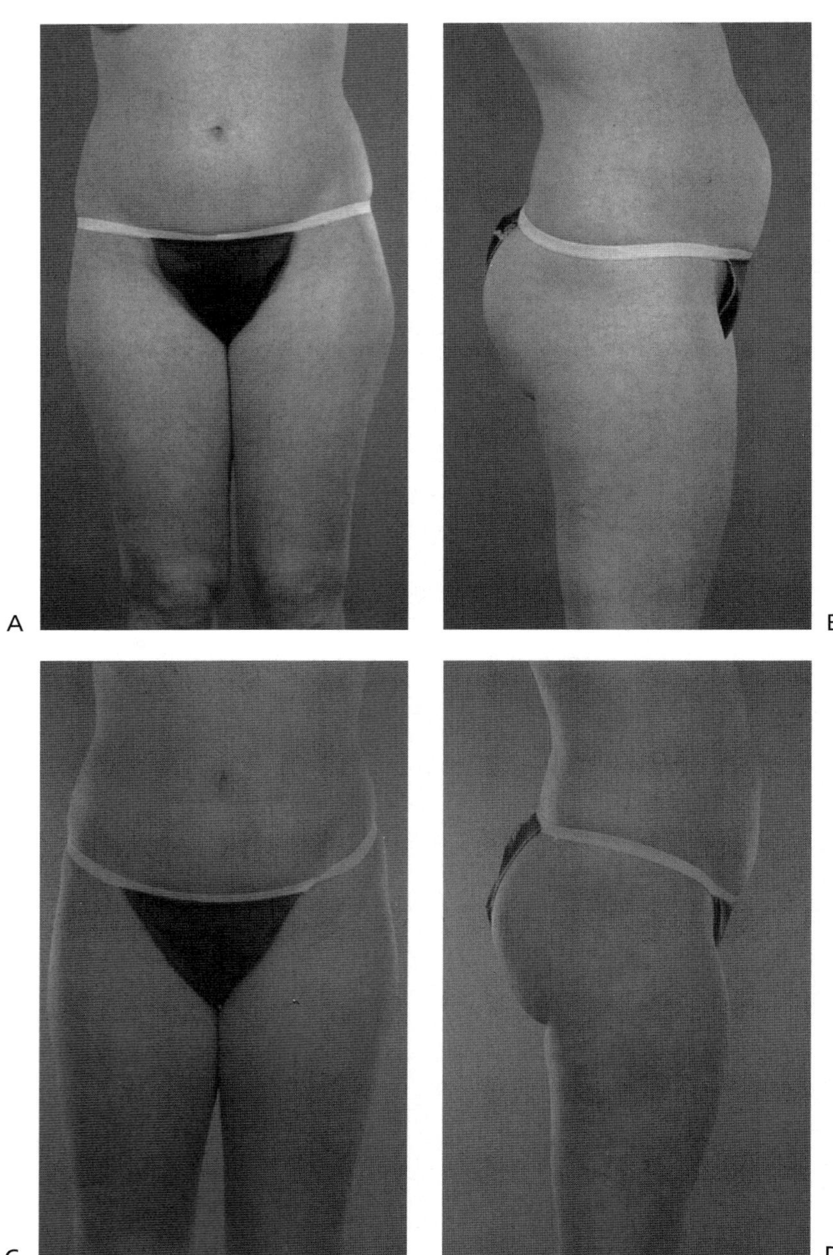

FIGURE 19-4. A: Preoperative view for endoscopic abdominoplasty. **B:** No improvement observed due to presence of excess supraumbilical skin. **C,D:** Loss of abdominal contouring also due to early postoperative trauma with loss of muscle plication. Patient will have conversion to full abdominoplasty including replication. (Case courtesy of Dr. Grady Core.)

fullness compared with the lower abdomen. Most important, however, is an accurate and thorough preoperative assessment of the skin quality and quantity. The prime limitation of the endoscopic technique is that it cannot address skin excess. For the endoscopic abdominoplasty to be successful, the patient should have little to no excess skin and the skin should be smooth. Extensive fatty deposits associated with excess skin will be unable to sufficiently retract with this procedure and may be treated best with more conventional techniques. It seems then that proper patient selection is critical to avoiding unsatisfactory outcomes with endoscopic abdominoplasty. Those with excess or poor quality skin should be appropriately excluded (Figs. 19-4 and 19-5).

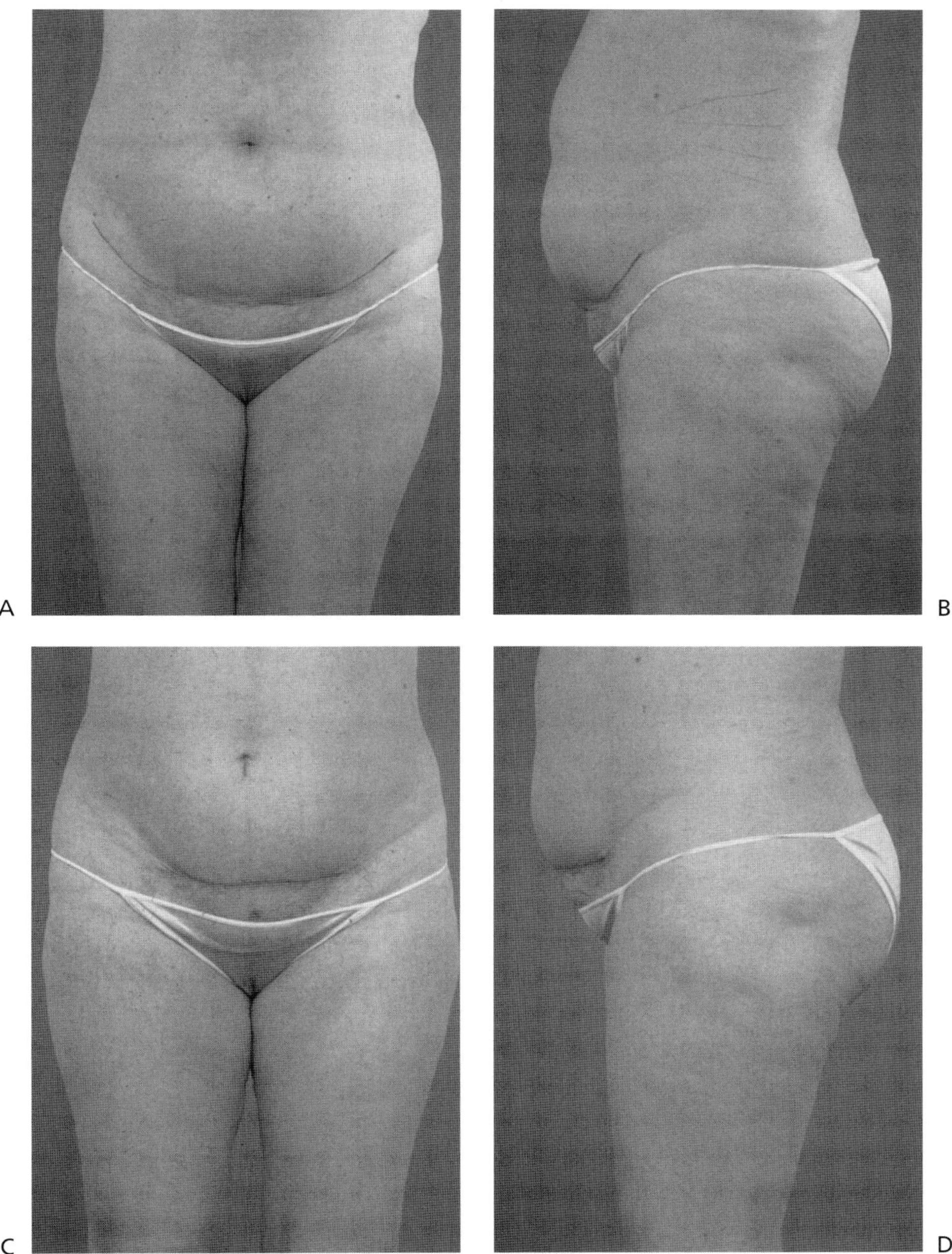

FIGURE 19-5. A: Preoperative views of a patient who was not a candidate for abdominoplasty due to her heavy smoking. **B:** No significant improvement was observed due to presence of excess skin and fat. She underwent revision with open abdominoplasty. (Case courtesy of Dr. Grady Core.)

FACIAL FRACTURES

The smaller incisions and limited dissection associated with endoscopic techniques in facial rejuvenation surgery naturally have prompted recent experimentation in applying them to the facial trauma population. However, the smaller incisions that make these minimal access techniques appealing simultaneously present some technical limitations. The complexity of these endoscopic techniques often translates into longer operating time and additional cost to the institution. Swelling and hemorrhage seen in this population can make endoscopic techniques particularly difficult.

Access to the frontal sinus is achieved through three incisions along the anterior hairline. Wide subperiosteal dissection is performed down to the level of the supraorbital rim and across the nasofrontal suture. Microplates are introduced through the incision and fixed percutaneously using overlying small stab incisions. In theory, avoidance of a coronal incision should minimize forehead numbness and swelling. Current problems include more difficult disimpaction and manipulation of bony fragments, which often means increased operating room time.

Access to the zygomatic arch is accomplished with a preauricular incision and upper buccal sulcus incision. Subperiosteal dissection proceeds along the deep temporal fascia, with care taken to avoid the temporal fat pad. Miniplate fixation of the arch is performed through percutaneous stab incisions. In 1995, Kobayashi et al. (14) described a technique of endoscopic zygoma repair, although placement of plates and screws was difficult through scalp and intraoral incisions. Saltz and Cheng (15) described a technique to repair *in situ* comminuted depressed zygomatic arch fractures that failed to reduce after the Gilles maneuver. A special trocar stabilizes the zygomatic arch fragments while allowing drilling and plate fixation through one small incision. This is introduced through a scalp incision in a similar technique as described for the endobrow (15). Lee et al. (16) reported a combined cadaveric and clinical study on endoscopic zygomatic fracture repair. In 15 patients with a unilateral comminuted fracture, four-point rigid fixation was achieved with limited access incisions. Frontalis function was impaired in one patient, but nerve function returned within 1 week. The cadaveric portion of the study reproduced the ability to restore arch anatomy, with preservation of the frontal branch of the facial nerve. In his recent series of 25 endoscopically repaired arches, seven were for Le Fort III fractures and 18 were for complex zygomatic complex injuries. Eight of the 25 arches developed postoperative frontal branch paralysis; all were recovering spontaneously and completely by the tenth postoperative week. The incidence of this temporary complication can be minimized by gentle traction and dissection in a plane hugging the deep temporal fascia (17). A recognized complication is temporal hollowing secondary to fat atrophy from injury to the middle temporal vessels supplying the fat pad. This can result from aggressive dissection in the fat pad in an effort to avoid injury to the facial nerve. This can be minimized by performing dissection superficial to the deep temporal fascia to the upper border of the arch, with the arch then dissected in a subperiosteal plane to minimize risk of nerve injury (Fig. 19-6).

Many techniques have been described to approach the subcondylar region. However, there is still hesitation about the use these approaches because of the risk of facial nerve injury, scarring, and difficult visualization. Jacobovicz et al. (18) described the first case report in which an endoscope was used to facilitate reduction and fixation of a displaced subcondylar fracture. Their technique involved an intraoral incision along the buccal sulcus of the posterior mandible, through which soft tissues were elevated in a subperiosteal plane. To avoid the facial nerve, the path of the trocar first was created with blunt dissection through the parotid and masseter. Dissection of the condylar segment was performed under endoscopic magnification. In this way, the risk of facial nerve transection was minimized and facial scarring limited. Subsequently, Chen et al. (19) reported a series of eight patients who underwent endoscopically assisted repair of mandibular subcondylar fractures. All patients recovered normal range of motion within 2 months without facial palsy or lip numbness. Lee has reviewed his series of 41 repairs (20). The complications in 41 endoscopic subcondylar fracture repairs generally resulted from either inadequate reduction of the fracture, paralysis, or late-presenting temporomandibular joint osteoarthritis. There were two cases of inadequate reduction breakdown: one case of plate fracture with complete loss of fracture reduction in a noncompliant edentulous patient, and one case of high condylar neck fracture where intraoperative reduction was achieved but not fixated because of the high fracture position, with subsequent loss of reduction despite mandibular maxillary fixation (MMF). One case of temporary facial paralysis (facial nerve palsy) resolved spontaneously and completely by the sixth postoperative week. This patient also had the complication of degenerative TMJ changes that appeared radiographically 2 years after surgery.

To minimize the risk of complications, it is crucial to evaluate the fracture and patient characteristics to determine the patient's suitability to undergo treatment. Fracture repair is dependent on the ability to manipulate a fracture reduction and the application of hardware to maintain position. However, fracture repair may not be achieved easily with fracture characteristics such as comminution, medial override of the condylar pole to the ascending ramus, and high location of the fractures. Therefore, we have found it necessary to evaluate fractures preoperatively with high-resolution computed tomographic images to determine the exact details of the fracture alignment. Approximately 10% of injuries are too proximal, comminuted, or medially overridden to such an extent as to preclude endoscopic repair. These fractures are beyond our endoscopic abilities.

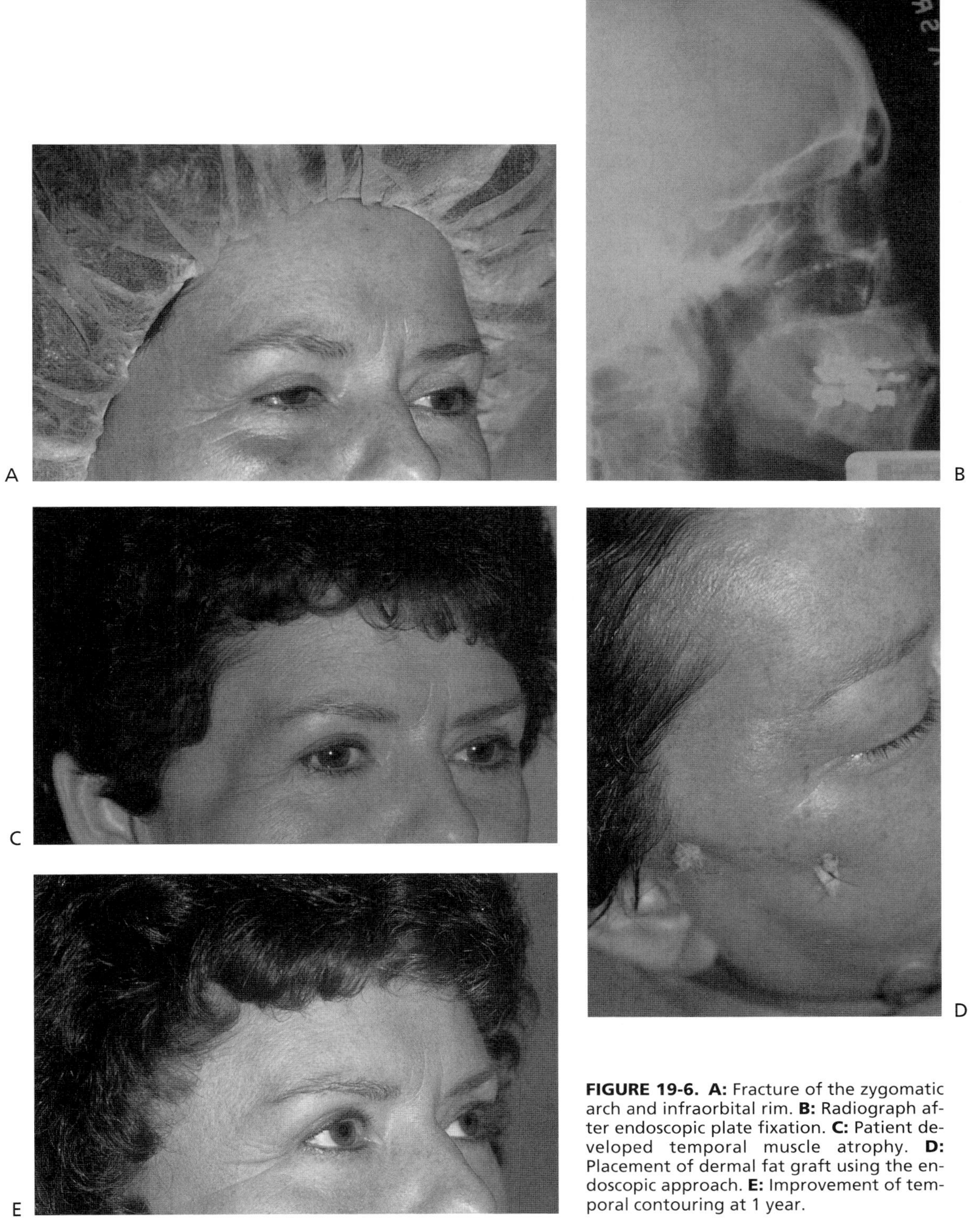

FIGURE 19-6. A: Fracture of the zygomatic arch and infraorbital rim. **B:** Radiograph after endoscopic plate fixation. **C:** Patient developed temporal muscle atrophy. **D:** Placement of dermal fat graft using the endoscopic approach. **E:** Improvement of temporal contouring at 1 year.

Although open surgical repair is considered, the vast majority are treated with functional rehabilitation to assist the patient to adapt to the altered mandibular form (20).

Repair of complex midfacial injuries necessitates anatomic reduction and fixation through adequate surgical exposure. A stable zygomatic arch is critical for facial stability and structural support, whereas integrity of orbital volume is necessary to avoid enophthalmos, diplopia, and cosmetic deformity. Traditional incisions include coronal incision for arch exposure and eyelid incision for orbital exploration. Potential complications with these techniques include injury to the frontal branch of the facial nerve, scarring, alopecia, ectropion, blood loss, and periorbital edema. Lee described a case report of endoscopic assisted repair of the arch and orbital floor through preauricular and buccal sulcus incisions (20). The only complication was a temporary ipsilateral palsy of the frontal branch of the facial nerve, which resolved by the sixth postoperative week.

ENDOSCOPIC SINUS SURGERY

Endoscopic sinus surgery (ESS) has revolutionized the surgical approach to sinus disease. The complications can be divided by anatomic region and include intranasal, periorbital/orbital, intracranial, and systemic.

Intranasal Complications

The most common complication of ESS is the formation of synechiae. It often is caused by the opposing raw surfaces of the middle turbinate and the ethmoid cavity. Stammberger (21) reported an incidence of 8%. Most of the adhesions can be lysed carefully in the early postoperative period. Other less common complications include closure of the maxillary anthrotomy and nasal lacrimal duct injury.

Periorbital/Orbital Complications

Lid edema, ecchymosis, and emphysema are related to the disruption of the lamina papyracea and subsequent orbital bleeding. Retrobulbar hemorrhage is a less common complication. Although less common, retrobulbar hematoma is a catastrophic complication prompting close observation of visual acuity and ocular pressure in the early postoperative period, as these are the early signs. Optic nerve injury can result in permanent blindness. Stankiewicz (22) suggested that inadequate intraoperative visualization and disorientation secondary to bleeding, as well as poor understanding of the anatomy, are potential causes of this complication. (Medial rectus or superior oblique muscle damage can be observed by direct trauma to the medial wall of the orbit.) Postoperative management of these patients will depend upon the presence of entrapment or transection of the muscle and associated nerve (22). Detailed preoperative preparation of patients, rigorous control of intraoperative bleeding, and adequate lighting during the procedure seem to be key aspects in the prevention of periorbital/orbital complications. Neuman and colleagues (23) emphasize that controlling hypertension during general anesthesia, in combination with strict orientation to the intrasinus anatomy, permit a safe surgical procedure. They also present a detailed orbital bleed/visual change algorithm that should be well known by surgeons performing ESS.

Intracranial Complications

Fortunately, intracranial complications of ESS occur infrequently. Cerebrospinal fluid leak is a rare event. A complete understanding of the anatomy and good visualization will avoid this complication. Multiple methods have been advocated for the intraoperative management of CSF (24–26). Brain penetration with parenchymal injury occurs uncommonly. Excessive intraoperative bleeding is a consequence of medications, preoperative bleeding diathesis, hypertension, or inflamed mucosa. A partial turbinate resection may cause delayed hemorrhage. Internal carotid artery injury, although rare, can be life threatening. It should be managed with sphenoid and intranasal packing followed by emergent angiography and neurosurgical consultation (24).

Systemic Complications

Infection and sepsis can occur with ESS. Toxic shock syndrome caused by *Staphylococcus aureus* bacteria has been associated with this procedure. Specifically, it has been reported with the use of nasal packing during sinus surgery (24). Bacitracin ointment is recommended as an effective prophylactic antibiotic against the bacteria.

It appears that the complications associated with ESS have increased due to the large number of procedures performed. Disorientation and the learning curve for this procedure are the main causes for the complications. Lack of knowledge about sinus anatomy, poor lighting, and poor vision secondary to hemorrhage can lead to disastrous consequences. ESS requires a thorough knowledge of the anatomy and adequate training by the endoscopic surgeon.

CARPAL TUNNEL RELEASE

The main advantage of endoscopic carpal tunnel release (ECTR) is found early in the recovery process, with an earlier return to work translating into a cost saving. It often is considered a more difficult procedure with greater potential for serious complications. Several published case reports substantiate this by describing vascular, tendinous, and neurologic complications associated with this technique. In 1999, Straub (27) reported his experience with 1,000 consecutive cases of ECTR. There were no major complications. Two patients developed a stitch abscess, which resolved with suture removal, and one developed hematoma, which resolved without additional intervention. Overall, 92% of patients stated they had satisfactory results. Various factors including preoperative weakness, widened two-point discrimination, abnormal ulnar nerve conduction studies, fibromyalgia, and involvement in litigation were associated with increased likelihood of unfavorable results.

Bsecкstyns and Sorensen (28) analyzed 54 publications with regard to reported rates of complications after ECTR. This analysis revealed a higher rate of nerve damage related to ECTR, although most resolved after a few months and probably were due to neuropraxia following instrumentation. Nonetheless, the risk of transient nerve disturbances was 4.3% in prospective randomized studies and 1.8% in retrospective controlled studies versus 0.9% and 0% in open carpal tunnel reduction (OCTR). The most serious complication was permanent nerve damage, with an overall occurrence of 0.3% after ECTR, a rate comparable to that reported with OCTR.

Palmer and Joivanen (29) reported results from their retrospective study that attempted to determine the frequency and type of complications resulting from ECTR and OCTR that were treated by members of the American Society for Surgery of the Hand between 1990 and 1995. They found surprisingly high numbers of complications associated with both ECTR and OCTR: 100 median nerve and 88 ulnar nerve lacerations were reported in ECTR versus 147 median and 29 ulnar nerve lacerations in OCTR; and 121 vessel lacerations were noted in the ECTR group versus 34 in the OCTR group. The authors concluded that it is advisable to release the tourniquet to diagnose an arterial laceration and avoid postoperative hematoma.

Shinya et al. (30) performed single-portal ECTR in 107 hands on 88 patients. They described 11 complications, including incomplete release, postoperative scarring around the nerves, laceration of the superficial palmar arch, reflex sympathetic dystrophy, palmar fasciitis, and wound inflammation. It now is realized that incomplete release is preventable by diligently checking for residual fibers after transecting the flexor retinaculum. Once the distal edges are divided, they must be reinspected and any remaining bands divided.

The small wound at the wrist may be irritated by retraction during passage of various instruments. This may predispose the wound to inflammation. Absorbable suture, which may cause a reaction, should be avoided.

Overall, complications can be avoided with proper training, careful technique, and conversion to OCTR when endoscopic visibility is poor, anatomy is abnormal, or the carpal tunnel is tight.

TISSUE HARVESTING

Endoscopic techniques have been used extensively to harvest tissue for reconstructive surgery. The use of these tissues without the conventional pattern of scarring and the decrease in donor site morbidity make this application very useful.

Vein Harvesting

Endoscopic vein harvesting has its greatest applications in cardiothoracic and peripheral vascular surgery, allowing significant reduction in morbidity and scarring. Very often, cardiac and vascular patients complain of the long saphenous donor site as the primary source of morbidity, which includes a painful incision and prolonged edema. Endoscopic harvesting can significantly reduce these problems as well as the scarring associated with open vein harvesting. Lundsen and Eaves reported that endoscopic harvesting of the saphenous vein significantly reduces postoperative pain and swelling (12). Complications included a graft that failed to mature and skin ischemia over a small area overlying the vein tract. New instrumentation and modification of this technique will make endoscopic vein harvesting an easier and safer procedure.

Nerve Harvesting

Jones and Howell described their experience in endoscopic nerve harvesting that includes the sural nerve in the leg and medial and lateral antebrachial cutaneous nerves in the forearm (12). The endoscopic harvest eliminated the lengthy scars and reduced potential wound healing problems and hypertrophic scars. In their hands, the nerve grafts were subjected to less trauma than the stair-step technique. No serious complications were seen. However, the authors recommended limiting the entrance incisions to the mid leg and performing the endoscopic dissection from proximal to distal to minimize wound healing problems at the distal incision.

Muscle Harvesting

The MD Anderson and Emory groups have pioneered the techniques of endoscopic harvesting of the rectus abdominis and latissimus dorsi muscles. Many of the technical difficulties encountered were attributed to instrument design. The advantages include a shorter operative time, smaller scars, and reduction in donor site wound healing problems. More sophisticated customized instrumentation will facilitate the endoscopic approach for muscle harvesting.

Omentum-Jejunum Harvesting

Saltz (31) reported endoscopic harvesting of omentum and jejunum free flaps, two very useful flaps in reconstructive surgery. The original description included exteriorization of the omental tissue before ligation of the vascular branches and isolation of the right gastroepiploic pedicle. However, this caused more trauma to the omental tissue and a large abdominal scar. The technique then was modified by more meticulous dissection of the greater curvature of the stomach using endoscopic vessel clips, which minimized the manipulation of the omental tissue and vessels, shortened the abdominal scar, and decreased the operative time. Once again, the complications were related to instrumentation and the learning curve required to safely perform the procedure. The laparoscopy instruments were not delicate enough for microscopic vessel manipulation, with potential intimal damage affecting the final outcome. One harvested omental flap was lost due to damage to the microcirculation during harvesting. The abdominal scar can be very small once the surgeon masters the technique (Fig. 19-7). Combining the procedures with a general surgical team may be necessary if the plastic surgeon has not been trained in laparoscopy. For free jejunal harvesting, it may be preferable to exteriorize the proximal and distal segments to facilitate completion of the intestinal anastomosis.

A
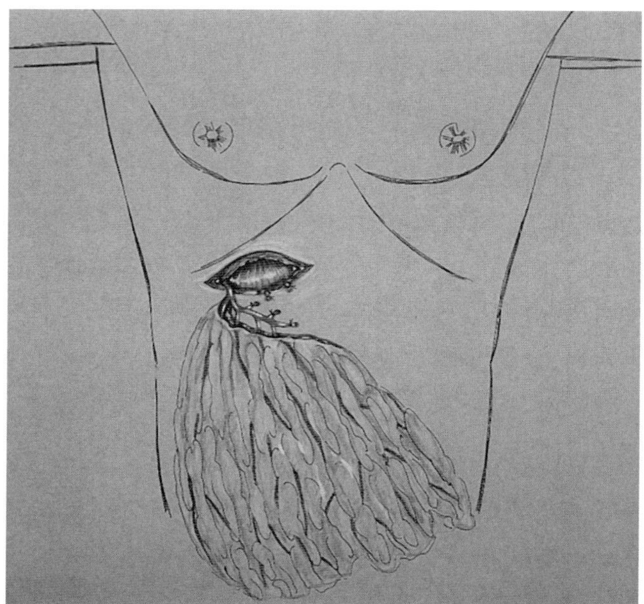

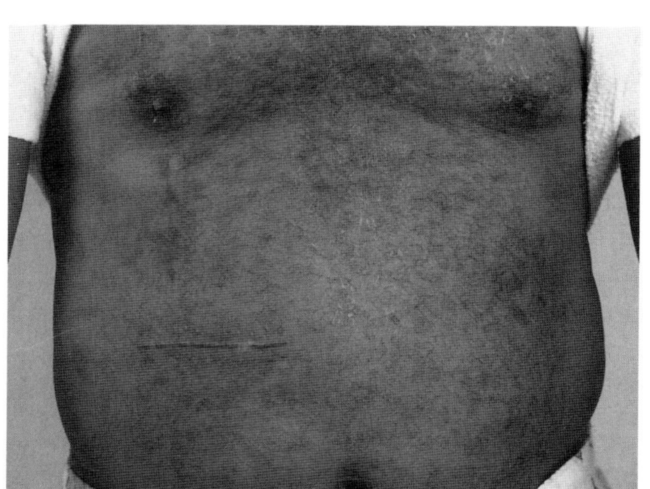
B

C
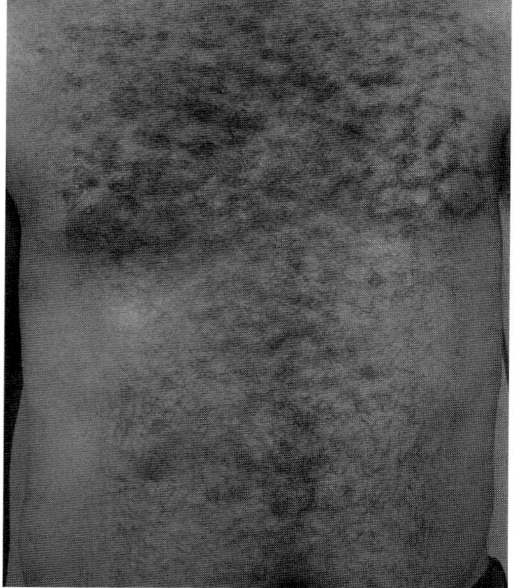

FIGURE 19-7. A: Original technique described for endoscopic omental harvesting with exteriorization and extraabdominal vessel ligation. **B:** Large abdominal scar. **C:** Modification of technique with intraabdominal endoscopic vessel ligation, resulting in smaller abdominal scar.

TISSUE EXPANSION

Endoscopy appears to provide many advantages for tissue expansion surgery. It allows one to introduce expanders through mini-incisions placed in a remote site and to obtain magnified endoscopic visualization during dissection of the pocket, resulting in minimal trauma to adjacent structures during the endo insertion of the expander. During the expansion period, endoscopic surgical revision can be done if necessary. Endoscopic diagnosis and correction of problems related to the implant, tubing valve, or the capsule permits continuation of the expansion without any loss of expanded tissue. Before tissue expander removal, endoscopy allows manipulation of the capsule to increase the gain achieved by the final intraoperative expansion.

The disadvantages of endoscopic expansion surgery include the loss of the traditional three-dimensional approach and the learning curve of working in a two-dimensional field, along with loss of direct contact with the tissues and limited mobility. The learning curve will delay some of the procedures, there may be possible inadvertent injury to the expander system, and there is a higher cost associated with the procedure due to new instrumentation and equipment. The use of CO_2 for creation of the optical cavity in the pocket is still very controversial. Complications of subcutaneous emphysema, hypercarbia, pneumothorax, and gas embolism have been reported in gynecologic and gastrointestinal procedures. The use of CO_2 should be restricted to only very large expanded areas, where one cannot build the optical pocket using safer and simpler methods, such the endoscope hood, intraoperative expander, or sternal traction devices (32).

CONCLUSIONS

This chapter provided a guide to the most common endoscopic plastic surgery techniques, their complications, and fundamental principles to avoid these complications. Plastic surgeons will benefit from familiarizing themselves with the new endoscopic procedures, basic equipment, potential complications, and means to avoid them. The necessity of basic training with cadavers and black boxes cannot be overemphasized, especially for surgeons who have no experience with endoscopy surgery during their residency. The goal of diminished scars and morbidity should be borne in mind during preoperative evaluation to determine where to place incisions and how to develop the optical cavity. The development of new instrumentation has allowed plastic surgeons to perform faster and safer endoscopic procedures with fewer complications. Also, by training operating room personnel and assisting them in arranging the operating room correctly, the plastic surgeon can avoid potential problems during the procedure and ultimately decrease the complication rate. For more complex intraabdominal and reconstructive procedures, plastic surgeons are strongly encouraged to work with general surgeons who are familiar with the equipment and laparoscopic techniques.

Plastic and reconstructive surgeons are still seeking outcome studies with comparative data to establish the effectiveness of endoscopic techniques and to allow comparison with open procedures based on cost, operative risk, and long-lasting effects. Although endoscopy provides a new and powerful tool for plastic surgeons, it also creates the potential for new problems.

ACKNOWLEDGMENTS

The authors thank Drs. Grady Core and Chen Lee for their contributions to the chapter and Ms. Christie Klungervik for preparing the manuscript.

REFERENCES

1. Core GB, Vasconez LO, Askren C, et al. Coronal facelift with endoscopic techniques. *Plast Surg Forum* 1992;15:227–228.
2. Swift RW, Nolan WB, Aston SJ, et al. Endoscopic brow lift: objective results after one year. *Aesthetic Surg J* 1999;19:287–292.
3. Sasaki GH. Comparison of open and endoscopic forehead lifts: a preliminary evaluation by questionnaire response. Presented at the Endoscopy in Plastic Surgery: A Consensus Multidisciplinary Symposium, Birmingham, Alabama, July 20–24, 1994.
4. Saltz R, Ramirez O, Vasconez W. Endoscopic Browlift: 6 Years and 800 Cases Later. IPRAS, San Francisco, California, 1999.
5. Daniel RK, Tirkantis B. Endoscopic forehead lift: an operative technique. *Plast Reconstr Surg* 1996;98:1148–1157.
6. Lorenc ZP, Ivy E, Aston SJ. Neurosensory preservation in endoscopic foreheadplasty. *Aesthetic Plast Surg* 195;19:411–413.
7. Isse NG. Endoscopic facial rejuvenation: endoforehead, the functional lift—case reports. *Aesthetic Plast Surg* 1994;18:21–29.
8. Knize DM. A study of the supraorbital nerve. *Plast Reconstr Surg* 1995;96:564–569.
9. Slade CS, Cohen SP. Elicitation of the oculocardiac reflex during endoscopic forehead lift surgery. *Plast Reconstr Surg* 1999;104:1828–1830.
10. Faria-Correa MA. Endoscopic abdominoplasty, mastopexy and breast reduction. *Clin Plast Surg* 1995;22:723–745.
11. Ho LCY. Endoscopic assisted transaxillary augmentation mammoplasty. *Br J Plast Surg* 1993;76:332.
12. Bostwick J III, Eaves FF III, Nahai F. *Endoscopic plastic surgery.* St. Louis: Quality Medical Publishing, 1995
13. Eaves FF, Nahai F, Bostwick J. Endoscopic abdominoplasty and endoscopically assisted miniabdominoplasty. *Clin Plast Surg* 1996;23:599–616.
14. Kobayashi S, Sakai Y, Yamada A, et al. Approaching the zygoma with an endoscope. *J Craniofac Surg* 1995;6:519.
15. Saltz R, Cheng L. Application of minimal access and endoscopic techniques in the management of facial fractures. Instructional Course for Plastic Surgery Educational Foundation, New Orleans, Louisiana, October 25, 1999.
16. Lee CH, Lee C, Trabulsy PP, et al. A cadaveric and clinical evaluation of endoscopically assisted zygomatic fracture repair. *Plast Reconstr Surg* 1998;101:333–345.

17. Lee C, Stiebel M, Young DM. Cranial nerve VII region of the traumatized facial skeleton: optimizing fracture repair with the endoscope. *J Trauma* 2000;48:423–431.
18. Jacobovicz J, Lee C, Trabulsy PP. Endoscopic repair of mandibular subcondylar fractures. *Plast Reconstr Surg* 1998;101:437–441.
19. Chen CT, Lai JP, Jung TC, et al. Endoscopically assisted mandibular subcondylar fractures repair. *Plast Reconstr Surg* 1999;103:60–65.
20. Lee C, Jacobovicz J, Mueller RV. Endoscopic repair of a complex midfacial fracture. *J Craniofac Surg* 1997;8:170–174.
21. Stammberger H. Results, problems and complications. In: Stammberger H, Hawke M, eds. *Functional endoscopic sinus surgery. The Messerklinger technique.* Philadelphia: BC Decker, 1991:459–477.
22. Stankiewicz JA. Blindness and intranasal endoscope ethmoidectomy: prevention and management. *Otolaryngol Head Neck Surg* 1998;101:320–329.
23. Neuman TR, Turner WJ, Davidson TM. Complications of endoscopic surgery. *ENT J* 1994;73:585–590.
24. Stankiewicz JA. Cerebrospinal fluid fistula and endoscopic sinus surgery. *Laryngoscope* 1991;101:250–256.
25. Mattox DE, Kennedy DW. Endoscopic management of cerebrospinal fluid leaks and cephaloceles. *Laryngoscope* 1990;100:857–862.
26. Wiesman RA. Septal chondromucosal flap with preservation of septal integrity. *Laryngoscope* 1989;99:267–271.
27. Straub TA. Endoscopic carpal tunnel release: a prospective analysis of factors associated with unsatisfactory results. *Arthroscopy* 15 (3), 269-274 1999.
28. Bsecskstyns ME, Sorensen AI. Does endoscopic carpal tunnel release have a higher rate of complications than open carpal tunnel release? An analysis of published series. *Br J Hand Surg* 1999;24:9–15.
29. Palmer AK, Joivanen DA. Complications of endoscopic and open carpal tunnel release. *Am J Hand Surg* 1999;24:561–565.
30. Shinya K, Lanzetta M, Conolly WB. Risk and complications in endoscopic carpal tunnel release. *Br J Hand Surg* 1995;20:222–227.
31. Saltz R. Endoscopic harvest of the omental and jejunal free flaps. *Clin Plast Surg* 1995;22:747.
32. Saltz R, Anger J. Endoscopic placement of tissue expanders. In: Ramirez OM, Daniel RK, eds. *Endoscopic plastic surgery.* New York: Springer-Verlag, 1996.

Discussion

ENDOSCOPY

FOAD NAHAI

The mere reduction of scar is not in and of itself an advance unless the results and morbidity match those of similar "open" procedures.

Over the past several years or so, I often have started my presentations on endoscopic plastic surgery with this quote. Now with more than 7 years of experience, we can respond to that quote. My own personal experience and that reported by Drs. Saltz and Boehm in their chapter confirm that the results of most endoscopic plastic surgery procedures match or surpass those with open techniques, with equal or lower morbidity. In fact, if we consider scar reduction as an improvement in the result, then it would be fair to say that the results surpass those with open techniques.

Why do we as plastic surgeons make skin incisions? We make skin incisions to access the deeper tissues, we make skin incisions to resect skin, or we make skin incisions to do both! If skin excision is not necessary for a procedure and is only made for access, then endoscopic procedures can and should produce equal results with shorter scars and perhaps less morbidity. The key is the need for skin excision, and it must be remembered that inelastic, stretched, or damaged skin will not contract and there is no substitute under those circumstances for skin excision.

The initial enthusiasm phase for endoscopic plastic surgery has passed and the evaluation phase is in progress. We now are in a position to comment on a variety of aesthetic and reconstructive endoscopic plastic surgery procedures. I believe that the pendulum has settled, that endoscopy has found its role in aesthetic plastic surgery, and that its place in reconstructive surgery continues to evolve. This evolution is firmly dependent on advances and modifications in instrumentation and technique.

In the spring of 1996, Eaves et al. with the Emory Group reviewed the first 1,000 endoscopic cases that we had performed in 693 patients (F.E. Eaves III, J. Bostwick III, and F. Nahai, *personal communication* 1996). The overall complication rate was 5% or less, with no deaths, permanent

F. Nahai: Division of Plastic Surgery, Emory University; and Paces Plastic Surgery & Recovery Center, Atlanta, Georgia

nerve injuries, skin or body cavity perforations, or misadventures. The published series quoted by Saltz and Boehm also confirms this low complication rate.

ENDOSCOPIC BROWLIFT

The endoscopic browlift is by far the most common and almost universally accepted endoscopic procedure that has proven to be safe and effective. In the series reviewed by Eaves, we had a 1% rate of transient frontal nerve branch paralysis. Since then, a review of a personal series of over 200 endoscopic browlifts reveals no permanent or transient frontal branch nerve palsy. As cited by the authors, we also have seen alopecia at the transcutaneous screw fixation sites, but unlike Swift et al. (1), we have seen it only in 10% or fewer of our patients and unlike Daniel and Tirkantis (2), these were not temporary and some required excision of the alopecia. Like Dr. Aston and his group (1), I also have abandoned external screws in favor of cortical tunnel fixation, with no related complications to date.

Temporary sensory changes in the distribution of the supra orbital nerve has been seen in 10% to 15%, with no permanent sensory loss.

There are reported complications, unique to the endoscopic browlift, that are not seen with open techniques. Fortunately, these complications are extremely rare, and so far I have not seen any in my personal practice. These complications include skin perforation, cautery-related skin burns, and bone bleeding from screw fixation and cortical tunnel sites and even sagittal sinus injuries.

These rare complications not withstanding, I believe that in most patients the endoscopic forehead lift has resulted in equal or more "natural results" than the open technique, with less morbidity. However, there does remain a small group of patients, e.g., those with heavy brows, those with significant asymmetry, and some men, in whom the open approach may be more suitable.

ENDOSCOPIC FACELIFT AND NECKLIFT

Although Saltz and Boehm do not comment on endoscopic facelifts and necklifts, I have had some experience. Again, I reiterate that inelastic and damaged skin must be excised, and there is no substitute for skin excision. Given this, there are a few patients in whom the deeper tissues can be rearranged endoscopically, especially in the neck, without making long access incisions. In this small group of patients, good-to-excellent results equaling the open technique can be achieved. However, candidates for these procedures are younger and few and far between. In my experience, the hematoma rate with endoscopic necklifts has been double that with the open technique.

ENDOSCOPIC BREAST SURGERY

The endoscope has proven useful for transaxillary, inframammary, and even transumbilical breast augmentation. In breast augmentation, the use of the endoscope is not to reduce scar. In fact, the incision length usually is not reduced. However, especially through the transaxillary route, the endoscope allows direct visualization with control of the dissection, which enables the surgeon to precisely dissect the breast pocket, especially medially and inferiorly. This has significantly eliminated implant malposition, which is not unusual with transaxillary subpectoral breast augmentation. Complications and morbidity have been similar to those seen with traditional breast augmentation procedures. However, the risk of skin burns at the skin incision site due to faulty or damaged insulation on the cautery dissector has been reported and is easily avoided by careful examination of the instrumentation. Although unusual with open or endoscopic techniques, intrathoracic penetration during endoscopic breast procedures has been reported.

As for endoscopic breast reduction and mastopexy, these techniques are yet to be proven. There may be a role for the endoscopic approach for small reductions and mastopexies; however, this role remains to be defined.

The role of the endoscope in breast mass excision and male gynecomastia also is being established at the current time. It appears that equal or superior results are attainable, with minimal scarring and without any new or unusual complications.

ENDOSCOPIC ABDOMINOPLASTY

The combination of liposuction and endoscopic repair of abdominal laxity is an attractive one. However, candidates for this procedure are few and far between. Most women presenting for abdominoplasty have irreparably damaged, stretched skin with striae that will require skin excision. However, there is a small group with limited excess skin of normal elasticity and limited fat excess with diastasis who are ideal for this procedure. In this group of patients, complications have been minimal, with results that match those of open abdominoplasties. There is limited experience to date with endoscopic ventral hernia repair in men.

RECONSTRUCTIVE ENDOSCOPIC PLASTIC SURGERY

The role of endoscopic procedures in reconstructive plastic surgery continues to emerge. This emergence has been slower than that seen with aesthetic plastic surgery, mainly because of the complex instrumentation and surgical techniques required for reconstructive endoscopic procedures. The development of the instrumentation has been rather slow. However, there is promise in the area of facial fractures and tissue harvest, as reported in this chapter.

The placement of tissue expanders has been made safer and morbidity reduced through the application of endoscopic techniques. Through small remote incision sites, the dissection can be performed so that rapid expansion can proceed without the risk of stretching adjacent, long access incisions.

CONCLUSIONS

Although some aesthetic endoscopic procedures (e.g., endoscopic forehead lift and augmentation) have become established, are generally accepted, and have almost universal application, most reconstructive endoscopic procedures are still evolving. Hard data comparing results and morbidity between endoscopic and open procedures are not yet available for all areas. However, I believe it safe to conclude from this early experience that the morbidity from endoscopic procedures is equal to, or perhaps even less than, those seen with comparable open techniques. We must recognize there are some unique complications, including skin burns and body cavity and organ perforations, not normally associated with comparable open techniques. These "sensational complications" are extremely rare and even more rarely reported! Their true incidence is unknown.

REFERENCES

1. Swift RW, Nolan WB, Aston SJ, et al. Endoscopic brow lift: objective results after one year. *Aesthetic Surg J* 1999;19:287–-1999.
2. Daniel RK, Tirkantis B. Endoscopic forehead lift: an operative technique. *Plast Reconstr Surg* 1996;98:1148–1157.

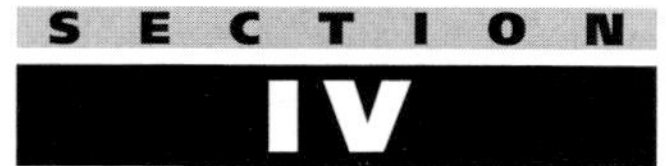

SKIN AND ADNEXA

20

VASCULAR MALFORMATIONS

JOHN B. MULLIKEN
PATRICIA E. BURROWS

In 1914, before a large audience in Philadelphia, the Bostonian Ernest Amory Codman chided his fellow surgeons to acknowledge their less-than-perfect outcomes. He had the temerity to suggest that every hospital be responsible for recording what happens to patients in the hands of every staff surgeon and for comparing these "end results" with those of other institutions. Today, E.A. Codman is the acknowledged father of clinical data collection, registries for specific disorders, and outcome analysis (including assessment by the patients) (1), yet his vision of documenting clinical effectiveness has only begun to be realized.

Codman classified complications, poor results, and deaths as the result of an error in diagnosis (E-d), error in judgment (E-j), error in technique (E-t), or lack of care of equipment (E-c). He insisted these categories be differentiated from a faulty outcome that was a consequence of a patient's unconquerable disease (P-d). This same accounting must be made by the conscience of every surgeon whose patient has an unfavorable result. To date, Codman's schema guides discussion on surgical rounds and in mortality conferences. His classification also serves as the outline for this chapter on adverse results in the management of vascular malformations. Category E-c is excluded because it has not been contributory to problems in these patients.

The field of vascular anomalies lies in the interface between many medical and surgical disciplines. It is well recognized that no one specialist has sufficient knowledge and expertise to diagnose and treat the various forms of vascular malformations in all organ systems. This chapter was written by a plastic surgeon and an interventional radiologist, two colleagues who work together daily on a vascular anomalies team. The patients presented herein were selected from the files of our Vascular Anomalies Center.

J. B. Mulliken: Department of Surgery, Harvard Medical School; and Division of Plastic Surgery, Children's Hospital, Boston, Massachusetts

P. E. Burrows: Department of Radiology, Harvard Medical School and Children's Hospital, Boston, Massachusetts

ERRORS IN DIAGNOSIS

Clinical Diagnosis

The majority of mistakes that occur in the clinical diagnosis of vascular malformations usually can be traced to improper use of words that constitute obsolete classifications (2). The admixed descriptive and histologic nosologies that evolved in the 19th century fail to discriminate between disparate vascular lesions. The word "hemangioma" still is used indiscriminately for lesions that regress as well as for those that progress. The most pertinacious is "cavernous hemangioma"—there is no such entity. The lesion is either a deep (subcutaneous) hemangioma or a venous malformation (VM). A vascular lesion that enlarges in an adult most likely is a malformation. However, there are very rare vascular tumors of adulthood that are labeled by the pathologist as "hemangioma" or "hemangioendothelioma" (3). It is important to underscore that these tumors do not spontaneously regress, as does hemangioma of infancy.

A biologic classification of vascular anomalies, introduced in 1982, is based on cellular features as correlated with clinical characteristics and natural history (2). This system was accepted at the 1996 biennial meeting of the International Society for the Study of Vascular Anomalies in Rome (3). In this schema, there are two major categories of vascular anomalies in infancy and childhood: *tumors* and *malformations.*

Hemangioma is by far the most common vascular neoplasm. Hemangiomas exhibit rapid postnatal growth (the proliferating phase) during infancy and slow regression (involuting phase) that continues until late childhood (involuted phase). Banal hemangioma does not cause platelet trapping (Kasabach-Merritt phenomenon). This life-threatening coagulopathy is associated with more aggressive infantile vascular tumors, kaposiform hemangioendothelioma, and congenital tufted angioma. Other, very rare, vascular tumors of infancy are hemangiopericytoma and angiosarcoma (Table 20-1) (3).

Vascular malformations arise from developmental errors (4). They are structural anomalies, composed of thin-walled channels with dysplastic smooth muscle and lined by quiescent endothelium. They enlarge in proportion to the growth of the patient. They do not regress, and they often expand

TABLE 20-1. VASCULAR ANOMALIES

Tumor	Malformation
Hemangioma	Slow-flow
Hemangioendotheliomas	Capillary (CM) telangiectases
Hemangiopericytoma	Lymphatic malformation (LM)
Angiosarcoma	Venous malformation (VM)
	Fast-flow
	Arterial (AM)
	Aneurysm
	Ectasia
	Stenosis
	Arteriovenous fistula (AVF)
	Arteriovenous malformation (AVM)
	Complex-combined
	Slow-flow
	Klippel-Trenaunay syndrome (CLVM)
	Fast-flow
	Parkes Weber syndrome (CAVF, CAVM)

(although the mechanisms probably differ in the various vessel types). Vascular malformations are subcategorized according to channel morphology and rheology as either *slow-flow* (capillary, lymphatic, venous) or *fast-flow* (arterial). Combined vascular anomalies also can be slow-flow or fast-flow, and these frequently are associated with soft tissue and skeletal overgrowth (Table 20-1).

In addition to improper terminology, vascular anomalies often are mislabeled because they all look quite similar, presenting in various shades of blue, pink, purple, or red. History and clinical findings permit an accurate distinction between a vascular tumor and vascular malformation in over 90% of patients. By definition, the word *congenital* means present at birth. The word *acquired* is used variably; it usually refers to cutaneous lesions that manifest after 1 year of age. However, the nidus for a vascular anomaly can arise *in utero* and not become clinically evident until years later. Although many vascular malformations are "congenital," the presence of a vascular lesion at birth is not necessarily diagnostic. About 30% of hemangiomas evidence a premonitory natal sign, e.g., a macular erythematous stain, papule, pale spot, telangiectasia, or pseudoecchymotic patch. However, 2 weeks is the median age for the first appearance of most cutaneous hemangiomas. Deep cutaneous hemangiomas or visceral tumors tend to manifest weeks to months later. In rare instances, hemangioma can arise *in utero* and present fully grown at birth. Such tumors are termed *congenital hemangioma.* They often regress rapidly, before 1 year (5).

Time is always on the side of the physician struggling to diagnose a vascular birthmark. If the lesion begins to regress after the child is 1 year old, it is hemangioma. If it does not, the lesion quite likely is a vascular malformation. Often, the parents of an infant with a vascular birthmark cannot wait for a retrospective diagnosis. They struggle with their reactions to the birth of a blemished child. Furthermore, the parents are barraged by comments by strangers. Parents need to understand the diagnosis, prognosis, and plan for treatment. If history and clinical examination are inconclusive, the next step is radiologic imaging.

Radiologic Diagnosis

Radiologic imaging is used either to clarify an uncertain clinical diagnosis or to delineate the extent of the lesion and its rheologic characteristics. Each technique has its specific applications and limitations. The reliability of a particular radiologic modality is dependent on the way it is used and the experience of the operator and the radiologist who interprets the study. Although the typical imaging findings of different types of vascular anomalies are generally well known, there are no controlled studies comparing the accuracy of ultrasonography, magnetic resonance imaging (MRI), computed tomography (CT), and angiography.

Ultrasonography with Doppler Investigation

This is the most rapid and inexpensive modality. It is particularly useful in determining the flow characteristics of superficial vascular anomalies. In particular, fast-flow lesions can be differentiated from slow-flow lesions, and the parenchymal component of hemangioma usually can be recognized (6). Ultrasonography is the most operator dependent of the imaging techniques and has limited capacity to evaluate the extent of a lesion.

Magnetic Resonance Imaging

MRI is the most accurate and useful single modality to determine the type of tissue(s), flow characteristics, and size of a vascular anomaly (7,8), but appropriate imaging sequences must be done. These include T2-weighted sequences to show the limits of the lesion, and T1-weighted sequences, without and with contrast medium, to show distortion of normal fat, to show flow voids, and to distinguish blood-filled slow-flow malformations from other fluid-filled lesions. Gradient-recalled echo sequences or magnetic resonance (MR) angiography should always be performed as part of the initial investigation to determine the presence or absence of fast-flow vessels. Adjunctive sequences include MR venography in patients with combined vascular anomalies, e.g., Klippel-Trenaunay syndrome (CLVM) and diffuse venous anomalies, and MR lymphangiography for diffuse lymphatic malformation (LM) or unexplained edema. An additional benefit of MRI over ultrasonography is its capacity to evaluate adjacent structures. This is especially important in demonstrating functional changes, such as airway displacement or obstruction, and the presence or absence of aberrant vessels and other associated malformative anomalies.

Computed Tomography

CT is inferior to MRI for visualizing soft tissue lesions, because differentiation of vascular tissue is less marked. However, CT is especially applicable for evaluating vascular anomalies of the lungs, abdomen, and skeleton.

Contrast Angiography

Conventional angiography and venography are used to delineate specific vascular lesions (8). Venography is the best method for evaluating the deep venous system in patients with combined vascular anomalies or diffuse VMs of the limbs. Angiography is used to investigate fast-flow lesions, i.e., arteriovenous fistulae (AVF), arteriovenous malformation (AVM), and microshunting that can occur in combined vascular anomalies. It provides a precise demonstration of the angioarchitecture of fast-flow vascular anomalies. Such information usually is required only if invasive treatment is planned. Thus, angiography usually is combined with a primary or preoperative embolization.

Radiologic Misdiagnosis

There are several reasons for misdiagnosis of a vascular anomaly by radiologic imaging. Mistakes usually are the result of a radiologist's inexperience and the use of inappropriate imaging techniques or sequences. The most common incorrect applications of these modalities are errors of omission are as follows:

1. Lack of spectral analysis or color Doppler assessment during ultrasonography
2. Failure to include contrast medium and/or fat suppression on postcontrast T1-weighted and T2-weighted sequences of superficial lesions
3. No gradient-recalled echo sequences on MRI
4. Discontinuation of filming before the venous phase during arteriography.

The most common reasons for misinterpretation of a technically adequate imaging study are:

1. Incorrect terminology
2. Assumption that a high-flow enhancing lesion in an infant is "hemangioma"
3. Assumption that all high-flow vascular lesions are AVMs
4. Mistaking a lesion with dilated venous channels as AVM
5. Misinterpretation of phleboliths (signal voids) on MRI for dilated vessels (flow voids).

Accurate Diagnosis is Interdisciplinary

Sixty percent of patients referred to our weekly vascular anomalies conference for consultation (*in absentia*) have been given an incorrect diagnosis, either clinical, radiologic, or both. The most common mistake is using the term "cavernous hemangioma" for a VM. The second most frequent error also is terminologic, that is, calling LM either "cystic hygroma" or "lymphangioma." Proper nomenclature for vascular anomalies is not just semantics. Over 90% of patients sent with an incorrect diagnosis received improper therapy. The most common therapeutic error is administration of an antiangiogenic drug (corticosteroid or interferon) to treat a VM or an LM. There are numerous examples in which a child with a hypervascular malignant tumor was given a drug for "hemangioma" or was misdiagnosed as a vascular malformation.

Biopsy of a vascular lesion is necessary if there is even the slightest suspicion of a malignancy, i.e., whenever the history or the clinical or radiologic findings are ambiguous or atypical. The opposite situation also occurs, i.e., a vascular malformation (especially a VM) is misdiagnosed as a sarcoma. This obviously causes unnecessary parental anxiety.

Examples of Errors in Diagnosis

Examples of errors in diagnosis are shown in Figs. 20-1 through 20-5.

ERRORS IN JUDGMENT

E-js are common. Often they are cloaked as an E-t or relegated to the less embarrassing category of P-d. These mistakes usually are the result of inexperience. Perforce, experience only comes after having committed many errors. E-js are diverse, making them difficult to categorize. Many of these mistakes can be traced back to failure to follow general surgical principles.

Examples of Errors in Judgment

Examples of errors in judgment are shown in Figs. 20-6 through 20-9.

ERRORS IN TECHNIQUE

Endovascular Procedures

The term *embolization* usually is reserved for occlusion of blood vessels using material injected through a catheter, which typically is introduced through the femoral artery. The term *sclerotherapy* denotes the injection of an irritating drug directly into a vascular anomaly, such as a venous varicosity, VM, or AVM. As with surgical procedures, techniques and results of embolization and sclerotherapy vary widely from center to center, depending on the training and the experience of the operator, the types of vascular anomalies, and the nature of the embolic devices and sclerosants.

Embolization

A number of embolic devices and materials are available; the choice depends on the type and size of vessels to be occluded

A

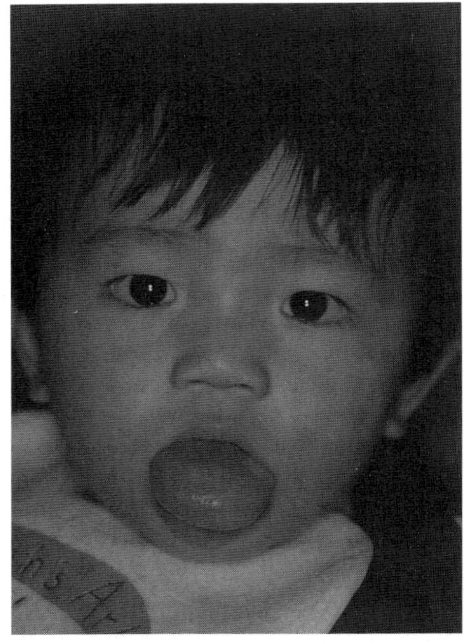

FIGURE 20-1. Arteriovenous malformation of the anterior tongue, misdiagnosed as "hemangioma." **A:** Fourteen-month-old infant with episodic bleeding from a vascular lesion in the anterior tongue. Partial resection and histopathologic diagnosis of "capillary hemangioma." **B:** Sagittal T2-weighted magnetic resonance image shows hyperintense vascular mass with prominent flow voids: dilated lingual artery (LA) and lingual vein (LV). **C:** Axial T1-weighted magnetic resonance image with fat suppression (and intravenous gadolinium) demonstrates diffuse enhancement of mass (M). Note prominent flow voids (*arrows*) representing dilated branches of lingual artery. Addendum: Lingual angiography also consistent with "hemangioma." Lesion embolized and was partially resected. Histology confirmed arteriovenous malformation.

B

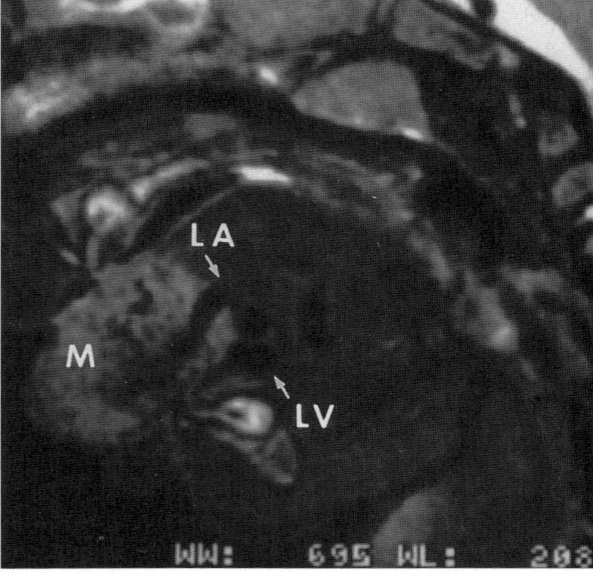

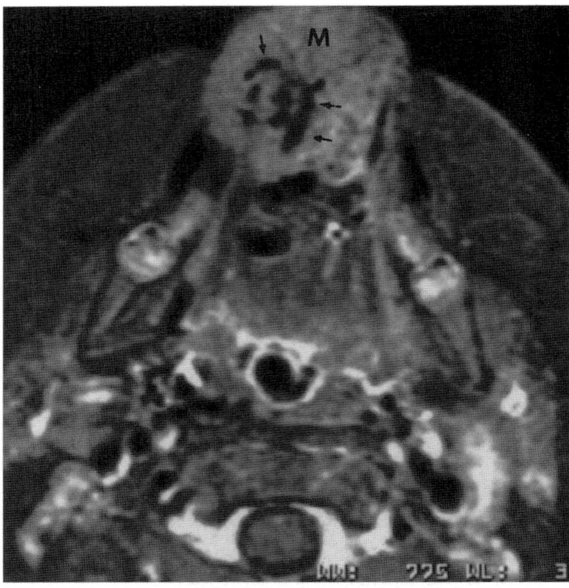

C

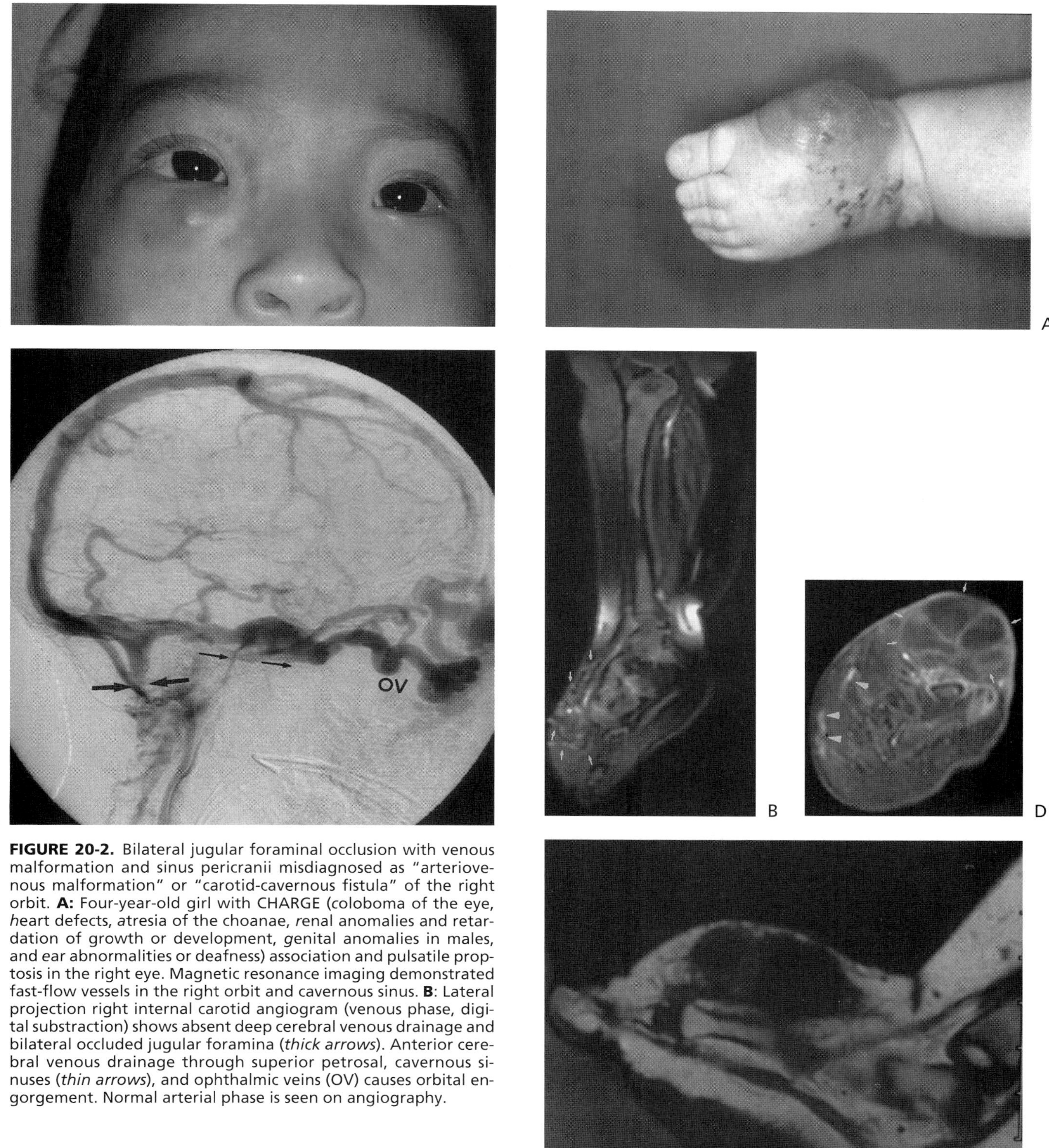

FIGURE 20-2. Bilateral jugular foraminal occlusion with venous malformation and sinus pericranii misdiagnosed as "arteriovenous malformation" or "carotid-cavernous fistula" of the right orbit. **A:** Four-year-old girl with CHARGE (*c*oloboma of the eye, *h*eart defects, *a*tresia of the choanae, *r*enal anomalies and retardation of growth or development, *g*enital anomalies in males, and *e*ar abnormalities or deafness) association and pulsatile proptosis in the right eye. Magnetic resonance imaging demonstrated fast-flow vessels in the right orbit and cavernous sinus. **B**: Lateral projection right internal carotid angiogram (venous phase, digital substraction) shows absent deep cerebral venous drainage and bilateral occluded jugular foramina (*thick arrows*). Anterior cerebral venous drainage through superior petrosal, cavernous sinuses (*thin arrows*), and ophthalmic veins (OV) causes orbital engorgement. Normal arterial phase is seen on angiography.

FIGURE 20-3. Angiosarcoma arising in slow-flow anomaly (LVM) in an infant with Aicardi syndrome. **A:** Punctate stains and vesicles consistent with LVM dorsum of the foot (note hemispheric mass). **B:** Sagittal T2-weighted image (with fat suppression) of the lower limb at age 8 months shows hypertensive linear channels (*arrows*), which were interpreted as veins or dilated lymphatics in subcutaneous tissue. **C:** At age 1 year, the dorsal mass is enlarged. Sagittal T1-weighted image shows focal, subcutaneous cystic areas. **D:** Axial T1-weighted sequence at the metatarsals shows rim enhancement of focal soft tissue masses (*arrows*) and dilated veins in subcutis (*arrowheads*). Addendum: Early magnetic resonance imaging and physical features are consistent with lymphatic malformation (LM). Dorsal mass is enlarged, prompting histologic examination. Another published case report of LM evolving to angiosarcoma in Aicardi syndrome is Tsao Cy, Sommer A, Hamoudi AB. Aicardi syndrome metastatic angiosarcome of the leg and scalp lipoma. *Am J Med Genet*, 1993;45:594.

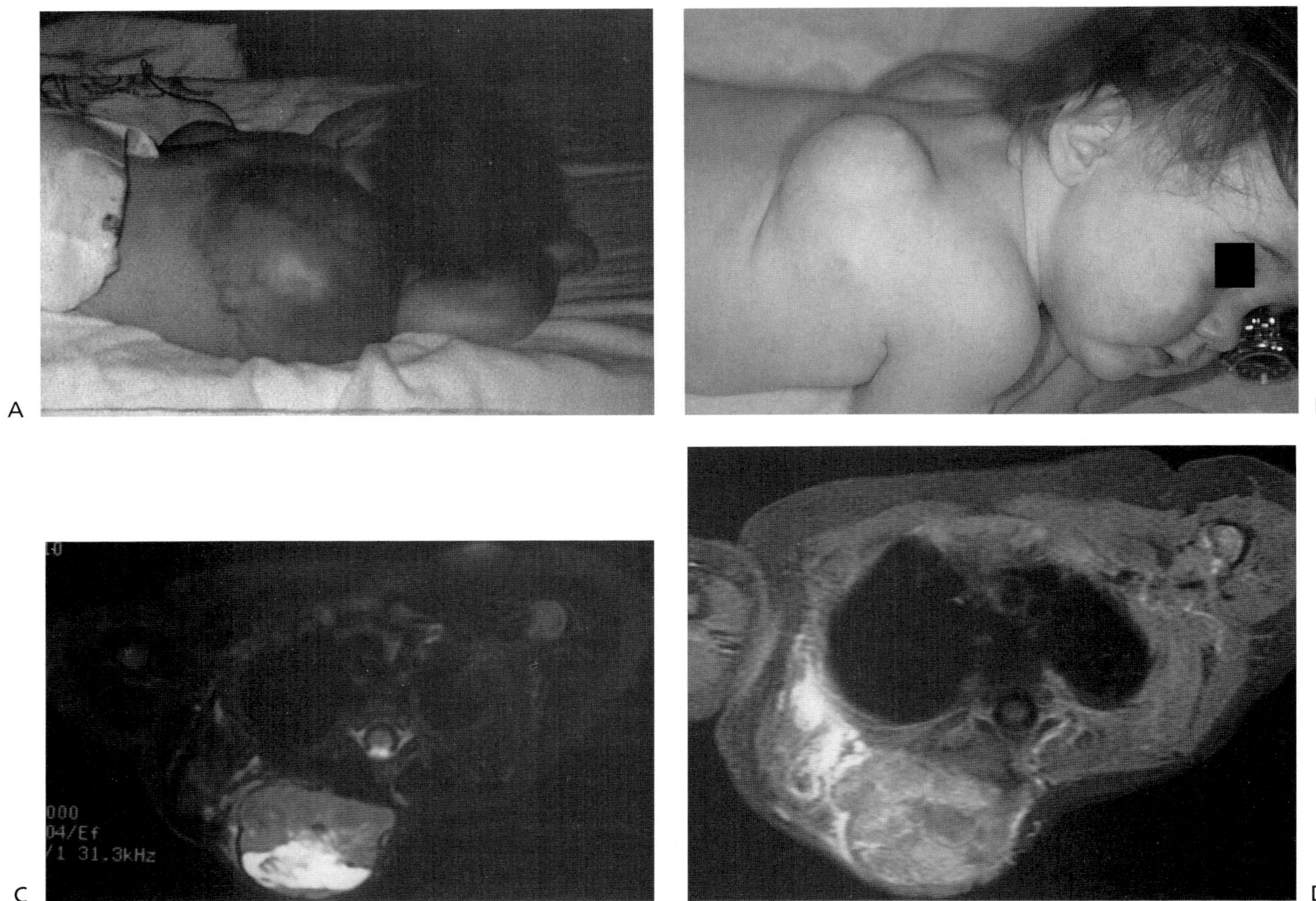

FIGURE 20-4. Thoracic infantile fibrosarcoma masquerading as "hemangioma." **A:** Infant with congenital vascular mass over the scapula. Magnetic resonance image reads as "hemangioma". **B:** Shrinkage of tumor after 6 months of corticosteroids and interferon. **C:** At age 1 year, another axial T2-weighted magnetic resonance image through the thoracic inlet shows soft tissue tumor with heterogeneous signal and focal cystic components. **D:** Axial T1-weighted magnetic resonance image (with gadolinium) demonstrates inhomogeneous enhancement consistent with sarcoma (biopsy confirmed).

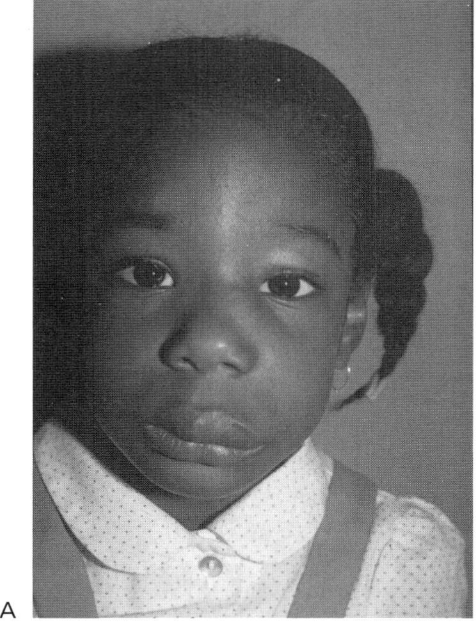

A

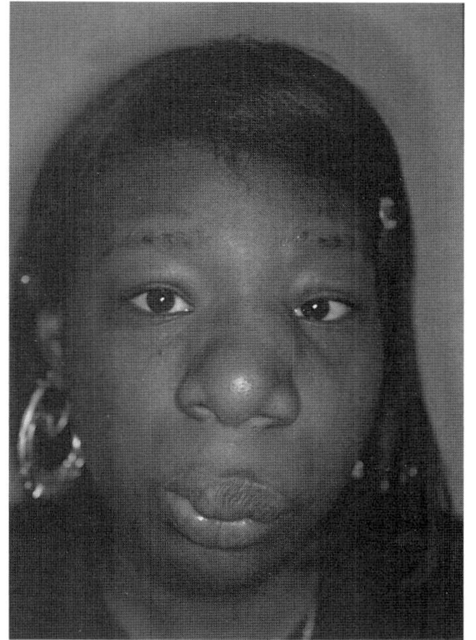

B

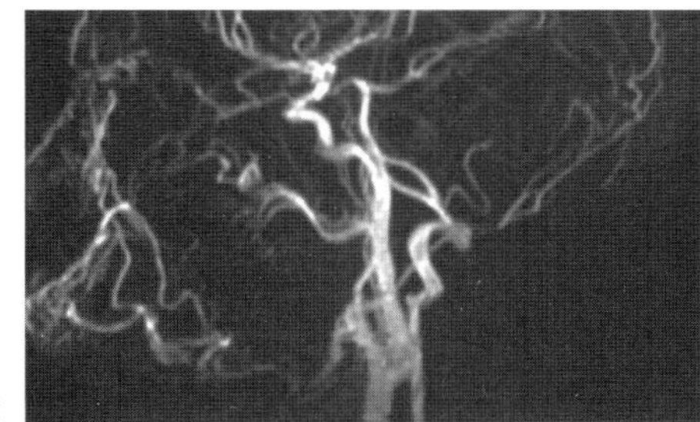

C

FIGURE 20-5. Facial arteriovenous malformation (AVM) misdiagnosed as lymphatic malformation since childhood. **A:** Eight-year-old girl with enlarged left cheek and lip. Clinical diagnosis was "lymphatic anomaly." **B**: Twelve years later, fast-flow lesion was detected by Doppler examination. **C:** Magnetic resonance angiography demonstrates nasolabial AVM supplied primarily by the facial artery.

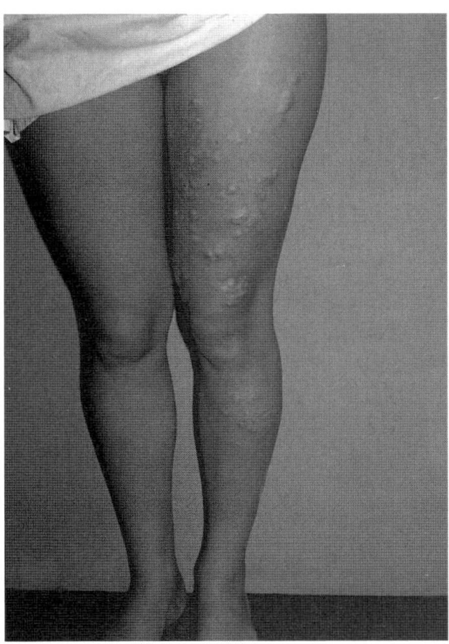

FIGURE 20-6. Multiple localized scars secondary to laser therapy for cutaneous venous anomalies of left lower limb.

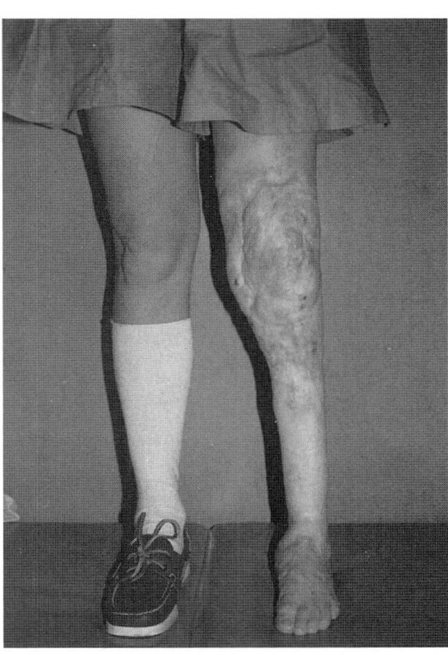

FIGURE 20-7. Young woman with scarring, atrophy, and paralysis of the left lower limb caused by bleeding into the sciatic nerve during partial resection of venous malformation of the knee.

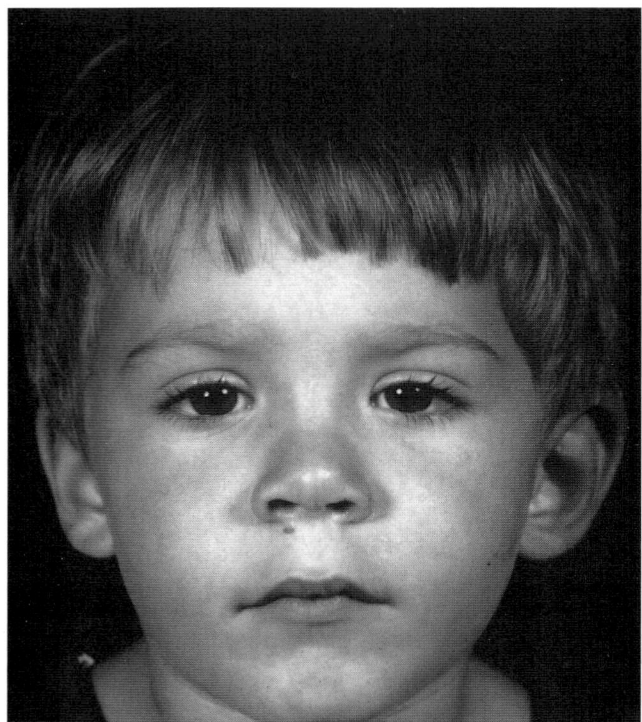

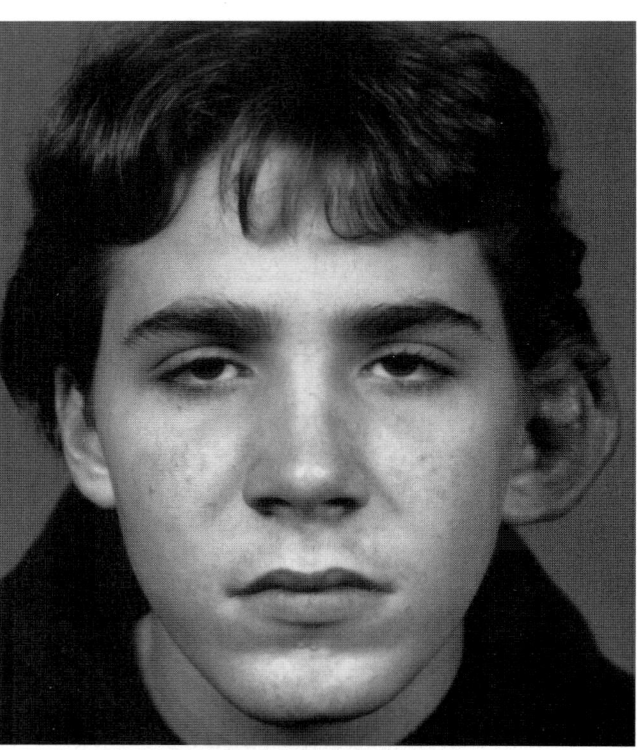

FIGURE 20-8. A: Two-year-old boy with warm, red left ear, noted since birth. There are pulsations but no bruit (stage I arteriovenous malformation [AVM]). **B:** Ill-advised proximal ligation of the superficial temporal artery was performed at age 5 years. Now at age 14 years, stage III auricular AVM.

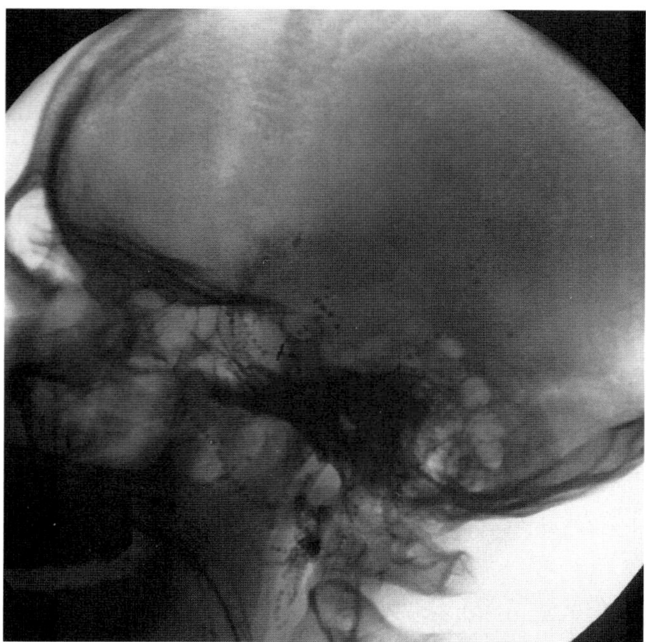

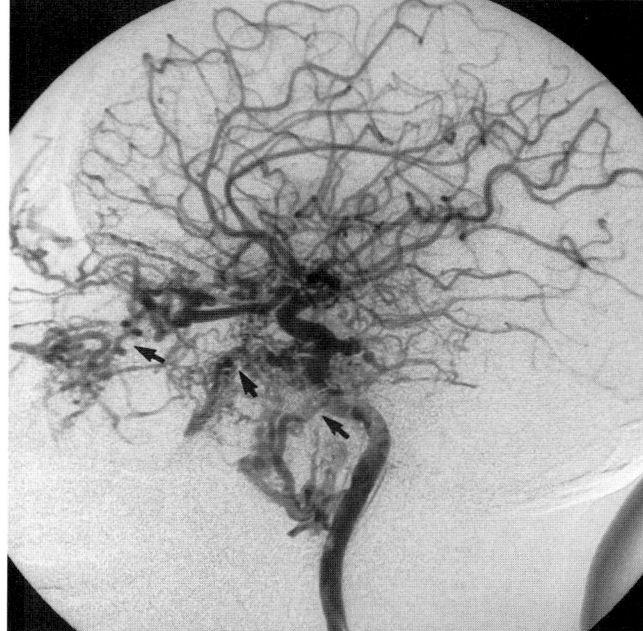

FIGURE 20-9. Stage III facial arteriovenous malformation (AVM) improperly treated by proximal arterial embolization. **A:** Lateral facial radiograph shows proximally located microspheres in the external carotid artery and branches. **B:** Internal carotid angiogram (lateral projection) demonstrates extensive collaterals (*arrows*) from ophthalmic and internal carotid arteries feeding the AVM.

and purpose of embolization (9–11). Preoperative devascularization of a hypervascular tumor or AVM is best accomplished using calibrated polyvinyl alcohol foam (Ivalon) particles with/without Gelfoam pledgets, delivered by superselective catheterization of feeding arteries. There is also a role for *N*-butyl-2-cyanoacrylate, a fast-polymerizing tissue adhesive that can be injected through a microcatheter. Microcoils are used for preoperative occlusion of large, direct, arteriovenous connections. With appropriate technique and selection of proper particle size, preoperative embolization rarely results in major morbidity. Ischemic pain in the distribution of embolization can be minimized by the use of systemic corticosteroid and by performing the embolization within 24 to 48 hours of the surgical resection. There is the potential for ischemic complications in nontarget areas, such as stroke or visual scotomata in patients undergoing head/neck embolization. All catheter procedures have the risk of hemorrhage or thrombosis at the cannulation site. Embolization must be superselective, directed toward destruction of the central portion ("nidus") of the AVM. For primary treatment (without planned resection) permanent, usually liquid agents, e.g., tissue adhesive or alcohol, must be delivered precisely into the nidus. Nevertheless, such aggressive therapy is associated with morbidity in the range from 10% to 30%, including tissue necrosis, neural injury, excessive swelling resulting in tissue damage, thromboembolism, cardiac arrhythmia, pulmonary hypertension, and death.

Proximal occlusion of a main arterial trunk upstream from a high-flow lesion should never be done. Interventional radiologists with inadequate training or experience with vascular malformations may think that occluding a proximal feeding artery will result in immediate hemodynamic improvement. In fact, just as after arterial ligation, there is worsening tissue ischemia and rapid formation of collaterals. Furthermore, proximal occlusion severely compromises the ability to treat the lesion, in the future, by superselective embolization.

With very fast-flow lesions, embolic devices or material may pass through the arteriovenous shunts, resulting in venous occlusion or pulmonary embolism. Also, unsuccessful deployment of coils, detachable balloons, or tissue adhesive can cause vascular occlusion in nontarget organs. Microcatheters can become glued in place during embolization with tissue adhesive, especially in occlusion of intracranial lesions.

Sclerotherapy

There are several sclerosants used to thrombose and shrink venous anomalies, including sodium tetradecyl sulfate (Sotradecol 1% and 3%), absolute ethanol, and Ethibloc (a vegetable protein, dissolved in oleum and mixed with alcohol, used in Europe but not available in the United States). Because Sotradecol and Ethibloc produce minimal discomfort during injection, they can be used after local anesthesia and sedation. Injection of alcohol is more painful and requires general anesthesia. Ethanol also produces more swelling and can result in transient or permanent neural injury. All sclerosants have the potential to cause swelling, deep venous thrombosis, thromboembolism, and cutaneous necrosis (12). In patients with VMs undergoing sclerotherapy, cutaneous necrosis usually occurs at the site of the dermal involvement, although it also can result from penetra-

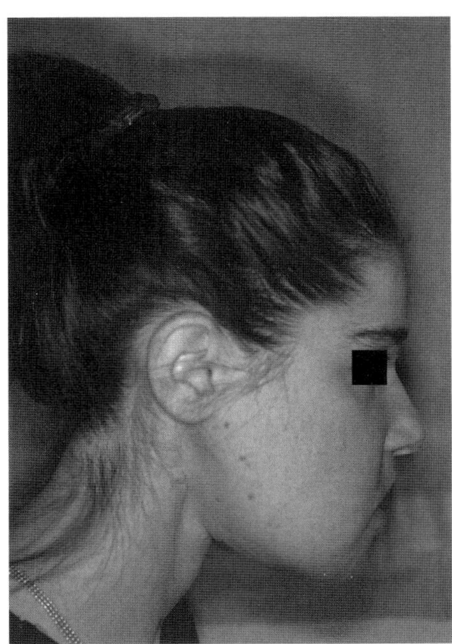

FIGURE 20-10. Distortion of the cervicofacial profile caused by overresection of a lymphatic malformation performed in infancy, accentuated by lower facial hypertrophy.

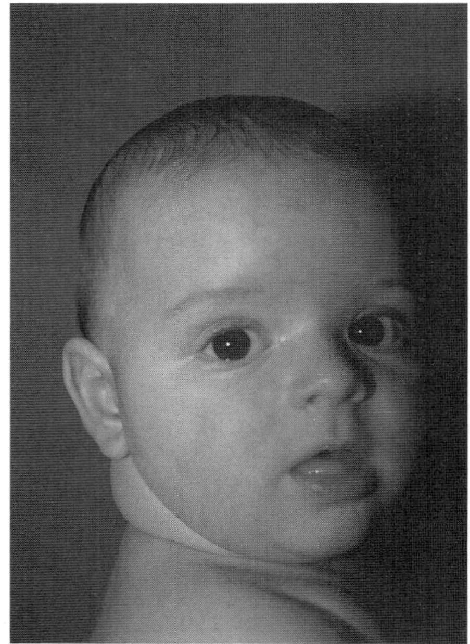
A

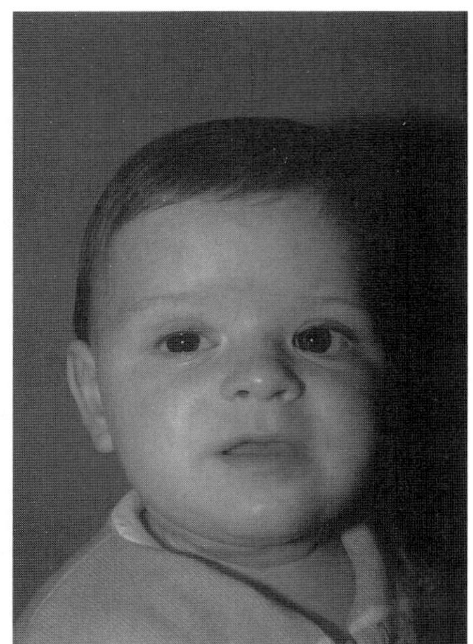
B

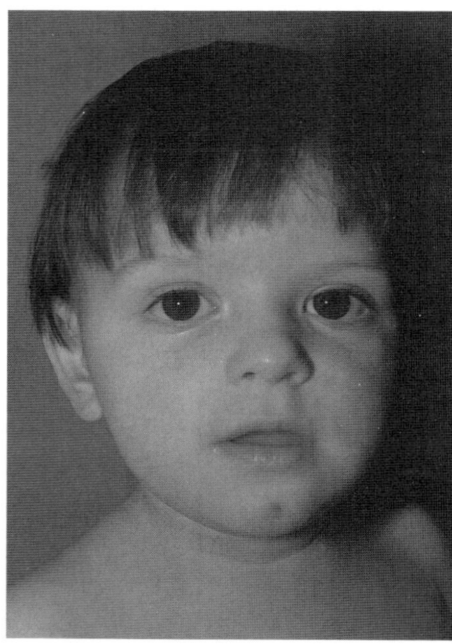
C

FIGURE 20-11. A: Infant with right cervical lymphatic malformation (LM). **B:** Sympathetic trunk divided during resection; Note ptosis (also miosis). **C:** Sympathetic chain repaired at injury; autonomic function returned 1 year later. Note that other nerves at risk for injury during resection of cervical LM are the marginal mandibular, lingual, hypoglossal, vagus, phrenic, and accessory.

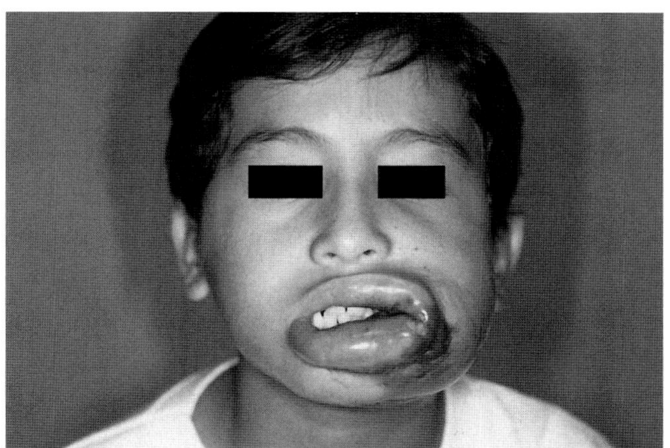
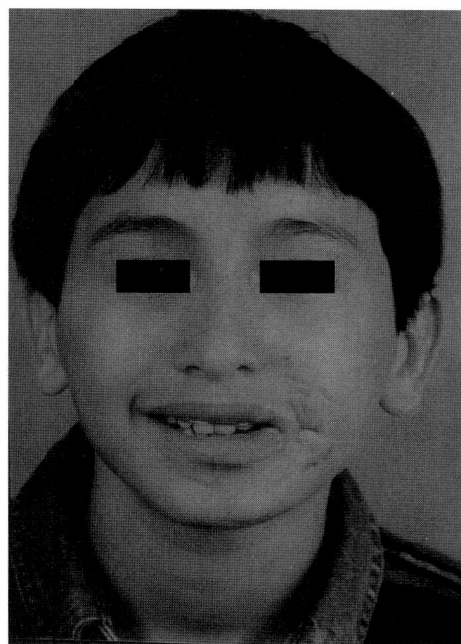

FIGURE 20-12. A: Full-thickness cutaneous necrosis 24 hours after ethanol injection for venous malformation of the cheek. **B:** Scarring 6 months later.

tion of small cutaneous veins in areas of normal skin. Sclerosing agents also cause hemoglobinuria, secondary to hemolysis; however, this is tolerated if the patient is well hydrated. Ethanol has been associated with electromechanical dissociation and cardiovascular collapse; therefore, careful patient monitoring is mandatory.

Operative Procedures

The decision to resect a vascular malformation is based on either a functional problem or aesthetic concern. The indications and possible complications must be understood clearly by the surgeon and the patient. All parties must agree as to the indications for a procedure, whether is to be undertaken in order to improve function, change contour, or control pain. Another important decision in the logic track is whether the procedure involves an attempt to remove all, or only part, of the lesion. The operative strategy for a resecting a vascular malformation can be likened to that for a tumor. However, unlike monobloc extirpation of a malignant tumor, the specimen can be divided and removed "piecemeal," thus sparing important anatomical structures. Whenever possible, the surgeon should try to remove the entire lesion in a single procedure. Indeed, this is the surgical goal in dealing with a fast-flow lesion. However, it often is not possible when operating on lymphatic, venous, and combined anomalies. Slow-flow vascular anomalies can be extensive and, in these instances, the best approach is staged resection, focusing on a particular anatomical region during each procedure. This recommendation particularly applies to lymphatic anomalies. VMs are amenable to partial resection without provoking subsequent expansion of remaining abnormal tissue. In general, sclerotherapy is done before resection of a VM.

The surgeon must be wary of exhibiting a Genghis Khan complex, i.e., "Give me a sword and I can conquer the world." The fast-flow vascular anomalies, in particular, can be treacherous, and often many are best left alone. Some vascular malformations are surgically incurable.

Examples of Errors in Technique

Examples of errors in technique are shown in Figs. 20-10 through 20-12.

PATIENT'S DISEASE

Every type of vascular malformation has its particular proclivity for complications. These untoward events cover in the entire spectrum of problems that can befall tissues, from infection, bleeding, and regrowth, to necrosis and scarring.

Capillary Malformation

Capillary malformation (the 19th century term is *port-wine stain*) is best treated with pulsed dye laser. Most reports claim an approximately 70% response; however, for many patients, the capillary malformation fails to lighten even after multiple laser sessions. Results in the lateral face are better than in the central face or the extremities. Facial stains that also involve the mucosa are especially poor responders. This is presumed to be the result of deep vascular channels, beyond the laser beam. Furthermore, laser photocoagulation is not permanent; reappearance of the stain is well recognized. Ulceration, once commonly seen with the argon laser, is a rare complication of current lasers. If ulceration is deep, this may result in shallow pock-like scarring and/or depigmentation.

Lymphatic Malformation

The two most common complications in a patient with an LM are intralesional bleeding and cellulitis. These are also common untoward occurrences after sclerotherapy or surgical resection. Both bleeding and infection cause acute swelling and induration. Ecchymosis signals the presence of intralesional blood. Usually the local/generalized signs of sepsis serve to differentiate infection from hematoma. Antibiotics should be considered if there is a large collection of blood because of hematoma's known propensity to potentiate secondary infection. For local cellulitis, oral antibiotics may suffice if given early enough. All too often, however, prolonged intravenous antibiotic therapy is needed, and, even so, persistent or recurrent infection is common. There may be a role for prophylactic antibiotics in patients who experience repeated bouts of infection. If an abscess can be documented (by MRI or tagged white blood cell scan), needle aspiration may be useful.

Surgical excision of an LM usually is incomplete. The best strategy is staged resection, attempting to do as complete a removal as possible in a single anatomical region (2). Long-term suction drainage is a postoperative routine to minimize formation of seroma. Nevertheless, the incidence of late fluid collection (or leakage) and wound infection is high.

There is a long-standing debate as to whether the remaining LM will grow back. It is well recognized that any transected lymphatic channel (be it normal or abnormal) will "regenerate." Thus, there must be some regrowth of lymphatic channels into the site after incomplete resection. There also is a pernicious tendency for lymphatic regeneration within the surgical entry wound, forming mucosal or cutaneous vesicles in the scar. These vesicles tend to ooze and bleed, and they are difficult to eradicate. Injection with sodium tetradecyl sulfate (Sotradecol 1%) or CO_2 laser phototherapy can be useful to shrink these vesicles.

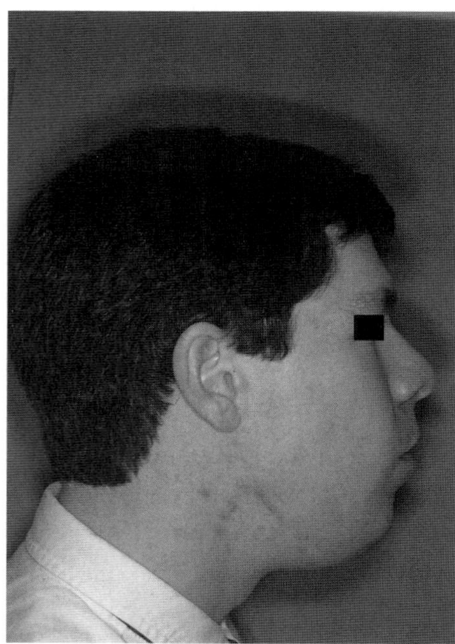

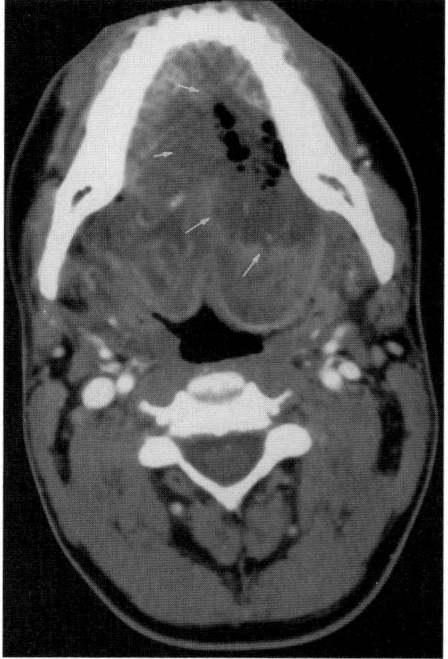

FIGURE 20-13. Cervicolingual lymphatic malformation (LM) with abscess after sclerotherapy. **A:** Thirty-year-old man with cervical LM and long history of recurrent infection and difficulty swallowing/speaking. **B:** Axial computed tomographic image (after intravenous contrast) shows focal collection of fluid/gas (*arrows*) on the floor of the mouth.

Although resection still is considered the best strategy in the management of a lymphatic anomaly, there is increasing interest in use of sclerotherapy. Injection of an irritating solution to shrink LMs has a long history of checkered success. We find that sclerotherapy is most effective for macrocystic LMs, which are the very lesions that are most amenable to surgical removal. Furthermore, multiple injections and scarring can make eventual surgical removal more difficult. We use sclerotherapy for LMs that extend to areas that are difficult to surgically approach, e.g., the parapharynx, pterygoid fossa, and floor of the mouth, and for cysts that appear after partial resection.

Venous Malformation

Slow-flow anomalies can be composed of both abnormal lymphatic and venous channels. This is not surprising, because lymphatics are known to bud from veins during embryonic vascular development. Coagulopathy is a potential problem in these extensive combined slow-flow anomalies (LVMs) or large VMs. Stasis within the anomalous channels probably is the primary event leading to localized intravascular coagulopathy. This complication should be considered in any patient with a vascular anomaly and a history of bleeding or recurrent localized thrombosis. Low-grade dis-

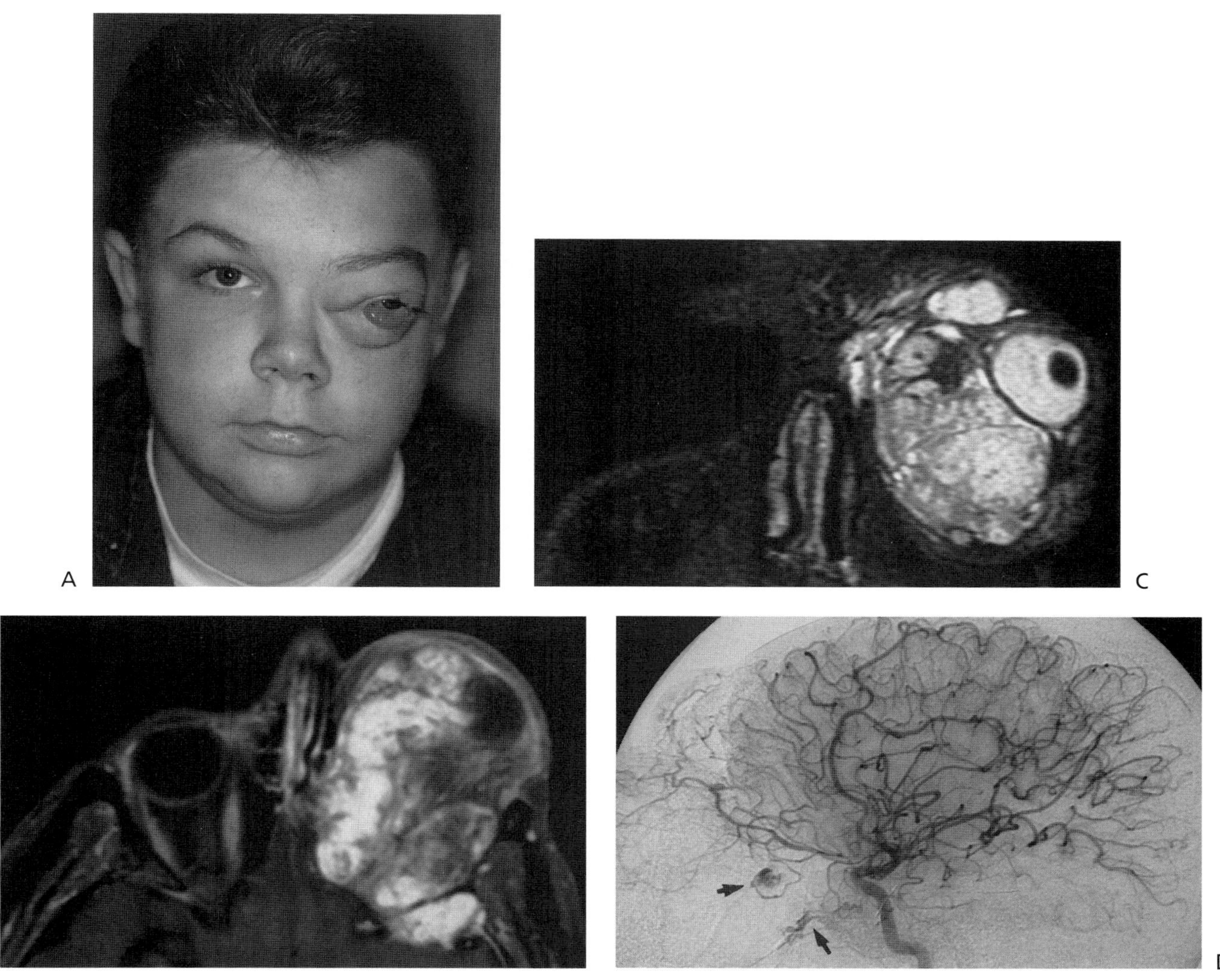

FIGURE 20-14. Orbital lymphatic malformation (LM) with arteriolymphatic shunting. **A:** Fifteen-year-old boy with LM of the left orbit presented with proptosis and progressive visual loss. **B:** Coronal T2-weighted magnetic resonance image shows extensive hypertense septated lesion (LM) displacing the globe. **C:** Axial T1-weighted magnetic resonance image (with intravenous gadolinium) shows contrast enhancement in part of the lesion. **D:** Internal carotid angiography (lateral digital subtraction technique) reveals arterial shunting (*arrows*) into the orbital LM.

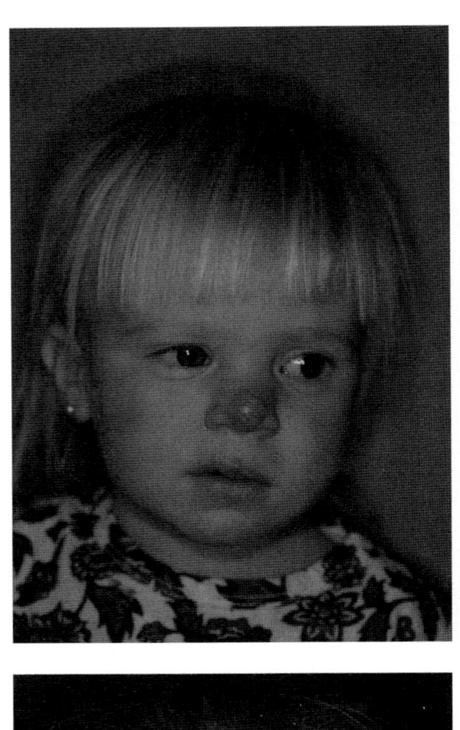
A

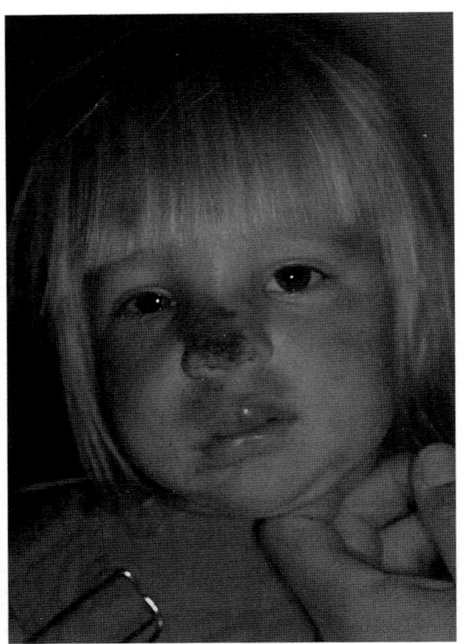
B

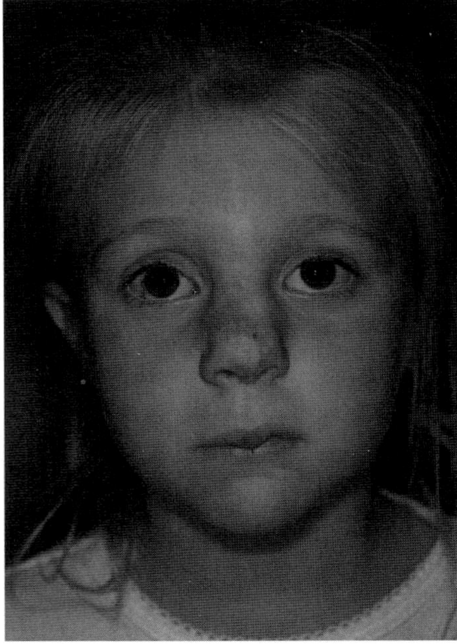
C

FIGURE 20-15. Six-year-old girl with naso-orbital venous malformation (VM) and scarring secondary to sclerotherapy. **A:** VM nose after multiple laser treatments, with diagnosis of "hemangioma." **B:** Acute ulceration after sclerotherapy with ethanol. **C:** Scarring of the nasal tip.

seminated intravascular coagulopathy probably is more common than is documented. Hematologic evaluation is necessary before any procedure, radiotherapeutic or surgical, is performed on these patients. We witnessed two fatalities due to massive pulmonary embolism that followed several days after a prolonged operation. Intraoperative and postoperative hemorrhage, the converse complication, also must be considered. The ideal perioperative management of these patients is unclear. Low-molecular-weight dextran injections should be given perioperatively to decrease thrombotic tendency and improve hemostasis. Heparin must be stopped 24 hours before an operation.

Sclerotherapy is the primary treatment for VM (12,13). A bright blue color signifies a VM lying just below the epidermal layer or mucosal surface. In these instances, injection of a strong sclerosant is likely to cause full-thickness destruction of tissue. The generally accepted incidence of ulceration is 7% to 10%. There typically is cutaneous expansion overlying a VM, so that with healing of such an ulceration, wound contraction often results in an improved contour of the affected area. Hypertrophic scarring also can occur.

The most frustrating outcome after multiple sclerotherapeutic sessions for VM is recanalization and reexpansion. In the past, we delayed surgical resection until several months after the last sclerotherapy. More recently, we have resected the sclerosed VM at an earlier time, before recanalization occurs.

Arteriovenous Malformation

The most common disappointment after resection of AVM is persistent anomalous tissue and early and late recurrence. The strategy guiding therapy of AVM is that cure is possible if the "nidus" first is selectively embolized, followed by total extirpation. The theory is that if the primary vessels are removed, the secondarily involved vessels (collaterals) will revert to normal (14). Embolization is done 24 to 36 hours preoperatively to reduce bleeding; this probably does not diminish the extent of resection required. Intraoperative determination of the completeness of resection is crucial. This is aided by study of the preoperative magnetic resonance images and angiograms. Intraoperatively, the surgeon can listen with a Doppler device, although this is unrewarding if all the feeding vessels have been properly embolized. Intraoperative frozen sectioning is difficult and time consuming. The most helpful predictor as to whether or not the resection is adequate is the type of bleeding observed at the resection margins.

As a general rule, closure of the defect after resection of an AVM should not be done with local tissue (with or without preliminary expansion) unless complete removal is certain. The exception is the rare possibility of removing a small, quiescent AVM. If "cure" is the goal and if there is any question as to adequacy of extirpation, the surgeon should consider temporary primary closure with a skin graft. If there is no evidence of recurrence after 6 to 12 months, more definitive closure can proceed (e.g., with local tissue,

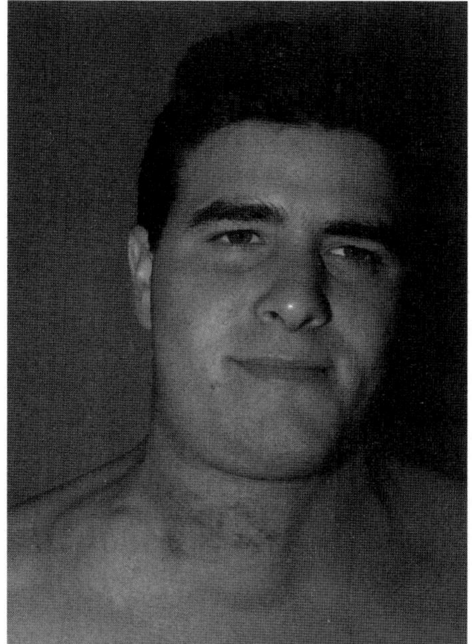

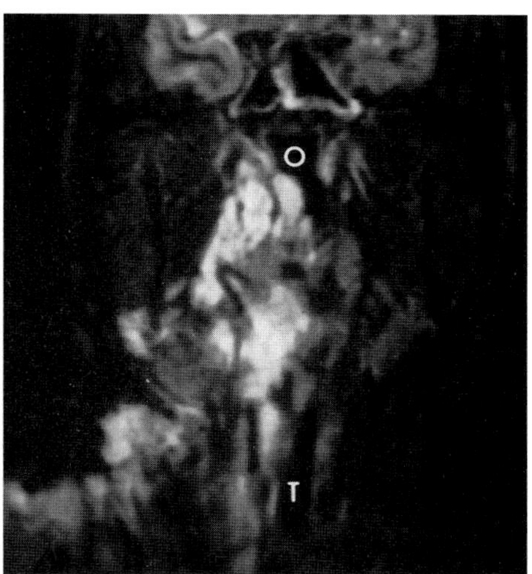

FIGURE 20-16. Extensive cervicothoracic venous malformation (VM) with airway obstruction. **A:** Twenty-two-year-old man performing the Valsalva maneuver to demonstrate VM. He must sleep on four to five pillows. **B:** Coronal T2-weighted magnetic resonance image demonstrates VM indentation and displacement oropharynx (O) and trachea (T).

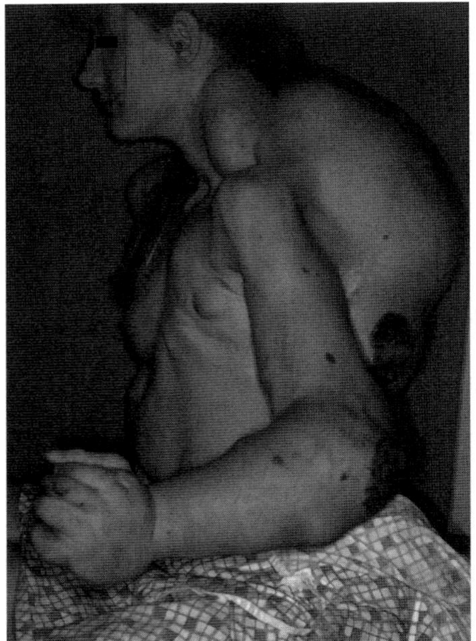

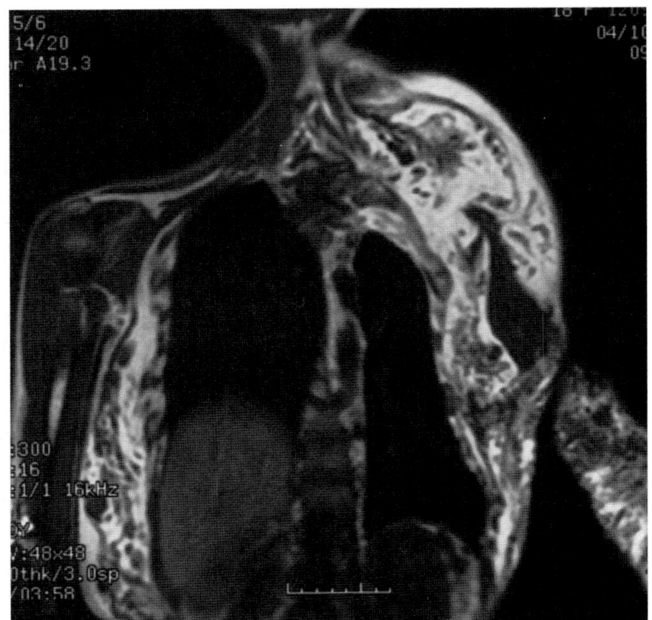

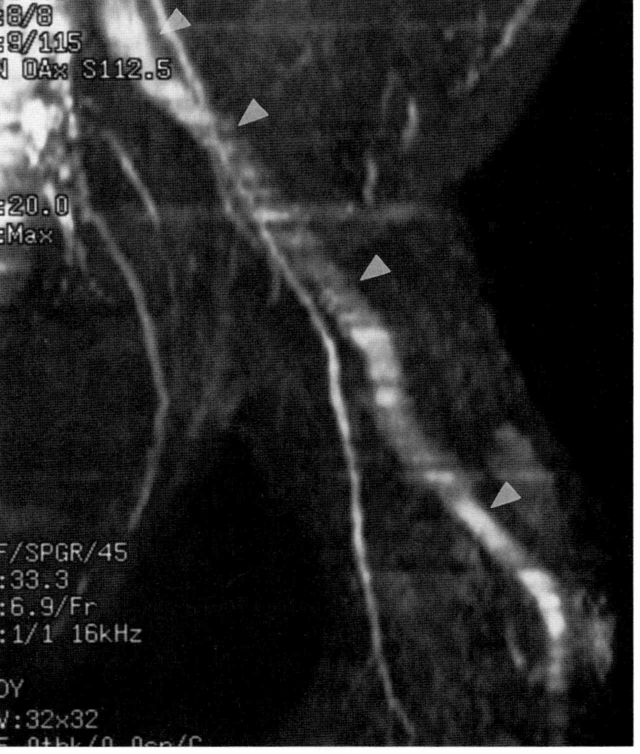

FIGURE 20-17. Fatal pulmonary embolism in a 15-year-old girl with truncal and upper extremity CLVM (Klippel-Trenaunay syndrome). **A:** Surgical resection of the posterior thoracic combined slow-flow vascular anomaly was complicated by wound hematoma, secondary to coagulopathy. **B:** Thoracic coronal T1-weighted magnetic resonance image demonstrates extensive soft tissue masses composed of fatty and slow-flow vascular tissues. **C:** Upper limb magnetic resonance venogram shows markedly dilated deep vein (*arrowheads*), the presumed source of pulmonary embolus.

cutaneous expansion, or free-tissue transfer). For large defects of complex configuration and surfaces, those for which primary closure is needed, tissue transfer with microvascular anastomoses is the best strategy. There is a working hypothesis that closure of such a defect with a microvascular flap changes the local flow dynamics and minimizes the chances for recurrence. This hypothesis has not been proven. We have documented reappearance of AVM with "invasion" of a microvascular flap. Unfortunately, AVM has a perverse tendency to reappear, even many years later.

Examples of Patient's Disease

Examples of patient's disease are shown in Figs. 20-13 through 20-17.

CONCLUSIONS

Patients with vascular anomalies endure not only the complications of their particular disorder, but also iatrogenic problems resulting from well-intentioned therapeutic efforts. All too often, these patients become discouraged either because of confusion about the diagnosis or after suffering the consequences of ill-conceived intervention. Thus, these patients become medical nomads, wandering from one physician to another, searching for someone who understands their problem. Physicians with a special interest in vascular anomalies are beginning to organize in the large referral centers. These teams rarely engender battles over turf. Most physicians are eager to send their patients for consultation, either because the condition seems too "complicated" (even "insolvable") or as an opportunity to share their ideas, experience, and frustration. A vascular anomalies center is a refuge for these migratory patients, a setting for accurate diagnosis, appropriate management, and focused research. Cure may not always be possible. However, in such an interdisciplinary setting, complications and imperfect outcomes are minimized and new therapies can be evaluated carefully.

REFERENCES

1. Passaro E Jr, Organ CH Jr. Ernest A. Codman: The improper Bostonian. *Bull Am Coll Surg* 1999;84:16–22.
2. Mulliken JB, Young AE. *Vascular birthmarks: hemangiomas and malformations.* Philadelphia: WB Saunders, 1988.
3. Enjolras O, Mulliken JB. Vascular tumors and vascular malformations (new issues). In: James WD, Cockerell CJ, Dzubow LM, et al., eds. *Adv Dermato* 1997;13:375–422.
4. Vikkula M, Boon LM, Mulliken JB, et al. Molecular basis of vascular anomalies. *Trends Cardiovasc Med* 1998;8:281–292.
5. Boon LM, Enjolras O, Mulliken JB. Congenital hemangioma: evidence of accelerated involution. *J Pediatr* 1966;128:329–335.
6. Paltiel H, Burrows PE, Kozakewich H PW, et al. Soft-tissue vascular anomalies: utility of US for diagnosis. *Radiology* 2000;214:747–754.
7. Meyer JS, Hoffer FA, Barnes BD, et al. Biological classification of soft-tissue vascular anomalies: MR correlation. *AJR* 1991;157: 559–564.
8. Burrows PE, Laor T, Paltiel H, et al. Diagnostic imaging in the evaluation of vascular birthmarks. *Dermatol Clin* 1998;16: 455–488.
9. Burrows PE, Fellows KE. Techniques for management of pediatric vascular anomalies. In: Cope C, ed. *Current techniques in interventional radiology,* 2nd ed. Philadelphia: Current Science, 1995:11–27.
10. Yakes WF, Rossi P, Odink H. Arteriovenous malformation management. *Cardiovasc Interv Radiol* 1996;19:65–71.
11. Dickey KW, Pollak JS, Meier CH III, et al. Management of large high-flow arteriovenous malformations of the shoulder and upper extremity with transcatheter embolotherapy. *J Vasc Interv Radiol* 1995;6:765–773.
12. Berenguer B, Burrows PE, Zurakowski D, et al. Sclerotherapy of craniofacial venous malformations: complications and results. *Plast Reconstr Surg* 1999;104:1.
13. Yakes WF. Extremity venous malformations: diagnosis and management. *Semin Interv Radiol* 1994;11:332.
14. Kohout MP, Hansen M, Pribaz JJ, et al. Arteriovenous malformations of the head and neck: natural history and management. *Plast Reconstr Surg* 1998;102:643.

Discussion

VASCULAR MALFORMATIONS

H. BRUCE WILLIAMS

Vascular neoplasms and malformations both represent an enigma to the medical practitioner. Their pathogenesis is unclear, and their pattern of evolution remains incompletely explained, yet they constitute the largest group of tumors, hamartomas, and malformations in childhood and later life. Most hemangiomas will completely involute and disappear, whereas others with a remarkably similar histologic appearance will remain as permanent blemishes (1).

Drs. Mulliken and Burrows have added important information in their chapter, which will help greatly in the avoidance of unfavorable results when such lesions are treated. In the landmark article based on endothelial characteristics, Mulliken and Glowacki (2) provide us with a clearer understanding and a classification of the various vascular lesions. Their ingenious decision to separate the lesions into hemangiomas and malformations has been propagated through the literature as we practitioners attempt to maintain the quality of care for children and adults who are afflicted with these conditions. Even though this classification has been available for the past 18 years, many clinicians and even pathologists continue to group all vascular lesions into hemangiomas, lymphangiomas, or mixed hemangiolymphangiomas. In addition, many pathologists regard the so-called hemangioma as a vascular hamartoma that is not far removed from a vascular malformation, so it would appear that both pathologists and clinicians need further reeducation for a universal adoption of this classification.

ERRORS IN DIAGNOSIS

The high percentage of missed diagnoses of vascular lesions in children also is evident in our Vascular and Limb Asymmetry Clinic at The Montreal Children's Hospital. However, even if the referring diagnosis is incorrect, it rarely alters the correct treatment procedure. For example, it is highly unlikely that a child referred by a pediatrician with a diagnosis of a cavernous hemangioma would have different treatment even if the diagnosis was given correctly as a venous malformation. Of more importance, it is essential to differentiate benign vascular lesions from malignant conditions. In my experience, I have encountered patients who have prolonged conservative treatment (benign neglect) for malignant lesions, such as rhabdomyosarcoma, and who have been incorrectly labeled as hemangiomas. Even with benign conditions, I have seen a number of children with lymphatic malformations who have undergone incorrect steroid therapy that would be of no benefit and possibly could cause secondary effects.

LYMPHATIC MALFORMATIONS

Treatment of lymphatic malformations should be based on their embryologic development. Much of the surgical treatment that is prevalent in the literature is based on incorrect information.

The lymphatics develop in close relationship with the venous system and can be identified in the embryo at the end of the fifth week, which is about 2 weeks later than the first signs of the developing cardiovascular system. The two theories of origin are (1) centrifugal and (2) centripetal (3). The centrifugal theory states that the lymphatic vessels are outgrowths of endothelium from the lymph sacs and veins into the surrounding mesenchyme. Sabin (4) did her work with intricate Indian ink injections in pigs, and this was supported by Lewis (5), who, using the rabbit in the animal model, believed that the lymphatics separated from the parent veins at the 16- to 20-mm stage and made new connections at 30 mm. Working with cats, Huntington and McClure (6) believed that the primitive lymphatic channels developed in the mesenchymal tissue and later made contact after coalescing with the venous system. Regardless of their origin, the lymphatic vessels develop from two paired and two unpaired lymph sacs. The two paired jugular lymph sacs appear between the internal jugular veins (precardinal veins) and subclavian veins at 10 mm or 6 weeks of embryonic development. The paired posterior sacs form at the bifurcation of the femoral and sciatic veins, and they link together by the ninth week or 30-mm stage of embryonic development. The unpaired lymph sacs are located at the root of the

H.B. Williams: Department of Surgery, McGill University and Montreal Children's Hospital, Montreal, Quebec, Canada

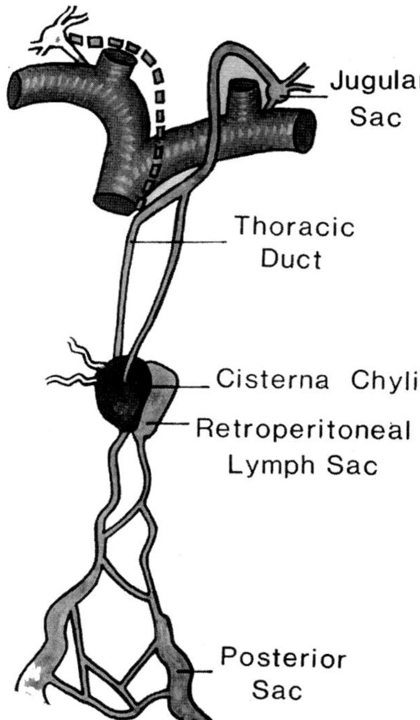

FIGURE 20D-1. Embryonic lymphatic system with two paired sacs (jugular and posterior) and two unpaired sacs (cisterna chyli and retroperitoneal). (Modified from Sabin FR. The development of the lymphatic system. In: Keibel F, Mall FP, eds. *Manual of human embryology, vol. 2.* Philadelphia: JB Lippincott Co., 1912. From Williams HB, ed. *Embryology and classification of lymphatic abnormalities.* St. Louis: CV Mosby, 1983, with permission.)

mesentery (retroperitoneal) and the cisterna chyli, which is dorsal to the aorta and appears at about the same time.

Transport in the lymphatic system, if it has a normal embryologic development, extends from the subepithelial, subdermal, and subcutaneous layers into the lymphatic main trunks (Fig. 20D-1). The main trunks then communicate with the collecting system from the extremities and trunk to drain through the thoracic duct from the inferior right and superior left draining systems, with the connecting portion crossing at the fourth to sixth thoracic vertebrae (Fig. 20D-2). The lymphatic drainage then enters the junction area of the internal jugular and subclavian veins. After the ninth week of embryonic development, the jugular lymph sacs and the cisterna chyli cease to enlarge and eventually become mere dilations of the thoracic duct.

Lymphatic abnormalities on an embryologic basis are classified as follows:

1. Lymphangioma (capillary simplex or macrocystic)
2. Lymphangioma circumscriptum
3. Cystic hygroma
4. Lymphedema
5. Lymphangiectasia.

Lymphangioma simplex most likely represents an error in development at the subepithelial level. The larger macrocystic lymphangiomas are similarly related to errors in development at the subdermal or subcutaneous level, whereas cystic hygromas are likely related to a developmental defect or lack of communication in the major lymphatic trunks or lymphatic sacs. The common occurrence of cystic hygromas in the cervical region, axilla, and groin might indicate an error in development in the jugular or posterior lymphatic sacs at embryonic development. Mesenteric cysts also may represent errors in development in the retroperitoneal sac or cisterna chyli. It is my opinion that cystic hygromas only occur at the juncture of the main lymphatic trunks and the venous system.

As a further extension, congenital lymphedema (Milroy disease), lymphedema praecox, or lymphedema tarda is characterized by hypoplasia of the lymphatics either at the periphery or in the draining lymphatic trunks, or it may be a combination of these two factors. Lymphangiectasia is believed to be a developmental error in which the normal regression of connective tissue elements around the lymphatics fails to occur in the embryo, thus leading to obstruction and an inability to communicate with the larger lymphatics that drain each specific area. Therefore, it represents an error in both the development and in the connection of embryonic lymphatics. Histologic examination of lymphangiectasia shows dilated lymphatics, with cystic spaces in many involved organs such as the lungs, liver, and intestinal tract. There seems

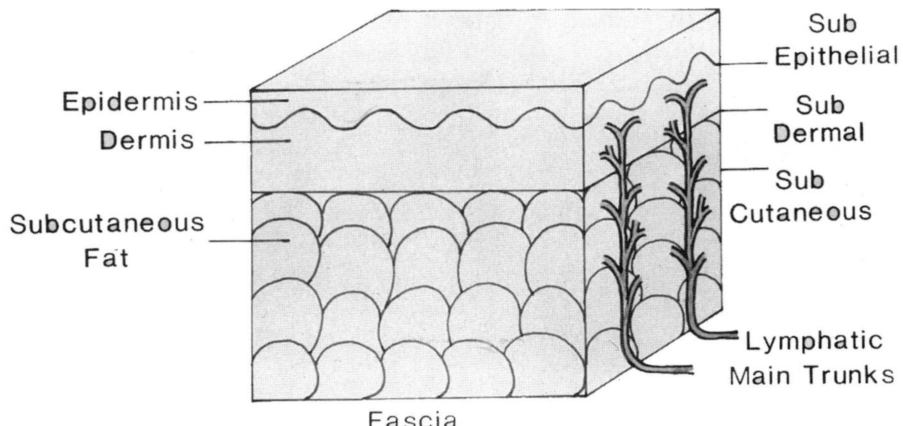

FIGURE 20D-2. Levels of lymphatic drainage. Errors in development at the subepithelial level might result in capillary lymphangiomas. However, macrocystic lymphatic malformations likely result from errors at the subdermal or subcutaneous level, and cystic hygromas are related to developmental defects in the major lymphatic trunks or sacs. (From Williams HB, ed. *Embryology and classification of lymphatic abnormalities.* St. Louis: CV Mosby, 1983, with permission.)

little doubt that the clinical conditions of lymphangiomas, lymphedema, and lymphangiectasia probably represent gradations in severity in embryologic maldevelopment of the lymphatic system.

REGRESSION OF CYSTIC HYGROMAS

Regression or spontaneous involution of lymphatic malformations is extremely rare, except for cystic hygromas. Lymphangiomas at either the superficial or deep tissues usually require surgery for complete removal. Management of lymphangioma circumscriptum is extremely difficult, as many of the deeper lymphatic channels extend through the fascia and even the muscle layers. On the other hand, it is my firm opinion that most cystic hygromas commonly seen in the cervical area will regress spontaneously without surgical treatment (Fig. 20D-3). It is extremely important to rule out involvement of the respiratory tract, and aspiration of the cystic hygroma may be required to relieve pressure on the trachea. Certainly, children with intraluminal lymphangiomatous changes in their respiratory tract need special attention. If there is doubt, then at the time of aspiration, a small biopsy of the lesion is taken just under the ear lobule to confirm the diagnosis. Two or three aspirations may be necessary in the first few weeks of life. In most cases, there is a gradual reduction in size of the lesion. Most patients show complete disappearance of the lesion by 1 year of age. It is unknown whether the cystic hygroma actually disappears or if, in fact, it collapses and has some potential of regrowth or filling in the future. This has not been seen in our cases. It is my belief that early surgery on cystic hygromas often will worsen the condition and encourage persistence of the lesion even if no complications (facial palsy, etc.) have been encountered in the surgical procedure.

COMBINED EMBOLIZATION AND SURGERY

The use of superselective angiography techniques by skilled radiologists has developed into an important facet in the management of children and adults with vascular malformations. It is our preference to have the embolization performed 5 to 7 days before the surgical procedure rather than at 24 to 48 hours. The marked tissue edema and induration following the embolization is most acute up to 2 to 3 days, and surgery is easier after this period of time.

Management of massive, rapidly growing, high-flow lesions has been improved with preoperative embolization followed with surgical excision. Adjunctive treatment using hypotension, cooling, bypass procedures, and possibly cardiac arrest also improves results in selected cases. I categorize these lesions as malignant benign disease, and they are extremely difficult and some times impossible to treat if complete excisions are considered as the endpoint. With my colleague Dr. Lucie Lessard and our skilled interventional radiologists and anesthetists at The Montreal Children's Hospital, we have achieved some success with cardiac bypass procedures and ancillary modalities (7). Most patients were treated with cardiac bypass alone, but some had cardiac arrest that allowed rapid removal of the lesion with minimal blood loss. There is no doubt that major complications might arise with this form of treatment, but to date our results are encouraging. No other form of treatment offers the same possibility of complete eradication of the malformation.

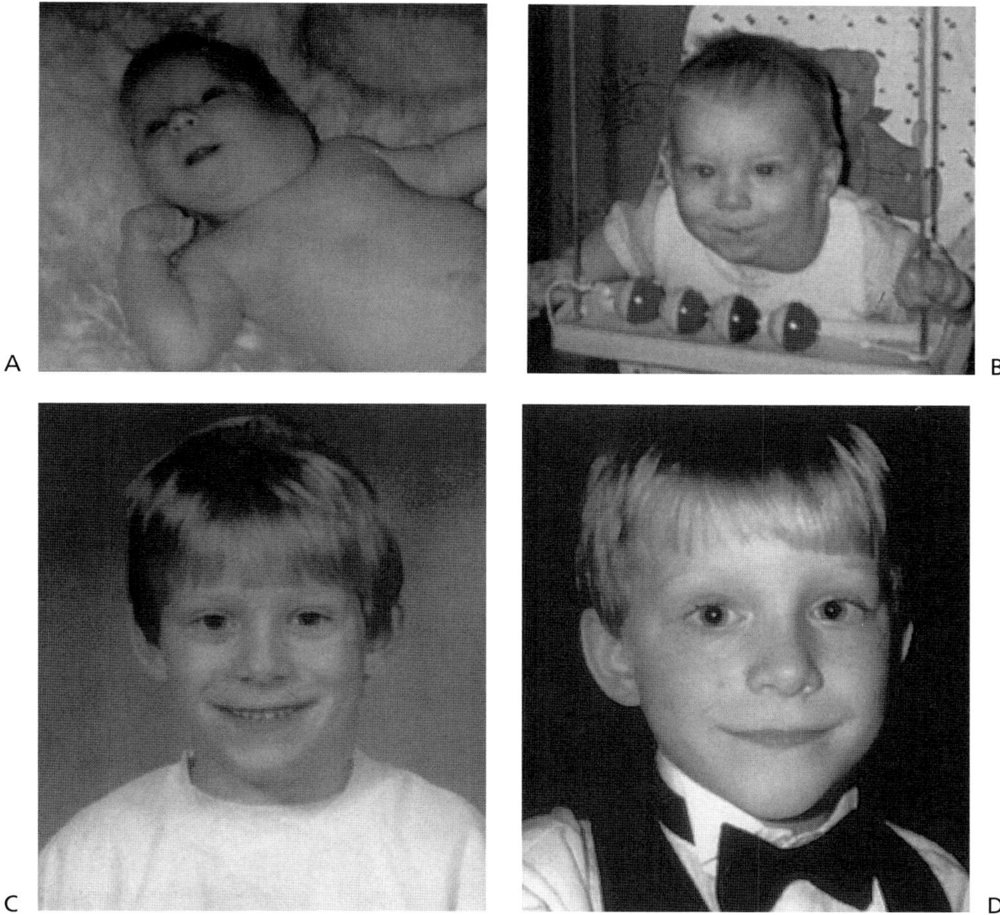

FIGURE 20D-3. A: Newborn with large cystic hygroma in the left cervical region. **B:** Early regression of the lesion at 5 months. **C:** Child at 5 years of age with no evidence of residual lesion (no treatment). **D:** Child at 8 years of age showing no evidence of the malformation.

PROXIMAL VESSEL OCCLUSION

I agree completely with the authors that proximal occlusion of a main arterial upstream from a high-flow vascular lesion should never be done. With the increasing sophistication of superselective angiography and embolization, this procedure should be eliminated from our surgical armamentarium.

VENOUS MALFORMATIONS

These persistent and unsightly malformations are extremely difficult to treat, and surgical excision usually is not completely successful. Many patients are first seen with painful nodules within the malformation. In my opinion, this is most likely localized thrombophlebitis from either trauma or vascular stasis. Treatment usually is conservative, although short-term heparin therapy might be of benefit.

SPECIALIZED CLINICS

A multispecialty surgical and medical clinic is essential for modern treatment of children and adults with vascular malformations. These clinics require input from pediatricians, radiologists, dermatologists, orthopedic surgeons, and plastic surgeons. Not all patients are cured even with these interdisciplinary clinics, but the treatment possibilities are expanded for improved patient care. Hopefully, using input from all involved specialists, the unfavorable results that have been seen too often in the past will be minimized and the outcome studies will be more favorable.

REFERENCES

1. Williams HB. Vascular malformations. *Clin Plast Surg* 1980; 7:397.
2. Mulliken JB, Glowacki J. Hemangiomas and vascular malformations in infants and children: a classification based on endothelial characteristics. *Plast Reconstr Surg* 1982;69:412.
3. Williams HB. Embryology and classification of lymphatic abnormalities. In: Williams HB, ed. *Melanotic lesions and vascular malformations.* St. Louis: CV Mosby, 1983:175–185.
4. Sabin FR. On the origin of the lymphatic system from the veins and the development of the lymph hearts and thoracic duct in the pig. *Am J Anat* 1902;1:367.
5. Lewis FT. The development of the lymphatic system in rabbits. *Am J Anat* 1905;5:95.
6. Huntington GS, McClure CFW. The anatomy and development of the jugular lymph sac in the domestic cat. *Am J Anat* 1910;10:177.
7. Lessard ML, Dobell ARL, Williams HB, et al. Resection with cardiac bypass for facial vascular malformations. International Proceedings of the V International Congress, Scientific Program, International Society of Craniofacial Surgery, 1995:5 Oaxaca, Mexico.

21

BURN RECONSTRUCTION

BRUCE M. ACHAUER
VICTORIA M. VANDERKAM

Writing a chapter about preventing unfavorable results in burn reconstruction is virtually an oxymoron. Most of the outcomes are highly unfavorable compared with normal appearance. The only chapter that would truly answer that goal would be a treatise on burn prevention. My personal feeling is that the only time we successfully surgically treat a burn patient is when we are able to totally excise the burn scar and leave only a linear surgical scar. When the patient no longer has a burn scar, he or she has been removed from the roll of burn patients. Fortunately, the expectations of success for burn reconstruction are considerably lower than in other fields of plastic surgery. At least the expectations for the surgeon are lowered. The patient's expectations may not be lower! Clearly, we have a long way to go. It is fortunate that other fields of plastic surgery, such as aesthetic, congenital, head and neck, and craniofacial, are fertile grounds for new concepts and techniques. This trend continues to raise not only our expectations but also our results. Although there are some situations that are particular to burn patients, in most cases technology can be transferred successfully.

There are some general principles for burn reconstruction. In most cases, we cannot totally eliminate burn scars, but we can minimize the amount of scarring (type, location, texture, and pigmentation). There is a reconstructive ladder that should be followed (Table 21-1). As stated, we can excise the burn scar and replace it with normal adjacent tissue. This is our first choice. The simplest form of this treatment is excision and direct closure. The next rung on the reconstructive ladder would be a local flap using adjacent tissue, advancing and rotating it onto a burned area and thereby replacing the burn scar with normal tissue. This rung can be exploited dramatically by the use of tissue expansion.

The next choice would be grafts, either sheet graft or full-thickness grafts, and then finally distant flaps. Each of these techniques will be discussed in terms of how they relate to burn patients and how they are used to minimize the risks of untoward results.

B. M. Achauer and V. M. VanderKam: Division of Plastic Surgery, University of California Irvine, Medical Center, Orange, California

EXCISION AND LOCAL FLAPS

The amount of tissue that can be excised directly can be estimated. Staged scar excision probably is preferable to tissue expansion if only two stages are needed, because tissue expansion involves at least two stages. Staged excision has definite limitations. This is especially true on the face, where there is a tendency to produce scleral show, which produces an unnatural result. This technique must not be overused. Staged excisions used to be our mainstay for burn scar alopecia of the scalp. This technique has been largely supplanted by tissue expansion. Simple triangular transposition flaps, with normal tissue adjacent to burn scar, can be very useful to break up a linear scar contraction. Z-plasties are quite risky if flaps involve burn scar tissue. Scars do not do well when they are undermined and transplanted and used as flaps. However, one-half of a Z-plasty, or more simply a local transposition flap, does almost as well at interposing elastic, unburned skin. This will correct some axillary contracture bands or contractures along the wrist and the areas of the hand. Local flaps also should be considered a high priority for facial scars. In these situations, scar flaps might be useful if the entire face is scarred.

Another specific example for local flaps would be for web space contractures in the hand. Standard Z-plasties can be used if there is normal tissue on each side of the scar band. However, for most web space contractures, particularly those involved in the second, third, or fourth web space, a V-M plasty works well. This series of local flaps does not involve any undermining; therefore, scarred flaps can be used just as readily as normal tissue.

Tissue Expansion

Although tissue expansion has a relatively high rate of complications, and this is exacerbated in burn patients, the technique has become very important for the burn patient. In dealing with burn scar deformities, one needs to be creative and aggressive as far as the use of tissue expansion. Often you have to use them in places and in ways that might not be considered ideal for other problems. The ability to resurface an area with local flap tissue with no donor defect is a

TABLE 21-1. RECONSTRUCTIVE LADDER

1. Excision and local flaps
2. Skin grafts
   A. Split-thickness skin graft
   B. Full-thickness skin graft
3. Distant flaps
   A. Pedicle
   B. Free

great advantage. The benefit usually is worth the trouble it takes to accomplish the goal. Skin expansion has made it possible to reconstruct virtually an entire scalp, most of the face, and even large areas on the trunk and extremity with absolutely normal local tissue. All of this can be accomplished without a donor defect. Successful outcomes in tissue expansion depend on patience. One needs to get the patient enthusiastic about the process and accepting of minor setbacks, such as loss of an expander, deflation, or infection. Careful planning of the placement of the tissue expanders is important. An expander cannot be placed underneath a burn scar. The process of expansion cannot separate normal skin from a burn scar. It is better to be conservative and make some progress with each tissue expander, even if it means having to do it a second or even a third time. Burn patients appreciate the elimination of their burn scar. Once they understand the process, they usually are willing to undergo multiple tissue expansion sessions to achieve the results. The most common source of unfavorable results is due to technical shortcomings during surgery, in particular, if expansion is done too close to the burn scar or if burn scar is included in the expanded area. It is worthwhile to wait at least 2 weeks after surgery, until the wound is well healed, to initiate expansion. It is better to go slowly and expand a few more times than to rush to surgery and be required to pull the skin tighter than is desirable. Flap ischemia is rarely a problem, but an overtight closure can result in loss of flap circulation as well as dehiscence of the wound. Tissue expansion is particularly risky in the lower extremities (Fig. 21-1). The use of tissue expansion has become a mainstay in reconstruction of burn patients. With careful attention to planning, surgical details, and the expansion process, very worthwhile results can be achieved.

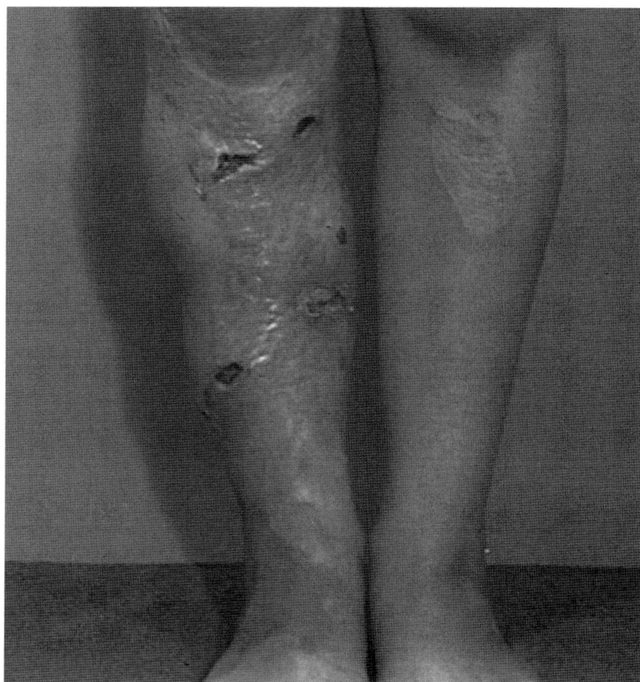

FIGURE 21-1. Tissue expansion in the lower extremity resulting in wound dehiscence.

SKIN GRAFTS

Skin grafts have been a mainstay of burn reconstruction for many years. Both split-thickness and full-thickness skin grafts have application to the burn patient.

Split-thickness Skin Grafts

In areas of hypertrophic scarring where tissue expansion is not possible, replacement with a good-quality medium-to-thick split-thickness sheet graft is an excellent reconstructive alternative. In addition, relatively poor skin grafts, especially within an aesthetic unit, can be excised and replaced with a split-thickness skin graft with excellent effect. Areas of chronic irritation and breakdown that require slightly thicker skin can be repaired with overgrafting. Using this concept, thin layers of tissue are removed and a skin graft applied, resulting in a thicker dermis. Skin grafts, however, are becoming less popular due to the aesthetic shortcomings of skin grafts. They also always look like a graft and are never quite the same color or texture of the skin next to them. Another problem with skin grafts is the donor site. Many people, particularly children, are very prone to hypertrophic scars in the donor site. This is especially true if one wants a thicker graft for a reconstructive procedure. One way to minimize this problem is to use dermis from another source. A number of skin substitutes have been developed recently, including freeze-dried human cadaver dermis (AlloDerm, Integra, and Dermagraf TC). When using these types of products, the offending scar is removed, the dermal substitute is placed, and a very thin skin graft is placed over the dermal substitute. This has the advantage of a thick dermis, which produces a higher-quality skin graft and reduces donor site morbidity because of the thinness of the autograft.

Full-thickness Skin Grafts

Full-thickness skin grafts have been an important part of burn reconstruction since they were introduced in 1875 by

Wolfe (1,2) for burn scar reconstruction of the eyelid. Full-thickness skin grafts are still the best for eyelids, particularly lower eyelids. In our experience, full-thickness skin graft is the best reconstruction for the lower lip area. Of course, the thicker the skin graft, the more meticulous the surgical technique needs to be. Adequate immobilization is important. A pressure dressing of some sort (a foam-rubber sponge) is needed for areas that are quite mobile. Special care needs to be taken, for example, if the lower lip is being done. A nasogastric feeding tube is inserted. The patient basically takes no food by mouth for about 1 week. This can be accomplished relatively easily as an outpatient. It simply means that all nourishment is given by the tube. Full-thickness skin grafts also are very useful in the hand, particularly for palmar contractures. Nasal ectropion can be treated with aesthetic unit full-thickness skin grafts. A turned-down flap is created to reconstruct the lining side of the nostril, and the entire tip of the nostril is constructed of a full-thickness skin graft. In general, full-thickness skin grafts are not used for acute burns because of a limited supply of donor sites.

DISTANT FLAPS

Distant flaps have a role in burn reconstruction. The main shortcoming of distant flaps is the introduction of skin that is of a different color and texture than the recipient site. However, in creating new structures, a flap is necessary. Distant flaps are very important in managing acute electrical burns and deformities where entire structures are lost. Examples of this would be for the reconstruction of an ear or nose. Distant flaps also are crucial in acute burn situations for covering exposed structures such as tendons and joints. Rose (3) has written about the use of distant flaps for facial reconstruction combined with makeup. He is a strong advocate of free flaps, which he uses effectively.

Many years ago, Gillies described the pedicled back flap for total facial reconstruction. Angrigiana (4) has developed this into a free flap for entire face reconstruction. His results are indeed exciting. The major problem with flaps is that they are thicker than the native tissue and tend to mask facial expression and normal facial angles and contours.

Pigmentation

Pigmentation problems are common in the burn patient. Both hyperpigmentation and hypopigmentation occur and usually coexist. Hyperpigmentation is difficult to treat; however, it often improves with time (Fig. 21-2). Bleaching agents, such as 4% hydroquinone or Kligman's formula, can be applied. Some patients will respond to laser treatment. Several lasers, including the quality-switched ruby, alexandrite, and neodymium:yttrium aluminum garnet (Nd:YAG), have been suggested for the treatment of hyperpigmentation. More work still needs to be done in this area.

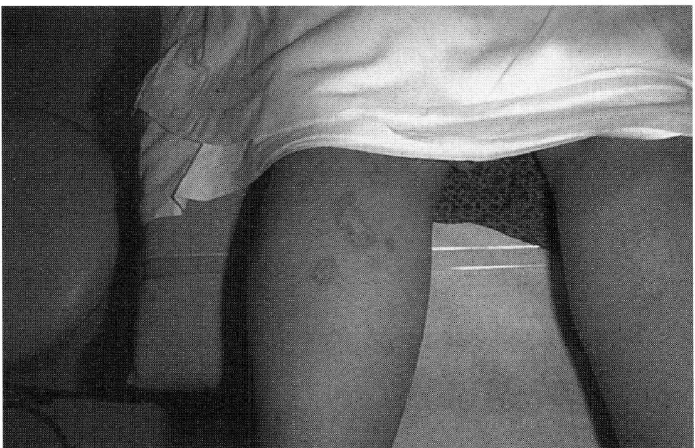

FIGURE 21-2. Example of hyperpigmentation that can result after a burn injury.

In many instances, hyperpigmentation is a permanent situation for which there is no solution.

Hypopigmentation also can be of great concern. To some people, makeup is not an option. They may desire a permanent solution. Tattooing has been reported (5). This technique has been frustrating in my experience. Tattoo pigment normally is deposited in dermis. Because scars do not have a dermal layer, a permanent color change is less likely. There will be initial take-up of the pigment, but the pigment dissipates after a few months or years. Melanocyte transplantation can be used for more permanent restoration of pigment. This procedure involves dermabrasion (or an alternate method of removing the epidermis) of the hypopigmented area. An ultrathin skin graft of epidermis is taken from a donor site. This extremely thin, virtually transparent skin graft is harvested and placed in the denuded area. This procedure successfully transplants melanocytes and can permanently eliminate hypopigmentation (6). In most cases, patients are not willing to undergo a skin graft procedure. However, if a patient is extremely concerned about hypopigmentation, this is an option. Due to the very thin nature of the skin graft, there is minimal donor site morbidity. It is a relatively uncomplicated and reliable form of treatment.

Scar Management

Nonsurgical methods to control hypertrophic scars are known to most plastic surgeons. Because of the extent of the scar, compression garments usually are prescribed for burn patients. Silicone inserts can be used to augmented garments. Silicone sheeting can be used by itself. Topical steroids, such as flurandrenolide (Cordran) tape, clobetasol propionate (Temovate), or triamcinolone, are used. Steroid injections also are used for specific problem scars. For a patient with extensive burns or sensitive burn scars, steroid injections are impractical. Lasers have been advocated for scars. There are some clinical studies demonstrating that scars can be improved by laser treatment (7). A 585-nm laser will provide the benefits of decreased redness and increased pliability. Multiple treatments often are required. Preliminary work shows some promise for the prevention of hypertrophic scar with the 585-nm wavelength. Two or three treatments are done in the early phases of wound healing in an effort to decrease the microvasculature of the skin. The role of this therapy in burn patients is not well determined at this time, but it might be helpful in some cases (8).

AVOIDING COMPLICATIONS OF SPECIFIC ANATOMICAL AREAS

Scalp

Tissue expanders have totally changed the potential for scalp reconstruction. They are the treatment of choice. They allow one to expand normal scalp without leaving a donor defect. The scalp can be expanded multiple times. As little as one-third of scalp can be expanded to efficiently cover the remainder of the surface area of the scalp. Hair restoration surgery may be applicable, but because of scars, small flaps are more risky and hair transplants do not do as well in scarred areas as in normal tissue. Micrografts should be considered for finishing touches on a particular hairline.

Eyelids

Many texts advocate the use of early tarsorrhaphies, particularly to prevent exposure of the eyelids. Tarsorrhaphies always distort the remaining eyelid anatomy and rarely are effective in protecting the eye for any length of time. Due to the constant motion in the eyelids, the sutures tear through, resulting in significant loss of eyelid tissue. Ectropion is corrected with release and skin graft. Full-thickness skin grafts are used for the lower eyelid. Extensive releases are done, and upper and lower lids are done at different settings. This is important to ensure proper correction.

Eyebrows

Eyebrows are a low priority. Most women can do well with cosmetics or tattooing. However, in extensively burned faces, a more dramatic feature is required. A scalp island flap based on the superficial temporal artery and vein can be used to construct a bushy eyebrow. These do not always work, nor are they a complete success. This procedure is reserved for special cases.

Face

Facial aesthetic units are an important consideration in planning reconstruction. Resurfacing of a face could be done with a good-quality, thick split-thickness skin graft respecting the aesthetic units. This may require the sacrifice of some normal tissue. This is a relatively simple technique and often is all that is required.

A large full-thickness graft was popularized by Feldman (9). With local flaps, local tissue is an excellent choice. Even scar tissue can be used in small local flaps. These could be very appropriate if they are being placed in an area of scar tissue, and they tend to blend in well. Small transposition flaps may provide more normal relationships, and landmarks can be established. Tissue expansion may be used for the periphery of the face, sideburn areas, cheeks, and mandibular margins. Using normal skin in the neck and submental area is useful for facial reconstruction. There are limits on the face. When reconstructing the face, one must be careful not to create an ectropion of the lower eyelid. The lower lip also can be pulled down; therefore, the key is to not advance the flap beyond the mental labial fold.

Full-face reconstruction could be done with total facial flaps, as proposed by Angrigiana (4), or by regional units and free flaps, as proposed by Rose (3). Lips and the chin almost always require full-thickness skin grafts. These two areas are quite mobile, and they often are soiled with saliva. A feeding tube is placed for about 1 week. The patient can be instructed on its use and can easily do feedings at home. The skin graft should take well within about 7 days.

Neck

Treating neck scar contracture bands and deformities is always a challenge. Traditionally, a split-thickness skin graft has been used. This works well, but it requires splinting and therapy afterwards. There is often the appearance of a patch. My treatment of choice is tissue expansion of any usable skin. This usually is done on both sides. Burned neck skin is replaced with normal skin. Repeated expansions may be required. They are quite effective, although they almost always are thicker than the ideal. If there is insufficient tissue on the lateral aspect of the neck, then an importation of tissue, such as the free flap, is required.

Breasts

The overlying principle in treating burned breasts is to be very conservative debriding in the area of the breast bud, behind the nipple. Preservation of the breast bud is essential to normal breast development in the future. This type of injury frequently occurs in toddlers or during early childhood. After puberty, problems can be identified and treated. As breast tissue emerges, scars may require release. If a more extensive release is required, a skin graft may be used.

Upper Extremities

Release of the elbow still is done primarily by repair with split skin grafts. If only a small area is involved, a full-thickness skin graft may be appropriate. For contractures of the hand, local flaps are used whenever possible. The most common problem requiring surgery is web space contracture. These may be treated effectively with local flaps. Our preference is the V-M plasty for web spaces 2, 3, and 4. Z-plasty is used

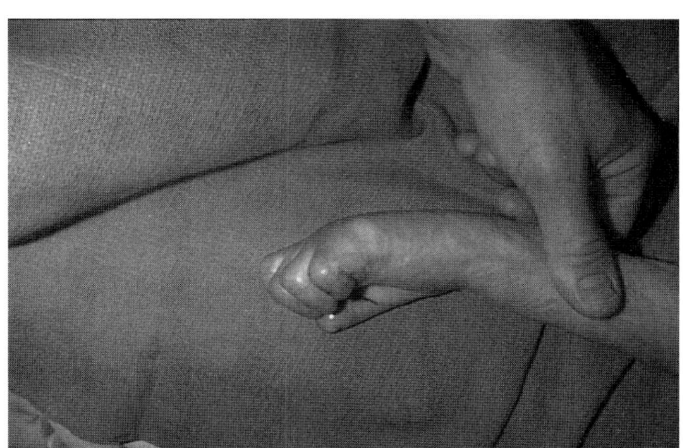

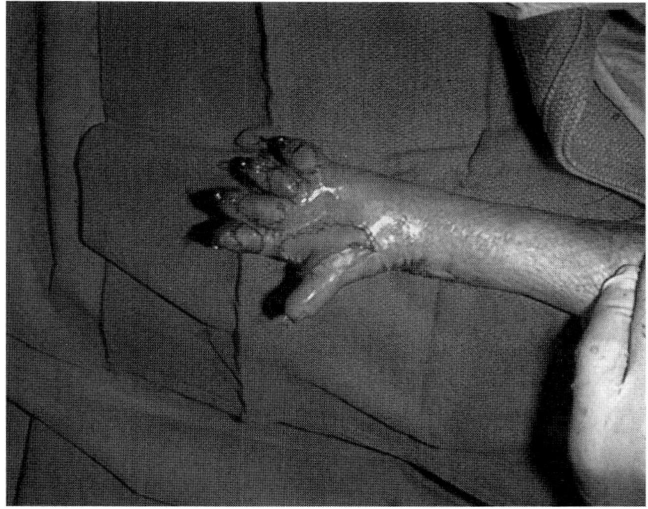

FIGURE 21-3. A: Severe contracture of the hand. **B:** Hand shown after release, skin grafts, and insertion of K-wires.

for the first web space. Severe contractures of the hand require multiple releases, skin grafting, and immobilization with K-wires (Fig. 21-3). The nailfold can be reconstructed with bilateral flaps from either side of the finger (10).

Abdomen

Extensive scarring of the abdomen results in a deformity known as the "hourglass deformity." This is caused by a circular contracture deformity of the trunk involving the upper abdomen and contracture of the lower chest and back. This debilitating deformity decreases ones ability to breathe or to exercise and perform activities of daily living. Multiple contracture releases with grafting are necessary to correct this deformity (Fig. 21-4).

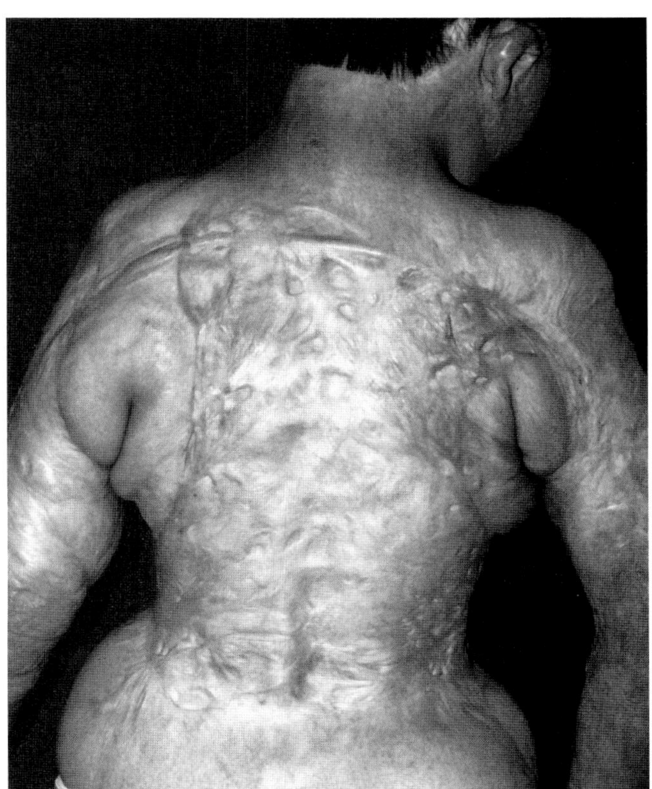

FIGURE 21-4. A: Anterior view of an "hourglass deformity" in a 13-year-old boy. **B:** Posterior view of the same deformity.

Groin

Skin contracture or webbing across the perineum is a common outcome of perineal burns. These contractures may be released and repaired using extensive Z-plasties and/or split-thickness skin grafts. The extremities must be maintained in abduction until the grafts are healed. This requires bilateral casting with a spreading bar. Pressure garments are used after cast removal and maintained for 6 to 12 months.

Lower Extremities

Deep burns of the lower extremity are devastating injuries requiring free-flap coverage. Microsurgery has enabled the use of free flaps, which can cover exposed tendon, bone, or cartilage. This single-stage procedure is preferable to a multistage pedicle flap transfer procedure. Unstable scars may be improved with overgrafting. The unstable scar is surgically excised, removing the epithelium and leaving as much tissue as possible. A medium-to-thick split-thickness skin graft is placed over the wound and immobilized. This process is repeated to achieve further gain.

Feet

When the dorsum of the foot is burned, an extension deformity of the metatarsal-phalangeal (MP) joint may occur. Treatment consists of release with transverse incisions and split-thickness skin grafts. Immobilization with K-wires and splinting may be needed until the skin graft take is certain.

REFERENCES

1. Wolfe JR. A new method of performing plastic operations. *BMJ* 1875;2:360.
2. Wolfe JR. Plastic operation on the eyelid. *Glasgow MJ., M.S.*, 1876;8:420.
3. Rose EH. Aesthetic restoration of the severely disfigured face in burn victims: a comprehensive strategy. *Plast Reconstr Surg* 1995;96:1573–1585.
4. Angrigiana C. Total face reconstruction with one free flap. *Plast Reconstr Surg* 1997;99:1566–1575.
5. El-Bishry MA, Nassar AM, El-Maghraby MZ. Tattooing, a new hope for secondary leukoderma. *Scand J Plast Reconstr Surg* 1979:13:147–153.
6. Kahn AM, Cohen MJ, Kaplan L. Treatment for depigmentation resulting from burn injuries. *J Burn Care Rehabil* 1991;12: 468–473.
7. Alster TS. Improvement of erythematous and hypertrophic scars by the 585 nm flashlamp-pumped pulsed dye laser. *Ann Plast Surg* 1995;32:186.
8. Achauer BM, VanderKam VM. Pulsed dye laser treatment for prevention of hypertrophic burn scars. *Proceedings of the 29th Annual Meeting of the American Burn Association* 1997;18:S121.
9. Feldman JJ. Reconstruction of the burned face in children. In: Serafin D, Georgian NG, eds. *Pediatric plastic surgery.* St. Louis: CV Mosby, 1984:552–632.
10. Achauer BM, Welk RA. One stage reconstruction of the postburn nailfold contracture. *Plast Reconstr Surg* 1990;85:937–941.

Discussion

BURN RECONSTRUCTION

ROGER E. SALISBURY

It is noteworthy that the chapter by Achauer and VanderKam is refreshingly direct and honest, reflecting Dr. Achauer's many years as a respected surgeon in the burn community. The readers should note that there are none of the traditionally wonderful before and after pictures reflecting Dr. Achauer's surgical expertise. The authors have tried to indicate that the state of the art at this time leaves much to be desired. The best of hands often results in improvements that are quite modest. The authors discussed each area of the body with the individual problems inherent to surgery, and they addressed the multiple techniques that are presently available for the control of scar, most of which are highly unsatisfactory in the patient and the surgeon's view. The simple truth is that all of these measures are merely temporizing alternatives until we develop laboratory techniques that faithfully reproduce a person's own skin and can be used in reconstruction. It is most encouraging that this reality may not be too far in the distant future. The technology exists to grow sheets of skin in the laboratory, and we rou-

R. E. Salisbury: New York Medical College, and The Burn Center, Westchester Medical Center, Valhalla, New York

tinely use these skin sheets to cover large, otherwise lethal burn wounds. Rather than use a host of unsatisfactory reconstructive procedures, the plan of the future will be to excise the unsightly scar and cover the resultant wound with an allograft dermis and good-quality epidermis that has been grown in the laboratory. There will be multiple variants of this approach, but the philosophy will always be the same: to use some small piece of the patient's own skin as a template for reproduction.

In the meantime, a far greater concern is the planning of patient's reconstruction. Preventable complications not addressed by the authors include the inability of physicians to develop a plan to address an individual patient's multitude of problems. Burn care has become so sophisticated that, in the best centers, patients are routinely surviving with 80% full-thickness burns. Dr. Herndon at the Galveston's Shrine has reported on long-term rehabilitation efforts in a series of children with burns of greater than 90% full thickness. Far too often, these survivors become professional patients. They drift from surgeon to surgeon, seeking the Holy Grail. Bits and pieces are done over period of years. The journey ends when the patient and/or the surgeons become tired of the quest, but the result usually is extremely unsatisfactory for both.

To give the patient the best chance for a reasonable result, it is our practice to document in writing at the initial evaluation all of the patient's cosmetic and functional deformities. During the initial consultation, the patient is made aware of the limitations of the current state of the art. Unless there is full communication and disclosure, trust will be broken and the surgical procedures will have been done in vain. Of course, patients hear what they want to hear and "hopes springs eternal," but it is the surgeon's responsibility to explain to the patient what realistically can be expected from surgical intervention. Once all of the patient's functional and cosmetic deformities are committed to paper, then the team can discuss with the patient what is his or her primary concern. The patient certainly can and should have some control over the sequence of reconstruction, and this measure of control is helpful in achieving cooperation. It is important to remember that these patients did not have any control over their acute care, and they appreciate the opportunity to be part of the surgical plan. The procedures then can be grouped to minimize hospitalization, anesthesias, and surgical periods of confinement. It is extraordinary how often patients are told that their reconstruction will take years before completion. This message usually is delivered to their lawyers, who are seeking to achieve a large settlement and drive up the cost of care. The reality is that this type of thinking only produces a professional patient and does absolutely nothing to rehabilitate an individual. The entire process of the reconstruction should be a time-related phenomenon. Specifically, the patient should know that a cluster of operations can be done in one hospitalization, followed by the next series of procedures several months later, and so forth. The patient can be given a very good idea of how long the entire process will take. Operations that are compatible can be clustered and done by a team. It is my personal belief that, unless severely burned, an individual should be reconstructed at a center where teams can operate in tandem. Specifically, part of the plastic surgery team can correct problems of the face while another team operates on an extremity. An upper and lower extremity can be done at the same time. It usually is not advisable to do both upper extremities at the same time because the patient then becomes helpless. On rare occasions, we have broken this rule in order to honor the request of the patient and the patient's own time schedule for reconstruction. In this aggressive manner, multiple defects can be corrected under one anesthesia, with only a few days of hospitalization, and the entire period of rehabilitation can be shortened dramatically. This type of planning will cut cost significantly, which is of appeal to insurers and usually wins their support. In summary, the most unfavorable result is lack of success that makes the surgeon and/or the patient believe that their efforts have been in vain. This type of extensive preoperative planning, clustering of surgical procedures, and thoughtful use of time and personnel is the best way to achieve results that please everyone. In the last 19 years, we have not had an increased incidence of failure or complications as a result of this type of plan.

In summary, I believe that Achauer and VanderKam addressed honestly and fairly all of the problems that confront burn reconstructive surgeons. They succinctly pointed out the shortcomings in the results that plague this particular type of reconstruction as opposed to our other areas of plastic surgery. It is hoped that by the time the next edition of this book is published, better answers can be given.

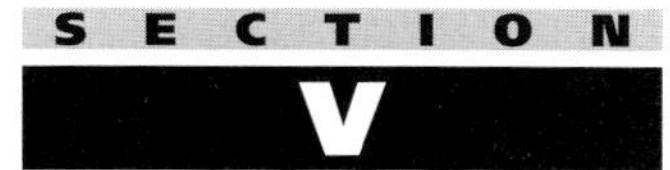

HEAD AND NECK

22

CLEFT LIP AND PALATE

MIMIS N. COHEN
BONNIE E. SMITH

Cleft lip and cleft palate are the most common congenital anomalies, affecting approximately one in 750 newborns each year. These patients require the care of several specialists and may require a number of surgical procedures from infancy to adulthood to achieve adequate functional and aesthetic habilitation. Such habilitation not only provides improved facial appearance, but also provides improvements in dental and occlusal relations, speech, hearing, and psychosocial status.

The need for long-term multidisciplinary management for children born with clefts of the lip and palate has been well recognized. Management by a team has become the standard of cleft care. Members of the team are responsible for the longitudinal evaluation and coordinated care of these patients. Such comprehensive care is designed to meet each patient's multiple and complex needs, as well as the needs of their families. Teams provide interactive encounters between professionals representing a variety of disciplines. Team members meet to communicate, collaborate, and consolidate knowledge. From these meetings, plans are made for present and future care based on each patient's individual needs as well as the team's treatment philosophy and protocols. A prime responsibility of each cleft team also includes careful record keeping. Collected data must be studied and analyzed periodically to fully appreciate outcome of protocols and surgical procedures, and to modify or improve them accordingly.

Evaluation of results after cleft lip and palate repair is not always easy; several weaknesses have been identified in most retrospective or prospective studies. For example, many studies include only a small number of patients, with multifaceted problems related to the deformity, as well as significant variations in treatment protocol, timing for each procedure, surgical technique, skills of the individual surgeon(s), and relatively short follow-up period. Results for each intervention, such as speech outcome after palatoplasty or effects of surgical procedures on maxillofacial growth, cannot be evaluated for several years. The vast majority of current studies rely primarily on subjective, not objective, evaluation. Furthermore, evaluation of facial features using only photographs may not be the most appropriate way to judge a surgical outcome given, that only static results are displayed and possible asymmetries or irregularities during animation cannot be detected. The need for well-planned and well-designed, ethical, multicenter, prospective long-term studies has been recognized. Such studies could provide us with quantifiable, nonbiased data and assist us in improving patient care by addressing remaining controversial issues, such as appropriate timing for specific surgical procedures as well as selection of the best possible surgical technique. Long-term effects of each procedure may be predicted more accurately as well (1,2). Until such studies are completed, we must rely on the results of existing, primarily retrospective studies as well as honest evaluation and analysis of our own results to provide the best possible care for our patients.

Existing parameters for evaluation and treatment of patients with cleft lip/palate and other craniofacial anomalies are based on fundamental principles regarding the optimal treatment of such patients, regardless of the specific type of disorder (3). These guidelines provide an excellent framework of care and include recommendations regarding interdisciplinary teams and longitudinal patient evaluation and treatment in the neonatal period, infancy, and adolescence by each team's specialist. With improved knowledge and experience of health-care professionals, appropriate coordination of care, cooperation among specialists, close monitoring, and analysis of short-term and long-term results, as well as adequate funding to cover all necessary services and management of patients with facial clefts, could improve further and superior habilitation could be achieved.

The establishment of a large number of cleft/craniofacial teams has resulted in a dramatic improvement in cleft care and in refinements of surgical techniques due to many years of collective experience and extensive long-term follow-up studies from these teams. However, despite this progress,

M. N. Cohen: Divisions of Plastic Surgery, University of Illinois at Chicago and Cook County Hospital, Chicago, Illinois

B. E. Smith: Department of Surgery, University of Illinois; and the Division of Speech Pathology, University of Illinois Hospital, Chicago, Illinois

several children with facial clefts still receive inferior care. Such inadequate care results from diagnostic errors, failure to recognize and treat the full spectrum of problems associated with facial clefting, unnecessary and poorly timed treatment, and inappropriate or poorly performed procedures.

Lack of adequate funding by some states or refusal to cover specific services by some managed care organizations and other insurance carriers comprise additional reasons for suboptimal care and inadequate habilitation of children with facial clefts. Examples include denial for coverage of secondary procedures, speech therapy, and dental and/or psychological care. The state of California recently passed a law prohibiting health maintenance organizations from denying patients' reconstructive surgery to correct birth defects or disfigurements due to disease or trauma. In 1998, the Treatment of Children with Deformities Act was introduced in the U.S. House of Representatives, and it is hoped that such legislation will soon be passed to secure constitutional necessary care for children with clefts as well as other craniofacial anomalies.

CLEFT LIP

The objectives of primary cleft lip repair are to reestablish anatomy and symmetry of the upper lip and to improve form and function. In 1953, Steffensen (4) established five criteria for satisfactory cleft lip repair that, to this day, represent the foundation for every successful repair:

1. Accurate skin, muscle, and mucous membrane union
2. Slight eversion of the lip
3. Symmetrical nostril floors
4. Symmetrical vermilion border
5. Minimal scar.

With accumulated experience and knowledge as well as evaluation of long-term results, several other criteria were added. Attention currently is given to mobilization of the orbicularis oris fibers from their initial oblique orientation and their junction in the appropriate horizontal position. More accurate reconstruction of the cupid's bow and alignment of the vermilion (dry lip) and the mucosa (moist lip) also are achieved. Correction of the nasal deformity has been incorporated into cleft lip repair. Nostril symmetry as well as adequate tip projection are addressed during the initial procedure. Techniques that are more likely to result in a short lip, such as the straight-line closure, or a long lip, such as the LeMesurier technique, have been virtually abandoned. They have been replaced by more dependable and elegant techniques, such as the rotation and advancement technique or the triangular flap technique and their respective modifications.

The value of preoperative orthopedics in the final outcome of lip repair is still debated. Repositioning of the maxillary alveolar segments in a more anatomically correct position theoretically can facilitate a tension-free closure, but it also could allow for a simultaneous periosteoplasty. Such an approach might result in a better appearance of the lip alveolus and nose and potentially reduce the total number of secondary procedures (5,6). Intermediate results in a limited number of patients appear promising, but final long-term results of such interventions and their effects on maxillofacial growth still are not available.

In contrast, the use of preoperative orthopedics in bilateral clefts with repositioning of the premaxilla is more widely accepted, particularly when the premaxilla is protruding significantly. Several techniques have been described to achieve premaxillary reposition. In our center, we use a premaxillary position appliance, fabricated by our prosthodontist, which is extremely helpful in the downward and backward movement of the premaxilla. Its cost is minimal, there is no need for pins or other invasive devices, and negative effects on facial growth and development have not been observed with its use. Several weeks of treatment are necessary to achieve a favorable reposition of the premaxilla and improved alignment with the maxillary segments before lip repair (7).

Residual Cleft Lip Deformities

Secondary operations are required to correct deformities that were not addressed in the primary procedure and to improve residual functional and aesthetic deformities that persist after the cleft lip repair. These procedures have been described at length in various textbooks and articles (8–11). Only a few surgeons have reported on the actual average number of procedures required to achieve the best possible results in patients with cleft lip and palate. Bardach et al. (12) reported an average of 1.82 lip revisions per patient in a study of 45 children with unilateral cleft lip and palate. Cohen et al. (13) reported an average of 1.13 revisional procedures for children with unilateral cleft lip and 2.17 lip revisions for bilateral clefts.

A revisional lip surgery should only be decided after extensive consultation with the family and the child or adolescent and with a clear understanding of their needs and expectations. Objectives of the procedure(s) and the surgical plan and possible outcome should be outlined. False expectations should be dispelled. Timing for the secondary surgery can affect the outcome and should be taken into consideration. Surgical procedures should be postponed when the adolescent is not interested or even refuses to have them, even when parents desire them. On the other hand, some procedures might be scheduled earlier than anticipated if there is evidence of a negative psychological effect of the deformity on the child. Finally, when possible, procedures should be bundled together to reduce time away from school or work, to reduce additional psychological trauma from multiple interventions, and to control cost (14).

Residual deformities might vary significantly in degree of severity from minor ones that require only limited procedures for correction of the deformity, to major asymmetries and deformities that require complete redo of the lip repair. Such deformities result from errors of planning and errors in technique, or they are due to inherent tissue deficiencies, maxillofacial changes, or scar contractures (Fig. 22-1). It is beyond the scope of this chapter to catalog all residual deformities encountered after repair of unilateral or bilateral clefts of the lip and to describe all the techniques and modifications available to correct such deformities. Only the most common deformities will be presented, and treatment will be suggested with time-honored and reliable techniques.

As a basic rule, the entire lip, alveolus, and nose should be carefully evaluated before each revision. The deformity should be analyzed and all contributing factors to the deformity should be taken into consideration. All necessary soft tissue landmarks should be well marked and measured, and each surgical procedure should be planned to specifically address the residual deformity(s). Careful planning, appropriate timing, and execution are extremely important, because failure of the revisionary procedure to correct the deformity will result in additional scarring and possible tissue loss that could reduce further the chances for adequate habilitation.

Scars

Wide, poorly healed scars of the upper lip with unsightly stitch marks across the scar currently are rarely seen. They are primarily due to technical errors, such as poor handling of the tissues, closure under tension, and use of large sutures tightly tied and left in place too long. Such problems could have been avoided in the majority of cases if the surgeon had used well-accepted fine basic plastic surgery techniques with meticulous tissue handling and a tension-free closure using fine suture material. Other aggravating factors for scarring include perioperative bleeding, infection around the suture line, and dehiscence. One should be able to differentiate these unsightly scars from the hypertrophic scars that form without apparent cause. Such scar hypertrophy usually fades away slowly, several months or even years after the lip repair, without the need for additional surgical intervention.

Timing for scar revision is important to the final outcome. The surgeon should wait at least several months or even several years to allow the scar to mature before embarking on any revision. After careful evaluation of the problem, appropriate surgical procedures should be planned. All the important upper lip landmarks should be kept in mind, marked, and measured to avoid distortion of the lip by the revisional procedure. Elliptical excision of the scar, precise reapproximation, and closure after limited undermining at the level above the orbicularis oris is the simplest solution. This technique, however, can only be applied for relatively narrow scars. Excision of wider scars might result in wider defects that, when closed primarily, could result in undue tension and tightness across the lip, narrowing of the nostril sill, and a shorter or a longer lip. To avoid these unfavorable results, the surgeon needs to appropriately rearrange the tissues on either side of the scar with Z-plasties or wave-lines. W-plasties have been recommended by some surgeons. This design, as stated by Borges, will require excision of additional healthy skin and would increase further the already high transverse tension of the repaired upper lip. Furthermore, each segment of the zigzag scar would lie almost perpendicular to the normally vertical relaxed skin tension lines and give a poor aesthetic result (10). Dermabrasion is helpful in some cases, but the use of this technique is limited and primarily recommended for improvement of residual surface irregularities.

Mucocutaneous Deformities

These deformities are seen in the mucocutaneous junction and result from poor alignment of the white roll during the initial lip repair. Accurate placement of the first skin suture at the white roll, under loupe magnification if needed, will assist in preventing this problem. This deformity can be primarily corrected with an elliptical or rhomboid excision of the scar and accurate reapproximation of the mucocutaneous junction. A quadrilateral flap technique also can be applied (9). As an alternative, a small Z-plasty can be used to allow for interposition of a vermilion and a skin flap and ultimately results in realignment of the mucocutaneous line.

Vermilion and Free-border Deformities

Lack of bulk or poor alignment of the vermilion can cause several deformities. Lack of bulk is primarily due to inherent tissue deficiency, inappropriate planning, and dehiscence or failure to approximate the lower portion of the orbicularis oris muscle during the initial lip repair. To correct such residual deformities, the scar of the vermilion border should be incised or excised, and the orbicularis fibers should be identified after limited undermining and approximated with several absorbable sutures. The mucosa and vermilion then should be approximated carefully with eversion of the margins. If additional bulk is needed, small local filler grafts can be used. Such grafts include demucosalized or subcutaneous tissue flaps or autogenous fascial grafts. Care should be taken to avoid overcorrection, which is an equally unsightly deformity.

Small whistling deformities of the lip resulting primarily from scar contracture in the area of the vermilion and the mucosa of the lip can be corrected with Z-plasties by placing the central limb of the Z on the existing scar. A central whistling deformity with good height of the lip is seen primarily after repair of bilateral clefts of the lip. For this deformity, the bilateral pendulum flap technique, as described by Kapetansky (15), is considered to be a reasonable choice.

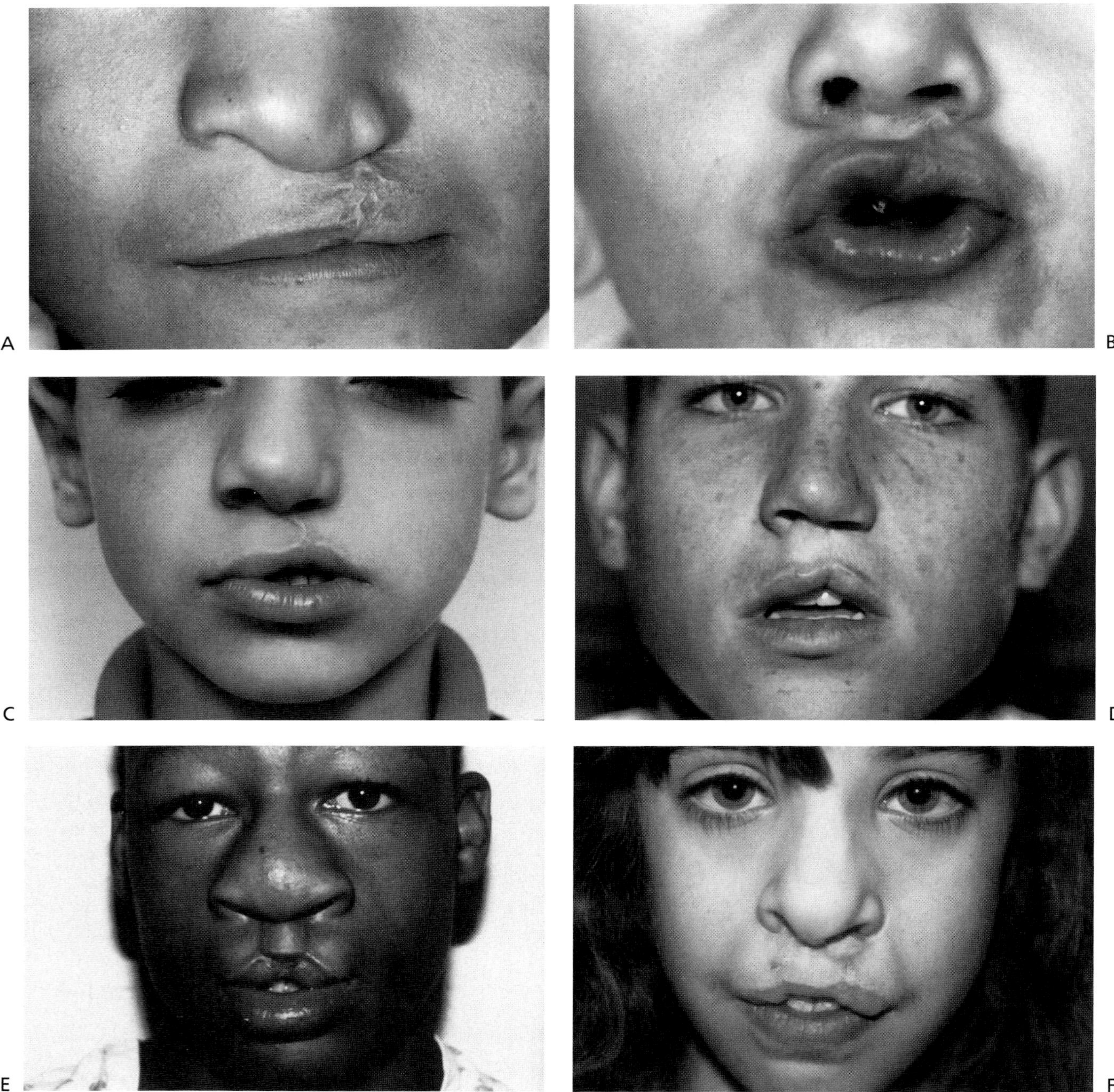

FIGURE 22-1. Residual cleft lip deformities. **A:** Significant scarring and residual stitch marks across the repaired lip. There is poor alignment of the lip segments and a significant residual nasal deformity. **B:** Whistling deformity due to incomplete approximation or dehiscence of the lower portion of the orbicularis oris muscle. **C:** Moderately short lip after complete unilateral cleft lip repair. **D:** Significantly short lip after straight-line closure and poor alignment of the vermilion border. **E:** Significant residual deformities after bilateral lip repair with short philtrum, poor alignment of the lateral segments, and lack of mobilization and approximation of the orbicularis oris. **F:** Significant residual deformity after bilateral cleft lip repair with very wide and short philtrum, discrepancy between the philtrum, and the lateral segments. The orbicularis muscle fibers are bulging under the lateral segments, presumably because they were not mobilized or joined in the midline. Poor scarring is noted.

The flaps are marked on the vermilion and mucosa of each lateral segment. After excision of the central lip scar, appropriate undermining of the orbicularis on either side, and a lateral back cut, the musculovermilion flaps are mobilized and sutured in the midline. Thus, the continuity of the orbicularis muscle is reconstituted, adequate bulk for the central portion of the lip is provided, and harmony of the upper lip is achieved.

Some scar contractures extend to the oral mucosa and labial sulcus. They need to be released in order to correct the retraction of the lip margin. In the vast majority of cases with unilateral cleft lip, release can be achieved with various Z-plasty or V-Y designs, which will allow for the lip to unfold to a more normal position. Mucosal or skin grafts are not necessary in most cases. Every effort should be made, however, to achieve full mucosa reapproximation, because any raw surface will heal by secondary intention and will result in further scar contracture (Fig. 22-2). In bilateral clefts of the lip, the soft tissue requirements in the area of the upper labial sulcus might be different, and patients might still present after lip repair with a totally absent sulcus. In such instances, the lip will appear short and retracted, showing the premaxilla and the incisors. Complete release of the soft tissues from the premaxilla will be necessary to correct this problem. In smaller defects, coverage can be achieved with various local mucosal flaps. If the defect is relatively large, however, the raw area will have to be resurfaced with a skin or mucosal graft. To achieve a successful outcome, one should avoid denuding the premaxilla from its periosteum, completely release the lip, suture the graft in place with absorbable sutures, and stabilize it with a small stent for 2 to 3 weeks (Fig. 22-3).

Orbicularis Deformities

Reconstruction of the orbicularis oris muscle currently is incorporated into the vast majority of unilateral and bilateral cleft lip repair techniques. To achieve proper repair, one needs to detach the lateral segment of the muscle from its abnormal attachment in the base of the nose, adequately

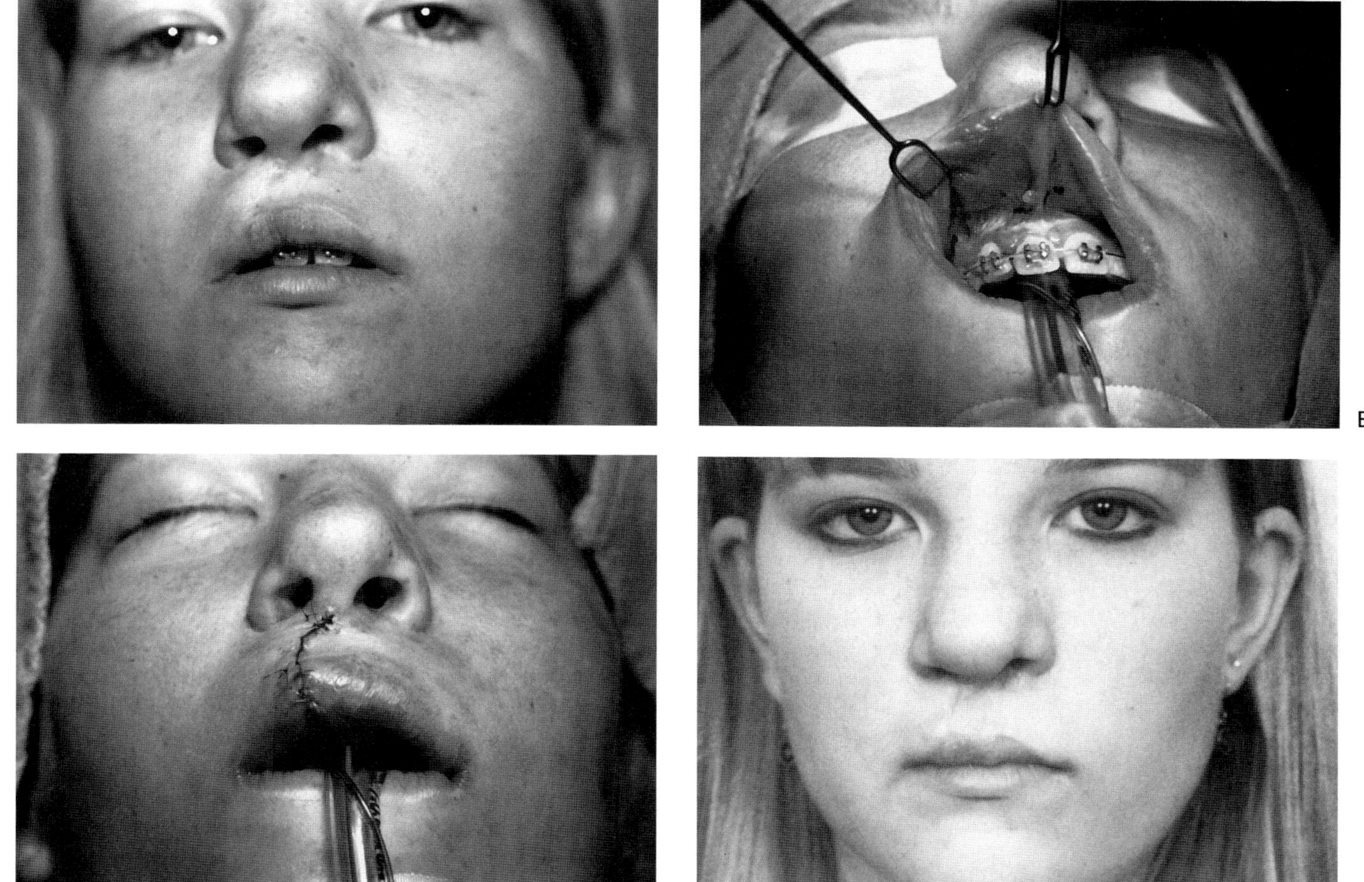

FIGURE 22-2. A: Deficiency of the vermilion border and bulge of the orbicularis oris muscle lateral to the lip scar. **B:** Intraoral scarring and contracture of the mucosa accentuate the deformity. **C:** Lip revision with excision of scar, reapproximation of the orbicularis fibers, and release of the mucosal scar with a V-Y design. **D:** Final result after correction of the deformity.

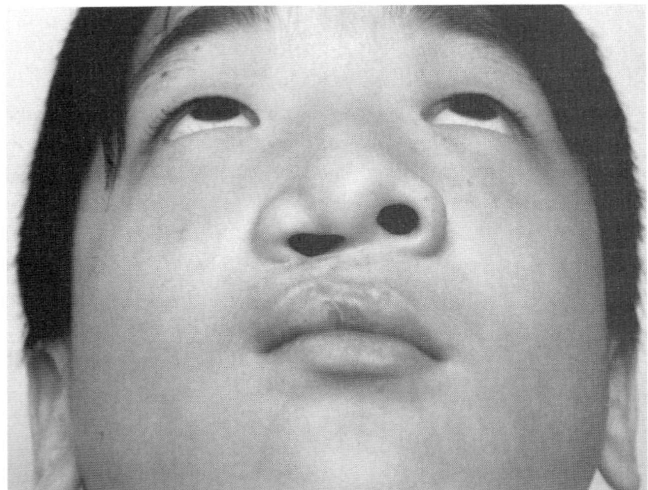

A

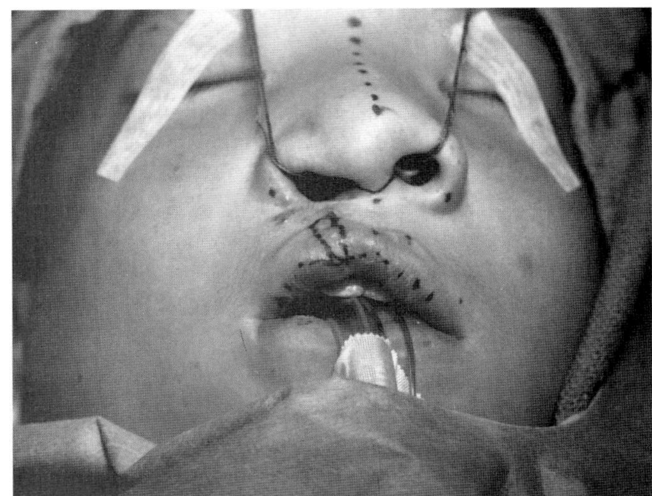

B

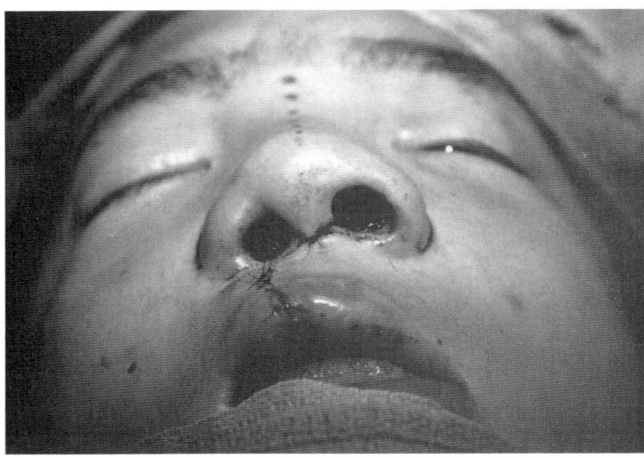

C

FIGURE 22-3. A,B: Residual lip and nasal deformity after unilateral cleft lip repair with poor alignment of the orbicularis oris, lack of bulk in the vermilion, depression and scarring of the nostril sill, and depression and lateral deflection of the lower alar cartilage with nostril asymmetry. After upper lip marking, 3 mm of excess tissue was noted in the upper lip. **C:** Excess tissue was excised. The lower fibers of the orbicularis oris were reapproximated and the nasal deformity was corrected through an open rhinoplasty approach.

mobilize both segments of the muscle, and suture them together the entire length of the muscle with absorbable sutures. Failure to reconstruct the muscular sling, and partial or complete dehiscence of the muscle repair will result in unsightly bulging of the muscle on either side of the lip scar or depressions and asymmetries that are accentuated further during animation and give the lip an unnatural look. For small deformities, the lip scar can be incised or excised, and the muscle fibers identified, freed from their abnormal attachments, and sutured together without tension. When a significant deformity exists, such as the one seen in some bilateral repairs requiring skin and mucosal excision in addition to the muscle realignment and approximation, then a total lip repair should be planned and all elements of the lip should be repositioned correctly. All upper lip landmarks need to be marked again, as for a primary repair, and special attention should be given to the width and length of the philtrum in rapport to the lateral lip segments (Fig. 22-4).

Long Lip

An excessively long lip on the cleft side after lip repair is truly technique related. Both LeMesurier and the initial Tennison repair techniques resulted in long lips. The LeMesurier technique is no longer used, whereas the triangular flap technique was modified by Musgrave and Garratt (16), Brauer and Cronin (17), and others. They suggested the design of the lip repair should be 1 mm shorter than the noncleft side to overcome this problem.

Correction of long lip is difficult. If the discrepancy is not significant, then it can be corrected with an appropriate tissue excision just below the nostril sill. If a significant deformity is present, the old scar should be excised, and the lip completely divided and repaired again after appropriate marking and measurement of all landmarks. Long lips also can be encountered after a bilateral cleft lip repair. In such instances, if the deformity is symmetrical, it can be corrected with subalar resection of an appropriate amount of tissue. Asymmetrical deformities after bilateral cleft lip repair con-

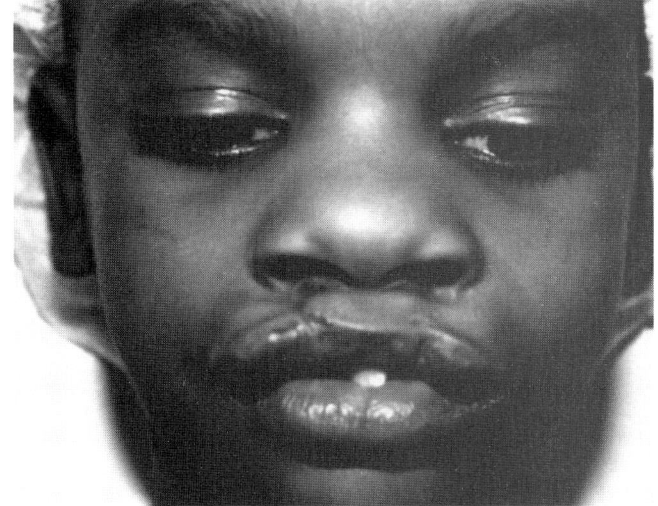

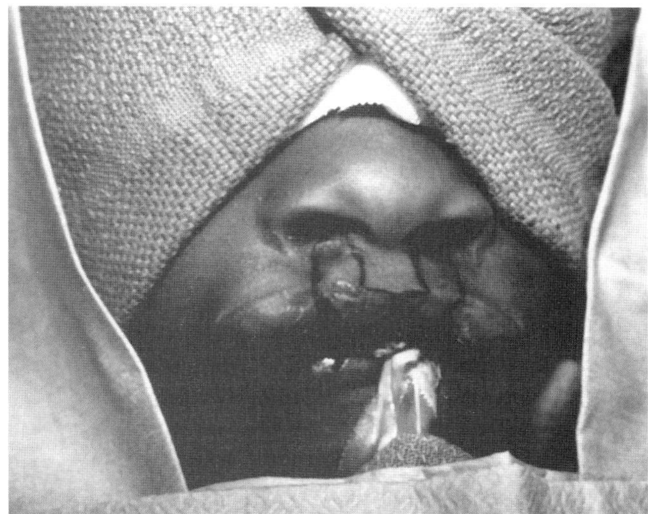

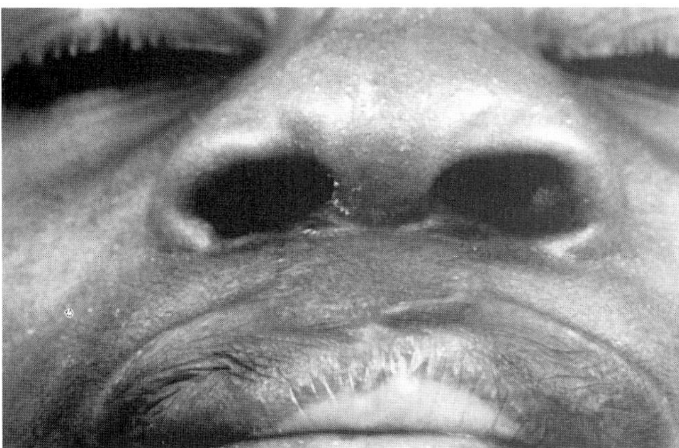

FIGURE 22-4. A: Significant residual deformity after repair of bilateral cleft lip with very large philtrum (2.2 cm), lack of mobilization and junction of the orbicular oris muscle fibers, and a whistling deformity. **B:** Markings of the proposed philtrum, 1 cm wide, and the excess skin and vermilion. **C:** Final result several years after reconstruction.

stitute a more complex problem. Unless the deformity is minimal, a total lip repair will be required for their correction. After appropriate measurement of all elements of the upper lip and excision of all excess tissues, reconstruction of the upper lip should be undertaken with accurate approximation of all anatomical layers.

Short Lip

A short lip results primarily from straight-line closure or from inadequate rotation and advancement techniques. Small discrepancies might result simply from skin contracture and can be corrected with elliptical or diamond-shaped excisions or excisions of the entire scar and closure after minimal undermining. If needed, Z-plasties can be designed and incorporated with the repair. The drawback to such approaches is the small gain of length that can be expected and the addition of a Z-scar on the lip. If a significant discrepancy exists, the only solution is to redo the lip repair. As with other deformities, the surgeon should evaluate carefully all possible coexisting elements of the deformity and, if possible, attempt to correct them all in one operation.

Tight Upper Lip

This deformity is encountered primarily in patients with bilateral clefts or soft tissue deficiency, but it also can be seen in some severe unilateral cases. The best solution for this problem is soft tissue replacement with a lip-switch technique. Because of the nature of the procedure and the temporary junction of the lips, this procedure is not recommended for very young children. Accurate placement of the flap in the center of the lip is extremely important in order to simulate the philtrum and place the final scars on the philtrum columns. The dimensions of the flap should be adequately planned to fit well in the upper lip to release the tightness and provide a balanced profile (Fig. 22-5). In the

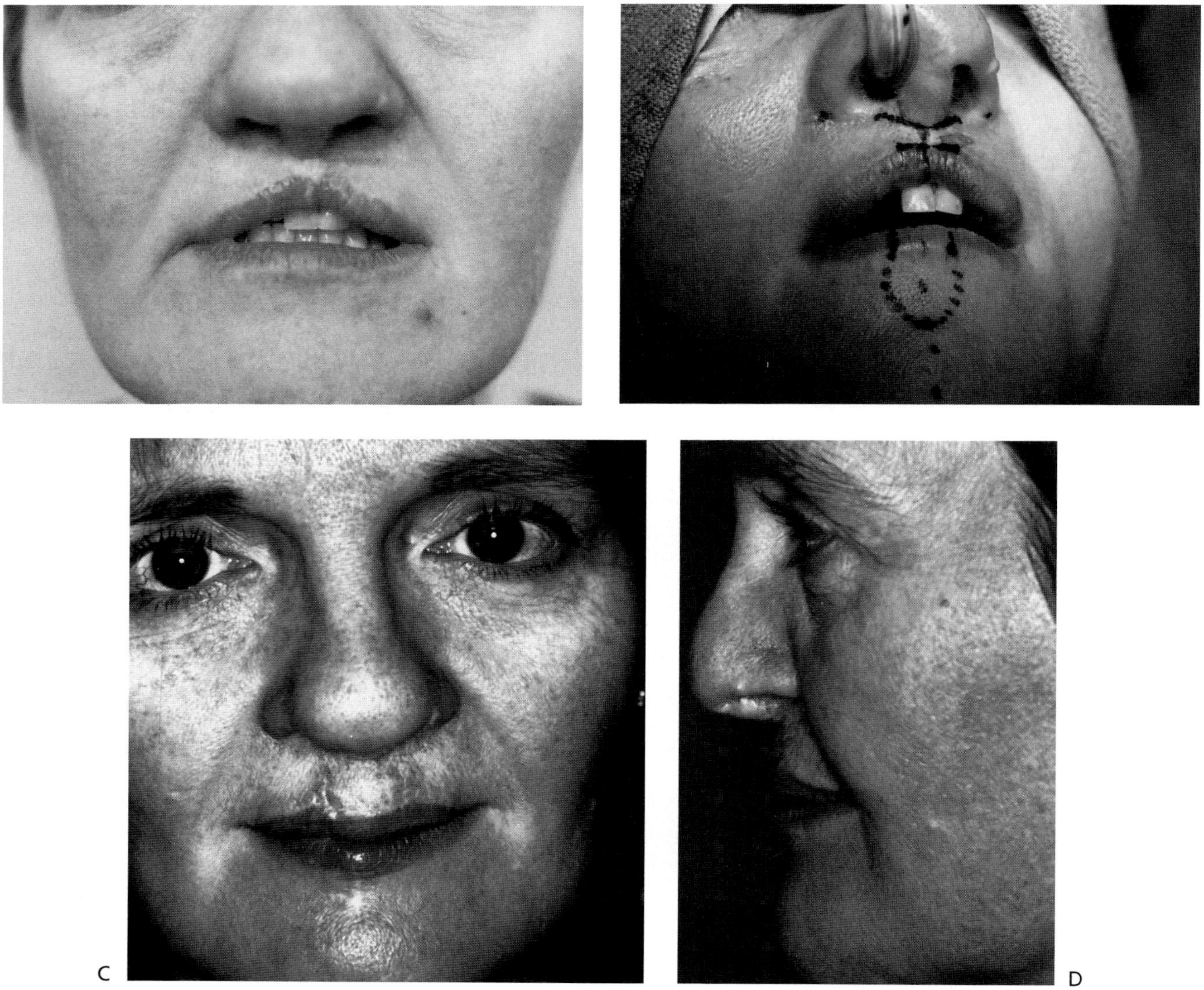

FIGURE 22-5. A: Very short and tight upper lip after bilateral cleft lip repair. **B:** Design of an Abbe flap on the lower lip. **C,D:** Final result with improved balance and symmetry of the upper lip.

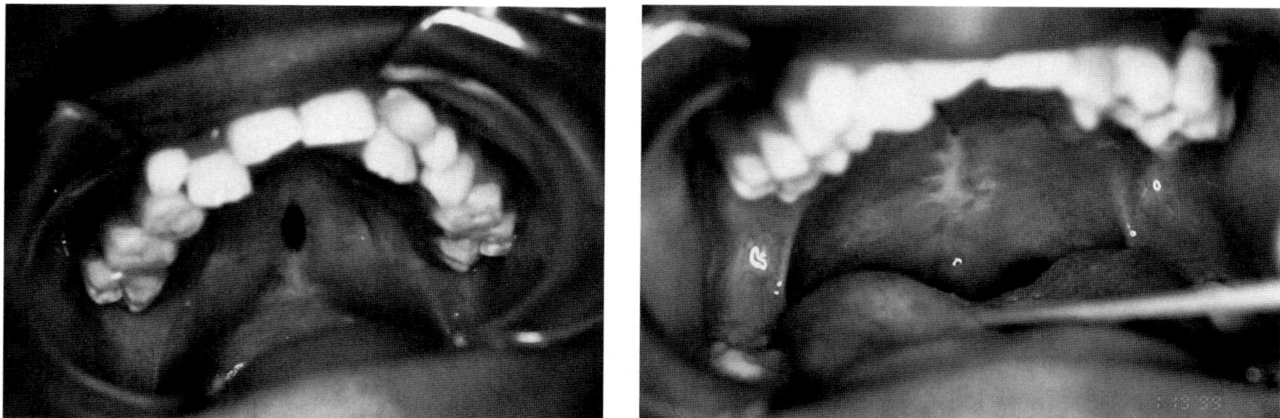

FIGURE 22-6. A: Palatal fistula in the junction between soft and hard palate. Note that the levator muscle fibers have not been dissected and released from their abnormal attachment in the posterior aspect of the hard palate. **B:** Postoperative view several months after fistula repair. Bilateral mucoperiosteal flaps were elevated, the muscles were completely released and approximated in the midline, and the fistula was closed in layers under no tension.

unilateral cases, placement of the flap in the location of the lip scar can correct the tightness but does not significantly improve the appearance of the lip. Millard (18) recommended placement of midline Abbe flaps in unilateral clefts as with bilateral clefts. After release of the tightness of the lip, a revision of the initial scar, if needed, could provide more optimal results.

CLEFT PALATE

The primary objective of cleft palate surgery is to reestablish the anatomy of the hard and soft palate as close to normal as possible, provide an adequate mechanism for velopharyngeal function for speech, and improve middle ear function. Regardless of surgical technique, the surgeon should plan to provide a palate of adequate length, reconstitute the muscular velopharyngeal sling, and approximate the tissues without tension to achieve the best functional results.

Timing for cleft palate repair has become a controversial issue, because the effects of palatal surgery on facial growth need to be considered. In the past, to avoid detrimental effects on growth, surgeons advocated delayed closure of the entire palate or early repair of the soft palate only and management of the hard palate prosthetically for several years. The majority of the patients treated with this protocol had almost normal facial growth but significant speech problems that were very difficult or almost impossible to correct (19).

Since the landmark publication by Dorf and Curtin (20) in 1982, a number of investigators have reported their findings on the effects of early palatoplasty (before the child's first birthday) on speech and facial growth. The vast majority of authors agree that proper speech production should be given priority; however, one should always be aware of the potential detrimental iatrogenic effects of palatoplasty on facial growth. Careful palatal dissection techniques should be used, causing as little trauma to the tissues as possible. The flaps should be approximated without undue tension, and large raw surfaces, which would subsequently heal with additional scarring, should be avoided. There currently is much evidence suggesting that early cleft palate repair (within the first year of life) results in better speech, especially for patients with more extensive clefts (21–24). Velopharyngeal competence is thought to be achieved more often when initial cleft repair is completed early.

Berkowitz (25) suggests a more cautious approach, particularly for patients with wide clefts of the palate. According to Berkowitz: "Attainment of normal speech, facial and palatal development and dental occlusion is possible without compromising one objective for another. Although speech development may benefit from early palatal closure, there are instances when the cleft space is very wide. In these instances, cleft closure should be postponed until the child is older to permit additional palatal growth and allow for a more conservative palatal surgery. Non-physiologic surgery causes facial and palatal deformation due to the destruction of blood supply and scar formation." To avoid these consequences, he recommends that timing of palatal closure be related to the anatomical and functional findings in the individual and not determined by age alone.

Further longitudinal studies are necessary to fully clarify these issues. Based on the existing information, however, it seems reasonable to recommend early palate repair in the majority of cases to achieve the best possible speech results. Potential effect of such interventions on maxillofacial growth should not be overlooked but taken into consideration and closely monitored.

PALATOPLASTY FAILURES

Despite advances in palatoplasty techniques and better understanding of their effects on speech and facial growth, several complications or failures requiring additional surgery still are encountered. The most significant ones include (i) palatal fistulas and (ii) velopharyngeal incompetence.

Palatal Fistulas

The reported incidence of palatal fistula formation after palatoplasty ranges from 0% to 34% (26). Incidence seems to be independent of the surgical technique used for the palatoplasty but is significantly higher in bilateral than in unilateral cases. Palatal fistulas represent failures of the surgical technique. They might be due to several factors, including poor design of the palatoplasty or problems in execution of the surgical procedure. This includes incomplete dissection of the flaps, poor handling of the tissues, closure under undue tension, failure to achieve a three-layered closure in the soft palate and a two-layered closure in the hard palate, postoperative bleeding between the oral and nasal layers, and/or infections. Some anterior fistulas just behind the premaxilla are found in patients with very wide bilateral clefts in whom a paucity of soft tissues might have been left unrepaired at the time of primary palatoplasty because of inability for tissue approximation in the area. Alveolar clefts also are left untreated by surgeons who prefer secondary to primary bone grafting.

Fistulas may be evident immediately after the palatoplasty, but they also may develop several years later at the time of orthodontic treatment and arch expansion. Larger fistulas may become symptomatic, resulting in nasal regurgitation of saliva and food particles. They might affect speech production, resulting in hypernasality, nasal emission, and articulation disturbances secondary to deviations in tongue placement during speech production in response to the fistula.

Some surgeons suggest that asymptomatic fistulas should

not be closed, whereas others recommend closure of even small fistulas given that regurgitation of food and liquids into the nasal cavity might result in constant irritation of the nasal mucosa. This may cause swelling, occasional bleeding, and potential effects on breathing, speech, or oronasal hygiene. I recommend waiting for several months after the palatoplasty before embarking on closure of a palatal fistula, because the tissues around the fistula initially are inflamed and friable in the early postoperative period, and any closure attempt might be destined to fail.

Some authors report a high rate of failure after repair of a palatal fistula, whereas others report a high success rate (27–29). Better understanding of the timing and mechanics of fistula repair enables us to achieve a high rate of success and significantly reduces the possibility of recurrence. Large fistulas should be closed as soon as possible to prevent regurgitation and improve speech and oronasal hygiene. If there is evidence of a negative effect on speech but the surgeon feels that the timing is not appropriate for fistula closure, an obturator should be fabricated until the time of definitive repair. An example of such a case is the young patient with a bilateral cleft with poor alignment of the maxillary segments and the premaxilla. This patient ultimately will require extensive orthodontic treatment and maxillary osteotomy(s) to correct the skeletal deformity. In this case, one should wait for completion of the orthodontic treatment and repair the fistula simultaneously with the maxillary surgery or setback of the premaxilla.

Each area of the palate has different requirements with respect to fistula closure. The surgeon first should decide if the available surrounding tissues are adequate for the closure or if additional tissues, brought primarily from other areas of the oral cavity, are necessary. Distant flaps or even free flaps, although technically feasible, are seldom needed to assist in closure of palatal fistulas. One should evaluate if adequate dissection and mobilization of the muscles was performed during the initial surgery and whether some muscle fibers still remain attached to the posterior edge of the hard palate. Whenever possible, speech should be evaluated before fistula repair.

When a small fistula is present in the soft palate, but palatal length and movement of the soft palate are judged to be adequate with no evidence of velopharyngeal insufficiency (VPI), the fistula can be closed with a relatively straightforward procedure without extensive dissection. The margins of the fistula should be excised sharply and the palatal scar incised anteriorly and posteriorly to the fistula to allow for visualization and mobilization of the nasal lining around the fistula and a tension-free, layered closure. This probably will not work for larger fistulas of the soft palate extending to the junction between hard and soft palate, because there is virtually no elasticity of the tissues of the hard palate. Attempting to close the fistula after excision of its margins might result in undue tension with subsequent failure. In such cases, lateral relaxing incisions with undermining and mobilization of the mucoperiosteum of the hard palate will allow for a tension-free closure in the vast majority of cases (Fig. 22-6). For very large fistulas in this area and when VPI also is present, one might combine fistula closure with a pharyngeal flap to provide for additional support and closure.

Fistulas of the hard palate represent a different challenge. Several surgeons have suggested the use of local turnover flaps from the periphery of the fistula for nasal lining closure and the use of local rotation or transposition flaps of palatal mucoperiosteum for oral coverage. These flaps can be successful on occasion, especially when dealing with small defects. For larger defects, however, I prefer to redo the palatoplasty with complete mobilization of bilateral palatal flaps on either side of the fistula, complete identification of the extent of the fistula, repair of the nasal lining directly or with

A

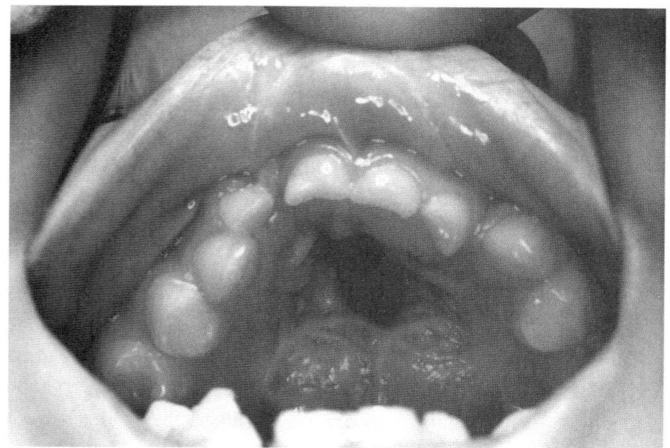

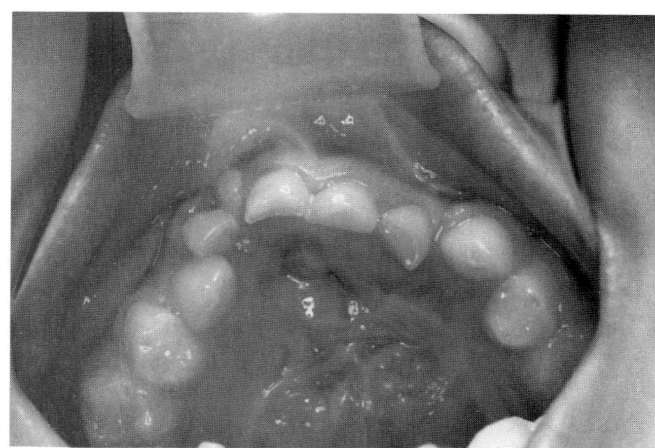

B

FIGURE 22-7. A: Large palatal fistula in the hard palate after repair of a bilateral cleft lip and palate. **B:** Complete closure was achieved with elevation of bilateral palatal mucoperiosteal flaps, closure of the nasal floor with vomer flaps, and approximation of the palatal flaps in the midline without tension.

the use of vomer flaps, if needed, and reapproximation of the palatal flaps in the midline without tension (Fig. 22-7).

Larger anterior palatal fistulas that have not been treated previously or that represent failures of previous attempts and result in stiffness, lack of elasticity, and hardness of the palatal tissues might require additional tissue for closure. Anteriorly or posteriorly based tongue flaps can be extremely helpful in the management of such difficult cases (30). Two stages are required with this technique, with a 2- to 3-week interval. Eating or speaking is not significantly restricted during the interim period. As with every surgical procedure, planning is extremely important with a tongue flap. The extent of the fistula should be delineated completely. In the majority of cases and when it is feasible, turnover flaps from the margins of the fistula should be used to achieve full closure of the floor of the nasal cavity. The palatal tissues around the fistula should be undermined circumferentially for a few millimeters to allow for adequate insetting and suturing of the tongue flap around the defect. I prefer anteriorly based flaps designed on either side of the midline. They must be a little wider than the size of the defect and 5 to 6 cm long, to prevent tethering of the tongue during speech or eating. The flap is about 0.5 cm thick and consists of mucosa and muscle fibers. The donor site is closed primarily, almost to the base of the flap. The flap then is inset around the margins of the fistula using absorbable mattress sutures. There is no need for maxillomandibular fixation for the period until division of the pedicle. After 2 to 3 weeks, the pedicle is divided and the posterior aspect of the flap is inset in the posterior area of the fistula after freshening of the palatal margins. The remaining pedicle is discarded, and additional sutures are placed to completely repair the defect on the tongue (Fig. 22-8). There have been no problems with tongue mobility or swallowing after this procedure; however, there have been some isolated reports of negative effects of tongue flaps on speech sound articulation. This may occur primarily with bulky flaps, which interfere with the position of the tongue during speech. This should be prevented by careful planning, design, and inset of the flap.

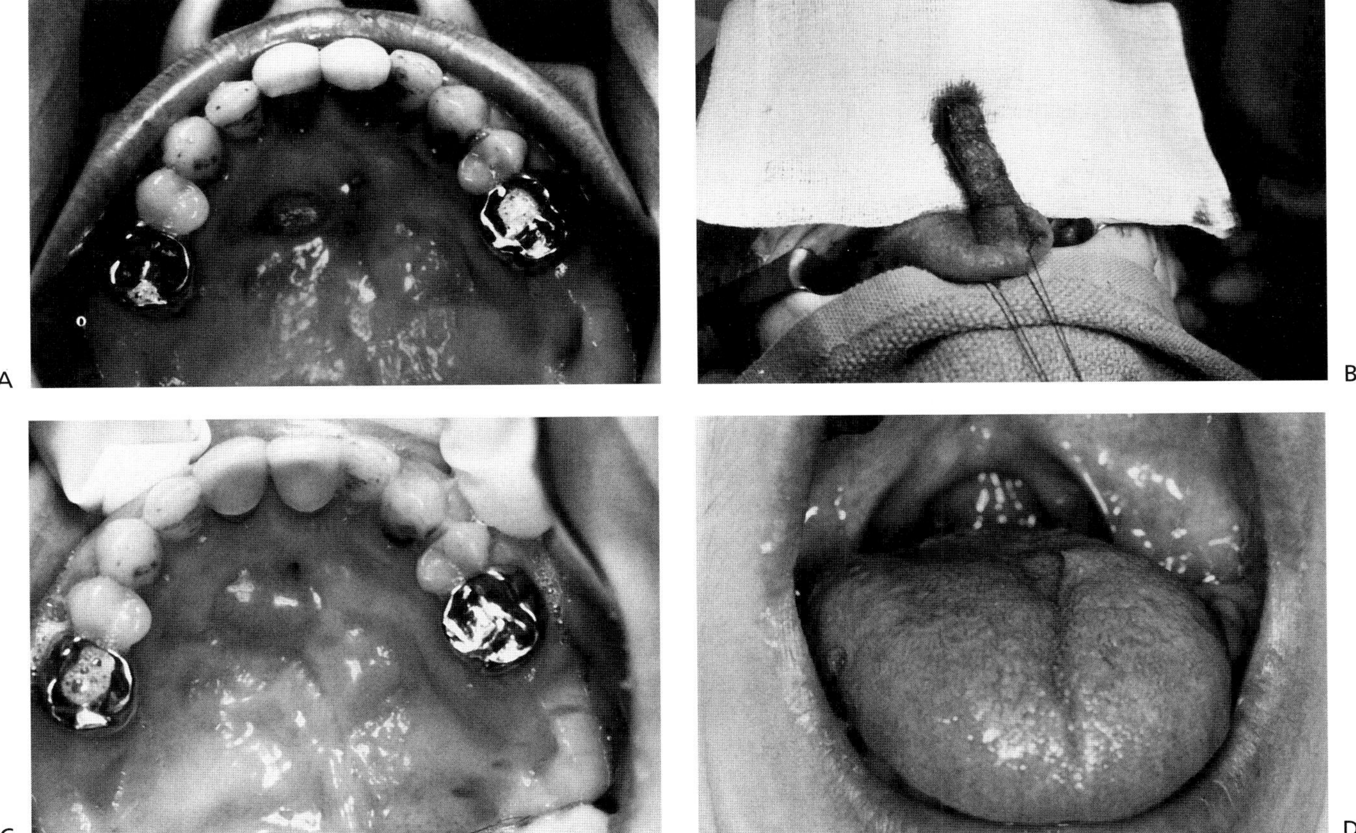

FIGURE 22-8. A: Significant palatal defect after extrusion and infection of a palatal bone graft. The palatal tissues were very thin and friable and did not allow for closure of the defect with local tissues. After debridement of all necrotic and scarred tissues, a 2–4 cm defect was created. **B,C:** Anteriorly based tongue flap was elevated and inset in the defect. Its pedicle was divided after 10 days and the flap was sutured around the margins of the defect, providing stable coverage. **D:** Good postoperative movement of the tongue without residual donor site deformity.

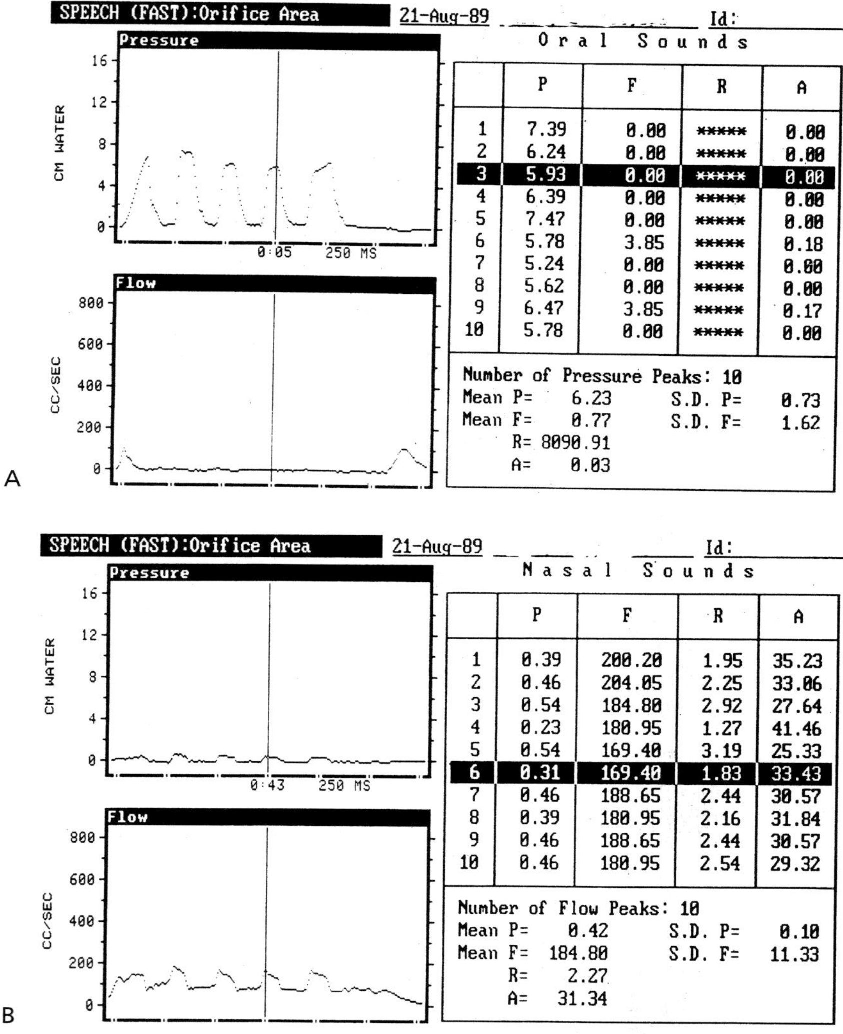

FIGURE 22-9. Graphic records **(left)** of oronasal pressures **(top)**. nasal airflow rates **(bottom)**, and corresponding numerical values **(right)** for pressure (P, in cm H_2O), flow (F, in cc/s), resistance (R, in cm H_2O/LPS), and velopharyngeal areas (A, in mm^2) for **(A)** normal repetitions of *oral* consonant-vowel syllables, such as /pi/; **(B)** normal repetitions of *nasal* consonant-vowel syllables, such as /mi/; *(continued)*

Velopharyngeal Disturbances

Despite better understanding of the physiology of speech, the effects of early palate repair on speech outcome, and the improvement of surgical techniques, an average of 20% of patients will have residual VPI after cleft palate repair. This rate does not seem to be influenced significantly by the surgical technique used for the palatoplasty.

Important to the management of VPI is the accurate diagnosis of the disorder and its impact on speech production. Techniques and measurements used to assess velopharyngeal function generally can be classified into three categories: (i) perceptual, including listener evaluations of speech production; (ii) anatomical, including evaluation of velopharyngeal and nasal structures; and (iii) physiologic, including assessment of velopharyngeal and nasal function. Many measurement approaches provide information in more than one of these areas, and a complete diagnostic evaluation should provide information in each category (31).

Patient History

Before testing, an extensive case history should be obtained, especially noting clefting or VPI in family members, a history of adenotonsillectomy or other orofacial and nasal procedures, a history of feeding or swallowing problems, including nasal regurgitation of liquids, a history of speech problems, and a history of frequent ear infections. If physical management of the velopharyngeal valve is anticipated, we include questions to determine whether nasal airway obstruction exists, as indicated by the presence of decreased exercise tolerance, eating or swallowing problems, arrested growth, snoring, frequent awakenings at night, decreased sensations of smell and taste, frequent colds, and hyponasal speech. These responses and the results of other diagnostic tests determine whether the nasal airway needs to be managed to increase patency before an additional resistive load, such as a pharyngeal flap, is introduced into the airway.

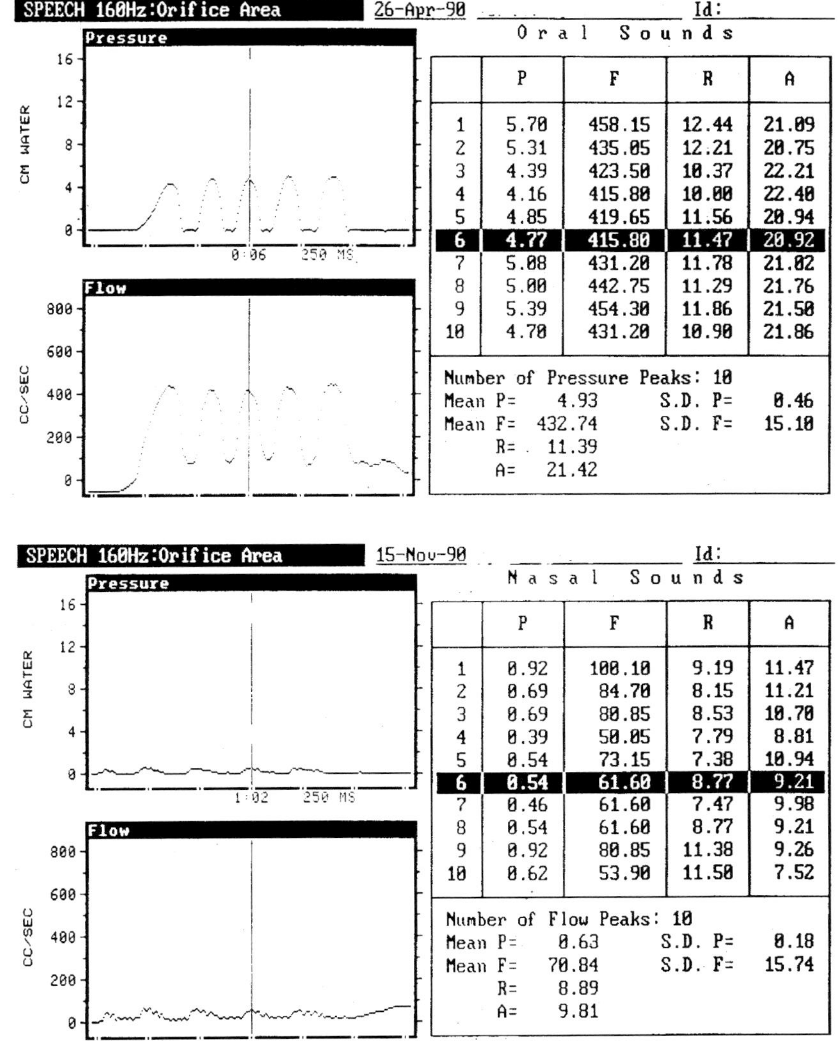

Oral Sounds

	P	F	R	A
1	5.70	458.15	12.44	21.09
2	5.31	435.05	12.21	20.75
3	4.39	423.50	10.37	22.21
4	4.16	415.80	10.00	22.40
5	4.85	419.65	11.56	20.94
6	4.77	415.80	11.47	20.92
7	5.08	431.20	11.78	21.02
8	5.00	442.75	11.29	21.76
9	5.39	454.30	11.86	21.50
10	4.70	431.20	10.90	21.86

Number of Pressure Peaks: 10
Mean P= 4.93 S.D. P= 0.46
Mean F= 432.74 S.D. F= 15.10
R= 11.39
A= 21.42

Nasal Sounds

	P	F	R	A
1	0.92	100.10	9.19	11.47
2	0.69	84.70	8.15	11.21
3	0.69	80.85	8.53	10.70
4	0.39	50.05	7.79	8.81
5	0.54	73.15	7.38	10.94
6	0.54	61.60	8.77	9.21
7	0.46	61.60	7.47	9.98
8	0.54	61.60	8.77	9.21
9	0.92	80.85	11.38	9.26
10	0.62	53.90	11.50	7.52

Number of Flow Peaks: 10
Mean P= 0.63 S.D. P= 0.18
Mean F= 70.84 S.D. F= 15.74
R= 8.89
A= 9.81

FIGURE 22-9. **(C)** *(Continued)* repetitions of oral consonant-vowel syllables produced by a person with velopharyngeal insufficiency; and **(D)** repetitions of nasal consonant-vowel syllables produced by a person with nasal (velopharyngeal) obstruction.

Perceptual Evaluation

Judgments of speech made by an experienced speech-language pathologist are an essential part of the evaluation of velopharyngeal function for speech. These judgments include the results of standardized speech sound (articulation) testing and ratings of oronasal resonance balance. We usually begin administering standardized articulation tests when the patient is between 2 and 3 years of age. We complete articulation testing to determine whether speech sound errors related to VPI exist. Such errors include weak production of plosive and fricative consonants, nasal emission of air during consonant sound production, and substitution of compensatory articulations for particular consonant sounds. Assessment of oronasal resonance balance includes judgments regarding the presence of consistent or inconsistent mild, moderate, or severe hypernasality. When the nasal airway is obstructed, mild, moderate, or severe hyponasality may be present.

Anatomical Evaluation

An intraoral examination is our first step in obtaining anatomical information about the velopharyngeal structures. This examination provides information about the presence, location, and size of palatal fistulas, the size of the tonsils, and the status of dentition/occlusion. It also provides impressions about length, movement, and symmetry of the velum and direction, degree, and symmetry of visualized pharyngeal wall movement. A rhinoscopic examination is performed to note the presence of hypertrophic turbinates, septal deviation, and nasal congestion or obstruction. If a reconstructive procedure such as a pharyngeal flap has been performed, the intraoral examination should provide impressions about the width and position of the base of the flap, size of ports, and degree of flap motion, if visualized.

Direct anatomical evaluation is complemented by several radiographic and endoscopic studies that provide static and dynamic anatomical information during speech and assist us in the final diagnosis and prescription for the best possible management. Such studies include cephalometric radiographs, videofluoroscopy, and nasopharyngoscopy. Through these studies, the entire velopharyngeal mechanism is evaluated extensively at rest and during speech production. This includes obtaining information about the depth of the nasopharynx, the movement of the velum and the pharyngeal walls, the position of contact or lack of contact between the velum and pharyngeal walls during speech, presence of Passavant ridge, size of residual velopharyngeal gap, and symmetry or asymmetry in movement. If a previous flap or pharyngoplasty is in place, residual incompetence of the ports or obstructions can be visualized and documented.

Physiologic Evaluation

Our most frequently used physiologic test, which provides information during both speech production and nasal respiration, is aerodynamic assessment. Specifically, we use the pressure-flow technique described by Warren and DuBois (32) to determine the presence and magnitude of velopharyngeal opening during speech production. We also use this method to determine whether velopharyngeal obstruction exists, i.e., too little velopharyngeal opening during production of nasal sounds (Fig. 22-9). Our normative and patient data led us to develop four categories for velopharyngeal function: one typical category (which consists of pressure-flow patterns generated by normal-sounding speakers) and three atypical categories (open—associated with excessive

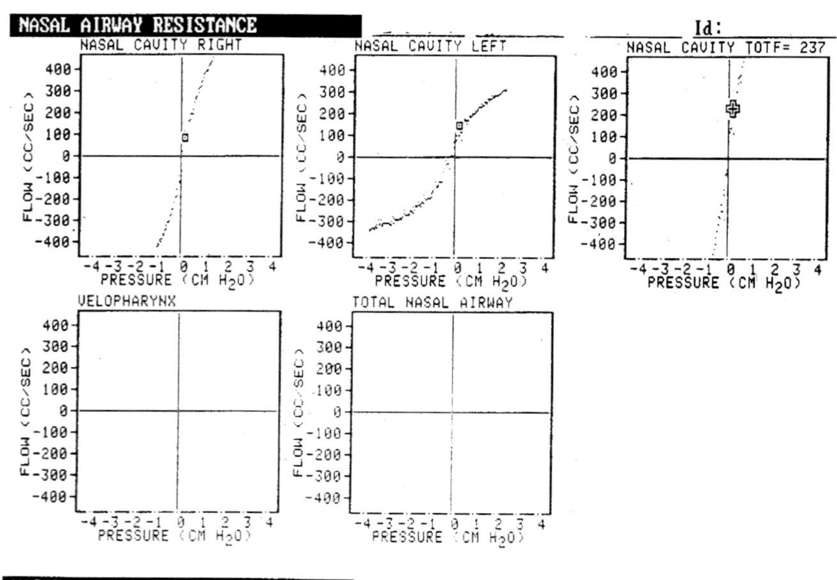

NASAL AIRWAY RESISTANCE

Id:

Nasal Cavity Total flow= 237.18 cc/sec

	P	F	R	A
Nasal Cavity Right	0.19	89.74	2.12	22.62
Nasal Cavity Left	0.19	147.44	1.29	37.17
Nasal Cavity Total	0.19	237.18	0.80	59.79
Velopharynx	*****	*******	0.00	*****
Total Nasal Airway	0.19	237.18	0.80	59.79

NCR= 0.80 (100% contribution)
VPR= 0.00 (0% contribution)

NAR= 0.80

P: Pressure in cm H2O
F: Flow in cc/sec
R: Resistance in cm H2O/L/sec
A: Area in mm^2

B

FIGURE 22-10. Pressure-flow plots **(A,C)** and corresponding numerical data **(B,D)** obtained using component rhinomanometry during nasal breathing by a pediatric patient before **(A,B)** and after *(continued)*

velopharyngeal opening during oral sounds; closed—associated with too little opening during nasal sounds; and mixed—having characteristics of both open and closed categories) (33).

We also use aerodynamic assessment to obtain information about nasal airway patency during nasal respiration. To obtain this information, we use component rhinomanometry. This approach provides nasal airway resistance data. It also provides calculation of the nasal cross-sectional areas using Warren's approach. Using component rhinomanometry, we obtain resistance and area data for the nasal cavities, velopharynx, and total nasal airway (34).

We also may use the Nasometer (Kay Elemetrics Corp.) to quantify changes in acoustic energy that occur with a greater or lesser degree of coupling between the oral and nasal cavities. In individuals with VPI, excessive nasal cavity energy (an elevated nasalance score) is registered during production of oral sounds. In individuals with velopharyngeal obstruction, insufficient nasal cavity energy (a low nasalance score) is registered during production of nasal sounds. These data are used in conjunction with other anatomical and physiologic information to make management decisions and/or evaluate the outcome of surgery (Fig. 22-10).

Procedures to Correct Velopharyngeal Insufficiency

At the current time, velopharyngeal incompetence most frequently is managed surgically with two procedures and their perspective modifications: (i) pharyngeal flap and (ii) sphincter pharyngoplasty.

Whereas these two types of procedures are widely used, a small number of surgeons still recommend augmentation of the posterior pharyngeal wall with various autogenous or alloplastic materials for management of mild VPI, with small gaps between the soft palate and the posterior pharyngeal

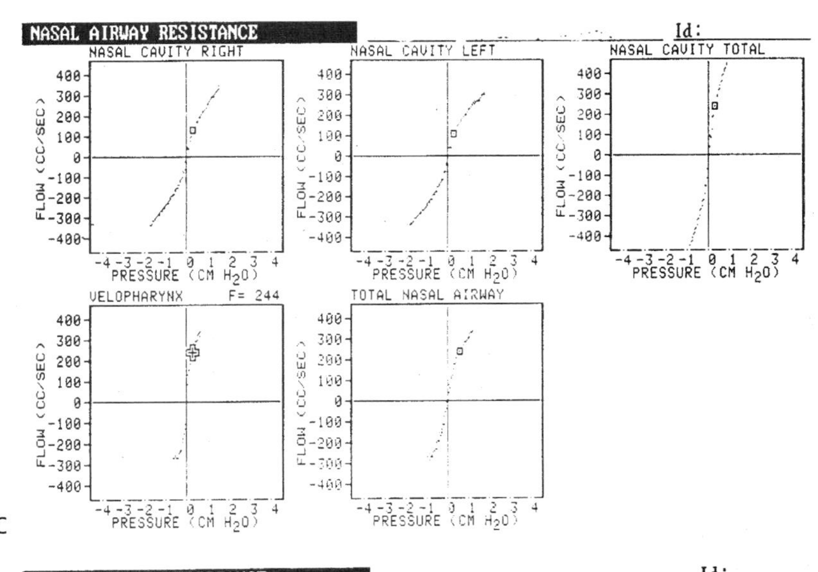

NASAL AIRWAY RESISTANCE

Id:

Velopharyngeal flow= 243.59 cc/sec

	P	F	R	A
Nasal Cavity Right	0.35	134.62	2.60	25.01
Nasal Cavity Left	0.35	108.97	3.21	20.24
Nasal Cavity Total	0.35	243.59	1.44	45.25
Velopharynx	0.31	243.59	1.27	40.08
Total Nasal Airway	0.66	243.59	2.71	32.95

NCR= 1.44 (53% contribution)
VPR= 1.27 (47% contribution)

D NAR= 2.71

P: Pressure in cm H_2O
F: Flow in cc/sec
R: Resistance in cm H_2O/L/sec
A: Area in mm^2

FIGURE 22-10. (C,D) *(Continued)* successful pharyngeal flap surgery. Note a small resistive load is added at the level of the velopharynx secondary to the presence of the pharyngeal flap. A successful speech result for oral and nasal sounds following surgery is shown in Figs. 22-9A and B, respectively.

wall. Prosthetic rehabilitation currently is reserved for surgical failures or for patients with significant medical problems who are not considered candidates for a surgical procedure.

Pharyngeal Flap

The pharyngeal flap is a widely accepted procedure for management of patients with VPI. In the past, some surgeons recommended the use of primary flaps in conjunction with palatoplasty. However, most surgeons currently agree that pharyngeal flaps generally should be performed as a secondary procedure when needed. This practice allows the team to complete an extensive evaluation, determining velopharyngeal form and function, and to prescribe the most appropriate management based on each patient's individual needs.

There are two designs for the flap, a superiorly and an inferiorly based flap. The vast majority of surgeons currently prefer the use of a superiorly based flap, because this design allows for more natural movement of the palate in a posterior and superior plane toward the tubercle of the axis. Unfortunately, there is no standardized procedure under the term superiorly based pharyngeal flap, and several technical variations that could have some effect on the final outcome of the procedure are included under this term. These technical variations include division of the soft palate to insert the flap versus the sandwich technique with separation of the palatal layers with an incision in the posterior free border of the palate and introduction of the flap through this opening. Lining of the raw undersurface of the flap with posteriorly based mucosal flaps obtained from the nasal surface of the palate is recommended by the majority of surgeons in order to prevent contracture and narrowing or "tubing" of the flap and subsequent increase in port size. Others surgeons, particularly those who promote the sandwich technique, do not believe in the importance of lining and demonstrate successful results without lining of the raw surface. The size of the ports is another area of controversy. Some surgeons recommend the lateral port control technique using appropriately sized catheters to precisely tailor the size of the ports, whereas others do not recommend this technique. Finally, several surgeons recommend the immediate approximation of the donor site defect of the posterior pharyngeal wall, claiming that such practice reduces the danger of postoperative bleeding and speeds up the healing period. Others recommend leaving the donor site open, allowing it to heal in a secondary intention for fear of interference with the anatomy of the pharynx that could accentuate potential episodes of airway obstruction in the immediate postoperative period.

With advances in pediatric anesthesia, better understanding of the anatomy, improvement of techniques, and, above all, increased awareness of the potential serious problems associated with the pharyngeal flap procedure, the intraoperative and perioperative complications of this procedure have decreased significantly, but some serious complications are still encountered. Death due to obstruction is an extremely rare complication, but occasional operative and postoperative bleeding and acute airway obstruction can be anticipated (35–37). The prime source of bleeding has been the donor site in the posterior pharyngeal wall. Infiltration of the donor site with vasoconstrictives facilitates dissection and reduces bleeding during surgery, but one should be very careful of mucosal and muscular bleeders that retract away from the wound margins. Packing of the donor site followed by meticulous hemostasis before insetting of the flap is considered extremely important. Some authors believe that suturing the donor site of the pharyngeal wall might be an additional beneficial step in controlling potential bleeding, whereas others do not believe that there is any benefit to suturing the donor site defect.

According to several series, the incidence of acute airway obstruction due to bleeding, tissue swelling, or inappropriate position of the flap has decreased significantly. In the past, tracheostomy was recommended to facilitate pharyngeal flap surgery or manage airway obstruction. It currently is recognized that, in the vast majority of patients, some degree of transient obstruction will be present immediately after surgery. Such obstruction can be identified clinically and with polysomnographic sleep studies and monitoring of the arterial saturation. Most of the obstructive signs and symptoms resolve in the vast majority of patients a few days or months after surgery (38,39).

Because transient obstruction of various degrees has been well documented, we believe that it is extremely important to carefully monitor these patients in the immediate postoperative period. Despite changes in the health care system with reduction of inpatient days, it is recommended that all patients be hospitalized after pharyngeal flap operation and monitored closely for signs of obstruction. Nasopharyngeal airway tubes are recommended to improve breathing in the perioperative period. In extreme cases, reintubation may be necessary to control the airway.

Results After Pharyngeal Flap Surgery

Several long-term studies evaluating the long-term effects of pharyngeal flap surgery on breathing and speech have been reported (40–42). The reported success rates range from 40% to 90%. This vast discrepancy in outcome can be explained in several ways. Different groups of patients are included in the studies; thus, patients with various forms of clefts or even patients without clefts are considered together in the available studies. Age at the time of the procedure varies from very young to adulthood, but it is well understood that the effect of a pharyngeal flap performed in adults is significantly inferior than the effect of the same procedure performed in children. Also, most studies are retrospective, and important data might be missing from the preoperative or postoperative evaluation.

The modalities used to evaluate postoperative improvement in speech vary as well. Some studies rely on perceptual (subjective) judgment of speech, whereas others include direct evaluation of the modified anatomy of the nasopharynx during speech with nasopharyngoscopy or videofluoroscopy and/or objective assessment of velopharyngeal function using aerodynamic or acoustic assessments. Interpretation of the findings of these tests is controversial. Some authors consider the elimination of hypernasality as the sole criterion for success and do not consider hyponasality as a failure. Thus, the reported percentages for success of this procedure are affected greatly by the methodology of evaluation and interpretation of findings. We use both breathing and speech outcomes to judge success of pharyngeal flap surgery.

Pharyngeal Flap Failures

Persistent Hypernasality

Persistent hypernasality after pharyngeal flap surgery is primarily due to partial or complete detachment of the flap, contracture and narrowing of the flap with residual widening of the ports, or poor design and inappropriate placement of the flap. Each of these conditions can result in deficient ports on one or both sides of the flap.

Established hypernasality several months or years after pharyngeal flap surgery requires extensive evaluation before treatment. Once the reasons for hypernasality are established, revision of the size of the port(s) is recommended. Several procedures have been reported for correction of residual hypernasality, including the following:

1. Augmentation of the flap with additional tissue from the posterior pharyngeal wall or the palate (43)
2. Alteration of the size of the ports with rearrangement of tissues using various Z-plasties and other techniques (44)
3. Division of the old flap and new pharyngeal flap (45) or pharyngoplasty.

Several reports have described various innovative techniques. Unfortunately, the number of patients included in these studies is small and the conclusions drawn are not always warranted. For relatively small defects, I prefer tissue rearrangement using local flaps based on existing tissues (Fig. 22-11). For larger defects, additional flaps from the posterior pharyngeal wall can be used to reduce the size of the port(s). For very large defects, I prefer to divide the old flap and use a new one based on the scarred posterior pharyngeal wall. Close cooperation with a speech pathologist is necessary to successfully manage these patients. Postoperative speech therapy might be required to correct habitual speech production errors.

Persistent Hyponasality

Persistent airway obstruction is a serious complication of flap surgery that could have detrimental effects on the patient's health. Symptoms may vary in degree and include hyponasality, snoring, sleep–wake disturbances, loss of olfactory acuity, rhinorrhea, epistaxis, pain following the distribution of the trigeminal nerve, and intranasal or sinus infections. Obstruction might have significant effects on dentofacial growth and even significant systemic effect on the cardiopulmonary and other systems. The exact incidence of this complication is not known, because several investigators do not even consider airway obstruction to be a failure of pharyngeal flap surgery. Complete obstruction and pharyngeal scarring are extremely difficult to treat. Even with prolonged stenting of the newly created ports, scarring and contracture may recur.

Milder hyponasality without other clinical symptoms might be considered an acceptable result. However, when the hyponasality significantly interferes with speech, intelligibility and/or a acceptability, or the patient's general condition, revision of the ports is recommended. Prior to any surgical procedure, extensive multispecialty evaluation again

A

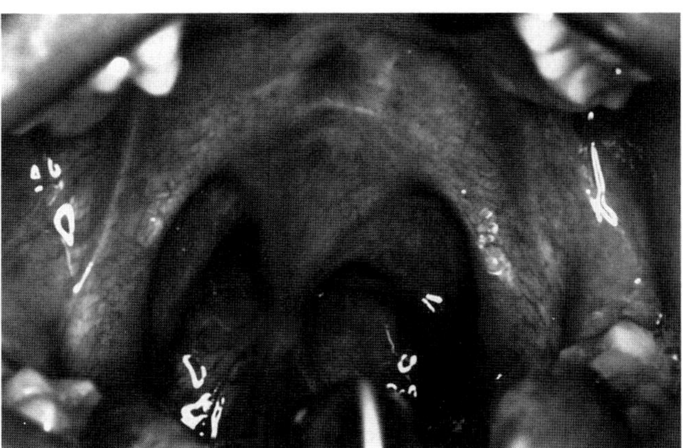

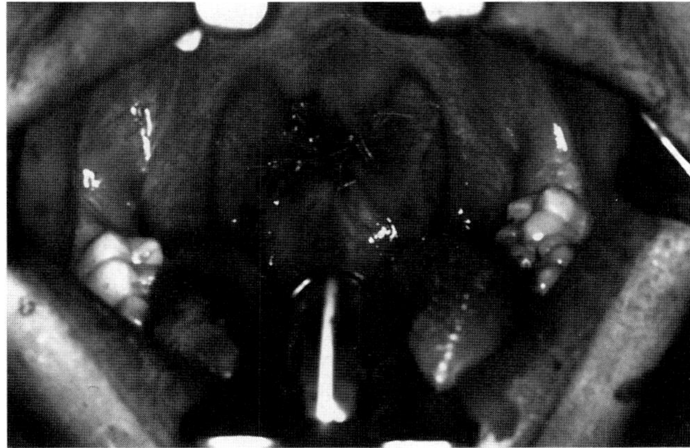

B

FIGURE 22-11. A: Residual velopharyngeal insufficiency (VPI) after superiorly based pharyngeal flap. Note large ports on either side of the flap. **B:** Reduction of port sizes was achieved with bilateral Z-plasties in the superior area of the ports.

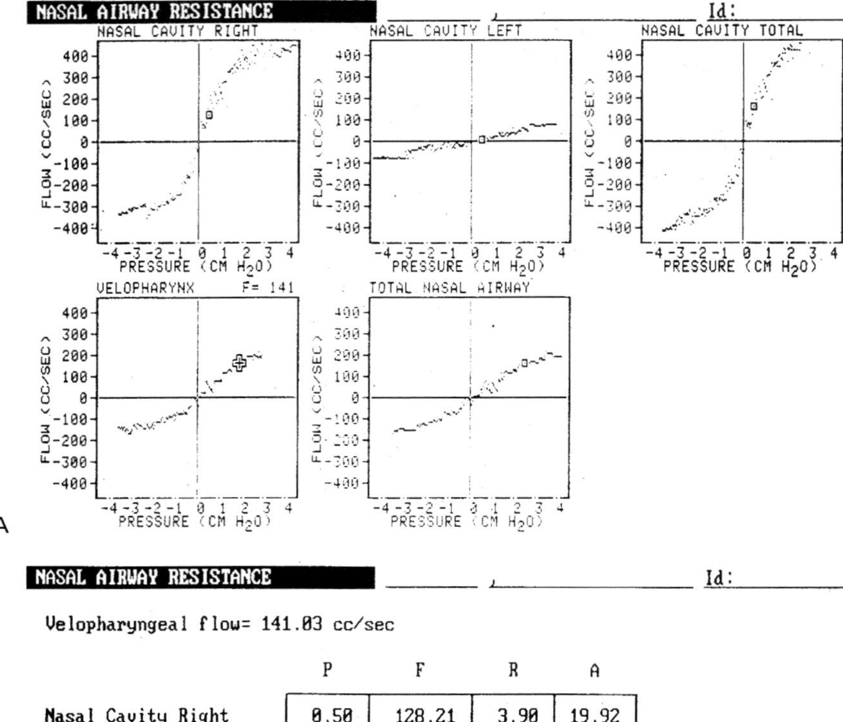

NASAL AIRWAY RESISTANCE Id:

Velopharyngeal flow= 141.03 cc/sec

	P	F	R	A
Nasal Cavity Right	0.50	128.21	3.90	19.92
Nasal Cavity Left	0.50	12.82	39.00	1.99
Nasal Cavity Total	0.50	141.03	3.55	21.91
Velopharynx	2.96	141.03	20.99	9.01
Total Nasal Airway	3.46	141.03	24.54	8.33

NCR= 3.55 (14% contribution)
VPR= 20.99 (86% contribution)

B NAR= 24.54

P: Pressure in cm H_2O
F: Flow in cc/sec
R: Resistance in cm H_2O/L/sec
A: Area in mm^2

FIGURE 22-12. Pressure-flow plots **(A,C)** and corresponding numerical data **(B,D)** obtained using component rhinomanometry during nasal breathing by a pediatric patient before **(A,B)** and after *(continued)*

is necessary to fully understand the problem and prescribe the most appropriate treatment (Fig. 22-12). Because there is no appropriate formula for the recommended size of the ports, the surgeon should be very careful to avoid overcorrection, creating ports that are too large and result in deterioration of speech and recurrence of hypernasality.

Direct excisions of a portion of the flap around the port can be performed. Every effort should be made to cover all the raw surfaces and avoid subsequent scarring and contracture. Local Z-plasties have been recommended as for correction of hypernasality, but outcomes are not always predictable. Caouette-Laberge et al. (46) reported on nine patients with obstruction after pharyngeal flap surgery who underwent complete transection of the flap at its base. Three patients required a second intervention, and one of these patients required a third procedure to correct recurrent velopharyngeal obstruction. Only one patient developed moderately hypernasal speech after this procedure. In the majority of patients, an adhesion ultimately formed between the transected flap and the posterior pharyngeal wall. This nasopharyngoscopic finding might explain why hypernasality is not encountered more often after division of the flap (46).

Despite its drawbacks, pharyngeal flap surgery remains an important procedure for the management and habilitation of patients with VPI, as long as the indications for the procedure are well understood and the patients have undergone extensive preoperative evaluation, which includes perceptual and instrumental evaluation, including visualization of the anatomy of the pharynx with attention to the adequate movement of the lateral pharyngeal walls. Attention should be given to all surgical details as well as postoperative follow-up. Other prerequisites for long-term success include the patient's adequate hearing, appropriate learning level, and postoperative speech therapy to assist in the correction of articulation problems, including compensatory strategies following surgery.

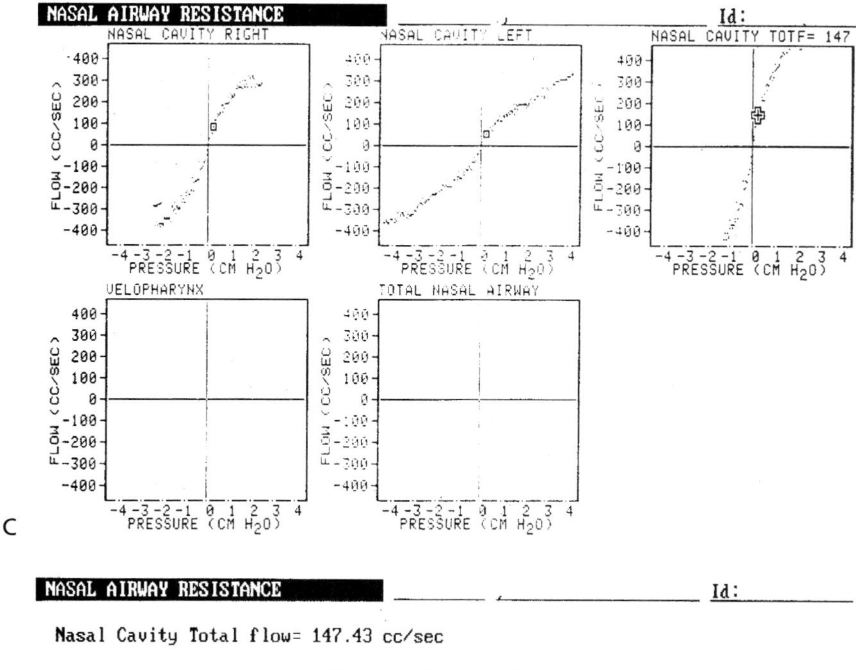

C

NASAL AIRWAY RESISTANCE Id:

Nasal Cavity Total flow= 147.43 cc/sec

	P	F	R	A
Nasal Cavity Right	0.27	89.74	3.01	18.98
Nasal Cavity Left	0.27	57.69	4.68	12.20
Nasal Cavity Total	0.27	147.43	1.83	31.18
Velopharynx	*****	*******	*****	*****
Total Nasal Airway	0.27	147.43	1.83	31.18

NCR= 1.83
VPR= *****

NAR= 1.83

P: Pressure in cm H2O
F: Flow in cc/sec
R: Resistance in cm H2O/L/sec
A: Area in mm²

D

FIGURE 22-12. *(Continued)* **(C,D)** successful surgery to correct nasal airway obstruction secondary to pharyngeal flap surgery. Note the elimination of velopharyngeal or flap resistive load after surgery.

Sphincter Pharyngoplasty

Sphincter pharyngoplasty was first described by Hines in 1950, but it only gained popularity 18 years later after the publication of a variation of this technique by Orticochea. He coined the term *dynamic muscle sphincter* and used the posterior faucial pillars with the underlying palatopharyngeus muscles for construction of the sphincter. The two flaps were inset to a short, inferiorly based pharyngeal flap in the oropharynx. Jackson modified this design and suggested suturing of the flaps to a more superior position on the nasopharynx. The importance of a higher site of inset for the flaps on the pharynx in the area of the attempted velopharyngeal contact, which was identified before the procedure using lateral radiographic evaluations, was stressed by Riski et al. (47). The two flaps initially were joined together in the midline. However, such a design does not always provide for adequate tightness of the sphincter; thus, overlap of the two flaps and suturing of their tips to the opposite side currently is recommended. As with other procedures, extensive preoperative evaluation and planning are necessary. Some authors recommend this procedure for all patients with velopharyngeal incompetence, whereas others suggest that a pharyngoplasty should be reserved for patients with good palatal movement and without a large velopharyngeal gap.

Attention to the technical details during pharyngoplasty will significantly influence the outcome. The flaps should be elevated sharply and should include as much muscle as possible. They should be inset high up in the pharyngeal wall at the level of the axis. To achieve good exposure of the nasopharynx, the soft palate should be retracted superiorly. This will allow for the incision of the posterior pharyngeal wall to be placed at the highest possible level and the suturing of the flaps accurately into the desired position under direct vision. Overlapping of the flaps rather than joining them in the midline seems to be important in the creation of a competent sphincter. One should avoid undue tension during flap approximation, which could result in partial or complete dehiscence of the flaps or obstruction with hyponasality. Life-threatening bleeding has not been a problem with pharyngoplasties as with pharyngeal flaps. Perioperative nasal airway obstruction and obstructive sleep apnea can occur, and the surgeon should be prepared to manage these situations. Witt et al. (48) reported a 13% incidence of perioperative obstruction in a series of 58 patients who underwent sphincter pharyngoplasty to correct postpalatoplasty VPI. Five patients had micrognathia with or without an identified syndrome, and three had a history of perinatal respiratory and/or feeding difficulties without micrognathia. In six patients, the airway dysfunction resolved within 3 days postoperatively; two patients required readmission and continuous positive airway pressure for several weeks prior to resolution of the obstructive syndromes. Both of these patients were found to have hyponasal speech postoperatively, which indicates they might have had an overcorrected sphincter in the first place. In any event, these findings demonstrate that the surgeon should carefully evaluate these patients in the immediate postoperative period. Despite pressure from insurance carriers, patients undergoing sphincter pharyngoplasties should be hospitalized for postoperative observation and should be managed aggressively as soon as symptoms of airway obstruction become evident.

Success rates of sphincter pharyngoplasties are high, ranging from 80% to 90%, according to various reports. Low insertion of the flaps has been identified as the most significant reason for failure. Flap dehiscence can contribute to failure. This dehiscence can be due to technical error. It also has been encountered in patients with previous tonsillectomies, because this procedure can lead to atrophy and scarring of the palatopharyngeus muscles, which might undermine the integrity and adequate function of the pharyngoplasty (49–51).

Persistent hypernasality after pharyngoplasty requires special attention. Extensive evaluation by the plastic surgeon and the speech pathologist is necessary before embarking on revisional surgery. If significant scarring is present from dehiscence of the flaps, contractures in the area of the donor site, or other reasons, the chances for success of any additional procedure may be diminished. If the central port is too large and a deficient sphincter is present, one should attempt to tighten it after partial or complete mobilization of the flaps from their attachments in the posterior pharyngeal wall. This procedure might be tedious, because after dehiscence and scarring, it could be difficult to reelevate the flaps and reuse them. In such cases, one may elect to use a superiorly based pharyngeal flap or a retropharyngeal implant to assist in velopharyngeal closure. Partial obstruction of the nasopharynx could pose a significant problem. Obstruction might result in several symptoms in addition to hyponasality, as noted earlier. The severity of these symptoms should be evaluated carefully.

Before any intervention, the surgeon must extensively discuss the procedure with the patient and the family and explain the pros and cons of the revision. One should always bear in mind the risk of transforming an overcorrected sphincter into a deficient one, with the significant effects on speech and return to hypernasality. Revision of the port should be done primarily in the "nondynamic" area of the sphincter, on the posterior pharyngeal wall. Partial mobilization and retroposition of the flaps, if feasible, may provide improved results. Every effort should be made to cover all the raw surfaces, because scarring in these areas may result in additional contracture and accentuation of the obstruction. For extreme cases, take-down of the flap may be recommended. This could be followed by a pharyngeal flap surgery if persistent VPI is identified.

SECONDARY BONE GRAFTING OF RESIDUAL ALVEOLAR CLEFTS

Reconstruction of the alveolar process and the hypoplastic maxilla by secondary bone grafting of the residual bony cleft and simultaneous closure of the coexisting oronasal communication in the transitional dentition stage is a time-honored procedure. Since Boyne and Sands first recommended use of particle cancellous bone grafts for the procedure in conjunction with orthodontic treatment, the value of the procedure has been demonstrated in several long-term studies (52). Several short-term and long-term reconstructive and aesthetic goals are achieved with secondary bone grafting of the maxilla and closure of residual alveolar fistulas. The most important goals are summarized in Table 22-1. Only when all or the majority of these goals are achieved should the reconstructive procedure be considered successful.

To achieve a consistently good result and reduce the incidence of complications, some well-defined principles need to be considered, including close cooperation with the surgeon and the orthodontist, timing of the procedure, type of bone graft, and flap selection.

TABLE 22-1. GOALS OF SECONDARY BONE GRAFTING OF RESIDUAL ALVEOLAR CLEFTS

Closure of oronasal fistula
Improvement of oral and nasal hygiene
Stabilization of maxillary segments
Preservation of adjacent teeth
Bony support of adjacent teeth
Tooth eruption through graft
Orthodontic movement of teeth
Reduction of need for prosthetic appliances
Improvement of nasal and facial symmetry and appearance
Increased alar support and projection
Improved appearance of the alveolus and nasal vestibule

Planning and Timing of the Procedure

Planning of the procedure and close cooperation with the orthodontist are prerequisites for success. The decision for and timing of surgical treatment should be based on a combination of developmental, orthodontic, and surgical factors. Dental rather than the chronologic age of the patient is the primary factor guiding the decision regarding the timing of a bone grafting procedure. Ideally, this procedure should be performed at the early transitional dentition stage, after eruption of the permanent central or lateral incisors but before eruption of the permanent cleft-side canine. If performed when the patient is at this age, there will be no adverse effects on the growth of the maxillofacial skeleton. Semb (53) evaluated the long-term results of secondary bone grafting in 28 patients, comparing preoperative cephalograms to those obtained after age 16 years. There was no evidence of any disturbance of the anteroposterior or vertical maxillary growth in patients of this sample. On the contrary, bone grafting was associated with increased upper facial height and, when performed early, was associated with a slightly greater maxillary protrusion. These findings support the hypothesis that bone grafting of alveolar clefts after age 8 has little or no adverse effect on maxillary growth.

Unfortunately, there are several conflicting reports on the effects of alveolar bone graft on the growth of the maxillofacial skeleton. This is due to the great variety of protocols and surgical techniques, along with their modifications, that currently are used. As a result, additional parameters are constantly introduced that make evaluation and comparison of results very difficult to almost impossible. Yet, based on currently available information, it is reasonable to state that secondary bone grafting at the stage of transitional dentition has no deleterious effects on the growth of the midface or the face in general.

Technical Considerations

Initially, blocks of bone from the ilium or the rib were used because the prime reason for bone grafting was to achieve stability of the maxillary segment and prevent maxillary collapse. With accumulated experience, however, it became apparent that superior results could be obtained when only cancellous bone particles were used instead of bony blocks. These particles can incorporate faster than the cortical grafts or blocks of bone, will remodel nicely with the rest of the maxilla, and will permit dental eruption through their substance.

Currently, most surgeons favor the use of bone particles harvested from the ilium for the bone grafting of residual alveolar clefts. A few surgeons still favor the use of grafts from the calvarium, tibia, rib, or mandible, and they report equally good results. Based on findings with various bone grafts from previous long-term studies and on our own comparative study between patients who received iliac or cranial bone grafts, we believe that the source of bone graft does not significantly influence the success or failure of this procedure. The use of cancellous bone particles only and close adherence to well-accepted steps of the procedure are, by far, the most important factors influencing the successful outcome and total habilitation of these patients (54).

Several local mucosal flaps have been reported to cover the bone graft, and very little attention was given to fully understand their importance and contribution to a successful outcome. It currently is well accepted that gingival mucoperiosteal flaps are superior to any other mucosal flap for coverage of bone grafts in the area of alveolar clefts (55). They are well vascularized, have a broad base, and can be mobilized medially to provide tension-free coverage over the bone graft. Because reconstruction is achieved with tissue of similar color, thickness, and texture to the surrounding alveolus, the final aesthetic appearance of the reconstructed area is superior. Furthermore, teeth are programmed to erupt through keratinized gingiva and will not erupt spontaneously through oral mucosa (Fig. 22-13).

Consistently successful bone grafting of residual maxillary and alveolar clefts requires several well-defined steps. Gingival mucoperiosteal flaps are designed on either side of the cleft and raised slowly to completely expose the bony cleft. All soft tissue from the margins of the bony defect should be stripped. When a palatal fistula also is present, it must be closed by raising bilateral palatal flaps and approximating them without tension. The soft tissue of the floor of the nose then should be repaired. Thus, a watertight pocket is created for placement of the bone graft. The cancellous bone chips are packed tightly within the defect to fill the bony cleft and restore thickness and height of the nasal floor and the maxilla as close to normal as possible. Any perma-

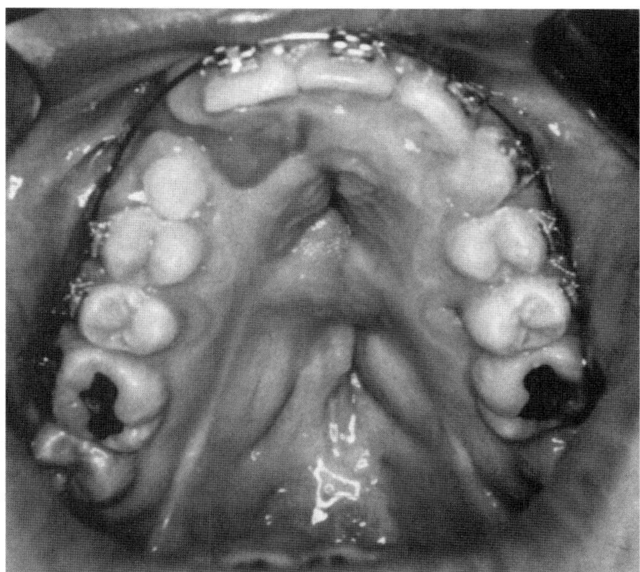

FIGURE 22-13. Patient who underwent coverage of the bone graft with a labial flap. Note the difference in appearance from the surrounding tissues. The cleft canine, although present, could not erupt through the flap. Surgical uncovering was required.

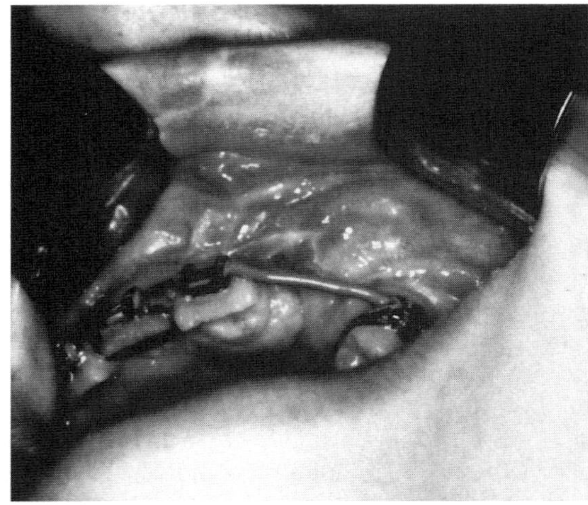

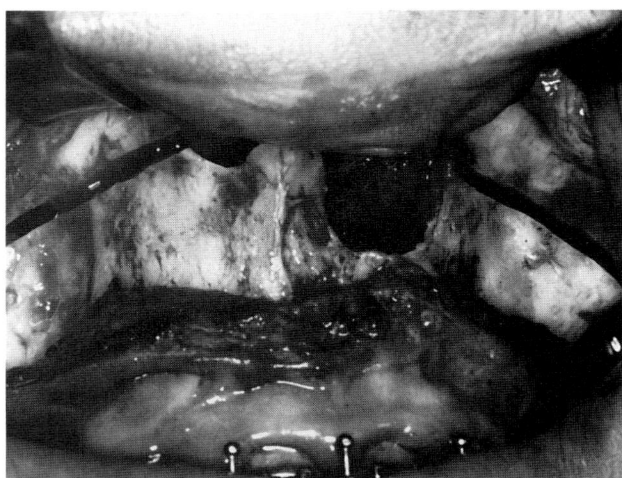

FIGURE 22-14. A: Residual notching of the alveolus after bone graft. **B:** Residual bony defect at the pyriform aperture and the floor of the nose, depicted at the time of a Le Fort osteotomy. This resulted presumably from inadequate placement of the graft in these areas. Residual lack of support and depression of the nostril on the cleft side were present.

nent tooth erupting through the cleft should be covered with a bone graft. The surgeon should carefully reconstruct the maxilla and the alveolar ridge by placing the bone graft along the cleft from the nasal floor to the level of the alveolar ridge. This should be done to provide better support to the teeth adjacent to the cleft and to the teeth that eventually will erupt through the graft. An unattractive notching of the alveolus will be prevented. Additionally, bone particles should be placed in the hypoplastic pyriform aperture of the maxilla to provide support for the nasal bone, raise the depressed nostril and sill, improve symmetry, and facilitate future correction of the residual cleft nasal deformity (56).

Finally, the previously raised gingival mucoperiosteal flaps should be sutured together and inferiorly to the palate, without tension, to provide complete coverage of the bone graft. Eight to ten weeks after the procedure, additional orthodontic treatment can be undertaken, if necessary.

Outcome: Unfavorable Results

With close cooperation between the plastic surgeon and the orthodontist, timely reconstruction, and adherence to the above-mentioned surgical principles, a very high success rate is expected. Complications arise primarily from inadequate use of bone or exposure of the bone graft in the oral or nasal cavity, which might result in partial or complete resorption of the bone graft (Figs. 22-14, 22-15).

In a retrospective study of 138 patients, we did not encounter any major flap dehiscence or bone graft loss in unilateral cases (57). However, there was a 10% incidence of par-

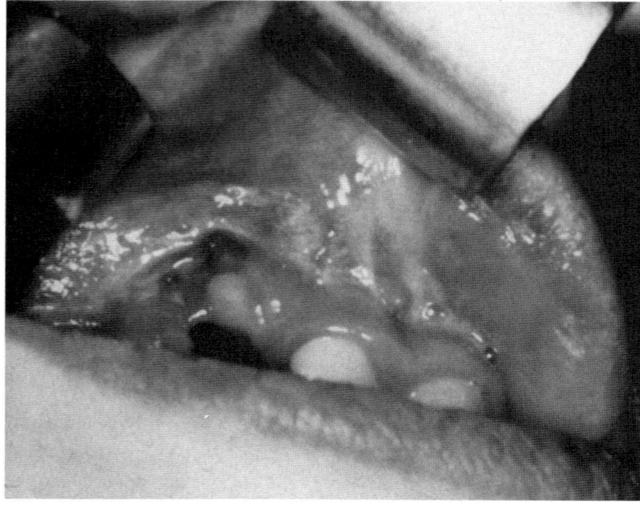

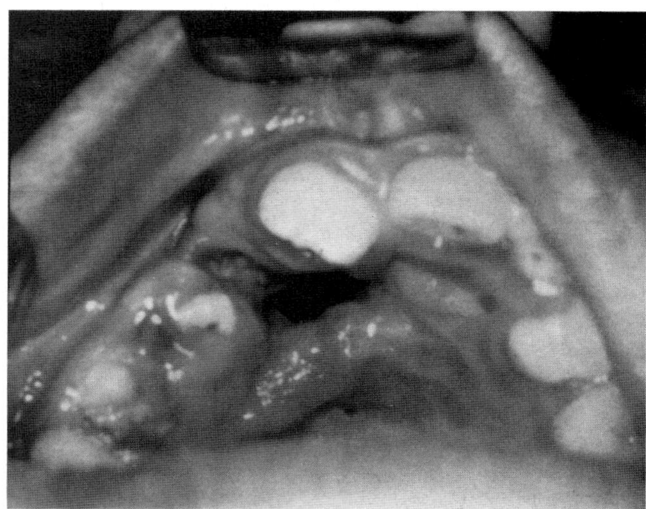

FIGURE 22-15. A,B: Partial loss of the bone graft due to soft tissue dehiscence in the alveolus and the palate and exposure of the graft.

tial dehiscence in the repair of the nasal mucosa or palate in bilateral cases, which resulted in partial or complete loss of the bone graft. Two patients with complete loss of the bone graft were successfully bone grafted again. Eight more patients with unilateral clefts developed minor intraoral dehiscences that were treated conservatively and did not result in significant bone graft loss. In 9% of the cases, we encountered partial resorption of the lowest portion of the graft, without bone exposure, which resulted in an unattractive notch in the alveolus. Ninety-five percent of teeth, when present, erupted spontaneously through the bone graft without the need for surgical exposure. Postoperative orthodontic treatment was required in all patients to achieve full alignment of the newly erupted teeth with the adjacent ones to close existing spaces and to complete the symmetry of the maxilla.

Because the main reason for failure is soft tissue deficiency, one should not attempt further bone grafting until fresh tissue can be brought in to provide coverage of the bone graft. Significant tissue deficiency in the palate can be addressed primarily with a tongue flap. Various designs of labial mucosal flaps can be used in the area of the alveolus. Scarred and deficient soft tissue in the floor of the nose presents with a more difficult problem that becomes even worse after failed previous attempts. In all these instances, prosthetic rehabilitation can provide adequate habilitation and should be considered.

SECONDARY CORRECTION OF CLEFT NASAL DEFORMITY

Initial correction of unilateral and bilateral cleft lip nasal deformities currently is incorporated with the lip repair. Thus, facial symmetry and harmony are restored early on, and children with clefts of the lip are given the opportunity to develop without the psychological burden of a nasal deformity. Several surgeons demonstrated that early intervention produces overall long-lasting improvement in nasal symmetry and appearance without detrimental effects on nasal or facial growth (58,59). Despite the use of these advanced techniques, a number of patients still will require a definitive secondary procedure to restore symmetry and improve function (60,61).

The classic secondary nasal deformity associated with unilateral clefts of the lip is caused by factors intrinsic to the nasal structures, such as deformed, depressed, and laterally deflected lower alar cartilages, a deviated septum, an asymmetrical nasal tip, columella, and nostrils, and asymmetrical and deviated nasal bones and nasal pyramid. The deformity is accentuated by extrinsic skeletal factors such as maxillary hypoplasia of the lower maxillary and alveolar process, a coexisting cleft of the maxilla, and the subsequent lack of bony support of the nasal base. The secondary nasal deformity associated with a bilateral cleft lip differs distinctly from the unilateral deformity. The nose is flat, lacking projection; the alar domes are laterally displaced; the columella is short; and the nostrils flare laterally, with a longitudinal rather than an oblique inclination. The deformity is accentuated further by a degree of maxillary hypoplasia and the presence of maxillary and alveolar clefts.

The severity of the residual nasal deformity varies, depending on the initial deformity and the degree, if any, of nasal and maxillary correction and repositioning performed during the initial lip repair or during subsequent revisions. Previous procedures and scarring produce an additional "iatrogenic" deformity that also needs to be considered. Such deformities may include malpositioning of the alar base, depression of the nostril sill, an excessively large or small nostril, or external scars (Fig. 22-16). A significant number of patients with residual cleft nasal deformities may demonstrate a degree of nasal obstruction as well. This obstruction might be due to several factors or a combination of factors, such as septal deviation, skeletal deformities, hypertrophy of the turbinates, and intranasal swelling or scarring. Thus, in addition to the extensive external evaluation and analysis of the nasal deformity, a rhinoscopic evaluation is extremely important to evaluate preexisting scars, septal deviations, previous cartilage resections, turbinate hypertrophy, and the condition of the nasal mucosa. Contributing factors to intranasal pathology, such as palatal or oronasal communications or airway obstruction due to an obstructive pharyngeal flap or a pharyngoplasty, should be evaluated and recorded.

The treatment plan for correction of the residual nasal deformity should be individualized based on extensive evaluation and analysis of the existing deformity. All contributing factors to the deformity should be addressed, and every effort should be made to correct the aesthetic as well as the functional aspects of the deformity. The final correction of the nasal deformity should be deferred until after orthodontic alignment of the maxilla, bone grafting of the hypoplastic maxilla, maxillary cleft, and alveolus, and closure of the coexisting oronasal fistula(s).

There are several distinct advantages to this approach:

1. In patients with unilateral clefts, the maxillary platform assumes a symmetrical position after realignment of its segments and bone grafting of the maxillary cleft and the hypoplastic area of the pyriform aperture. The depressed unsupported nostril is raised to a level similar to that of the contralateral side.
2. In patients with bilateral clefts, after the premaxilla is realigned with the lateral segments and the maxillary clefts are bone grafted, both nostrils are supported and raised, and the nasolabial angle is improved.
3. After closure of residual oronasal fistulas and reestablishment of the natural barrier between the oral and nasal cavities, regurgitation of food and saliva is controlled and irritation of the nasal mucosa is eliminated. More accurate evaluation of the intranasal abnormalities is feasible, leading to more appropriate and successful management of the various components of any coexisting airway obstruction.

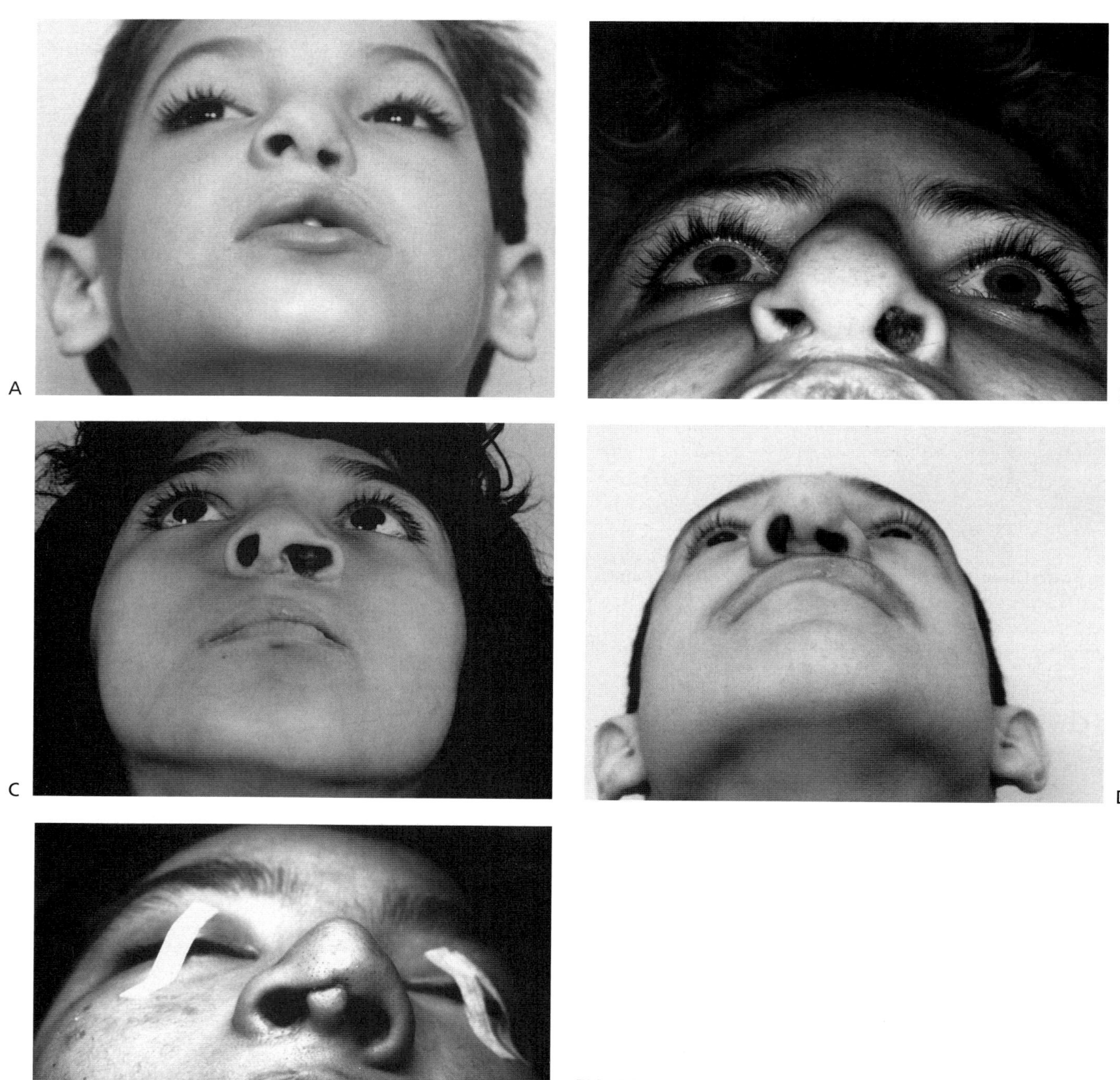

FIGURE 22-16. Various degrees of residual cleft nasal deformities. **A:** Smaller size nostril on the cleft side after repair of a unilateral cleft lip. **B:** Smaller size nostril on the right side after repair of a bilateral cleft lip. **C:** Cleft-side nostril significantly larger than the normal size. **D:** Discrepancy in size and shape of nostrils after correction of a unilateral cleft lip nasal deformity. **E:** Iatrogenic deformity with poorly placed scar on the columella.

The traditional principles and techniques of rhinoplasty apply to correction of cleft nasal deformity. However, successful outcome is not always as predictable as with cosmetic rhinoplasties, due to several factors including the existing nasal asymmetry, inherent tissue deficiencies of soft tissues and cartilage, hypoplasia of the maxilla, iatrogenic deformities, and scarring from previous procedures as well as the coexisting nasal obstructions. A myriad of surgical techniques and modifications has been reported to manage the initial cleft nasal deformity or the residual secondary deformities. It is not the purpose of this chapter to present all such procedures.

After careful evaluation and analysis, the surgeon should use the most appropriate technique designed to correct a given deformity(s) and relieve the nasal obstruction, if present. Although a closed rhinoplasty approach can be used for minor or moderate deformities, we prefer the open rhinoplasty approach for most significant deformities. This approach allows for direct visualization of the deformity and more accurate correction. Repositioning of the alar cartilages and domes, placement of cartilage grafts when needed, and overall establishment of symmetry is facilitated greatly under direct vision. A coexisting septal deviation can be managed accurately through this approach without the need for other incisions in the nasal mucosa (62). To achieve nasal tip symmetry when small discrepancies are present between the alar cartilages, we mobilize the depressed dome and suture it to the contralateral one with a few interrupted clear nylon sutures. When the discrepancy is more significant, with lateral flaring of the lateral crus, this maneuver alone is not sufficient to produce long-lasting symmetry because the lateral crus on the cleft side is tethered during medial mobilization of the dome. A lining deficiency also might be present. In these patients, we dissect the lateral crus with its mucosal lining as a medially based flap. This is achieved easily by extending the lateral infracartilaginous incision around the lateral border of the alar cartilage and back along its cephalic border. With this maneuver, the alar cartilage can be mobilized freely in a more medial and superior position and sutured to the contralateral alar cartilage. Additional height is gained in the area of the medial crus, and the domes are secured at an equal height to produce symmetry. The residual lateral mucosal defect left after this mobilization usually is closed in a V-Y manner. If there is considerable shortage of lining because of scarring or resection from previous procedures, we use a composite graft from the ear to resurface this intranasal defect. The advantage of using a composite graft rather than skin grafts is that the underlying cartilage acts as a splint and prevents contracture of the skin graft. Any additional asymmetry between the alar cartilages is corrected with appropriate cephalic cartilage resections and scoring of the lateral crus or with the addition of cartilaginous tip grafts.

In many patients, the tip of the nose lacks adequate projection. In such cases, a cartilaginous strut harvested primarily from the septum is used to provide support to the tip and increase projection. A pocket is dissected between the medial crura to the area of the nasal spine, and all fibrofatty tissue between the crura is removed. The graft is designed to be long enough to extend from the nasal spine to just above the nasal tip. It is secured to the medial crura with two or three permanent clear nylon sutures. One should keep in mind that the medial crura of the alar cartilages have a natural flare. Therefore, all sutures should be placed through the cephalic border of these cartilages to retain the flaring of the medial crura and the shape of the columella. Additional tip projection and improved tip contour and symmetry, when necessary, can be achieved with tip grafts. Conchal cartilage grafts are primarily recommended and secured in place with interrupted clear nylon sutures. Any residual depressions of the alar cartilages are corrected with small local cartilaginous grafts, and asymmetries of the upper lateral cartilage are managed by limited resections or placement of additional grafts (Fig. 22-17).

Deviation of the nasal bony pyramid will require bilateral osteotomies for correction. Septal deviations need appropriate management as well. The nasal skin is draped over the reconstructed bony and cartilaginous skeleton. The columellar incision is closed in a V-Y manner, which can provide a gain of 0.5 to 0.8 cm in length for the columella, when needed.

As soon as the incisions are closed, attention is directed to the symmetry of the nasal base. Small discrepancies in size are corrected by local excisions in the floor of the nostril. These excisions involve skin only and should be closed with care to avoid notching in the area of the nostril sill. For greater discrepancies, completely detach the cleft-side nostril and set it in a more appropriate position and level. With accurate preoperative evaluation and measurement, one can not only correct the nostril flaring but also reposition the entire nostril in a symmetrical plane with the noncleft side. If the circumference of the nostril is found to be greater than that of the noncleft-side nostril, an appropriate resection is carried out in addition to the repositioning. A more difficult condition to correct is a cleft-side nostril that is smaller than the normal nostril. In such cases, the nostril is completely detached and an appropriate composite graft from the ear is used to achieve symmetry.

Correction of Nasal Obstruction

The information gained from preoperative clinical and rhinomanometric evaluation assists the surgeon in formulating and individualizing a plan of action for correction of nasal airway obstruction. Component rhinomanometry and other testing can demonstrate the level of obstruction. Attention then is directed toward the septum, the inferior turbinates, and, if necessary, to a potentially obstructive pharyngeal flap or pharyngoplasty.

When an open rhinoplasty is used, the septum is exposed after lateral reflection of the medial crura of the alar cartilages. The mucoperichondrium on either side of the septum is dissected from the cartilage to completely expose the surface of the cartilage up to the perpendicular plate of the ethmoid bone, the crest of the maxilla, the vomer, and the anterior nasal spine. Thus, the septal anatomy and configuration are

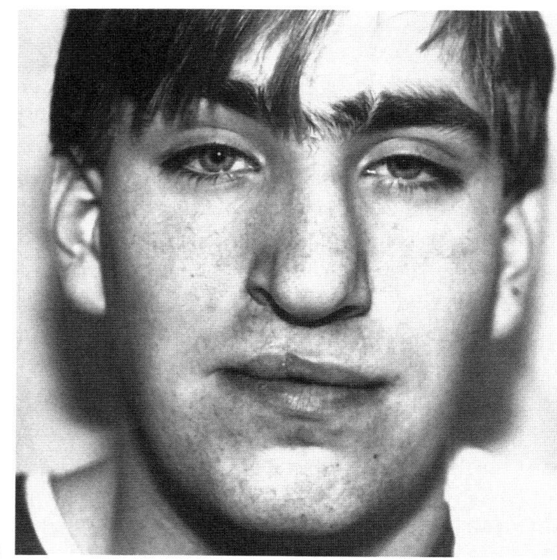

A

FIGURE 22-17. A: Residual cleft nasal deformity with nasal deviation and asymmetry. **B,C:** Preoperative views demonstrating a significant nasal and septal deviation. Nasal obstruction was present. **D,E:** Postoperative views after septoplasty, bilateral turbinectomies, and correction of the nasal deformity through an open rhinoplasty approach. Airway obstruction was corrected and appearance was improved significantly.

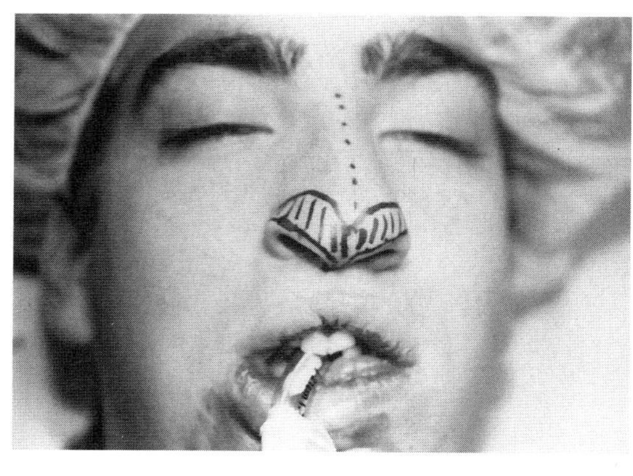

B

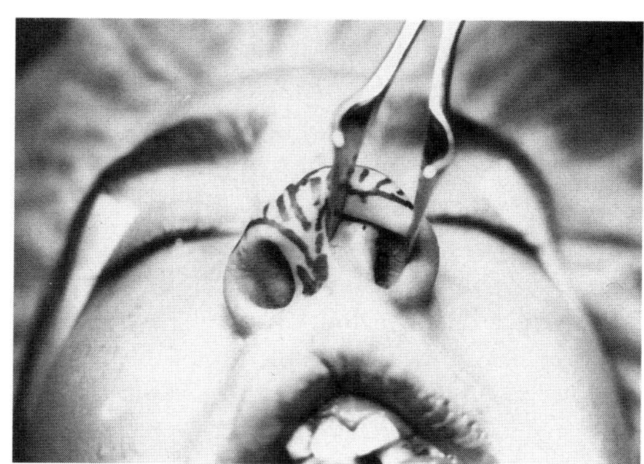

C

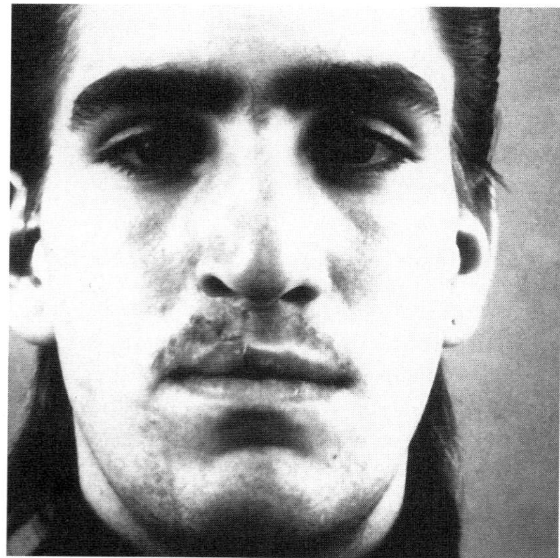

D

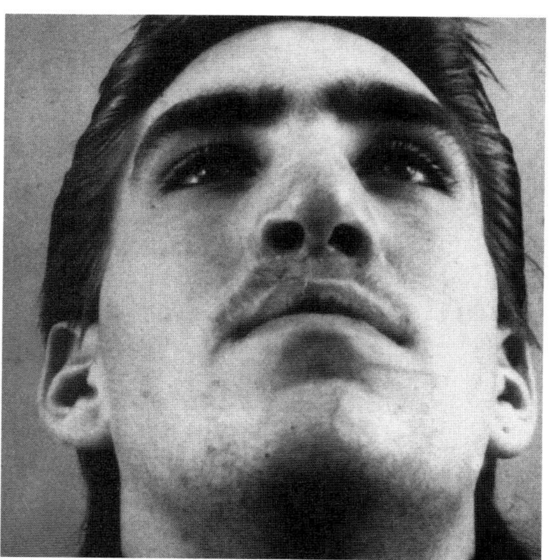

E

visualized and managed directly. In most patients with nasal deformities from a unilateral cleft lip, there is some degree of deviation of the septum. In some patients, only the deviated caudal portion of the septum needs to be managed; in others, the entire septum requires manipulation to alleviate nasal airway obstruction. The caudal portion of the septum typically deviates toward the noncleft side. To reposition it in the midline, one should completely free it from the nasal spine and the maxilla and score the concave surface of the cartilage. If the septal deformity is severe and cannot be corrected with these techniques, a resection should be performed, leaving an L-shaped portion of the septum for nasal support. Additional obstructive factors might be present, such as a deviated perpendicular plate and bony spears in the crest of the maxilla. Such bony irregularities should be treated by direct excisions.

Hypertrophy of the inferior turbinate processes must be evaluated and treated accordingly. Obstruction caused primarily by mucosal swelling can be relieved by excision of the redundant mucosa. However, when inferior turbinate hypertrophy is caused by mucosal swelling and bony hypertrophy, an *en bloc* resection of the inferior portion of the turbinate process should be performed. The surgeon should carefully evaluate the remaining portion of the turbinate process and remove any additional segment causing obstruction. These resections should be done with extreme care to avoid overresection of the inferior turbinate process that may lead to atrophic rhinitis. All visible bleeding points should be cauterized. If an obstruction persists, an outfracture of the remaining portion of the turbinate process may be helpful (Figs. 22-18 and 22-19).

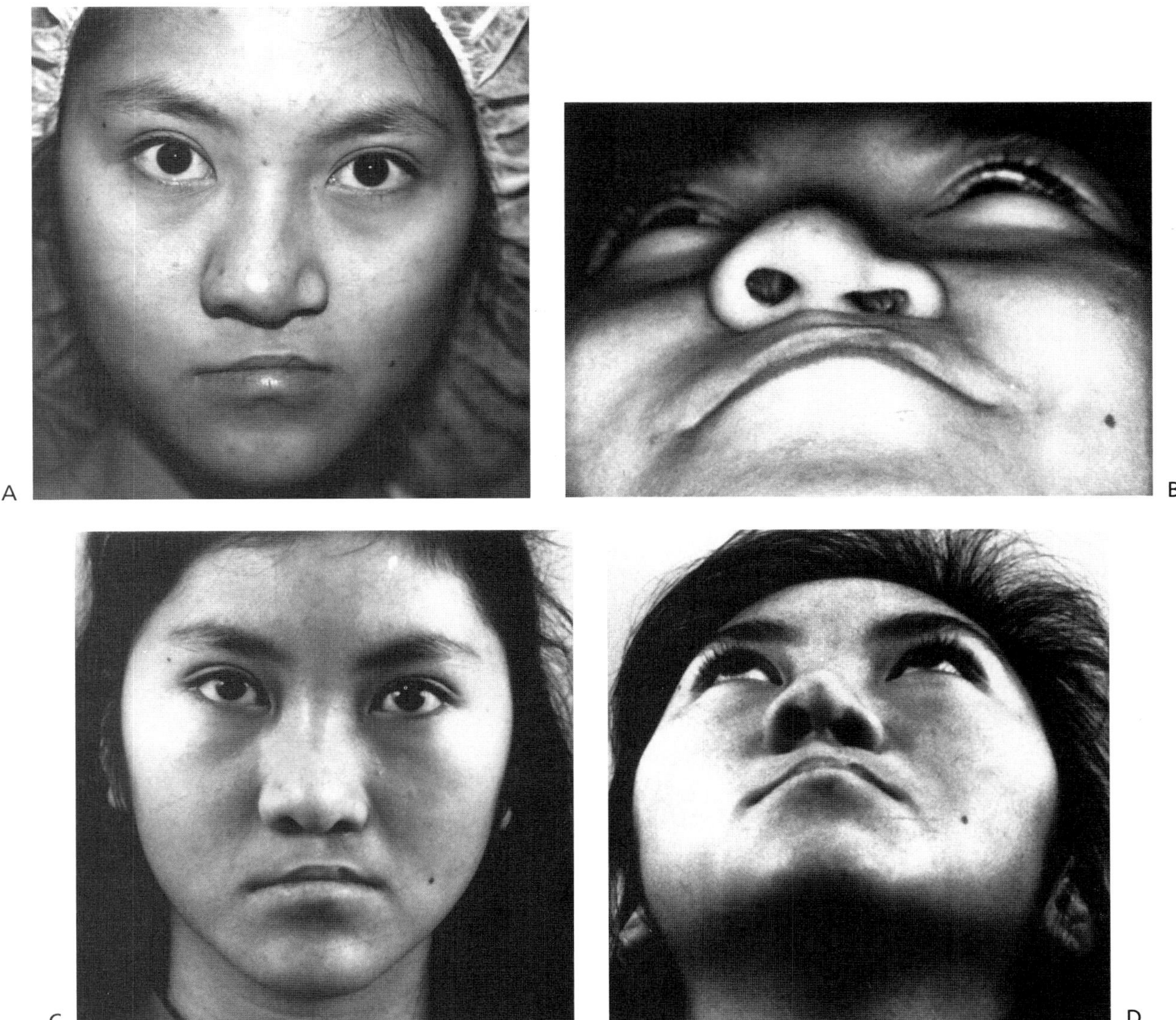

FIGURE 22-18. A,B: Preoperative views of 15-year-old patient with residual nasal deformity after unilateral cleft lip repair. Note the deviation and asymmetry. **C,D:** Postoperative views at 17 years of age. Symmetry was achieved, the nasal deviation was corrected, and tip projection was augmented. Septoplasty and partial bilateral inferior turbinectomies were necessary to relieve airway obstruction.

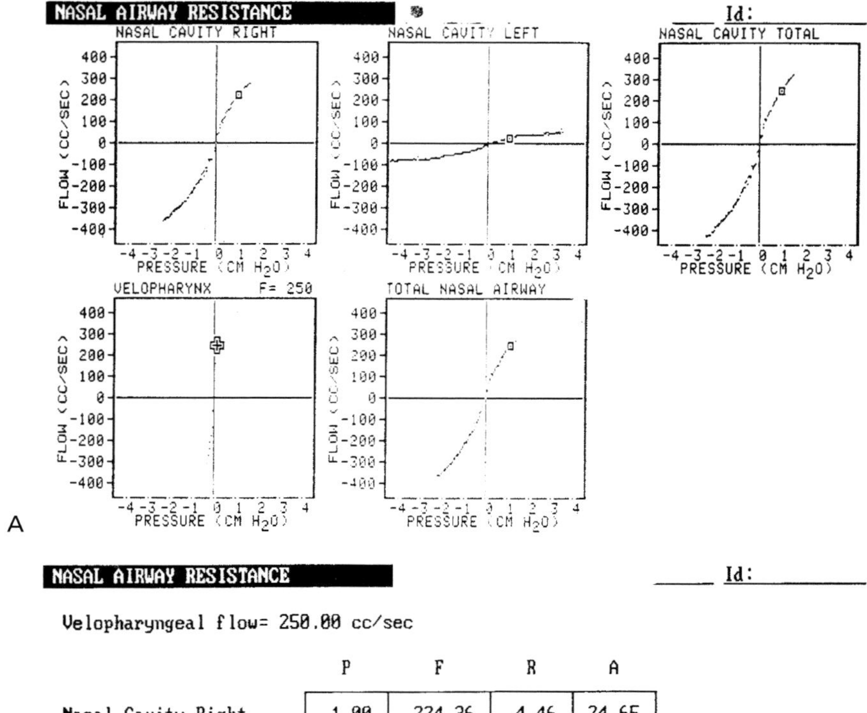

NASAL AIRWAY RESISTANCE Id:

Velopharyngeal flow= 250.00 cc/sec

	P	F	R	A
Nasal Cavity Right	1.00	224.36	4.46	24.65
Nasal Cavity Left	1.00	25.64	39.00	2.82
Nasal Cavity Total	1.00	250.00	4.00	27.47
Velopharynx	0.15	250.00	0.60	70.93
Total Nasal Airway	1.15	250.00	4.60	25.62

NCR= 4.00 (87% contribution)
VPR= 0.60 (13% contribution)

NAR= 4.60

P: Pressure in cm H_2O
F: Flow in cc/sec
R: Resistance in cm H_2O/L/sec
A: Area in mm^2

B

FIGURE 22-19. Pressure-flow plots **(A,C)** and corresponding numerical data **(B,D)** obtained using component rhinomanometry during nasal breathing by the patient shown in Fig. 22-18 before **(A,B)** *(continued)*

As noted earlier, preoperative rhinomanometric studies along with direct evaluation provide invaluable information about the contribution of a pharyngeal flap to airway obstruction. If this obstruction is clinically significant, it is managed in the same setting as discussed previously.

Nasal Deformity from a Bilateral Cleft Lip

When planning for correction of the nasal deformity from a bilateral cleft lip, the surgeon should evaluate the adequacy of skin coverage or the need for additional skin in the area of the columella. With improved surgical techniques for management of the primary lip deformity and incorporation of a columella-lengthening procedure in the treatment plan, fewer patients require columellar grafts to increase length in this area. When needed, a forked flap from the lip is incorporated into the design of open rhinoplasty to provide additional skin coverage of the columella.

I approach the nasal deformities associated with bilateral cleft lips as I do deformities of unilateral clefts, primarily through an open rhinoplasty. After skeletonization and exposure, the fibrofatty tissues between the domes and the medial crura are excised and the domes are mobilized medially and stabilized with clear 5-0 nylon sutures. Additional projection is achieved, as described for unilateral deformities, by placement of a columellar strut graft harvested from the septum and/or onlay cartilage tip grafts. All grafts should be secured in place with permanent sutures. When irregularities or asymmetries of the alar cartilages or the upper lateral cartilages are encountered, they are corrected by local resections, additional grafting, or scoring.

Bilateral osteotomies are indicated when the nasal pyramid is found to be wide or when skeletal asymmetry is present. Additionally, in a number of patients with nasal deformities from bilateral cleft lip, a dorsal augmentation with onlay cartilage or bone grafts is necessary to increase projec-

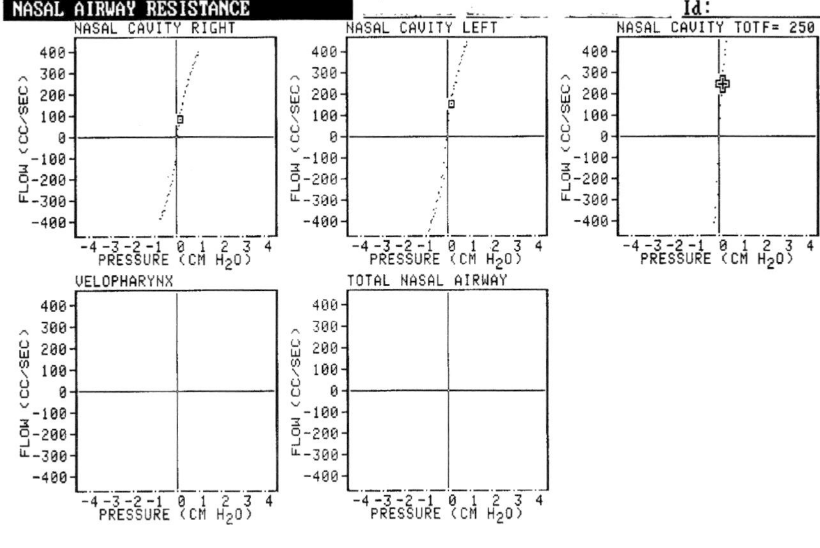

C

NASAL AIRWAY RESISTANCE Id:

Nasal Cavity Total flow= 250.00 cc/sec

	P	F	R	A
Nasal Cavity Right	0.19	89.74	2.12	22.62
Nasal Cavity Left	0.19	160.26	1.19	40.40
Nasal Cavity Total	0.19	250.00	0.76	63.02
Velopharynx	*****	*******	0.00	*****
Total Nasal Airway	0.19	250.00	0.76	63.02

NCR= 0.76 (100% contribution)
VPR= 0.00 (0% contribution)
NAR= 0.76

P: Pressure in cm H2O
F: Flow in cc/sec
R: Resistance in cm H2O/L/sec
A: Area in mm²

D

FIGURE 22-19. *(Continued)* and after **(C,D)** successful surgery to correct left nasal cavity obstruction. Such surgery would not be expected to have an effect on velopharyngeal measurements during speech.

tion and improve facial harmony. Most patients are treated by an onlay septal cartilage graft, but when a considerable augmentation is necessary, I prefer to use a bone graft taken from the calvarium or rib. The columellar incision is closed with interrupted 6-0 nylon sutures in a V-Y manner to increase length. Excess flaring of the nostrils may persist despite medial mobilization of the lateral alar cartilage and increased nasal tip projection with grafts. In these patients, the shape and size of the nostrils can be modified additionally with appropriate alar resections. These resections are designed according to the deformity and can be symmetrical or asymmetrical.

Despite extensive evaluation, analysis, planning, and careful execution, a number of patients will have suboptimal aesthetic and functional results. Patients who have undergone multiple previous procedures with extensive tissue resections and scarring will have worse results than patients who present with minimal nasal deformity or scarring. This is because most of these patients present with tissue deficiencies of skin, lining, and/or cartilage, and skin or nasal vestibular scars and contractures. Patients previously treated with alloplastic implants might have additional scarring and thinning of the overlying skin.

By far the most difficult area to correct is the asymmetry of the nostrils. Careful evaluation of postoperative results in many publications will reveal a degree of residual asymmetry in the worm's-eye views in a significant number of patients despite near-normal appearance in all other views. Other commonly encountered residual deformities include asymmetrical tip projection, lack of adequate tip projection, persistent lateral flaring of the nostril, asymmetry and shortness of the columella, and persistent skeletal deviations.

Some of these deformities, particularly the significant ones, should be corrected to improve form and function. The surgeon should exercise judgment and caution as with other secondary deformities associated with cleft lip and palate. A decision for surgery should be made only when there is reasonable expectation for improvement. Small deformities after reconstructive procedures should be accepted, because further surgical procedures will produce additional scarring and result in little or no improvement while subjecting the patient and his family to the additional emotional trauma.

In contrast, residual airway obstructions after correction of cleft nasal deformities should be evaluated and treated when appropriate. Unfortunately, the vast majority of publications deal primarily with the aesthetic improvement of the nasal deformity. Very little attention is given to the simultaneous correction of nasal obstruction, and little information is given about the functional outcome following these procedures. In a small study of 25 consecutive patients, we found significant improvement of airway patency in 80% of the patients. This improvement was not only subjective, but objective, based on comparison of preoperative and postoperative rhinomanometric results (63). Three patients (11%) with a pharyngeal flap in place had only modest improvement. The residual postoperative airway obstruction in these patients was attributed to the flap; however, no attempt was made to revise the ports because the patients' preoperative speech was judged to be very good. Any intervention in the ports could have resulted in a deterioration in speech. Finally, two patients had no functional improvement; they both had several previous procedures with significant intranasal scarring and cartilage and mucosal loss.

In conclusion, superior results can be achieved with appropriate and extensive evaluation, short and long-term planning with optimal timing for each procedure, and close cooperation among various members of the cleft team. If additional surgical procedures are necessary to improve function and appearance or manage unfavorable results, it is important for the surgeon to understand the limitations of each technique for the specific patient and discuss these limitations with the patient and the family. Although some residual deformities can be corrected with an additional touchup procedure, one should be careful to avoid multiple revisions in a short period of time that might result in additional scarring with little chance for further improvement.

REFERENCES

1. Roberts CT, Semb G, Shaw WC. Strategies for the advancement of surgical methods in cleft lip and palate. *Cleft Palate Craniofac J* 1991;28:141–149.
2. Witt PD, Marsh JL. Advances in assessing outcome of surgical repair of cleft lip and cleft palate. *Plast Reconstr Surg* 1997;100:1907–1917.
3. Parameters for evaluation and treatment of patients with cleft lip/palate or other craniofacial anomalies. *Cleft Palate Craniofac J* 1993;30[Suppl]: S1–16.
4. Steffensen WH. Further experience with the rectangular flap operation for clef t lip repair. *Plast Reconstr Surg* 1953;11:49.
5. Millard DR Jr, Latham RA. Improved primary surgical and dental treatment of clefts. *Plast Reconstr Surg* 1990;86:856–871.
6. Millard DR Jr, Morovic CG. Primary unilateral cleft nose correction: a 10-year follow-up. *Plast Reconstr Surg* 1998;102: 1331–1338.
7. Figueroa AA, Reisberg DJ, Polley JW, et al. Intraoral appliance modification to retract the perimaxilla in patients with bilateral cleft lip. *Cleft Palate Craniofac J*1993;33:497–500.
8. Jackson IT, Fasching MC. Secondary deformities of cleft lip, nose and palate. In: McCarthy J, ed. *Plastic surgery.* Philadelphia: WB Saunders, 1990:2771–2877.
9. Lewis MB. Secondary soft tissue procedures for cleft lip and palate. In: Cohen M, ed. *Mastery of plastic and reconstructive surgery.* Boston: Little, Brown and Company, 1994:605–618.
10. Millard DR Jr. *Cleft craft. The evolution of its surgery,* vol. I. Boston: Little, Brown and Company, 1976:527–628.
11. Millard DR Jr. *Cleft craft. The evolution of its surgery,* vol. II. Boston: Little, Brown and Company, 1977:421–475.
12. Bardach J, Morris H, Olin W, et al. Late results of multidisciplinary management of unilateral cleft lip and palate. *Ann Plast Surg* 1984;12:235–242.
13. Cohen SR, Corrigan M, Wilmot J, et al. Cumulative operative procedures in patients aged 14 years and older with unilateral or bilateral cleft lip and palate. *Plast Reconstr Surg* 1995;96: 267–271.
14. Marsh JL. When is enough enough? Secondary surgery for cleft lip and palate patients. *Clin Plast Surg* 1990;17:37–47.
15. Kapetansky DI. Double pendulum flap for whistling deformities in bilateral cleft lips. *Plast Reconstr Surg* 1971;47:321–323.
16. Musgrave RH, Garrett WS Jr. The unilateral cleft lip. In: Converse JM, ed. *Reconstructive plastic surgery,* vol. 4. Philadelphia: WB Saunders, 1977:2016–2047.
17. Brauer RO, Cronin TD. The Tennison lip repair revisited. *Plast Reconstr Surg* 1983;71:633–640.
18. Millard DR Jr. Shaping and positioning the lip-switch flap in unilateral clefts. In: Millard DR Jr, ed. *Cleft craft: the evolution of ITS surgery, vol. I.* Boston: Little, Brown and Company, 1976:593–628.
19. Bardach J, Morris HL, Olin WH. Late results of primary veloplasty: the Marburg project. *Plast Reconstr Surg* 1984;73: 207–215.
20. Dorf DS, Curtin JW. Early cleft palate repair and speech outcome. *Plast Reconstr Surg* 1982;70:74.
21. Rohrich RJ, Byrd HS. Optimal timing of cleft palate closure: speech, facial growth and hearing considerations. *Clin Plast Surg* 1990;17:27–36.
22. Rohrich RJ, Rowsell AR, Johns DF, et al. Timing of hard palate closure: a critical long-term analysis. *Plast Reconstr Surg* 1996;98:236–246.
23. Randall P, LaRossa DD, Fakhraee SM, et al. Cleft palate closure at 3 to 7 months of age: a preliminary report. *Plast Reconstr Surg* 1983;71:624–628.
24. Haapanen ML, Rantala SL. Correlation between the age at repair and speech outcome in patients with isolated cleft palate. *Scand J Plast Reconstr Hand Surg* 1992;26:71.
25. Berkowitz S. Lip and palate surgery. In: Berkowitz S, ed. *Cleft lip and palate, vol. I.* San Diego: Singular Publishing Group, 1996:65–101.
26. Cohen SR, Kalinowski J, LaRossa D, et al. Cleft palate fistulas: a multivariate statistical analysis of prevalence, etiology and surgical management. *Plast Reconstr Surg* 1991;87:1041–1047.
27. Schultz RC. Management and timing of cleft palate fistula repair. *Plast Reconstr Surg* 1986;78:739–745.
28. Abyholm FE, Borchgrevink HC, Eskeland G: Palatal Fistulae Following Cleft Palate Surgery. Scand. *J Plast Reconstr Surg* 13:295–300, 1979.
29. Lehman JA. Closure of palatal fistulas. *Op Tech Plast Reconstr Surg* 1995;2:255–262.

30. Guerrero-Santos J, Altamarino ST. The use of lingual flaps in repair of fistulas of the hard palate. *Plast Reconstr Surg* 1966;38:123–128.
31. Smith BE, Guyette TW. Velopharyngeal insufficiency. In: Cohen M, ed. *Mastery of plastic and reconstructive surgery,* vol. I. Boston: Little, Brown and Company, 1994:619–631.
32. Warren DW, DuBois AB. A pressure-flow technique for measuring velopharyngeal orifice area during continuous speech. *Cleft Palate J* 1964;1:52–71.
33. Andreassen ML, Smith BE, Guyette TW. Pressure flow measurements for selected oral and nasal sound segments produced by normal adults. *Cleft Palate Craniofac J* 1992;29:1–9.
34. Smith BE, Guyette TW. Component approach for partitioning nasal airway resistance: pharyngeal flap case studies. *Cleft Palate Craniofac J* 1993;30:78–81.
35. Graham WP III, Hamilton R, Randall P, et al. Complications following posterior pharyngeal flap surgery. *Cleft Palate J* 1973;10:176–180.
36. Valnicek SM, Zuker RM, Halpern LM, et al. Perioperative complications of superior pharyngeal flap surgery in children. *Plast Reconstr Surg* 1994;93:954–958.
37. Fraulin FOG, Valnicek SM, Zuker RM. Decreasing the perioperative complications associated with the superior pharyngeal flap operation. *Plast Reconstr Surg* 1998;102:10–18.
38. Sirois M, Caouette-Laberge L, Spier S, et al. Sleep apnea following a pharyngeal flap: a feared complication. *Plast Reconstr Surg* 1994;93:943–947.
39. Lesavoy MA, Borud LJ, Thorson T, et al. Upper airway obstruction after pharyngeal flap surgery. *Ann Plast Surg* 1996;36:26–32.
40. Vedung S. Pharyngeal flap after one- and two-stage repair of the cleft palate: a 25-year review of 520 patients. *Cleft Palate Craniofac J* 1995;32:206–215.
41. Morris HL, Bardach J, Jones D, et al. Clinical results of pharyngeal flap surgery: the Iowa experience. *Plast Reconstr Surg* 1995;95:652–662.
42. Smith BE, Skef Z, Cohen M, et al. Aerodynamic assessment of the results of pharyngeal flap surgery: a preliminary investigation. *Plast Reconstr Surg* 1986;76:402–408.
43. Barone CM, Sprintzen RJ, Strauch B, et al. Pharyngeal flap revisions: flap elevation from scarred posterior pharynx. *Plast Reconstr Surg* 1994;93:279–284.
44. Barot LR, Cohen MA, LaRossa D. Surgical indications and techniques for posterior pharyngeal flap revision. *Ann Plast Surg* 1986;16:527–531.
45. Owsley JQ, Lawson LI, Ghierici GJ. The redo pharyngeal flap. *Plast Reconstr Surg* 1976;57:180–185.
46. Caouette-Laberge L, Egerszegi EP, deRemont AM, et al. Long-term follow-up after division of a pharyngeal for severe nasal obstruction. *Cleft Palate Craniofac J* 1992;29:27–31.
47. Riski JE, Serafin O, Riefkohl R, et al. A rationale for modifying the site of insertion of orticochea pharyngoplasty. *Plast Reconstr Surg* 1984;73:882–890.
48. Witt PD, Marsh JL, Muntz HR, et al. Acute obstructive sleep apnea as a complication of sphincter pharyngoplasty. *Cleft Palate Craniofac J* 1996;33:183–189,.
49. Orticochea M. A review of 236 cleft palate patients treated with dynamic muscle sphincter. *Plast Reconstr Surg* 1983;71: 180–186.
50. Riski JE, Ruff GL, Georgiade GS, et al. Evaluation of failed sphincter pharyngoplasties. *Ann Plast Surg* 1992;28:545–553.
51. Witt PD, Myckatyn T, Marsh JL. Salvaging the failed pharyngoplasty: intervention outcome. *Cleft Palate Craniofac J* 1998; 35:447–453.
52. Abyholm FE, Bergland O, Semb G. Secondary bone grafting of alveolar clefts. *Scand J Plast Reconstr Surg* 1981;15:127–140.
53. Semb G. Effect of alveolar bone grafting on maxillary growth in unilateral cleft lip and palate patients. *Cleft Palate J* 1988;25: 288–299.
54. Cohen M, Figueroa AA, Haviv Y, et al. Iliac versus cranial bone for secondary grafting of residual alveolar clefts. *Plast Reconstr Surg* 1989;83:812–819.
55. Cohen M, Figueroa AA, Aduss H. The role of gingival mucoperiosteal flap in the repair of alveolar clefts. *Plast Reconstr Surg* 1989;83:817–819.
56. Cohen M. Secondary bone grafting of residual alveolar clefts. In: Cohen M, ed. *Mastery of plastic and reconstructive surgery.* Boston: Little, Brown and Company, 1994:669–681..
57. Cohen M, Polley JW, Figueroa AA. Secondary (intermediate) alveolar bone grafting. *Clin Plast Surg* 1993;20:691–705.
58. McComb HK, Coughlan BA. Primary repair of the unilateral cleft lip nose: completion of a longitudinal study. *Cleft Palate Craniofac J* 1996;33:23–31.
59. Salyer KA. Primary correction of the unilateral cleft lip nose: a 15-year experience. *Plast Reconstr Surg* 1986;77:558–566.
60. Millard DR Jr. *Cleft graft: the evolution of its surgery,* vol. I. *The unilateral deformity.* Boston: Little, Brown and Company, 1976:629–732.
61. Millard DR. *Cleft graft: the evolution of its surgery,* vol. II. *The bilateral and nose deformities.* Boston: Little, Brown and Company, 1977:477–591.
62. Cohen M. Secondary correction of the nasal deformity associated with cleft lip. In: Cohen M, ed. *Mastery of plastic and reconstructive surgery.* Boston: Little, Brown and Company, 1994:702–719.
63. Cohen M, Smith BE, Guyette T, et al. Functional and aesthetic correction of cleft nasal deformities. In: *Transactions of the International Congress of Cleft Palate and Related Anomalies.* Singapore, 1997:249–252.

Discussion

CLEFT LIP AND PALATE

JEFFREY L. MARSH

The variables that may affect outcome in cleft lip and palate surgery include the initial dysmorphology, biology of the patient, type of intervention, timing of intervention, and unanticipatable postintervention events. Of these, the care provider cannot affect unanticipatable untoward events, such as the patient who, after lip revision, falls on the face several days postoperatively, causing traumatic dehiscence. Similarly, care providers have little influence over unfavorable wound healing characteristics of specific patients, such as a propensity for hypertrophic scar. Nor can the care provider affect hereditary mandibular prognathism, which results in a class III dentoskeletal relationship even when maxillary growth impairment has been minimal. Although it may seem that care providers also have no influence over the extent of the cleft, presurgical manipulations of hard and soft tissues of the face and mouth can alter the unoperated anatomy of the cleft: this concept will be addressed further later. The type of intervention and the timing of intervention, then, remain the major variables for which the decisions of the care provider primarily affect outcome (1,2).

Successful management of cleft lip/palate (CLP), as for any complex problem, requires an initial enumeration of goals and the means of their achievement (Table 22D-1). For cleft lip and its accompanying nasal deformity, this means restoration of anatomical and functional normalcy. For cleft palate, this means restoration of static separation between the nasal and oral cavities, as well as functional separation, i.e., velopharyngeal closure, for swallowing and speech, and minimal impairment of dentoskeletal development. Furthermore, successful management seems to require a set treatment protocol, executed by a few well-trained and experienced providers in a cleft center with sufficient volume to maintain clinical skills and conduct meaningful outcomes assessments (3–5). The decisions made regarding the type of intervention and the timing of intervention (6) can affect each of these goals in a positive or negative fashion. Conscious recognition of these effects by the care provider(s) before each intervention hopefully will maximize beneficial effects and minimize detrimental effects. This "conscious recognition" is the philosophy that guides my personal treatment of clefts and my education of residents in cleft care.

Assessment of the morbidity of the unfavorable result in cleft surgery is not merely documentation of the persistence of stigmatization. It also must include consideration of the need for additional intervention and the costs of that intervention. The intervention may be surgical or nonsurgical, and its costs include money, time, pain and suffering, and interference with daily life. It was still commonplace into the 1980s to encounter individuals with clefts who had undergone 20 or more operations, had been in speech therapy from preschool into high school, had been in orthodontic appliances starting with the eruption of their 6-year molars, and who were still not destigmatized! Maximum intervention did not yield maximum results; rather, it often produced diminishing returns. Comparison of outcomes must not only consider specific aspects such as lip/nose appearance, palatal integrity, velopharyngeal function, and dentoskeletal development, but also the amount of intervention required to achieve those results. When results can be demonstrated to be similar, the protocol requiring the least intervention and consumption of resources should be preferred.

It is easy to discuss the unfavorable results of cleft repair for patients treated at "St. Elsewhere"; it is more difficult to assess one's own results. Aside from the obvious contaminant of personal bias in self-assessment, there are other unbiased factors that confound assessment. With respect to the patient, the most significant are the need for passage of time until speech can be assessed, perceptually and then instrumentally; for dentoskeletal development to have matured sufficiently, as to make a major change in the occlusion or skeleton unlikely; and for the patient to become old enough to be empowered to make decisions regarding lip and nose revision surgery. This means that the cleft surgeon must remain in one geographic location and must serve a geographically stable population (7–12). Whereas the former constraint may be realistic for many surgeons, the latter may not be, depending on where that surgeon practices. With respect to the surgery performed, most significant are the consistency of the procedure and the preoperative and postoperative documentation. If the surgeon does not use a specific treatment protocol, it is unlikely that sufficient numbers

J. L. Marsh: Washington University School of Medicine, and Division of Pediatric Plastic Surgery, Department of Surgery, St. Louis Children's Hospital, St. Louis, Missouri

TABLE 22D-1. GOALS OF CLEFT CARE

	Goal	Means
Cleft lip	Lip normalcy	Lip repair
	Nose normalcy	Nasal repair
Cleft palate	Palatal integrity	Palate repair
	Effective velopharyngeal function	Palate repair
	Normal occlusion	Alveolar management
	Normal facial skeletal growth	Soft and hard tissue management

will be accumulated to allow meaningful outcome assessment. Even with standardized protocols, it may be difficult for an individual surgeon, at least in the United States, to acquire sufficient numbers of patients with clefts because of the nature of our health care system (Shaw 1996, #5). Given that the effect of initial cleft extent on outcome is poorly understood, the adequacy of sample size to make results statistically valid is unclear. Furthermore, is a sufficient sample size for assessment of lip or nose appearance the same for assessment of velopharyngeal function or dentoskeletal development? Until these questions are answered, it will be difficult for the contemplative cleft surgeon to interpret outcome reports (13).

CLEFT LIP

Cleft lip surgery has evolved from mere obliteration of the soft tissue defect, to construction of an anatomically correct lip with respect first to surface features, next to muscular function, and most recently to correction of the associated nasal deformity. Unsatisfactory lip repairs may result from a poorly conceived, poorly executed, or incompletely performed operation. The surgeon of cleft lips must be able to plan spatially, deconstruct aberrant anatomy, and reconstruct normal anatomy from rearranged tissues. The challenge of cleft lip repair is compounded by the extent of the disruption of the underlying skeleton. Is the alveolus cleft? Is the premaxilla rotated out of the facial plane? Is the ipsilateral hemimaxilla retruded? Is the secondary palate cleft? Although it is possible to repair a cleft lip without consideration of the underlying skeleton, to do so is less than optimal in my opinion. Since the 1950s, some cleft care providers have noted a relationship between hard and soft tissue management for clefts of the primary palate (lip+alveolus+anterior hard palate ventral to the incisive foramen). Although the approach to hard and soft tissue management among these providers varies in specifics, the general concept is uniform: alignment of the premaxilla into the facial plane and restoration of the U-shaped maxillary alveolar arch with prevention of intercanine collapse improves the quality of lip repair (14–17).

From 1978 to 1980, I performed one-stage rotation-advancement repair of all cleft lips without consideration of any associated maxillary deformity. Of those patients, many had subsequent lip revisions that required take-down and rerepair due to lip height asymmetries. Beginning in 1980, our cleft team decided to change the approach to complete cleft lip and palate due to the stimulus of a new orthodontist who had been trained by Dr. Sheldon Rosenstein and exposed to the surgical approach of Dr. Desmond Kernahan. Our version of the Kernahan-Rosenstein approach consisted of initial lip adhesion with placement of a passive alveolar molding plate at about 6 weeks of age, followed by definitive Millard rotation-advancement lip repair at about 7 months of age (18). The alveolar molding plate was retained until palatoplasty at about 14 months of age. We chose not to perform the infantile alveolar bone graft advocated by Kernahan because we had reservations about possible effect of such grafts, as well as gingivoperiosteoplasty, on maxillary growth. We felt that restoration of a complete arch, with abutting premaxillary and lesser segment alveolar cleft surfaces, would be physically stable. All patients were documented with standard pretreatment facial and intraoral photographs and a maxillary impression. They have been followed serially with additional documentation at regular intervals. A preliminary lip adhesion without alveolar molding plate was performed for clefts of the primary palate only if the premaxilla was rotated out of the plane of the face. If the premaxilla was within the plane of the face, a one-stage definitive Millard cheiloplasty was performed. By 1984, when the orthodontist who stimulated this change in treatment protocol left our team, I had noted a favorable difference in the facial appearance of my cleft cases whose lip was repaired following initiation of the protocol compared with to those I repaired before. Lip take-downs had ceased, and if lip revision was performed it was a minor touchup in conjunction with alveolar bone grafting, optimizing that anesthesia, rather than as a "necessity" prior to entering school. The positive change in lip/nose appearance associated with the lip adhesion/alveolar molding plate protocol prompted me to seek a new dental provider who could fabricate the molding plate. For those who read this chapter and are not familiar with the subject of "maxillary orthopedics," it should be noted that it is an emotion-laden subject that has, does, and probably will continue to generate heated discussion among cleft providers (19,20).

The persistent attachment of our cleft team to normalization, as much as possible, of the maxillary alveolar arch before definitive lip repair in unilateral and bilateral CLP is based on the facial appearance of children so treated (Fig. 22D-1). As of September 1, 1999, 209 cases of unilateral and 53 cases of bilateral CLP have been entered into this protocol. Objective assessments of maxillary arch morphology (21), dentoskeletal development, and facial appearance are in progress. Of these, there are 22 patients who are at least 14 years of age. Their dentoskeletal status is as follows:

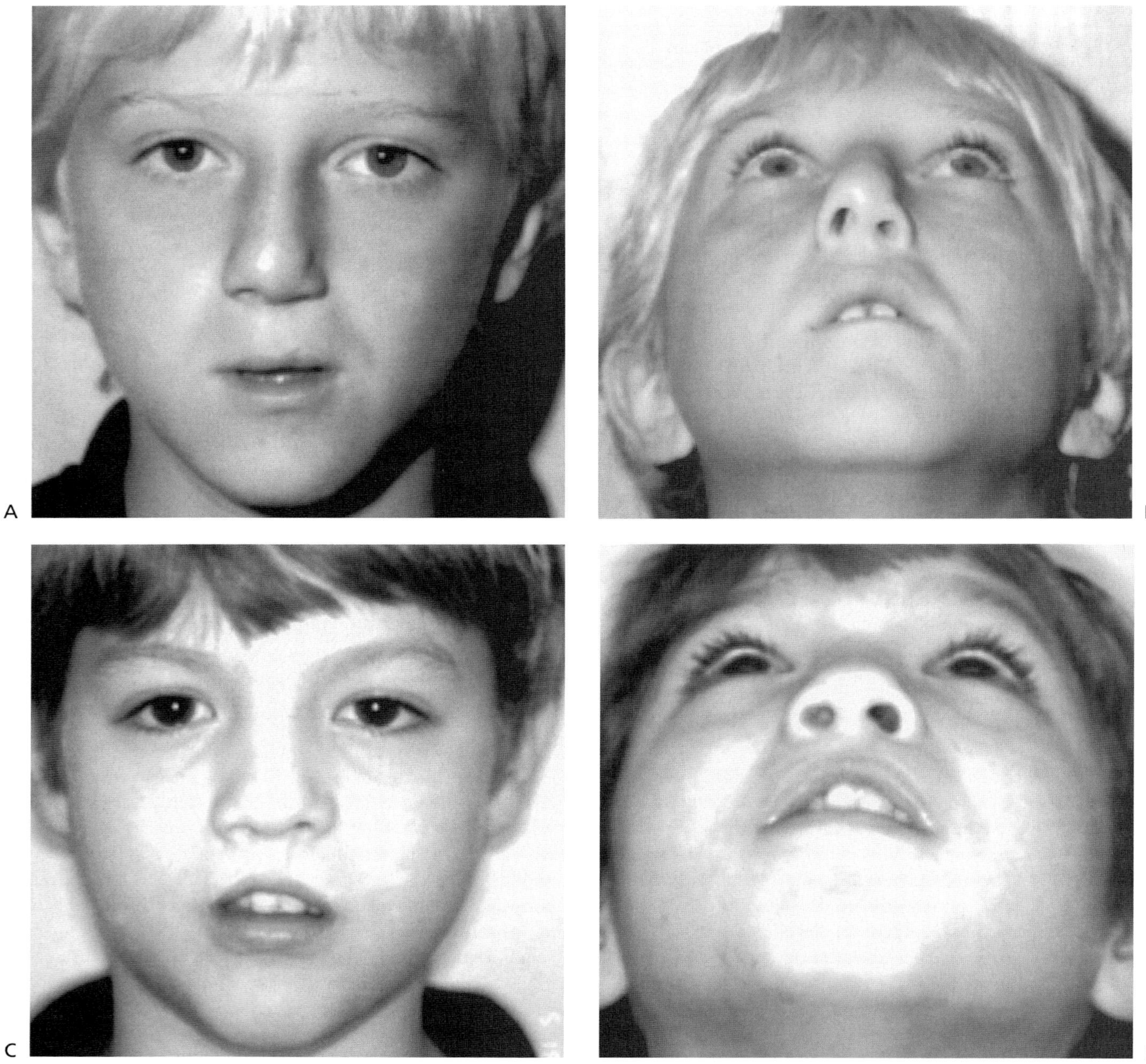

FIGURE 22D-1. A,B: A 10-year, 8-month-old boy status post repair left complete unilateral cleft lip/palate (CLP) performed elsewhere, with one-stage definitive cheiloplasty at age 2 months; velar repair and lip revision at 16 months; and anterior palatoplasty and lip revision at 2 years 8 months; and a pharyngeal flap for VPD and nasal revision at 5 years 8 months. There were no maxillary orthopedics or orthodontics. Note nasal tip deviation to the left, recession of the left alar–facial junction, and left malar flattening. **C,D:** An 11-year, 8-month-old boy status post repair left complete unilateral CLP performed by our cleft team, with lip adhesion and placement of a passive alveolar molding plate at age 6 weeks; definitive cheiloplasty at 7 months; discontinuation of the molding plate and one-stage palatoplasty at 14 months; autogenous posterior pharyngeal wall augmentation for VPI at 6 years 5 months; and autogenous iliac cancellous bone grafting of the alveolar cleft at 8 years 10 months after first-stage orthodontics. No nasal revision or maxillary/malar augmentation has been performed. Compare nasal and facial symmetry to the asymmetry shown in *A*.

unilateral CLP (n = 15)—class I = 20%, class II = 33%, class III = 47% (2 of whom have undergone LF I maxillary advancement); bilateral CLP (n = 7)—class I = 14%, class II = 29%, class III = 57%.

Because not all patients presenting for care to a cleft team will have had their care initiated by the team according to the principles that team believes produce the best outcome (6), secondary revisional intervention will be required. (Of 640 patients with cleft lip and/or palate I have treated since 1978, 63% were referred as unoperated infants; the remainder were had already undergone lip and/or palate repair.) At our team, the type, extent, and timing of such revisions are dependent on the magnitude of the residual deformity, the age of the patient, and the morbidity of the deformity. When there has been minimal surgery and the cleft is only partially repaired, recreation of the defect with definitive repair according to the principles of our team is performed. When the lip and the palate have been repaired and there are no major functional or psychosocial problems associated with the cleft, revision is deferred until desired by the patient and family or the patient is undergoing anesthesia for some other necessary procedure, e.g., alveolar bone grafting. If, however, a major functional or psychosocial problem is identified, revision usually is recommended at that time. We empower the older child and teenager regarding decisions for lip and/or nose revision (Figs. 22D-2 and 22D-3) (22)

My personal management of the nasal deformity associated with cleft lip has varied during the past 21 years of my tenure. An initial enthusiasm for primary nasal alar reconstruction using circumferential intranasal incisions was dampened quickly by iatrogenic nares stenoses. Because of the difficulty in correcting such stenoses, I deferred alar manipulation until mid-childhood, when the deformity was corrected in conjunction with alveolar bone grafting (23). Following exposure to the excellent results obtained with primary alar reconstruction by Dr. Samuel Noordhoof and his associates (24), I introduced his procedure to our cleft care protocol in 1993 and have continued its use to this day. This technique, which separates the nasal skin from the alar cartilage/nares lining with subcutaneous dissection, avoids circumferential intranasal incisions and excessive resection of nasal floor tissue, and, more recently, includes postoperative nares stenting with Silastic stents, has proved efficacious. Secondary nasal tip and ventral septum corrections are performed in conjunction with alveolar bone grafting in mid-childhood, if desired by the patient. Although the child is not empowered to reject alveolar bone grafting, I encourage parents to empower their child to make the decision regarding nose and concurrent lip revisions. Definitive nasal reconstruction, including full septoplasty and osteotomies as needed, is deferred until completion of facial maturation. Destigmatization of the nasal deformity of CLP is more difficult when the underlying skeleton is displaced. In such cases, dentoskeletal reconstruction precedes nasal reconstruction. If dentoskeletal reconstruction either is not indicated or is rejected by the patient, augmentation of the skeleton beneath the alar–facial junction remains an option.

CLEFT PALATE

Since the mid-19th century, the basic objective of cleft palate repair has been establishment of the static physical separation of the nasal and oral cavities that failed to occur *in utero*. Failure of the surgical attempt to achieve this separation is either dehiscence, which implies complete breakdown of the repair, or fistula, which implies partial breakdown. Although dehiscence is a very uncommon event, postoperative fistulas still occur. Rerepair of dehiscence is mandated once the subacute phase of healing is complete; repair of a fistula depends on whether or not it is symptomatic with respect to nasal regurgitation during eating or impaired speech. The literature on palatal fistulas can be confusing, because some authors fail to distinguish between the opening that results from breakdown of a palatal repair and that which persists from an unrepaired portion of the alveolus or hard palate. Because there is no standard jargon to distinguish between these two uses of the noun "fistula," I refer to them as either "inadvertent" or "intentional." The inadvertent fistula is a true surgical complication that often heals with scar tissue. It is less malleable and less well vascularized than virgin palatal tissue and thus more likely to break down with subsequent attempts at rerepair. Repair of such fistulas may require introduction of well-vascularized tissue via local (e.g., buccal mucosa) or distant (e.g., tongue) flaps. The intentional fistula is not a complication, and the virgin tissue that surrounds it should be as healthy as the tissue used for the initial palatoplasty. Such fistulas may become symptomatic with orthodontic maxillary expansion during mixed dentition in anticipation of alveolar bone grafting. This was common in our patients before introduction of the Oslo vomer flap (25) in primary palatoplasty at our cleft center in 1997. Such alveolar-nasal and anterior palatal fistulas are repaired synchronously with the alveolar bone grafting and accompanying gingivoperiosteoplasty in our practice.

As surgeons gained proficiency in the repair of cleft palate, it was recognized that a percentage of patients continued to have problems with speech intelligibility and that inability to functionally close the nasal from oral cavities at the velopharynx was a major cause of this impaired intelligibility. It was hypothesized that dorsal displacement of the soft palate would resolve this problem. A series of operations have been, and continue to be, proposed to either retroposition or lengthen the soft palate. Although many surgeons advocate their preferred form of palatal lengthening, whether such procedures are truly efficacious remains to be demonstrated in a rigorous fashion. Aggressive attempts to "push back" the mucoperiosteum of the hard palate and thus leave the ventral hard palate bone denuded seem to be

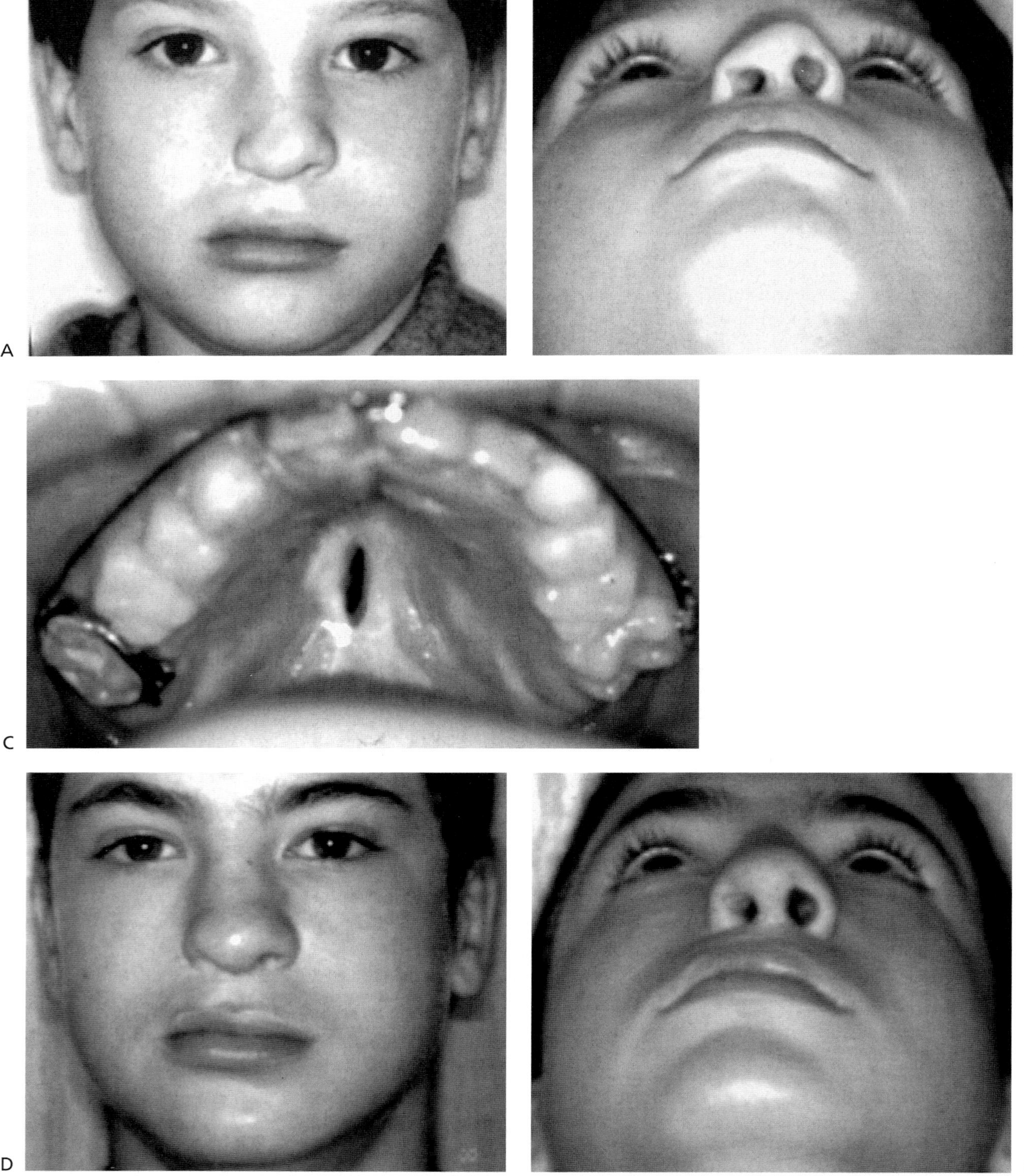

FIGURE 22D-2. **A–C:** A 9-year, 6-month-old boy status post repair left complete unilateral cleft lip/palate performed elsewhere, with one-stage definitive cheiloplasty at age 3 months; anterior palatoplasty with vomer flaps and buccal flap repair of alveolar ridge cleft at 16 months; posterior palatoplasty and cleft lip and nose revisions at 21 months; repair of palatal fistula, lip revision, and Teflon injection into the posterior pharyngeal wall for VPD at 2 years 11 months; and revision lip and alveolus soft tissue at 5 years 4 months. He has residual nasal deformity and a recurrent mid-palatal fistula as well as inability to effectively close his velopharyngeal port. **D,E:** At age 15 years 4 months status post synchronous repair palatal fistula, autogenous rib cancellous alveolar bone graft, repair alveolar-nasal fistula, sphincter pharyngoplasty, and nasal reconstruction, including an autologous auricular cartilage graft performed at age 9 years 9 months. He has no concerns regarding his appearance. His speech is completely intelligible without velopharyngeal dysfunction. His nasal airway is patent. His dentoskeletal relationship is class I. A dental implant is planned for his missing maxillary lateral incisor.

associated with increased incidence of palatal fistulas, deformation of the maxillary arch, and, perhaps, maxillary retrusion.

That certain palatal operations produced undesired maxillary deformations and growth impairments has been recognized since at least the early 20th century. Study of populations in less developed countries of adults with cleft palate, some of whom underwent surgical palatoplasty in childhood and others who remained unoperated, have documented the deleterious effect of palatal surgery in childhood upon maxillary ventral development (26,27). Similar findings were documented in medically sophisticated countries by comparing dentoskeletal development of individuals with clefts with those without clefts (28). Recognition of the negative iatrogenic effects of palatal surgery upon the maxilla prompted many surgeons to abandon those palatoplasty procedures associated with gross maxillary impairment in preference of those operations that demonstrated lesser degrees of detriment. However, some surgeons advocated deferral of repair of the hard palate, at least until late childhood or even later. Although this seems a reasonable approach to the problem, it has not only failed to avoid maxillary retrusion, but more ominously it has markedly increased the need for secondary velopharyngeal management (29). Although comparative weighting of the morbidity of dentoskeletal deformity versus velopharyngeal dysfunction (VPD) has not been reported, most contemporary cleft surgeons in the United States emphasize speech over growth and perform one-stage palate repair within the first 18 months of life. Since 1978, I have performed the so-called "two-flap" palatoplasty on 518 patients. Of these patients, 52% still are followed by our cleft team; the rest have reached dentoskeletal maturity and graduated or left our care. It will take another decade of follow-up, at which time I shall be approaching retirement, before I accurately know the incidence of significant dentoskeletal impairment in patients whose palatoplasty I performed.

VELOPHARYNGEAL DYSFUNCTION

When it is determined that a patient has VPD that is uncorrectable by speech therapy, the therapeutic options are prosthetic or surgical velopharyngeal management (30). The efficacy of such therapies has been reported by many authors, including myself. Interpretation of those reports can be difficult at times due to incomplete or absence definition of the criteria for "success." Complete separation of the nasal from the oral pharynges at the velopharynx will eliminate excessive nasal resonance and turbulence, but at what cost? Can a patient who can no longer breath through the nose, clear nasal secretions into the pharynx, and properly resonate vowel and nasalized consonant phonemes be said to have a surgical success? And what if impairment of sleep or sleep apnea has been induced? The morbidity of operations for VPD with respect to the upper airway has only recently attracted attention. Furthermore, if there has been a diminution in VPD by instrumental assessments but the patient still is stigmatized by abnormal velopharyngeal function, is the operation a "success"?

The approach to VPD management of our cleft team has changed over the past 2 decades due to the introduction of additional diagnostic procedures and new operations. Initially, we treated patients with VPD unresponsive to speech therapy with either a speech prosthesis or a pharyngeal flap. Speech prostheses were prescribed for patients who already had compromised upper airways, progressive neurologic disorders, other medical conditions that precluded surgery, or an aversion to surgery. The remainder received superiorly based, lined, lateral port controlled pharyngeal flaps. In 1989, the recruitment of a new plastic surgeon brought the operation of sphincter pharyngoplasty to our cleft team. Observation of that surgeon's results at postintervention staffings (see later) convinced me to add the procedure to my armamentarium. Over the past decade, sphincter pharyngoplasty has become the most common form of VPD management at our center. It is prescribed for all patients requiring or electing surgical management, with the exception of those with a narrow-to-moderate sagittal or circular closure gap. The patient with good lateral pharyngeal wall motion receives superiorly based, lined, narrow- or moderate-width pharyngeal flap. The criteria for prosthetic management have remained constant, with the exception of the compromised upper airway, where we now perform sphincter pharyngoplasty on patients with a history of glossoptosis secondary to mandibular hypoplasia, provided they do not have a very positive Muller's test. We observed a small number of patients with perioperative obstructive sleep apnea that was treated with nocturnal positive pressure via face mask and resolved within the first week postoperatively in all but one patient (31).

In 1984, a formal velopharyngeal diagnostic laboratory was established at our center. Speech videofluoroscopy was joined by fiberoptic nasoendoscopy, recorded on videotape, which replaced rigid endoscopy, viewed only by the endoscopist. Interdisciplinary (speech/language pathology, otolaryngology, prosthodontics, and plastic surgery) staffing of the videotapes of the speech perceptual, fluoroscopic, and endoscopic velopharyngeal assessments was initiated to determine anatomical function, recommend intervention, and assess intervention outcome (32). Patients referred for speech prostheses underwent definitive fitting of the prosthesis using nasoendoscopy. Not only were patients evaluated before intervention, but also at 3 and 12 months after intervention (the 12-month postintervention endoscopic and fluoroscopic evaluations were eliminated after several years' experience that documented the stability of the 3-month assessment). The postintervention evaluations taught us much about the perception of the prosthodontist or the surgeon with respect to his or her specific interven-

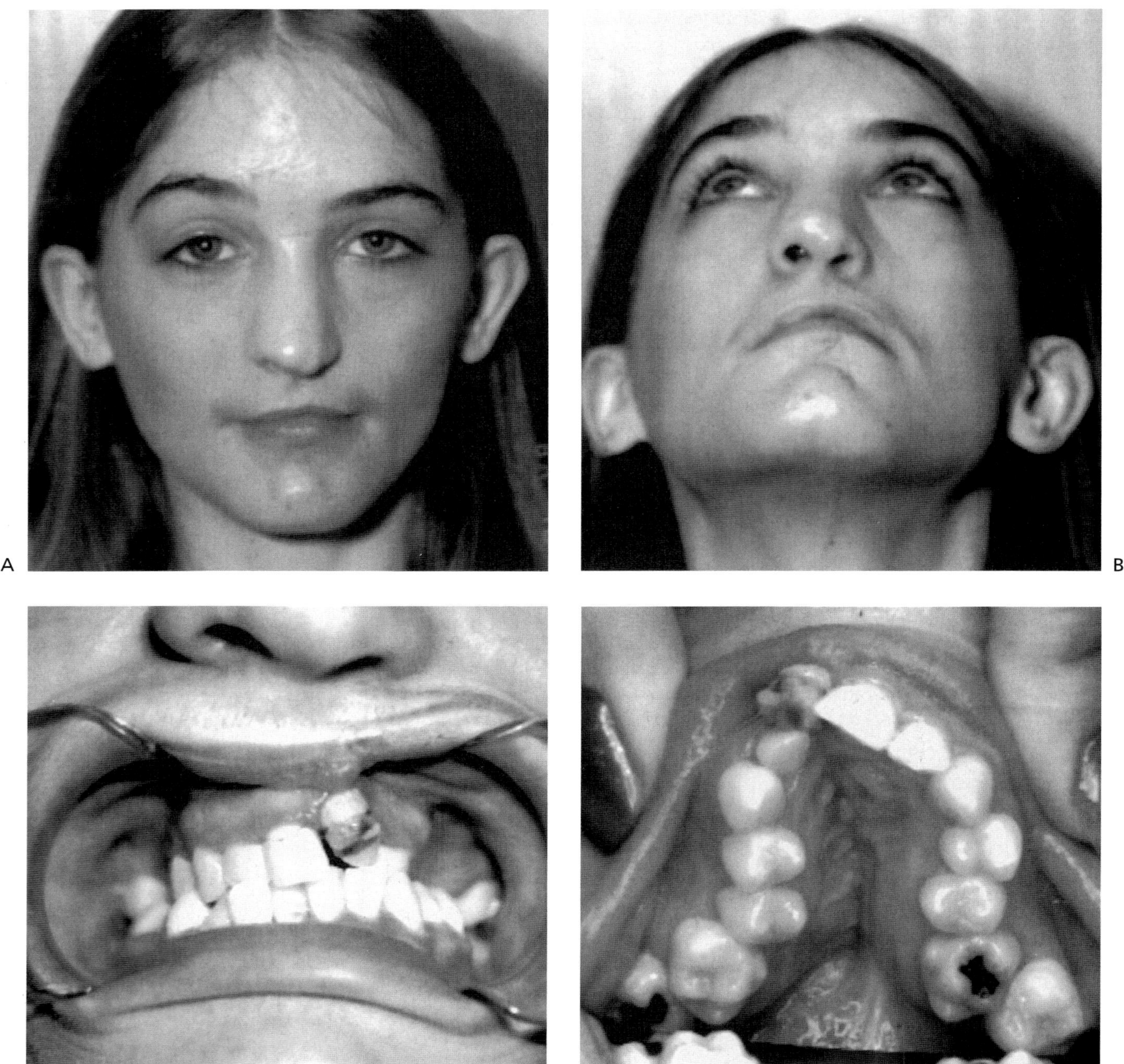

FIGURE 22D-3. A–D: A 16-year, 8-month-old girl status post repair left complete unilateral cleft lip/palate performed elsewhere, with lip repair in "infancy" and "island flap pushback" palatoplasty at age 24 months. Note asymmetry of the nasal tip and lip, with elevation of the left cupid's bow peak, retruded upper lip, protrusive lower lip, and malocclusion with severe iatrogenic palatal deformity. *(continued)*

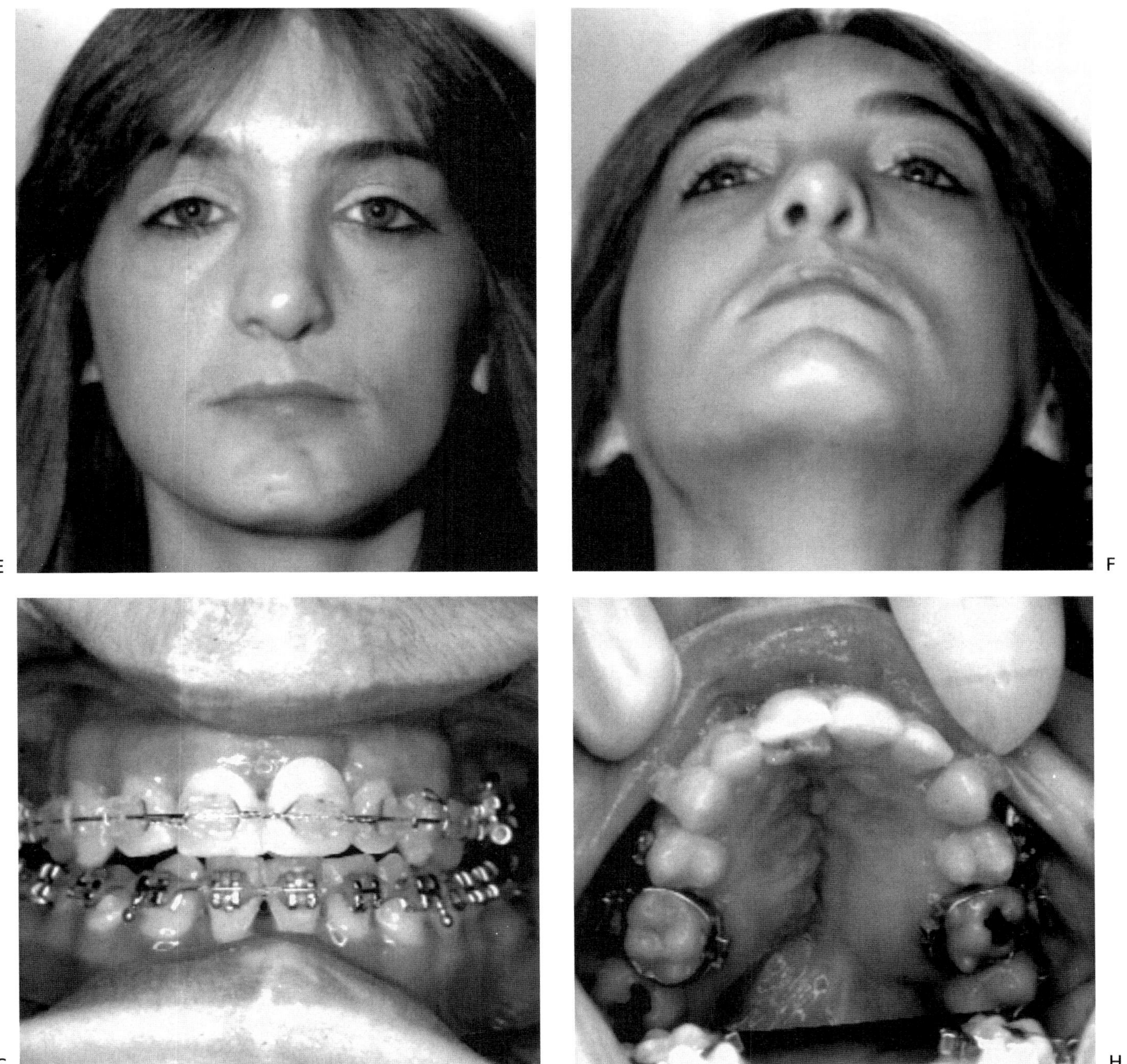

FIGURE 22D-3. *(Continued)* **E–H:** At age 20 years 8 months status post synchronous lip revision, nasal revision, and repair of alveolar-nasal fistula at age 16 years 10 months and subsequent cross-lip flap and pharyngeal flap for VPI performed at 20 years 4 months by myself. Maxillary arch morphology was restored by orthodontics alone.

tions and the reality of the intervention. The introduction of accurate functional information into the feedback loop allowed us to improve the success of initial prosthetic fittings as well as operations. Furthermore, it facilitates secondary management of failed velopharyngeal interventions, whether prosthetic or surgical (33). Inappropriate size or position of the velopharyngeal obturator, insufficient elevation of the velar lift, excessively patent pharyngeal flap lateral ports or sphincter pharyngoplasty central port, or dehiscence of the surgical flaps all can be identified and an appropriate remedy prescribed. This interdisciplinary process remains an integral part of our weekly cleft team conferences, where an average of four patients are reviewed per session.

CONCLUSIONS

Experience with my own patients for over 22 years at one tertiary cleft center, treated both from infancy and upon secondary referral, has demonstrated to me the importance of the first intervention. Much like a chess game, the first move is the most important move, for it sets the stage for all subsequent moves. Ideally, the initial intervention should minimize the need for subsequent interventions and maximize the benefit while diminishing the morbidity of each intervention. The initial intervention should be conservative, because destruction of essential tissue is almost irreversible. Although salvage is possible for patients with undesirable results, it requires careful assessment of needs and expectations so that rehabilitation, rather than additional disappointment, is delivered.

REFERENCES

1. Friede H. Growth sites and growth mechanisms at risk in cleft lip and palate. *Acta Odontol Scand* 1998;56:346–351.
2. Semb G, Shaw WC. Facial growth after different methods of surgical intervention in patients with cleft lip and palate. *Acta Odontol Scand* 1998;56:352-355.
3. Strauss RP. The organization and delivery of craniofacial health services: the state of the art. *Cleft Palate Craniofac J* 1999; 36:189—195.
4. Murray J. *Cleft lip and/or palate: report of a CSAG committee.* London: Department of Health, The United Kingdom, 1998.
5. Shaw WC, Williams AC, Sandy JR, et al. Minimum standards for the management of cleft lip and palate: efforts to close the audit loop. Royal College of Surgeons of England [see Comments]. *Ann R Coll Surg Engl* 1996;78:110–114.
6. Marsh JL. *Decision making in plastic surgery.* St. Louis: CV Mosby, 1992.
7. Henkel KO, Gundlach K, Saka B. Incidence of secondary lip surgeries as a function of cleft type and severity: one center's experience. *Cleft Palate Craniofac J* 1998;35:310–312.
8. Friede H, Priede D, Moller M, et al. Comparisons of facial growth in patients with unilateral cleft lip and palate treated by different regimens for two-stage palatal repair. *Scand J Plast Reconstr Surg Hand Surg* 1999;33:73–81.
9. McComb HK, Coghlan BA. Primary repair of the unilateral cleft lip nose: completion of a longitudinal study. *Cleft Palate Craniofac J* 1996;33:23–30; discussion 31.
10. Witt PD, Wahlen JC, Marsh JL, et al. The effect of surgeon experience on velopharyngeal functional outcome following palatoplasty: is there a learning curve? *Plast Reconstr Surg* 1998; 102:1375–1384.
11. Witt PD, Cohen DT, Muntz HR, et al. Long-term stability of postpalatoplasty perceptual speech ratings: a prospective study. *Ann Plast Surg* 1999;43:246–251.
12. Mackay D, Mazahari M, Graham WP, et al. Incidence of operative procedures on cleft lip and palate patients. *Ann Plast Surg* 1999;42:445–448.
13. Witt PD, Marsh JL. Advances in assessing outcome of surgical repair of cleft lip and cleft palate. *Plast Reconstr Surg* 1997; 100:1907–1917.
14. Huebener DV, Marsh JL. Alveolar molding appliances in the treatment of cleft lip and palate infants. In: Bardach J, Morris HL, eds. *Multidisciplinary management of cleft lip and palate.* Philadelphia: WB Saunders, 1990:601–606.
15. Cutting C, Grayson B, Brecht L, et al. Presurgical columellar elongation and primary retrograde nasal reconstruction in one-stage bilateral cleft lip and nose repair. *Plast Reconstr Surg* 1998;101:630–639.
16. Bennun RD, Perandones C, Sepliarsky VA, et al. Nonsurgical correction of nasal deformity in unilateral complete cleft lip: a 6-year follow-up. *Plast Reconstr Surg* 1999;104:616–630.
17. Millard DR, Latham R, Huifen X, et al. Cleft lip and palate treated by presurgical orthopedics, gingivoperiosteoplasty, and lip adhesion (POPLA) compared with previous lip adhesion method: a preliminary study of serial dental casts. *Plast Reconstr Surg* 1999;103:1630–1644.
18. Rosenstein SW, Monroe CW, Kernahan DA, et al. The case of early bone grafting in cleft lip and cleft palate. *Plast Reconstr Surg* 1982;70:297–309.
19. Sierra FJ, Turner C. Maxillary orthopedics in the presurgical management of infants with cleft lip and palate. *Pediatr Dent* 1995;17:419–423.
20. Huebener DV, Liu JR. Maxillary orthopedics. *Clin Plast Surg* 1993;20:723–732.
21. Prasad CN, Marsh JL, Long RE, et al. Quantitative 3D maxillary arch evaluation of two different infant managements for unilateral cleft lip and palate. *Cleft Palate Craniofac J* 2000;37: 562–570.
22. Marsh JL. When is enough enough? Secondary surgery for cleft lip and palate patients. *Clin Plast Surg* 1990;17:37–47.
23. Kane AA, Pilgram TK, Moshiri M, et al. Long-term outcome of cleft lip nasal reconstruction in childhood. *Plast Reconstr Surg* 2000;105:1600-1608.
24. Yeow VK, Chen PK, Chen YR, et al. The use of nasal splints in the primary management of unilateral cleft nasal deformity. *Plast Reconstr Surg* 1999;103:1347–1354.
25. Dahl E, Hanusardottir B, Bergland O. A comparison of occlusions in two groups of children whose clefts were repaired by three different surgical procedures. *Cleft Palate J* 1981;18:122–127.
26. Mars M, James DR, Lamabadusuriya SP. The Sri Lankan Cleft Lip and Palate Project: the unoperated cleft lip and palate. *Cleft Palate J* 1990;27:3–6.
27. McCance AM, Roberts-Harry D, Sherriff M, Mars M, Houston NJ. Sri Lankan cleft lip and palate study model analysis: clefts of the secondary palate. *Cleft Palate Craniofac J* 1993;30: 227–230.
28. Hermann NV, Jensen BL, Dahl E, et al. Craniofacial comparisons in 22-month-old lip-operated children with unilateral complete cleft lip and palate and unilateral incomplete cleft lip. *Cleft Palate Craniofac J* 2000;37:303–317.

29. Bardach J, Morris HL, Olin WH. Late results of primary veloplasty: the Marburg Project. *Plast Reconstr Surg* 1984;73:207–218.
30. Marsh JL. Cleft palate and velopharyngeal dysfunction. *Clin Commun Disord* 1991;1:29–34.
31. Witt PD, Marsh JL, Muntz HR, et al. Acute obstructive sleep apnea as a complication of sphincter pharyngoplasty. *Cleft Palate Craniofacial J* 1996;33:183–189.
32. D'Antonio LL, Marsh JL, Province MA, et al. Reliability of flexible fiberoptic nasopharyngoscopy for evaluation of velopharyngeal function in a clinical population. *Cleft Palate J* 1989; 26:217–225.
33. Witt PD, Myckatyn T, Marsh JL. Salvaging the failed pharyngoplasty: intervention outcome. *Cleft Palate Craniofac J* 1998; 35:447–453.

23

SECONDARY OROFACIAL CLEFT DEFORMITIES

JOHN W. POLLEY
ALVARO A. FIGUEROA
MICHAEL S. HOHLASTOS

Orofacial clefting is one of the most common facial anomalies seen by craniofacial teams. The combined incidence of unilateral and bilateral cleft lip and palate is estimated to be between 1 in every 700 to 850 live births. Most cleft lip and palate treatment protocols include closure of the soft tissue lip defect within the first 3 to 6 months, and closure of the hard and soft palatal clefts within the first 6 to 24 months of life (1,2). Despite contemporary techniques for surgical correction of cleft lip and palate defects, secondary revisions are common, and the requirement for further soft palatal and pharyngeal surgery to correct problems of velopharyngeal incompetence is not uncommon (roughly 10% to 15%) (3). Even with successful surgical closure of the congenital cleft of the lip, hard and soft palate, and alveolar cleft, developmental craniofacial growth in these patients is frequently abnormal. The dysplastic development of the maxillofacial skeleton usually includes deficiencies in the sagittal, vertical, and transverse planes of the maxilla. When bone grafting of the alveolar cleft is performed, in either infancy or later during the period of transitional dentition, this process can also potentially negatively affect the sagittal and vertical growth components of the maxilla (1). It has been estimated that as many as 50% of all patients with clefting have a significant deficiency in the sagittal development of the maxilla, such that they may be candidates for surgical maxillary advancement at the Le Fort I level (1,2). In addition, many of these patients present with residual oronasal fistulas, dental anomalies, and secondary nasal and lip deformities. The purpose of this chapter is to discuss the current treatment modalities available for patients with orofacial clefting and residual secondary skeletal and soft tissue deformities.

J. W. Polley and Alvaro A. Figueroa: Department of Plastic and Reconstructive Surgery, Rush Craniofacial Center, Rush-Presbyterian–St. Luke's Medical Center; and Department of Surgery, Cook County Hospital, Chicago, Illinois

M. S. Hohlastos: Rush Craniofacial Center, Rush-Presbyterian–St. Luke's Medical Center, Chicago, Illinois

EVALUATION OF THE PATIENT WITH SECONDARY CLEFT FACIAL DEFORMITIES

All patients with secondary cleft lip and palate deformities should be examined by an experienced craniofacial team, comprising of, at least, an orthodontist, a surgeon, and a speech pathologist. A complete history is taken, including the type and extent of the orofacial cleft, and the techniques and timing of methods previously used to close the lip and palatal defects. It is extremely important for the surgeons to know about any additional surgeries, such as alveolar bone grafting, pharyngoplasties, or fistula closures. The history of dental care and prior orthodontic treatment must be documented. The speech pathologist will be interested in a prior history of speech therapy, including its extent and duration.

The most important aspect of the workup of a patient with secondary cleft lip and palate deformities is the clinical examination. Study of the full face from the frontal view, both lateral views, and oblique and worm's-eye views is extremely important in determining the extent of secondary deformities. Special attention must be given to the facial profile in terms of overall convexity and lip-to-nose, lip-to-lip, and lip-to-chin relationships. From the frontal view, evaluation of the lip itself includes the scar and its elasticity, and symmetry of the Cupid's bow. Analysis of lip-to-lip and lip-to-tooth relationships and of dental and skeletal midlines is also essential in planning treatment. The degree of paranasal and malar projection should be noted. Moderate to severe deficiencies in the paranasal region and in the malar regions bilaterally are common in patients with orofacial clefting. These regions, in addition to the position of the maxillary dental arch, must be addressed.

Intraoral examination includes an assessment of dental and gingival health; dental abnormalities, including absent or aberrant dentition, which is extremely common in patients with clefting; and residual fistulas in the labial, alveolar, and palatal regions. The size of the dental arch of the maxilla is important to determine, in addition to the quality of the soft tissues of the hard and soft palate and posterior pharynx. Occlusal relationships, crossbite, overjet, and overbite are all recorded.

The speech pathologist will perform a complete speech examination, including studies of nasal air flow. In addition, any patient under consideration for possible maxillary advancement should undergo a preoperative nasopharyngoscopy for evaluation of the velopharyngeal mechanism. This is extremely important because sagittal advancements of the maxilla can adversely affect the competency of the velopharyngeal mechanism.

Radiographic examination includes frontal and lateral cephalometry and a Panorex. Facial and intraoral photography and video imaging are all-important aspects of the initial evaluation.

Following the full evaluation, a problem list and treatment plan are formulated for each patient. Soft tissue abnormalities of the nose and secondary nasal deformities are also important to integrate into the treatment plan. In patients with secondary cleft lip and palate deformities, the central problem is focused around the maxillary hypoplasia. Sagittal deficiency of the maxilla is the most recognizable deformity in these patients. Frequently, however, deficiencies in the vertical position of the maxilla and transverse dental arch relationships are also present. All must be recognized, evaluated, and planned for accordingly. Crossbites, malocclusions, residual oronasal and palatal fistulas, and dental abnormalities are all associated with the varied degrees of maxillary hypoplasia. The degree of maxillary bony deficiency still remaining in many of these patients needs to be recognized. Frequently, despite prior alveolar bone grafting, the patient may still have bony deficiency of a significant degree in both the alveolar region and the piriform aperture and palatal region of the cleft. Such a deficiency results in a lack of support of the soft tissues of the upper lip, nasal vestibules, and nasal alae and must be recognized and addressed. An overall flattening of the face, including the paranasal regions and malar prominence, is also common in these patients. Treatment planning for secondary deformities focuses on correction of the maxillary hypoplasia and any associated abnormal findings.

Until recently, maxillary hypoplasia could be treated safely only after the patient had reached skeletal maturity (4,5), generally at 14 to 16 years in girls and slightly later in boys. The foundation for maxillary rehabilitation in these patients has been the Le Fort I osteotomy, in conjunction with presurgical orthodontics. Although this treatment plan can be successful in patients with moderate maxillary deficiency, for more severe cases of sagittal deficiency of the maxilla, the long-term relapse rates with traditional surgery have been extremely high, in the 20% to 40% range (4–8). In addition, a tremendous drawback of our traditional treatment modalities for secondary cleft deformities has been our inability to address midface deficiency problems during the childhood years. This situation has now been dramatically changed by our ability to perform maxillary advancement surgery with distraction osteogenesis. Utilizing an external approach, we are able to control the sagittal and vertical advancement of the maxilla fully in patients with clefting in a totally predictable fashion. Through slow, rhythmic advancement of the maxilla with distraction osteogenesis utilizing an external framework, we can virtually advance the maxilla to an unlimited degree in the sagittal plane reliably and precisely. With the availability of the technique of rigid external distraction, it is no longer necessary to delay the required treatment for secondary cleft lip and palate deformities in the childhood years. Rigid external distraction is becoming the recognized procedure of choice for maxillary advancement in children (9–11).

TREATMENT OF SECONDARY CLEFT DEFORMITIES IN CHILDREN AGES 5 TO 14

In the pediatric age range (full primary dentition and older), maxillary distraction osteogenesis is the treatment of choice for maxillary hypoplasia secondary to orofacial clefting (9–11). This minimally invasive treatment modality utilizing rigid external distraction is eminently suitable for young patients during the period of skeletal and dental maturation (Figs. 23-1 through 23-3). The essence of the treatment is a high Le Fort I osteotomy followed by a period of slow, rhythmic maxillary distraction accomplished by means of an external framework and an intraoral appliance. The patient wears the halo framework, which causes no pain, while a

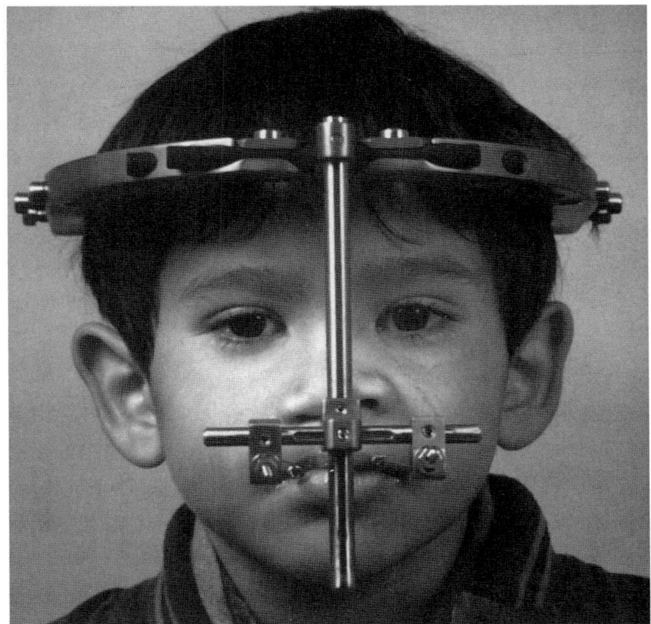

FIGURE 23-1. A 5-year-old boy with cleft maxillary hypoplasia undergoing correction of a midface deformity with rigid external distraction *(RED)*. The RED device and the distraction process itself cause no discomfort, even to a very young patient.

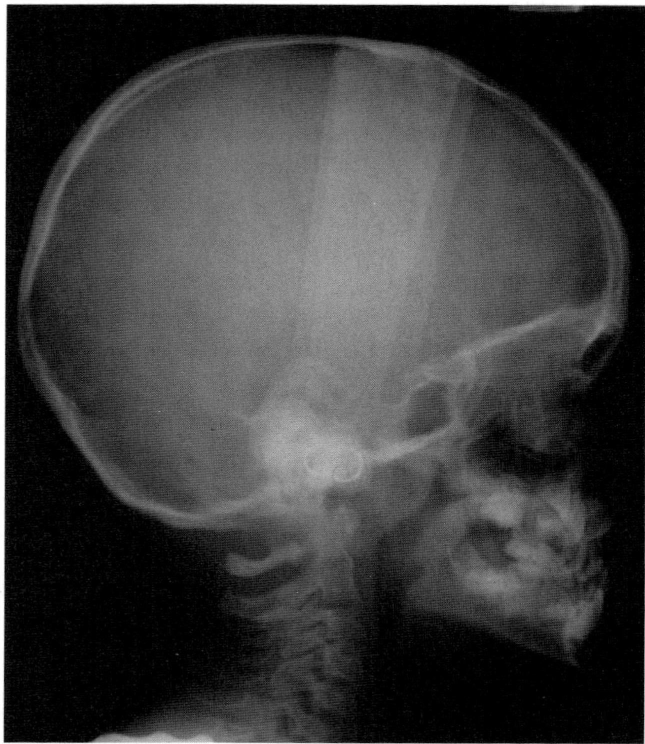

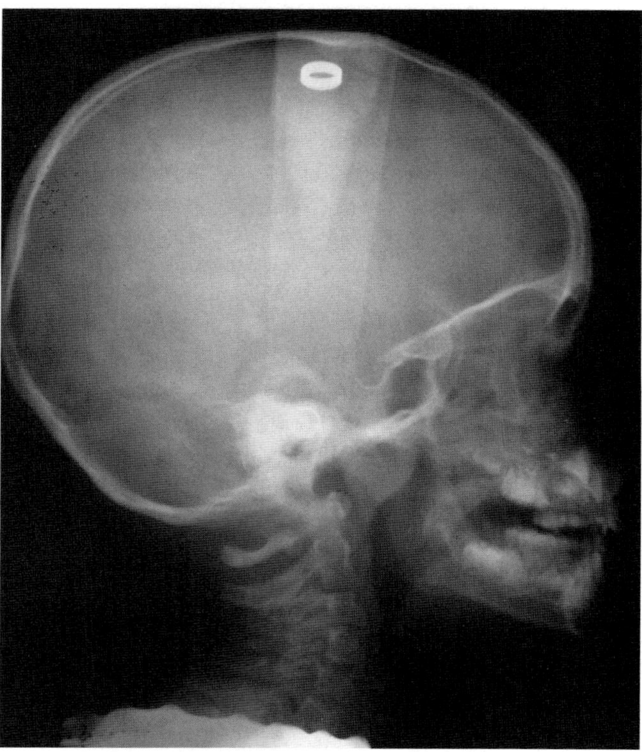

FIGURE 23-2. A: Pre-distraction lateral cephalogram of a 5-year-old patient with concave skeletal profile secondary to orofacial clefting. **B:** The 1-year postdistraction lateral cephalogram for this patient. Notice the convexity of the skeletal profile, with maintenance of the sagittal position of the maxilla. The small bone markers were placed for cephalometric landmark identification.

family member gradually distracts the maxilla forward under the guidance and observation of the treating physician.

For the surgeon, a key element to the procedure is to determine the level of the transverse portion of the Le Fort I osteotomy (10). This determination is based on two factors: (a) the position of unerupted tooth buds within the maxilla, and (b) the desired aesthetic changes required for each patient in terms of paranasal and malar projection. All patients undergo a high Le Fort I osteotomy. In younger patients, special care and consideration are taken not to damage any permanent tooth buds within the maxilla. This can easily be accomplished by preoperative study of the panoramic radiograph and by careful observation of the surface markings of the maxilla at the time of surgery. In younger patients, the transverse osteotomy frequently lies just below the level of the infraorbital rim. The lateral extent of the osteotomy can be carried up onto the malar bone to allow for a sagittal advancement of this region to correct sagittal malar deficiency. With external distraction, the surgeon does not need to worry about the placement of rigid internal fixation hardware or internal distraction devices, and is free to design the osteotomy based on the aesthetic requirement of the patient. This is a tremendous advantage because it allows for full correction of the facial disfigurement through the Le Fort I osteotomy.

The linkage between the distraction device and the maxillofacial skeleton is through the intraoral splint. The splint is readily manufactured from standard orthodontic supplies and includes a lingual and labial arch wire and maxillary molar bands (9,10). Labial hooks from the device are bent down and around the upper lip, with the end eyelet placed at the center of rotation of the maxilla. From this eyelet, a 25-gauge stainless steel wire connects the splint to the activation mechanism of the distraction device. The parents are then given an activating screwdriver and instructed regarding the rate and rhythm of advancement. Patients are seen weekly during active distraction, and changes in the vertical position of the distraction vectors and in the rate of advancement are made on a weekly basis. With the use of this technique, complete rigid control over the movement of the maxilla is ensured, along with the ability to adjust the vectors of distraction throughout the period of active distraction. Consistent, predictable results can now be obtained in this difficult group of children with maxillary hypoplasia secondary to orofacial clefting. The results are extremely stable, with little or no sagittal relapse seen at 12-month follow-up.

The surgery for maxillary distraction osteogenesis is performed either on an outpatient basis or during a 24-hour admission with virtually no morbidity. No blood transfusions,

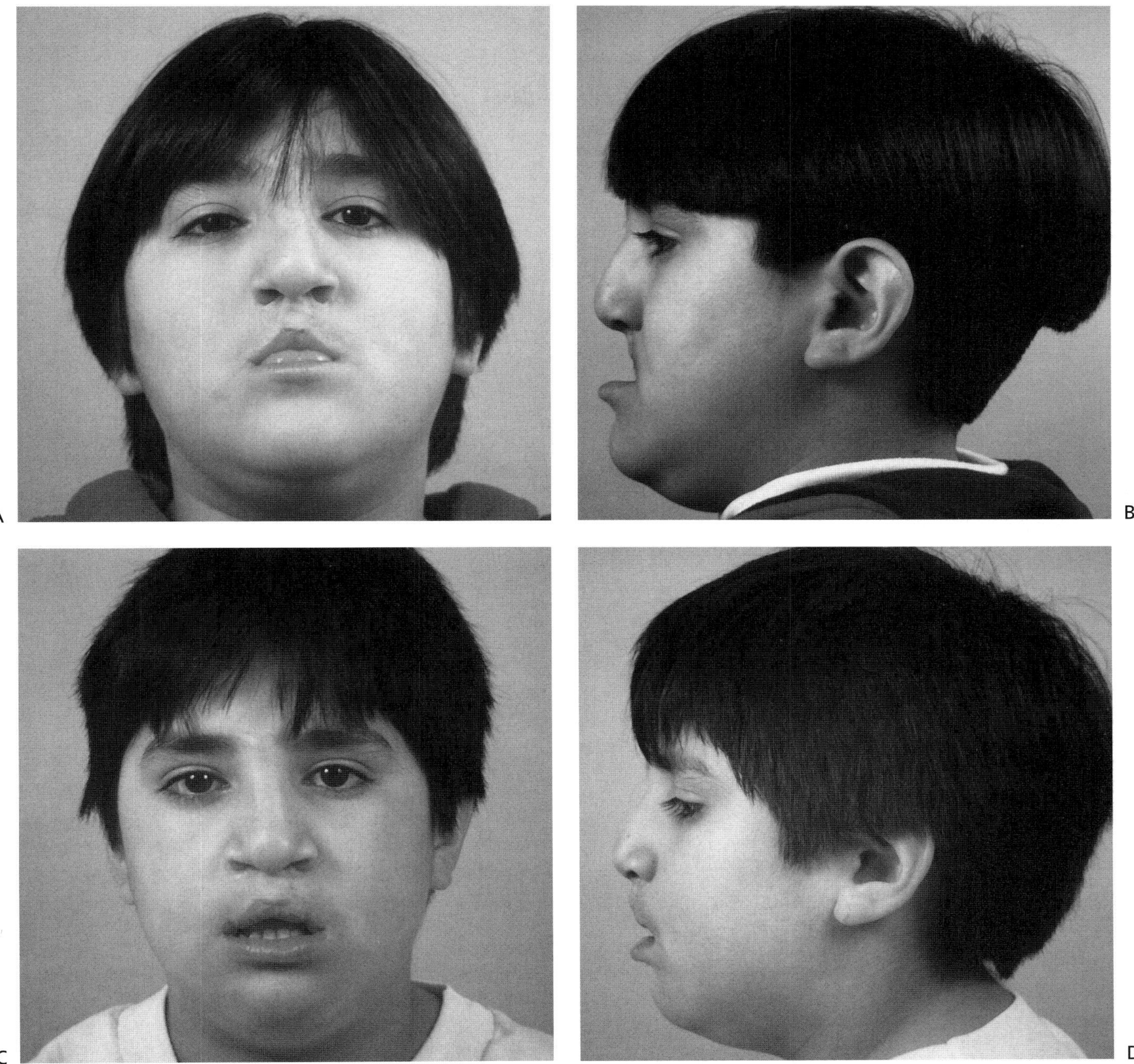

FIGURE 23-3. Pre-distraction **(A,B)** and post-distraction **(C,D)** frontal and lateral views of a young patient with severe bilateral cleft lip and palate deformities and midface hypoplasia. The patient underwent a three-piece Le Fort I maxillary osteotomy followed by maxillary distraction with a rigid external device. Note the post-distraction change in facial convexity and the positive change in lip-to-nose relationships. *(continued)*

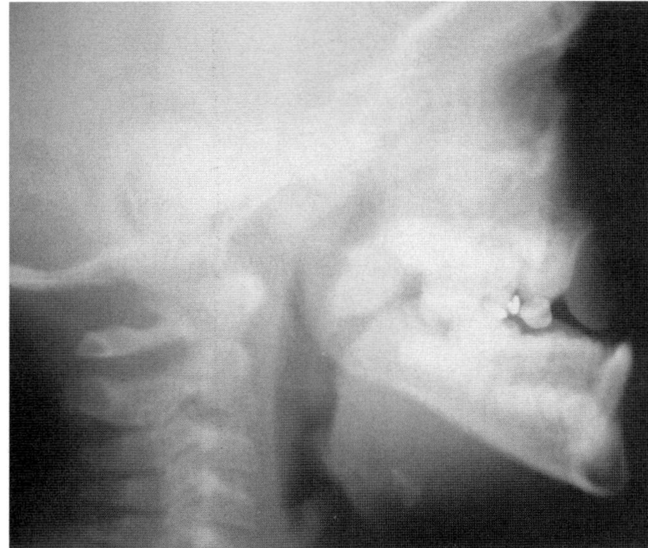

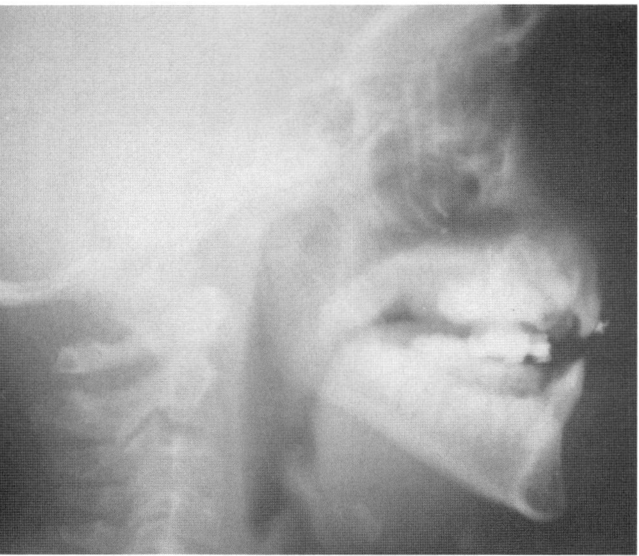

E F

FIGURE 23-3. *(Continued)* **E,F:** Pre-distraction and 1-year post-distraction lateral cephalograms for the patient. Note the change in the sagittal projection of the maxilla after the distraction, in addition to the opening of the posterior pharyngeal airway.

bone grafting, rigid internal fixation devices, or intermaxillary fixation has been required in these patients. The device is extremely well tolerated and can be removed without anesthesia following the completion of distraction in the clinic.

TREATMENT OF SECONDARY CLEFT DEFORMITY IN THE MATURE PATIENT

For patients in their middle to late teenage years or older who present with secondary cleft lip and palate deformities and maxillary hypoplasia, treatment planning allows for the use of either distraction osteogenesis or more traditional orthognathic surgical procedures. The decision regarding which surgical modality to utilize should be based on the treating team's experience and the deformity of the patient. In addition to perioperative morbidity, the biggest disadvantage of traditional orthognathic surgery for sagittal advancements of the maxilla in patients with cleft deformities has been the significant rate of long-term sagittal relapse. Even in the best of hands, maxillary sagittal relapse in these patients at 1 year after surgery generally is in the range of 20% to 40% (4–8). In patients who require minimal or modest sagittal advancement, traditional surgical approaches with rigid internal fixation and bone grafting can provide satisfactory solutions. In adult patients with moderate to severe midface hypoplasia, distraction osteogenesis with rigid external distraction should be considered as a viable treatment plan. It has been our observation that after more than 12 months, sagittal relapse has been minimal in patients who have undergone maxillary distraction with rigid external distraction in excess of 10 mm. The orthotopic bone that forms gradually during the distraction process has proved extremely stable in the long term. Other important considerations for adult patients who require correction of maxillary deficiency secondary to cleft lip and palate deformities include the degree of presurgical malar and paranasal hypoplasia. Because the osteotomy in patients undergoing rigid external distraction can be performed at a very high level, better facial convexity can be achieved with distraction osteogenesis than with traditional orthognathic surgery. All these factors need to be considered and discussed with the family when a treatment modality is chosen for an adult patient with cleft maxillary deficiencies. Correction of malocclusions, closure of oronasal fistulas, and maxillary bone grafting in these patients can be performed either at the time of Le Fort I osteotomy surgery or as a secondary procedure according to the overall treatment plan for each patient. It is also important to plan soft tissue lip and nasal rehabilitation for these patients when a final treatment plan is prepared.

CONCLUSION

Maxillary deficiencies in secondary deformities related to cleft lip and palate have traditionally been difficult to correct fully. Treatment with bone grafting and rigid internal fixation to produce large sagittal advancements of the maxilla has often resulted in compromising aesthetic results and significant rates of sagittal relapse. In addition, traditional approaches have not been applicable in children. With the use of rigid external distraction, we can now successfully and predictably treat children with a minimally invasive procedure that causes virtually no morbidity. The technique of distraction can also be applied in adult patients, in whom problems with long skeletal stability are also a real concern. With the utilization of the full techniques of traditional surgery and maxillary distraction osteogenesis, all patients with secondary cleft deficiencies can now anticipate excellent functional and morphologic outcomes.

REFERENCES

1. Ross RB. Treatment variables affecting facial growth in complete unilateral cleft lip and palate: an overview of treatment and facial growth. *Cleft Palate J* 1987;24:5–71.
2. Semb G. A study of facial growth in patients with unilateral cleft lip and palate treated by the Oslo CLP team. *Cleft Palate Craniofac J* 1991;28:1–21.
3. Witzel MA, Vallino LD. Speech problems in patients with dentofacial and craniofacial deformities. In: Bell WH, ed. *Modern practice in orthognathic and reconstructive surgery,* vol. 3. Philadelphia: WB Saunders, 1992:1686–1699.
4. Erbe M, Stoelinga PJW, Leenen RJ. Long-term results of segmental repositioning of the maxilla in cleft palate patients without previously grafted alveolopalatal clefts. *J Craniomaxillofac Surg* 1996;24:109–117.
5. Cheung LK, Sammam N, Hiu E, et al. The 3-dimensional stability of maxillary osteotomies in cleft patients with residual alveolar clefts. *Br J Oral Maxillofac Surg* 1994;32:6–12.
6. Hochban W, Gans C, Austermann KH. Long-term results after maxillary advancement in patients with clefts. *Cleft Palate Craniofac J* 1993;30:237–243.
7. Posnick JC, Dagys AP. Skeletal stability and relapse patterns after Le Fort I maxillary osteotomy fixed with miniplates. The unilateral cleft lip and palate deformity. *J Plast Reconstr Surg* 1994;94:924–932.
8. Eskenazi LB, Schendel S. An analysis of Le Fort I maxillary advancement in cleft lip and palate patients. *J Plast Reconstr Surg* 1992;90:779–786.
9. Polley JW, Figueroa AA. Management of severe maxillary deficiency in childhood and adolescence through distraction osteogenesis with an external, adjustable, rigid distraction device. *J Craniofac Surg* 1997;8:181–185.
10. Polley JW, Figueroa AA. Rigid external distraction: its application in cleft maxillary deformities. *Plast Reconstr Surg* 1998;102:1360–1372.
11. Polley JW, Figueroa AA. Maxillary distraction osteogenesis with rigid external distraction. *Atlas Oral Maxillofac Surg Clin North Am* 1999;7:15–28.

Discussion

SECONDARY OROFACIAL CLEFT DEFORMITIES

JEFFREY C. POSNICK
RAMON L. RUIZ

The authors state that the purpose of their book chapter is to review "current treatment modalities available for patients with orofacial clefting and residual secondary skeletal and soft tissue deformities." Their premise is that (a) with the use of the techniques of external distraction, it is *no longer necessary* to delay definitive treatment for patients with secondary cleft lip and palate deformities—that these corrections can now be (definitively) made in the childhood years; and (b) with the use of an external distraction approach, it is possible to *fully control* the sagittal and vertical advancement of the maxilla (after Le Fort I osteotomy) in the cleft patient in a *totally* predictable fashion with *virtually no morbidity* and as a *minimally invasive procedure.*

The authors summarize the advantages of their external distraction approach to reconstructing the maxilla in patients with cleft deformities as follows: (a) The approach is "minimally invasive"; (b) it is "highly suitable for use in young patients"; (c) "the halo framework causes no pain"; (d) "the surgeon is free to design the osteotomy based on aesthetics"; (e) the results of the external distraction approach are extremely stable; and (f) use of the external distraction approach causes "virtually no morbidity."

An unfortunate fact is that when the distraction approach is used to manage the jaw and dental deformities of a patient with clefting, many of the advantages of the classic approach are lost. These advantages include the following:

J. C. Posnick and R. L. Ruiz: Posnick Center for Facial Plastic Surgery, Chevy Chase, Maryland

1. With the classic approach, a planned and successfully executed procedure achieves ideal results (preferred facial aesthetics and occlusion) immediately, in the operating room.
2. Patients with cleft lip and palate often present with multiple residual problems, including oronasal fistula; cleft dental gap(s); bone defects of the alveolar ridge, hard palate, and floor of the nose; different degrees of hypoplasia in each maxillary segment; maxillary transverse constriction; mandibular disproportion and asymmetry; chin disproportion; extra or rudimentary teeth; and nasal obstructive breathing caused by septal and turbinate abnormalities. With the classic approach, these problems can be corrected simultaneously.
3. After surgery, only limited cooperation by the patient and family is required because no office procedures or technical maneuvers are necessary to complete the reconstruction.
4. The patient is much more comfortable after surgery because no external appliances (external hardware or halo head frame) or bandages are required.
5. No scalp or facial scars are produced.

During the past several years, Polley and associates have enumerated six theoretical advantages of the external distraction approach over classic techniques (1–3). Each of these six hoped-for advantages should be considered in detail in an attempt to separate fact from fantasy.

STATED ADVANTAGE 1

When the maxilla is advanced at the Le Fort I level in a cleft patient with the external distraction approach, velopharyngeal function is not disturbed. Polley initially stated that external distraction would provide a way to avoid velopharyngeal dysfunction when maxillary advancement was required in cleft patients. We now know that this is *not* the case. Hung et al. (4) recently presented their long-term results in a series of 30 patients with cleft lip and palate who presented with midface retrusion. These patients underwent Le Fort I advancement during childhood (ages 9 through 14) with use of the external distraction approach. As part of the protocol, each patient underwent a clinical assessment of speech, nasopharyngoscopy, and video fluoroscopy before and after the surgical procedure. The patients were categorized as having either adequate, marginal, or inadequate velopharyngeal closure. Each patient underwent a similar evaluation 1 to 2 years after surgery. In 60% of their patients, at least mild deterioration in velopharyngeal function was noted. The authors concluded that "... use of the external distraction approach to gradually reposition the maxilla at the Le Fort I level in the cleft patient resulted in alteration of velopharyngeal function in a similar way to the classical approach."

STATED ADVANTAGE 2

The secondary deformities of the cleft patient can be simultaneously managed with the external distraction approach. Unfortunately, with use of the external distraction approach, it has *not* been possible to manage the multiple residual skeletal and dental problems often seen in the presenting cleft patient (fistulas; cleft dental gap(s); bony defects; differential segmental hypoplasia of the upper jaw, including constriction of the arch width; intranasal deformities; disproportion of the mandible, chin, or both). It is for this reason that Chen and colleagues (5,6) have abandoned use of the external distraction approach to resolve these problems. They are attempting to develop an interdental (intraoral) distraction device to reposition the cleft maxillary segments independently. Unfortunately, to date, their technique still does not allow for meticulous repair of the dental, skeletal, and intranasal deformities of the cleft patient. The classic techniques previously described remain the gold standard to resolve the multiple residual dental, skeletal, and intranasal problems of the patient with cleft deformities (7–12).

STATED ADVANTAGE 3

When the external distraction approach is used to advance the upper jaw, soft tissue volume (skin, subcutaneous tissue, muscle) is created. Beginning in 1992, advocates of the distraction technique had hoped that the movement of the bone segments over several weeks would "create" soft tissue volume (skin, subcutaneous tissue, muscle, adipose, and nerve) (13,14). Unfortunately, this hoped-for advantage has *not* been documented through clinical studies. The rapid stretching of the soft tissues, in the range of 5 to 15 mm during 1 to 3 weeks (typical distraction protocol), is likely to be just that (stretching), and not the creation of soft tissues. However, it is recognized that when classic techniques are used to correct maxillofacial skeletal disproportion, the facial soft tissue envelope will redrape in a more normal way (9–11). The same should be true when the distraction approach is used.

STATED ADVANTAGE 4

Maxillary advancement carried out with the external distraction approach in cleft patients results in absolute stability (no relapse occurs). Polley and colleagues initially hoped that their external distraction approach would completely prevent skeletal relapse. In a recent presentation in abstract form (15), measured relapse at cephalometric point ANS in cleft patients managed with external distraction was similar to that in patients managed with classic Le Fort I osteotomy stabilized with miniplates and screws. Eskenazi and Schendel (16) and Posnick and colleagues (17,18) have independently documented 1-year relapse rates after Le Fort I advancements in cleft patients to be in the range of 1% to 12%. Initial information would indicate that the external distraction approach, like other forms of skeletal repositioning, can and does result in relapse/bony remodeling in some patients.

STATED ADVANTAGE 5

The external distraction approach is a noninvasive and nonsurgical method to resolve the cleft patient's dentofacial deformities without causing morbidity. It is now recognized that the external distraction approach is *not* a nonsurgical approach. A death has even been reported in one patient in whom the halo type of external distraction device was used to move the midface forward. A full and complete Le Fort I osteotomy and disimpaction are required, just as with the classic techniques. General anesthesia is required; similar incisions must be made, and during osteotomy and disimpaction, blood is lost and fluids must be replaced. The same forms of morbidity and complications can occur with the distraction approach, including devitalization of bone segments and teeth, infection, airway difficulties, hemorrhage, nonunion, malunion, facial sensory loss, permanent scarring, periodontal problems, less than ideal aesthetic results, and poor occlusion. When classic techniques are used, the incidence of most of these complications in the hands of experienced surgeons is extremely low (12).

STATED ADVANTAGE 6

The external distraction approach "allows you to operate on the young cleft patient" and correct the secondary skeletal deformities once and for all. A major talking point for Polley and colleagues is that the external distraction approach allows the surgeon to correct the maxillary deficiency problem for the cleft patient in childhood rather then "needing to wait until skeletal maturity." The logic of this thinking is difficult to follow. The authors describe a distraction technique in which the same complete (Le Fort I) osteotomy and disimpaction of the maxilla are required as in the classic approach. The surgeon's choice of whether to reposition the maxilla immediately in the operating room (classic technique) or to reposition it gradually during several weeks (distraction approach) would *not* be expected to influence the basic biology as to whether the healed maxilla will, over time, grow according to a "normal" facial pattern.

If the growth of the clefted, surgically treated, and now healed maxilla does not keep pace, it will be disproportional to the growth of the "normal" mandible. Once the mandible has finished growing, the maxilla, which has not kept up, will again be at least horizontally, if not also vertically and transversely, deficient.

In 1990, Wolford et al. (19,20) published their long-term results in a consecutive series of cleft patients in whom "significant" maxillary hypoplasia had been recognized during childhood. They hoped that after completion of a Le Fort I osteotomy and repositioning of the upper jaw, the maxilla would continue to grow and that preferred facial aesthetics and a precise occlusion would be maintained at the time of skeletal maturity. Unfortunately, they did not find this to be the case. A retrospective study evaluated preoperative and postoperative growth in 12 maxillary-deficient cleft patients who underwent orthognathic surgery (all performed by Wolford). The study included six unilateral and six bilateral cleft patients whose average age was 12 years and 7 months (range, 9 to 15 years) and whose average follow-up was 3 years and 1 month. For each patient, preoperative, immediately postoperative, and late postoperative cephalometric radiographs were obtained and analyzed. The patients were grouped and evaluated according to age, cleft type, proportionate or disproportionate presurgical growth pattern, and the presence of a pharyngeal flap. A variety of cephalometric parameters were analyzed, and their findings included the following: (a) In 92% of the studied patients, anteroposterior maxillary growth was decreased in comparison with presurgical growth. (b) In 83% of the studied patients, dental compensations in the form of maxillary incisor angulation developed to mask the ongoing jaw discrepancy. (c) Proportionate facial growers before surgery became disproportionate facial growers after surgery, showing a tendency toward development of a skeletal class III pattern. (d) Patients studied postoperatively tended to become predominantly vertical growers (along with maxillary horizontally deficient growth patterns). (e) Studied patients who had a pharyngeal flap in place tended to have more deficient horizontal growth and increased vertical growth over time. Wolford concluded that the maxillary-deficient cleft patient who undergoes a Le Fort I osteotomy with advancement in childhood demonstrates an unfavorable growth pattern over time. He believes that if maxillary surgery is undertaken in these patients before the completion of facial growth, they will require overcorrection, and they must clearly understand that additional orthognathic surgery is likely to be necessary when they reach skeletal maturity.

In addition to Wolford's clinical research, four independent animal studies were conducted at three separate centers to answer the question of what are the effects of a Le Fort I (type) osteotomy on subsequent dentofacial growth when it is carried out during childhood or early adolescence (21–24). In each study, the data confirmed that a restrictive midface growth pattern results from the procedure.

The decision to surgically improve the cleft patient's horizontal maxillary hypoplasia during childhood (before skeletal

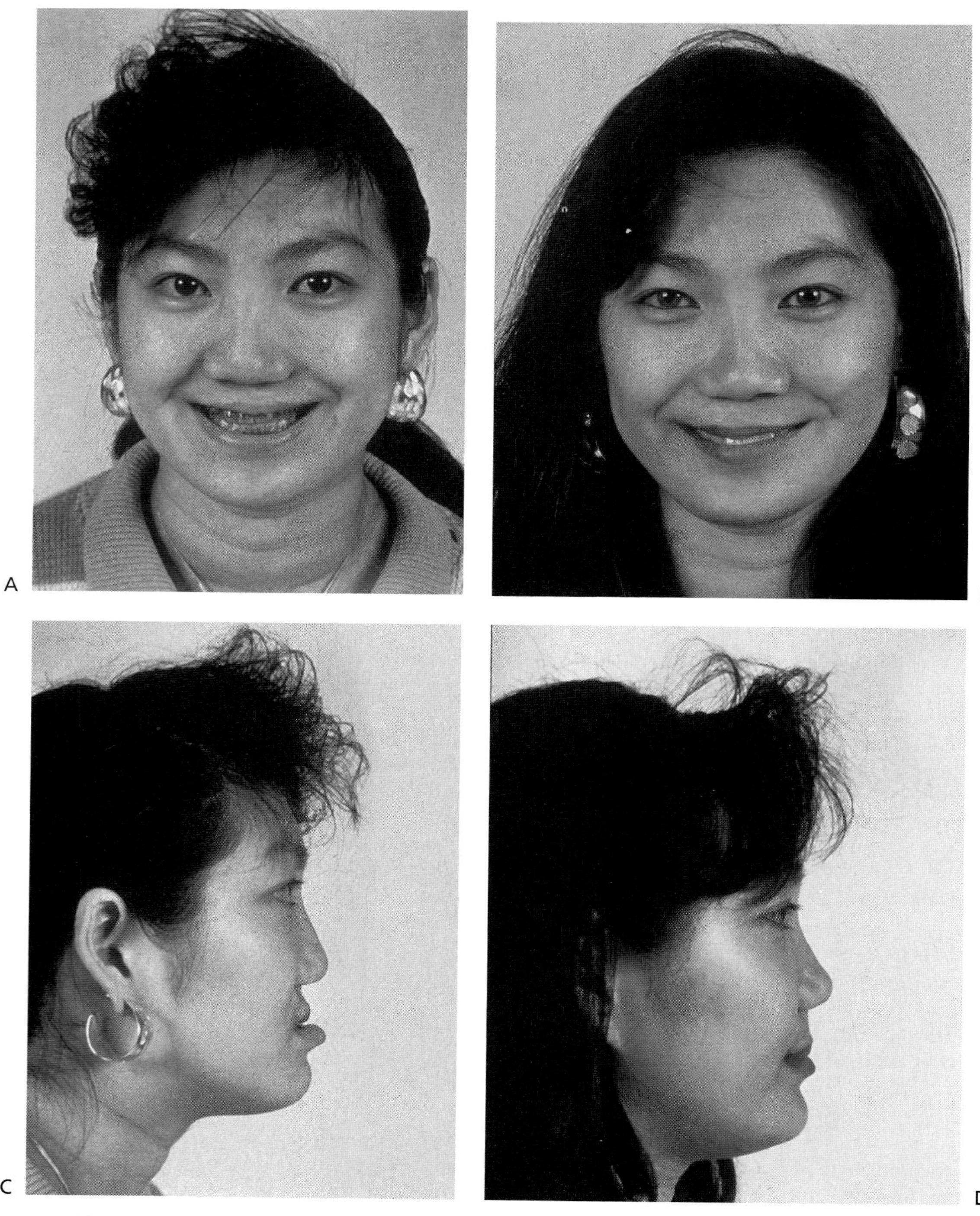

FIGURE 23D-1. A 16-year-old girl born with unilateral cleft lip and palate. She was treated by a combined orthodontic and orthognathic surgical approach, including a modified Le Fort I osteotomy in two segments (differential repositioning of the segments; correction of occlusal canting; and closure of oronasal fistula, alveolar defect, and cleft-dental gap), bilateral sagittal split osteotomies of the mandible (correction of asymmetry), and osteoplastic genioplasty (vertical reduction and horizontal advancement). Stabilization was accomplished with iliac graft and miniplate and screw fixation. **A:** Frontal view with smile before surgery. **B:** Frontal view with smile after reconstruction. **C:** Profile view before surgery. **D:** Profile view after reconstruction. *(continued)*

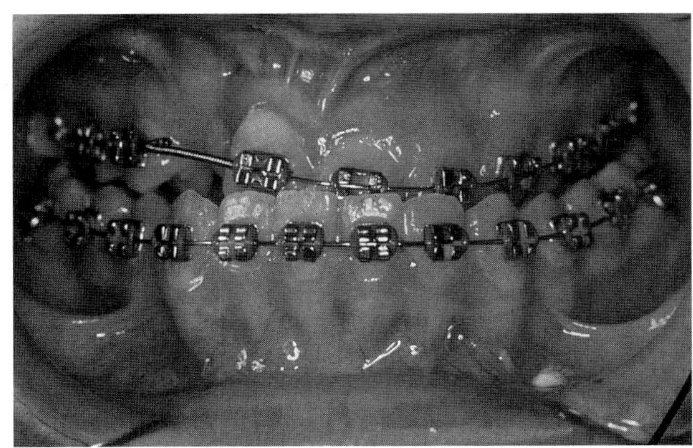
E

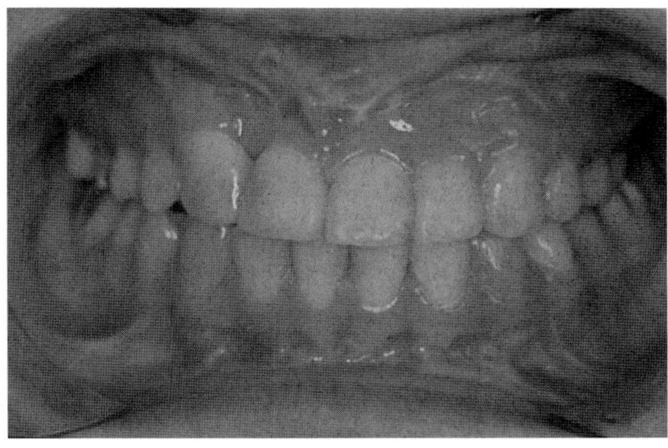
F

FIGURE 23D-1. *(Continued)* **E:** Occlusal view before surgery. **F:** Occlusal view after reconstruction. (From Posnick JC, Tompson B. Cleft-orthognathic surgery: complications and long-term results. *Plast Reconstr Surg* 1995;96:255–266, with permission.)

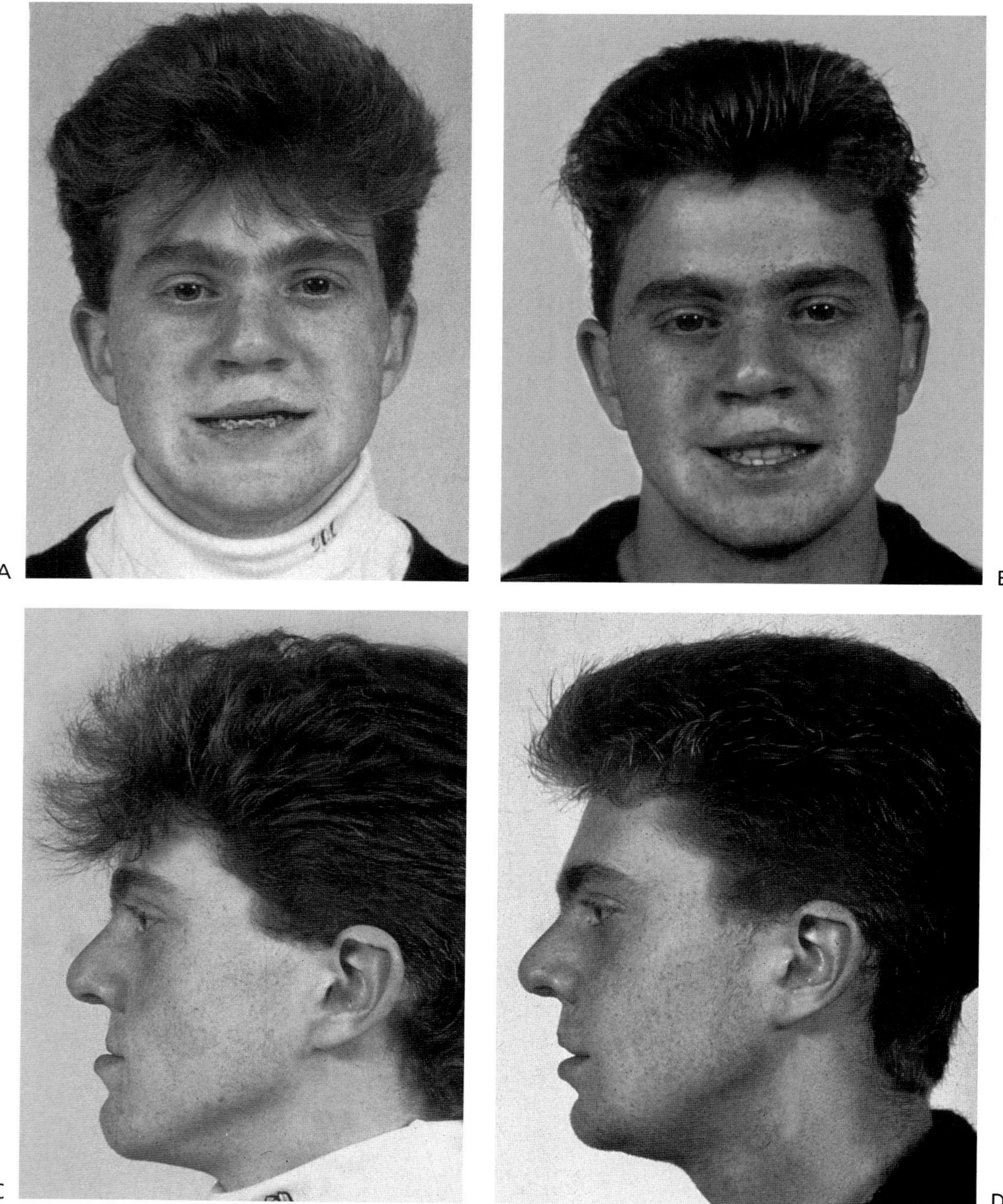

FIGURE 23D-2. An 18-year-old boy, born with bilateral cleft lip and palate, was treated by a combined orthodontic and orthognathic surgical approach, including a modified Le Fort I osteotomy in three segments (differential repositioning of the segments; closure of oronasal fistula, alveolar defects, and cleft-dental gaps; and stabilization of the premaxilla), bilateral sagittal split osteotomies of the mandible (correction of asymmetry), and an osteoplastic genioplasty (vertical reduction and horizontal advancement). Stabilization was accomplished with iliac bone graft and miniplate and screw fixation. **A:** Frontal view with smile before surgery. **B:** Frontal view with smile after reconstruction. **C:** Profile view before surgery. **D:** Profile view after reconstruction. *(continued)*

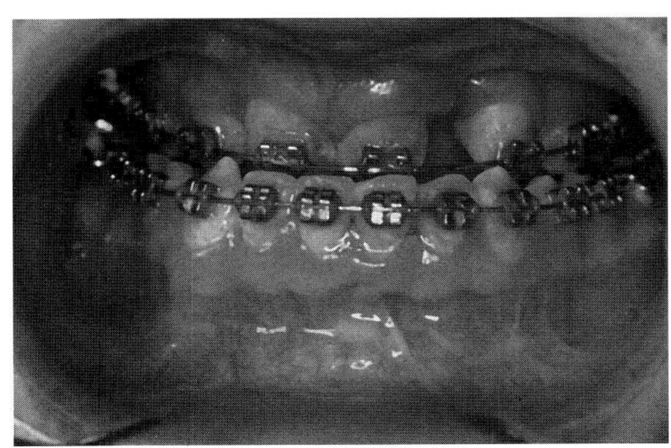
E

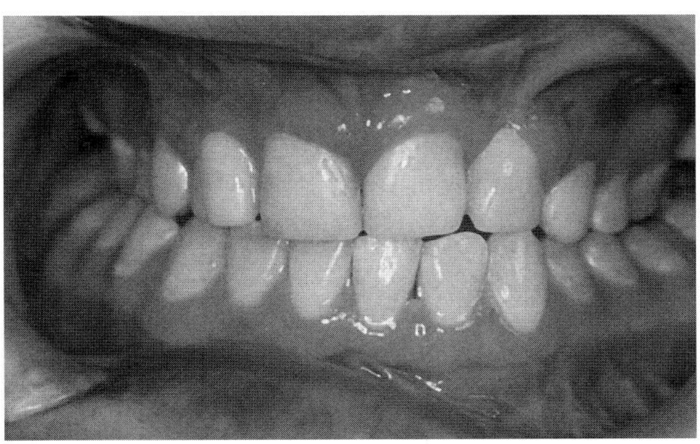
F

FIGURE 23D-2. *(Continued)* **E:** Occlusal view before surgery. **F:** Occlusal view after reconstruction. (From Posnick JC, Tompson B. Modification of the maxillary Le Fort I osteotomy in cleft-orthognathic surgery: the BCLP deformity. *J Oral Maxillofac Surg* 1993;51:2–11, with permission.)

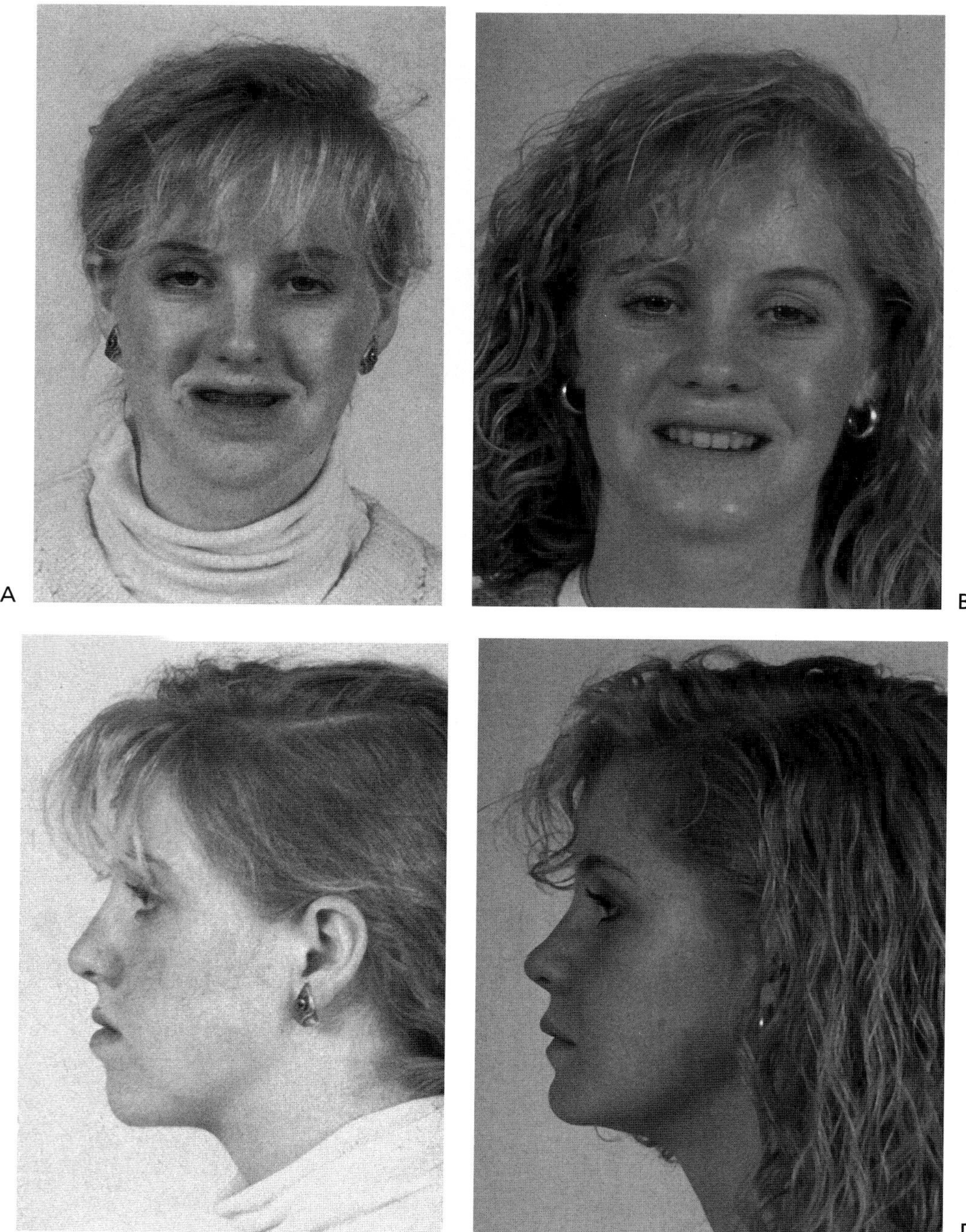

FIGURE 23D-3. A 16-year-old girl born with isolated cleft palate. She was treated by a combined orthodontic and orthognathic surgical approach, including a Le Fort I osteotomy (horizontal advancement) and an osteoplastic genioplasty (vertical reduction and horizontal advancement). Stabilization was accomplished with miniplates and screws. **A:** Frontal view with smile before surgery. **B:** Frontal view with smile after reconstruction. **C:** Profile view before surgery. **D:** Profile view after reconstruction. *(continued)*

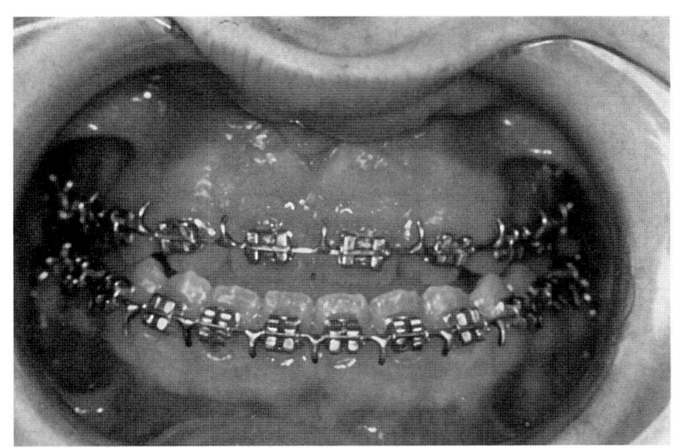
E

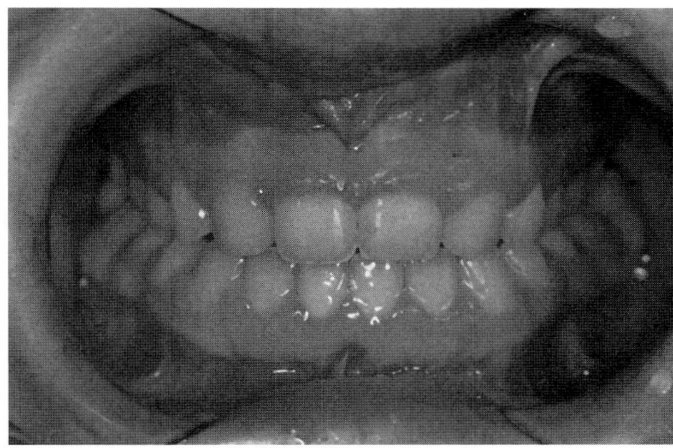
F

FIGURE 23D-3. *(Continued)* **E:** Occlusal view before surgery. **F:** Occlusal view after reconstruction. (From Posnick JC. Cleft-orthognathic surgery: the isolated cleft palate deformity. In: Posnick JC, ed. *Craniofacial and maxillofacial surgery in children and young adults.* Philadelphia: WB Saunders, 2000:951–978, with permission.)

maturity) must be made by the family only after complete disclosure consent. The decision of whether to do so by classic techniques (Figs. 23D-1 through 23D-3) or by a distraction approach should depend on the patient's overall deformities and the parents' preference. The surgeon must appreciate that the operated and anomalous maxilla cannot be expected to grow normally. Overcorrection is not likely to be adequate or precise in the long run. The surgeon should also explain to the family their child's spectrum of residual maxillofacial deformities (if any) and suggest a plan to resolve them, including alternative approaches.

CONCLUSION

The successful rehabilitation of a child born with cleft lip and palate requires close cooperation among the specialists who care for the cleft patient. Each clinician is involved at different stages of the patient's growth and development. A coordinated approach is necessary to help the child achieve ideal speech, occlusion, facial appearance, and self-esteem. Unnecessary, unproductive, and unproven interventions, whether speech therapy, orthodontic or prosthetic treatment, or surgical procedures, should be avoided because they exhaust the patient, family, and health care system, produce unfulfilled expectations, and often introduce secondary deformities that may limit the eventual success of rehabilitation. Maximizing the patient's ability to pursue and achieve personal success during their life without special regard to the original cleft lip or palate malformation is the ultimate objective.

REFERENCES

1. Polley JW, Figueroa AA. Rigid external distraction: its application in cleft maxillary deformities. *Plast Reconstr Surg* 1998;102:289–311.
2. Figueroa AA, Polley JW. Management of severe cleft maxillary deficiency with distraction osteogenesis: procedure and results. *Am J Orthod Dentofacial Orthop* 1999;115:1–12.
3. Figueroa AA, Polley JW, Ko EWC. Maxillary distraction for the management of cleft maxillary hypoplasia with a rigid external distraction system. *Semin Orthod* 1999;5:46–51.
4. Hung KF, Chen PKT, Lo LJ, et al. Alteration of the velopharyngeal functions after rigid midface distraction. *Proceedings of the International Society of Craniofacial Surgery VIIIth International Congress,* Taipei, Taiwan, November 1999, p 42(abst).
5. Chen PKT, Liou EJW, Hung KF, et al. Lengthening of hypoplastic maxilla in cleft patients using interdental distraction osteogenesis and rapid orthodontic tooth movement. *Proceedings of the International Society of Craniofacial Surgery VIIIth International Congress,* Taipei, Taiwan, November 1999, p 28(abst).
6. Liou EJW, Chen PKT, Hung KF, et al. Approximate alveolar cleft or oronasal fistula using interdental distraction osteogenesis and rapid orthodontic tooth movement. *Proceedings of the International Society of Craniofacial Surgery VIIIth International Congress,* Taipei, Taiwan, November 1999, p 29(abst).
7. Posnick JC. The staging of cleft lip and palate reconstruction: infancy through adolescence. In: Posnick JC, ed. *Craniofacial and maxillofacial surgery in children and young adults.* Philadelphia: WB Saunders, 2000:785–826.
8. Posnick JC. Cleft lip and palate: bone grafting and management of residual oro-nasal fistula. In: Posnick JC, ed. *Craniofacial and maxillofacial surgery in children and young adults.* Philadelphia: WB Saunders, 2000:827–859.
9. Posnick JC. Cleft-orthognathic surgery: the unilateral cleft lip and palate deformity. In: Posnick JC, ed. *Craniofacial and maxillofacial surgery in children and young adults.* Philadelphia: WB Saunders, 2000:860–907.
10. Posnick JC. Cleft-orthognathic surgery: the bilateral cleft lip and palate deformity. In: Posnick JC, ed. *Craniofacial and maxillofacial surgery in children and young adults.* Philadelphia: WB Saunders, 2000:908–950.
11. Posnick JC. Cleft-orthognathic surgery: the isolated cleft palate deformity. In: Posnick JC, ed. *Craniofacial and maxillofacial surgery in children and young adults.* Philadelphia: WB Saunders, 2000:951–978.
12. Posnick JC, Tompson B. Cleft-orthognathic surgery: complications and long-term results. *Plast Reconstr Surg* 1995;96: 255–266.
13. McCarthy JG, Schreiber J, Karp N, et al. Lengthening the human mandible by gradual distraction. *Plast Reconstr Surg* 1992;89:1–8.
14. McCarthy JG. Mandibular bone lengthening. *Op Tech Plast Reconstr Surg* 1994;1:99–104.
15. Polley JW, Figueroa AA, Ko W. Rigid external distraction, long-term follow-up. *Proceedings of the International Society of Craniofacial Surgery VIIIth International Congress,* Taipei, Taiwan, November 1999, p 39(abst).
16. Eskenazi LB, Schendel SA. An analysis of Le Fort I maxillary advancement in cleft lip and palate patients. *Plast Reconstr Surg* 1992;90:779–786.
17. Posnick JC, Dagys AP. Skeletal stability and relapse patterns after Le Fort I osteotomy fixed with miniplates: the unilateral cleft lip and palate deformity. *Plast Reconstr Surg* 1994;94:924–932.
18. Posnick JC, Taylor M. Skeletal stability and relapse patterns after Le Fort I osteotomy using miniplate fixation in patients with isolated cleft palate. *Plast Reconstr Surg* 1994;94:51–58.
19. Wolford LM, Cooper RL. Orthognathic surgery in the growing cleft patient and its effect on growth. American Association of Oral and Maxillofacial Surgeons Annual Scientific Sessions, Anaheim, September 1987(abst).
20. Wolford LM, Cooper RL, El Deeb M. Orthognathic surgery in the young cleft patient and the effect on growth. American Cleft Palate-Craniofacial Association Annual Meeting, St. Louis, May 1990(abst).
21. Shapiro PA, Kokich VG, Hohl TH, et al. The effects of early Le Fort I osteotomies on craniofacial growth of juvenile *Macaca nemestrina* monkeys. *Am J Orthod* 1981;79:492–499.
22. Nanda R, Sugawara J, Topazian RG. Effect of maxillary osteotomy on subsequent craniofacial growth in adolescent monkeys. *Am J Orthod* 1983;83:391–407.
23. Nanda R, Bouayad O, Topazian RG. Facial growth subsequent to Le Fort I osteotomies in adolescent monkeys. *J Oral Maxillofac Surg* 1987;45:123–136.
24. Tanne K, Nanda R, Sakuda M. Longitudinal study on craniofacial growth following Le Fort I maxillary osteotomies in adolescent monkeys. *J Osaka University Dental School* 1989;29:33–40.

24

CRANIOSYNOSTOSIS

DANIEL MARCHAC
DOMINIQUE RENIER
ERIC ARNAUD

The premature synostosis of cranial sutures is responsible for both functional and morphologic problems. The restriction of skull growth can result in an increase in intracranial pressure that is associated with mental disturbances and visual problems. The various distortions of the cranium affect the development of the forehead and orbital region; in addition, facial growth is restricted in complex cases of faciocraniosynostoses.

Traditional neurosurgical treatments—represented by more or less extensive craniectomies and elevation of bone flaps—too often resulted in a need for early reintervention to manage recurrent synostosis, with poor aesthetic effects. During the 1970s, a radically different approach was introduced by the senior authors of this chapter, in which the craniofacial principles developed by Paul Tessier (1,2) were adapted to the treatment of craniosynostosis in infants and children (3–6). This new approach has gained wide acceptance. Twenty years later, it is interesting to evaluate the early and late results of frontocranial remodeling. This chapter describes the major problems encountered during a 20-year experience (7), based on retrospective and prospective evaluations, and offers suggestions on how to treat and avoid the major problems associated with craniofacial surgery for craniosynostosis in infancy (8).

PRINCIPLES OF CRANIOSYNOSTOSIS TREATMENT

The general principle of treatment for craniosynostosis in infancy is to restore the normal anatomy by elevating, adjusting, and repositioning the distorted portion of the frontocranial area. After mobilization, the supraorbital rim and bone flaps are fixed with various techniques, including wires or plates that are either metallic or resorbable. In infants, the rapidly expanding brain promotes skull remodeling by pushing the bone forward (the floating forehead principle) (4,9) or by expanding the skull after a simple craniectomy, even if the major growth mechanism is a periosteal resorption-apposition phenomenon.

The various types of frontocranial remodeling initially described to treat the different craniosynostoses are still in use, with minor modifications (7,10). The operations are technically more complicated and require a longer operative time than the classic neurosurgical approach, and complications and unfavorable results must be evaluated.

OPERATED CASES AND FOLLOW-UP

Since 1976, the year in which the craniofacial team (D. Marchac and D. Renier) was formed in the neurosurgical department of the Hôpital Necker-Enfants Malades, 1,111 cases of nonsyndromic craniosynostosis have been operated on according to craniofacial principles, among a total of 1,563 cases examined.

The patients were followed at the craniofacial clinic and were systematically checked at regular intervals until 16 years of age. At each visit, a complete examination was performed, and the functional and morphologic problems encountered were assessed.

Regarding functional results, patients were specifically screened for mental problems (by a specialized psychological team), visual disturbances, hydrocephaly, epilepsy, occurrence of new synostoses, and recurrence of previous synostoses.

To evaluate the morphologic results, a simple scale was used based on the need for further surgical procedures, ranging from 1 (excellent) to 4 (bad).

1. Excellent (no visible anomalies or sequelae)
2. Good (minor anomalies with minor surgery optional)
3. Poor (incomplete result, revision required)
4. Bad (major deformity, no improvement)

We evaluated only the operated frontocranial area; we did not take into account any lower facial anomalies. However, other existing anomalies were assessed.

D. Marchac, D. Renier, and E. Arnaud: Craniofacial Unit, Pediatric Neurosurgical Department, Hôpital Necker-Enfants Malades, Paris, France

TABLE 24-1. OPERATIONS PERFORMED WITH MEANS OF FIXATION

CST	No. Cases	Age (y)	Surgery			Osteosynthesis				
			Forehead	Vault	Craniectomy	Not Used	Wire	Absorbable Suture	Plate	Undefined
SCA	255	0.9	100	64	91	90	45	73	—	47
TRIG	80	0.9	76	2	—	—	—	—	—	
PLG	133	1.1	131	2	—	1	116	15	—	1
BRA	61	0.9	56	4	1	3	49	7	10	
OXY	40	5.1	26	11	3	6	25	1	—	8
COM	39	9	27	11	1	3	22	7	—	7
	608									

CST, craniosynostosis; SCA, scaphocephaly; TRIG, trigonocephaly; PLG, plagiocephaly; BRA, brachycephaly; OXY, oxycephaly; COM, complex or unclassified.

RESULTS

Herein we present an analysis of 760 cases with a mean follow-up of 7.8 years. The results are summarized in Tables 24-1 through 24-6.

In Table 24-1, the type of procedure performed (fronto-orbital remodeling, vault flaps, or craniectomy) is presented, in addition to the type of osteosynthesis used. Table 24-2 shows the results of skull ossification. Altogether, the reported rate of lack of ossification after surgery for craniosynostosis was 6.8% (Fig. 24-1). The results of a prior study indicated that fixation of the fronto-orbital rim advancement with a resorbable thread may lead to an increased rate of resorption of the bony pieces, and therefore this technique is not used any longer (11). Palpation of metallic wires through the skin is common but is not a major concern because few of them need to be removed (< 3%). Some lack of ossification was noted in the oldest children or when craniectomies were performed. Metallic plates were used only in a few cases of brachycephaly (10 cases) and were abandoned because of migration.

In Table 24-3, a complete list of functional problems is presented. As expected, the poorest mental outcomes are in the cases with the highest intracranial pressures (oxycephaly and other unclassified forms) (12–15). Cases of trigonocephaly and brachycephaly, which may be inherited, have lower mental outcome scores in comparison with the others. The incidence of *de novo* synostosis (new suture affected) is particularly frequent after extended craniectomies have been performed, such as H-craniectomies for scaphocephaly, which may be associated with bicoronal synostosis (14%). The recurrence rate of craniosynostosis (i.e., an affected suture affected again; 2.1%) was higher in the group with multiple craniosynostoses (7.7%). The occurrence of neurologic problems, such as hydrocephaly, epilepsy, and visual disturbances, was sporadic in this study; the rate was, in fact, remarkably low for isolated craniosynostosis (16,17).

Morphologic evaluation according to our classification is reported in Table 24-4. In our series, no patients were given a grade of 4, which means that a significant improvement was always noted. Excellent and good results represented 94.2% of the cases; results were excellent in two-thirds of the cases. The rate of secondary surgery for morphologic reasons was low, and secondary surgery was performed mostly for minor deformities (grade 2). In 5.7% of the cases, major revision surgery had to be performed (Figs. 24-2 and 24-3). For cases of complex synostosis, the rate of unsatisfactory results was 25.7% (grade 3). In this series, patients with oxycephaly who were operated on late in life did not require major surgery for unfavorable results.

The number of patients requiring multiple procedures is presented in Table 24-5. In 8 of 608 patients evaluated,

TABLE 24-2. SKULL OSSIFICATION AFTER SURGERY FOR CRANIOSYNOSTOSIS

CST	No. Cases	Age (y)	Bony Problems		
			Lack of Ossification	Partial Resorption	Material Palpated
SCA	255	0.9	10	3	6
TRIG	80	0.9	1	1	2
PLG	133	1.1	2	8	7
BRA	61	0.9	3	6	2
OXY	40	5.1	1	1	1
COM	39	9	4	2	
	608		21 (3.4%)	21 (3.4%)	18 (3%)

CST, craniosynostosis; SCA, scaphocephaly; TRIG, trigonocephaly; PLG, plagiocephaly; BRA, brachycephaly; OXY, oxycephaly; COM, complex or unclassified.

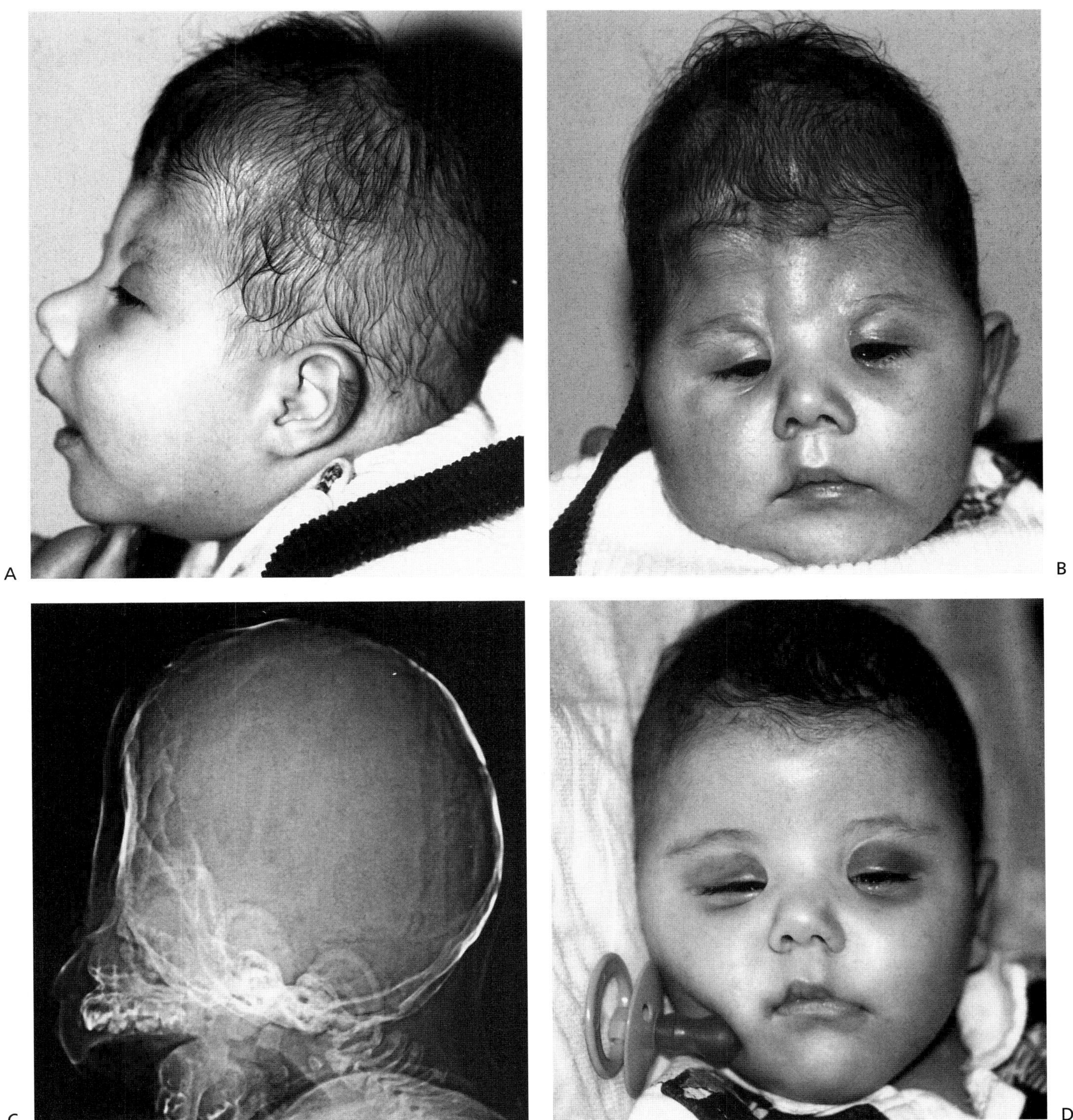

FIGURE 24-1. Lack of ossification. **A,B,C:** An infant presenting with multiple craniosynostoses (coronal and sagittal) in addition to a severely retruded forehead. *(continued)*

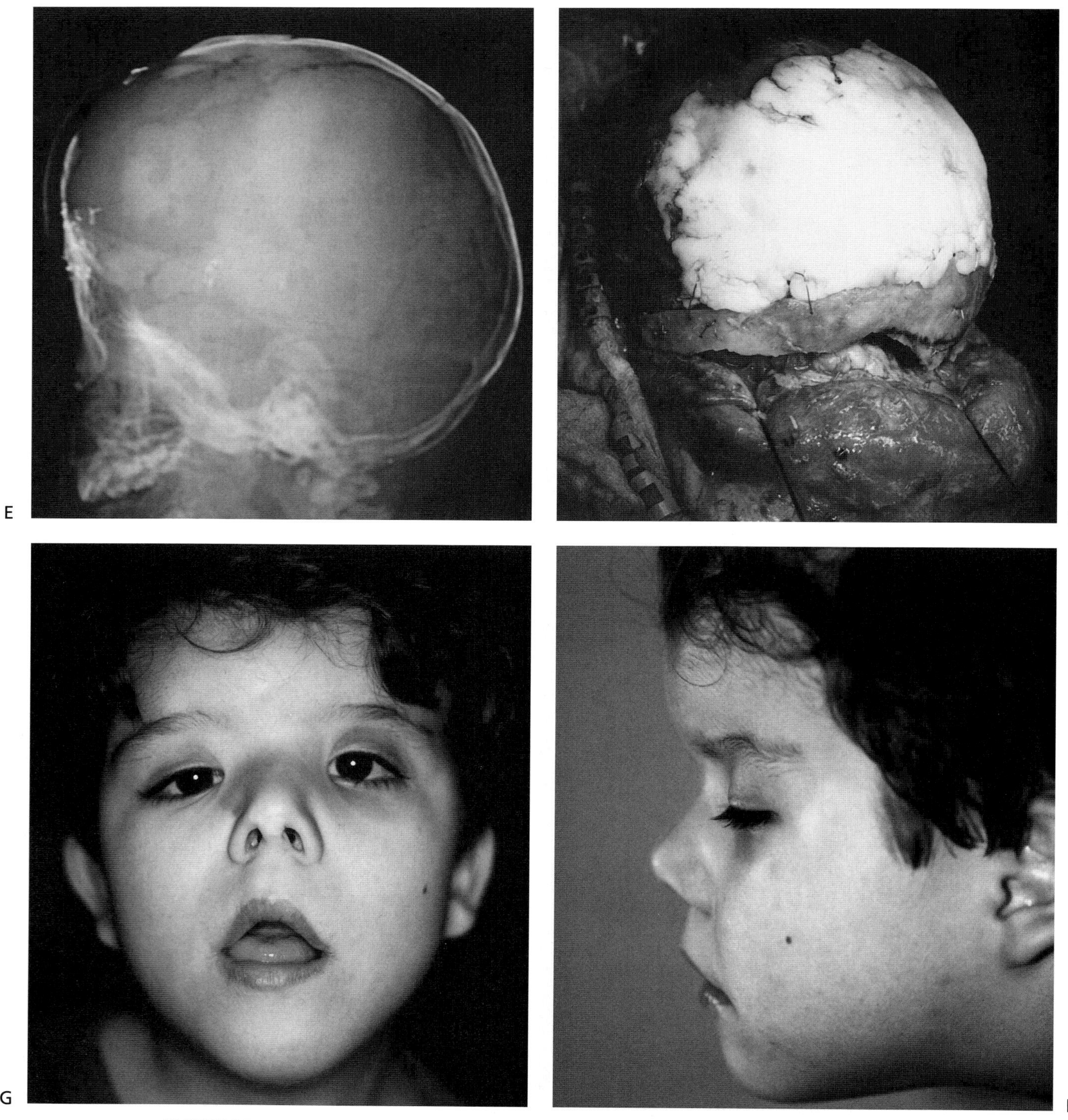

FIGURE 24-1. *Continued.* **D,E:** After frontocranial remodeling at 6 months, the shape is satisfactory but the frontal area has not reossified. **F:** A methylmethacrylate implant is placed above the supraorbital bar. **G,H:** Stable result 4 years later.

TABLE 24-3. NEUROFUNCTIONAL PROBLEMS AFTER SURGERY FOR CRANIOSYNOSTOSIS

CST	No. Cases	Follow-up (y)	Hydrocephaly	Visual Disturbances	Epilepsy	Evolutive Synostosis	Reccurrent Synostosis	Mental Outcome
SCA	255	6.1	4	1	3	36 (14%)	4	105
TRI	80	7.1	—	—	—	5 (6.2%)	2	96
PLG	133	8.1	—	2	—	—	1	104
BRA	61	8.1	1	—	1	—	2	97
OXY	40	7.1	—	2	—	—	1	88
COM	39	8.1	—	1	1	3 (7.7%)	3	96
	608					7.2%	2.1%	

CST, craniosynostosis; SCA, scaphocephaly; TRIG, trigonocephaly; PLG, plagiocephaly; BRA brachycephaly; OXY, oxycephaly; COM, complex or unclassified.

TABLE 24-4. MORPHOLOGIC EVALUATION AFTER SURGERY FOR CRANIOSYNOSTOSIS

CST	No. Cases	Follow-up (y)	Morphologic Evaluation Score[a]			
			1	2	3	4
SCA	244	6.1	190	47	7 (2.9%)	—
TRI	78	7.1	53	21	4 (5.1%)	—
PLG	133	8.1	77	49	7 (5.3%)	—
BRA	59	8.1	32	21	6 (10.2%)	—
OXY	32	7.1	26	6	—	—
COM	35	8.1	10	16	9 (25.7%)	—
	581		66.7%	27.5%	5.7%	

[a] 1, excellent; 2, good; 3, poor; 4, bad.
CST, craniosynostosis; SCA, scaphocephaly; TRIG, trigonocephaly; PLG, plagiocephaly; BRA, brachycephaly; OXY, oxycephaly; COM, complex or unclassified.

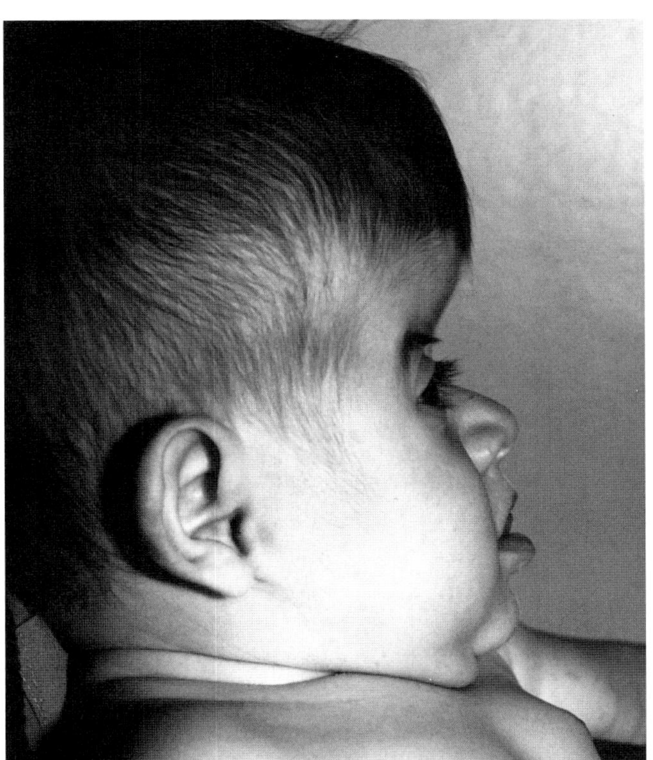
A

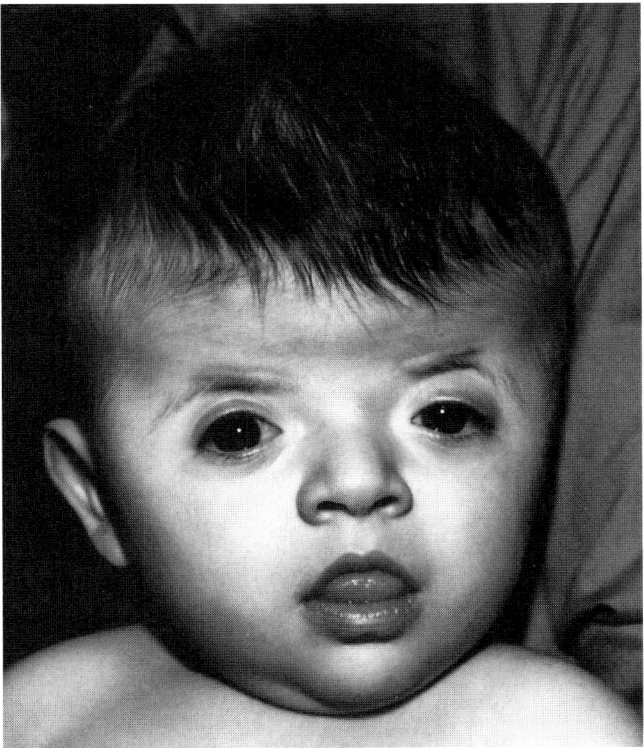
B

FIGURE 24-2. Secondary frontocranial remodeling. **A,B:** An infant presenting with a severe brachycephaly (coronal synostosis) before early frontocranial remodeling. *(continued)*

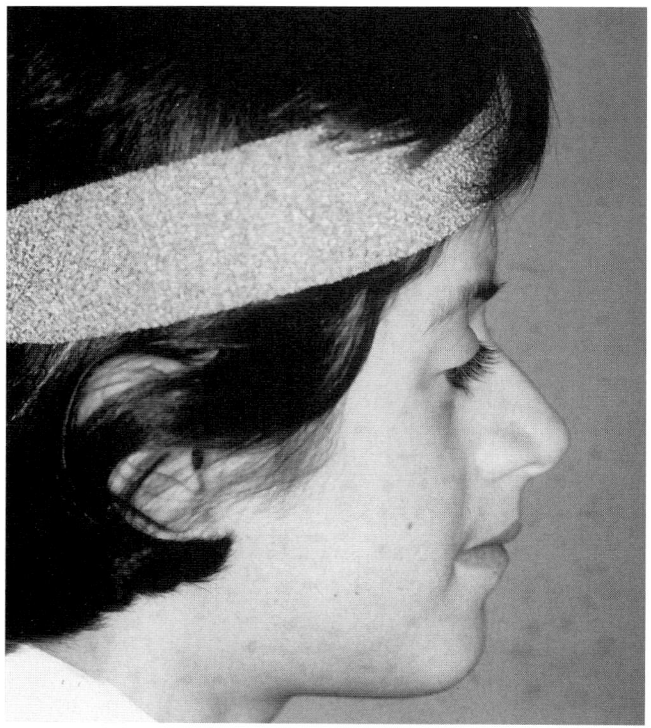

C

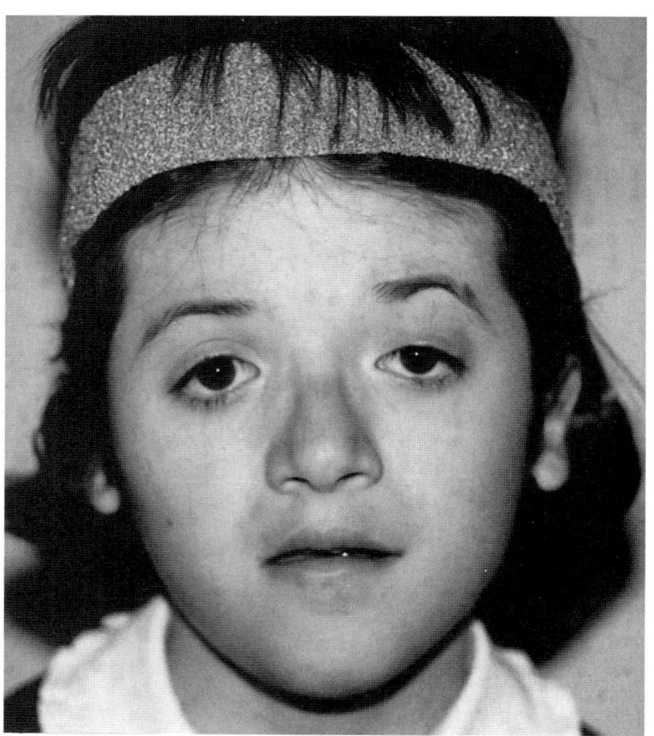

D

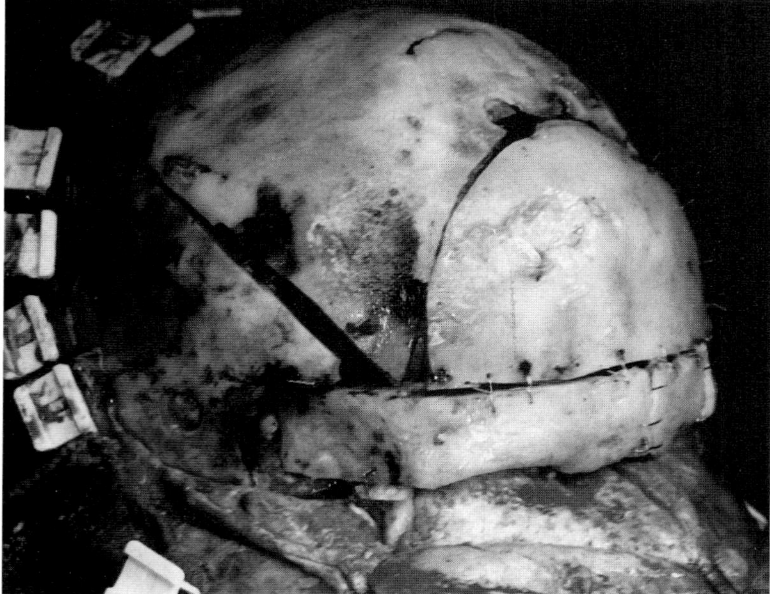

E

FIGURE 24-2. *Continued.* **C,D,E:** At 10 years of age, presenting with a retruded and flat forehead. A secondary advancement and remodeling are performed. *(continued)*

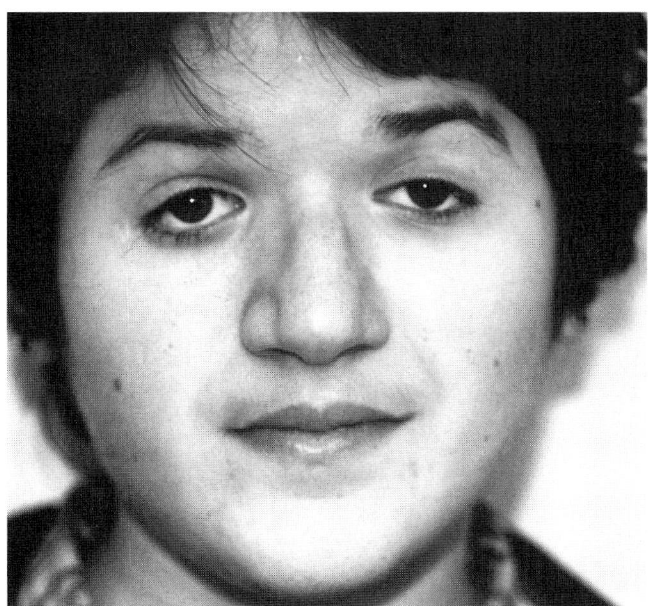

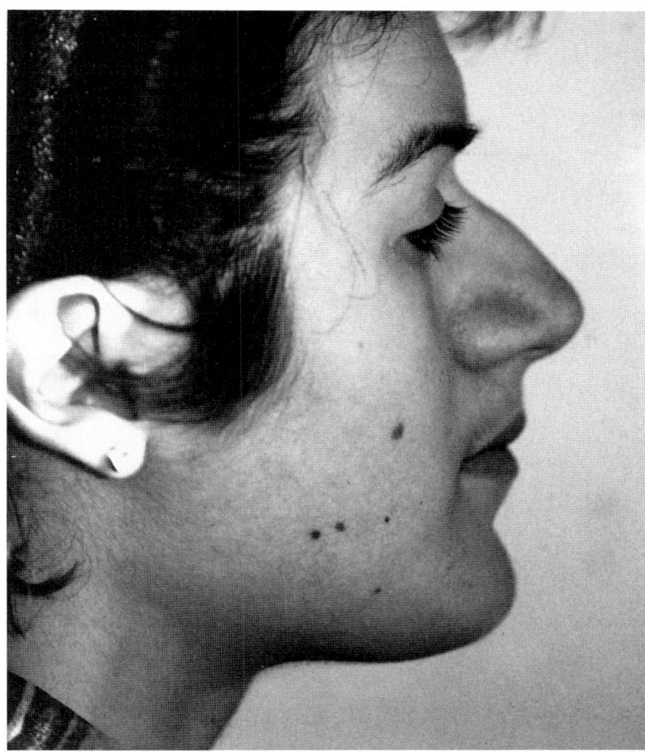

F G

FIGURE 24-2. *Continued.* **F,G:** At 15 years of age, stable result. *(continued)*

three procedures were needed; they represented 3% of the brachycephaly cases and 5% of the complex synostosis cases. In the latter, recurrence was linked to increased intracranial pressure. Among patients with all types of craniosynostosis, 7.6% had to be operated on twice. The reasons for secondary surgery are indicated in Table 24-6. The majority of these reoperations were cranioplasties, performed to fill a bony defect resulting from lack of ossification after advancement or from bony resorption. The rate of reintervention for unfavorable morphologic results was only 1.8%, and it was 2.1% for recurrence of symptoms.

Functional Problems

The recurrence of craniosynostosis or incomplete primary release of the skull was the major cause of recurrence of increased intracranial pressure (15). Standard roentgenograms usually showed the recurrence of a fingerprint pattern in the skull, which was most frequent in multiple craniosynostoses, such as in unclassified cases or cases of faciocraniosynostosis. Mental outcome was not clearly correlated with intracranial pressure. In most cases, the mental status was identical before and after surgery, and

TABLE 24-5. NUMBER OF MULTIPLE PROCEDURES FOR CORRECTION OF CRANIOSYNOSTOSIS

CST	No. Cases	Age (y)	No. Procedures		
2 3	>3				
SCA	255	11	10 (3.9%)	2 (0.7%)	—
TRIG	80	11	3 (3.7%)	—	—
PLG	133	1.1	10 (7.5%)	2 (1.5%)	—
BRA	61	11	10 (16.4%)	2 (3.3%)	—
OXY	40	5.1	2 (5%)	—	—
COM	39	9	11 (28.2%)	2 (5.1%)	—
	608		7.6%	1.3%	0

CST, craniosynostosis; SCA, scaphocephaly; TRIG, trigonocephaly; PLG, plagiocephaly; BRA, brachycephaly; OXY, oxycephaly; COM, complex or unclassified.

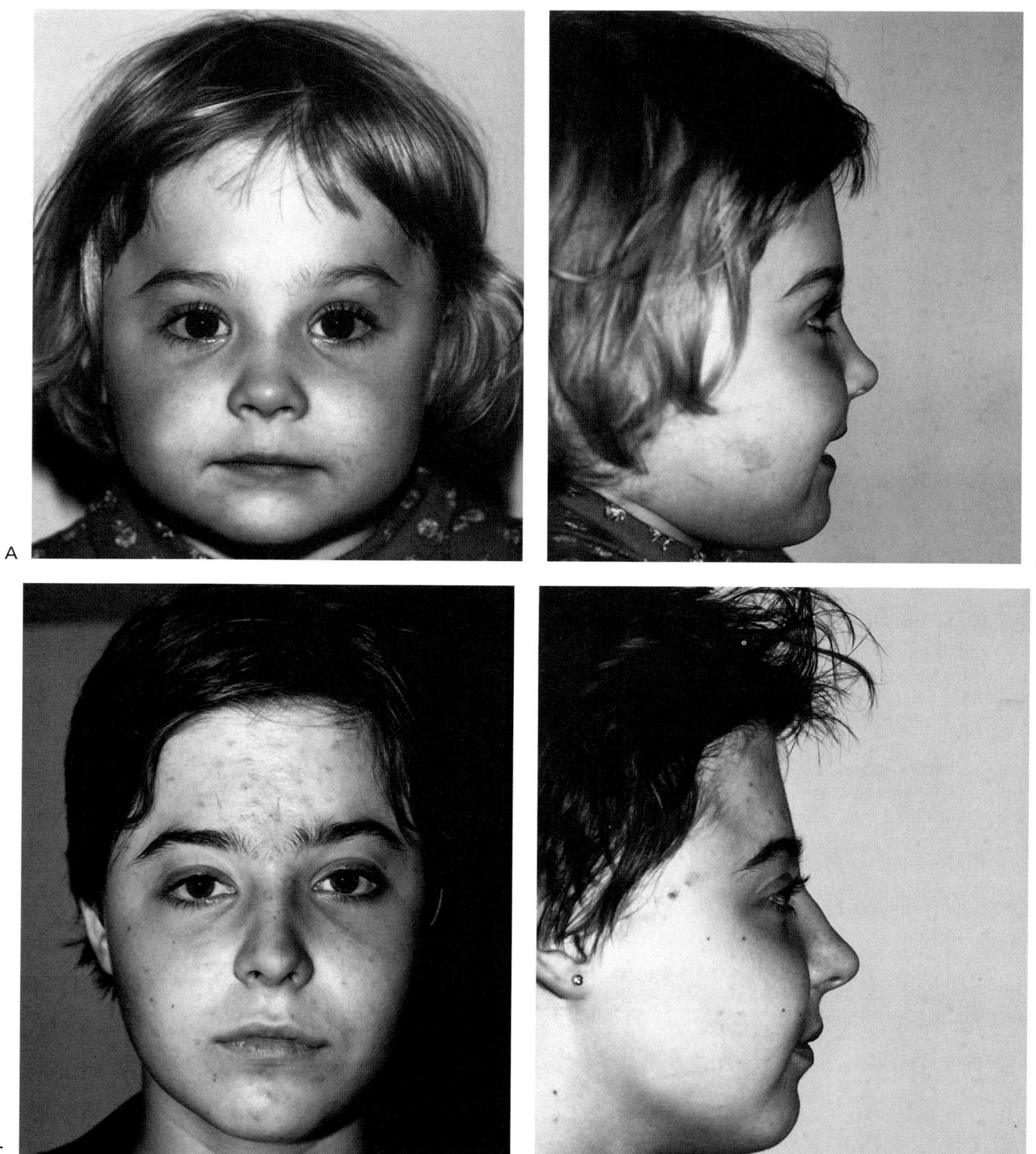

FIGURE 24-3. Secondary deformities after trigonocephaly. **A,B:** At age 2, after trigonocephaly correction at 6 months of age. **C,D:** At age 15, the forehead is slightly retruded and flat. It is also narrow at the temporal level. *(continued)*

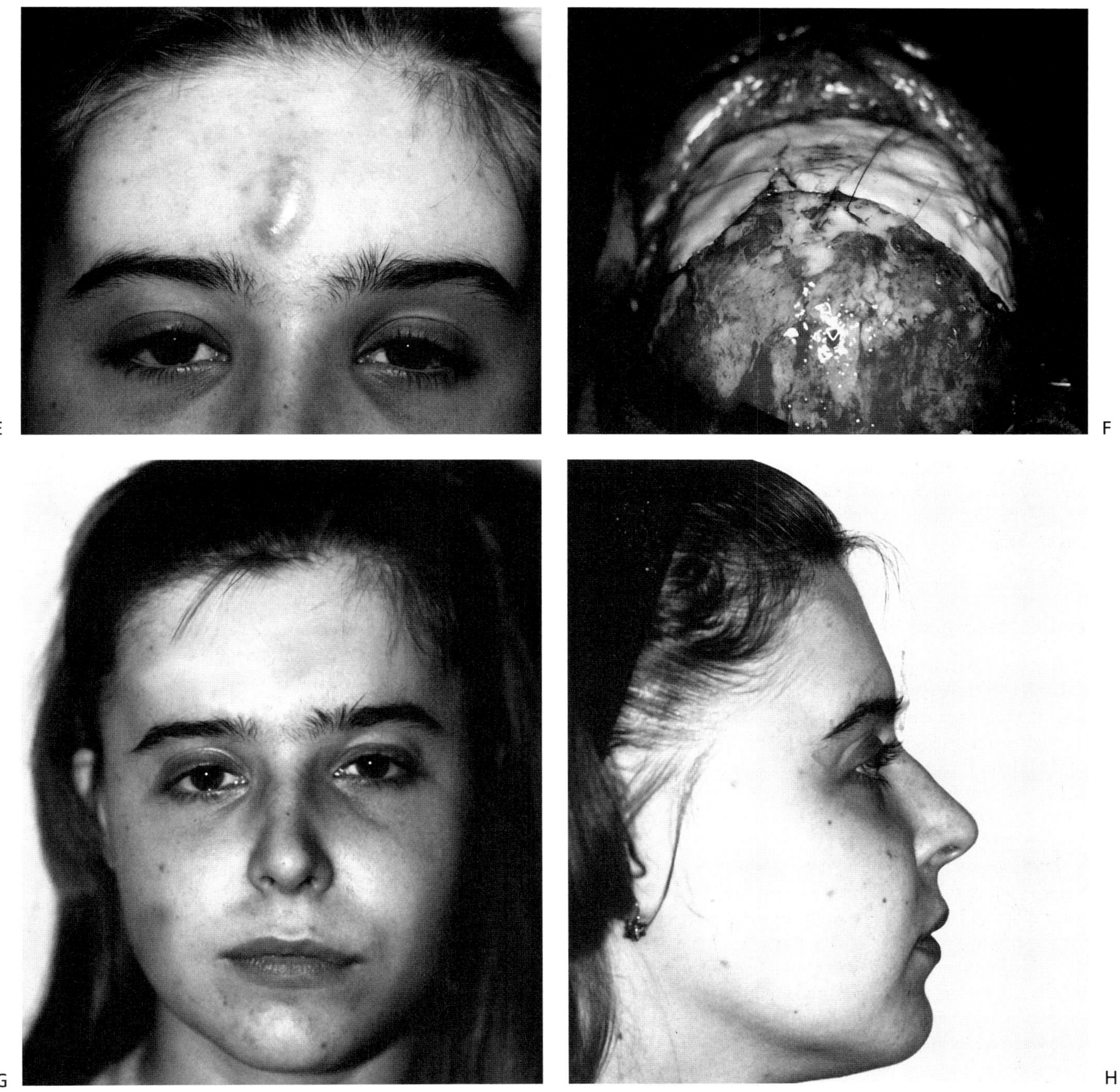

FIGURE 24-3. *Continued.* **E:** Frontal inflammation after injection of coral granules. **F:** Application of methylmethacrylate implant fixed with wires 4 years later. **G,H:** At age 22, after the frontal onlay.

early procedures appeared to prevent a deterioration of mental status. The occurrence of hydrocephaly, visual disturbances, or epilepsy was not correlated with any specific type of operation but was linked to the preoperative neurologic status (18,14,17).

The incidence of *de novo* synostosis should also be discussed. It was particularly high in scaphocephaly, in which bicoronal synostosis could appear, but this was a radiologic diagnosis without clinical relevance. An evolving synostosis following the treatment of scaphocephaly raises the question of latent faciocraniosynostosis, with no midface hypoplasia yet evidenced.

TABLE 24-6. INDICATIONS FOR SECONDARY CORRECTION IN CRANIOSYNOSTOSIS

CST	No. Cases	Age (y)	Recurrent Synostosis	Cranioplasty	Morphologically Unacceptable
SCA	255	11	4	9	1
TRIG	80	11	2	1	1
PLG	133	1.1	1	8	4
BRA	61	11	2	13	1
OXY	40	5.1	1	1	—
COM	39	9	3	6	4
	608		2.1%	6.2%	1.8%

CST, craniosynostosis; SCA, scaphocephaly; TRIG, trigonocephaly; PLG, plagiocephaly; BRA, brachycephaly; OXY, oxycephaly; COM, complex or unclassified.

Cranio-orbital Morphologic Problems

Morphologic problems can be divided into two groups: early, resulting mainly from technical mistakes or complications that it should be possible to avoid, and intermediate- and long-term, which represent the disappointing outcome of a well-performed operation (evidence of the limitations of the procedure) or an unfavorable outcome caused by external factors.

Early Unfavorable Results

Inadequate correction of a deformity can be observed immediately after surgery. It can result from an error in evaluating the required displacement of the bony structures, an asymmetrical correction, or a failure to reposition the temporal muscle. It can also be caused by a secondary displacement. This can happen if the fixation is inadequate or after trauma (in our series, one patient fell, and another sustained a blow to the forehead).

Fixation was initially obtained with wires. Miniplates provide a more stable fixation, but we were always reluctant to use them in infants, and we limited their use to fixation of the supraorbital bar in cases of brachycephaly. We quickly stopped even that practice because of observed significant migration of the miniplates. Now that absorbable miniplates are available, we should be able to obtain very stable fixation in most cases.

Lack of ossification is a second early unfavorable result. In infants, wide defects can be left open after remodeling because spontaneous reossification is usually rapid. After 2 years of age, one cannot count on spontaneous reossification, and all defects are closed with bone grafts and a mixture of bone dust and fibrin glue.

In infants, the usual reossification may not occur, or the displaced bone flaps may be resorbed; in older children, resorption of the flaps and graft failure can occur, usually after an episode of mild infection. The clinical picture is one of a small hematoma or seroma or, in some cases, just a mildly elevated temperature and some redness. The problem appears to resolve with antibiotic treatment, with or without irrigation, but in the following months, the bony defect becomes apparent; its size can vary from a few centimeters to half the cranial vault. When large defects appear, an implant must sometimes be used to protect the brain (Fig. 24-1).

Intermediate- and Long-term Unfavorable Results

Even when results after the first year appear favorable, with a normal or nearly normal appearance, a deterioration can develop during craniofacial growth. The supraorbital bar can appear retruded, sometimes asymmetrically. The frontal bone can become tilted backward or appear a little narrow. Irregularities may also appear on the forehead (Fig. 24-2).

Depression of the temporal fossae is frequent in our se-

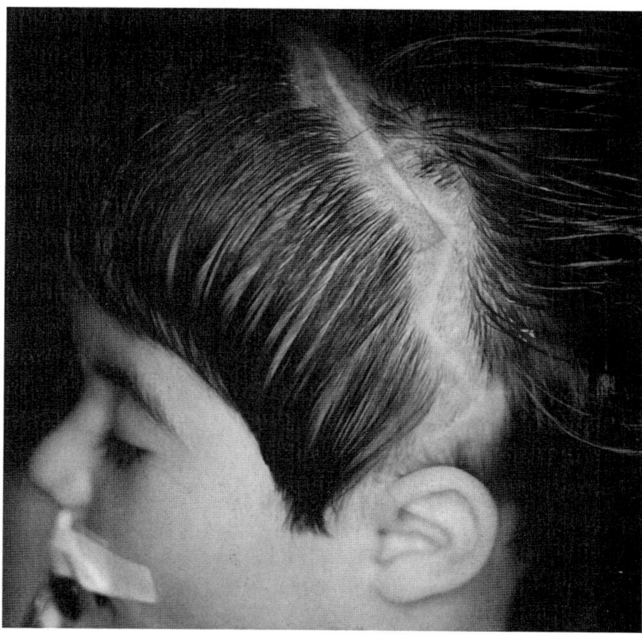

FIGURE 24-4. A zigzag scar in the temporal area is much less visible than a linear scar.

ries of fronto-orbital advancements for plagiocephaly (unilateral) or trigonocephaly (bilateral) (Fig. 24-3).

Orbital asymmetry is possible in cases of major plagiocephaly but is seen especially in complex cases of asymmetry in which several sutures are fused, including the coronal suture. In these complex cases, the synostoses are more likely to recur.

Finally, a widening of the coronal scar is frequent. It is all the more visible when a linear coronal approach has been used, which is what we did until a few years ago. We now use a zigzag incision in the temporal areas, which allows the scar to be hidden more satisfactorily (Fig. 24-4).

TREATMENT

Although the treatment of complications and unfavorable results of craniofacial surgery is highly complex and should be individualized for each patient, we arbitrarily divide complications into short- and intermediate-term complications and late complications.

Short- and Intermediate-term Complications

- Functional problem with normal shape
- Functional problem with abnormal shape
- Minor morphologic problems
- Lack of ossification of the skull—cranial defects

Functional Problem with Normal Shape

If after fronto-orbital remodeling the morphologic status is satisfactory but the intracranial pressure is increased, a limited decompressive craniectomy is indicated; the elevation of two parietal flaps (one on each side) is a simple option to decrease the intracranial pressure. In some instances, especially complex craniosynostoses, decompressive surgery is indicated more than once. The treatment of hydrocephalus by valve derivation is sometimes necessary.

Functional Problem with Abnormal Shape

In cases of both increased intracranial pressure and a morphologic problem, major corrective surgery may be indicated. This may involve reshaping of the fronto-orbital region and expansion of the cranial vault. The best fixation is achieved with miniplates and screws, preferably absorbable plates in younger patients.

Minor Morphologic Problems

According to the significance of the supraorbital bar retrusion, a slight readvancement of the supraorbital bar or an external remodeling can be performed. Sometimes, irregularities of the vault also have to be corrected by remodeling.

Lack of Ossification of the Skull—Cranial Defects

When a small bony defect is observed after frontocranial remodeling for craniosynostosis, one first waits to see if any spontaneous reossification occurs. In infants, one waits until 2 years of age, eventually protecting the brain with a helmet if the defect is large and the child active.

In older children (up to the age of 4 years), if the defect is small, one also waits at least 1 year because spontaneous reossification sometimes occurs.

Cranioplasty is considered only when one is certain that ossification will not occur, except in some exceptional cases in which the extent of the defect or difficulties in follow-up leads one to operate earlier.

The ideal repair is with autologous bone, but its availability is limited in infants and young children.

Before the age of 2 years, spontaneous reossification of the skull can normally be expected. If the frontal remodeling for craniosynostosis has been followed by a bone defect—usually in the laterofrontal areas—because of a mild infection or another incident, it is perfectly logical to repair the defects. Eventually, the entire upper forehead may have to be reconstructed with a bone graft taken from posterior areas untouched during the first operation. The posterior area can be left open and reossifies.

After 2 years of age, one can harvest a moderate-sized (e.g., 6 × 4 cm) fragment of the skull to repair the defect. The donor area is filled with bone fragments and bone dust mixed with fibrin glue, and reossification usually occurs satisfactorily.

The ideal situation is to split the calvarium. It is sometimes possible to do this in a child more than 4 years old, but one usually has to wait until 10 to 12 years of age to be able to split the calvarium. One therefore cannot take a graft from the vault if a significant defect has to be reconstructed.

The harvesting of several ribs or of iliac bone can be considered, but scars and morbidity can be significant factors, and the supply is limited in children. We prefer to use other materials in this situation.

Like others, we have utilized homografts of the cranial vault, obtained from bone resection or cadavers. They were irradiated before use. Despite a certain but limited number of favorable outcomes, we have abandoned this technique because the number of cases in which progressive resorption occurred was much too high.

In the future, bone substitutes may be useful (18), but for the present, we utilize implants.

Titanium plates have been used on a few occasions, but we have been using methylmethacrylate implants routinely for the past 20 years. If the adjustment and immobilization are perfect (we fix them with embedded wires), tolerance of these implants has been remarkably good in our series.

In young children, we use implants in two circumstances: (a) for a defect of limited size if bone splitting is not possible; and (b) in a very large defect, even in infants, when protection of the brain seems necessary, as a temporary measure until autologous bone becomes available (Fig. 24-1).

The optimal thickness of the implant should be taken into account when cranioplasties are performed with methylmethacrylate. A thickness of 3 to 4 mm is best; if the implant is thinner than that, the piece will be fragile and unable to resist trauma; if it is too thick, exothermia during curing and closure of the scalp can be difficult. With perfect immobilization, the success rate with these implants is very high (90%).

Late Deformities

Frontocranial Problems

Minor Defects

A moderate depression of the temporal fossae may be noted, or a slight recession of parts of the forehead or supraorbital rim.

It seems tempting to correct these minor deformities with a minor procedure, and for several years we injected coral granules with a syringe through a very short incision placed in the hairline. Coral granules are equivalent to hydroxyapatite granules. We had some initially satisfactory results (19), but these deteriorated with time, and inflammation and infection developed in some cases (Figs. 24-3E and 24-5).

At present, we prefer to reopen the coronal scar and correct the contour anomaly under direct vision. One often has to perform some burring of the bone when placing an implant. Our favorite implant material is methylmethacrylate, molded *in situ* and securely immobilized by embedded wires or screws (Fig. 24-3F).

Besides the bony contour, the position of the eyebrows and lateral canthi can benefit from a revision.

In plagiocephaly, the nose can deviate toward the affected side. A classic rhinoplasty can be sufficient to correct this in moderate cases, but sometimes a paranasal osteotomy is necessary to reposition a deviated nasal root on the midline.

Significant Frontocranial Anomalies

When the frontocranial shape is not satisfactory after growth is complete, an evaluation of the scope of the required correction is made. High-quality imaging, with computed tomography and three-dimensional reformatting, is very helpful in analyzing the intracranial status, sinuses, and bony defects and irregularities (20–22).

If a forehead remodeling seems advisable, with elevation of a frontal flap and the supraorbital bar, the risks associated with this reoperation should be evaluated with the neurosurgeons (Fig. 24-2).

If it seems better to avoid an intracranial operation, an onlay implant can be considered, combined with burring of any irregularities. Sometimes, an excessively developed frontal sinus leads to a fairly noticeable contour deformity and correction is required (Fig. 24-6). The methylmethacrylate implants are carefully molded to produce the desired contour and are immobilized as well as possible with embedded wires or screws.

If the deformity is significant and the patient has no history of intracranial problems, a complete remodeling is performed, according to the same original principles, by elevation and repositioning of the frontocranial bone segment in the proper position. Adherences and small bony defects make the reoperation more demanding than the initial operation, but the difficulty of this secondary procedure is very much linked to the quality of the first operation. When the first operation has been well executed, the secondary operation is usually performed without significant problems because all the anatomical elements are in place.

On the other hand, when the first operation has not been performed according to the craniofacial principles of careful handling and reconstruction, secondary repair can be difficult and even dangerous because numerous dural tears are then difficult to avoid. This is the reason why Tessier used to advise neurosurgeons to avoid touching the supraorbital bar during the primary treatment of craniosynostosis (8,23,24).

During the secondary operation, the frontal sinus is often opened. The portion of the sinus included in the supraorbital bar is cranialized, with removal of the posterior bone and the mucosa. The mucosa of the lower nasal section is pushed down, and a bone graft closes the sinus, like a roof (Fig. 24-6).

Temporal Deformities

Unfortunately, we have quite frequently observed temporal deformities in the long-term follow-up of patients who have undergone frontocranial remodeling for craniosynostosis. We correct these now with an onlay of methylmethacrylate (Fig. 24-3).

Orbital Asymmetry

If orbital asymmetry is minor, affecting only the supraorbital rim, it is corrected as described above. If an actual dystopia is present, in which one entire orbit is higher than the other, as in some severe cases of plagiocephaly, an *en bloc* displacement of the affected orbit should be considered. Usually, this procedure involves lowering the orbit on the affected side; lowering the roof is combined with an intracranial approach and resection of a segment of the malar bone and maxilla.

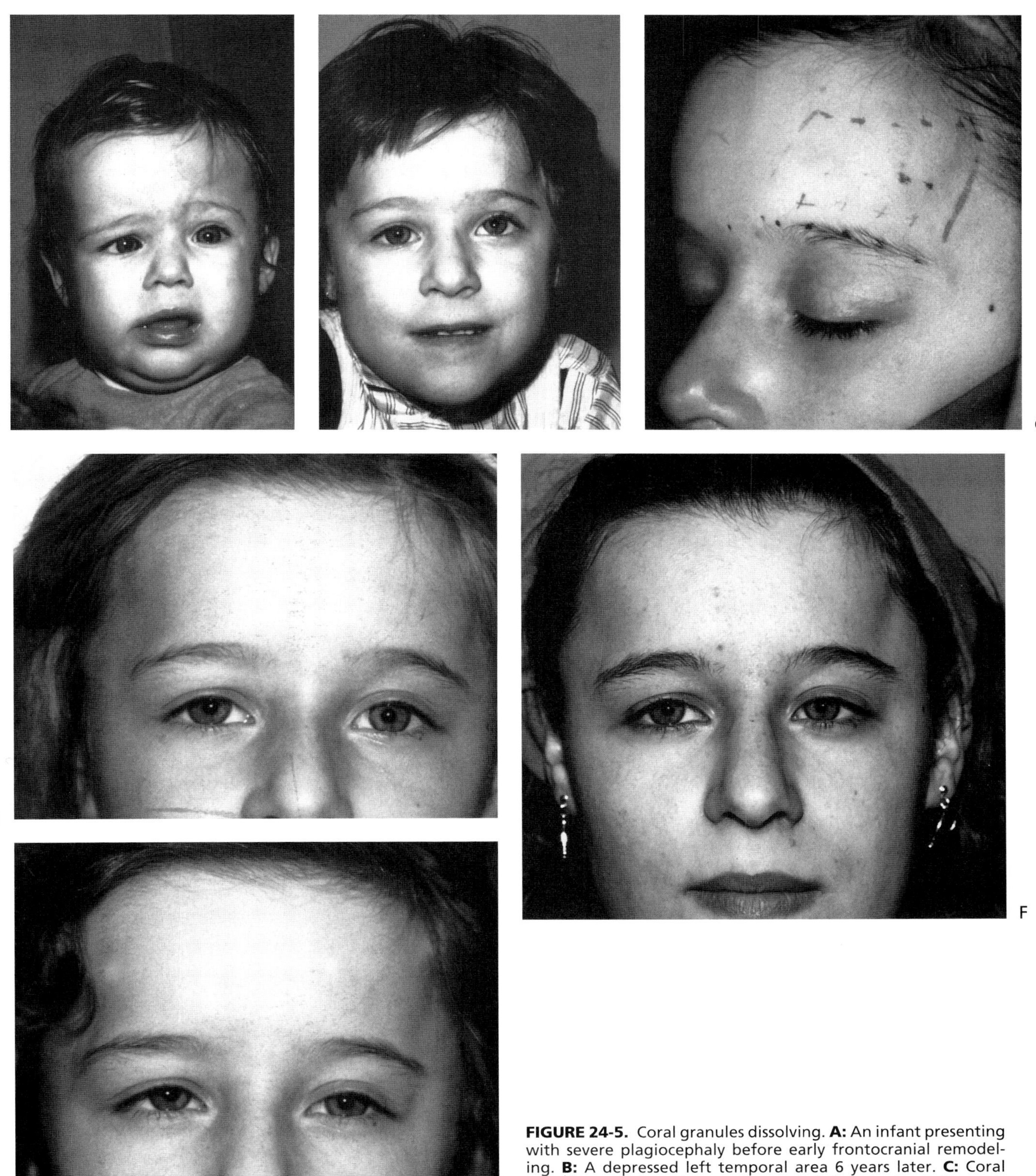

FIGURE 24-5. Coral granules dissolving. **A:** An infant presenting with severe plagiocephaly before early frontocranial remodeling. **B:** A depressed left temporal area 6 years later. **C:** Coral granules are injected. **D:** At 3-month follow-up. **E:** At 6-month follow-up. **F:** Recurrence of the depression 3 years after injection.

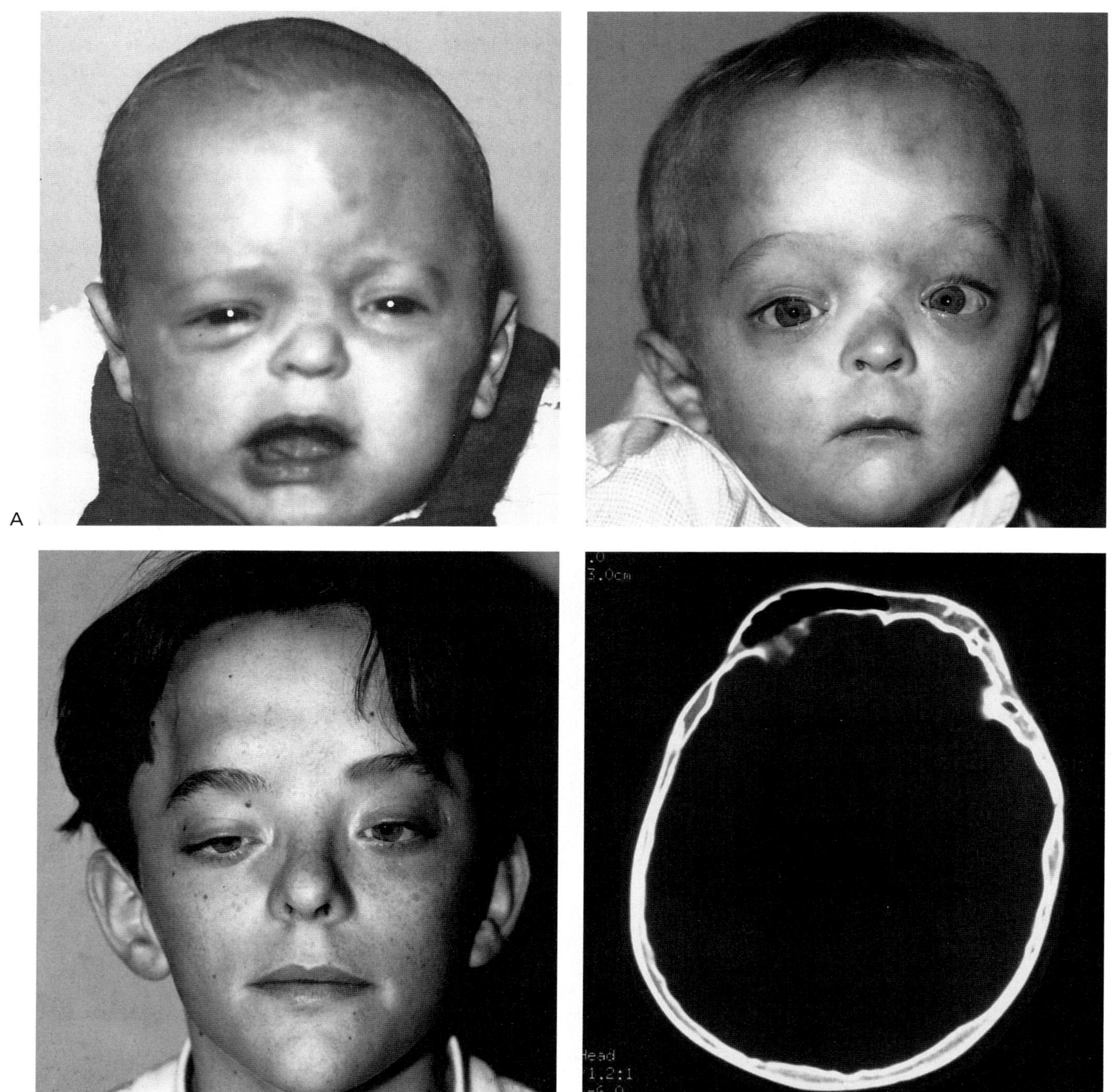

FIGURE 24-6. Frontal sinus development. **A:** An infant presenting with severe plagiocephaly (synostosis of the left coronal suture). **B:** At 1 year of age, after early frontocranial remodeling. **C:** At age 15, the forehead is very irregular. **D:** Roentgenogram showing overdevelopment of the frontal sinus. *(continued)*

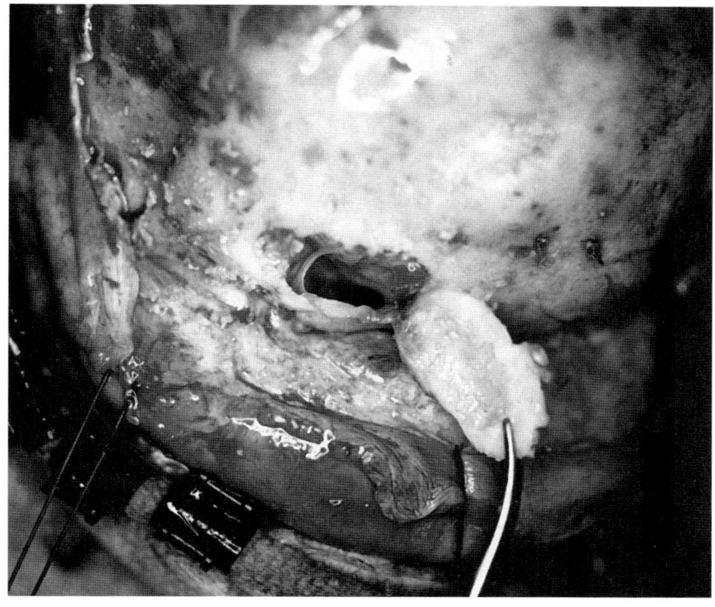
E

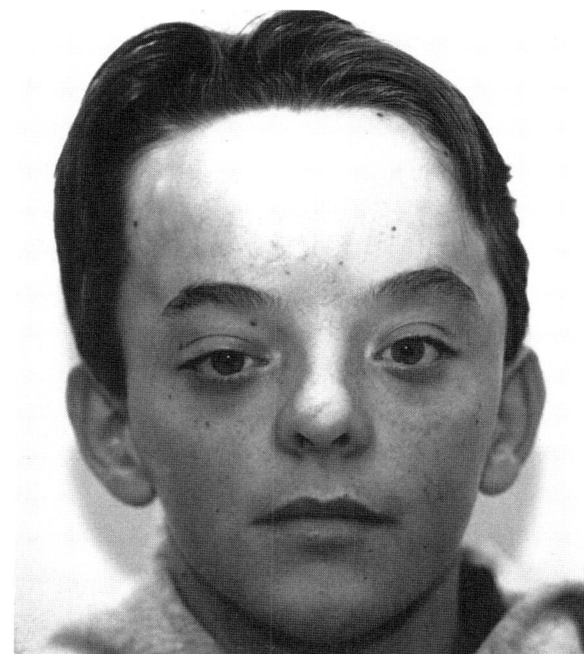
G

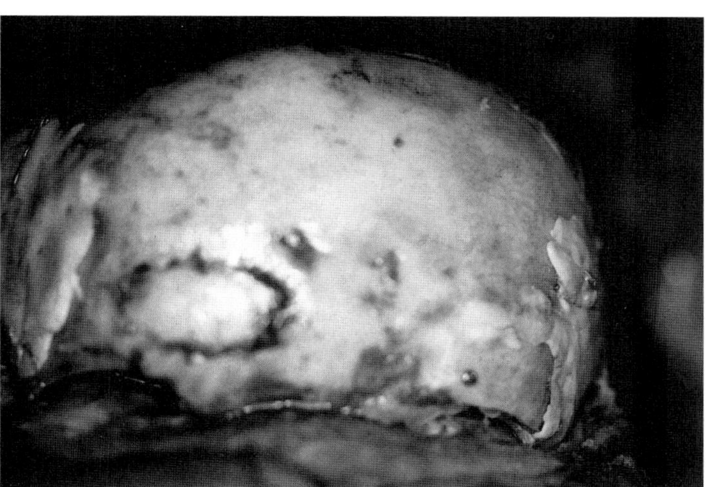
F

FIGURE 24-6. *Continued.* **E,F:** Retropositioning of the anterior wall of the frontal sinus and implant apposition. **G:** After correction.

Canthopexies

A lateral canthopexy is frequently necessary. It can be performed through a coronal approach if that approach has been used, or through a palpebral approach if the problem is limited. Freeing of the septal insertions of the lower orbital rim and fixation of the lateral canthal tissues to the inner side of the lateral orbital rim in a higher position with nonabsorbable sutures is very effective.

Ptosis

Unilateral and occasionally bilateral ptosis can be observed. The location of the supraorbital rim must be evaluated first. If it is recessed, it must be corrected because a recessed supraorbital rim can be responsible for ptosis.

When the levator is functional, a transpalpebral shortening is our operation of choice. When the levator is nonfunctional, suspension to the frontalis muscle with temporal aponeurosis or fascia lata grafts or lowering of the frontal muscle is performed.

Coronal Scars

A coronal scar can be visible through short hair, even if it is not very wide. If enlarged, the scar is of course still more evident, especially when the hair is wet.

In cases of laxity, revision can be performed by excision, which is followed by careful approximation after undermining. One should be careful to incise parallel to the hair follicles. If no laxity is present, a skin expander can be utilized,

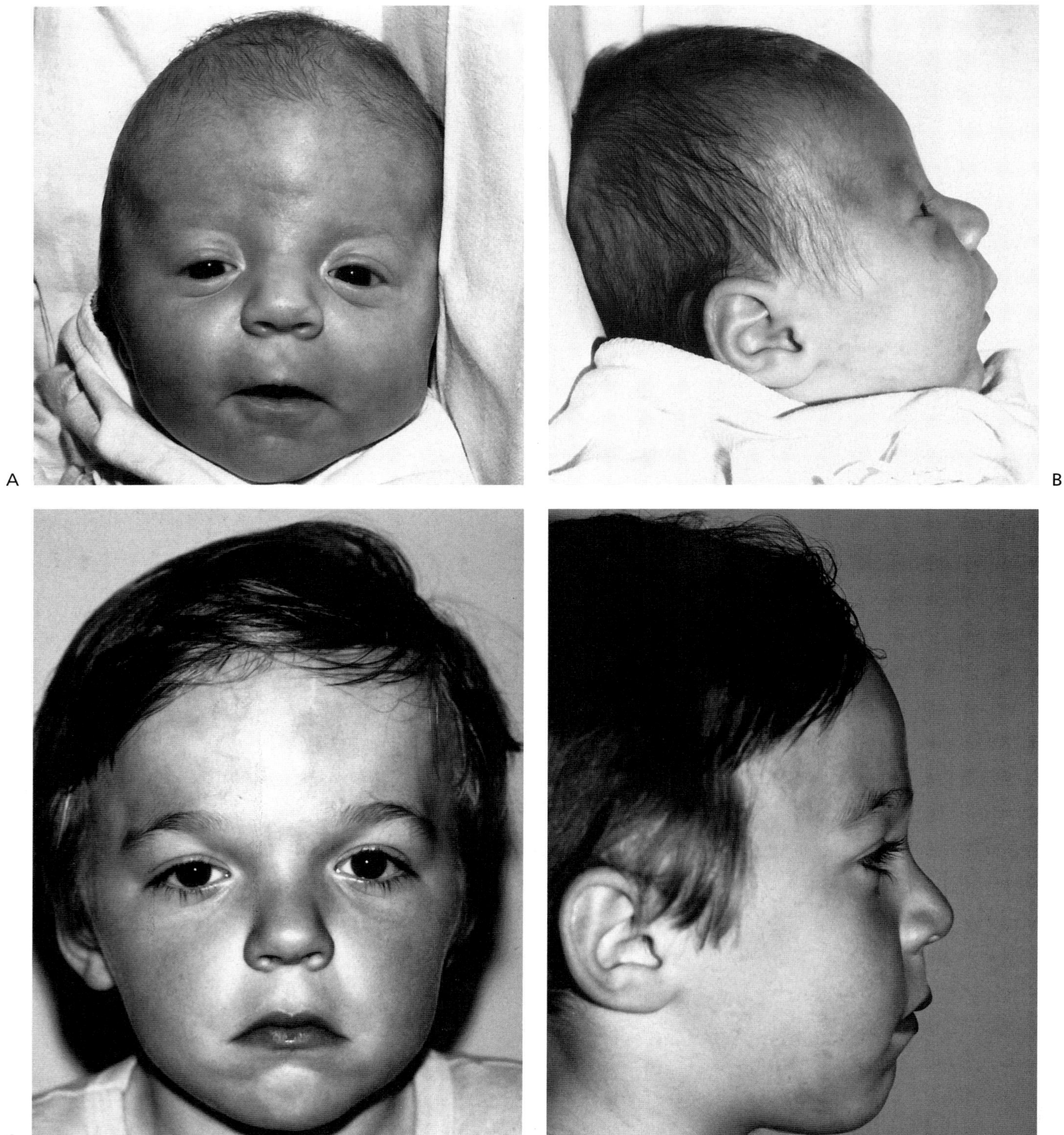

FIGURE 24-7. Final revisions. **A,B:** An infant presenting with brachycephaly. **C,D:** At 4 years of age, the result is satisfactory. *(continued)*

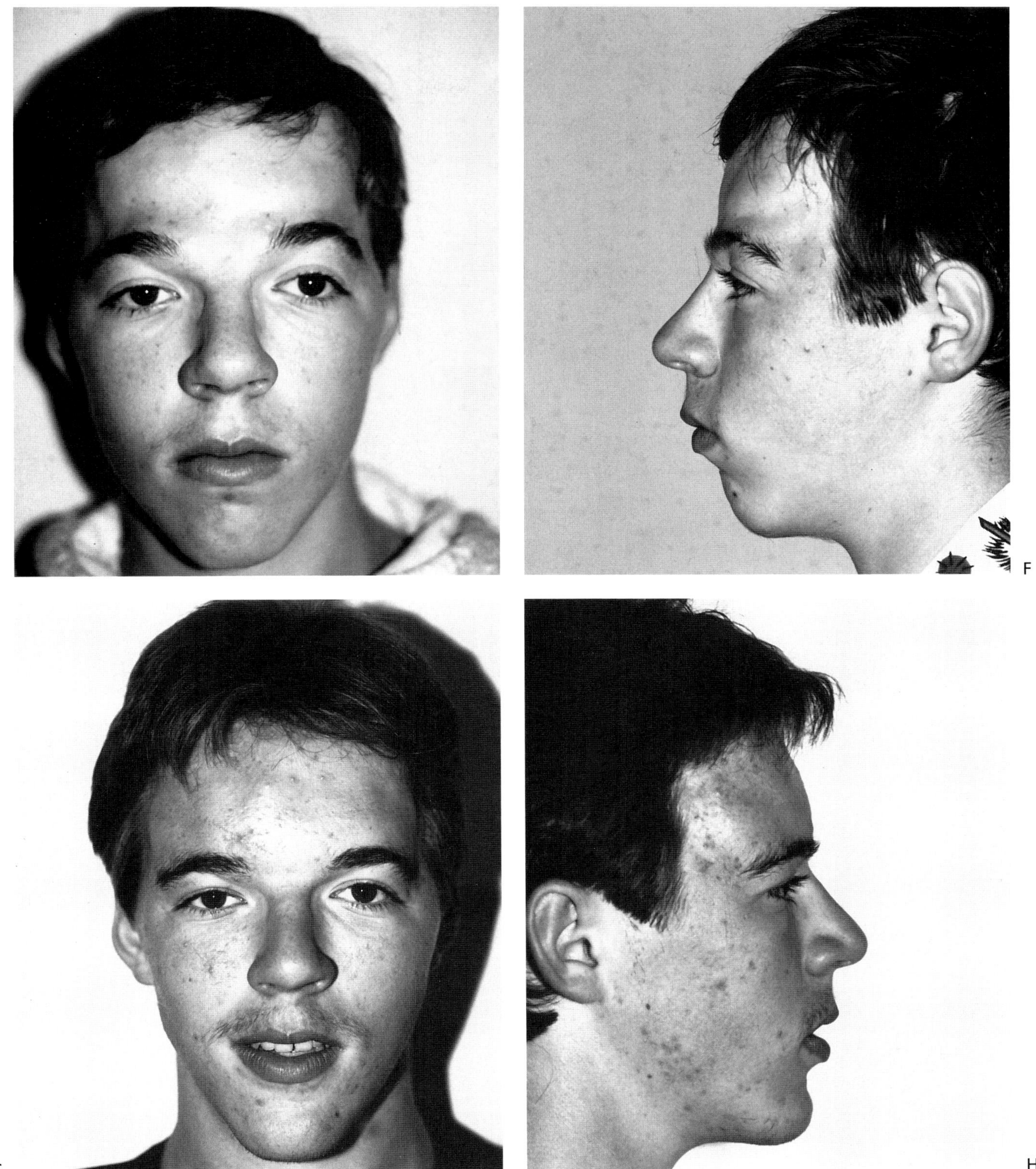

FIGURE 24-7. *Continued.* **E,F:** At 15 years of age, the forehead is slightly retruded and irregular. **G,H:** After frontal methylmethacrylate implant, rhinoplasty, and genioplasty.

which also makes it possible to perform several plasties, especially at the temporal level (Fig. 24-4).

Other Procedures

At adolescence, when facial growth is complete, an evaluation of facial harmony is performed by the craniofacial team.

Besides revision of the frontal area, discussed above, rhinoplasty, genioplasty, or an orthognathic operation may be proposed to obtain the best possible final result (Fig. 24-7).

AVOIDANCE OF PROBLEMS

Surgical treatment of craniosynostoses should be performed by a trained team. Neurosurgeons, who formerly treated craniosynostoses with older techniques, are less familiar than

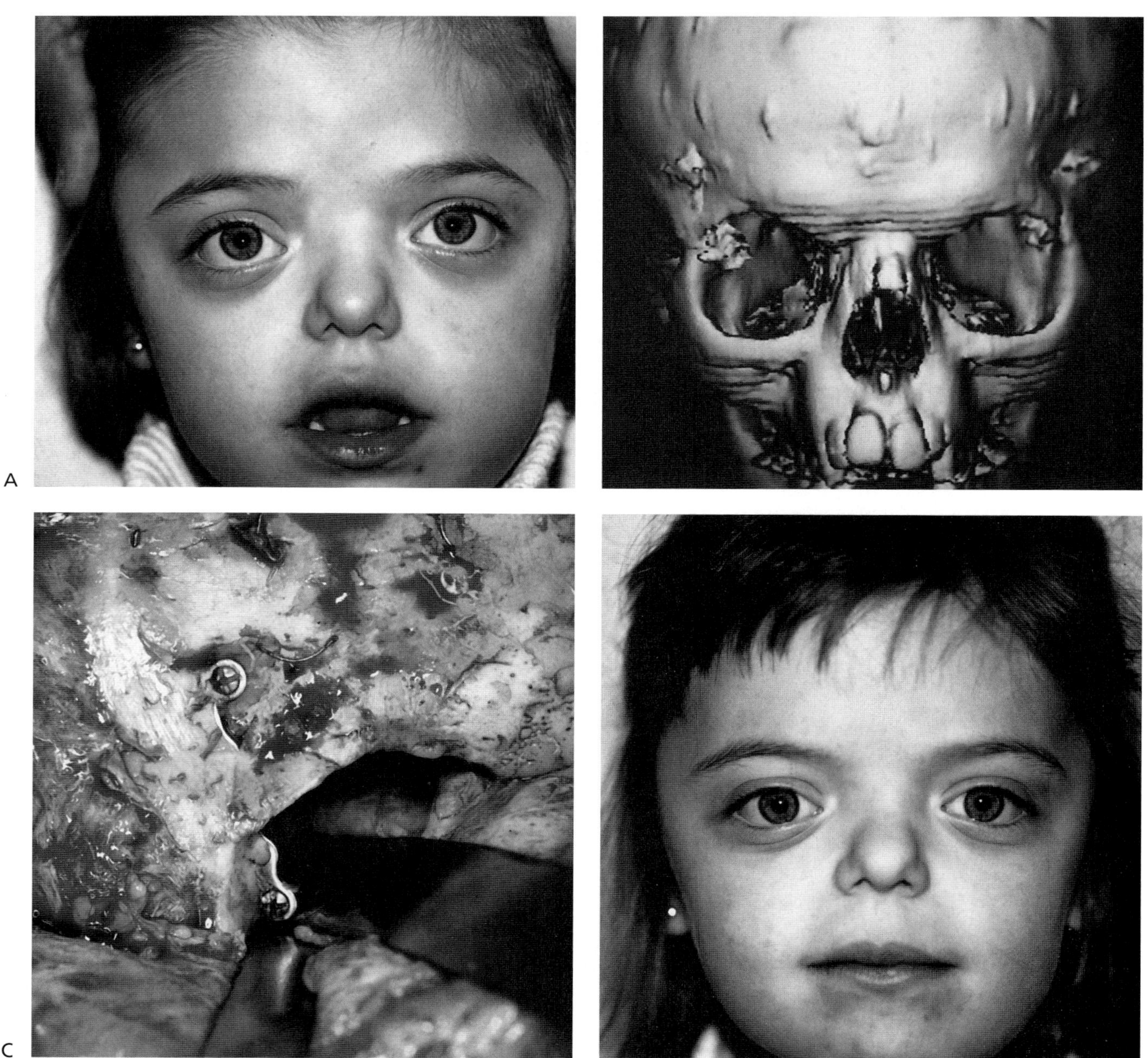

FIGURE 24-8. Migration of miniplates. **A:** A 6-year-old girl presenting with right exophthalmos. She underwent an early correction of brachycephaly, including fixation with miniplates. **B:** The three-dimensional reformatting shows an anomaly of the right orbit. **C:** The miniplate has migrated intraorbitally. **D:** After removal of the miniplate.

plastic surgeons with shape evaluation and bone remodeling. Plastic surgeons trained in craniofacial surgery do not have the neurosurgical knowledge and skills required for brain surgery. Therefore, we strongly recommend the association of a craniofacial plastic surgeon and a pediatric neurosurgeon to treat patients as safely and effectively as possible (24). A pediatric anesthesiologist is, of course, mandatory.

Good imaging with computed tomography and three-dimensional reformatting is useful to evaluate the deformity and plan the surgical treatment. In exceptional cases, a plastic model derived from the computed tomogram can be used to plan the repair.

Surgical techniques are now well-known, with variations by different teams. The principle is always to reconstruct a normal anatomy *as far as possible.*

Strict asepsis should be practiced during surgery, with complete separation of the midface, nostrils, and mouth from the intracranial field.

The incision of the skin should be carefully planned to avoid a visible coronal scar, as follows:

- In the temporal area, the incision is zigzagged to avoid a vertical segment (Fig. 24-4).
- The incision is first made with a classic scalpel perpendicular to the hair shafts, and cauterization with the fine Colorado tip is used only at a deeper level to avoid damaging the hair follicles.
- The periosteum is carefully preserved and the temporal muscle elevated along with the periosteum.
- The remodeling and rearrangement of bony pieces are tailored to each individual case according to the surgical evaluation. Fixation in the proper position is of paramount importance, especially in cases of advancement or corrections of asymmetry. We use steel wires routinely. Metallic miniplates are to be avoided in infants because they migrate during the resorption-apposition process (Fig. 24-8). Absorbable miniplates provide excellent stability and appear to be a satisfactory solution to the fixation problem in infants and young children, provided that follow-up in large series indicates good resorption without an inflammatory reaction.
- Antibiotic therapy is not routinely prescribed in isolated craniosynostosis. It is given only if a risk factor for infection is present.
- Dressings should be carefully applied. Special care should be taken to avoid excessive pressure in the reconstructed areas.
- Careful follow-up during the first postoperative week is mandatory, with particular care taken to detect any fever and collections of blood or fluid.

CONCLUSION

During a follow-up of more than 20 years, the results of applying craniofacial principles to the primary and secondary treatment of craniosynostosis have been evaluated. Satisfactory functional and morphologic results have been achieved in a large majority of operated patients (94.2%), in whom significant revision has not been required.

Further improvement in techniques should increase this percentage in the future.

REFERENCES

1. Tessier P. Ostéotomies totales de la face. Syndrome de Crouzon, syndrome d'Apert, oxycéphalies, turricéphalies. *Ann Chir Plast* 1967;12:273.
2. Tessier P. Relationship of craniostenoses to craniofacial dysostoses and to faciostenosis. *Plast Reconstr Surg*1971;48:224–237.
3. Marchac D, Cophignon J, Van der Meulen J, et al. À propos des ostéotomies d'avancement du crâne et de la face. *Ann Chir Plast* 1974;19:311–323.
4. Marchac D, Renier D. Le front flottant, traitement précoce des faciocraniosynostoses. *Ann Chir Plast* 1979;24:121–126.
5. Marchac D, Renier D. *Craniofacial surgery for craniosynostosis.* Boston: Little, Brown and Company, 1982.
6. Marchac D, Renier D. Treatment of craniosynostosis in infancy. *Clin Plast Surg* 1987;14:61–72.
7. Marchac D, Renier D, Broumand S. Timing of treatment for craniosynostosis and faciocraniosynostosis: a 20-year experience. *Br J Plast Surg* 1994;47:211–222.
8. Whitaker LA, Munro IR, Salyer K, et al. Combined report of problems and complications in 793 craniofacial operations. *Plast Reconstr Surg* 1979;64:198–203.
9. Marchac D, Renier D, Jones B. Experience with the floating forehead. *Br J Plast Surg* 1987;41:1–15.
10. McCarthy JG, Epstein F, Sadove M, et al. Early surgery for craniofacial synostosis: an eight-year experience. *Plast Reconstr Surg* 1984;73:521–530.
11. Prévot M, Renier D, Marchac D. Lack of ossification after cranioplasty for craniosynostosis: a review of relevant factors in 592 consecutive patients. *J Craniofac Surg* 1993;4:247–254.
12. Renier D, Sainte-Rose C, Marchac D, et al. Intracranial pressure in craniosynostosis. *J Neurosurg* 1982;57:370–377.
13. Arnaud E, Renier D, Marchac D. Prognosis for mental function in scaphocephaly. *J Neurosurg* 1995;83:476–479.
14. Bottero L, Lajeunie E, Arnaud E, et al. Functional outcome after surgery for trigonocephaly. *Plast Reconstr Surg* 1998;102: 952–958.
15. Gault DT, Renier D, Marchac D, et al. Intracranial pressure and intracranial volume in children with craniosynostosis. *Plast Reconstr Surg* 1992;90:377–381.
16. Cinalli G, Kollar E, Sainte-Rose C, et al. Hydrocephalus and craniosynostosis. In: Marchac D, ed. *Craniofacial surgery.* Bologna, Italy: Monduzzi, 1996:101–104.
17. Dollfus L, Vinikoff L, Renier D, et al. Insidious craniosynostosis and chronic papilledema in childhood. *Am J Ophthalmol* 1996;122:910–911.
18. Arnaud E, Molina F, Mendoza M, et al. Bone substitute in defects of the cephalic skeleton: preliminary reports of a clinical trial. In: Marchac D, ed. *Proceedings of the Sixth Congress of the International Society of Craniofacial Surgery.* Bologna, Italy: Monduzzi, 1996:19–20.
19. Marchac D, Sandor G. Use of coral granules in the craniofacial skeleton. *J Craniofacial Surg* 1994;5:213–217.
20. Arnaud E, Renier D, Marchac D. The development of the frontal sinus after frontocranial remodeling for craniosynostosis in infancy. *J Craniofac Surg* 1994;5:1–12.
21. Arnaud E, Renier D, Marchac D. The glabellar morphology after

frontocranial remodeling for craniosynostosis in infancy. *J Craniofac Surg* 1994;5:13–18.
22. Marchac D, Renier D, Arnaud E. Evaluation of the effect of early mobilization of the supraorbital bar on the frontal sinus and frontal growth. *Plast Reconstr Surg* 1995;5:802–811.
23. Marchac D, Renier D, Guerrero P. Lethal complications after craniofacial surgery. In: Marchac D, ed. *Proceedings of the Sixth Congress of the International Society of Craniofacial Surgery.* Bologna, Italy: Monduzzi, 1996:225–230.
24. Tessier P. The scope and principles, dangers and limitations and the need for special training in orbitocranial surgery. In: Hueston JT, ed. *Transactions of the Fifth International Congress of Plastic and Reconstructive Surgery,* Melbourne, Australia, 1971. Boston: Butterworth-Heineman, 1971:903–929.

Discussion

CRANIOSYNOSTOSIS

JOHN A. PERSING

Drs. Marchac, Renier, and Arnaud are members of an experienced and innovative craniofacial team that has been responsible for a number of advances in the understanding and management of children with craniosynostosis. They have developed successful techniques that are used throughout the world today, and they also regularly evaluate the results of their efforts.

Begun at the most superficial aspects of the cranium and extended inward, zigzag coronal incisions to expose the surface of the skull do appear to be less noticeable in the temporal region. This is true not necessarily because the scar is any narrower than in a vertically oriented (coronal) incision, but because the obliquely oriented pattern of the hair shafts is more likely to camouflage the scar by overlapping rather than paralleling it.

On entering the skull, one might be able to reduce some of the negative effects of periorbital congenital anomaly by adhering to the principles used in trauma surgery. Specifically, in patients with orbital-nasal-ethmoid fractures, one does not elevate the medial canthus from the bone to reduce the fracture. This practice consistently leads to a rounding out of the medial canthus (or telecanthus) by reducing the strength of the attachment of the medial canthus to bone, even with suture refixation of the tendon. Similarly, a temporal depression after a frontal orbital craniotomy may be the result of a reduced adherence to bone of the temporalis muscle, whose contraction force is certainly much greater than that of the orbicularis muscle for the medial canthal tendon detachment. We now believe that postoperative temporal hollowing following orbital rim advancement can be obviated by elevating the squamous portion of the temporal bone with its overlying temporalis muscle as a single unit. In this way, the strong attachments to the bone are maintained so that detachment of the muscle postoperatively and depression in this area are minimized (1).

J. A. Persing: Department of Plastic Surgery, Yale University School of Medicine, New Haven, Connecticut; and Department of Plastic Surgery, Yale-New Haven Hospital, New Haven Connecticut

The more complex the cranial deformity, the more comprehensive the treatment approach often must be. For instance, we use the technique pioneered by Marchac and Renier (2,3) for patients with a late presentation of sagittal synostosis. Whole-vault cranioplasty regularly gives the best results for them. We dissect in a supraperiosteal plane, as do the authors, to reduce blood loss and maintain the bone segment orientation provided by the adherence of periosteum to bone. This practice shortens operative time and increases the quality of results. Our goal is to normalize the skull shape as much as possible and to release the restriction to growth at the fused suture. We refrain from using metallic fixation plates in infancy because, as has been noted (4), plates translocate internally during subsequent growth of the skull. The rigid profile of these plates may produce a future health risk to children in whom they have been placed, at least conceptually. However, current reviews of the incidence of complications as a result of plate migration have not shown any increase in seizures, brain injury, or death related to them (4). Long-term observation of patients who have received metallic fixation plates and screws in infancy will be necessary to determine whether these devices ultimately should be removed.

It should be noted also that although the authors describe

the use of wires when stable fixation is required, the Yale craniofacial team uses wires only for *temporary* fixation in younger children. Wires migrate internally at about the same rate as the metallic plates (4). Therefore, our goal is to try to avoid the use of permanent metallic materials in the fixation of an infant's skull altogether. Once the skull bone is stabilized, intraoperatively, a bioabsorbable plate system is used to fix the bone and replace the wire.

In performing craniotomies for various forms of craniosynostosis, as the authors report, the surgeon must tailor the approach to each individual patient. No one approach is uniformly successful in all patients. However, we have been able to reduce the likelihood of reoperation, particularly in patients with bilateral coronal synostosis [in which the authors have noted their greatest percentage of unsatisfactory results (10%) and reoperative procedures (16%)], by using a more comprehensive approach than fronto-orbital advancement alone. Because much of the residual deformity associated with an incompletely corrected bilateral coronal synostosis patient is related to inadequate lengthening of the anterior posterior axis of the skull and inadequate reduction of the height of the skull, an approach that simultaneously achieves both goals in infancy is desirable. With use of the modified prone position (5), the barrel stave osteotomy or whole-vault approach (6,7) has been more successful in the hands of our team (Figs. 24D-1 and 24D-2). To achieve the best results, we believe that a wide range of remodeling of skull bone should be combined with an *active* reduction of the abnormally long dimension of the skull. In bilateral coronal synostosis, it is the vertical dimension that needs to be reduced. In sagittal synostosis, the abnormally long dimension is the anteroposterior axis of the skull. This approach was initially used in patients with sagittal synostosis by Jane et al. (8) in the π procedure. We use modifications of this procedure today (3,9).

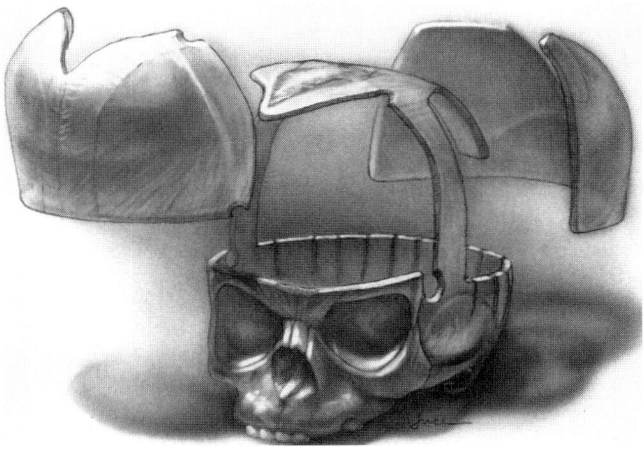

FIGURE 24D-1. Bilateral coronal synostosis. A bilateral parieto-occipital bone graft is developed posteriorly with a bone bridge between the two hemicrania located below the level of the torcula. A barrel stave osteotomy is performed on the remaining occipital bone.

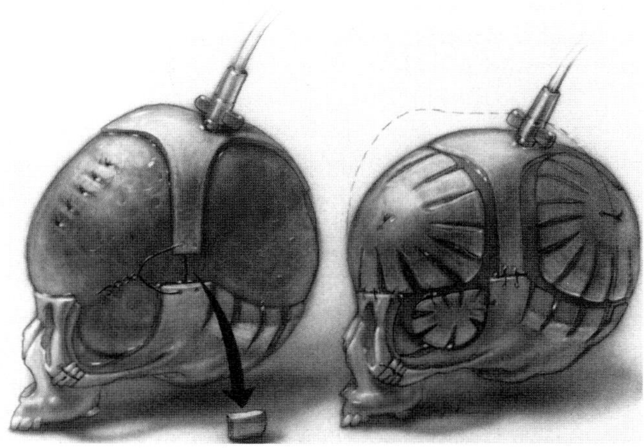

FIGURE 24D-2. The height of the skull is reduced by removing a segment of parietal bone at the inferior portion of the parietal strut. The basal and parietal bone segments are cinched together while the intracranial pressure is monitored. The frontal and temporal bone grafts are reattached to the skull, but the parieto-occipital bone flap is allowed to float, with attachments only to the underlying dura.

We agree with Drs. Marchac, Renier, and Arnaud that patients with unilateral coronal synostosis and an asymmetric skull deformity pose the most formidable challenge to surgeons attempting to achieve a completely normal skull structure postoperatively. During development, growth forces appear to be imbalanced. To try to reduce the asymmetry, the surgeon modifies the depressed or hypoplastic segment by cutting, elevating, and remodeling it. Although this practice has the beneficial effect of reshaping the malformed portion of the skull (e.g., the orbital rim), it also has the negative effect of devascularizing the bone segment. Reduced blood supply is not conducive to the enhanced bone growth that is necessary if the growth of the affected portion of the skull is to "catch up" to the growth of the normal or expanded portions. As a result, an approach has evolved in which both orbital rims, for instance, are elevated and reshaped to enhance postoperative symmetry. This approach is intended to exert the same perioperative influences on growth (positive and negative) in both sides of the skull, so that asymmetry in subsequent growth will be less. It is our belief that the main uncorrected influence on asymmetrical growth is the torquing of forces associated with an asymmetrical skull base. Although the cranial base resists restructuring, even the most vital structures can be repositioned provided it is carried out slowly, particularly when distraction devices are employed in the base of the skull, as has been done experimentally (10).

Postoperative cranial defects are a problem virtually all surgeons encounter eventually, regardless of the surgical techniques used. The schema that the authors have proposed is very similar to the program that my colleagues and I use. Like the authors, we have tried (hydroxyapatite) coral mixed with fibrin glue and have obtained unsatisfactory results. However, I have been very pleased with the use of hydroxyapatite cement, in cases in which a minor degree of bony deformity is evident and in which contour irregularity is not associated with a concern about structural stability, to protect the brain. Here, hydroxyapatite is a very effective means to fill in contour irregularities. The drawbacks are the need for direct exposure to manipulate the cement to a proper form and to drain the operative site. Used in this way, hydroxyapatite cement offers the advantage of bone ingrowth, which stabilizes the implant. Stabilization provides, at least conceptually, a greater resistance to displacement and infection if contamination occurs later on in life.

As stated above, when cranial defects are relatively large (≥3 cm in diameter) and the brain must be protected, hydroxyapatite cement alone is not sufficient. In this situation, either a combination of titanium mesh and hydroxyapatite cement or acrylic cement, with or without the mesh may be used (as the authors describe) to achieve a solid and cosmetically normal skull contour. When implant materials are properly secured, are placed in a location where the overlying soft tissue has good vascularity, and are not communicating with the sinuses or encircling a bone graft, acrylic has been very successful in providing long-term correction of contour depressions in the skull.

The authors also note a relatively high incidence of lack of ossification of bone gaps following cranioplasty. Our team has also experienced this problem, and because we are unable to define completely how bone develops in craniosynostosis, we too are unable to explain why bone sometimes does not regrow as expected. Perhaps scarring between the osteogenic layers (dura and periosteum), either from infection or hemorrhage, as the authors suggest, plays a role. We have found certain practices in handling bone grafts effective in enhancing their viability. Once the bone graft is removed from the skull, it is wrapped in blood-soaked sponges that are kept moist with (but not immersed in) saline solution. We use no bacitracin in the bathing solution because it is toxic to osteoblasts.

To this point, we have not encountered (or recognized clinically) an infection at the operative site in a patient with nonsyndromic craniosynostosis. However, we have encountered patients with large hematomas or seromas; these may cause scarring and diminished osteogenic potential in the periosteum and dura. Like the authors, we are unimpressed with the purported advantages of banked cadaveric bone; in our experience, it dissolves with time. An implant (acrylic) as a temporary spacer to fill a bone defect is the mode that we would use in infants. Defects are reconstructed at skull maturity and the development of substantial bilaminar structure of the skull.

Another aspect of surgery for cranial defects relates to time at which defects in bone should be filled in "completely" with bone grafts. Although individual patients vary to some degree, we use the age of 1 year, not 2 years as the authors report, as the "cutoff" point at which bone gaps larger than 5 to 10 mm are filled in with either bone dust or split calvarial bone. The bone becomes relatively brittle at this stage (age of 1 year) in comparison with the bone of a younger child. The osteogenic potential is different in the surrounding mesenchymal tissues, as has now been clarified in cytokine studies of bone regeneration in the dura and periosteum (11,12).

As the authors describe, one may be able to split calvarial bone at age 4, but reliable solid segments of bone are infrequently obtained until later. However, rather than letting children go to age 10 with a cranial defect or resigning them to an acrylic implant, we routinely have the patient undergo computed tomography yearly to determine the size of the tables of the skull and the diploic space. If bone window computed tomography reveals a definable diploic space in the bone, the patient is referred for a split calvarial bone graft rather than reconstruction of the defect with synthetic materials.

The authors' observations and recommendations regarding the treatment of craniosynostosis deformities are based on an extensive clinical experience that allows them to judge when to employ minor augmentative procedures or major procedures in skull reconstruction. Every deformity in the skull should be evaluated according to its significance and severity. The location of the deformity also should be taken into account because a larger deformity behind the hairline is often less of an issue than a lesser deformity in a more cosmetically sensitive area. Complete reconstruction of the skull is not recommended except in residual or "introduced" major deformities. Operative risks, including dural tear and the potential for cortical brain damage, must be weighed against the potential long-term success of augmentative approaches in which either biomaterials or synthetics are used. I strongly endorse the conservative approach advocated by the authors. As the authors state, the surgeon's wishes to achieve perfection in every case must be balanced against the risks of the operative procedure being considered. Drs. Marchac, Renier and Arnaud and their colleagues have for many years been able to do this successfully.

REFERENCES

1. Persing JA, Mayer PA, Spinelli HM, et al. Prevention of "temporal hollowing" following fronto-orbital advancement for craniosynostosis. *J Craniofacial Surg* 1994;5:271–274.
2. Marchac D, Renier D. *Craniofacial surgery for craniosynostosis.* Boston: Little, Brown and Company, 1982:1–207.
3. Persing JA, Jane JA, Edgerton MT, eds. *Scientific foundations and surgical treatment for craniosynostosis.* Baltimore: Williams & Wilkins, 1989.
4. Persing JA, Posnick J, Magge S, et al. Cranial plate and screw fixation in infancy: an assessment of risk. *J Craniofac Surg* 1996;7:267–270.

5. Park TS, Harris M, Broaddus WC, et al. Vacuum-stiffened beanbag for cranial remodeling procedures in modified prone position. *J Neurosurg* 1989;71:623–625.
6. Persing JA, Edgerton MT, Park TS, et al. Barrel stave osteotomy for correction of turribrachycephaly. *Ann Plast Surg* 1987; 18:488–493.
7. Persing JA, Jane JA, Delashaw JB. Treatment of bilateral coronal synostosis in infancy: a holistic approach. *J Neurosurg* 72:171-175, 1990.
8. Jane JA, Edgerton MT, Futrell JW, Park TS: Immediate correction of sagittal synostosis. *J Neurosurg* 1978;49:705–710.
9. Vollmer DG, Persing JA, Park TS, et al. The variants of sagittal synostosis: strategies for surgical corrections. *J Neurosurg* 1984;61:337–562.
10. Persing JA, Morgan EP, Cronin AJ, et al. Skull base expansion: craniofacial effects. *Plast Reconstr Surg* 1991;187:1028–1033.
11. Opperman LA, Sweeney TM, Redmon J, et al. Tissue interactions with underlying dura mater inhibit osseous obliteration of developing cranial sutures. *Dev Dyn* 1993;198:312–322.
12. Hobar PC, Schreiber JS, McCarthy JG, et al. The role of the dura in cranial bone regeneration in the immature animal. *Plast Reconstr Surg* 1993;92:405–410.

25

ORBITAL HYPERTELORISM

STEVEN R. COHEN

In 1924, Greig (1) published an extensive article on hypertelorism in which he described the anatomic features of an affected skull in great detail. For Greig, hypertelorism meant wide-set eyes. He left no standards or instructions about precisely what to measure. Contemporary clinical treatment of hypertelorism originated in the early 1970s (2). Paralleling the development of surgical techniques were improvements in the classification of orbital hypertelorism and rare craniofacial clefts, one of the major causes of increased interorbital distance. Tessier and associates (3) in 1967 made a major breakthrough when they recognized that an intracranial approach is essential to ensure the safety and efficacy of the definitive corrective procedure. They performed intracranial and extracranial osteotomies of the orbital walls, roof, and floor and resected a central segment from the nasofrontal area and the floor of the anterior cranial fossa. The functional orbit on each side was mobilized after circumferential elevation of the periorbita respecting the apex of the orbit and optic nerve as well as the nasolacrimal duct. Tessier's original approach included a second-stage procedure in which the cribriform plate and nasal septum were resected and the orbital osteotomies performed. Converse and associates (4) in 1970 developed a one-stage procedure with osteotomy, similar to those of Tessier, except that the cribriform plate and olfactory function were preserved. Long-term studies by McCarthy (5) demonstrated little change in gustatory or olfactory function after correction of orbital hypertelorism by this technique. Psillakis and associates (6) modified the Converse technique by leaving a central T-shaped segment of bone in the nasofrontal region to serve as a bony platform for reconstructing the nose. The extracranial or subcranial approach to orbital hypertelorism was originally utilized by Converse and Smith (7) in 1962 and Schmid (8) in 1968 and involved either the medial orbital wall alone or the medial portions of the roof and floor of the orbits, representing an extensive type of paranasal osteotomy. Improved results have been obtained in patients with a moderate degree of orbital hypertelorism by means of a U-shaped osteotomy that involves both walls and floor but spares the roof of the orbit (9). In 1971, Tessier (10) described the single-stage frontofacial advancement, in which the fronto-orbital bandeau was advanced as a separate element in conjunction with a Le Fort III complex below and the frontal bone above. Seven years later, Ortiz Monasterio et al. (11) developed a monobloc osteotomy to advance the orbits and midface in one unit, combined with frontal bone repositioning to correct Crouzon deformity. In 1979, Van der Meulen (12) described the medial fasciotomy " . . . for the correction of midline facial clefting." Van der Meulen split the monobloc osteotomy vertically in the midline, removing the central nasal and ethmoid bone and moving the two halves of the face together to correct orbital hypertelorism. To correct the midface dysplasia and associated orbital hypertelorism in patients with Apert syndrome, Tessier refined the vertical splitting and reshaping of the monobloc segment, thus correcting the midface deformity in three dimensions in a procedure now known as *facial bipartition.*

S. R. Cohen: Department of Surgery, Division of Craniofacial Surgery, Children's Hospital of San Diego, and Department of Surgery, University of California San Diego Medical Center, San Diego, California

NORMAL PRENATAL AND POSTNATAL CHANGES IN INTEROCULAR DISTANCE

During intrauterine life, the relative position of the eyes changes dramatically, the widely divergent embryonic appearance gradually assuming the convergent appearance seen at birth (13). Convergence can be measured in changes of the angle of the optic nerves in fetuses of different ages. If two straight lines are extended from the center of the optic chiasm to the points at which the optic nerves exit the eye globes, an angle is formed at the chiasm that can be measured. At 2 months *in utero,* the optic angle is 180 degrees, and by 3 months it has converged to 105 degrees. At birth, the optic angle is 70 degrees, and in adult life it decreases to 68 degrees (13). Postnatal development of the interorbital distance is complex. On the one hand, the distance between the orbits increases; on the other hand, the optic angle decreases from 71 to 68 degrees (13). The interorbital distance is increased gradually by a number of factors acting synchronously and in concert. These include the following (13): (a) early enlargement of the neurocranium with passive growth of the metopic suture; (b) early growth of the frontal ethmoidal suture; (c) anteroposterior growth of the cranial base at the ethmoidal and sphenofrontal suture; (d) passive growth at the internasal and frontomaxillary suture; and (e) bone apposition on the medial orbital walls with resorption on their underlying surfaces.

The paranasal sinuses—frontal, ethmoidal, sphenoidal, and maxillary—develop as outpouchings from the walls of the nasal cavity (13). The ethmoidal air cells are interposed between the orbits. At birth, they occupy most of the lateral nasal walls. By age 10, the anterior and posterior ethmoidal cells grow toward the cribiform plate and encroach on the frontal and sphenoidal sinuses. Ford (14) suggested that the increase in interorbital distance resulted from pneumatization of the paranasal sinuses. Interorbital growth is 50% completed by 3 years of age (13).

DEFINITIONS AND MEASUREMENTS

The word *hypertelorism* is derived from the Greek and refers to an abnormally increased distance between any bilateral structures. Normal interocular distance, primary telecanthus, hypertelorism, and secondary telecanthus are illustrated in Fig. 25-1. Bony interorbital measurements of ra-

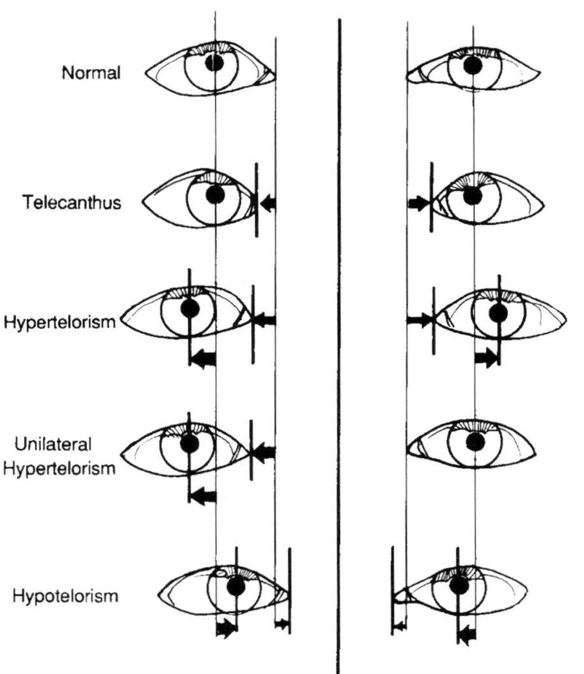

FIGURE 25-1. Primary telecanthus, secondary telecanthus, and hypertelorism. **A:** Normal interocular distance. **B:** Primary telecanthus. Inner canthi are far apart, although outer canthi are normally spaced. Note how vertical line through lacrimal punctum cuts cornea. **C:** True ocular hypertelorism. Both inner and outer canthi are abnormally far apart. **D:** True ocular hypertelorism together with secondary telecanthus. Note how vertical line through lacrimal punctum cuts cornea.

TABLE 25-1. DEFINITIONS AND MEASUREMENTS OF HYPERTELORISM

Ocular hypertelorism—Increased distance between the inner canthi and between the outer canthi. The term *hypertelorism* has come to refer specifically to the eyes. However, it actually means an abnormally wide distance between any two bilateral structures, such as nipples or kidneys. Technically, the term *ocular* is required.

Bony interorbital distance (BIOD)—The distance between orbits on radiographs taken at the most medial point on each orbit. There is also a radiographic measurement for outer orbital distance.

Telorbitism—Increased distance between the bony orbits.

Dystopia canthorum—Lateral displacement of the inner canthi together with lateral displacement of the lacrimal puncta.

Telecanthus—Increased distance between the medial canthi.

Primary telecanthus—Increased distance between the medial canthi with normal outer canthal distance and/or interpupillary distance.

Secondary telecanthus—Disproportionate increase in distance between the medial canthi with ocular hypertelorism.

Inner canthal distance (ICD)—Distance between the two medial canthi, technically called *inter-inner canthal distance*. The medial canthal point is anthropometrically called *endocanthion*. Some authors call the inner canthal distance *interocular distance*.

Outer canthal distance (OCD)—Distance between the two lateral canthi, technically called *inter-outer canthal distance*. The lateral canthal point is anthropometrically called *ectocanthion*. The outer canthal distance is called *biorbital distance* by some authors.

Interpupillary distance (IPD)—Distance between the pupils. Direct and indirect methods are available for this measurement.

Canthal index—The ratio of inner canthal distance to outer canthal distance, the ratio being multiplied by 100. Some authors call this the *intercanthal index*.

Orbital index—Ratio of medial bony interorbital distance to lateral bony interorbital distance, the ratio being multiplied by 100.

Bitemporal/inner canthal index—Ratio of the maximal bitemporal diameter across the orbits to the inner canthal distance, the ratio being multiplied by 100. Sometimes called the *eyespan-eyespace index* or *interocular-biorbital index*.

Inner canthal/head circumference index—The ratio of the inner canthal distance to the head circumference, the ratio being multiplied by 100. Sometimes called *circumference-interorbital index* or *inner canthal index*.

Interpupillary/head breadth ratio—Ratio of interpupillary distance to the head breadth—sometimes called *interocular-head breadth ratio*.

First-degree hypertelorism—Surgical definition in which the BIOD equals 30 to 34 mm. Not true orbital hypertelorism but euryopia or telecanthus.

Second-degree hypertelorism—Surgical definition. BIOD > 34 cm. True hypertelorism with wide face, but orbits nearly normal in orientation and shape.

Third-degree hypertelorism—Surgical definition. BIOD > 40 mm. True hypertelorism with wide face, orbits lateralized and oval in shape, and ethmoid prolapsed.

Traumatic telecanthus—Bony fracture, usually producing unilateral telecanthus.

diographic or computed tomographic (CT) images are the most accurate. The canthal index may be useful for consultations by correspondence when measurements are not available, but facial photographs are provided. A list of definitions is provided in Table 25-1.

As emphasized by Tessier (15), orbital hypertelorism is not a syndrome but rather a physical finding associated with other cranial and facial malformations. Various prenatal clefts and premature synostoses of the craniofacial sutures are the principal causes of orbital hypertelorism. Tessier (16) classified orbital clefts into 15 types, anatomically arranged around the orbit. A meningoencephalocele is a congenital herniation of brain and meninges through a craniofacial skeletal defect. Meningoencephaloceles may be subdivided into occipital, parietal, basal, and sincipital. The latter group is further subdivided into frontoethmoidal, interfrontal, and craniofacial clefts. The skeletal and soft tissue morphology of frontoethmoidal meningoencephaloceles was described by David and associates (17) with three-dimensional CT reconstructions. In all cases, the cranial end of the defect is a hole in the anterior cranial fossa at the site of the foramen caecum at the junction of the frontal ethmoid bones. The facial component of the defect determines the subclassification: nasofrontal, nasoethmoidal, or naso-orbital. In the nasofrontal type, the facial defect is at the junction of the frontal and nasal bones. In the nasoethmoidal type, the facial defect lies between the nasal bones and nasal cartilages. Naso-orbital meningoencephaloceles present on the face through holes in the medial orbital wall. Hypertelorism is present in all patients, but is not as severe as that observed in midline clefts. Dermoid cysts and glial tumors of the root of the nose result from cranial clefts that can be associated with orbital hypertelorism. Patients with craniofacial synostosis, especially Apert syndrome, show some element of orbital hypertelorism, and a medial translocation of the orbits, in addition to correction of the midface hypoplasia, is often indicated. Moss (18) also demonstrated a significantly increased interorbital distance in a radiographic study of a population of patients with cleft lip and palate. Some of the syndromes associated with hypertelorism are listed in Table 25-2.

TABLE 25-2. SOME SYNDROMES ASSOCIATED WITH HYPERTELORISM

Frontonasal dysplasia
Craniofrontonasal dysplasia
Brachycephalofrontonasal dysplasia
Acrofrontofacionasal dysostosis
Frontofacionasal dysplasia
Greig cephalopolysyndactyly
Naguib syndrome
Nasopalpebral lipoma-coloboma syndrome
Noonan syndrome
Opitz BBB/G syndrome
Aarskog syndrome
Leopard syndrome
Waardenburg's syndrome, type 1
Blepharonasofacial syndrome
Sotos' syndrome
Bannayan-Riley-Ruvalcaba syndrome
Robinow's syndrome
Apert syndrome
Pfeiffer's syndrome
Cloverleaf skull
Nevoid basal cell carcinoma syndrome
Craniometaphyseal dysplasia
Craniodiaphyseal dysplasia

PATHOGENESIS

Hypertelorism is known to be causally heterogenous (Table 25-2). As noted by Cohen et al. (13), because different causes do not lead to a common pathogenetic pathway, hypertelorism is not a single malformation, sequence, or developmental field. It is both pathogenetically and causally heterogenous. For example, Apert syndrome, frontonasal dysplasia, and Waardenburg syndrome, type 1, produce "wide-set" eyes in different ways.

Several theories of pathogenesis have been advanced. Mann (19) suggested that hypertelorism results from early ossification of the lesser wings of the sphenoid, which fixes the orbits in fetal position. A common anatomical finding in many cases of hypertelorism is a marked increase in the horizontal width of the ethmoid sinuses. Median bony facial clefting in the frontonasal region is common in severe instances of frontonasal dysplasia. If the nasal capsule fails to develop properly, the primitive brain vesicle fills the space normally occupied by the capsule to produce anterior cranium bifidum, a morphokinetic arrest in the position of the eyes, and a lack of elevation of the nasal tip. Frank encephalocele in the midline can produce the same type of morphokinetic arrest found in frontonasal dysplasia. Less commonly, frontal teratoma, frontal lipoma, hamartoma, intracranial cyst, or some intrinsic cartilaginous defect affecting the nasal capsule can produce hypertelorism.

Hypertelorism of lesser degrees occurs in Apert syndrome, in which the cribriform plate of the ethmoid bone is prolapsed between the orbits. The mechanism causing hypertelorism is related to disturbances in cranial base formation. When patients with cleft lip and palate show evidence of hypertelorism, the pathogenesis appears to be related to a developmental field defect.

A number of abnormalities can be associated with hypertelorism, including nonprotruding lipomas of the corpus callosum, calcification of the falx cerebri, duplication of the crista galli, wrinkling of the nose, and tissue tags of the nose (13). Most are associated with frontonasal dysplasia, but their significance is presently unknown.

Experimental models have been produced by various teratogenic agents in animals. Burke and Sadler (20) concluded that cell death of midline mesenchyme induced by diazo-oxo-norleucine in the frontonasal process and neuroepithelium together with an increased facial width were the underlying factors producing a frontonasal dysplasia-like condition in mice. Darab et al. (21) used methotrexate to induce a frontonasal dysplasia-like condition in mice. The pathogenesis was attributed to damage to embryonic blood vessels of the frontonasal prominences, which resulted in a paucity of mesenchyme and distension of the neural tube.

PATHOLOGIC ANATOMY

McCarthy et al. (22) nicely summarize the pathologic anatomy of orbital hypertelorism. The principal anatomic abnormality associated with the increase in interorbital distance is felt to be horizontal widening of the ethmoid sinuses. The increase in width is usually limited to the anterior part of the ethmoid sinuses and does not affect the posterior ethmoidal cells and sphenoid sinus. The cribriform plate is usually not significantly increased in width. When the roof of each ethmoidal mass is prolapsed, the cribriform plate can be depressed to a point 20 mm below the orbital roof, the normal distance being 10 mm. This anatomical finding is a major contraindication to the use of a subcranial or extracranial surgical approach to the deformity.

The olfactory grooves can be enlarged and rounded and the crista galli duplicated or absent. The sphenoid bone, including the portion on the lesser wing about the optic foramen, usually shows no abnormalities.

The frontal bone is usually affected. The glabella may be less prominent and may be the site of a meningoencephalocele defect. The skeletal framework between the orbits adapts to the enlarged interorbital space and varies in structure. The nasal bones may be small; the frontal processes of the maxilla greatly widened; the lateral cartilages larger; the nasal bones, lateral cartilages, and septum duplicated; and the alar cartilages of the bifid nasal tip enlarged. Hyperplasia of the subcutaneous layer in the naso-orbital area is a peculiar yet almost constant finding.

Whitaker et al. (23) described a variety of abnormalities of the lacrimal apparatus in patients with orbital hypertelorism. These include obstruction of the nasolacrimal ducts and absent puncta. The bilateral exotropia commonly seen in orbital hypertelorism accentuates the deformity. Convergence in binocular vision is not possible in the more severe forms. The extraocular muscle dysfunction may also be associated with craniofacial deformities.

CLASSIFICATION

Definitions of hypertelorism are listed in Table 25-1 and Fig. 25-1.

On the basis of Gunter's work, Tessier classified orbital hypertelorism according to the interorbital distance: first-degree, 30 to 34 mm; second-degree, more than 34 mm with normal shape and orientation of the orbits; third-degree, more than 40 mm.

OPERATIVE PROCEDURES

The design of osteotomies and the nature of soft tissue surgical procedures depend on the clinical and radiologic evaluation. Depending on the degree of hypertelorism, an extracranial or intracranial approach may be chosen. A subcranial procedure alone may be indicated in first-degree hypertelorism when the cribriform plate is not prolapsed inferiorly into the interorbital space. The types of osteotomies now employed are the result of a progressive evolution of techniques during the last 30 years. Converse and Smith (24) were really the first to describe an operation based on their experience in the treatment of malunion of naso-orbital fractures with telecanthus. An osteotomy of the entire medial orbital wall was performed, including the anterior lacrimal crest, so that the medial wall with the attached canthi was displaced toward the midline. The dorsum of the nose was augmented with autogenous iliac bone graft. This type of operation was only partly successful because it failed to achieve any significant displacement of the functional orbital volume. In 1972, Tessier (25) reported a slight modification of this operation, noting that the subcranial procedure failed because only a portion of the orbit was mobilized. Schmid (26) in 1968 reported a nearly circumferential orbital osteotomy to correct unilateral orbital hypertelorism. This was possible because the patient had an unusually large frontal sinus that permitted the roof osteotomy. In 1967, Tessier et al. (27) made a major breakthrough by recognizing that the intracranial approach is essential to ensure the safety and efficacy of definitive correction. Performing intracranial and extracranial osteotomies of the orbital walls, roof, and floor, they resected a central segment from the nasofrontal area and the floor of the anterior cranial fossa to permit mobilization of the entire orbit. The operative approach of Tessier and colleagues (27) comprised two stages. Converse and associates (28) in 1970 developed a one-stage procedure with osteotomies similar to those of Tessier, except the cribriform plate and olfactory function were preserved.

Extracranial (Subcranial) Approach

In patients with relatively minor degrees of hypertelorism, a subcranial approach may be indicated (Fig. 25-2). In children who have mild frontonasal dysplasia, hypertrophy of the ethmoid sinuses, and mild hypertelorism resulting from chronic sinusitis, some children who have hypertelorism associated with cleft lip and palate, and patients who have

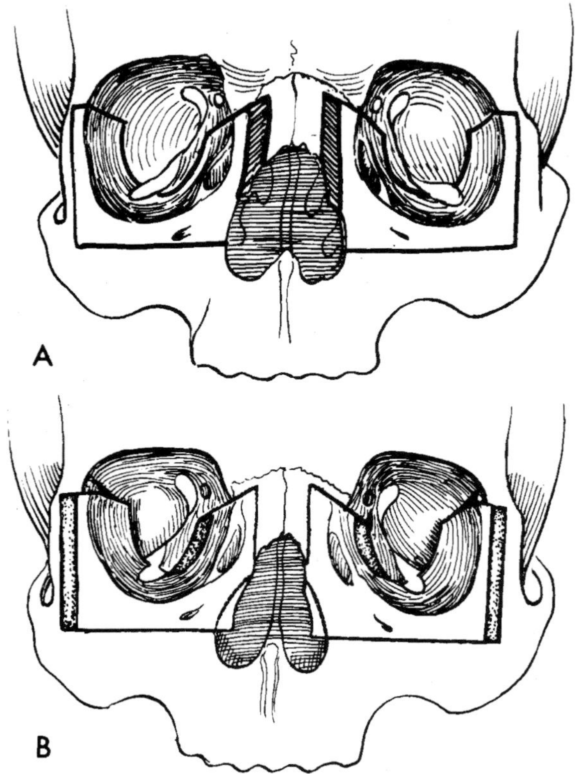

FIGURE 25-2. Subcranial approach to correct milder cases of hypertelorism.

posttraumatic widening of the interorbital distance secondary to naso-orbital ethmoid fractures, a subcranial approach may be appropriate. The type of osteotomy to be utilized is determined by a precise clinical evaluation. When a subcranial approach is being considered, a range of osteotomies can be used: medial orbital osteotomies involving medial translocation of the inferior orbital rim and floor to bilateral subcranial U-shaped osteotomies including medial translocation of the entire zygoma extending upward along the lateral orbital rim and occasionally including the lateral aspect of the orbital roof, depending on aesthetic needs (Fig. 25-3). For children with hypertelorism associated with hypoplasia of the nasal dorsum, as in Binder's syndrome, medial orbital osteotomies can include the nasomaxillary buttresses of the maxilla to permit central facial advancement with simultaneous correction of mild hypertelorism and cranial bone grafting to the nasal dorsum.

Intracranial Approach

The classic combined intracranial and extracranial treatment of hypertelorism involves a combined neurosurgical and craniofacial approach (Fig. 25-4). The techniques and details of the operation have been well illustrated by several authors. A coronal incision is utilized for exposure. We no longer detach the medial canthi or utilize a subciliary or transconjunctival approach to the orbit. Rather, the upper

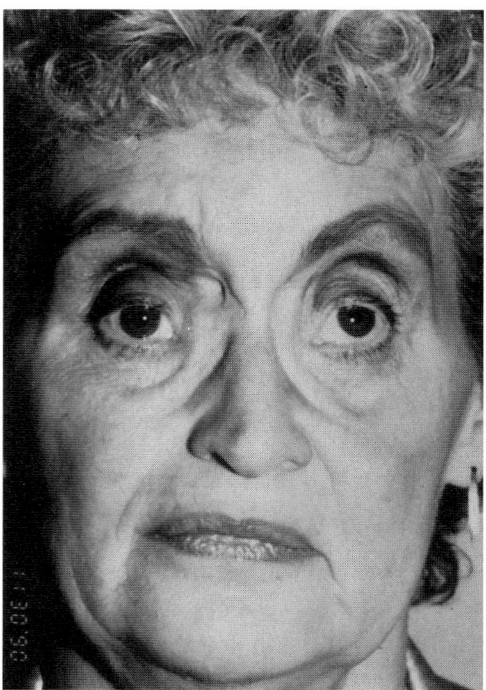

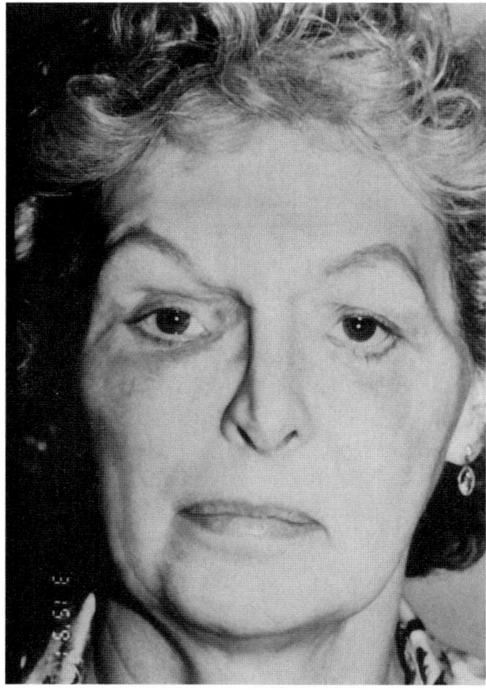

FIGURE 25-3. Left: Preoperative frontal photograph of elderly woman with posttraumatic telecanthus and malar dystopia. **Right:** Result after bilateral subcranial osteotomies, which included the zygoma, to reposition the medial canthi.

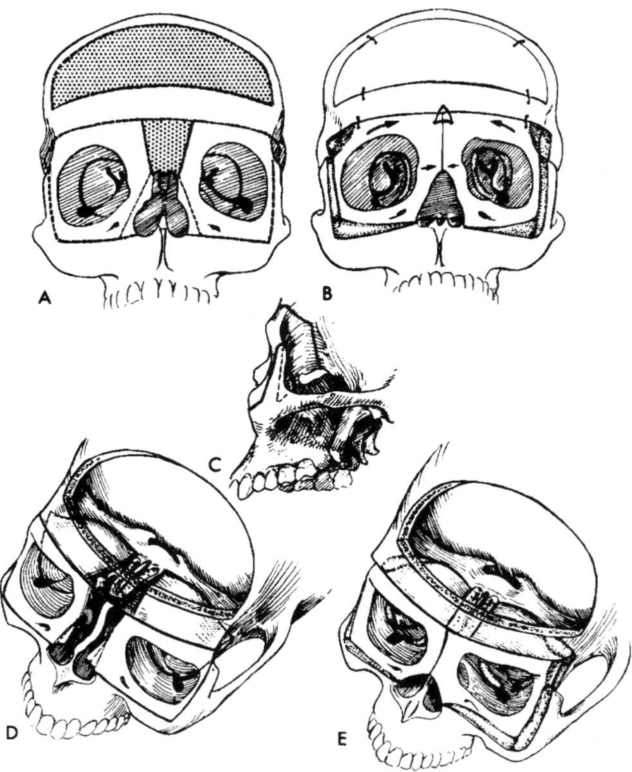

FIGURE 25-4. Intracranial "box" orbital osteotomies.

buccal sulcus incision is dissected to the inferior orbital rim, and with the use of Obwegeser and malleable retractors, the periorbita is pulled away from the anterior aspects of the orbital floor and superior orbital rim. The neurosurgeon at this point proceeds with frontal craniotomy, and exposure of the anterior cranial fossa down to the level of the cribriform plate is carried out. The crista galli may be duplicated and, to increase exposure, it is occasionally necessary to resect it. The plastic surgeon continues the dissection circumferentially around the orbits, staying in the subperiosteal plane. The proximal portion of the zygomatic arch and the zygomatic body are exposed. The attachment of the canthal tendon is preserved, if possible. If not, it is taken down and reattached at the end of the case. The upper buccal sulcus incision is made and, as previously mentioned, the dissection is carried out to expose the inferior orbital foramen and nerve up to the junction with the nasal process. Once exposure has been obtained, a reciprocating saw is utilized to sever the junction of the zygomatic arch and body. In patients with a normal bizygomatic width, the osteotomy is carried out more proximally in the substance of the zygomatic body to prevent undue narrowing of the face at the bizygomatic distance (Fig. 25-5). In patients with nasofrontal dysplasia, a brachycephalic appearance is not unusual, and generally the osteotomy is carried out at the junction of the zygomatic arch and body, as noted above.

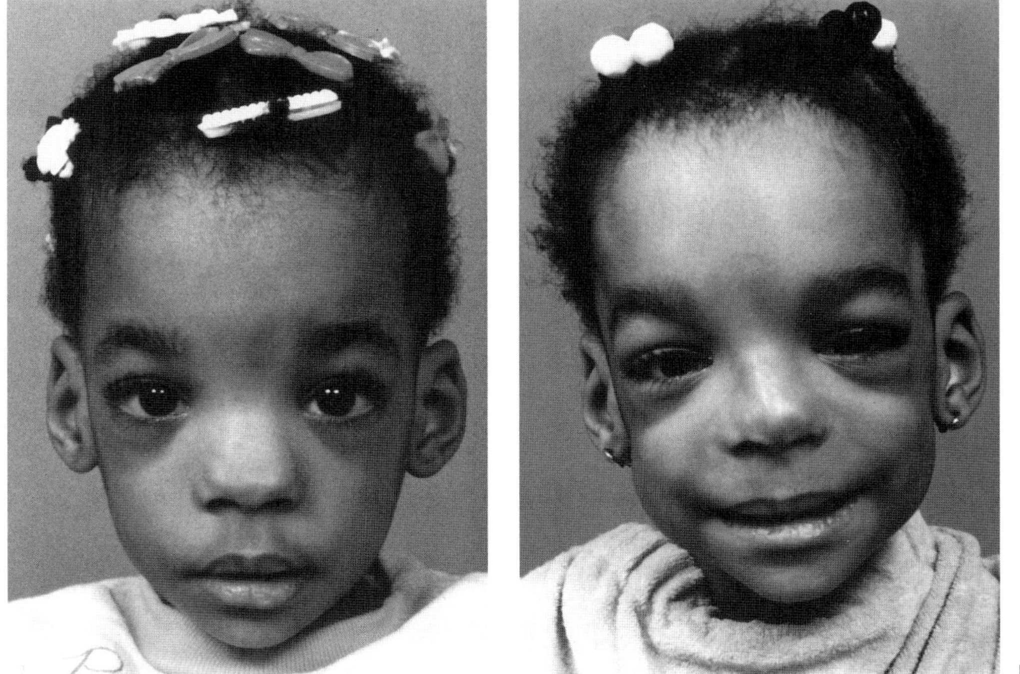

FIGURE 25-5. A: Three-year-old child with frontonasal dysplasia and hypertelorism. **B:** Postoperative result following intracranial "box" osteotomies. Because of the narrow bizygomatic distance, osteotomy was performed through body of zygomas.

The lateral orbital rim is cut along its attachment to the sphenoid, beginning at the anterior aspect of the inferior oral fissure. This osteotomy is extended up along the junction of the zygoma and greater wing of the sphenoid, and then intracranially along the orbital roof just anterior to the cribriform plate. The same maneuver is performed on the opposite side. Then, with 3-mm osteotomes, the inferior orbital floor is cut from the anterior medial aspect of the inferior orbital fissure to the posterior lacrimal crest and from the medial naso-orbital osteotomy, just above the cribriform, along the medial orbital wall, to the posterior lacrimal crest. This completes the circumferential osteotomies of the orbit. With either a reciprocating or oscillating saw, the inferior cut across the maxilla is kept as close to the inferior orbital foramen as possible to avoid injury to the erupting dentition. This osteotomy is carried medially into the piriform aperture. Once the osteotomy is completed on the opposite side, the interorbital distance is remeasured, and the appropriate amount of bone to be resected is recorded.

Either a paramedian or median osteotomy is performed along the supraorbital bar through the nasal dorsum. These sections of bone are then removed and the enlarged ethmoidal air cells exonerated on each side. If the septum is bifid, the skeletal framework is resected, with preservation of the mucous membrane lining. Care is taken to maintain the olfactory mucosa by preserving the cribriform plate, in addition to the mucosa of the upper portion of the nasal septum and the mucosa overlying the superior turbinate. Gradually displacing the two orbital box osteotomies medially will determine points of interference that prevent ideal reduction of the fragments in the midline. Typically, additional septum is resected, as well as the medial aspects of the inferior orbital rim and nasal processes of the maxilla. It is important following reduction of the osteotomies in the midline to inspect the piriform aperture and ensure that sufficient opening is present to permit adequate air flow. The segments are then displaced to the midline in the nasofrontal region and stabilized with a titanium microplate or a 26-gauge wire. The placement of the wire should be as far posterior as possible to control the posterior aspects of the naso-orbital maxillary osteotomies. This controls medial canthal drift, which frequently compromises the results of treatment. In patients with an antimongoloid tilt to the orbit or in patients with unilateral orbital dystopia and hypertelorism, adjustments must be made to move the orbital boxes independently. Reciprocal removal of bone from the superior orbital rim is necessary to permit these rotations. In addition, the boxes may be bent in the midline to improve the curvature of the central face and malar regions. Once the osteotomy has been stabilized in the midline, lateral stabilization at the zygomatic arches is carried out with placement of interposition bone grafts. Further stabilization at the inferior orbital rim along the nasomaxillary buttress region is performed with bone grafts and rigid fixation. The nasal deformities are addressed with cranial bone grafts and an open rhinoplasty approach (Fig. 25-6), which is described later in the chapter.

A 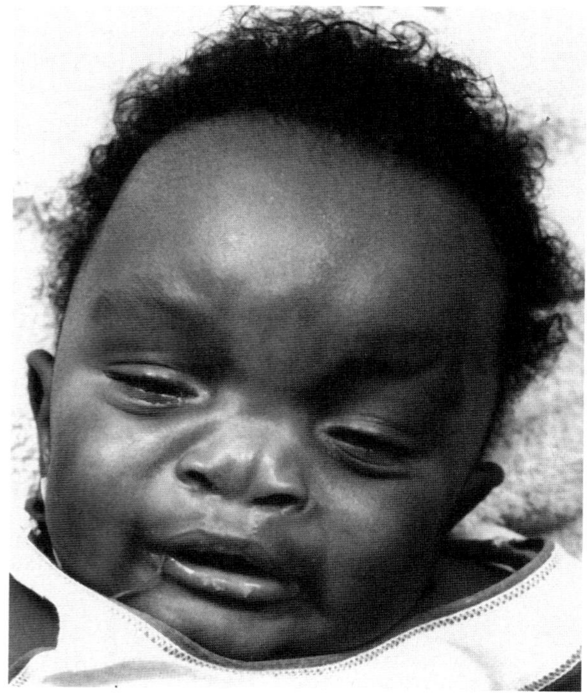

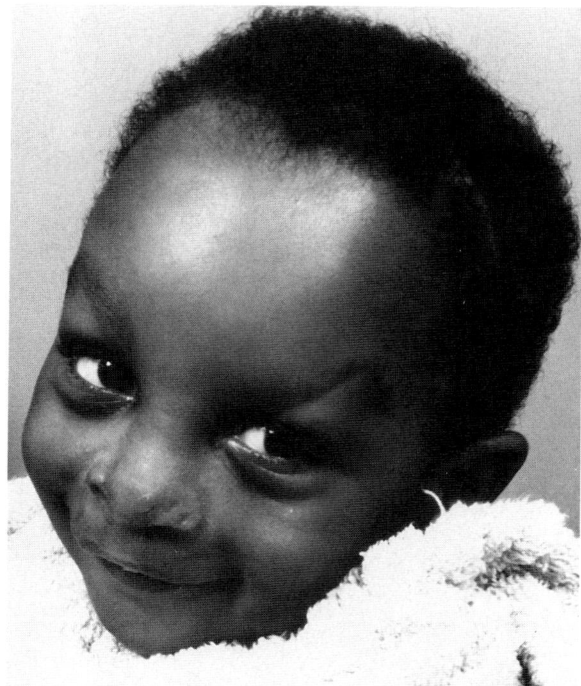 B

FIGURE 25-6. A: Three-year-old child with hypertelorism and bilateral cleft lip and palate. **B:** Result after intracranial "box" osteotomies and nasal repair with midface degloving approach.

Facial Bipartition

The above-described "orbital box" osteotomies are successful in correcting hypertelorism in many cases, especially if occlusion is normal. In patients with Apert syndrome, some variants of frontonasal dysplasia, or other forms of hypertelorism with transverse compromise of the maxillary dimensions, hypertelorism is best addressed by a facial bipartition (Fig. 25-7). The facial bipartition segments the face by means of a wedge ostectomy of the median portions of the supraorbital bar and nasal dorsum. The resultant reduction of the midline osteotomies permits correction of hypertelorism, reestablishment of the proper orbital plane, relocation of the lateral canthi to a more normal position relative to the medial canthi, and reshaping of the flat brachycephalic face by bending of facial halves. A coronal incision is made and frontal craniotomy carried out. The anterior cranial fossa and cribriform region are exposed by the neurosurgeon. The osteotomy is begun by severing the junction of the zygomatic arch and body with a reciprocating saw. The lateral orbital rim is then cut with a reciprocating saw along its junction with the greater wing of the sphenoid. The osteotomy is carried intracranially along the orbital roof to a point just above the cribriform. The same osteotomy is performed on the contralateral side. With the small, 3-mm osteotomes, intraorbital osteotomies are carried out. At this point, through the upper buccal sulcus incision, bilateral pterygoid maxillary osteotomies are performed with a curved osteotome. Rowe-Killey forceps are inserted in the nose or along the floor of the nose through the piriform apertures and, with use of an acrylic palatal splint to prevent uncontrolled midline fracture, the monobloc segment is down-fractured. As the down-fracture begins, the vomer is severed from its attachments with a guarded osteotome from above to permit full mobilization of the face. Once this is completed, the interorbital distance is measured and the appropriate median osteotomy planned. A reciprocating saw is utilized to make the median osteotomy, which is completed at the occlusal level with a small, 3-mm osteotome along the palate and interdental space. The face is now in two halves and may be reduced in the midline. Ethmoid air cells and septum are resected carefully to permit medial translocation and adequate reduction. A slight bevel placed on the median osteotomy will allow for proper facial bending and good coaptation of the two facial halves in the midline. The midline is stabilized with a transnasal 26-gauge wire or a Microplus titanium plate. The lateral zygoma is plated to the arch, and interposition bone grafts are placed. Occasionally, an interdental wire is necessary between the upper incisors to prevent undue transverse expansion of the palate if this is not desired. Generally, the palatal region will widen; hence, the need for a Dorrance-style palatal incision to permit easier transverse movement of the palatal segments. The mucoperiosteum of the palate is closed at the conclusion of the procedure.

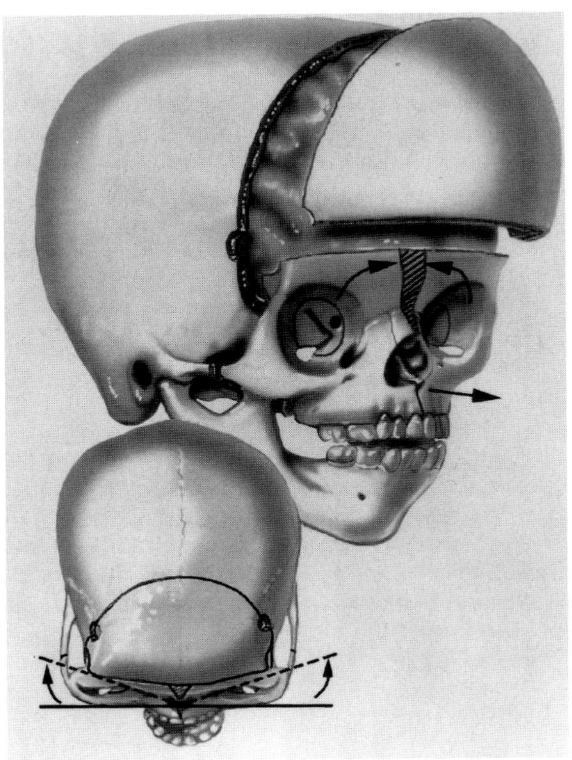

FIGURE 25-7. Monobloc with facial bipartition.

When conventional monobloc advancement is combined with facial bipartition, the nasofrontal opening needs to be addressed with care. A pericranial flap is preserved at the initial dissection, and this is "mailed" through a slot between the supraorbital bar and replaced, recontoured forehead. This is inset along the nasofrontal opening, and fibrin glue is used to seal the area. On occasion, a lumbar shunt may be necessary for temporary postoperative drainage. If no nasofrontal gap is created, the pericranial flap and fibrin glue are still used unless distraction osteogenesis is planned (29) (Fig. 25-8). In these cases, distraction is delayed 5 to 7 days postoperatively to allow for the regrowth of mucosa in the nasofrontal area.

Operative Approach to the Nose

The nasal deformity in patients with nasofrontal encephaloceles is variable. In older patients, orbital translocation by means of a box-type osteotomy may be required. In these cases, cranial bone grafting to the nose is almost always necessary. In milder cases of nasofrontal encephalocele, once the encephalocele is resected and the sack removed as well as is possible from the nasal tissues, we prefer to augment the nasal dorsum and not resect skin, permitting shrinkage of the excess. Secondary surgery may be necessary for further nasodorsal augmentation and possibly skin resection if shrinkage is inadequate. The medial canthal tendons are handled in milder cases of encephalocele by means of a su-

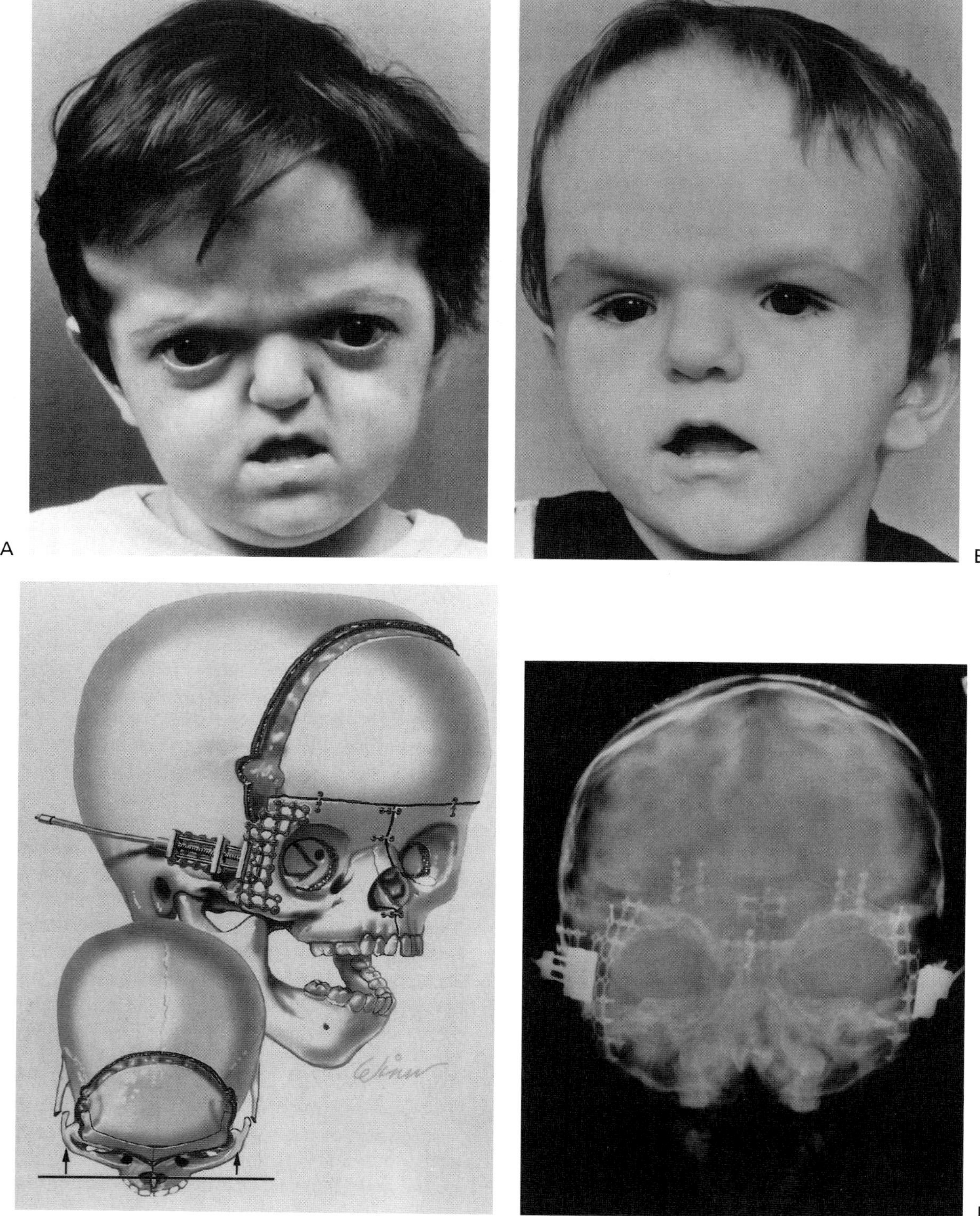

FIGURE 25-8. A: Four-year-old boy with Apert syndrome. **B:** Postoperative result after facial bipartition and monobloc distraction. **C:** Artist's depiction of facial bipartition with monobloc distraction. **D:** Immediate postoperative roentgenogram showing midline stabilization following monobloc distraction with facial bipartition.

turing technique. Because encephalocele repair is often carried out within the first week of life, the tendons may be grasped directly through small incisions with a 4-0 clear nylon suture. If a K-wire is attached to a drill, it can be inserted into the drill in a reverse fashion. In this way, transnasal drilling is possible with the eyelet of the needle directed toward the contralateral side. Each suture can be grasped by passing it through the eyelet of the Keith needle and pulling across to the contralateral side. We have found this technique to be quite helpful in younger children undergoing medial canthopexy. In addition, the transnasal canthopexy can be carried out without the need for a skin incision by means of the same technique with a dissolvable horizontal mattress suture placed directly through the skin in the canthal region. The horizontal mattress should be sufficiently broad to include the medial canthus and some of the surrounding soft tissue to prevent residual telecanthus.

Nasal Deformity

The nasal deformities associated with hypertelorism are largely related to the underlying diagnosis. However, the appearance of the nose is often the ultimate determinant of a successfully aesthetic outcome in hypertelorism repair. As Tessier (15) has emphasized, "Surgery for hypertelorism is surgery of the nose." In patients with syndromic craniosynostosis, the nose frequently requires additional augmentation by means of a cantilever cranial bone graft. We prefer to attach a T-shaped titanium or Vitallium plate to the bone graft, then shape the graft with a cutting burr. A bend is placed in the fixation plate, and the graft is inserted along the nose in a subperiosteal fashion. As one pushes the plate against the glabella, additional height of the nasal tip can be obtained. This process is fine-tuned by bending the plate until the desired projection is apparent. Depending on the degree of abnormality and age of the patient, an open rhinoplasty can be employed. An open rhinoplasty is approached with a stair-step columellar incision. The lower lateral cartilages are mobilized and brought over the cranial bone graft for further tip augmentation. In this way, a soft, more natural-appearing tip will be produced.

In patients with cleft lip and palate and associated hypertelorism, either an open rhinoplasty is utilized (unilateral cleft lip and palate deformity), or midface degloving (bilateral cleft lip and palate deformity) is performed to gain access to the nasal cartilaginous skeleton and septum (Fig. 25-6). With facial bipartition, the vomer is severed during the down-fracture. The septoplasty must take this into consideration to preserve sufficient dorsal and caudal cartilage. Most patients require nasal augmentation, generally with cranial bone. The nasal augmentation can be increased to improve residual telecanthus.

In children with cleft lip and palate, once the cartilages are reshaped, an effort is made to bring them above the bone graft. Occasionally, a drill hole directly into the tip of the nasal bone graft is necessary to support the alar cartilages. Care should be taken not to rotate the alar cartilages too far cephalad because an open and unattractive nasolabial angle with nostril show will result. Once the nasal bone graft is placed, the medial canthi can be dealt with. If the bony interorbital distance has been corrected but residual telecanthus is present, medial canthopexy may be necessary. A small external incision is made, the medial canthal tendon is detached from its bony attachment, and a suture or wire is placed directly into the tendon. It is important to burr a bony fenestration posterior and superior to the lacrimal groove to permit a transnasal canthopexy with snug seating of the canthal tendon against the naso-orbital skeleton. If necessary, the lateral canthi can be suspended by means of nylon sutures or fine wire through drill holes placed on the inner aspect of the lateral orbital rims. The lateral canthal tendon should be 1 to 2 mm above the medial canthal tendon in most Caucasian patients. Techniques for medial canthal repositioning have included transnasal wiring and direct suture fixation to either a Mitek anchor or a Sherlock screw.

Distraction Osteogenesis with Facial Bipartition

Increasingly, midfacial distraction is carried out for patients with syndromic craniosynostosis. The objection to this technique is that without selective segmental osteotomies, one will simply distract a broad, flat face with orbital hypertelorism in a number of cases of Apert or Crouzon syndrome. We have developed a technique in which facial bipartition can be carried out simultaneously with monobloc distraction. Satisfactory results have been achieved in seven patients by means of this technique (Fig. 25-8). The facial bipartition is performed in the exact same fashion as conventional bipartition. Typically, a nasal bone graft is not placed at the initial procedure. At the time of distraction device removal, should placement of a bone graft or treatment of residual telecanthus be necessary, both these procedures can be carried out during device removal.

AVOIDANCE AND TREATMENT OF COMPLICATIONS

Complications of craniofacial surgical procedures in general are less common than initially reported by Whitaker and associates (30) in 1979. In their report, an international, retrospective analysis of data from 793 patients at six centers, the mortality rate was 1.6%. The deaths were related to inadequate blood replacement, cerebral edema, respiratory obstruction, and sepsis. The infection rate was higher (6.2%) after an intracranial procedure. Two patients had decreased vision in one eye. No instances of brain damage were noted, but nine patients required an additional operation for cerebral spinal fluid leakage. Other problems reported included loss of bone grafts, excessive blood loss, ectropion, ptosis, nasolacrimal obstruction, and bone donor site morbidity, including pneumothorax, contour irregularities, and pain. The article of Tessier that appeared in *Plastic and Reconstructive Surgery* in January of 1974 (16) reviewed 65 patients undergoing hypertelorism correction. Two of these patients died, one because of insufficient blood replacement and the other because of cerebral edema. Ulceration of the cornea occurred in three cases. Sequestration of the nasal bone graft occurred in two cases, and partial resorption of the cranial bone graft to the nose occurred in six cases. Bone necrosis at the frontal flap occurred in one case as a result of infection from the frontal sinus. Sequestration of the rib grafts in a cranioplasty occurred in one case because of infection from the frontal sinus. Diplopia occurred in one patient, permanent anesthesia of the infraorbital nerve occurred in four patients, and true partial relapse, possibly explained by secondary growth of the ethmoid or frontal sinus, occurred in two cases. From careful observation of his 65 cases, Tessier developed a number of personal observations and improvements regarding the problem of hypertelorism.

Deformities of the cribiform plate were found in approximately 60% of the cases of third-degree hypertelorism. In these cases, preservation of the olfactory nerves was difficult or impractical. Paramedian resections on either side of the nose, as described by Converse may be used especially if the nose is not bifid (22). Because the intraorbital distance is increased on both sides of the nose, it seems logical to perform the resections in this region. A narrow nasofrontal bridge in the shape of a keel must be left intact.

Tessier (16) preserves what he calls a "frontal crown," which is a strip of the frontal bandeau that is left above the orbital frames and below the frontal craniotomy. By placing a midline reference and having the frontal crown serve as a horizontal reference, the distance that each orbit is translocated medially can be ascertained with precision. In addition, if unilateral orbital dystopia is present or asymmetrical movements of the two orbits are required, the frontal crown can serve as a horizontal and vertical reference to improve symmetrical outcomes. Lastly, the frontal crown serves as a sagittal reference to prevent displacement of the superior orbital roof anteriorly; this produces enophthalmos, which can be a difficult problem to correct (Fig. 25-9).

An important component of the treatment of hypertelorism is the selection of a cranial or subcranial route for correction. This choice is not entirely determined by the degree of orbital hypertelorism. The extent of prolapse of the cribriform plate is one determining factor because of the risk for dural injury and the inability to bring the orbits closer together. Control with the subcranial route is more hazardous. Factors that influence the choice, therefore, are the degree of ethmoidal prolapse and orbital hypertelorism, the presence of frontal deformities and vertical asymmetry of the orbits, and deformity the frontal bone. Provided that these situations are accounted for in preoperative planning, the extracranial route can be extremely effective.

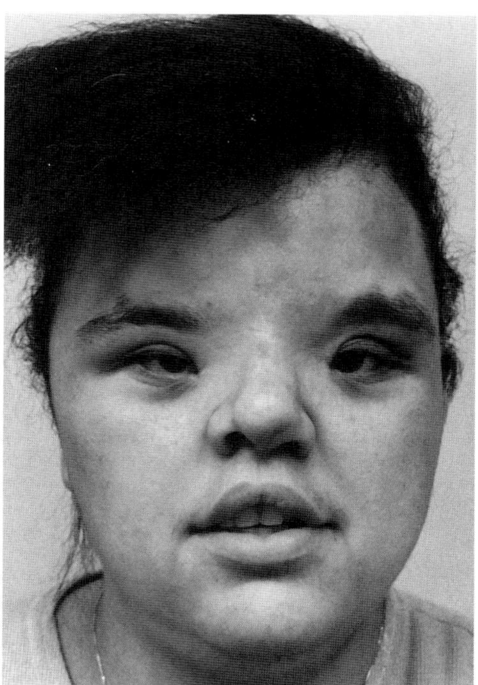

FIGURE 25-9. After patient underwent orbital "box" osteotomies at an outside institution, postoperative enophthalmos developed, as shown in this photograph.

When the distance between the eyebrows is relatively normal, the median incision can be restricted to the nasal bridge and the median forehead incision can be omitted. At the frontonasal angle, a Z-plasty will bring the eyebrows closer together and lengthen the nose, thereby serving to prevent the formation of epicanthal folds, shortening the intercanthal distance, and providing additional support for the canthopexies (16). Midline and forehead scars can be avoided in most cases and it may be preferable to do this on a secondary procedure.

Partial resorption of bone grafts, especially in the nasal area, can be prevented by rigidly fixing the graft to the frontal bone, using an auxiliary strut into the anterior nasal spine to support the nasodorsal graft, ensuring a wide area of contact between the graft and the remnants of the nasal skeleton, covering the frontal process of the maxilla and the nasal bone grafts with additional sheets of bone, and preventing dead space by suspending the nasal mucosa to the main graft and filling any defects with cancellous bone.

Postoperative depression in the temporal regions can result from medial displacement of the orbits. This can be prevented by advancement of the entire temporal muscle or its anterior part after vertical section of its aponeurosis (16).

Infections of the frontal sinus can be prevented by complete resection of its posterior wall and mucosa and plugging of the nasofrontal ducts (i.e., cranialization of the frontal sinus) (16).

The temporal lobe can be damaged in some cases during osteotomy of the lateral orbital wall. Preliminary protection of the temporal lobe is obtained before this osteotomy. Some of the observations made by Tessier (16) after analyzing his own cases have been presented. His work continues to stand as a landmark and gold standard toward which others must reach to achieve similar outcomes.

Adverse outcomes and complications related to hypertelorism repair can be grouped into several categories. These are best separated into preoperative causes, intraoperative problems, early postoperative complications, and later complications and residual deformities.

Preoperative Causes of Complications

Adverse outcomes related to preoperative causes are generally secondary to errors in preoperative planning. Choice of the proper operation is the most critical factor in this regard. Appropriate frontal and profile analysis is essential in the treatment of any craniofacial deformity. It is imperative that an accurate diagnosis be made and a proper treatment plan established before a surgical treatment of hypertelorism is undertaken. The cause of the hypertelorism should be determined. The timing of treatment in patients with craniosynostosis may vary depending on whether their problem is frontonasal dysplasia or encephalocele. In general, we prefer to address nasofrontal encephalocele shortly after birth to prevent cerebral spinal fluid leaks and neurologic complications. The operations are technically quite simple to perform, and removal of the supraorbital bar, along with the frontal bone, affords the neurosurgeon excellent exposure. Once the encephalocele sack is ligated and the dura repaired or patched, the nasal contents of the encephalocele sack are removed, generally with a pituitary rongeur under direct vision or occasionally with endoscopic assistance. Not all cases of encephalocele require orbital translocation for correction. Smaller encephaloceles can generally be treated by medial canthopexies and cranial bone grafting to the nose to correct the associated hypertelorism. Secondary deformities are generally related to telecanthus and inadequate nasodorsal projection.

In more severe cases, facial bipartition or orbital box osteotomy should be chosen. It is critical in these cases to anticipate potential instability along the zygomatic–frontal and zygomatic–maxillary sutures, and consideration should be given to preplating these areas before the down-fracture. In patients with craniosynostosis, facial bipartition is generally the procedure of choice. A transverse collapse of the maxilla is present in many patients with Apert or significant Crouzon deformities, and they benefit from the expansion provided by the bipartition procedure. In addition, the flat facial plane can be bent to reestablish a more normal projection. Midface advancement is anticipated between the ages of 4 to 7 years. We have recently performed facial bipartition in conjunction with monobloc distraction with excellent results (29).

We generally prefer to treat patients with nasofrontal dysplasia at about 3 years of age. Orbital growth and growth of the globe are nearly complete, and the bone is sturdy. In more severe cases, earlier operation should be considered. In patients with nasofrontal dysplasia, the anterior hairline and abnormally large and inferiorly displaced "widow's peak" must be addressed, in addition to the increased distance between the eyebrows and the nasal shortening. When the distance between the eyebrows is substantial, a Z-plasty performed in the nasofrontal region can bring them together and lengthen the nose. Additional median resection of the nasal tissues is frequently necessary. In most cases, we prefer to perform the nasal soft tissue resection secondarily to see if the excess skin will shrink following correction. Simple secondary procedures with additional bone grafting to correct the telecanthus or, more rarely, a Mustardé procedure can be carried out.

It is critical to address orbital dystopia in treatment planning. Frequently, patients have asymmetrical hypertelorism with dystopia. In these cases, a facial bipartition can be satisfactorily performed, provided a differential wedge of bone is removed to allow more rotation of the dystopic orbit. Box osteotomies can also be used to correct orbital dystopia and are extremely useful, especially when the occlusion is normal.

Preoperative occlusion is an important factor in determining the choice of osteotomy. If the occlusion is normal, we often choose a box osteotomy. In addition, if a unilateral or bilateral cleft is associated with hypertelorism, we prefer box osteotomies, or some variation thereof, rather than facial bipartition.

Intraoperative Problems

The most frequently encountered intraoperative problems of consequence are neurosurgical. Dural tears with cerebral spinal fluid leaks can be difficult to control. If the dura is impossible to suture and patch or if a cerebral spinal fluid leak develops postoperatively, temporary lumbar drainage can be considered. Generally, after 2 to 3 days, the leak will seal. The nasofrontal region can be handled by "mailing" a galeal frontalis flap through a slot between the frontal bone and bandeau. This can be layered along the nasofrontal region. When a frontal sinus is present, cranialization of the frontal sinus with plugging of the nasofrontal ducts is indicated to prevent postoperative epidural infections.

It is critical to monitor blood loss during surgery. The blood volume in infants and young children is quite small, and careful and prompt replacement is required. We check with the anesthesiologist at appropriate intervals, usually before an osteotomy or down-fracture, whether blood replacement is adequate.

Most patients are intubated orally, and a circummandibular wire is utilized to stabilize the endotracheal tube. To check occlusion, the tube is displaced behind the retromolar trigonal area and temporarily released from the circummandibular fixation. Soft corneal protectors are applied, although temporary tarsorrhaphies can also be carried out. The eyes are generously lubricated and, at the conclusion of the procedure, rinsed copiously with balanced salt solution. Some authors advocate prophylactic intubation of the nasolacrimal system.

The technical aspects of the procedure are critical to a successful outcome. Although we routinely do not detach the medial canthi, if residual telecanthus is present after medial translocation of the orbits and cranial bone grafting, canthopexies are performed. In these cases, a nasal splint is used postoperatively to assist in tissue redraping. Occasionally, we have used silicone naso-orbital splints for further support. These are stabilized through transnasal wires.

The nose can be approached in several ways. In patients with bilateral cleft lip and palate and nasofrontal dysplasia, and in selected patients with hypertelorism and craniosynostosis, a midface degloving approach is utilized to access the nasal tip. The technique involves the placement of circumferential nasal incisions and a small V-shaped incision on the nasal floor to prevent stricture. In conjunction with an upper buccal sulcus incision, this can be dissected to raise the entire upper lip over the nasal cartilaginous and bony skeleton. The technique can also provide an especially helpful exposure in children undergoing orbital box-type osteotomies.

Depending on the amount of blood lost and the length of the procedure, a decision must be made intraoperatively regarding the need for postoperative ventilation. Approximately 70% of our patients are extubated following the procedure. These children are observed closely in the recovery room, and if signs of respiratory distress are noted, reintubation is promptly carried out. We routinely ventilate patients undergoing facial bipartition for 24 hours postoperatively. Depending on tongue edema and intraoral secretions, a decision is then made to wean them from the ventilator on the first or second postoperative day. We routinely paralyze and sedate those children who require postoperative ventilation. This practice makes it impossible to perform a postoperative neurologic examination, so postoperative CT is performed in these cases routinely either the night of surgery or the first postoperative morning.

Postoperative Complications

The usual surgical complications can occur, such as bleeding and infection. Unless the midface has been simultaneously advanced, infection is actually quite rare in our experience. As soon as the patient is able to communicate, vision is checked. The occlusion is also inspected. Significant malocclusion may indicate displacement of the osteotomy. Other problems, such as abnormalities of extraocular motion, enophthalmos or exophthalmos, and nasolacrimal duct dysfunction, generally appear within the first 30 days following surgery. Cerebrospinal fluid leakage is usually an indication for lumbar drainage. We have not yet had to reoperate on a child to seal a cerebrospinal fluid leak.

Late Problems

Injury to the erupting dentition may not be detected for a number of years. In patients who have undergone facial bipartition, malocclusion generally consists of an overexpanded maxillary transverse dimension and a diastasis between the maxillary front teeth. The diastasis is easily corrected by orthodontics once bony healing has occurred. We generally prefer to wait 6 months before undertaking orthodontic treatment. It is rare for the transverse maxillary dimensions to remain abnormal, and they tend to collapse with time.

The biggest problems related to hypertelorism repair in our experience are residual aesthetic deformities and a tendency for hypertelorism or, more likely, telecanthus to recur. In addition, temporal and frontal bone abnormalities become more evident as time goes on and underlying bony resorption occurs. We prefer to wait a minimum of 6 months to a year before correcting temporal depressions or frontal bone abnormalities. Currently, our preferred technique of secondary cranial reconstruction involves the use of hydroxyapatite cement (Fig. 25-10). Telecanthus must be distinguished from increased interorbital distance. Depending on the clinical and radiologic findings, several steps may be necessary. It is rare for a reoperation of the same magnitude as the initial procedure to be required. Medial orbital osteotomies can be carried out in some cases, especially if residual increases in bony interorbital distance are present. Our mainstay of treatment, however, is cranial bone grafting of the nose, transnasal medial canthopexy, or both (Fig. 25-11). Adding additional bone to the nose takes up the extra tissue in the medial canthal regions and often is the only step necessary for correction. It is important to balance the nasofrontal junction and graft or recontour the glabella when indicated. Occasionally, Mustardé procedures are necessary to correct telecanthus. These are generally performed simultaneously with medial canthopexies. Repeated medial canthopexies are also necessary in many patients. When these are carried out, a small incision is made and the medial canthal tendon identified. The tendon is then labeled with either a 4-0 wire or 3-0 nylon suture. The wires or sutures are passed transnasally and twisted under direct vision. A bony fenestration is performed superior and well posterior to the lacrimal groove to seat the canthi as posteriorly and medially as possible.

Posnick et al. (31) reported on a quantitative CT assessment of patients undergoing monobloc and facial bipartition osteotomies. In patients undergoing frontal bipartition osteotomy with advancement of the monobloc segment, CT measurements early after the operation and 1 year later

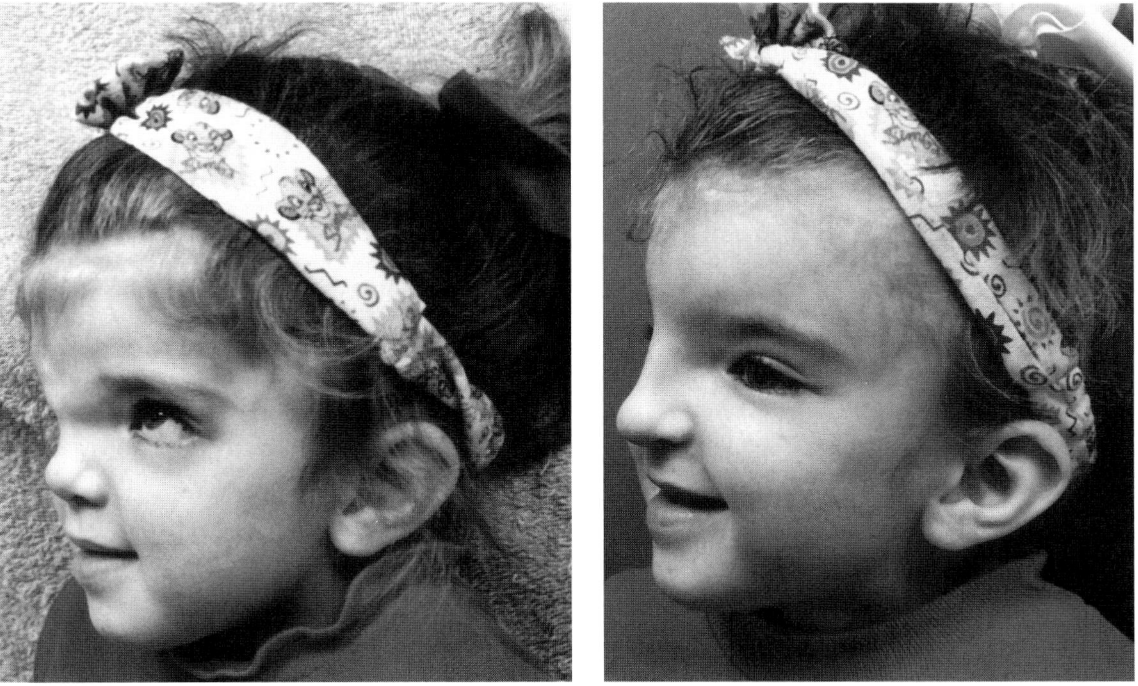

FIGURE 25-10. A: Young girl with partial resorption of frontal and temporal bone grafts after facial bipartition. **B:** Correction of contour deformities with hydroxyapatite cement.

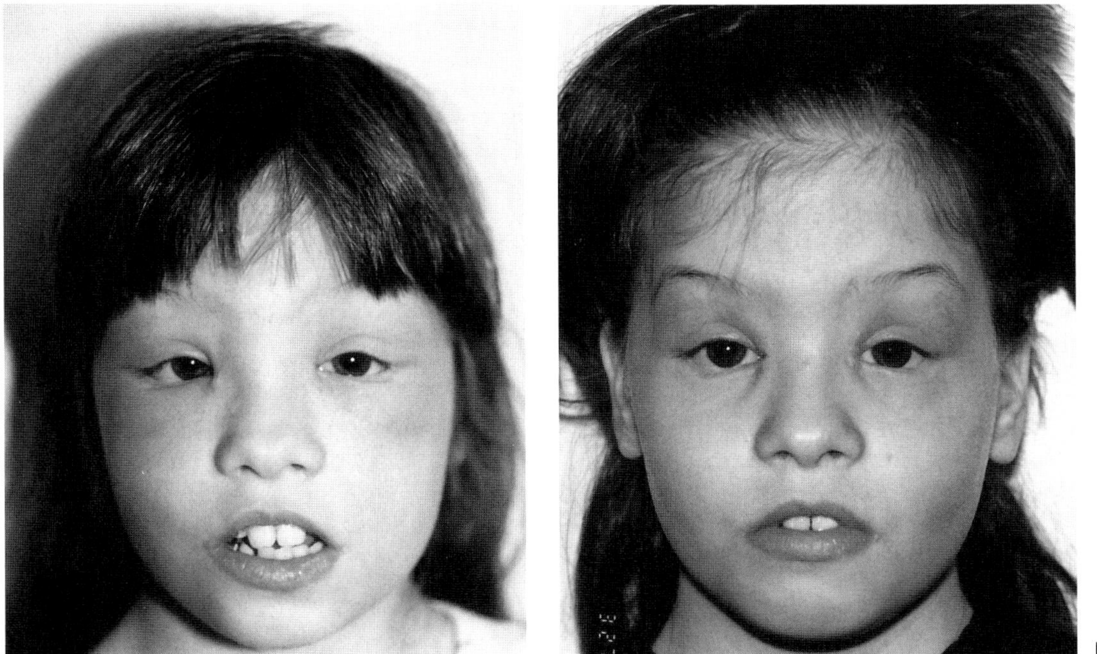

FIGURE 25-11. A: Seven-year-old girl after orbital "box" osteotomies with postoperative telecanthus. **B:** Telecanthus diminished by cranial bone graft to nose.

showed an improvement in the direction of the normal range. When compared with those of age-matched controls, the orbital measurements reflected correction of the hypertelorism. The anterior interorbital distance early after the operation was 106%, and later it was 105% of normal. The middle interorbital distance initially improved to 106% and later to 100% of normal. The distance between the lateral orbital walls stabilized at 108% and the intertemporal width at 115% of normal, an improvement over the preoperative values of 125% of normal. In patients undergoing facial bipartition osteotomy without advancement for the correction of hypertelorism, assessment of the results early after operation and 1 year later showed improvement in the orbital measurements, although the hypertelorism was not completely corrected. The anterior interorbital distance stabilized at 123% of normal, the middle interorbital distance initially approached 117% and later improved to 114% of normal, and the distance between the lateral orbital walls was corrected to 102% of normal.

McCarthy et al. (32) evaluated a series of 20 patients under 5.3 years of age who underwent correction of orbital hypertelorism. The patients were followed on average for 5 years, and six of the patients were followed in excess of 7 years with clinical and cephalometric parameters. The study demonstrated that the procedure can be safely performed at an early age and that results are aesthetically desirable. Clinical or cephalometric evidence of skeletal orbital relapse was minimal except in three patients. During the period of postoperative study, nasomaxillary growth and development proceeded as expected, except in those patients with associated clefting. All patients demonstrated an increased cranial width preoperatively and postoperatively, but bigonial and bimastoid measurements were generally within normal range. Excessive resection of nasoglabellar skin at the time of hypertelorism correction appeared to affect nasal development adversely. The bony interorbital distance was measured preoperatively on a posteroanterior cephalogram and intraoperatively with calipers. The intraoperative measurements were chosen if the values did not coincide with the cephalometric values. The average preoperative bony interorbital distance was 32 mm as measured intraoperatively with calipers. The average reduction intraoperatively was 16.1 mm. These authors typically recommended treatment to a bony interorbital distance of 14 mm. The results were compared with standards, and the patients were grouped according to the severity of their hypertelorism (i.e., first-degree, interorbital distance between 30 and 34 mm; second-degree, interorbital distance > 34 mm but < 40 mm; third-degree, interorbital distance of 30 mm). In the first-degree group, five of the seven patients were within two standard deviations of the mean according to their most recent cephalograms. In the second-degree group, six of the eight patients were within two standard deviations of the mean, and in the third-degree group, five of five patients were within two standard deviations of the mean. It is noteworthy that both patients in the first-degree group who were two standard deviations outside the mean had undergone predominantly unilateral or asymmetrical corrections. Overall, 16 of the 20 patients (80%) were within two standard deviations of the mean according to their most recent cephalometric examination. Primary iliac or rib graft reconstruction of the nose at the time of hypertelorism correction was performed in 16 of their 20 patients. Although subsequent reconstructive rhinoplasty was performed in all cases, secondary bone reconstruction was performed only in 5 of the 20 patients. Each of these five patients had undergone primary bone graft reconstruction. One of their patients required bone graft nasal reconstruction on four separate occasions. Primary transnasal medial canthopexy was performed in 16 of their 20 patients. Subsequent medial or lateral canthopexy was required in 12 of the 20 patients, including three of the four patients who did not undergo canthopexy at the original operation. Two or more canthal reconstructions were performed in 8 of the 20 patients (40%). In terms of facial aesthetics, the most important finding was that excessive soft tissue resection along the nasal dorsum and naso-orbital valley at the time of orbital translocation appears to interfere with nasal development and results in foreshortening of the nose. This problem was noted in six of their patients, four of whom subsequently required surgical lengthening of the nose.

The morbidity and mortality in this group of 20 patients were also reported. No deaths occurred. Infection occurred in two patients, one a limited bicoronal wound infection that resolved with intravenous antibiotic therapy. In the second case of infection, bilateral infraorbital abscesses developed that required surgical drainage and debridement of the orbital bone grafts. Cerebral spinal fluid rhinorrhea occurred in two patients. One required a lumboperitoneal injection, and the other required temporary spinal drainage to close the leak. Mulliken et al. (33) noted that relapse in interorbital distance tended to be related to a relatively greater preoperative interorbital measurement rather than to the age of the patient at the time of surgery, the orbital configuration, or the diagnosis. Their study also suggested that corrective hypertelorism surgery performed in children may interfere with anterior facial growth. This finding has not been confirmed by McCarthy et al. (32) or Tulasne (34).

In a study of patients with orbital hypertelorism who underwent corrective surgery, exotropia or exophoria was noted preoperatively in the majority (35). A trend toward esotropia was observed in the postoperative period. The strabismus appeared to stabilize approximately 6 months after surgery. Accordingly, surgery to correct strabismus should be deferred for a minimum of 6 months after the orbital translocation procedure.

REFERENCES

1. Greig DM. Hypertelorism: a hitherto undifferentiated congenital craniofacial deformity. *Edinburgh Med J* 1924;31:560.

2. McCarthy JG. The concept of a craniofacial anomalies center. *Clin Plast Surg* 1976;3:611–620.
3. Tessier P, Guiot G, Rougerie J, et al. Ostéotomies cranio-naso-orbitales. Hypertélorisme. *Ann Chir Plast* 1967;12:103–118.
4. Converse JM, Ransohoff J, Mathews ES, et al. Ocular hypertelorism and pseudohypertelorism: advances in surgical treatment. *Plast Reconstr Surg* 1970;45:1–13.
5. McCarthy JG. A study of gustatory (taste) and olfactory function in craniofacial anomalies. *Plast Reconstr Surg* 1979;64:52–58.
6. Psillakis JM, Zanini SA, Godoy R, et al. Orbital hypertelorism: modification of the craniofacial osteotomy line. *J Maxillofac Surg* 1981;9:10.
7. Converse JM, Smith B. An operation for congenital and traumatic hypertelorism. In: Troutman RC, Converse JM, Smith B, eds. *Plastic and reconstructive surgery of the eye and adnexa.* London: Butterworth-Heineman, 1962.
8. Schmid E. Surgical management of hypertelorism. In: Longacre JJ, ed. *Craniofacial anomalies: pathogenesis and repair.* Philadelphia: JB Lippincott Co, 1968:155.
9. Tessier P, Guiot G, Derome P. Orbital hypertelorism. II. Definitive treatment of orbital hypertelorism by craniofacial or by extracranial osteotomies. *Scand J Plast Reconstr Surg* 1973; 7:39–58.
10. Tessier P. The definitive plastic surgical treatment of the severe facial deformities of craniofacial dysostosis, Crouzon's and Apert's disease. *Plast Reconstr Surg* 1971;48:419–442.
11. Ortiz Monasterio F, Fuente del Campo A, Carillo A. Advancement of the orbits and the midface in one piece, combined with frontal repositioning, for the correction of Crouzon's deformity. *Plast Reconstr Surg* 1978;61:507–516.
12. van der Meulen JC. Medial fasciotomy. *Br J Plast Surg* 1979;32:339–342.
13. Cohen MM, Richieri-Costa A, Guion-Almeida M, et al. Hypertelorism: interorbital growth, measurements, and pathogenetic considerations. *Int J Oral Maxillofac Surg* 1995;24: 387–395.
14. Ford HER. Growth of the cranial base. *Am J Orthod* 1958;44:498–506.
15. Tessier P. Experiences in the treatment of orbital hypertelorism. Presented at the Annual Meeting of the American Society of Plastic and Reconstructive Surgeons, September 20, 1972, Las Vegas, Nevada.
16. Tessier P. Experiences in the treatment of orbital hypertelorism. *Plast Reconstr Surg* 1974;53:1–18.
17. David DJ, Sheffield L, Simpson D, et al. Frontoethmoidal meningoencephaloceles: morphology and treatment. *Br J Plast Surg* 1984;37:271–284.
18. Moss ML. Hypertelorism and cleft palate deformity. *Acta Anat* 1965;61:547–557.
19. Mann I. *Developmental abnormalities of the eye.* London: Cambridge University Press, 1970.
20. Burck D, Sadler TW. Morphogenesis of median facial clefts in mice treated with diazo-oxo-norleucine (DON). *Teratology* 1983;27:385–394.
21. Darab DJ, Minkoff R, Sciote J, et al. Pathogenesis of median facial clefts treated with methotrexate. *Teratology* 1987;36:77–86.
22. McCarthy JG, Thorne CHM, Wood-Smith D. Principles of craniofacial surgery: orbital hypertelorism. *Craniofacial Anomalies* 60:2974–3012.
23. Whitaker LA, Katowitz JA, Randall P. The nasolacrimal apparatus in congenital facial anomalies. *J Maxillofac Surg* 1974; 2:59–63.
24. Converse JM, Smith B. An operation for congenital and traumatic hypertelorism. In: Troutman RC, Converse JM, Smith B, eds. *Plastic and reconstructive surgery of the eye and adnexa.* London: Butterworth-Heineman, 1962.
25. Tessier P. Orbital hypertelorism. I. Successive surgical attempts, material and methods, causes and mechanisms. *Scand J Plast Surg* 1972;6:135–155.
26. Schmid E. Surgical management of hypertelorism. In: Longacre JJ, ed. *Craniofacial anomalies: pathogenesis and repair.* Philadelphia: JB Lippincott Co, 1968:155.
27. Tessier P, Guiot G, Rougerie J, et al. Ostéotomies cranio-naso-orbitales. Hypertélorisme. *Ann Chir Plast* 1967;12:103–118.
28. Converse JM, Ransohoff J, Mathews ES, et al. Ocular hypertelorism and pseudohypertelorism: advances in surgical treatment. *Plast Reconstr Surg* 1970;45:1–13.
29. Cohen SR, Boydston W, Burstein FD, et al. Monobloc distraction osteogenesis during infancy: report of a case and presentation of a new device. *Plast Reconstr Surg* 1998;101:1919–1924.
30. Whitaker LA, Munro IR, Salyer KE, et al. Combined report of problems and complications in 793 craniofacial operations. *Plast Reconstr Surg* 1979;64:198.
31. Posnick JC, Waitzman A, Armstrong D, et al. Monobloc and facial bipartition osteotomies: quantitative assessment of presenting deformity and surgical results based on computed tomography scans. *J Oral Maxillofac Surg* 1995;53:358–367.
32. McCarthy JG, LaTrenta GS, Breitbart AS, et al. Hypertelorism correction in the young child. *Plast Reconstr Surg* 1990; 86:214–225.
33. Mulliken JB, Kaban LB, Evans CA, et al. Facial skeletal changes following hypertelorism correction. *Plast Reconstr Surg* 1986;77:7.
34. Tulasne JF. Maxillary growth following total septal reconstruction in telorbitism. In: Caronni EP, ed. *Craniofacial surgery.* Boston: Little, Brown and Company, 1985:176–189.
35. Choy AE, Margolis S, Breinin GM, et al. Analysis of preoperative and postoperative extraocular muscle function in surgical translocation of bony orbits: a preliminary report. In: Converse JM, McCarthy JG, Wood-Smith D, eds. *Symposium on diagnosis and treatment of craniofacial anomalies.* St. Louis: Mosby, 1979.

Discussion

ORBITAL HYPERTELORISM

FERNANDO ORTIZ MONASTERIO

Based on his experience in the treatment of craniofacial trauma and tumors, Paul Tessier in 1967 made a transcendental contribution to the correction of many severe craniofacial malformations. Neurosurgery was a well-established specialty offering safe, systematic access to the cranial cavity. Maxillofacial surgery also encompassed a well-developed territory limited to the upper and lower jaws. Between these two areas was the bony orbit, a sort of "no man's land" where only timid forays had been attempted (1).

Tessier extended neurosurgery to the orbit and maxilla. He showed that the orbits could be mobilized in every direction and that is is possible to work simultaneously on the maxilla, orbits, nose, and cranium. Craniofacial surgery was born. It was only logical that the correction of hypertelorism would be among the early surgical techniques developed in this new field.

Three decades later, surgical procedures to correct hypertelorism have been refined and modified. Several options are available for different types of malformations of varying degrees of severity. Complications are infrequent and skeletal alterations are predictable, but optimal aesthetic results cannot be obtained in all patients.

Dr. Cohen has written an excellent and well-documented review of the subject, from the early attempts to the present time. The indications for the different osteotomies according the type of deformity are analyzed in detail based on his extensive personal experience. The timing of surgery, relapses of malformations, soft tissue problems, and nasal correction are discussed, and surgical sequelae are presented thoughtfully. This comprehensive chapter offers the reader an overview of the pathology and treatment of hypertelorism.

In accordance with the basic concept of this book, which is to analyze "unfavorable results in plastic surgery," I feel it is pertinent to make some observations about the indications for the different osteotomies, long-term outcomes, nasal corrections, and final aesthetic results. These are based on experience during the last 27 years in treating 167 patients with hypertelorism. Included in this series are seven patients with Apert syndrome and two with Crouzon syndrome in whom the correction of hypertelorism was performed simultaneously with a monobloc advancement. Except for three patients with pharyngeal encephaloceles and two others with large frontal encephaloceles presenting as true hypertelorism, our patients with frontoethmoidal encephaloceles have been excluded from the series. This distinction is made because all of them presented with a lateral displacement of the medial orbital wall that was not associated with lateralization of the entire orbit. It should also be noted that the nasal deformity in this group is entirely different. Practically all patients with hypertelorism, regardless of type, have a short nose, in contrast to patients with nasoethmoidal encephaloceles, whose noses are elongated. True hypertelorism related to incomplete medial rotation of the orbits may sometimes be associated with frontal cranial defects and encephaloceles, as has been observed in some of the cases of Tessier et al. (2) and David et al. (3) in addition to those in our series.

Furthermore, orbital translocations performed in some patients with frontoethmoidal encephaloceles early in our work resulted in hypotelorism, and I believe that this result has also been demonstrated in cases published by other surgeons (3–5).

F. Ortiz Monasterio: School of Medicine, Universidad Nacional Autónoma de México; Professor of Plastic Surgery, Department of Plastic & Reconstructive Surgery, Hospital General "Manuel Gea Gonzalez," Mexico City, Mexico

OSTEOTOMIES

In a few cases of minimal hypertelorism associated with a broad nose, the medial orbital walls were mobilized medially after a bony resection of the midline (6). In other grade 1 cases, ethmoid resections and subcranial U-shaped osteotomies of the orbit were carried out, with sparing of the roofs. In the rest of our patients, up to 1980, a "box osteotomy" of the orbits was performed through the intracranial route. This procedure corrected the orbital malposition without elongating the nose and the midface skeleton. Most of the patients in this group required horizontal maxillary osteotomies later in life to correct the short midface. All the patients who originally presented with an anterior open bite required prolonged orthodontic treatment and oblique bilateral maxillary osteotomies to achieve a normal central vertical dimension. Minor to moderate impairment in anteroposterior growth of the maxilla was observed when a box osteotomy was performed at an early age (3 to 8 years), and this also required surgical correction (Figs. 25D-1 and 25D-2).

After 1980, we preferred to carry out a monoblock facial bipartition in most patients, advancing only the lateral part of the orbits when necessary (7). This group included all cases with craniofrontonasal dysplasia, midline and lateral clefts, or unilateral and bilateral clefts of the lip and palate (in which the facial halves are already separated by the cleft).

A cephalometric analytic system was developed by our

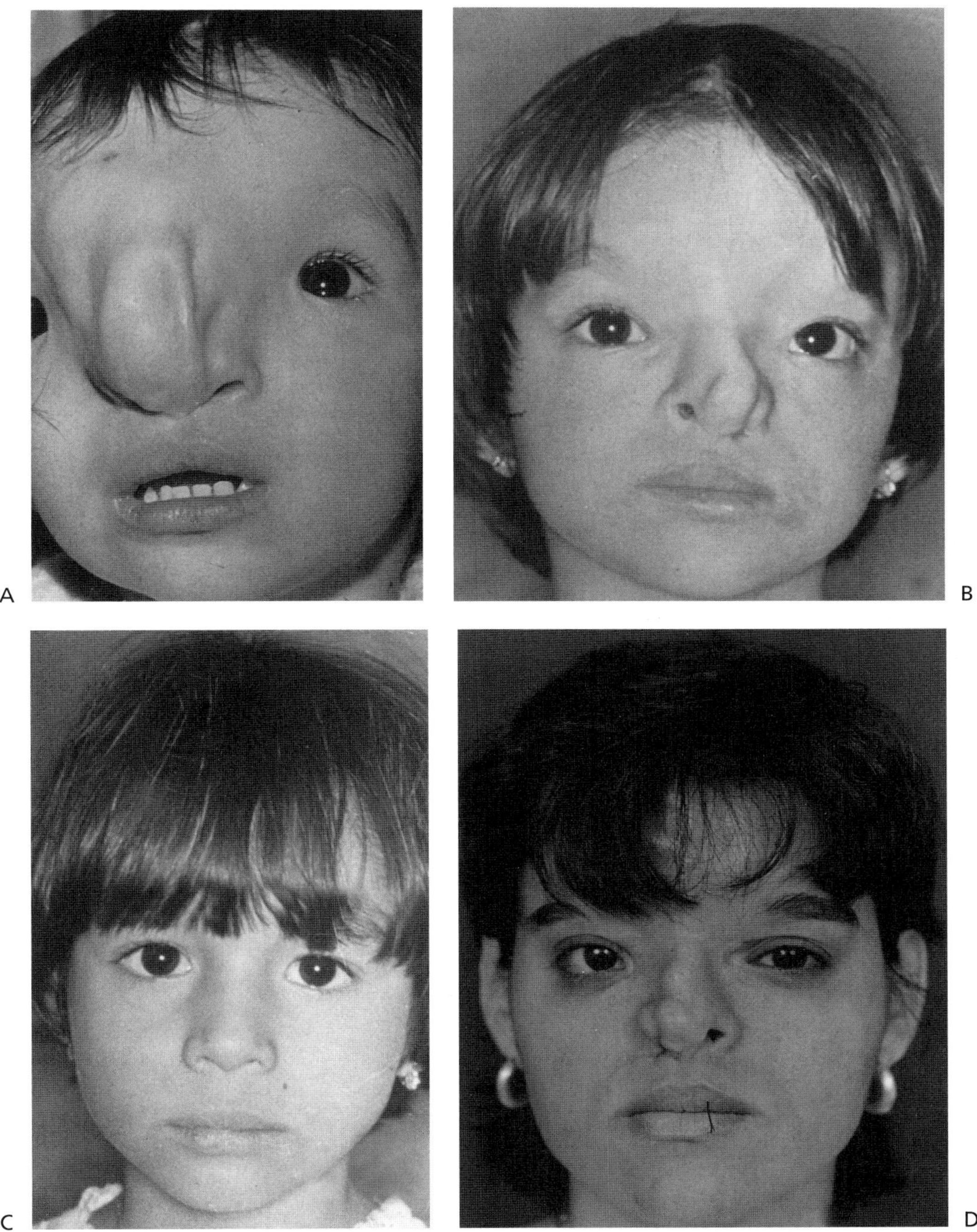

FIGURE 25D-1. A: Preoperative photograph of 3-year-old child with grade 3 hypertelorism, frontal bone defect, and encephalocele. **B:** Photograph 3 years postoperatively at age 6 after box osteotomy showing telecanthus, nasal deformity, and short midface. **C:** The twin sister of the patient in A and B demonstrating normal facial vertical growth. *(continued)*

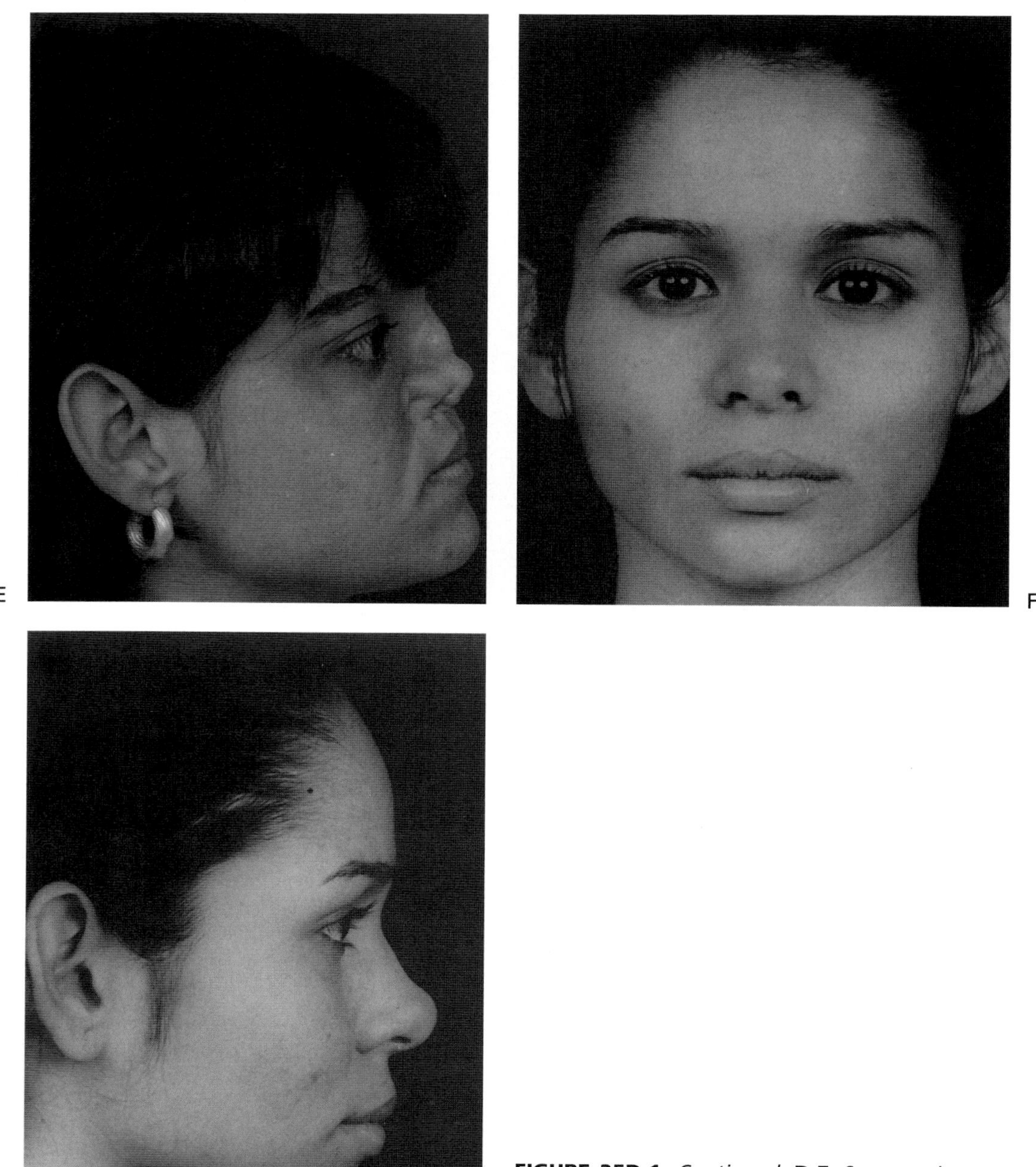

FIGURE 25D-1. *Continued.* **D,E:** Same patient at age 23 (20 years after surgery) showing inadequate vertical and sagittal maxillary growth. **F,G:** The twin sister at the same age.

group (8,9) to determine the exact amount of central bone resection and the extent of orbital mobilization and facial elongation that would be required (Fig. 25D-3). Lateral expansion of the dental arch is prevented by extending the resection of the nasal spine at its junction with the bony palate. Incisions of the palatal mucosa are eliminated by dissecting a subperiosteal tunnel at the midline and inserting a narrow malleable retractor for protection. We have had no relapses after elongation of the facial skeleton. The sagittal growth of the maxilla is normal in this group in comparison with the deficit found when a box osteotomy was used by our group (10) and others (11,12).

Subcranial facial bipartitions sparing the orbital roof were performed in three adult patients with craniofrontonasal dysplasia, and the results were excellent. The extracranial approach was utilized to avoid a frontal craniectomy. We feel that this is an aesthetic operation, and we try to eliminate the potential complications, such as bone resorption, inherent in any major craniectomy in adults.

As stated by Dr. Cohen, despite careful planning and

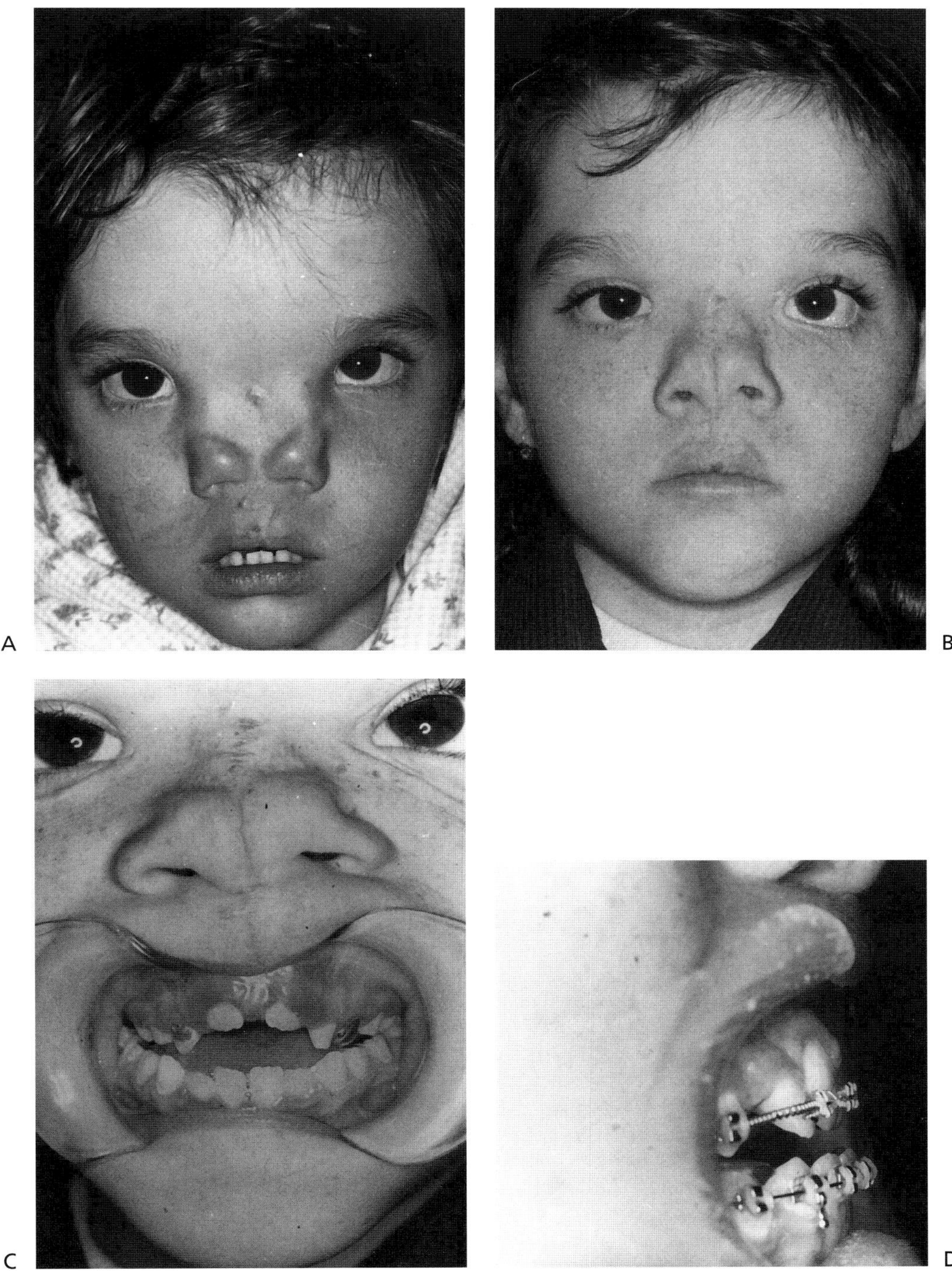

FIGURE 25D-2. A: Preoperative photograph of 3-year-old girl with 0-14 cleft (median cleft of the lip had been repaired). **B:** Photograph 3 years postoperatively at age 6 after box osteotomy. **C:** Same patient at age 6 showing anterior open bite and deficient vertical growth at center of the face. **D:** The anterior open bite and deficient sagittal growth of each maxilla persisted at age 14 and required maxillary osteotomies.

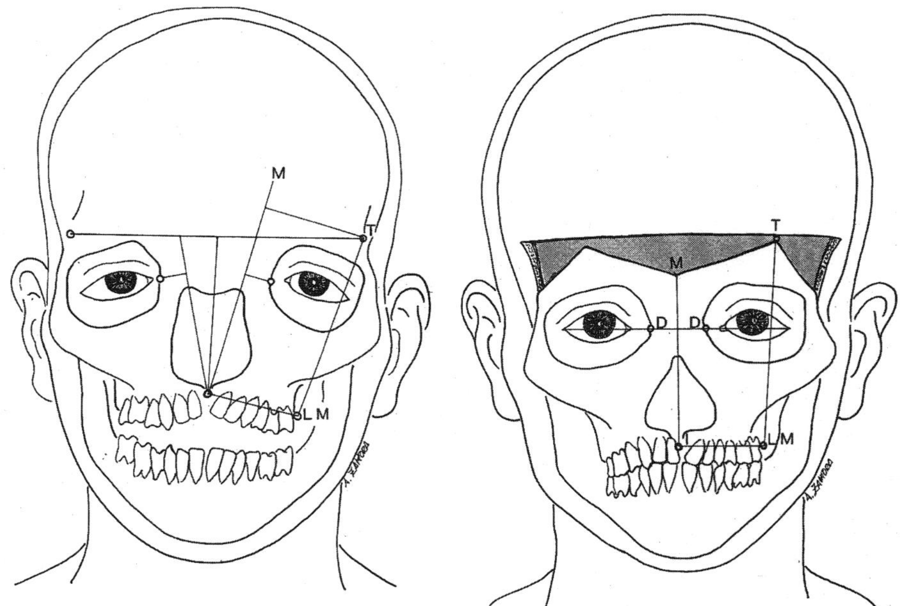

FIGURE 25D-3. Tracing on anteroposterior cephalometry. The following points are located: *I*, interincisor; *LM*, lateral maxillary; *T*, temporal; *D*, dacrion; *S*, sagittal. The following planes are traced: *TT*, temporal; *SI*, sagittal; *LMT*, lateral facial; *LMJ*, maxillary; *DD*, intercrestal. The ideal distance from the lacrimal crest to the midline is marked on each side on the intercrestal plane, *M*. A line is traced from *I* to *D* and extended beyond the temporal plane on each side. A line parallel to the maxillary plane *(LMT)* is traced on each side from point *T* to the extension of line *IM*. The distance from the intersection of these two lines to the temporal plane corresponds to the elongation that will be obtained at the center of the face *(right)*. Position of the two halves of the face after medial mobilization. The bony defect created below the temporal plane *(TT)* represents the facial elongation and corresponds (in an inverted position) to the anterior open bite. (Modified from Ortiz Monasterio F, Medina O, Musolas A. Geometrical planning for the correction of orbital hypertelorism. *Plast Reconstr Surg* 1990;86:650–657, with permission.)

meticulous technique, many patients require repeated secondary procedures to correct telecanthus. I thoroughly agree with him that the most unfavorable results are related to the nasal correction, so that secondary surgery is required in all patients except those with minimal degrees of hypertelorism.

Eliminating excess skin at the glabellar area results in vertical midline scars that are acceptable in most patients, but elongation of the nose with a Z-plasty diminishes the aesthetic result. Despite the rigid fixation of cranial bone grafts to the dorsum, resorption was observed in some of our cases, as reported by Cohen. For the secondary dorsal augmentation, we prefer to use costal cartilage grafts at the present time. A thin Kirschner wire is inserted into the cartilage to prevent warping.

Many of our patients with third-degree hypertelorism had single or multiple soft tissue clefts, often bilateral, and severe nasal malformations that ranged from bifidity to complete separation of the two halves of the nose, and from nasal hypoplasia to complete arrhinia. The No. 2 and No. 3 clefts (Tessier classification) varied from alar retractions to unilateral hypoplasia to hemiarrhinia. In the early stages of our work, we used local flaps followed by numerous secondary procedures, with disappointing aesthetic results. Multiple Z-plasties in which tissues were borrowed from neighboring areas resulted in a patchwork effect, with flaps of different colors and textures crossing the limits of the aesthetic units (4).

We feel that the concept of aesthetic units and subunits is of primary importance in nasal reconstruction, and that flaps extending beyond the boundaries of these units should be avoided. In the last 10 years, we have used frontal flaps, sometimes with previous tissue expansion to reconstruct the nasal units. These procedures are performed simultaneously with the primary osteotomies to achieve a more comprehensive reconstruction at the first stage of the treatment. With good skin coverage, it is much easier to build a good structural support. Forehead skin expansion before the orbital facial mobilization did not affect the cranial and orbital osteotomies (9).

Despite enormous advances in the treatment of hypertelorism, described in this excellent chapter by Dr. Cohen, the final aesthetic outcome is still limited in some respects. Most problems can be corrected subsequently, but we must accept that the repair of these complex malformations is rarely a one-stage procedure and that secondary procedures are generally required.

REFERENCES

1. Guiot G, Rougerie J, Tessier P. La groffe dermique. Procédé de protection cérebro-méningée et de blindage duramérien. *Ann Chir Plast* 1967;12:94.
2. Tessier P, Guiot G, Rougerie J, et al. Ostéotomies cranio-naso-orbitales. Hypertélorisme. *Ann Chir Plast* 1967;12:103.
3. David DJ, Sheffield L, Simpson D, et al. Frontoethmoidal meningoencephaloceles: morphology and treatment. *Br J Plast Surg* 1984;37;271.
4. Ortiz Monasterio F, Fuente del Campo A. Nasal correction in hypertelorism. *Scand J Plast Reconstr Surg* 1981;15:277–286.
5. Tessier P. Orbital hypertelorism. 1. Successive surgical attempts, material and methods, causes and mechanisms. *Scand J Plast Surg* 1972;6:135.
6. Ortiz Monasterio F. Surgical correction of the bifid nose. In: Brent B, ed. *The artistry of reconstructive surgery.* St. Louis: Mosby, 1983:57–62.
7. Van der Muelen JC. Medial fasciotomy. *Br J Plast Surg* 1979;32:339.
8. Ortiz Monasterio F, Medina O, Musolas A. Geometrical planning for the correction of orbital hypertelorism. *Plast Reconstr Surg* 1990;86:650–657.
9. Ortiz Monasterio F, Molina F. Orbital hypertelorism. *CI Plast Surg* 1994;21:599–612.
10. Ortiz Monasterio F, Molina F, Sigler A, et al. Maxillary growth in children after early facial bipartition. *J Craniofac Surg* 1996;6:440–448.
11. Mulliken JB, Kaban LB, Evans CA, et al. Facial skeletal changes following hypertelorism correction. *Plast Reconstr Surg* 1986;77:7.
12. Tulasne JF. Maxillary growth following total septal reconstruction in teleorbitism. In: Caronni EP, ed. *Craniofacial surgery.* Boston: Little, Brown and Company, 1985:176–189.

26

ORTHOGNATHIC SURGERY

HARVEY M. ROSEN

To discuss the unfavorable result in orthognathic surgery, one must first have a clear understanding of the goals or objectives of orthognathic surgical procedures. Simply stated, if the goals are not achieved, then the result must be considered unfavorable. Therefore, it becomes imperative that goals be clearly defined. Accordingly, a significant part of this chapter is devoted to a discussion of what one should be attempting to accomplish in orthognathic surgery.

TREATMENT PLANNING GOALS

Historically, orthognathic surgical procedures attempted to address the issues of stability and aesthetics. Concerns regarding stability were related to establishing a functional occlusal result, and concerns about aesthetics focused on normalizing facial proportions.

Although the traditional goals were commendable, this approach to treatment planning was always conceptually flawed for two primary reasons. The first was that the best possible aesthetic result was not necessarily synonymous with what was considered to be the most stable correction. Thus, the dual goals of stability and aesthetics were frequently competing goals, and more often than not, aesthetics were sacrificed in an effort to enhance skeletal stability. For instance, a class III skeletal patient was frequently treated with mandibular setback surgery regardless of the aesthetic consequences because for many years, particularly during the 1970s and early 1980s, mandibular setback surgery was considered to produce a more stable result than maxillary advancement surgery.

The second flaw in traditional surgical goals was that aesthetic judgments were to a large extent based on normative data taken from skeletal and soft tissue cephalometric analyses. The problem with this approach is that normalcy is not synonymous with beauty. Imagine the many patients we see in our practices who have normal facial proportions and yet are not considered beautiful. On the other hand, we are aware of strikingly attractive people who have facial measurements and proportions that fall outside the normal ranges. It begins to be easy to understand why the traditional approach to treatment planning, which involved a balance between aesthetics and stability and in which aesthetic decisions were based on normative cephalometric data, was conceptually flawed.

Beginning in the 1980s, advances in technology and biomaterials became available to surgeons that should have dramatically influenced our treatment planning goals. Without question, the most important of these was rigid internal fixation, which came into routine use. Rigid fixation has significantly reduced the mean rates of relapse in many types of orthognathic procedures. More importantly, it has made the results of procedures much more predictable (i.e., the expected range of degrees of skeletal relapse has been dramatically narrowed). Enhanced predictability has been demonstrated for maxillary impaction and maxillary advancement surgery based on the Le Fort I osteotomy (1,2) and for mandibular advancement surgery based on the sagittal split ramus osteotomy (3). Most recently, it has been demonstrated for mandibular advancement surgery in which the distal mandibular segment is subjected to significant counterclockwise rotational movement, the mandibular osteotomy being the point of rotation (4,5). This type of procedure was formerly considered ill-advised because high rates of relapse were associated with its use. However, rigid fixation has made the results of the procedure predictable.

The only procedure in which gross skeletal stability continued to be a problem despite rigid fixation was inferior maxillary repositioning, which is performed to correct a short face. The instability was primarily related to the inevitable resorption of autogenous bone grafts placed into the osteotomy gap secondary to the compressive forces of mastication. The advent of porous block hydroxyapatite, a nonresorbable bone graft substitute, solved this problem. When the use of this material was combined with rigid fixation, stable results following vertical elongation of the maxilla were consistently achieved (2,6).

Rigid fixation techniques and bone graft substitutes should have dramatically changed our entire perception of orthognathic surgery and its goals. The treatment planning

H. M. Rosen: Department of Surgery, University of Pennsylvania, Philadelphia, Pennsylvania; Division of Plastic Surgery, Pennsylvania Hospital, Philadelphia, Pennsylvania

pendulum has now swung in the direction of aesthetic enhancement and away from stability concerns. The primary emphasis on the occlusal result can no longer be justified (i.e., it is clearly no longer acceptable to sacrifice facial aesthetics in an effort to restore a normal occlusion). Most importantly, however, for the purposes of treatment planning, orthognathic surgery should be considered aesthetic surgery. One can now offer patients a surgical treatment plan that appears to be in their best interest aethetically without worrying that what is being offered is inherently unstable. The occlusal result should now be considered as a means to achieving the aesthetic result rather than as an end in itself. Accordingly, this discussion focuses on the unfavorable aesthetic result in orthognathic surgery. Although operative complications and unstable occlusal results must also be considered unfavorable, they are beyond the scope of this chapter.

TREATMENT PLANNING METHODOLOGY

If one plans to adopt this approach to treatment planning, how can one continue to rely on skeletal diagnoses to plan treatment? Skeletal diagnoses are derived from skeletal cephalometric analyses (7,8) that are compared with normative data derived from "normal" persons, not necessarily persons who would be considered attractive or beautiful. It is worthwhile to repeat that normalcy is not necessarily beauty. Additionally, skeletal data are limited to the midsagittal plane and provide no information regarding the soft tissues. Cephalometric analyses of soft tissues (9) may be more clinically relevant than skeletal analyses, but they too lack clinical significance. They are deficient in that they are limited to the sagittal midline and, most importantly, are taken from "normal" individuals.

Despite all the imaging technology that is available today, the best possible approach to aesthetic treatment planning relies on clinical examination of the patient. From this is derived a through description of the facial morphology. The clinical examination is meant to be a qualitative, visual assessment of the patient's face and how one can best alter it to achieve the maximum aesthetic benefits. The word *qualitative* is used to emphasize the fact that the visual impression of the facial morphology may be quite different from what would be indicated by quantitative measurements. For instance, a lower face that is quantitatively long relative to the midface may not appear excessively long. It is very important that morphologic assessment take into account the dynamic interrelationship between the underlying skeletal foundation and the overlying soft tissue, and how each can affect the appearance of the other.

A description of the facial morphology should, at a minimum, include the following: In the frontal view, overall facial symmetry and vertical proportionality should be assessed. Although asymmetries in the upper face are important, those of the lower face are more clinically relevant in jaw surgery. A qualitative determination of the height of the lower face, visualized from the menton to the subnasale, relative to that of the midface, visualized from the subnasale to the glabella, is then undertaken. Although quantitative measurements can be obtained, it is the qualitative visual assessment of whether the lower face appears too long or too short that is most relevant. Other assessments in the frontal view that relate to vertical proportionality include circumoral lip strain, the depth and definition of the labiomental fold, and the position of the incisal edge of the maxillary teeth relative to the vermilion edge.

In the lateral view, the two basic visual assessments are overall facial divergence and facial convexity or concavity. Facial divergence is determined by the position of the soft tissue pogonion relative to a vertical line dropped from the glabella. If the chin point is posterior to this line, the face diverges posteriorly. If it appears to be anterior to this line, the face diverges anteriorly. Normal degrees of facial divergence have been described both anthropometrically (10) and cephalometrically (9). Anthropometric mean values of facial divergence in normal North American male and female Caucasians are negative; the facial profile is posteriorly divergent. Anterior divergent profiles are typically not seen in either sex until one deviates from the mean values by two standard deviations. Cephalometric mean values usually place the pogonion in a neutral position (i.e., the position of the soft tissue chin point relative to a vertical line from the glabella is within a range of values from plus 4 mm to minus 4 mm).

Overall facial convexity or concavity describes the profile by a line connecting the glabella to the subnasale and the subnasale to the pogonion. These points can produce a line that is straight, concave, or convex. Additionally, the parasagittal profile should be qualitatively described—that is, are the sagittal relationships of the soft tissues from the infraorbital area to the paranasal area to the parasymphyseal area convex or concave in appearance? The most aesthetically pleasing profiles are convex both in the midsagittal and parasagittal planes.

The last factor in the description of the overall facial morphology is an assessment of the overlying soft tissues. Most pertinent is a qualitative assessment of the support of the soft tissues afforded by the underlying skeletal foundation. Are the soft tissues redundant or deficient relative to skeletal volumes? Are the soft tissues thin, delicate, and refined, or are they thick and fleshy? All these soft tissues qualities significantly affect the overall visual impression of the face. An impression of angularity, definition, and highlighting is created when the facial mask is well supported by the skeletal foundation. With a lack of skeletal support, these features are absent, and in the extreme, the face may be described as amorphous.

These basic concepts are critically important in treatment planning because the support of the facial soft tissues is the single most important factor in determining the aesthetic success or failure of many orthognathic surgical procedures. For this reason, the normative cephalometric and anthropometric data previously described should be largely ignored in surgical planning. On the contrary, the most predictable way to achieve soft tissue support is to achieve adequate (not necessarily normative) projection of the middle and lower face and adequate height of the lower face. In this context, *adequate* means that skeletal segments are displaced as much as necessary to achieve the desired soft tissue support. Ironically, therefore, soft tissue goals influence, and in certain circumstances dictate, skeletal proportions. This concept is distinctly different from the traditional one of orthognathic surgery, in which one tries to achieve normal facial measurements and proportions and, in so doing, hopes that the soft tissues will respond favorably. The traditional approach to treatment planning is at best naïve because the soft tissue responses to many types of skeletal displacement made in an effort to achieve facial normalcy are unpredictable and unreliable. Accordingly, it is advisable to set qualitative goals for the soft tissue and then use these goals to determine skeletal displacements and, therefore, facial proportionality (11,12).

In summary, the aesthetic goals of orthognathic surgery are to achieve (a) good support of the soft tissues by the underlying skeletal foundation, (b) adequate projection of the middle and lower face, and (c) adequate height of the lower face. The first goal is accomplished by achieving the second and third goals. By understanding these goals, one can more readily appreciate what constitutes the unfavorable result in orthognathic surgery, why it occurs, and how to avoid it. As with any unfavorable result, avoidance is far preferable to treatment because the latter entails secondary jaw surgery, an option not to be relished by either patient or surgeon.

SAMPLE CASES

The philosophy of treatment planning previously described is illustrated by the patient in Fig. 26-1, who presented for surgical correction of a class III malocclusion. In the frontal view, one can describe the appearance as symmetrical with normal vertical proportions (i.e., the height of the lower face approximates that of the midface). The nasal base is excessively wide. The profile is described as one of neutral divergence (soft tissue chin point falls on a vertical line dropped from the glabella) with overall slight convexity. The soft tissues, however, are inadequately supported by the underlying skeletal foundation despite the fact that the patient displays "normal" facial proportions in both the vertical and sagittal planes. Note the lack of zygomatic highlighting and submalar hollowing. Jowls and submental fullness are associated with poor definition along the inferior border of the mandible. The face lacks refinement and definition. Following presurgical orthodontics, the class III occlusal relationship will allow for a modest, 4-mm advancement of the maxilla, which is inadequate to achieve the soft tissue goals of enhanced skeletal support, angularity, and highlighting. Accordingly, surgical correction will involve advancement of both maxilla and mandible in addition to the chin. This will be carried out despite the fact that the preoperative position of the chin is normal relative to the glabella. In addition, the maxilla and chin will be inferiorly repositioned as they are advanced, despite the fact that the preoperative vertical proportions are normal. Soft tissue goals are dictating the skeletal displacements and, therefore, the facial proportions.

Postoperatively, improvement in the soft tissue definition is marked, with a well-defined zygomatic complex, submalar hollowing, and elimination of the jowls. This has been achieved by creating vertical facial disproportion (i.e., the lower face is now quantitatively too long relative to the midface). In the lateral view, enhanced definition of the inferior border of the mandible and angularity in the cervical mandibular region are noted. However, the projection of the middle and lower face is now excessive, at least in comparison with normative standards (i.e., sagittal disproportion has been created). This case nicely illustrates how soft tissue considerations have dictated skeletal proportions.

The result in Fig. 26-1 is in marked contrast to the one seen in Fig. 26-2. This patient also underwent correction of a class III malocclusion, which in this instance involved mandibular setback surgery performed by another surgeon. Facial aesthetic considerations have been completely sacrificed in an effort to restore a normal occlusion. Secondary to an excessive reduction in the overall skeletal volume, soft tissue support is now inadequate. The result is soft tissue excess and a total absence of facial definition and angularity. A gross disequilibrium between soft tissue mass and skeletal mass has been produced. This patient clearly should have been treated with maxillary advancement surgery. Although the case is an extreme illustration of this principle, more subtle examples of the same phenomenon are frequently observed in orthognathic surgery.

The patient in Fig. 26-3 was treated by me. She was to undergo surgical correction of a class I anterior open bite. She has a long lower face with secondary lip strain. Surgical correction will involve posterior maxillary impaction, allowing the mandible to autorotate at the condyle to close the open bite, and vertical reduction genioplasty. Overall, the height of the lower face will be decreased by 8 mm. Postoperatively, the anterior open bite has been totally corrected. In the frontal view, the aesthetic result is acceptable, with an obvious reduction in the height of the lower face and elimination of the lip strain. However, in the lateral view, note the accumulation of soft tissue in the midcheek region just lateral to the nasolabial fold. This represents relative soft tissue excess in the region secondary to skeletal re-

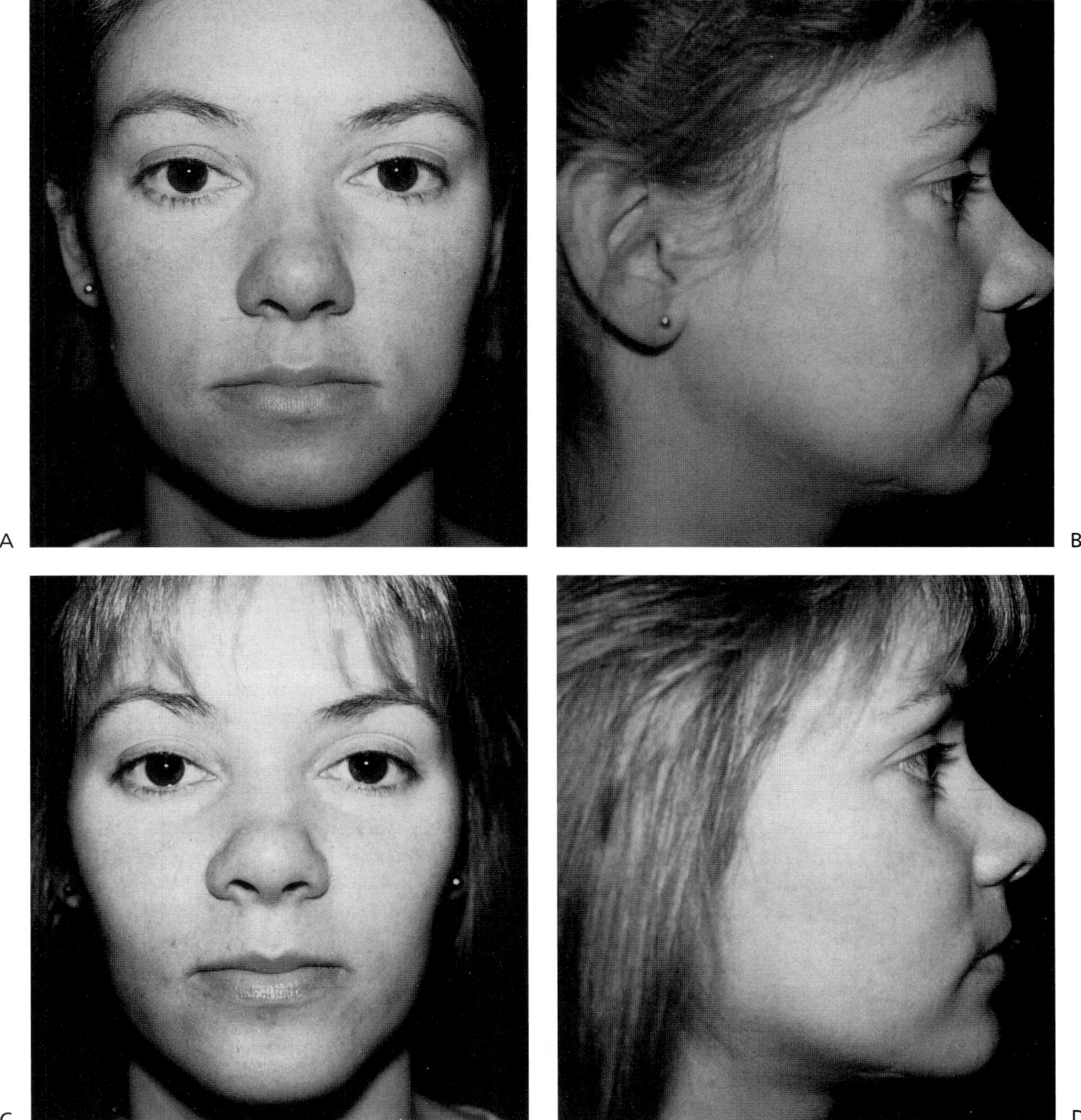

FIGURE 26-1. A,B: A class III patient with so-called normal facial proportionality (i.e., in the vertical dimension, the lower face is equal to the midface, and in the sagittal dimension, neutral divergence is combined with midsagittal convexity). Soft tissue support is inadequate, with an absence of definition and angularity. Note the lack of zygomatic definition and the presence of jowls and submental fullness. Surgical correction will entail overcorrection in both the vertical and sagittal dimensions to create a quantitatively long lower face and excessive projection of the midface and lower face. In this way, skeletal support of the soft tissues is enhanced. **C,D:** In the postoperative views, note the marked improvement in skeletal support of the soft tissues, with a more angular, defined appearance. *(continued)*

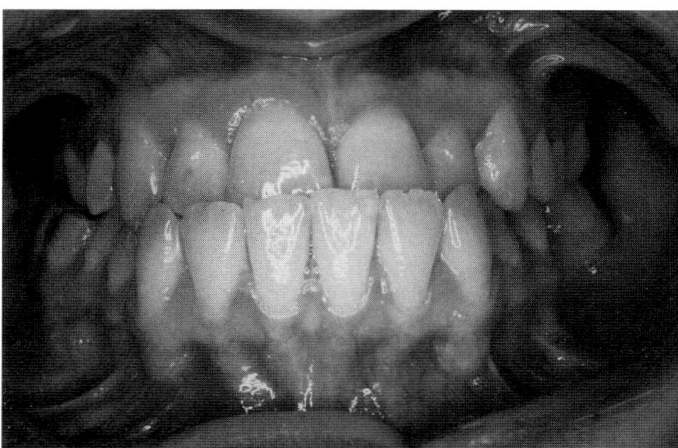
E

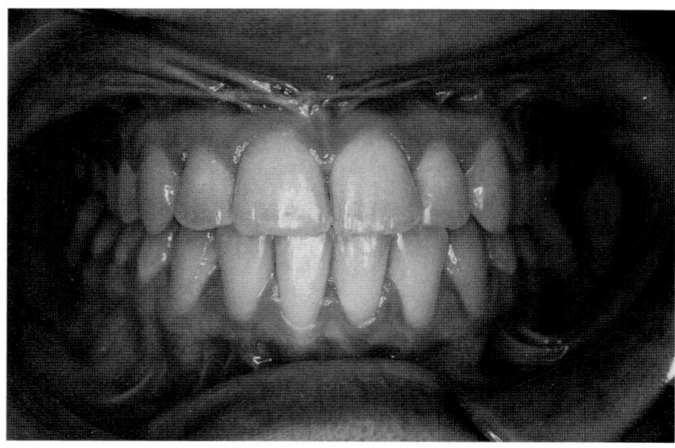
F

FIGURE 26-1. *Continued.* **E,F:** The preoperative and postoperative occlusions. (From Rosen H. Facial skeletal expansion: treatment strategies and rationale. *Plast Reconstr Surg* 1992;89:798, with permission.)

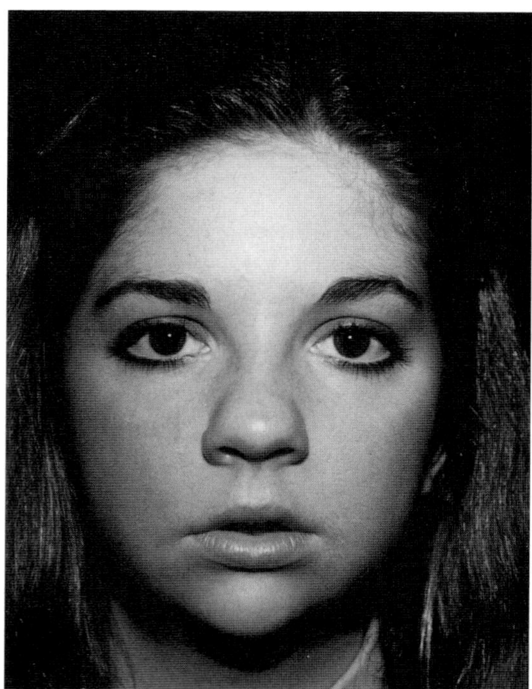
A

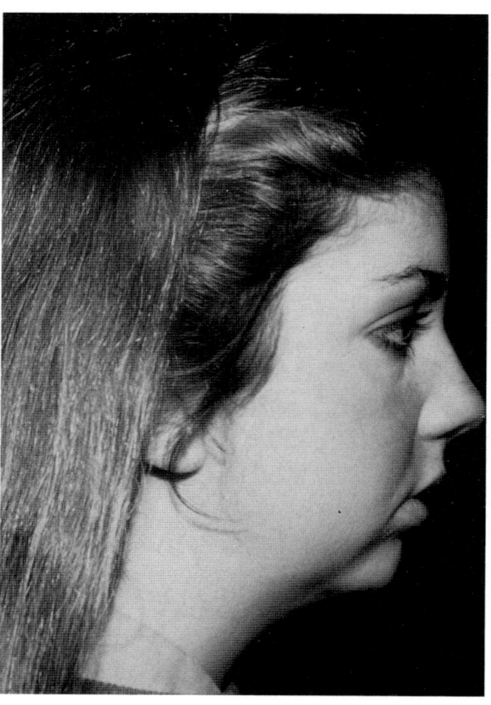
B

FIGURE 26-2. A,B: This patient underwent mandibular setback surgery to correct a class III malocclusion. Note the severe lack of skeletal support and soft tissue excess secondary to an overreduction in facial skeletal volume. She would have been aesthetically better served with a maxillary advancement procedure to correct her class III malocclusion. (From Rosen H. *Aesthetic perspectives in jaw surgery.* New York: Springer-Verlag, 1998:17, with permission.)

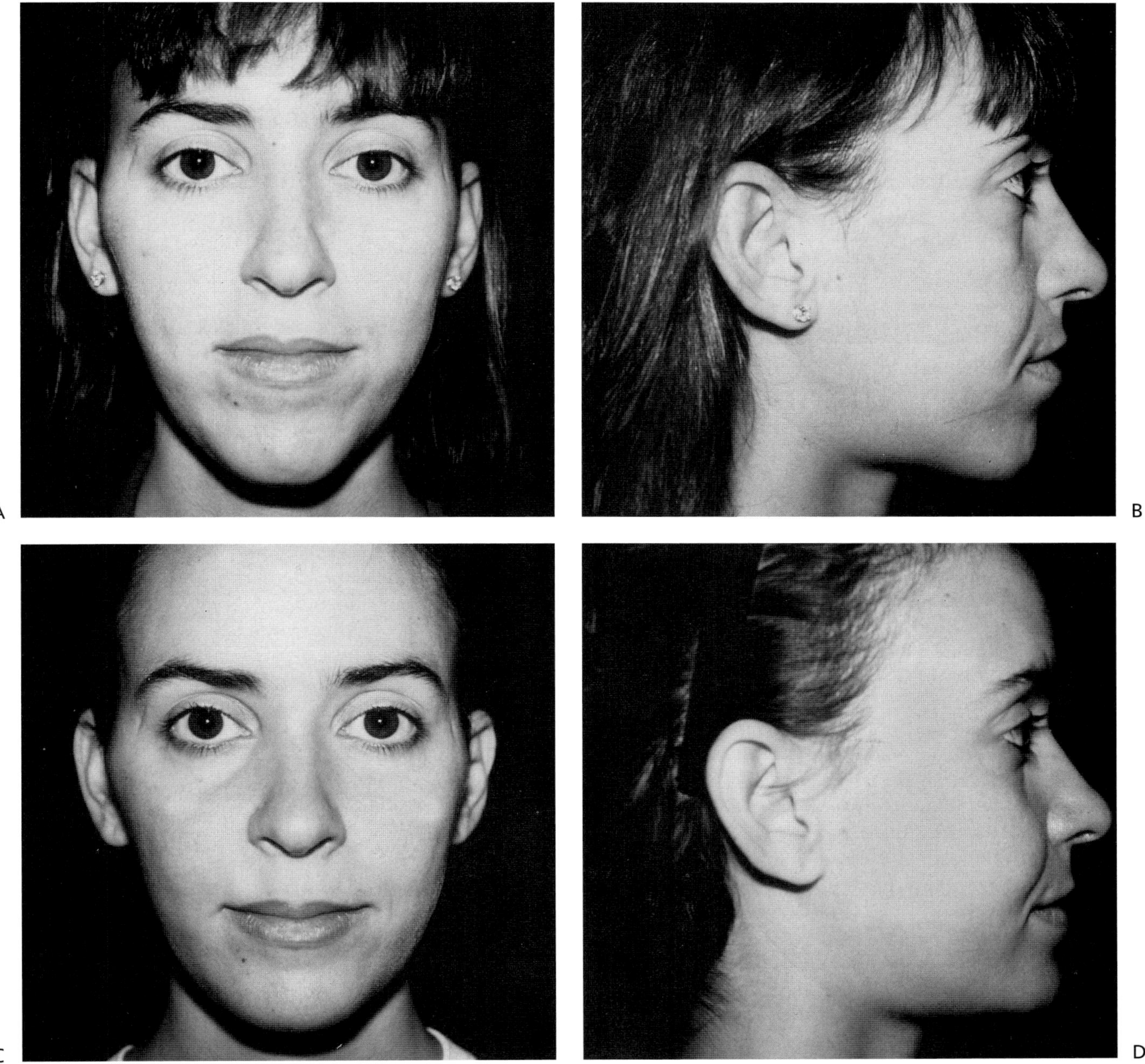

FIGURE 26-3. A,B: A patient with a long face and an anterior open bite who is to undergo superior repositioning of the maxilla and vertical reduction genioplasty. **C,D:** The postoperative frontal view demonstrates an aesthetic result, but the lateral view reveals a relative soft tissue excess in the region of the malar fat pad with secondary deepening of the nasolabial fold. *(continued)*

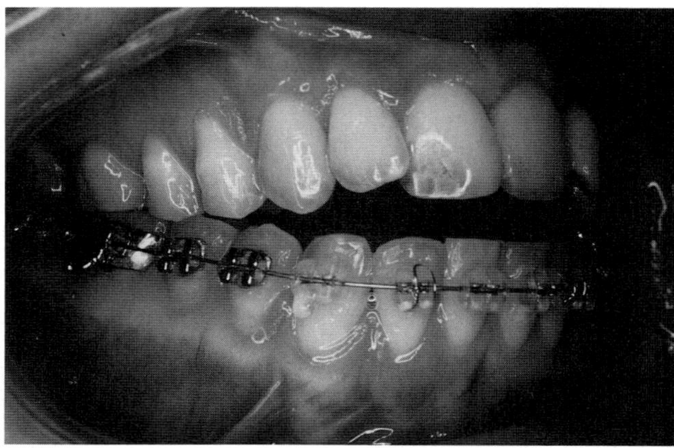

E

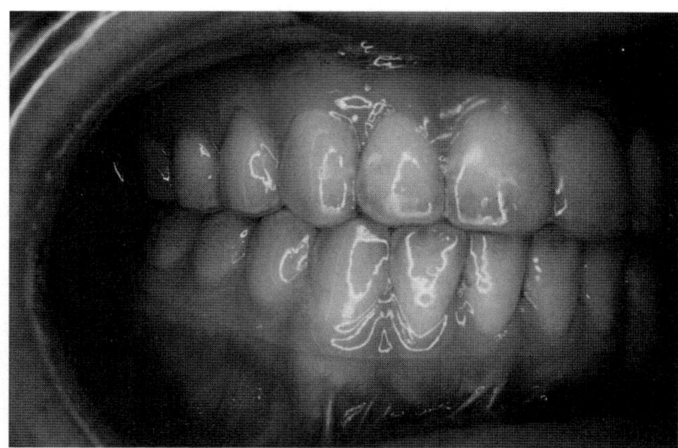

F

FIGURE 26-3. *Continued.* **E,F:** The preoperative and postoperative occlusions. (From Rosen H. *Aesthetic perspectives in jaw surgery.* New York: Springer-Verlag, 1998:18, with permission.)

duction in the vertical dimension, which has clearly exceeded the ability of the soft tissues to contract, so that deepening of the nasolabial fold is now apparent. This undesirable soft tissue response to reduction of the facial skeleton in the vertical dimension is not infrequently observed following the surgical correction of a long face.

SKELETAL EXPANSION VERSUS SKELETAL CONTRACTION

The underlying principle being described is that a decrease in volume of the facial skeleton (i.e., skeletal contraction) causes a relative excess of soft tissue because the ability of the soft tissues to contract is finite. A reduction in foundational support results in a loss of facial definition and angularity. This detrimental response of the soft tissues to skeletal contraction has been well documented. Sheen (13) has described the phenomenon in the nasal tip and area above the tip following a reduction rhinoplasty. Vanderdusen and Egyedi (14) observed it in the face and upper lip following maxillary setback surgery. Kawamoto (15) and Rosen (16) have noted the soft tissue response as a limiting factor in reduction genioplasty and mandibular setback surgery. Friehofer (17) stated this to be reason for a prematurely aged appearance after posterior repositioning of the anterior maxilla.

On the other hand, the soft tissue response to increases in volume of the facial skeleton (i.e., skeletal expansion) is typically favorable. As the facial skeleton is expanded, the support of the facial soft tissues is enhanced, and any soft tissue excess is minimized. As a result, overall facial definition, highlighting, and angularity are improved.

Accordingly, when given the aesthetic option either to expand or contract the facial skeletal volume, one should always opt to expand it. This choice is supported by two compelling arguments: (a) Expansion can now be accomplished with a reasonable degree of clinical predictability as it relates to skeletal relapse, and (b) the soft tissue response to skeletal enlargement is predictable and favorable. In turn, the aesthetic goals of orthognathic surgery are met—to provide a well-supported facial mask by achieving adequate projection of the middle and lower face and adequate height of the lower face. If these goals are not achieved, the aesthetic result in orthognathic surgery will be unfavorable.

ROLE OF FACIAL DISPROPORTION

Expansion of the facial skeleton in an effort to provide adequate support of the soft tissues may result in facial disproportion, at least in comparison with normative standards, in both the sagittal and vertical dimensions. One must therefore address the following question: Can excessive projection of the middle and lower face (sagittal disproportion) and excessive height of the lower face relative to the midface (vertical disproportion) be attractive?

Projection of the middle and lower face beyond normative standards, or excessive anterior facial divergence, can be attractive provided it is accompanied by the following: (a) an overall convex profile in the midsagittal plane; (b) a convex soft tissue relationship in the parasagittal plane from the infraorbital region to the paranasal region to the parasymphyseal region; (c) a relatively normal relationship of maxilla and mandible, as evidenced by the sagittal positions of the upper and lower lips relative to each other (ideally, the upper vermilion should be slightly in advance of the lower vermilion or, at the very least, equally prominent); (d) adequate projection of the nasal dorsum and nasal tip. Because the apparent size of the nose diminishes as one moves the middle and lower face forward, nasal projection must be adequate to accommodate forward movement of the upper and lower jaw. If not, the nose will appear too small.

In Fig. 26-4, preoperative and postoperative lateral pho-

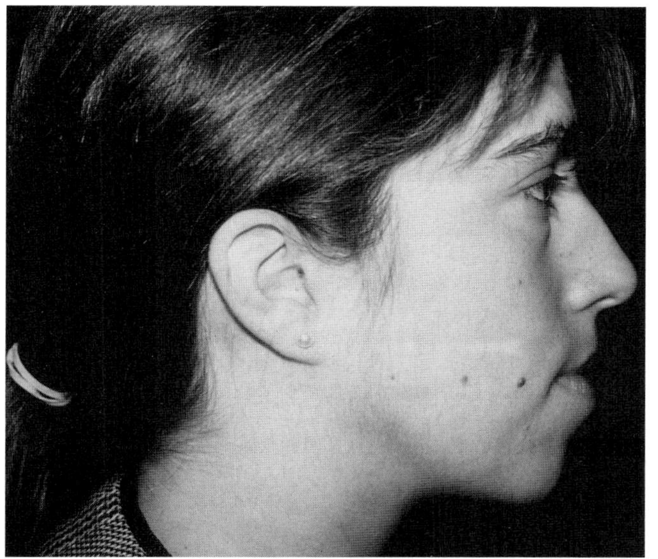

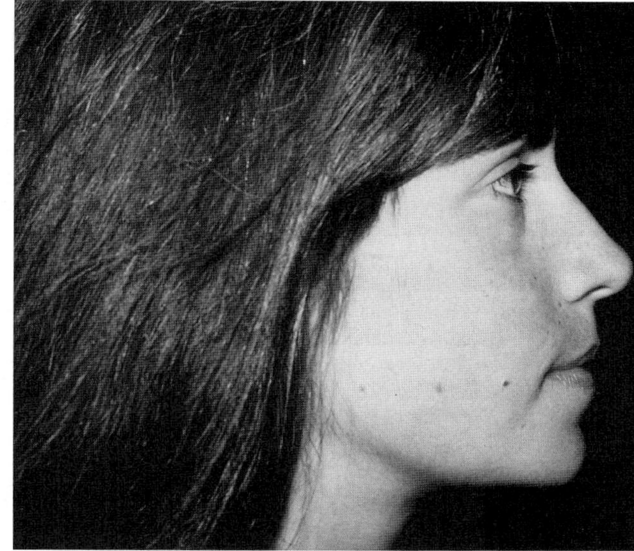

FIGURE 26-4. A: Patient with a class III anterior open bite treated with advancement of both the maxilla and mandible in addition to the chin. **B:** The postoperative view reveals excessive anterior facial divergence, but with overall facial convexity in the midsagittal and parasagittal planes, good labial relations, and adequate projection of the nasal dorsum and nasal tip. (From Rosen H. *Aesthetic perspectives in jaw surgery.* New York: Springer-Verlag, 1998:27, with permission.)

tographs are shown of a patient who was overcorrected in the sagittal dimension to correct a class III anterior open bite. Projection of the middle and lower face is now excessive in comparison with normative standards. Note the exaggerated overall anterior facial divergence. However, this degree of facial divergence is attractive because it is accompanied by an overall convex profile in both the sagittal and parasagittal planes, a good labial relationship, and adequate projection of the nose.

Excessive height in the lower face relative to the midface may also be attractive provided it is not accompanied by the aesthetic stigmata or visual signs of a long lower face. These stigmata include (a) excessive lip strain to achieve lip seal, (b) excessive gingival show during a full smile, and (c) an absent or exceedingly shallow labiomental fold. Figure 26-5 shows before and after frontal photographs of a patient who presented for surgical correction of a short face. This patient was intentionally overcorrected to achieve a quantitatively long lower face. Despite the quantitative vertical excess of the lower facial third relative to the midface, her appearance is now very attractive because it is not accompanied by any of the visual stigmata of a long face. There is no lip strain with attempted lip closure; if the patient were to smile, there would be no excessive gingival show, and the labiomental fold, although less deep postoperatively, has been well preserved. It is important to note that overcorrection of the vertical dimension was carried out in an effort to enhance skeletal support of the soft tissues.

The depth and definition of the labiomental fold are significant in the visual perception of the height of the lower facial third. The fold runs perpendicular to the long axis of the lower face, and therefore it breaks the vertical axis of the lower face and deemphasizes the visual impression of vertical facial excess. A shallow or absent fold emphasizes the vertical axis of the lower face.

It should be evident that facial disproportion in both the sagittal and vertical dimensions can be attractive. Despite this fact, however, most of the unfavorable aesthetic results that we continue to see in orthognathic surgery are a consequence of this basic principle having been ignored. Perhaps it is because surgeons do not feel comfortable with the idea of making faces disproportionately large. Most still feel more secure relying on traditional standards of facial normalcy, and therefore they continue to use normative anthropometric and cephalometric data in treatment planning. Consequently, the overwhelming tendency is either to overcontract or to underexpand facial skeletal volume. The soft tissue response to surgery is therefore inadequate, and an unfavorable aesthetic outcome results.

To appreciate the prevalence of these unfavorable outcomes, one can merely categorize the different dentofacial deformities that are surgically treated. The first morphologic type is the class II patient presenting with excessive facial convexity and a posteriorly divergent profile. These patients are typically underexpanded by inadequate anterior repositioning of the mandible. Adequate projection of the lower face relative to the soft tissue requirement is never achieved. To avoid this outcome, it is frequently necessary to perform double jaw surgery to advance the maxilla as well as the mandible, or to use counterclockwise rotational vectors to flatten the occlusal plane. The second type is the class III patient with a flat or concave profile and an anteriorly diver-

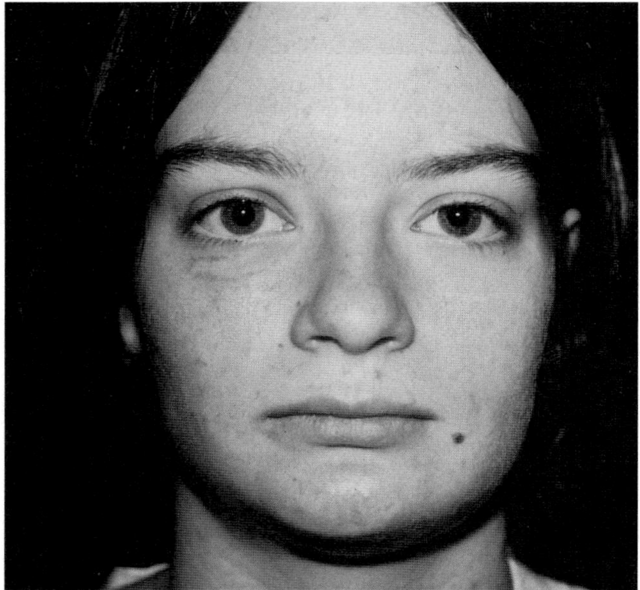

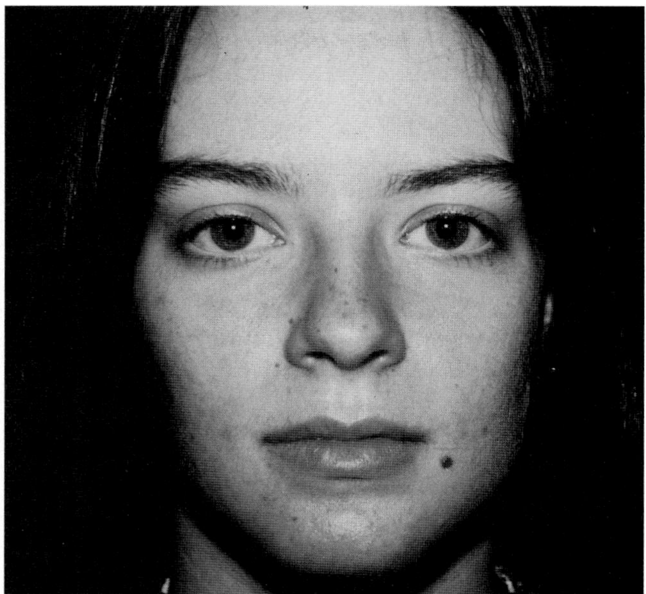

FIGURE 26-5. A: A class II patient with a short face. She will undergo surgical correction involving vertical elongation of the maxilla, mandible, and chin in addition to advancement of the mandible. Intentional vertical overcorrection is planned. **B:** The postoperative appearance is characterized by quantitative vertical excess in the lower third of the face. However, lip strain is absent, gingival show is not excessive when the patient smiles, and the labiomental fold is well defined. Although the lower face is now long, it does not appear to be so. This surgical plan was undertaken to maximize skeletal support of the soft tissues. Soft tissue considerations have dictated skeletal displacements. (From Rosen H. *Aesthetic perspectives in jaw surgery.* New York: Springer-Verlag, 1998:29, with permission.)

gent face. Historically, these patients have typically been overcontracted because excessive reliance is placed on mandibular setback surgery by itself or in combination with some maxillary procedure. Again the result is inadequate projection of the mandible and lower face with a subsequent lack of skeletal support. The third type is the patient with a short face. It is very common for these patients to be under-expanded surgically. They remain undercorrected, and inadequate height of the lower face results in deficient soft tissue support. The last morphologic type is the patient with a long face. The tendency to overcontract the facial skeleton is most commonly observed in this group of patients. Aesthetic disasters are created in which the patients appear older and possibly even edentulous. One must remember that the aging process is associated with a decrease in the vertical dimension of the lower face. With this type of patient, the prudent aesthetic course of action is to leave the patient undercorrected and minimize contraction of the facial skeleton in the vertical dimension. It is often appropriate to over-expand in the sagittal dimension and achieve excessive facial projection to compensate for what is lost in skeletal volume in the vertical dimension.

It is important to remember that the common denominator among all these categories is the potential for creating disequilibrium between skeletal and soft tissue volumes.

CONCLUSION

In summary, the three underlying principles of aesthetic surgical treatment planning are the following: (a) Support of the facial soft tissues is a critical factor in achieving a favorable aesthetic outcome in orthognathic surgery. The soft tissue goal must influence and in certain circumstances dictate the extent of skeletal displacements. (b) In achieving soft tissue goals, results are generally more predictable if skeletal volume is expanded rather than contracted. (c) Efforts to expand the facial skeleton may result in disproportion of the facial skeleton, which can potentially be extremely attractive.

Utilization of these aesthetic principles will help avoid the unfavorable aesthetic outcome in orthognathic surgery.

REFERENCES

1. Carpenter CW, Nanda RS, Currier GF. The skeletal stability of Le Fort I downfracture osteotomies with rigid fixation. *J Oral Maxillofac Surg* 1989;47:922.
2. Wardrop RW, Wolford LM. Maxillary stability following downgraft and/or advancement procedures with stabilization using rigid fixation and porous block hydroxyapatite implants. *J Oral Maxillofac Surg* 1989;47:336.

3. Kierl MJ, Nanda RS, Currier GF. A 3-year evaluation of skeletal stability of mandibular advancement with rigid fixation. *J Oral Maxillofac Surg* 1990;48:587.
4. Rosen H. Occlusal plane rotation: aesthetic enhancement in mandibular micrognathia. *Plast Reconstr Surg* 1993;91:1231.
5. Wolford LM, Chervello PD, Hilliard FW. Occlusal plane alterations in orthognathic surgery. *J Oral Maxillofac Surg* 1993; 51:730.
6. Rosen H. Definitive surgical correction of vertical maxillary deficiency. *Plast Reconstr Surg* 1990;85:215.
7. Ricketts RM. Cephalometric analysis and synthesis. *Angle Orthod* 1961;31:141.
8. Steiner CC. The use of cephalometrics as an aid to planning and assessing orthodontic treatment. *Am J Orthod* 1960;46:721.
9. Legan HL, Burstone CJ. Soft tissue cephalometric analysis for orthognathic surgery. *J Oral Surg* 1980;38:744.
10. Farkas LG, Sohm P, Kolar JC, et al. Inclinations of the facial profile: art versus reality. *Plast Reconstr Surg* 1985;75:509.
11. Rosen H. Facial skeletal expansion: treatment strategies and rationale. *Plast Reconstr Surg* 1992;89:798.
12. Rosen H. Aesthetics in facial skeletal surgery. *Perspect Plast Surg* 1993;6:1.
13. Sheen JH. *Aesthetic rhinoplasty.* St. Louis: Mosby, 1978:370.
14. van der Deusen FN, Egyedi P. Premature aging of the face after orthognathic surgery. *J Craniofac Surg* 1990;18:335.
15. Kawamoto HK Jr. Discussion of reduction mentoplasty. *Plast Reconstr Surg* 1982;70:151.
16. Rosen H. Maxillary advancement for mandibular prognathism: indications and rationale. *Plast Reconstr Surg* 1991;87: 823.
17. Friehofer HP. Reversing segmental osteotomies of the upper jaw. *Plast Reconstr Surg* 1995;96:88.

Discussion

ORTHOGNATHIC SURGERY

JONATHAN S. JACOBS

To describe the unfavorable result in orthognathic surgery, one must consider the miscalculations made and complications that arise during surgery separately from those associated with assessment and treatment. As Dr. Rosen has so ably described, the advent of rigid fixation devices and reliable and well-tolerated interpositional materials has reduced operative complications. Long-term problems after surgery are more frequent when miscalculations are made during assessment. It should be noted, however, that the idea of aesthetics as the primary focus in this type of surgery is far from universally accepted. It should also be kept in mind that significant improvements in function are gained by the appropriate alignment of dental arches and the restoration of normal functional occlusion. In addition, long-term function of the temporomandibular joint is better after the normalization of occlusion. Although no data are available to indicate a direct relationship between malfunction of the occlusion and malfunction of the joint, the teleologic reasoning that normal functioning of both is important to long-term stability is strong. Dr. Rosen's chapter emphasizes the aesthetic deliberations that are appropriate in regard to these patients. Briefly, it is also appropriate to review the complications that can occur during surgery, revisit the issues raised in regard to aesthetics with a small difference in emphasis, and consider the patients who present with bimaxillary prognathism who do not fall into the categories he describes in his chapter.

In regard to operative considerations, three procedures have emerged that can be used to treat a great majority of patients presenting with dentofacial deformities. With the help of understanding and able orthodontists, who can both prepare patients for surgical correction and complete the occlusal correction postoperatively, most deformities are treatable with a relatively limited surgical armamentarium. These procedures include Le Fort I osteotomy for the maxilla and a variation that will allow expansion when necessary, sagittal split osteotomy for the mandible (usually for advancement and sometimes for retrusion), and genioplasty for alignment of the chin in three dimensions.

Le Fort I has become the mainstay for the surgical correction of maxillary deformity. It is a reliable procedure, and with bone plate fixation, relapses are usually limited. The

Jonathan S. Jacobs: Department of Surgery, Eastern Virginia Medical School, Norfolk, Virginia; Surgical Executive Committee, Sentara Leigh Hospital, Sentara Hospitals—Norfolk, Norfolk, Virginia

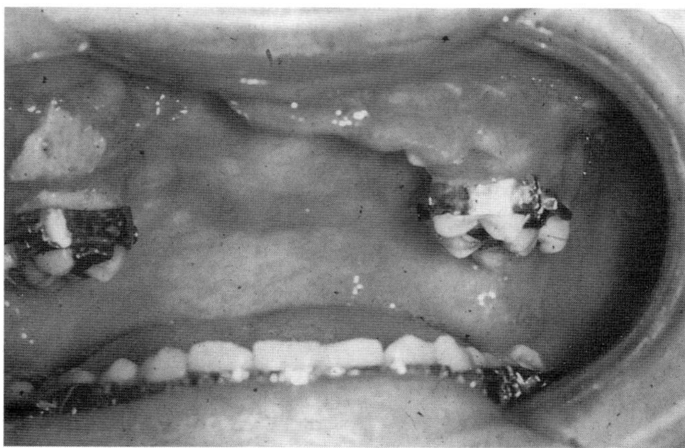

FIGURE 26D-1. This patient underwent multiple-part Le Fort I osteotomy. Intrusion of the segments against an intact nasal septum and midline palate caused stripping of the palatal mucosa and loss of vitality in the anterior segments.

tendency to relapse is greatest when down-fracture is performed to add height or when a patient with a cleft deformity and a scarred lip and palate requires exaggerated advancements. As noted, the use of interpositional materials, either bone graft or hydroxyapatite, has helped in regard to relapse. However, our concern about exceeding freeway space in these patients is still pertinent. *Freeway space* is described as the vertical space between the maxillary and mandibular occlusal surfaces when the muscles of mastication are at physiologic rest. Exceeding this physiologic rest position is theorized to be a cause of relapse. Operative complications with Le Fort I are rarely seen but can involve the loss of significant volume of blood during down-fracture and a disruption of the pterygoid plexus of veins and greater palatine artery. Anesthesia may cause long-term problems in the gingiva and palatal soft tissue. With poorly designed osteotomies, even bone and teeth may be lost, and in the worst scenarios, this loss may result in oroantral or nasal fistulas. Figure 26D-1 shows a patient treated for maxillary intrusion by a multiple-part Le Fort I osteotomy in a horseshoe configuration. Because the nasal septum and midline palate were not trimmed appropriately, stripping of the palatal mucosal attachments and loss of vitality in the anterior maxilla resulted. Poor operative design or poor execution can lead to surgical disaster in such procedures. The relapse rates for Le Fort I osteotomy are low in general, and complications are rarely reported as significant, except in the already noted circumstance of down-fracture with interposition and excessive impingement on the freeway space.

For sagittal split osteotomy, similar operative admonitions are appropriate. Most importantly, damage to the inferior alveolar nerve and lip anesthesia are still reported in 20% to 50% of cases, and hypoesthesia in the region of distribution of this nerve may be permanent. Instances of damage to other nerves are rare; however, Fig. 26D-2A

A

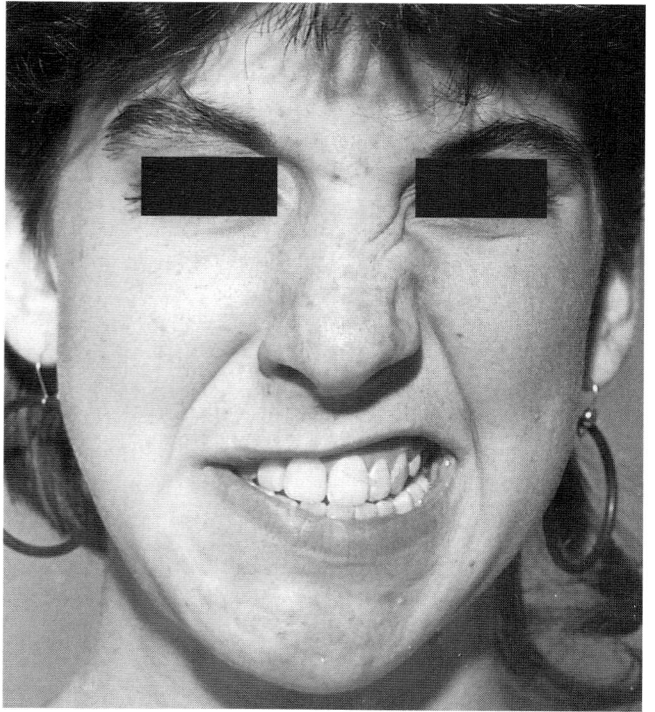

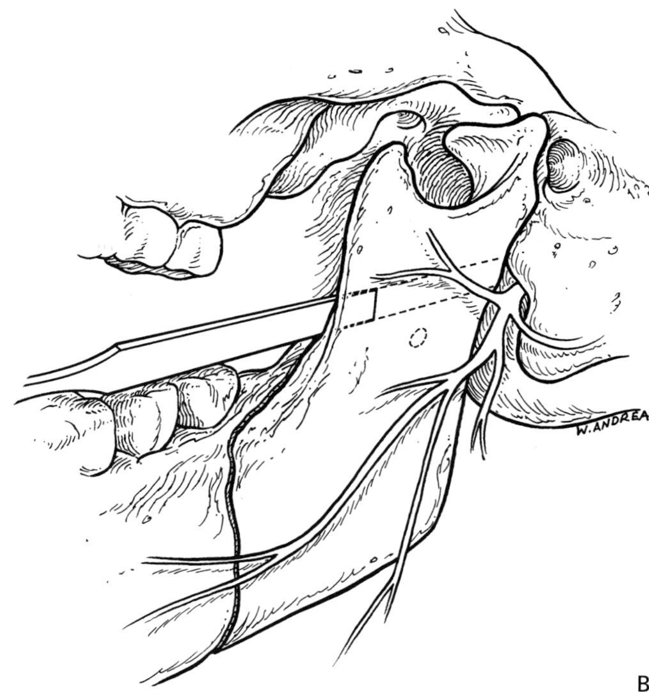

B

FIGURE 26D-2. A,B: In this patient, the horizontal osteotomy at the ramus was taken posteriorly with an osteotome to disrupt the main trunk of the facial nerve. (Courtesy of Dr. Julia Terzis.)

demonstrates a patient in whom a horizontal osteotomy at the ramus was taken posteriorly with an osteotome to disrupt the main trunk of the facial nerve (Fig. 26D-2B). This is an example of poor operative execution and subsequent complication. The patient was seen secondarily for readvancement of the mandible at the time of staged facial nerve repair. The tendency to relapse after sagittal split osteotomy is more common if advancement has been performed. The use of bone screw fixation has prevented initial relapse. Frequently, relapse is hidden by dental compensation and postoperative orthodontics. In larger advancements, relapse is still reported as 20% to 30% of the mandibular position. Relapse has also been associated with advancement combined with maxillary intrusion, which places undue tension on the suprahyoid musculature. It should be emphasized that although screw fixation of the mandible at the sagittal split osteotomy has lessened initial retropositioning, long-term results remain commensurate with those achieved when simple wire fixation and intermaxillary fixation were used. Operative complications in the mandible with this osteotomy rarely cause a loss of vascularity in dento-osseous structures, but inappropriate splits with instability of the proximal segments may develop. In addition, possible damage to the facial artery at the time of the vertical osteotomy may lead to excessive bleeding and postoperative hematoma.

With genioplasty, operative complications are again rare, but disruption of the mental nerve and subsequent permanent lip anesthesia can occur. More frequently, a failure of symmetry may be seen when the distal segment has not been aligned in an appropriate fashion. Even more often, as emphasized by Dr. Rosen, complications are caused by poor assessment and subsequent alterations in appearance. Figure 26D-3 shows a patient whose chin segment was inappropriately advanced. She is left with an exaggerated labiomental fold and severe prominence at the pogonion ("witch's chin"). This situation could have been avoided with better preoperative assessment and planning. Simple advancement genioplasty is inappropriate when the labiomental fold is already deep.

The assessment of patients with dentofacial deformities who are candidates for orthognathic correction has been emphasized. However, it must be maintained that although we seek to match skeletal changes to soft tissue needs for the sake of aesthetics, normative values taken from cephalometric and anthropometric evaluations still provide a guideline and basis for assessment. Let us not be too cavalier in regard to discarding normative values because they are not aesthetic values, a philosophy that is hard to justify. The example of the patient with mandibular prognathism corrected inappropriately in the mandible rather than in the maxilla is classic. We have come to realize, with Dr. Rosen's help, that the class III patient with malocclusion should almost always be corrected in the maxilla. However, for some patients, two-

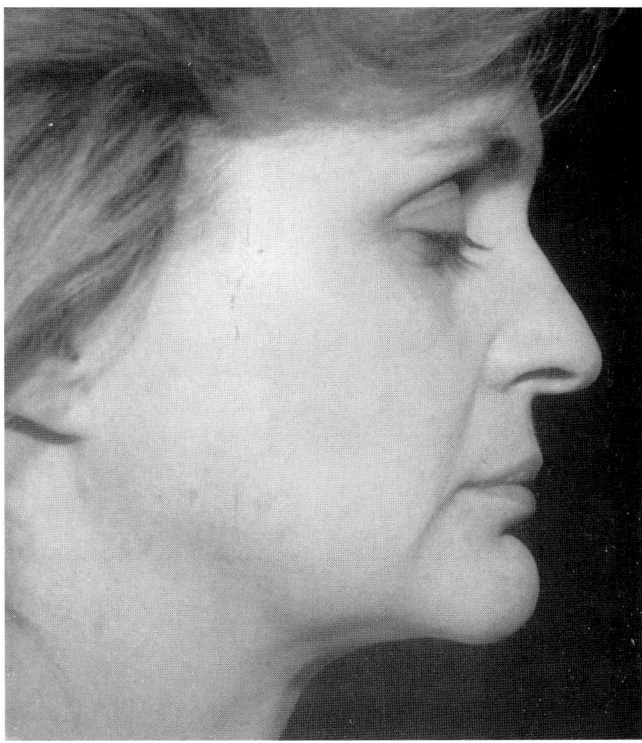

FIGURE 26D-3. Inappropriate genioplasty with advancement has resulted in exaggeration of the labiomental fold.

jaw surgery is appropriate. Figure 26D-4 shows a young woman with mandibular prognathism treated by both maxillary advancement and mandibular setback to lessen the chin prominence. At the same time, overlying bone grafts were used to fill the soft tissue envelope over the malar region and lessen the nasal prominence to yield a very satisfactory postoperative appearance and good occlusal correction. These assessments and decisions obviously must be individualized and made with careful consideration of the patient's needs and understanding of the expected change in appearance. Dr. Rosen's basic premise—that young faces are full faces and that aging can be delayed by filling the soft tissue envelope with the skeleton—is accurate and represents a major contribution to this field.

One must also include in a consideration of facial aesthetics those patients presenting with bimaxillary prognathism. These patients, usually African-American or Asian, are afforded more appropriate aesthetic corrections when their facial skeletons are straightened and some diminution of the prognathism is obtained. Figure 26D-5 shows a young woman whose bimaxillary prognathism has been corrected with closure of an anterior open bite to achieve a straighter facial profile. Lessening the convexity yields a more aesthetic facial skeleton. In addition to correcting the dentofacial functional problem, the chin point is advanced

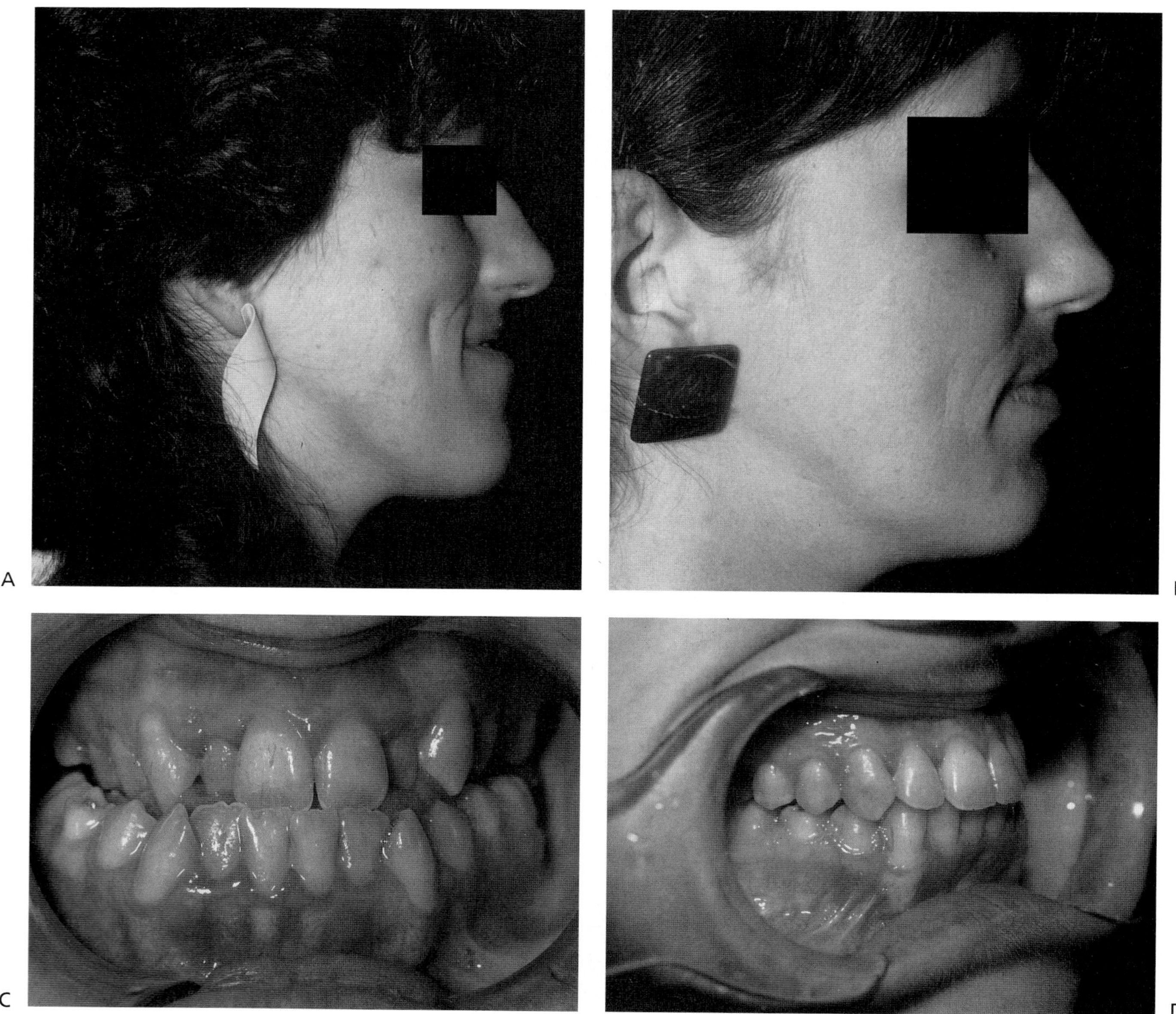

FIGURE 26D-4. **A:** Preoperative facial profile demonstrating a retrognathic maxilla with prominent chin. **B:** Postoperative correction with combined maxillary advancement and mandibular setback. **C:** Preoperative occlusion before orthodontic treatment. **D:** Postoperative correction of occlusion by combined orthodontics, maxillary advancement, and mandibular setback.

to deepen the labiomental fold and add angularity to the facial configuration.

In summary, unsatisfactory outcomes in orthognathic surgery can result for several reasons. However, such surgery offers an opportunity to create significant changes in the facial configuration and is a potent tool for achieving aesthetic improvements. The appearance of Caucasian patients is generally improved when maxillary and mandibular advancements are undertaken. However, the constraints of existing soft tissue structures and their ability to withstand such advancements must be kept in mind. The issue of too much deepening at the labiomental fold is important. The needs of male versus female patients in this type of advancement also must be considered. Female patients obviously benefit from less projection at the pogonion, and appropriate preoperative plans should be made. However, patients who present with bimaxillary prognathism are best treated by straightening the facial profile. They also should be counseled about the anticipated postoperative results and possible failure of the soft tissue to adapt to skeletal changes (al-

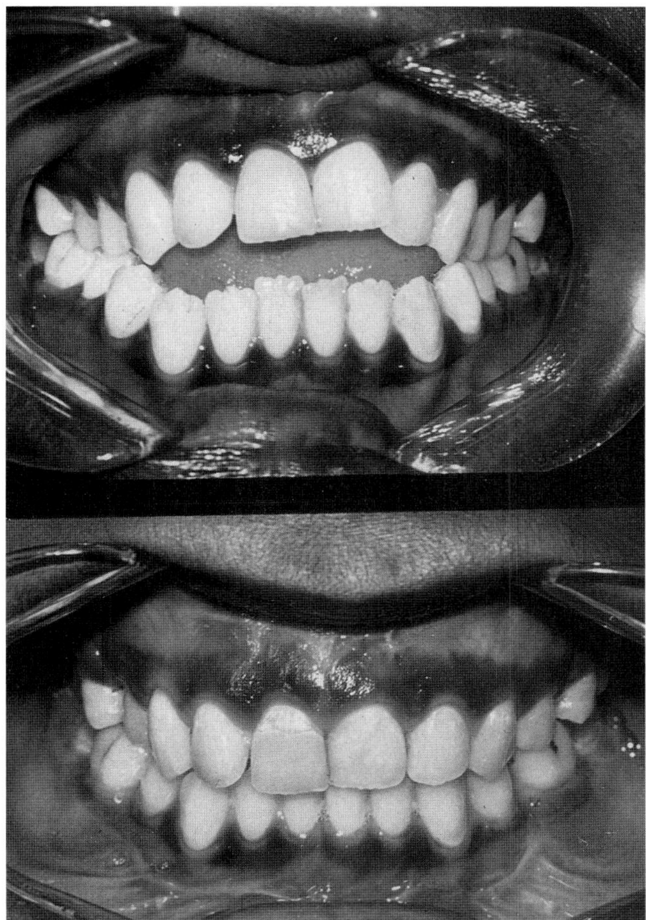

A

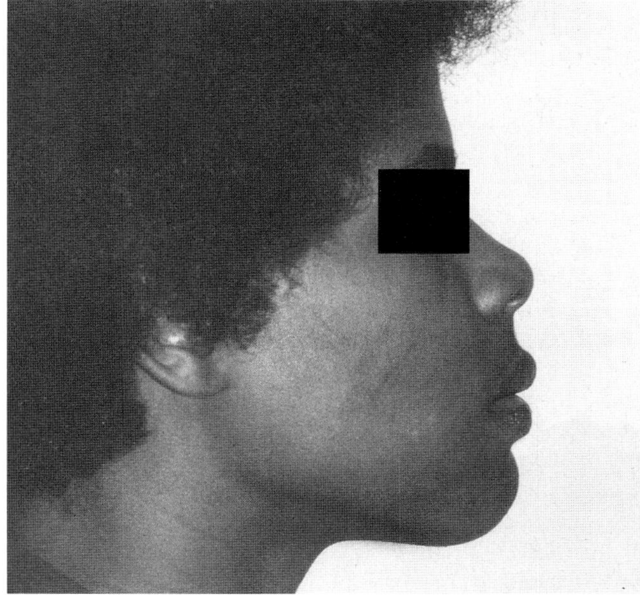

B

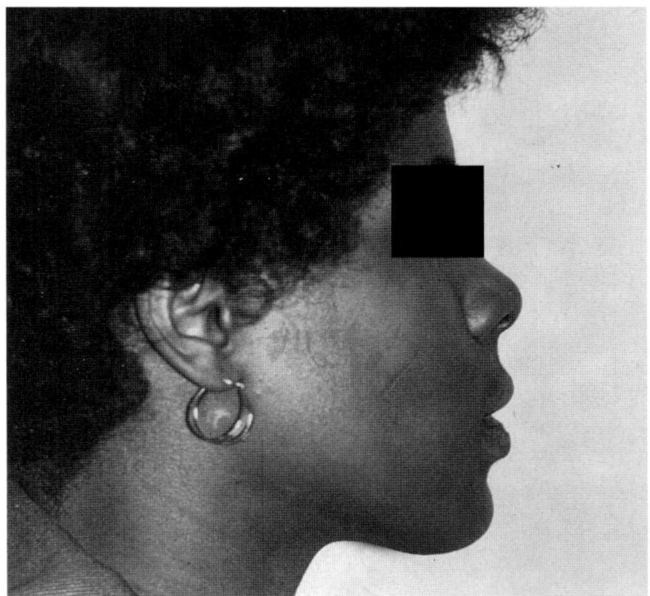

C

FIGURE 26D-5. A: Preoperative and postoperative occlusal correction with setback for profile advancement. **B:** Preoperative correction for bimaxillary prognathism. **C:** Postoperative correction of bimaxillary prognathism and open bite with setback procedures to straighten profile.

though this is rare). Operative complications may be disastrous in these procedures, but with appropriate planning and execution, they are unusual.

This treatise by Dr. Rosen provides us with an admirable game plan for restoring the facial appearance of patients who present with dentofacial deformities. However, we must maintain a functional perspective in this work. The procedures described are laudable in that they enable one to improve a patient's appearance, but they are often necessary because of the patient's lack of appropriate function.

27

AURICULAR RECONSTRUCTION

BURTON D. BRENT

Any technically demanding surgery is beset with possible unfavorable results and disastrous complications. As one of the more challenging tasks in plastic surgery, reconstruction of the auricle often serves as an example of the above. With this in mind, the author wishes to outline measures with which to avoid the common pitfalls of auricular reconstruction and to prescribe prudent steps in managing problems once they have occurred.

INITIAL PLANNING AND PREPARATION

A favorable result of auricular reconstruction can be attained by selection of a sound procedure, good preparation of the surgeon, and enlightenment of the family with realistic goals. A realistic goal is a constructed ear of reasonable size and contour that is well positioned in relation to the contralateral auricle and surrounding topographical landmarks. However, a reconstructed ear will be firmer, relatively immobile, and less delicate than the opposite, normal ear. If the family and surgeon accept these limitations, then the child has an excellent chance of growing up normally without self-consciousness.

All the options and alternatives of ear reconstruction should be discussed with the family. In contrast to homologous cartilage, which is absorbed (1), and alloplastic frameworks, which often fail (2), autogenous cartilage produces favorable results, is subject to few complications, and withstands trauma (3,4). I have not been impressed with the recently developed Medpor implants (5), having seen multiple framework exposures and draining sinuses associated with the use of this material; I feel that it fares no better than other alloplastic materials. I have seen silicone ear frameworks lost to even minor trauma up to 12 years after implantation. On the other hand, after the 10th postoperative day, I have never lost an autogenous ear framework. To date, more than 70 of my reconstructed ears have survived major trauma (6).

Burton D. Brent: El Camino Hospital, Mountainview, California; and Stanford University Medical Center, Palo Alto, California

Prostheses are occasionally applied in adult trauma cases, but their use in children is limited because of the risk for dislodgement during normal energetic activities, which causes great emotional stress.

Surgery of the middle ear should be addressed thoroughly during the initial consultation. To ensure that the gains of middle ear surgery outweigh the risks and complications of the procedure itself, I reserve this surgery for cases of bilateral microtia and selected unilateral cases in which the patient is highly motivated and the radiologic evidence indicates middle ear development. Then, it must be thoughtfully planned in a "team approach" (4) with an otologist who is competent and experienced in atresia surgery. The auricle must be constructed first because once an attempt has been made to open the ear, invaluable virgin skin becomes damaged and scarred, and the chances of obtaining an excellent auricular construction are hampered severely.

In the team approach, the plastic surgeon initiates the middle ear procedure by lifting the surgically constructed auricle from its bed while carefully preserving connective tissue on the undersurface of the framework. Next, the otologist takes over, first drilling a bony canal, completing the ossiculoplasty, and then repairing the tympanum with a temporal fascial graft. Finally, the plastic surgeon resumes by excising soft tissues to exteriorize the meatus through the conchal region and harvesting a skin graft that the otologist uses to line the new canal and complete the repair (4).

PREOPERATIVE PLANNING

As preoperative preparation, the surgeon must practice carving numerous frameworks from cadaver cartilage long before sculpting cartilage in living patients. The surest path to an unfavorable result is to "practice" on patients. The successful grafting of a well-sculpted cartilage framework is the foundation for a sound ear repair. When this is accomplished as the first surgical stage, one can take advantage of the optimal circulation and elasticity of inviolate virgin skin. For this reason, I avoid initial repositioning of vestige remnants, as resulting scars can inhibit circulation and restrict the elasticity of the skin and its ability to accommodate a three-dimensional framework (7). Secondary procedures, such as lobule rotation, tragus construction, and sulcus grafting, take place after sound healing of the "foundation." Shortcuts with so-called one-stage repairs (8) are risky and produce ears that inevitably require further detailing to achieve a quality result (9).

Age of the Patient

The age at which to begin surgery is determined by the patient's size and psychological considerations. Because rib cartilages are usually insufficient for framework fabrication before the age of 5 1/2 or 6 years, and because psychological disturbances are rarely encountered before age 6 or 7, I prefer to postpone surgery until age 6. It should be emphasized that the first attempt is the best opportunity for a good reconstruction; therefore, one should not handicap oneself technically by beginning too soon, when skimpy rib cartilages will inhibit sculpting a good framework. Conversely, one ought not procrastinate until psychological disturbances develop.

Location of the Ear

One of the most frequent complications of ear construction is poor placement. Because it is far easier to prevent than to correct this complication, special care should be taken initially to avoid it. Careful preoperative planning is mandatory to ensure that both ears are at the same level, that the crus helices are at the same distance from the lateral canthi, and that the axis of the ear is roughly parallel to the nasal profile (10,11).

The greatest force working against one's goal to place the ear properly is the patient's hairline; the desire to avoid hairy skin over the superior helix may cause the surgeon to place the ear too low. One rarely, if ever, sees an ear framework placed too high.

In the operating room, still another complication arises when the posterior hairline acts as a constricting band at the juncture of the thin, hairless retroauricular skin and the thick skin of the scalp. This tends to displace the framework anteriorly and can best be avoided by limiting the anterior dissection of the cutaneous pocket and by carefully checking the framework position before closing the incision and applying the head dressing.

Positioning the ear is straightforward and easy to plan in pure microtia, but much more difficult in severe hemifacial microsomia. Not only are the facial halves unequal in height; the anteroposterior dimensions of the affected side are also foreshortened. In these patients, the height of the new ear is best planned by lining up the new ear with the upper pole of the normal ear—its distance from the lateral canthus is somewhat arbitrary.

In pure microtia, the vestige-to-canthus distance mirrors the helical root-to-canthus distance of the opposite, normal side. However, in severe hemifacial microsomia, the vestige is much closer to the eye. If one places the anterior margin of the new ear at the vestige site, then the ear appears to be too close to the eye; if one uses the measured distance of the normal side as a guide, then the ear appears to be too far back on the head. In these patients, I find it best to compromise by selecting a point halfway between the two positions.

When both auricular construction and bony repairs are planned, then careful, integrated timing is essential. Most often, the family pushes for the ear repair to begin first, which helpfully ensures that virginal, unscarred skin will be available to the auricular surgeon. However, craniomaxillofacial surgeons argue that if they first correct the facial asymmetry, ear placement is made easier (12). I find this initial correction unnecessary when the guidelines previously described are followed.

If the bony work is done first, it is imperative that the location of scars be peripheral to the proposed auricular site. When a coronal incision is used to approach the upper face or to harvest cranial bone grafts, special care must be taken that the scar does not lie within the region of the future upper helix.

Low Hairline

As mentioned, one should ignore the hairline and place the framework in its proper position; the auricular hair can be dealt with at a later date. One method is to excise the hairy skin, taking great care to preserve connective tissue over the underlying cartilage framework, and then resurface the defect with a full-thickness skin graft (usually taken from the contralateral retroauricular sulcus for an optimal color match). To avoid a "patchwork" appearance completely, auricular hair can be managed by electrolysis (13,14) or laser (15). The formal is prickly and bothersome to children, whereas the latter is still in the developmental stage and does not provide a *permanent* solution to date (16).

While planning preoperatively, if I sense a tight skin pocket and a hairline that will cover half the new ear, then I may consider a primary fascial flap (7). Although it entails an extensive operation, a fascial flap represents "two operations in one" in that it permits one to place an ear framework while simultaneously dealing with a low hairline and shortage of skin.

Obtaining the Rib Graft

To ensure that optimal material is obtained for the living sculpture, I always harvest the rib cartilage myself. To conserve anesthesia time, my assistant closes the chest wound while I fabricate the framework. When this approach is used, the entire operation (rib harvest, framework fabrication, and insertion of the framework beneath the auricular skin) routinely takes less than 3 hours.

When grafting cartilage, I prescribe intraoperative antibiotics as a prophylactic measure, and continue to prescribe them for several days after the procedure. In subsequent stages of ear repair, I do not administer antibiotics except when elevating and grafting the ear of an adolescent patient with intractable acne.

The two most common complications that arise when a rib cartilage graft is harvested are pneumothorax and atelectasis. A pneumothorax should cause no alarm because an actual air leak is not created. Therefore, the iatrogenically introduced air needs only to be realized and extracted before the chest wound is closed. As a final precaution, a portable chest roentgenogram is taken in the operating room before extubation (17).

Atelectasis is best prevented through candid preoperative preparation of the patient and vigorous postoperative respiratory therapy. When admitted to the hospital, the patient should be motivated to practice with the Triflow spirometer as if it were a toy. Postoperatively, the patient must be encouraged to use it despite any discomfort that may be experienced.

FRAMEWORK FABRICATION AND IMPLANTATION

Carving Process

It is essential to keep the cartilage moist during the actual carving process to avoid desiccation. This makes the cartilage as slippery as a bar of soap, and I have had several frameworks actually slip from my hands onto the floor. Although this mishap was a cause for concern, in each case the framework was swirled in antibiotic-containing saline solution before being inserted into the cutaneous auricular pocket, and no postoperative complications ensued.

One common complication that has been reported after implantation of an autogenous rib cartilage framework is extrusion of the wire sutures used to fasten the framework together (18). For this reason, I switched to the use of clear nylon years ago. This suture material rarely has caused problems.

Cutaneous Pocket

Because the details of a sculpted framework would be obliterated if covered by a thick flap, a thin cutaneous pocket must be created. Great care must be taken not to damage the subdermal vascular plexus. The framework is introduced only after precise hemostasis has been obtained and the skin tension appraised carefully. The use of epinephrine should be strictly avoided; in that way, any flap blanching that occurs indicates a discrepancy between the three-dimensional framework and the created two-dimensional cutaneous pocket. If the skin tension is unsatisfactory, then either the pocket must be enlarged or the bulk of the framework must be reduced.

Finally, the skin is coapted to the framework by means of a small infusion catheter and vacuum drain system. In the

A

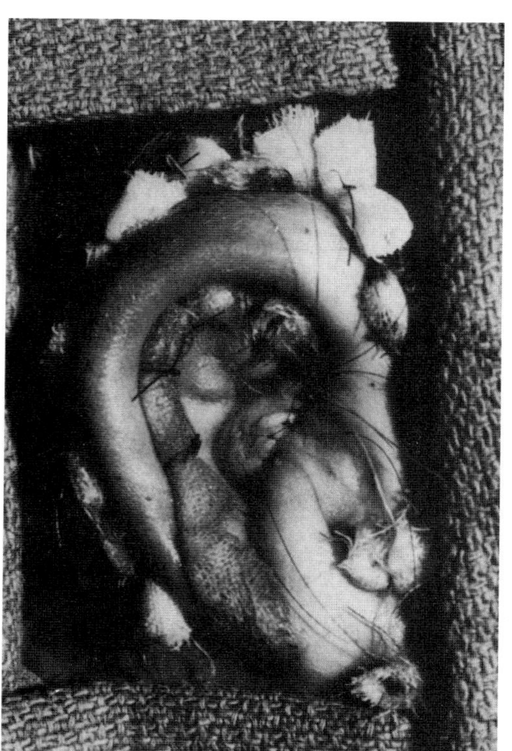

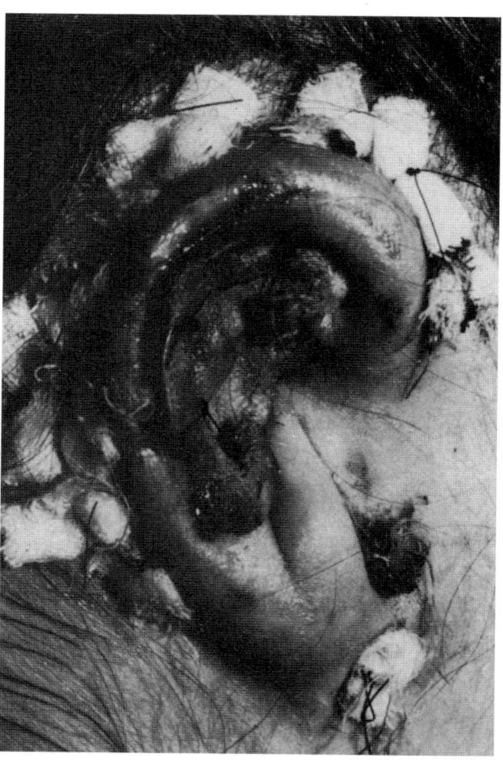

B

FIGURE 27-1. Skin necrosis resulting from tight bolster sutures. **A:** Repair of microtic ear with cartilage graft. Skin coaptation maintained with bolster sutures. **B:** Skin necrosis with cartilage exposure, 5 days postoperatively. The framework subsequently was lost to infection. *(continued)*

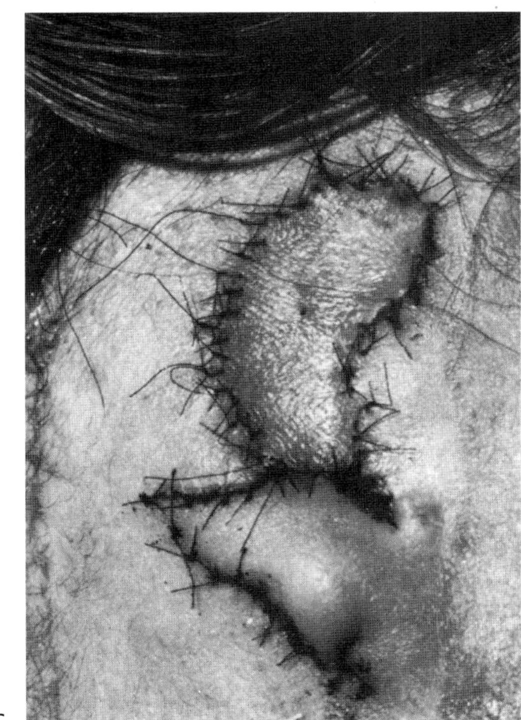

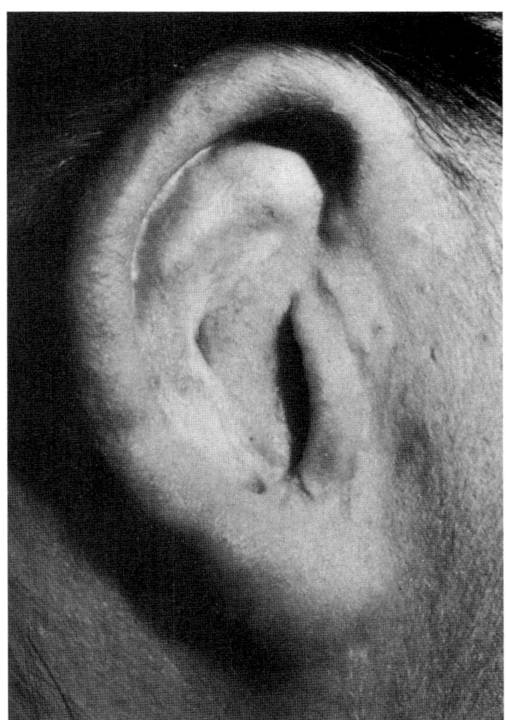

FIGURE 27-1. *Continued.* **C:** Auricular region resurfaced with full-thickness skin graft. The lobule has been preserved. **D:** Reconstruction with a second rib cartilage graft 1 year later. The tragus has been constructed with a composite graft from the contralateral concha.

author's experience, this suction method has reduced the incidence of infection and skin necrosis, which previously were a significant threat when compression mattress sutures were used (Fig. 27-1). This vacuum system creates a continuous suction that not only coapts the nourishing skin flap to the carved cartilage but also prevents the formation of disastrous hematomas.

OTHER STAGES OF AURICULAR CONSTRUCTION

For proper healing to take place, a minimum of several months is allowed between the staged surgeries. During this extra time, swelling subsides, the circulation improves, and the tissues settle down. There is no such thing as waiting too long between surgical stages, and it would not matter even if one waited years! Basically, I like to allow at least 2 months between the rib cartilage graft and the earlobe transposition procedure, then 3 months between the other operations. In certain instances, I wait even longer between stages to ensure the optimal condition of tissues.

POSTOPERATIVE COMPLICATIONS

As mentioned, when I first began reconstructing ears, I used compression mattress sutures to coapt the skin to the helical cartilage (19), and auricular complications were common. Infections, skin losses, or both developed in 5 of the 15 cases performed with this older method (33%). Since the discontinuation of bolster sutures and initiation of the suction drain, auricular complications have been rare. In more than 1,200 cases, only three cases of infection, three of hematoma, and five of skin loss with cartilage exposure have occurred—for a total complication rate of less than 1% (9). Most were preventable.

Hematoma

Hematoma is best prevented by gaining precise hemostasis and utilizing suction drains. Pressure head dressings are no substitute for these measures and in fact are contraindicated. In addition to preventing flap adherence and subsequent revascularization of the cartilage graft, hematoma leads to infection. Once encountered, it should be evacuated quickly and hemostasis ascertained. Two of the three aforementioned hematomas in my personal practice occurred early in my experience, when I used only one drain tube. These were both in older patients on adult wards where nurses were not familiar with the test tube routine, and steadily filling vacuum test tubes went unnoticed until it was too late. Although both these hematomas were successfully evacuated without loss of the framework (Fig. 27-2), I now use two drain tubes and hospitalize all my patients on the pediatric ward, where the nurses are thoroughly familiar with the importance of maintaining a good vacuum.

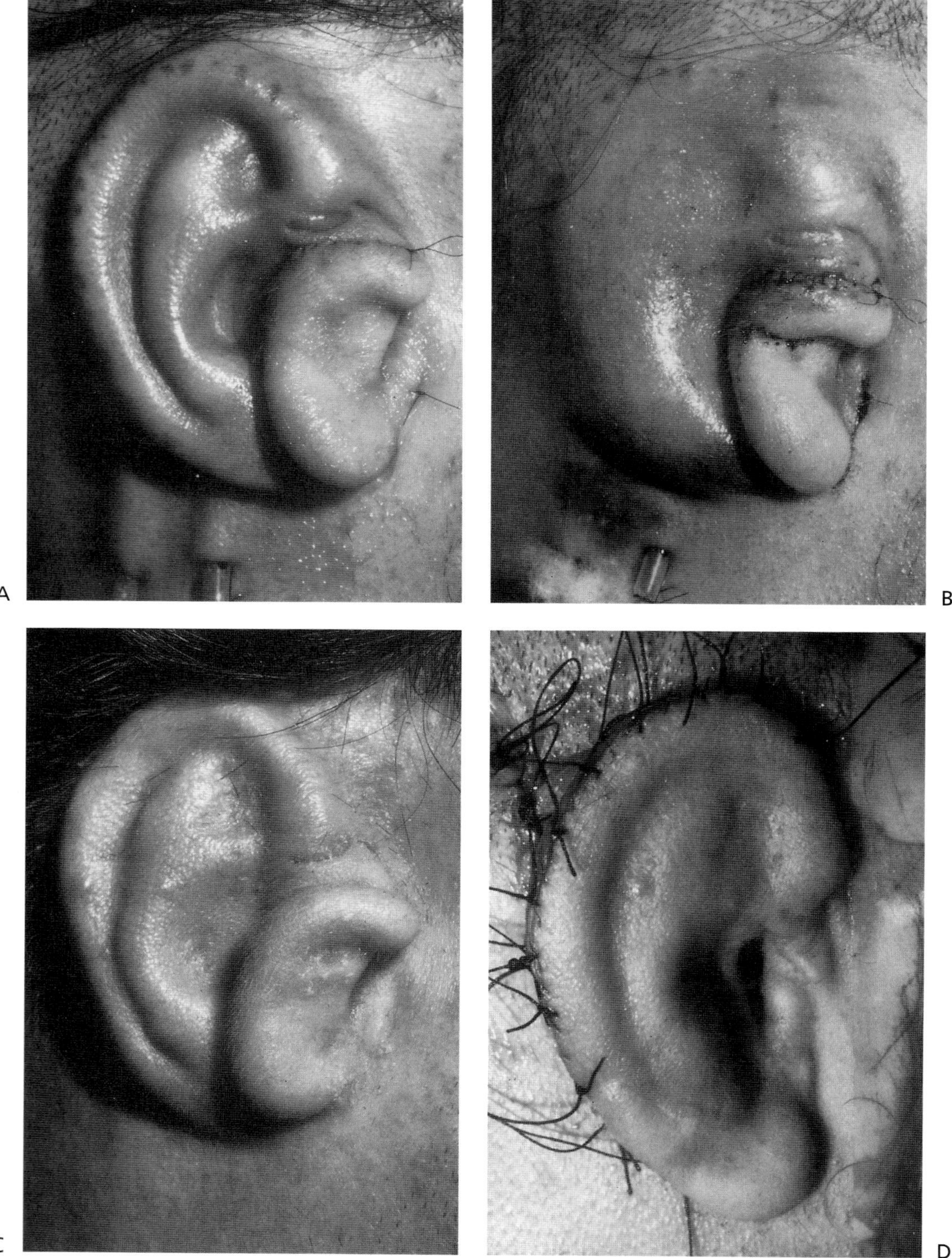

FIGURE 27-2. Hematoma. **A:** Immediate postoperative appearance of microtia repair with sculpted rib cartilage graft. **B:** Early postoperative hematoma resulting from loss of vacuum (see text). **C:** Healed ear after evacuation of hematoma. **D:** Appearance of ear after earlobe transposition and lifting with skin graft.

Skin Loss with Cartilage Exposure

When alloplastic materials are used, the framework can become exposed through mere attenuation of skin over the frame. I have not seen this happen with an autogenous framework. Therefore, when cartilage becomes exposed, it is secondary to primary cutaneous damage. The vascular damage that precedes skin breakdown is caused by either subdermal vascular damage during flap dissection, undue tension after framework insertion, or tight head dressings (Fig. 27-3A).

Two of the five cases of cartilage exposure I have encountered in my practice (since discontinuing compressive bolster sutures) were caused when parents tightly reapplied a loose head dressing. I successfully repaired these with small rotational scalp or fascial flaps (Fig. 27-3B). To prevent this risk, I no longer allow parents to change ear dressings.

Whatever the cause, the treatment must be prompt. The exposed cartilage must be covered with a generous amount of antibiotic ointment and dressed appropriately to avoid desiccation. The next step takes place in the operating room, where the wound edges are debrided and the defect closed appropriately.

Whereas a small cartilage exposure can be covered by primary skin closure, most defects require flap coverage. Transposition skin flaps are most suitable for these defects, even though they carry hair-bearing skin to the ear (Fig. 27-3C). The hair problem can be dealt with later by returning the flap and leaving protective connective tissue covering the framework via the "crane principle" (20) (Fig. 27-3D). The resurfacing is accomplished simultaneously with an appropriate skin graft (Figs. 27-3 E,F and 27-4).

Occasionally, the skin loss may be great enough to warrant the use of a temporoparietal fascial flap for adequate coverage. In this case, a skin graft is placed directly on the fascial flap after it is secured over the exposed framework.

Infection

One of the most dreaded complications of this surgery is postoperative infection. Prophylactic measures include administering antibiotics before, during, and after surgery, and postponing the auricular scrub and preparation until after the framework fabrication is complete so that no long time elapses between scrub and pocket dissection.

Despite attentive precautions and meticulous technique, infections do occur occasionally. Fortunately, the incidence of infection is significantly lower when autogenous cartilage frameworks are used than when inorganic materials are implanted. Likewise, autogenous tissue responds better to therapy than an alloplastic implant does.

In most cases, early infection is manifested not by auricular pain or fever but by local erythema, edema, subtle fluctuation, or a combination thereof. Therefore, frequent ob-

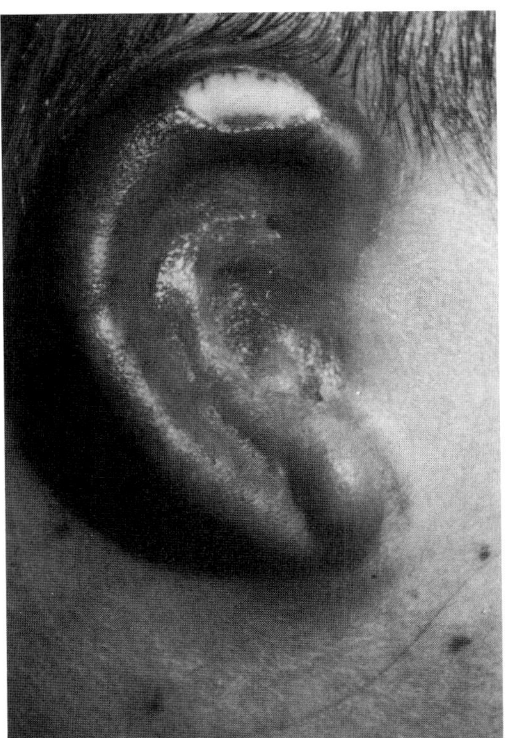

A

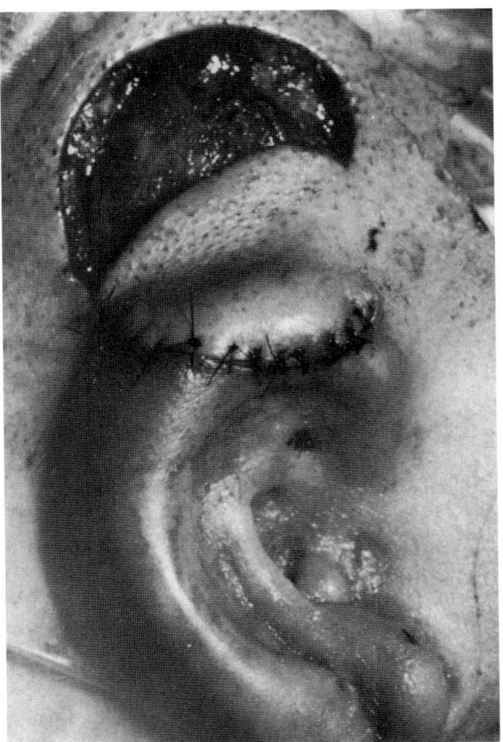

B

FIGURE 27-3. Management of exposed cartilage graft. **A:** Skin necrosis with cartilage exposure resulting from tight dressing applied by mother, 7 days postoperatively. **B:** Rotational skin flap. The donor defect will be covered by a skin graft. *(continued)*

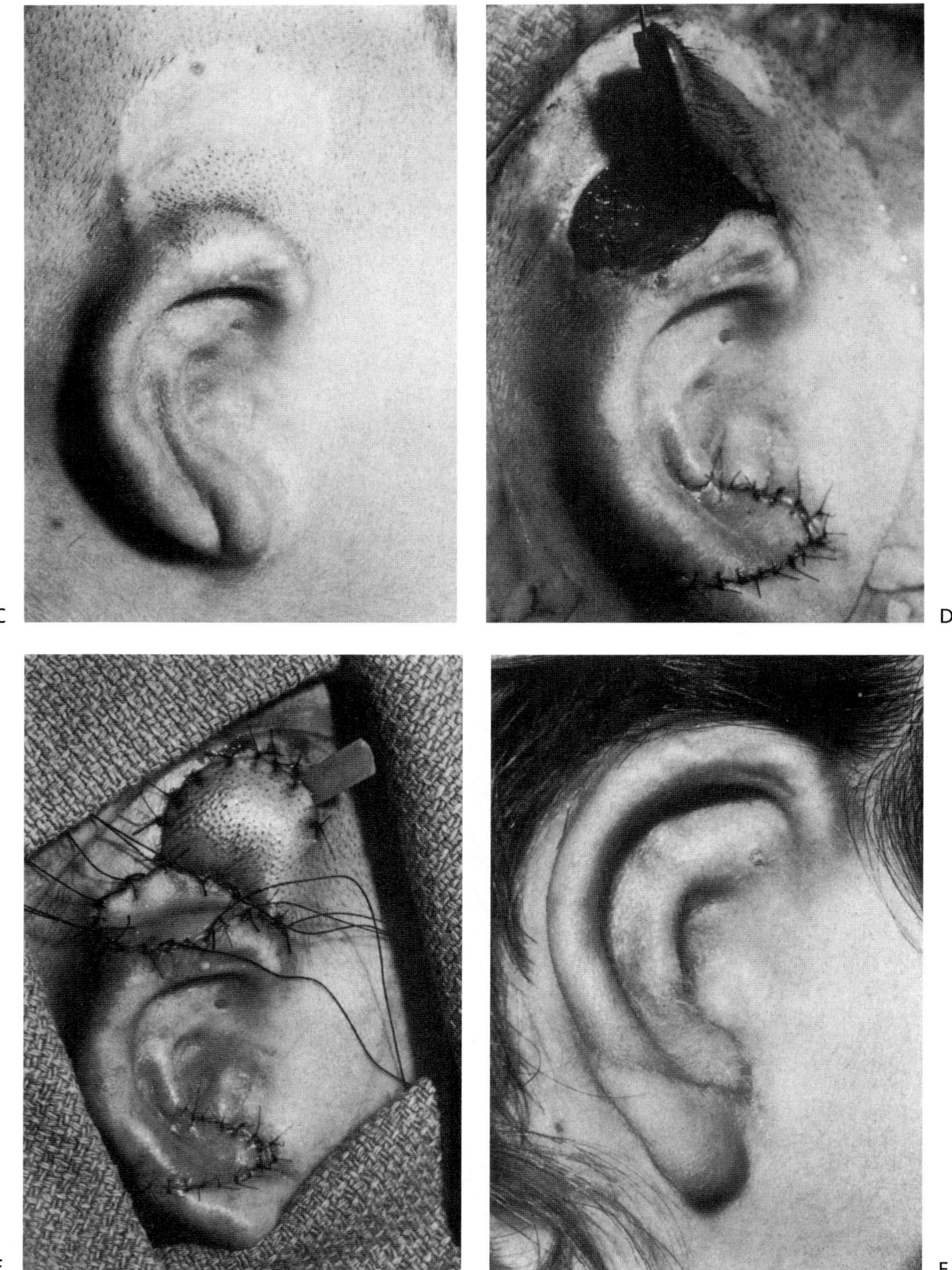

FIGURE 27-3. *Continued.* **C:** Healed repair. Note that hair-bearing skin has necessarily been transported to the auricle. **D,E:** Management of auricular hair by the "crane principle." The hair-bearing flap is elevated, and subcutaneous tissue has been retained over the cartilage framework. The flap has been returned to its original site by excising the temporary split-skin graft; a full-thickness graft (contralateral retroauricular) has been placed on the helical region. Note that the lobule has been simultaneously transposed. **F:** Result achieved.

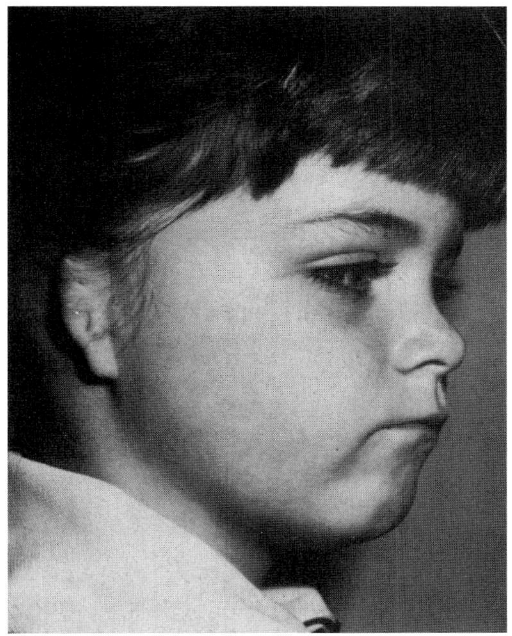
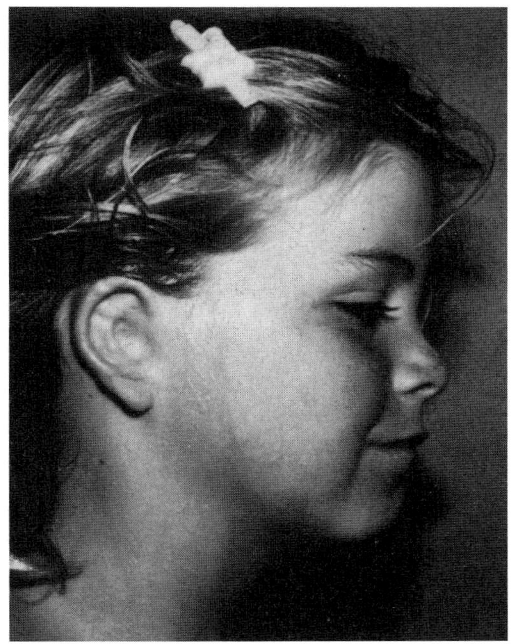

A B

FIGURE 27-4. Repair of microtic ear (same patient as in Fig. 27-3). **A:** Five-year-old child with microtia. **B:** Result following salvage of complication illustrated in Fig. 27-3.

servation and immediate, aggressive therapy can prevent overwhelming infection.

When an infection is suspected, continuous antibiotic drip irrigation should be started via an irrigation drain placed under the flap. When sensitivity studies become available from the initial culture, both the antibiotic irrigation and the systemic therapy are adjusted accordingly. Cronin (21) used this particular technique to manage infections in his Silastic framework reconstructions.

The three infections that occurred in my personal practice were all in patients with vestigial canal remnants, and all involved unusual bacterial organisms commonly found there. I now aggressively prepare all auricular canals with full-strength Betadine "paint" solution,[1] be they vestigial remnants in congenital microtia, normal canals in traumatic reconstructions, or normal canals in patients undergoing aesthetic otoplasty. On completing each case, I flush the canal thoroughly with saline solution; I have noted no untoward effects from the iodine. Although statistical luck may have been more of a factor than this precaution, I am pleased to report that no rib cartilage graft infections have occurred in my patients since I began this routine 15 years ago (approximately 1,000 frameworks) (6).

DRESSINGS, PROTECTION, ACTIVITIES

Dressings are designed to be protective but not constricting. As previously mentioned, I have experienced two cases of framework exposure that were caused by tight dressings applied without my knowledge by parents (Fig. 27-3A). The dressing should serve merely as a "bumper guard" and should be discarded 10 to 14 days after surgery. Conspicuous headgear is unnecessary and calls attention to the problem for which surgery has been undertaken.

Unlike alloplastic ear frameworks, autogenous auricular constructions tolerate significant trauma (22). I have had numerous patients withstand significant, if not dramatic, trauma to reconstructed auricles, such as a dog bite, a bee sting, blunt trauma from a soccer ball, a scratch from a sibling, and the line drive of a baseball to the antihelix (4,6).

RECONSTRUCTION ANEW

Because of previous surgical failure, the plastic surgeon is commonly confronted with a mass of scar tissue in the auricular region (Fig. 27-5A). In the early history of ear reconstruction, the only solution was to excise all scar tissue, resurface with a skin graft, and await a long maturation period before starting over (23), at which time one was faced with an inelastic two-dimensional pocket that could not safely accommodate a projecting three-dimensional framework.

An encouraging solution to this difficult problem has been to mobilize large temporoparietal fascial flaps as a cover tissue for a new cartilage framework (24,25). With this technique, the fascial flap is draped over the framework, then covered with a skin graft (Fig. 27-5 B–F). Although a fine salvage technique, this procedure is a major undertaking; it

[1]Betadine solution, povidone-iodine, 10%.

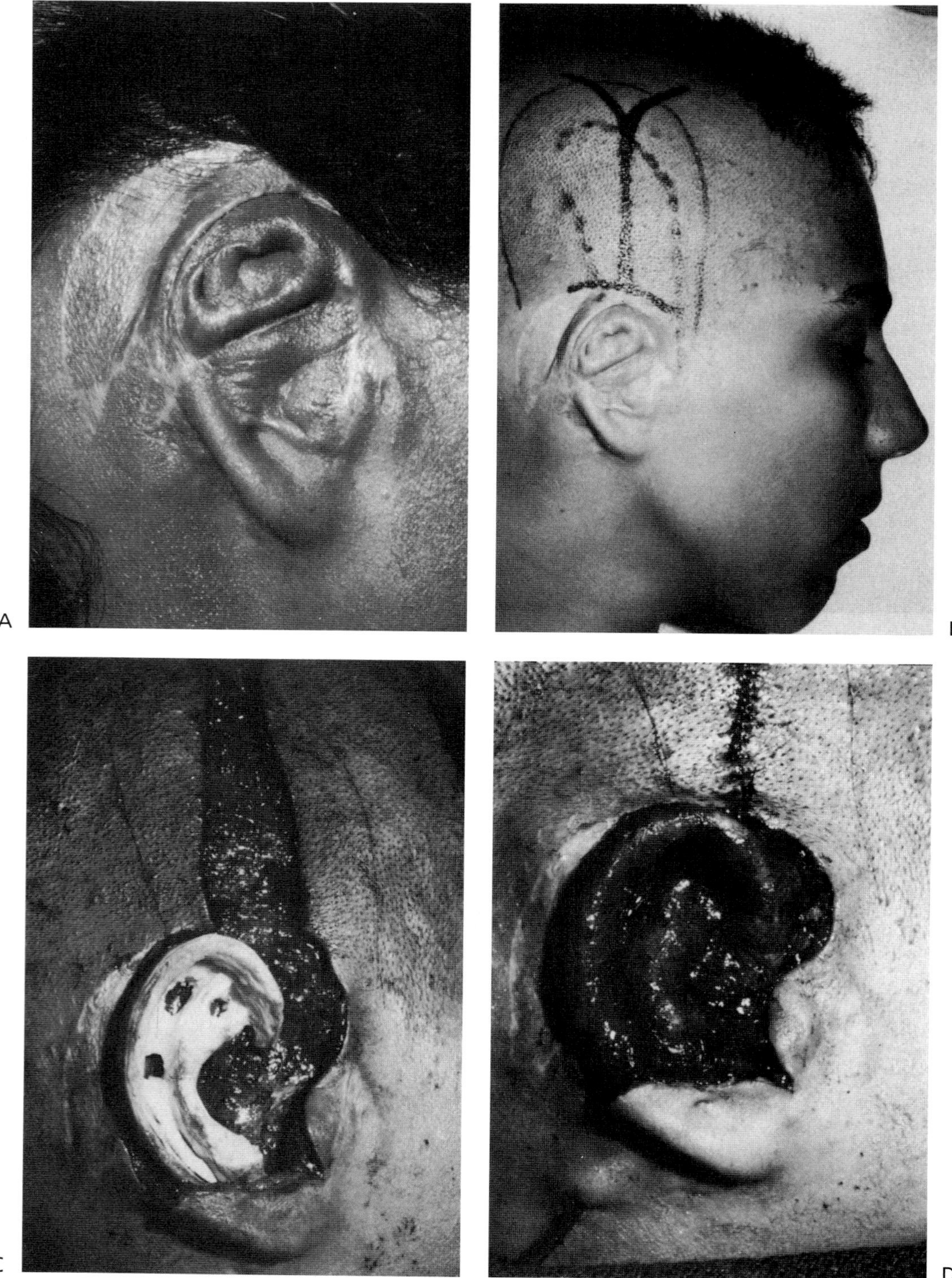

FIGURE 27-5. Secondary ear reconstruction with rib cartilage graft and temporoparietal fascial flap. **A:** Previous repair of microtic ear with Silastic framework. Note multiple scars, skin grafts, and irregularities. **B:** Planning of temporoparietal fascial flap. The flap has been outlined, the dopplered vessels are indicated, and the Y-shaped incision is drawn. **C:** Excision of scarred auricular mass, including Silastic framework. A rib cartilage graft is placed; the lobule has been retained, and the scalp dissection has begun. **D:** Draping of fascial flap over cartilage framework. *(continued)*

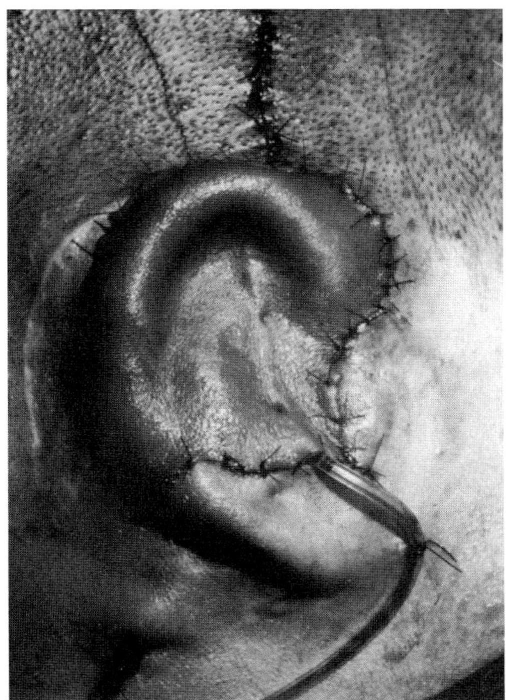

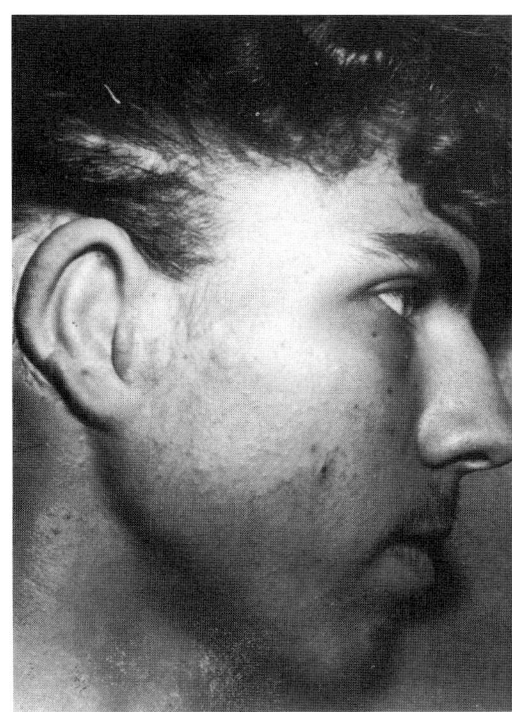

E F

FIGURE 27-5. *Continued.* **E:** Skin graft applied over fascia, immediately postoperatively. **F:** Result achieved, 1 year postoperatively. Tragus has been constructed with composite graft from contralateral auricle. (From Brent B, Byrd HS. Secondary ear reconstruction with cartilage grafts covered by axial, random, and free flaps of temporoparietal fascia. *Plast Reconstr Surg* 1983;72:141, with permission.)

should not be attempted without prior experience and confidence in managing virgin microtia.

CONCLUSION

Surgical construction of the auricle is an exacting discipline. To achieve favorable results, one must adhere strictly to sound surgical principles and be fortified with careful preparation, confidence, and, most importantly, a long-range game plan for each particular reconstruction. It is essential that the surgeon be confident in anticipating any complication that may arise and prepared to manage it if it does.

The author has presented a collection of trials, tribulations, and pitfalls in managing total ear reconstruction. It is hoped that they will not dampen enthusiasm but rather serve to forewarn and fortify the practitioner of auricular surgery.

REFERENCES

1. Steffensen WH. Comments on reconstruction of the external ear. *Plast Reconstr Surg* 1955;16:194.
2. Tanzer RC. Discussion of Silastic framework complications. In: Tanzer RC, Edgerton MT, eds. *Symposium on reconstruction of the auricle.* St. Louis: Mosby, 1974.
3. Brent B. The correction of microtia with autogenous cartilage grafts: I. The classic deformity. *Plast Reconstr Surg* 1980;66:1.
4. Brent B. Auricular repair with autogenous rib cartilage grafts: two decades of experience with 600 cases. *Plast Reconstr Surg* 1992;90:355.
5. Wellisz T. Reconstruction of the burned external ear with a Medpor porous polyethylene pivoting helix framework. *Plast Reconstr Surg* 1993;91:811.
6. Brent B. Technical advances in ear reconstruction with autogenous rib cartilage grafts—personal experience with 1,200 cases. *Plast Reconstr Surg* 1999;104:319–334.
7. Brent B. The correction of microtia with autogenous cartilage grafts: II. Atypical and complex deformities. *Plast Reconstr Surg* 1980;66:13.
8. Song Y, Song Y. An improved one-stage total ear reconstruction procedure. *Plast Reconstr Surg* 1983;71:615.
9. Brent B. Discussion of Song Y, Song Y. An improved one-stage total ear reconstruction procedure. *Plast Reconstr Surg* 1983; 71:623.
10. Broadbent TR, Mathews VL. Artistic relationships in surface anatomy of the face: application to reconstructive surgery. *Plast Reconstr Surg* 1957;20:1.
11. Gorney M, Murphy S, Falces E. Spliced autogenous conchal cartilage in secondary ear reconstruction. *Plast Reconstr Surg* 1971;47:432.
12. Lauritzen C, Munro IR, Ross RB. Classification and treatment of hemifacial microsomia. *Scand J Plast Reconstr Surg* 1985;19:33.
13. Converse JM. Discussion of deepilation. In: Tanzer RC, Edgerton MT, eds. *Symposium on reconstruction of the auricle.* St. Louis: Mosby, 1974:246.

14. Richards RN, McKenzie MA, Meharg GE. Electroepilation (electrolysis) in hirsutism: 35,000 hours' experience on the face and neck. *J Am Acad Dermatol* 1986;15:693.
15. Lask G, Elman M, Slatkine M. Laser-assisted hair removal by selective photothermolysis. Preliminary results. *Dermatol Surg* 1997;23:737–739.
16. Nanni CA, Alster TS. Optimizing treatment parameters for hair removal using a topical carbon-based solution and 1064-nm Q-switched neodymium:YAG laser energy. *Arch Dermatol* 1997; 133:1546–1549.
17. Brent B. Reconstruction of the ear. In: Grabb WC, Smith JW, eds. *Plastic surgery. A concise guide to clinical practice,* 5th ed. Boston: Little, Brown and Company, 1997:413–429.
18. Tanzer RC. Total reconstruction of the auricle. The evolution of a plan of treatment. *Plast Reconstr Surg* 1971;47:523.
19. Tanzer RC. Total reconstruction of the external ear. *Plast Reconstr Surg* 1959;23:1.
20. Millard DR. The crane principle for the transport of subcutaneous tissue. *Plast Reconstr Surg* 1969;43:451.
21. Cronin TD. Use of a Silastic frame for total and subtotal reconstruction of the external ear: preliminary report. *Plast Reconstr Surg* 1966;37:399.
22. Brent B. Total auricular construction with sculpted costal cartilage. In: Brent B, ed. *The artistry of reconstructive surgery.* St. Louis: Mosby, 1987:113–127.
23. Tanzer RC. Secondary reconstruction of the auricle. In: Tanzer RC, Edgerton MT, eds. *Symposium on reconstruction of the auricle.* St. Louis: Mosby, 1974:238.
24. Brent B, Byrd HS. Secondary ear reconstruction with cartilage grafts covered by axial, random, and free flaps of temporoparietal fascia. *Plast Reconstr Surg* 1983;72:141.
25. Brent B. Auricular reconstruction with fascial transposition flaps. In: Brent B, ed. *The artistry of reconstructive surgery.* St. Louis: Mosby, 1987:129–138.

Discussion

AURICULAR RECONSTRUCTION

SATORU NAGATA

It is well-known that primary auricular reconstruction is a technically demanding operation in which precision and technique are required, especially because the skin surface area is insufficient to cover the fabricated costal cartilage framework (1–5). Furthermore, the possibility of postoperative complications, such as vascular compromise, resorption of the cartilage framework, protrusion of the cartilage framework, and infection, must be considered, as stated by Dr. Brent. When the management of postoperative complications fails or when one is faced with an unfavorable result of a primary auricular reconstruction, the ultimate solution is to perform a secondary auricular reconstruction, which is an extremely difficult and challenging procedure (5,6).

In a secondary auricular reconstruction, the surgeon is faced with massive scarring, an insufficient skin surface area to cover the three-dimensional costal cartilage framework, and complications such as a severed superficial temporal artery. Therefore, the surgeon must be extremely careful and plan for the secondary procedure precisely (5,6).

For both primary and secondary auricular reconstructions, I utilize a two-stage auricular reconstruction procedure that I introduced previously (1–4,6–9). Secondary auricular reconstruction is far more difficult than primary auricular reconstruction (3,4,7).

PREOPERATIVE PLANNING FOR THE FIRST-STAGE OPERATION

Preoperative planning for a secondary auricular reconstruction is extremely important, as it is in all auricular reconstructions. Preoperative planning for the first-stage auricular reconstruction includes the following:

1. Determining the proper anatomical location for the reconstructed auricle
2. Determining how much tensile skin can be salvaged and how much skin surface area will be insufficient to cover the new three-dimensional framework
3. Determining the amount of costal cartilage that will be needed to fabricate the new three-dimensional framework
4. Assessing the status of the local circulation at the surgical site

S. Nagata: Department of Reconstructive Plastic Surgery, Chiba Tokushukai Hospital, Funabashi, Chiba, Japan

5. Selecting the fascia flap
6. Considering miscellaneous factors

SURGICAL PROCEDURE FOR THE FIRST-STAGE OPERATION

The first-stage operation in auricular reconstruction consists of fabricating and grafting the three-dimensional framework (1–4,5,6,8).

First, the proper anatomical location for the reconstructed auricle must be determined. At our institution, we utilize a transparent film template to select the anatomical location for the reconstruction (presented at the 12th International Confederation for Plastic Reconstructive and Aesthetic Surgery in San Francisco, June 28 to 30, 1999). Next, the outline for the first-stage operation is plotted. The costal cartilage framework from the primary auricular reconstruction is removed, and all scar tissue is excised completely. In unilateral cases, the costal cartilage is harvested and the three-dimensional frame is fabricated, but in bilateral cases, we must salvage the costal cartilage framework and fabricate a new three-dimensional framework. Ultradelicate split-thickness scalp skin is harvested, and the temporoparietal fascia flap is then elevated. The fabricated three-dimensional framework is placed in the proper anatomical location and covered with the temporoparietal fascia flap, and the skin surface area is covered with the ultradelicate split-thickness scalp skin. Next, bolster sutures are applied. I have been using this procedure for more than 10 years, and no postoperative complications or problems have developed. I have used suction drains, but the overall appearance of the reconstructed auricle is flat, and detailed definition of the auricle is difficult to attain, especially in cases of secondary auricular reconstruction.

SURGICAL PROCEDURE FOR THE SECOND-STAGE OPERATION

In the second-stage operation, the reconstructed auricle is projected (6).

For the second stage of the auricular reconstruction, the ultradelicate split-thickness scalp skin is harvested, and the deep temporoparietal fascia flap, which includes the periosteum in the distal portion, is elevated. The costal cartilage block for projection of the auricle is shaped to the eminentia conchae. The costal cartilage block is grafted and covered with a deep temporoparietal fascia flap followed by the ultradelicate split-thickness scalp skin.

COMPLICATED SECONDARY AURICULAR RECONSTRUCTION

Any secondary auricular reconstruction poses a formidable challenge to the reconstructive plastic surgeon, and these cases can be further complicated by a low hairline, a severed superficial temporal artery, and excessive and massive scarring at the surgical site (5,6).

A, B

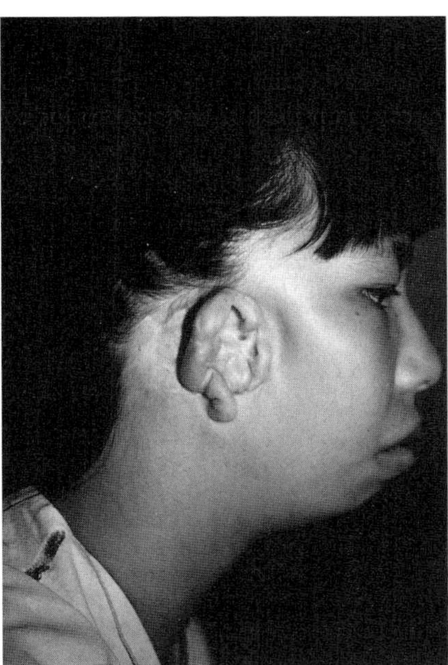

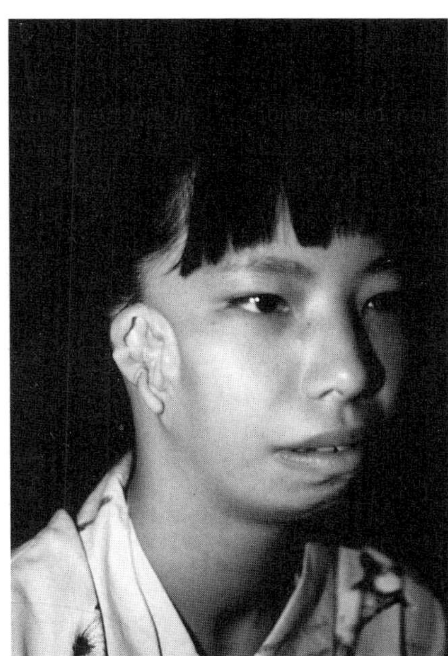

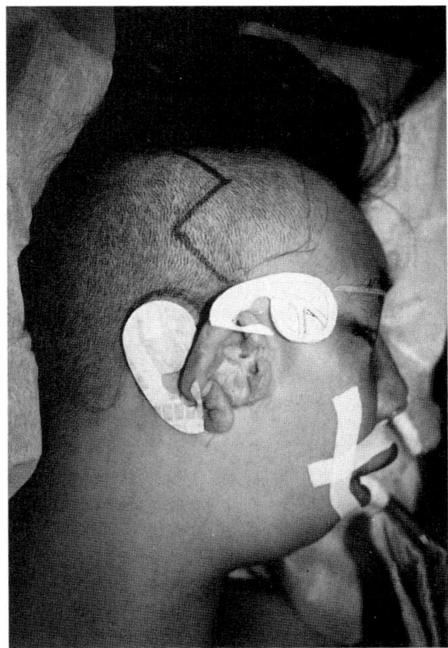

C

FIGURE 27D-1. An unfavorable result of a primary auricular reconstruction in a case of bilateral hemifacial microsomia with bilateral microtia, further complicated by a low hairline. **A,B:** Preoperative appearance. Note extensive scarring, deep indentation anterior to the constructed auricle, incorrect anatomical location of the constructed auricle, and abnormal hairline (no bangs or sideburns). **C:** Determination of the proper anatomical location where the auricle is to be reconstructed. *(continued)*

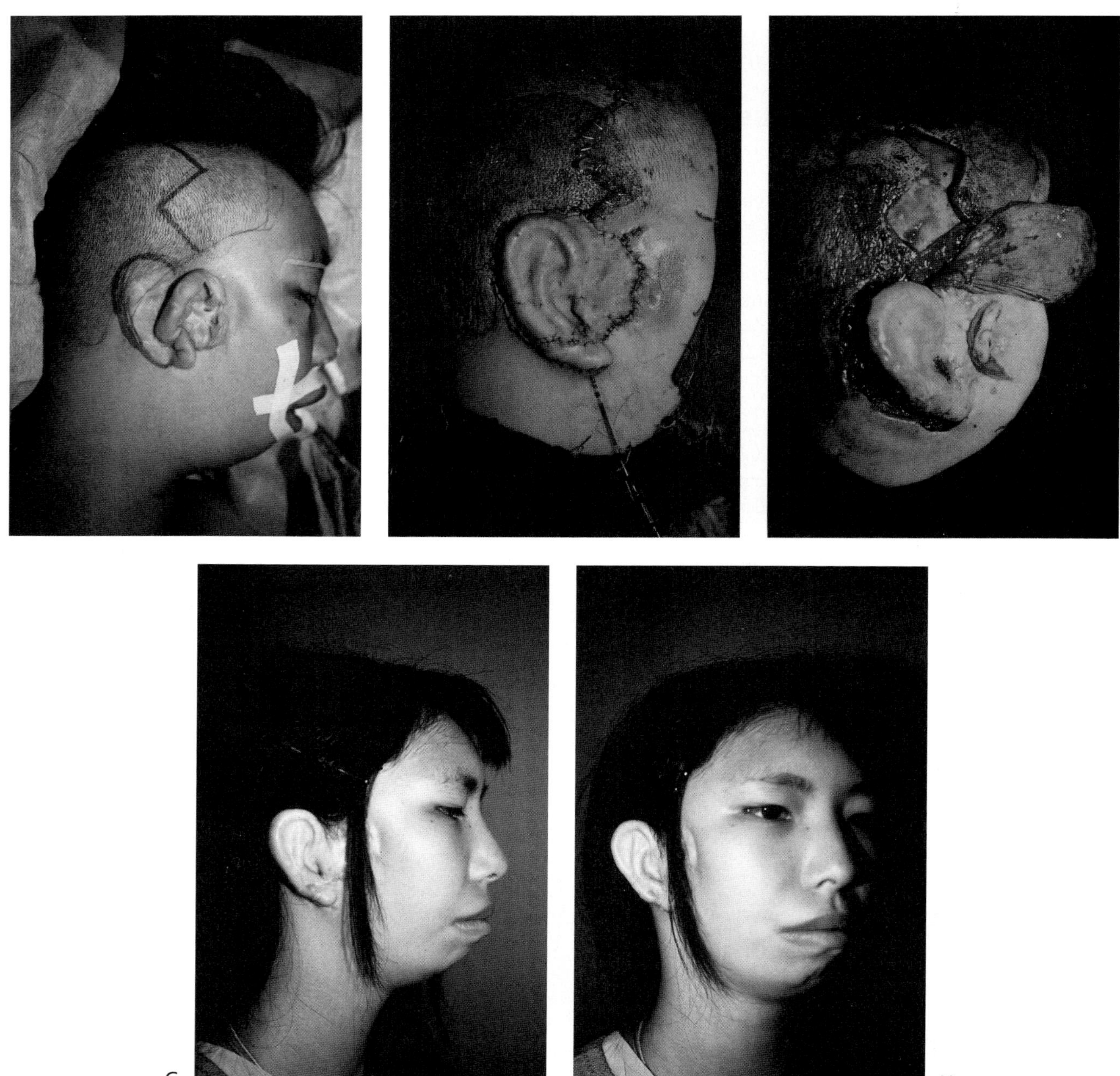

FIGURE 27D-1. *Continued.* **D:** Outline of the first-stage operation; note the low hairline. **E:** Appearance immediately after the first-stage operation. **F:** Intraoperative appearance during the second-stage operation, with the costal cartilage block for auricular projection and the deep temporoparietal fascia flap *(DTF).* **G,H:** Postoperative appearance after the two-stage secondary auricular reconstruction. The reconstructed auricle is well maintained and projected.

REPRESENTATIVE CASES

Case 1

The first case is a patient with bilateral hemifacial microsomia and an unfavorable result of primary auricular reconstruction (Fig. 27D-1A,B). The reconstructed auricle is located in a deep indentation and anterior to the normal anatomical location. There are no bangs or sideburns, and massive scarring is present (Fig. 27-D1A–D). The proper anatomical location is shown and outlined (Fig. 27D-1C,D). This case is further complicated by a low hairline (Fig. 27D-1D). Epilation is performed during the first-stage operation. Figure 27D-1E shows the patient's appearance immediately after the first-stage operation, before the application of bolster sutures. The temporoparietal fascia flap has been utilized during this stage. The removed cartilage is used to fill the indentation formed after removal of the cartilage framework. The second-stage operation is the projection of the recon-

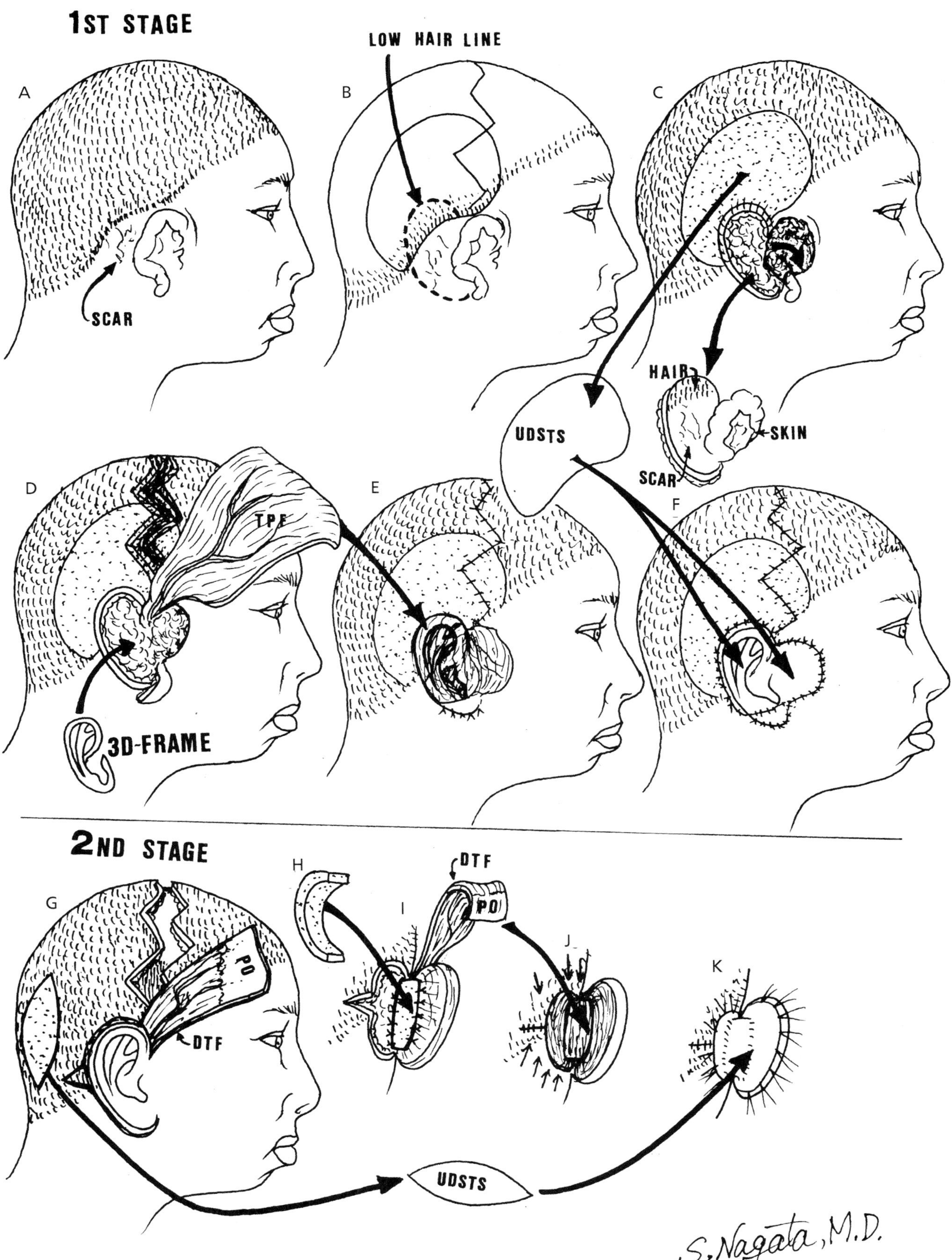

FIGURE 27D-2. Schematic illustration of the two-stage secondary auricular reconstruction performed in Case 1. **A–F:** Schematic illustration of the first-stage operation. **G–K:** Schematic illustration of the second-stage operation.

structed auricle. A costal cartilage block shaped to the eminentia conchae and a deep temporoparietal fascia flap are used to cover the posterior aspect of the projected auricle (Fig. 27D-1F). After the second-stage operation, the reconstructed auricle is well projected and maintained, and no postoperative complications are present (Fig. 27D-1G,H).

A schematic illustration of the surgical procedure for this case appears in Fig. 27D-2. In the first-stage operation (Fig. 27D-2A–F), massive scarring is present posterior to the constructed auricle in the area that corresponds to the surgical site for the secondary auricular reconstruction (Fig. 27D-2A). The outline for the first-stage operation is plotted. Note the proper anatomical location of the auricle to be reconstructed. This case is further complicated by a low hairline (Fig. 27D-2B). The ultradelicate split-thickness scalp skin is harvested, the costal cartilage framework from the first-stage operation is re-

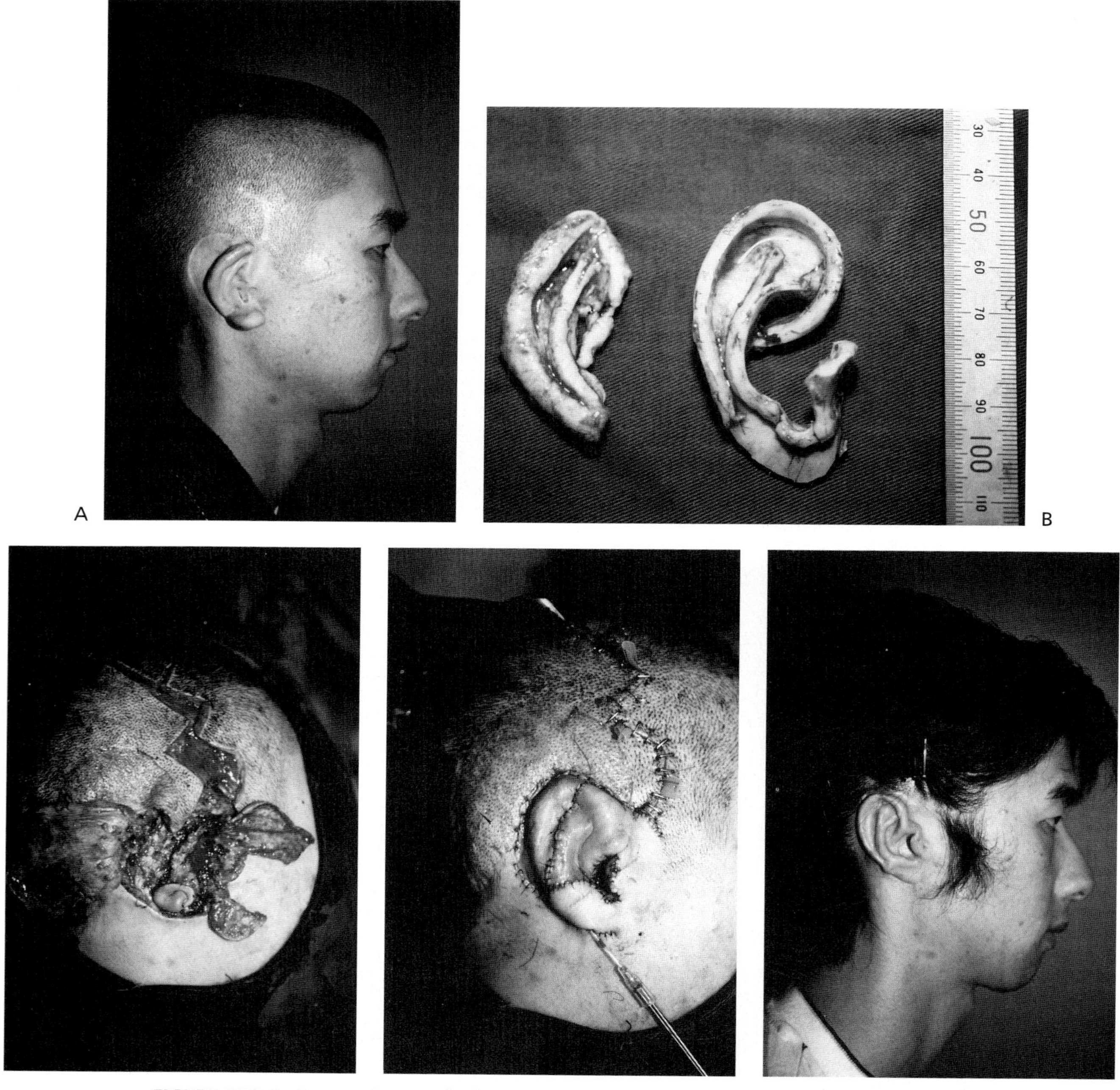

FIGURE 27D-3. A secondary auricular reconstruction with a severed superficial temporal artery *(STA)*. A: Preoperative appearance. Note that the STA was severed during the first auricular reconstruction. **B:** The removed costal cartilage framework *(left)* and the newly fabricated three-dimensional costal cartilage framework *(right)*. **C:** Intraoperative appearance during the first-stage operation. Elevation of the temporoparietal fascia flap *(TPF)* with a posterior pedicle and a postauricular subcutaneous pedicle. **D:** Appearance immediately after the first-stage operation. **E:** Appearance immediately before the second-stage operation. *(continued)*

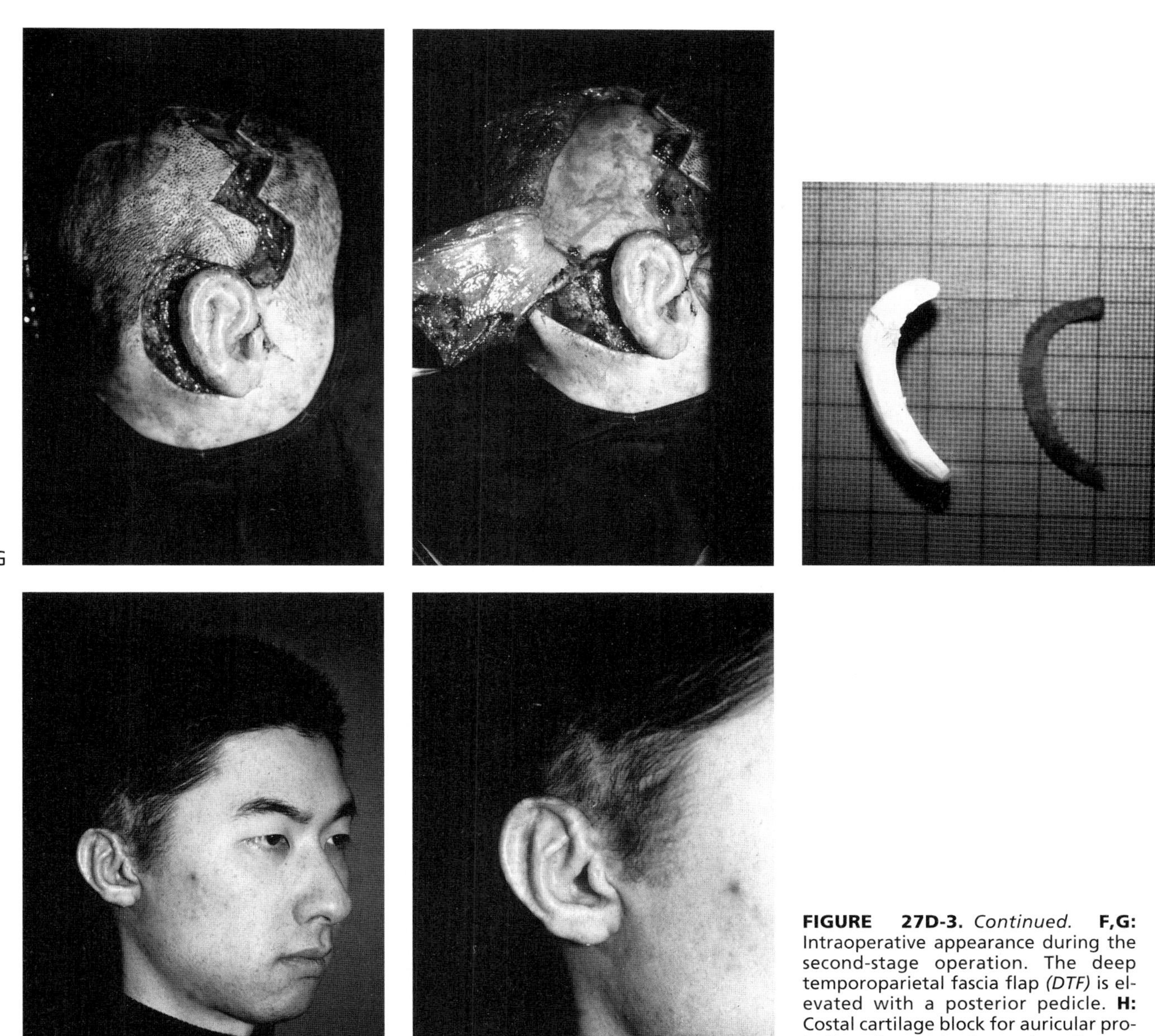

FIGURE 27D-3. *Continued.* **F,G:** Intraoperative appearance during the second-stage operation. The deep temporoparietal fascia flap *(DTF)* is elevated with a posterior pedicle. **H:** Costal cartilage block for auricular projection shaped to the eminentia conchae. **I,J:** Postoperative appearance after the two-stage secondary auricular reconstruction. The reconstructed auricle is well maintained and projected.

moved, all scar tissue is excised, and epilation is accomplished by removing the hair-bearing layer (Fig. 27D-2C). The temporoparietal fascia flap is elevated to cover the fabricated three-dimensional frame after it has been placed in the proper anatomical location (Fig. 27D-2D). The insufficient skin surface area of the three-dimensional frame and the area anterior to the grafted three-dimensional frame are covered with the temporoparietal fascia flap (Fig. 27D-2E). The final procedure before the application of bolster sutures is to cover the raw surface of the temporoparietal fascia flap with the harvested ultradelicate split-thickness scalp skin (Fig. 27D-2F). The second-stage operation (Fig. 27D-2G–K) is the projection of the reconstructed auricle. For the second-stage operation, the ultradelicate split-thickness scalp skin is harvested in a spindle shape and the deep temporoparietal fascia flap is elevated (Fig. 27D-2G). The costal cartilage shaped to the eminentia conchae is grafted to the posterior surface of the reconstructed auricle and the mastoid surface (Fig. 27D-2H and Fig. 27D-2I) and then covered with the deep temporoparietal fascia flap (Fig. 27D-2J). The final procedure is to cover the posterior surface of the projected auricle with the spindle-shaped ultradelicate split-thickness scalp skin (Fig. 27D-2K).

Case 2

Case 2 is a secondary auricular reconstruction. The superficial temporal artery was severed during the first reconstruction, and massive scarring is present (Fig. 27D-3A). The three-dimensional frame is fabricated according to the dimensions of the opposite, normal auricle. Note the difference in the shapes of the removed costal cartilage framework (Fig. 27D-3B, left) and the newly fabricated three-dimensional framework (Fig. 27D-3B, right). Because of the severed superficial temporal artery, the temporoparietal fascia flap is elevated with a posterior pedicle, and the circular skin at the inferior region of the surgical site is left attached to serve as a subcutaneous pedicle (Fig. 27D-3C). Immediately after the first-stage operation, the subcutaneous pedicle is

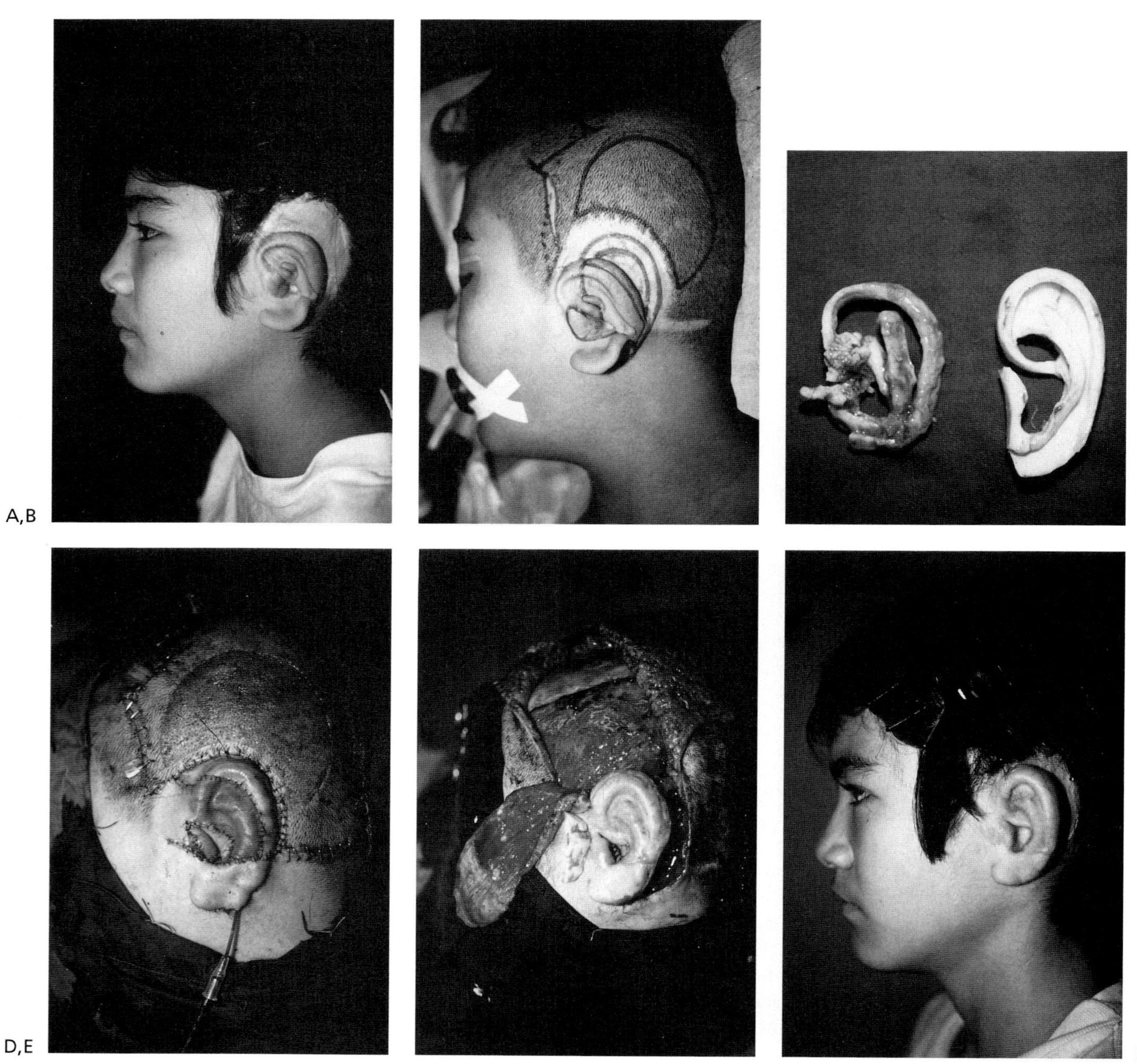

FIGURE 27D-4. Secondary auricular reconstruction for unfavorable results of a primary auricular reconstruction. **A:** Preoperative appearance. The skin posterior to the constructed auricle is a skin graft from the groin area. **B:** Outline for the first-stage operation. The constructed auricle is not in the proper anatomical location—it is anterior and inferior to the normal anatomical location. **C:** The removed costal cartilage framework and three-dimensional framework. **D:** Appearance immediately after the first-stage operation. The postauricular subcutaneous pedicle flap was utilized in the tragal region along with an ultradelicate split-thickness scalp skin *(UDSTS)*. **E:** Intraoperative appearance during the second-stage operation with the elevated deep temporoparietal fascia flap *(DTF)* and costal cartilage block for auricular projection. *(continued)*

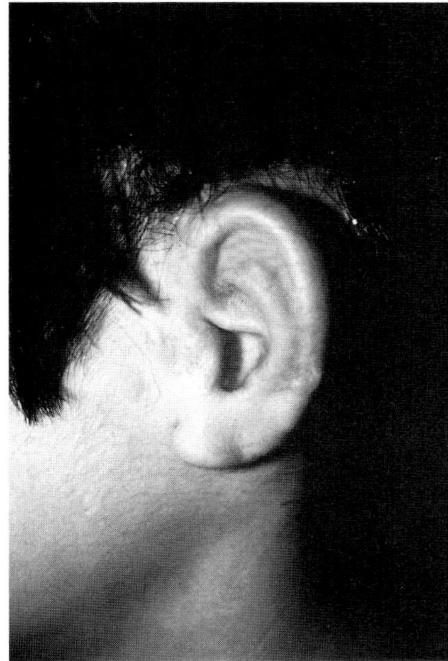
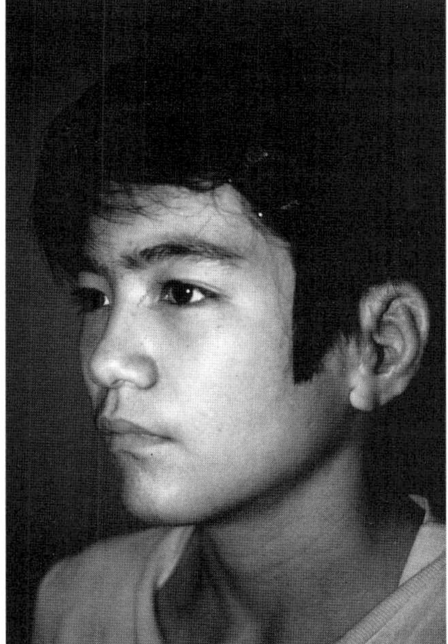
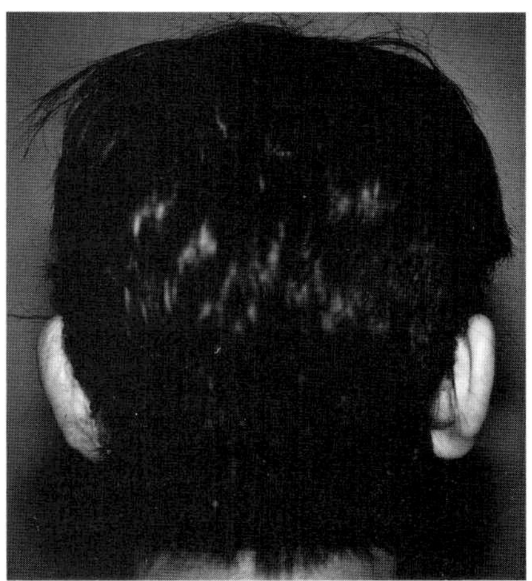

G,H I

FIGURE 27D-4. *Continued.* **F,G:** Lateral view after the two-stage secondary auricular reconstruction. **H:** Anterolateral angle view. **I:** Posterior view. The reconstructed auricle is well maintained and projected.

located in the conchal region (Fig. 27D-3D). The appearance immediately before the second-stage operation is shown in Fig. 27D-3E, the intraoperative appearance during the second-stage operation in Fig. 27D-3F, and the deep temporoparietal fascia flap elevated with a posterior pedicle in Fig. 27D-3G. The fabricated costal cartilage block shaped to the eminentia conchae is shown in Fig. 27D-3H. After the second-stage operation, the projected auricle is well maintained, and no postoperative complications or problems are present (Fig. 27D-3I,J).

Case 3

Case 3 shows extensive and massive scarring. The color of a skin graft from the groin area located posterior and superior to the constructed auricle is mismatched (Fig. 27D-4A). The outline for the first-stage operation reveals that the constructed auricle is anterior and inferior to the normal anatomical location, and a scar is present in the hair-bearing skin anterior and superior to the outline of the surgical site (Fig. 27D-4B). The difference between the removed costal cartilage framework and the newly fabricated three-dimensional frame is apparent in Fig. 27D-4C. The appearance immediately before the bolster sutures is shown in Fig. 27D-4D. The ultradelicate split-thickness scalp skin, temporoparietal fascia flap, and postauricular pedicle flap were utilized during the first-stage operation. Figure 27D-4E shows the intraoperative appearance with the costal cartilage block and elevated deep temporoparietal fascia flap. The postoperative appearance after the second-stage operation is shown in Fig. 27D-4F–H, and the posterior view in Fig. 27D-4I shows that the projected auricle is well maintained and that no postoperative complications or problems are present.

CONCLUSION

Total or subtotal auricular reconstruction is a difficult and challenging surgical procedure. Multiple factors affect the success of auricular reconstruction: preoperative planning; the availability of a properly trained, skilled, and experienced reconstructive plastic surgeon; and the ability of the surgeon to perform recovery procedures when faced with postoperative complications or problems. When any one of these factors is lacking, it is difficult to achieve a satisfactory result, and the final result can be disastrous.

Many pitfalls are involved in total and subtotal auricular reconstruction with the use of autogenous costal cartilage. In auricular reconstructions for congenital defects such as microtia, the surgeon focuses on constructing an auricle that resembles a normal auricle as closely as possible. In addition, management of the donor site must be considered in planning an auricular reconstruction. The surgeon may be able to correct one anatomical defect but may also create another, such as a chest wall deformity at the site where the costal cartilages were harvested (10).

For an auricular reconstruction to succeed, the surgeon must consider all the factors previously mentioned. Furthermore, psychological and sociological factors must be considered in treating the patient and dealing with family members. The patient's parents often ask that the surgery be performed as soon as possible, or at least before the child enters elementary school. If this type of surgery is performed prematurely, the result can be disastrous; therefore, it is extremely important for the surgeon to explain thoroughly what the patient and family members can expect. We perform auricular reconstructions in children with congenital deformities or other problems at the age of 10 years. The reason for this is that 95% of the adult auricular size has been attained at the age of 10 years, and the costal cartilage mass is usually sufficient to fabricate the three-dimensional frame (5). The costal cartilage of a very young patient (< 6 or 7 years old) may be more prone to resorption because it is often thin and flimsy.

Extreme care must be exercised in auricular reconstruction, as in all types of surgery, to avoid postoperative complications, problems, and unfavorable results.

REFERENCES

1. Nagata S. New method of total reconstruction of the auricle for microtia. *Plast Reconstr Surg* 1993;92:187–201.
2. Nagata S. The modification stages involved in the total reconstruction of the auricle: part I. The modification in the grafting of the three-dimensional costal cartilage framework (3-D frame) for the lobule type microtia. *Plast Reconstr Surg* 1994;93:221–230.
3. Nagata S. The modification stages involved in the total reconstruction of the auricle: part II. The modification in the grafting of the three-dimensional costal cartilage framework (3-D Frame) for the concha type microtia. *Plast Reconstr Surg* 1994;93:231–242.
4. Nagata S. The modification stages involved in the total reconstruction of the auricle: part III. The modification in the grafting of the three-dimensional costal cartilage framework (3-D frame) for the small concha type microtia. *Plast Reconstr Surg* 1994; 93:243–253.
5. Nagata S. Microtia: auricular reconstruction. In: *Plastic surgery: indications, options, outcomes.* St. Louis: Mosby, 2000:1028–1056.
6. Nagata S. Secondary auricular reconstruction for unfavorable microtia results: utilizing the temporoparietal and innominate fascia flaps. *Plast Reconstr Surg* 1994;93:254–265.
7. Nagata S. The modification stages involved in the total reconstruction of the auricle: part IV. The modification in the ear elevation of the constructed auricle. *Plast Reconstr Surg* 1994; 93:254–266.
8. Nagata S. Total auricular reconstruction with a three-dimensional costal cartilage framework. *Ann Chir Plast Esthet* 1995; 40:371–403.
9. Nagata S. Ear reconstruction utilizing three-dimensional costal cartilage framework. In: *Salyer and Bardach's atlas of craniofacial and cleft surgery,* vol. 2. 1999:410–415.
10. Nagamizu H, Nagata S. Minimization of postoperative problems at the donor site after cartilage resection. *Transactions of the 11th Congress of the International Confederation for Plastic, Reconstructive and Aesthetic Surgery,* May 1995: Yokohama, Japan, pp 423–424.

28

OTOPLASTY

SAMUEL STAL
MICHAEL KLEBUC
MELVIN SPIRA

The image of the first dressing change is deeply emblazoned in the public consciousness. The surgeon removes heavy bandages to reveal a beautiful silhouette where just days before trauma and disfigurement had prevailed. This expediency is seldom enjoyed in plastic surgical pursuits with the exception of otoplasty. Surgical correction of the prominent ear can produce an immediate and permanent result that provides great satisfaction to both patient and surgeon (Fig. 28-1). Otoplasty is an effective and trouble-free procedure if the surgeon is cognizant of the prospective complications, which often prove difficult to correct and are better avoided via appropriate patient selection, careful preoperative analysis, and attention to intraoperative details. The errors of omission or commission leading to the unfavorable result in otoplasty can be categorized as occurring during (a) preoperative planning, (b) intraoperative execution, or (c) postoperative management (1).

PREOPERATIVE PLANNING AND SELECTION

The unfavorable result in otoplasty is the product of a domino effect that often begins with the preoperative assessment. The prominent ear is usually the product of incomplete folding of the scapha, which produces a poorly defined or absent antihelix in concert with an excessively tall or large posterior conchal wall. These anomalies may exist together or in isolation and are frequently associated with a host of secondary deformities, including (a) an overprojected lobule, (b) an excessively prominent helical root, and (c) insufficient curling of the helix. Subsequently, otoplasty is not a "one size fits all" procedure; rather, it must be tailored to the individual deformity after careful analysis. Familiarity with standard external ear morphometrics facilitates the preoperative evaluation. On the frontal view, the ear occupies a zone extending from the brow superiorly to the base of the columella inferiorly. On lateral inspection, it should lie a single ear length behind the lateral orbital rim (6.5 to 7.5 cm) with its vertical axis inclined 15 to 30 degrees posteriorly (2). The width of the ear is typically 50% to 60% of its height; the average width is 3 to 4.5 cm, and the average height is 5.5 to 6.5 cm. The helical rim measures approximately 10% of the vertical height (7 mm) and protrudes 10 to 12 mm at the helical apex, 16 to 18 mm at the midpoint, and 20 to 22 mm at the lobule (3,4). Protrusion is further quantified by the cephaloauricular and scaphoconchal angles. The auricle is considered prominent when the cephaloauricular angle is greater than 25 degrees in males and 21 degrees in females, or when the scaphoconchal angle exceeds 90 degrees (5). A standardized data sheet compiled during the preoperative visit can prove useful in facilitating an analytical evaluation (Fig. 28-2).

Up to 85% of cartilaginous ear growth (approximately 5.5 cm of length) is completed by 3 to 4 years of age, so that otoplasty is ideally performed in the interval between 3 years of age and the initiation of kindergarten. If the child exhibits behavioral problems (enuresis, social withdrawal, acting out), then a psychological evaluation is obtained (6). Additionally, prominent ears are frequently asymmetrical with regard to size, position, and degree of protrusion. It is imperative to point out these discrepancies to the patients and their families preoperatively because they will certainly become recognized during the postoperative scrutiny and attributed to surgical inaccuracy. Asymmetry is the concern of the patient preoperatively and of the surgeon postoperatively (7).

In preparation for surgery, the child and family are instructed to wash the hair and face with medicated soap 48, 24, and 12 hours before surgery. The surgical skin preparation is undertaken by swabbing Betadine in the external auditory canal in an attempt to minimize potential *Pseudomonas* colonization. Intraoperative antibiotics are given intravenously and continued in oral form for 7 days postoperatively. The hair can be directed away from the surgical field with transparent 10 × 10-cm plastic drapes. The drapes should provide an unfettered view of both ears.

S. Stal, M. Klebuc, and M. Spira: Department of Plastic Surgery, Baylor College of Medicine; and Department of Plastic Surgery Texas Children's Hospital, Houston, Texas

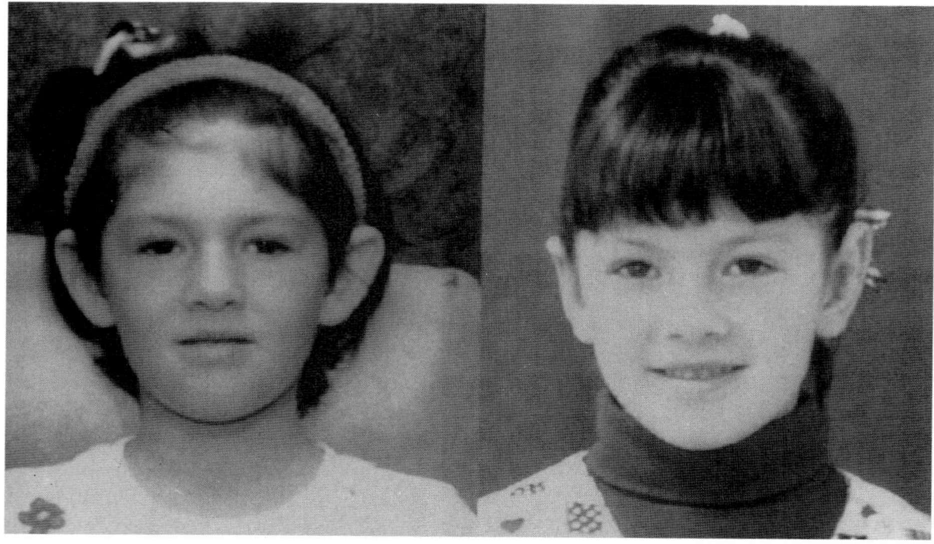

FIGURE 28-1. Left: Five-year-old child preoperatively. **Right:** One year after otoplasty.

OTOPLASTY EVALUATION

Texas Children's Hospital
Samuel Stal, M.D.
Clinical Care Center, Suite 330
6621 Fannin Street
(713) 770-3180
FAX: (713) 770-3192

Patient Name: ______________________

Date of Birth: ______________________

Date of Exam: ______________________

❒ Male ❒Female

Patient Information:
Prominent ears are congenital in origin. Correction of a congenital abnormality is considered reconstructive in nature.
Normal Ear Protrusion from post-auricular scalp to lateral aspect of superior helix 1.5-2.0cm.
Normal conchal-scaphal angle is approximatley 90 degrees.

Primary Complaint

- ❒ External Deformity
- ❒ Internal Deformity
  - ❒ Unilateral
  - ❒ Bilateral
    - ❒ Left
    - ❒ Right

Etiology

- ❒ Trauma (documented)

  __________Age at trauma
- ❒ Congenital
  - ❒ Prominent
  - ❒ Microtia
  - ❒ Cup ear
  - ❒ Cryptocia

Diagnosis

- ❒ Within normal limits
- ❒ Protruding ears,cong. 744.29
- ❒ Congential malformation 744.3
- ❒ Acquired deformity 872.10
- ❒ Microtia 744.23
- ❒ Atresia 744.02

____
Samuel Stal, M.D.
Chief, Plastic Surgery Texas Children's Hospital

PHYSICAL EXAMINATION

Left

Abnormal areas

- ❒ None
- ❒ Antihelix absent
- ❒. Antehelix weak
- ❒ Concha/Conchal Angle_____
- ❒ Ear Lobe
- ❒ Root of helix
- ❒ Extra Crus

____

____

Right

Abnormal areas

- ❒ None
- ❒ Antihelix absent
- ❒ Antihelix waek
- ❒ Concha/Conchal Angle_____
- ❒ Ear Lobe
- ❒ Root of helix
- ❒ Extra Crus

____

____

Medical History As Related by Parents/Patient to Physician

Ridicule by peers	❒ Yes ❒ No
Low self image reg. appearance	❒ Yes ❒ No
Hearing problems	❒ Yes ❒ No
Chronic Ear Infection	❒ Yes ❒ No
Allergy symptoms	❒ Yes ❒ No
Bleeding Problems	❒ Yes ❒ No
Wears Eyeglasses	❒ Yes ❒ No
Scar Formation	❒ Yes ❒ No
Use of Apirin Products	❒ Yes ❒ No
Hair covers ears	❒ Yes ❒ No

Recommendation

- ❒ No intervention
- ❒ Referral to Otolaryngologist
- ❒ Delay surgical correction in favor of growth/after age 5
- ❒ Otoplasty 69300/50
  - ❒ Scaphal Folding
  - ❒ Conchal Reduction
  - ❒ Conchal Setback
  - ❒ Lobule Setback
  - ❒ Mustarde Sutures
  - ❒ Hatch Maneuver
- ❒ Otoplasty w/skin graft 69399
- ❒ Otoplasty/ear cartilage graft 21230
- ❒ Adjacent tissue transfer 14060
- ❒ Psychological Evaluation
- ❒ Outcome Evaluation
- ❒ Social Services Referral

FIGURE 28-2. Otoplasty check-off list.

DECISIONS DURING SURGERY THAT INFLUENCE DEFORMITY

The surgical goal is to produce an ear with a soft, naturally curved neoantihelix that does not obscure the helical rim on the front view. Deviation from these objectives is frequently manifest in residual deformity, including the following: (a) telephone ear, (b) reverse telephone ear, (c) postlike ear (vertical antihelix), (d) external auditory canal stenosis, (e) variegation of the scapha, (e) postauricular bowstring formation, and (f) an overzealous "pinned back, operated" appearance (8,9).

Telephone Ear Deformity

The telephone ear deformity is characterized by a residual protuberance of the lobule and helical root relative to an apparently excessively set-back middle segment (Fig. 28-3). The deformity has two possible causes. It may arise from excessive conchal recession, inadequate correction of the upper and lower poles, or both. In the case of the former, overzealous excision of the conchal cartilage and postauricular muscle and fibrofatty tissue may be the causative factor. If suture techniques alone are employed, then sequencing in terms of placement and tying becomes an issue of significance. Concha-mastoid sutures should be utilized to establish a new conchal position before Mustardé sutures are tied (10,11). Gauging the effect and vector of pull of the sutures with noncommittal single half hitch knots is a good preventative strategy. Overcorrection of the middle third is further avoided by tying the middle suture last (Fig. 28-4). Additionally, attention should be focused initially on the most prominent ear, with the less deformed auricle tailored to the contralateral result.

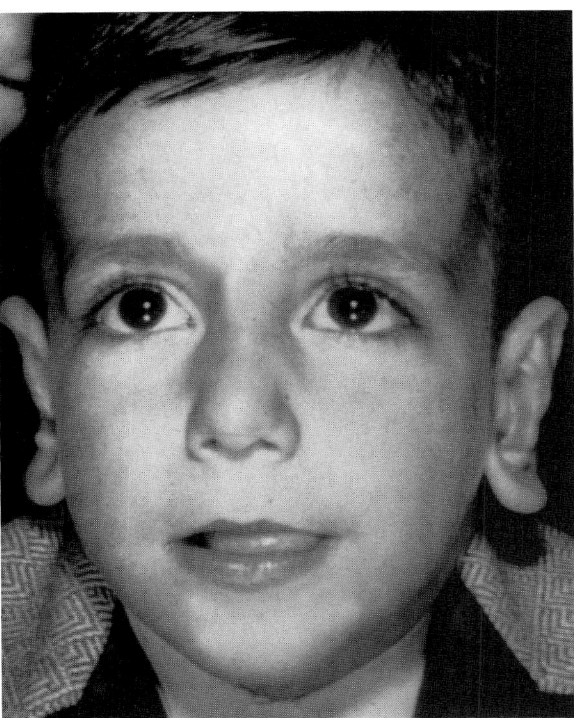

FIGURE 28-3. Child with classic telephone deformity.

Root of Helix Prominence

If the central zone of the helical rim occupies a position between 1.8 and 2.0 cm from the mastoid skin, then the telephone ear deformity represents a relative undercorrection of the helical root and lobule. *A Hatch suture is an effective means of correcting the laterally projecting helical root with an increased temporal-helical angle* (1,7,12). This is accomplished by creating a longitudinal incision along the medial edge of the helical root as it merges with the scalp. Scissor dissection is employed to expose the helical cartilage and temporal fascia, after which the helical root is fixed to the underlying fascia with two 4-0 Mersaline sutures on a round knot-cutting needle (Fig. 28-5). This serves to draw the upper auricle close to the scalp in the large ear. On occasion, the maneuver produces cartilage buckling or skin redundancy, which is remedied by a V-shaped excision of skin and cartilage.

Lobule

Residual lobular prominence is also a frequent contributor to the telephone ear deformity. In a review of 100 consecutive otoplasties, Beernink et al. (13) found residual prominence of the lobule in 86% of subjects treated with Mustardé and Furnas sutures in isolation. *These residual deformities can be dealt with efficaciously by retropositioning the helical tail or by utilizing variously patterned skin excisions and suture-positioning techniques.*

Helical tail repositioning, as described by Webster (14), is a technique used to contour the lower third of the ear. However, we do not use it because by manipulating the tail of the helix posteriorly, secondary deformities can be created. Unlike the upper two-thirds of the ear, where posterior skin excision produces a transient setback, the prominent lobule can be corrected by a series of skin excisions or suture plication techniques. Relapse can develop during the following year as the elastic recoil of the cartilage stretches the residual postauricular skin. The more malleable lobule can be permanently repositioned with the use of excision and direct closure of posterior lobular skin and fibrofatty tissue in V-shaped, heart-shaped, eccentric elliptical, and Z-plasty patterns (7).

Spira et al. (15) and Furnas (10) have described a series of suture plication techniques to correct residual lobular prominence. Spira and colleagues employ an eccentric posterior skin excision in conjunction with an anchor suture (Fig. 28-6). A 4-0 white Mersaline suture is placed between the dermis of the lateral edge of the soft tissue excision and the conchal cartilage near the postauricular sulcus or mastoid periosteum. Suture tightening approximates the wedge

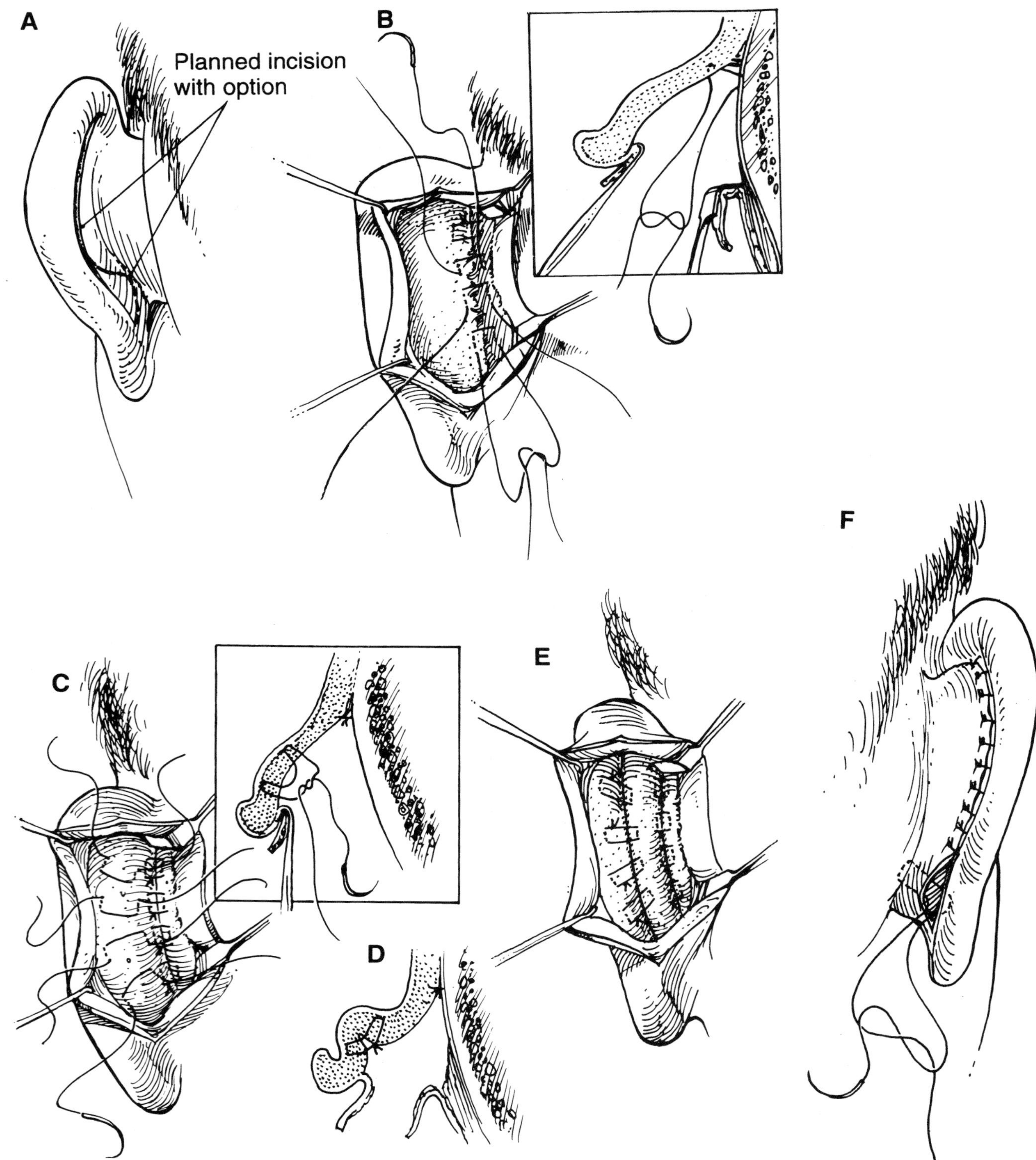

FIGURE 28-4. A–F: Recommended suture technique.

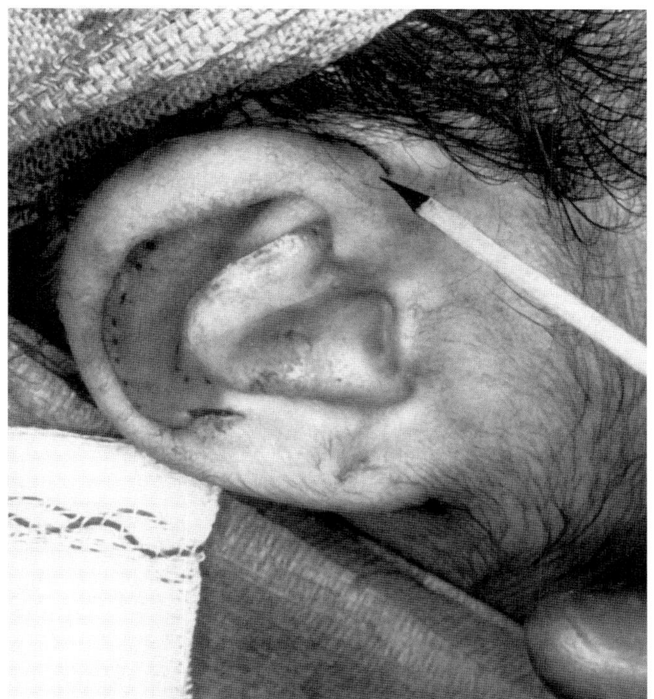

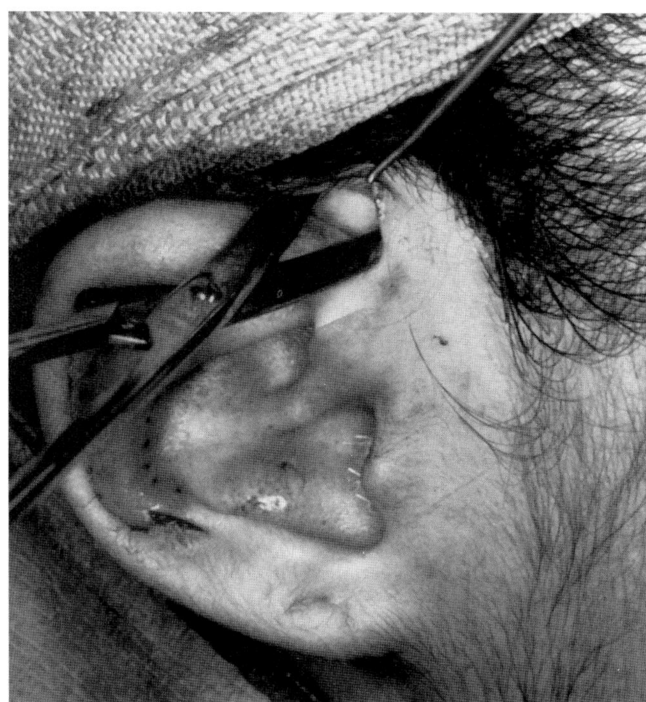

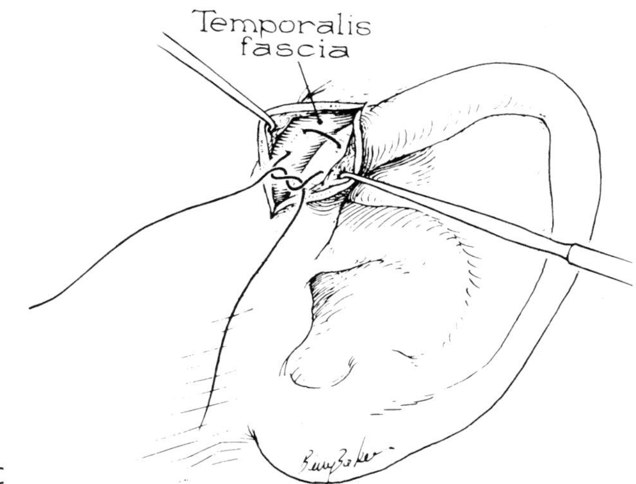

FIGURE 28-5. A–C: Hatch maneuver to set back root of helix prominence.

excision and retropositions the lobule. Furnas (10) describes a solitary lobe-muscle suture to fix the fibrofatty tissue of the lobule to the insertion of the sternocleidomastoid muscle.

Reverse Telephone Ear and Narrowing of the External Auditory Canal

The reverse telephone ear deformity is a relative prominence of the concha or central third of the ear. The deformity may result from overcorrection of the upper and lower poles; however, *inadequate conchal setback is the more common inciting factor.* Excessive conchal prominence may result when the Mustardé sutures are tied before the concha is sutured into its new position. Additionally, when the conchal height exceeds 2.5 cm, then Furnas sutures (concha-mastoid) alone may produce foreword rotation and narrowing of the external auditory meatus, which forces the surgeon to accept a suboptimal setback. Meatal narrowing can be reduced by positioning the concha-mastoid sutures in a strict anteroposterior orientation, which serves to draw the cartilage directly backward (16,17). If suture reorientation is ineffective, then creation of a postauricular pocket or Spira's trapdoor conchal flap or direct excision of conchal cartilage via an anterior or posterior approach can yield the desired setback and avoid the undercorrected middle third (reverse telephone ear) (Fig. 28-7).

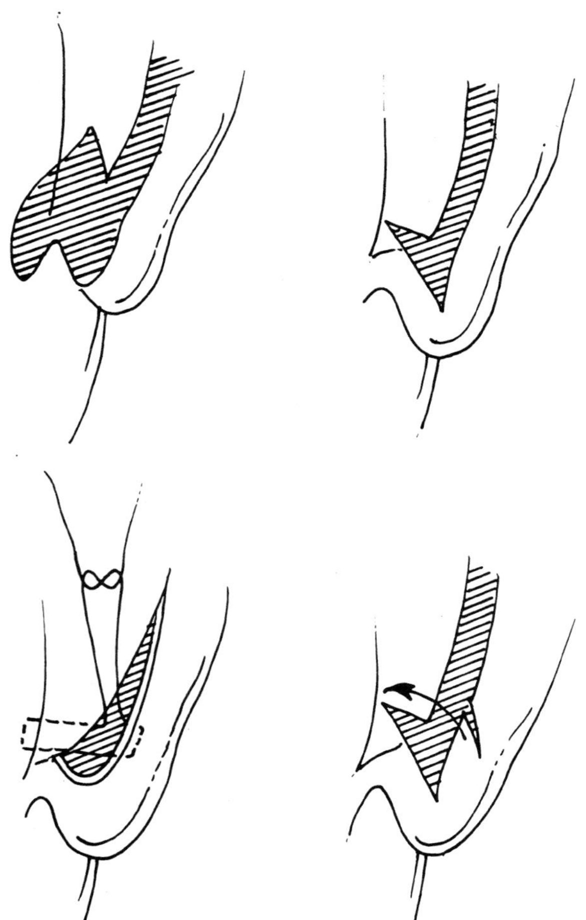

FIGURE 28-6. Spira technique for lobule setback.

Post Ear Deformity

In general, nature abhors straight lines. On the lateral view, the naturally appearing ear follows this principle, with the helix and antihelix charting a gentle C-shaped course. The "post ear" deformity is a telltale sign of an operated ear (Fig. 28-8). The antihelix has a distinct vertical orientation, and the ear appears rigid and abnormally elongated. The deformity is a result of inaccurate scaphoconchal suture placement or misdirected cartilage scoring. *The post ear can be minimized by orienting the Mustardé sutures radially* (Fig. 28-9). This serves to bend the neoantihelix around a central fulcrum and overcomes the vertical folding produced when horizontally oriented sutures are employed (18). Additionally, care should be taken to score the anterior cartilage in a curvilinear fashion. Vertically oriented cartilage scoring produces a straight linear weakness and preferential folding into a postlike contour.

Recurrence

Suture techniques for correcting the prominent ear have proved reliable, and recurrence has been 1.8% to 3% in young children (11,19). Our experience has shown high rates of recurrence with minor complications with sutures alone, and reprotrusion rates of up to 1.5% in older children (> 6 years old) and adults (7,20). The increasing failure rate parallels the loss of pliability that accompanies cartilage maturation. *Greater control over rigid adult cartilage is achieved by scoring on the anterior surface of the antihelix with a Dingman otobrader* (21). The cartilage is exposed via a short incision at the base of the antihelix. The anterior surface of the cartilage, in the region of the neoantihelix, is abraded until the desired position can be maintained with light digital pressure. This maneuver serves to guard against recurrence. Relying on skin resection alone to set back the superior two thirds of the ear is associated with a high rate of long-term failure.

Proper selection of suture type, quantity, and placement is also integral to a lasting result. Nonabsorbable sutures, such as 4-O white Mersaline, on a half-round atraumatic needle should be used. A minimum of four concha-scapha and three concha-mastoid sutures are utilized. The suture

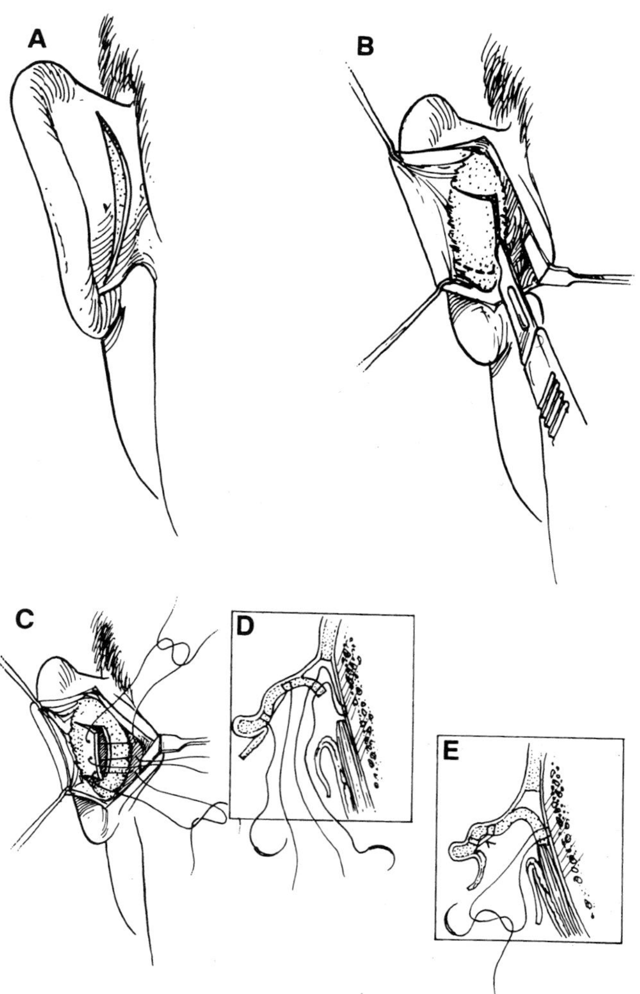

FIGURE 28-7. Spira-Stal concha flap technique to prevent canal narrowing.

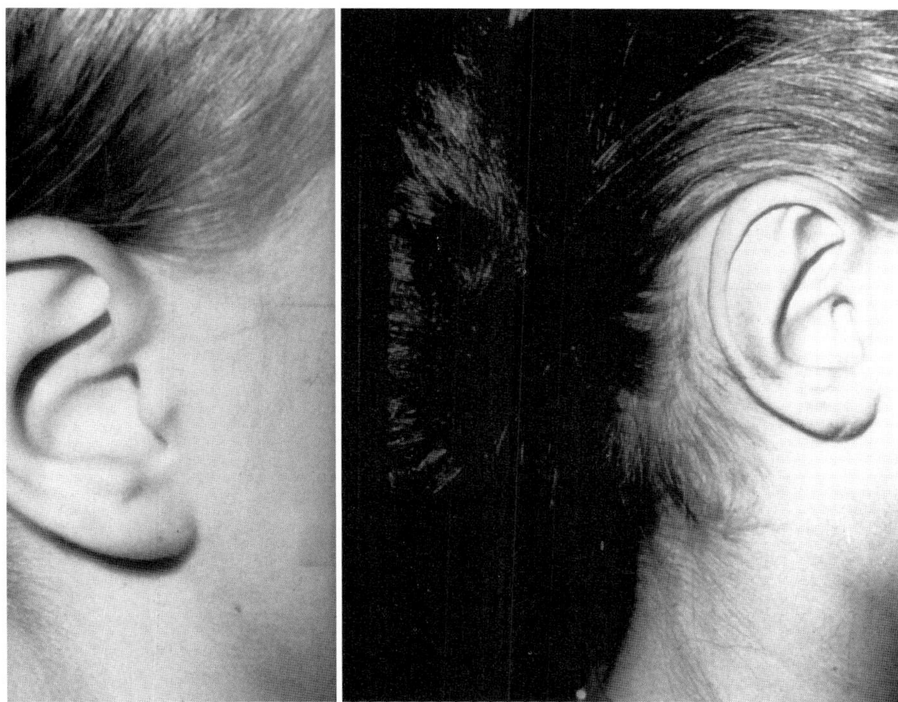

FIGURE 28-8. Post ear deformity.

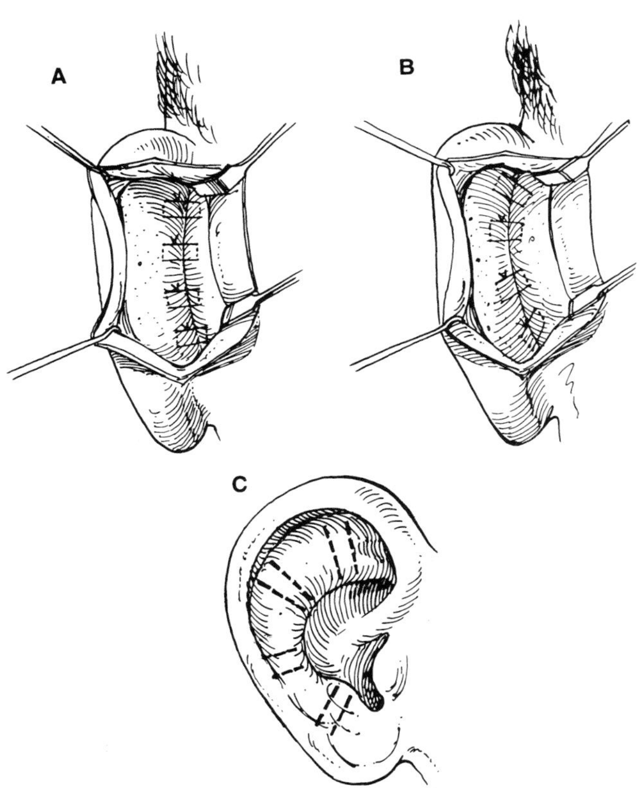

FIGURE 28-9. Example of correct orientation of Mustardé sutures.

purchase should incorporate cartilage and both perichondrial layers without breaching the skin of the anterior ear. The possibility of anterior suture exposure can be lessened by infiltrating the anterior conchal skin with local anesthetic. A clean posterior dissection will avoid the incorporation of perichondrial remnants into the suture knots, which is associated with loosening.

A bulky mastoid dressing in the immediate postoperative period and the use of a daytime sports headband for 3 weeks and a stockinet or elastic fishnet gauge cap nocturnally for a minimum of a month will reduce the risk of traumatic recurrence.

Bowstringing

A visible bridging of sutures beneath the thin postauricular skin is always present to some degree because the spanning sutures are placed under tension over and across a distance devoid of any overlying subcutaneous tissue (Fig. 28-10). When present, it is usually well tolerated by the patient unless infection, difficulty in wearing glasses, or hygiene problems develop. The deformity is usually well hidden and nontender, and routine correction is unjustified unless sutures extrude or cause painful granulomas or hygiene issues, which can be addressed in the office. Six months after surgery, sutures can be removed as needed, and the ear position will be stable. The bowstring deformity is largely overcome by avoiding any posterior skin excision techniques in the upper two thirds and approaching the ear via a posterior incision. The retained excess soft tissue, which is wrinkled initially but smoothes out eventually, serves to

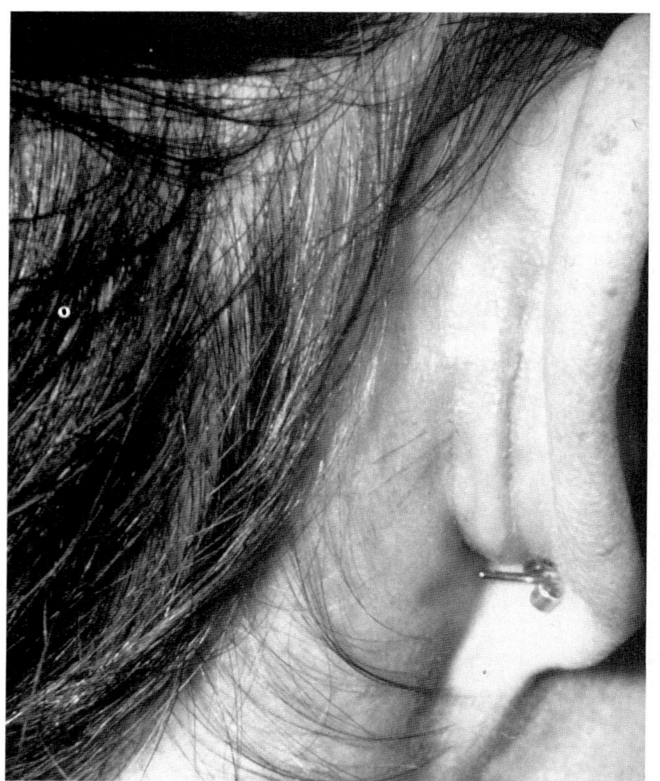
A

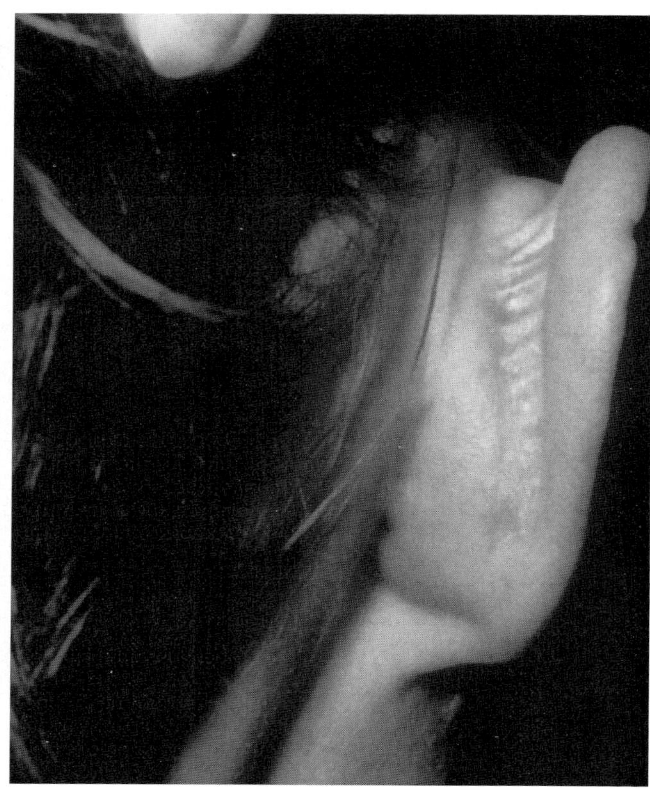
B

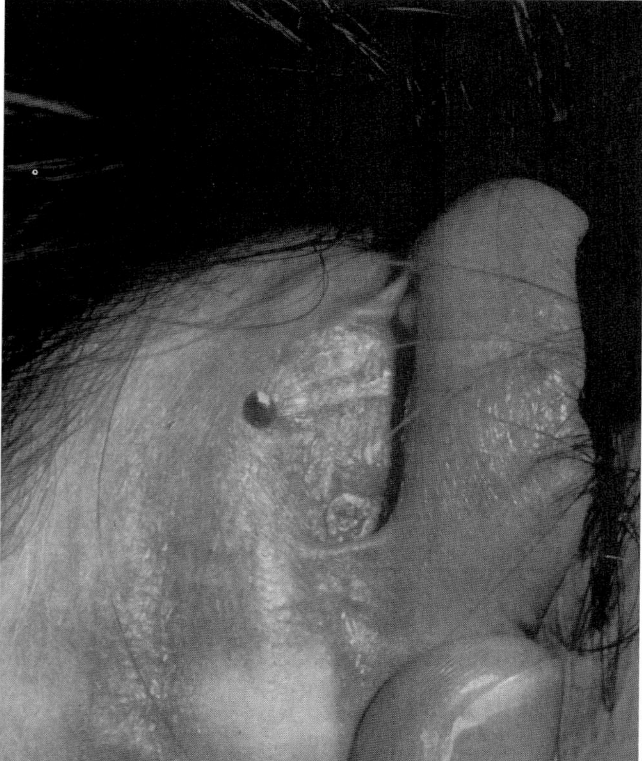
C

FIGURE 28-10. Bowstringing of posterior suture. **A:** Minimal. **B:** Moderate. **C:** Severe with crusting.

camouflage the underlying sutures and reduces the rates of granuloma formation and suture extrusion (22).

Variegation of the Scapha and Antihelix Deformity

Imprecise scapha-concha suture placement can be manifested as a rippled deformity along the scapha and neoantihelix. On average, three to four obliquely oriented Mustardé sutures are used. The suture purchase should include approximately 0.4 mm of cartilage and should be separated from the adjacent suture by no more than 4 mm if horizontal furrowing is to be avoided (11). A neoantihelical roll of appropriate width is obtained by separating the scapha and concha suture bites by a span of 6 to 8 mm. *Care should be taken to avoid overtightening these sutures to a point at which the helix is obscured in the front view to produce a "pinned back," overcorrected appearance* (Fig. 28-11). Cartilage incision and excision and tubing techniques were key components of older procedures and frequently produced sharp edges with a distinct "operated" appearance (23,24).

POSTOPERATIVE COMPLICATIONS

In the acute postoperative period (24 to 48 hours), *the rapid onset of persistent, unilateral pain is a marker for ominous underlying processes.* The dressings should be promptly removed because a concealed hematoma, folded part, allergic reaction, or infection may lurk within (9).

Approximately 2 weeks after surgery, an additional series of "late onset" complications come into play. Granulomas, keloid scars, asymmetry, suture fistulas, and suture bridging are rising concerns.

Bleeding and Hematoma

Hematoma formation, usually but not always heralded by pain and a blood-stained dressing, is an infrequent complication and may result from a surgical error, including improper dressings. Dissection should follow the relatively avascular tissue planes, and meticulous hemostasis should be achieved with a needle-tip cautery. The posterior skin incisions are not closed on either ear until the procedure is nearing completion and a final inspection demonstrates a dry field. Local anesthetic containing 1/100,000 epinephrine is employed conservatively (approximately 5 mL) to prevent rebound hemorrhage after the vasoconstrictive effects dissipate. *A conforming mastoid dressing of moist cotton wadding to preserve the convolutions of the anterior ear, buttressed posteriorly by layered gauze pads, provides the desired compression, absorption, and protection.* Inspection of the ears at 24 to 48 hours without removal of the operative dressing is paramount.

A 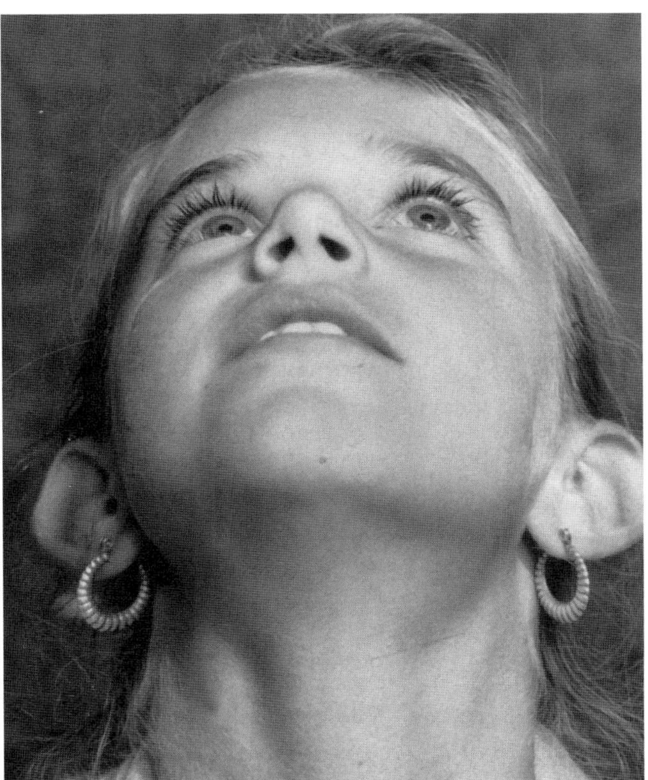

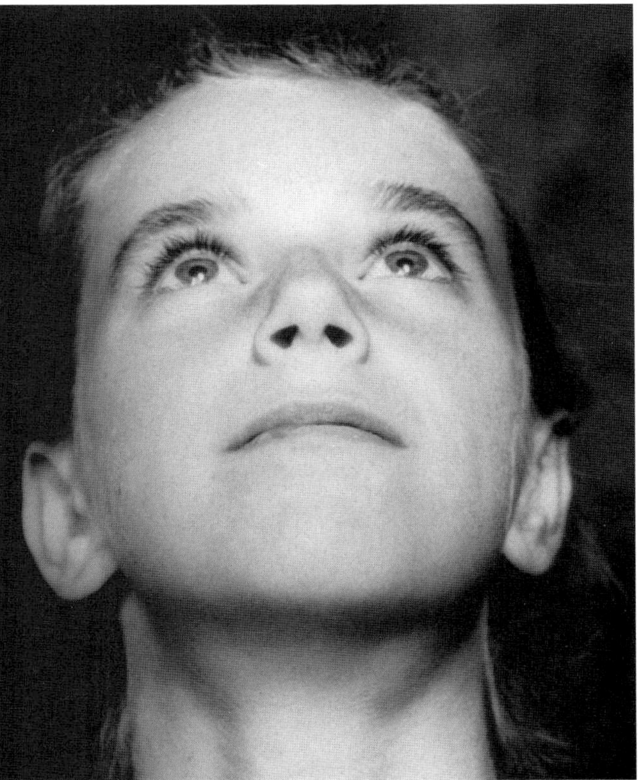 B

FIGURE 28-11. Ten-year-old child preoperatively and 1 year postoperatively with overcorrection. **A:** Preoperative basal view. **B:** Postoperative basal view. *(continued)*

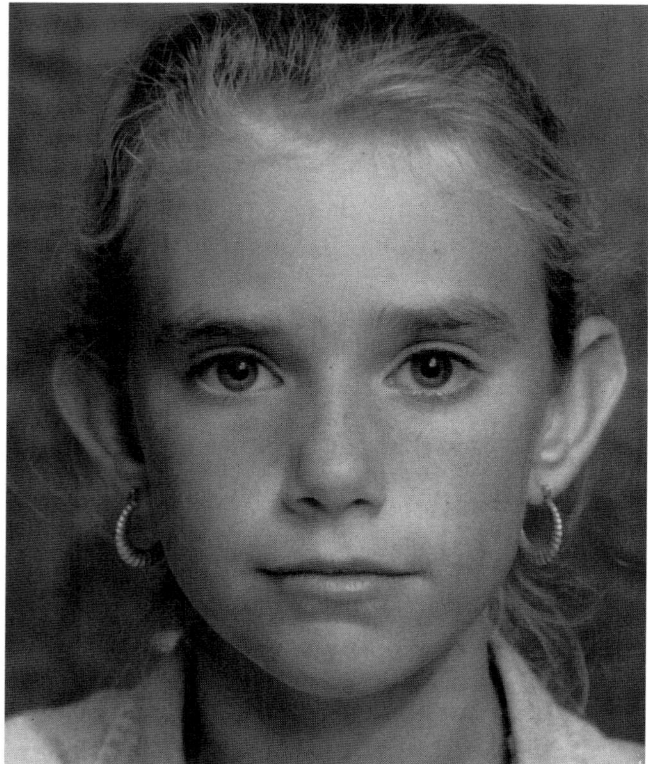
C

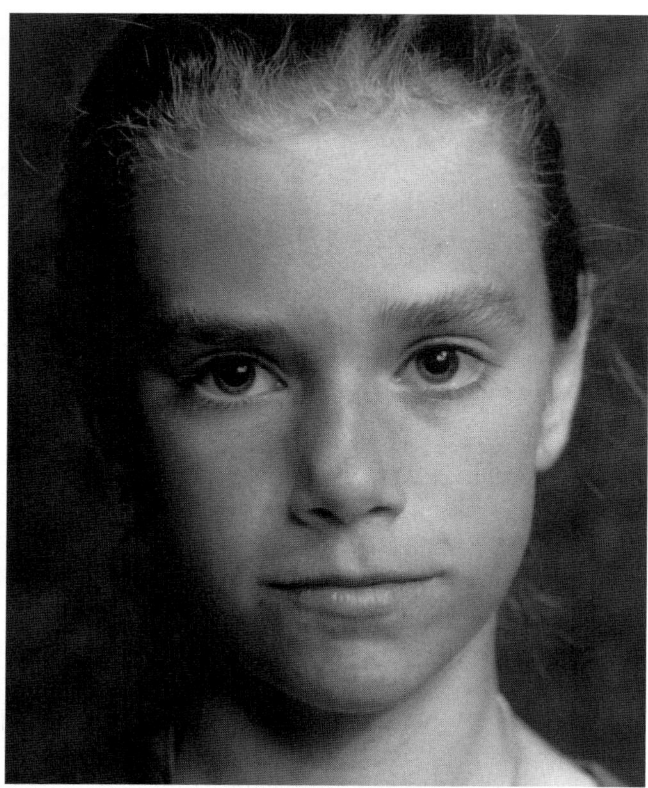
D

FIGURE 28-11. *Continued.* **C:** Preoperative anteroposterior view. **D:** Postoperative anteroposterior view.

Hematomas should be promptly evacuated in the operating room to avoid the development of skin necrosis. Small Penrose or rubber band drains are utilized in conjunction with a mild compressive dressing and broad-spectrum antibiotics.

Infection and Chondritis

Infection culminating in frank chondritis with a severe Bramanert deformity is the most dreaded complication in otoplasty (Fig. 28-12). The onset of unilateral pain on the third or fourth postoperative day should raise suspicion of an underlying infection, and the dressing should be promptly removed. *If an underlying cellulitis is present without associated fluctuance, the patient should be admitted for empirical intravenous antibiotics.* Laudable pus is drained in the operating room, and copious lavage is utilized. A specimen should be collected for Gram's stain, and intravenous antibiotics should be initiated that will cover *Pseudomonas aeruginosa, Staphylococcus aureus,* and *Streptococcus,* which are the usual causative organisms (25,26). The wound is loosely approximated with tacking sutures and dressings soaked in saline solution are initiated. Alternately, a fine fenestrated drain can be placed under the skin flap and used to irrigate the wound with antibiotic solution (7). If the infection does not resolve promptly, then all suture material should be removed and the reprotrusion corrected in 4 to 6 months. If true chondritis develops, then all devitalized cartilage must be debrided and a secondary reconstruction performed in several months. Several enthusiastic clinical and basic scientific reports have described the use of electrical currents to enhance the transcutaneous delivery of antibiotics to the burned ear (iontophoresis) (27,28). This technique would seem to hold promise in treating postoperative chondritis. Additionally, patients are instructed to avoid swimming pools for a minimum of 4 weeks after surgery because early swimming has been associated with the development of pseudomonal infection in our series (two cases).

Skin Necrosis

The ear is repositioned by means of sutures and cartilage scoring, and the surgical dressing should support this positioning. Tight dressings cannot produce a lasting relocation, and skin necrosis is the consequence of excessive pressure. Skin loss is also associated with hematoma formation, infection, traumatic surgical technique, excessive use of cautery, and folded parts.

Skin necrosis can be addressed in several ways. Small regions can be treated with drying agents (Betadine, Mercurochrome) to cause eventual separation of the stable eschar from the underlying regenerated tissue. Oral antibi-

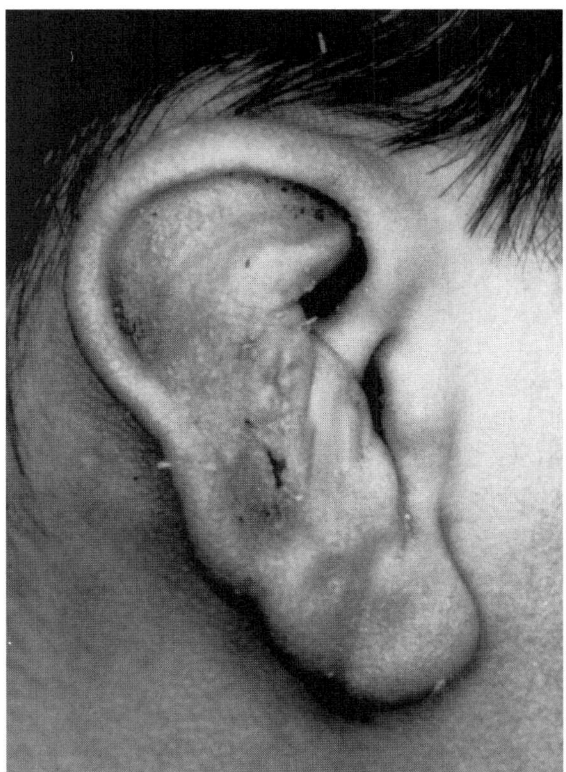
A

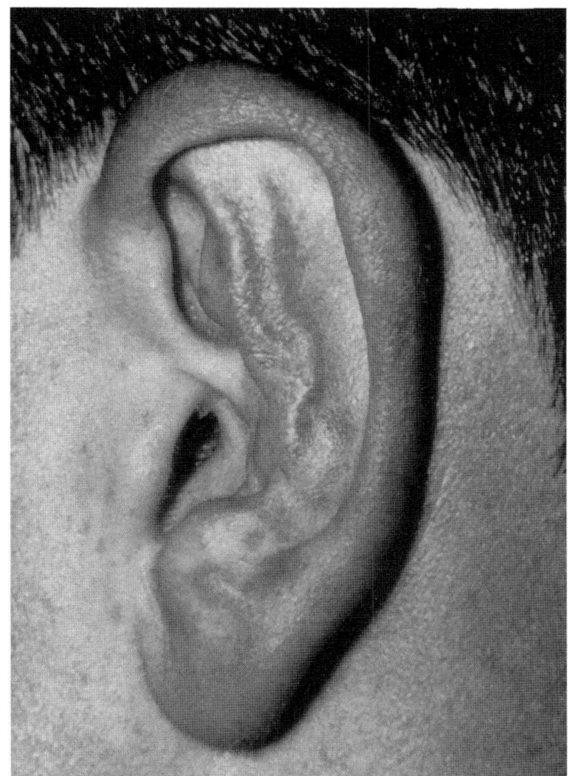
B

FIGURE 28-12. A,B: Patient after severe infection with cartilage resorption.

otics are provided to limit the possibility of chondritis. Larger regions of skin loss are treated with topical agents (Sulfamylon, Bactroban) and nonadherent dressings in conjunction with intravenous antibiotics. Often, a small, resistant defect will close spontaneously. Debridement, if undertaken, should be very conservative. Additionally, a temporal skin dressing of a xenograft or allograft can prevent cartilage desiccation and enhance local immunologic activity while the milieu of the wound improves. If perichondrium or granulation tissue is not present in a resultant full-thickness skin loss, then local flap coverage is preferred over skin grafting (29). Additionally, debridement of cartilage may expose the deep surface of the opposite skin surface and facilitate skin graft placement. Iontophoresis and hydrogel dressings also may play a role in managing these problems.

Allergic Reactions

Pruritus and contact dermatitis may develop in response to local "caine"-containing anesthetics, antibiotic ointments (neomycin and sulfonamides), iodine, mercury-containing antiseptics, lanolin, and additives such as methylparaben (30). The process is treated by removal of the dressings, gentle cleansing, application of moist dressings soaked in saline solution, and the administration of systemic antihistamines. The process is usually self-limiting without permanent sequelae.

Hypertrophic Scars and Keloids

Keloid scar formation and hypertrophic scarring develop in approximately 2% of patients who undergo otoplasty, especially young, darkly pigmented persons (Fig. 28-13). Excessive resection of posterior ear skin resulting in a tight closure and possible infection is an important, yet controllable, factor. Anterior conchal incisions are avoided in dark-skinned patients to avoid this potential complication and the darkening of scars with sun exposure (1). Excessive scarring has been successfully treated with several modalities. A response can be achieved with monthly infiltration of triamcinolone (40 mg/mL) in aliquots of 0.25 to 0.5 mL (7). Local pressure with customized soft rubber splints (thermoplastic) may work synergistically with steroid injection. Recalcitrant scarring is treated with excision, tension-free closure, and low-dose radiation in the perioperative period. Postauricular full-thickness grafts may be required.

Suture Granuloma and Extrusion

The development of the bowstring deformity and later suture extrusion or granuloma formation is significantly reduced by limiting postauricular skin excision. Skin is excised only in elderly patients with excessive redundancy, in whom the likelihood of normal recoil and contraction is limited. Additionally, sutures should be oriented with the knots

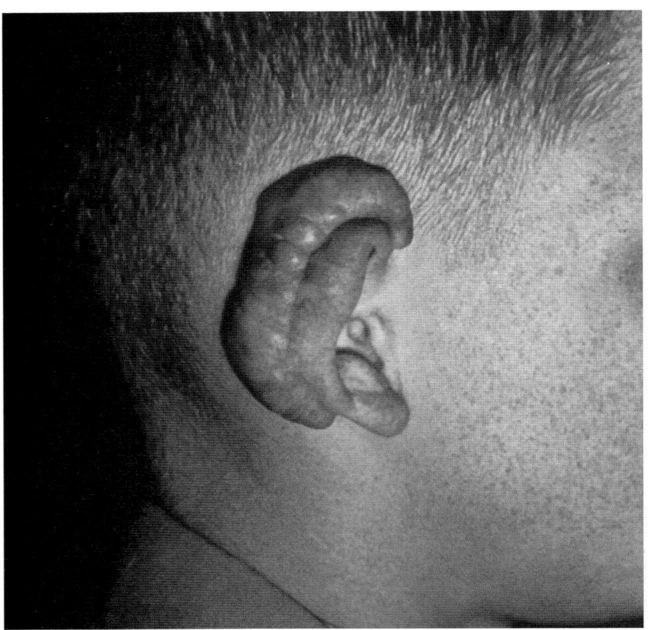

FIGURE 28-13. Rare example of severe keloid.

along the deep surface of the wound. If exposure or granulomas develop 6 months after surgery, then the offending suture can be removed with little or no effect on ear position.

Hypesthesia and Dysesthesia

Sensory changes are not uncommon, especially when posterior auricular muscle excision has been performed to enhance conchal setback. Gradual return of sensation is the rule, and reassurance goes a long way toward resolving the problem. Sensory reeducation, similar to that employed after digital nerve, repair may be beneficial.

CONCLUSION

Otoplasty is an effective, reliable procedure that requires attention to detail. The avoidance of complications by careful preoperative analysis and an algorithmic approach to surgery is paramount because revisions often improve the situation but seldom yield an ideal surgical result (Fig. 28-14). We are fortunate as surgeons in that unless the complication is severe, necessitating additional surgery or treatment in the immediate postoperative period, the complication is well tolerated by the patient (Fig. 28-15). Unlike deformities in other areas, where asymmetry is for more noticeable and under great scrutiny (eyes, nose, breasts), most ear deformities are not seen by patients. They appreciate that an ear is well set back, reasonably symmetrical, and within the boundaries of normalcy. Still, we, as both artists and scientists, need to strive for predictable,

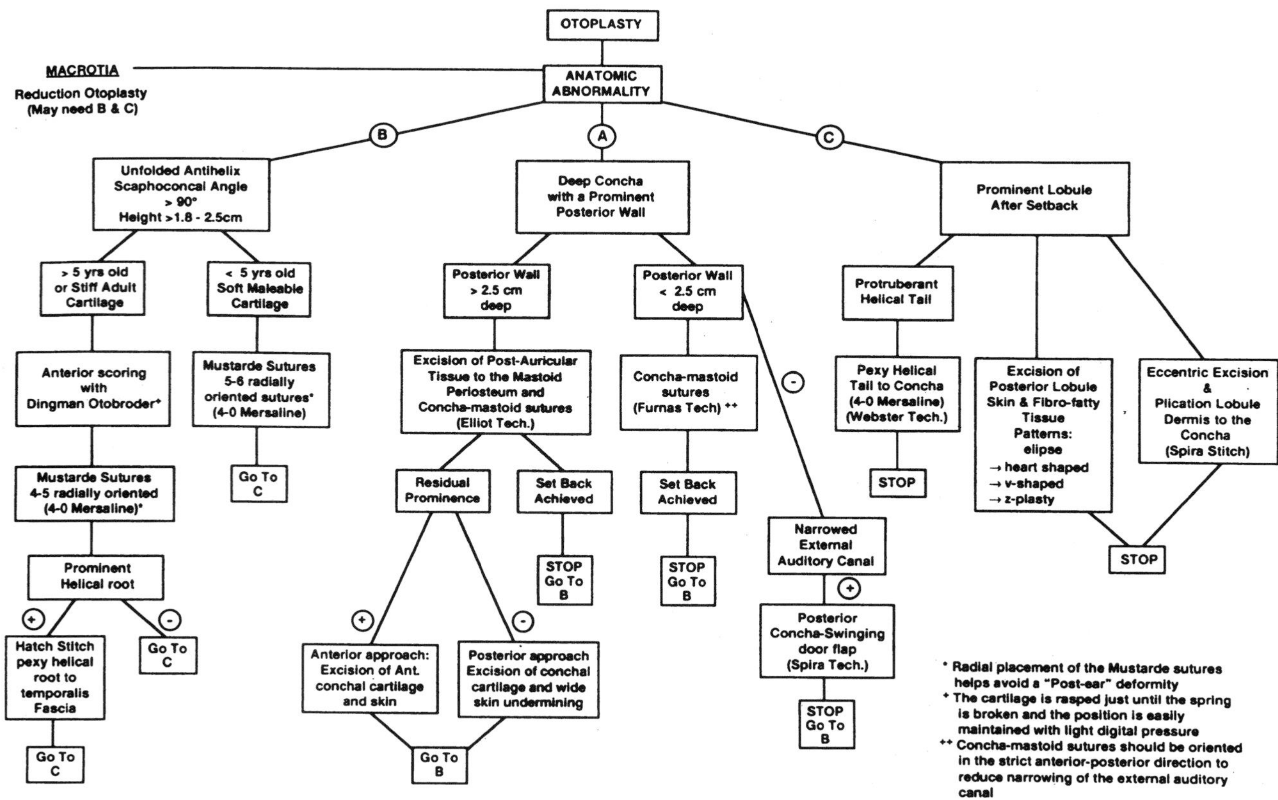

FIGURE 28-14. Algorithm for otoplasty.

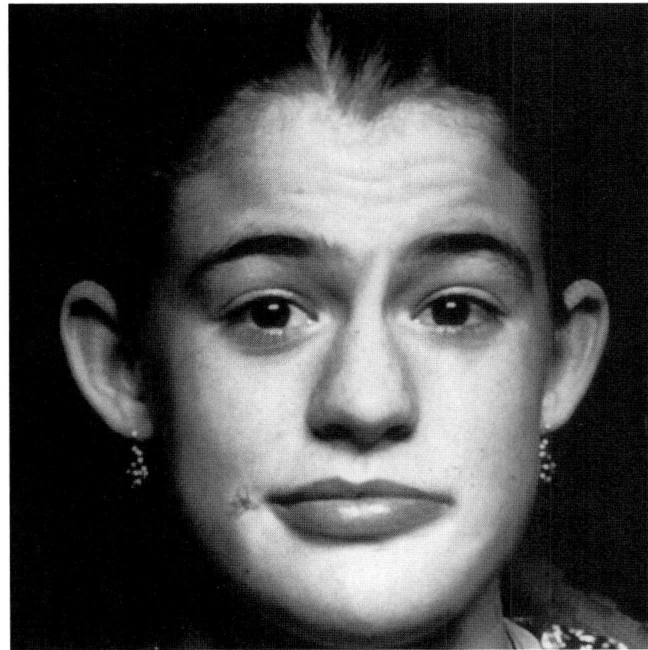
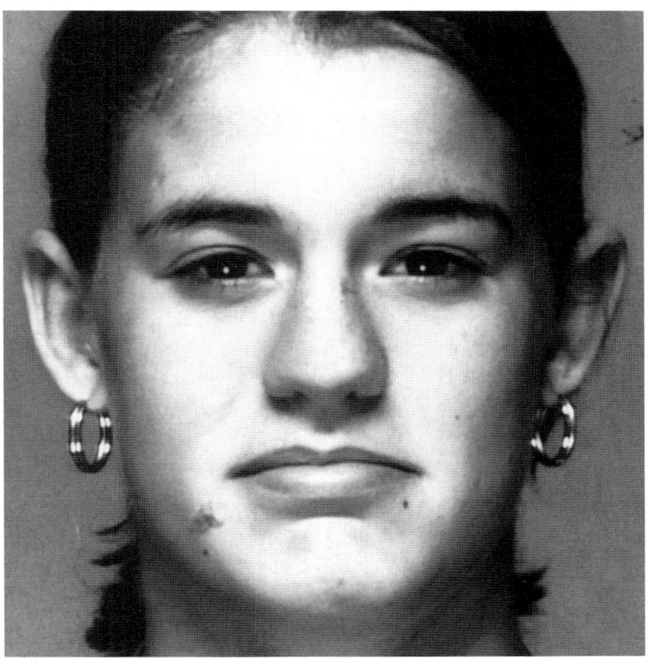

FIGURE 28-15. Thirteen-year-old preoperatively and postoperatively with natural setback. **A:** Preoperative anteroposterior view. **B:** Postoperative anteroposterior view.

anatomically pleasing, and symmetrical results (Fig. 28-15).

REFERENCES

1. Stal S, Klebuc M, Spira M. An algorithm for otoplasty. *Operative Techniques in Plastic and Reconstructive Surgery* 1997;4:88–103.
2. Tolleth H. Artistic anatomy, dimensions, and proportions of the external ear. *Clin Plast Surg* 1978;5:337–345.
3. Tanzer RC. An analysis of ear reconstruction. *Plast Reconstr Surg* 1963;31:16–30.
4. Adamson JE, Horton CE, Crawford HH. The growth pattern of the external ear. *Plast Reconstr Surg* 1965;36:466–470.
5. Farkas LG. Growth of normal and reconstructed auricles. In: Tanzer RC, Edgerton MT, eds. *Symposium on reconstruction of the auricle.* St. Louis: Mosby, 1974:24–32.
6. MacGregor F. Ear deformities: social and psychological implications. *Clin Plast Surg* 1978;5:347–350.
7. Spira M. Reduction otoplasty. In: Goldwyn RM, ed. *The unfavorable result in plastic surgery: avoidance and treatment,* 2nd ed. Boston: Little, Brown and Company, 1984:307–323.
8. Stal S, Spira M. Long-term results in otoplasty. *Fac Plast Surg* 1985;2:153–165.
9. Elliot RA. Complications in the treatment of prominent ears. *Clin Plast Surg* 1978;5:479–490.
10. Furnas DW. Correction of prominent ears with multiple sutures. *Clin Plast Surg* 1978;5:491–495.
11. Mustardé JC. The correction of prominent ears using simple mattress sutures. *Br J Plast Surg* 1962;5:170–176.
12. Hatch MD. Common problems of otoplasty. *J Int Coll Surg* 1958;30:171–178.
13. Beernink JH, Blocksma R, Moore WD. The role of the helical tail in cosmetic otoplasty. *Plast Reconstr Surg* 1979;64:115–117.
14. Webster GV. The tail of the helix as a key to otoplasty. *Plast Reconstr Surg* 1969;44:455–461.
15. Spira M, McCrea R, Gerow FJ, et al. Correction of the principal deformities causing protruding ears. *Plast Reconstr Surg* 1969;44:150–154.
16. Furnas DW. Correction of prominent ears by concha-mastoid sutures. *Plast Reconstr Surg* 1968;42:189–193.
17. Elliot RA. Aesthetic surgery of the ears. In: Gerogiade SG, Georgiade NG, Riefkohl R, et al., eds. *Textbook of plastic, maxillofacial and reconstructive surgery.* Baltimore: Williams & Wilkins, 1992:729–736.
18. Johnson PE. Otoplasty: shaping the antihelix. *Aesthetic Plast Surg* 1994;18:71–74.
19. Pitanguy I, Muller P, Piccolo N, et al. The treatment of prominent ears: a 25-year survey of the island technique. *Aesthetic Plast Surg* 1987;11:87–93.
20. Pilz S, Hintringer T, Bauer M. Otoplasty using a spherical metal head dermabrader to form a retroauricular furrow: five-year results. *Aesthetic Plast Surg* 1995;19:83–91.
21. Stenstöm SJ. A "natural" technique for correction of congenitally prominent ears. *Plast Reconstr Surg* 1963;32:509–518.
22. Weerda H, Siegert R. Complications in otoplastic surgery and their treatment. *Fac Plast Surg* 1994;10:287–297.
23. Converse JM, Nigro A, Wilson FA, et al. A technique for surgical correction of lop ears. *Plast Reconstr Surg* 1955;15:411–418.
24. Rogers BO. A medical "first": Ely's operation to correct protruding ears. *Aesthetic Plast Surg* 1987;11:71–72.
25. Turkeltaub SH, Habal MB. Acute *Pseudomonas* chondritis as a sequel to ear piercing. *Ann Plast Surg* 1990;24:279–281.

26. Bentrem DJ, Bill TJ, Harvey H, et al. Chondritis of the ear: a late sequela of deep partial-thickness burns of the face. *J Emerg Med* 1996;14:469–471.
27. Rigano W, Yanik M, Barone FA, et al. Antibiotic iontophoresis in the management of burned ears. *J Burn Care Rehabil* 1992;13;407–409.
28. Kaweski S, Baldwin RC, Wong RK, et al. Diffusion versus iontophoresis in the transport of gentamicin in the burned rabbit ear model. *Plast Reconstr Surg* 1993;92:1342–1349.
29. Walter C, Nolst Trenitè GJ. Revision otoplasty and special problems. *Fac Plast Surg* 1994;10:298–308.
30. Goodman LS, Gilman A. *The pharmacological basis of therapeutics: a textbook of pharmacology, toxicology and therapeutics for physicians and medical students.* New York: Macmillan, 1997.

Discussion

OTOPLASTY

A. MICHAEL SADOVE

Drs. Stal, Klebuc, and Spira have logically and thoroughly covered potential pitfalls in otoplasty. They point out that the procedure is largely problem-free. It should also be mentioned that this group of patients (much like patients with macromastia) are so relieved to have the source of their ridicule reduced that they are largely tolerant of all but the most unfavorable outcomes.

Unfortunately, with increasing restriction of health care dollars, otoplasty has moved to an almost entirely "self-funded" procedure. For this reason, along with an ever-increasing emphasis by other surgical disciplines on cosmetic surgery, the average plastic surgeon may not perform otoplasty on a regular basis. This fact may lead to the problem that the authors emphasize—failure to make the proper preoperative assessment. Much as in rhinoplasty or cleft lip repair, we may have a general approach that we utilize, but we must customize this technique to each patient's anatomical needs rather than attempt a "one size fits all" approach. To avoid such a "trap," it is essential that the surgeon critically analyze the individual anatomical variations that cause the patient to deviate from the aesthetic ideal. Failure to take the time or acquire the knowledge and experience to make this analysis may cause an unfavorable outcome, even if all the technical elements are executed to perfection. Therefore, failure to diagnose is one of the primary causes of unfavorable results in otoplasty.

The authors state that unfavorable results may result from errors in preoperative planning. I would like to comment on several of their observations. As they suggest, 4 years is in general the ideal age for the procedure. However, if palpation of the cartilage reveals it to be soft and malleable, then delaying surgery may be advisable, particularly if a Mustardé technique is to be utilized. Drs. Stal, Klebuc, and Spira also point out the need for careful preoperative preparation and draping of the patient to avoid chondritis (one of the most feared complications of otoplasty). I have used a technique that is helpful in allowing good visualization while eliminating hair from the field (1).

Decisions made *during* surgery can also lead to an unfavorable result. The authors provide many useful suggestions to avoid these problems. One of their interesting points is that residual prominence of the lobule may be seen in many of the patients treated with Mustardé or Furnas procedures (2). I agree with this observation and would suggest a suture technique that we have found very useful in preventing this problem (Figs. 28D-1 and 28D-2).

The final group of problems addressed by the authors are those that arise in the postoperative period. Again, Drs. Stal, Klebuc, and Spira provide many insightful comments on the most frequent problems that can occur and how to avoid them. In my experience, suture granulomas have been the most bothersome. My impression is that 4-0 Mersaline may not be the optimal suture for reshaping the antihelix. I have utilized 5-0 Gore-Tex sutures more recently, with a corresponding decrease in suture-related problems. Although these sutures may become exposed, they appear to remain softer and be less reactive than Mersaline sutures.

As stated in my introduction, Drs. Stal, Klebuc, and Spira have very logically and thoroughly addressed the potential problems associated with otoplasty, leaving very little to add. All surgeons would do well to read and reread their

A. M. Sadove: Department of Plastic Surgery, Indiana University School of Medicine, Indianapolis, Indiana

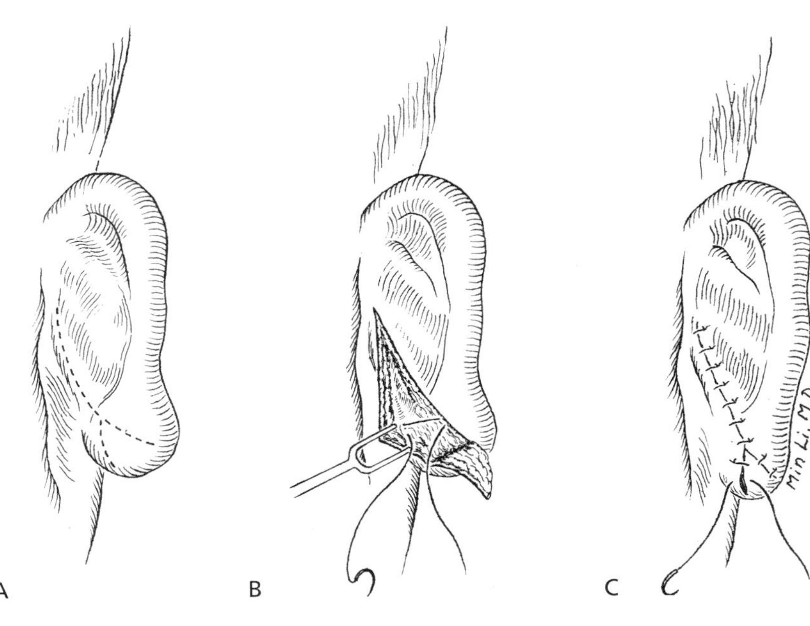

FIGURE 28D-1. A: Lobule repositioning technique: anteriorly positioned lobule. **B:** The suture is tied down to the mastoid fascia or ear cartilage. **C:** Suture closure of the lobule excision.

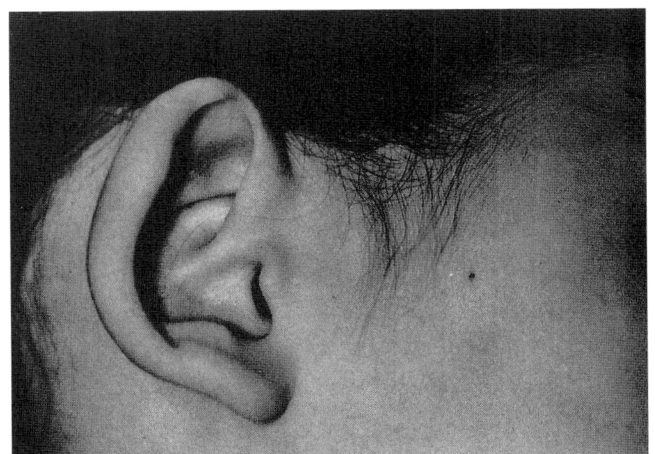

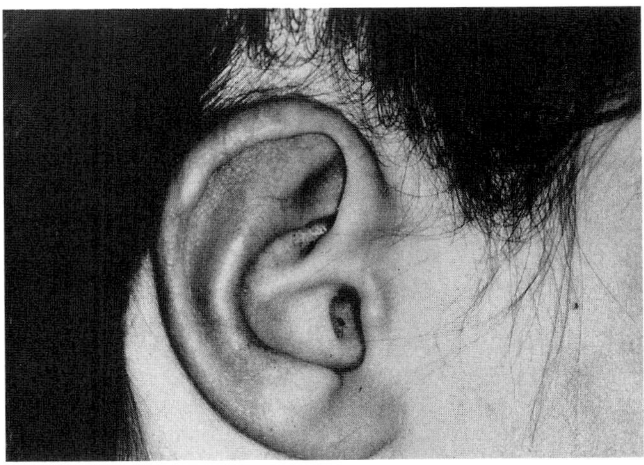

FIGURE 28D-2. Close-up of otoplasty patient **(A)** before and **(B)** after.

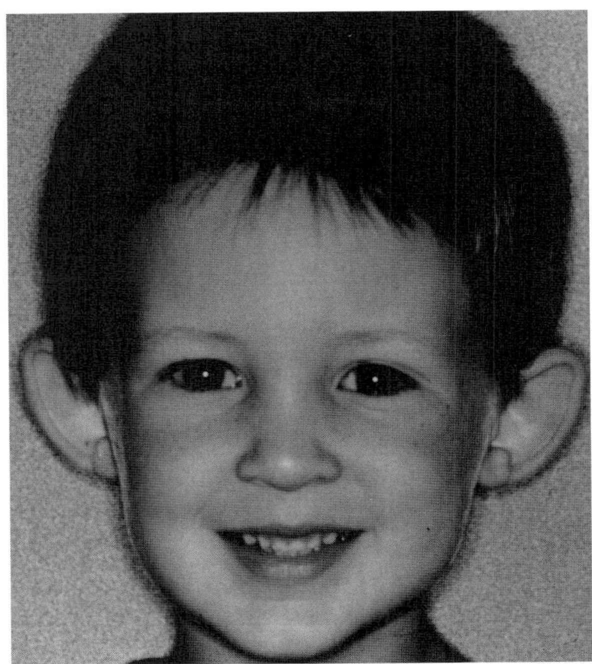

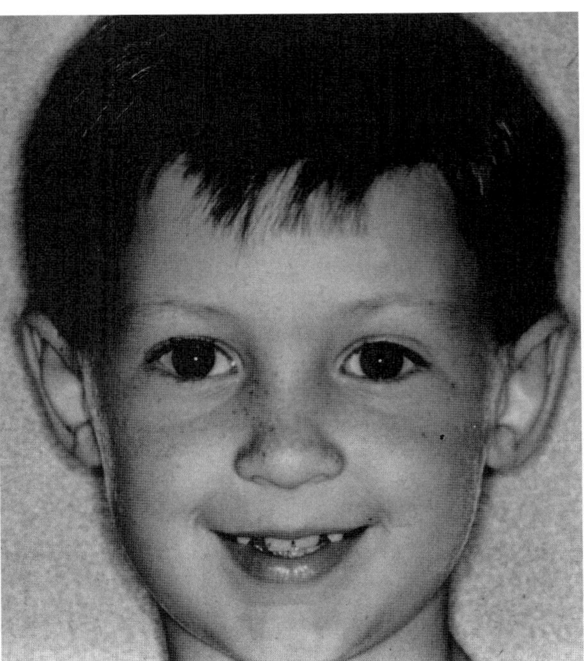

FIGURE 28D-3. Otoplasty patient **(A)** before and **(B)** after.

insightful overview. It would be a useful exercise for us all to follow patients through adolescence to observe our long-term results. As a group, plastic surgeons are self-analytical and critical, and it is this honest postoperative self-assessment that will continue to push our quest for improved outcomes in our otoplasty patients (Figs. 28D-3).

REFERENCES

1. Eppley BL, Colville C, Sadove AM. An improved draping method for otoplastic surgery. *Aesthetic Plast Surg* 1990;14:293–294.
2. Sadove AM, Eppley BL. Lobule repositioning in aesthetic plastic surgery. *Operative Techniques in Plastic and Reconstructive Surgery* 1997;4:129–133.

29

SOFT TISSUE INJURIES

HENRY C. VASCONEZ

Good judgment comes from experience, and experience comes from poor judgment.
—Anonymous

One thorn of experience is worth a whole wilderness of warning.
—James Russell Lowell

Soft tissue injuries of the face are very common and extremely obvious. The face is, without a doubt, the main injury site that prompts a patient or family member specifically to request a plastic surgeon for evaluation and management. The reason is clear. Probably more than in any other part of the body, an unfavorable result on the face can lead to catastrophic results from both an aesthetic and functional point of view. These results can require frequent office visits and the utilization of a series of measures, initially conservative and progressively more invasive, aimed at modifying or revising scars, restoring functional competence, and providing psychological counseling and support to the patient. Undoubtedly, prevention is the preferred route to success, but this is sometimes not possible or evident only retrospectively.

A classification of soft tissue injuries to the face should include elements of etiology, location, size and severity, and associated injuries (1,2). Such injuries can range from a simple contusion or abrasion, to a puncture or laceration, to a major avulsion with or without soft tissue deficit. Various tissue elements may be involved, including skin, subcutaneous fat, fascia, muscle, nerves, vessels, and glands. Injuries can be caused by blunt, sharp, thermal, or blast trauma. The timing and approach to repair and the postoperative care can seriously affect the final result. Soft tissue injuries are often associated with facial fractures, and both must be repaired in concert so that an optimal result can be obtained. In this chapter, we concentrate on the repair of the soft tissue component, as fracture management is discussed in subsequent chapters in this section.

ASSESSMENT OF FACIAL INJURIES

Proper treatment depends on a correct diagnosis and a thorough assessment of the injured patient. After life-threatening injuries have been resolved and the patient has been stabilized, a detailed survey of the specific regions of the head and neck can take place, including the scalp, face, and neck. Along with this examination, a basic history is established, including time and mechanism of injury, present and past associated illnesses, current medications, allergies, immunization status, and other pertinent information. Such a survey, although important, can often be difficult to obtain depending on the general condition of the patient and the degree of facial trauma. This is a common problem that can lead to unfavorable results. A familiar scenario may involve the following: you are consulted for a patient involved in a motor vehicle accident late at night. Multiple facial and scalp lacerations are present, which are covered with gauze soaked with saline solution and are now saturated with blood and clots. The patient is wearing a soft neck collar until cervical injury can be ruled out, which makes it difficult to evaluate any chin laceration and possible mandible fracture. The history of the accident is sparse except for information provided by the emergency medical team, and no family members or friends are present. Evidence of long bone fractures is apparent, and the right lower extremity is in temporary traction. The patient requires computed tomography (CT) to rule out intraabdominal and thoracic injuries and is uncooperative, in pain, and inebriated. The temptation is to manage the wounds quickly in the emergency room under poor lighting with inadequate supplies and assistance before the patient is scurried to the dark quarters of the radiology suite. Unfortunately, 3 weeks or 3 months later, this patient could come into the office with severe residual facial scarring, muscle weakness, and difficulty closing an eye. What this scenario tries to highlight is that the expedient treatment may appear the best course of action at times but is commonly the source of unfavorable results and residual problems that are difficult to manage later. Soft tissue wounds that cannot be properly and definitively treated initially can wait until a better time is available. The wounds can be temporarily closed or even left open for up to 24 hours on a face covered with moist dressings. We insist on optimal conditions to excise a mole on the temple. So too, we should optimize the conditions under which we repair difficult and complex wounds on the face.

H. C. Vasconez: Department of Surgery and Pediatrics, Division of Plastic Surgery, University of Kentucky School of Medicine, Lexington, Kentucky

The assessment and treatment are usually performed in the emergency room, but in more complex cases, an operating room setting will be required. Appropriate anesthesia and sedation should be administered according to the extent of injury, particularly in children. After bleeding is carefully controlled, the wounds are cleaned of debris and foreign material; grossly devitalized tissue is also debrided. Hair should be shaved sparingly only to ensure an even closure and never on the eyebrow because it takes so long to grow back and growth may be inconsistent. The wound is thoroughly inspected to determine the tissues and structures involved, including vessels, nerves, muscles, glands, ducts, and other pertinent anatomy. Systemic antibiotics are administered in clearly contaminated wounds, in animal and human bites, and when a significant delay in treatment has occurred. Wounds open for more than 6 to 8 hours in other parts of the body may have to be left open to prevent infection, but on the face and scalp, they can be closed with good results even up to 24 hours after injury because of the rich blood supply to the area.

Proper and complete documentation is important for many reasons. A thorough description of the type and severity of the injury, debridement and closure technique, and dressing and postoperative care is very useful in follow-up and evaluation of the outcome. It will also further aid in an analysis of complications or medicolegal consequences. Pictures or even drawings at the time of initial injury or inspection and throughout the course of treatment are invaluable. A picture is worth a thousand words from a trial lawyer.

APPROACH TO PEDIATRIC PATIENTS

Lacerations in children account for up to 40% of emergency department visits in the United States (3,4). They are located on the face or scalp 60% of the time (5). These common injuries represent a technical and emotional challenge to the health care team, not to mention an extremely frightening and stressful situation for the child and parent. Proper preparation and explanation to the patient and parent will reap benefits in the long run.

When possible, an appropriate relationship with the child and parent should be established at the outset. The age of the patient will determine the methods used to obtain a history and physical examination and to formulate a treatment plan. Infants are usually best examined and treated in the presence of the parent. In the case of toddlers or preschoolers, a nonthreatening environment must be established in the presence of the parent, but children of this age may ultimately respond better to a brief separation during treatment. Older children and adolescents may require some control of the situation in which their autonomy is respected and they are able to make certain choices. Kindness and patience are almost always more rewarding than roughness and expediency and provide a basis for a more favorable result.

In the process of obtaining the history of an injury for a pediatric patient, special attention should be given to the immunization status (to consider prophylaxis), mechanism of injury, and the possibility of child abuse. This is sometimes a very subtle and very delicate subject. If suspicion arises because of the nature, location, or circumstances of the injury, social services should be enlisted to investigate the case further. This subject should not be broached directly at the time treatment is being administered, nor should judgmental comments be offered at this time.

The parents require special attention, including an explanation of the injuries and the results that can be anticipated. They should understand that scars are permanent but that they will improve with time and can be revised in the future. Falsely raising expectations can in itself lead to an unhappy situation that is hard to resolve later. The parents should understand the proposed treatment of the wound, including the need for appropriate anesthesia, wound cleansing, and repair. They should be properly instructed about the postoperative care of the wounds and should know what to look for and whom to call in case of problems. We provide patients and parents with written follow-up instructions and phone numbers, which are otherwise easily forgotten after the fact.

SEDATION AND ANESTHESIA

A calm, cooperative patient during the repair of a facial laceration is an essential element of a favorable result. Sometimes, general anesthesia is necessary because of the age of the patient, the extent and complexity of the injury, or the presence of associated surgical problems. Most facial soft tissue wounds, however, can be managed with local anesthesia and additional sedation, depending again on the condition of the patient and the extent of the injury.

A child may not cooperate because of pain, fear, or simply an inability to remain still. The mention of needles and further probing and stimulation will of course aggravate the situation. A varying degree of sedation and analgesia is required to get the job done appropriately. Too much time and effort are wasted when this simple point is not heeded. An adult is usually able to tolerate most manipulations with just infiltration of local anesthesia, although at times some sedation and analgesia may also be necessary.

When sedation is indicated, light or conscious sedation is preferable. The protective reflexes and a patent airway are maintained, and patients breathe on their own. They are able to respond to verbal commands. Appropriate equipment for monitoring and resuscitation is necessary in case the sedation becomes deep or the patient suffers an adverse event. The American Society of Anesthesiologists and the American Academy of Pediatrics have established guidelines for the proper use of conscious sedation and analgesia and for patient discharge in an outpatient setting outside the operating room (6).

The choice and amount of sedation and pain medication will depend on several factors, including the level of consciousness of the patient. The route of administration is also important. The intravenous route is faster and makes it easy to titrate doses, but access is required and problems can develop more quickly. Oral, intranasal, rectal, and intramuscular routes are other possibilities. The surgeon should be familiar with dosage and administration based on weight and age and the potential side effects of the drugs given.

Morphine, meperidine, and fentanyl are common opioid narcotics used for pain control. Fentanyl has the advantage of a rapid onset of action, a short duration of action, and predictability. Naloxone can reverse the effects of overdose. It is much more expensive than morphine but 100 times more potent. A short-acting benzodiazepine such as midazolam can be given in combination for more extensive wounds. Careful titration is necessary because of the increased risk for respiratory depression. Careful monitoring of vital signs and pulse oximetry are essential. More extensive or complex wounds may be better addressed and managed in the operating room, where an anesthesiologist and better lighting and equipment are available.

Midazolam alone is often used, especially in children. It provides effective sedation, a reduction of anxiety, and anterograde amnesia. It can be administered intravenously, orally, or intranasally. Intranasal drops can sting and be irritating but are generally effective. A new formulation is available in a sweet syrup that makes it more appealing to children than the intravenous route for shorter procedures. In case of oversedation, the reversal agent flumazenil is effective.

A particularly useful drug for more invasive and painful procedures, especially in children, is ketamine. It is actually a dissociative anesthetic that produces profound analgesia while the pharyngolaryngeal reflexes and a patent airway are preserved. Skeletal tone is nearly normal, and some increased secretions may be noted. Its safety and effectiveness are well proven when it is given in appropriate doses with good monitoring. Its hallucinatory aftereffects can generally be controlled by administering smaller doses or by combining it with other sedatives, such as midazolam.

Notwithstanding good sedation and an optimal environment, local or regional anesthesia is a mainstay of effective repair. Several topical anesthetics are available that may be helpful, but they require a good deal of patience to use and results are often inconsistent. They have the advantage that they do not distort the wound. They can have a vasoconstricting effect, and the parent can participate in the procedure. An infiltrative anesthetic is usually necessary to cleanse and debride a wound fully and to perform a repair.

Lidocaine is the most popular local anesthetic used because of its rapid onset of action, good diffusion, and long history of safety. When it is combined with epinephrine, its duration of action is increased, and it produces vasoconstriction at the site that greatly improves visibility during technical repair. The onset of action of lidocaine is almost immediate, but at least 5 to 7 minutes is necessary for epinephrine to produce full vasoconstriction. Bupivacaine is an amide local anesthetic similar to lidocaine, but its onset of action is much longer (8 to 12 minutes). Its duration of action is also much longer (4 to 8 hours), and therefore it is more desirable in certain cases. The combination of lidocaine and bupivacaine should be used with caution because they have additive toxic side effects.

Local anesthetics are stored in an acidic solution to ensure stability and to lengthen shelf life. When injected, they cause pain, and they must be neutralized in the tissues to produce a nerve blockade. To avoid this problem, it is helpful to buffer the lidocaine/epinephrine solution with sodium bicarbonate solution, usually in a 1:10 ratio (1 mEq of bicarbonate per milliliter with 9 mL of 1% lidocaine with or without epinephrine). This greatly reduces the sting of injection and the time to the onset of anesthesia. It is also helpful to use a needle with a small diameter, such as a 27- or 30-gauge needle, to lessen the pain and improve the accuracy of the local injection.

Whenever possible, regional nerve block anesthesia is useful in the face. An extensive area can be anesthetized with minimal distortion of the wound. A thorough understanding of the anatomy of the sensory nerves of the face, primarily the distribution of the branches of the trigeminal nerve, is required. The more popular locations include the supratrochlear and supraorbital nerves, which supply the forehead and anterior scalp; the infraorbital nerve at the medial base of the orbit, which supplies the midface, lateral nose, and ipsilateral upper dentition and lip; and the mental nerve, which exits the mandible just below the second bicuspid and supplies much of the lower portion of the chin and lower lip. Further infiltration in the lateral face and the malar, periocular, and auricular regions is required to obtain more complete anesthesia.

GENERAL TECHNIQUES OF WOUND CLOSURE

Proper instrumentation and suture materials are important in the treatment of all wounds, but particularly those of the face. Staples are quick and effective in the scalp and are easy to remove. They have no place in the closure of most lacerations on the face. Absorbable sutures are used in the deeper layers, such as fascia and fat, to approximate the tissues, and fine monofilament nonabsorbable suture is used to close the skin. Fine fast-absorbing gut can be used to close skin in infants and small children so that sutures do not have to be removed. This can also be accomplished by using a subcuticular or intradermal suture technique with absorbable sutures. Such a practice will leave a firm incision site and scar for several weeks that is best treated with massage, but ultimately, the result will be as good as when the wound is closed with percutaneous pull-out sutures. Suture choice depends on the characteristics of the wound and the suture material. A contaminated wound on the face is best treated with a few deep monofilament absorbable sutures and an interrupted percutaneous skin closure with a monofilament suture. If drainage of blood, serum, or pus is required subsequently, individual sutures can be removed without disrupting the entire wound. In relatively clean wounds, the braided absorbable polymer sutures [polyglycolic acid (Dexon) and polyglactin 910 (Vicryl)] are very effective for deeper planes and subcuticular closures. The newer monofilament absorbable sutures [polyglyconate (Maxon), polydioxanone (PDS), and Monocryl] maintain their tensile strength longer and may be associated with less tissue reaction and less potential for infection, but they are more expensive and somewhat more difficult to handle. Improvements in suture materials and needle configuration are making the newer sutures increasingly more popular.

The nonabsorbable sutures are best used for external skin closure or internal fixation, in which a more permanent hold is desirable. They may be indicated in a medial or lateral canthopexy in an upper eyelid laceration or ptosis repair, or in cartilage fixation in the nose or ear. Nylon, dyed or undyed, is the most commonly used suture in this group. It causes little tissue reaction and has good tensile strength, but knot security is relatively poor and at least four throws are required, including a surgeon's knot. Polypropylene [Prolene (Ethicon)] causes little tissue reaction and has excellent tensile strength, but knot security is even less than with nylon, with a high degree of memory. It is good for subcuticular pull-out sutures, such as are used in the upper and lower eyelids. Silk and braided nylon sutures are less useful than in prior years but have excellent handling characteristics. They are useful in repairing wounds close to the eye because their soft consistency prevents undue irritation to the nearby globe structures.

A new and developing area in wound closure is the introduction of tissue adhesives. The Food and Drug Administration has recently approved the use of *N*-butyl-2-cyanoacrylate [Dermabond (Ethicon)] for the closure of skin lacerations. Advantages are that wound closure takes less time, and little or no anesthesia is required. The advantages in children are obvious, and in patients with small, uncomplicated, linear lacerations. A small learning curve in the use of the product has been noted, and the risk for wound dehiscence in the first few days is greater than with suture closure. After 1 week, no significant difference in tensile or bursting strength is found between the two methods. Cyanoacrylates can be irritating to the deeper tissues, and its use should be restricted to the skin surfaces. The results of studies of its potential to cause carcinogenesis have been inconclusive, and carcinogenesis has been demonstrated only in the rat model. Its use is indicated in short linear or curvilinear lacerations under minimal tension that require few or no deep sutures and have no evidence of infection. Caution should be taken near the eye. Although cyanoacrylate is used for corneal repair, inadvertent adhesion of the eyelids or other adnexal structures may occur.

Fibrin glue or sealant is a biologic adhesive that has also been recently approved in the United States by the Food and Drug Administration for tissue adhesion. It is more commonly used at this time for hemostasis and the adhesion of both split-thickness and full-thickness grafts. A preparation [Tisseel VH (Baxter)] is now commercially available that comes in a kit of component materials ready for mixing and application (7). The components include the following:

1. Freeze-dried, vapor-heated human fibrinogen concentrate obtained from pooled plasma
2. Freeze-dried, vapor-heated human thrombin, also from pooled plasma
3. Calcium chloride solution
4. Solution of aprotinin, which is a fibrinolysis inhibitor of bovine origin

The fibrinogen and thrombin solutions are highly concentrated and can produce a very reliable mixture in a short period of time. Although the solutions are screened carefully for viral and other infectious agents, because they are plasma-derived products, the potential to transmit disease still exists. This potential also is present with the homologous preparation made from cryoprecipitate. The Aprotinin solution can potentially cause sensitization because of its bovine origin. As the price of the product begins to drop, it should become more widely acceptable and applicable for skin grafts and deeper tissue wounds of the face.

REMOVAL OF SUTURES AND POSTOPERATIVE CARE

Sutures on the face should generally be removed sooner than those in other parts of the body because of faster healing and the propensity for conspicuous, hypertrophic scarring. Eyelid skin is very thin, and sutures should come out in 3 to 4 days. For sutures on other parts of the face, 4 to 6 days is recommended. External sutures that are removed this early do not usually leave marks or "tracks." Subcuticular or pull-out sutures are alternatives, especially in children or when sutures must remain for a longer period of time. Skin tapes or strips are very useful to keep the scar from spreading or even pulling apart after the sutures are removed. They also apply pressure on the healing scar that aids in softening and flattening the scar. The patient is then instructed to massage the scar with any lotion of choice. Vitamin E lotions seem to work well, although the massage itself is probably the more important feature. If after all this care the scar takes on a very reddened and prominent appearance, we have had some initial success with the use of pulsed dye vascular laser as early as 2 to 3 weeks after initial repair. It is useful as long as the scar is erythematous and seems to soften the scar considerably.

Repaired wounds on the face can be left open and should be kept clean. Antibiotic ointment for the first few days is used to protect the wound and to keep it moist. Gentle washing is permitted usually after 24 hours, after which the wound is patted dry and ointment applied. The physician should be alerted if any signs of infection develop.

The patient should always be forewarned about the possibility of unsightly scars and the possible need for modulation or revision in the future. The common unfavorable result in soft tissue injuries to the face is the scar that the patient did not expect. The patient may feel that plastic surgery was either not performed or performed poorly because an unsightly scar is present. Constant warning and reassurance about scars are necessary so that surprises are minimal and the patient can cooperate in later care.

SPECIFIC ANATOMIC REGIONS

Scalp

The scalp has a relatively large surface area that is often injured in motor vehicle accidents and other blunt trauma. Accounts of total or subtotal scalping injuries have been reported; usually, hair becomes caught in a moving object and the scalp is avulsed. Replantation should always be considered as an option. Lacerations are very common in this area and can bleed profusely because of the rich blood supply of the scalp. The scalp is usually hair-bearing and thick; the initial letters of the names of its five known layers form the acronym "SCALP":

1. Skin
2. Connective fat and fascial layer
3. Aponeurotic muscle layer (galea)
4. Loose areolar tissue
5. Periosteum

Bleeding should be controlled initially because it may be profuse and can cause hemodynamic compromise. The wound should then be anesthetized with a solution of lidocaine and epinephrine if possible; this also aids in hemostasis. The wound is carefully inspected and palpated for the presence of foreign material or fractures, and the findings are corroborated by radiography or scanning. The wound is then irrigated and debrided, particularly in cases of stellate lacerations with irregular margins. Judicious trimming is advised because the soft tissues of the scalp are not as redundant or flexible as other areas, and closure may become difficult (Fig. 29-1A). Contused scalp tissue in less than optimal condition usually heals well and should be left preserved. Infection is very rare because of the rich vascularity, but hematomas are common, so hemostasis is important. Hair is not cut or shaved except at times around the wound

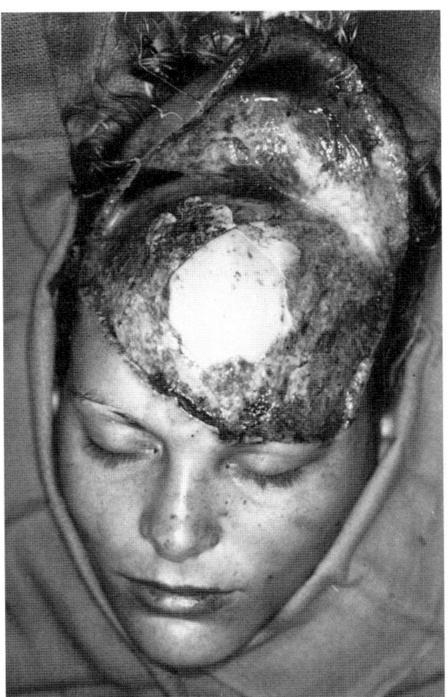
A

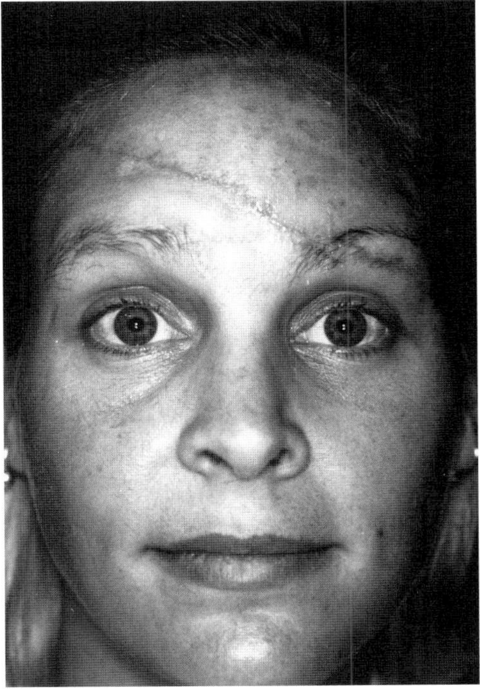
B

FIGURE 29-1. A: An extensive subtotal scalp avulsion in a 25-year-old woman hurled from the back seat of a car. With meticulous approximation of reference points, including the eyebrow, it should be possible to avoid future problems. **B:** Good healing 6 weeks later. Frontal nerve branch was repaired initially but is still somewhat weak. Insensate forehead is improving slowly.

to facilitate full evaluation of the injury and repair. Close shaving may actually increase the chance of infection (8).

Deep to the galeal aponeurotic layer are emissary veins that course through the bone to the intracranial structures. Deep, contaminated lacerations should be carefully cleaned; the galea should be closed and the patient placed on antibiotics to avoid infection, which could include osteomyelitis or a brain abscess.

The scalp can be closed with sutures or staples with comparable results, and the scar will commonly heal well and be hidden. Scar alopecia can be a problem and can usually be avoided by beveling the edges such that the hair follicles grow up into the scar. Male patients at some point during their life will undergo some degree of balding according to familial patterns. The location and characteristics of the scar may be of significant concern in these cases.

A compression bandage may be necessary in extensive cases to reduce the incidence of hematoma or seroma, but otherwise, because of the presence of hair, an antibiotic ointment on the suture line is sufficient for wound management. The stitches or staples can be removed in 7 to 10 days. Numbness and paresthesias are common, although in most cases temporary (Fig. 29-1B).

Forehead and Eyebrows

The upper third of the face is commonly injured in automobile accidents. The subsequent repair of injuries can be favorable in this area if they run parallel to the furrows or skin tension lines. Otherwise, they can be very obtrusive. When the eyebrow is lacerated, it should not be shaved and the repair should be as precise as possible. The hair shafts should be used as reference points because any discrepancy will be obvious. If debridement is necessary in this area, it should be carried out parallel to the hair follicles so that a minimum of hair is lost and the scar is better concealed.

Sutures in this area are removed in 3 to 5 days. The wounds are cleaned daily with a mild soap and water and are usually left open to air. Antibiotic ointment is applied for the first few days. As in other areas of the face, special protection from the sun for up to a year is important to avoid unsightly pigmentation.

If the laceration is deep to the frontalis muscle or other small muscles around the eyebrow, they should be repaired to maintain animation and prevent spreading or depression of the scar. Motor and sensory nerves may also be injured and should be repaired with appropriate magnification. If this is not possible at the time of injury, it should be addressed secondarily at a later time.

A common injury to the forehead is blunt trauma from an automobile collision or a fall. One or multiple stellate lacerations and abrasions can be caused by a shattered windshield, dashboard, or other flying object. If a myriad of shallow cuts and gouges are present that are less than 5 mm in width, it is better to let these heal secondarily and address the scars later. The patient should be advised that scar revisions may well be required in the future. Dermabrasion or in some cases carbon dioxide laser resurfacing may be used to smooth out these areas. Commonly, foreign bodies such as glass will need to be removed as well as possible. Tattoos caused by road rash or other embedded particles may be present, and if they cannot be removed safely at the initial setting, later revision will also be required. Larger superficial flaps are closed with simple percutaneous sutures and a minimum of deep stitches. Irregular or jagged edges should be trimmed if sufficient tissue is available close primarily. If tissue loss is significant, such that primary closure is not possible or closure will produce a marked deformity or asymmetry, the option of skin grafting should be considered. Another option is to leave the wound open and allow it to heal by contracture and secondary intention. Goldwyn and Rueckert (9) have clearly shown the value and applicability of healing by secondary intention in sizable defects, not only on the forehead but also on other parts of the face. Circumstances and the condition of the patient may warrant this approach so that the patient is not placed at undue risk.

Eyelids

Lacerations or injuries to the eyelids or periorbital structures can be among the most challenging and complex to manage because of the large number of structures involved. Injuries to the globe can be present in cases of even relatively minor trauma and must be ruled out initially. Fluorescein examination of the cornea to look for abrasions, cuts, or foreign bodies is quite useful. Further injuries to the globe require an ophthalmologic consultation.

The examination of avulsions or complex lacerations of the upper or lower eyelids requires careful attention to detail and a thorough knowledge of the anatomy, and loupe magnification is required for repair. When the lid margin and tarsus are involved, these should be approximated with precise alignment, with care taken not to evert or invert the lashes or leave an opportunity for notching. In the upper eyelid, damage to the levator complex can lead to ptosis, and a careful repair is important (Fig. 29-2). Damage to other extraocular muscles, which can lead to strabismus, diplopia, and other complications, must be addressed by an ophthalmologist. Injury to the medial and lateral canthal segments requires repair. Visualization and comparison with the uninjured eye are necessary to obtain symmetry. Normally, the lateral canthus is located 4 to 6 mm more cephalad than the medial canthus. When the medial canthus is injured, inspection or exploration of the lacrimal apparatus may be required. When the punctum or canalicular system is violated, excessive tearing or epiphora may be present. Careful repair of these structures should be performed. Judicious manipulation or intubation of the lacrimal system is necessary to avoid further injury. The inferior punctum and canaliculus

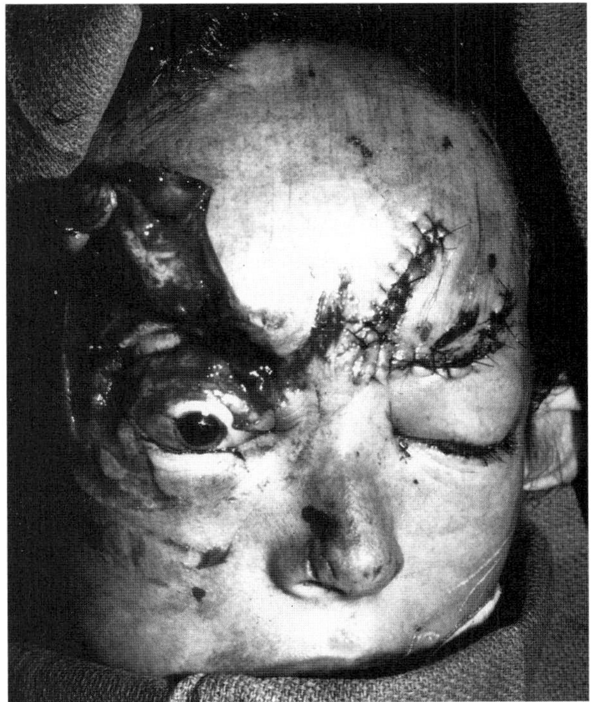
A

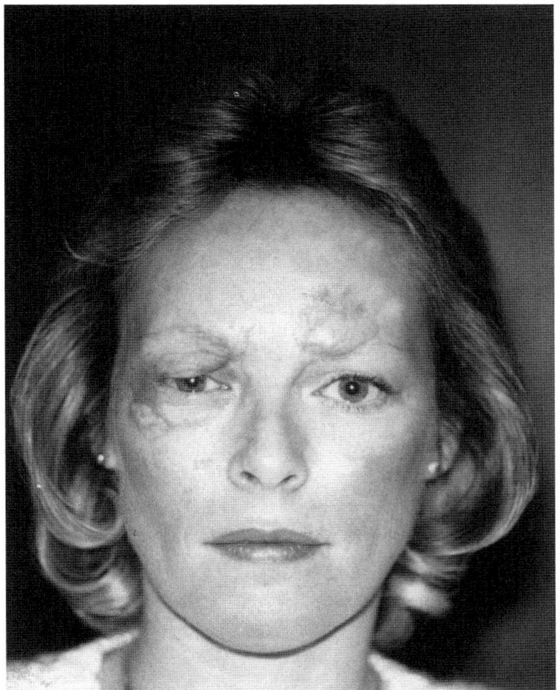
B

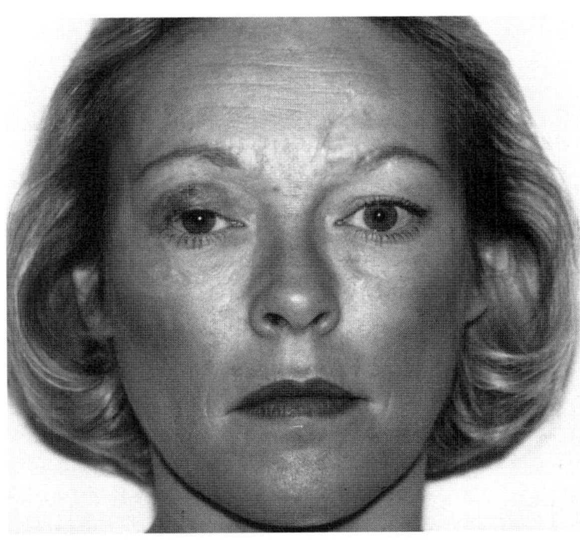
C

FIGURE 29-2. A: A 37-year-old woman with severe avulsion and lacerations sustained in a motor vehicle collision; the globe was spared, but loss of tissue requires skin grafting and secondary closure. **B:** Six months after injury, ptosis of right upper eyelid and prominent scars are still present, even with vigorous conservative management. **C:** Two years after injury. Patient has undergone ptosis repair, dermabrasion, and revision of scars, and uses makeup sensibly.

drain up to 90% of tears. In a repair of this structure, a stent of 3-0, 4-0, or 5-0 nylon can be used to keep the canalicular system open during healing. In more distal injuries to the sac or lacrimal duct, especially in conjunction with orbital fractures, a more conservative approach is employed. If the patient still complains of epiphora, a dacryocystorhinostomy may be indicated once all wounds have healed and at least 6 weeks have elapsed since the initial repair.

When tissue is lost or the closure is too tight, flap rotation or skin grafting is necessary to prevent lid retraction and potential exposure keratitis. A full-thickness skin graft is preferred and is commonly taken from the contralateral upper eyelid if possible. Preauricular or retroauricular skin is also useful. A bolster or a biologic adhesive is placed to keep the graft immobilized.

Aftercare consists of gentle daily washing and the application of antibiotic ointment. Sutures are removed early, at 3 to 4 days. Soft massage of the scars is begun as soon as the patient can tolerate it. This helps reduce swelling and smooth out the scars. It can also help relieve mild retraction or contractures of the lids. A tincture of time with conservative management may be quite beneficial in this area (Fig. 29-2C).

Cheeks

The midface or cheek region is commonly injured. The superficial structures, like other areas of the face, should be repaired with precision and usually heal well. The deeper structures in this area are of greater concern in regard to long-term problems. Injury to the parotid gland and branches of the facial nerve can cause significant residual problems. A salivary leak or collection and varying degrees of facial paralysis can complicate an otherwise simple facial cut (Fig. 29-3).

The parotid gland lies anterior and inferior to the ear between the mandible and the sternocleidomastoid muscle. It is deep to the superficial fascia of the face, and in its midst lie the main branches of the facial nerve as they course to their target organs. The course of the main parotid duct (Stensen's duct) is superficial to the masseter muscle; the duct then pierces the thin buccinator muscle and opens into

A

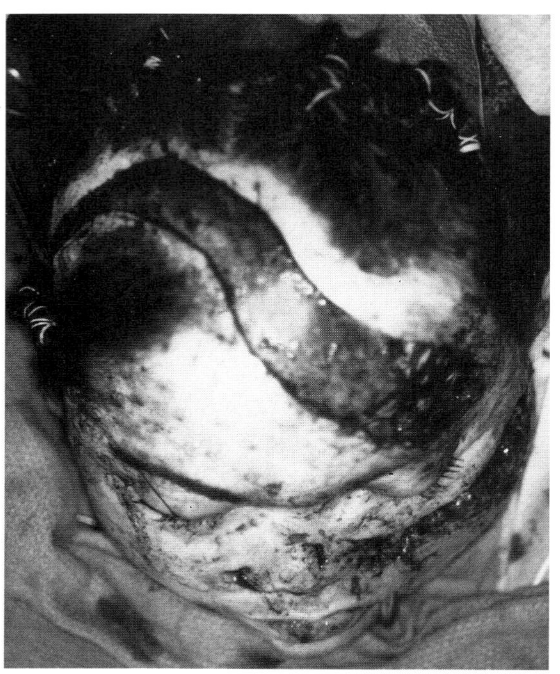

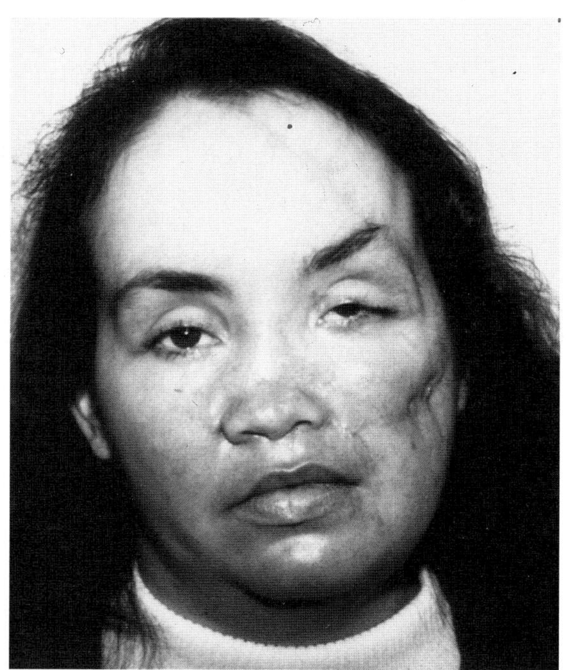

B

C

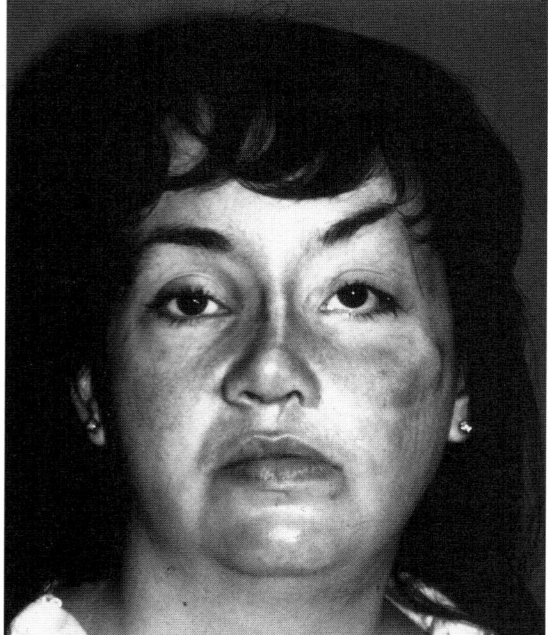

FIGURE 29-3. A: A 28-year-old woman suffered severe facial trauma in an automobile accident, including Le Fort III fractures and extensive lacerations. These resulted in a dishpan facial deformity and enucleation of the left eye. **B:** A cantilever nasal bone graft failed, and serious scarring complicated the subsequent result. **C:** A repeated nasal cartilage graft, malar augmentation, left eyelid and prosthetic reconstruction, and scar revisions have yielded favorable results.

the oral cavity just opposite the crown of the second upper molar. In cases of injury, some blood staining may be noted at this opening in the mouth, or clear salivary fluid leaking in the wound. Usually, it is not readily evident, and if injury is suspected, a formal exploration is required. Major ductal injury can be assessed by intubating the papillary opening in the mouth with a flexible catheter or a fine lacrimal tube. Gentle advancement is indicated to avoid a false passage. If a complete or partial cut is found, it should be repaired with fine absorbable suture. A plastic stent may be left in place for a few days to ensure patency. If injury to the duct has been substantial, with loss of tissue, the proximal stump can be ligated. The parotid gland will undergo gradual atrophy. Close to Stensen's duct are the buccal branches of the facial nerve. They are commonly also injured in such circumstances and should be repaired if possible. Superficial rents in the gland without major ductal injury may result in salivary leaks for a period of days, but these will eventually resolve.

Injury to one or more branches of the facial nerve should be diagnosed by physical examination. An unconscious or uncooperative patient makes this examination difficult. The location and depth of injuries can help with the diagnosis in most cases. Whenever possible, immediate repair should be performed with loupe or microscope assistance. The zygomaticotemporal branches are particularly important in protecting the globe from exposure keratitis. Exploration within 72 hours is helpful to locate distal nerve fibers because wallerian degeneration has not yet ablated distal nerve stimulation. If repair is not possible initially, the stumps should be tagged for future identification.

Nose

This central structure is composed of many soft tissue and bone elements. The cartilage and bony skeleton are easily and often injured. The proper nasal bones are the most commonly fractured bones in the facial skeleton. Along with these, the chondro-osseous septum is also fractured, and the typical saddle deformity is the result. Intranasal examination with a speculum is essential to rule out a septal hematoma that can lead to chondromalacia or necrosis of the septum and subsequent nasal collapse if not drained expeditiously. Once the airway and skeletal structures have been addressed, attention can be directed to the soft tissues. A minimum of deep sutures are placed and the edges are well approximated to avoid depressions or trapdoor deformities (Fig. 29-4).

Full-thickness tears or avulsions require meticulous layered closure if a satisfactory result is to be obtained. The mucosa is repaired while a patent airway is maintained. All exposed cartilage is covered or judiciously trimmed to avoid chondritis and scarring. The skin envelope is then approximated anatomically. The alar rims need to be well aligned and slightly everted to avoid notching. A tension-free closure is necessary to prevent deformity or breakdown. If tissue has been lost, skin grafting or delayed closure with a facial flap should be considered. Packing the nasal airway is useful in septal injuries but otherwise optional. Antibiotics are given to patients with extensive injuries that involve bone and cartilage.

Lips

The lips are composed of skin, vermilion, and mucosa of varying degrees of keratinization and melanization. They

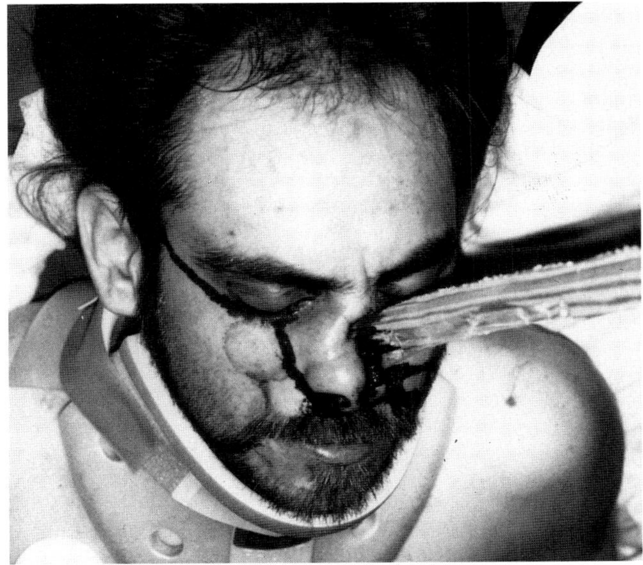
A

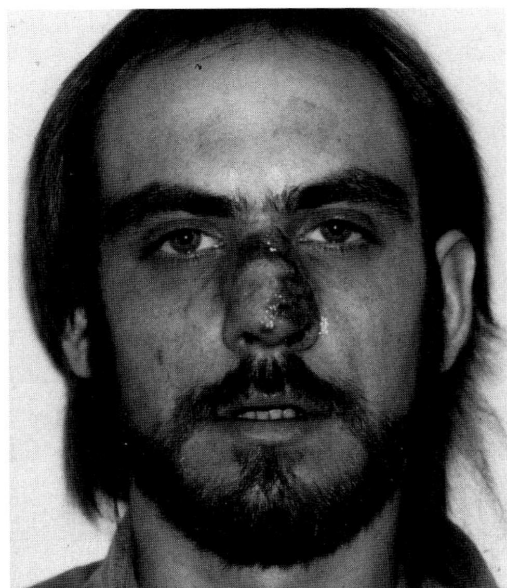
B

FIGURE 29-4. A: A 32-year-old lumber mill worker suffered an impalement injury to the nose with a large wooden splinter. This penetrated the parapharyngeal space but fortunately spared the major neck vessels. **B:** The proper nasal bones were repaired and splinted, as were the cartilage structures. Abraded and crushed nasal skin was approximated and left to heal. *(continued)*

C

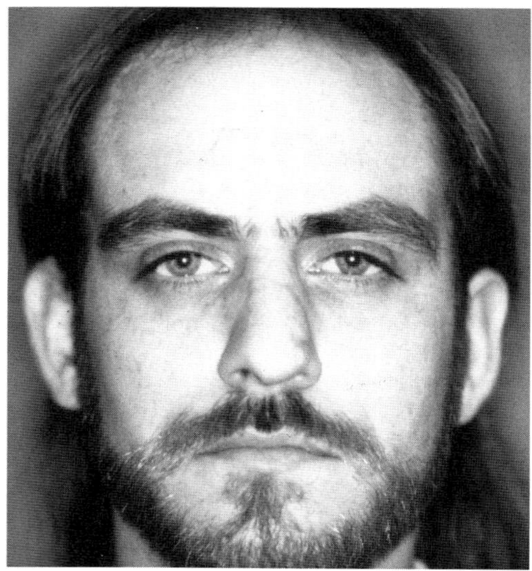

FIGURE 29-4. *Continued.* **C:** One year after injury, the patient has a good airway and a healed nasal skin envelope.

A

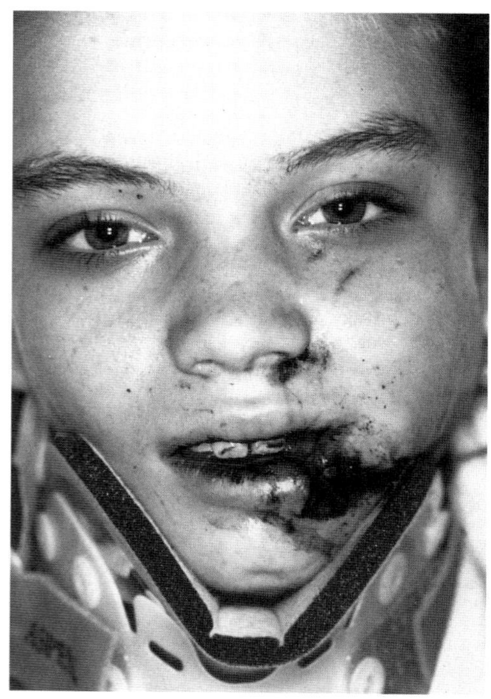

B

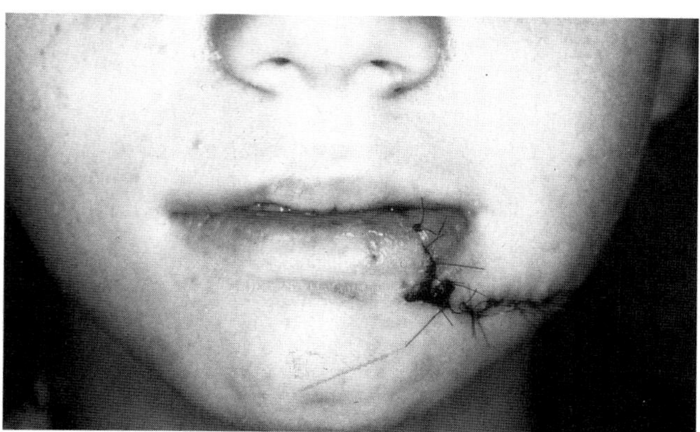

C

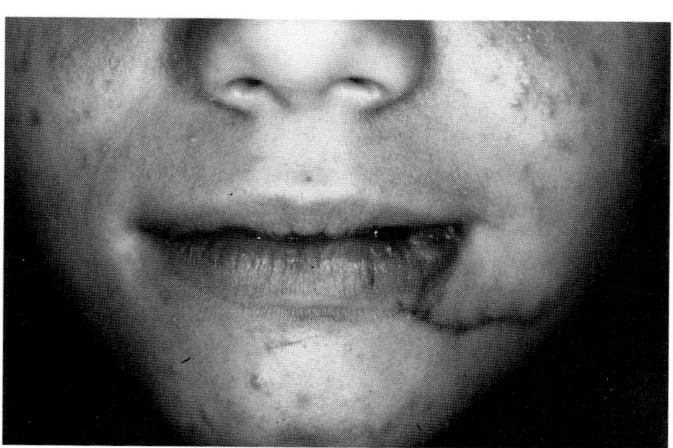

FIGURE 29-5. A: A 13-year-old girl on a bicycle fell and injured her lip and dentoalveolar maxilla. **B:** She underwent interdental fixation and careful repair of the vermilion-cutaneous region. **C:** After 4 months, the scar has healed reasonably well. Massage and actinic protection were recommended. Dermabrasion or pulsed dye laser may be useful later if thick scarring persists.

also contain muscle, salivary glands, and connective tissue. Repair of lacerations is carried out in layers. Of primary importance is the precise approximation of the vermilion-cutaneous border. As in a cleft lip repair, even a slight discrepancy can be very obvious and the focus of considerable distress. This border or "white roll" should be carefully marked or tattooed if possible before any local anesthetic is injected so that it will be fully preserved (Fig. 29-5). A superficial reference suture is placed at the juncture that will orient the subsequent closure of the lip. Careful approximation of the orbicularis oris muscle will restore function and avoid stretching of the scar and occasional "lumps" of muscle on either side of the scar. The philtral dimple, columns, and Cupid's bow are all characteristic features that require precise apposition and reconstruction if a satisfactory result is to be obtained. To prevent distortion of the lip structures, regional blocks of the infraorbital or mental nerves should be used minimally in these areas.

Dental puncture wounds are usually treated conservatively, especially in the intraoral region of the lip. A few simple sutures can be placed in the skin, and the internal mucosa is left open to drain. Teeth or fragments must be removed from the wound to avoid infection.

When the angles or commissures of the lips are involved, a careful layered closure is essential to achieve an adequate functional and cosmetic result. Just lateral to the buccal angle is the modiolus, which is a dense, compact, mobile, fibromuscular mass that is extremely important in the animation of the face and the function of the oral cavity. A series of facial muscles converge at this site to produce a three-dimensional mobility combining elevation, depression, retraction, and protraction. Proper and anatomical repair of this complex becomes crucial to the normal appearance and function of the lips, cheeks, and oral cavity.

Ears

The ear consists of a characteristic convoluted cartilaginous framework covered by densely adherent skin. Trauma to the ear can result in tears, crush injuries, avulsions, and partial or complete amputations. Hematomas are common, and if they are not drained expeditiously, they can produce long-lasting deformities, such as cauliflower ears, that result from pressure necrosis of the underlying cartilage. Exposed cartilage should be covered quickly or carefully dressed until coverage is feasible to avoid desiccation or infection with subsequent chondritis. Because of the rich blood supply, partial avulsions or amputations, even with relatively narrow pedicles, can usually be repaired successfully by careful anatomic approximation. Complete amputations of the ear are best treated with replantation if possible (10). Small vessels and traumatized soft tissues make this is one of the more demanding microsurgical procedures. If replantation is successful, it can produce an excellent cosmetic result. Heparinization, medicinal leeches, or vein grafts are often necessary (11). In partial or complete amputations in which microsurgical repair is not possible, burying the deepithelialized segment of the cartilage in a retroauricular pocket has been successful (12). Immediate coverage of the cartilage with local flaps or the superficial temporal fascia are other treatment options.

In cases of complex lacerations, debridement should be performed carefully and conservatively and proper attention given to the unique topography of the structures involved. Perichondrial and cutaneous sutures are usually sufficient for approximation. Sutures through the cartilage may cut the tissue and should be used sparingly and with care. The anterior and posterior skin surfaces of the ear are closed independently and the edges somewhat everted to avoid notching.

The ear is usually dressed open with antibiotic ointment. A protective cupped cover is advisable in children to avoid subsequent trauma. Frequent evaluation to look for hematoma or infection is useful to prevent future problems. Sutures are removed at around 5 days.

When large segments of the pinna are lost at the time of the injury or during subsequent exposure or infection, then delayed reconstruction with costal cartilage should be the procedure of choice. Reconstruction of helical defects and others in the margin of the ear can be performed with several techniques, including that suggested by Antia (13).

ANIMAL AND HUMAN BITES

The chances of being bitten by an animal or another human during one's lifetime is 50% (14). More than 80% of bites are inflicted by dogs, cats, and humans, in that order. Children are most often affected, and the younger the victim, the more likely the location is the face or scalp (15). Most of the estimated 2 million annual bites are trivial and go unreported, but those for which medical attention is sought include punctures, abrasions, cuts, and avulsions with or without loss of tissue (16). The incidence of serious and even fatal dog bites is rising, especially as large and aggressive breeds are more often being raised for sport and home protection. Other animals, such as skunks, bats, foxes, and various rodents, are much less frequent sources of bites, but they are much more likely to carry rabies, and victims should be treated appropriately. The factors involved in the treatment of bites include the source, location and type of wound, age of the patient, treatment delay, associated injuries, and other medical conditions.

Most wound infections from dog and cat bites are polymicrobial, both aerobic and anaerobic. A wealth of other contaminant microorganisms do not cause disease except in the susceptible and immunocompromised patient. The most clinically relevant bacterial species in dog and cat bites are the aerobes *Staphylococcus aureus, Pasteurella multocida,* and *Streptococcus* species and the anaerobic *Bacteroides* species. Patients with deep, contaminated wounds, cellulitis or frank infection, or significant risk factors should be treated with a combination of wound irrigation, debridement, and broad-spectrum antibiotics. The most effective antibiotics in this setting are ampicillin/sulbactam (Unasyn), given intravenously, and amoxicillin/clavulanate (Augmentin), given orally, depending on the severity of the wound. The microbiology of human bites is even more complex and florid. In addition to *Staphylococcus* and *Streptococcus* species, *Eikenella corrodens* is present in up to 29% of positive cultures. Anaerobic organisms are also common in human bites, including *Peptostreptococcus* and *Bacteroides* species. Fortunately, the same broad-spectrum antibiotics are effective for human bites as for dog and cat bites—namely, ampicillin/sulbactam and amoxicillin/clavulanate. Rare microorganisms that have been isolated from human bites include hepatitis B and C viruses, herpes simplex virus, *Clostridium tetani, Mycobacterium tuberculosis,* and *Treponema pallidum.*

Management of the wound depends on its nature, severity, and location, and on the characteristics of the patient. Proper tetanus immunization should be ascertained. Superficial cuts or abrasions on the face without treatment delay require simple cleansing and minimal suture approximation. More extensive wounds require thorough cleansing, judicious debridement, and careful skin approximation with a minimum of deep sutures. Puncture wounds present special problems because they may penetrate more deeply than is apparent. It should be kept in mind that the upper and lower jaws often produce external and internal puncture wounds that must be irrigated and debrided appropriately. The time factor is also important in avoiding future problems. Animal and human bites of the trunk and extremities untreated for longer than 8 to 12 hours should be left open. Bites on the face and scalp are an exception because of the rich vascularity in these areas and the concern for cosmesis. Wounds can be treated with copious pressure irrigation, debridement, and loose superficial closure up to 24 hours after injury. The use of prophylactic antibiotics on bite wounds to the face is controversial and depends on the judgment of the surgeon. Studies have shown good results with both regimens (17). Although infection is rare on the face, it can occur if proper attention is not paid to the individual characteristics of the wound and the patient.

The possibility of contracting rabies in this country is very rare, even after a bite from a rabid animal. However, proper guidelines should be followed because of the uniformly fatal course of the disease. Worldwide, the dog is the major animal reservoir for rabies and causes more than 20,000 deaths per year. In the United States, less than one death is reported annually, and the common vectors are skunks, raccoons, and bats. In the majority of dog and cat bites, provided the animal is known, vaccinated, otherwise healthy, and able to be observed for 10 days, no postexposure prophylaxis is necessary unless symptoms develop in the animal. If the animal is unknown or unavailable for observation or is suspected of having rabies, public health officials should be consulted and both passive and active immunization begun immediately. In cases of bites from skunks, raccoons, bats, or other animals suspected of being vectors in the geographic region, immunization is also begun immediately (18). The public health department should be involved in all these suspect cases. To date, no cases of rabies development have been reported in the United States after appropriate recommended immunization.

CONCLUSION

Soft tissue injuries of the face are common. Careful assessment and surgical technique and close follow-up are required to obtain a good result of treatment and reduce the danger of an unexpected or unfavorable outcome. Analysis of the injury, including location, size, depth, and associated injuries, aids in the formulation of a surgical plan. A keen appreciation of the aesthetic units of the face and skin tension lines is important in bringing together a complex laceration. An understanding of the functional consequences of the wound will provide a proper perspective regarding overall management and outcome. Thorough communication with the informed patient and family regarding these issues and the healing process is necessary for a trusting and cooperative relationship. Adequate follow-up should be available for as long as necessary, and the physician must remain sensitive to the patient's concerns. In a difficult case or one that is not going well, a second opinion from a more experienced colleague can be beneficial. Surgeons usually gain the respect of their patients when they admit their limitations (19). Despite all appropriate efforts, unfavorable results and outcomes cannot be avoided or eliminated altogether. If and when such results occur, the surgeon should be able to manage them with appropriate surgical and nonsurgical measures in a timely fashion.

REFERENCES

1. Schultz RC. Facial injuries, 3rd ed. Chicago: Year Book, 1988: 24–43.
2. Lee RH, Gamble WB, Robertson B, et al. The MCFONTZL classification system for soft-tissue injuries to the face. *Plast Reconstr Surg* 1999;103:1150–1157.
3. Izant RJ, Hubay CA. Annual injury of 15,000,000 children: a limited study of childhood accidental injury and death. *J Trauma* 1966;6:65–74.
4. Trott AT. *Wounds and lacerations: emergency care and closure,* 2nd ed. St. Louis: Mosby, 1997:38.
5. Baker MD, Selbst SM, Lanuti M. Lacerations in urban children. *Am J Dis Child* 1990;144:87–92.
6. American Academy of Pediatrics. Guidelines for monitoring and management of pediatric patients during and after sedation for diagnostic and therapeutic procedures. *Pediatrics* 1992;89: 257–262.

7. Schlag G. Immuno's fibrin sealant: the European experience. Symposium on Fibrin Sealant: Characteristics and Clinical Uses, Uniformed Services University of the Health Sciences, Bethesda, Maryland, December 8–9, 1994(abst).
8. Seropian R, Reynolds B. Wound infections after preoperative depilatory versus razor preparation. *Am J Surg* 1971;121: 251–254.
9. Goldwyn RM, Rueckert F. The value of healing by secondary intention for sizable defects of the face. *Arch Surg* 1977; 112:285.
10. Kind GM, Buncke GM, Placik OJ, et al. Total ear replantation. *Plast Reconstr Surg* 1997;99:1858–1867.
11. Sadove RC. Successful replantation of a totally amputated ear. *Ann Plast Surg* 1990;24:366–370.
12. Pribaz JJ, Crespo LD, Orgill DP, et al. Ear replantation without microsurgery. *Plast Reconstr Surg* 1997;99:1868–1872.
13. Antia NH, Buch VI. Chondrocutaneous advancement flap for the marginal defect of the ear. *Plast Reconstr Surg* 1967;39: 472–477.
14. Goldstein EJ. Bite wounds and infection. *Clin Infect Dis* 1992;14:633–640.
15. Chun Y, Berkelhamer JE, Herold TE. Dog bites in children less than 4 years old. *Pediatrics* 1982;69:119–120.
16. Griego RD, Rosen T, Orengo IF, et al. Dog, cat, and human bites: a review. *J Am Acad Dermatol* 1995;33:1019–1029.
17. Guy RJ, Zook EG. Successful treatment of acute head and neck dog bite wounds without antibiotics. *Ann Plast Surg* 1986;17: 45–48.
18. Centers for Disease Control. Rabies prevention—United States, 1991: recommendations of the ACIP. *MMWR Morb Mortal Wkly Rep* 1991;40(RR-3):1–18.
19. Goldwyn RM. The unfavorable result in plastic surgery: avoidance and treatment, 2nd ed. Boston: Little, Brown and Company, 1984:7.

Discussion

SOFT TISSUE INJURIES

MIMIS N. COHEN

Soft tissue injuries of the head and neck result primarily from accidents at home or work, sports and other recreational activities, motor vehicle accidents, violence, and animal or human bites. Such injuries range in severity from minor abrasions and lacerations to complex lacerations and wounds with damage to several important structures and significant tissue loss. The management of such injuries ranges from cleansing and dressing of a single wound to complex reconstructive procedures, including vascular and nerve repair, soft tissue reconstruction with flaps, or replantation of parts under magnification or with microsurgical techniques.

Soft tissue injuries and their treatment occupy a prominent place in the plastic surgery literature. Several books are dedicated to the subject (1–3). Additionally, hundreds of thousands of pages in textbooks and journals deal with the details of managing various soft tissue injuries in the emergency department, office, or operating room. Postoperative follow-up and the prevention and management of unfavorable results with revisional procedures have also been addressed in detail (4–7).

M. N. Cohen: Divisions of Plastic Surgery, University of Illinois at Chicago and Cook County Hospital, Chicago, Illinois

To manage patients with soft tissue injuries successfully, achieve the best possible functional and aesthetic results, and reduce the incidence of complications or unfavorable results and the subsequent time needed for convalescence, the surgeon should have an extensive knowledge of the anatomy of the area involved and understand the specific problems related to the injury of each anatomic unit and subunit. In addition to the basic surgical principles of managing trauma victims, the principles of local and regional anesthesia and sedation, and those of antibiotic administration, the surgeon who deals with patients with soft tissue injuries should have a detailed knowledge and experience in the management, repair, and reconstruction of various types of injuries by means of appropriate, well-planned, and well-designed surgical techniques.

It has been well accepted that adequate early treatment minimizes late deformities and produces superior results. Unfortunately, early definitive repair is not always possible. Several factors need to be taken into consideration, including the nature and extent of the injury, the patient's general condition, coexisting serious injuries, the time interval between injury and repair, and the surgeon's personal experience and preference.

In addition, the surgeon should be aware of potential social issues associated with the injury, such as child abuse and home violence, and the potential medical and legal implications of an injury. Adequate description and documentation of the injury in the patient's chart with appropriate drawings and photographs, a detailed explanation of the rationale for the management plan, and a discussion with the patient and other family members about the possible outcome or potential need for additional surgery in the future are of the utmost importance. A legal suit for malpractice, criminal investigation or prosecution, and industrial or other compensation may depend on evidence from such notes, not only when the potential for litigation is obvious, but also in several unexpected situations.

Dr. Vasconez has handled a difficult and demanding topic very well and has covered in detail the most appropriate management strategies for the care of various injuries according to their anatomic location. Adherence to these basic principles can ensure, as much as possible, a successful outcome and reduce the potential for unfavorable results. It is beyond the scope of Dr. Vasconez' chapter to discuss in detail every potential complication in each anatomic location of the head and neck and describe all the available techniques for revisionary reconstructive surgery. This would be impossible, given the extent and complexity of the topic and the available space in the book. Furthermore, several other chapters in the book deal with unfavorable results of wound healing, scar revision, and soft tissue reconstruction.

Several principles of the management of patients with soft tissue injuries to the head and neck area should be further discussed, stressed, and reiterated:

During the initial careful assessment of a wound and evaluation of the mechanism and extent of injury, it is of the utmost important to appreciate the patient's general condition and potentially coexisting injuries fully if one is to formulate an appropriate timetable and treatment plan.

Wound size and location can be deceiving. On the one hand, a small laceration to the cheek may have resulted in an injury to the facial nerve (Fig. 29D-1), and timely appropriate management will be required in the operating room for nerve and soft tissue repair. On the other, multiple gaping lacerations (Fig. 29D-2) may have spared all vital structures, and it will be possible to repair them under local or general anesthesia with excellent outcome and minimal residual deformity.

The presence of a foreign body may not always be obvious, as in the case of a patient who has walked through a glass door. A high index of suspicion is therefore necessary. Wounds should not be closed until the surgeon has made certain that a foreign body does not remain in the wound.

The clinical evaluation reveals clues about potential underlying facial fractures. If a fracture is suspected, appropriate x-rays, scans, or images should be ordered and reviewed by the surgeon before wound repair is undertaken. Occasionally, the plastic surgeon will be called in to repair the facial injuries of a patient undergoing an emergency procedure by another service. Although this practice cannot be totally condemned, it should be recognized that it entails several medical and legal dangers. Because the plastic surgeon has not had the opportunity to evaluate the patient fully before the administration of anesthesia, there is a strong possibility that some injuries have not been docu-

A

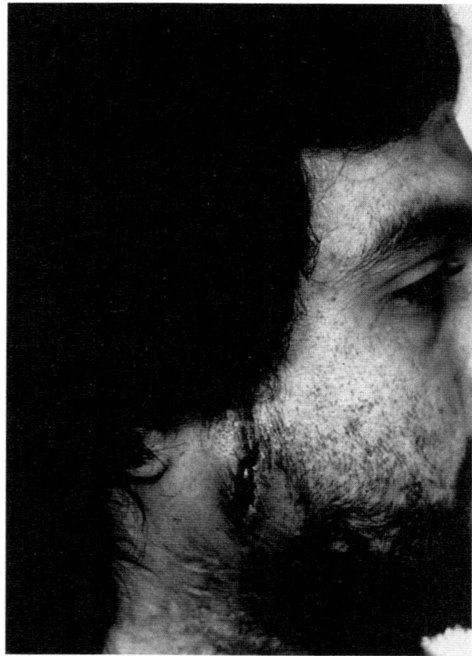

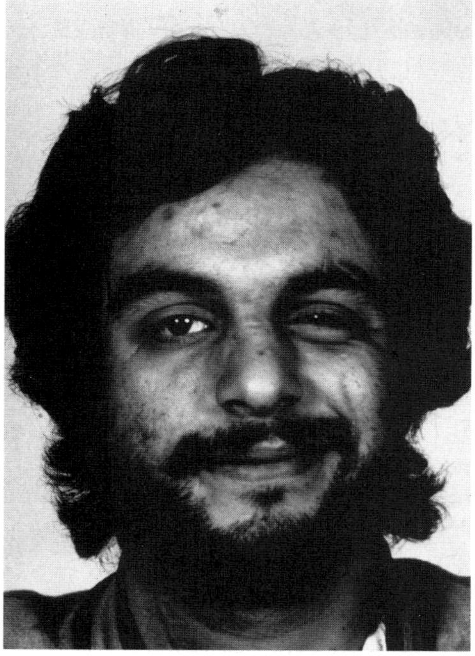

B

FIGURE 29D-1. A: Small facial laceration of the right cheek treated with wound packing in the emergency department. **B:** The injury to the main trunk of the facial nerve was missed until the follow-up visit several days later.

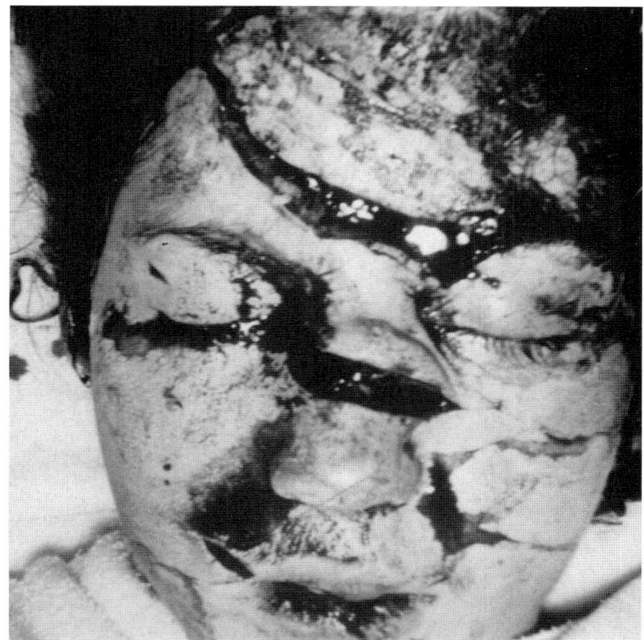
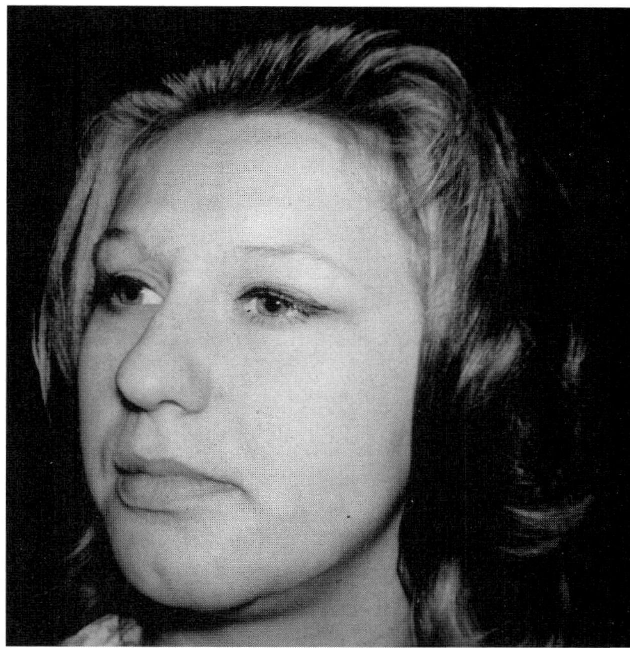

A B

FIGURE 29D-2. A: Multiple soft tissue lacerations and avulsions of the face after a motor vehicle accident. Despite the extent of the injury, no vital structures were damaged. **B:** Result 1 year after initial repair. No revisions were needed.

mented and will be missed or not repaired. This scenario pertains primarily to an injured branch of the facial nerve or a coexisting facial fracture.

The issue of timing of the repair of facial injuries merits some additional discussion. Although it is true that facial injuries should be repaired as early as possible, the cutoff of 24 hours should not be used in a dogmatic fashion. Clean lacerations can be successfully repaired even several days after the injury. On the other hand, contused, crushed, or mangled wounds tend to swell early or become infected; they should either be repaired during the first few hours after the injury or managed with local care and repaired with late primary closure as soon as the swelling or infection has subsided several days after the injury. Copious irrigation and debridement of the wound margins will be necessary before repair (8). The same rules apply for wounds from animal or human bites. The surgeon should exercise clinical judgment based on the condition and appearance of the wound rather than unscientific "dogma" or taboos to determine the timing of a repair.

The management of patients who present with facial injuries and tissue loss also needs to be addressed. If a small amount of tissue is lost, the defect can be repaired, in the majority of cases, with limited undermining of the surrounding tissues. Distortion of facial features and closure under tension should be avoided at any cost because the subsequent deformity may be difficult to correct with revisionary surgery.

Z-plasties and other techniques of tissue rearrangement should be avoided in most emergency situations, in particular if a patient presents with contusions, avulsions, or any kind of tissue damage in the periphery of the wound. Although such injuries do not result in obviously devitalized tissues, they may have produced a degree of ischemia that can influence and impair primary healing. Even in a patient who presents with an unfavorable wound orientation perpendicular to the lines of facial expression, one should not be tempted to reorient the final scar by means of a Z-plasty or other tissue rearrangement procedures in the emergency setting because such practice may result in further tissue loss and an unattractive scar. Adequate debridement and primary closure should be the procedure of choice when possible. Secondary scar revisions to improve function and appearance can be performed, if necessary, at a later time on an elective basis with more predictable results.

When primary closure is not possible, the surgeon may elect to stabilize the wound temporarily and cover it with a skin graft, deferring a major flap procedure for the future. Such an approach has the advantage of preventing significant wound contracture and tissue distortion during the early period after injury. A final reconstruction can then be carried out some months after the injury, with well-planned and well-designed flaps providing superior results.

One area that deserves special attention is the orbit, specifically traumatic defects of the eyelids. Partial or complete loss of an eyelid results in exposure and possible permanent damage of the globe. Losses of up to 25% of the upper or lower lid can be directly approximated with a layered closure. Larger defects of the upper lid require some form of reconstruction, including lateral cantholysis and a flap from the lower lid based on the marginal artery. Large defects of

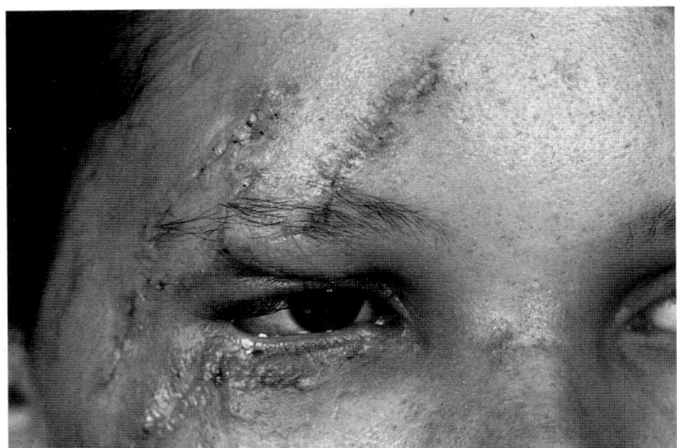

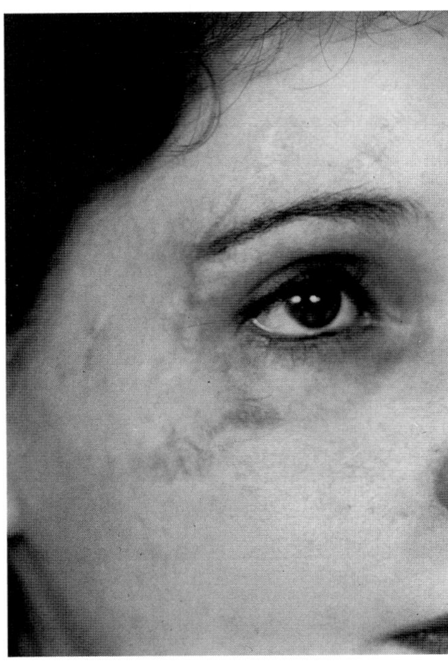

FIGURE 29D-3. A: Young woman with multiple lacerations on the forehead and lower eyelid was treated in the emergency department. The patient was extremely unhappy with the early outcome and requested an immediate revision. After lengthy discussions, she was able to understand the rationale for waiting a few months and agreed to the delay. **B:** Same patient 16 months after the initial injury. A Z-plasty was performed 9 months after the injury to correct the lower lid ectropion. The other injuries did not require revision.

the lower lid can be reconstructed with a combination of a chondromucosal graft and a cheek advancement flap or with other reconstructive procedures (9).

Patients and their families should be given detailed instructions about wound care. Close follow-up is essential to identify and treat postoperative complications in a timely fashion. Patients and their families also need to be informed about the process of wound healing and the necessary time interval for scar maturation. Hypertrophic scarring is common in the early stages of healing, particularly in children. Patients must be reassured that the appearance and color of the scar will improve with time (Fig. 29D-3). Massaging the scar and using a sunblock are helpful during the first months after an injury and should be recommended. The possibility of keloid formation or an unfavorable result that will require revision should be discussed at the time of the initial repair. The timing of a potential revision should also be discussed in detail and documented in the chart. Such practice, in most instances, will enable patients and their families to understand better the complexity of wound healing and the need to wait for scar maturation before any secondary procedure is undertaken.

Finally, detailed communication, close follow-up, and reassurance can be very helpful in preventing false expectations that can result in an unhappy patient and the possibility of unnecessary litigation.

REFERENCES

1. David DJ, Simpson DA, eds. *Craniomaxillofacial trauma,* vols 1 and 2. New York: Churchill Livingstone, 1995.
2. Rowe NL, Williams JLR, eds. *Maxillofacial injuries,* vols 1 and 2. New York: Churchill Livingstone, 1985.
3. Schultz RC. Facial injuries. In: Converse JM. 3rd ed. Chicago: Year Book, 1988.
4. Cohen M, ed. *Mastery of plastic and reconstructive surgery,* vols 1–3. Boston: Little, Brown and Company, 1994.
5. Aston SJ, Beasley RW, Thorne CHM, eds. *Grabb and Smith's plastic surgery,* 5th ed. Philadelphia: Lippincott–Raven Publishers, 1997.
6. McCarthy JG, ed. *Plastic surgery,* vols 1–8. Philadelphia: WB Saunders, 1990.
7. Georgiade GS, Georgide NG, Riefkohl R, et al., eds. *Textbook of plastic maxillofacial and reconstructive surgery,* 2nd ed. Baltimore: Williams & Wilkins, 1992.
8. Kajanjian VH, Converse JM. Early treatment of facial injuries. In: Kajanjian VH, Converse JM, eds. *Surgical treatment of facial injuries,* 3rd ed. Baltimore: Williams & Wilkins Co., 1974:86–131.
9. Jelks GW, Jelks EB. Reconstruction of the eyelids. In: Cohen M, ed. *Mastery of plastic and reconstructive surgery.* Boston: Little, Brown and Company, 1994:864–882.

30

FRACTURES OF THE JAWS

KARSTEN K.H. GUNDLACH

Unfavorable results following treatment of fractures of the jaws may be due to either diagnostic errors or inadequate management, including medication and incomplete follow-up (1–5). In addition, there are unfavorable conditions to begin with, where optimum results are almost impossible to achieve because of the nature of the injuries.

Long-term results must be evaluated with respect to function and aesthetics to adequately discuss the unfavorable outcome resulting from treatment of fractures of the jaws. It seems appropriate to first present the classification of facial, maxillary, and mandibular fractures, dislocations, distortions, and contusions that will be used in this chapter.

CLASSIFICATION OF FACIAL FRACTURES

There are numerous ways to classify fractures of the facial bones, including the jaws. To make it easier for the reader, the following simple classification is used in this chapter (Table 30-1). The face is divided into upper, middle, and lower thirds. Fractures of the upper third include fractures of the frontal bones, frontal sinuses, and anterior base of skull. They will not be discussed here.

Fractures of the middle third of the face include central, centrolateral, and lateral fractures. In this chapter, only those fractures that involve occlusion of teeth, such as Le Fort I, II, and III fractures (6–8), as well as sagittal palatal or maxillary fractures, will be discussed.

Dentoalveolar fractures, such as fractures of the alveolar bone (including involvement of the teeth), and injuries to the teeth are considered separately because they occur in either jaw or possibly in both jaws simultaneously.

Fractures of the lower third are fractures of the mandible. They can be subdivided into more than ten different types. For simplicity, only three groups are used here, namely, fractures of the horizontal ramus, fractures of the ascending ramus, and fractures of the condyle and glenoid fossa. The first group includes all fractures located in the dentition-bearing part of the lower jaw, as well as those of the edentulous body of the mandible. The second group covers fractures of the angle, the ascending ramus proper, and the coronoid process. Fractures of the condylar head and neck, as well as fractures of the temporal fossa, form the third group. Injuries of the temporomandibular joint (TMJ) resulting from blunt trauma and not leading to a fracture also will be included in this part of the chapter.

K. K. H. Gundlach: Department of Maxillofacial and Facial Plastic Surgery, Rostock University and University Hospital Rostock, Rostock, Germany

PRINCIPLES OF TREATMENT

General Rules for Diagnosis and Surgical Treatment

When a patient with maxillofacial trauma initially is evaluated, he should be examined according to a rigid checklist. This list should be short and simple, so that it can be memorized and used in every single case and in all circumstances, because facial trauma complications frequently occur as a result of inadequate primary diagnosis (Tables 30-2 and 30-3).

Every physical examination should follow the same routine program and begin with a general examination of the integrity of all facial, intranasal, and intraoral soft tissues, as well as of the external auditory canals. This is followed by testing the function of the cranial nerves and the mobility of the globes. Palpation of bony contours and checking for pain to pressure, for bony steps or irregularities, and for pathologic mobility should follow (Fig. 30-1). The function of the TMJ is studied next. This diagnostic screening ends with an examination of all teeth, inspection of the marginal periodontium, and investigation of possible sites of fractures of upper and lower alveolar bones.

Appropriate radiologic evaluation assists in understanding the extent of injury and evaluating coexisting conditions. The final treatment plan should be formulated after appropriate consultations. Every effort should be made to coordinate care with other specialists, as needed.

Surgical repair also should follow routine guidelines. Reconstruction of hard tissue should be given priority over repair of soft tissue injuries. When taking care of panfacial

TABLE 30-1. GENERAL CLASSIFICATION OF TRAUMA TO THE FACIAL SKELETON

A. Fractures of the skull base and upper third of face
B. Fractures of the middle third of face
   1. Central region
      a. Fractures of the nasal bones and/or nasal septum
      b. Naso-orbital fractures
      c. Maxillary fractures including Le Fort I and Le Fort II type fractures
   2. Centrolateral region
      a. Le Fort III type fractures
   3. Lateral region
      a. Fractures of the orbit (orbital rim, orbital walls)
      b. Fractures of the zygoma
      c. Fractures of the zygomatic arch
C. Dentoalveolar fractures
      a. Fractures of the alveolar bone
      b. Localized injuries of the teeth
D. Fractures of the mandible (lower third of face)
      a. Fractures of the (dentition-bearing) body of the mandible
      b. Fractures of the angle, ascending ramus, and coronoid process of the mandible
      c. Fractures of the condyle and the glenoid fossa
E. Dislocation, meniscal injury, distortion, and contusion of the temporomandibular joint

fractures, the orbits should be reconstructed first. Normal occlusion should be restored and secured before reestablishing mandibular continuity, including plating of condylar fractures, when needed. Bone plates must be applied to the correct site, sparing, for instance, the mandibular canal with its content. Optimum plate contouring when using conventional bone plates with bicortical screws and consideration of the lines of equal tension in the mandible when using miniplates or monocortical screws are prerequisites for success osteosynthesis.

When plating the maxilla, the nasomaxillary and zygomaticomaxillary buttresses are the most important pillars of

TABLE 30-2. CHECKLIST FOR EVALUATION OF PATIENTS WITH FACIAL TRAUMA

- Evaluate soft tissue of the face, nasal and oral cavities, as well as external auditory canal
- Examine function of all cranial nerves, including reaction of pupils, sensibility of facial skin, mobility of facial muscles, and ability to hear on both sides
- Palpate contours of bony skeleton (especially orbital rims, nose, malar bones, and zygomatic arches, as well the inferior border of the mandible) and check for irregularities
- Test physiologic mobility of lower jaw (i.e., temporomandibular joint) and press the chin into a posterosuperior direction guiding the condyles into the fossae
- Look for any pathologic mobility of the mandible by using both hands or introducing a small spatula into suspicious interdental spaces
- Examine all 32 teeth (chipped, mobile, missing, dental restorations complete) and their gingival collar

TABLE 30-3. MANAGEMENT OF PANFACIAL FRACTURES

1. Life-saving measures first
2. Neurosurgical interventions when needed
3. Ophthalmologic procedures for globe injuries
4. Reconstruction of the facial skeleton in the following order:
   Reduction and stabilization of orbital bones
   Reestablishment of dental occlusion
   Restoration of mandibular continuity
   Reconstruction of maxilla and nose
5. Soft tissue repair including
   Repair of nerve injuries and ducts
   Direct repair using local or distant flaps
6. Postoperative monitoring to prevent and treat airway obstruction, bleeding, neurologic sequelae, and infection

the midface that require reconstruction with miniplates. It is extremely important to always ensure continuous *cooling* of the low-speed drill, because high speed produces high temperatures that can damage osteocytes. Devitalized bone in turn leads to early loosening of screws, loss of stability, and infection of the bones. When using a plating system, it is necessary to use enough screws (at least two on either side of the fracture plus at least one in every small fragment interposed) to ensure maximum stability. This is essential for optimum fracture healing (Fig. 30-2). Finally, the plates must be long enough to completely cover the whole fracture site. Utmost care must be taken not to place a screw—not even "just the tip" of a screw—into the line of a fracture, as such practice could greatly increase the chance of bone infection. It is of major importance to maintain as many bony fragments as possible, as only then one is able to reestablish midfacial height by reconstructing the maxilla and nasal

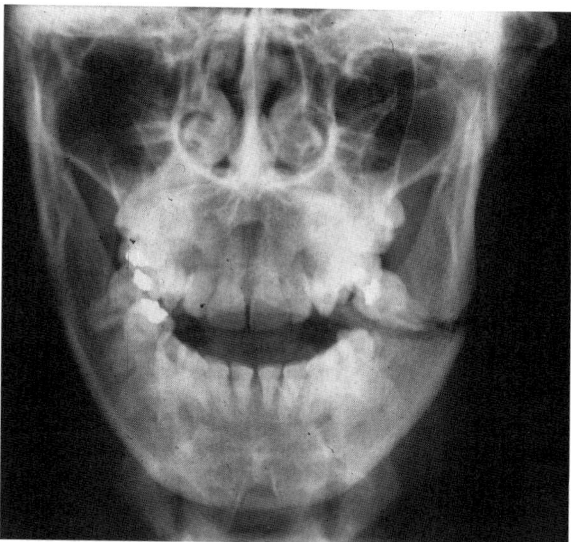

FIGURE 30-1. Plain head radiograph (anteroposterior view) of a 33-year-old woman exhibiting fresh mandibular fracture at left angle and old fracture at left mandibular neck. There was a bony step but no pain on digital pressure.

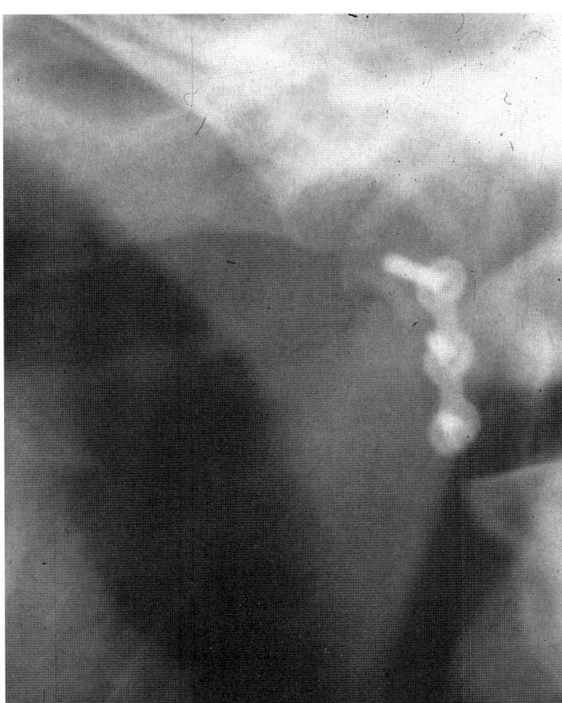

FIGURE 30-2. Section of orthopantomogram depicting dislocated mandibular head following osteosynthesis with only three screws.

bones. If significant bony gaps are present, liberal use of bone grafts is recommended to reestablish continuity, promote healing, and maintain facial dimensions.

Finally, soft tissue repair should be undertaken. If adequate soft tissue is available after debridement of all devitalized tissue, primary closure should be performed. When local tissue is not adequate for tension-free closure, local, regional, and even free flaps must be used. Soft tissue repair should include, when needed, microsurgical suturing of nerves and lacrimal and salivary ducts (Table 30-3).

General Rules for Evaluation

The goals of treatment of any type of maxillofacial trauma include restoration of facial function and facial aesthetics.

TABLE 30-4. FACTORS IMPORTANT FOR FUNCTION OF THE JAWS AND SURROUNDING TISSUES

- Function of all cranial nerves (especially I, II, III, IV, V, VI, VII, VIII)
- Free upper airway and adequate drainage of paranasal sinuses, including integrity and appropriate position of nasal septum
- Integrity of lacrimal and salivary ducts
- Function of temporomandibular joints (especially maximum interincisal distance, laterotrusion, and protrusion)
- Occlusion and integrity of teeth, including form and vitality of teeth
- Growth and development (in pediatric patients)

TABLE 30-5. ADDITIONAL FACTORS IMPORTANT FOR AESTHETICS OF THE JAWS AND SURROUNDING TISSUES

- Integrity of skin and "invisibility" of scars
- Symmetry and harmony of skeletal and soft tissue proportions in all three dimensions, especially of the glabella and nose, content of the orbits, middle third of the face and malar bones, as well as shape, projection, and growth of mandible
- Color and alignment of teeth

When considering all aspects relevant to the function and aesthetics of the face and jaws, there are two lists that are helpful in planning the individual treatment of a patient with fresh maxillofacial injuries and in avoiding unnecessary additional harm to the patient during treatment. Because these lists (Tables 30-4 and 30-5) also are useful for evaluating outcome following treatment of fractures of the jaws and determining possible unfavorable results, they are used as guidelines when discussing every individual type of fracture in this chapter.

DETAILED DISCUSSION OF UNFAVORABLE RESULTS FOLLOWING TREATMENT AND THERAPY OF JAW FRACTURES

In diversion from the general classification of facial bone fractures listed in Table 30-1, this detailed discussion begins with the most cranially located fractures of the upper jaws, as described in 1901 by Rene Le Fort (6–8). Discussion of maxillary, mandibular, and alveolar (and dental) fractures follows.

Special Aspects of Le Fort III and Le Fort II Fractures

When treating subcranial fractures located at the plane of cleavage between the neurocranium and face, the timing and approaches may vary considerably and should be individualized for each patient (9,10). Unfavorable conditions and unfavorable results, however, can be discussed, regardless of the treatment method chosen.

Preoperative or intraoperative, and rarely postoperative, pharyngeal, palatal, or *nasal hemorrhage* is a presenting symptom and complication of all fractures of the middle third of the face. Anterior nasal hemorrhage and bleeding from the palatine vessels most often is neither hazardous nor life threatening. An anterior nasal packing or a deep suture (or vessel clip) at the greater palatine foramen normally will suffice.

As an emergency measure, placement of an anterior and posterior nasal pack, in addition to and directly following oral intubation, is the easiest and most often successful technique used for uncontrollable nasopharyngeal bleeding.

However, rapid "impaction" of the loose maxillary block and stabilization at the time of surgery or simple subcutaneous wire suspension after upper dental arch bar application may be necessary, in addition to nasal packing, to control bleeding.

Secondary hemorrhage from posttraumatic or postoperative infection may require a second-look operation, with clipping or tying of the bleeding vessel. In addition, one should determine that the laboratory values of all clotting factors are normal.

Anosmia is a rare postoperative sequela and normally cannot be attributed to treatment modalities. However, smelling capacity needs to be checked preoperatively for legal reasons. There is no treatment for anosmia when the upper airway is patent.

Loss of vision, impeded ocular rotation, and reactions of the pupils to light and accommodation are important symptoms that need to be recognized before surgery. Injuries to the globes, eyelids, and lacrimal ducts also should be determined preoperatively. When reconstructing the orbital rim and orbital walls, one has not only to remove small bony fragments, possibly piercing the extraocular muscles, but also to reshape the orbit completely in order to recreate its proper form, volume, and position.

Next to infection, *intraorbital hemorrhage* is the foremost danger in the postoperative phase. Retrobulbar hematoma, including the orbital apex syndrome (involvement of cranial nerves II, III, IV, V, VI) and the superior orbital fissure syndrome (cranial nerves III, IV, V, VI), may be caused by injury to either the posterior ethmoidal or the infraorbital artery during surgery. Such bleeding may lead to blindness if the increased pressure is not recognized early. Hemophilia and von Willebrand-Jürgens syndrome should be considered and looked for, especially in the first 24 hours after surgery. In any event, immediate drainage is mandatory.

Enophthalmos and inward displacement of the content of the orbit by more than 3 mm resulting in diplopia are typical conditions often noted several weeks postoperatively (Fig. 30-3). Occasionally it is seen immediately after injury and must be followed closely. Displacement of the globe may be the result of incomplete reconstruction of all four orbital walls or imperfect leveling of the orbital floor (11). In both cases, the result is an orbit that is too wide for the intraorbital content. Reconstruction using cartilage grafts has proven to work nicely. As a rule of thumb, 0.5 mL of graft volume will bring the eyeball forward by about 1 mm. Bone grafts also can be used to reconstruct the anatomy and contour of the orbit. Enophthalmos may be accompanied by *ptosis* of the eyelid, which most often is corrected simply by treating enophthalmos successfully.

Diplopia persisting even after perfect reconstruction of the bony orbit and release of muscular adhesions may be due to primary damage to the cranial nerves or the extraocular muscles, or both. Posttraumatic scarring of these muscles is a typical cause for this type of complication. As postoperative muscle imbalance may persist for 3 to 6 months, repair by shortening or lengthening the ocular muscles should be considered only 6 to 12 months after the final maxillofacial surgical procedure.

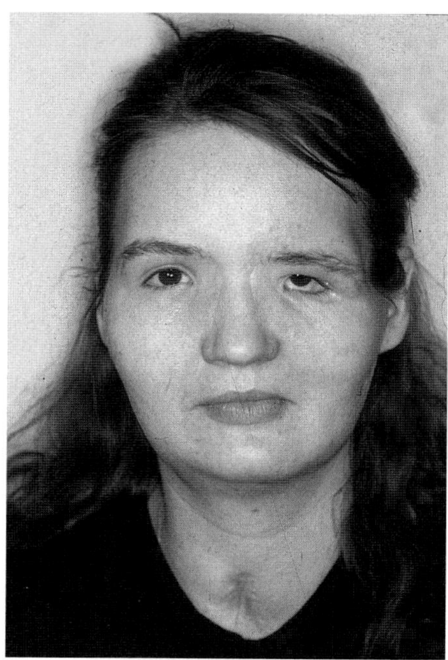

FIGURE 30-3. A 30-year-woman with enophthalmos and downward displacement of the zygoma and globe following a fall from a balcony.

Hypesthesia, paresthesia, and *anesthesia* of the branches of the trigeminal nerve are problems encountered posttraumatically or postoperatively. Decompression of the nerve during exploration and reduction of the fracture may be helpful in those cases where the fracture line runs through the foramen; however, decompression does not necessarily improve sensibility.

Infections such as an *orbital abscess* or *phlegmon* must be treated immediately by incision and drainage to prevent extension of the infection into the brain, damage to the plate, and blindness (Fig. 30-4). Other types of infections, *foreign bodies,* and postoperative sinusitis, as well as *mucoceles* (Fig. 30-5), are possible complications. Predisposing factors include preexisting sinusitis that has not been treated, impeded nasal airway passage, and free air circulation to the paranasal sinuses. Routine operations such as antrostomy, foreign body extraction, rhinoplasty, and septal reconstruction are the treatments of choice.

Tetanus booster vaccination is recommended for all soft tissue injuries.

Repair of an anterior *septal perforation* may be necessary if the patient is bothered by an inspiratory noise. Laceration or *obstruction of the lacrimal duct* is another problem sometimes encountered following polytrauma to the face. Elimination of long-lasting epiphora, the overflow of tears, is very difficult. Any type of repair or dacryocystorhino-

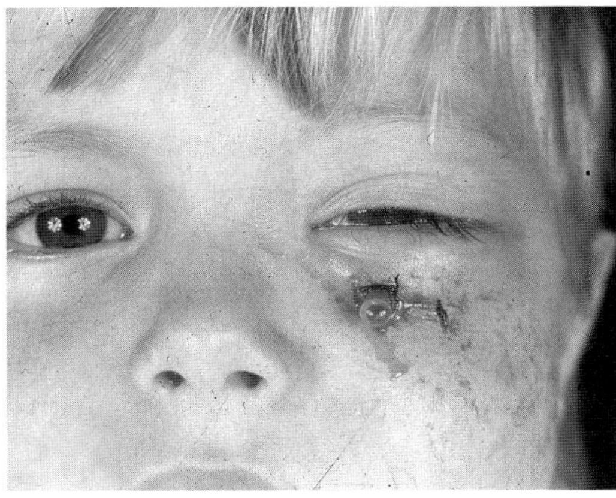

FIGURE 30-4. A 9-year-old boy with orbital abscess treated by incision and drainage.

stomy is recommended to address this problem. However, our experience with this type of complication is limited.

For functional disorders of the TMJ, occlusion, and mandibular growth, the reader is referred to the relevant sections later in this chapter. *Obvious scars* are the result of facial laceration, inappropriate design of the lines of incision, wound infection, or specific reaction of the skin of the individual patient.

For primary repair of Le Fort III and/or Le Fort II fractures, as well as repair of residual deformities, the following four approaches are recommended: (i) bicoronal incision, (ii) periorbital (especially lateral eyebrow and subciliary incision), (iii) transoral upper buccal sulcus approach, and (iv) approach through wounds or preexisting scars (9–11).

If scar revision is necessary, it should be performed several months after the initial repair. When the lower lid is too short, everted, or fixed to the bony infraorbital rim (Fig. 30-6), grafting of fat and/or full-thickness skin may be indicated in conjunction with surgical revision.

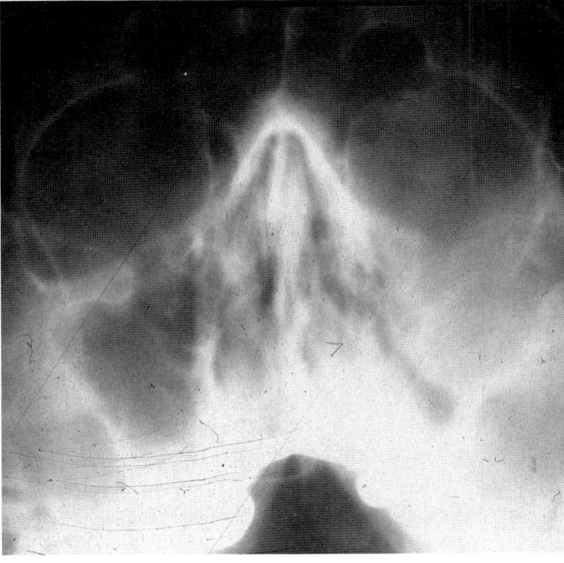

FIGURE 30-5. Radiogram (Waters view) of mucocele of the left maxillary sinus.

It is difficult to achieve symmetry and harmony of skeletal proportions in all three dimensions in every individual case. Diminished vertical dimension of the middle third of the face, a depressed zygomatic arch (especially with impingement on the coronoid), aesthetically unacceptable steps, or enophthalmos are classic indications for surgical treatment (Figs. 30-3 and 30-7). Removal of bony surplus, classic Le Fort I, II, or III osteotomies in conjunction with typical orthognathic surgery, repositioning of malunited fragments and of fractured osteosynthesis material, as well as inlay and onlay bone grafts, are methods used to treat asymmetry.

Preoperative photographs, lateral head radiographs, three-dimensional computed tomographic (CT) visualization, and hard foam models made by computer-aided design/modeling (using the patient's CT data) are helpful in planning the appropriate method for individual repair (Fig. 30-7).

Special Aspects of Le Fort I and Other Types of Maxillary Fractures

Subzygomatic central fractures of the maxilla, i.e., complete or incomplete separation of the inferior segment composed of the upper alveolar arch, the palatine vault, and part of the pterygoid process, are discussed in this section. Le Fort I fracture corresponds to the so-called Guérin fracture, which may be either incomplete or unilateral. Therefore, median or paramedian sagittal fractures also are found in this group of patients. This type of trauma formerly was treated by a combination of suspension wires, upper and lower arch bars with intermaxillary fixation, and possibly an additional palatal acrylic plate to maintain and stabilize the palatal vault. This method of therapy has been discontinued, and

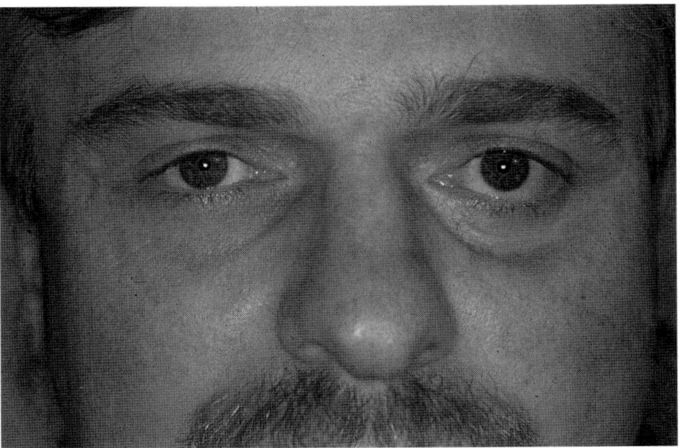

FIGURE 30-6. A 36-year-old man with left lower eyelid fixed by scar tissue to infraorbital rim after repair of a blow-out fracture.

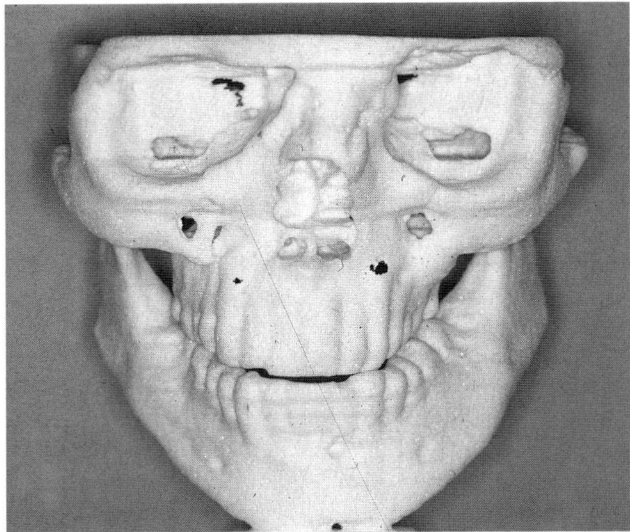

A

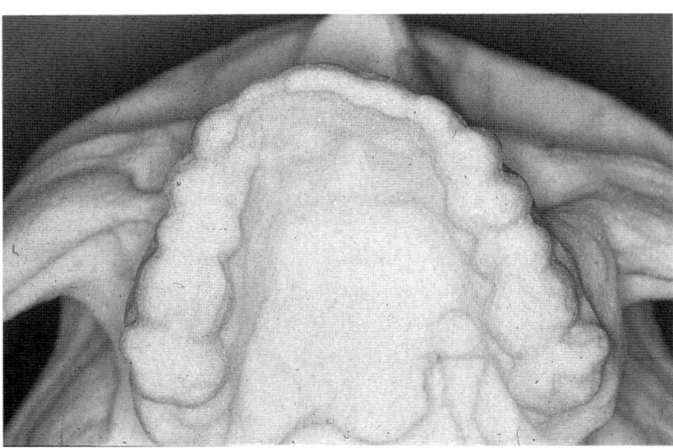

B

FIGURE 30-7. A,B: Styrofoam model of 20-year-old woman demonstrating displacement of the upper jaw and deformed upper dental arch after a motor vehicle accident.

miniplate and microplate osteosynthesis is used instead (9–11). The unfavorable results and their treatment are as follows: preoperative, intraoperative, and postoperative nasal, palatal, or nasopharyngeal *hemorrhage* is treated in the same manner as Le Fort II and Le Fort III fractures. Injury to branches of the trigeminal nerve, especially sensory loss of the infraorbital, incisal, or palatine *nerves*, is encountered in some cases. Treatment of anesthesia, hypesthesia, or paresthesia of the infraorbital nerve was discussed in the previous section, but therapeutic measures to enhance poor or deficient sensibility of the nerves supplying the palatal mucosa currently are not known. Functional disorders of the TMJ, impairment of growth, malocclusion, and problems with the teeth are discussed later in this chapter. Loss of tissue and bone in the upper jaw will lead to *fistulas and deformities* if they are not treated adequately (Fig. 30-8). I have not yet experienced any case where partial necrosis of the maxilla was a sequela of trauma. However, in the pertinent literature on the treatment of sagittal fractures of the palate,

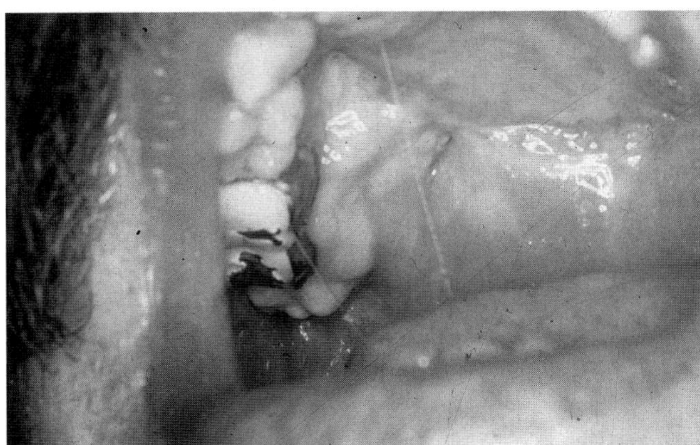

FIGURE 30-8. A 38-year-old man with palatal fistula close to tooth number 16 following alveolar bone fracture and tissue loss due to a car accident.

particular attention is paid to the blood supply of the upper jaw. Plating palatal fractures by using the Le Fort I approach should only be done if arterial blood supply of the broken maxilla is guaranteed after down fracture.

Overt fistulas and defects must be closed using standard procedures known from cleft palate repair as well as reconstructive measures following tumor surgery. Such procedures include local flaps and temporalis muscle or temporal fascia flaps, bone transplantation, and dental implants, if necessary.

Loss of tissue or *scarring* in the upper labial sulcus may result in dysfunction or unaesthetic appearance of the upper lip. In isolated cases, the external nasal aperture may exhibit an unaesthetic flaring of the alae nasi posttraumatically. In such patients, buccal advancement, redraping of the gingiva and labial mucosa, and so-called alar pinch suture may be the easiest measures for repair. Sometimes secondary vestibuloplasty, buccal flaps, or tongue flaps may be used. The latter often can be performed at the same time as when the hardware (wires, screws, and plates) is removed, approximately 6 months after primary repair.

Special Aspects of Mandibular Fractures

It was noted earlier that there are several ways to classify fractures of the lower jaw (9,10). When discussing unfavorable results, it seems appropriate to use the classification presented in Table 30-1.

For fractures of the body of the mandible, mostly bearing teeth, treatment must begin with ensuring good occlusion by means of dental arch bars plus intermaxillary fixation (12). At the present time, bone plating is the next surgical step (13,14).

Fractures of the angle and the ascending ramus are treated in the same way. On the one side, occlusion and unimpaired function of the TMJ are most important; therefore, intermaxillary fixation is a prerequisite to repair, even though the fracture does not directly affect dentition. On the other side, application of arch bars (12) is especially simple in those cases, as the dental arches are intact and repositioning of fragments is only necessary at the time of bone plating in the operating room.

Fractures of the coronoid process are treated either the same way as other fractures of the ascending ramus or not at all. There is no danger of adverse sequelae following nonrepair of isolated fractures of the coronoid process.

In contrast, there are well-known and disagreeable sequelae that can occur after trauma to the TMJ complex. Severely dislocated fractures, especially fracture dislocations of the condyle, will lead to limitation of mediotrusion, symmetrical protrusion, and maximum interincisal distance. Therefore, surgical treatment with open reduction and fixation with bone plates or resorbable pins is being used more frequently for such trauma.

A typical problem in bilateral, compound, or comminuted fractures is the danger of obstruction of the *upper airways*. Bleeding, obstruction by foreign bodies (such as pieces of the denture, teeth, or loose bone fragments), and displacement of soft tissue (such as the tongue) need to be looked for and managed. First aid includes clearing the mouth and throat with a finger, placing an oropharyngeal or nasopharyngeal airway tube, and rolling the patient into a semiprone position. Endotracheal intubation or even tracheotomy, if deemed necessary, should be considered to avoid a fatal outcome.

Infection is always a danger, and antibiotics must be given in all cases of open fractures and where fracture lines are located in close proximity to teeth.

Osteomyelitis of the mandible (Fig. 30-9) is a possible complication that should be avoided by all means using early rigid fixation, ample soft tissue coverage, and appropriate antibiotics. Any fracture site that is continuously discharging pus should be considered infected. When such a complication occurs, I recommend the following five steps for treatment: (i) culture and sensitivity testing once a week for specific and long-term antibiotic therapy; (ii) removal of all infected material, foreign bodies, and sequestra, as well as teeth in the line of fracture; (iii) stabilization first by means of intermaxillary fixation or pin fixation if no other means are feasible; (iv) sometimes decortication according to Mowlem to enhance access of blood perfusion to the infected body of the mandible, which may be helpful; and (v) transplantation of cancellous bone in combination with rigid fixation by means of bone plates, if necessary, to manage residual bony gaps. One should try to use either an intraoral or an extraoral approach only to maximize the chances for the take of the graft.

Nonunion and *pseudarthrosis* (Fig. 30-9) are typical unfavorable long-term results of mandibular fracture healing. Treatment is rather straightforward. First, occlusion should be reestablished and secured by rigid fixation. Then—at the same time—a cancellous bone graft is fixed and stabilized between the two mandibular bone stumps by means of rigid bone plating. It is best to first scrape both stumps with a rongeur and to induce bleeding to enhance the chances for the take of the graft.

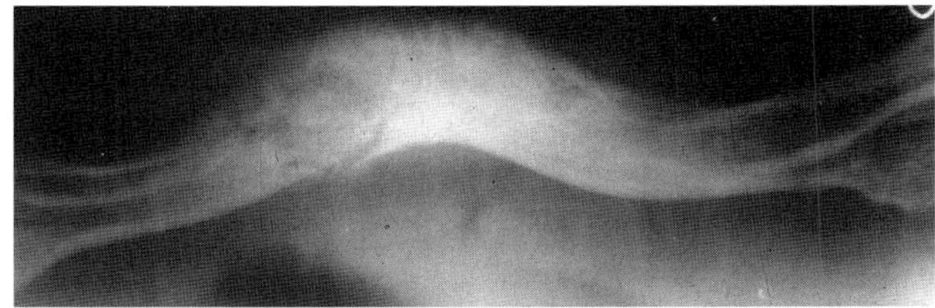

A

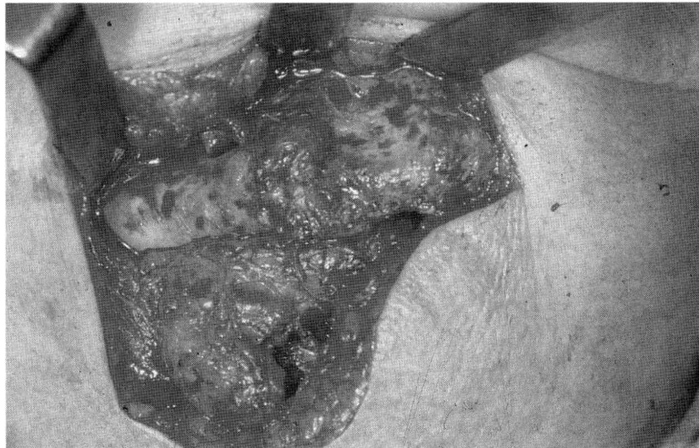

B

FIGURE 30-9. A 79-year-old woman with osteomyelitis and pseudoarthrosis following fracture of the mandible. **A:** Radiogram (status X, a special type of panoramic radio-graphic technique). **B:** Intraoperative view.

When doing so, careful attention should be paid to the integrity of the inferior alveolar nerve (and possibly the facial and the lingual nerves) by painstakingly dissecting it out of the scar tissue before proceeding with the operation. When drilling the holes, one should take care not to injure any root of the teeth or the inferior alveolar canal. Gross comminution and significant bony loss due to trauma are other indications for bone grafts. In such cases, primary bone grafting is the treatment of choice. One prerequisite for this procedure is good soft tissue coverage. If this is not guaranteed, it is possible first to stabilize the fracture and allow the bone to heal. Such a procedure can be followed by distraction osteogenesis to reestablish good occlusion, an anatomical form, and contour.

Extreme atrophic mandibles are difficult to treat when fractured (Fig. 30-10). Several aspects must be considered when such a problem is encountered. The fragments should not be denuded from the periosteum, as done otherwise. The holes should be drilled through the periosteal layer, and plates (and screws) are placed on top of the periosteum. The bone plates used should be extra long to provide better stability. It should be remembered that the holes drilled to place a screw are themselves decreasing the strength and stability of the mandible. In addition, the drill holes must not injure the inferior alveolar nerve. Onlay bone grafts can be used to enhance bone healing and stability, when needed.

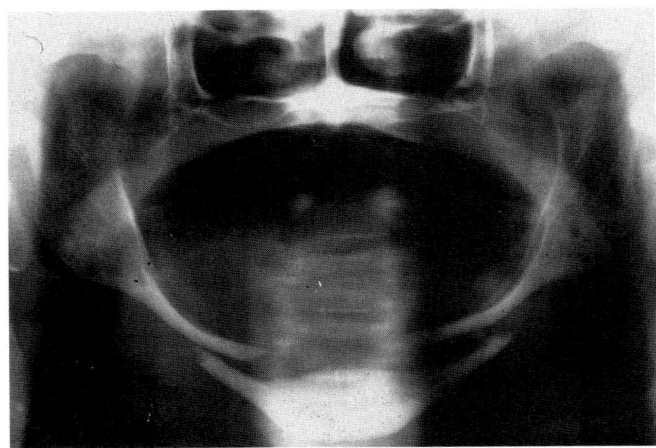

FIGURE 30-10. Orthopantomogram of a 75-year-old woman with bilateral mandibular fractures. The lower jaw is extremely atrophic (thin).

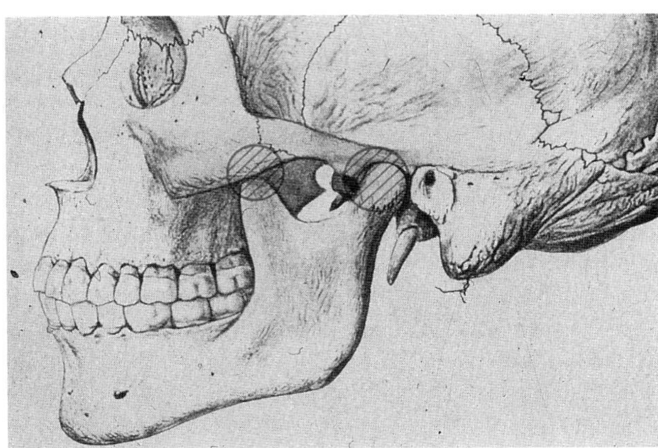

FIGURE 30-11. Sketch indicating two typical locations for ankylosis of mandible (lateral aspect): coronoid process and condylar process (temporomandibular joint).

Anesthesia, hypesthesia, painful hypesthesia, and paresthesia of the *mental nerve* are classic unfavorable results following mandibular fractures (and mandibular osteosynthesis). Before any surgical intervention, consider the following: normally the inferior alveolar nerve will recover within a year if proper repositioning of the mandibular fragments has been achieved and continuity of the bony mandibular canal has been reestablished. If continuity of the inferior alveolar nerve itself is interrupted and optimum conditions for the mandibular canal cannot be achieved, then microsurgical repair may be considered. Here, a nerve graft and possibly paramandibular deviation of the nerve are measures to be discussed, but they are not performed routinely to treat these complaints. In contrast, painful hypesthesia is a serious condition in which microsurgical revision and excision of a traumatic neuroma, followed by reconstruction using a nerve graft, are routine measures. One should always take care not to injure the alveolar nerve in its canal during osteosynthesis. Therefore, the plates should be placed either well below the canal when bicortical screws for compression osteosynthesis are used or above the canal and below the dental root tips when the monocortical miniplate technique is used.

Good function of the TMJ is a prerequisite for perfect rehabilitation following fracture of the mandible. There are several possibilities for impairment of TMJ function. Differential diagnosis should include preexisting ankylosis of the TMJ; defects of the condyle, posttraumatic internal derangement, and arthrosis (compare section E in Table 30-1); impingement on the coronoid; and scarring and/or myositis ossificans of the masticatory muscles.

Ankylosis is a problem in diacapitular fractures and cases of hemarthrosis, when intermaxillary fixation was maintained for too long (Fig. 30-11). In these cases, remobilization should begin 3 to 7 days after immobilization, if ever possible. When ankylosis is likely to occur, immediate training to move the mandible and open the mouth should be instituted. Widening the maximum interincisal distance with the patient under general anesthesia and inserting an intermaxillary acrylic block to guarantee a wide opening may be indicated (15). Mouth opening training should follow on the third day post-anesthesia and controlled for months. If ankylosis is already manifest, surgical repair should be performed as soon as possible. Although various techniques are advocated, we have achieved very good results by inserting a Silastic sheet or block for 6 months. First, the joint space obliterated by bone needs to be opened, then that space needs to be widened until the chin is located in the midline again, and finally the Silastic block is inserted before the skin is closed in layers. Such an operation should be followed by training joint function, as described earlier. Six months later, the foreign material is removed and the condyle can be reconstructed using a rib graft.

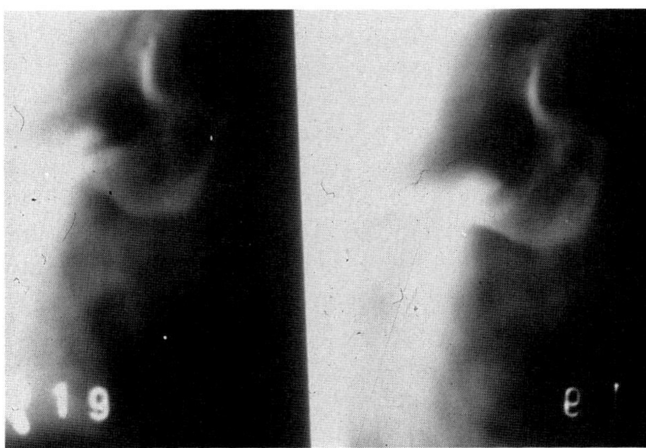

FIGURE 30-12. Two planes of classic radiographic tomogram depicting elongated coronoid (on the left side) hitting the zygoma (right side) when the patient attempts to open the mouth.

Defects of the condyle can be reconstructed using a rib graft carrying a small amount of cartilage.

Internal derangement and *degenerative arthrosis* are typical sequelae following fractures or blunt trauma to the TMJ. These conditions should be mentioned when an expert's opinion is requested. In addition, they are well-known disorders that can occur without any knowledge of major trauma. They should be treated as follows. When possible, the disc should be repositioned, but this is not always feasible. Here again, inserting a Silastic sheet for 6 months has proved to be a successful method. After the foreign material is removed 6 months postoperatively, the newly created scar tissue surrounding the Silastic material is left in place and acts as an artificial disc.

Impingement on the coronoid (Fig. 30-12), possibly pseudarthrosis between the coronoid process and the zygomatic arch (Fig. 30-11) or even the temporal bone, is treated by resection of the bone that interferes with mandibular mobility. In some cases, a displaced and malunited zygoma results in impingement on the coronoid. In such cases, repositioning of the zygoma will correct the problem. In any case, well-controlled training of mouth opening is a necessary adjunct to surgery. This also is true when there is ankylosis between the mandible and the pterygoid plate, as seen in two of our patients (Fig. 30-13).

Scarring of the masticatory muscles and posttraumatic ossifying myositis are rare postoperative complications. I have encountered this condition twice in my career (Fig. 30-14). In both cases, excision of the calcified scar-like tissue and postoperative exercises cured the limitation of motion successfully.

It is well known that *mandibular growth* in children may be impaired by trauma to the condyle (Fig. 30-15). The reason probably is not that any kind of "growth center" is disturbed, as still can be read in many old textbooks. Today, most authorities believe that function is steering and stimulating growth in the craniomaxillofacial complex. In the case of a fractured condyle, when the mandibular head is dislocated, the insertion of the lateral pterygoid muscle is dislocated as well. Thus, the action of the whole muscle is not effective, and the mobility of the whole mandible and consequently the stimulation of growth are hindered grossly. This, in turn, leads to asymmetrical development of first the lower and then the middle third of the face. This is why I personally advocate open reduction and internal fixation by means of bone plates in children (ages 8 years and older) with fracture dislocations of the condyle. Such an approach not only enables physiologic growth, but it also takes care of and helps to ensure symmetry and harmony of mandibular proportions in juveniles.

Major disturbances of the symmetry and proportions of the craniomaxillofacial complex in all three dimensions, as well as minor disturbances in dental occlusion and postoperative problems with the teeth, are discussed later.

Scars resulting from trauma are treated using routine measures, as with other scars of the body. If an extraoral incision is necessary to approaching a mandibular fracture, it should be placed into inconspicuous submandibular folds or in the preauricular area. In both areas, injury to any branch of the facial nerve should be carefully avoided. The facial nerve can be traumatized at the time of the initial injury and should be treated at the time of primary repair using microsurgical techniques.

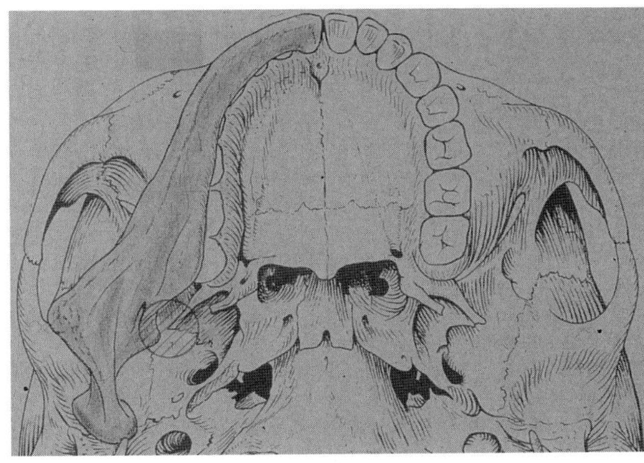

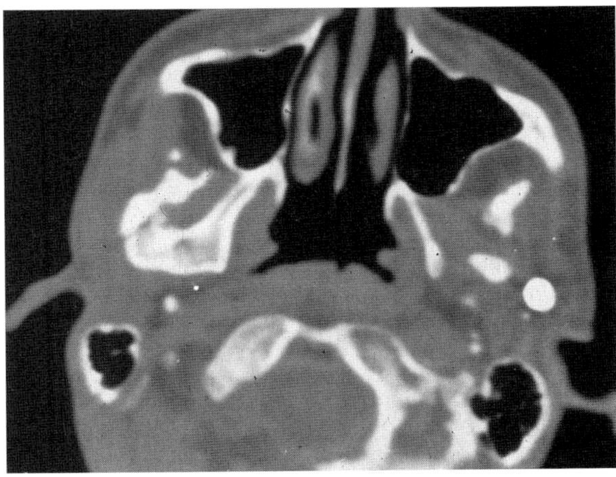

FIGURE 30-13. Ankylosis between the medial aspect of the mandible and the lateral pterygoid plate. **A:** Sketch (view from below). **B:** Computed tomographic scan of 20-year-old man exhibiting massive bony ankylosis on his right side.

Unfavorable Results in Dental Occlusion Resulting from Dentoalveolar, Complex, Comminuted, or Combined Fractures of the Jaws

Malocclusion can be found in patients with or without a medical history of fractures of the jaws. However, if malocclusion is of a posttraumatic nature, it needs to be taken seriously and corrected. As with upper airways and vision, dental occlusion is an important criterion for optimum posttraumatic function (Fig. 30-7). Perfect occlusion goes hand in hand with facial aesthetics and the well-being of the patient.

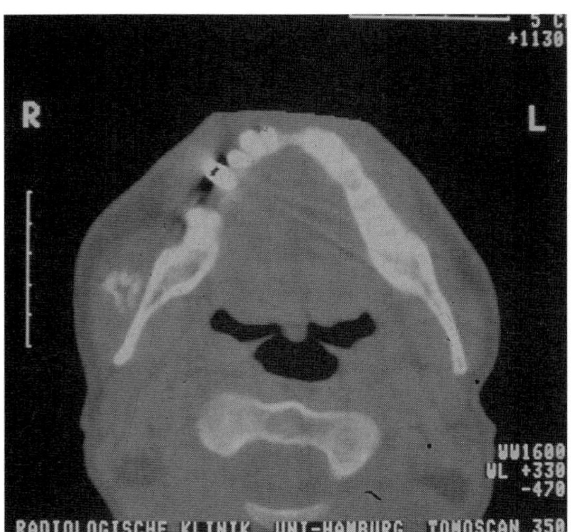

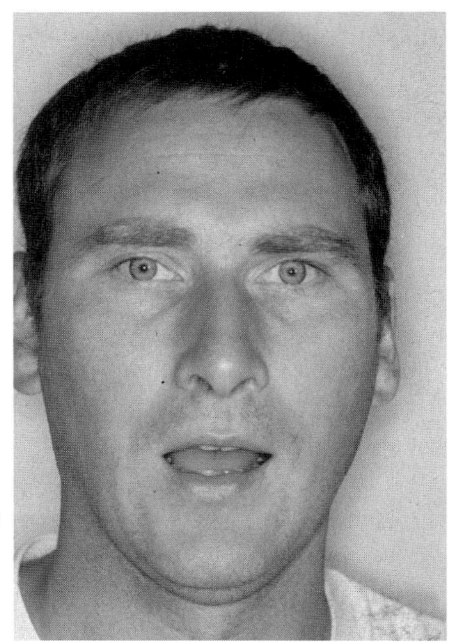

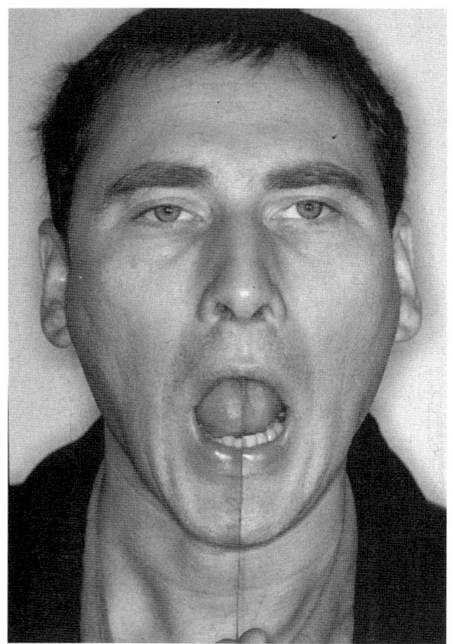

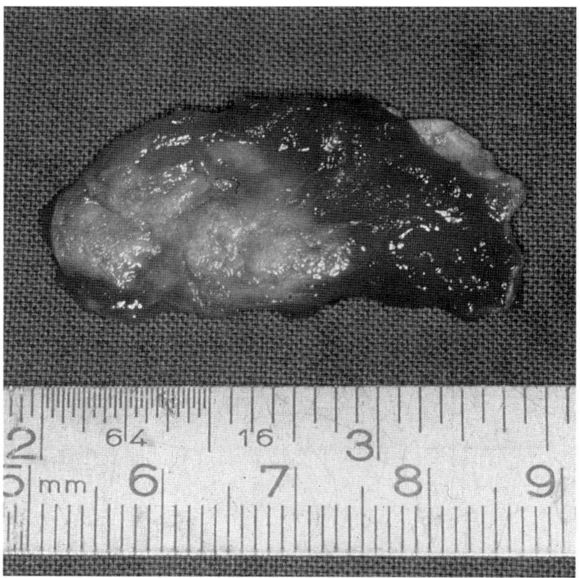

FIGURE 30-14. Ossifying myositis. **A:** Computed tomographic scan of a 66-year-old man with calcification in the right masseter muscle. **B:** A 33-year-old man with restricted mouth opening (before surgery). **C:** Same patient with wide open mouth after surgery. **D:** Piece of calcified muscle removed from right temporal muscle.

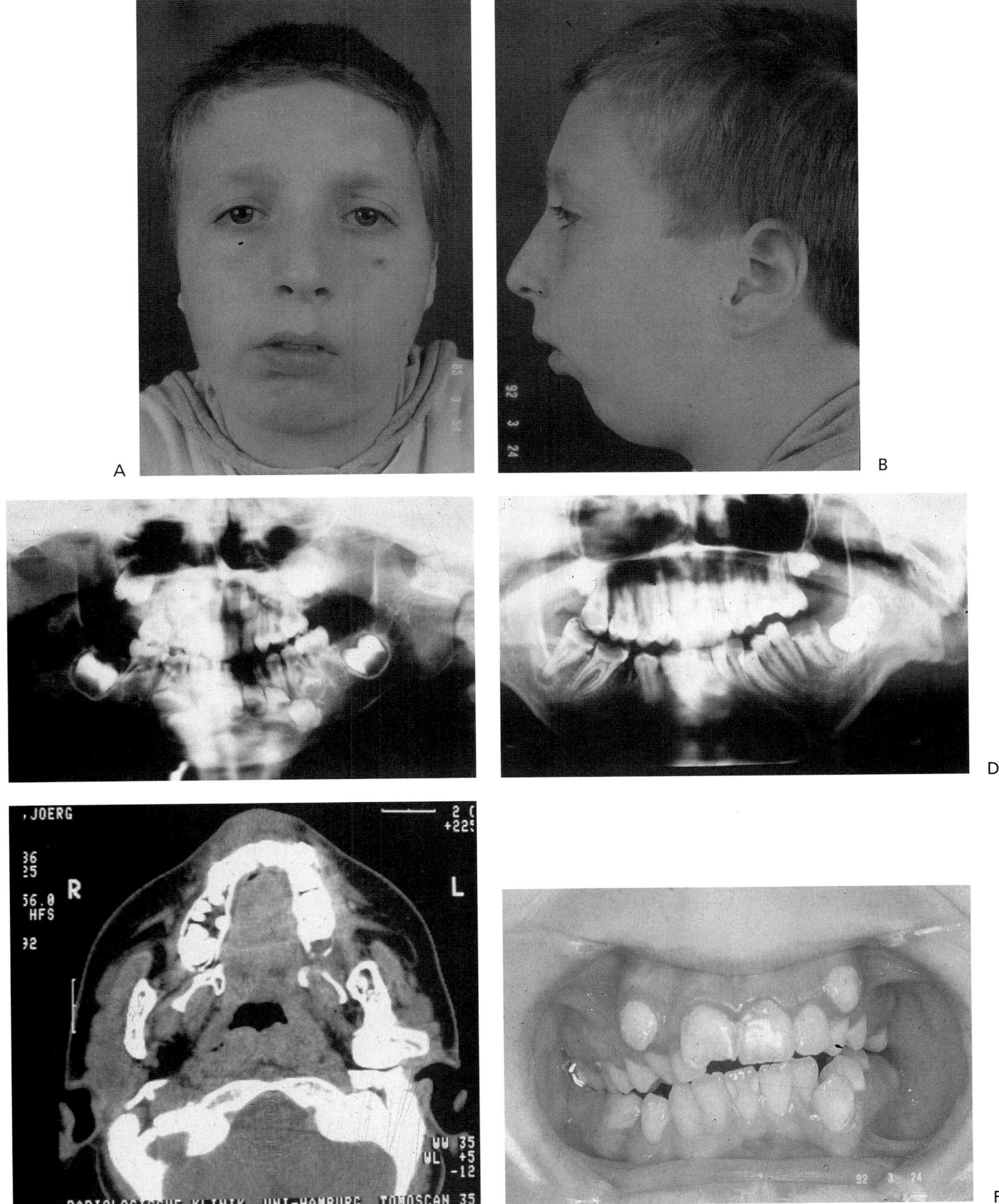

FIGURE 30-15. **A:** A 15-year-old boy with a chin deviation to the left as a result of retarded mandibular growth. **B:** Result after bony ankylosis of the temporomandibular joint (TMJ). **C:** Panoramic radiograph depicting early posttraumatic ankylosis of the left TMJ after inadequate treatment of a left condylar fracture. **D:** Preoperative panoramic radiograph 10 years after injury. **E:** Preoperative computed tomographic scan depicting the ankylosis. **F:** Occlusion with maximum interincisal distance before surgery. *(continued)*

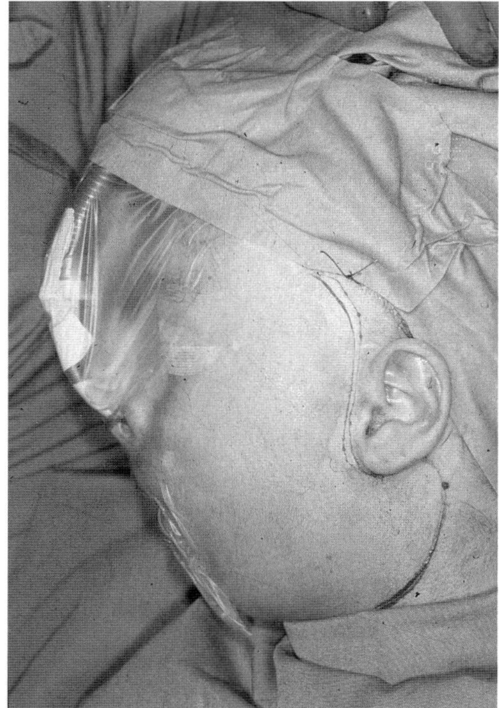
G

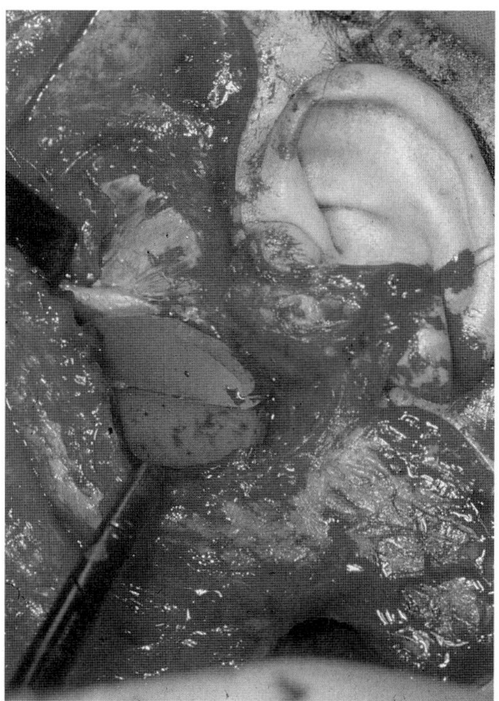
H

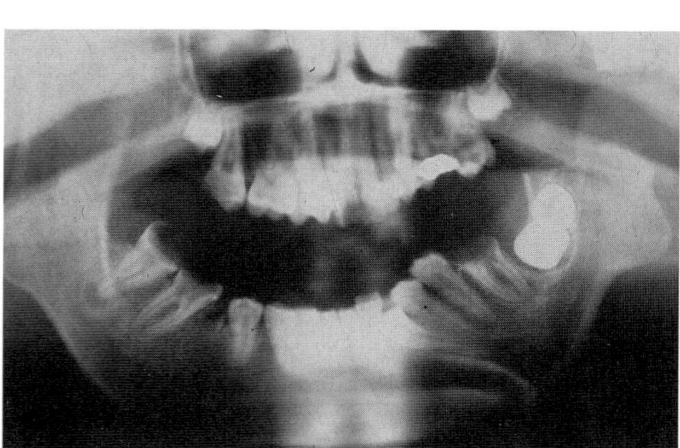
I

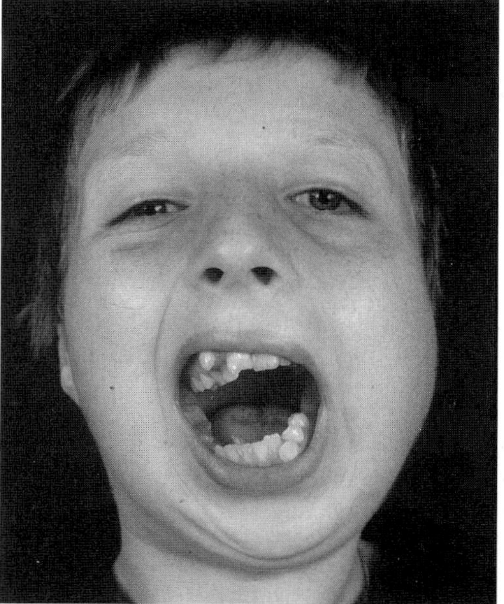
J

FIGURE 30-15. *Continued.* **G:** Preauricular incision with markings for possible extension. **H:** Intraoperative view: two blocks of Silastic *in situ* after osteotomy. **I:** Postoperative panoramic radiograph depicting two Silastic blocks between fossa and ascending ramus on the left. **J:** Maximum interincisal distance after surgery. Note the improvement in facial symmetry while occlusion planes are still oblique in both jaws.

Malocclusion can result from malalignment of just a single tooth or of a small or a larger segment of the alveolar process, or from malunion of one or more fractures in either one or even in both jaws. It may be the result of bone loss, be a sequela of posttraumatic infection, or result from nonunion of a fracture. Malocclusion is an unfavorable result, and it should be avoided and prevented by all means. Maximum stability of the fractures is the catchword, and the measures to this end are dental arch bars and intermaxillary fixation (9,10,12) applied during the operation plus bone plating (Fig. 30-16). Postoperatively, most often it is possible to release intermaxillary fixation. Of all current techniques, compression osteosynthesis with bicortical screws leads to maximum stability, which is most important for the mandible. There is one disadvantage for the inexperienced surgeon: even minor displacement of fragments cannot be corrected by function and muscle pull. Miniplate fixation is not as strong and should be used with caution (Fig. 30-17). Axial compression is not recommended for use in the middle third of the face, and miniplating is unanimously considered the therapy of choice for fractures of the maxilla.

Dental arch compression, laterognathia and cross bite, maxillary or mandibular prognathia or retrognathia (i.e., the classic "dish face"), open bite, maxillary impaction rather than maxillary vertical excess, and all combinations of dysgnathia are typical posttraumatic disfigurements that require simple orthodontic or combined orthodontic plus surgical orthognathic treatment (Fig. 30-18). These various types of acquired malocclusion call for various types of osteotomies. Median osteotomy of the mandible, surgical measures for rapid palatal expansion, anterior (16–18) as well as posterior (19), multiple piece, and total maxillary osteotomies of the Le Fort I, II, or III type (17,20) are possible. They should be followed by miniplate osteosynthesis and can be combined with bone grafting, if necessary. In the mandible, one may choose from anterior segmental osteotomies (21–23), bone cuts at the posterior part of the mandibular body (24–26), and various types of ramus osteotomies (17,19,27–30). They should be followed by rigid internal fixation. Bimaxillary osteotomies are another good method to correct posttraumatic malocclusion.

At the current time, distraction osteogenesis of the upper or lower jaw is a more sophisticated treatment for dysgnathia, disfigurement, and dysfunction. Limited experience is available, but with appropriate patient selection, planning, and execution, the initial results appear good.

Camouflage surgery in terms of bone or cartilage grafts only corrects problems related to *aesthetic facial disharmony*. It may help the patient's self-confidence, but malocclusion is not treated by such procedures.

Fractures of the alveolar bone are simple to treat, and long-term complications are rare if stabilization is ensured. If the alveolar process is dentate and the bone is adherent to teeth or mucosa, or both, application of arch bars for splinting the teeth and suturing the mucosa laceration is a sufficient form of treatment. If the alveolar process is edentulous, then most often single-layer suturing of the gingiva will suffice.

Finally, loss of tooth vitality is considered. Infected or abscessed teeth should be removed before osteosynthesis to prevent osteomyelitis (Fig. 30-19). Poor oral hygiene, gingivitis, and marginal periodontitis are other factors predis-

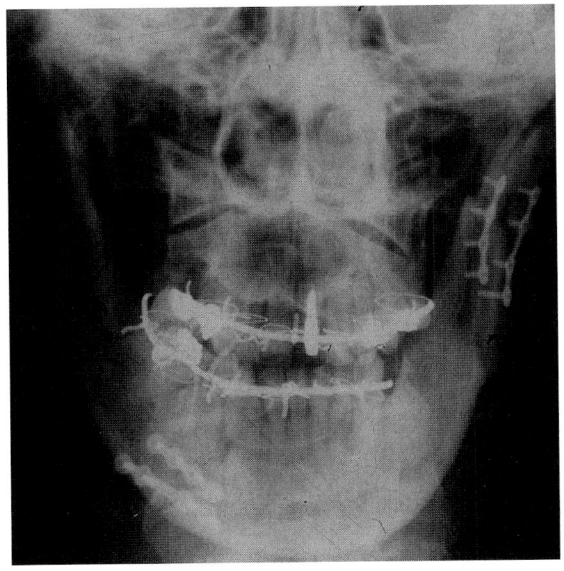

A

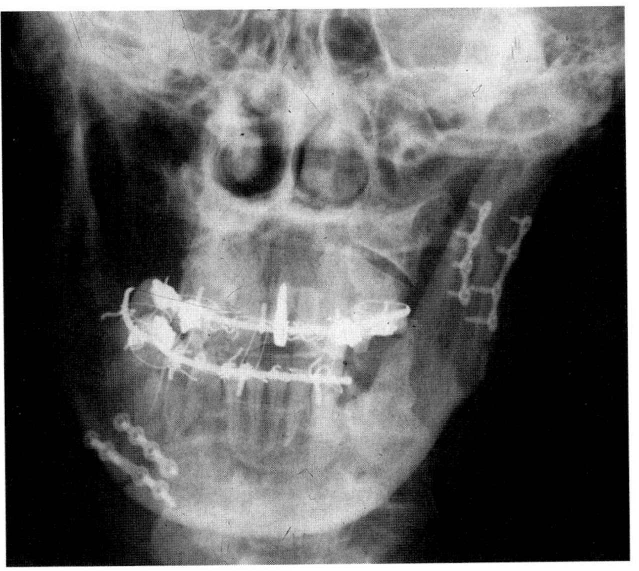

B

FIGURE 30-16. Head radiograph (anteroposterior view) of a 36-year-old man. **A:** Malocclusion after poor reconstruction of ascending ramus after osteosynthesis of a bilateral fracture of the mandible. **B:** Good occlusion after reosteosynthesis with midlines of lower and upper dental arch corresponding.

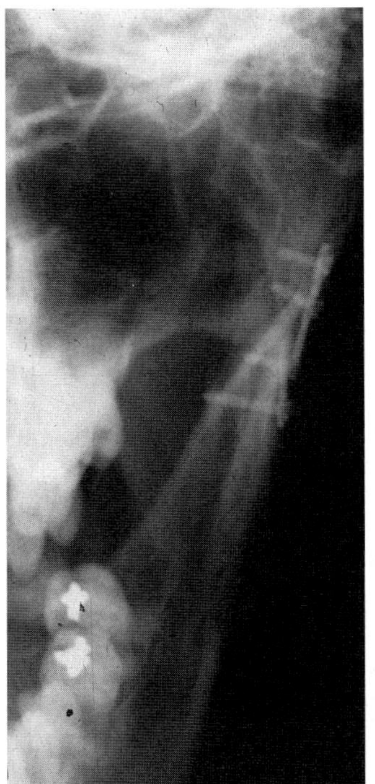

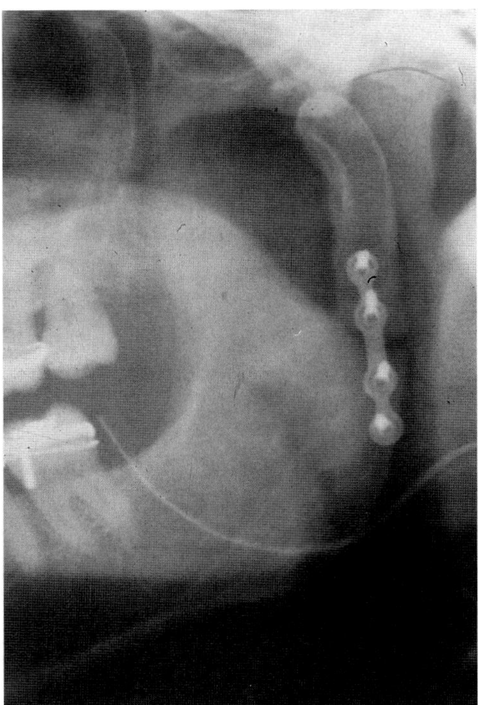

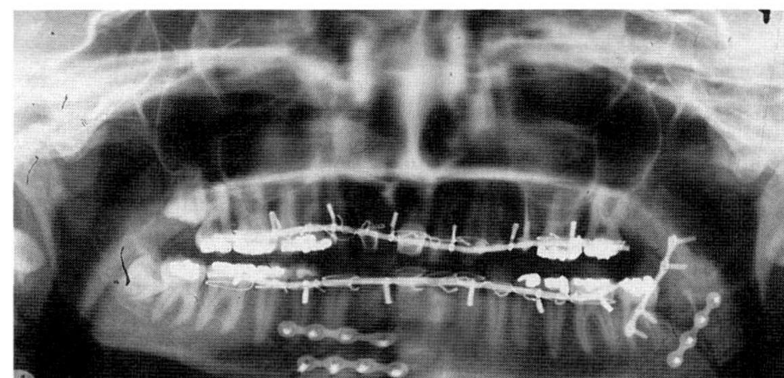

FIGURE 30-17. A: Section of radiograph (anteroposterior view) of a broken miniplate after osteosynthesis of a condylar fracture. **B:** Section of an orthopantomogram showing dislocated condyle after miniplate osteosynthesis. **C:** Orthopantomogram showing dislocated ascending ramus occurring after osteosynthesis with two miniplates on either side of the mandible in a case of bilateral fracture.

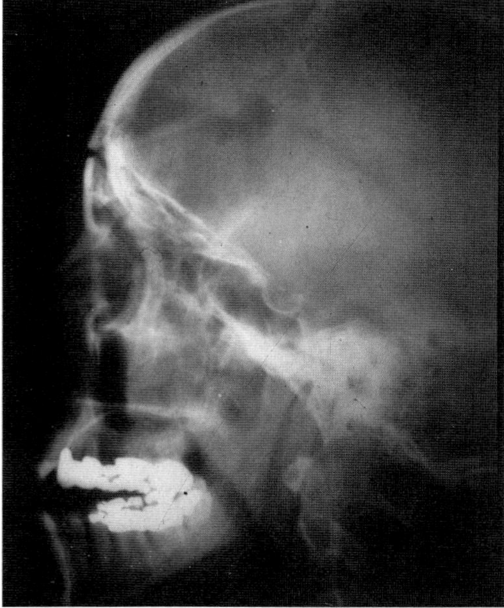

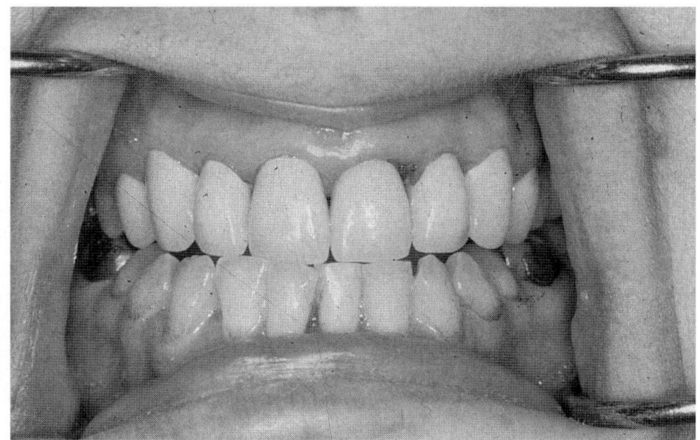

FIGURE 30-18. A: Posttraumatic lateral view of a 33-year-old woman with Le Fort II fracture malunited and displaced after a car accident and inadequate conservative treatment. **B:** Malocclusion with edge-to-edge bite. *(continued)*

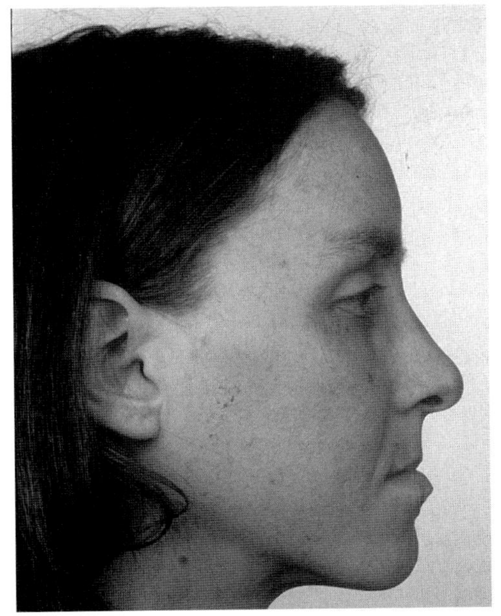

C

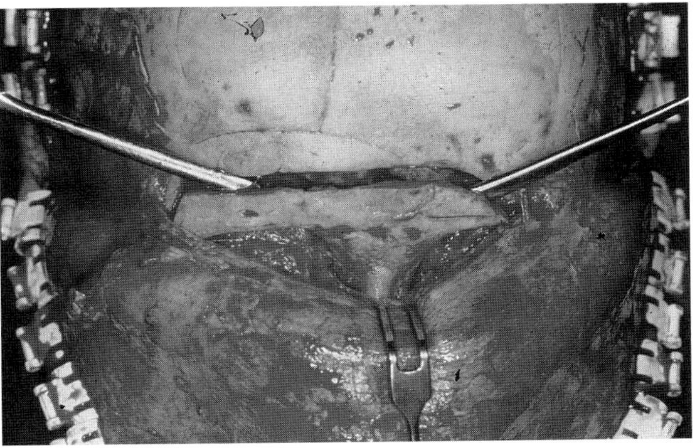

D

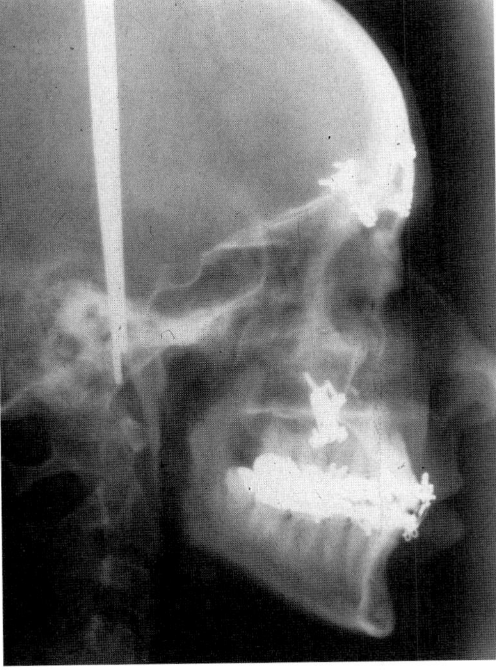

E

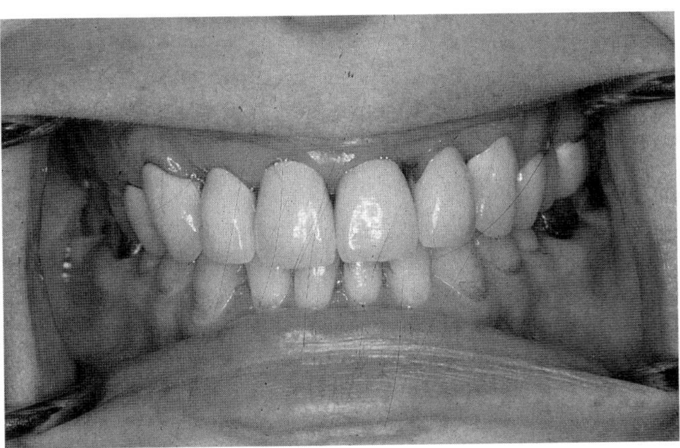

F

FIGURE 30-18. *Continued.* **C:** Significant retrusion of the midface. **D:** Intraoperative disimpaction and repositioning of the maxilla. **E:** Postoperative lateral radiograph with miniplates and arch bars still in place. *(continued)*

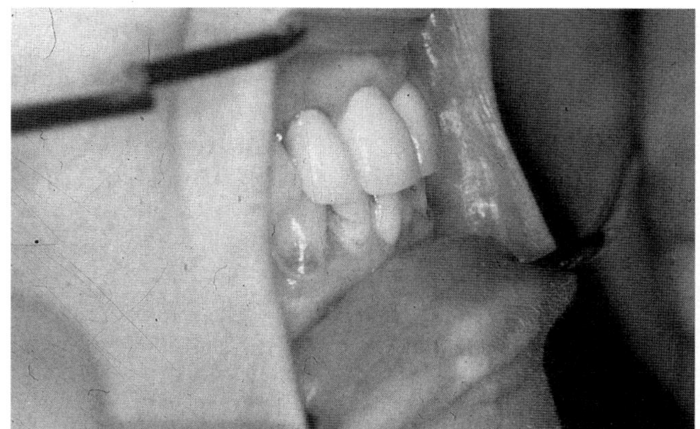
G

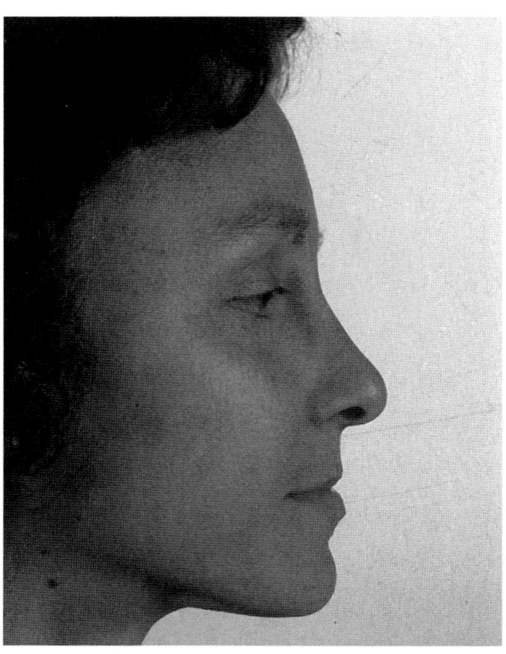
H

FIGURE 30-18. *Continued.* **F,G:** Occlusion 14 months after surgery with normal over jet. **H:** Lateral view of the patient 14 months after surgery. Note the significant improvement of the midfacial profile.

posing to infection of a fracture. Impacted teeth should be extracted, if they are in the line of the fracture, if they interfere with bone fragment reduction, or if removal is indicated in any way.

Dislocated avulsed teeth, complicated crown fractures with pulp exposed, and fractured or retained roots are problems that should be treated in the following manner. Teeth with exposed pulps require endodontic treatment. Loosened or partially displaced teeth require splinting. Completely avulsed teeth can be repositioned and splinted, unless they are located in the fracture line. Exarticulated teeth and teeth with fractured or isolated retained roots must be removed, if they are located in the fracture line, in order to avoid infection.

Devitalization or discoloration, or both, of teeth as a long-term unfavorable result may have several causes: crown infraction or dental concussion with consecutive pulp necrosis, internal resorption, or iatrogenic interference with the vascular supply of a tooth during osteosynthesis. Discoloration should be treated during long-term follow-up with sensitivity testing and roentgenograms. Endodontic treatment is the therapy of choice.

To avoid traumatic or iatrogenic injury to tooth buds in children with fractures of the jaws, the use of monocortical instead of bicortical screws is recommended in the pediatric population.

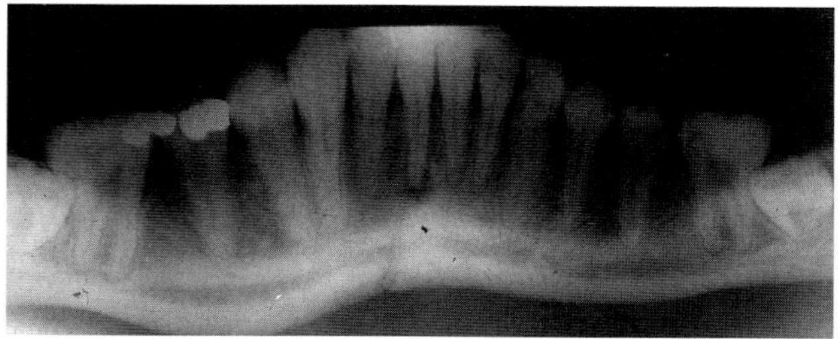

FIGURE 30-19. Status 7× (special panoramic technique) of mandible exhibiting periapical granuloma in the line of a fracture in a 34-year-old woman.

REFERENCES

1. Dingman RO, Izenberg PH. Complications of facial trauma. In: Conley JJ, ed. *Complications of head and neck surgery.* Philadelphia: WB Saunders, 1979:353–400.
2. Schuchardt K, ed. *Die operative Behandlung der Verletzungen des Gesichtschädels, Fortschr. Kiefer- u. Gesichtschir., vol. 19.* Stuttgart: Thieme, 1975.
3. Pfeifer G, Schwenzer N, eds. *Aufklärung, Fehler und Gefahren in der Mund-Kiefer-Gesichtschirurgie; Fortschr. Kiefer- u. Gesichts-Chir., vol. 30.* Stuttgart: Thieme, 1985.
4. Schwenzer N, Pfeifer G, eds. *Traumatologie des Mittelgesichts, Fortschr. Kiefer- u. Gesichtschir., vol. 36.* Stuttgart: Thieme, 1991.
5. Mathog RH. Complications of surgery for facial fractures. In: Weissler MC, Pillsbury HC III, eds. *Complications of head and neck surgery.* New York: Thieme, 1995.
6. Le Fort R. Experimental study on fractures of the upper jaw, part I, *Rev Chir* 1901;23:208–227.
7. Le Fort R. Experimental study on fractures of the upper jaw, part II. *Rev Chir* 1901;23:360.
8. Le Fort R. Experimental study on fractures of the upper jaw, part III. *Rev Chir* 1901;23:479–507.
9. Ewers R, Wild K, Wild M, et al. Traumatologie. In: Hausamen JE, Machtens E, Reuther J, eds. *Mund-, Kiefer- und*

Gesichtschirurgie, Kirschnersche allgemeine und spezielle Operationslehre, vol. II, 3rd ed. Berlin: Springer Verlag, 1995:211–298.
10. Horch HH, Herzog M. Traumatologie des Gesichtsschädels. In: Horch HH, ed. *Mund-Kiefer-Gesichtschirurgie I, Praxis der Zahnheilkunde, vol. 10/I,* 3rd ed. Munich: Urban & Schwarzenberg, 1997:53–163.
11. Gundlach KKH, Pfeifer G. Residual deformities, fractures of the zygomatic complex. In: Williams JLL, ed. *Rowe and Williams' maxillofacial injuries, vol. 2,* 2nd ed. Edinburgh: Churchill Livingstone, 1994:976–986.
12. Hopkins R. Mandibular fractures: treatment by closed reduction and indirect skeletal fixation. In: Williams JLL, ed. *Rowe and Williams' maxillofacial injuries, vol. 2,* 2nd ed. Edinburgh: Churchill Livingstone, 1994:283–327.
13. Gundlach KKH. Fractures of the mandible. In: Cohen M, ed. *Mastery of plastic and reconstructive surgery, vol. 2.* Boston: Little, Brown and Company, 1994:1165–1180.
14. Luhr HG. Principles of rigid bony fixation of the craniofacial skeleton. In: Cohen M, ed. *Mastery of plastic and reconstructive surgery, vol. 1.* Boston: Little, Brown and Company, 1994: 169–200.
15. Gundlach KKH. Long-term results following derangement of the temporomandibular joint. *J Craniomaxillofac Surg* 1990; 18:206–209.
16. Cohn-Stock G. Die chirurgische Immediatregulierung der Kiefer, speziell die chirurgische Behandlung der Prognathie. *Vjschr Zahnheilkd* 1921:37:320–354.
17. Wassmund M. *Lehrbuch der praktischen Chirurgie des Mundes und der Kiefer, vol. I.* Leipzig: Meusser, 1935:245–308.
18. Wunderer S. Die Prognathieoperation mittels frontal gestieltem Maxillafragment. *Österreich Z Stomatol* 1962;59:98.
19. Schuchardt K. Ein Beitrag zur chirurgischen Kieferorthopädie unter Berücksichtigung ihrer Bedeutung für die Behandlung angeborener und erworbener Kieferdeformitäten bei Soldaten. *Dtsch Zahn Mund Kieferheilkd* 1942;9:73.
20. Tessier P. Osteotomies totales de la face: syndrome de Crouzon, syndrome d'Apert, oxycephalies, scaphocéphalies. *Ann Chir Plast* 1967;12:273.
21. Hullihen SR. Case of elongation of the under jaw and distortion of the face and neck, caused by a burn, successfully treated. *Am J Dent Sci* 1849;9:157.
22. Hofer O. Die operative Behandlung der alveolären Retraktion des Unterkiefers und ihre Anwendungsmöglichkeit für Prognathien u. Mikrogenien. *Dtsch Zahn Mund Kieferheilkd* 1942;9:121.
23. Köle H. Bewährte form- und funktionsändernde chirurgische Eingriffe am Kausystem. *Österreich Z Stomatol* 1967;64:297.
24. Blair VP. Operations on jaw bones and face: study of aetiology and pathological anatomy of developmental malrelations of maxilla and mandible to each other and to facial outline and of operative treatment when beyond the scope of the orthodontist. *Gynecol Obstet* 1907;4:67–78.
25. Dingman RO. Surgical correction of mandibular prognathism, an improved method. *Am J Orthodont* 1944;30:683.
26. Delaire J. Sagittal splitting of the body of the mandible (Mehnert's technique) for correction of open bite and deep over bite. *J Maxillofac Surg* 1977;5:142.
27. Converse JM, Shapiro H. Treatment of developmental malformations of the jaw. *Plast Reconstr Surg* 1952;10:473.
28. Kazanjian VH. Surgical correction of mandibular prognathism. *Int J Orthodont* 1932;18:1224.
29. Obwegeser H. The indications for surgical correction of mandibular deformity by sagittal splitting technique. *Br J Oral Surg* 1963;1:157.
30. Trauner R. Eine neue Operationsmethode bei der Progenie. *Dtsch Zahn Mund Kieferheilkd* 1967;49:77.

Discussion

FRACTURES OF THE JAWS

SETH R. THALLER

Adverse outcomes arising during the management of jaw fractures may occur as a result of routine therapy, insufficient or improper treatment, iatrogenic errors, or lack of treatment. Complications may be subdivided further into acute complications, which primarily consist of airway compromise and hemorrhage; intermediate complications, which include improper fracture reduction, bone loss, bony displacement, and comminution, injury to the dentition and its supporting structures, soft tissue interposition between healing fracture segments, wound infection, and unrecognized concomitant fractures; and late complications, include malocclusion, delayed union, nonunion, malunion, osteomyelitis, tooth loss, temporomandibular joint (TMJ) ankylosis, and other related TMJ problems. A number of factors have been found to contribute to the development of these untoward sequelae complications, such as oral sepsis,

S. R. Thaller: Division of Plastic Surgery, University of Miami School of Medicine; and Division of Plastic Surgery, Jackson Memorial Hospital, Miami, Florida

teeth located in the line of fracture, bony displacement and comminution, underlying systemic diseases, fractures within the region of the mandibular angle, fractures involving the edentulous mandibles, subcondylar fractures, and pediatric jaw fractures. It must be stressed that even when all sound basic surgical principles are followed closely, unfavorable results still can occur in a relatively small group of patients who have sustained jaw fractures. In fact, it is quite fascinating that most jaw fractures are able to go on to uneventful recovery despite the distracting forces of rather strong muscles and the inhospitable milieu of the oral environment bathing the healing bony segments.

Bony injuries to the jaws should always be managed in an orderly and systematic manner. Definitive repair should be performed only after the patient's general status has been carefully documented and life-threatening problems satisfactorily addressed. A rigid checklist as suggested by Dr. Gundlach is extremely important, because complications frequently occur secondary to inadequate primary diagnosis. All concomitant injuries to the dentition and supporting structures must be attended to simultaneously. This aids in reestablishing the preinjury dental occlusion and function. These two goals remain the primary objective of all jaw fracture management. In general, I suggest using closed reduction techniques for grossly comminuted fractures when the overlying periosteum is intact, for pediatric fractures, and in the management of the majority of condylar fractures. Open approaches, on the other hand, may be used appropriately in the management of displaced fractures involving the angle or parasymphyseal region, inadequate outcomes from closed reduction techniques, and panfacial fractures where satisfactory vertical height must be achieved by adequate anatomical reduction of the condyles. When open reduction and internal fixation are used, a number of authors have reported a lower risk of complications when utilizing rigid fixation with miniplates and screws, thereby avoiding prolonged use of maxillomandibular fixation (1–10). In addition, it is important to point out that the reconstructive surgeon should adhere closely to Dr. Gundlach's guidelines for using rigid fixation and the additional need to obtain satisfactory soft tissue coverage of the hardware. By following these basic tenets, reconstructive surgeons will be able to restore facial function and aesthetics.

Dr. Gundlach provides the reader with a comprehensive discussion of the special aspects of Le Fort fractures and details associated complications.

I will try to limit my discussion to special aspects of mandibular fractures. General treatment modalities are directed toward restoring preinjury occlusion and function.

Infection remains the most commonly encountered complication in the management of mandibular fractures. Reported incidence ranges from 0.4% to 32% (11). A number of predisposing etiologic factors have been described (12). Chole and James (13) reported a high incidence of infection, approaching 50%, when preoperative antibiotics were not administered. Therefore, antibiotic coverage is strongly recommended prophylactically and once infection has occurred. Successful therapy is directed toward appropriate administration of systemic antibiotics following cultures and sensitivity, removal of all foreign bodies and bony sequestra, and maintenance of appropriate stabilization, preferably with rigid fixation. Fractures located within the mandibular angle have been associated with an increased occurrence of untoward results (14,15). Ellis and Walker (16) reported that, over a 10-year period, fractures of the mandibular angle were plagued with the highest complication rate, and they proposed that open reduction with rigid fixation was associated with the lowest incidence of complications. I agree wholeheartedly with this statement (8,9). Similar experiences have been reported by other authors (15–19). Considerable controversy surrounds the treatment of teeth located in the line of fracture (20) and fractures in edentulous jaws (21). Most authors agree that a conservative approach should be taken for management of teeth located in the line of fracture and dental extraction reserved for cases where the teeth are extremely mobile, there is exposure of the root, or these teeth directly interfere with anatomical fracture reduction (20). When the tooth is to be maintained, systemic antibiotics must be administered. Rigid fixation should be used, and the patient should be closely observed for the possibility of infection.

Fractures of the atrophic mandible are relatively uncommon and represent approximately 1% of all mandible fractures (22). However, treatment modalities are fraught with significant difficulties. Consensus regarding treatment modalities remains controversial (23–25). Compared to other treatments, osteosynthesis with rigid fixation has produced the most acceptable results (23,24). This technique is recommended for management of fractures of the atrophic mandible (23,26). However, as reported by Luhr et al. (24), it is extremely important to avoid extensive periosteal degloving and the surgeon must position the rigid fixation in a supraperiosteal location. One must remember that it is extremely important to establish appropriate maxillomandibular relationships in edentulous fractures (27). Another adjunct to treatment as aptly described by Dr. Gundlach is bone grafting to enhance healing and stability of fracture segments as required in certain circumstances.

Management of infection requires immediate systemic antibiotic therapy and incision and drainage of the soft tissue. If the source of the infection is a carious tooth, extraction and systemic antibiotics, preferably with penicillin, should be instituted. James (28) reported an infection rate of 7% in a prospective study of 422 fractures. In 50% of these cases, there was a fractured or carious tooth. It is important to stress that rigid internal fixation must be maintained with appropriate systemic antibiotic coverage until full bony reconstitution of the bony fracture segments is completed (30). Following this, the hardware can be removed in a secondary procedure.

On the other hand, if the infection continues and osteomyelitis develops, leading to altered vascularity and eventual ischemia, more extensive therapy is necessary. The mainstay of treatment includes comprehensive bony and soft tissue debridement and adequate stabilization with long-term administration of systemic antibiotics.

According to Spiessel (29), nonunion develops when a bony fracture does not unite within 6 months of fracture. On the other hand, delayed union is defined as the absence of bony consolidation within 6 to 12 weeks (17). The most frequent contributing factors causing delayed union and nonunion are persistent bony mobility, alcohol and drug abuse, associated systemic illness, anatomical location of the fracture, teeth located in the line of fracture, and occurrence of postsurgical infections (30). Management requires comprehensive evaluation to determine the initiating causes and thorough debridement back to normal bleeding bone, instillation of appropriate fixation, and possible bone grafting.

Malunion, which may cause both functional and aesthetic impairments, occurs in approximately 0% to 4.2% of all cases (31). Causes include inadequate reduction or immobilization, poor patient compliance, and inappropriate implementation of the rigid internal fixation. Satisfactory correction requires orderly and comprehensive preoperative preparation, including a thorough clinical examination with photographs, dental models, and radiologic documentation, followed by refracture, repositioning of these bony segments, bone grafting (32), and rigid fixation in an appropriate anatomical position.

As Dr. Gundlach points out, good function of the TMJ is a prerequisite for successful rehabilitation following mandibular fracture repair. There are a number of causes for impairment of the TMJ, and Dr. Gundlach provides an excellent differential diagnosis. Previous authors provided the absolute indications for open reduction of condylar fractures (33–35), which include displacement of the bony segments into the middle cranial fossa, persistent malocclusion following adequate conservative management, and foreign bodies in the joint space (36). The most serious complication is the development of ankylosis, which is a relatively rare occurrence in 0.2% to 0.4% of all condylar fractures (31). This untoward sequelae occurs primarily in fractures located in close proximity to the glenoid fossa or in younger patients who have been placed in prolonged intervals of maxillomandibular fixation. Surgical management of ankylosis includes osteotomies, autologous joint replacement, and interposition grafts of soft tissue. The best treatment is prevention, which requires early remobilization and postoperative physical therapy. Regardless of surgical technique, recurrence remains the most problematic unfavorable result.

Pediatric facial bone fractures remain a rather infrequent occurrence when compared to the overall incidence of adult facial bone fractures (37–40). This is related to the bony architecture of the child and a relative protected environment. Pediatric jaw fractures should be treated according to the identical tenets related to facial fractures in older age groups. Initial therapy should always be directed toward maintenance of an adequate airway and control of hemorrhage, as well as attending to all associated injuries. It is important to note that associated injuries are seen more commonly in children; therefore, the initial examiner must always be aware of these potential life-threatening injuries (41). Choice of treatment modalities are dependent on the state of the child's dentition (42). For the most part, closed reduction techniques should be used. Even displaced bony segments remodel relatively well (40) and, therefore, do not necessarily require extensive exposure and use of rigid fixation. Reconstructive surgeons can use open techniques for those patients who failed conservative therapy because of potential damage to the tooth buds and potential adverse effects on future growth and development (40,42,43). Although consensus regarding treatment of condylar fractures in this age group has been controversial, conservative therapy with early motion to prevent the onset of ankylosis should be the primary therapeutic mode (44).

In the future, many of the controversial areas in the management of mandibular fracture will be settled by evolving technologies. For the treatment of subcondylar fractures, endoscopic repair will alleviate the risk posed to the facial nerve by necessary surgical exposure (45,46,47). This technique allows adequate visualization and permits direct manipulation of fractured facial bone segments (48) and has demonstrated excellent clinical application and results. The second area is the utilization of biodegradable plates and screws, which has shown a predictable short-term stability pattern that is comparable to titanium fixation (49,50) and will remove the potential adverse effects caused by nonresorbable hardware.

REFERENCES

1. Hoffman W, Barton R, Price M, et al. Rigid internal fixation vs. traditional techniques for treatment of mandible fractures. *J Trauma* 1990;30:1032.
2. Leach J, Truelson J. Traditional methods vs. rigid internal fixation of mandible fractures. *Arch Otolaryngol Head Neck Surg* 1995;121:750.
3. Ardary W. Plate and screw fixation in the management of mandible fractures. *Clin Plast Surg* 1989;16:61.
4. Terris D, Lalakea M, Tuffo K, et al. Mandible fracture repair: specific indications for newer techniques. *Otolaryngol Head Neck Surg* 1994;111:751.
5. El-Degwi A, Mathog R. Mandible fractures—medical and economic considerations. *Otolaryngol Head Neck Surg* 1993; 108:213.
6. Reinhart E, Reuther J, Michel C, et al. Treatment outcome and complications of surgical and conservative management of mandibular fractures. *Fortschr Kiefer Gesichtschir* 1996;41:64.
7. Bilkay U, Gurler T, Bilkay U, et al. Comparison of fixation methods in treating mandibular fractures: scintigraphic evaluation. *J Craniofac Surg* 1997;8:270.
8. Schortinghuis J, Bos R, Vissink A. Complications of internal fixation of maxillofacial fractures with microplates. *J Oral Maxillofac Surg* 1999;57:130.

9. Brown J, Grew N, Taylor C, et al. Intermaxillary fixation compared to miniplate osteosynthesis in the management of fractured mandible: an audit. *Br J Oral Maxillofac Surg* 1991;29:308.
10. Davies B, Cederna J, Guyuron B. Noncompression unicortical miniplate osteosynthesis of mandibular fractures. *Ann Plast Surg* 1992;28:414.
11. Bouhlogyros P. A retrospective study of 1521 mandibular fractures. *J Oral Maxillofac Surg* 1990;43:597.
12. Punjabi A, Thaller S. Complications of mandibular fractures. *Op Tech Pediatr Reconstr Surg* 1998;5:266.
13. Chole R, James Y. Antibiotic prophylaxis for facial fractures. *Arch Otolaryngol Head Neck Surg* 1987;113;1055.
14. Iizuka T, Lindqvist C, Hallikainen D, et al. Infection after rigid internal fixation of mandibular fractures: a clinical and radiologic study. *J Oral Maxillofac Surg* 1991;49:585.
15. Schierle H, Schmelzeisen R, Rahn B. Experimental studies of the biomechanical stability of different miniplate configurations for the mandibular angle. *Fortschr Kiefer Gesichtschir* 1996;41:166.
16. Ellis E, Walker L. Treatment of mandibular angle fractures using one noncompression miniplate. *J Oral Maxillofac Surg* 1996; 54:864.
17. Potter J, Ellis E. Treatment of mandibular angle fractures with a malleable noncompression miniplate. *J Oral Maxillofac Surg* 1999;57:288.
18. Levy F, Smith R, Odland R, et al. Monocortical miniplate fixation of mandibular angle fractures. *Arch Otolaryngol Head Neck Surg* 1991;117:149.
19. Ellis E. Treatment methods for fractures of the mandibular angle. *Int J Oral Maxillofac Surg* 1999;28:243.
20. Thaller S, Mabourakh S. Teeth located in the line of mandibular fracture. *J Craniofac Surg* 1994;5:16.
21. Thaller S. Fractures of the edentulous mandible: a retrospective review. *J Craniofac Surg* 1993;4:91.
22. Newman L. The role of autogenous primary rib grafts in treating fractures of the atrophic edentulous mandible. *Br J Oral Maxillofac Surg* 1995;33:381.
23. Luhr H, Reidick T, Merten H. Fractures of the atrophic mandible—a challenge for therapy. *Fortschr Kiefer Gesichtschir* 1996;41:151.
24. Luhr H, Reidick T, Merten H. Results of treatment of fractures of the atrophic edentulous mandible by compression plating: a retrospective evaluation of 84 cases. *J Oral Maxillofac Surg* 1996;54:250.
25. Eyrich G, Gratz K, Sailer H. Surgical treatment of the edentulous mandible. *J Oral Maxillofac Surg* 1997;55:1081.
26. Iatrou I, Samaras C, Theologie-Lygidakis N. Miniplate osteosynthesis for fractures of the edentulous mandible: a clinical study 1989–96. *J Craniomaxillofac Surg* 1998;26:400.
27. Crawley W, Azman P, Clark N, et al. The edentulous Le Fort fracture. *J Craniofac Surg* 1997;8:298.
28. James R. Prospective study of mandibular fractures. *J Oral Surg* 1981;39:275.
29. Spiessl B. *Internal fixation of the mandible: a manual of AO/ASIF principles.* New York: Springer-Verlag, 1988:212–284.
30. Haug R, Schwimmer A. Fibrous union of the mandible: a review of 27 patients. *J Oral Maxillofac Surg* 1994;52:832.
31. Koury L, Pogrell A, Perrot D. *Complications in oral and maxillofacial surgery.* Philadelphia: WB Saunders, 1997:121–146.
32. Thaller S, Reavie D. Refracture reposition of mandibular malunion. *Ann Plast Surg* 1990;25:188.
33. Santler G, Karcher H, Ruda C, et al. Fractures of the condylar process: surgical vs. non-surgical treatment. *J Oral Maxillofac Surg* 1999;57:392.
34. Moritz M, Niederdellman H, Dammer R. Mandibular condyle fractures: conservative treatment versus surgical treatment. *Rev Stomatol Chir Maxillofac* 1994;95:268.
35. Pereira M, Marques A, Ishizuka M, et al. Surgical treatment of the fractured and dislocated condylar process of the mandible. *J Craniomaxillofac Surg* 1995;23:369.
36. Chuong R, Piper M. Open reduction of condylar fractures of the mandible in conjunction with repair of discal injury. *J Oral Maxillofac Surg* 1988;46:257.
37. MacLennan D. Fractures of the mandible in children under the age of six years. *Br J Plast Surg* 1956;9:125.
38. Kazanjian V, Converse J. *The surgical treatment of facial injuries.* Baltimore: Williams & Wilkins, 1949:100.
39. Hagan E, Huelke D. Analysis of 319 case reports of mandibular fractures. *J Oral Surg Anesthet Hosp Dent Serv* 1961;19:93.
40. Spring P, Cote D. Pediatric maxillofacial fractures. *J La State Med Soc* 1996;148:199.
41. Cossio I, Galvez F, Gutierrez-Perez J, et al. Mandibular fractures in children. A retrospective study of 99 fractures in 59 patients. *Int J Oral Maxillofac Surg* 1994;23:329.
42. Thaller S, Marbourakh S. Pediatric mandible fractures. *Ann Plast Surg* 1991;26:511.
43. Schweinfurth J, Koltai P. Pediatric mandibular fractures. *Fac Plast Surg* 1998;14:31.
44. Strobl H, Emshoff R, Rother G. Conservative treatment of unilateral condylar fractures in children: a long-term clinical and radiologic follow-up of 55 patients. *Int J Oral Maxillofac Surg* 1999;28:95.
45. Jacoboviccz J, Lee C, Trabulsy P. Endoscopic repair of mandibular subcondylar fractures. *Plast Reconstr Surg* 1998;101:437.
46. Lauer G, Schmelzeisen R. Endoscope-assisted fixation of mandibular condylar process fractures. *J Oral Maxillofac Surg* 1999;57:36.
47. Park D, Lee J, Song C, et al. Endoscopic application in aesthetic and reconstructive facial bone surgery. *Plast Reconstr Surg* 1998;102:1199.
48. Lee C, Mueller R, Lee K, et al. Endoscopic subcondylar fracture repair: functional, aesthetic, and radiographic outcomes. *Plast Reconstr Surg* 1998;102:1434.
49. Kallela I, Iizuka T, Salo A, et al. Lag-screw fixation of anterior mandibular fractures using biodegradable polylactide screws: a preliminary report. *J Oral Maxillofac Surg* 1999;57:113.
50. Haers P, Sailer H. Biodegradable self-reinforced poly-LDL-lactide plates and screws in bimaxillary orthognathic surgery: short-term skeletal stability and material related failures. *J Craniomaxillofac Surg* 1998;26:363.

31

FACIAL FRACTURES

PAUL N. MANSON

Complications from facial fractures occur because of misdiagnosis, incomplete reduction, loss of fixation, infection, poor union, formation of excessive scar tissue, or the accidental effects of the injury. Inadequate physical diagnosis and imaging contribute to misdiagnosis, setting the stage for errors. Complications can be minimized by an accurate physical examination, refined imaging, and development of a thorough preoperative plan. In no case, however, can complications be entirely prevented, as many of them are secondary to the severity of the injury itself (1). Expectant observation permits early identification of complications and thus their early treatment. A plan for management of each tissue component following a complication will minimize adverse change. Both bone and soft tissue treatment then may be incorporated into the definitive plan for management of the complications and for reconstruction (2).

GENERAL PRINCIPLES

Bone Position

In any anatomical area of the face, malposition of a facial bone must be identified and characterized fully in terms of its relationship at each of its buttress articulations to the adjacent skeleton (2–5). A detailed description of the anatomy of buttress articulations is provided in the literature for each anatomical area and for each buttress articulation (4–11). Suffice it to say that exposing some of the buttresses of a displaced bone segment often may achieve sufficient exposure to permit realignment, but, conceptually, all of the buttress articulations for a given anatomical area (a full exposure) should be considered in each instance (2).

Justification for partial (incomplete) exposure may be provided by less severe injuries. Anatomically, the face is divided into areas of the frontal skull and supraorbital regions, the upper midface (consisting of the bilateral zygomas and the central nasoethmoidal area), the occlusion (consisting of the alveolar arches of the maxilla and the mandible), and the basal mandible (consisting of horizontal and vertical segments) (Fig. 31-1) (12). In reoperative fracture management, malposition of each anatomical segment at each of its buttress articulations is considered individually; then the need for an osteotomy in each area is analyzed. Although minimal deformities can be managed by onlay grafting of bone or alloplastic material, a wise conceptual framework includes consideration for both osteotomy and onlay grafting in revisional fracture work, as a portion of the original bone mass may have resorbed, or it may have to be altered in surface contour or shape for contour restoration or a bone graft provided to ensure bone union (11,13,14). Therefore, each anatomical area conceptually needs two types of evaluations: (i) osteotomy and repositioning; and (ii) augmentation or replacement of any deficient or missing portions of the facial skeleton (2,12,13). Bone grafts can be harvested from the calvarium, rib, or iliac crest, as required (15). Bone graft take is improved by rigid fixation (16).

Incisions for secondary surgical repair may include new elective, previous incisions, and old lacerations or scars. Separate "stealth" access incisions sometimes are preferred, such as the use of a conjunctival incision after a previous cutaneous subciliary incision. Emphasis is placed on "stealth incisions," which minimize cutaneous scarring (2); an intraoral or transconjunctival incision will minimize cutaneous scarring (2,4). In some cases, endoscopic approaches are acceptable for facial injury management. Further, the use of a conjunctival incision, where a previous lower lid skin incision has been performed, will minimize the chance of ectropion or scleral show by avoiding the previous scar plane (3,17,18).

In general, five incisions provide exposure to any area of the craniofacial skeleton (10). The coronal incision provides access to the upper face and the upper medial and lateral orbit. The transconjunctival incision with lateral canthotomy provides access to the upper maxilla and lower orbit, including the lower medial and lateral orbit (19). The maxillary and mandibular gingival buccal sulcus degloving incisions provide access to the lower maxilla, the Le Fort I level to the inferior orbital rim, and the anterior horizontal por-

P. N. Manson: Division of Plastic Surgery, The Johns Hopkins Hospital, Baltimore, Maryland, and the University of Maryland, Shock Trauma Unit, Baltimore, Maryland

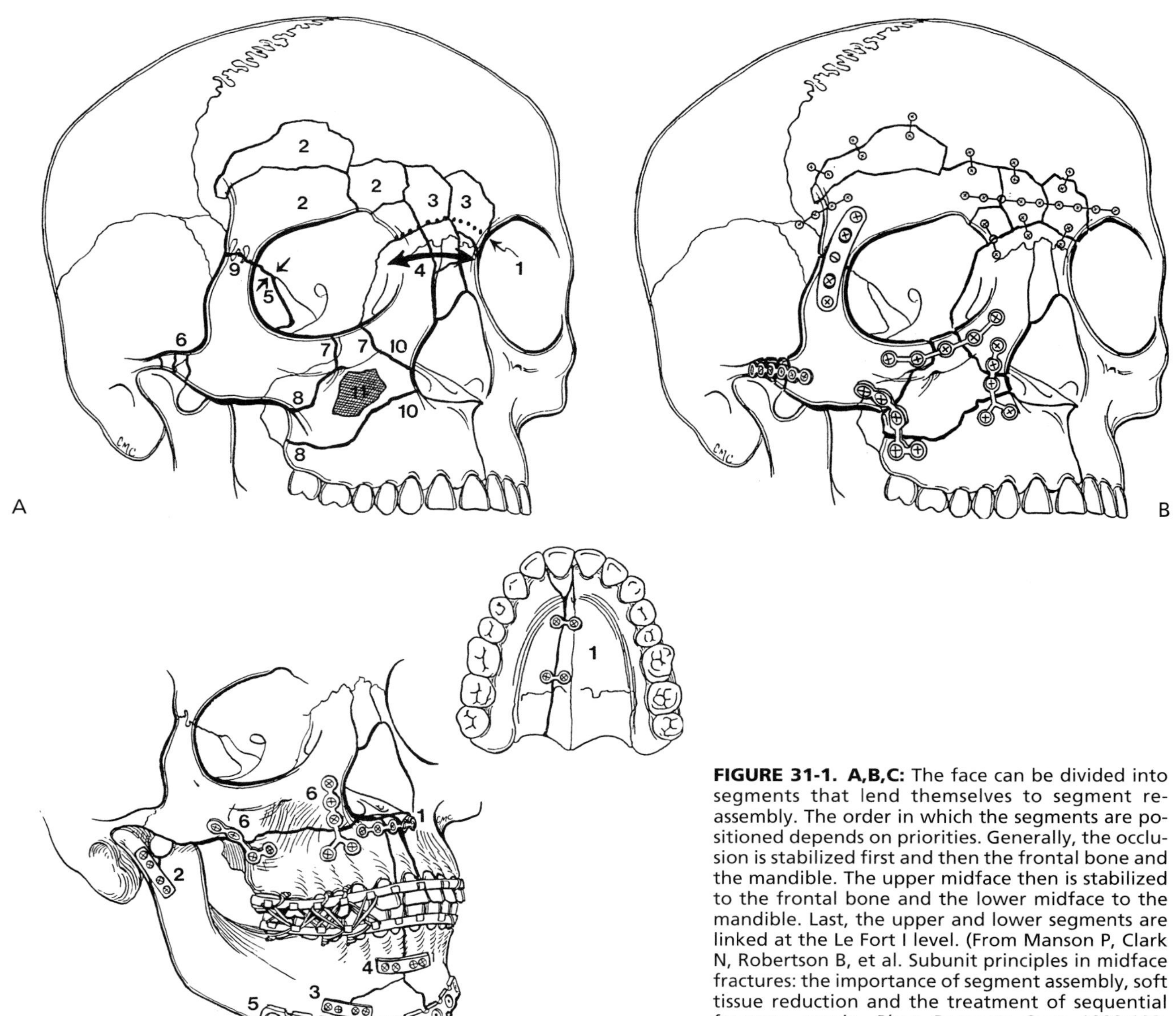

FIGURE 31-1. A,B,C: The face can be divided into segments that lend themselves to segment reassembly. The order in which the segments are positioned depends on priorities. Generally, the occlusion is stabilized first and then the frontal bone and the mandible. The upper midface then is stabilized to the frontal bone and the lower midface to the mandible. Last, the upper and lower segments are linked at the Le Fort I level. (From Manson P, Clark N, Robertson B, et al. Subunit principles in midface fractures: the importance of segment assembly, soft tissue reduction and the treatment of sequential fracture repair. *Plast Reconstr Surg* 1999;103:1287–1306, with permission.)

tion of the mandible and mandibular angle, respectively (19). The preauricular and retromandibular incisions provide access to the vertical portion of the mandible (19). Thorough subperiosteal degloving of the involved bone segments through these incisions permits accurate analysis of bone position and alignment for planning repositioning after osteotomy (13,19). Generally, the osteotomies should travel through previous fracture lines, unless a different osteotomy pattern has been predicated based on the result of computed tomographic (CT) scan (5,9), dental model, or cephalometric analysis. Once the bone segment is repositioned, the whole area's volume and the junctions of the segment are inspected for the need for contour or interpositional grafts. Bone grafts supplement, add contour, or fill in gaps between repositioned buttress segments (13). After the hard tissue (bone) reconstruction is completed, the facial soft tissue is repositioned in its proper location on the bone fragments (13). In secondary repairs, the soft tissue must be thoroughly degloved from all areas in order to allow for free repositioning of bone segments (15,20). The soft tissue then can be inspected for thickness and mobility. The periosteum may need to be resected to permit mobility and the soft tissue thinned by resection or thickened by the addition of a flap (20). The soft tissue then is repaired in terms of its layers (muscle, periosteum, and skin) and repositioned by reattachment to the reconstructed facial skeleton at multiple locations to simultaneously guarantee it thickness (layered closure) and position (reattachment) (20–24).

Hemorrhage

Life-threatening bleeding from facial fractures usually responds to anterior posterior nasal packing. Coagulation factors should be assessed, and the maxilla stabilized by intermaxillary fixation (IMF). Interventional radiology may embolically occlude the vessel if specific. Ligation of both the external carotid and superficial temporal arteries may be attempted as a last resort.

Airway

Facial fractures involving the nose or occlusion potentially impair the airway. Any fractures involving the occlusion also may cause aspiration by interfering with the control of swallowing and management of secretions. Intubation is the surest control of airway protection and may be accomplished orally or nasally. In those patients who are comatose or who have a chest injury, a tracheostomy should be considered if IMF is necessary. Tracheostomies should be done with horizontal incisions to minimize scarring.

Tracheostomy scar revisions should be planned to reapproximate the muscle, fat, and skin in separate layers to achieve a flat wound without skin adherence to deeper structures. The direction of the scar should be horizontal, if possible.

ANALYSIS OF COMPLICATIONS BY ANATOMICAL REGION

Frontal Bone Fractures

Many frontal bone fractures are open through the skin externally and communicate with the sinuses and nose internally (25); therefore, there is an inherent predisposition to infection from contamination and sinus obstruction (3,5,26,27). Frontal sinus or frontal bone fragments can be replaced after debridement and repositioning; if excessively small or deformed, they are prone to contour irregularity and may better be replaced by a larger bone graft as a single piece reconstruction (26,28–33).

If there is "dead space" between the reconstructed frontal bone and the brain, and especially if the dead space communicates with residual sinus defects or with the nasal cavity, an infection is more likely to occur (26,34). In the event of infection, local drainage and antibiotics are instituted, and a CT scan is performed to identify any sinus obstruction (35). If the infection is more than superficial or soft tissue infection does not clear, it is likely that removal of nonvascularized bone fragments will be required. At the time of the original repair, it may have been possible to fill the sinus cavity with particulate bone graft and to incorporate a soft tissue flap into the area of the anterior cranial base defect, which reduces the possibility of communication with the nose. Any remnants of residual frontal-nasal duct are cleaned of mucosa and the nasofrontal ducts plugged, so that frontal bone reconstruction will not be risked by a persistent communication with the nose. All residual frontal sinus mucosa should be debrided and replaced frontal bone fragments burred to eliminate any traces of mucosa or granulation tissue (Fig. 31-2). After the initial bone and sinus debridement, any cerebrospinal fluid fistula should be closed (30). The dural closure may need to be reinforced with a fascia lata patch if the leak is in the floor of the anterior cranial fossa and has existed for a period of time. In the face of low-grade postoperative infection following bone replacement, considerable resorption of frontal bone may occur and require secondary cranioplasty (Fig. 31-3A). Before a secondary cranioplasty is accomplished, a period of time free of infection, generally 6 to 12 months, should elapse. An intact layer of bone between the cranial vault and the nose or sinuses at the level of the anterior cranial base should be confirmed before secondary reconstruction. In some cases, the bone of the anterior cranial fossa may need to be augmented to seal the intracranial cavity from the nose either prior to or at the time of cranioplasty (30–33).

Loss of frontal bone can be managed by secondary cranioplasty, using autogenous or alloplastic materials (Figs. 31-3B–31-3D) (36,37). Secondary cranioplasty may be accomplished with calvarial, rib, or iliac bone, or with artificial

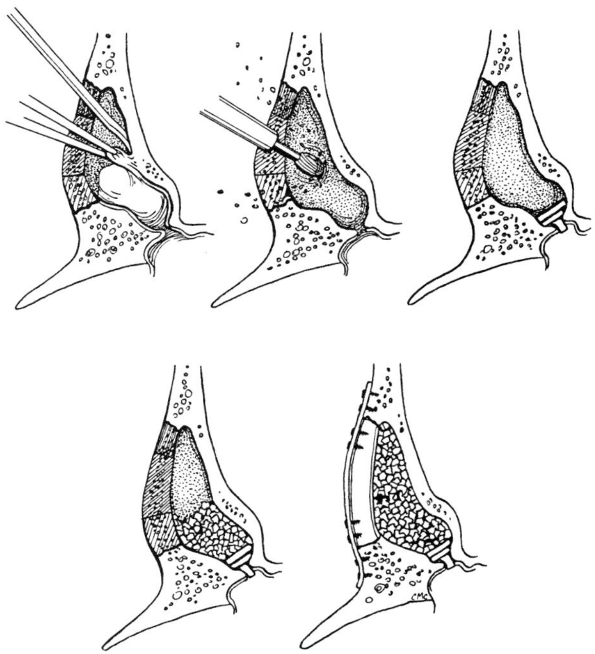

FIGURE 31-2. Frontal sinus mucosa must be meticulously removed from the walls of the sinus and bone fragments. The bone should be burred to eliminate any mucosa that extends along intracalvarial veins. The bone then is replaced and the sinus filled with particulate bone graft. (From Manson P. Reoperative facial fracture repair. In: Grotting J, ed. *Reoperative aesthetic and reconstructive plastic surgery.* St. Louis: Quality Medical Publishing, 1995:701, with permission.)

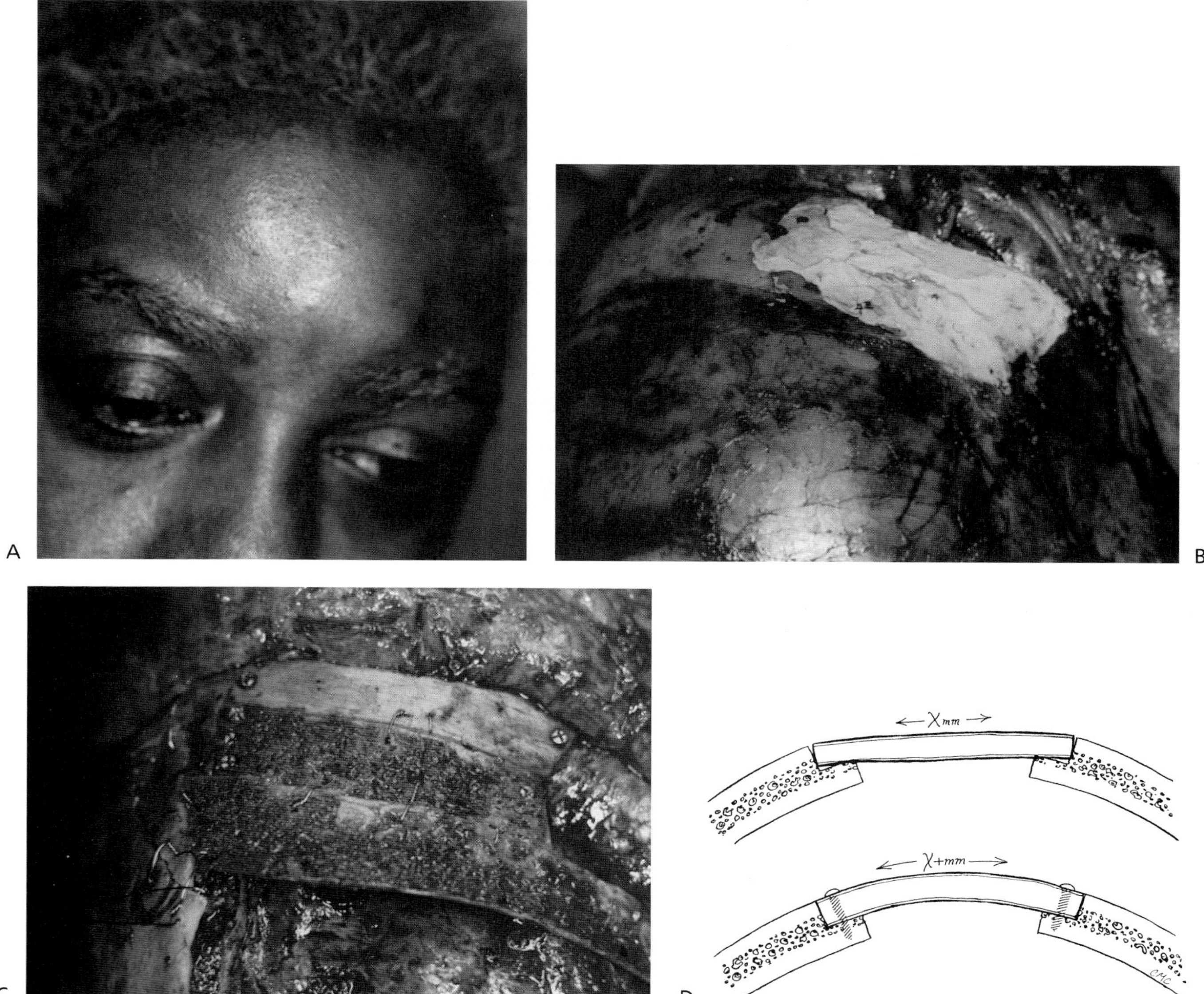

FIGURE 31-3. A: Frontal bone irregularity is common after partial resorption. Resorption is accelerated by low-grade infections that sometimes slowly create considerable deformity. **B:** Hydroxyapatite cement can be used secondarily for frontal bone recontouring. **C:** Split ribs can be anchored in a trough and placed under slight tension, so that they create a bowed arch in the recipient area. They also can be anchored with plate and screw fixation. **D:** More length is needed if an arch structure of the forehead is to be accomplished.

material if the location is not adjacent to a sinus or mastoid (a bone layer should be present between the sinus and the planned alloplastic reconstruction) and if all evidence of infection has been absent for a period of 6 months.

An extensive bone cranioplasty can be accomplished either with split rib or with bone harvested from the parietal calvarial region (36). The segment to be used should have a curvature similar to that desired in the recipient area (36,37). A full-thickness craniotomy is performed, the calvarium is split, and the lower half of bone is returned to the donor site. The upper layer of the donor segment is placed in the recipient site and contoured appropriately. Bone shavings obtained from the craniotomy are used to fill in the osteotomy sites, or hydroxyapatite cement can be used to smooth small bone gaps or surface irregularities.

The aesthetic result may be improved by onlay of hydroxyapatite cement in the area of the donor or the recipient site (36–38). Bone grafts also are useful to convert a multiple segment reconstruction to a smooth, one-piece bone segment. Any communication with a sinus or the nose must be managed by sinus obliteration or partition from the intracranial cavity with bone or vascularized soft tissue. A small galeal flap may be easily turned into the region, but damaged sinus mucosa or devascularized bone must be thoroughly removed before flap or bone obliteration. The frontal sinus ostea may each be bone graft obliterated with a suitably carved piece of calvarial bone. For frontal bone replacement, ribs may be split and placed under slight tension so that they create a bowed arch in the recipient area, and anchored with plate and screw fixation (Fig. 31-3B).

When fractures simultaneously involve the orbital roof and frontal bar area, the orbital roof and frontal region must be assessed for contour and projection. It is common to reconstruct the superior orbital roof in a location that is positioned too inferiorly. This downward displacement of the roof decreases the space available for the globe and forces it downward and forward (Fig. 31-4). The appearance of the pro-optotic eye should not be confused with that secondary to orbital dystopia, which creates an inferiorly positioned globe that usually is *recessed* (or enophthalmic) in terms of globe prominence. Accurate analysis of plain films, patient measurements, and axial and coronal CT scans permits planning of a properly shaped orbital reconstruction. Usually, an intracranial correction of a depressed orbital roof is required. The new roof should be affixed to the frontal bar intracranially to reduce the possibility of constricting the orbit.

Contour problems of the frontal bone are caused most frequently by bone irregularity occurring at fracture sites, osteotomies, bur holes, partially resorbed bone or bone grafts, or visible and palpable plates. In contour problems, the involved areas should be exposed, the plates removed, and contours of the bone smoothed with a bur. If additional contour is needed, hydroxyapatite cement and methylmethacrylate are ideal materials for onlay cranioplasty. They can be used to fill in bur holes or osteotomy sites to create a regular, smooth contour. The Norian Craniofacial Repair System (CRS) material is convenient to use, sets in a wet environment, and is reasonably simple to contour with a shaping bit or by sanding (with a bovie cleaning pad). If Norian CRS is used in a large area of absent bone and placed directly on pulsating dura, it cures as multiple small particles because of motion. A rigid metal grid must first be placed into the bone defect against the dura to keep the dura level and eliminate dural pulsations, which cause the material to cure as multiple fragments with migration and splintering. The Norian material also may be used to contour small soft tissue defects by augmenting the bone in that region. Logistically, this is a more difficult reconstructive maneuver. The issues regarding the choice of alloplastic versus autogenous material relate to the preferences of the surgeon and the desire to minimize either the long-term chance of infection with alloplastic materials or the chance of irregularity from partial resorption ("take") of bone. There are arguments for and against the use of each material that are cogent and defendable.

A

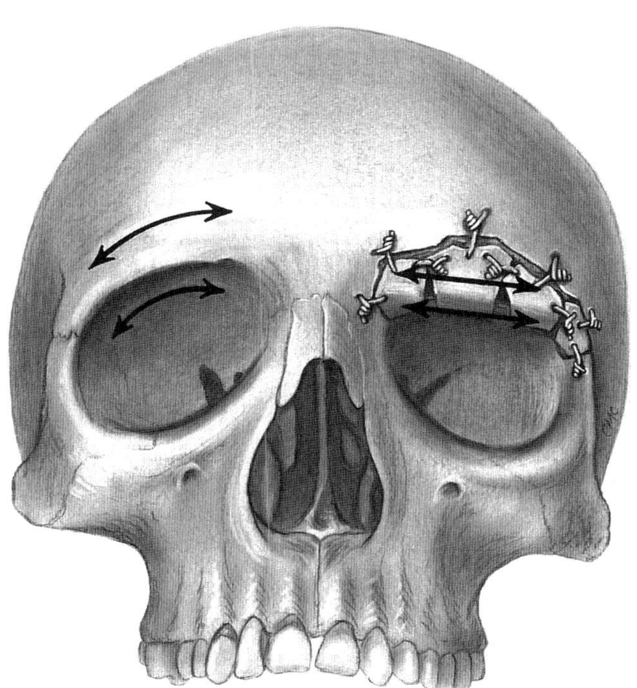

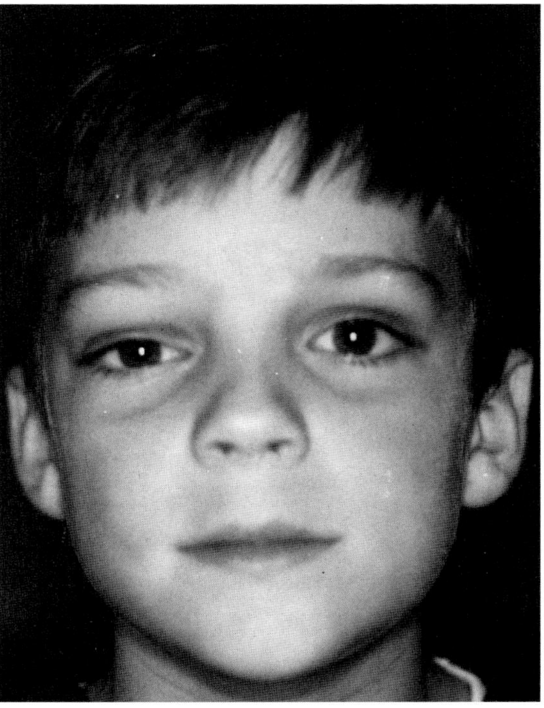

B

FIGURE 31-4. **A:** Reconstructing the orbital roof too inferiorly creates a pro-optic position of the globe. Artists concept of sagging rim and roof. (Copyright Johns Hopkins Plastic Surgery.) **B:** Clinical photograph of patient with roof pressing globe inferiorly.

Obstruction of Frontal or Ethmoid Sinuses

In the face of frontal or ethmoid sinus obstruction (air–fluid levels) and even in the absence of clinical infection, the sinus cavity must be assumed to have inadequate drainage and should be considered for bone obliteration or cranialization in the case of the frontal sinus and, in the case of the ethmoids, partial ethmoidectomy and obliteration (Fig. 31-2) (26,28). The obliterative procedure consists of opening the obstructed area and removing crushed bone fragments with mucosal removal. In the case of the frontal sinus, mucosal removal is performed and the mucosa dissected down into the nasofrontal duct. Any remaining sinus walls are burred to eliminate areas where mucosa invaginates along the veins that penetrate the diploë of the calvarium (26,28). The nasofrontal duct is plugged with a carved external table calvarial bone graft (Fig. 31-2). In the absence of clinical infection, as in the case of a sterile mucocele, the sinus may be filled with cancellous bone from the iliac crest. Despite its advocates, hydroxyapatite cement has a yet unproved record for sinus obliteration after thorough mucosal removal. However, this material can be used to replace missing frontal bone or smooth irregularities. In the case of infection, the source of the infection must be eliminated and the infection allowed to clear before any formal bone grafting, cranioplasty, or reconstruction is contemplated. Many advocate a period of 6 months to 1 year (36,37) as the interval between infection and reconstruction, in order to eradicate sinus disease before definitive treatment. Nasal airway obstruction should be corrected before sinus obliteration or cranial reconstruction.

Frontal sinus mucocele is an unusual complication in treated frontal sinus fractures. This condition occurs following untreated frontal sinus fractures (39). It generally produces pressure symptoms and usually is sterile expanding toward the orbit and the brain. Generally, mucoceles represent sterile obstructed mucosal secretions. Mucoceles require the same treatment as an obstructed frontal sinus with mucosal removal, duct obliteration with bone, and reconstruction of the walls of the orbit and nose by bone graft, partitioning of the frontal sinus from the nose by bone graft, bone obliteration of the frontal sinus, and cranioplasty. For sinus cavity obliteration, iliac crest particulate marrow grafts seem much more vigorous bone producers than are external table calvarial shavings. In cases where a soft tissue flap is deemed appropriate for improved seal between the sinus and nasal cavity, a galeal frontalis flap may be harvested, vascularized by the supraorbital and supratrochlear arteries. However, the use of a galeal flap thins the forehead skin and itself may create an additional forehead contour deformity.

In any planned reentry into the frontal cranial and cranial base area, the level of the brain should be established in relationship to the nose and the orbits in a coronal CT scan, as previous injury and bone loss may allow the brain to prolapse inferiorly behind the nose, where it may inadvertently be injured by intranasal instrumentation. Similarly, bone defects often exist in the orbital roof, and attempts at subperiosteal dissection in the area of a roof defect may find the elevator beneath the dura or in the frontal lobe by accident. The use of a frontal bone flap allows safe visualization of the orbital roof from two exposures, intracranial and extracranial. Safe access to the back of the nose, the supraorbital-ethmoid, and orbital roof is provided.

The position of a displaced orbital roof fracture may explain ocular dystopia (Fig. 31-4A,B). Preinjury photographs should be reviewed to confirm the eye position before the accident. In reconstructing the roof of the orbit, one should remember that the orbital roof has a convex curvature arching superiorly from medial to lateral and superiorly from anterior to posterior (Fig. 31-5). This double curvature must be reconstructed, and one of the easiest ways to reconstruct the roof is to place a bone graft external to the orbital roof defect from an intracranial approach. The frontal bone and intracranial bone grafts may be stabilized with a 1.0 or 1.3 micro system (1). Large plates are not required, because there are insignificant muscular forces on the skull. One should re-

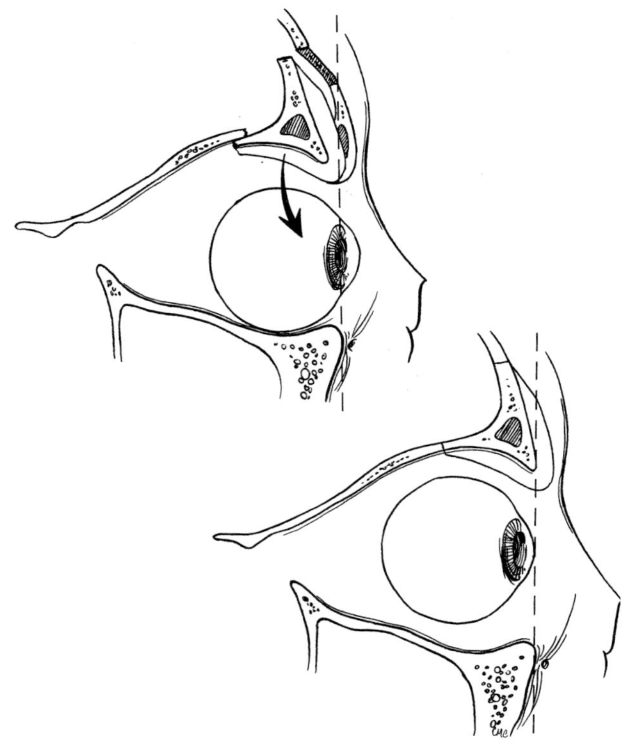

FIGURE 31-5. The orbital roof has a complex curvature, consisting of two superiorly convex superior arches from anterior to posterior and from medial to lateral. This double curvature must be reconstructed from an intracranial approach. (From Manson P. Reoperative facial fracture repair. In: Grotting J, ed. Reoperative aesthetic and reconstructive plastic surgery. St. Louis: Quality Medical Publishing, 1995:702, with permission.)

call, however, that bone grafts secured with rigid fixation have a better "take" than bone grafts that are not rigidly fixed (16). Secure fixation also prevents bone graft displacement.

Reconstruction of the orbital roof prevents the possibility of pulsating exophthalmos from the transmission of brain pulsations to the globe.

In the case of a frontal sinus infection, a biopsy of the tissue in the area will distinguish the conditions of mucosal regrowth or residual mucosa and that of granulation tissue. In each case, the infected abortive products of incomplete healing and all mucosa and devascularized bone (chronic osteitis) must be removed and the infection studied to identify the reason for the complication. In late reconstructions of the skull base, it is my preference to line the skull base defect with iliac crest bone grafts to create a solid bone partition between the sinuses, nose, and intracranial cavity. Before this is done, any nasal airway obstruction should be eliminated, such as that from a deviated septum, chronic sinus disease, or turbinate hypertrophy, which would otherwise predispose to sinusitis and infection in the frontal and ethmoid sinuses that will contaminate the intracranial reconstruction.

Hematoma

Hematoma beneath a coronal incision masquerades as postoperative swelling. The failure of the significant swelling to improve on the third postoperative day should suggest the presence of a hematoma. Palpably increased thickness is apparent and the skin may pit with pressure. Hematoma should be evacuated, as it will not be long until infection colonizes the clotted blood and converts the collection to an abscess (40). Even in the absence of infection, fibrosis and scar organization will affect the postoperative aesthetic result.

Small areas of frontal bone that are exposed postoperatively through a small wound dehiscence generally may be managed expectantly. If a bone defect does not close, the bone may be burred to the point of bleeding or a small bone segment removed, and the skin closed by advancement or a thin skin graft laid on the bleeding bone area. This "temporizing technique" often will prevent remobilization of the entire coronal flap, which again devascularizes the entire bone reconstruction. If the exposed bone is burred to bleeding tissue, even a small, thin skin graft may be applied directly to the bleeding bone. It can be serially excised in the future. Remobilizing an entire scalp flap devascularizes all the bone and may convert a small nonhealing area to a large devascularized region prone to infection. If the patient does not have signs of sepsis, extensive procedures for small problems are ill advised.

Injuries of the Nasoethmoidal Orbital Region

The central portion of the midface, the nasoethmoidal orbital region, presents the most complex reconstructive challenge in all facial injuries (Fig. 31-1) (41–43). Here, the results of initially inadequate treatment are the least reversible of any facial region (41,42). Complications occurring from nasoethmoidal fractures include telecanthus, enophthalmos, nasal septal perforation, shortened or retruded nose, a short palpebral fissure, dramatic thickening of the skin of the nasal orbital valley, globe displacement, and nasal airway obstruction. The errors that relate to complications include failure to make an accurate diagnosis, failure to adequately reduce and stabilize bone fragments, loss of fixation or stripping of the medial canthal ligament, unsatisfactory positioning of the medial canthal ligament, failure to correct the orbital volume, dehiscence of the medial canthal ligament after the reduction, lacrimal obstruction, and failure to stabilize or reconstruct the nasal skeleton and nasal septum (34). Loss of nasal lining creates a setup for infection, especially if nasal bone grafts are exposed intra nasally (44). Consideration for primary nasal lining replacement with a galeal frontalis flap should be performed in a patient with shredded nasal lining who is to have primary bone grafting. Lacrimal obstruction usually is produced by malpositioned bone in the area of the nasolacrimal duct (44). It also may be produced by direct transection of the lacrimal duct system or lacrimal canaliculus, which secondarily is best managed by dacryocystorhinostomy. Most of these patients with soft tissue injury to the lacrimal system have cutaneous lacerations. Obstruction of the nasolacrimal duct or sac may present as an abscess in the inferomedial orbit that requires drainage. When the infection has cleared, a formal dacryocystorhinostomy should be accomplished (42).

The emphasis in nasoethmoidal fractures should be on early definitive reduction of bone with specific management of the canthus and the canthal ligament-bearing bone fragment (42). In most nasoethmoidal fractures, the canthus remains attached to a relatively large bony fragment of the medial orbital rim. The lower two-thirds of the medial orbital rim have been identified as the "central fragment," meaning this fragment provides the control maneuver to canthal repositioning because it contains the attachment of the canthal ligament (42). Repositioning the central bone fragment repositions the medial canthal ligament. It is easy to partially strip this ligament; detaching the area of the canthal attachment as the transition from periosteum to canthal ligament attachment is so gradual that it is imperceptible (45). If the canthal ligament is inadvertently partially or totally stripped, or if the segments of the central fragment are so small that they require stripping of the canthus to accomplish a bone reduction, then the canthus must be reattached to a site posterior and superior to the lacrimal fossa *after* the bone reduction and just *before* closing the coronal incisions (46). This is best done with a separate set of transnasal wires passed from the opposite deep medial orbit through the frontal process of the maxilla posterior and superior to the lacrimal fossa. The wires are connected to the canthus with a nonabsorbable suture, which has been passed directly through the medial canthal tendon via a 3-mm external incision 2 mm medial to the medial eyelid commissure and then passed into the orbit to be connected to the transnasal wires. This mechanism of fixation creates the proper force and vectors to keep the eyelids tangent to the globe and to produce a properly oriented and posteriorly directed medial canthal reattachment. There is no canthal reconstruction technique that re-creates the complex anatomy of the canthus, so it should not be detached, if possible. Neither transnasal reduction of the central bone fragments nor medial canthoplasty should be accomplished anterior to the bony lacrimal fossa, as a splayed "telecanthic" architecture of the canthus will occur by lateral rotation of the canthal-bearing bone fragments (Fig. 31-6).

Any significant injury of the central midface should always be suspect for including a nasoethmoidal orbital component. The bimanual examination, where the tip of a clamp is placed inside the nose directly opposite the medial canthal ligament and a palpating finger is placed deeply over the canthus (46), allows mobility of the central fragment to be detected by moving the canthal-bearing bone fragment between the index finger and the clamp. This maneuver is the most accurate way to identify and confirm the presence of a mobile nasoethmoidal fracture that requires reduction. On CT scan, four fractures (5) must surround the central fragment: involvement of the nose, the ethmoid, the inferior orbital rim, and the internal angular process of the frontal bone/frontal process of the maxilla. These isolate the central fragment from the adjacent bone and create the simplest combination of fractures required to produce instability of the medial canthal ligament (the definition of a nasoethmoidal orbital fracture). One of the most frequent problems leading to inaccurate reduction of a nasoethmoidal fracture is inadequate exposure (47). Conceptually, any nasoethmoidal orbital fracture requires 3 incisions for exposure: a coronal, a lower eyelid, and a gingivobuccal sulcus incision (42). Failure to expose, reduce and stabilize all of the peripheral buttresses of the nasoethmoidal fragment inevitably results in poor alignment. It is not generally appreciated that the height of the mid nose is controlled by reduction of the bone along the pyriform aperture. Improvement of nasal height and contour needs to be obtained with bone grafts when the septum has been telescoped, but there is no substitute for the accurate reassembly of the basic nasal skeleton, and for stabilizing the existing nasal skeleton to the adjacent maxilla and frontal bone which we call ?junctional? rigid fixation (42). The best results occur when considerable time has been spent piecing segments of the nasal skeleton together with fine wires (2). The final addition of a straight dorsal bone graft on top of the re-assembled nasal framework results in a stately nasal appearance, with good height, smooth dorsal contour, admirable projection and correct nasal width. The soft tissue must be held against this framework during healing through the use of temporary external bolsters (42). These bolsters merely hold the skin to the nose and have nothing to do with the canthal ligament reduction.

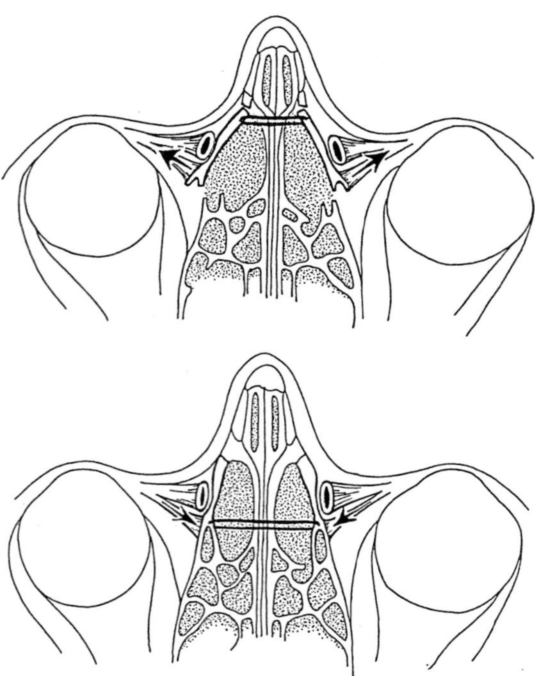

FIGURE 31-6. If a transnasal reduction is performed anterior to the canthal ligament, the posterior aspect of the frontal process of the maxilla may rotate, splay, and create telecanthus. (From Markowitz B, Manson P. Management of the medical canthal tendon in nasoethmoid orbital fractures: the importance of the central fragment in treatment and classifications. Plast Reconstr Surg 1991;87:843–883, with permission.)

It should be emphasized that it is easier to obtain a good result in a nasoethmoidal fracture reduction when it is performed within 48 hours of the injury (19). Fractures treated two weeks after the injury are prone to canthal dehiscence because of softening of the canthal tendon. Sutures in the friable tendon pull out easily.

In fractures treated late, the bone fragments must be stripped more thoroughly to accomplish a reduction. The soft tissue has already developed a "memory" and thickening by deposition of internal scar tissue in the wrong position; therefore, it is more difficult to reposition. The shortened nose may require a perinasal osteotomy with dorsal nasal bone grafts, caudal bone or cartilage grafts, and tip grafts to lengthen and augment the existing nasal bony and cartilaginous skeleton. To gain nasal length, the septum may need to be sectioned from the maxilla and vomer inferiorly and the cranial base superiorly. The septum then may be tilted downward and forward. Spreader grafts may be required to increase the thickness of the middle nasal vault to improve respiratory obstruction at the internal nasal valve. Significant nasoethmoidal orbital fractures are always accompanied by significant septal fractures; often a septal perforation exists. Usually, no attempt should be made to close septal perforations, as they are difficult to repair and may not be symptomatic. The respiratory obstruction needs to be managed by nasal septal resection and correction of any turbinate hypertrophy with turbinate out fracture, turbinate cautery, or, less commonly, turbinate resection. The scars from cutaneous lacerations sometimes provide the ability to enter the nose for a direct secondary inspection and repair. In secondary nasoethmoidal repairs, where thick soft tissue obscures the nasal orbital valley, the excess soft tissue needs to be resected to reduce thickness to its proper dimension (13). Soft tissue thinning begins with a periosteal resection and proceeds as needed. The lacrimal system must be cannulated if the pericanthal soft tissue needs to be thinned to avoid accidental injury of this important structure (13). Primarily or secondarily, the use of Doyle nasal splints postoperatively helps to keep the nasal mucosa approximated to the septum in the internal nose and preserves the nasal airway.

Nasal Fractures

Nasal fractures have both functional and esthetic sequelae (48). Initially, the fractures generally demonstrate either lateral and/or posterior dislocation. Functional airway obstruction may be minimized by repositioning the septum with an Asch forceps and by splinting the septum with Doyle nasal splints. Any residual nasal airway obstruction is best managed 3 to 6 months after the fracture, when healing has occurred, making secondary operations more predictable. A septal resection, turbinate out fracture, resection, and/or cautery could be required. Spreader grafts may be necessary if the upper lateral cartilage–septal junction has been disturbed, creating narrowing of the internal nasal valve. In secondary surgery, the deviated portion of the septum is resected, leaving at least a 1- to 1.5-cm dorsal and caudal strut. To straighten a deviated nose, the septum is scored to create a curvature away from the side of deviation (it should be scored on the concave side). It also may be necessary to move, in a converse "swinging door" fashion, the residual septum back in line with the vomer and nasal spine. The septum may be sutured to the spine to prevent its recurrent dislocation (14). When the septal cartilage is weak, it may tend to lean to one side; in this case, it requires a cartilage graft to strengthen it and create more buttressing support for the inherent weakness of the material.

The bony nasal pyramid generally demonstrates two types of deviation: lateral and posterior. Lateral deviations persist because of insufficient mobilization (completion of fractures), incomplete reduction of the bony displacement at the time of closed reduction, or warping forces, generated by cartilage damage, that cause postoperative deviation with healing. The deviated bony nose must be subjected to osteotomies medially and laterally, accompanied by septal repositioning, resection of the distorted portion of the septum, and septal contouring to thoroughly mobilize the nose and septum simultaneously, which replaces the deviated septal structures toward the midline. Any internal "spring" forces that could re-create displacement must be minimized.

Three common errors are committed in acute nasal fracture reductions. The first error is insufficient mobilization of the fractures in order to complete greenstick fractures, which must include those involving the septum as well as the nasal bones. Failure to completely mobilize the nasal bones bilaterally, so one may freely dislocate the mobilized nose and literally rest it toward either cheek, will set the stage for recurrent nasal deviation, as cartilage warps during healing.

The second error is failure to perceive a significant loss of dorsal height or caudal nasal projection. This is caused by septal or nasal bone overriding, creating a loss of bone and cartilage support through bony retrusion and septal collapse. Usually, these fractures cannot be fully reduced by closed or open reduction techniques in the absence of bone or cartilage grafting. They are initially generally allowed to heal, unless it is considered that acute bone or cartilage grafting should be performed to limit contraction of soft tissue that would secondarily reduce the possibility of full nasal skeletal volume correction. Late correction of loss of dorsal height calls for mobilization of the soft tissue, and dorsal and caudal cartilage and bone grafting, with or without osteotomies, depending on whether or not narrowing of the nasal bones is required. Open rhinoplasty often is helpful, but the design of the incision must respect the presence of lacerations that may influence the skin circulation. Generally, nasal fractures that display loss of height demonstrate a slightly widened nose, as the nose flattens and sinks posteriorly.

The comminuted posteriorly impacted nasal fracture will increase its width, widen, and sink backward. These fractures literally are a "bag of bones" that must be initially stabilized by a specific closed reduction technique. Our recommendation in this situation is to pass No. 28 wires percutaneously with a spinal or a curved Mayo needle across the middle aspect of the nasal fracture and below the nasal bones, just over the pyriform aperture. If a wire can be passed anterior and caudal to the canthus from one side of the nose to the other, good proximal control of nasal width is obtained. The wires are "walked" through the nasal fracture sites, passed across the nose, passed through the skin, and then threaded through Xeroform-wrapped orthopedic felt external nasal splints. The wires can be tightened over the padded bolsters, increasing the height and narrowing the width of the nose. Internal nasal Doyle, Xomed, and Mirocel splints may be inserted to preserve the nasal airway. These splints should be left in place for 1 week. It must be emphasized that daily observation and cleaning by the *surgeon* is required underneath any external bolsters if skin necrosis is to be prevented and cutaneous infection is to be monitored. It has been our experience that nursing personnel are incapable of ensuring that circulation is intact and infection is absent, as they desire not to hurt the patient, which is a necessity in the inspection. Only the specialized interest and knowledge of the surgeon will permit the aggressive inspection techniques needed to detect skin conditions under the bolster. Invasive skin infection with ulceration may occur rapidly under any tight compression bolster placed on facial skin.

Late correction of the short nose involves osteotomies that essentially dissect or section the septum at the superior and inferior portions of the nose. As the nose is tilted downward, which requires complete mobilization of the nasal bones, external skin, internal lining, and nasal septum, the lining and septal defects are left superiorly, which are stabilized by bone grafts. Fortunately, this superior (dependently drained) lining defect seldom results in bone graft loss. If nasal lining replacement is required, one can mobilize a galeal frontalis flap, transposing it into the area of absent lining, which solves the lining deficit.

Secondary rhinoplasty in comminuted nasal fractures may be a difficult operation because of irregularity of soft tissue and bone. Considerable thought must be given to the use of incisions, such as in open rhinoplasty, so that the tip framework is not devascularized by previous limitations imposed on the circulation by scars or lacerations.

Orbital Fractures

Orbital fractures are common because of the prominent position the orbit occupies in the midfacial skeleton. The magnitude of orbital fractures varies considerably from simple inferior blow-out fractures to a disruption of the entire anterior and middle orbital sections (13,48,49). The most important prerequisite for a successful outcome is knowledge of the orbital anatomy, specifically internal orbital contours and wall positions (50,51). Orbital injuries commonly damage the globe (52–54). Although many of these injuries are minor, they must be noted and treated. Visual acuity must be checked in each patient.

The pattern of orbital fractures is best revealed by high-resolution CT scans performed in axial and coronal planes with both bone and soft tissue windows (5,35). Three-dimensional CT scans are helpful in cases of late facial asymmetry, but they do not provide the specific detail generated in two-dimensional scans for precise wall identification and internal orbital wall reconstruction (55). When analyzing scans, one is searching for volume discrepancies, either increased or decreased orbital volume, which will lead to the conditions of exophthalmos and enophthalmos, and evidence of entrapment or incarceration of either the extraocular muscle system or the musculofibrous ligament system described by Koorneef (56). The musculofibrous ligament system is a system of fine ligament fibers that link the globe, extraocular muscles, and periosteum extending through the fat to the muscles, globes, and orbital walls. Because all the orbital contents are interconnected, one can impair the motion of an extraocular muscle simply by entrapping a portion of the musculofibrous ligament system, such as the inferior extracoronal fat. From anterior to posterior, the bony orbit has an anterior rim, a middle third, and a posterior section (5). In general, significantly displaced fractures are confined to the anterior and middle segments.

Orbital Bony Anatomy

The orbital rim section is thick, whereas the middle third of the orbit is thinner. The posterior third of orbit is thicker bone and not usually subject to displacement. In effect, the anterior and middle sections of the orbit absorb fracture forces and protect the posterior third from displacement (57–59). In the anterior third of the orbit are the nasoethmoidal section medially, the supraorbital section superiorly, and the zygomatic section laterally and inferiorly. In the middle section of the orbit are located the roof, lateral wall, floor, and medial wall. One must note the curving contours of the middle third of the normal orbit. The lateral wall is straight and reaches the posterior orbit between the superior and inferior fissures. The roof has a double arching superior curvature from anterior to posterior and from medial to lateral. Both the floor and medial wall have a bulge that projects inward, constricting the orbit projecting toward the globe immediately behind the axis of the globe. These constrictions in effect push the globe forward, and they hold extramuscular cone fat in the superior orbit against the upper lid. It is this precise area of floor reconstruction that corrects a supratarsal depression in the upper lid. This inferomedial bony orbital "bulge" is supported by a buttress that extends to the middle turbinate. If damaged, this buttress must be created by floor support.

Reconstructions of the orbit must involve knowledge of the common patterns of fracture displacement and their effects on orbital volume (57,58,60). "Blow-in" (orbital volume construction) and "blow-out" (orbital volume expansion) fractures should be corrected for volume change. The accuracy with which the elliptical diameter of the rim and the accuracy with which the internal orbital walls are constructed will determine the proper position of the globe (61,62). An error of only several millimeters will yield enophthalmos (49,60). It is postulated that every 1 mm of enophthalmos relates to 1 mL of orbital volume increase and that a 2-cm area of orbital wall displaced 3 mm will create orbital enlargement sufficient that globe displacement occurs. It must be emphasized that the shape of the reconstructed orbit controls the position and the appearance of the eye and the periorbita; thus, orbital bone volume and orbital bone shape both are important components of reconstruction (6–8,13). Ninety percent of orbital fractures initially do not induce much orbital fat atrophy; therefore, accurate assembly of the bony walls of the orbit will yield an appropriate eye position in most patients (13,49). Assuming the orbit is a modified cone, increasing the radius of the cone, that is, displacing a segment of the rim, will have a marked effect on orbital volume increase, as the volume of a cone-shaped structure is π $r^2 \times 1/2h$, where r is the radius (Fig. 31-7). Merely displacing one of the internal walls alone adds a linear addition to volume, but the volume addition is not as powerful as increasing the radius of the base (rim), by virtue of the fact that any increase in the radius is squared in the final volume calculation (63–65). Because the volume of the orbit is about 30 mL, small increases (2 to 3 mL or 10%) in orbital volume will begin to produce enophthalmos or globe positional change. Therefore, the adjustment of the orbital volume requires at least as precise an adjustment as setting the occlusion, for instance, where the multiple facets available on the teeth result in precise positioning when placed in IMF. The alignment guides within the orbit are not as clear as the occlusal facets of the teeth, and yet the alignment requirements are as precise and underappreciated by most clinicians.

Medial wall orbital fractures often symmetrically displace (or thin the thickness of) the ethmoid cells. The ethmoid cells are accurately visualized on axial CT scans, and they are reconstructed by adding bone graft over the depressed ethmoid region. In viewing this area in the operating room, it must be appreciated that the medial orbital wall may be symmetrically depressed inward even though disrupted fractures are not seen. The symmetrical ethmoid compression needs to be treated with bone grafting. Often, these medial fractures connect with an inferior floor fracture in the inferomedial portion of the orbit. It is in this area (the inferomedial orbit) where it is difficult to achieve stable bone grafts for correction of orbital volume because of the frequent lack of bone support. In reconstructing the orbit, one must remember that, beyond the initial concavity behind the orbital rim, the orbital floor inclines upward at a 30-degree angle from anterior to posterior. As one travels from lateral to medial across the orbital floor, the orbital floor begins to incline superiorly at a 45-degree angle to meet the medial wall, and it is in this area, just behind the globe, that the inferior and medial walls have the internal "bulge" that needs to be reconstructed (the buttress here essentially needs to be replaced by a stable inferomedial support to stabilize the reconstruction) (52).

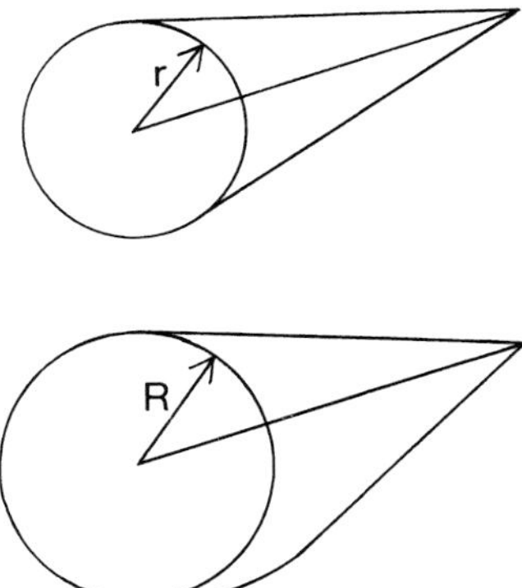

FIGURE 31-7. The orbit is roughly a conical structure, where the radius of the anterior orbit is related to the volume by the formula $\pi r2 \times 1/2h = V$. Increasing the radius has an dramatic effect on volume increase as compared with simply increasing the height, because the radius is squared in the calculation, and the height is a simple linear factor. (From Manson P. Reoperative facial fracture repair. In: Grotting J, ed. *Reoperative aesthetic and reconstructive plastic surgery.* St. Louis: Quality Medical Publishing, 1995:716, with permission.)

At the time of surgical correction, confirmation of the proper vertical level of the globe has an accurate relationship to late postoperative appearance. The globe should, however, in most cases appear anteriorly overcorrected, as swelling causes a relative exophthalmos to be present around the time of injury and the swelling may be increased by the dissection in long operations.

In general, in primary fracture repair, we emphasize an anatomical reconstruction of the orbital walls and rim (60). Secondary operations for globe positional change or enophthalmos may have to emphasize an overcorrection in cases that have fat atrophy (2,14,60). Because the amount of fat atrophy cannot be predicted at the time of primary fracture repair, it is not necessary to routinely overcorrect globe position for this possibility, because most of the patients will not experience significant fat atrophy.

Internal orbital bone grafts or reconstructive materials should be fixed to stable sections of the orbital walls via the lag or "tandem" screw technique, or with a small microplate to ensure table position and prevent migration (66). It is known that bone grafts have increased "take" when they are stabilized by rigid fixation (19). Metallic plates also have been specifically designed for fracture repair and may be used without bone grafts (66,67). The three most prevalent areas where undercorrection occurs are in the size of the orbital rim (too large), of the inferomedial orbit, and the area of the inferior orbital fissure (13,49). The latter area should routinely be obliterated by a bone graft, when it is fractured in primary or secondary reconstruction. It is important that the lateral wall of the orbit be reconstructed as a straight line (13,49). The greater wing of the sphenoid must be aligned with the orbital process of the zygoma. Small (3 mm) differences in rim position may result in an extra 5 mL of orbital volume, which may mean 4 mL or more of enophthalmos, which is a significant amount. Therefore, emphasis on precise positioning in orbital rim reconstruction needs to be stressed.

In patients presenting for secondary correction of globe positional disturbances, a thorough CT scan is used to analyze the displacement of each component of the rim and internal orbital walls (13,48,49,68–70). A thorough physical examination documents (in millimeters) the position of the globe relative to the midline of the nose and relative to the eye on the other side, as well as the number of millimeters of rim displacement. The combination of the physical examination and the CT scan is used to predict which maneuvers, such as additional bone grafting or osteotomy, are needed to correct the globe position in each orbital section. Generally, 3 to 6 months should elapse before all of the induration from the primary injury has dissipated; then, the results of secondary surgery will become more predictable because the soft tissue is more flexible and does not oppose repositioning. Although bone is preferred for primary reconstruction of major orbital defects, bone is subject to some resorption (71) and is a secondary choice to Medpor or polyethylene for small orbital fractures or in secondary reconstruction. Infection and/or late bleeding around alloplastic implants complicated a few implants on long-term follow-up (50,51).

Visual Disturbances

Orbital fractures are commonly associated with visual disturbances and globe positional change. The relationship between globe positional change and double vision is not precisely known; however, in general, it is believed that over 5 mm of vertical globe positional change is necessary to produce double vision. Therefore, one should not promise patients that double vision will be corrected based on a planned repositioning of the globe. Most double vision is, in fact, due to muscular contusion and scarring. Postoperative visual acuity and diplopia problems may only be evaluated accurately when compared with preoperative visual acuity and diplopia measurements. Preoperative measurements are essential for medical record documentation. Therefore, the absence of preinjury measurements makes it difficult to establish the cause of the condition. Further, any secondary surgery must always be performed with this knowledge, and a thorough ophthalmologic examination is required before any patient is subjected to secondary orbital surgery.

Visual Acuity Changes

Any change in visual acuity must be assumed to be optic nerve contusion or vascular impairment of the nerve or sensitive visual system (48,72–77). Thorough CT scans of the posterior portion of the orbit and the optic canal may or may not demonstrate fractures of the optic canal or retrobulbar hematoma. MRI may detect edema, hematoma, and other conditions (76,7). Most patients with visual acuity change and presumed optic nerve damage initially are treated with megadose steroid administration (medical optic nerve decompression). In the absence of improvement or if further deterioration occurs, surgical optic nerve decompression is advocated, as is drainage of retrobulbar hematoma, lateral canthotomy, and soft tissue decompression. In many studies, it has been difficult to prove that vision is routinely improved when surgical decompression of the optic nerve is added; however, there are exceptions and some vigorous advocates of surgical decompression (84). In our unit, surgical decompression is reserved for those who deteriorate or who have no light perception and no response to medical optic nerve decompression alone. In patients with light perception and decreased vision, considerable improvement was obtained without surgical decompression of the optic nerve by medical optic nerve decompression. In total unilateral visual loss, surgical decompression of the optic nerve seems to have little additional risk and may have occasional benefit (79). The optic nerve usually is approached through the medial aspect of the orbit within the ethmoid sinus, releasing the tight bony ring of the optic canal anteriorly and performing a full decompression of the entire canal. The optic nerve sheath should be incised under direct vision, and use of an operating microscope is recommended.

Double Vision

Most double vision, particularly that accompanying inferior blow-out fractures, is due to muscular contusion (57,58,68,80). In some patients, a trapping of fat adjacent to the muscles creates restriction of the extraocular muscle system (81). This is a portion of the comprehensive orbital fibrous connective tissue network described by Koorneef (56,82,83). Small fascial connections link all intraorbital soft tissue structures, and entrapment of the orbital fat may restrict the action of an extraocular muscle. This condition can be determined preoperatively by a forced duction examination. A drop of anesthetic is placed in the inferior lid cul-de-sac, the insertion of the inferior rectus onto the globe is grasped, and the globe is rotated. Any increase in force required to rotate the globe means that the muscle is either contused (and shortened) or trapped. In a late case, a positive duction test also may mean that there has been fibrosis, where the limitation is due to internal muscular scarring. If the forced duction examination demonstrates limited motility and the CT scan confirms an area of soft tissue incarceration, evidence is present to justify operative intervention for the purpose of improving extraocular muscle function. Although Putterman et al. (59) demonstrated that many patients with acute muscle restriction will slowly resolve their diplopia, it is our feeling that these patients now have surgical indications for release where the improvement to be obtained balances the risk (49). Early release presumably allows better muscle motion and permits muscle fiber scarring to occur in an anatomical position, where presumably more muscle movement is possible. Therefore, the therapeutic benefit of early release of the musculofibrous ligament system conceptually is only maximally achieved in the immediate postinjury period (49,56).

At the time of operation, after the area of entrapment has been released surgically, it is appropriate to again perform ductions to determine whether there is improvement (2,49). The lack of improvement after a thorough release emphasizes the presence of extraocular muscle contusion and fibrosis. Therefore, one can compare the preoperative forced duction with the intraoperative forced duction and, following bone graft or alloplast reconstruction of the walls of the orbit, an additional duction examination is performed to assess whether or not the reconstruction materials have worsened the extraocular motility. Only by having the information of several motility examinations clearly in mind can we fully analyze the status of the extraocular muscle system (13,49,56).

The presence of the extraocular muscles immediately adjacent to the walls of the orbit behind the globe should prompt surgeons to dissect carefully in these areas under direct vision with magnification. One usually can see the muscles in deep orbital reconstruction if careful dissection is performed (49).

A situation exists in acute orbital fractures where an extraocular muscle may be "scissored" (that is, the muscle itself is trapped) in a small fracture. These patients cannot look up at all, and decompression should be accomplished *immediately* in these patients to preserve the function of the muscle. Finally, it should be noted that soft tissue edema also produces adverse effects on motility, and it is common in longer operations to notice that the motility examination decreases as the length of the operation increases and as additional wall reconstruction materials are forced against the orbital soft tissue (66).

In the course of operations, strong retraction should not be used on an intraorbital retractor. If incisions and dissection are performed properly, the retractors may be laid in the orbit and simply supported with light finger pressure. The use of strong traction on the eyelids or globe may tear or necrose the eyelid margin, which contributes scarring, scleral show, or ectropion. Strong retraction may produce excess globe pressure that impairs central retinal artery perfusion. The use of strong traction on the globe may damage muscles and increase globe pressure. Strong traction is *never* necessary for exposure if incisions and dissection are adequate (66).

Management of postoperative diplopia usually is conservative. A CT scan performed with axial and coronal sections may demonstrate, with bone and soft tissue windows, each extraocular muscle along its entire course. Duction examinations also are helpful. It is rare that secondary orbital repair surgery should be undertaken for postoperative diplopia unless specific indications exist, such as incomplete exploration and incomplete release of a previous incarceration of the extraocular muscle system in a fracture. Most diplopia will be improved by late eye muscle surgery and not by late fracture reduction or muscle lysis. Any secondary orbital reconstruction, however, should always precede any eye muscle correction by a period of healing, often 6 months.

Ptosis and the Superior Orbital Fissure Syndrome

Ptosis and the superior orbital fissure syndrome (ptosis, ophthalmoplegia, and sensory defects in cranial nerve VI) (75,84,85) are caused by blunt injuries in the posterosuperior orbit that damage nerves traveling through the superior orbital fissure. There may or may not be fractures involving the superior orbital fissure. Although the Japanese have advocated decompression of the superior orbital fissure, decompressions have not been popular in North America (85). The use of medical-dose steroids would seem to be indicated and, if a fracture repair is contemplated, simultaneous attention to decompression can be given. A period of 6 months should elapse before any lid procedures for ptosis correction are considered, as spontaneous improvement is common. Traumatic injuries may disrupt the levator aponeurosis, particularly in older individuals in whom the levator is fragile because it has been thinned by aging changes. These patients, of course, are candidates for surgical levator repair.

Lacrimal Obstruction

Most lacrimal obstructions occur because of direct damage to the bony lacrimal canal where displacement of the bone causes lacrimal canal obstruction (16). Soft tissue canalicular injury of significance usually is accompanied by a cutaneous laceration. Studies have shown that attempts to intubate the lacrimal system at the time of injury to improve function are not helpful and may further damage the system. Precise repositioning of bone fragments is the best preventive treatment for lacrimal obstruction. If lacrimal obstruction occurs, it is best managed by a secondary dacryocystorhinostomy. Abscess formation is possible when lacrimal obstruction exists and presents over the canalicular system. Drainage of the mass occurring at the inferomedial orbit and antibiotics are indicated. A secondary dacryocystorhinostomy should also be performed.

Lid and Canthal Malposition

Possibly the most distressing postoperative complications are related to malposition of the lids and canthal structures (86). Many operations for orbital fracture reduction require a lower lid incision. The inferior lid is prone to malposition with scleral show and ectropion. Most studies emphasized that the lower the incision is in the lid, the less the chance of ectropion, but the more visible the incision (18,87). The use of skin muscle flaps (as compared with skin flaps) decreases the incidence of ectropion, as does the use of conjunctival incisions. Scar contracture and orbicularis muscle denervation set the stage for lid position abnormalities in subciliary incisions. Two factors are important: (i) damage to the orbicularis muscle and orbital septum, or simply surgical dissection, which creates fibrosis and contracture, pulling the lid downward; and (ii) denervation of the pretarsal portion of the orbicularis muscle, which has an action (when it contracts) to force the lower lid upward. When the pretarsal muscle is taken off the tarsus, it is denervated and reinnervation may be incomplete. Therefore, surgeons who prefer subciliary incisions emphasize that the first portion of a subciliary dissection should be a "skin-only" flap with dissection transecting the muscle inferior to the tarsal plate. Conceptually, this "stepped" dissection preserves the innervation of the pretarsal orbicularis. An orbital rim incision should be made in eyelid skin (not cheek skin), as any incision is visible in cheek skin. Generally, the extension of incisions in the mid or lower lid lateral to the midpupillary line makes the eyelids more prone to edema and increases the visibility of the scar. The midtarsal incision seems to be a compromise between a rim incision and a subciliary incision: it begins medially, just inferior to the lacrimal system, and crosses the lower edge of the tarsal plate (87). The transconjunctival incision may be located either inferior to the tarsal plate or in the fornix. The fornix incision is less traumatic to the orbital septum (86). Conceptually, an incision high in the conjunctiva may create almost the same septal fibrosis as a transcutaneous incision by scarring produced along the border of the orbital septum and orbicularis oculi muscle.

Lid support consists of the traction provided by the medial and lateral canthi and tarsal plate, and the upper orbicularis forcing the lid upward. Lid support also is dependent on the positioning of the fixed length of periosteum and orbital septum (which connect lower lid structures to the bone) to the orbital rim. It also depends on upward force of contraction of the orbicularis muscle and the elastic fibers of the lids. Therefore, all of these factors must be defined when lid positional abnormalities are encountered, to define the etiology of the problem. The medial canthus has three limbs that surround the lacrimal fossa (46). The anterior limb extends anterior to the lacrimal system and up the nasal side wall, and the posterior limb keeps the eyelid tangent to the globe. Similarly, the lateral canthus has two limbs (88), the deeper of which attaches to the Whitnall tubercle and, by virtue of this posterior connection, the eyelid margin is maintained tangent to the globe. When one is reattaching canthal ligament structures, it is common to direct the lateral canthus to a point above and behind its normal attachment, as a single vector of traction is being used to reconstruct a three-dimensional structure. The lateral canthus generally should be vectored almost to the zygomaticofrontal suture, or at least attached as high as the superior level of the pupil and just inside the internal aspect of the lateral orbital rim (89,90).

The medial canthus should be directed to a point posterior and superior to the upper edge of the lacrimal fossa (42). Drill holes are placed and two wires are connected to a nonabsorbable suture placed in the canthus through an external incision. The suture, by virtue of the wire connection, is pulled toward the medial orbital rim and may be tightened or released quite easily to check alignment. To secure the transnasal wires, they are tied around a screw in the frontal bone (glabella) or placed through a hole in a plate used for fracture reduction. Secondarily, canthi may be freely repositioned *only* following wide subperiosteal dissection, which releases abnormal attachments and fibrosis and permits tension-free repositioning. The periosteum may have to be resected to permit increased flexibility of soft tissue.

At least 10% of patients having lower eyelid subciliary incisions will experience scleral show and ectropion (91). Entropion is less common and usually is the result of an incision too close to the lower lid ciliary margin. Entropion is produced by scarring within the posterior lamella, which turns the lid inward and inverts it. Elderly individuals (and those with very lax lower lids) should have skin incisions placed over the inferior orbital rim. Otherwise, consideration must be given to a simultaneous procedure that improves lower eyelid elasticity, such as horizontal lid shortening or canthopexy.

Use of the transconjunctival fornix incision is complicated by the least lower eyelid retraction (68). Most inferior orbital access incisions dissect the external lamella from the internal lamella of the lid, which increases the potential for scar contracture and surgical damage to the septum. Additionally, the use of titanium plates on the inferior orbital rim creates soft tissue fibrosis that contributes to septal and lid shortening. Placing the inferior orbital rim plate below the prominence of the inferior orbital rim (Fig. 31-8) is one option for decreasing metallic structures along the rim that contribute to inflammation. Finally, when extensive dissections have mobilized the entire soft tissue of the cheek off the maxilla and zygoma, the cheek tissue must be repositioned and anchored to the bone (21–23). When making an incision in the periosteum over the lower anterior face of the inferior orbital rim, it is our practice to mark each of the incised periosteal edges with a silk suture so that they may be precisely identified at the time of closure.

The initial management of scleral show or ectropion should include massage, squinching exercises to strengthen the orbicularis oculi muscle, and warm compresses, which stimulate circulation and make the lid more flexible. In the presence of corneal drying, urgent protection of the cornea must be provided by tarsorrhaphy or skin graft with canthoplasty for severe ectropion. In the absence of corneal exposure, at least 6 months should be permitted for the lid to complete the cycle of healing and resolution of induration, during which the contracture and lid abnormality may entirely resolve. When a lid position abnormality exists, one should analyze the position of the lower orbital rim, the position of the canthi, and the location and severity of fibrosis within the lid (anterior or posterior lamella) (63–65,92). If the lid is grasped with forceps, it should be able to be elevated over the superior margin of the pupil in a normal, flexible lid. When this cannot be done, fibrosis and contracture have restricted the lamella, and these structures need to be released (93). Opinion is divided on whether spacers or grafts (65,92) should be placed into a contracture of the posterior lamella (Fig. 31-8) (48). Some favor placing a thin

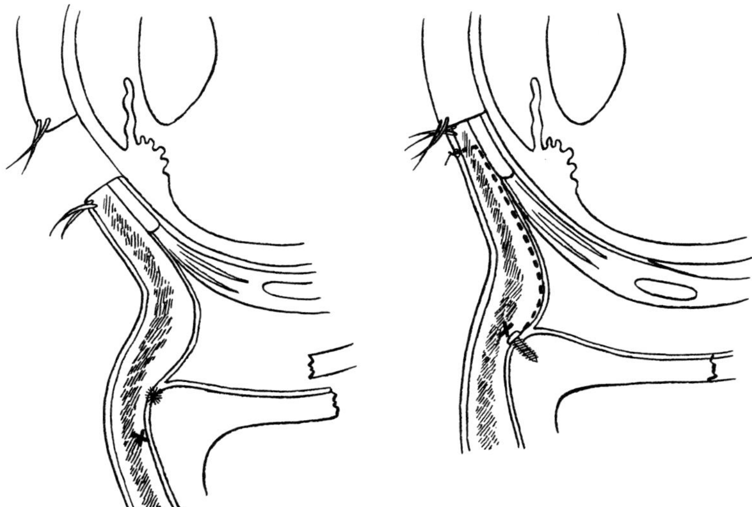

FIGURE 31-8. Lid contractures must be analyzed for defects in the anterior or posterior lamella. Repositioning of the soft tissue that slipped onto the inferior orbital rim and malar eminence.

carved wafer of nasal cartilage graft to support the tarsus in a superior position. In the face of internal lamellar contracture with conjunctival fibrosis, a graft of palatal or buccal mucosa may be added. A decision has to be made whether there is adequate skin in the anterior lamella; otherwise, a skin graft may need to be used (Fig. 31-9). In dissecting the contracture, it is wise to perform a skin-only flap initially for 6 to 8 mm and then extend the dissection beneath the orbicularis muscle inferior to the tarsus. This would allow one to skin graft the superior portion of the orbicularis oculi, if necessary. After the fibrosis and contractures are released, the decision about what grafts are necessary may be made. The cutaneous incisions are closed after cartilage or soft tissue grafts are added internally, and the lid is held superiorly for several days with two Frost traction or two intermarginal sutures. Intermarginal sutures should be placed through a rubber bolster, which stays for 1 week, to minimize the chance of pressure necrosis of the delicate skin of the lid margin. These sutures encourage superior positioning of the lower lid. In cases where the entire soft tissue of the cheek has slipped inferiorly, the whole soft tissue envelope must be redissected to the gingival margin and then anchored securely to the body of the zygoma and to the inferior orbital rim, releasing any cheek contracture by periosteal resection. The periosteum of the cheek may need to be scored or completely resected to permit free movement.

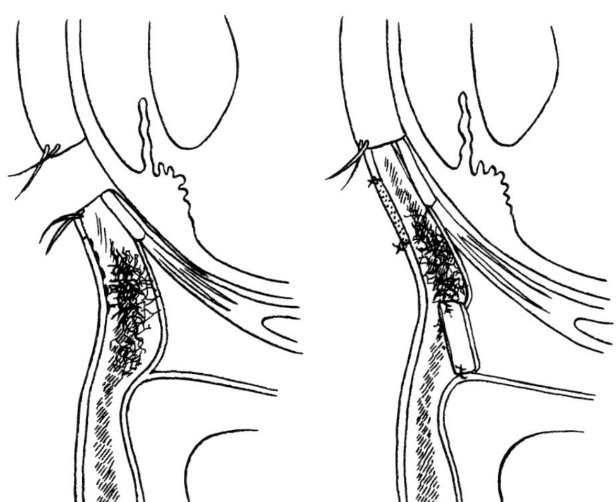

FIGURE 31-9. Anterior and posterior lamella contracture requires release and perhaps splinting with a thin (tarsal thickness) cartilage graft posteriorly and a skin graft anteriorly. Anterior lamella contracture may require a skin graft, which can be placed on the preserved tarsal orbicularis oculi muscle. (From Manson P. Reoperative facial fracture repair. In: Grotting J, ed. *Reoperative aesthetic and reconstructive plastic surgery*. St. Louis: Quality Medical Publishing, 1995:728, with permission.)

Retrobulbar Hematoma

Retrobulbar hematoma is an accumulation of blood in the intraconal compartment produced by an episode of bleeding behind the globe (94). The bleeding may contribute to vascular spasm or create excessive pressure that may slow circulation in the ophthalmic or retinal arteries or veins or slow the circulation to critical capillary beds that perfuse portions of the optic nerve (75,77,95). Two areas of the optic nerve may receive decreased circulation initiated by spasm or pressure from a retrobulbar hematoma. The pressure should be relieved *immediately* by release of all cutaneous sutures and section of the lateral canthal ligament. Thereafter, a CT scan should be obtained in an optic nerve protocol format. The bony reduction may need to be disassembled and bone grafts removed to decrease pressure. The removal of intraorbital grafts releases pressure, as does evacuation of hematoma. Urgent ophthalmologic consultation is obtained, and when the pressure is relieved, the vision usually will return. It has been postulated that "watershed areas" of the optic nerve circulation may tolerate absent circulation for about 2 hours, so urgency is imperative if vision is to be salvaged. Incisions may be opened immediately and the lateral canthus released. Anterior chamber paracentesis should not be attempted without expert ophthalmologic consultation.

Orbital Cellulitis

Orbital cellulitis is a serious condition that requires prompt treatment (96). Any increased pressure should be dealt with by opening skin sutures and sectioning the lateral canthus. The cause of the orbital cellulitis usually is spread of infection from a sinus obstruction, such as an ethmoid or frontal sinus obstruction or an infected hematoma, and urgent drainage of any collection under pressure is indicated. Immediate operative intervention to eliminate the focus of the infection is essential. Culture-specific antibiotics are used. The vision must be monitored carefully throughout this period. Steroids are not indicated unless vision is compromised. Their use must be considered carefully, as they are believed to impair response to infection, but they may act to preserve capillary circulation and limit reactive edema. Blindness has occurred with orbital cellulitis (97).

Zygomatic Fractures

Zygomatic fracture malposition is common following midface fracture treatment (98). Usually, the malposition is related to the failure to expose all of the zygomatic buttresses when performing fracture reduction (99). Consequently, good alignment is not achieved. Conceptually, as with the nasoethmoid, three incisions are required for full zygomatic exposure: the coronal incision, a lower lid incision of some type, and a gingivobuccal sulcus incision (9,97,100). Currently, it is popular to treat zygoma fractures with limited approaches to minimize cutaneous scars, such as those present with lower lid incisions. Limited incisions are an entirely appropriate approach for simple zygoma fractures; however, the approach requires skill and judgment. The most appropriate fractures for treatment by limited approaches are those that are greensticked at the zygomaticofrontal suture, those that do not display a significant intraorbital component, and those that are not comminuted at the inferior orbital rim (14,97). Because many zygoma fractures are medially displaced, when they are reduced, a significant dehiscence of the orbital floor may occur whereas previously, the "telescoped" fracture edges prevented prolapse of intraorbital contents and functional orbital volume increase.

Based on experience, a classification may be developed for zygomatic displacement that predicts which incisions usually are necessary for accurate reduction of a fracture (9). For instance, when the zygomatic arch is laterally displaced, a coronal incision usually is required to accurately reduce the fracture (10,14,97), because the periosteum of the arch is torn in lateral displacements and stability cannot be achieved after closed reduction (9). However, the coronal incision may create temporal contour deformity from fat atrophy or plate prominence (2,13,15,24). On the other hand, medially displaced arch fractures generally respond to closed reduction, with satisfactory stability. Thus, these fractures may be treated with anterior alone approaches, such as the combination of lower lid and gingivobuccal sulcus incisions. Conceptually, each zygoma fracture must be assessed at six areas of alignment with adjacent bones, including the greater wing of the sphenoid (10,13). The structural relationships of the zygoma to bones in the internal lateral and posterior orbit also provide helpful guides to predicting what reduction maneuvers are necessary. An accurate analysis of each area of alignment is also essential when planning a zygomatic osteotomy. Generally, the most common abnormality experienced following zygoma fracture treatment is a flattening of the malar eminence. This occurs because the malar eminence is not tipped up at the time of fracture reduction and held while plate and screw fixation is applied. Reduction of the malar eminence may be accomplished percutaneously through the skin of the malar eminence with a small external incision through which a Carroll-Girard screw is placed into the zygoma. Otherwise, a bone hook can be placed under the malar eminence through a buccal incision. The next most common abnormality is an inferior positioning of the orbital rim, which leads to enlargement of the orbit, a lower position of the lower eyelid, and enophthalmos. These deformities usually are accompanied by lateral canthal dystopia. The best way to prevent zygomatic fracture malposition is to simultaneously assess the alignment of the zygoma (which is being obtained at the time of open reduction through multiple approaches), with all of its adjacent bones (19). First, stainless steel interfragment wires are placed to temporarily reduce the fractures at the zygomaticofrontal suture, the inferior orbital rim, and perhaps in the arch, as positioning guides. A complete zygoma open reduction requires multiple approaches, and one can only visualize one approach at a time. The wires provide temporary fixation and alignment. Initial wire fixation minimizes the displacement that may occur when working in another area and yet still presents the option for some flexible movement to reach final bone position. Therefore, one may finely adjust zygoma position with these wires in place, knowing that one is not significantly displacing fracture sites in the other exposure areas. This sequential reduction permits the most accurate final positioning for stabilization by plates and screws.

Late Deformity

Conceptually, small postoperative deficiencies of projection of the malar prominence can be managed by simple augmentation with alloplastic materials through an intraoral approach. More extensive zygomatic deformities will require a complete osteotomy and usually simultaneous bone grafting, as the shape or contour of the zygoma often is different following a fracture and the fracture sites often have remodeled. The design of the osteotomy is based on the requirements of repositioning and may be total or subtotal, depending on the deformity observed. Bone grafts often may have to be added to complete reconstruction of bone deficiencies. Malar fractures associated with exophthalmos require an expansion of orbital volume (69,101).

Infraorbital Nerve Numbness

Infraorbital nerve numbness is a component of almost every zygomatic or inferior orbital fracture. The symptom requires specific decompression of the infraorbital foramen at the time of zygomatic fracture repair and decompression should be accomplished in late osteotomy if numbness is a symptom. This is a very important step in fractures that are medially dislocated. Generally, hypesthesia of the lip, ipsilateral nose, and anterior teeth improves over a 1-year period. In those with chronic pain, dilute triamcinolone acetonide (Kenalog) may be injected near the infraorbital nerve foramen. More extensive neurolysis or nerve decompressions have been partially successful.

Le Fort Fractures

Le Fort fractures involve various segments of the midfacial skeleton alone or in combination (10). The most minor midfacial fractures consist of alveolar fractures of the maxilla. These fractures usually are stabilized with an arch bar that may be acrylated for support (4,19). If the fracture is open, it is easy and very desirable to openly reduce the bone through the laceration. For the alveolar ridge, unicortical plates and screws avoid damage to tooth roots. The common problem with alveolar fractures is premature occlusal contact secondary to interposition of soft tissue or callus in the fracture site. Conceptually, this might require an open removal of the interposed soft tissue or muscle or completion of a greenstick fracture. Late tooth loss in alveolar segment fractures is common, and patients should be warned to expect this (2,102). Another (more sophisticated) method to stabilize an alveolar fracture consists of the application of orthodontic bands cemented onto the teeth, which are more convenient for the patient and more comfortable than an arch bar. All premature occlusal contact must be prevented in order to avoid tooth loss (8).

Fractures of the palate are frequent in high-energy, lower midface trauma. The segments consist of portions of the maxillary alveolus (103). Many palatal fractures are accompanied by a complete fracture at the Le Fort I level. About half of these fractures are accompanied by lacerations of the lip and roof of the mouth. Therefore, it is easy to expose the fracture segments by stripping 1 cm of mucoperiosteum (102,103). In younger individuals and in teenagers, the fracture may be a true midline palatal fracture. In older individuals, the fracture usually parallels the palatal midline or the alveolus. The fracture may be exposed by developing mucoperiosteal flaps, sufficient that two three-hole plates may be placed, one toward the anterior and one toward the posterior aspect of the palatal vault fracture. Next, the anterior margin of the fracture at the pyriform aperture should be reduced and stabilized with a five-hole plate (Fig. 31-10). This plate may be purchased with short screws, if it is necessary to avoid tooth roots. The palatal vault and the maxillary arch stabilization thus are complete, reconstructing the dental-bearing portion of the maxilla as a one-piece fragment that can be managed like a noncomminuted Le Fort I fracture. Application of an arch bar to the dentition usually precedes fixation in the roof of the mouth and at the pyriform aperture; in effect, the arch bar provides a "tension band" across the maxillary dentition. Thus, four fixation maneuvers are available to stabilize the split palate fracture: vault, pyriform aperture, arch bars, and splint. The fourth maneuver is a palatal splint, which can be used to improve dental occlusion or the stability of the fixation. The splint is constructed from dental models in which the alveolar segments have been repositioned at the fracture sites. Comminuted palatal fractures are more difficult to manage with vault plate and screw fixation and are best managed with a splint, arch bars, and alveolar ridge stabilization.

Reconstruction of the maxillary dental arch should precede reconstruction of the mandible, as the key to mandibular width is an intact maxillary dental arch. There is no other absolute guide to mandibular width that is as precise as the intact or anatomically reconstructed maxilla.

Le Fort fractures are suspected when there are signs of a bilateral midface fracture. In the case of a Le Fort I, the presence of the fracture is signaled by malocclusion, maxillary mobility, or bilateral air–fluid levels of the maxillary sinus (93,102,103). High Le Fort fractures that are impacted and subtly displaced are more difficult to diagnose and may be easily missed. Generally, these "greensticked" high Le Fort fractures can be managed by application of arch bars and institution of elastic traction alone (without an open reduction) (6,7). If this maneuver does not satisfactorily stabilize normal occlusion, an osteotomy at the Le Fort I level should be performed (most impacted Le Fort fractures are actually high Le Fort II or III fractures) (102–105). The reason for performing an osteotomy at the Le Fort I level is that it is more straightforward and predictable, and it avoids completion of a fracture by force application within the orbits, which may cause fractures to extend to the cranial base or optic foramen and produce visual loss or cerebrospinal fluid leak (13). Impacted lower Le Fort fractures should have completion of the maxillary fracture at the Le Fort I level, and the patient should be placed in IMF in normal occlusion and plate and screw fixation completed at the four anterior maxillary buttresses (8). Bone grafts should span any bone gap and should cover the maxillary sinuses. Any patient with a bilateral periorbital ecchymosis should be suspected of having a Le Fort fracture. It is possible, in im-

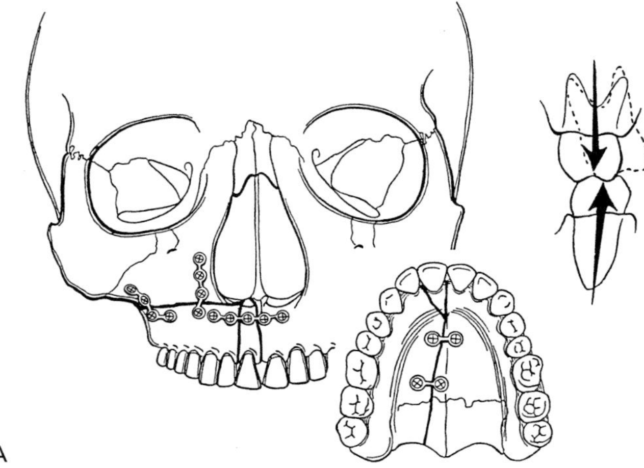

FIGURE 31-10. Sagittal fractures of the maxilla can be stabilized by palatal vault stabilization and stabilization at the pyriform aperture. **A:** Artist's depiction of palatal vault stabilization. **B:** Clinical view of stabilization in the palatal vault. **C:** View of stabilization at the pyriform aperture. (From Hendrickson M, Clark N, Manson P. Sagittal fractures of the maxilla: classification and treatment. *Plast Reconstr Surg* 1998;101:319–332, with permission.)

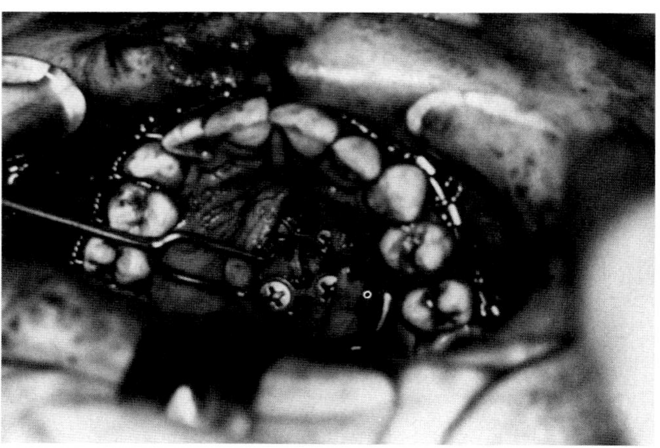

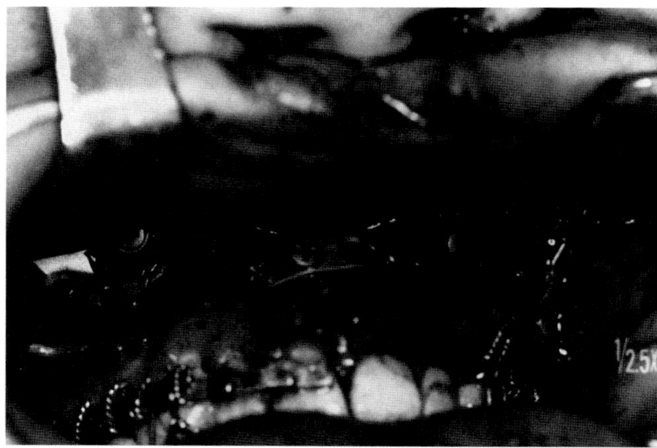

pacted Le Fort II or III fracture treatment, to dislocate the mandible, as there is laxity in the attachments of the mandible at the temporomandibular joint (TMJ), and the mandible may be easily displaced forward, forcing it into occlusion with an impacted and slightly anteriorly displaced maxilla (Fig. 31-11). Once the IMF is released, the condyles of the mandible resume their normal position in the condylar fossae, and the teeth are in malocclusion with an anterior open bite and a class II occlusion. Therefore, the impacted or incompletely mobilized maxilla is prone to malocclusion. In the reduction of Le Fort fractures, initial disimpaction and mobilization of the maxilla should be accomplished so that the maxilla may be freely placed, without any resistance, in normal occlusion with the mandible and the mandibular condyles seated in the condylar fossa.

Bone Loss at the Le Fort I Level

In cases where there is bone loss at the Le Fort I level, the anterior maxillary wall and the buttresses should be bone grafted for stability. In the absence of bone graft, plates and screws may loosen over time, and fibrous union produces malocclusion and malunion. The bone of the Le Fort I level is thin and is prone to microfractures and screw loosening. At the end of every Le Fort or mandibular fracture open reduction, the IMF should be released, the mandibular condyles seated in the condylar fossa by placing pressure against the inferior aspect of the mandibular angles, and the mandible brought into occlusion with the maxilla. This maneuver checks the occlusion at rest. If the occlusion is not correct, the plates and screws need to removed and reapplied with the mandible in proper condylar position and the maxilla freely mobilized.

Facial Height in the Face of Bone Loss

In the face of extensive bone loss at the Le Fort I level in all buttresses, sometimes it is difficult to select proper buttress height. Usually, if the components of one buttress are present and are reassembled, reconstruction of one buttress provides a clue to the height required in the other three anterior Le Fort I level buttresses. If none of the buttresses can be reassembled anatomically by repositioning their component parts, lip-tooth position is the best clue to midface height. An old picture gives a clue to facial height and lip tooth position. Absent or deficient maxillary buttresses or anterior maxillary wall segments require bone grafting as well as plate and screw fixation.

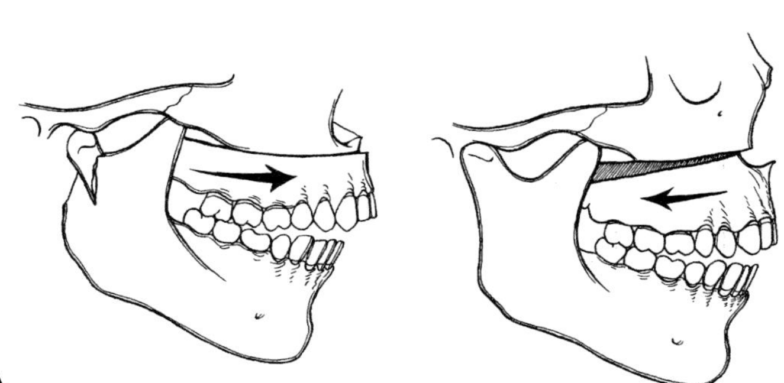

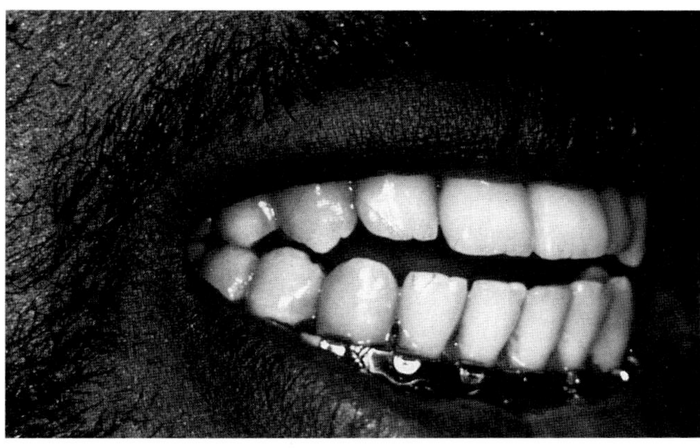

FIGURE 31-11. Impacted Le Fort fractures can easily be mistreated by dislocating the mandible forward to meet the impacted, dislocated maxilla. **A: Right:** The mandible can be dragged forward in the glenoid fossa to an impacted anteriorly dislocated maxilla. When the intermaxillary fixation (IMF) is released, the mandible returns to its normal position, creating an anterior open bite and malocclusion. **Left:** The combination of subcondylar and Le Fort fractures requires fixation of both structures, the mandible, and malocclusion. **B:** Anterior open bite and malocclusion created by reseating of a mandible in the condylar fossa after release of IMF. Its original placement in IMF to an impacted Le Fort fracture created initial occlusal alignment at the expense of condylar displacement. (From Manson P. Reoperative facial fracture repair. In: Grotting J, ed. *Reoperative aesthetic and reconstructive plastic surgery.* St. Louis: Quality Medical Publishing, 1995, with permission.)

Late management of the short midface or maxilla with malocclusion is by maxillary osteotomy (Fig. 31-12) and down-graft. Usually, patients require preoperative and postoperative orthodontics. Detailed analysis by dental models, cephalometrograms, and CT scans to determine precisely what changes need to be accomplished is a requirement for success.

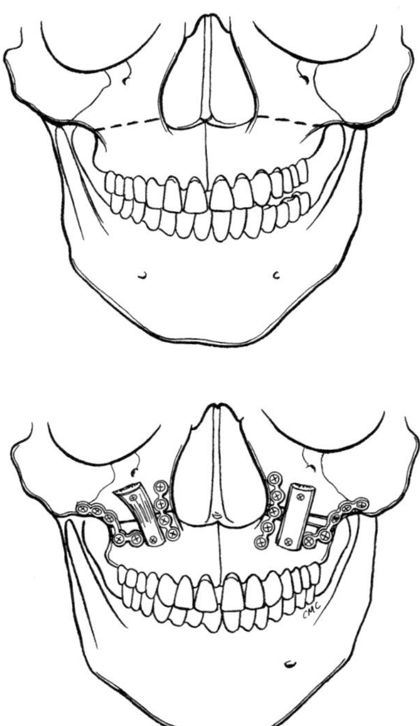

FIGURE 31-12. Maxillary osteotomy can be used to reposition the maxilla, which is in malocclusion with the mandible. In general, bone grafts are required on at least one side.

Edentulous Le Fort Fractures

Edentulous Le Fort fractures represent fractures occurring in bone that has an underlying "bone disease" yielding alveolar ridge resorption and loss of teeth (8,105). Prophylactic bone grafting is recommended for these fractures to provide extra bone for good osseous union. Additionally, the pyriform aperture area and anterior maxilla often have atrophied, so that placing augmentation bone grafts in these areas tends to improve the appearance of the patient, as well as provide extra bone for healing. Placing bone grafts in these areas may interfere with the fit and seal of previously constructed dentures, and patients must be so informed. In order to find solid bone for fixation in edentulous Le Fort fractures, it often is necessary to bring the reduction plate down to the basal bone of the maxillary alveolus. Such a low fixation point often produces interference with wearing of the denture by changing the contour of the alveolar ridge. Fixation hardware may have to be removed or bone grafts remodeled or partially removed before denture use. Sensitive or prominent plates also should be removed following fracture treatment, as they are uncomfortable and will result in plate exposure through the mechanism of mucosal trauma.

Comminuted Le Fort and Panfacial Fracture Treatment

In comminuted Le Fort fractures (2), it is difficult to stabilize the maxilla as securely as desired. Plates may become loose because the bone is thin, and there may be microfractures in the bone that is used for fixation, which yields loose screws. In these cases, considerable stability is achieved by a short period of IMF. Two to three weeks in IMF generally provides an initial period of stability and soft tissue rest, after which motion may be instituted, watching the occlusion carefully to make sure that no shift occurs. A soft diet is permitted at the time of mobilization.

Frequently, malocclusion results from inadequate application of arch bars or from establishing initially unsatisfactory occlusal relationships. Loose or improperly applied arch bars permit the possibility of segment movement and permit migration of the dental segments. The application of rigid fixation when the arch bars are loose may stabilize the fractures in the wrong position.

Complex Le Fort Fractures

Importance of "Washouts" in Le Fort Fracture Treatment

Complex Le Fort fractures represent severe injuries where there is much soft tissue and bone damage (2). These patients easily tolerate return to the operating room at 48-hour intervals for a "washout," where the sinuses are irrigated, the oral hygiene is improved, the teeth are cleansed, hematomas are drained, the nose is suctioned free of all clot and inspissated material, the arch bars are retightened, and the proper occlusal relationships are confirmed. Such cleansings minimize infection and are used in significant combined soft tissue and bony injuries routinely in our unit. They initially were advocated in shotgun injuries, but they are useful in a variety of high-energy facial injuries.

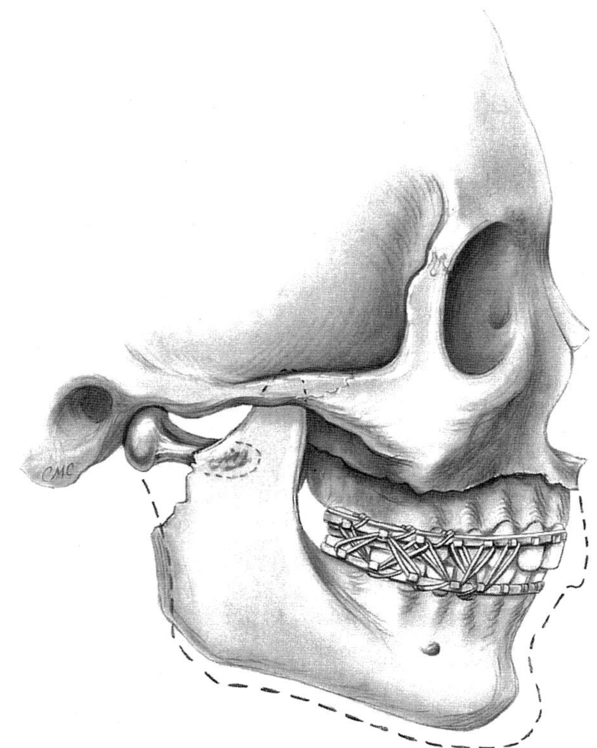

FIGURE 31-13. The maxilla may displace differently, depending on the reduction maneuvers used. In the absence of intermaxillary fixation, the maxilla drops posteriorly and inferiorly. It is easier to bring the maxilla forward than it is superiorly after partial healing has occurred. When a shortened ramus is not addressed in concomitant mandibular and loose Le Fort fractures, the entire complex of the lower maxilla and mandible may shorten and retrude, producing a short, retruded lower facial third. (From Manson P, Crawley W. Midface fractures: advantages of immediate reconstruction and bone grafting. Plast Reconstr Surg 1985;76:1, with permission.)

Combined Le Fort and Vertical Ramus Fractures

The lower maxilla (Le Fort I level) represents thin bone and cannot be relied on to support a mandibular fracture, particularly when a loose ramus (mandibular low subcondylar) fracture that one is trying to treat closed displaces the maxilla through the forces of the strong mandibular musculature (2). The vertical height of the ramus in subcondylar fractures is not necessarily guaranteed by anterior maxillary buttress plate and screw fixation. Shortening of the maxilla posteriorly and superior migration of the occlusal plane may be experienced (Fig. 31-13). The only accurate way to guarantee proper mandibular ramus height is through an open reduction of the mandible, which should be considered especially when loose maxillary fractures accompany a loose mandibular fracture where there has been a simultaneous reduction of ramus height.

Postoperatively, the treatment of a shortened ramus with a tilted occlusal plane requires a simultaneous two-jaw procedure, a bilateral sagittal split osteotomy of the mandible and genioplasty, and a Le Fort I osteotomy of the maxilla with bone grafting on at least one side. A prerequisite to the success of this plan is good TMJ function. The two-jaw osteotomy is a formidable procedure in these patients. If they are not symptomatic with malocclusion, some may be treated by ignoring the occlusal cant, masking the deformity by camouflage asymmetrical genioplasty.

The superior aspect of Le Fort fractures consists of zygomatic and nasoethmoidal components. These fractures were discussed previously, and the treatment of complications in these areas is addressed under the individual components of the zygoma, orbit, nose, and nasoethmoidal area.

The zygomatic arch is an important landmark in midfacial reconstruction, especially the comminuted midface. It represents one of the only good "sagittal" buttresses of the midface (2). Its importance, however, and its singular use as a guide to midface position have been overemphasized. Lateral displacement of the zygomatic arch in a CT scan implies a higher-energy fracture that usually benefits from open reduction (1,9,100). The zygomatic arch is flat in its midportion and should be reconstructed anatomically as a flat structure by the use of plates and screws applied on the lateral surface of the arch. This fixation needs to be strong, and a special thin but strong plate, the Zydaption plate (Synthes), has been manufactured for this role. This fixation is strong enough to hold any arch straight, thereby correcting the anterior projection of the body of the zygoma. The plate needed is thin but stiff to guarantee this position without producing contour deformity. Zygomatic arch fractures that are dislocated medially usually can be managed with a closed reduction of the arch (Gillies reduction) with exposure, open reduction, and rigid fixation of the anterior zygomatic buttresses. When drilling in the zygomatic arch, one should bear in mind the location of the glenoid fossa to avoid screw penetration of the TMJ or the condyle of the mandible. As zygomatic arch fragments are reduced and positioned medially, the greater wing of the sphenoid and orbital process of the zygoma come into alignment and the projection of the malar eminence is corrected. Proper restoration of zygomatic projection requires an arch reduction that is brought to its full length, and the reduction of the zygomatic arch is confirmed by looking inside the lateral portion of the orbit to confirm alignment of the sphenoid and orbital process of the zygoma. One therefore needs to periodically look inside the orbit as one is performing arch open reduction to confirm that proper midface width and arch length are obtained.

Midface lengthening may occur either at the Le Fort I level, where the maxilla generally descends posteriorly and begins to heal in an elongated position, creating an anterior open bite, or through the orbit. An anterior open bite and edge incisor occlusion (Fig. 31-14) are the first signs of posterior and inferior maxillary movement. Both of these situations occur mostly in delayed fracture treatment, where the fractures have begun to heal in a lengthened position, where IMF has not initially been utilized. Alternately, such displacement may be noted when comminuted Le Fort fractures are stabilized without IMF postoperatively. In this regard, the patient's preinjury appearance needs to be carefully scrutinized and compared with the reduction result achieved, especially with regard to midface length and lip-tooth relationships.

In planning osteotomies on fractures that demonstrate malposition or retrusion, conceptually one should always plan for bone grafts, which probably will be required at least on one side. Usually an osteotomy alone is not enough to guarantee proper projection and position, as the bone has partially resorbed and requires onlay and inlay bone grafting as well as osteotomy. In fractures of the maxilla that are short, the need for bone buttressing and supplemental bone grafts is obvious to reinforce the thin maxillary walls in their newly reconstructed position, and one may exceptionally need distraction techniques. One may expect a degree of relapse after elective down-graft or advancement maxillary procedures, as one does in elective maxillary osteotomies. Generally, patients should be prepared to undergo preoperative and postoperative orthodontic treatment to obtain the best result and occlusal relationships in maxillary osteotomies.

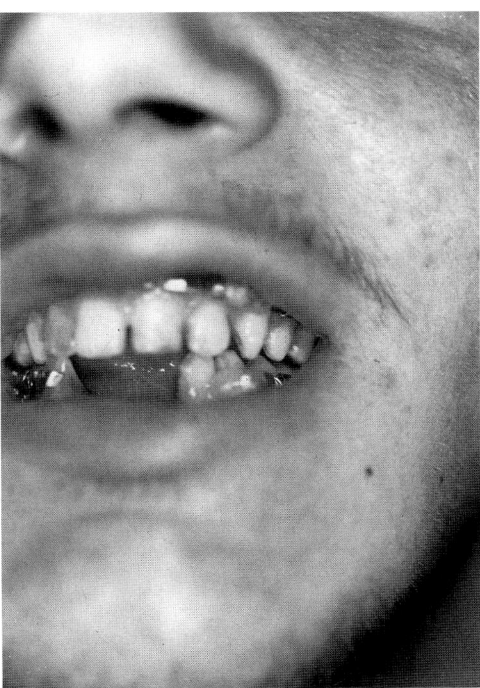

FIGURE 31-14. An open bite at the cuspids and edge incisor occlusion are the first signs of maxillary retrusion if it is occurring following release of intermaxillary fixation. Anterior open bite is observed by loss of cuspid contact.

Malocclusion noted early after initial fracture repair sometimes can be corrected by elastic traction (Fig. 31-15). Once the maxilla has begun to heal, however, one may extrude or extract teeth rather than move the bone segment. The malpositioned bone segment should be remobilized in a return to the operating room, removing the plates and screws, mobilizing the bone, and repositioning the plates. If malocclusion is noted 4 or more weeks after fracture treatment and does not respond to elastic traction under close observation, an elective osteotomy or maxillary mobilization may be required. It may or may not be advisable to allow the patient to heal initially, acquiring more range of mandibular motion and TMJ function. One then may proceed with an elective osteotomy after orthodontic correction has been instituted and full TMJ function achieved. Orthodontics sometimes can completely manage a minor occlusion or occlusal discrepancy, but the range of orthodontic correction is only millimeters. Orthodontics is best suited for small horizontal movements and manages anterior open bite correction with more difficulty.

Mandibular Fractures

Mandibular fractures often are multiple and, as such, frequently involve both the horizontal and vertical portions of

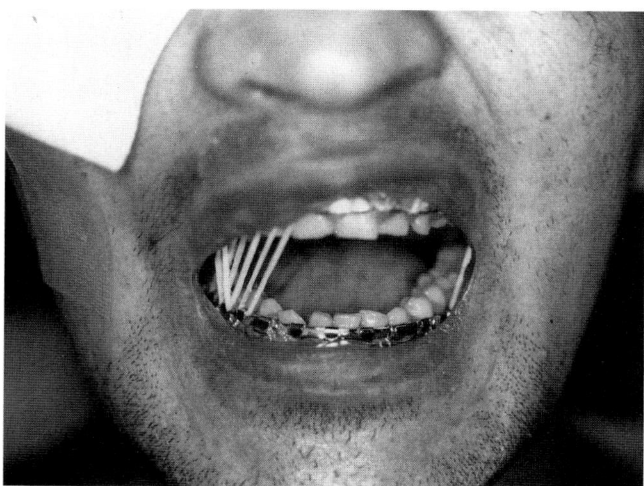

FIGURE 31-15. Elastic traction may restore occlusion that has only recently deviated. In established malocclusion, elastic traction will only extrude teeth as the bone has healed.

the mandible. Frequent mandibular complications are infection (106), malocclusion, TMJ pain, limitation of oral opening, plate removal, motor or sensory damage, scarring, delayed healing, and malunion (106–109). Generally, complications are proportionate to the severity of the fracture and are more common with open fractures that involve the dentition. Complication rates of 10% to 15% are common.

One of the most common reasons for poor results in mandibular fracture treatment is the initial failure to establish a satisfactory occlusion (110). Often, application of inadequate or unstable IMF is the cause. A loose or inaccurate occlusion established at the time of open reduction will only worsen with time. The second and third most common problems are inadequate fixation of a mandibular fracture and fixation in malreduction (112–115). Fractures of the horizontal portion of the mandible often are more complex on the internal aspect of the mandible; therefore, a false sense of security may be obtained by viewing the outer cortex alone in reduction. A complete analysis of the patterns of the mandible fracture is easily provided by a CT scan and indicates the exact length of comminuted bone, which must be avoided in placement of secure screws (110,113,116). Secure fixation screws must be outside the zone of comminution to be stable; normally, fixation in the horizontal mandible consists of a superior border plate with unicortical screws and an inferior border plate that is anchored by bicortical screws. Use of 2.0-mm plates and screws in mandibular fracture treatment is appropriate in noncomminuted, nondefect, noninfected fractures treated early, and in fractures in cooperative patients where one may consistently and carefully monitor the occlusion postoperatively. The use of small plates (117) is not indicated in comminuted mandibular fractures, mandibular fractures that are going to used as a basis for complex midface fracture treatment, or those that have a bone defect (93), or when subcondylar fractures are going to be treated closed.

Conceptually, at least two solid screws should be present on each side of the fracture in solid bone beyond any comminuted fracture area. If one of these screws becomes loose, however, secure fracture fixation cannot be maintained. Therefore, placement of three good bicortical screws to each side of the fracture provides a measure of security. In defect fractures where there is comminuted or missing bone, the "tumor bridging" rule is used, and solid bone beyond the fractures on each side is used for fixation of four screws. The "four-screw large plate" rule also applies to thinner mandibles, where there is inadequate bone for bone buttressing such as the edentulous atrophic mandible. The use of compression plates in mandibular fracture treatment is theoretically attractive; however, in practice, the varying obliquity of the fracture planes and the changes in occlusion that these small compression movements may cause to occur through these variable planes of action make the use of the compression technique unpredictable with respect to subtle changes in occlusion. Abnormal forces on the occlusion generate undesirable displacement and may adversely affect bone healing by compressing and injuring cells at the edges of the bone defect (118). It is our opinion that it is advantageous not to use compression, but merely stable bicortical fixation with plates of the reconstruction type, solidly purchasing two to three bicortical screws to each side of the fragment. The use of compression obviously has no place in bone defect or in comminuted mandibular fracture treatment, which requires a larger plate with four screws to each side of the fracture. Further, the occlusal results with rigid plates are generally inferior to those obtained with more malleable plates. especially when practitioners have less experience because of the finesse required in the bending of rigid plates (109,119).

Patients with infection should be managed by dependent drainage, irrigation, and antibiotics (106). If this does not solve the problem, removal of loose teeth, loose fixation hardware, and/or dead bone may be required, bridging any bone defect with a longer plate or perhaps using external fixation. Mandibular fractures sometimes involve infected, unstable, or periodontically involved teeth; these teeth are better extracted at the time of treatment. Otherwise, teeth usually may be preserved in a fracture line if they are unfractured and have solid, intact roots. Third molars should be removed if they are easily accessible or infected. Antibiotics are instituted in all fractures of the horizontal mandible involving the dentition, especially in those that are infected. They should be maintained until the infection resolves and should be culture specific. One must be careful to detect and manage infections before spread occurs into the deep planes of the neck, which may create significant sepsis.

Although some practitioners recommend (117) immediate rigid fixation and bone grafting for bone gaps created by infection, the wound must be clean, the oral lining intact, and invasive infection cleared. Our own experience favors delayed wound closure, a period of absent problems, and delayed grafting.

Nonunion

Nonunion occurs in about 3% of mandible fractures (120–123). Delayed treatment, teeth in the fracture line, alcohol and drug abuse, early removal of MMF, and multiple fractures are prerequisites to the complication. Fractures of the body, angle, and symphysis are the three most common areas observed, in that order. Treatment delay is the most important cause of infection and nonunion. Vascular compromise to the bone is the usual issue in nonunion of fractures. Clinical nonunion is less common at this time, because it often is masked by the presence of rigid fixation (121–126). It is managed by resection of the area of nonunion to healthy bleeding bone and by bone grafting (preferably extra orally) under protection from stable internal fixation, which means a rigid plate of "defect bridging" strength with four solid bicortical screws in the proximal and distal fragments.

A wound that is closed and has been clear of infection is a classic prerequisite for success (127,128) of a subsequent bone graft. In edentulous mandible fractures, there is an increased frequency of nonunion, especially if the height of the mandible is less than 1 cm.

Internal Anatomy of Fracture Reduction

In multiple-segment mandible fractures, and particularly if one is treating simultaneous fractures in the vertical ramus closed, it is easy to induce a deformity in the horizontal portion of the mandible. Specifically, in combined symphysis and subcondylar fractures, the lateral mandibular segments tend to lean, canting toward the tongue, opening the occlusion on the lingual aspect (2,10). This creates a lingual open bite, laterally flaring the mandibular angles; the deformity is aggravated by the application of tight arch bars, whereby the lateral segments of the mandible are literally forced into a lingual cant by excessive tightening of the IMF loops.

In significant malocclusion, malalignment can only be corrected by refracture (125,126). This kind of malalignment is prevented in combined symphysis and condylar fractures at the time of open reduction by watching the alignment of the external cortex of the mandibular symphysis, while pushing in on the mandibular angles and condylar heads. When the anterior cortex at the symphysis just begins to gap, the lingual symphyseal mandibular cortex is approximated and forced together by the pressure applied at the mandibular angle and condyle regions. This reduction maneuver also uprights the lateral mandibular dentition. A longer plate across the symphysis is required to guarantee that the mandibular angles remain medially positioned, achieving the thin bigonial distance of the mandible posteriorly. It is recommended that plates applied to the mandible initially be overbent by 3 mm over the fracture; their lowest surface should remain away from the fracture site by 2 to 3 mm (129). Theoretically, this overbending (projection off the fracture site) improves the ability to approximate the lingual cortex after tightening the screws (110–112,114,130).

Generally, high condylar fractures should be treated closed, with early mandibular mobilization and guiding elastics to close the open bite. Training elastics are important, and the application of nighttime elastics gives the patient a period of rest in occlusion, in effect lengthening the ramus. Arch bars can be stabilized by skeletal wires if postoperative elastics are to be used over the anterior (incisor) dentition, when the teeth are missing, or in children. When the fracture is lower in the neck or the upper ramus, the chance of experiencing a complication from reduced ramus height is increased (110). Some of these fractures require open reduction (113,115). Fractures with poor contract between proximal and distal bone fragments and those with more displacement should be considered for open reduction (130–132). Patients with complete dislocation of the condyle also may benefit from open reduction, especially when an accompanying horizontal mandibular fracture is complicated. When the condyle fracture is bilateral or when the mandible is being used as the basis for Le Fort fracture treatment, a rigid reconstruction of the entire mandible, which requires open reduction of the lower subcondylar fractures, always is desirable. When combined mandibular and subcondylar fractures exist, the anterior sections of the arch bars should be supported by skeletal wires, so that anterior elastics can be applied to close the bite, if necessary, without developing extrusion forces on the anterior incisor teeth. These strong, supported arch bars allow considerable flexibility in the application of elastic traction anywhere along the dental arch. The open management of condylar fractures is highly controversial: one trades the external scar and the risk of nerve damage of extraoral approaches to slightly better occlusion and aesthetics (130–132). Intraoral approaches now are endoscopically assisted with specific instrumentation and presumably decrease the nerve damage. The late management of condylar fracture malunion with malocclusion is best managed by standard Le Fort I or bilateral sagittal split osteotomies of the mandible if condylar function is good. Reoperation on joint fractures is fraught with problems, and standard orthognathic procedures give better results. No osteotomies should be performed when range of motion of the mandible is poor and active TMJ rehabilitation should be engaged. In rare cases, a costochondral graft must be considered for joint replacement.

If the condylar disc is displaced or damaged, it can be repaired and replaced with sutures. If it requires replacement, a vascularized temporoparietal fascial flap can be interposed into the joint to act as a disc reconstruction. Most condylar disc derangements will respond to physiotherapy or endoscopic surgery.

In exposure of the mandible intraorally, considerable effort should be directed to repair of the muscle incision in order to reposition the soft tissue properly on the mandible. Otherwise, the soft tissue "sags," and an ectropion of the lower lip, for instance, may result from failure to reconstruct the mentalis muscle attachment in the course of closure of the incision. It is difficult to secondarily reposition a contracted malpositioned lower lip with incompetence. One begins by degloving the mandible, releasing any soft tissue contracture, and refixing the soft tissue to the facial skeleton in a superior position. Gravity and internal soft tissue scarring, however, tend to cause the deformity to recur.

Mandibular alveolar fractures, when they accompany mandible fractures, need to be managed with a specific technique as well, repositioning and stabilizing them in order to avoid malocclusion (2). Again, if the fracture is viewed through a laceration, an open reduction facilitates repositioning, and small unicortical plates and screws may stabilize these fractures. Initially, repositioning first smaller alveolar fragments on the larger fragments in comminuted fracture treatment allows the large fragments to be reassembled with considerable precision.

Fractures in Children

In general, fractures in children should be treated as early as possible because of their rapid bone healing (10,19,35). In the mandible and maxilla, care needs to be taken to avoid injury to tooth buds when placing fixation devices because the tooth buds are plentiful and easily injured (3,20). It has been difficult to quantitate any clinical adverse effect of the use of metal plates on growth, but these devices cause 5% growth restriction in animals. Generally, there has been slow transition to the use of resorbable plates in children, although titanium plates have been used frequently and do not seem to be complicated by clinical reports of growth disturbance. Because of the shape of children's teeth, it is difficult to stability ligate arch bars to the dentition, and arch bars should be stabilized by skeletal wires attached to the mandible and the maxilla. The facial fracture pattern in children favors the frontal bone, nose, and mandible. Sinus development then creates a fracture pattern similar to that in the adult. Fractures in children occasionally are complicated by growth disturbances. Condylar and naso-orbital fractures before age 5 years are most prone to late growth retardation.

Gunshot, Shotgun, and Avulsive Wounds

Generally, low-caliber gunshot wounds can be managed as facial fractures with overlying lacerations (133). The exception is mandibular fractures in which bone loss occurs and where immediate bone grafting or replacement of the comminuted fragments is subject to a high rate of loss of these nonvital bone fragments. Bone grafting in the mandible usually should be performed as a delayed procedure. The initial replacement of comminuted bone fragments should be performed only if the surgeon is willing to remove these in about one-half of cases. If the bone pieces survive, the patient may avoid a secondary procedure, but poor union and infection are common, and bone resorption may be masked by a rigid fixation plate. When more extensive combined bone and soft tissue loss occurs, all bones and soft tissue injuries initially should be stabilized by open reduction of bone and soft tissue closure. Bone gaps should be spanned by rigid fixation. The patient should be returned to the operating room at 48-hour intervals to confirm the absence of infection and hematoma, and to perform serial debridement of devitalized tissue. Once no further devascularized tissue is seen, definitive soft tissue or soft tissue and bone reconstruction may commence. At the initial operation, existing bone is stabilized in anatomical position. Additional bone and soft tissue can be added when the wound is clean. Expansion of the soft tissue envelope must be maintained by primary bone stabilization in anatomical position and skin-to-skin or skin-to-mucosa closure. This serial debridement protocol maximizes the ability to achieve anatomical reduction of existing bone and soft tissue without infection. When mandibular bone defects exceed 6 cm, free vascularized bone transfers are preferable to nonvascularized grafts. Generally, the use of omental flaps for reconstruction of soft tissue loss or for coverage of nonvascularized bone does not prevent the necessity to perform a "designer free flap" for reconstruction of an area. Vascularized omental grafts should be considered only as a temporizing maneuver, but they may salvage some exposed bone and provide temporary closure. Continued maintenance of bone and soft tissue expansion and the early carefully planned replacement of missing bone and soft tissue allow the achievement of maximal functional and aesthetic results.

CONCLUSION

Complications can be minimized by making the correct diagnosis, pursuing adequate exposure, achieving accurate bone reduction, and reclosing and replacing the soft tissue. When complications occur, deliberate analysis of their mechanism allows for development of the most straightforward plan for correction. Because the face is important in appearance and communication, the precise repair of facial injuries minimizes the psychosocial sequelae of the injury.

REFERENCES

1. Rudderman R, Mullen R. Biomechanics of the facial skeleton. *Clin Plast Surg* 1992;19:11.
2. Manson P, Clark N, Robertson B, et al. Subunit principles in midface fractures: the importance of sagittal buttresses, soft tissue reductions and sequencing treatment of segmental fractures. *Plast Reconstr Surg* 1999;103:1287–1306.

3. Manson PN. Facial fractures. In: *Perspectives in plastic surgery, vol. 2.* St. Louis: Quality Medical Publishing, 1998:I-36.
4. Manson PN. Dimensional analysis of the facial skeleton. *Prob Plast Surg* 1991;1:213.
5. Manson PN, Markowitz B, Mirvis S, et al. Toward CT based facial fracture treatment. *Plast Reconstr Surg* 1990;84:202.
6. Manson PN, Hoopes JE, Su CT. Structural pillars of the facial skeleton: an approach to the management of LeFort fractures. *Plast Reconstr Surg* 1980;66:54.
7. Gruss JS, MacKinnon SE. Complex maxillary fractures: role of buttress reconstruction and immediate bone grafts. *Plast Reconstr Surg* 1986;78:9.
8. Manson PN, Crawley WA, Yaremchuk MJ, et al. Midface fractures: advantages of immediate extended open reduction and bone grafting. *Plast Reconstr Surg* 1985;76:1.
9. Gruss JS, Van-Wyck L, Phillips JH, et al. The importance of the zygomatic arch in complex midfacial fracture repair and correction of post traumatic orbito-zygomatic deformities. *Plast Reconstr Surg* 1990;85:878.
10. Gruss JS, Bubak PJ, Egbert M. Craniofacial fractures: an algorithm to optimize results. *Clin Plast Surg* 1992;19:195.
11. Tessier P. Complications of facial trauma: principles of later reconstruction. *Ann Plast Surg* 1986;17:411.
12. Manson PN, Clark N, Robertson B, et al. Comprehensive management of pan-facial fractures. *J Craniomaxillofac Trauma* 1995;1:43–56.
13. Manson PN. Re-operative facial fracture surgery. In: Grotting J, ed. *Re-operative plastic surgery.* St. Louis: Quality Medical Publishing, 1995.
14. Wheeler ES, Kawamoto HK, Zarem HA. Bone grafts for nasal reconstruction. *Plast Reconstr Surg* 1982;69:9–18.
15. Cohen SR, Kawamoto H. Analysis and treatment of established post traumatic facial deformities. *Plast Reconstr Surg* 1992; 90:574.
16. Kawamoto HK Jr. Late posttraumatic enophthalmos. A correctable deformity? *Plast Reconstr Surg* 1982;69:423.
17. Manson PN, Clark N, Robertson B, et al. Comprehensive management of pan facial fractures. *J Craniofac Trauma* 1995;1:43.
18. Bahr N, Baganlisa F, Schlegel G. A comparison of transcutaneous incisions used for exposure of the orbital rim and orbital floor: a retrospective study. *Plast Reconstr Surg* 1992;90:85.
19. Phillips J, Gruss J, Wells M. Periosteal suspension of the lower eyelid and cheek following subciliary exposure of facial fractures. *Plast Reconstr Surg* 1991;88:145.
20. Yaremchuk M, Kim W. Soft tissue alterations associated with acute extended open reduction and internal fixation of the orbital fractures. *J Craniofac Surg* 1992;3:134.
21. Hardesty RA, Marsh JL. Craniofacial onlay bone grafting: a prospective evaluation of graft morphology, orientation, and embryonic origin. *Plast Reconstr Surg* 1990;85:1.
22. Antonyshyn OM, Gruss JS, Galbraith DJ, et al. Complex orbital fractures: a critical analysis of immediate bone graft reconstruction. *Ann Plast Surg* 1989;22:220–235.
23. Dawar M, Antonyshyn OM. Long term results following immediate reconstruction of orbital fractures. A critical morphometric analysis. *Can J Plast Surg* 1993;1:24–29.
24. Lacey M, Antonyshyn O, MacGregor JH. Temporal contour deformity after coronal flap elevation: an anatomical study. *J Craniofac Surg* 1994;5:223.
25. Manson PN. Cranial-orbital fractures. *Clin Oral Surg* 1990;2:121–143.
26. Luce EA. Frontal sinus fractures: guidelines to management. *Plast Reconstr Surg* 1987;80:500–510.
27. Wolfe SA, Johnson P. Frontal sinus injuries: primary care and management of late complications. *Plast Reconstr Surg* 1988; 82:781–791.
28. Rohrich RJ, Hollier LH. Management of frontal sinus fractures. Changing concepts. *Clin Plast Surg* 1992;19:219–232.
29. Duvall AJ, Porto DP, Lyons D, et al. Frontal sinus fractures: analysis of treatment results. *Arch Otolaryngol Head Neck Surg* 1987;114:933–935.
30. Larabee WF, Travis LW, Tabb HG. Frontal sinus fractures—their suppurative complications and surgical management. *Laryngoscope* 1980;90:1810–1813.
31. Stanley RB. Management of severe frontobasilar skull fractures. *Otolaryngol Clin North Am* 1991;24:139–150.
32. Gilklich RE, Lazor JB. The subcranial approach to trauma of the anterior cranial base: preliminary report. *J Craniomaxillofac Trauma* 1995;1:56–62.
33. Markowitz BL, Manson PN. Discussion of frontal basilar trauma: classification and treatment. *Plast Reconstr Surg* 1995;99:1322–1323.
34. Gruss JS. Fronto-naso-orbital trauma. *Clin Plast Surg* 1982;9:577.
35. Gruss JS, Pollock RS, Phillips JH, et al. Combined injuries of the cranium and face. *Br J Plast Surg* 1989;42:385.
36. Manson PN, Crawley WA, Hoopes JE. Frontal cranioplasty: risk factors and choice of cranial vault reconstructive material. *Plast Reconstr Surg* 1986;77:888–904.
37. Rish BL, Dillon JD, Meirowsky AM, et al. Cranioplasty: a review of 1030 cases of penetrating head injury. *Neurosurgery* 1979;4:381–385.
38. Zide MF, Kent JN, Machado L. Hydroxyapatite cranioplasty directly over dura. *J Oral Maxillofac Surg* 1987;45:481–486.
39. Stanley RB Jr. Fractures of frontal sinuses. *Clin Plast Surg* 1989;16:115–123.
40. Ardekian L, Samet N, Shoshani Y, et al. Life threatening bleeding following maxillofacial trauma. *J Craniomaxillofac Surg* 1993;21:336–338.
41. Leipziger LS, Manson PN. Nasoethmoid orbital fractures. Current concepts and management principles. *Clin Plast Surg* 1992;19:167–193.
42. Markowitz BL, Manson PN, Sargent LA, et al. Management of medial canthal tendon in naso-ethmoid orbital fractures: the importance of the central fragment in classification and treatment. *Plast Reconstr Surg* 1991;87:843.
43. Sargent LA. Nasoethmoid orbital fractures. *Probl Plast Reconstr Surg* 1991;1:426–445.
44. Gruss JS, Hurwitz JJ, Nik NA, et al. The pattern and incidence of nasolacrimal injury in naso-orbital-ethmoid fractures: the role of delayed assessment and dacryocystorhinostomy. *Br J Plast Surg* 1985;38:116–121.
45. Peter H, Freihofer HMP. Experience with transnasal canthopexy. *J Maxillofac Surg* 1980;8:119–124.
46. Paskert JP, Manson PN. The bimanual examination for assessing instability in naso-orbito-ethmoidal injuries. *Plast Reconstr Surg* 1989;83:165–167.
47. Sargent L. Acute management of nasoethmoid fractures. *Op Tech Plast Surg* 1998;5:213–223.
48. Antonsyhyn O, Gruss JS, Galbraith DJ, et al. Complex orbital fractures: a critical analysis of immediate bone graft reconstruction. *Ann Plast Surg* 1989;22:220.
49. Manson PN, Iliff N. Management of blow out fractures of the orbital floor. *Surv Ophthalmol* 1991;35:280.
50. Aronowitz JA, Freeman BS, Spira M. Long term stability of Teflon orbital implants. *Plast Reconstr Surg* 1986;78:166–173.
51. Weintraub B, Cucin RL, Jacobs M. Extrusion of an infected orbital-floor prosthesis after 15 years. *Plast Reconstr Surg* 1981;68:586–587.
52. Petro J, Tooze FM, Bales CR, et al. Ocular injuries associated with peripheral fractures. *J Trauma* 1979;19:730–733.
53. al-Qurainy IA, Dutton GN, Ilankovan V, et al. Midfacial frac-

tures and the eye. The development of a system for detecting patients at risk of eye injury: a prospective study. *Br J Oral Maxillofac Surg* 1991;29:368–369.
54. Grossman MD, Roberts DM, Barr CC. Ophthalmic aspects of orbital injury. A comprehensive diagnostic and management approach. *Clin Plast Surg* 1992;19:71–85.
55. Marsh J, Gado M. The longitudinal orbital CT projection. A versatile image for orbital assessment. *Plast Reconstr Surg* 1983;71:308–317.
56. Koorneef L. Current concepts on the management of orbital blow -out fractures. *Ann Plast Surg* 1982;9:814–900.
57. Manson PN, Clifford CM, Su CT, et al. Mechanisms of global support and posttraumatic enophthalmos. I. The anatomy of the ligament sling and its relation to intramuscular cone orbital fat. *Plast Reconstr Surg* 1986;77:193.
58. Manson PN, Grivas A, Rosenbaum A, et al. Studies on enophthalmos II. The measurement of orbital injuries and their treatment by quantitative computed tomography. *Plast Reconstr Surg* 1986;77:203.
59. Putterman AM. Stevens T, Urist MJ. Nonsurgical management of blowout fractures of the orbital floor. *Trans Am Acad Ophthalmol Otolaryngol* 1974;77:650.
60. Pearl RM. Surgical management of volumetric changes in the bony orbit. *Ann Plast Surg* 1995;19 349.
61. Converse JM, Smith B. Enophthalmos and diplopia in fractures of the orbit floor. *Br J Plast Surg* 1957;9:265–274.
62. Converse JM, Smith B, Obear MF, et al. Orbital blow-out fractures. A ten year survey. *Plast Reconstr Surg* 1967;39:20–36.
63. Shorr N, Fallor M. "Madame Butterfly" procedure: combined cheek and lateral canthal suspension procedure for post blepharoplasty "round eye" and lower eyelid retraction. *Ophthalmic Plast Reconstr Surg* 1985:1:229.
64. Holds JB, Anderson RL, Theise SM. Lower eyelid retraction: a minimal incision surgical approach to retractor lysis. *Ophthalmic Surg* 1990;21:767–771.
65. Bartley GB, Kay PP. Posterior lamellar eyelid reconstruction with hard palate mucosa grafting. *Am J Ophthalmol* 1989; 107:609–612.
66. Manson PN, Glassman D, Iliff NT, et al. Rigid fixation of orbital fractures. *Plast Reconstr Surg* 1990;86:1103–1109.
67. Grant MP, Iliff NT, Manson PN. Strategies for the correction of the treatment of enophthalmos. *Clin Plast Surg* 1997;24:539.
68. Manson PN, Iliff NT. Post traumatic enophthalmos. In: Marsh J, ed. *Current therapy in plastic and reconstructive surgery, vol. 1, no. 1.* Philadelphia: WB Saunders, 1987:113.
69. Antonyshyn O, Gruss JS, Cassle EE. Blow-in fractures of the orbit. *Plast Reconstr Surg* 1989;84:10–20.
70. Bite U, Jackson IT, Forbes GS, et al. Orbital volume measurements using three dimensional imaging. *Plast Reconstr Surg* 1985;75:502.
71. Romano J, Iliff N, Manson P. Use of Medpore high density polyethylene implants in 140 patients. *J Craniofac Surg* 1993; 4:142–147.
72. Anderson RL, Panje WR, Gross CE. Optic nerve blindness following blunt forehead trauma. *Ophthalmology* 1975;14: 474–481.
73. Fukado Y. Results of 400 cases of surgical decompression of the optic nerve. *Mod Probl Ophthalmol* 1975;14:474–481.
74. Yanagihara N, Murakami S, Nishihara S. Temporal bone fractures inducing facial nerve paralysis: a new classification and its clinical significance. *Ear Nose Throat J* 1997;76:79–80,83-86.
75. Kline LB, Morawitz RB, Swaid SN. Indirect injury of optic nerve. *Neurosurgery* 1984;14:756–764.
76. Stanley RB Jr, Sires BS, Funk GF, et al. Management of displaced lateral orbital wall fractures associated with visual ocular motility disturbances. *Plast Reconstr Surg* 1998;102:972.
77. Habal MB. Reflections on traumatic neuropathy. *J Craniofac Surg* 1997;8:356.
78. Girotto J, Davidson J, Wheatley M, et al. Blindness as a complication of LeFort osteotomies: the role of atypical fracture patterns and distortion of the optic canal. *Plast Reconstr Surg* 1998;102:1409–1421.
79. Anderson RL, Panje WR, Gross CE. Optic nerve blindness following blunt forehead trauma. *Ophthalmology* 1982;89:445.
80. Marin P, Love T, Carpenter R, et al. Complications of orbital reconstruction: misplacement of bone grafts within the intramuscular cone. *Plast Reconstr Surg* 1998;101:1323,1327.
81. Fujino T, Makino K. Entrapment mechanisms and ocular injury in orbital blow-out fractures. *Plast Reconstr Surg* 1980;65:571.
82. Koorneef L. *Sectional anatomy of the orbit.* Amsterdam: Aeolus Press, 1981:1.
83. Koorneef L. *Spatial aspects of the orbital musculo-fibrous tissue in man.* Amsterdam: Swets and Zeitinglinger, 1977.
84. Kurza A, Patel M. Superior orbital fissure syndrome associated with fractures of the zygoma and orbit. *Plast Reconstr Surg* 1979;64:715–719.
85. Dufresne CR, Manson PN, Iliff NT. Early and late complications of orbital fractures. *Clin Plast Surg* 1988;15:239–253.
86. Manson PN, Ruas EJ, Iliff NT. Deep orbital reconstruction for the correction of post traumatic enophthalmos. *Clin Plast Surg* 1987;14:113–121.
87. Wolfe SA, Davidson J. Avoidance of lower lid contraction in surgical approaches to the lower orbit. *Op Tech Plast Reconstr Surg* 1998;5:201–212.
88. Gioia VM, Linberg JV, McCormick SA. The anatomy of the lateral canthal tendon. *Arch Ophthalmol* 1987;105:529–532.
89. Glat PM, Jelks GW, Jelks EB, et al. Evolution of the lateral canthoplasty. Techniques and indications. *Plast Reconstr Surg* 1997;100:1396–1408.
90. Jelks GW, Glat PM, Jelks EB, et al. The inferior retinacular lateral canthoplasty: a new technique. *Plast Reconstr Surg* 1997;100:1262–1270.
91. Whitaker L. Selective alteration of palpebral fissure form by lateral canthoplasty. *Plast Reconstr Surg* 1984;74:611–619.
92. Siegel RF. Palatal grafts for eyelid reconstruction. *Plast Reconstr Surg* 1985;76:411–414.
93. Jackson IT. Classification and treatment of orbito-zygomatic and orbito-ethmoid fractures: the place of bone grafting and plate fixation. *Clin Plast Surg* 1989;16:77.
94. Ord RA. Post-operative retrobulbar hemorrhage and blindness complicating trauma surgery. *Br J Oral Surg* 1981;19:202.
95. Nicholson DH, Guzak SW. Visual loss complicating repair of orbital floor fractures. *Arch Ophthalmol* 1971;86:369.
96. Allen MV, Cohen IK, Grimson B, et al. Orbital cellulitis secondary to dacryocystitis following blepharoplasty. *Ann Ophthalmol* 1985;17:498–499.
97. Rohrich RJ, Hollier LH, Watumull D. Optimizing the treatment of orbito-zygomatic fractures. *Clin Plast Surg* 1992; 19:149.
98. Ellis E, El-Attar A, Moos KF. An analysis of 2,067 cases of zygomatico-orbital fractures. *J Oral Maxillofac Surg* 1985;43:428.
99. Tajima S, Sugimoto C, Jajino R, et al. Surgical treatment of malunited fractures of zygoma with diplopia and with comments on blow out fractures. *J Maxillofac Surg* 1974;2:201.
100. Stanley RB Jr. Reconstruction of midface vertical dimension following LeFort fracture treatment. *Arch Otolaryngol* 1984; 110:571.
101. Manson P, Glassman D, Vander Kolk D, et al. Rigid stabilization of sagittal fractures of the maxilla and palate. *Plast Reconstr Surg* 1990;85:711.
102. Hendrickson M, Clark N, Manson P. Sagittal fractures of the

maxilla: classification and treatment. *Plast Reconstr Surg* 1998;101:319–332.
103. Manson PN. Some thoughts on classification and treatment of LeFort fractures. *Ann Plast Surg* 1986;17:356.
104. Sofferman RA, Danielson PA, Quatela WA, et al. Retrospective analysis of surgically treated LeFort fractures. *Arch Otolaryngol* 1983;190:446.
105. Crawley W, Azman P, Clark N, et al. The edentulous LeFort fracture. *J Craniofac Surg* 1997;8:298.
106. Izuka T, Lindqvist C, Hallikainen D, et al. Infection after rigid internal fixation of mandibular fractures: a clinical and radiological study. *J Oral Maxillofac Surg* 1991;49:585–593.
107. Moreno JC, Fernandez A, Ortiz J, et al. Complications rates associated with different treatments for mandible fractures. *J Oral Maxillofacial Surg* 2000;58:273–280.
108. Teenier TJ, Smith BR. Management of complications associated with mandible and maxillofacial surgery. *Clin Am* 1997;5:181–209.
109. Ellis E III, Walker L. Treatment of mandibular angle fractures using two noncompression miniplates. *J Oral Maxillofac Surg* 1994;52:1032–1037.
110. Klotch DW, Lundy B. Condylar neck fractures of the mandible. *Otolaryngol Clin North Am* 1991;24:181–194.
111. Zide MF, Kent JN. Indications for open reduction of mandible condyle fractures. *J Oral Maxilofac Surg* 1983;41:89–98.
112. Ellis E III, Dean J. Rigid fixation of mandibular condyle fractures. *Oral Surg Oral Med Oral Pathol* 1993;76:6–15.
113. Raveh J, Vuillemin T, Laedrach K. Open reduction of the dislocated fractured condylar process: indications and surgical procedures. *J Oral Maxillofac Surg* 1989;47:120–126.
114. Walker RV. Condylar fractures: nonsurgical management. *J Oral Maxillofac Surg* 1994;52:1185–1188.
115. Konstantinovic VS, Dimtrijevic B. Surgical versus conservative treatment of unilateral condylar process fractures: clinical and radiographic evaluation of 80 patients. *J Oral Maxillofac Surg* 1992;50:349–352.
116. Silennoinen U, Iizuka T, Oikarinen K, et al. Analysis of possible factors leading to problems after nonsurgical treatment of condylar fractures. *J Oral Maxillofac Surg* 1994;42:793–799.
117. Johansson B, Krekmanov L, Tomsson M. Miniplate osteosynthesis of infected mandible fractures. *J Craniomaxillofac Surg* 1988;16:22–27.
118. Lazow SK. The mandible fracture: a treatment protocol. *J Craniomaxillofac Trauma* 1996;2:24–30.
119. Kearns GJ, Perrott DH, Kaban LB. Rigid fixation of mandibular fractures: does operator experience reduce complications? *J Oral Maxillofac Surg* 1994;52:226–232.
120. Becking A, Zijderveld S, Tuinzing D. Management of post traumatic malocclusion caused by condylar process fractures. *J Oral Maxillofacial Surg* 1998;56:1370,1374.
121. Bochlogyros PN. Nonunion of fractures of the mandible. *J Maxillofac Surg* 1985;13:189–193.
122. Haug RH, Schwimmer A. Fibrous union of the mandible: a review of 27 patients. *J Oral Maxillofac Surg* 1994;52:832–839.
123. Mathog RH, Boies LR Jr. Nonunion of the mandible. *Laryngoscope* 1976;86908–920.
124. Bruce RA, Strachan DS. Fractures of the edentulous mandible. The Chalmer, J. Lyons Academy Study. *J Oral Surg* 1976;34: 973–979.
125. Rubens BC, Stoelinga PJ, Weaver TH, et al. Management of malunited mandibular fractures. *Int J Oral Maxillofac Surg* 1990;19:22–25.
126. MacIntosh RB. The case for autogenous reconstruction of the adult temporomandibular joint. In: Worthington P, Evans JR, eds. *Controversies in oral and maxillofacial surgery.* Philadelphia: WB Saunders, 1994.
127. Ellis E, Throckmorton G. Facial symmetry after closed and open treatment of fractures of the mandibular condylar process. *J Oral Maxillofac Surg* 2000;58:719–728.
128. Luhr HG, Redick T, Merten HA. Results of treatment of fractures of the atrophic edentulous mandible by compression plating. *J Oral Maxillofac Surg* 1996;54:250.
129. Haug R. The effect of screw number and length on the two methods of tension band plating. *J Oral Maxillofac Surg* 1993;51:159.
130. Ellis E, Simon P, Throckmorton G. Occlusal results after open or closed treatment of fractures of the condylar process. *J Oral Maxillofac Surg* 2000;58:260–268.
131. Ellis E, Throckmorton G, Palmieri C. Open treatment of condylar process fractures: assessment of adequacy of repositioning and maintenance of stability. *J Oral Maxillofac Surg* 2000;58:27–34.
132. Bruce RA, Ellis E. The second Chalmers J. Lyons Academy Study of fractures of the edentulous mandible. *J Oral M axillofac Surg* 1993;51:904.
133. Gruss J, Antonshyn O, Phillips J. Early definitive bone and soft tissue reconstruction of major wounds of the face. *Plast Reconstr Surg* 1991;87:436–450.

Discussion

FACIAL FRACTURES

JOSEPH L. DAW, JR

A thorough and comprehensive review on the prevention, recognition, and management of complications related to the treatment of facial fractures has been lacking. Paul Manson, one of the preeminent clinicians and innovators in craniomaxillofacial trauma, has eliminated this void through this chapter. He provides numerous clinical and surgical "pearls" that only may be gained through a tremendous experience such as his. One of the most important points that was continually stressed throughout the chapter was adherence to the most basic principles of craniofacial surgery: providing wide exposures for evaluation and access to the fractures, thereby allowing for accurate reduction of the displaced fracture segments. All too often, compromised results are seen after attempts at repair through limited incisions and inadequate, nonanatomical reductions. Another principle discussed, but one that I felt could have been emphasized more, was primary bone grafting in the initial fracture repair (1,2). Liberal use of primary bone grafts for comminuted fractures at sites such as the frontal sinus, naso-orbitoethmoid region, and anterior wall of the maxillary sinus will maintain the proper position of the soft tissue envelope. Outcomes will be improved, and nonunion and late deformities may be prevented.

For frontal bone fractures involving the sinus, management is directed toward preventing infection and restoring the anatomical contour of the forehead. When these fractures are severely comminuted, it usually is best to reconstruct the area with a single split cranial bone graft. This will provide a more stable repair and a better contour of the forehead. As the forces on this area are negligible, stabilization should be achieved using a microplating system to minimize the profile of the fixation devices. Long-term follow-up of patients with frontal sinus fractures is necessary, as untoward sequelae such as a mucocele or mucopyocele may not present clinically until 5 or 10 years after injury or postoperatively. Secondary reconstruction of posttraumatic deformities of the forehead may be accomplished with autologous bone or alloplastic materials. Hydroxyapatite and calcium phosphate cements, as well as computer-aided design/computer-aided manufacture (CAD/CAM) custom implants, have improved our ability to reconstruct these defects. However, before secondary repair, communication between the nasal cavity and the brain must be eliminated, and there should be an absence of infection for at least 6 months (3). Briefly, use of a closed suction drain when a coronal approach is used for 1 or 2 days is simple and creates little discomfort and inconvenience for the patient.

As Dr. Manson mentions, naso-orbitoethmoid fractures are the most difficult facial fractures to treat and have the greatest propensity toward unfavorable results. Traumatic telecanthus may occur if the injury is not diagnosed properly and is left untreated (2). It also may occur after nonanatomical fracture reduction or improper medial canthopexy. The positioning of the medial canthal complex superior and posterior to the lacrimal fossa cannot be overly emphasized. For secondary correction, I also try to overcorrect its position medially, as there is often some degree of canthal drift. This is done by drilling a 2-mm hole in the bone at the site of attachment, which will allow the complex to be pulled further medially. Saddle nose deformity is best treated by its prevention through accurate reduction and stabilization of the naso-orbital skeleton and nasal septum (2). In contrast to Dr. Manson, I prefer to use microplates for this purpose. Primary bone grafting of the nasal dorsum should be used liberally. Once contraction of the soft tissue envelope occurs, the deformity is much more difficult to correct and the patient is left with a short nose.

Isolated nasal fractures are very common and frequently require secondary revision. Frontal impact fractures have a higher incidence of reoperation as opposed to lateral force fractures (4). Thus, patients should be forewarned of the potential need for secondary surgery, both from a cosmetic and a functional perspective. The errors of omission described by Dr. Manson in treating nasal fractures should be well understood and avoided when managing them.

The discussion on zygomatico-orbital fractures is the most complete. First and foremost, one must rule out any

J. L. Daw, Jr.: Division of Plastic Surgery, Craniofacial Center, University of Illinois at Chicago, Chicago, Illinois

associated injuries to the globe. Occasionally, physical findings relating to ocular injuries are subtle and difficult to identify by nonophthalmologists (5). For this reason and medicolegally, ocular examination performed by an ophthalmologist for all fractures involving the orbit is prudent. This is followed up with another examination by the ophthalmologist approximately 4 weeks postoperatively.

Successful repair of orbital fractures cannot be obtained without an appreciation of orbital anatomy, volume, and contours of the walls of the orbit. Dr. Manson does an outstanding job of bringing these concepts to light. The inclination of the inferomedial aspect of the orbit is a site that is especially likely to be improperly restored, leading to increased orbital volume and enophthalmos or dystopia of the globes. Use of the lateral wall of the orbit as a guide to accurate anatomical reduction of zygoma fractures will improve the likelihood of a desired outcome. With regard to zygomaticomaxillary fractures, exposure and plating of the zygomatic arch may be necessary to recreate the preinjury sagittal projection of the malar eminence and the proper transverse facial dimension (6).

Choice of surgical approach and surgical technique are especially important in preventing complications when gaining access to the orbital floor and inferior rim. The transconjunctival incision continues to gain popularity, but it is not free of complications. It would have been interesting to know whether Dr. Manson advocates a preseptal or a postseptal approach. When using a subciliary incision, several maneuvers may be instituted to reduce the incidence of scleral show. Use of a Frost suture/tarsorrhaphy or eye patch for approximately 5 days will assist in keeping the lower eyelid extended during the early healing period. A very efficacious technique to prevent lower lid retraction after repair of zygoma fractures, particularly when an extensive subperiosteal dissection is required, is suspension of the malar fat pad and periosteum superiorly to either the inferior orbital rim (7) or the temporalis fascia in the manner of a subperiosteal midface suspension. Evaluation of lower lid tone preoperatively will allow one to anticipate a tendency toward increase scleral show or ectropion. Ancillary procedures, such as lateral canthopexy or lower lid shortening, then can be discussed with the patient preoperatively and incorporated in the fracture repair.

Care must be taken to avoid iatrogenic injury to the globe during fracture repair. Particularly, one must readily recognize the occurrence of a corneal abrasion and treat accordingly. Chronic and recurrent corneal ulcerations may result if not diagnosed. Postoperative diplopia usually is self-limiting, improving with resolution of surgery-induced edema. In cases in which it is severe and persistent, short-term high-dose steroids may be useful. One must resist the temptation to return to the operating room and allow for a period of several weeks' observation. Continued diplopia with or without pain on vertical gaze may represent persistent entrapment and warrant reoperation. Computed tomography or magnetic resonance imaging may help define the problem.

In the section on Le Fort fractures, a brief discussion on alveolar fractures is provided. Although not mentioned in the section on mandible fractures, the issues are the same. Most plastic surgeons will not be called upon to manage isolated alveolar fractures, but they often occur along with Le Fort or mandibular fractures. An important point to consider is the management of subluxated teeth that are contained within the alveolar segment or in association with a jaw fracture involving the occlusion. Circumdental wires must be placed above the height of contour of the cingulum of the anterior teeth in order to fully seat them into the tooth socket and adequately immobilize them. If the wire is placed below the height of contour, then the tooth may be displaced slightly out of the socket, resulting in a premature occlusal contact and traumatic occlusal forces. If premature contacts persist despite appropriate maneuvers to reduce the alveolar fracture, occlusal equilibration must be carried out. In addition to potential loss of teeth, patients should be warned about the possible need for root canal therapy, which may not arise until years later.

Loss of teeth due to traumatic avulsion or root fracture may occur with alveolar, maxillary, and mandibular fractures. If the tooth or teeth cannot be accounted for, a chest x-ray should be obtained to identify an aspirated foreign body in the bronchopulmonary tree. Tooth loss, especially of the anterior teeth, compromises facial aesthetics and can be difficult for patients to accept psychologically. Absence of teeth in the alveolar bone leads to resorption. However, the bone may be maintained with placement of osseointegrated implants (Fig. 31D-1) and the cosmetic result of the dental rehabilitation improved (8). Placement of dental implants should be carried out as soon as the soft tissue has fully healed. If resorption of the alveolar process has already set in, then bone grafting or distraction of the alveolus itself may allow for satisfactory bone volume to accept dental implants.

Any fracture involving the occlusion (all Le Fort fractures and all mandibular fractures) must include as the initial treatment the placement of the teeth in maximal intercuspation according to the preinjury occlusion and stabilized with maxillomandibular fixation (MMF). Omitting this step or removal of the arch bars at the completion of the case should be condemned. Postoperatively, patients usually are placed in light elastics similar to protocols used in orthognathic surgery. If there is any instability, then more secure MMF with heavier elastics or stainless steel wires should be used. Even if MMF is not initially used postoperatively, the need for arch bars remains in case there is an unanticipated shifting of segments or change in the occlusion. Institution of MMF then may be necessary to manage this problem. Most persistent occlusal discrepancies in the late postoperative period are amenable to either occlusal equilibration or orthodontic therapy. Orthognathic surgery is very uncommon but occasionally necessary.

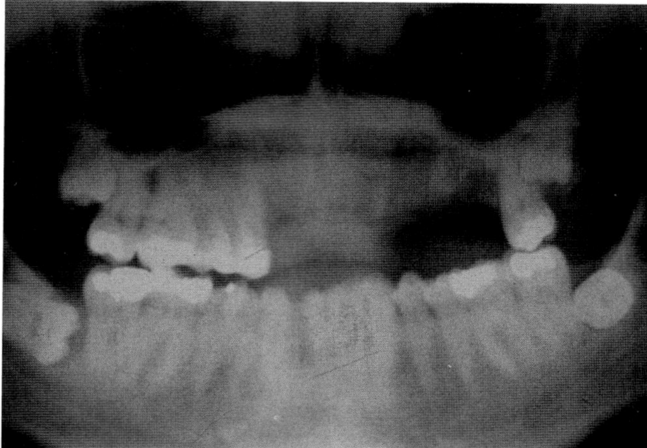

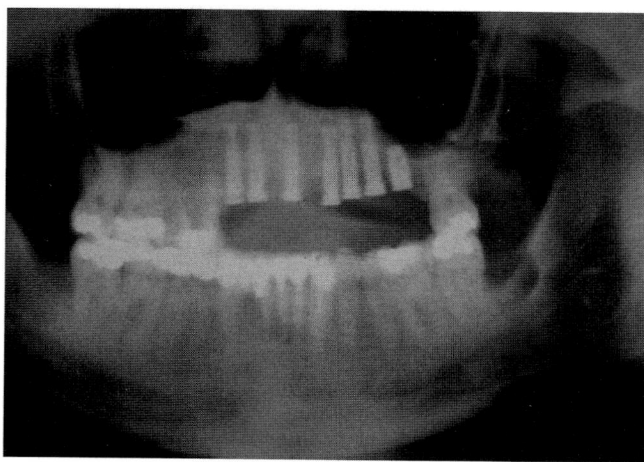

FIGURE 31D-1. Postextraction Panorex radiograph **(left)** of a patient with dentoalveolar fractures in which the teeth were not salvageable. Postoperative Panorex radiograph **(right)** showing placement of multiple osseointegrated implants.

In the treatment of mandible fractures, a common deficiency seen is improper placement of arch bars, usually too loosely applied. This may result in an inaccurate and unstable reduction. Grasping the arch bar with a wire twister and rotating it should demonstrate no mobility. This should be confirmed in the office during follow-up visits and wires tightened as necessary. I agree with the use of 2.0-mm plates and screws in stabilizing fracture segments, as long as the prerequisites mentioned are followed. More often, though, I will use a larger plate, but I avoid the use of compression. Using compression has resulted in too frequent shifts in the occlusion intraoperatively, resulting in reapplication of the plate and lengthening the operative time. An important technical point mentioned was the overcontouring of the inferior border plates to provide a 1- to 2-mm gap when applied to the buccal cortex. This will allow for accurate reduction of the lingual cortex when the screws are tightened.

By definition, any fracture involving a tooth is an open fracture regardless of the absence of a gingival or mucosal laceration at the location of the fracture. Therefore, antibiotic therapy is required. Management of teeth in the line of fracture, especially third molars, is a concept that causes some confusion. Routine removal of third molars is not necessary. Indications for their removal includes fracture of the tooth root, gross caries, and interference with anatomical reduction of the bony segments. An increased incidence of infection has been reported with tooth extraction in the line of mandibular fracture (9). In addition, the retained tooth may aid in stabilizing the reduced segments. They can be removed after fracture healing is complete.

When an infection or abscess develops at the site of a mandible fracture in which rigid internal fixation has been used, it must be treated aggressively. Drainage and irrigation of the site and inspection of the plate for complete stability should be carried out. Stable plates may be left in place until healing is complete, with the patient on antibiotic therapy (10). Intravenous antibiotic therapy is given until control of the infection is certain.

Pediatric facial fractures are uncommon compared to adult fractures. When they occur, they can be intimidating to the surgeon. Fracture healing occurs much more rapidly in the young child, so treatment must not be delayed. Most mandible fractures can be treated with a lingual splint secured with circummandibular wires, Ivy loops, and MMF (difficult in the mixed dentition), or an arch bar constructed by a dentist or orthodontist anchored to the molars by cemented bands. Orbital roof fractures are more unique to pediatric patients due to the small size of the face in relation to the cranium and the lack of pneumatization of the frontal sinuses. Operative repair via a frontal craniotomy may be necessary to prevent orbital volume discrepancies, orbital dystopia, pulsatile exophthalmos, and a traumatic encephalocele (11). When internal fixation is required for repair of pediatric facial fractures, resorbable systems can be used in most circumstances.

This chapter has provided a very comprehensive review of complications that may occur as a result of facial fractures and their treatment. Thus, anyone treating facial fractures should be familiar with these complications and their management. Understanding and anticipating complications will allow the surgeon to provide thorough informed consent to the patient and avoid "surprises" postoperatively. Another important point is to develop a good working relationship with a dentist and an ophthalmologist. Because facial fractures often involve the teeth/occlusion and the eyes, their collaboration in treatment is helpful for you and beneficial to the patient. Finally, one must face up to their complications and intervene if necessary because they usually are not going to disappear over time.

REFERENCES

1. Gruss JS. Complex craniomaxillofacial trauma: evolving concepts in management. A trauma unit's experience—1989 Fraser B. Gurd Lecture. *J Trauma* 1990;30:377–383.
2. Gruss JS. Complex nasoethmoid-orbital and midfacial fractures: role of craniofacial surgical techniques and immediate bone grafting. *Ann Plast Surg* 1986;17:377–390.
3. Manson PN, Crawley WA, Hoopes JE. Frontal cranioplasty: risk factors and choice of cranial vault reconstructive material. *Plast Reconstr Surg* 1986;77:888–900.
4. Daw JL, Lewis VL. Lateral force compared with frontal impact nasal fractures: need for reoperation. *J Craniomaxillofac Trauma* 1995;1:50–55.
5. Ioannides C, Treffers W, Rutten M, et al. Ocular injuries associated with fractures involving the orbit. *J Craniomaxillofac Surg* 1988;16:157–159.
6. Gruss JS, Van Wyck L, Phillips JH, et al. The importance of the zygomatic arch in complex midfacial fracture repair and correction of posttraumatic orbitozygomatic deformities. *Plast Reconstr Surg* 1990;85:878–890.
7. Phillips JH, Gruss JS, Wells, MD, et al. Periosteal suspension of the lower eyelid and cheek following subciliary exposure of facial fractures. *Plast Reconstr Surg* 1991;88:145–148.
8. Barber HD, Betts NJ. Rehabilitation of maxillofacial trauma patients with dental implants. *Implant Dent* 1993;2:191–193.
9. Iizuka T, Lindqvist C, Hallikainen D, et al. Infection after rigid internal fixation of mandibular fractures: a clinical and radiologic study. *J Oral Maxillofac Surg* 1991;49:585–593.
10. Koury M, Ellis E. Rigid internal fixation for the treatment of infected mandibular fractures. *J Oral Maxillofac Surg* 1992;50:434–443.
11. Messinger A, Radkowski MA, Greenwald MJ, et al. Orbital roof fractures in the pediatric population. *Plast Reconstr Surg* 1989;84:213–216.

32

PAROTID TUMOR SURGERY

PAUL M. GLAT
MARK S. GRANICK

The treatment of choice for parotid tumors, benign or malignant, is parotidectomy in one form or another. The potential complications after parotid gland surgery are many. Careful surgical planning and meticulous surgical technique can help decrease these complications to a minimum. It is important to understand the cause of these complications so that they may be avoided.

DIAGNOSIS

The diagnosis of parotid tumor usually is simple. The vast majority of parotid tumors present as asymptomatic masses (Fig. 32-1). Clinical examination of the patient generally is sufficient to determine if a mass is in the parotid. Sophisticated imaging techniques, such as magnetic resonance imaging or computed tomography, can be performed if there is any question as to the exact location or extent of a parotid area lesion. Fine needle aspiration biopsy is a reliable technique for obtaining a presumptive tissue diagnosis; however, all parotid tumors should be removed regardless of the fine needle aspiration biopsy results. When in doubt, proceed on the assumption that the mass is a parotid tumor so that the surgeon is completely prepared.

PREOPERATIVE DISCUSSION

After the diagnosis and the decision for surgery have been made, the patient must be completely informed about the potential complications of the surgery. In particular, the facial nerve must be discussed in detail. The possibility of facial nerve paresis or paralysis must be presented, and the long-term sequelae of this problem must be discussed. Patients often have concerns that are not readily apparent (Fig. 32-2). All other potential problems should be discussed as well.

P. M. Glat: Department of Surgery, Division of Plastic Surgery, MCP-Hahnemann University; and Division of Plastic Surgery, St. Christopher's Hospital for Children, Philadelphia, Pennsylvania

M. S. Granick: Department of Surgery, MCP—Hahnemann University; and Division of Plastic Surgery, Medical College of Pennsylvania Hospital and Hannemann Hospital, Philadelphia, Pennsylvania

SURGICAL TECHNIQUE

The majority of unfavorable results after surgery on the parotid gland arise from inadequate operations performed by inexperienced surgeons. A thorough understanding of the anatomy and of the surgical technique is imperative to facilitate the surgery and minimize complications (1).

The purpose of this chapter is not to present operative techniques, but there are some important points of technique that can help lead to a brief and safe operation. The preferred type of anesthesia is general anesthesia, although the procedure using local anesthesia. Infiltration of large amounts of local anesthetics can make visualization more difficult. Any movement of the patient can lead to inadvertent nerve injury.

In the operating room, both the anesthesiologist and surgeon should have complete access to the head and neck. Both eyes should be protected to avoid corneal abrasion. Petrolatum gauze can be placed in the external auditory canal to prevent blood from collecting in the canal. The anesthesiologist must avoid paralytic agents after induction, so that the facial nerve can be stimulated.

Either an extended facelift type of incision or a preauricular/lateral neck crease incision can be utilized (2). The incision should be generous in order to provide wide exposure that will allow easy and safe identification of the facial nerve. Bipolar cautery should be used exclusively to reduce the risk of damage to the facial nerve branches.

The facial flap is raised at the level just above the parotid fascia. The superficial musculoaponeurotic system is included in the skin flap. The flap can be raised sharply up to the peripheral borders of the gland. Beyond that, the nerve branches are at risk during dissection. After raising the flap, the gland is widely separated from its posterior attachment to the external ear cartilage and the sternocleidomastoid muscle. Those branches of the great auricular nerve that penetrate the gland are divided, but those to the ear lobule are left intact.

At this point, it is necessary to identify the facial nerve. The nerve trunk can be isolated at its exit from the stylomastoid foramen before entering the posterior gland.

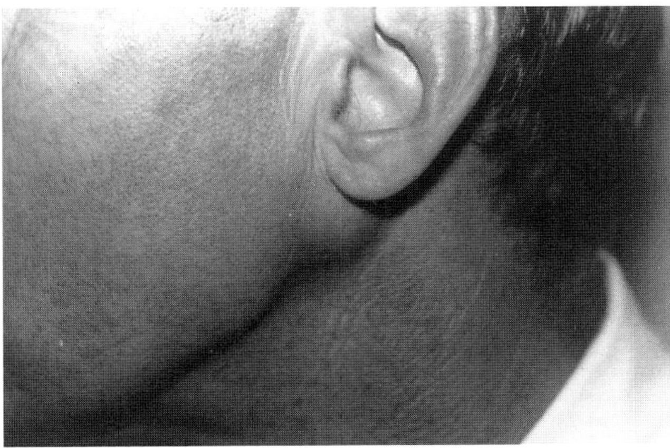

FIGURE 32-1. Parotid tumors typically present as asymptomatic masses present for 1 year or more.

Alternatively, as the authors prefer, the peripheral branches are identified and traced retrograde through the gland substance. The nerve is dissected using loupe magnification and delicate technique. The fibers are bluntly separated from the parenchyma and the glandular tissue tested for nerve stimulation by gentle compression. The glandular tissue is sharply divided and the lateral lobe is removed. If the deep lobe is to be removed, the nerve branches are individually elevated with nerve hooks and the remaining gland is removed.

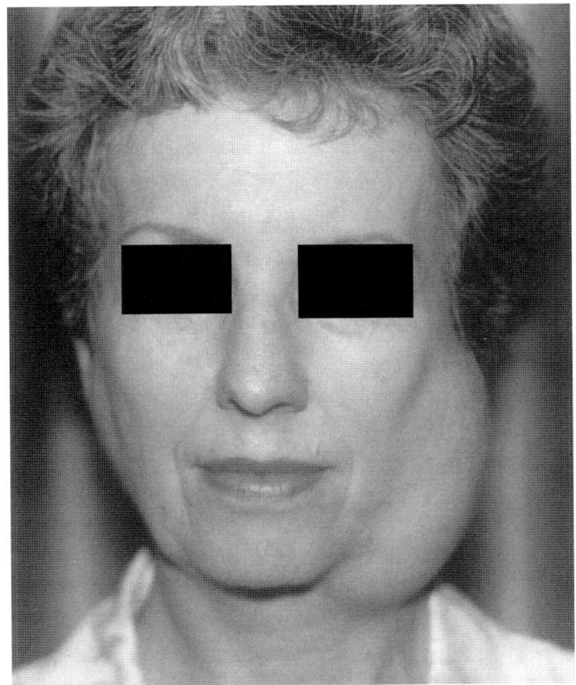

FIGURE 32-2. Patient with a large parotid tumor. This patient was apprised of all the risks of injury to the facial nerve and the potential need for nerve resection and neck dissection. She refused surgery because she could not accept a preauricular scar.

Care must be taken to maintain tumor integrity. Rupture of a benign mixed tumor will cause seeding of the tumor and increase the risk of recurrence.

The skin flap then is closed over a small suction drain. We routinely obtain a frozen section analysis at the time of surgery (3). This additional information assists in decision making regarding the extent of the surgery.

COMPLICATIONS

Tumor Recurrence

The most frequent and one of the worst complications after parotid tumor surgery is recurrence of the tumor. The best way to prevent this is the proper performance of an adequate operation at the first opportunity. Superficial parotidectomy is performed for all tumors in the superficial part of the gland. Malignant tumors generally require total parotidectomy. Rupture of the tumor and incomplete removal are risk factors for recurrence (Fig. 32-3). The facial nerve should only be intentionally sacrificed if there is malignant tumor invading or encapsulating the nerve.

Facial Nerve Damage

To prevent postoperative facial nerve palsy, the facial nerve trunk or branches must be identified and exposed early in the procedure. However, sometimes injury to the nerve is unavoidable, even with benign tumors, especially in cases where the tumor is large or is located in the deep lobe of the gland. Inadvertent transection of the nerve is unacceptable, but traction injuries and local trauma are common problems. Gentle dissection and retraction of the nerve minimize this disturbing complication. However, postoperative facial paresis is a relatively common and potentially serious prob-

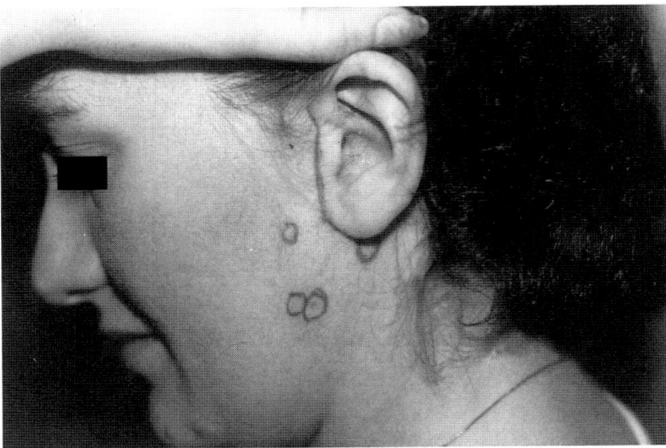

FIGURE 32-3. Young woman 5 years after parotidectomy for a benign mixed tumor. The tumor ruptured during excision, and the patient developed multiple tumor recurrences. Each circle represents a separate palpable tumor recurrence.

lem, even if temporary. The patient must be well aware of the sequelae before undergoing the surgery.

Previous reports listed the incidence of 10% to 40% for temporary paresis and less than 20% for permanent palsy (4). These data include all types of tumors, benign and malignant. One would expect lower incidences in benign tumors confined to the superficial lobe. However, even in these cases, there is a significant incidence of facial nerve injury. Two factors have been noted as potential etiologies for nerve injury. One is direct blunt trauma with contusion of the nerve, and the other is ischemic anoxia of the nerve after it has been separated from the gland (4).

Several studies documented lower incidences of facial nerve palsy after parotidectomy. One study advocated use of the operative microscope for dissection of the nerve (4). This study reported an incidence of 4% to 40% for temporary paresis and 0% for permanent palsy. Moreover, the cases with temporary palsy all recovered within 3 months after surgery. This suggests that the damage to the facial nerve was mainly due to trauma. Other studies documented similar results, with an initial rate of 29% to 46% for postoperative weakness and permanent weakness in 4% to 6% (5,6).

Intraoperative facial nerve monitoring also has been suggested as beneficial for protecting the peripheral nerve branches during revision parotidectomy. One study documented an improvement in the incidence of early temporary weakness of the facial nerve with continuous facial nerve monitoring (7). However, there was no difference in the rate of permanent facial nerve palsy. Whether the added time and expense of this procedure are of benefit to the patient is unclear and requires further investigation.

If the main trunk of the facial nerve is transected, either purposely or inadvertently, prompt repair using microsurgical techniques should be performed.

If a portion of the nerve is resected, we prefer to perform an autogenous nerve graft at the time of the initial operation (Fig. 32-4). The great auricular nerve is an easily obtained donor nerve with minimal donor site morbidity.

Long-term sequelae of permanent facial nerve palsy should be addressed surgically. The goals are to restore the function of eyelid closure and oral continence. The mimetic muscles of the face are important for cosmesis. Facial reanimation can be performed through a vast panoply of techniques (1).

Frey Syndrome

Frey syndrome was first described in 1923 by a French neurologist. It was initially called the auriculotemporal nerve syndrome and later became known as gustatory sweating.

Gustatory sweating is a well-known sequela after parotid surgery. The reported incidence varies enormously, ranging from 2% to 80%, but almost all patients will have an abnormal starch iodine test up to 12 months after surgery. Fortunately, only 5% to 10% have symptomatic complaints (8). Patients can become socially debilitated by episodes of unilateral gustatory hyperhidrosis, pain, or flushing over the cutaneous distribution of the auriculotemporal nerve. At this time the most widely accepted theory for the pathophysiology of Frey syndrome is the aberrant regeneration theory. In this theory, autonomic fibers from the parotid gland, when damaged by surgery or trauma, regrow into the sheath of the severed auriculotemporal nerve, causing the syndrome (9).

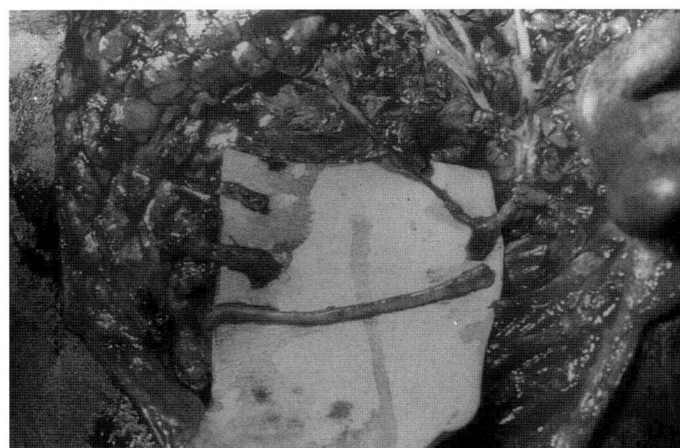

FIGURE 32-4. The main trunk of the facial nerve was excised in this patient due to involvement with an undifferentiated mucoepidermoid carcinoma. The great auricular nerve was harvested and is shown as a cable graft.

Numerous articles have reported on the treatment, both surgical and nonsurgical, of Frey syndrome. These include medications such as topical anticholinergics and systemic atropine, and surgery such as tympanic neurectomy, insertion of fascial lata grafts or muscle flaps, and reelevation of the skin flap. None of these methods have proven very effective. Recent reports, however, have shown an 80% to 100% disappearance of symptoms with the use of botulinum toxin in patients with Frey syndrome (10,11). In our experience, topical antiperspirants usually are easy to use and effective.

There are a number of surgical options to prevent the late onset of Frey syndrome. These studies suggest that the syndrome can be avoided at the time of parotidectomy by using the superficial musculoaponeurotic system as an interposing flap to interrupt the anastomotic communications with the sweat glands (Fig. 32-5). This also provides improvement in the aesthetic result after parotidectomy by providing more bulk. These studies reported a much improved rate of gustatory sweating after parotidectomy of 0% to 6% (12–15). Temporoparietal fascial flaps at the time of surgery or the use of dermal allograft also have been suggested as preventive measures.

Great Auricular Nerve Injury

Facial and auriculotemporal nerve injuries receive the majority of attention after parotidectomy. A lesion of the great auricular nerve normally is not regarded as significant, but damage to this nerve can give rise to sensorineural sequelae,

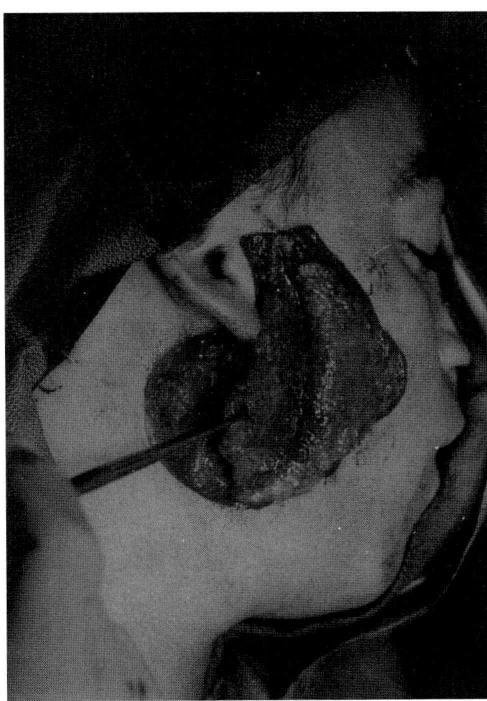

FIGURE 32-5. The superficial musculoaponeurotic system flap is shown interposed between the parotidectomy bed and the skin flap in a successful attempt to prevent Frey syndrome.

including a lack of or an alteration of sensation to the ear lobe. The cheek usually is hypesthetic for 3 to 6 months postoperatively. This can be quite uncomfortable, even painful. These sequelae can be avoided by preserving the posterior branch of the great auricular nerve (16). The anterior branches innervate the parotid gland and are routinely transected. Neuromas of the great auricular nerve are rare but can occur as a painful mass overlying the sternocleidomastoid muscle.

Salivary Fistula/Sialocele

Fistulas occurring after parotid surgery are relatively rare. Many wounds leak for a few days, but a true persistent fistula is uncommon. Sialoceles are similarly uncommon and self-limited. These pools and leaks of saliva are treated with aspiration, local pressure, and avoidance of sialagogues. If a fistula persists, the drainage site and the residual gland should be excised and the duct explored and religated.

Postoperative Bleeding

Parotidectomy is the most common head and neck procedure associated with postoperative bleeding, which is reported to occur in 2.7% of patients after this procedure (17). It can be minimized by meticulous hemostasis and careful surgical technique. The difficulty with hemostasis is the proximity of the nerve to the bleeding sites. Bipolar cautery or surgical ties limit the risk of nerve trauma.

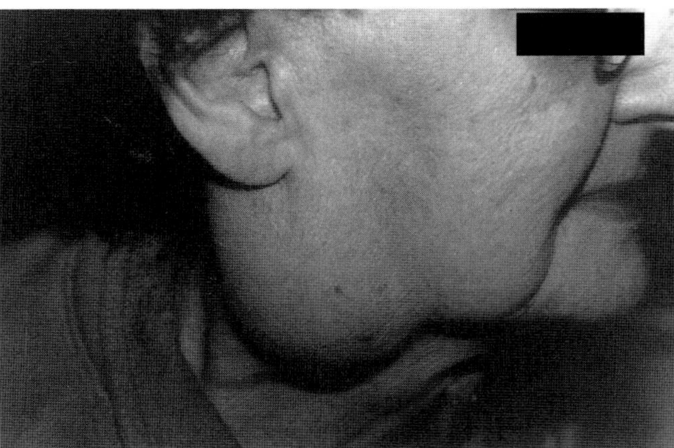

A

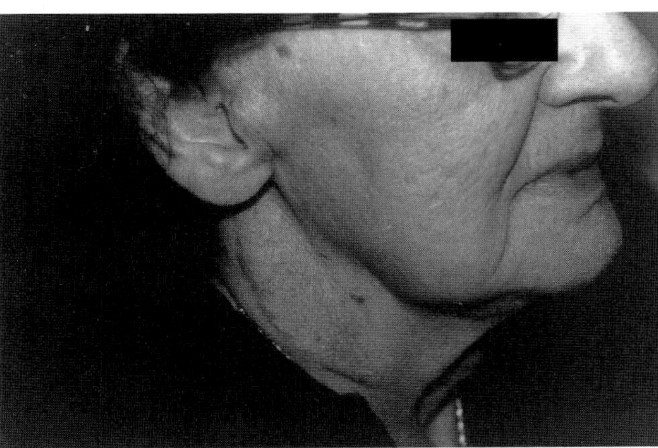

B

FIGURE 32-6. A: Preoperative large parotid tumor. **B:** Postoperative defect in the same patient.

Postoperative Deformity

Patients who have large tumors or glands may develop significant facial asymmetry postoperatively (Fig. 32-6). Although the preauricular area cannot be visualized simultaneously on both sides, patients and careful observers may notice a hollow appearance on the operated side. This asymmetry can be corrected, in part, by interposing a temporoparietal fascial flap or a piece of dermal allograft over the excision site before skin closure.

REFERENCES

1. Granick MS, Hanna DC. Surgical management of salivary disease. In: Granick MS, Hanna DC, eds. *Management of salivary gland lesions.* Baltimore: Williams & Wilkins, 1992:145–174.
2. Granick MS, Hanna DC. Salivary glands. In: Nora PF, ed. *Operative surgery.* Philadelphia: WB Saunders, 1990:172–182.
3. Granick MS, Hanna DC, Erickson ER. Accuracy of frozen section diagnosis in salivary gland lesions. *Head Neck Surg* 1985;7:465–467.
4. Watanabe Y, Ishikawa M, Shojaku H, et al. Facial nerve palsy as a complication of parotid gland surgery and its prevention. *Acta Otolaryngol (Stockh)* 1993;[Suppl 504]:137–139.
5. Bron LP, O'Brien CJ. Facial nerve function after parotidectomy. *Arch Otolaryngol Head Neck Surg* 1997;123:1091–1096.

6. Mehle ME, Kraus DH, Wood BG, et al. Facial nerve morbidity following parotid surgery for benign disease: The Cleveland Clinic Foundation experience. *Laryngoscope* 1993;103:386–388.
7. Terrell JE, Kileny PR, Yian C, et al. Clinical outcome of continuous facial nerve monitoring during primary parotidectomy. *Arch Otolaryngol Head Neck Surg* 1997;123:1081–1087.
8. Linder TE, Huber A, Schmid S. Frey's syndrome after parotidectomy: a retrospective and prospective analysis. *Laryngoscope* 1997;107:1496–1501.
9. Farrell ML, Kalnins IK. Frey's syndrome following parotid surgery. *Aust N Z J Surg* 1991;61:295–301.
10. Bjerkhoel A, Trobbe O. Frey's syndrome: treatment with botulinum toxin. *J Laryngol Otol* 1997;111:839–844.
11. Laskawi R, Drobik C, Schonebeck C. Up-to-date report of botulinum toxin type A treatment in patients with gustatory sweating (Frey's syndrome). *Laryngoscope* 1998;108:381–384.
12. Bonnano PC, Casson PR. Frey's syndrome: a preventable phenomenon. *Plast Reconstr Surg* 1992;89:452–456.
13. Allison GR, Rappaport I. Prevention of Frey's syndrome with superficial musculoaponeurotic system interposition. *Am J Surg* 1993;166:407–410.
14. Moulton-Barrett R, Allison G, Rappaport I. Variation's in the use of SMAS (superficial musculoaponeurotic system) to prevent Frey's syndrome after parotidectomy. *Int Surg* 1996;81:174–176.
15. Yu LT, Hamilton R. Frey's syndrome: prevention with conservative parotidectomy and superficial musculoaponeurotic system preservation. *Ann Plast Surg* 1992;29:217–222.
16. Christensen NR, Jacobsen SD. Parotidectomy: preserving the posterior branch of the great auricular nerve. *J Laryngol Otol* 1997;111:556–559.
17. Matory YL, Spiro RH. Wound bleeding after head and neck surgery. *J Surg Oncol* 1993;53:17–19.

Discussion

PAROTID TUMOR SURGERY

JATIN P. SHAH

The authors of this chapter have provided a comprehensive coverage of the anticipated unfavorable results of parotid gland surgery, their prevention and management, along with a succinct bibliography of important contributions to the literature on the subject. The unfavorable results of parotid surgery can be classified into four categories: (i) postsurgical, (ii) functional, (iii) aesthetic, and (iv) oncologic.

Unfavorable postsurgical results generally are described under postoperative complications of surgery, such as development of hematoma, infection, and formation of a salivary fistula. The functional sequelae or results that are unfavorable include facial nerve paresis or paralysis, development of Frey syndrome, development of numbness of the skin of the lower part of the external ear and adjacent region, and development of amputation neuroma secondary to transection of the greater auricular nerve. Unfavorable aesthetic results include poor healing of the scar and soft tissue deficit secondary to removal of the superficial lobe of the parotid gland. Finally, unfavorable oncologic results include development of recurrent tumor.

J. P. Shah: Department of Surgery, Weill Medical College of Cornell University; and Head and Neck Service, Department of Surgery, Memorial Sloan-Kettering Cancer Center, New York, New York

Avoidance of these unfavorable and unpleasant sequelae of parotid gland surgery requires careful preoperative planning, which includes thorough clinical evaluation, appropriate diagnostic imaging, and documentation of histologic diagnosis when deemed necessary (1). In addition to accurate and detailed clinical examination, appropriate imaging studies are indicated for ill-defined lesions and lesions suspected to be in the deep lobe of the parotid gland. Computed tomographic scan or magnetic resonance imaging scan generally are adequate and will demonstrate the anatomical location and extent of the tumor. Tumors may arise in the superficial lobe of the parotid gland, deep lobe of the parotid gland (salivary tissue medial to the plane of the facial nerve), or in accessory parotid tissue along the course of the Stensen's duct. Surgical approach to these tumors depends on the location and size of the tumor. Most parotid tumors located in the superficial lobe of the parotid gland are easily approached through a skin incision just anterior to the tragus in the skin crease in front of the external ear curving inferomedially behind the angle of the mandible and superimposing an upper neck skin crease, if necessary. A majority of deep lobe parotid tumors also can be excised through this surgical approach. Only rarely is it necessary to perform a mandibulotomy to gain access to the parapharyngeal location of a deep lobe parotid tumor. Superior extension of the skin incision along the sideburn and with a right angled extension anteriorly is required to gain exposure to the anterior aspect of the parotid gland, particularly for tumors in the accessory parotid tissue along the Stensen's duct.

Preoperative discussion with the patient and a truthful and honest assessment of the hazards of parotid surgery in relation to the facial nerve are vitally important. The patient needs to understand the complexity of the surgical procedure and the potential risks of injury and/or the need to sacrifice the facial nerve and the sequelae of such surgical procedure in detail. Unhappiness on the part of a majority of patients during the postoperative period can be avoided by such a detailed preoperative discussion and gaining the confidence of the patient in the ability of the surgeon to conduct an appropriate surgical procedure.

Meticulous surgical technique and attention to detail are crucial to the conduct of a safe surgical procedure (2). Use of anatomical landmarks for identification of the main trunk of the facial nerve and sensitivity on the part of the surgeon in preserving the posterior branch of the greater auricular nerve are essential to avoid unpleasant functional sequelae. Accurate placement of the incision in the skin creases is crucial to an aesthetically pleasing scar. I prefer elevation of the skin flap and dissection of the parotid tissue away from the nerve with the use of electrocautery. It is important to remember that cavalier use of electrocautery can cause inadvertent thermal injury to the nerve leading to facial paralysis. However, judicious use of the electrocautery is safe. Generally, use of bipolar electrocautery is preferred for securing absolute hemostasis. Absolute hemostasis during the entire course of the operation is crucial to the safe conduct of the operative procedure. The skin flap is elevated deep to the superficial musculoaponeurotic layer just over the parotid fascia. Leaving the superficial musculoaponeurotic layer on the skin flap reduces the soft tissue deficit in the parotid bed and is also claimed to reduce the risk of Frey syndrome. During elevation of the skin flap, meticulous attention to detail should be paid to identification of the greater auricular nerve and its branches. If it has a sizable posterior branch, it should be preserved to retain sensation of the lower half of the external ear.

Dissection of the facial nerve may be performed in antegrade or retrograde fashion. Generally, antegrade dissection is recommended with identification of the main trunk of the facial nerve first and its dissection to identify its main divisions and peripheral branches. The anatomical landmarks used for identification of the facial nerve are the superior border of the posterior belly of the digastric muscle, the tip of the mastoid process, and the anteroinferior portion of the cartilaginous auditory canal. Where these three landmarks meet, the facial nerve exits from the stylomastoid foramen and enters the parotid gland. Once the main trunk is identified, dissection proceeds along the peripheral divisions of the facial nerve. The usual technique of dissection requires that the parotid tissue be spread open over the nerve, keeping the nerve under direct vision at all times while the superficial parotid tissue is divided. Blunt dissection should be avoided at all times and frankly should be condemned because it will cause "neurapraxia" secondary to blunt trauma to the nerve. Similarly, excessive retraction of the superficial lobe by the surgical assistant will cause "stretch neurapraxia" to the facial nerve, and this also should be avoided. Although electrocautery may be used judiciously during the operation, its use should be avoided when dissection is in the immediate vicinity of the facial nerve. On the other hand, fine bleeding points in the vicinity of the nerve can be adequately controlled with judicious use of the bipolar electrocautery. A bipolar scissors can be used with advantage during this phase of the dissection. If the peripheral branches of the facial nerve are too small and are not easily recognizable without the aid of optical magnification, then the use of loupes or a microscope is encouraged. Similarly, if the operating surgeon is inexperienced or not confident in identification of the facial nerve or its branches, then a nerve stimulator may be used to identify the branches of the facial nerve. Generally, in a fresh surgical field (first surgical procedure on the parotid gland), a nerve stimulator is rarely required. I personally prefer that the patient be completely paralyzed to avoid any movement of the facial muscles during the surgical procedure. On the other hand, others recommend that the patient not be paralyzed with muscle relaxants so that a nerve stimulator can be used to identify the nerve during the course of the dissection. Continuous facial nerve monitoring can be used but is seldom necessary for routine parotid surgery. It is expensive, time consuming, and generally not cost effective.

Patients whose tumors are located immediately overlying the main trunk of the facial nerve generally are not suitable candidates for antegrade dissection of the facial nerve. In these instances, retrograde dissection of the facial nerve is undertaken. It generally is easy to identify the zygomatic or buccal branches of the facial nerve to begin the dissection in a retrograde fashion, carefully following each of the other branches up to the main trunk of the facial nerve. At this juncture. the tumor is easily lifted off the lateral aspect of the main trunk of the facial nerve with the superficial lobe in a *mono bloc* fashion.

Rupture of the tumor due to rough manipulation, excessive traction, or digital dissection should be avoided, because it has been associated with an increased risk of local recurrence. The extent of parotid tissue resection depends on the size, location, extent, and pathology of the tumor being removed. The majority of the tumors located in the superficial lobe of the parotid gland will require a complete superficial lobectomy with dissection and preservation of the facial nerve. This maneuver will allow the remaining minimal amounts of parotid tissue deep to the facial nerve to undergo fibrosis and reduce the risk of parotid fistula. Partial parotidectomy without identification of the facial nerve is to be condemned, because it increases the risk of injury to the facial nerve and the risk of postoperative parotid fistula. In addition, partial parotidectomy or local excision of a parotid tumor leads to an unacceptably high risk of local recurrence. The only exceptions to this rule are Warthin's tumors, which usually are located at the periphery of the tail of the parotid gland, and accessory parotid tumors. Warthin tumors can be excised without dissection of the facial nerve or disturbance to the integrity of the parotid gland. Similarly, accessory parotid tumors generally are not contiguous with the main parotid gland and often can be adequately excised without disturbing the main mass of the superficial lobe of the parotid gland. It is important, however, to remember that the buccal branch of the facial nerve should be carefully identified and preserved during excision of the accessory parotid tumor.

Inadvertent injury and transection of the facial nerve should be immediately identified and promptly corrected by nerve suture. Use of the operating microscope is strongly encouraged for nerve repair. Similarly, use of the operating microscope and nerve stimulator are encouraged during reoperative surgery on the parotid gland. Identification and preservation of the facial nerve and its branches are difficult due to fibrosis in the parotid bed; therefore optimal magnification and nerve stimulator can assist the operating surgeon in identifying and preserving the nerve. Similarly, if resection of any part of the facial nerve is required for a curative surgical resection, then a nerve graft should be considered immediately. Primary nerve grafting is ideal for accurate anatomical repair and excellent long-term results. A sural nerve graft or graft from the cutaneous branches of the cervical plexus can be used. Accurate neural anastomosis is best performed with the use of the operating microscope.

Finally, drainage of the wound following parotid surgery is recommended to minimize the risk of postoperative hematoma. Although suction drains can be used, I prefer a Penrose drain with light pressure dressing. Improper placement of the suction drain over the facial nerve can produce suction damage and neurapraxia to the facial nerve leading to paresis or paralysis. If suction drains are used, they should not overlie any part of the facial nerve; their proper placement is crucial. Meticulous closure of the skin incision with accurate approximation of the skin edges and a fine nonabsorbable suture material are all essential for an aesthetically pleasing scar. Nearly all unfavorable results of parotid surgery can be avoided by accurate preoperative diagnosis, detailed preoperative discussion with the patient, and exercise of attention to detail in execution of the surgical procedure with meticulous surgical technique. Despite these precautions, some patients will have results that are unfavorable and unanticipated, and appropriate management should be initiated as soon as possible.

REFERENCES

1. Shah JP, Ihde JK. Salivary gland tumors. *Curr Probl Surg* 1990;12:755–843.
2. Shah JP. *Head and neck surgery,* 2nd ed. St. Louis: Mosby, 1996.

33

OROPHARYNGEAL RECONSTRUCTION

JOHN JOSEPH COLEMAN III

There have been enormous improvements in reconstruction of the head and neck in the last 15 years. Elucidation of the musculocutaneous concept and refinement in microsurgical techniques have changed our approach, which once was characterized by long delays to secondary reconstruction by multiple staged local or locoregional flaps. Currently, reconstruction is achieved primarily in one stage, at the time of the extirpative procedure. Despite these advances, there is still a high complication rate with such procedures in the pharynx and in other areas of the head and neck. Many of these problems resolve without further surgery. Because of this and the variety of the techniques available, a more aggressive approach to extensive primary disease has been fostered. Moreover, surgery on recurrent disease that previously was rarely performed is now more common, with excellent evidence of palliation and sometimes a cure.

In the United States, the most common problem requiring surgical reconstruction of the pharynx is malignancy. Squamous cell carcinoma of the oropharynx and larynx usually requires surgery and adjuvant radiotherapy for its treatment because patients commonly are at late stage of the disease at presentation (1). Although traumatic penetration, iatrogenic caustic ingestion, infection, and congenital problems (tracheoesophageal fistula, cleft palate) occasionally may demand pharyngeal reconstruction, the overwhelming majority of cases are secondary to resection of squamous cell carcinoma in adults or the less common tumors of childhood, such as rhabdomyosarcoma. The associated requirements of surgical access for resection or cervical lymphadenectomy and preoperative or postoperative radiotherapy further complicate the reconstruction and increase the likelihood of complications (2).

Unfavorable results in pharynx reconstruction mirror the general complications potential to all head and neck surgery (Tables 33-1 and 33-2). There are, however, several complications that are particularly relevant to this site, including (i) recurrence of disease; (ii) flap failure; (iii) partial wound necrosis, infection, and fistula; (iv) failure to restore function or impairment of existing function (i.e., dysphagia and aspiration); and (v) necessity for an unplanned second procedure. There are three general methods of reconstruction that are used for pharyngeal reconstruction: (i) local or locoregional skin flaps, (ii) musculocutaneous flaps primarily from the thorax, and (iii) free-tissue transfer. Each of these methods has certain advantages and disadvantages and may be appropriate for some defects and not for others. After an initial discussion of the general principles for avoidance of unfavorable results, including the complication of recurrent disease, we examine these problems specifically with regard to each of the techniques.

Unfavorable results may occur due to errors in judgment or technical flaws in preoperative assessment and operative planning, during the execution of the procedures, or in the postoperative care of the patient (3).

PREOPERATIVE ASSESSMENT AND PLANNING

Head and neck surgery, and thus surgery on the pharynx, has evolved into a multidisciplinary approach frequently using the skills of surgeons from various backgrounds (general surgery, otolaryngology, plastic surgery) in varying roles, as well as medical oncologists and radiotherapists. Cancer of the pharynx still usually is diagnosed at an advanced stage of disease and requires at least surgery and radiotherapy. There has been some success with organ-preserving chemotherapy with cisplatin and 5-fluorouracil, followed by or concurrent with radiotherapy, with surgery remaining a salvage option. However, most patients require surgery and subsequent radiotherapy or undergo surgery after failure of an attempt at definitive radiotherapy. Detailed knowledge by the plastic surgeon of the principles of multidisciplinary cancer therapy is critical to avoid complications. This knowledge must embrace in detail the general principles and tissue effects of radiotherapy to the head and neck. In addition to general principles, the specific knowledge of the patient's previous history—including previous operative therapy; timing, amount, delivery ports, fractionation, and source of radio-

J. J. Coleman III: Department of Surgery, Indiana University School of Medicine; and Division of Plastic Surgery, Indiana University Medical Center, Indianapolis, Indiana

TABLE 33-1. COMPLICATIONS OF HEAD AND NECK SURGERY

- I. Anatomical
  - A. Nerve palsies
    1. Accessory
    2. Cervical plexus motor branches
    3. Phrenic
    4. Vagus
    5. Recurrent laryngeal
    6. Facial
    7. Marginal mandibular
    8. Hypoglossal
    9. Lingual
    10. Mental
    11. Inferior alveolar
    12. Mylohyoid
  - B. Thoracic duct injury
- II. Physiologic
  - A. Hypothyroidism
  - B. Hypoparathyroidism
  - C. Intracerebral edema
  - D. Lymphedema
  - E. Parotid disorders
- III. Technical
  - A. Respiratory
    1. Pneumothorax
    2. Acute upper airway obstruction
       - a. Hematoma
    3. Tracheostomy complications
       - a. Subcutaneous emphysema
       - b. Tracheoinnominate artery fistula
  - B. Infection
    1. Wound infection
    2. Osteomyelitis-osteoradionecrosis
    3. Carotid hemorrhage
  - C. Ischemic
    1. Suture line breakdown
    2. Flap necrosis
    3. Carotid hemorrhage
- IV. Functional
  - A. Chronic airway obstruction
  - B. Aspiration pneumonia
  - C. Dysphagia
  - D. Dysphonia
  - E. Mental depression

Adapted from Coleman JJ. Complications in head and neck surgery. *Surg Clin North Am* 1986;66:149–167.

TABLE 33-2. CATASTROPHIC COMPLICATIONS OF HEAD AND NECK SURGERY

Hypoparathyroidism-tetany
Acute airway obstruction
Carotid hemorrhage
Carotid exposure in an irradiated neck
Oropharyngocutaneous fistula in an irradiated neck
Major flap necrosis in an irradiated neck
Bilateral recurrent laryngeal nerve palsy
Tracheoinnominate fistula

Adapted from Coleman JJ. Complications in head and neck surgery. *Surg Clin North Am* 1986;66:149–167.

therapy; and the potential need for postoperative adjuvant radiotherapy—is necessary. Radiotherapy has well-documented tissue effects in the head (4) and neck, and numerous authors have documented an increased risk of complications when operating in the previously irradiated head and neck (Tables 33-3 and 33-4) (5).

Fibrosis of skin connective tissue and muscle and accelerated atherosclerosis of the local tissue blood supply and the external and internal carotid system demand careful preoperative assessment by the reconstructive surgeon. Although the choice of a recipient vessel in the head and neck for microvascular reconstruction of the pharynx ultimately must be made based on observed pulsatile flow after it has been divided in the neck, careful preoperative assessment and history taking may steer the reconstructive surgeon to a blood supply out of the field of radiation, such as the transverse cervical vessels. Occasionally, preoperative angiography or ultrasound analysis of the veins in the neck is useful in identifying a patient's jugular vein or suggesting adequate flow through the carotid system. Usually, however, careful history and physical examination, noting symptoms of carotid insufficiency such as transient ischemic attacks or history of stroke and the finding of a palpable pulse in the neck and at the mandibular notch, are sufficient to plan microvascular reconstruction.

The plastic surgeon as an extirpative or reconstructive surgeon must be familiar with the oncologic principles and procedures specific to pharynx resection. Knowledge of the American Joint Committee on Cancer staging system for cancer at this site, as well as the special methods of physical examination and indirect and direct laryngoscopy, allows proper treatment planning and reproducible communication with other members of the multidisciplinary team. Failure to evaluate the patient properly before surgery may result in inadequate resection, which in turn may result in persistence or recurrence of disease. In addition to physical examination, computerized axial tomography is useful for assessment of extension of pharyngeal tumors into the mandible or larynx framework. Magnetic resonance imaging is more sensitive and specific for the degree of soft tissue spread and the extension of tumor into the cranial nerves.

The hierarchy of priorities for treatment of all disease—survival, function, appearance, and efficiency (or the ability to deliver the therapy and restore the patient to the best stage possible in a period commensurate with the natural history of his disease)—applies to pharyngeal disorders. Survival usually lies within the domain of resection, but function, appearance, and efficiency are very much dependent on the talents and choices of the reconstructive surgeon. Careful preoperative analysis of existing function with careful notation of any presurgical dysfunction is critical to operative planning and execution. Review of radiologic studies, including magnetic resonance imaging, computerized axial tomography, and fluoroscopy, as well as indirect or direct laryngoscopy, will allow such assessment and oper-

TABLE 33-3. TOLERANCE DOSES OF VARIOUS TISSUES OF THE HEAD AND NECK BASED ON A LARGE VOLUME OF TREATMENT

Tissue	TD_5/5 cGy	TD_{50}/5 cGy	Complication
Skin	5,500	7,000	Necrosis/ulcer
Larynx	5,000	7,000	Edema, cartilage necrosis
Esophagus	5,500	6,800	Stricture, perforation
Jejunum	4,000	5,500	Obstruction, perforation
Brachial plexus	6,000	7,500	Neuropathy
Spinal cord	4,700	7,000	Myelitis/necrosis
Thyroid	4,500	8,000	Thyroiditis, hypothyroidism
Parotid	3,200	4,600	Xerostomia
Brain	4,500	6,000	Necrosis
Temporomandibular joint	6,000	7,200	Ankylosis
Stomach	5,000	6,500	Ulcer/perforation

ative planning. Knowledge of the physiologic functions of the upper aerodigestive tract is critical.

The pharynx is the continuation of the alimentary canal that lies between the oral cavity and the cervical esophagus. The pharynx may be anatomically subdivided into the nasopharynx, the oropharynx, and the hypopharynx. Stated simply, each of these subunits contributes to the main function of the pharynx: the correct and appropriate transit of air to the larynx and lungs and food to the esophagus and stomach. Like the rest of the alimentary tract, it is a mucosal tube encircled by muscles that, in some areas, are more prominent than in others and that primarily serve as sphincters, but also as elevators and depressors. The intricate synergistic action of the muscles of the tongue, palate, pharynx, and larynx allows the efficient and semiautomatic passage of air in and out of the lungs and food through the alimentary canal without mixing the two streams. When air is inhaled the larynx is low in the neck, the cords are open, the epiglottis is at its normal elevated position, and the palate is low, with the superior pharyngeal constrictor muscles relaxed. A similar position of these structures characterizes exhalation of air. The modification of breathing that results in speech requires that the palatal muscles (part of the oropharynx) contract or relax, obstructing the flow of air from the nasopharynx and nasal cavity and directing it through the mouth, where it is modulated by the tongue, buccal muscles, teeth, and lips to produce speech. During swallowing, the base of the tongue elevates, pushing the food backward and up; the palate rises, obturating the nasopharynx; and the superior constrictor initially relaxes, allowing ingress of the bolus to the hypopharynx, and then contracts, stripping it down. As the food bolus passes to the pharynx with the tongue pushing it down, the larynx rises to meet the relatively fixed position of the epiglottis, which bars the entry of the bolus into the lungs and the inferior pharyngeal constrictor, the cricopharyngeus muscle relaxes, allowing passage into the esophagus, where a peristaltic wave carries it to the stomach (6).

TABLE 33-4. TUMOR LETHAL DOSES FOR VARIOUS MALIGNANCIES BY PRIMARY STAGE AND HISTOLOGY

Tumor	Tumor Lethal Dose (cGy)
Seminoma	3,500
Neuroblastoma	3,500
Hodgkin disease	4,500
Basal cell carcinoma	4,500
Subclinical lymph node metastasis of squamous cell carcinoma	5,000
T1 larynx	6,000–6,500
T2 oral cavity	7,000–7,500
T2 pharynx	7,000–7,500
Sarcoma	8,000+
T3 oral cavity	8,000+

Adapted from Coleman JJ. Management of radiation-induced soft tissue injury to the head and neck. *Clin Plast Surg* 1993; 20:491–505.

Thus, the two main vegetative functions of humans, respiration and alimentation, depend on this complex sequence of events that is part voluntary and part automatic. Any disruption of the structure of this area or the nerve supply to it can have devastating effects, resulting in dysphagia, the inability to swallow, or airway obstruction or dysfunction that, in turn, may result in acute or chronic aspiration, pneumonia, or death. Although both routes can be bypassed (tracheostomy and enterostomy), quality-of-life concerns suggest that because of oral alimentation and speech, either laryngeal or alaryngeal functioning be restored whenever possible. Although reconstruction of the larynx is imperfect at present, a tubular conduit to replace the pharynx almost always is possible. Such a conduit should allow free passage of solid food and interfere as little as possible with remaining functional structures (larynx, tongue, palate) (7).

The number of methods of head and neck reconstruction have proliferated in the past 20 years. In 1969, only local flaps, prefabricated and waltzed, thoracoepigastric flaps, and the deltopectoral flap were available for pharyngeal reconstruction (8–10). By 1979, the pectoralis major and other thoracic musculocutaneous flaps were well established, and there were a few reports of free-tissue transfer, especially of the jejunum. By 1989, free-tissue transfer was well established as a superior method of reconstruction, and the ensuing years have seen further analysis of the advantages and disadvantages of the various methods and refinements used to improve function and appearance and reduce the cost and duration of hospitalization (11). This flowering of techniques and the subsequent benefits demand that the reconstructive surgeon have intimate familiarity with all methods, local, musculocutaneous, and microvascular. The "one-trick pony" surgeon whose repertoire is limited to the deltopectoral and pectoralis major flaps should not undertake pharyngeal reconstruction.

In the recent past, reconstruction was delayed from 2 to 5 years after resective surgery and radiotherapy to assure a cure of the malignancy. Because of the high risk of a second primary disease and the miserable functional state and appearance of the patient and encouraged by improvement in technique and analysis of data showing no survival advantage to this approach, the present evidence suggests that most patients be treated by definitive surgical resection, synchronous single-stage reconstruction, and postoperative adjuvant radiotherapy. To avoid excessively prolonged operative procedures, many surgical teams choose to perform the extirpative and reconstructive procedures simultaneously, raising the flap and repairing as much of the donor site as possible while the tumor extirpation and lymphadenectomy is performed, after which the transfer of the flap is completed. This simultaneous approach increases the necessity of comprehensive preoperative planning, awareness of possible changes in the plan that could occur during surgery (resection of mandible, larynx, tongue base, etc.), and excellent communication between the extirpative and reconstructive surgeons. Failure of any one of these elements may result in inappropriate choice of technique and catastrophe to the patient (12).

For whatever reason, various attributes have been attached to surgeons, surgical procedures, or approaches that have confused analysis and impaired results, sometimes even leading to personal, departmental, or institutional confrontation. Such attitudes have suggested that the resection, and thus the resective surgeon, was more important (virile, macho)—perhaps because of the relationship of resection to survival. Reconstructive surgery, radiotherapy, and other aspects of patient care were relegated to a lower echelon in this feudal, although prevalent, mentality. Fortunately, this concept seems to be waning, although it still is visible in local, national, and international arenas. Attention to patients, surgical results, quality-of-life outcomes, and a gradually increasing recognition by physicians of interdependency in multidisciplinary care have mitigated this thinking considerably and fostered a system of mutual respect for the specific skills and abilities that result in improved patient care. Such spirit is relevant to the preoperative assessment, intraoperative manipulation, and postoperative care of the patient who undergoes pharyngeal reconstruction. Although the resection should not be compromised to fit the reconstructive technique, the old concept of "we'll make the hole and then call you so you can come in and fix it" is obsolete and dangerous. Similarly, the attitude that all technical skill resides in the hands of the reconstructive surgeon is destructive to team effort.

INTRAOPERATIVE CONSIDERATIONS

The position of the patient on the operating room table, the placement of the endotracheal tube, and the placement of the drapes all greatly affect the ability of the reconstructive surgeon to obtain access to the affected site of the pharynx and to one or both necks. Many pharynx problems require removal or significant compromise of the larynx and, thus, the oronasal route of respiration. In such cases, a preoperative tracheostomy with placement of a flexible anode tube facilitates exposure to the pharynx and the neck. A long connecting tube to the anesthesia machine allows the airway to be placed across the chest and down the tucked or slightly extended arm contralateral to the side of the pharyngeal lesion. This allows access to both necks and the ability to move the head from side to side without interfering with, or the possibility of disturbing, the airway during the procedure. When tracheostomy is not part of the procedure and only one side of the pharynx and neck is involved, an oral tube with similar positioning is possible. If both necks are within the field and no tracheostomy is performed, a nasal right-angled tube brought over the head on a long connector to the anesthesia machine is satisfactory. It must be taped carefully to allow mobility of the head during surgery. It is critical to position the airway appropriately, because dislodgment can be catastrophic and because microvascular reconstruction requires the positioning of one surgeon on each side of the neck such that each can rest his arms in a place where he can perform the microvascular anastomosis (Fig. 33-1).

Although a clear operative plan usually is developed before surgery, it is wise to "prepare for the worst, hope for the best." The draping of the patient is relevant to this maxim. For access to the pharynx, both necks and most of the face should be in the sterile field. This is accomplished by the use of a head drape and towel sewn or stapled along both trapezius muscles from head to coracoacromial joint. The ipsilateral chest should be included in the field in case a pectoralis major flap is necessary. The arm, leg, or abdomen is appropriately prepped and draped to ensure that there is no contamination of this separate field from the oropharyngeal surgery site. If the endotracheal tube or airway tubing transgresses the field, it can be draped out with towels or sterile adhesive plastic to minimize contamination. Obviously, such elaborate preparation requires both excellent communication among the extirpative surgeon, the reconstructive

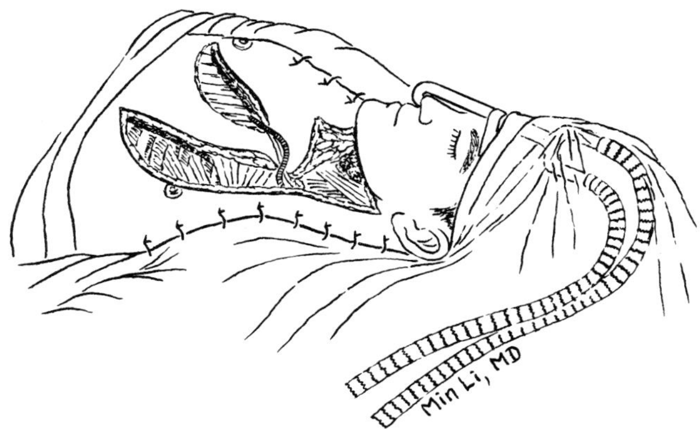

FIGURE 33-1. Position of the nasotracheal tube for pharynx reconstruction will allow the reconstructive surgeon access to both sides of the neck. Wide draping to expose the entire neck, face, and thorax facilitates access to the pharynx and both necks.

surgeon, and the anesthesiologist and the presence of a member of the reconstructive team at the time of positioning, prepping, and draping.

The increasing incidence of simultaneous surgery has increased the importance of proper positioning at the time of surgery. Although this occasionally requires some ingenuity and considerable respect for colleagues' personal space, it almost always is possible to arrange two teams of surgeons and nurses appropriately for the most efficient care (Fig. 33-2).

A slight degree of reverse Trendelenburg positioning is helpful in controlling blood loss during surgery, although care must be observed for orthostatic hypotension or, if the jugular vein is opened, for air embolus to the brain. Access to the mouth and nose is important for potential endoscopy or to test the integrity of the pharyngeal suture line.

Communication during the operation is important, just as it is in the preoperative period. Any change in the plan by the extirpative surgeon must be communicated to the re-

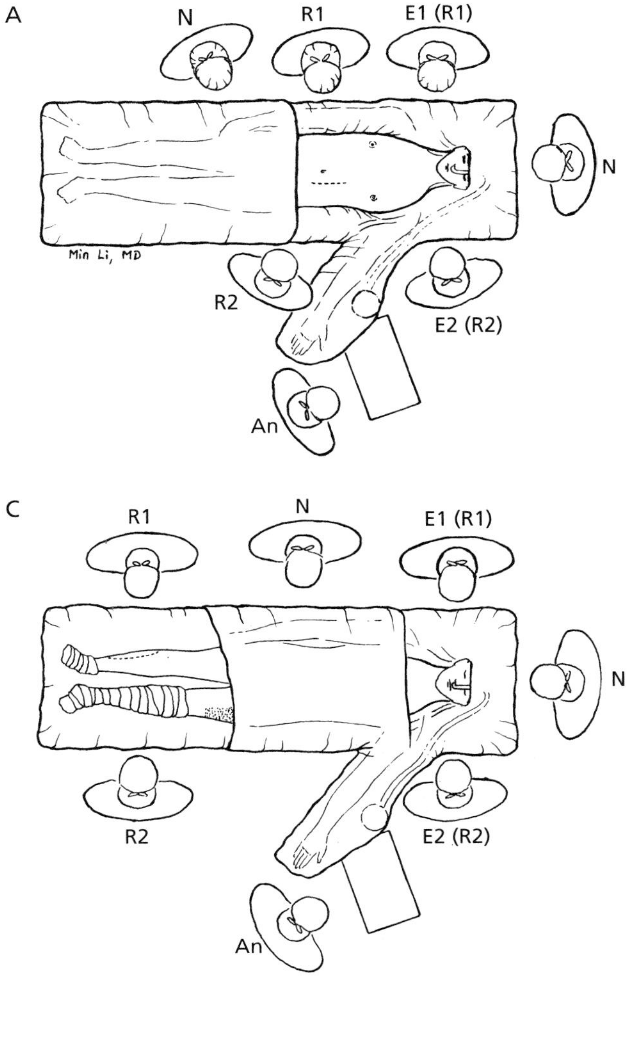

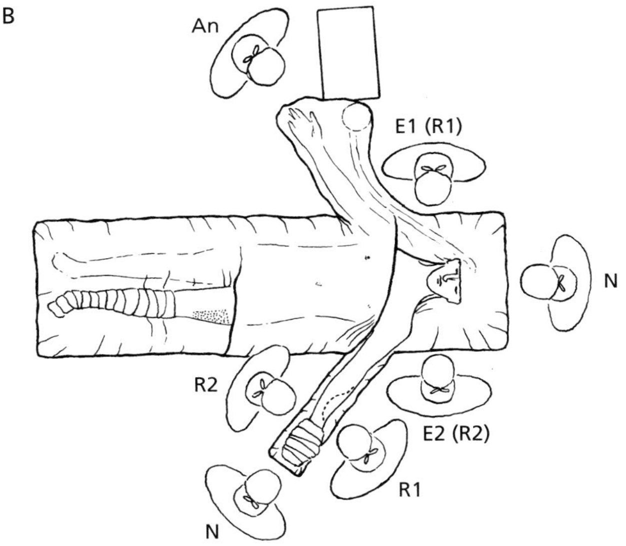

FIGURE 33-2. Careful positioning of each member of the surgical team will allow simultaneous tumor extirpation and flap harvest. **A:** Pharynx resection and jejunal free autograft reconstruction. **B:** Pharynx resection and radial forearm free autograft reconstruction. **C:** Pharynx resection and fibula free autograft reconstruction.

constructive surgeon. This is particularly crucial in simultaneous procedures. The unexpected necessity of removing further adjacent structures, such as the mandible, larynx, or base of the tongue, may drastically change the reconstructive plan. Although it usually is possible to avoid such situations, the reconstructive surgeon must anticipate and, whenever possible, prospectively prepare for them. In most cases, designing the reconstructive method somewhat larger than the requirement will provide the flexibility to revise it to the appropriate size at the time of inset.

Another important line of communication is between the surgeon and the anesthesiologist. Many operations on the pharynx are lengthy, but maintenance of homeostasis requires constant observation. The surgeon must be constantly aware of the patient's blood pressure and pulse to ensure tissue perfusion, urine output, and airway stability. Preoperative communication will prevent attempts at intravenous access in the neck and use of nitrous oxide, which may distend the bowel. Constant intraoperative vigilance and dialogue decreases the need for pressors or other pharmacologic manipulations that may impair flap perfusion. During these long procedures, there may be a tendency toward unbalanced fluid administration. This can result in either hypotension, which usually is treated emergently with pressors, or overhydration, which may cause increased bleeding, edema, and other problems both during the procedure and in the postoperative period. Again, mutual respect and tactful communication of individual observations and needs among the treating physicians results in the best patient outcomes.

Perhaps the most common mistake in pharyngeal surgery is the attempt to perform a complex reconstruction without adequate exposure. This manifests most frequently during the inset of the flap and in the dissection of the recipient vessels in the neck. Inadequate visualization of the suture line between reconstruction and native tongue or pharynx will result in leakage of salivary contents, anaerobic proliferation of bacteria, abscess or secondary infection, fistula, and possible vascular thrombosis and flap loss. This is most common at the cephalad inset of the flap along the base of tongue or at the triple-point site of primary closure of the pharynx and tongue base. Direct visualization and careful suturing technique are necessary to avoid this problem. When access to the superior pharynx or tongue base is difficult, mandibulotomy and extension of the pharyngotomy may be useful (Fig. 33-3). Whenever possible, a double-layer closure of suture lines with interrupted absorbable sutures is indicated.

When microvascular reconstruction is chosen for the pharyngeal reconstruction, the recipient vessels must be positioned at the most favorable site for microvascular anastomosis with the greatest ease to the surgeon. If the external carotid and jugular systems are to be used, a rapid and simple exposure is possible. Dissection along the medial (anterior) border of the sternocleidomastoid muscle from the parotid gland to the lower third with exposure of the posterior belly of the digastric muscle will allow removal of minimal lymphatic tissue and exposure of the jugular vein and external carotid system. The facial artery ascends into the submandibular triangle at a very constant position beneath the digastric muscle, approximately one-third of the way between the tendon and the muscle's origin on the mastoid process. It courses medially and anteriorly through the submandibular gland, from which it can easily be dissected. By clipping several small branches and parts of the ranine plexus of veins, it can be mobilized beneath the digastric and placed on top of the sternocleidomastoid muscle for easy microvascular anastomosis. Through this approach, the occipital and lingual vessels similarly are available. Dissection of the fascial envelope of the jugular vein from the carotid and deep structures of the neck allows easy retraction with vessel loops in a superficial direction to facilitate visualization and easy access for end-to-side anastomosis or with division of one of its large cephalad branches (anterior or posterior facial) for end-to-end anastomosis. Prospective communication with the extirpative surgeon or actual dissection by the reconstructive surgeon allows preservation of the external jugular vein if the internal jugular is involved in the resection. When adequate vessels are not present in the carotid jugular system, the transverse cervical vessels usually are available in the base of the neck. Dissection along the posterior border of the sternocleidomastoid muscle in the posterior triangle exposes the posterior belly of the omohyoid. This can be retracted or divided, revealing the transverse cervical vessels. There is an ascending and transverse branch of the artery, and either may be used. Considerable vessel length can be achieved by dissection back to the subclavian. This allows transposition to the surface of the sternocleidomastoid muscle and facilitates anastomosis, avoiding the difficulty of suturing in a deep hole late in a lengthy procedure. The artery may demonstrate spasm in the exposure. If there is no obvious obstruction from adventitial hematoma or atherosclerosis, application of papaverine and water sponges, dissection of the adventitia, ligation of small side branches, and placement of an Acland clamp on the end of the vessel and observing it in a warm environment almost always result in pulsatile flow, which is the requirement for anastomosis. Flap choice, flap design, recipient vessel choice, and preparation and dissection of donor pedicle almost always allow direct anastomosis, whether the jejunum radial forearm or other skin flap or fibula flap is used for pharynx reconstruction. Use of vein grafts, which greatly increase the risk of flap failure and the necessity for secondary procedures, is virtually never necessary.

A successful operation is the sum of a number of different steps. Although some are trivial, omission can result in significant consequence. Planning the position of the vascular pedicle is part of the initial design, but it also is important to check its position at the end of the operation, whether using a microvascular or pedicle flap. Most pha-

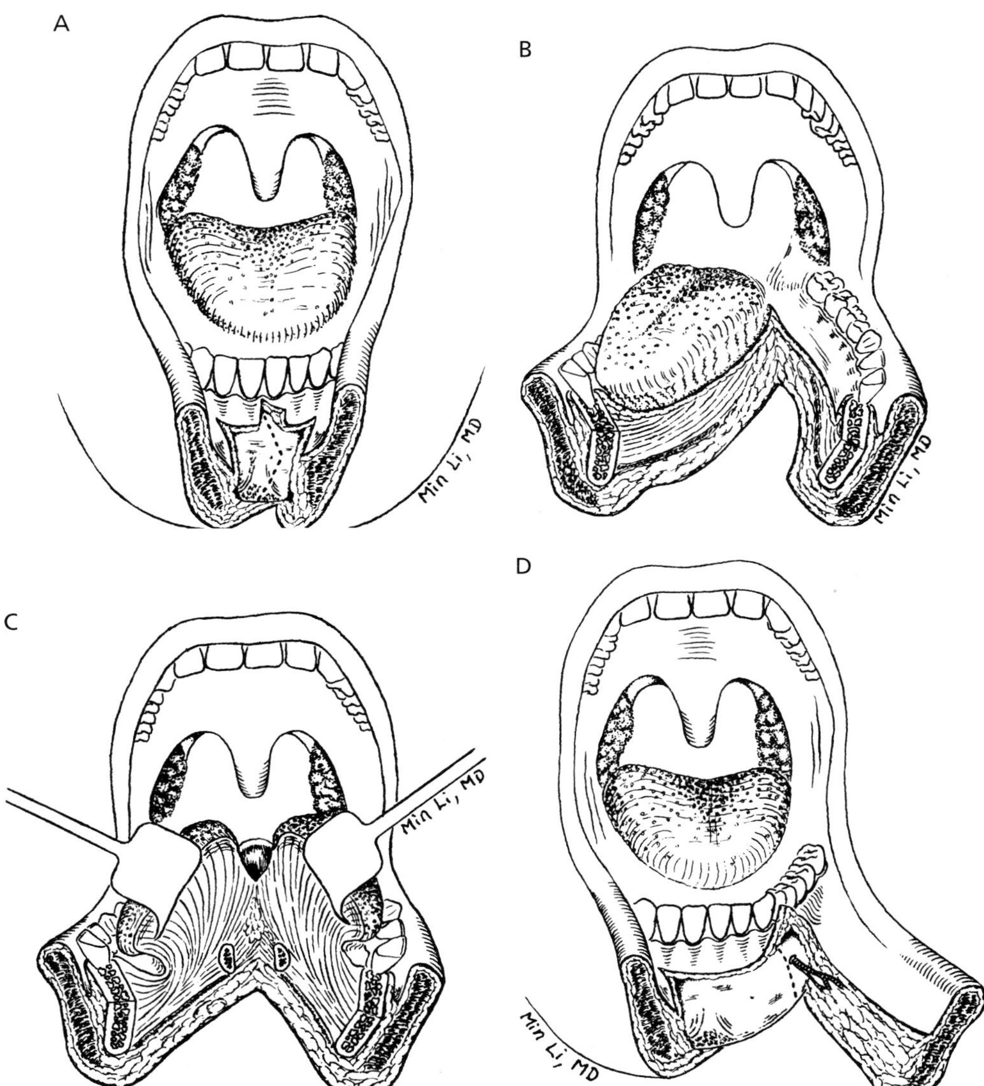

FIGURE 33-3. Access to the cephalad and posterior aspects of the pharynx may require extended pharyngotomy and even mandibulotomy. **A:** The median labial midline mandibulotomy (Trotter) creates minimal dysfunction (lip or dental anesthesia) and leaves an excellent postoperative aesthetic result. **B:** The incision is carried along the lingual alveolar sulcus, taking care not to injure the hypoglossal or lingual nerves to provide better visualization of the base of the tongue or posterior pharynx. **C:** An alternative approach is directly through the midline of the tongue, where there is a relatively avascular plane. Because the tongue is bilaterally innervated and perfused, there is minimal disruption of function. **D:** The mandibulotomy for pharyngeal reconstruction may be made through the body of the mandible, preferably mesial to the mental nerves.

ryngeal reconstructions are performed with the neck hyperextended in a cephalad and lateral position. A vascular pedicle of seemingly ideal length may, in fact, be too long and redundant, resulting in kinking when the neck is flexed or in the neutral position. Before closure of the skin flaps, the position of the vascular pedicle must be observed with the neck moved through its full range of motion. If the pedicle is too short, it may be possible to divide some structures, such as the parotid fascia or sternocleidomastoid or digastric muscles, to provide a more direct route to the flap and defect. If the pedicle is too long, it may be placed in a more favorable position by anchoring it and fixing a side of the branch or a piece of adventitia to an underlying structure to avoid kinking and thrombosis. If this is not possible or if the pedicle is twisted, it should be divided and the anastomosis should be performed again.

Leakage of salivary contents into the neck may occur through the suture line. The oropharynx is a complex, three-dimensional structure, and what seems like an intact suture line may, in fact, have a defect where a suture pulled through or was poorly thrown. Before closure of the neck flaps, the suture line must be checked to ensure that it is watertight and will remain so under the pressure generated during swallowing. Placement of the tip of a rubber bulb syringe that contains 120 mL of saline through one nostril while occluding both nostrils and the mouth allows injection of an adequate amount of saline to distend the pharynx and demonstrate any leaks. These leaks should be sutured, and the suture line should be inspected again before closure of the neck (Fig. 33-4).

Pharyngeal reconstruction operations often require broad elevation of skin flaps in a compact area where soft tissue and oral contents regularly mix. Despite careful technique and the relatively copious blood supply to the head and neck, the potential for contamination that results in invasive infection is real, and tube drainage is an important adjunct in pharyngeal reconstruction. Soft suction tubes allow an egress of pus, should infection occur, and should be placed where they will not apply suction to the pharyngeal suture line or vascular pedicle with the neck in its full range of motion. Dislodgment of the drains into a dangerous position can be prevented by suturing the drains at the appropriate site with 5-0 catgut suture. They should be applied to wall suction and, after several days, to bulb suction. Contamination of the flap donor site by tumor or bacteria from the extirpative site should be prevented by the establishment of separate sterile fields at the beginning of the reconstruction, use of separate instrument trays, and care throughout the reconstruction to avoid cross contamination. At completion of the reconstruction or before closure of the donor site, both areas should be irrigated copiously with sterile water or saline. Whenever possible, as much of the donor site should be closed as early as possible to avoid potential operative or airborne contamination.

Pharyngeal surgery, particularly when combined with resection and reconstruction with microvascular free autograft, can be a complex and lengthy procedure. Critical and delicate portions of the operation may necessarily be performed near the end of this long haul and require careful attention and flawless technique. A team that includes nurses with the requisite skill and adequate physical stamina must be assembled to perform these procedures. If such individuals are not available for the team, there will be a high incidence of unfavorable results.

Postoperative care begins as the patient is prepared to leave the operating room. During these often prolonged procedures, there may be a tendency to overhydrate the patient. The head and neck and pharynx do not have the surface area of the thoracic or abdominal cavities; thus, the extent of insensible fluid loss is significantly less. This also is true during the recovery period. Careful assessment of fluid needs, monitoring of urine output, and physical examination decrease the likelihood of excessive or inadequate fluid administration, which in turn minimize problems such as local edema in the head and neck that may cause wound disruption or compression of the vascular pedicle.

Wound dressings of the neck must be applied carefully, because they have the potential to create two significant problems. First, occlusive dressings may mask hematoma or edema that could compromise the airway or vascular pedicle. Second, circumferential dressings, tape, or ribbon used to stabilize the tracheostomy or the endotracheal tube may shift when the patient changes position, causing a tight band in the neck that may compress the vascular pedicle of either a pedicle flap or a microvascular autograft. Direct suturing of the tracheostomy tube to the central neck area and cir-

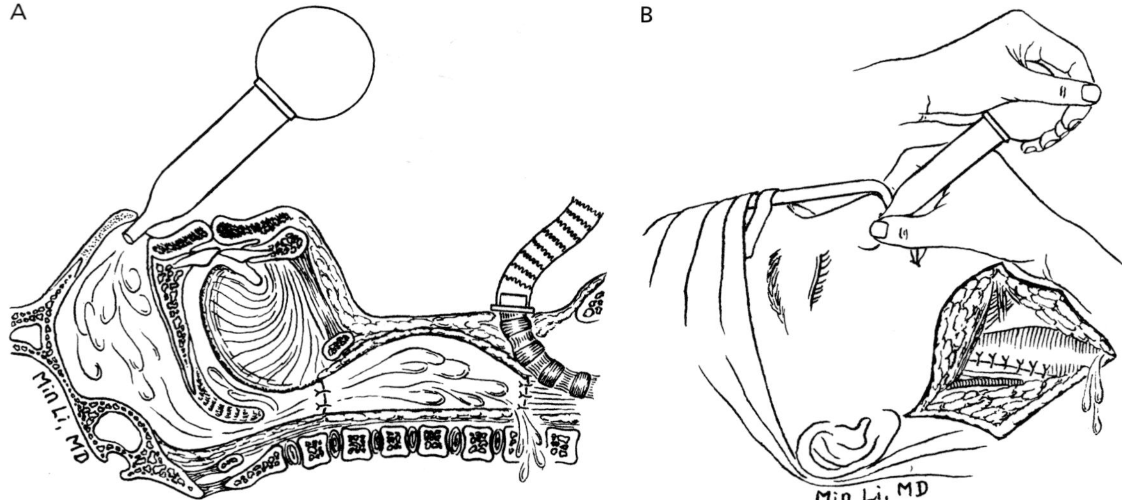

FIGURE 33-4. Method of testing integrity of the pharyngeal suture line. **A:** A bulb syringe with approximately 100 mL of saline is inserted snugly into one nostril. **B:** Injection of adequate fluid volume under enough pressure to distend the pharynx will allow identification of potential leak areas.

cumdental or mandibular wiring of the endotracheal tube will fix the tube without endangering the pharynx reconstruction. Similarly, a thick layer of antibiotic ointment over the suture line is an adequate occlusive dressing in the face and neck and will allow constant observation of the wound and surrounding areas. Monitoring of the reconstruction of the pharynx can be a challenge, because in many cases there is no visible portion of the flap. For both thoracic musculocutaneous flaps and free-tissue transfers, direct visualization usually can be obtained by flexible laryngoscopy through the nose, but this is somewhat cumbersome for routine use. Doppler ultrasound monitoring of blood flow also is useful, although it is not as sensitive as some of the implantable flow meters, oxygen tension monitors, or heat probes that have been described. A number of authors have suggested exteriorizing a portion of the reconstruction for monitoring purposes (13). Whenever possible, it is our practice to leave a small segment of the skin suture line open and packed with lubricated gauze. After several days of direct inspection, this is closed by tying the previously placed untied sutures. Obviously, general physical examination looking for erythema, wound drainage, foul odor, or other signs of problems also is important. Whatever method of monitoring is chosen, prompt action is necessary if a problem is identified. Uncontrolled infection in the neck can cause vascular thrombosis (flap, jugular, carotid), wound breakdown, fistula, and death. Infection or even exposure of a radiated carotid artery should be considered a surgical emergency, treated by debridement with or without resection, and covered with well-vascularized tissue (14).

Postoperative care requires continued communication and participation among members of the multidisciplinary team, particularly the extirpative and reconstructive surgeons. In the immediate postoperative period and over the longer rehabilitation, unfavorable results are more likely to be avoided if there is regular assessment and joint participation by both of these members. It is inappropriate and not in the patient's best interest for the reconstructive surgeon to relinquish the acute or chronic postoperative care to other team members. Again, this requires dedication, flexibility, and tact on the part of all concerned.

SPECIFIC COMPLICATIONS BY TECHNIQUE

Flap Loss or Major Tissue Loss

Local or Locoregional Reconstructions

Virtually all flap loss in pharyngeal reconstructions is secondary to ischemia. In primary closure or local tissue rearrangement, such as cervical flaps, tongue flaps, or myomucosal flaps, tension at the suture line, twisting, or inappropriate positioning of the tissues or flap design are the usual causes of tissue ischemia. The history of preoperative radiotherapy can greatly increase these risks. All such reconstruction should be reserved for small defects, preferably in nonirradiated patients. Whenever a local flap is chosen, an attempt should be made to include an axial vascular supply, and two-layer closure should be performed. Bolstering a tenuous suture line with a muscle flap, such as with the platysma or sternocleidomastoid muscles, may prevent problems (Fig. 33-5).

Thoracic Musculocutaneous Flaps

Pharynx reconstruction with thoracic musculocutaneous flaps has a high complication rate and a significant total failure rate (15). Perhaps the most common problem that results in total failure is poor flap design and inadequate mobilization of the pedicle, resulting in kinking of the pedicle and venous outflow obstruction. There are specific anatomical relationships for both the pectoralis major latissimus dorsi musculocutaneous flaps that may predispose a patient to this result.

The vascular pedicle to the pectoralis major musculocutaneous flap originates from the axillary artery and vein and descends down the chest wall medial to the pectoralis minor muscle, giving numerous vascular and nerve branches to this muscle and the adjacent tissues that closely bind the pedicle to the chest wall. Unless all of these are divided in mobilizing the flap, the pedicle is held against the chest wall in its caudad descent from the axillary vessels, which at this point are cephalad to, or just beneath, the clavicle. On transposition into the neck or pharynx area, these vessels then make a 180-degree turn. Complete release of the fascia and dissection of the areolar tissue around the vessels will allow a much more direct pathway of the pedicle to and from the axillary vessels (Fig. 33-6).

The thoracodorsal vessels, the blood supply to the latissimus dorsi musculocutaneous flap, originate from the axillary vessels below the pectoralis major muscle, run across the axilla, and then branch on the deep surface of the muscle. When the latissimus dorsi musculocutaneous flap is used in pharynx or other types of head and neck reconstruction, the flap is transposed medially to the defect from a more lateral axilla. Furthermore, because the origin of the nutrient vessels is underneath and well medial to the humeral insertion of the pectoralis major muscle, the pedicle travels from medial to lateral and then back to medial again, creating an angulation in the pedicle that can be exacerbated further by extension of the neck or downward motion of the arm at the shoulder. This may cause venous thrombosis of the pedicle and complete flap loss. If the latissimus dorsi musculocutaneous flap is chosen as the method of reconstruction, care must be taken to divide the humeral insertion of the pectoralis muscle so that the pathway of the pedicle is direct from its lateral axillary origin to the medial oropharyngeal defect. This is important even when the latissimus dorsi musculocutaneous flap is used as a secondary procedure after a pectoralis major flap has failed, because there often remains a significant amount of the lateral pectoralis muscle, and its humeral in-

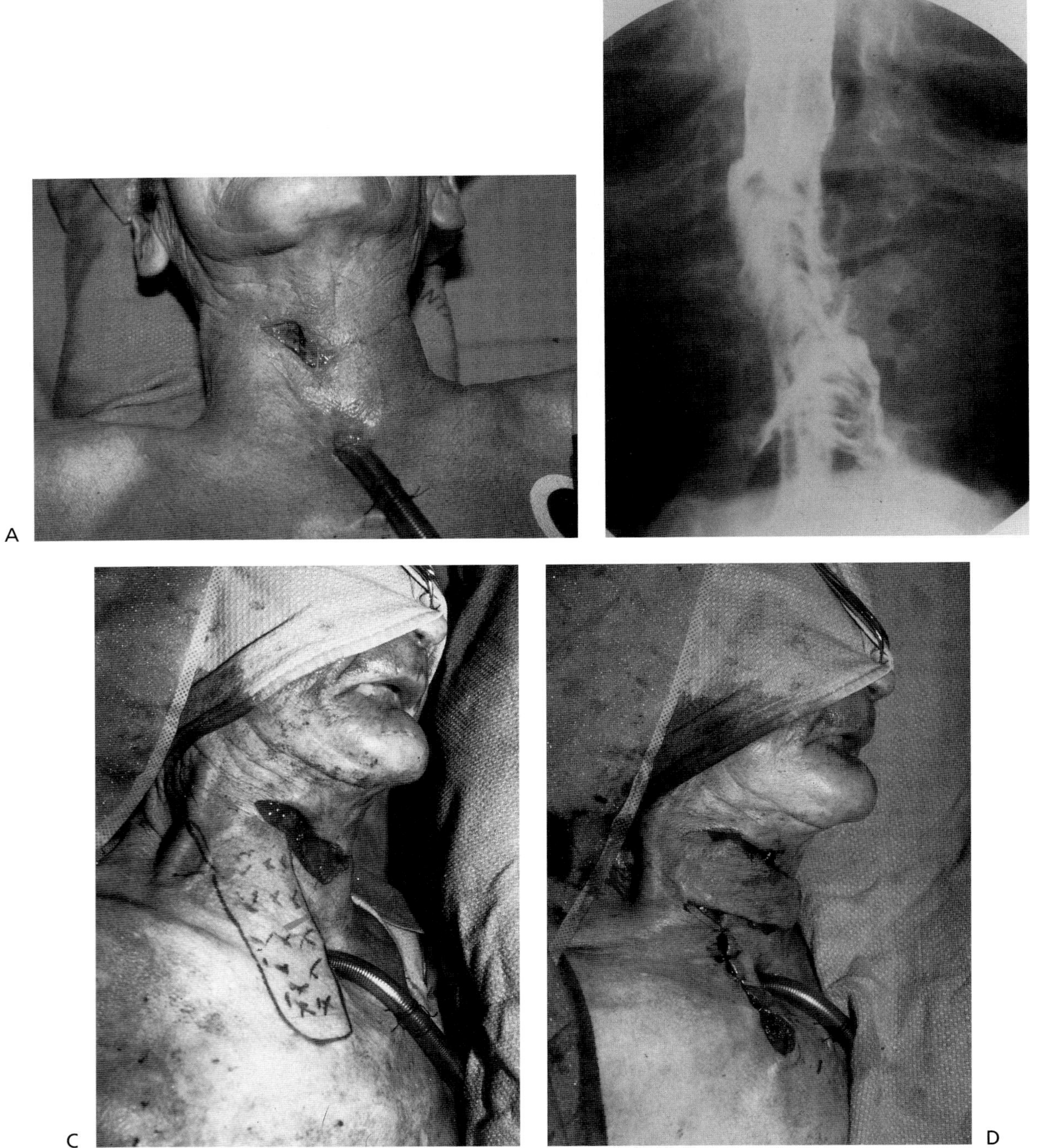

FIGURE 33-5. A,B: Pharyngeal fistula after reconstruction with jejunal free flap. **C:** Turnover flaps of mucosa were used to close the lumen of the neopharynx. A sternocleidomastoid flap was designed to bolster the suture line. **D:** Flap transposed over defect. *(continued)*

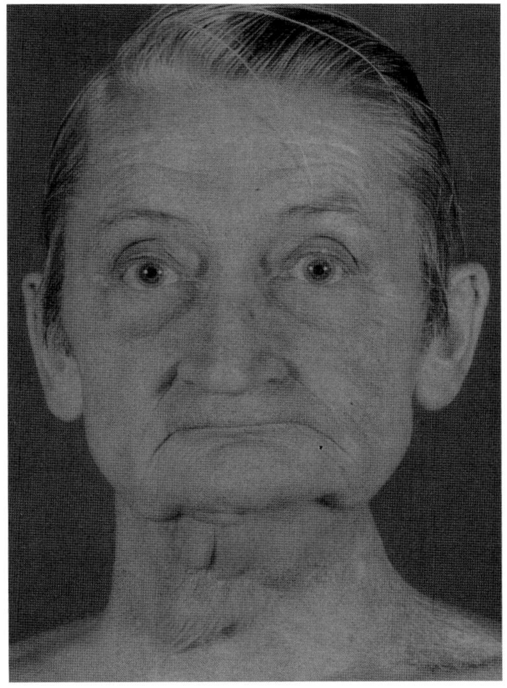

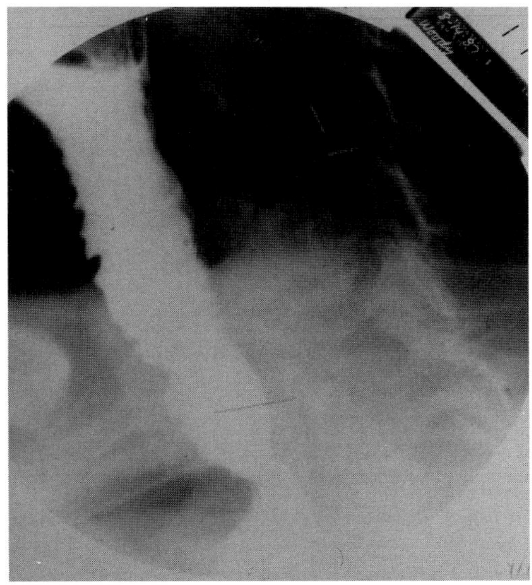

FIGURE 33-5. *Continued.* **E:** Three months after surgery. **F:** Alimentary continuity reestablished.

sertion is present (Fig. 33-7). Careful attention to the ultimate pathway of the vascular pedicle of the thoracic musculocutaneous flaps from the origin on the axillary and subclavian vessels to their inset in the pharyngeal defect to ensure a direct route that is not changed by motion of the thorax or shoulder girdle is critical in avoiding total or partial flap loss.

Free-tissue Transfer

Most large series in which free-tissue transfer for head and neck or oropharyngeal reconstruction is used show a roughly equal distribution of total flap necrosis caused by arterial thrombosis and venous thrombosis. To avoid arterial thrombosis, the recipient vessels must demonstrate pulsatile arterial flow before microvascular anastomosis. The use of interposition vein grafts seems to increase the risk of both arterial and venous thrombosis. Anastomotic suture technique and pedicle positioning are critical elements of successful free flap design and execution. The pathway to the inset flap from the recipient vessels must be direct and free from tensions or redundancy in all positions of the head and neck. Flap selection should consider the pedicle length. When a

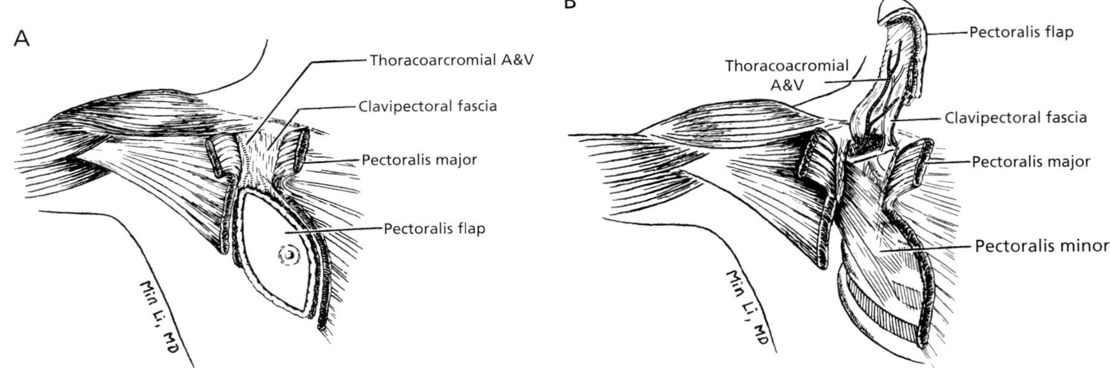

FIGURE 33-6. A: Anatomical relationships of the origin of the thoracoacromial pedicle at the axillary vessels. For the first several centimeters below the clavicle, it runs caudad through the clavipectoral fascia, which binds it tightly to the chest wall and gives multiple small vascular and neural branches to the pectoralis minor muscle at its insertion. **B:** The clavipectoral fascia and all branches to the pectoralis minor must be completely divided to allow the flap to be transposed into the pharynx and neck without kinking the pedicle.

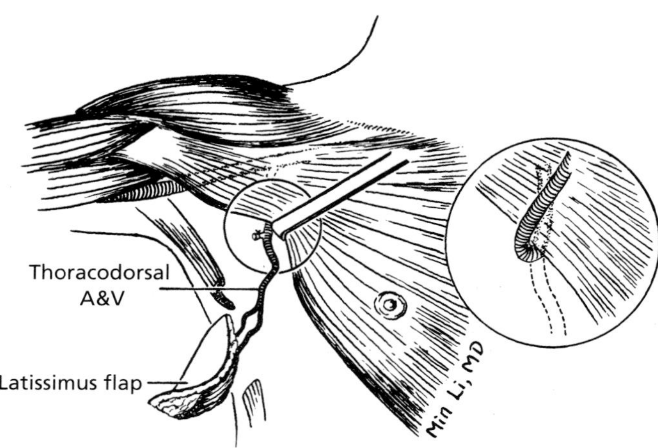

FIGURE 33-7. Anatomical relationship of the origin of the thoracodorsal pedicle at the axillary vessels behind the pectoralis major muscle. Unless the humeral insertion of the pectoralis muscle is divided, the vessels will be twisted when the flap is rotated by almost 180 degrees and transposed into the pharynx and neck (inset).

long pedicle is necessary, the gastroepiploic flap, the radial forearm flap, and the scapula flap with inclusion of the subscapular vessels are useful for pharynx reconstruction. Although probably most total flap losses are secondary to some intraoperative mistake or misadventure, there are occasional postoperative occurrences that may result in this problem. Unrecognized or untreated infection below the neck skin flaps usually secondary to a pharyngeal leak and subsequent abscess may cause progressive thrombosis of the tissues of the flap or acute thrombosis of the vascular pedicle. Adequate drainage at the time of surgery and careful wound monitoring should prevent this. Mechanical compression of the pedicle by circumferential dressings or excessive edema also may cause thrombosis and flap loss.

Wound Infection, Marginal Necrosis, and Fistula

Local and Locoregional Flaps

Although the skin of the face and neck is very well vascularized, the only axial blood supplies of any length are the superficial temporal vessels that supply the forehead flap and facial vessels that supply the nasolabial flap. Neither of these flaps is ideal for pharynx reconstruction. The deltopectoral flap described by Bakamjian (9) in 1965 resulted in a significant advance in pharynx and head and neck reconstruction, allowing relatively reliable two-stage reconstruction. Extension of the length beyond the anterior axillary line, however, requires a delay procedure. Because of the surgical approach necessary to perform pharynx surgery and the frequent accompaniment of radiotherapy, local cervical flaps are at high risk of distal ischemia, and thus the reconstruction is at risk of fistula or infection (16,17). Local and locoregional flaps should only be used for small defects where flap size can similarly be small. Delay procedures are appropriate whenever greater length is required. Perhaps the most appropriate role for local and locoregional skin and fasciocutaneous flaps at the present is the external coverage of a musculocutaneous flap, such as the pectoralis or sternocleidomastoid flap used to reconstruct a complex defect.

Thoracic Musculocutaneous Flaps

The major risk factors for development of these complications when using the thoracic musculocutaneous flap are technical inadequacy, such as misplaced or poorly placed suture; bacterial contamination and subsequent infection at the suture line; and distal ischemia of the flap resulting in suture line disruption. Although the thoracic site of origin for the pectoralis major latissimus dorsi and trapezius musculocutaneous flaps rarely is irradiated, the distal portion of the flap—especially if it extends beyond the muscle—usually is a random pattern skin flap and thus marginally perfused. When designing the flap, the skin island should be oriented over the largest possible number of perforating vessels from the muscle. In most Americans, even those with head and neck cancer, the skin and fat of the chest wall or the breasts are thick and the muscle is heavy (18). The effect of gravity tends to pull the flap back down toward the chest, thus increasing the mechanical stress on the suture line. Significant intraoral and pharyngeal pressures up to 120 cm H_2O are generated by the base of the tongue (19,20). When these pressures are added to the weight of the thoracic musculocutaneous flap, the force against the suture line can be great, thus increasing the risk of fistula. To mitigate the effect of the gravity when the pectoralis major musculocutaneous flap is used for pharynx reconstruction, the edges of the muscle flap suture line should be inset, not only to the mucosa but also to the prevertebral fascia, which is firm and tenacious, unlike the mucosa and submucosal tissue (Fig. 33-8). When the pharyngeal defect is circumferential, the posterior pharynx can be resurfaced with a split-thickness skin graft and the anterior 270 degrees of the pectoralis major flap with the edges sutured to the prevertebral fascia and the end of the tongue base, which will take much of the weight off the mobile tongue base.

Free-tissue Transfer

When designed correctly and successfully revascularized, free-tissue transfer should be homogeneously perfused thus avoiding the risk of distal ischemia. Before harvest of the jejunum, radial forearm, lateral arm, or other free flaps used in pharynx reconstruction, all edges of the flap should be observed for adequate bleeding. When the jejunum is chosen, the segment of tissue to be harvested is left *in situ* on its mesenteric branch while a jejunojejunostomy is performed to restore intestinal continuity. Any areas of dusky mucosa muscle or serosa should be resected along the mesenteric border, leaving only the well-perfused bowel. Most free-tis-

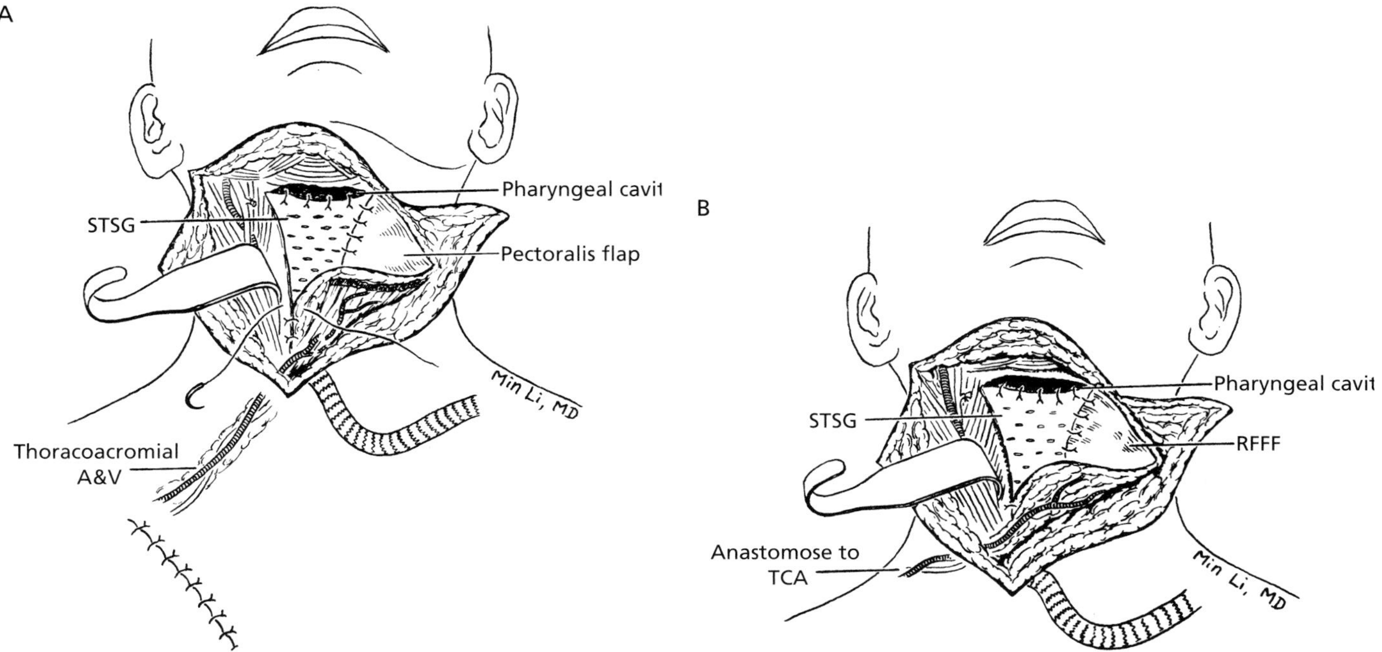

FIGURE 33-8. A: Method of Fabian (16) used for circumferential pharyngeal reconstruction with the pectoralis major musculocutaneous flap. Resurfacing the prevertebral fascia with a skin graft allows the edges of the pectoralis flap to be sutured to the lateral aspect of the prevertebral fascia, thus providing some rigidity against gravity in a fixed diameter of the lumen. **B:** A comparable method using the jejunum or radial forearm free flap has been successful in our hands in mitigating spasm in the jejunum and collapse of the tubular structure with radial forearm free autograft.

sue transfers are not as bulky and heavy as the thoracic musculocutaneous flaps, so the effects of gravity on the suture line are minimal (Fig. 33-9). Careful inset of the flaps and occasional anchoring of the flap to the prevertebral fascia will decrease the likelihood of mechanical dehiscence.

Avoidance of Secondary Procedures

Most local and locoregional flaps initially were used as staged procedures, which by definition required a second operation. Limiting the size and scope of their use decreases the risk of unplanned second or third operations. A number of series have demonstrated the superiority of free-tissue transfer over the pectoralis major in avoidance of secondary procedures (12,21). Because of its homogeneous blood supply and light weight, the jejunum is more likely to resolve fistulas spontaneously than the pectoralis major or gastric pullup or colon interposition, where distal ischemia and inadequate length of the reconstruction are the main problems (4).

Functional Disorders

The overwhelming cause of swallowing and speech dysfunction and aspiration secondary to inability to protect the laryngeal airway is the amount and type of tissue resected. Numerous studies have demonstrated that the amount of disruption of tongue function secondary to parenchymal or nerve resection determines the degree of interference with swallowing or speech. The amount of resection usually is dictated by the stage of the tumor and thus is independent of the reconstructive method. A desire to preserve the larynx must be based on a conscious preoperative estimate of the risk of aspiration pneumonitis. Radiotherapy either before or after surgery will decrease oral and oropharyngeal mobility because of destruction of salivary secretory units. The goal of pharyngeal reconstruction is to provide a large enough conduit to allow food passage.

Local and Locoregional Flaps

Because of their limited size and thus use, interference with function is not a major problem with this method of reconstruction. Poor choice of such techniques when more tissue is necessary may result in stricture or fistula and thus dysphagia.

Thoracic Musculocutaneous Flaps

The antecedent event in many cases of stenosis or stricture is fistula. The risk of subsequent dysphagia secondary to fistula was 80% in a series of pyriform sinus tumors requiring pharynx reconstruction (22); thus, avoidance of fistula is key in flap design. Positioning and anchoring the flap against gravity is important. The weight of the pectoralis musculocutaneous flap and where it is inset can result in pulling on the base of the tongue, dragging it back and limiting protrusion or even interfering with elevation of the larynx should it still be present. Similarly, if inset into the lateral pharyngeal wall or palatopharyngeal fold area, such a heavy flap can limit elevation of the palate, thus creating a secondary velopharyngeal insufficiency that may interfere with both speech and swallowing. Care must be taken to anchor the flap and inset it so that the residual function of remaining structures is not impaired. In pharyngoesophageal reconstruction, the distal anastomosis with the cervical esophagus frequently is the site of stenosis and subsequent dysphagia. The thick skin and subcutaneous fat of the thorax are a difficult match for the thin cervical esophageal wall. A number of methods of inset to decrease the risk of stenosis in this area have been described, most of which make use of one or more V-shaped enlargements of the esophagus.

Free-tissue Transfer

The light weight, the ability to shape to size, and the positioning limited only by pedicle length in the neck allow the jejunum or fasciocutaneous free autografts the latitude to fit

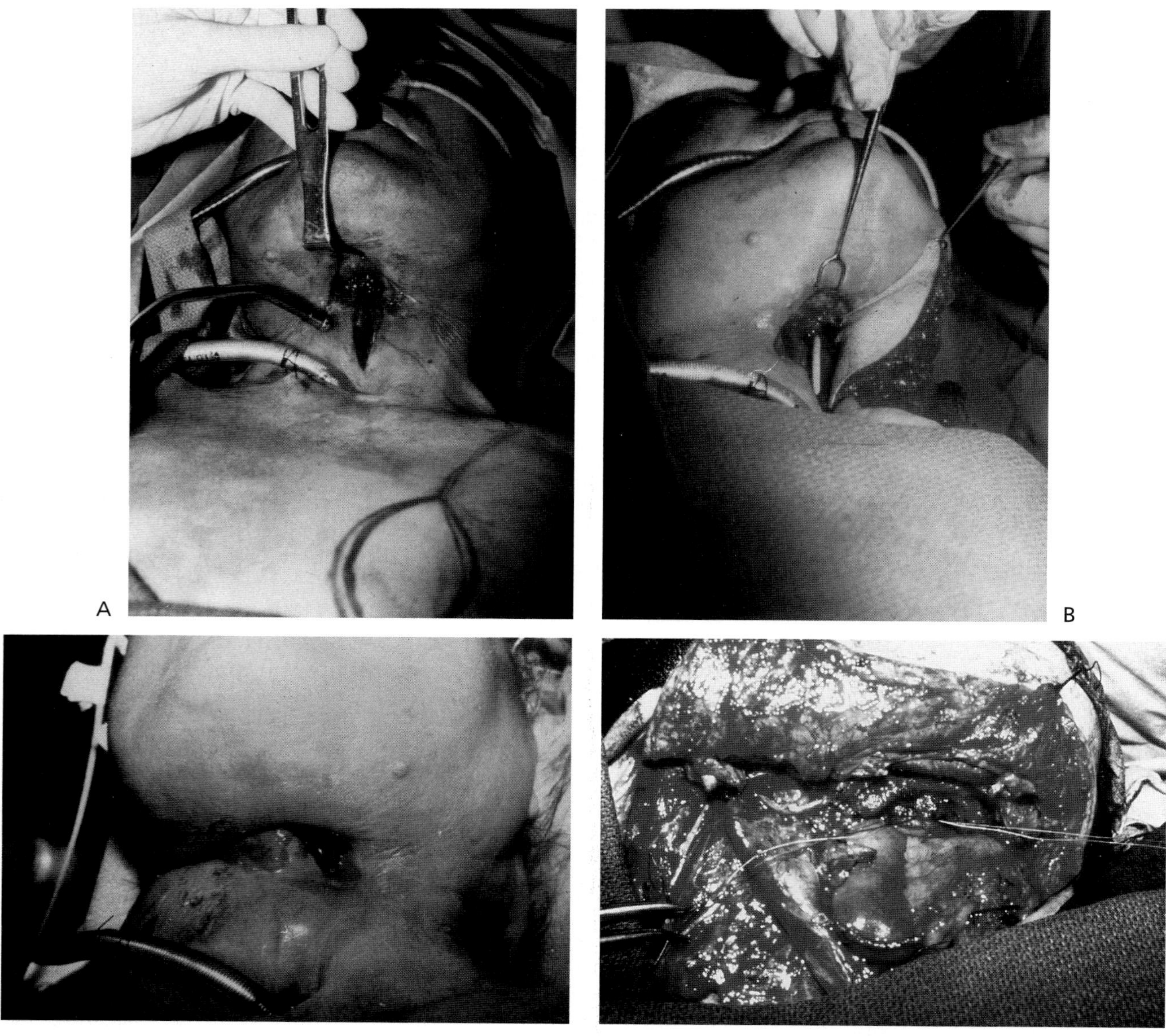

FIGURE 33-9. A: Fistula after laryngectomy for salvage of radiation failure for carcinoma of the larynx. **B:** Reconstruction with pectoralis major musculocutaneous flap. Note the bulk of the flap in this relatively thin patient. **C:** Pharyngocutaneous fistula from base of tongue down after reconstruction. **D:** Reconstruction of fistula with patch graft of revascularized jejunum. *(continued)*

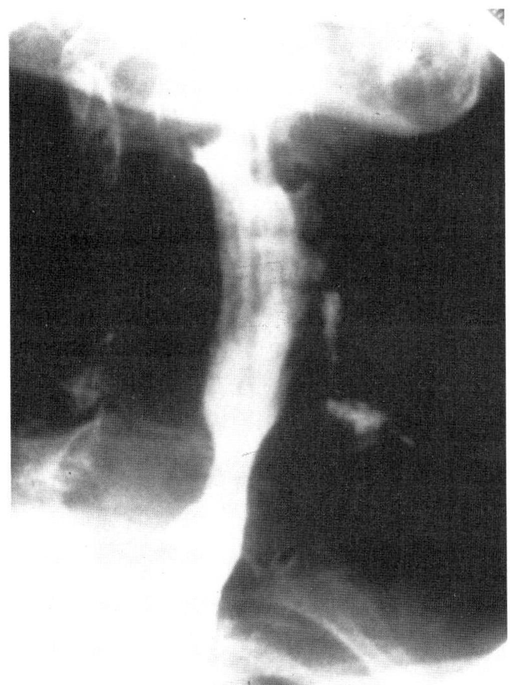

E

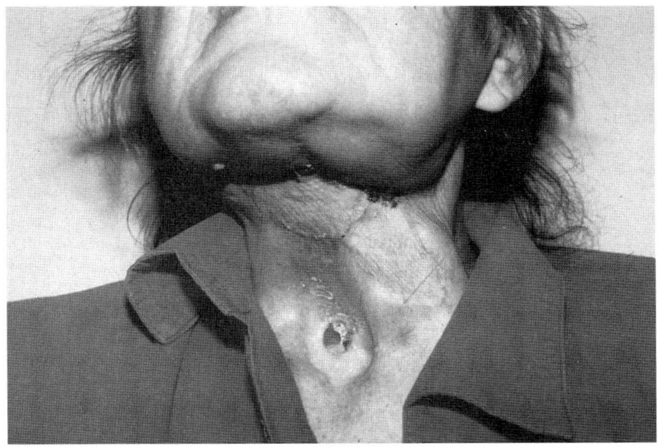

F

FIGURE 33-9. *Continued.* **E:** Alimentary continuity reestablished. **F:** Healed wound. The surface of the jejunum was covered with a split-thickness skin graft.

almost any defect without deforming it and without interfering with the function of remaining structures. The radial forearm and lateral arm flaps are particularly amenable to sensory innervation, and there is fairly convincing data that function in the oral cavity and oropharynx may be improved by anastomosis of a cutaneous sensory nerve in the flap to a sensory cranial nerve or branch of the cervical plexus. This is particularly appropriate when the flap is used to reconstruct the base of the tongue or lateral or posterior pharynx in an area contiguous to the intact larynx. The mobility of the tongue also will allow it to be transposed into the pharynx without tethering it too much. Sometimes it is useful when there is a large defect in the area of the vallecula to resurface the part immediately adjacent to the supraglottic larynx with the remaining sensate tongue, pulling it backward and down somewhat while lateralizing or moving more anterior the defect to be closed by the flap. As long as this does not narrow the laryngeal aditus, put excessive tension on the suture line, or tether the tongue too much, it may facilitate subsequent swallowing function and prevent aspiration. In the unusual circumstance where the larynx is left intact and the extent of the defect reaches above the level of the epiglottis, it is preferable to use a neurotized radial forearm or lateral arm flap for reconstruction. The secretory nature of the jejunum and its lack of sensation increase the risk of aspiration in such cases.

As previously noted, the goals for pharynx reconstruction with respect to swallowing are modest: to create a conduit of adequate size to accommodate a food bolus or to allow the expulsion of air as esophageal or tracheoesophageal speech. Flap design, size, and inset should reflect this. The jejunum, when used as a tube segment, should be sutured under slight tension to avoid redundancy, which may impair passage of the bolus. Neurectomy and myotomy of residual pharyngeal muscles or myotomy of the jejunum may prevent spasm and functional obstruction. A 270-degree reconstruction of a tubular defect with skin grafting of the posterior pharyngeal wall also may help maintain a wide conduit when using jejunum or fasciocutaneous flaps.

CONCLUSIONS

Despite an unfavorable local wound milieu, late-stage disease presentation, and complex functional requirements, unfavorable results can be avoided in pharyngeal reconstruction. The reconstructive surgeon must attain the following to achieve success with technique and with patients:

1. Knowledge of the complex anatomy and physiology of the area
2. Knowledge of the natural history and current therapy of malignancy of the upper aerodigestive tract
3. Familiarity with the general and specific effects of radiotherapy
4. Communication with the resecting surgeon in a multidisciplinary effort
5. Skill and familiarity with surgery in the area (Fig. 33-10)

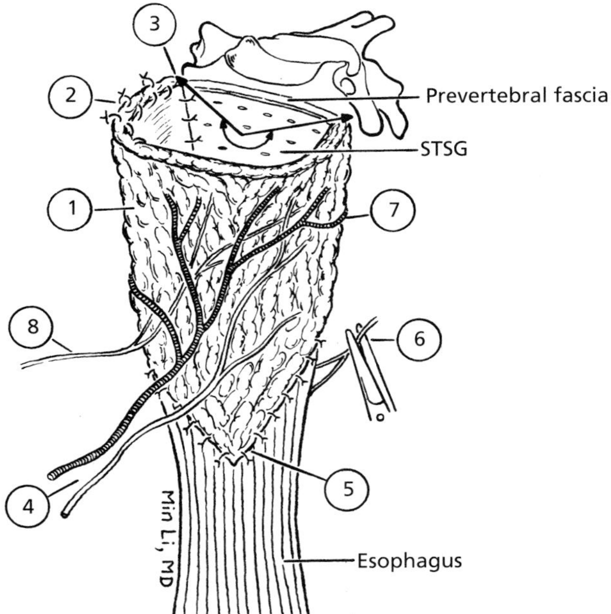

FIGURE 33-10. Technical methods to avoid unfavorable results in pharyngeal reconstruction. ***1:*** Choice of any of a number of lightweight well-vascularized free autografts. ***2:*** Two-layer closure at base of tongue with adequate visualization for placement of sutures. ***3:*** Suture graft to prevertebral fascia to stabilize and mitigate effects of tongue motion and gravity. Proper size of graft to avoid redundancy or excess tension. ***4:*** Safe positioning of vascular pedicle in the neck to avoid kinking on normal neck motion. ***5:*** Widely patent distal esophageal anastomosis. ***6:*** Myotomy and/or neurectomy to prevent spasm of residual cricopharyngeus of constrictor muscles. ***7:*** Careful preharvest evaluation of blood flow at the margins of the graft and preinset evaluation of blood flow and tissue integrity at the margin of the residual pharyngeal tissue to avoid local ischemia and suture line dehiscence. ***8:*** Sensory reinnervation to potentially improve swallowing and local sensation in the pharynx.

6. Skill and familiarity with numerous methods of reconstruction in the pharynx and head and neck (Table 33-5)
7. A multidisciplinary team to efficiently effect surgery follow-up and functional rehabilitation
8. Stamina, honesty, and compassion requisite to the problems encountered.

TABLE 33-5. COMMONLY EMPLOYED RECONSTRUCTIVE METHODS FOR PHARYNGEAL AND OTHER HEAD AND NECK DEFECTS

Local and Locoregional	Thoracic Musculocutaneous	Microvascular Autograft
Cervical facial	Pectoralis major	Jejunum
Deltopectoral	Latissimus dorsi	Gastro-omental
Platysma	Trapezius	Radial foreman
Sternocleidomastoid		Lateral arm
		Lateral thigh
		Rectus abdominis
		Latissimus dorsi

REFERENCES

1. Shah JP, Shaha AR, Spiro, RH et al. Carcinoma of the hypopharynx. *Am J Surg* 1976;132:439.
2. Larson DL, Lindberg RD, Lane E, et al. Major complications of radiotherapy in cancer of the oral cavity and oropharynx. A 10 year retrospective study. *Am J Surg* 1983;146:531–563.
3. Coleman JJ. Complications in head and neck surgery. *Surg Clin North Am* 1986;66:149–167.
4. Coleman JJ. Management of radiation-induced soft tissue injury to the head and neck. *Clin Plast Surg* 1993;20:491–505.
5. Johnson JT, Bloomer WD. Effect of prior radiotherapy on post-surgical wound infection. *Head Neck* 1989;11:132.
6. Logemann JA. *Evaluation and treatment of swallowing disorders.* San Diego: College-Hill Press, 1983.
7. Moreno-Osset E, Thomas-Ridocci M, Paris F, et al. Motor activity of esophageal substitute (stomach, jejunal, and colon segments). *Ann Thorac Surg* 1986;41:515.
8. Zovickian A. Pharyngeal fistulas: repair and prevention using mastoid-occiput based shoulder flaps. *Plast Reconstr Surg* 1957;19:355.
9. Bakamjian VY, Long M, Rigg B. Experience with the medially based deltopectoral flap in reconstructive surgery of the head and neck. *Br J Plast Surg* 1971;24:174.
10. Surkin MI, Lawson W, Biller H. Analysis of the methods of pharyngoesophageal reconstruction. *Head Neck Surg* 1984;6: 953–970.
11. Coleman JJ, Searles JM, Hester TR, et al. Ten years experience with the free jejunal autograft. *Am J Surg* 1987;154:394–398.
12. Coleman, JJ. Reconstruction of the pharynx after resection for cancer. *Ann Surg* 1989;209:554–561.
13. Coleman, JJ. Reconstruction of the pharynx and cervical esophagus with jejunal free autograft. *Probl Gen Surg* 1989;6:2.
14. Fabian RL. Pectoralis major myocutaneous flap reconstruction of the laryngopharynx and cervical esophagus. *Laryngoscope* 1988;98:1227
15. Shah JP, Haribhakji V, Loree TR, Sutaria P. Complications of the pectoralis major myocutaneous flap in head and neck reconstruction. *Am J Surg* 1990;160:352.
16. Brown P, Coleman JJ. The role of radiotherapy and musculocutaneous flaps in oropharyngocutaneous fistulas. *Am J Surg* 1988;156:256.
17. Lavelle RJ, Maw AR. The aetiology of postlaryngectomy pharyngo-cutaneous fistulae. *J Laryngol Otol* 1972;86:785.
18. Lau WF, Lam KH, Wei WI. Reconstruction of hypopharyngeal defects in cancer surgery: do we have a choice? *Am J Surg* 1987;154:374–380.
19. Cerenko D, McConnell FMS, Jackson RT. Quantitative assessment of pharyngeal bolus driving forces. *Otolaryngol Head Neck Surg* 1989;100:57–63.
20. McConnell FMS, Hester TR, Mendelsohn MS, et al. Manofluorography of deglutition after total laryngopharyngectomy. *Plast Reconstr Surg* 1988;81:346.
21. Carlson GW, Coleman JJ, Jurkiewicz MJ. Reconstruction of the hypopharynx and cervical esophagus. *Curr Probl Surg* 1993;30: 425–480.
22. McConnell FMS, Duck S, Hester TR. Hypopharyngeal stenosis. *Laryngoscope* 1984;94:1162–1165.

SUGGESTED READING

Coleman JJ. Treatment of the ruptured or exposed carotid artery: a rational approach. *South Med J* 1985;78:262–267.

Spiro RH, Shah JP, Strong EW, et al. Gastric transposition in head and neck surgery: indications, complications and expectations. *Am J Surg* 1983;146:483.

Discussion

OROPHARYNGEAL RECONSTRUCTION

ABHAY GUPTA
GREGORY R.D. EVANS

We would like to take this opportunity to commend Dr. Coleman on his well-organized and thorough review of the complications of oropharyngeal reconstruction and their treatment. Dr. Coleman discusses the various flaps commonly used in reconstruction of the oropharynx and separates them into locoregional, musculocutaneous, and free flaps. With each of these categories, he then outlines the possible unfavorable results under the headings of (i) flap loss or major tissue loss; (ii) wound infection, marginal necrosis, and fistula; and (iii) functional disorders. Finally, he presents his own approach to the management of these complications and suggests many preoperative and intraoperative precautions to help optimize flap survival and minimize complications. Dr. Coleman has brought to light many key points in his chapter. It is the purpose of this discussion to emphasize these points and present our own experience with reconstruction of the oropharynx at the University of Texas M.D. Anderson Cancer Center (UTMDACC). We then will discuss our own approach to the management of partial and complete circumferential defects of the oropharynx, including our indications for locoregional, musculocutaneous, or free flap reconstruction. In paralleling Dr. Coleman's chapter, we will exclude reconstruction of glossectomy defects.

We agree with Dr. Coleman that many unfavorable postoperative results can be avoided by careful preoperative assessment, which consists of a thorough history and physical examination and appropriate investigations, including various medical imaging modalities. Unfortunately, most patients with pharyngeal carcinoma present with advanced disease and will require both surgery and radiotherapy. Alternatively, patients may present with recurrent disease after failed surgery and/or adjuvant therapy. Therefore, it is essential that the reconstructive surgeon be cognizant of any previous operative details or radiation treatments, or any further planned radiotherapy, all of which may significantly affect planned reconstruction. The various effects of radiotherapy on tissue, as well as the increased risk of postoperative complications, have been well documented (1–4). Reconstruction in these cases must use healthy, well-vascularized tissue from nonirradiated donor sites, taking care to obliterate any dead space and avoid any tension during wound closure (4).

Many patients presenting with pharyngeal carcinoma have a history of heavy tobacco or alcohol abuse. Whenever possible, they should be encouraged to abstain from these substances before surgery. Any concurrent medical problems or malnutrition should be thoroughly assessed, corrected, or optimally preoperatively controlled. A careful history and physical examination will uncover any possible contraindications to various reconstructive options. For example, a patient with multiple previous laparotomies and possible intraabdominal adhesions would not be a good candidate for a free jejunal transfer. A history of stroke or transient ischemic attacks must be excluded, and the neck should be examined carefully at the initial consultation for the presence of reliable recipient vessels in case a free-tissue transfer is necessary. This involves inspection, auscultation, and palpation of the carotid and jugular systems. If there is any question regarding blood flow, further assessment is necessary with a duplex Doppler ultrasound. We believe that routine angiography of the neck vessels is rarely indicated.

Dr. Coleman's emphasis that the management of these patients should be a multidisciplinary team effort cannot be overstated. Surgeons trained in otolaryngology, general surgery, plastic surgery, and oral surgery or dentistry, as well as radiation therapists and medical oncologists, all are vital for the patient's treatment. All of these specialties should be directly involved in preoperative treatment planning to avoid any confusion and to optimize patient care. The reconstructive surgeon should review the preoperative imaging studies, including any computed tomographic or magnetic resonance imaging scans, and should be familiar with the general principles of tumor ablation, thus enabling rational reconstructive options anticipated by the resulting defect. Significant advances in reconstructive techniques avail-

A. Gupta: Department of Plastic Surgery, The University of Texas M.D. Anderson Cancer Center, Houston, Texas

G. R. D. Evans: Division of Plastic Surgery, The University of California, Irvine, California

able to surgeons have inherently led to more advanced tumor extirpative techniques, such that many oncologic surgeons now are more aggressive with tumor ablation than are the traditional approaches. Consequently, it is even more important that the extirpative and reconstructive surgical teams have continuing communication preoperatively and intraoperatively to optimize treatment results.

Proper positioning of the patient on the operating room table and placement of the drapes and endotracheal or tracheostomy tube must allow complete exposure and access to the entire operative field on both sides of the neck. The surgeon must be able to manipulate the head and neck intraoperatively. It is imperative that there be adequate room for the primary surgeon and any assistants to stand at the operative site, which often requires repositioning the operating room table relative to the anesthesia machine. As Dr. Coleman states, it is wise to "prepare for the worst [and] hope for the best"; therefore, adequate preparation of all possible donor sites for reconstructive flaps, including the chest and abdomen, and one thigh for skin grafting, is necessary. At UTMDACC, it is standard for a senior member of the reconstructive team to be present at the beginning of the case, to assist the extirpative team in the initial preparation and draping of the patient. In many situations, it is also possible for the reconstructive team to work simultaneously with the extirpative team, with two separate scrub nurses and instrument sets, allowing a significant portion of the flap to be raised during tumor ablation. This can often significantly decrease the patient's overall anesthesia time.

When free-tissue reconstruction is planned, proper preparation of the recipient vessels before completing flap elevation is essential. This is performed following tumor ablation by a member of the reconstructive team. Our preference is to use the external carotid artery and internal jugular vein for end-to-side anastomoses because of their ease of exposure and reliable blood flow. However, we agree with Dr. Coleman that the transverse cervical vessels may be a suitable alternative in selected circumstances. It is imperative to properly plan the position of the vascular pedicle during flap marking and elevation. The optimal site of vascular anastomoses to the neck vessels is based on anticipated flap position upon inset, avoiding any redundancy or kinking. As Dr. Coleman stresses, the flap pedicle must be examined carefully while moving the neck through a complete range of motion before final skin closure. In our experience, vein grafts have the potential to increase the risk of complications. We have found that, with careful planning and dissection of the flap pedicle, they are rarely necessary.

Our postoperative management is similar to that of Dr. Coleman. All patients are admitted to the surgical intensive care unit for a period of 1 to 2 days. Careful attention is given to accurate monitoring of fluid intake and output to ensure optimal hydration and thus maximize flow through our anastomoses. This is especially true for those vessels previously irradiated. Proper elevation and positioning of the head postoperatively and avoidance of any potentially constricting circumferential dressings around the neck, including tracheostomy ties, are essential precautions in postoperative management. Regular flap checks are performed hourly, assessing the color and refill of any visible portion skin paddle, as well as the Doppler flow signal over the pedicle. When a free jejunum is used, a portion of the jejunum is brought out through the neck wound and anchored to the skin to act as a monitor, allowing assessment of blood flow. In the case of buried flaps where there is no visible portion, we often use implantable Doppler probes (Cook-Schwartz). Patients eventually are transferred to our flap unit, where they usually stay for 3 to 5 days before being transferred to a regular bed or discharged home. Flap checks are continued and wounds are carefully examined daily to rule out hematoma or infection. Enteral feeds are started early postoperatively via a nasogastric tube, percutaneous gastrostomy, or jejunostomy tube, depending on the circumstances. Oral intake is commenced approximately 7 to 10 days postoperatively, or at 2 weeks if the patient has been previously irradiated. We usually order a modified barium swallow to check the flap inset for leaks and positioning of the jejunum before commencing oral intake; however, recent studies do not support the use of routine barium swallow prior to initiating oral intake (5).

Unfortunately, the 5-year survival rate for patients with locally advanced carcinoma of the pharynx and cervical esophagus is only 25% to 35%; hence, resection of the disease and reconstruction usually are considered palliative (6). Therefore, our approach to planning reconstructions in these patients is to choose a reliable one-stage procedure that has minimal morbidity and mortality but restores early swallowing. Generally, for a partial defect of the pharynx or cervical esophagus, we prefer to use a free radial forearm flap or a pectoralis major myocutaneous flap to act as a patch. For a complete circumferential defect, we primarily use a free jejunal transfer, provided there are no contraindications to its use. We rarely use the locoregional flaps mentioned by Dr. Coleman for reconstruction of oropharyngeal defects because, in our experience, they do not provide enough tissue bulk or vasculature and usually do not have adequate length to close the defect without significant tension. Furthermore, many of these flaps are within a previously irradiated field and thus are more prone to complications. We reserve the use of these flaps for small lower neck defects, for external coverage of another flap such as a free flap, or for salvage procedures after previous failed reconstruction. Similarly, we do not use latissimus dorsi flaps because of their inadequate reach to the oropharynx. One situation where local flaps, such as the sternocleidomastoid muscle, are helpful is in providing coverage of exposed vessels in the neck or for bolstering suture lines of another flap inset to decrease the risk of fistula formation.

For complete circumferential defects of the oropharynx and cervical esophagus, we have found the free jejunum transfer to be the best choice because it is a reliable, single-stage procedure that can be tailored to reconstruct almost any size defect and is well tolerated by postoperative radiation therapy (7). A recent review of the literature by Reece et al. (8) demonstrated a flap survival rate of 80% to 100%, with success rates greater than 94% in more recent series. The overall complication rate was between 47% and 68%, with fistula and stricture each accounting for 20% of the morbidity (6). A review of our own experience at UTM-DACC revealed a 97% flap survival rate and an overall morbidity rate of 57%. Fistula (19%) and stricture (15%) formation again were the most common complications. Donor site complications were present in 11% of our patients; the most common complication was small bowel obstruction. The overall perioperative mortality rate was 2% (8). Our operative technique for harvesting, transferring, and insetting the free jejunal flap has been described extensively in the past (7–9) and will not be discussed here, but we would like to present a few key steps that have been developed over the years to optimize reconstruction and limit morbidity.

Whenever possible, the reconstructive team starts exposing and elevating the jejunal flap while the extirpative team is working at the head and neck. At the time of flap harvest, we prefer to take a segment of jejunum that is 5 to 6 cm longer than the measured defect, to allow for a 3- to 4-cm monitor segment and an few extra centimeters of bowel in case further pharyngoesophageal resection is necessary due to positive margins. Care is taken to mark the proximal end of the jejunum with a serosal suture to ensure isoperistaltic inset. End-to-side anastomoses to the external carotid artery and internal jugular vein are our preference. The proximal bowel anastomosis is performed prior to revascularizing the flap, because this is often the most difficult part due to poor exposure, and this technique avoids later tension on our anastomoses. Furthermore, we do not have to contend with the bleeding, peristalsis, and mucus production that occur once the flap is revascularized. The proximal edge of the jejunum often is splayed open to widen the anastomosis and prevent stricture formation. We have found a marked decrease in our fistula rate since we started to perform the proximal bowel anastomosis using two layers of interrupted sutures, reinforcing our initial mucosal-serosal closure with a layer of serosal silk Lembert sutures. Following flap revascularization, before performing the distal bowel anastomosis, the dissected stump of the cervical esophagus is excised to within 1 to 2 cm of intact periesophageal tissue to ensure reliable blood supply of the distal stump. The distal anastomosis is performed after the neck is returned to a neutral position and any excess jejunum is excised to avoid redundancy and possible obstruction postoperatively. It is important to place the jejunum within the defect on some tension. In our experience, the majority of distal fistulas occur anteriorly, immediately adjacent to the superior edge of the tracheostomy stoma (8). To try to prevent this, we often place a small flap of mesentery between the distal bowel anastomosis and the tracheocutaneous suture line.

When reconstructing partial defects of the pharynx or esophagus, we primarily use a free radial forearm flap. Once the defect is created, a template is made and transferred to the forearm to mark out the flap based on the radial artery. We prefer to design and elevate the flap using the superficial system of veins for flap drainage. Whenever possible, the flap is neurotized by primary neurorrhaphy of the lateral antebrachial cutaneous nerve to a local sensory nerve in the neck, such as the lingual nerve or a branch of the cervical plexus. As with the free jejunum, we perform the inset of the flap first, before revascularization. This allows manipulation of the flap freely, without placing tension on the anastomoses, and allows proper positioning of the anastomoses based on how the flap is inset into the defect. This maneuver only adds 30 to 45 minutes to the overall ischemic time, which still is much less than 2 hours in duration. The flap is monitored postoperatively by Doppler examination using either a hand-held or implantable probe.

Many surgeons prefer to use a tubed radial forearm flap for reconstruction of a circumferential pharyngeal defect because of its superior postoperative voice rehabilitation. However, these flaps are associated with a much higher fistula rate than the jejunum, perhaps due to the additional longitudinal suture line (10,11). Therefore, we do not use this flap regularly for such a circumferential defect. If jejunal harvest is contraindicated, consideration for the radial forearm flap should be given. Similarly, for salvage of a failed free jejunum, we have used a tubed radial forearm if a repeat free jejunum transfer was contraindicated. For some patients in whom optimal speech rehabilitation is desired, we may opt to use a tubed radial forearm flap reconstruction and accept the higher risk of fistula formation (11).

One controversial area in oropharyngeal reconstruction that Dr. Coleman does not discuss is the situation where only a small strip of posterior pharyngeal mucosa remains after tumor ablation. Although some surgeons prefer to preserve this tissue and reconstruct the remaining pharynx, we favor excising this strip to create a circumferential defect and then reconstruct with a free jejunal transfer. We do not use the technique that Dr. Coleman describes of skin grafting the prevertebral fascia to reconstruct the posterior pharyngeal wall and then using a flap for the anterior 270 degrees.

Although not our first choice, we occasionally use a pectoralis major myocutaneous flap for pharyngeal reconstruction in select situations, such as heavily irradiated necks where vessel anastomosis is compromised or in patients in whom the neck skin flaps may become ischemic by the end of the ablation. One advantage of using a pectoralis major flap such situations is the ability of the cutaneous paddle to repair the pharyngeal defect while the muscle provides reliable soft tissue coverage of the exposed neck vessels. In some cases, we have used two pectoralis myocutaneous flaps placed back to back, using one to reconstruct the pharyngeal mucosa and the other to provide external coverage. This allows the skin paddle to be aligned, making a tube for the passage food or liquids. We also find the pectoralis flap to be a good option for salvage of failed reconstructions and for fistula repair. As Dr. Coleman states, this flap can be rather bulky and tends to fall inferiorly with the effects of gravity unless properly secured in the neck. This is a key step in trying to prevent tension on the flap inset and subsequent fistula formation.

We agree with Dr. Coleman's comments on the functional results of these various pharyngeal reconstructions with respect to speech and swallowing, with the exception of one statement made regarding innervated flaps. Dr. Coleman states, "there are fairly convincing data that function in the oral cavity and oropharynx may be improved by anastomosis of a cutaneous sensory nerve in the flap to a sensory cranial nerve or branch of the cervical plexus." Although there is much literature demonstrating that reinnervated free flaps to the head and neck recover excellent sensation, there are still no well-designed prospective trials demonstrating that this recovered sensation actually improves oropharyngeal function (12–14).

Dr. Coleman gives an excellent review of oropharyngeal reconstruction and presents many of his own precautions used to limit unfavorable results. In his closing statements, he lists several key points that any surgeon planning reconstruction of these defects should keep in mind both preoperatively and postoperatively. To his list, we would like to add one more important point. The reconstructive surgeon should always know the limitations of the flap being used and be able to adjust his or her plan accordingly in order to optimize results. Once again, we applaud Dr. Coleman on a very well-written and comprehensive chapter.

REFERENCES

1. Johnson JT, Bloomer WD. Effect of prior radiotherapy on postsurgical wound infection. *Head Neck* 1989;11:132–136.
2. Coleman JJ. Management of radiation-induced soft tissue injury to the head and neck. *Clin Plast Surg* 1993;20:491–505.
3. Bernstein EF, Sullivan FJ, Mitchell JB, et al. Biology of chronic radiation effect on tissues and wound healing. *Clin Plast Surg* 1993;20:435–453.
4. Miller MJ, Janjan NA. Treatment of injuries from radiation therapy. In: Kroll SS, ed. *Reconstructive plastic surgery for cancer.* St. Louis: Mosby, 1996:17–36.
5. Cordeiro PG, Shah K, Santamaria E, et al. Barium swallows after free jejunal transfer: should they be performed routinely? *Plast Reconstr Surg* 1999;103:1167–175.
6. Reece GP, Bengtson BP, Schusterman MA. Reconstruction of the pharynx and cervical esophagus using free jejunal transfer. *Clin Plast Surg* 1994;21:125–136.
7. Gallas MT, Lewin JS, Evans GRD. Outcome considerations in upper aerodigestive tract reconstruction. In: Achauer BM, Eriksson E, Guyuron B, et al., eds. *Plastic surgery: indications, operations, outcomes.* St. Louis: Mosby-Year Book Inc., 2000:1115–1128.
8. Reece GP, Schusterman MA, Miller MJ, et al. Morbidity and functional outcome of free jejunal transfer reconstruction for circumferential defects of the pharynx and cervical esophagus. *Plast Reconstr Surg* 1995;96:1307–1316.
9. Reece GP. Pharyngoesophageal reconstruction. In: Schusterman MA, ed. *Microsurgical reconstruction of the cancer patient.* Philadelphia: Lippincott-Raven Publishers, 1997:67–84.
10. Anthony JP, Singer MI, Mathes SJ. Pharyngoesophageal reconstruction using the tubed free radial forearm flap. *Clin Plast Surg* 1994;21:137–47.
11. Anthony JP, Neligan PC, Rotstein LE, et al. Reconstruction of partial laryngopharyngectomy defects. *Head Neck* 1997;19: 541–544.
12. Graham B, Dellon AL. Sensory recovery in innervated free tissue transfers. *J Reconstr Microsurg* 1995;11:157–166.
13. Vriens JP, Acosta R, Soutar DS, et al. Recovery of sensation in the radial forearm free flap in oral reconstruction. *Plast Reconstr Surg* 1996;98:649–656.
14. Kimata Y, Uchiyama K, Ebihara S, et al. Comparison of innervated and noninnervated free flaps in oral reconstruction. *Plast Reconstr Surg* 1999;104:1307–1313.

34

MANDIBULAR RECONSTRUCTION

J. BRIAN BOYD

Mandibular reconstruction plays a vital role in the rehabilitation of patients with oral cancer following ablative surgery. Until the advent of microvascular surgery and free-tissue transfer, results were uneven, particularly with the increasing adjunctive use of radiotherapy. In many cases, mandibular reconstruction was omitted altogether, and soft tissue alone was replaced. This situation is not considered here. In a consideration of how to avoid and treat unfavorable results, this chapter covers the outcomes and complications of mandibular reconstruction.

OUTCOMES OF MANDIBULAR RECONSTRUCTION

Outcomes of Conventional Bone Grafting

By the turn of the 20th century, surgeons were using a variety of nonvascularized autogenous bones, including the iliac crest, tibia, and calvarium, to reconstruct the mandible. The numbers of reconstructive options described merely emphasize the suboptimal outcome of any given technique. Bone grafts consisted of small or large corticocancellous blocks (1–3), or cancellous grafts housed in a metallic mesh (4). When these grafts were applied in irradiated beds, extrusion, infection, or resorption occurred in up to 50% of cases, with an overall complication rate near 80% (4).

To eliminate donor site morbidity, surgeons used allograft bone in mandibular reconstruction—again with unacceptably high failure rates in irradiated beds (5,6). They also subjected excised (autogenous) mandibles to various "purging" treatments—including the application of soldering irons or caustic materials, diathermy, and cryotherapy—in an attempt to kill neoplastic cells. The purified, lifeless bone was then recycled to act as a framework for creeping substitution. Investigators reported failure rates of 50% with techniques such as this (7).

Even with advances in excision, reconstruction, chemotherapy, and radiotherapy, patients with oral cancer now have an overall 5-year survival of only 40% (8). In patients whose life expectancy is so limited, reconstructive techniques with failure rates of 50% severely affect the quality of remaining life. The late 1960s and 1970s were a golden age for the discovery of regional flaps suitable for head and neck reconstruction. These flaps made use of undamaged, well-vascularized tissue in poorly healing radiated wounds, so that mandibular reconstruction was facilitated. However, donor morbidity, the uncertainty of "random" cutaneous components, bulky soft tissue, a limited arc of rotation, and poor bony vascularity prevented these regional skin, skin-muscle, and skin-muscle-bone (9,10) flaps from fulfilling their early potential. Even with rigid fixation, conventional bone grafts covered by regional flaps had an unacceptably high failure rate in the primary setting (11,12).

The success of "conventional" or nonvascularized bone grafting is related to defect size, vascularity of the bed, bacterial contamination, and rigidity of the fixation. The failure rate becomes unacceptably high in a defect larger than 6 cm; in an irradiated, contaminated, or fibrotic bed; when the defect communicates with the oral cavity, and when the synostosis is subject to movement. In other words, "conventional" bone grafting is risky in most of the situations encountered in modern head and neck surgery (4,13).

Although some have advocated combining repeated hyperbaric oxygen dives with "mesh and mush," corticocancellous blocks or medulla-packed cadaveric shells, results have not been reproducible, and the expense in terms of cost, quality of life, and time and effort required has not been justified. Conventional bone grafting is reasonable for the short lateral defect when it can be approached via an extraoral incision without a breach of the oral mucosa. Fixation should be rigid (reconstruction plate preferred) and bone contact should be exact and generous.

Outcomes of Alloplastic Reconstruction

To be successful, alloplastic reconstruction must provide rigid and durable mandibular fixation, prove resistant to the massive stresses and strains produced by normal chewing, and must not interfere with healing of the overlying soft tis-

J. B. Boyd: Department of Surgery, Ohio State University, Columbus, Ohio; and Department of Plastic Surgery, Cleveland Clinic Hospital, Fort Lauderdale, Florida

sue. Alloplastic materials must be covered with a well-vascularized mucosal replacement, usually either a regional or free flap.

The history of alloplastic mandibular reconstruction is littered with failures in regard to these requirements. Nevertheless, progress has been made, particularly in rigid fixation and implant osseointegration. Six or more stainless steel bicortical screws in each fragment can provide rigid fixation. Alternatively, three titanium screws integrated with the native mandibular bone can provide equal stability (14).

The problem lies in the metal plate itself—stainless steel or titanium—which, although strong enough to bear the weight of a human body, inevitably is weakened by the repeated stresses and strains of normally loaded mastication. In patients who have undergone alloplastic mandibular reconstruction and who continue to consume a normal diet and do not succumb to their disease, the plates often become fractured 2 to 3 years postoperatively (15–18) (Fig. 34-1A).

The interaction of metal and mucosa can prove equally infelicitous. Proximity of the plate to the oral lining, particularly at a suture line, often results in exposure (Fig. 34-1B). The solution lies in placing the plate far from skin or mucosa. Laborious attempts have been made to secure the plate low on the *medial* cortex, but this process is extremely tedious and requires complex instrumentation. To avoid contact with the oral mucosa and gain purchase on the densest bone, the plate is generally placed laterally along the lower border of the mandibular remnants.

The use of reconstruction plates has proved effective in elderly patients and those with a poor prognosis. However, a long-term study has shown that the outcome is suboptimal when the plate is used to reconstruct the anterior arch (C segment) (16). In the series in question, the failure rate was 35% when the plate was used anteriorly and only 5% when the flap was used laterally. Furthermore, the aesthetically debilitating condition of "lip and chin ptosis" (Fig. 34-2) often accompanied a technically "successful" anterior reconstruction. This technique is therefore recommended only for lateral defects.

Outcomes of Free Vascularized Bone Grafting

The use of complex free-tissue transfers for composite oromandibular defects previously repaired with soft tissue pedicled flaps alone has raised issues of cost-effectiveness, morbidity, and suitability, particularly in patients with a poor prognosis.

The most objective outcome is *survival* of the free-tissue transfer, which has been reported to be in the order of 93% to 100%. These figures are consistent with the survival rate of free flaps used in other parts of the body and are superior to the survival rate for replanted digits. Problems of vessel spasm encountered in replants and in free flaps in the lower leg are not seen in the head and neck. However, positional problems, external pressure, hematomas, kinking, and oral contamination can lead to vessel thrombosis in this area (Fig. 34-3).

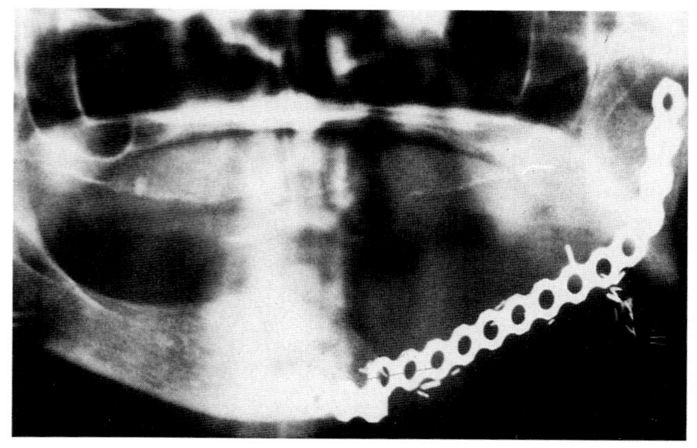

A

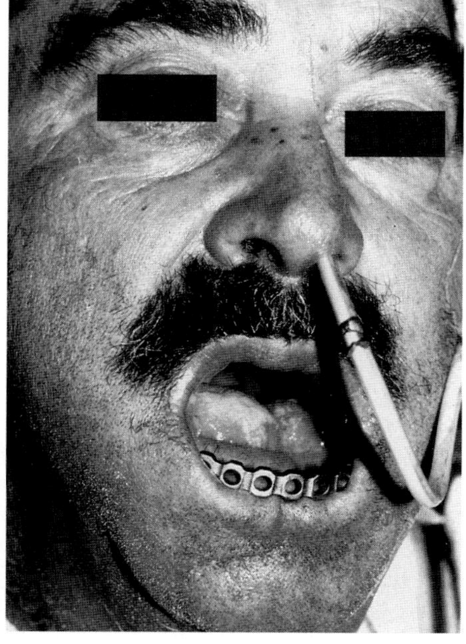

B

FIGURE 34-1. A: Plate fractured after 2 years of use in a patient with a poor prognosis at the time of diagnosis. The fracture is at the usual place—where the bone gives way to metal. Prolonged and repeated stress leads to metal fatigue. **B:** Intraoral mandibular plate exposure. Anterior reconstruction plates have a 35% failure (removal) rate. See text and Fig. 34-2 for an analysis of the forces responsible.

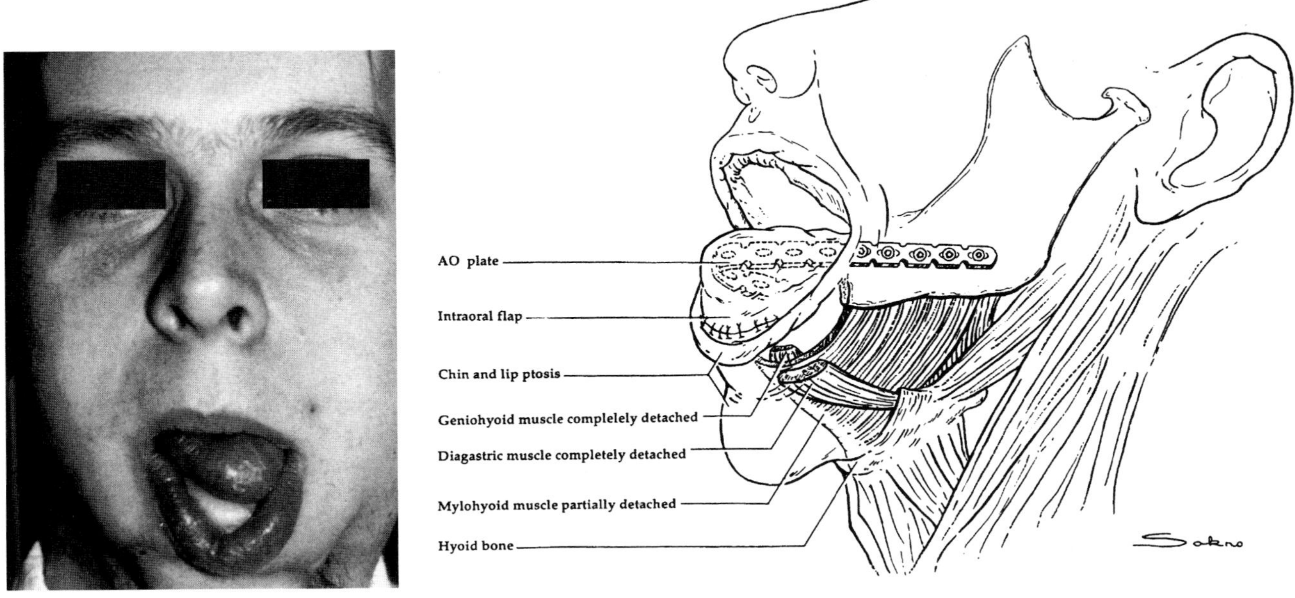

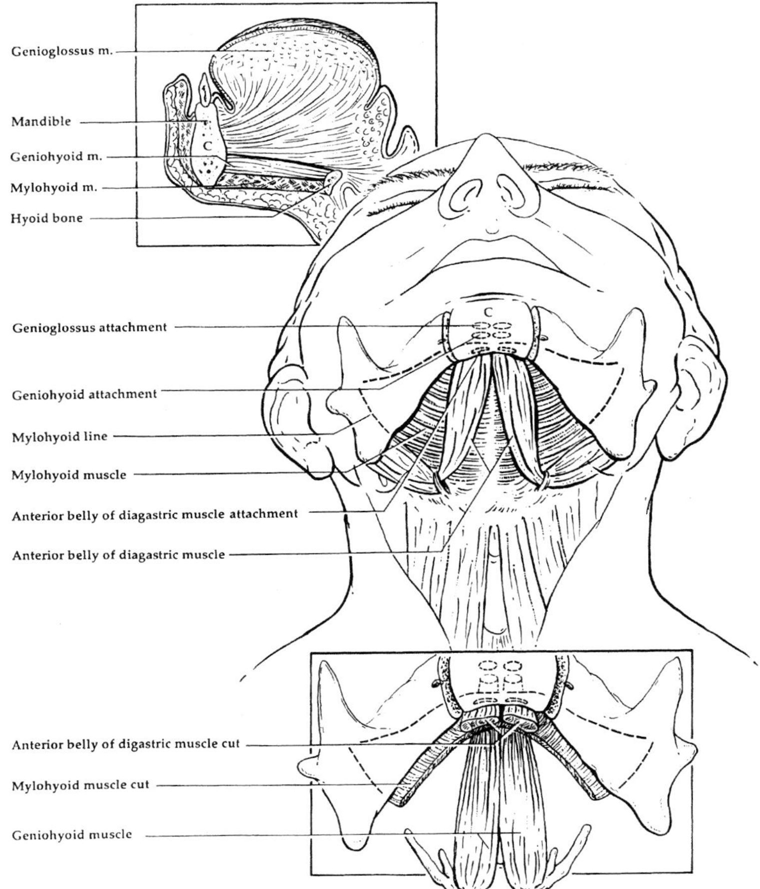

FIGURE 34-2. A,B: Lip and chin ptosis caused by loss of the critical C segment, resection or detachment of the submental musculature, degloving of the chin, lower lip paralysis, and gravity. **C:** Anatomy of the mentum and submental area. Note the muscular attachments to the central C segment. These may be detached or resected during ablative surgery for anterior floor of mouth lesions. The consequences are illustrated in A and B.

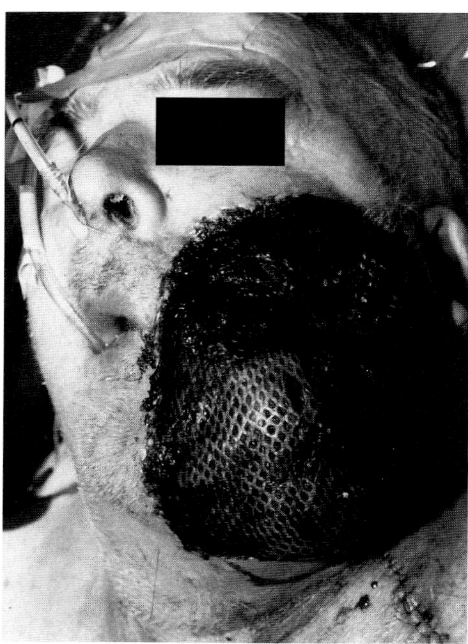

FIGURE 34-3. Failure of an osteocutaneous iliac crest free flap because of a kinked pedicle.

Flap survival, however, tells us nothing about flap effectiveness, either from a financial or a functional/aesthetic perspective. It does not really address the "unfavorable result." Many seminal articles have reviewed the outcome of free-flap mandibular reconstruction in terms of oral continence, masticatory function, speech, swallowing, and cosmesis, but only a few have compared the alternatives. Urken et al. (19) used a battery of tests to assess and compare overall well-being, cosmesis, deglutition, oral competence, speech, length of hospitalization, and dental rehabilitation in 10 reconstructed and 10 unreconstructed patients with lateral defects. They also measured masticatory function in terms of interincisal opening, bite force, chewing performance, and chewing stroke. The results showed a clear advantage for the reconstructed patients in almost all categories. However, the issue of cost was not considered. Talesnik et al. (20) compared the cost and outcome of osteocutaneous free-tissue transfer (iliac crest excluded) with pedicled soft tissue reconstruction for composite defects. Operating times were greatest for osteocutaneous free flaps, least for pedicled soft tissue flaps, and intermediate for soft tissue free flaps in conjunction with a plate. (Scapular flaps required the most time because simultaneous dissection could not be performed.) Surprisingly, blood loss was greatest in the pedicled group. Hospital stay was similar for all groups, but time spent in the intensive care unit was longest for osteocutaneous free flaps, the scapular flaps being the worst. Intensive care unit stay appeared to be proportional to operating time. The pedicled flaps were associated with a higher incidence of flap complications, including partial necrosis and fistulas, but pulmonary complications were more common with the free flaps (perhaps also related to longer operating time).

Aesthetically, the appearance of the patients receiving a plate and a free-tissue transfer was rated highest by patients and surgeons alike. Next came the patients with composite free flaps, whereas the appearance of the patients with pectoralis flaps was rated poorest. Many of these exhibited severe mandibular deviation to the affected side and flattening of the mandibular contour. Several patients requested further surgery to remedy their iatrogenic deformities.

Social function mirrored aesthetic outcome, with the plate group being most comfortable in public. Speech quality was not related to the extent or location of the osseous defect or to the form of reconstruction, but rather to the degree of scarring and mobility of the remaining tongue. Ease of swallowing and oral continence were similar in all groups, but the plate group and the free-tissue transfer group had a better tolerance to diet than the pectoralis major group.

Readmissions for complications and cancer recurrence were more frequent in the pectoralis musculocutaneous flap group, but the total cost of free osteocutaneous transfer was nonetheless higher. The total costs for the plate/flap group were on par with those of the pectoralis group. When individual flaps are considered, radial bone reconstructions were only a little more expensive than pectoralis reconstructions, whereas scapula reconstructions were the costliest. The fibula was intermediate. Clearly, costs relate to the duration of surgery, which affects intensive care recovery time and length of hospital stay.

In the era of managed care, a reconstruction that is not cost-effective is arguably an unfavorable result. However, the authors maintain that the superior aesthetic and functional outcomes of osteocutaneous transfers justify the additional costs, although they do advocate reducing costs by performing simultaneous dissection whenever possible and encouraging the use of intermediate care units and early discharge with home care. The results of using a pectoralis flap alone were considered unpredictable, whereas the plate/flap option was highly cost-effective.

Kroll et al. (21) looked at three groups of patients who underwent oromandibular resection: 20 underwent vascularized bone reconstruction, 15 received a metallic plate (plus either a pectoralis major or a radial forearm flap), and 15 underwent reconstruction with soft tissue alone. They found that when the reconstruction was performed with bone, immediate reconstruction was more cost-effective than delayed reconstruction and was associated with a lower complication rate. However, soft tissue reconstructions were less expensive than those involving vascularized bone, notwithstanding their inferior functional and cosmetic results, particularly in anterior defects. They also were associated with fewer complications. Plates had an unacceptably high failure rate when used to reconstruct the anterior arch.

Some of these findings are supported and amplified by another outcome study from the same center, in which free flaps for intraoral reconstruction were compared with pectoralis flaps used for the same purpose (22). In this study, defects involving the mandible were regrettably excluded. The mean costs of surgery were higher for free flaps but were more than offset by shorter hospital stays. Failure rates in the two groups were similar. However, it would be incorrect to extrapolate these findings to osteocutaneous free flaps because the addition of the osseous component increases donor site morbidity, magnifies the complexity of the surgery, and lengthens operating time, intensive care unit recovery time, and, presumably, hospital stay. These factors, as we have seen, serve to drive up costs. Rather, the findings are supportive of the plate/free-flap option, in which the osseous defect is addressed simply and accurately and little is added to a simple flap transfer.

Clinical nonunion with a vascularized bone graft results in additional hospitalization, further surgery, and an increase in suffering and "days of life lost" for patients whose days are already numbered. The costs associated with this course of events are also increased. Fortunately, primary union occurs in more than 90% of synostoses, whether so-called rigid or nonrigid methods of fixation are used (23). The only form of fixation that has been shown to be ineffective is the combination of miniplates with iliac crest. Although they hold well in the fibula, the screws cannot gain purchase on the soft, cancellous bone of the crest.

No large-scale outcome studies of the efficacy of reinnervated flaps in the mouth have been performed. In one series, 15 patients who received an innervated radial forearm flap were compared with 15 who received a noninnervated radial forearm flap and 15 who received a pectoralis major flap (24). With the reinnervated flaps, a level of sensation was achieved that was comparable to that in the contralateral, normal side of the mouth and significantly superior to that in forearm skin in its native site. The noninnervated flaps provided little or no measurable sensation. Exactly how this translates into improved speech, oral continence, mastication, and swallowing is a matter for detailed outcome review. It seems logical, however, that reinnervation in the mouth, as in the hand, must confer some functional benefit.

Finally, what patient factors militate against a good outcome in free osteocutaneous reconstruction of oromandibular defects? The use of irradiated vessels has been thought to increase the risks for thrombosis and flap failure. The evidence consists of "gut feeling" and the results of animal experiments of questionable clinical applicability. Two large clinical series (25,26), comprising 226 and 308 patients respectively, could not relate failure to previous irradiation. The first included a case-control study that related flap failure to only two factors: postoperative wound infection and *time interval* between radiation and surgery. In a multifactorial analysis of delayed reconstruction, tobacco use, alcohol consumption, and previous irradiation, the other study related flap loss only to previous surgery and the use of vein grafts. The use of vein grafts to bypass radiated vessels is therefore illogical.

COMPLICATIONS OF MANDIBULAR RECONSTRUCTION

As we have seen, until comparatively recently, the mainstay of reconstructive modalities was autologous bone grafting, supplemented when necessary by soft tissue cover in the form of local or regional flaps. This was associated with a high failure rate, particularly in irradiated beds and despite the occasional use of hyperbaric oxygen. When alloplastic methods were used, the outcome was similar. Microvascular surgery now plays an increasingly vital role in mandibular reconstruction (27). Both function and aesthetic appearance can be restored in a one-stage procedure, with rapid recovery and minimal morbidity. In comparison with local or regional flaps, free flaps are more effective in complex or extensive defects, have a better blood supply, are not restricted by the tyranny of the pedicle, and are associated with fewer complications. Nevertheless, complications still limit our success, constrain our enthusiasm, and help define the quality of life of our patients. In short, they are partially responsible for the unfavorable result in mandibular reconstruction.

Complications of mandibular reconstruction can be classified as general complications, anastomotic problems, and specific complications related to either the recipient site or the donor area.

General Complications

Complications Related to Age and Preexisting Medical Conditions

Many cancer patients are elderly and at higher risk for cardiac arrest, respiratory problems, deep vein thrombosis, pulmonary emboli, and wound complications (28,29). Elderly patients are also more prone to psychiatric sequelae. A careful preoperative anesthetic evaluation and the inclusion of an internist and a social worker on the team managing such patients are of great importance.

In an interesting study, Chick and associates (30) found that the rate of wound and medically related complications in a group of elderly patients undergoing free-flap transfer was nearly double the rate observed in a younger group. However, after correction for preexisting medical conditions, no significant differences were seen between the two groups. Singh et al. (31), in a study of 200 consecutive cases, noted that in patients over 70 years of age, operative time was related to the development of systemic complications, especially in patients with advanced Charlson grades. [Charlson staging (32) is based on 16 different medical conditions found to affect survival.]

A thorough preoperative assessment followed by the

treatment and stabilization of preexisting conditions helps to minimize general complications. The institution of adequate prophylaxis against infection and deep vein thrombosis is also important because oral contamination is invariably present, and pulmonary embolus is a leading cause of death in the postoperative phase. Because the patients are often debilitated, the antibiotic regimen should cover gram-negative organisms in addition to the normal oral contaminants. At this time, combinations of first-generation cephalosporins and metronidazole or of gentamicin and clindamycin are preferred. Subcutaneous injections of 5,000 units of heparin twice daily do not result in excessive bleeding during surgery and do help prevent deep vein thrombosis and pulmonary embolus. They may also serve to protect the microanastomoses from thrombosis, although this is open to question. In fact, the administration of systemic anticoagulants has not been shown to confer any beneficial effect on the patency of microvascular anastomoses in the uncomplicated clinical setting (33,34). Cross-matched blood should be available during surgery and an active respiratory protocol instituted in the postoperative phase. Finally, patients should resume ambulation as soon as their general condition permits.

Complications Related to Head and Neck Cancer

Malnutrition in patients undergoing mandibular reconstruction is not uncommon and predisposes them to postoperative wound problems and even mortality (35). Postoperative parotitis is a serious complication associated with increased age, cancer, dehydration, and poor oral hygiene. Preoperative assessment and correction of the nutritional status is essential in patients with head and neck cancer.

In general, patients should undergo a tracheostomy before major intraoral and hypopharyngeal surgery to avoid the disastrous consequences of airway loss in the immediate postoperative phase.

Complications Related to Duration of the Surgical Procedure

Free-flap reconstruction after ablative surgery of the head and neck can significantly prolong the duration of surgery, predisposing patients to complications such as pressure sores, deep vein thrombosis, positional nerve injuries, corneal desiccation, and hypothermia.

The operation should proceed quickly, with two teams available for simultaneous surgery of the donor and recipient sites. Invasive monitoring, proper positioning of the patient, eyelid margin suturing, and the liberal use of foam rubber padding and full-length warming blankets will help prevent the problems related to lengthy procedures.

Schusterman and Horndeski (36) investigated whether the lengthy operative time required for free flaps in head and neck reconstruction increase the risk for medical complications. Twenty consecutive free-flap patients were compared with 20 controls matched for age, preexisting medical condition, surgical site, and histology. The mean length of the procedure was 11.0 hours for the flap group and 6.95 hours for the control group. The mean occurrence of postoperative medical problems was 0.75 per patient for the flap group and 0.90 per patient for the control group. The results of this study clearly indicated that length of the procedure alone should not be the basis for the decision of whether or not to perform immediate microvascular reconstruction in patients with head and neck cancer. However, in the study of Singh et al. (31), an increased operative time was related to the development of systemic complications in patients over 70 years of age, especially those with advanced Charlson grades.

Microvascular Complications

In a review of the results of free-flap surgery, Shaw (37) noted that 10% of flaps required reexploration, with an overall failure rate of approximately 5% (Fig. 34-3). Similar or even higher success rates were reported in various series of free-flap reconstruction in the head and neck (38–40). A recent survey from a large microvascular center revealed an overall free-flap success rate of 98.8% (41); the rate of vessel thrombosis was lowest in reconstructions of the head and neck and highest in reconstructions of the lower limb. These success rates compare favorably with those for regional flaps in head and neck reconstruction (42,43). Factors relevant to the selection of recipient vessels in head and neck reconstructions are summarized in the next sections.

Timing of Reconstruction

The optimal time to select vessels at the recipient site is during cancer resection or immediately after trauma, when fibrosis or perivascular scarring is absent. Although Whitney et al. (44) found no difference in the success rates for simultaneous versus sequential multiple microvascular transplants in complex head and neck defects, most surgeons accept that secondary reconstruction presents a greater technical challenge because of the difficulty of releasing and accurately repositioning residual mandibular fragments and the danger of damaging the facial nerve while dissecting them out. Furthermore, with extensive ablations, recipient vessels are frequently unavailable or hard to locate.

Vessel Availability after Modified Neck Dissection

During the neck dissection, prospective recipient vessels should be preserved as much as possible. Ligation or clipping of vessels is better than the use of electrocautery. High ligation of the external carotid artery to gain additional length is safe, but clamping of the common carotid artery is contraindicated in most cancer patients because of the risk for stroke.

Atherosclerotic Vessels

Elderly cancer patients have thick-walled calcified vessels with loosely attached intima. Although techniques for microanastomosis are more demanding, the free-flap failure rate is not increased (45).

Preoperative Irradiation

Some experimental studies have demonstrated decreased patency rates in anastomosed irradiated vessels (4,46,47). Irradiated blood vessels in the human neck show diminished smooth-muscle density, endothelial cell dehiscence, vessel wall fibrosis, and fragile intima (23). Clinically, Tabah et al. (49) found that the rate of complete failure of free-tissue transfer in the head and neck was three times higher in previously irradiated patients than in nonirradiated patients. However, in the study of Kiener et al. (50), previous irradiation did not affect the success of subsequent microvascular reconstruction or the difficulty of such reconstruction in the head and neck, judged by operative time. In our case-control study of 226 irradiated and 108 nonirradiated cases of free flaps in the head and neck (25), no difference in anastomotic patency was found between the two groups. Only two factors correlated with anastomotic failure: lag time between radiation and subsequent surgery and the presence of infection.

Vascular Spasm

Spasm is much less problematic in head and neck blood vessels than in those of the extremities. However, vein grafts harvested from the lower limb for use in the neck are prone to spasm. Lo Gerto et al. (51) recommend hydrostatic distension as a means of preventing spasm in saphenous vein grafts.

Smoking

The majority of patients with head and neck cancer are smokers. The known vasoconstrictor effect of nicotine justifies its being prohibited for at least 2 weeks preoperatively and also during the first 2 weeks after surgery while the vascular repair site is being reendothelialized. Experimentally, intraarterial nicotine decreases blood flow in anastomosed rat femoral arteries, but no corresponding decrease in patency is observed (52). Clinically, the failure rate of elective free-tissue transfers in patients who are long-term smokers but have quit in the perioperative period is not increased in comparison with the failure rate patients who do not smoke. However, smokers do have a higher incidence of delayed wound healing (53).

Infection

Infection of the subcutaneous tissues of the neck, usually secondary to an intraoral dehiscence, is the most common cause of *late* anastomotic failure. Presumably, the infective process immediately adjacent to the vascular pedicle has a direct thrombogenic effect (25). Dehiscence is minimized by meticulous surgical closure of well-vascularized tissue. As previously discussed, antibiotic prophylaxis is also important.

Other Complications

If vessel anastomosis is performed with the patient's head turned to one side, a kinked vessel (Fig. 34-3) may develop during the postoperative period once the head is straightened. The vessels may also be compressed by drains and circumferential tracheostomy tapes. Postoperative ventilation with positive end-expiratory pressure may cause venous hypertension in the jugular vein draining the free flap (27). It is common for humidification masks to be placed over tracheostomy openings during the early postoperative phase. Condensation of humidified air on the neck produces cooling that leads to vasospasm and may induce thrombosis in the pedicle. The solution is to use a T piece with an extension tube to remove the excess humidified air in addition to the expired gases. Tapes used to secure these masks, like tracheotomy ties, may also compress the pedicle.

Complications Related to the Components of Mandibular Reconstruction

Intraoral Component

Intraoral structures are responsible for several functions, including speech, swallowing, and upper respiratory dynamics. Loss of these functions, which represents an unfavorable result, arises not only from the oromandibular resection itself but also from reconstruction with inadequate or poorly adaptive tissue. Bulky tissue can inhibit tongue mobility and masticatory function. Nowadays, thin flaps, such as the radial forearm flap, are generally used to avoid this problem (54,55).

Singh et al. (31) found that most complications at the recipient site were related to the junction of the free flap and recipient bed, and that they were more common in irradiated patients. Fistulas are more commonly seen following reconstructions of the floor of the mouth and part of the tongue than in composite resections involving the cheek or palate. Pooling of saliva and the deleterious effects of perpetual tongue motion are contributory factors. Watertight closure is essential to prevent fistulas that can lead to neck sepsis, secondary flap loss, carotid blowout, and osteoradionecrosis (in previously irradiated mandibles). For suture line competence to be maintained, the skin flap must have a good blood supply. The marginal necrosis commonly seen on the skin paddles of pectoralis major and deltopectoral flaps indicates suboptimal circulation. This problem has led to the increasing use of free flaps for the purposes of oral lining (Fig. 34-4).

"Functional" tongue reconstruction with a muscle-neurovascular flap harnessed to the hypoglossal nerve has recently been reported (56). Reconstruction of the total glossectomy defect with bulky tissue is said to allow better speech preservation than reconstruction with thin skin flaps (57), and it is hoped that preserving intraoral sensibility with the use of sensory innervated radial forearm flaps (connected to the lingual or inferior alveolar nerve) will decrease drooling and increase oral hygiene. Being able to recognize the presence of food or saliva in reconstructed parts of the mouth is the first prerequisite for clearance.

Osseous Reconstruction

The choice of the microvascular flap in mandibular reconstruction depends on the size of the defect, need for osteotomies, amount of adipose tissue, and requirement for soft tissue reconstruction. Donor site availability, the surgeon's preference, and the patient's prognosis and preference are secondary factors. Recipient site complications may be flap-specific or related to the resulting functional deficit.

The reliability of the skin paddle of the fibular osteocutaneous flap is now confirmed (58), and excellent clinical results have been observed (59).

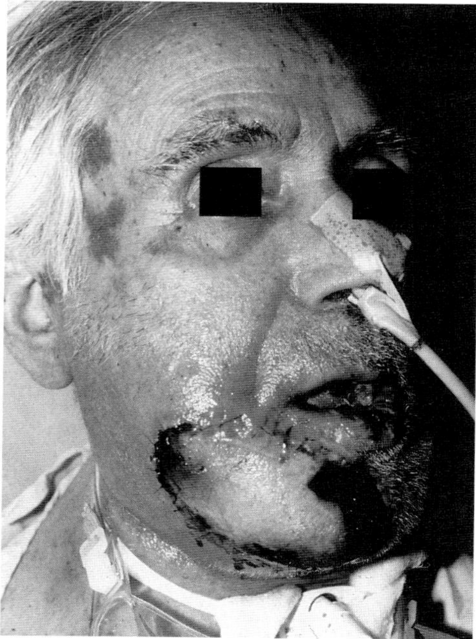

FIGURE 34-4. Marginal necrosis of the skin paddle of a fibula musculocutaneous flap. If planned correctly, the fibular osteocutaneous flap is very reliable. However, this skin flap was divided in two—one for lining and one for cover—and the external paddle was left with insufficient perfusion.

To ensure the reliability of the skin paddle of the osteocutaneous iliac crest (60), the soft tissue attachments to the bone (the "obligatory muscle cuff") should be maintained to preserve the perforating vessels. Therefore, the flap is often bulky, and secondary revision of the soft tissues is frequently required (61). The position of the skin paddle on the *outside* of the iliac crest makes it rather difficult to use for intraoral lining. Rotation of the paddle either under or over the reconstructed mandible leads to compression of the pedicle and unwanted tension on already tenuous vascular connections. This has led to partial flap loss and intraoral wound breakdown in nearly 25% of cases (61). Nevertheless, the skin paddle is safe, albeit bulky and of poor color match, when used externally (Fig. 34-5).

The free radial forearm osteocutaneous flap (62) has a thin, reliable skin paddle, but the length of bone available is limited and the bone thickness does not usually accommodate implant osseointegration. However, implants can be placed in the adjacent mandible. This flap should not be used after large-volume resections because it provides little bulk, so that a contour irregularity may result (Fig. 34-6). Other free flaps have been used in mandibular reconstruction with variable success (63–65). Most osteocutaneous flaps, with the possible exception of the scapular flap, provide a poor color match for facial skin (Figs. 34-5 and 34-7).

A recently developed alternative to mandibular reconstruction has been use of a reconstruction plate covered by a cutaneous free flap. This technique should be reserved for older patients and those with extensive malignancy and a poor prognosis. It should be limited to lateral mandibular defects [defects not containing the central segment bearing the canines and incisors (16,66)] because of the high incidence of plate extrusion (Fig. 34-1B) when it is used anteriorly (67). The complications specific to this method include plate exposure (intraorally and extraorally) (Fig. 34-2), cold intolerance, and stress fracture. Intraoral exposure frequently develops when dentures are worn directly over the plate.

As previously mentioned, the study of Kroll et al. (21) showed that immediate mandibular reconstruction with vascularized bone is more cost-effective than delayed reconstruction, and that the complication rates are lower.

When contralateral recipient neck vessels must be used, the location of the vascular pedicle of the flap must be oriented so as to avoid kinking of the vessels.

Other complications of mandibular reconstruction are related to functional loss. Securing the proximal and distal mandibular segments in a precise anatomical position to maintain normal occlusion is important and can be accomplished by means of temporary intermaxillary fixation or contouring a reconstructive plate to the mandible *before* the resection. Models constructed from roentgenograms and

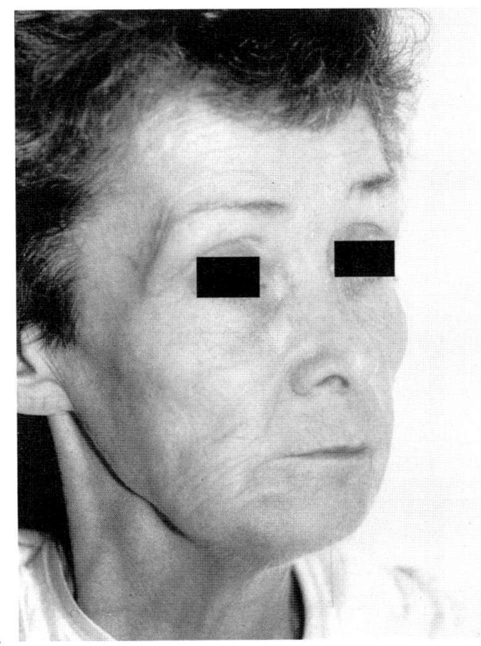

A

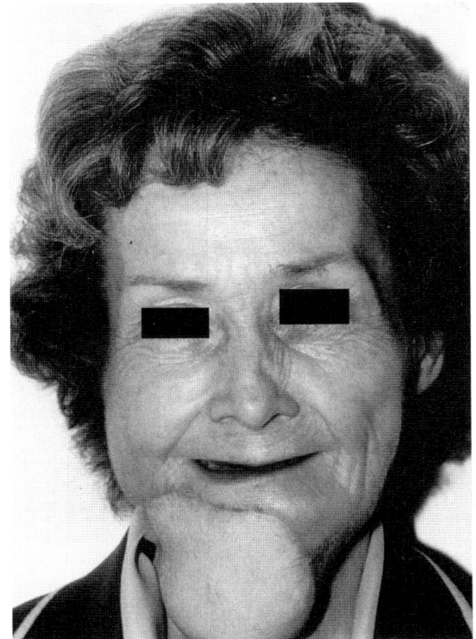

B

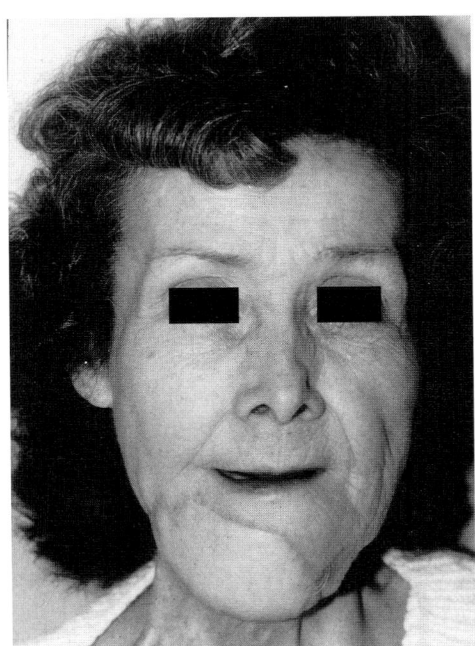

C

FIGURE 34-5. A,B: Lateral "through-and-through" reconstruction with use of a reinnervated radial forearm flap for lining and an iliac crest for structure and cover. Note the poor color match and bulkiness of the flap. **C:** This is easily debulked at a second stage and can be improved even further by overgrafting or other conventional techniques.

computed tomograms may also be useful. Nonunion or malunion should be avoided by using secure interosseous fixation and obtaining primary intraoral healing (23).

Anterior mandibular height is frequently lost after reconstruction of the anterior arch with a narrow bone graft, such as a radius or a fibula (Fig. 34-7). Normal anatomy calls for a double arch: a prominent one for the mentum and a retruded one for the alveolus. A fibula placed along the lower border would serve to restore normal chin projection but would be in the wrong position for implant osseointegration because the alveolus lies more posteriorly. Implants placed in the fibula would cause a class III malocclusion unless inclined sharply backward in a highly unstable position. Conversely, placement of a fibula in the alveolar position would facilitate osseointegration, but chin projection would be lacking, with an obvious contour defect.

The problem can be avoided by arranging for chin projection to maintain facial contour and using a dental prosthesis fixed to osseointegrated implants on either side to span the anterior arch and occupy the position of a normal alveolus. Otherwise, a double-barreled fibula graft can be used anteriorly, the upper one placed back to serve as an

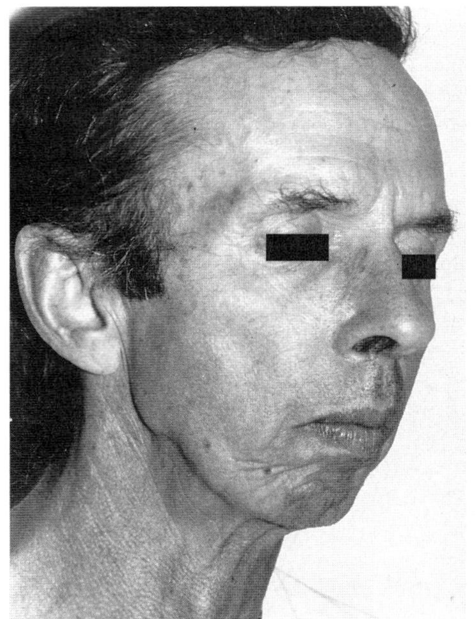

A

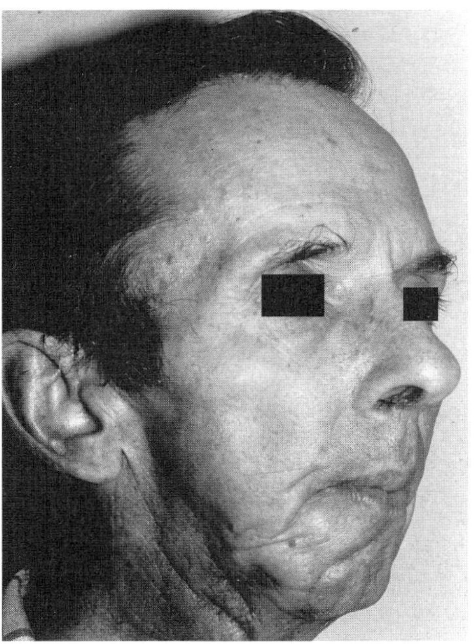

B

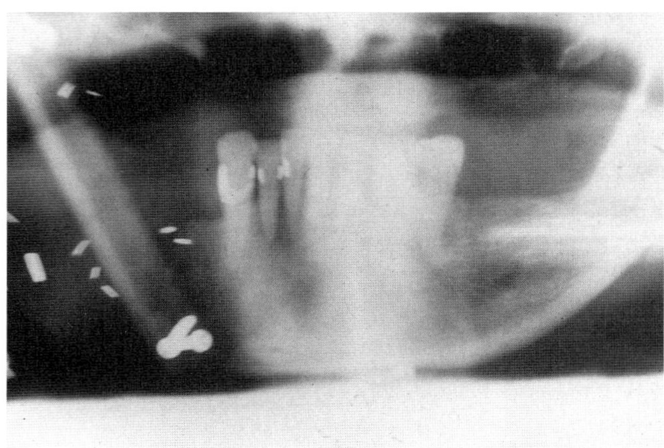

C

FIGURE 34-6. A,B,C: Preoperative and postoperative views of a lateral mandibular reconstruction with use of an unosteotomized radial strut. The patient has had solid union and good oral function since the arch was reconstructed. The loss of contour at the angle is considered a reasonable price to pay.

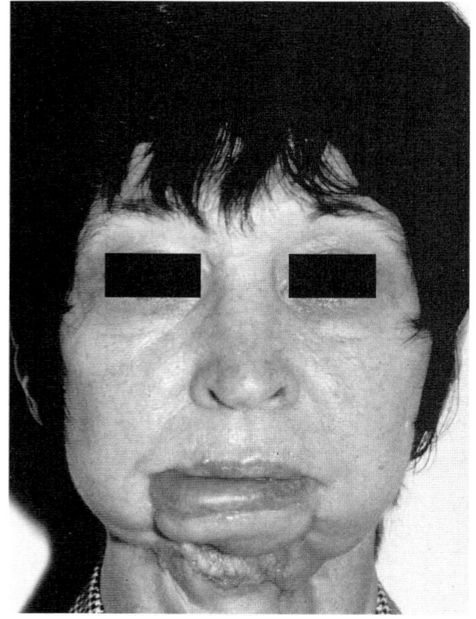

A

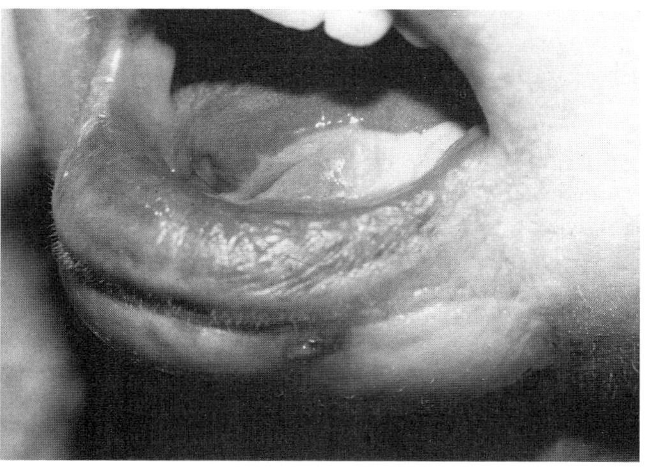

B

FIGURE 34-7. A,B: Anterior "through-and-through" defect reconstructed by a double-paddle radial osteocutaneous flap. Radius, like fibula, lacks vertical height; however, unlike fibula soft tissue, radius soft tissue lacks bulk. The result is a cosmetic and functional deficit. *(continued)*

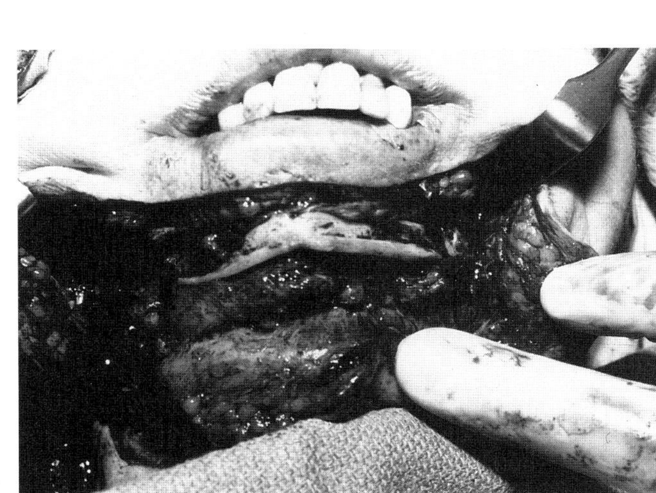
C

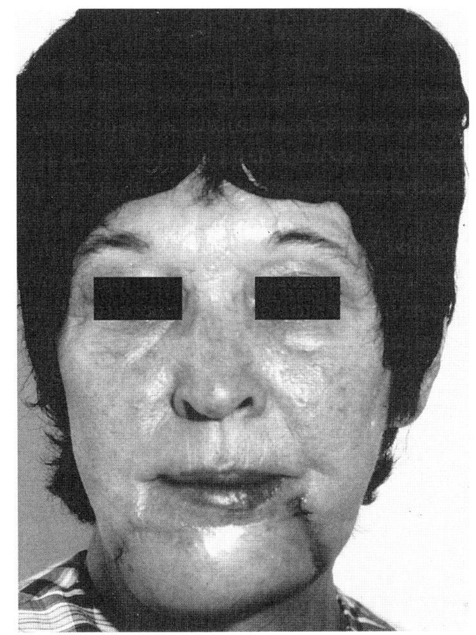
D

FIGURE 34-7. *Continued.* **C:** The bone is exposed and the osteotomy found to be solidly united. **D:** The addition of a vascularized iliac crest supplies vertical bony height and soft tissue bulk to produce a more acceptable result.

alveolus. This arrangement maintains mandibular height and allows the direct placement of implants for osseointegration. It also presents a significant technical challenge.

Complications related to the temporomandibular joint include ankylosis, dislocation, and pain. The original condyle should be retained whenever possible to preserve normal function. Even when the proximal synostosis consists of a single interosseous wire loop fixing a narrow condylar neck to a vascularized bone graft, the function remains surprisingly good. Sculpting a precise condylar replacement from one end of the vascularized graft, although artistically satisfying, frequently results in bony ankylosis and should be avoided. Dislocation is prevented by heavy suture suspension (to the zygomatic arch) or by reconstruction of the joint and surrounding ligaments (60).

The loss of vestibular sulcus and improper seating of dentures over the flap usually require secondary procedures. Alternatively, masticatory function can be restored with osseointegrated implants (68).

Simultaneous inferior alveolar nerve and osseous reconstruction of the mandible helps to restore sensation in the lower lip and avoid the complication of incontinent drooling (69).

When mandibular reconstruction involves the anterior segment of the arch [the C segment in the HCL classification (61,66)], the postoperative complication of *lip and chin ptosis* becomes a real possibility (Fig. 34-2). In this situation, the soft tissues slide downward off the reconstructed mentum to produce eversion of the lower lip and incontinence of saliva. If the patient is edentulous, the mandibular arch tends to rotate upward, causing the intraoral flap to become visible at rest and occasionally leading to wound breakdown in the anterior floor of mouth.

Several factors probably contribute:

1. Powerful mouth-opening muscles, the geniohyoid and the digastric, are attached to the inner inferior border of the C segment of the mandible (Fig. 34-2C). When the bone is resected, these are necessarily detached. They may even be partially removed as part of the soft tissue ablation (Fig. 34-2A,B). This has two effects. First, the mandible, free of its muscular tethering, tends to ride upward, especially if the patient is edentulous and overclosure is no longer limited by occlusion. Second, the detached muscles, now attached only to soft tissues, retract inferiorly and pull the same soft tissues with them. Even when the mandibular resection has been massive, good oral function can be maintained by preserving the C segment and its muscular attachments. When this is not possible, it is occasionally feasible to reattach either the submental musculature or the soft tissues of the chin to the reconstructed symphysis.
2. The detached soft tissues become ptotic, resembling the "witch's chin" seen occasionally after orthognathic and cosmetic surgery with overly zealous degloving of the mentum. (The mentum is, of course, automatically degloved in C resections.) Here, gravity plays a major role. Reattachment of the degloved soft tissues to the new mandible helps avoid this problem.
3. Bilateral neck dissections and extensive anterior ablative

surgery can destroy the lower branches of the facial nerve on both sides. Lack of good oral sphincter tone certainly contributes to a patulous and ptotic lower lip.

4. If during reconstruction a large "dead space" in the anterior floor of the mouth is not adequately filled with soft tissue, the resultant contracture tends either to distort the new bony arch or draw the soft tissues inferiorly, contributing to the same inferior displacement described above.

Clearly, these mechanisms all serve to make reconstruction of the C segment-*containing* defect (although it is possible, very few ablative defects are *purely* C segment) a daunting prospect. However, other factors contribute to a poor clinical outcome in these patients. Any resection of the anterior floor of mouth potentially involves the lower lip directly, particularly when skin is included, and this, in turn, can result in a loss of function and cosmesis even after the best reconstruction. With the division of the genioglossus and hyoglossus, the tongue tends to retract backward, and this retraction, combined with the fact that an insensate flap is lining the anterior floor of mouth, contributes to the "hot potato" voice frequently heard when the tracheostomy tube is finally removed. It may also lead to difficulties in deglutition.

To minimize the problems of lip and chin ptosis, the following precautions should be taken (Fig. 34-8):

1. Minimize stripping of the attached musculature before bony fixation.
2. If possible, reattach the submental musculature to the mandible.
3. Attach soft tissues of the degloved chin to the underlying reconstruction.

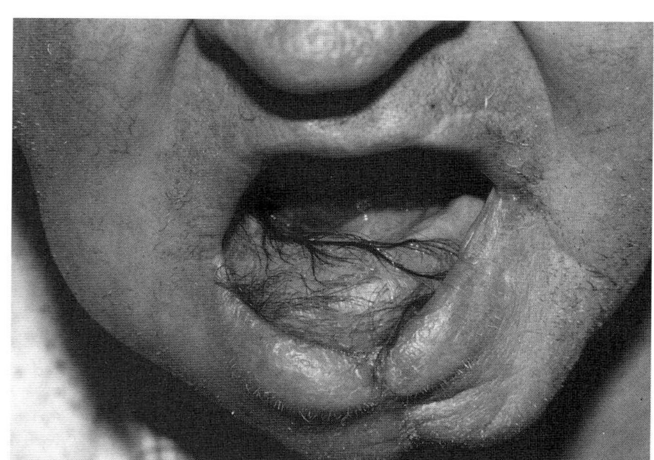

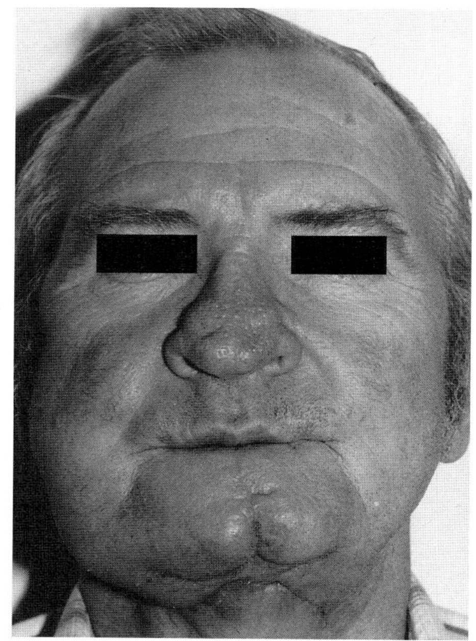

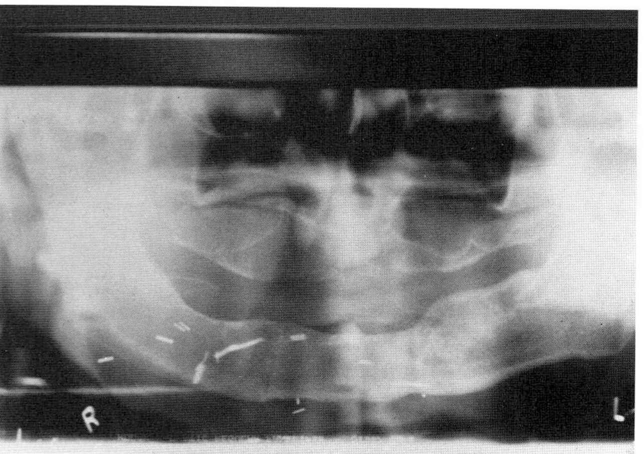

FIGURE 34-8. A: Lip and chin ptosis following anterior reconstruction of a composite defect with a radial forearm osteocutaneous flap. The patient was incontinent of food and saliva. **B,C:** Result of replacing the radial bone graft with a vascularized iliac crest and attaching the soft tissues of the skin to its anterior surface.

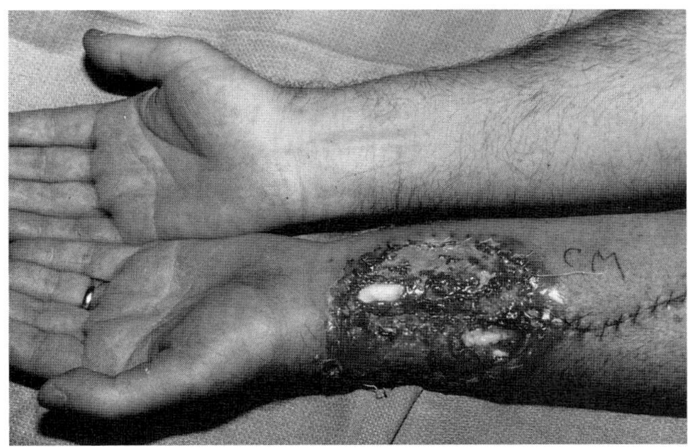

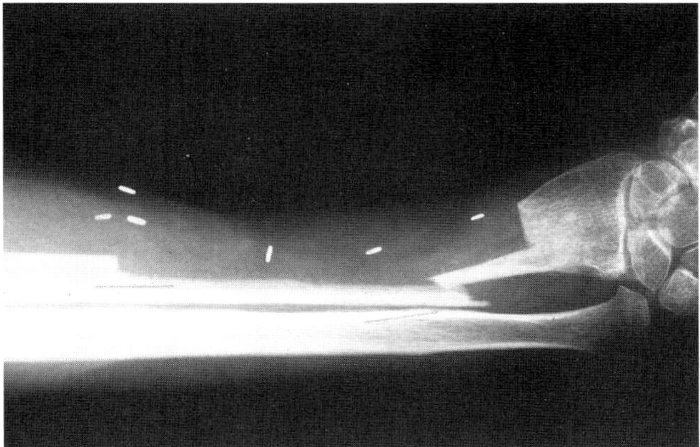

A B

FIGURE 34-9. A: Skin graft breakdown over a radial forearm donor site. **B:** Radius fracture following osteocutaneous forearm flap.

4. Accurately assess the volume of the soft tissue defect in the anterior floor of the mouth and fill it in with vascularized tissue.

Complications Related to Free-flap Donor Sites

The complications arising at favored free-flap donor sites have been analyzed in detail in a number of publications (27,70).

Osteocutaneous Flaps

Complications at the *radial forearm flap* donor site (71–74) include partial skin graft loss with tendon exposure (Fig. 34-9A), numbness in the distribution of the radial nerve, patient dissatisfaction with cosmetic appearance, decreased grip strength, limited range of movement, and intolerance to cold. The partial loss of skin graft that occurs in more than 30% of the patients can be prevented by meticulous attention to detail, with placement of the skin paddle over the middle and proximal forearm and avoidance of the radial border and volar wrist. However, the distal radial wrist is often the flap site of choice because of the thinness of the skin, ease of innervation, and location over the cephalic vein. Radius fracture following osteocutaneous forearm flap transfer (Fig. 34-9B) is prevented by beveling the osteotomy corners, removing no more than one-third of the radial cross section, and placing an above-elbow splint for 8 to 12 weeks (72).

Despite a satisfactory Allen's test result, acute ischemia of the hand resulting from the elevation of the forearm flap has been reported (75). This requires immediate recognition and reconstruction of the radial artery. It may also result from inadvertent injury to a *superficial ulnar artery* (76) while the tourniquet is up. Damage to the ulnar artery can be avoided by situating the skin paddle over the radial aspect of the wrist. Cold intolerance does not seem to be a major problem, even when the Allen's test result is equivocal preoperatively.

The *scapular flap* donor site (77) is known for its hypertrophic and spread scars. Shoulder stiffness is uncommon provided early mobilization and therapy are instituted. Seromas are common and are best avoided with closed suction drains.

Potential complications of the *dorsalis pedis flap* (63) include delayed wound healing, foot ischemia, and poor skin graft take (Fig. 34-10). The flap is contraindicated in elderly patients with peripheral vascular disease. Gait problems after harvesting the second metatarsal appear to be uncommon despite loss of the transverse plantar arch.

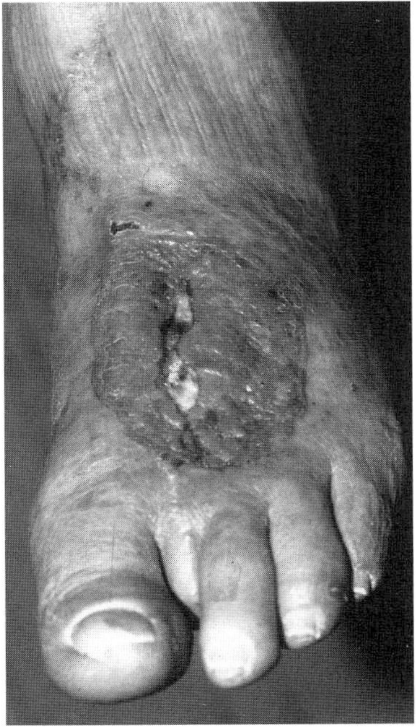

FIGURE 34-10. Skin graft breakdown on the dorsum of the foot following the harvest of a second metatarsal flap.

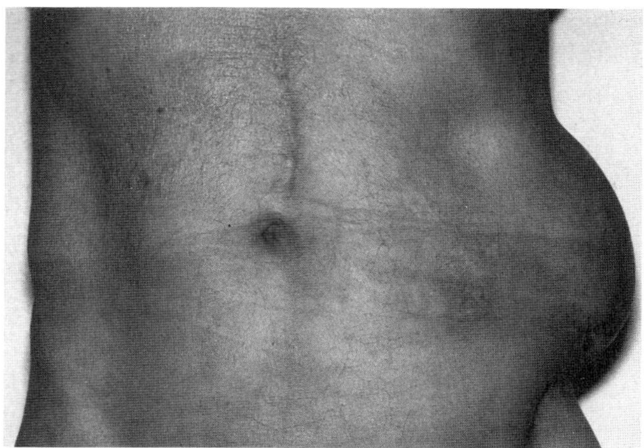

FIGURE 34-11. An incisional hernia several months after harvesting of an iliac crest osteocutaneous flap.

Numerous potential complications of the *iliac crest* donor site have been described (78), including pain, femoral nerve palsy, ileus, sensory changes, contour irregularity, poor scar, gait abnormality, hernia (Fig. 34-11), meralgia paresthetica, and impotence.

Most complications at the *fibula* donor site (59), such as peroneal nerve injury and ankle instability, can be avoided by leaving the upper and lower segments of the fibula *in situ.* Delayed skin healing is not uncommon, particularly if the wound is sutured under tension or if a skin graft is used. Preoperative angiograms are useful in ruling out potentially disastrous conditions, such as vascular anomalies and major vessel arteriopathy. Preoperative Doppler is also useful in locating the fasciocutaneous perforators for the skin island if one is required.

Muscle and Musculocutaneous Flaps

These flaps are occasionally used in conjunction with alloplastic methods and as part of extensive osteocutaneous reconstructions. *Rectus abdominis* donor site complications, such as abdominal wall weakness and hernia, are uncommon if a unilateral muscle flap is harvested (60,79). However, the use of synthetic mesh should be considered if a significant fascial defect is present.

The *latissimus dorsi flap* donor site is known for a high incidence of seroma. Shoulder function is generally not affected except in paraplegics and persons who engage in activities such as mountain climbing and competitive swimming (80). Other complications include contour deformity, stretched scar, and traction injury to the brachial plexus (81).

CONCLUSION

With meticulous technique, rigid fixation, a nonradiated bed, and the absence of oral contamination, "conventional" bone grafting has been successful in mandibular reconstruction, particularly if the defects are small. Conventional bone grafting in other situations has over the years been a major contributor to "the unfavorable result in mandibular reconstruction." However, the advent of free-tissue transfer has led to a proliferation of other "unfavorable results," ranging from anastomotic thrombosis to cold intolerance and from radial fracture to femoral paresis. However, the litany of misadventure described in this chapter serves to emphasize that this form of reconstruction is now widely used and generally accepted as the "gold standard" of mandibular replacement. The overall success rates, as we have seen, are better than 95%, and in the search for perfection, we are essentially increasing our critical awareness, cataloguing donor deficits, and analyzing the effects of prolonged anesthesia on potentially compromised patients.

As the art and science of mandibular reconstruction advance, we are becoming more and more critical of the aesthetic result. Where previously flap survival was the only issue, we are now disappointed when reconstructed mucosa has less sensation than a normal tongue. Where we were previously preoccupied with avoiding tube dependency and oral incontinence, it is no exaggeration to say that we are now concerned with the restoration of dentition, mastication, lispless phonation, and a "toothy" smile.

It is clear that a knowledge of the different modalities available will allow the reconstructive surgeon to tailor the procedure, not only to the defect but also to the disease and, most particularly, to the patient. The idea of managing all new patients with the same technique should be condemned, as should also be a refusal to consider new developments as they inevitably supersede, or perhaps complement, older methods. Mandibular reconstruction has come a long way in the last 20 years and has a long way to go, and for critical surgeons, an "unfavorable result" will always act as an impetus for further progress.

REFERENCES

1. Boyn PJ, Zaren H. Osseous reconstruction of the resected mandible. *Am J Surg* 1976;132:49–53.
2. Manchester WM. Immediate reconstruction of the mandible and temporomandibular joint. *Br J Plast Surg* 1965;18:291–303.
3. Millard DR, Dembrow V, Shocket E, et al. Immediate reconstruction of the resected mandibular arch. *Am J Surg* 1957;114:605–613.
4. Adamo A, Szal RL. Timing, results and complications of mandibular reconstructive surgery: report of 32 cases. *J Oral Surg* 1979;37:755–763.
5. Baker SR, Krause CJ, Panje WR. Radiation effects on microvascular anastomosis. *Arch Otolaryngol* 1978;104:103–107.
6. Mainous EG. Restoration of resected mandible by grafting with combination of mandible homograft and autogenous iliac marrow and postoperative treatment with hyperbaric oxygenation. *Oral Surg Med Oral Pathol* 1973;35:13–20.
7. Weaver AW, Smith DB. Frozen autogenous mandibular stent-graft for immediate reconstruction in oral cancer surgery. *Am J Surg* 1973;126:505–506.

8. Rice DH, Spiro RH. *Current concepts in head and neck cancer.* Atlanta: American Cancer Society, 1989:2–3.
9. Conley T. Use of composite flaps containing bone for major repairs in the head and neck. *Plast Reconstr Surg* 1972;49:522–526.
10. Cuono CB, Ariyan S. Immediate reconstruction of a composite mandibular defect with a regional osteo-musculo-cutaneous flap. *Plast Reconstr Surg* 1980;65:477–484.
11. Komisar A, Warman S, Danziger E. A critical analysis of immediate and delayed mandibular reconstruction using A-O plates. *Arch Otol Head Neck Surg* 1989;115:830–833.
12. Lawson W, Loscalzo L, Baek S, et al. Experience with immediate and delayed mandibular reconstruction. *Laryngoscope* 1982; 92:5–10.
13. Harrison DNF. Intraoral malignancy with special reference to jaw replacement. Problems of reconstruction following preoperative radiotherapy. *Proc R Soc Med* 1974;67:601–603.
14. Raveh J, Stich H, Sutter F, et al. Use of titanium-coated hollow screw and reconstruction system in bridging of lower jaw defects. *J Oral Maxillofac Surg* 1984;42:281–294.
15. Boyd JB. Use of reconstruction plates in conjunction with soft tissue free flaps for oromandibular reconstruction. *Clin Plast Surg* 1994;21:69–77.
16. Boyd B, Mulholland S, Davidson J, et al. The free flap and plate in oromandibular reconstruction: long-term review and indications. *Plast Reconstr Surg* 1994;95:1018–1028.
17. Davidson J, Boyd JB, Gullane PJ, et al. A comparison of the results following oromandibular reconstruction using a radial forearm flap with either radial bone or a reconstruction plate. *Plast Reconstr Surg* 1991;88:201–208.
18. Gullane PJ. Primary mandibular reconstruction: analysis of 64 cases and evaluation of interface radiation dosimetry on bridging plates. *Laryngoscope* 1991;101(6 Pt 2):1–24.
19. Urken ML, Weinberg H, Vickery C, et al. The neurofasciocutaneous radial forearm flap in head and neck reconstruction: a preliminary report. *Laryngoscope* 1990;100:161–173.
20. Talesnik A, Markowitz B, Calcaterra T, et al. Cost and outcome of osteocutaneous free tissue transfer versus pedicled soft tissue reconstruction for composite mandibular defects. *Plast Reconstr Surg* 1996;97:1167–1178.
21. Kroll SS, Schusterman MA, Reece GP. Costs and complications in mandibular reconstruction. *Ann Plast Surg* 1992;29:341–347.
22. Kroll S, Evans GRD, Goldberg D, et al. A comparison of resource costs for head and neck reconstruction with free and pectoralis major flaps. *Plast Reconstr Surg* 1997;99:1282–1286.
23. Boyd JB, Mulholland RS. Fixation of the vascularized bone graft in mandibular reconstruction. *Plast Reconstr Surg* 1993; 91:274–282.
24. Boyd JB, Mulholland S, Gullane P, et al. Reinnervated lateral antebrachial cutaneous neurosome flaps in oral reconstruction: are we making sense? *Plast Reconstr Surg* 1994;93:1350–1359; discussion 1360–1362.
25. Mulholland S, Boyd JB, McCabe S, et al. Recipient vessels in head and neck microsurgery: radiation effect and vessel access. *Plast Reconstr Surg* 1993;92:628–632.
26. Schusterman MA, Miller MJ, Reece GP, et al. A single center's experience with 308 free flaps for repair of head and neck cancer defects. *Plast Reconstr Surg* 1994;93:472–478; discussion 479–480.
27. Swartz WM, Banis Jr JC, eds. *Head and neck microsurgery.* Baltimore: Williams & Wilkins, 1992.
28. Djokovic JL, Hedley-Whyte J. Prediction of outcome of surgery and anesthesia in patients over 80. *JAMA* 1979;242:2301–2306.
29. Warnold I, Lundholm K. Clinical significance of preoperative nutritional status in 215 non-cancer patients. *Ann Surg* 1984;199:299–305.
30. Chick LR, Walton RL, Reus W, et al. Free flaps in the elderly. *Plast Reconstr Surg* 1992;90:87–94.
31. Singh B, Cordeiro PG, Santamaria E, et al. Factors associated with complications in microvascular reconstruction of head and neck defects. *Plast Reconstr Surg* 1999;103:403–411.
32. Charlson ME, Pompei P, Ales KL, et al. A new method of classifying prognostic co-morbidity in longitudinal studies: development and validation. *J Chronic Dis* 1987;40:373–383.
33. Johnson PC. Platelet-mediated thrombosis in microvascular surgery: new knowledge and strategies. *Plast Reconstr Surg* 1990;86:359–367.
34. Johnson PC, Barker JH. Thrombosis and antithrombotic therapy in microvascular surgery. *Clin Plast Surg* 1992;19:799–807.
35. Johnson WC, Ulrich F, Meguid MM, et al. Role of delayed hypersensitivity in predicting postoperative morbidity and mortality. *Am J Surg* 1979;137:536–542.
36. Schusterman MA, Horndeski G. Analysis of the morbidity associated with immediate microvascular reconstruction in head and neck cancer patients. *Head Neck* 1991;13:51–55.
37. Shaw WW. Microvascular free flaps: the first decade. *Clin Plast Surg* 1983;10:3–20.
38. Colen SR, Baker DC, Shaw WW. Microvascular flap reconstruction of the head and neck: an overview. *Clin Plast Surg* 1983;10:73–83.
39. Watkinson JC, Breach NM. Free flaps in head and neck reconstructive surgery: a review of 77 cases. *Clin Otolaryngol* 1991;16:350–353.
40. Zuker RM, Rosen IB, Palmer JA, et al. Microvascular free flaps in head and neck reconstruction. *Can J Surg* 180;23:157–162.
41. Khouri RK. Avoiding free flap failure. *Clin Plast Surg* 1992;19:773–781.
42. Larson DL, Goepfert H. Limitations of the sternocleidomastoid musculocutaneous flap in head and neck cancer reconstruction. *Plast Reconstr Surg* 1982;70:328–332.
43. Quillen CG. Latissimus dorsi musculocutaneous flaps in head and neck reconstruction. *Plast Reconstr Surg* 1979;63:664–670.
44. Whitney TM, Buncke HJ, Lineaweaver WC, et al. Multiple microvascular transplants: a preliminary report of simultaneous versus sequential reconstruction. *Ann Plast Surg* 1989;22:391–404.
45. Shestak KC, Jones NF. Microsurgical free tissue transfer in the elderly patient. *Plast Reconstr Surg* 1991;88:259–263.
46. Tan E, O'Brien B, Brennen M. Free flap transfer in rabbits using irradiated recipient vessels. *Br J Plast Surg* 1978;31:121–123.
47. Watson JS. Experimental microvascular anastomosis in radiated vessels. A study of the patency rate and the histopathology of healing. *Plast Reconstr Surg* 1979;63:525–533.
48. Guelinckx PJ, Boeckx WD, Fossion E, et al. Scanning electron microscopy or irradiated recipient blood vessels in head and neck free flaps. *Plast Reconstr Surg* 1984;74:217–226.
49. Tabah RJ, Flynn MB, Acland RD, et al. Microvascular free tissue transfer in head and neck and esophageal surgery. *Am J Surg* 1984;148:498–504.
50. Kiener JL, Hoffman WY, Mathes SJ. Influence of radiotherapy on microvascular reconstruction in the head and neck region. *Am J Surg* 1991;162:404–407.
51. Lo Gerto FW, Handerschild CC, Quist WC. A clinical technique for prevention of spasm and preservation of endothelium in saphenous vein grafts. *Arch Surg* 1984;119:1212–1214.
52. Lee MS. Effect of nicotine on blood flow and patency of experimental microvascular anastomosis. *Plast Reconstr Surg* 1987; 80:763(abst).
53. Reus WF III, Colen LB, Straker DJ. Tobacco smoking and complications in elective microsurgery. *Plast Reconstr Surg* 1992;89:490–494.
54. Soutar DS, Scheker LR, Tanner NSB, et al. The radial forearm flap: a versatile method for intraoral reconstruction. *Br J Plast Surg* 1983;36:1–8.
55. Stern JR, Keller AJ, Wenig BL. Evaluation of reconstructive tech-

niques for oropharyngeal defects. *Ann Plast Surg* 1989; 22:332–336.
56. Wolff KD, Grundmann A. The free vastus lateralis flap: an anatomic study with case reports. *Plast Reconstr Surg* 1992;89:469–475.
57. Salebian AH, Rappaport J, Allison G. Functional oromandibular reconstruction with the microvascular composite groin flap. *Plast Reconstr Surg* 1985;76:819–825.
58. Beppu M, Hamel DP, Johnston GHF, et al. The osteocutaneous fibula flap: an anatomical study. *J Reconstr Microsurg* 1992;8:215–223.
59. Hidalgo DA. Aesthetic improvements in free flap mandible reconstruction. *Plast Reconstr Surg* 1991;88:574–585.
60. Taylor GI, Townsend P, Corlett R. Superiority of the deep circumflex iliac vessels for free groin flaps: clinical work. *Plast Reconstr Surg* 1979;65:745–759.
61. Jewer DD, Boyd JB, Manktelow RT, et al. Orofacial and mandibular reconstruction with iliac crest free flap: a review of 60 cases and a new method of classification. *Plast Reconstr Surg* 1989;84:391–403.
62. Soutar DS, Widdowson WP. Immediate reconstruction of the mandible using a vascularized segment of radius. *Head Neck Surg* 1986;8:232–246.
63. MacLeod AM, Robinson DW. Reconstruction of defects involving the mandible and floor of mouth by free osteo-cutaneous flaps derived from the foot. *Br J Plast Surg* 1982;35:239–246.
64. Serafin D, Riefkohl R, Thomas I, et al. Vascularized rib-periosteal and osteocutaneous reconstruction of the maxilla and mandible. An assessment. *Plast Reconstr Surg* 1980;66:718–727.
65. Swartz WM, Banis JC, Newton ED, et al. The osteocutaneous scapular flap for mandibular and maxillary reconstruction. *Plast Reconstr Surg* 1986;77:530–545.
66. Boyd JB, Gullane PJ, Rotstein LE, et al. Classification of the mandibular defect. *Plast Reconstr Surg* 1993;92:1266–1275.
67. Schusterman MA, Reece GP, Kroll SS, et al. Use of the AO plate for immediate mandibular reconstruction in cancer patients. *Plast Reconstr Surg* 1991;88:588–593.
68. Riediger D. Restoration of masticatory function by microsurgically revascularized iliac crest bone grafts using enosseous implants. *Plast Reconstr Surg* 1988;81:861–876.
69. Wessberg GA, Wolford LM, Epker BN. Simultaneous inferior alveolar nerve graft and osseous reconstruction of the mandible. *J Oral Maxillofac Surg* 1982;40:384–390.
70. Colen SR, Shaw WW, McCarthy JG. Review of the morbidity of 300 free flap donor sites. *Plast Reconstr Surg* 1986;77:948–953.
71. Boorman JG, Brown JA, Sykes PJ. Morbidity in the forearm flap donor site. *Br J Plast Surg* 1987;40:207–212.
72. Swanson E, Boyd JB, Manktelow RT. The radial forearm flap: reconstructive applications and donor site defects in 35 consecutive patients. *Plast Reconstr Surg* 1990;85:258–266.
73. Swanson E, Boyd JB, Mulholland RS. The radial forearm flap: a biomechanical study of the osteotomized radius. *Plast Reconstr Surg* 1990;85:267–272.
74. Timmons MJ, Missooten FEM, Poole MD, et al. Complications of radial forearm donor sites. *Br J Plast Surg* 1986;39:176–178.
75. Jones BM, O'Brien CJ. Acute ischemia of the hand resulting from elevation of a radial forearm flap. *Br J Plast Surg* 1985; 38:396–397.
76. Fatah MF, Nancarrow JD, Murray DS. Raising the radial artery forearm flap: the superficial ulnar artery "trap." *Br J Plast Surg* 1985;38:394–395.
77. Gilbert A, Teot L. The free scapular flap. *Plast Reconstr Surg* 1982;69:601–604.
78. Forrest C, Boyd B, Manktelow R, et al. The free vascularized iliac crest tissue transfer: donor site complications associated with eighty-two cases. *Br J Plast Surg* 1992;45:89–93.
79. Meland NB, Fisher J, Irons GB, et al. Experience with 80 rectus abdominis free tissue transfers. *Plast Reconstr Surg* 1989; 83:481–487.
80. Russell RC, Pribaz J, Zook EG, et al. Functional evaluation of the latissimus dorsi donor site. *Plast Reconstr Surg* 1986;78:336–344.
81. Logan AM, Black MJM. Injury to the brachial plexus resulting from shoulder positioning during latissimus dorsi pedicle dissection. *Br J Plast Surg* 1985;38:380–382.

SUGGESTED READING

Defries HO, Marble HB, Snell KW. Reconstruction of the mandible. Use of a homograft combined with autogenous bone and marrow. *Arch Otolaryngol* 1971;93:426–432.

Smith A, Bowen VA, Boyd JB. Donor site deficit of the osteocutaneous radial forearm flap. *Ann Plast Surg* 1994;32:372–376.

Taylor GI, Corlett RJ, Boyd JB. The versatile deep inferior epigastric (inferior rectus abdominis) flap. *Br J Plast Surg* 1984;37:330–350.

Discussion

MANDIBULAR RECONSTRUCTION

BLAIR M. MEHLING
GREGORY R. D. EVANS

We would like to commend Dr. Boyd for presenting an objective review of the literature pertinent to the outcomes and complications of mandibular reconstruction. To achieve optimal results in our specialty, it is essential that we first have an unbiased appraisal of the factors contributing to unfavorable results. Dr. Boyd has made a significant contribution in this regard. Herein, we attempt to expand on this chapter by sharing the philosophy and approach to mandibular reconstruction of the Department of Plastic Surgery at the University of Texas M. D. Anderson Cancer Center (UTMDACC) in Houston. We first discuss our criteria for flap selection, then some technical points that have helped us to improve our results in this challenging field of reconstructive surgery.

In 1984, when the last edition of this textbook was published, the overwhelming majority of mandibular defects encountered at UTMDACC were reconstructed with varying combinations of plates, nonvascularized bone grafts, and local soft tissue flaps (primarily pectoralis major). In fact, before 1988, only 12 free flaps had been performed at UTMDACC for defects at *all* anatomic sites, including the mandible (1). Since then, more than 2,200 free-tissue transfers, approximately 434 of which were for mandibular reconstruction, have been performed at our institution. Obviously, much has changed during the past decade! Why? Because for the complex defects and irradiated tissues encountered in head and neck oncologic reconstruction, it has become increasingly apparent that a microsurgical approach produces better outcomes than traditional approaches, with lower morbidity (1,2). Despite the increased complexity and operating time inherent in this approach, in the long run it has also proved to be more cost-effective (3).

When we reflect on our experience with mandibular reconstruction at UTMDACC, we are left with the impression that, in the broadest sense, the majority of our "unfavorable results" have been caused by errors in either of two areas. First are errors in flap selection, the failure to match each individual patient with the proper flap from our reconstructive armamentarium. Second are technical errors, costly mistakes in the execution of these complex and unforgiving reconstructions. We address each of these separately below.

FLAP SELECTION

In our opinion, careful flap selection is the single most important determinant of success in mandibular reconstruction. Close preoperative collaboration with the ablative surgeon remains the crucial element in this process. Preoperatively, key issues to be considered include the patient's overall medical fitness and prognosis for long-term survival, the location and size of the projected bone defect, the location and size of any concomitant soft tissue defect, whether the patient has received or will be receiving radiotherapy, the prognosis and plan for dental rehabilitation, and the status of all potential flap donor sites.

The most important decision in the process of flap selection is not which specific anatomical donor site to use; rather, it is the much more fundamental decision of whether to select a flap that includes vascularized bone or a flap comprised of soft tissue alone. The consequences of errors in this decision (bone vs. no bone) generally are much graver for the patient than errors in the selection of a specific donor site (e.g., fibula vs. iliac crest). Although all the factors listed above come into play when this decision is made, defect location and patient prognosis generally are the most heavily weighted at our institution.

Anterior Defects

We agree with Dr. Boyd that defects of the anterior mandible, which includes the area bearing the incisors and canines (the C segment), represent an absolute indication for reconstruction with vascularized bone, irrespective of the patient's prognosis or dental status (4). The "Andy Gump" deformity that results from failure to restore bony continuity across this re-

B. M. Mehling: Department of Plastic Surgery, The University of Texas M. D. Anderson Cancer Center, Houston, Texas
G. R. D. Evans: Division of Plastic Surgery, The University of California, Irvine, California

gion adequately is crippling both functionally and aesthetically and severely affects quality of life for these patients. Our experience has paralleled Dr. Boyd's in this region, in that attempts at less complex reconstructions by bridging the defect with a plate and soft tissue flap have yielded an unacceptably high frequency of complications (5,6).

Lateral Defects

For segmental lateral defects (anterior to the ramus and not including the C segment) in patients with a favorable or indeterminate prognosis for long-term survival, we again strongly advocate the use of vascularized bone, transferred either as bone alone or as an osteocutaneous flap, depending on soft tissue requirements. In our hands, this method provides the most predictable and favorable long-term results and remains the "gold standard" against which other methods of reconstruction must be evaluated. However, it is not uncommon at our institution to encounter patients with lateral defects who have a poor prognosis for long-term survival. We sometimes use soft tissue free flaps alone for reconstruction in this group of patients, without attempting to bridge the bony defect with a reconstruction plate. The combination of a plate and a soft tissue flap (without bone) is in fact an uncommon method of reconstruction at UTMDACC. Although our early reports of the plate/soft tissue option for lateral defects were favorable, our subsequent experience has been that this technique represents a race between the demise of the patient and the demise of the hardware (5–8). The literature suggests that complication rates for this technique are generally below 10% for patients with a "poor prognosis" (7% in our own series). On the other hand, an excellent study by Dr. Boyd has demonstrated that when complications do occur, these patients pay dearly in terms of "days of life lost," spending more than a month of their final days hospitalized during attempts at salvaging a failed reconstruction (6). Furthermore, if they defy the odds and live long enough, eventual failure of the reconstruction is in our experience inevitable (8). The surprisingly good results we have achieved in this group of patients by omitting the plate and reconstructing with soft tissue alone have led us now to favor this approach over the plate/soft tissue option. For patients with an indeterminate prognosis, and for selected patients with a "poor prognosis" who in our opinion would benefit from the moderate improvements in aesthetics and function provided by restoring continuity between the posterior and central segments, we still feel that the osteocutaneous flap provides the most definitive and reliable means of reconstruction and eliminates the possibility of having one day to salvage a failed soft tissue/plate reconstruction.

Posterior Defects

Posterior defects (i.e., ramus, with or without condyle) represent an area of considerable controversy. The arguments in favor of restoring bony continuity in this region are less compelling from a functional standpoint, particularly when the condyle or the pterygomasseteric muscle sling that stabilizes this segment has been resected. When this is the case, we generally reserve attempts at reconstruction with vascularized bone for younger patients with a favorable long-term prognosis. For elderly patients, and patients whose prognosis is uncertain or poor, we typically use soft tissue free flaps alone for reconstruction, with satisfactory results (8).

If the pterygomasseteric muscle sling and condyle are preserved, our selection criteria are similar to those for patients with lateral defects—that is, vascularized bone is the preferred method of reconstruction provided that the prognosis and overall medical condition of the patient justify the added complexity and potential for complications of this approach (9). When they do not, we favor reconstruction with soft tissue alone.

Posterior defects that extend anteriorly (mesially) are considered according to the same criteria we use for lateral or anterior defects, depending on how far anteriorly they extend. When these defects include the condyle and are to be reconstructed with vascularized bone, no clear consensus exists regarding how far posteriorly the reconstruction should be extended. One approach is to stop posteriorly at the angle; another is also to attempt reconstruction of the ramus and temporomandibular joint. Although the latter approach generally produces slightly better aesthetics, it is controversial whether the results are functionally superior. When we choose to attempt reconstruction of the ramus and temporomandibular joint, our most common approach at the joint is to create a pseudarthrosis by suspending the blunted end of the bone flap from the periosteum of the condylar fossa with a large, nonabsorbable suture. We also aim to provide a soft tissue interposition by utilizing the periosteal cuff remaining from any discarded bone at the proximal end of the (fibula) flap. In our experience, more elegant temporomandibular joint reconstructions, in which costochondral grafts or grafts of the native condyle are utilized, have not yielded results superior to those obtained with the much simpler pseudarthrosis method, most likely because these methods do not work well in the setting of preoperative or postoperative radiotherapy. We therefore cannot justify the added operative time and complexity in what is already a long and complex procedure.

From the preceding discussion, it should be evident that in a significant proportion of the patients who undergo composite resections of the posterior and lateral mandible at UTMDACC, reconstructions are performed with soft tissue free flaps alone, with no attempt made to reconstitute the integrity of the mandibular arch. This reflects the relatively large proportion of patients who are referred to our institution with locally advanced (T3, T4) or recurrent tumors and, sadly, the grim prognosis of this population. It also reflects the balance that we have struck after a decade of attempting to optimize results while minimizing complications in this challenging group of patients. Although we strongly feel that the osteocutaneous free flap is the current gold standard in mandibular reconstruction, we feel equally strongly that vascularized bone is neither necessary nor appropriate for every patient who undergoes composite resection of the mandible. The added complexity and morbidity of this approach must be justified on a case-by-case basis. At UTMDACC, soft tissue free flaps have been found to have lower failure and complication rates overall than their vascularized bone counterparts (7,9). Furthermore, when appropriately selected, our patients have found the functional and aesthetic results achieved with this technique to be quite acceptable (8). A recent review of 58 posterior mandible reconstructions performed at our institution compared the aesthetic and functional outcomes of patients who underwent reconstruction with soft tissue or osteocutaneous free flaps (10). A computer-assisted soft tissue cephalometric analysis found the aesthetic superiority of the osteocutaneous flaps to be minimal, and a statistically significant difference for only one of the measured parameters—midline symmetry. Functional assessment demonstrated superiority of the osteocutaneous reconstructions in only 5 of 12 functional subcategories, and the improvements seen, although statistically significant, were modest. We are currently more closely analyzing these apparent functional differences. Preliminary results indicate that the larger associated soft tissue defects and the greater likelihood of condylar resection may account for the slightly poorer functional outcomes of the group with soft tissue flaps.

Once we have made the critical decision of whether a given patient will undergo reconstruction with a vascularized bone flap or soft tissue alone, the selection of a specific free-flap donor site is generally relatively straightforward. Our first choice by far when vascularized bone is required is the fibula osteocutaneous flap. We feel that this flap provides optimal tissue and intraoperative convenience at the lowest price in terms of donor and recipient site complications. Although the skin paddle available with the fibula flap is smaller than those of the flaps from some of the other common vascularized bone donor sites, provided that one is prepared to apply a skin graft to the donor defect on the leg, it is adequate for the great majority of intraoral defects encountered. When it is insufficient (usually in the setting of a combined intraoral and extraoral soft tissue defect), we first consider whether a local flap (pectoralis major, cervicofacial, deltopectoral) is available that will reliably satisfy the remainder of the soft tissue requirement. If not, we resort to an alternate osteocutaneous flap donor site (most commonly iliac crest) or, if a single site will not satisfy the requirements of the defect, a second free flap. When the fibula is selected as the preferred donor site, we do not routinely perform preoperative angiography unless the patient has abnormal pedal pulses or a history suggesting vasculopathy or prior trauma to the leg.

For soft tissue free-flap reconstructions of mandibular defects, we favor the rectus abdominis myocutaneous (RAM) flap. Although the radial forearm flap is the more commonly used "workhorse" flap for intraoral reconstruction, the RAM flap is frequently overlooked for this purpose and is often a better choice (8). Objectively, this flap has the highest survival rates and lowest complication rates of all the flaps used for head and neck reconstruction at our institution (9). Subjectively, this wonderfully versatile flap is often more favorably positioned for simultaneous harvest during head and neck surgery than the radial forearm flap, and considerably less aesthetic deformity is produced with the use of this donor site. Furthermore, the added bulk provided by the thicker skin and muscular component of the RAM flap is frequently advantageous in the setting of mandibular reconstruction. In obese patients, in whom flap bulk is excessive, we have still successfully used this flap on several occasions by discarding the skin paddle and either skin-grafting the rectus muscle or allowing it to become mucosalized intraorally, which takes place spontaneously.

TECHNICAL CONSIDERATIONS

At UTMDACC, immediate reconstruction of the mandible has yielded both lower complication rates and better cost efficiency than delayed reconstruction (7). This is no doubt largely related to our two-team approach, whereby the free flap is harvested during the tumor resection. A detailed summary of our preferred techniques for flap design and harvest at each of the donor sites commonly associated with mandibular reconstruction has been presented elsewhere and Dr. Boyd has done an admirable job of listing the pros and cons of each site (11). Accordingly, we do not address these issues here. We would emphasize, however, that when properly designed, with the flap axis over the posterior intermuscular septum and harvested with a cuff of flexor hallucis longus and soleus muscle, the skin paddle of the fibula osteocutaneous flap is highly reliable (12).

For vascularized bone reconstructions, our preferred method of bone graft fixation is a sturdy mandibular reconstruction plate. Recently, we have been using a newer "locking" version of this plate (Synthes Maxillofacial, Paoli, Pennsylvania) with good results. The locking plate has the added advantages of providing more secure fixation despite incomplete bony apposition to the plate, requiring fewer screws per fragment for secure fixation, and theoretically causing less periosteal compression (and therefore allowing better vascularity) in the bone flap. Whenever possible, we contour the plate to the exposed mandible and drill holes both proximal and distal to the area where the bony resection will be performed. This approach has three main advantages. First, it controls the position of the posterior segment and prevents postoperative malocclusion by reestablishing the patient's centric relation at the temporomandibular joint. Second, it provides a template that permits the bone flap to be shaped accurately with osteotomies and to be attached to the plate while it is perfused *in situ* at the donor site. In this way, ischemia time is shortened significantly. Third, the use of this plate obviates the need for intermaxillary fixation. When we are unable to fashion a reconstruction plate before the bony resection, we use intermaxillary fixation to maintain the centric relation, and we use roentgenography or a skull from the anatomy laboratory to provide a template for bone shaping. When intermaxillary fixation is not technically possible, we have controlled the position of the posterior segment by temporarily applying an external fixator before the bony resection. In our hands, these methods are less reliable and more time-consuming than the reconstruction plate, and they are considerably more likely to result in some degree of postoperative malocclusion.

When shaping bone, we favor closing wedge osteotomies to minimize gaps that could lead to nonunion. For the same reason, the ends of the bone flap are intentionally left a few millimeters long on the plate and burred down at the recipient site to maximize apposition between bone graft and native mandible.

We strongly advocate the use of high-flow recipient vessels. Our most common practice is end-to-side anastomosis to the internal jugular vein and external carotid artery. This approach has been facilitated by the head and neck surgeons who are our colleagues; they favor functional neck dissections over the traditional radical neck dissection. Like Dr. Boyd, we have not noted any increase in flap failure with the use of previously irradiated vessels in the neck, and we do not hesitate to use them unless severe scarring in the area would make their dissection treacherous (1,9,13).

The pedicle length of the fibula flap is virtually always adequate if we dissect the peroneal vessels all the way back to their point of bifurcation from the posterior tibials, and we design the flap to optimize the position of vessel emergence into the neck (11). A few centimeters of added "effective length" can also be gained by subperiosteally stripping the bone no more than 2 to 3 cm at its proximal end. We reiterate, however, that high-flow vessels of reasonable caliber at the recipient site are an absolute prerequisite for flap success, and if such vessels cannot be reached without vein grafts, we do not hesitate to use them.

Dr. Boyd gives an excellent description of the pathogenesis of postoperative lip and chin ptosis after the reconstruction of central defects, in addition to reasonable strategies to prevent this deformity. Although we have encountered this phenomenon, two other sequelae more commonly compromise the aesthetic results of our mandibular reconstructions with vascularized bone. The first of these is soft tissue hollowing in the submental and submandibular regions. This is usually the result of a true deficiency of soft tissue resulting from both the floor of mouth resection and the neck dissection. It is frequently exacerbated by the tissue scarring and fibrosis that develop after radiotherapy. It is best prevented by taking a relatively generous cuff of soleus and flexor hallucis longus with the fibula flap and using this soft tissue to replace the absent bulk in the submandibular region. In patients who will be undergoing radiotherapy, we usually aim for a slight initial overcorrection. The second adverse aesthetic sequela is a prognathic postoperative appearance. This frequently results from the combined effects of a high-profile reconstruction plate and edentulous segments after tooth extraction, which can cause lower lip retrusion or overrotation. Such an appearance can also be exacerbated by the aforementioned submandibular hollowing. It is usually most effectively addressed by restoring the occlusal surface through dental rehabilitation. Some authors have suggested preventing it by shifting the reconstruction plate posteriorly by one hole when it is set into the mandible. Although this approach is probably acceptable for the edentulous patient, we do not advocate it for patients with teeth because of the risk for disrupting the occlusal relationship.

Postoperatively, we emphatically agree with Dr. Boyd that systemic anticoagulants have not been shown to confer any beneficial effect on the patency of microvascular anastomoses in the uncomplicated clinical setting. Meticulous technique, not heparin or dextran, prevents thrombosis. Accordingly, we do not routinely administer postoperative anticoagulants of any type, including aspirin. Venous thromboembolism prophylaxis is provided through the use of pneumatic compression stockings alone. We do not warm the patient's room beyond a comfortable temperature, nor do we religiously avoid caffeine or follow special "flap diets." We monitor our flaps by hourly clinical assessment of color, capillary refill, and percutaneous "pencil" Doppler examination of a perforating vessel in the skin flap (marked by a single 6-0 suture). For buried bone flaps, or for skin paddles with an intraoral location too deep to be accessible, we are increasingly utilizing a 20-MHz implanted Doppler probe (Cook Vascular, Leechburg, Pennsylvania) placed around the flap vein. We do not routinely perform radionuclide bone scans in our patients because our experience has been that if the soft tissue component of an osteocutaneous reconstruction is viable, so is the bone—particularly in the case of a fibula flap. Whatever means of monitoring we choose, if there is *any* question of flap compromise, a return to the operating room is indicated. A brief exploration of the flap pedicle to verify that all is well is far less risky for the patient than a missed microvascular thrombosis.

Most of our patients have a swallowing assessment by a speech pathologist at 7 to 10 days postoperatively. If no problems with aspiration are noted and the intraoral skin paddle inset appears healthy, oral intake of fluids can be commenced at this time, with progression to a soft diet. As for dental rehabilitation with osseointegrated implants, only 12% of the patients who undergo mandibular reconstruction at UTMDACC currently receive this technology (14). Reasons for this include the limited life span of many of our patients, the frequent use of adjuvant radiotherapy and the associated risk for osteoradionecrosis, and last but not least, the high cost of the procedure (an average of $6,000 to $8,000 at our institution), which is borne almost exclusively by the patients themselves. Despite a considerable body of literature supporting improved patient outcomes after osseointegrated dental rehabilitation in a reconstructive setting, we have had very little success thus far in obtaining third party reimbursement for the procedure.

Clearly, we have come a long way in our efforts to reconstruct composite defects of the mandible in the 15 years that have passed since the last edition of this textbook. We cannot resist the temptation to end by speculating about where we will be 15 years from now. The field of tissue engineering holds exciting possibilities for the future and may one day provide us with the "ultimate" mandible reconstruction: an exact replica of the missing tissue that can be transferred with great reliability and little morbidity, and without the need to sacrifice tissue from another anatomical site. Although such an idea may seem farfetched today, we recall that not so long ago, the notion that free flaps would become our preferred means of mandibular reconstruction seemed equally preposterous. Tissue engineering is still in its infancy, however, and we have a long way to go before such ideas become reality. In the interim, we must continue to strive for excellence with our current methods of microsurgical mandibular reconstruction, always evaluating and learning from our results, both favorable and unfavorable.

REFERENCES

1. Schusterman MA, Miller MJ, Reece GP, et al. A single center's experience with 308 free flaps for repair of head and neck cancer defects. *Plast Reconstr Surg* 1994;93:472–480.
2. Kroll SS, Reece GP, Miller MJ, et al. Comparison of the rectus abdominis free flap with the pectoralis major myocutaneous flap for reconstructions in the head and neck. *Am J Surg* 1992;164:615–618.
3. Kroll SS, Evans GR, Goldberg D, et al. A comparison of resource costs for head and neck reconstruction with free and pectoralis major flaps. *Plast Reconstr Surg* 1997;99:1282–1286.
4. Boyd JB, Gullane PJ, Rotstein LE, et al. Classification of mandibular defects. *Plast Reconstr Surg* 1993;92:1266–1275.
5. Schusterman MA, Reece GP, Kroll SS, et al. Use of the AO plate for immediate mandibular reconstruction in cancer patients. *Plast Reconstr Surg* 1991;88:588–593.
6. Boyd JB, Mulholland RS, Davidson J, et al. The free flap and plate in oromandibular reconstruction: long-term review and indications. *Plast Reconstr Surg* 1995;95:1018–1028.
7. Kroll SS, Schusterman MA, Reece GP. Costs and complications in mandibular reconstruction. *Ann Plast Surg* 1992;29:341–347.
8. Kroll SS, Robb GL, Miller MJ, et al. Reconstruction of posterior mandibular defects with soft tissue using the rectus abdominis free flap. *Br J Plast Surg* 1998;51:503–507.
9. Kroll SS, Schusterman MA, Reece GP, et al. Choice of flap and incidence of free flap success. *Plast Reconstr Surg* 1996; 98:459–463.
10. Gallas MT, Miller MJ, King TW, et al. Flap selection for optimal functional and aesthetic reconstruction of the posterior mandible [Poster Presentation]. Annual meeting of the American Society for Reconstructive Microsurgery (ASRM), Miami, Florida, January 9, 2000.
11. Schusterman MA, ed. Microsurgical reconstruction of the cancer patient. Philadelphia: Lippincott–Raven Publishers, 1997.
12. Schusterman MA, Reece GP, Miller MJ, et al. The osteocutaneous free fibula flap: is the skin paddle reliable? *Plast Reconstr Surg* 1992;90:787–798.
13. Kroll SS, Robb GL, Reece GP, et al. Does prior irradiation increase the risk of total or partial free flap loss? *J Reconstr Microsurg* 1998;14:263–268.
14. Gurlek A, Miller MJ, Jacob RF, et al. Functional results of dental restoration with osseointegrated implants after mandible reconstruction. *Plast Reconstr Surg* 1998;101:650–659.

35

FACIAL AND NASAL RECONSTRUCTION

FREDERICK J. MENICK

The goals of an aesthetic reconstruction should be to blend scars, avoid a patchlike replacement of the defect, recreate landmark symmetry and match the contralateral normal face, establish three-dimensional contour and a facial shape, and minimize donor deformity (1).

Ultimately, a reconstruction should restore the face and the patient to function within society. To obtain such results, the surgeon must continually ask, "Where do I wish to go? How can I get there? What do I do to accomplish the task?" Poor results are usually caused by a failure of *vision,* a failure of *planning,* or a failure of *fabrication.*

VISION

Aristotle has said, "Art is the conceptualization of the final result before its realization in the material." Vision is intrinsic to every aspect of facial reconstruction. The short-term and long-term effects of each action must be considered at each step until the final product reflects the desired goal.

The primary function of the face is to look normal. Patients expect more than a healed wound. They wish to look normal—not horrible, peculiar, or even different. Plastic surgeons must respect the importance of facial reconstruction to the patient, to themselves, and to their specialty. We bear a great responsibility. A complex defect can overwhelm the surgeon, and when the surgeon fears making things worse or has limited expectations, the result is inaction or poor action. Although a patient's natural fears and anxieties, the costs of a procedure, scheduling problems, number of stages required, associated morbidity, and technical complexity may misdirect us, the surgeon's responsibility is to guide the patient through the process to normalcy.

Results must be measured by patient satisfaction and objective visual aesthetics, not by the amount of tissue transferred or tissue viability. The emphasis must shift from discussions of blood supply and anatomy to the visual aesthetic. There is a difference between "healed" and "restored," and a difference between technical complexity and visual aesthetic complexity. One might describe a modern tawdry movie romance as excitement without commitment. Similarly, a quick, superficial, and unfeeling approach to facial reconstruction will not truly satisfy the patient or the surgeon.

F. J. Menick: Private Practice, St. Joseph's Hospital, Tucson, Arizona

PSYCHOLOGY OF PERCEPTION

The face is a gestalt of color, contrasts, lines, and reflections that identify each of us as beautiful, ugly, normal or abnormal (2). Our eyes are not a lens, nor our brain photographic paper. The study of psychology reveals that when we view an object, our minds and eyes sort and select significant details from a myriad of colors, contrasts, forms, and motions that are visible to the eye. Consciously and unconsciously, the mind seeks answers to questions: Who or what am I looking at? Is that a nose or a lip? Attractive, grotesque, normal, or abnormal? If the basic components of an expected visual image are present, and if deficiencies are few, we quickly recognize the familiar. We assume the expected, even if on close inspection all the elements are not actually present. In contrast, we see the unexpected—the jarring abnormality that draws our utmost attention and critical analysis and causes us to recognize it immediately as abnormal.

The reconstructive surgeon must acknowledge that it is impossible to recreate Mother Nature. No combination of cover, lining, or support can be a nose, lip, or eyelid. A successful reconstruction is only a visual illusion. It must appear to be what it is not. So a surgeon must assemble a facsimile fabricated from otherwise expendable parts that appears to be normal in quality, outline, and contour. The surgeon must recreate an image that is recognized as familiar and that is not visually "unexpected"—the abnormal. We must supply the visual elements that make something familiarly "what it is" while avoiding the creation of distracting deficiencies or unexpected abnormalities that draw too close visual scrutiny.

Regional Units

The face is divided by ridges and valleys into slightly convex and slightly concave surfaces whose contour is determined by the underlying hard and soft tissues (Fig. 35-1). Each region has a specific skin quality (color, texture, thickness, character, type of hair), outline, and three-dimensional contour. Our eyes pass over the smooth, expansive surfaces of the face and light on the ridges and valleys that create facial landmarks and identify the characteristic parts. Although skin quality is important, contour, outline, and symmetry of landmarks are the primary determinants of "normal." Color or texture can be altered by makeup, but a contour abnormality cannot be camouflaged (except, for instance, by a moustache when a hair-bearing scalp flap is employed to resurface the upper lip in a man). Skin quality, although important, is secondary and varies from unit to unit and within units.

The forehead is divided into one large central and two lateral subunits by the contours formed by the bony buttresses of the temporal crest and zygomatic arches, which outline the superior and inferior boundaries of the lateral subunits. The skin of the forehead has a smooth, shiny, and tight character in both the central and lateral units.

The nose can be divided into the subunits of the dorsum, tip, and columella and the paired sidewalls, alae, and soft triangles. Although the valleys and ridges of contour define the nasal subunits, the nasal skin itself varies in texture and thickness over the nasal surface. The upper two-thirds of the nose is covered by thin, smooth, and mobile skin, whereas most of the lower one-third is thick and pitted except along the alar rims, inferior tip, and columella. The thick and thin zones of nasal skin do not correspond to subunit contour and outline, which are established by the shapes of underlying hard and soft tissues.

The subunits of the upper lip are defined by the contour changes of the nasolabial folds, philtrum columns, and midline depression to form two lateral and two medial subunits.

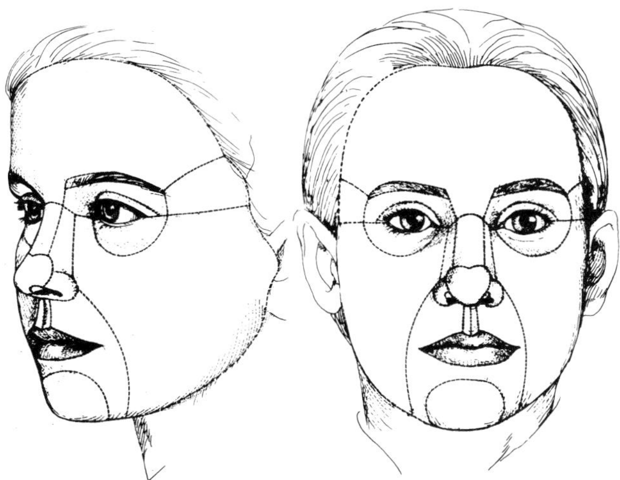

FIGURE 35-1. The facial units are adjacent concave and convex topographical areas of characteristic skin quality, outline, and contour. (From Menick FJ. Facial reconstruction in regional units. *Perspect Plast Surg* 1994;8,106, with permission.)

Within these boundaries, a hairless triangle of smooth skin is situated between the alar base and cheek and a hairless strip along the vermilion and white roll. Most of the upper lip is covered by matte hair in women and a beard in men.

The central facial units (nose, lip, eyelids) contribute most significantly to the visual facial gestalt. These midfacial units are contoured in a complex and subtle fashion. They are seen in primary gaze, and their contralateral normal subunits are available for critical comparison in almost all views. They are fixed units. Any expected alteration in size, shape, character, or symmetry creates an obvious discrepancy. These central landmarks are of primary visual interest, and their contributions to facial expression and motor function play an important role in the facial norm.

In contrast, the units of the facial periphery (forehead and cheek) act like a picture frame. They are largely flat, expansive surfaces of secondary interest. Their borders vary with age, sex, hairline position, hairstyle, and expression. Their dimensions and outlines are not fixed, varying from person to person and from time to time. The outline of their contralateral subunits cannot be simultaneously compared in any view. Although the central units must be reconstructed exactly, only gross abnormalities of a peripheral unit capture our attention. A discrepancy of unit outline is of lesser importance.

In the past, too much emphasis has been placed on analyzing defect dimensions (length, width, and depth of the wound), anatomical loss (cover, lining, or support), or donor blood supply (skin graft, random flap, axial flap, myocutaneous flap). The face is made up of regional units—topographical areas of characteristic skin quality, outline, and contour that define it. The surgeon must visualize the desired end result, not the defect. An examination of the wound provides anatomical information about the loss but not about the aesthetic requirements for an ideal reconstruction. With the normal desired result in mind, specific plans, priorities, materials, and methods of reconstruction must be developed to rebuild units. The reconstructive surgeon should spend less time visualizing the wound and more time "seeing" the normal that is missing and must be replaced. The reconstruction of a normal face depends on restoring normal skin quality and the outlines and contours that define the subunits while limiting unacceptable scarring.

PLANNING

When presented with a facial defect, surgeons must stop and think (3). Combining their visual aesthetic and a scientific knowledge of anatomy, wound healing, and tissue transfer, they must use direct observation, intuition, and imagination in an overall plan designed to achieve the desired goal (restoration of facial units). First mentally and then in actuality, each step is evaluated and modified to ensure the expected result. An imaginary outline of the entire reconstruction should be prepared as a road map preoperatively. Each surgical maneuver, revision, or complication must be reviewed. A logical explanation of each success or failure should be sought.

How to Plan

First, surgeons must know the normal. Then they must perform an examination and consider the patient's age, associated diseases, and goals; any past history of injury, surgery, smoking, and radiation; and any risk for local cancer recurrence. The defect is analyzed in terms of site, size, shape, depth, exposure of vital structures, tissue nonviability, and infection. The goal of reconstruction must be defined—a healed wound, functional restoration, or an aesthetic result. Is survival more important than aesthetics, the transfer of bulk tissue more important than finesse, or a healed wound more important than the restoration of normal?

With the desired end result in mind, the anatomical and aesthetic requirements of reconstruction must be determined. What is present? What is missing? What is available at the defect or donor sites that can be used to create what is wanted? Direct wound measurements, preoperative photographs and radiographs, and at times a facial moulage are combined to formulate a list of anatomical and aesthetic needs. This is best written down as part of a permanent plan and is often combined with personal drawings to form a record that can be turned to during each stage of the reconstruction. Anatomically, the wound requirements of cover, lining, and support are determined and the regional unit needs for skin quality, outline, and contour defined.

Surgical planning consists of a series of goals, priorities, and choices of materials, methods, stages, and timing. A series of surgical steps is planned to bring vision into reality. Most importantly, the surgeon must take the time to think. With the ultimate goal kept in mind, short-term and long-term objectives are determined.

False Principles

Traditionally, the primary goal of facial reconstruction was to achieve wound healing and defect closure. "Filling" was the priority. Certain reconstructive principles often misdirected the surgeon (Fig. 35-2):

1. *Design the flap from a pattern of the defect.* Unfortunately, a "hole" seldom represents what is missing. If contracted by a scar, the apparent defect appears smaller than its actual size. If enlarged by edema, local injection of anesthetic, or the tension of resting skin, it appears larger. Traditionally, skin grafts or flaps have been placed in existing defects. However, the ideal normal—not disease,

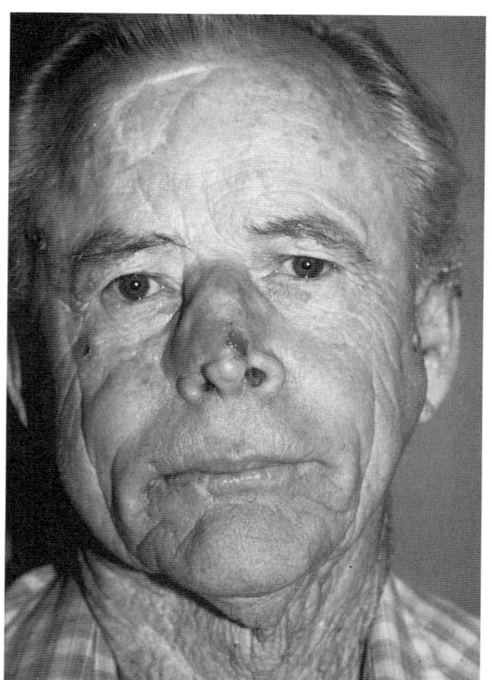

A

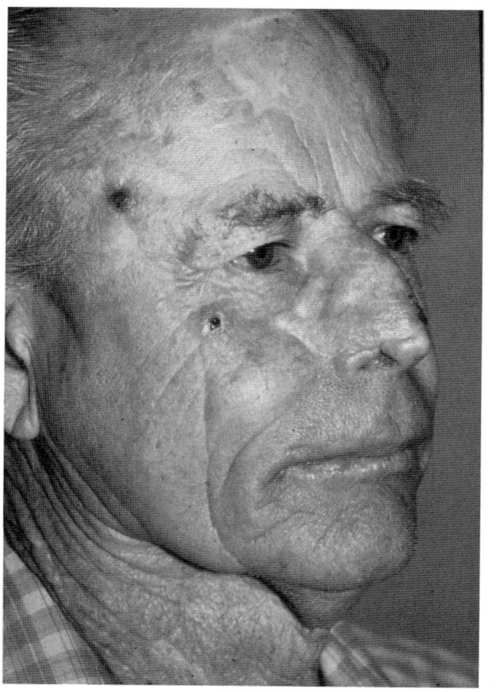

B

FIGURE 35-2. A,B: With the use of "false principles," a nasal defect encompassing parts of the bridge, tip, right sidewall, and cheek has been reconstructed by transferring a large forehead flap to fill the entire defect without wound modification. The reconstruction appears as a large, poorly formed patch within the central face. (From Menick FJ. Aesthetic refinements in the use of the forehead for nasal reconstruction. *Clin Plast Surg* 1990;17:607, with permission.)

injury, or congenital deficiency—determines tissue requirements, priorities, and techniques.

2. *Take extra tissue to be safe.* Taking extra tissue "for good measure" or because of fear for the vascularity of a flap only complicates the reconstruction. As the flap contracts, the excess tissue "trapdoors" and obliterates surface contour. Additional stages of reconstruction are then required to tailor the excess and contour the extra bulk.
3. *Make the flap smaller to preserve the donor site.* This approach nearly always makes the regional deformity worse. Restoration of the central facial units should be given the highest priority. If tissue is inadequately replaced in a midface defect, the reconstructed side will not match the contralateral normal side, and adjacent facial landmarks, such as the alar base or philtral column, will be distorted. When a forehead flap that is too small is transferred to the nose, the existent tip, alar margin, and alar base are displaced inward toward the defect. The nose becomes distorted and asymmetrical.
4. *Use a tissue expander to conserve the donor site.* The tissue expander creates the modern correlation—make the donor site "larger" to preserve it. Again, the priorities are confused. Preexpansion of a forehead flap for nasal reconstruction destroys the important qualities of thinness and softness in the flap and resurfaces the new nose with stretched skin, lined by a bed of scar that tends to contract. In an attempt to spare the forehead donor site, the priorities are confused. The nose is an uncompromising facial feature, whereas the forehead is a forgiving one. Shortchanging the nasal contour to spare the appearance of the forehead is a mistake. If necessary, tissue expansion or a whole-unit skin graft can be used to restore the forehead at a later stage. The surgeon should harvest whatever skin is necessary to reconstruct the nose, with little concern for the donor site. However, the expansive flat nature of the peripheral units (cheek or forehead) does lend itself to skin expansion for their own repair.
5. *One hole, one flap, one operation.* Composite defects are those that overlap two or more facial units. Frequently, a nasal defect extends into adjacent cheek or lip, producing a large, three-dimensional wound that encompasses several facial units. Often, the simplest and most obvious reconstructive solution is to fill the hole and replace missing bulk. Although a single defect can be filled with a single flap at a single operation, this approach may defeat the goal of restoring a normal appearance. First, resultant scars are obvious because they are not hidden within normal contour lines. The transferred tissue appears as a patch. Second, it is difficult to reproduce the delicate three-dimensional character of multiple units with a single flap. When a single flap spans several three-dimensional units, it takes a surgical shortcut across the face and fails to supply enough skin to resurface the complex topography. Secondary attempts to improve the result are permanently hampered by a net skin deficit. Third, myofibroblasts lie within a bed of scar beneath all healing flaps. The inevitable force of biologic wound contraction draws the overlying tissues into a domelike mass—the trapdoor effect. Wound contraction acts on a single large flap that overlies several facial units by pulling all tissues toward the common center. Delayed attempts to divide and shape the single, large, haphazard flap into individual convex or concave surfaces are rarely successful. Also, when the principle of one hole, one flap is applied to repair a full-thickness nasal defect (e.g., folding a forehead flap to supply both cover and lining), additional problems with flap vascularity, the inability to place a primary support framework, and bulkiness of folded tissues further complicate the situation.
6. *Place a supportive framework secondarily after soft tissue wound maturation.* Often, nasal cover and lining are supplied without initial support. Once the soft tissues have healed, large bone and cartilage tissues are placed to act as a cantilever graft to lift the dorsum and tip. Because of their bulk and the risk for extrusion, this framework is not placed primarily but is added months later in final touch-up operations. Surgeons are reluctant to place bone and cartilage grafts in the nose at the initial operation primarily because of the risk for lining flap necrosis, infection, and graft extrusion. Unfortunately, once gravity, tension, and the contracting effects of the healing process are completed, the soft tissue contour can rarely be regained. If missing, the normal cartilaginous framework of the dorsum, tip, ala, columella, and sidewall should be replaced at the primary operation as it was before it was damaged.
7. *The presence and number of scars determine the final result. Place incisions in existing scars. Minimize scars.* All wounds heal by scarring and all scars are visible. A fear of scarring has led to the use of one flap or graft to repair each defect, the avoidance of local tissue rearrangement and wound modification, and the use of distant, poorly matched tissue for facial reconstruction in the hope of limiting the number and length of local incisions and their resulting scars. However, a scar is not a deformity. A thin, flat scar within a normal contour line is largely invisible. In fact, existing scars can often be ignored and not reexcised. Instead, incisions should be placed in the normal facial contour lines, such as the alar crease, alar-labial fold, and nasolabial groove.
8. *Never throw anything away.* Surgeons are taught to preserve normal tissue. Although a dog-ear, a scrap of covering skin, or a bit of scar can be turned in for lining or subcutaneous bulk to great advantage, rarely is the wound altered and normal tissue discarded to improve the result and permit a more ideal unit reconstruction. When a defect encompasses only part of a facial unit and the defect is simply patched, the scars that surround the repair create unexpected lines of light and shadow that

do not follow the hills and valleys of normal contour. Although the scars fade somewhat with maturation, their reflection or depression distorts the final result forever if they are not positioned in the joins between units.

Subunit Principles

A reconstructive plan based on the psychology of perception, an understanding of wound healing, and the subunits of the face can produce better results (Fig. 35-3):

1. *The normal is recreated by establishing facial contour, highlights, and landmarks. The presence or absence of scars is of lesser importance.* Fastidious patients want not only a healed wound but a normal appearance. They want the missing part to be restored to its original color, texture, thickness, hair character, outline, and contour. Regional facial units must be restored.
2. *Restore units, not defects.* If a defect is simply filled without regard to facial subunits, a graft or flap will appear as a distracting patch within the unit. However, if defects are resurfaced in units, the segmental quality of the facial surface will be maintained. Flaps and grafts should be designed to replace topographical units. Unit replacement of missing tissue positions scars within the joins between adjacent units, harnesses the contractile force of the myofibroblast to help simulate the surface contour of surface units, and directs the choice of suitable donor tissues.
3. *Alter the site, size, outline, and depth of wounds to permit reconstruction of entire units.* The extent of destruction required to ablate a skin cancer does not necessarily equal the extent of reconstruction needed to restore facial aesthetics. The wound should be manipulated so that the reconstruction conforms to subunit principles. Frequently, the defect should be enlarged and the entire unit resurfaced rather than just part of it. If a defect encompasses more than one unit and extends into another, the wound margin may be advanced inward. This positions the final border scar along the expected border of adjacent units and allows reconstruction of the defect as a single unit. Another approach would be to enlarge the defect and resurface the involved units with a single flap, two separate flaps, or a flap and a skin graft, depending on the aesthetic requirements.
4. *Discard adjacent normal tissue to improve the result.* When more than 50% of the unit has been lost and the restoration of normal is the goal, it is appropriate to replace the entire unit, not merely patch the defect. This means that normal skin must be discarded within the unit and the wound enlarged. Border scars are thus positioned so that they reflect lines of light and cast linear shadows that mimic the normal ridges and valleys that separate topographical units. In the same way, like the trapdoor contraction that develops in a flap used to replace a convex unit such as the dorsum, tip, or ala of the nose, the resultant bulge will resemble the expected convexity of these subunits.
5. *Use exact patterns to design flaps.* Exact three-dimensional foil templates are made of the unit defect. If too much skin is supplied, it will contract postoperatively and obscure the detail created by any underlying support framework. If too little is supplied, it will be too tight and cause an underlying cartilage framework to collapse. Therefore, a three-dimensional foil pattern must be cut, bent, and crimped to fit the defect exactly.
6. *The contralateral normal or the ideal is used as a guide when possible.* Tissue must be replaced in the exact amount necessary to restore normal facial appearance. The contralateral normal unit or subunit can be used as a guide to create a template that exactly replaces the missing surface skin in quantity and outline. Remember that a wound may be expanded by edema, local anesthetic, or wound tension, or it may be contracted by scar, so that the true dimensions of the tissue loss will not be reflected. No extra tissue is taken, nor is the flap made smaller than needed to preserve the donor site.
7. *Integrate contour into the initial and all subsequent stages.* The underlying structure of hard and soft tissue creates the hills and valleys of the facial contours—the visual topographical patterns of regional units. An ideal contour must be a primary reconstructive objective and integrated into the initial and all subsequent reconstructive stages. An underlying framework must be assembled to form the contour of the expected facial feature. In nasal reconstruction, primary cartilage grafts are used to recreate the subsurface contours of a nose and to brace the soft tissue of cover and lining against contraction or collapse. During an intermediate stage, 3 weeks after transfer and before wound maturation, a forehead flap may be reelevated before its pedicle is divided; this allows the placement of additional grafts and extensive subcutaneous sculpturing of soft tissue and scar to improve the final nasal contour. Reexpansion of a previously placed covering flap that is fixed by a scar in a contracted position months later is difficult or impossible. Similarly, in cheek reconstruction, a fat flip-flap can be used to restore the missing soft tissue bulk required to recreate the gentle slope of the nasal-cheek join. When the nasolabial fold is destroyed by flap advancement, an incision can be made at the site of a new nasolabial fold and underlying soft tissue sculpted to create a visually correct nasolabial crease.
8. *Choose ideal donor materials and use an ideal method of transfer.* Traditionally, the choice of tissue transfer method has been based on wound vascularity and depth. Skin grafts are recommended to resurface well-vascularized superficial defects when only skin and a small amount of subcutaneous tissue are missing. Donor sites from above the clavicle seem best suited for facial repair. Skin flaps are used to resupply bulk to a deep defect or to

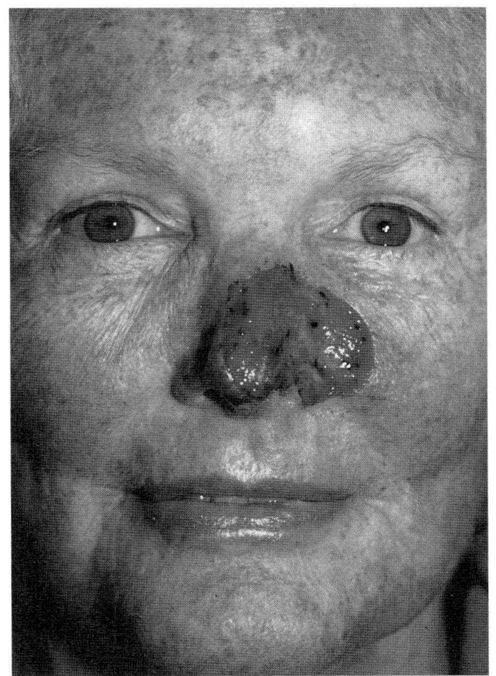

A

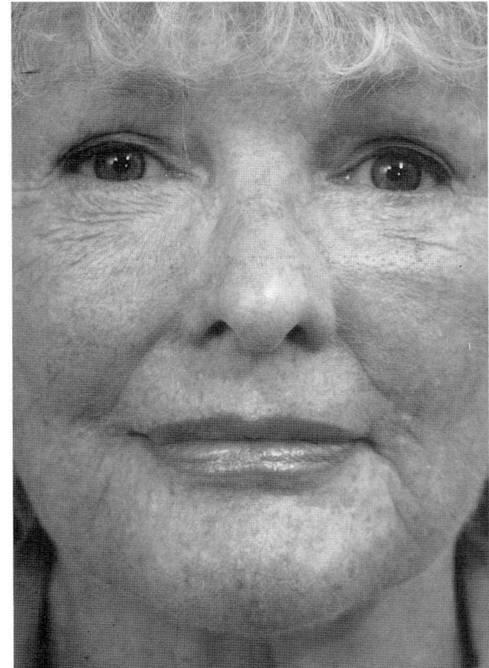

B

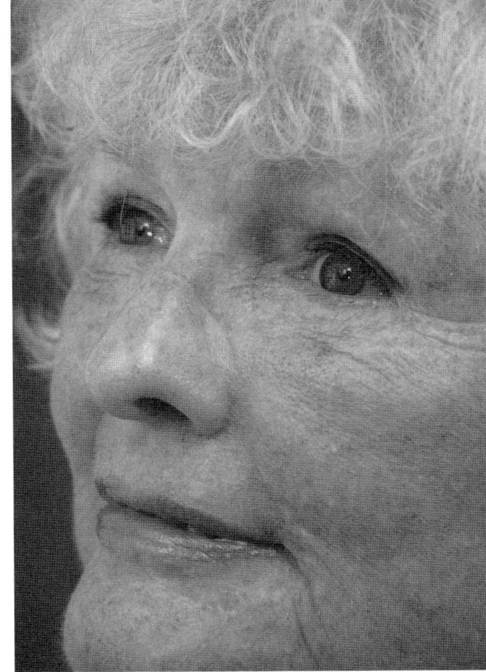

C

FIGURE 35-3. A–C: A similar defect is present after Mohs' excision of a basal cell carcinoma within parts of the dorsum, tip, left ala, and sidewall and extending onto the cheek. The use of subunit principles to reconstruct this woman's defect as individual units restored the appearance of normalcy. Cheek tissue was moved as a superiorly and laterally based flap to reconstruct the cheek as a separate unit, so that the final scars were left along the junction of the cheek and sidewall and within the nasolabial fold. A paramedian forehead flap was used to resurface the entire dorsum, sidewall, ala, and tip after excision of the adjacent normal skin that remained in those subunits after the Mohs' excision. Primary cartilage grafts and extensive subcutaneous sculpturing were used to restore support and a nasal shape. (From Menick FJ. Facial reconstruction in regional units. *Perspect Plast Surg* 1994;8,121, with permission.)

cover a poorly vascularized recipient bed or a wound with vital or support structures exposed or missing. Adjacent local skin is preferred to distant tissue.

A skin graft, even one from an appropriate donor site that is matched preoperatively to the recipient site, is subjected to transient ischemia during the period of skin graft take, so that unpredictable color and texture changes may occur after transfer. Postoperatively, skin grafts are typically shiny, atrophic, and either hypopigmented or hyperpigmented. Thus, a shiny, smooth skin graft might be a good choice to resurface a superficial defect within the shiny, nonpitted skin of the nasal sidewall or dorsum, but it will stand out as a mismatched patch if used within the pitted, sebaceous nasal tip, where a flap would be a better choice. Remember also that myofibroblasts lie within a sheet of scar between a skin graft or skin flap and its recipient bed. Although a skin graft may shrink within its boundaries, it does not rise above the surface level of the adjacent recipient skin. Flaps, however, have a tendency to "pincushion," assuming convex forms as they contract. For this reason, flaps are best employed to replace convex surfaces, whereas grafts are better for planar or concave recipient sites (Figs. 35-4 and 35-5).

Skin expansion is ideally used to supply skin to a flat sur-

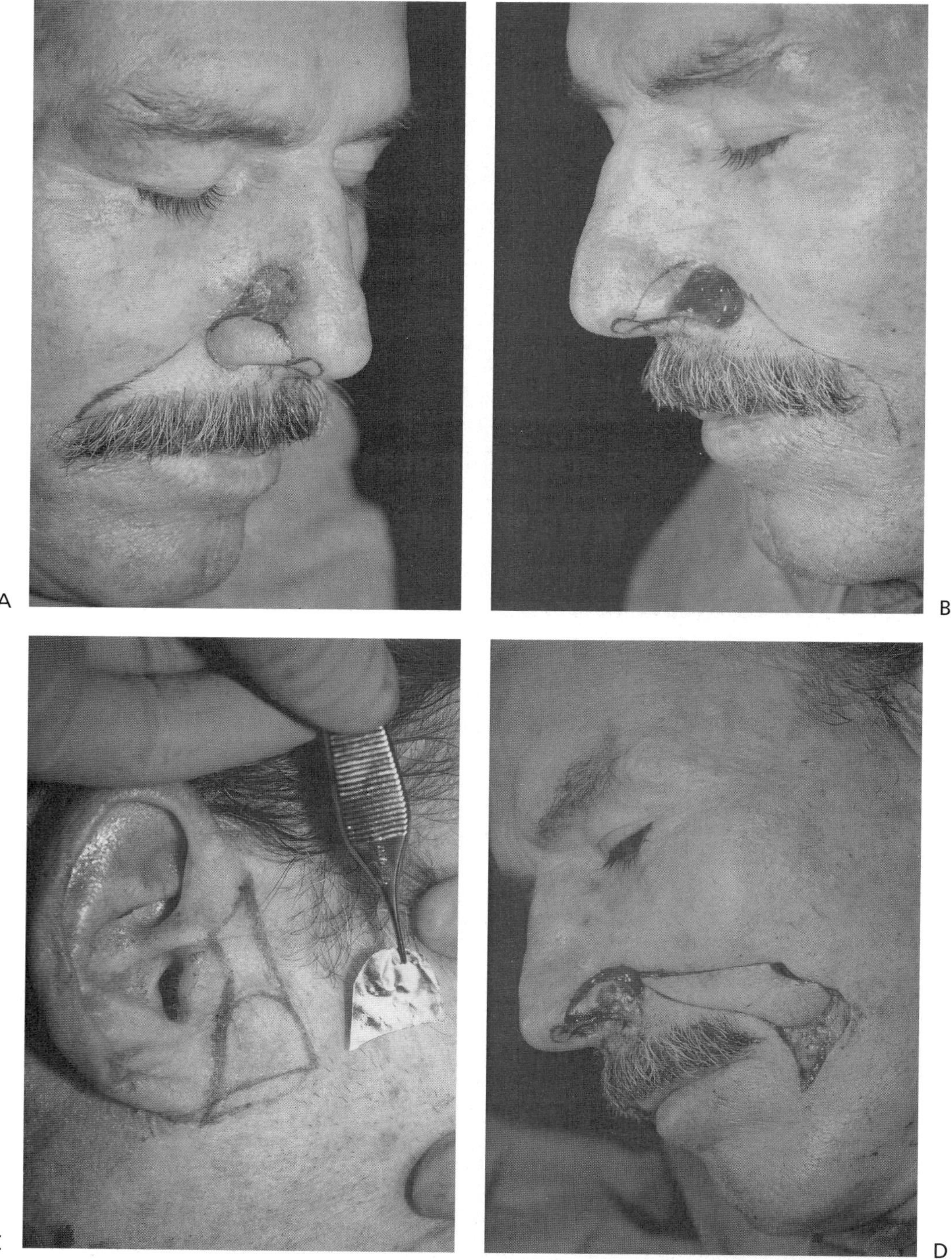

FIGURE 35-4. A–D: A full-thickness preauricular skin graft has been used to resurface the normal flat, shiny, and smooth right sidewall without regard to unit design. The left ala defect was enlarged by discarding adjacent normal skin, and a two-stage nasolabial flap was used simultaneously to resurface the left ala as a unit in this middle-aged man. (Courtesy of F. J. Menick, Tucson, Arizona.)

A

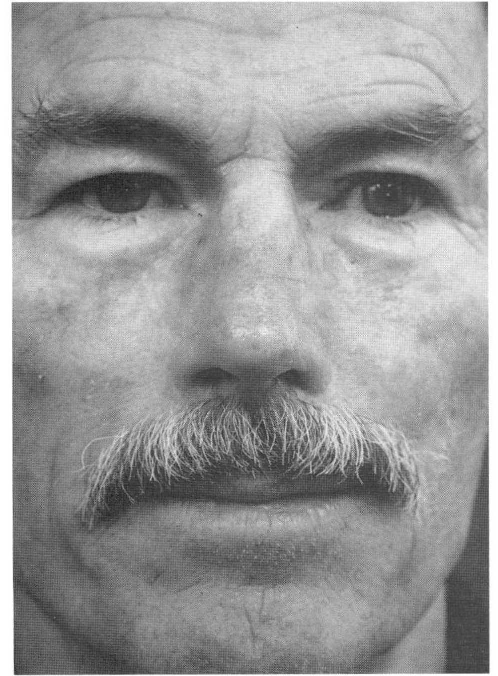

B

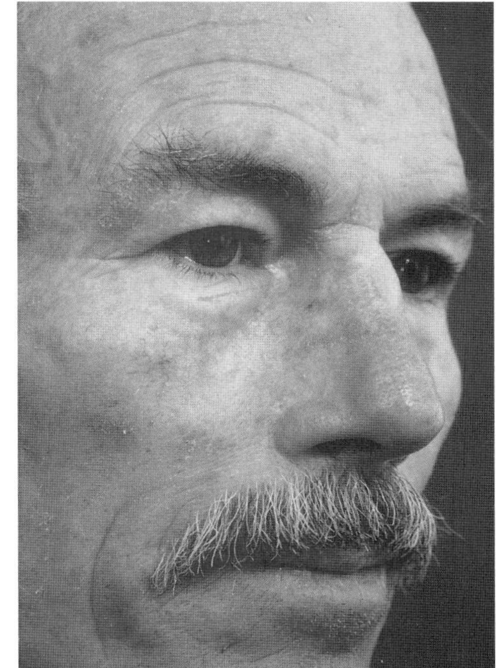

C

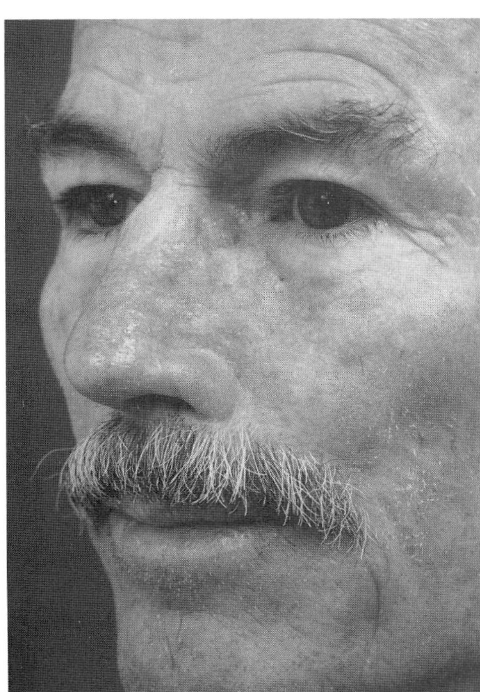

FIGURE 35-5. A–C: Postoperatively, the shiny, tight skin graft blends well within the right sidewall unit. The left ala appears normal because flap contraction and unit scar positioning have added to the expected alar convex contour and positioned the final scars in the alar unit joins. (Courtesy of F. J. Menick, Tucson, Arizona.)

face defect by simple advancement. It is less suited to reconstruction in areas containing mobile landmarks or requiring complex contour restoration with thin, conforming, noncontracting flaps. With these rules in mind, the surgeon can harness the forces of wound healing to obtain predictable surface skin quality and contour. The method of transfer most likely to restore the correct contour and skin quality of each unit defect is chosen based on the healing response of grafts and flaps.

Aesthetic reconstructive planning is a thoughtful, artistic process. Aesthetic judgment determines its success. Each action, choice of donor materials, technique, and stage creates an opportunity to improve or worsen the result. A step-by-step process must be outlined to achieve the end result. The plan is a group of related parts with priorities and possibilities. Each stage prepares for the next. Basic plastic surgery is combined with aesthetics. Speedy or technologically complex operations are useful only if they improve the final result.

FABRICATION

The surgeon has to "get the job done." Through a choice of technical options and maneuvers, the surgeon's vision and plan can be realized. Failures in fabrication are caused by the following:

1. A failure to take time. "If you won't take the time, you'll do the crime." A wound must be evaluated, a goal set, a plan outlined, and then the time taken to execute the final result. No one thanks you for finishing early and getting in a golf game. Patients are eternally grateful for a normal appearance.
2. A lack of attention to detail. Previously, surgeons measured themselves by the size of the defect or flap, the technical difficulty of transferring tissue, or the speed with which the reconstruction was completed. In fact, it is the minor nuances that separate the ordinary from the excellent end result. Delicacy and artistry are required.
3. Poor technical choices. The face is composed of anatomical layers of cover, lining, and support, and wounds can be closed by secondary healing, primary healing, skin grafts, or flaps. The surgeon's choices and methods of application must always keep the end goal in mind. Will your cover choice have the color and texture of the face? Will the lining be thick and stiff, bulging into the airways to cause obstruction or bulging outward to distort the nasal shape? Will the support framework re-create an artistic and delicate contour?
4. Poor fabrication skills. Tissues must be handled delicately and stitching performed with skill. Wounds must be manipulated so the defect is healed and the character of the associated unit restored.

First, the surgeon must re-create the defect. Debris and infected granulation tissue may have to be excised. Old scar may have to be released and the "normal" returned to its normal position. In composite three-dimensional defects, a stable platform should be established at a preliminary operation. If parts of the nose, cheek, and upper lip are missing, the cheek and upper lip should be reconstructed at a preliminary operation. If the nose is reconstructed simultaneously, the resolution of wound edema, gravity, and wound contracture will shift the cheek/lip platform on which the alar base sits. The nose, which must sit at a specific site and angle on the cheek/lip base, will become distorted over time.

Frequently, the site, size, or depth of a wound located in a central unit should be altered to improve the final result. The goal is to restore defects as units rather than as patches (4). Practically speaking, two design options can be considered. First, adjacent normal tissue within a normal unit may be discarded so that the defect itself is modified to a unit shape (Fig. 35-6). After resurfacing, the skin covering the entire unit will be of uniform quality. Unit resurfacing during the reconstruction of convex units harnesses myofibroblast contraction in the wound bed, which helps to control soft tissue contour by the trapdoor effect. In some cases, it is more useful to design the flap as a unit, rather than the defect itself (Fig. 35-7). A gaping wound of the upper lip does not reflect the actual tissue loss. When reconstructing the philtrum or lateral unit of the upper lip, the surgeon should design the flap based on the ideal or the contralateral normal unit. A cross-lipped Abbe flap based exactly on the ideal or on the contralateral normal unit, by its size and shape, will correctly position the landmarks of the alar base and philtral columns while positioning border scars within the joins between units. Replacement of up to one-half of the lateral upper lip or of the philtrum is performed as a topographical unit with an Abbe flap taken from the midline of the lower lip.

Recall that when the traditional cross-lipped Abbe flap was used to reconstruct the upper lip, only half of the defect was replaced, and the pedicle was positioned to straddle the defect. In this way, the surgeon inaccurately and incompletely replaced the upper lip tissue defect, distorting the nasolabial fold, philtral columns, and alar base; simultaneously, the surgeon distorted the lower lip malleolus and commissure on lower lip closure, creating lower lip asymmetry. Both design plans (designing the defect as a unit or the flap as a unit) are unrelated to old scar position or the borders of the original defect. Both control the end result by subunit design. Restoration of an exact outline is less important for defects that lie within peripheral units. Variabilities of outline are expected within the forehead and cheek units, and the approach to their reconstruction is less rigid (Fig. 35-8).

Templates are useful in the design of covering flaps, support grafts, and the positioning of reconstructed landmarks (Fig. 35-9). Foil patterns of the contralateral normal or the ideal subunit can be cut, bent, and crimped to reflect the unit exactly in quantity and outline. This pattern can then be flattened on the donor site and used as a guide to cover flap design. Support grafts of bone or cartilage can be fashioned based on templates to establish their correct size and shape. When a heminose is rebuilt on the cheek/lip platform, the position and width of the alar base and sill must be known to prevent malposition and asymmetry to the opposite side. A pattern of the opposite normal lip and ala can be designed and positioned on the reconstructed side to verify correct placement. Similarly, when the temple/sideburn hairline is restored by scalp flap advancement, a pattern of the opposite normal hairline is useful.

An important aspect of fabrication is the timing of reconstruction (5). Wounds can be restored primarily, in a delayed primary fashion, or secondarily. Such decisions are based on various factors: the patient's wishes, the time required for wound stabilization, the likelihood of cancer cure based on a Mohs' excision or permanent histologic margin check, monitoring for high-risk local recurrence, the time required for the patient to stop smoking, and the time needed to improve the skin of the recipient or donor sites by

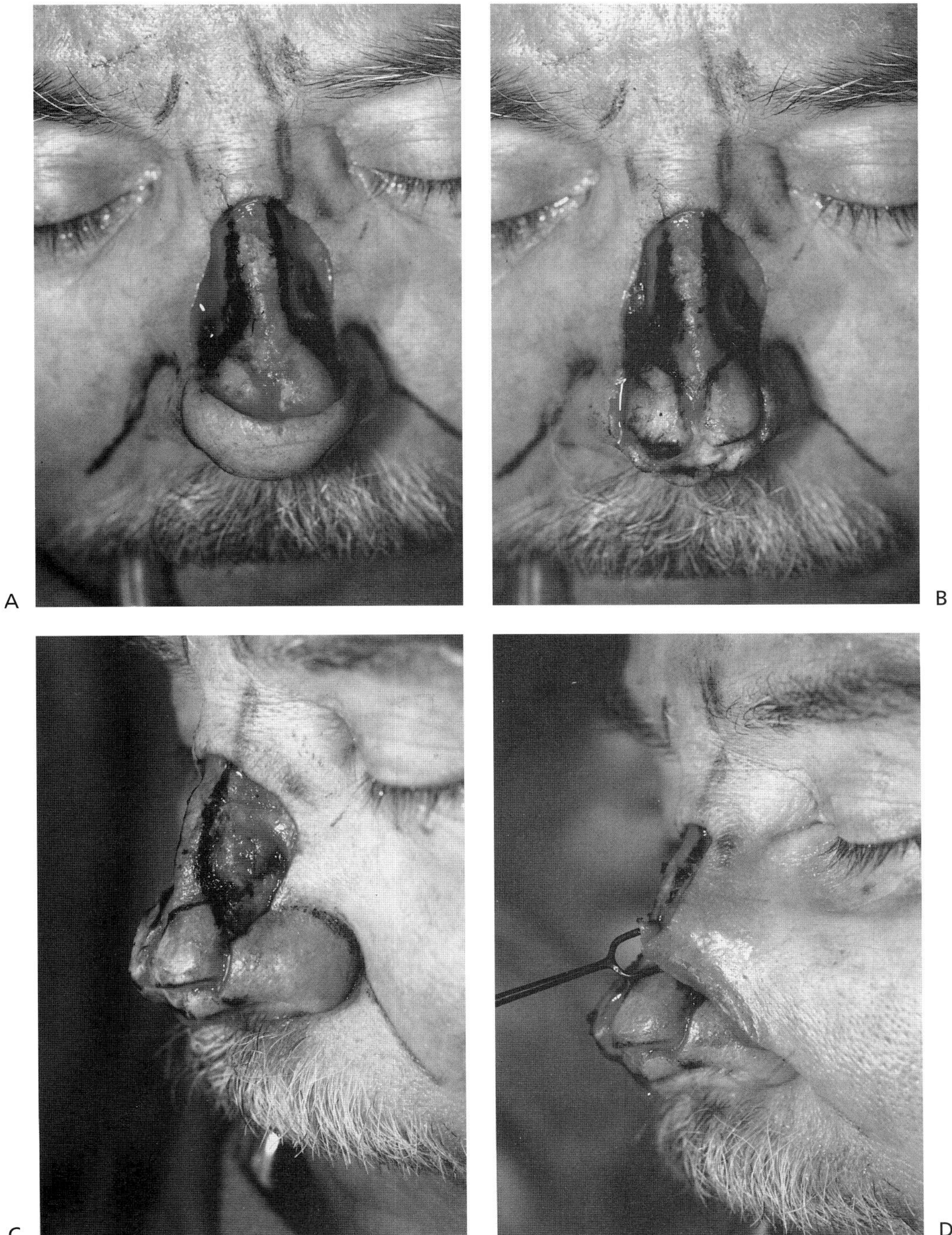

FIGURE 35-6. A,B: Restoring a unit outline—altering the wound, a subunit defect. A wound encompassing part of the dorsum, tip, and nasal sidewall is altered to conform to a unit defect. Adjacent normal skin of the tip is discarded so that no scar will remain across the normally smooth tip unit after forehead flap resurfacing. The defect is enlarged. **C,D:** The remaining sidewall cheek is advanced medially to cover that part of the defect within the sidewall unit. The defect is diminished in size but altered in outline. *(continued)*

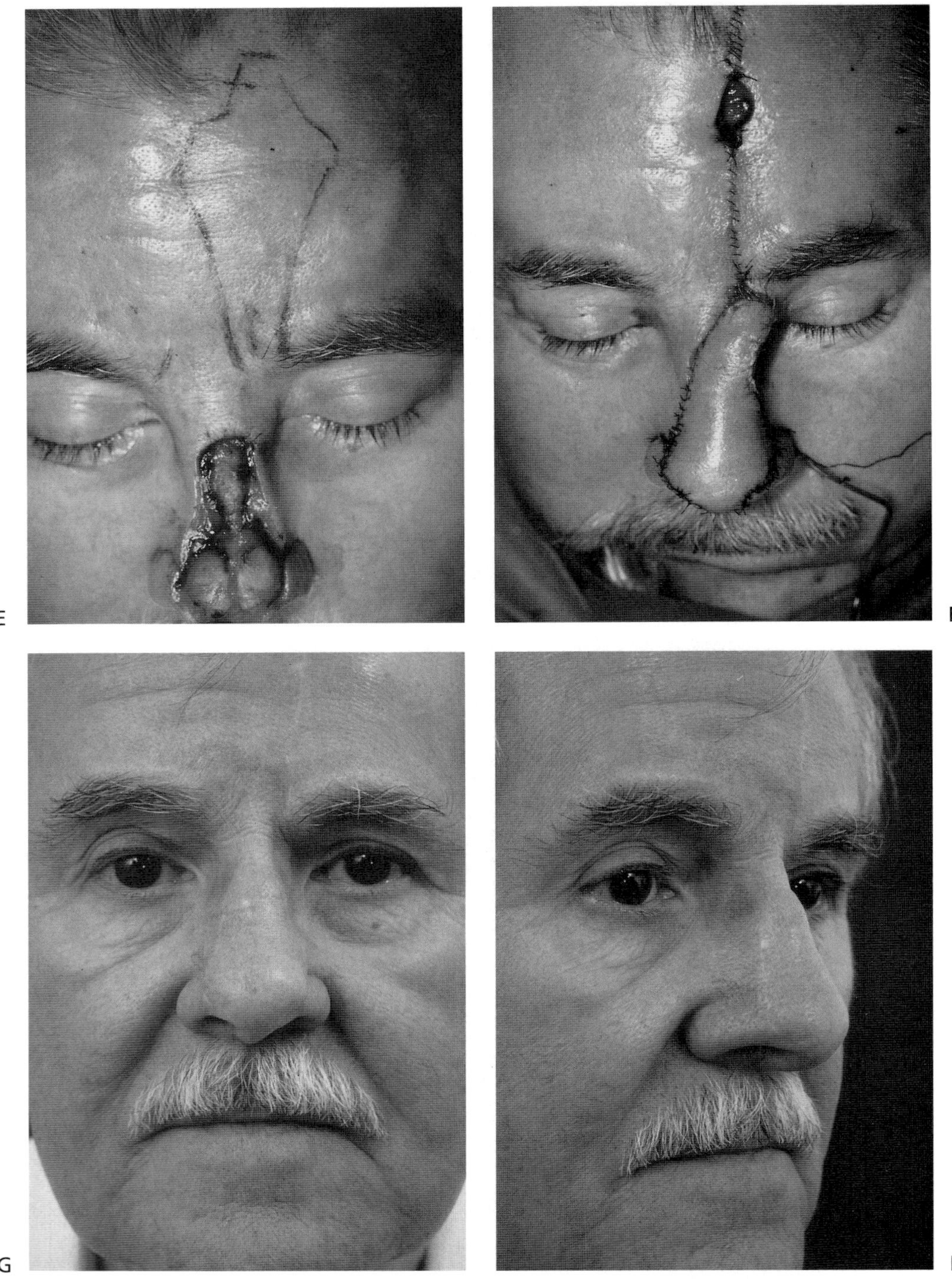

FIGURE 35-6. *Continued.* **E,F:** The wound now resembles a subunit defect of the tip and dorsum, which is resurfaced with a paramedian forehead flap. **G,H:** The final scars lie hidden in the joins between units. The convexity of the contracting flap has helped, rather than hurt, the end result. (Courtesy of F. J. Menick, Tucson, Arizona.)

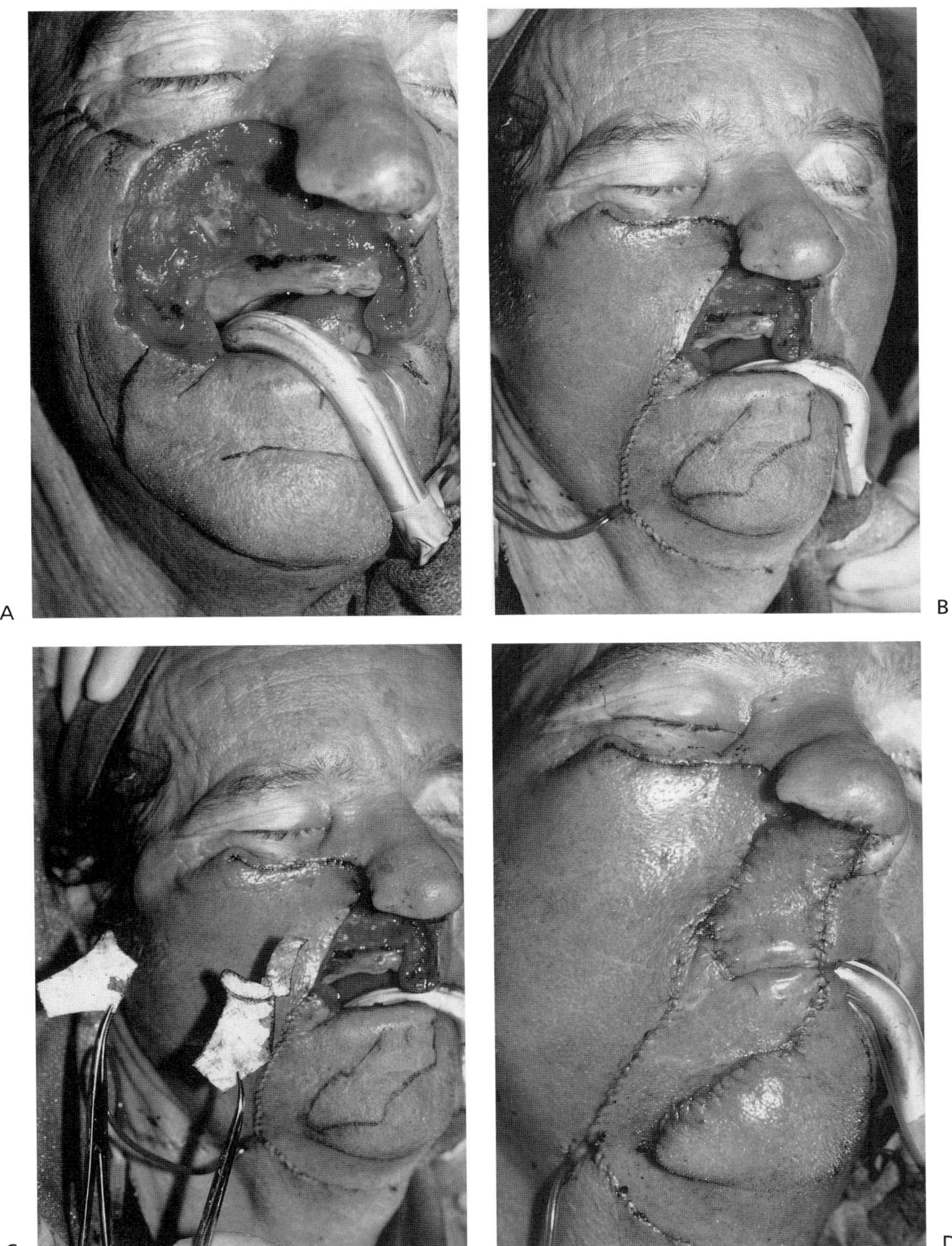

FIGURE 35-7. A–D: Altering the wound, the subunit flap. A massive defect of the medial cheek, more than half of the right upper lip, columella, and full-thickness right ala is present. First, the right cheek is incised along the nasolabial fold and into the submental crease and rotated up and medially to restore the cheek unit. Then, a subunit midline cross-lipped Abbe flap is designed according to a template based on the contralateral normal lateral lip unit. It is transposed on the inferior labial vessels to replace the right lateral upper lip unit, nostril, sill, and columella. At a subsequent operation, after the lip/cheek platform had settled, the right ala was reconstructed with a forehead flap. *(continued)*

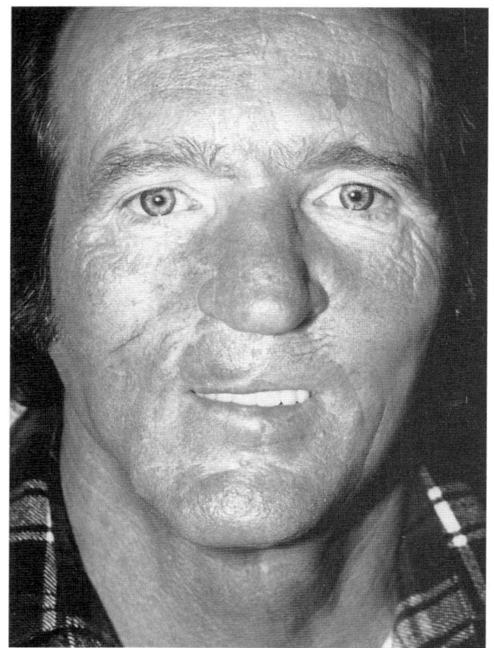

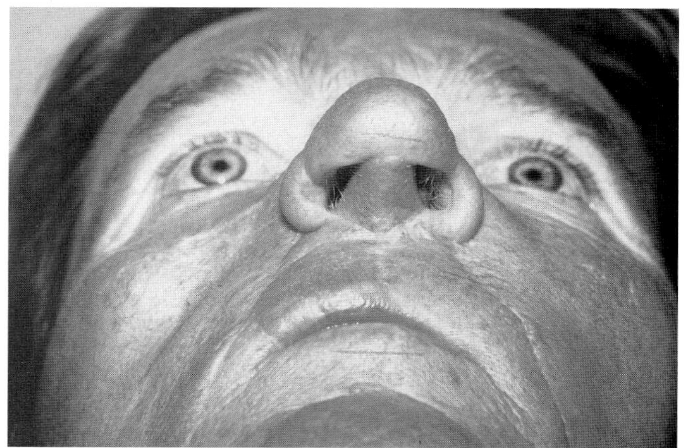

FIGURE 35-7. *Continued.* **E,F:** Postoperative result. The unit Abbe flap filled a gaping upper lip wound accurately and created upper lip balance. (From Menick FJ. Nasal reconstruction: creating a visual illusion. *Adv Plast Reconstr Surg* 1990:8,193, with permission.)

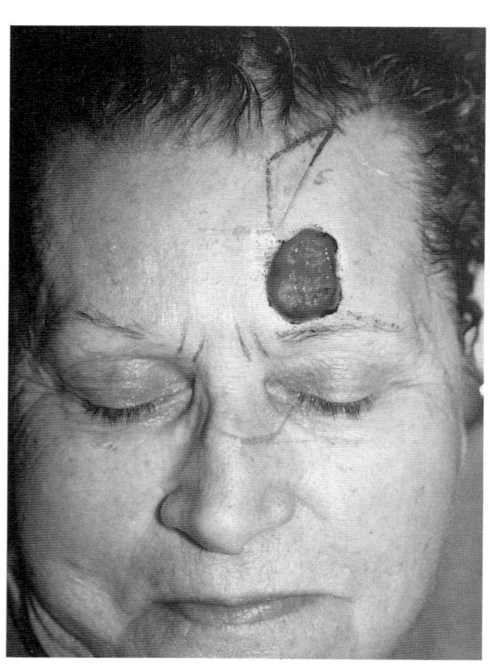

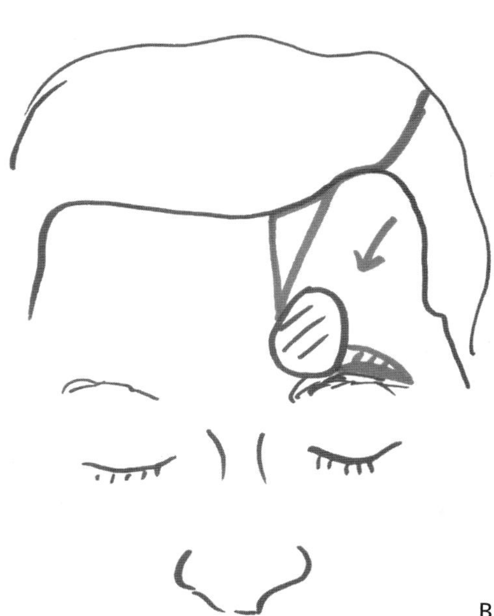

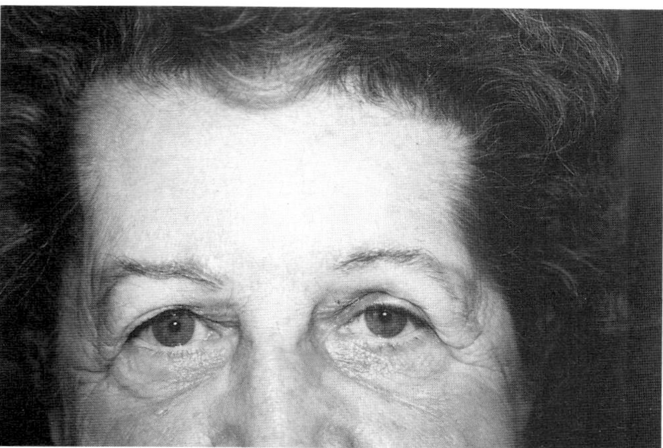

FIGURE 35-8. A,B: Reconstructing a defect within a peripheral unit. Because of unpredictable color and texture, a skin graft used to repair a defect within the forehead unit may appear as a patch. Large rotation flaps containing both forehead and scalp skin are available to close major forehead defects. The variable position of the hairline, which determines the height, width, and outline of the forehead unit, can be altered without creating a significant distortion in the borders of this peripheral, nonfixed unit. After excision of a basal cell carcinoma, less than half of the vertical dimension of the forehead is missing. Sufficient skin remains to allow ipsilateral rotation of the residual forehead skin and adjacent scalp to close both the defect and donor site primarily. A vertical incision is carried upward but does not pass directly into the scalp at the widow's peak. A hair-bearing step-off is avoided by following the hairline for a distance into the temple bay before the scalp is entered. On closure, the hair-bearing scalp slides along the junctional portion of the operative incision, which parallels the old hairline. Although the hairline is lowered on the operative site, a significant visible step-off distortion of the hairline is avoided. **C:** Postoperative result. The forgiving nature of the forehead unit permits such an alteration in its outline and height without a significant visible abnormality. Such an alteration is not permissible when a fixed central unit is restored. (From Menick FJ. Facial reconstruction in regional units. *Perspect Plast Surg* 1994;8,106, with permission.)

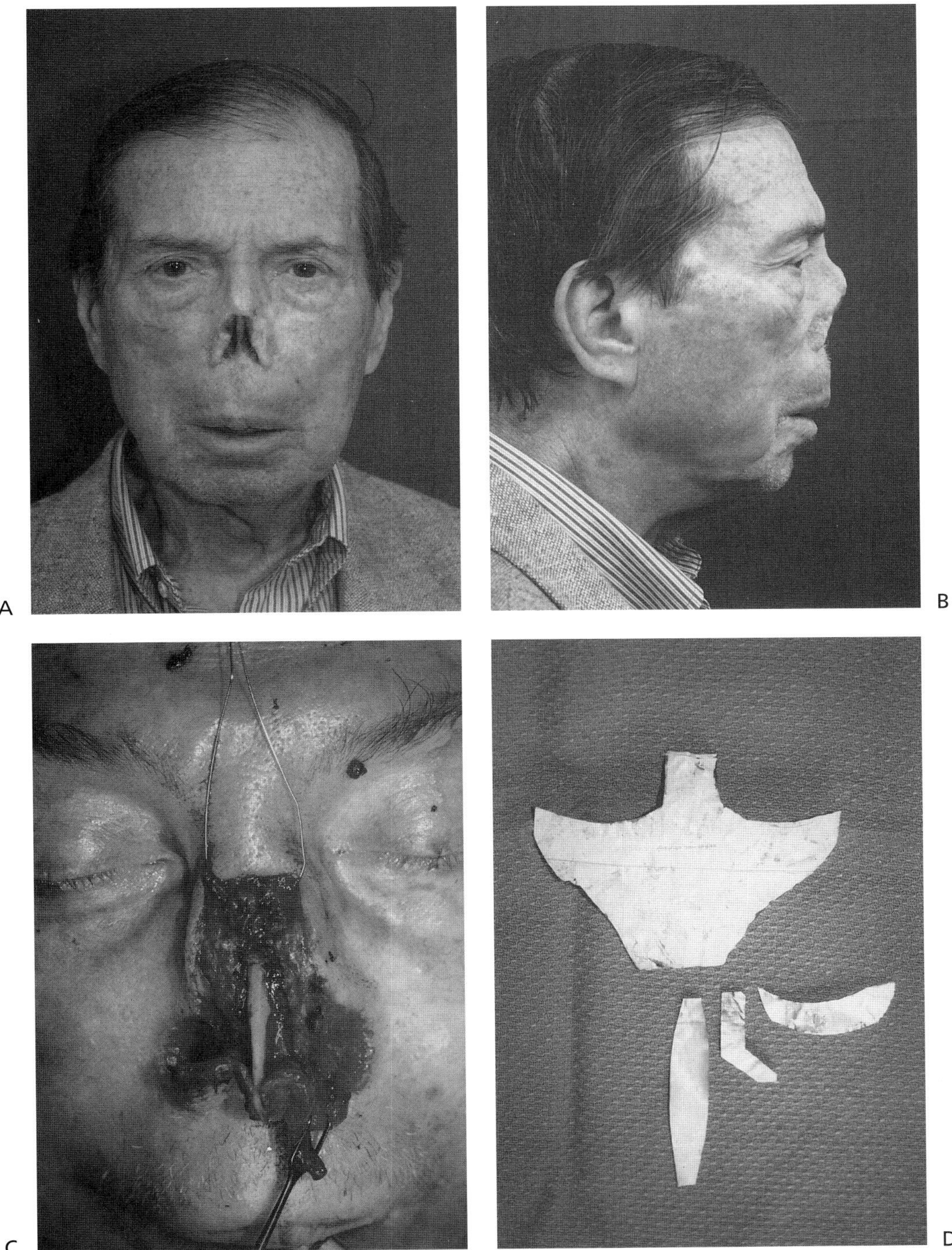

FIGURE 35-9. A–C: In this subtotal nasal loss, a central nasal scaffold and lining were restored with a composite septal flap hinged out of the piriform aperture based on the superior labial arteries. *(continued)*

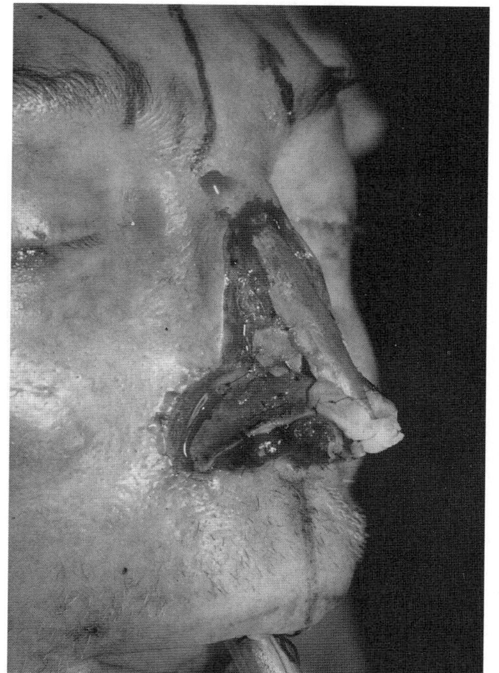

E

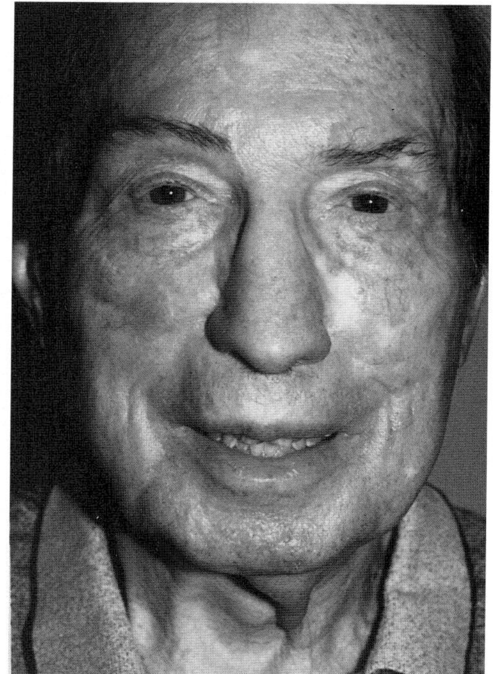

F

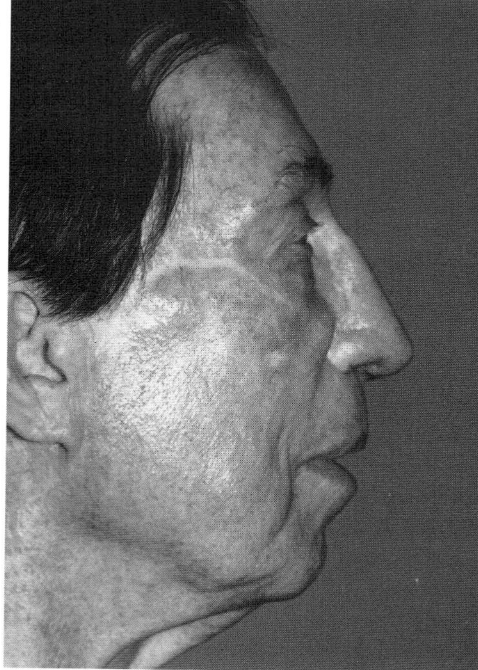

G

FIGURE 35-9. *Continued.* **D,E:** With the use of foil templates, patterns were fashioned to design the covering flap, and rib and ear cartilage grafts to restore the appropriate dorsal, tip, alar, and sidewall support framework. The reconstruction was covered with a forehead flap. **F,G:** Postoperative result. (Courtesy of Menick FJ, Tucson, Arizona.)

the use of tretinoin, 5-fluorouracil, or dermabrasion. A delay in reconstruction allows the patient and surgeon to consider the long-term goals of reconstruction, and the surgeon can explain the operative plan to the patient.

Time can be an ally. Some wounds heal secondarily. This is an excellent option for small or moderate defects of the forehead, where a tight, shiny scar created by secondary healing will blend in well with the tight, shiny peripheral unit. A granulating wound may allow a skin graft to be applied that might not have survived initially. Cover and lining flaps simply sewn together and allowed to heal permit the use of hinge-over covering flaps for lining at a later date. A delayed operation to increase the random blood supply of local flaps may increase flap safety or allow the fabrication of a composite flap to restore cover, lining, and support. Staged operations also permit the surgical repositioning of normal-to-normal and secure healing in position, the re-creation of a stable platform on which other three-dimensional features can be built, intermediate operations to allow soft tissue sculpturing before pedicle division, and the addition of delayed primary support grafts before the completion of wound healing. Staged operations may produce a better result in a shorter period of time than a single-stage operation that may require multiple late and neglected revisions.

The subunits of the face are restored by placing covering skin of the expected quality and by replacing the outline and symmetry of facial landmarks and three-dimensional contours. Quality is determined by choosing donor tissues for surface cover that match those of the recipient facial site. The end result is also determined by the method of tissue transfer, whether skin graft or flap. Local tissues are ideal for surface cover because of their excellent match but are often limited in quantity. The transfer of distant tissue by microvascular technique provides the advantages of rich vascularity, rapid transfer without delay, and almost unlimited bulk with excess available to reconstruct other facial parts, and it frequently frees the surgeon from the restraint of a distant pedicle. Unfortunately, distant tissue must often be transferred in stages or by complex techniques. Most importantly, distant skin is a poor match in quality to facial skin, and no distant tissue has a facial shape. Distant tissue moved by free-flap transfer can be used to close dead space, fill a cavity, protect vital structures, create a barrier between the central nervous system and an oral cavity, close a fistula, or build a stable platform. Distant tissue provides ideal "invisible" tissue for reconstruction but does not match the face. Therefore, local and distant tissue must often be combined. The reconstruction of a massive facial defect should be carried out in two stages (Fig. 35-10):

1. Bulk engineering (do not waste time). Supply bulk materials with distant tissue, initially ensure flap viability

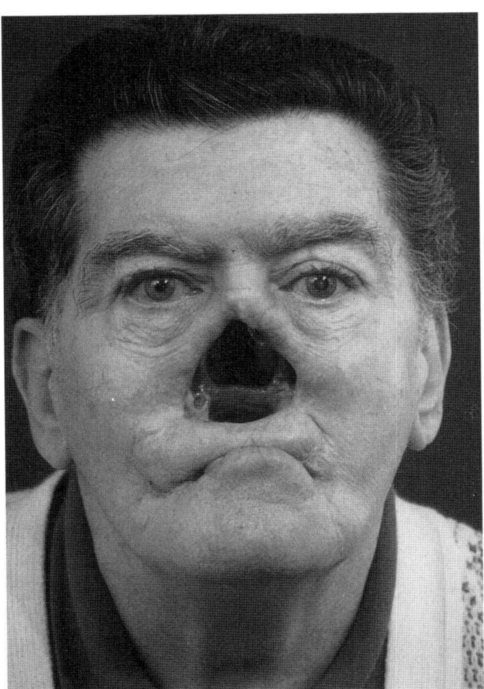
A

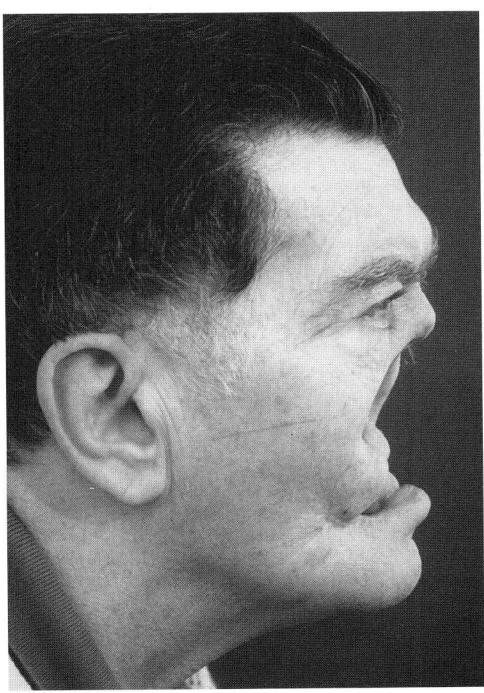
B

FIGURE 35-10. A,B: A massive facial defect remains after median maxillectomies, total rhinectomy, and excision of the upper lip for multiply recurrent squamous cell carcinoma of the septum that was unresponsive to multiple previous operations, radiation therapy, and chemotherapy. Previously placed and poorly designed fan flaps span the upper lip defect. The patient can neither talk nor take food orally and drools constantly. The anterior alveolar arch and hard palate are missing. *(continued)*

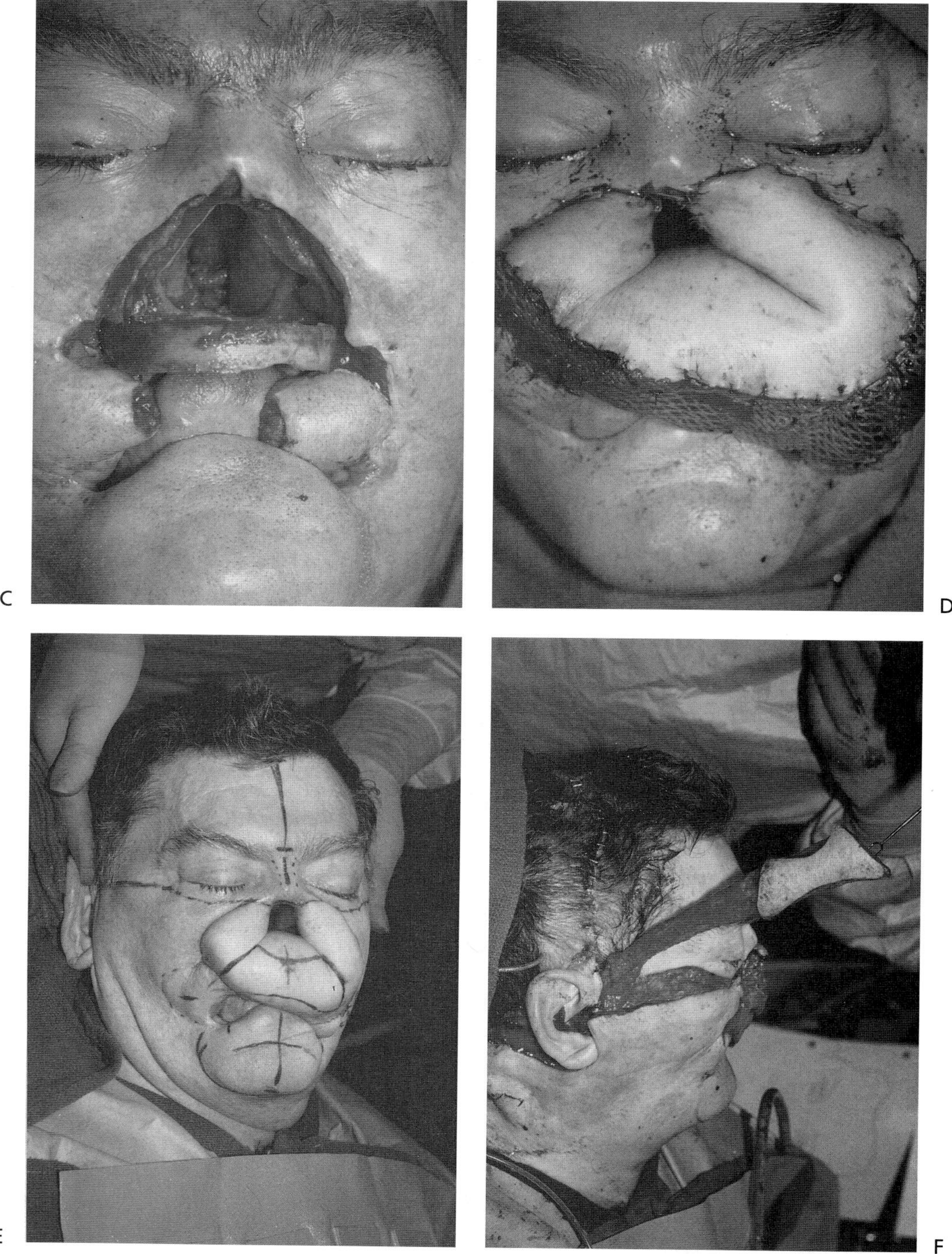

FIGURE 35-10. *Continued.* **C,D:** First, facial projection and a separation of the nose and mouth were obtained by positioning a bony rib strut arching between maxillary tuberosities and wrapped with a free latissimus dorsi myocutaneous flap and skin graft. The old fan flaps were returned to the lower lip. **E–G:** Later, the upper lip unit was resurfaced with a pedicled scalp flap passed under advancing cheek flaps to resurface the lip and cheek units. *(continued)*

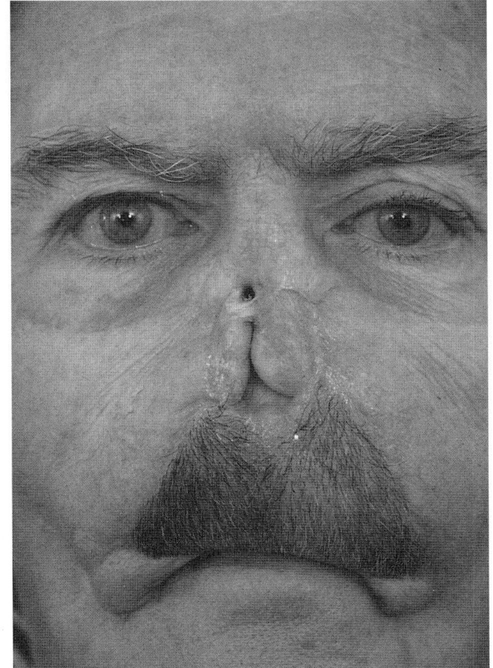

H

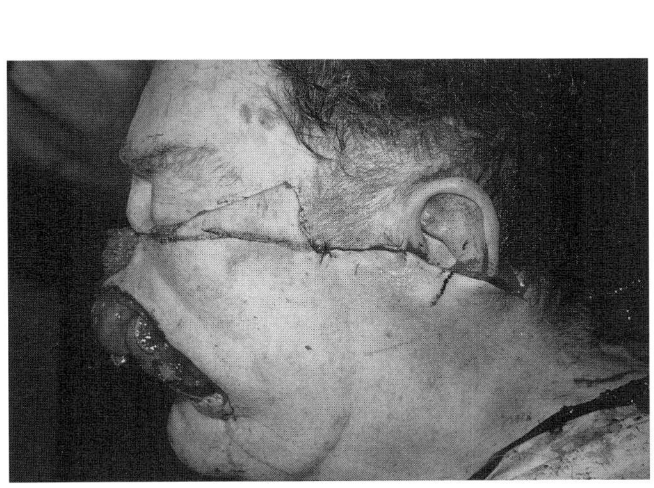

G

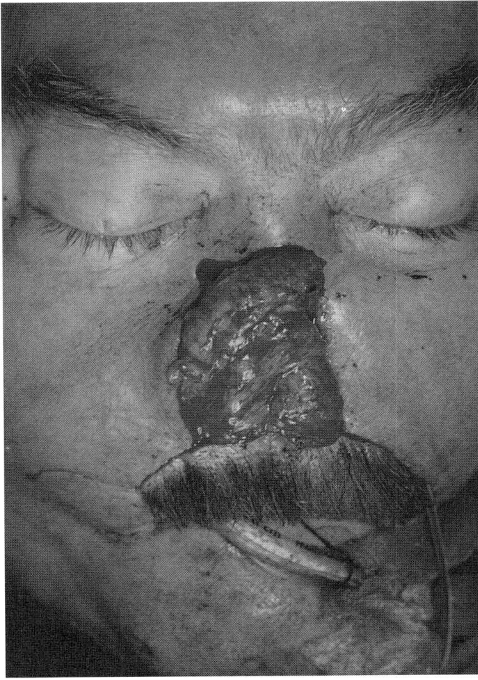

I

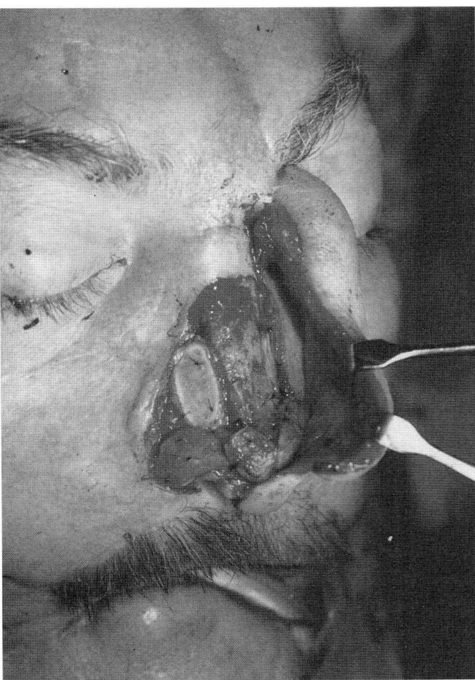

J

FIGURE 35-10. *Continued.* **H,I:** A stable facial platform was now available to support a three-dimensional nose. Subsequently, a free radial forearm flap was transferred, skin side inward, to establish a nasal lining. Its surface was temporarily skin-grafted. Once the viability of the flap was ensured, the covering skin graft was removed. A cantilever rib graft fixed to the residual nasal bones was placed and the reconstruction resurfaced with a forehead flap to restore nasal skin quality. **J:** Later, in a staged delayed primary fashion, rib and ear cartilage grafts were used to restore a subsurface architecture during an intermediate operation before pedicle division. Both cheek flaps were advanced to the expected junction of hair-bearing and non–hair-bearing upper lip skin. **J:** Later, in a staged delayed primary fashion, rib and ear cartilage grafts were used to restore a subsurface architecture during an intermediate operation before pedicle division. Both cheek flaps were advanced to the expected junction of hair-bearing and non–hair-bearing upper lip skin. *(continued)*

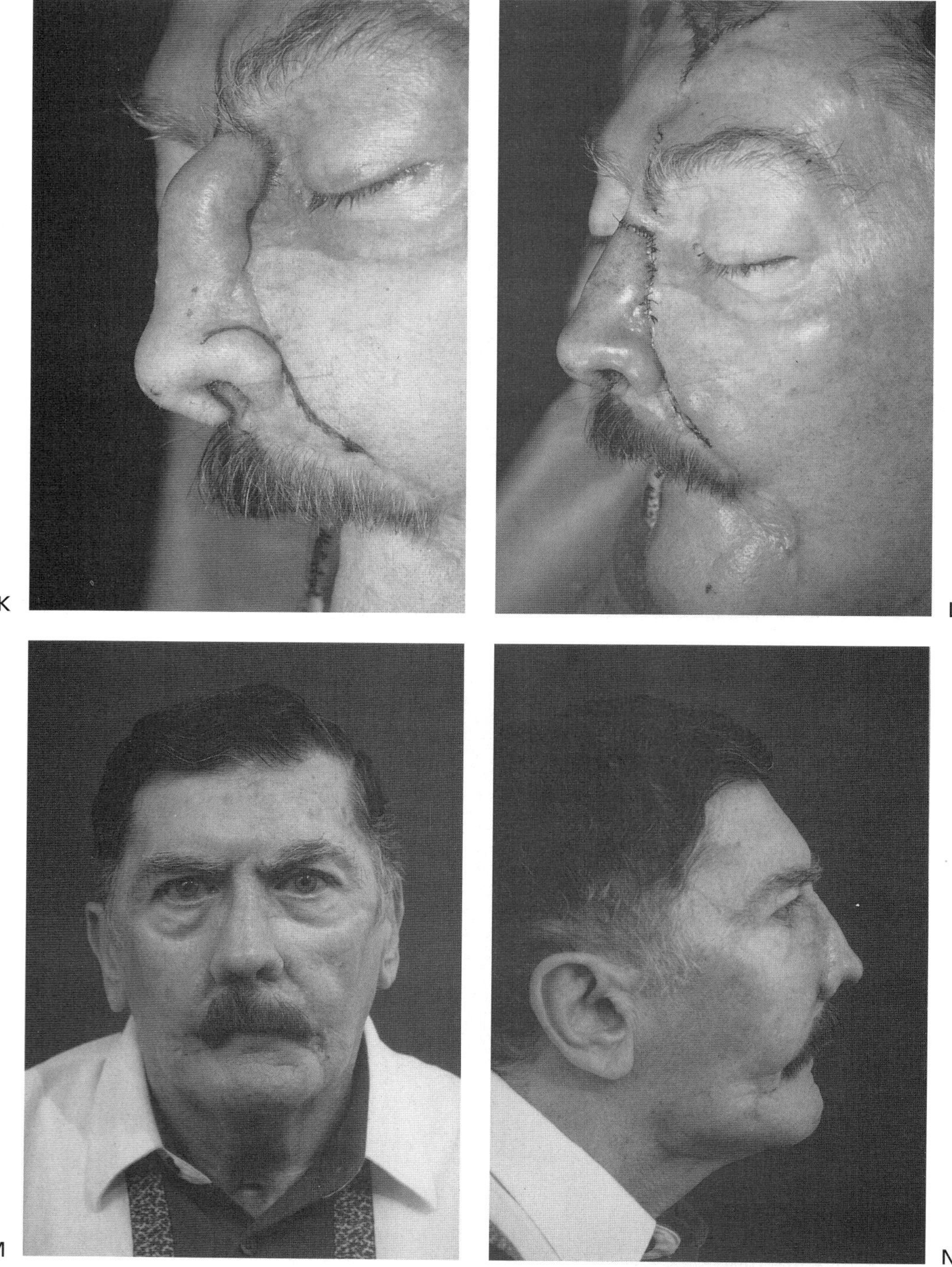

FIGURE 35-10. *Continued.* **K,L:** Later, at the time of forehead flap pedicle division, nasolabial folds were incised in an ideal position and soft tissue debulked to create the flat, hairless triangle of the upper lip and the nasolabial crease. **M,N:** Postoperative result. A normal face was reestablished by restoring the expected skin quality, outline, and three-dimensional contour of the facial units. Distant tissues provided vascularized hidden bulk and projection, and local tissue supplied surface skin that matched the face in color, texture, and hair-bearing quality. Primary support grafts and soft tissue sculpturing restored support and a three-dimensional shape. Scars lie hidden in final contour lines or unit joins. (From Menick FJ. Facial reconstruction with local and distant tissue: the interface of aesthetic and reconstructive surgery. *Plast Reconstr Surg* 1998;102:1424, with permission.)

and a healed inset, protect vital structures, revascularize the wound, and reconstruct the stable platform.
2. Finesse tailoring (apply subunit principles to restore facial skin quality, outline, and contour). Distant tissue should be used for "invisible" requirements (lining and support) but not to replace surface skin. Excessive bulk should be sculpted and either discarded or used for other purposes (lining and soft tissue contour). Conventional techniques and local grafts and flaps are employed to contour facial units and resurface individual regions at a separate stage.

CONCLUSION

In summary, the reconstructive surgeon must combine vision, planning, and fabrication to take charge of the wound. The reconstructive surgeon cannot prevent cancer or facial trauma and cannot control wound healing, scars, or the inherent sequelae associated with the transfer of a skin graft or flap. However, the surgeon can select the size, site, shape, and depth of a wound and choose the donor materials and methods of tissue transfer that are most likely to provide a good result. It is impossible to recreate the normal, but it is possible to assemble a facsimile that can appear normal. Aesthetic reconstruction is determined by vision, planning, and fabrication.

REFERENCES

1. Burget G, Menick FJ. *Aesthetic restoration of the nose.* St. Louis: Mosby, 1994.
2. Menick F. Artistry in aesthetic surgery: aesthetic perception and the subunit principle. *Clin Plast Surg* 1987;14:723.
3. Menick FJ. Aesthetic restoration of the face. In: Cohen M, ed. *Difficult wounds.* Philadelphia: JB Lippincott Co, 1989:455–480.
4. Menick FJ. Aesthetic refinements in the use of the forehead for nasal reconstruction: the paramedian forehead flap. *Clin Plast Surg* 1990;19:607–622.
5. Menick FJ. Principles of head and neck reconstruction. In: Cohen M, ed. *Mastery in surgery: plastic and reconstructive surgery.* Boston: Little, Brown and Company, 1994:842–905.

Discussion

FACIAL AND NASAL RECONSTRUCTION

ELLIOTT H. ROSE

Dr. Fred Menick has very elegantly described his systematic planning and execution of complex facial and nasal reconstructions of difficult defects, emphasizing the *aesthetic outcome* as a primary objective of facial restoration. In the final paragraph of the chapter, he relegates the role of microvascular free-tissue transfers to "bulk engineering," and dismisses them as being "too complex," providing a "poor color match, " lacking "facial shape," and suitable only for "invisible tissue reconstruction." Although I use contiguous local tissue rearrangement and smaller grafts in most of my facial reconstructions (believe it or not, I do not use a free flap for every facial defect), restoration in faces severely disfigured by major trauma, burns, or congenital deformities requires the replacement of *massive* blocks of tissue of similar texture and contour to achieve adequate facial balance, symmetry, and architecture. In massive defects, local flaps and scar releases with skin grafting are useful in mitigating the functional concerns of exposure keratitis, nostril stenosis, perioral and neck contractures, and exposed ear cartilages (1); however, with the exception of the forehead flap for total nasal reconstruction (when the tissue is neither burned nor scarred), these techniques of tissue rearrangement are *not* adequate to replace larger "aesthetic facial units." Feldman (2) has used "megaunits" in split-thickness skin grafts for cheek, neck, and nasal units. Even in the best of circumstances, these partial-thickness grafts, lacking substantial dermal and subcutaneous tissue elements, often adhere to the submuscular aponeurotic layer or the muscles of facial expression, yielding flat, "adynamic facies" with a corrugated, dry, thick surface texture (Table 35D-1). This type of surface is inadequate for skin moisturization

E. H. Rose: Division of Plastic Surgery, Mount Sinai Medical Center; and The Aesthetic Surgery Center, New York, New York

TABLE 35D-1. LIMITATIONS OF CONVENTIONAL TECHNIQUES OF POSTTRAUMATIC AND BURN RECONSTRUCTION IN SEVERELY DISFIGURED FACES

Limited availability of local tissue
Extensive hypertrophic or keloid scars
Thick, corrugated texture following skin grafting
Adynamic, "flat" facies
Poor motion of mimetic muscles of expression
Color mismatches
Indistinct demarcation of facial planes

Reprinted from Rose EH, ed. *Aesthetic facial restoration.* Philadelphia: Lippincott–Raven Publishers, 1998:2, with permission.

and corrective camouflage makeup, and gives the face a flaky, pasty, "caked on" look after flesh-colored foundation is applied.

The goals of a successfully integrated and architecturally pleasing facial reconstruction are the following: (a) aesthetic balance and symmetry; (b) distinct facial planes unmarred by conspicuous, distracting scars; (c) a "doughy" skin texture appropriate for the application of corrective camouflage makeup; and (d) natural, unfettered facial animation (3) (Table 35D-2). To achieve these goals, the meticulous technique of a microsurgeon and the artistry of a cosmetic surgeon must be combined. Because this work is neither strictly reconstructive nor *strictly* cosmetic, but rather borrows techniques and skills from each endeavor, the more appropriate terminology is *aesthetic facial restoration* (3).

COMPREHENSIVE STRATEGY OF AESTHETIC FACIAL RESTORATION

In 1985, while practicing in California, I was asked by Dr. Richard Grossman of the Sherman Oaks Burn Unit to integrate my interests in reconstructive microsurgery and facial cosmetic surgery with the newly emerging technology of computer imaging in an attempt to restore the faces of severely disfigured burn victims. From that initial encounter, a comprehensive strategy of aesthetic facial restoration has evolved, in which "prepatterned" microvascular tissue transfers are utilized that are extensively sculpted intraoperatively to match the shapes of facial aesthetic units (4). Seams are hidden inconspicuously at the junction of facial aesthetic units. Subtraction analysis software is used to define architectural imbalance, and osteoplastic modifications are aided by computer-generated models. State-of-the-art computer imaging "paint" software assists in the preoperative facial analysis and the "mapping" of planned hard and soft tissue surgical changes. In the early years, the color match of microvascular flaps from distant donor sites was less than optimal, but these limitations have been overcome by the skills of aestheticians, who custom-design flesh-colored foundations that make it possible to blend transferred tissues with the composite face most effectively (Table 35D-3).

TABLE 35D-2. GOALS OF FACIAL RECONSTRUCTION

Aesthetic balance and symmetry
Distinct facial planes unmarred by conspicuous scarring
"Doughy" skin texture appropriate for the application of corrective camouflage makeup
"Natural" facial animation

Reprinted from Rose EH, ed. *Aesthetic facial restoration.* Philadelphia: Lippincott–Raven Publishers 1998:3, with permission.

TABLE 35D-3. COMPREHENSIVE STRATEGY OF AESTHETIC FACIAL RESTORATION

"Prepatterned" microvascular tissue transfers to inset into aesthetic facial units
Three-dimensional software assessment of bony architectural abnormalities and fabrication of computer-generated acrylic models
State-of-the-art computer imaging to assist in preoperative planning of soft tissue modifications
Extensive intraoperative sculpting of tissue transfers to simulate facial contours
Application of flesh-colored corrective makeup to conceal scars and blend flap to rest of face
Microdermal pigmentation (tattooing of beard, lips, eyebrows, scars)
Integration of muscles of expression into flap transfers
Broad application of cosmetic ancillary procedures

Reprinted from Rose EH, ed. *Aesthetic facial restoration.* Philadelphia: Lippincott–Raven Publishers, 1998:3, with permission.

PREPATTERNED MICROVASCULAR TISSUE TRANSFER

The *key* to the artistic restoration of a disfigured facial unit is the precisely patterned and sculpted microvascular free-tissue transfer. In most centers, microvascular free flaps have achieved success rates above 96% (5–7). A tracing of the "target" facial element is transcribed through a transparent pattern centered over the vascular pedicle, auscultated at the donor site. The flap is debulked *in situ* to correspond to areas of desired thinness at the recipient site, with thickness preserved only along the course of the pedicle (Fig. 35D-1). At transfer, the precisely designed flap fits neatly into the recipient site to form a replica of the missing "puzzle piece" of the face (Figs. 35D-2 and 35D-3). The thinned undersurface adheres to the muscles of mimetic expression and allows freedom of excursion for naturally appearing facial animation. With the judicious application of flesh-colored camouflage makeup, scars are concealed, and the flap blends in with the overall facial harmony. Favored flaps for aesthetic facial reconstruction are the following: (a) scapular flap (cheeks, hemiface, forehead); (b) volar forearm flap (neck, upper lip, nose); (c)temporoparietal fascial/calvarial flap (ear, cheek,

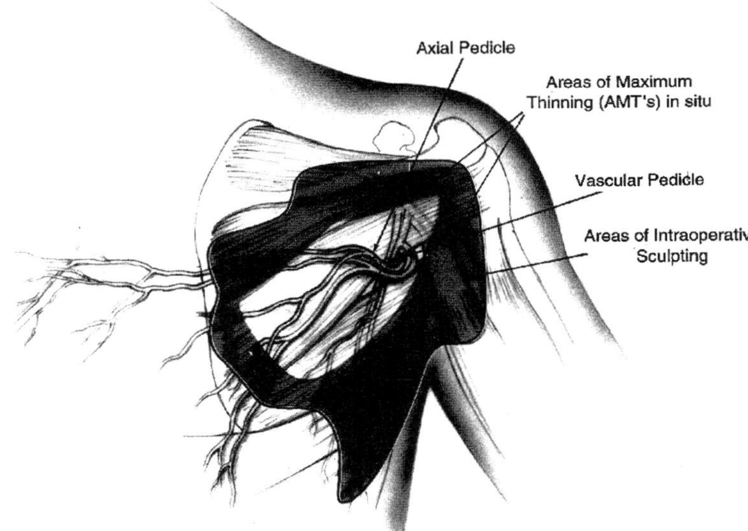

FIGURE 35D-1. Intraoperative sculpting. Prepatterned aesthetic facial unit is undermined *in situ* at subdermal plane to achieve proper thinness of facial contours. The flap is left thick beneath the axial pedicle, determined by Doppler auscultation. (From Rose EH, ed. *Aesthetic facial restoration.* Philadelphia: Lippincott–Raven Publishers, 1998:30, with permission.)

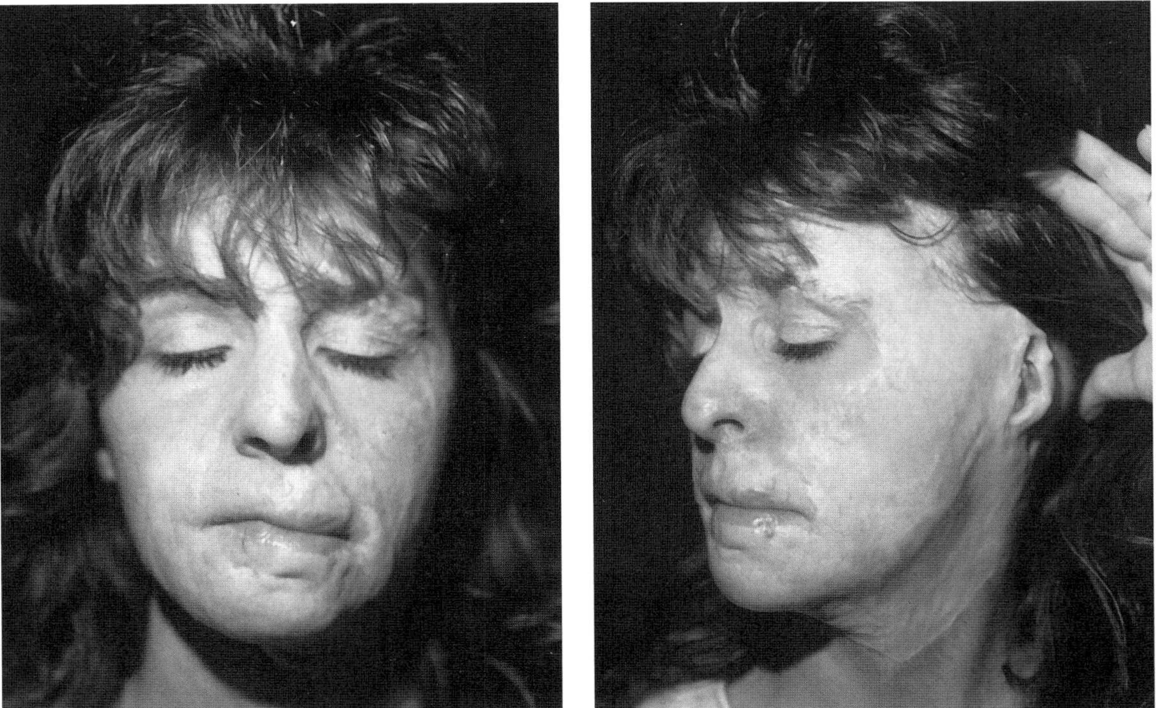

FIGURE 35D-2. A 19-year-old woman (patient 1) was engulfed in flames as a toddler when her nightgown caught fire. **A,B:** Preoperatively. Flat, adynamic face. *(continued)*

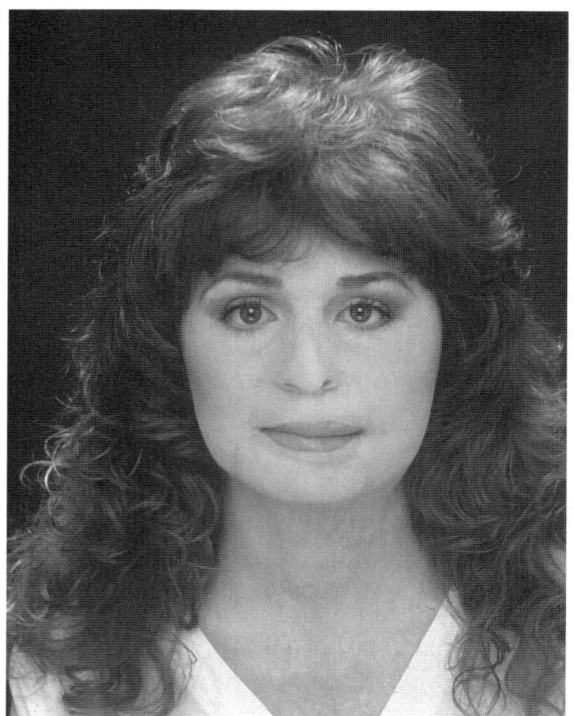

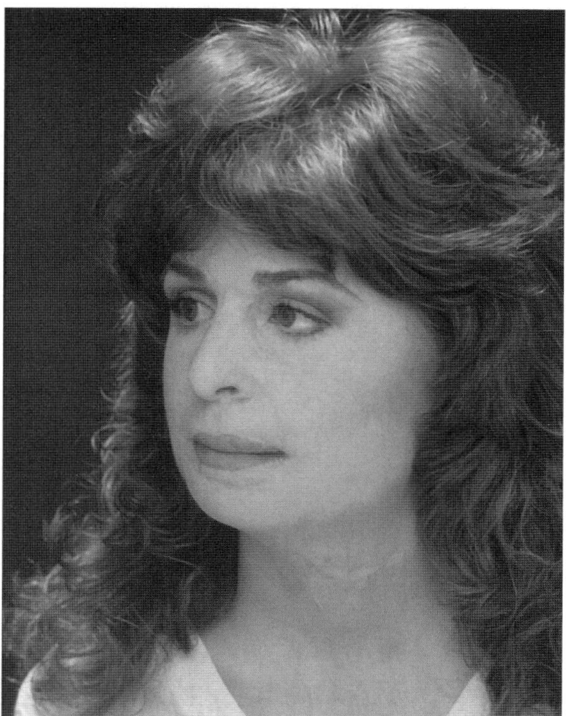

FIGURE 35D-2. *Continued.* **C,D:** Postoperatively, after restoration of left cheek by microvascular free-tissue transfer and right cheek advancement with placement of intraoperative tissue expander. Patient is wearing corrective makeup. (From Rose EH. Aesthetic restoration of the severely disfigured face in burn victims: a comprehensive strategy. *Plast Reconstr Surg* 1995;96:1573, with permission.)

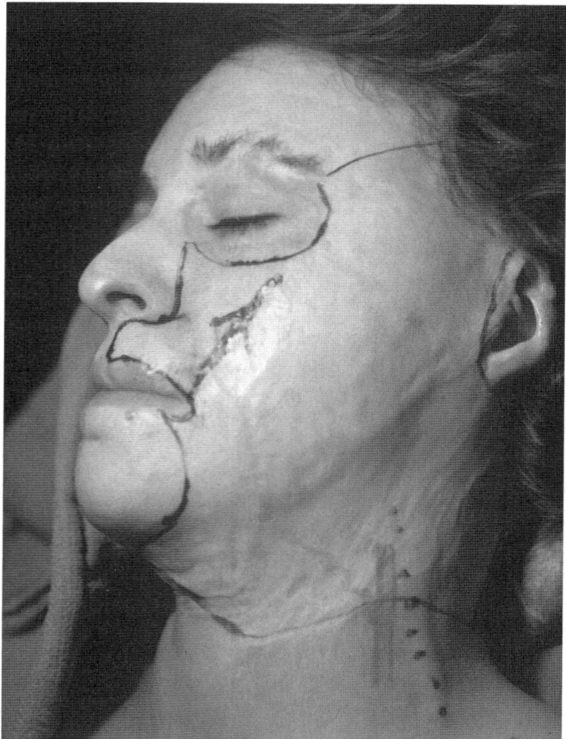

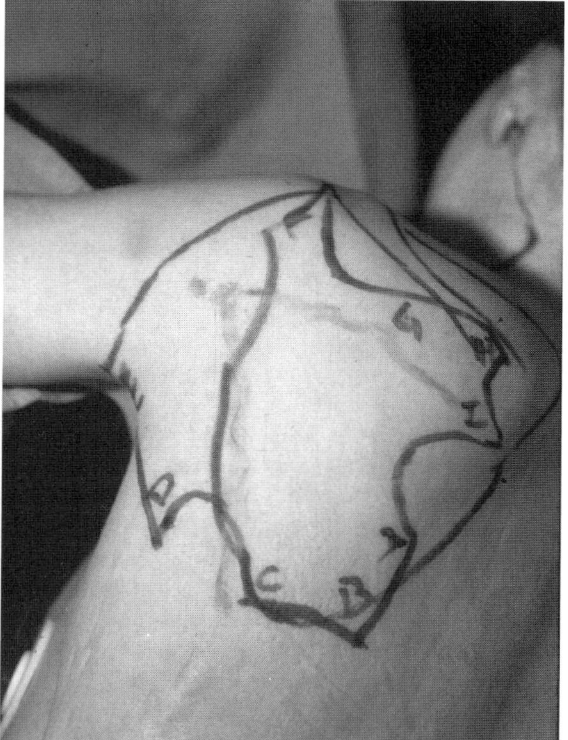

FIGURE 35D-3. Patient 1. **A:** Preparation of hemifacial defect. Tracing of cheek aesthetic unit. **B:** Prepatterned scapular flap corresponding to hemifacial unit. (From Rose EH. Aesthetic restoration of the severely disfigured face in burn victims: a comprehensive strategy. *Plast Reconstr Surg* 1995;96:1573, with permission.)

periorbital regions, jaw) (8); (d) vascularized forehead flap (nose); (e) fibular free flap (jaw); (f) dorsalis pedis/second metatarsal flap (nose). Priority is given to conditions warranting immediate functional correction (e.g., exposure keratitis, incompetent lip sphincter, nostril stenosis, perioral stenosis). Beyond that, top priority is given to the more peripheral elements of the face, such as the forehead, jaws, cheek, and neck (whereas Dr. Menick relegates these regions to the status of "largely flap, expansive surfaces of secondary interest"). Release of the deforming *centripetal vectors of force* allows more precise reconstruction of the central facial features (lips and nose, periorbital regions). Ear and scalp restorations are given the lowest priority. Architectural modifications are performed before or simultaneously with soft tissue restoration.

APPLICATION OF COMPUTER TECHNOLOGY IN FACIAL RESTORATION

Dr. Menick has emphasized the surgeon's "direct observation, intuition, and imagination" in the overall planning of facial restoration. Although I consider myself intuitive and very creative, I nevertheless do not trust my instincts or memory entirely and so avail myself of the most up-to-date computer technology for surgical planning, analysis, and retrieval of data.

Computer-generated Models

Complex facial defects with distorted skeletal architecture are an enigma to the reconstructive surgeon (Fig. 35D-4A). Without a "road map, " the design of alloplastic material or bone grafts is based on an educated guess regarding the geometric shape and dimensions of the contour abnormality. The use of three-dimensional images reformatted from two-dimensional computed tomographic (CT) data has greatly assisted in the precise assessment of the geometry of architectural defects, and has thereby improved accuracy in the surgical plane. Acrylic models, generated from computer data and available in the operating room, facilitate the fabrication of alloplastic implants as autogenous bone grafts for a precise fit in architectural augmentation (9).

Preoperative CT data, digitized in tape, are converted by Cemax 1500 hardware and software (Santa Clara, California) to a three-dimensional visualization of skull and bony facial anatomy. Unilateral facial architectural "puzzles" are solved by subtraction analysis from the normal side. The normal architectural anatomy of the face is electronically mirrored onto the abnormal side, shown as a different color on the screen, to fill the missing segment (Fig. 35D-4D). The encoded digital message is transmitted to a three-axis CNC milling machine to mold plastic "negatives" into which fast-drying acrylic is poured (accuracy is within 2%) (10) (Fig. 35D-4E). These acrylic templates have been used to generate precisely fitting alloplastic prostheses for orbitocranial reconstruction, and intraoperatively as a model to carve vascularized bone graft (Figs. 35D-4B, 4C and 35D-5) (9) or porous polyethylene onlay implants (Porex Surgical, College Park, Georgia).

Facial Video Imaging

Sophisticated "paint" software now available enables the plastic surgeon to manipulate soft tissue deformities visually

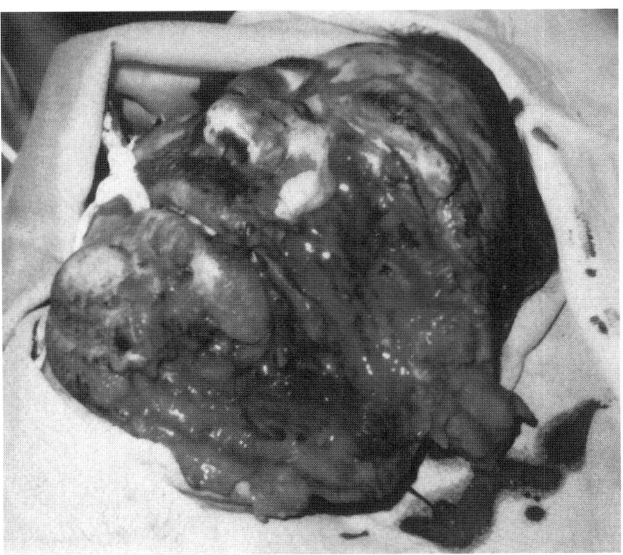
A

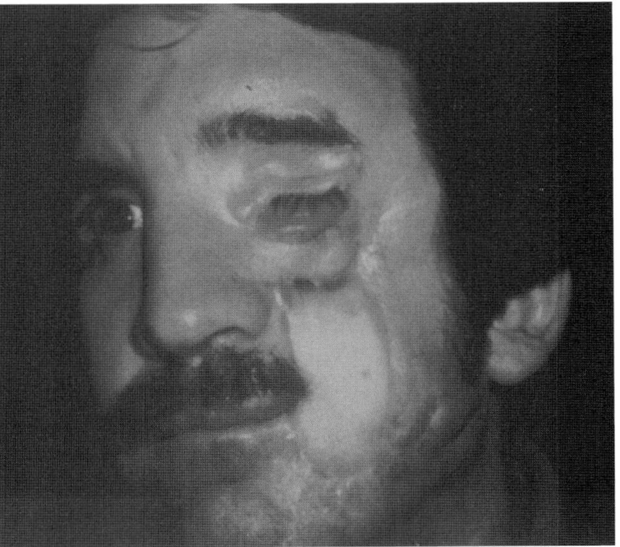
B

FIGURE 35D-4. Patient 2. **A:** Self-inflicted gunshot wound to the face in a 40-year-old Vietnam veteran has destroyed left orbital floor and eye. **B:** Intermediate stage after deep circumflex iliac artery *(DCIA)* osteocutaneous flap for jaw reconstruction and filling of cheek defect. *(continued)*

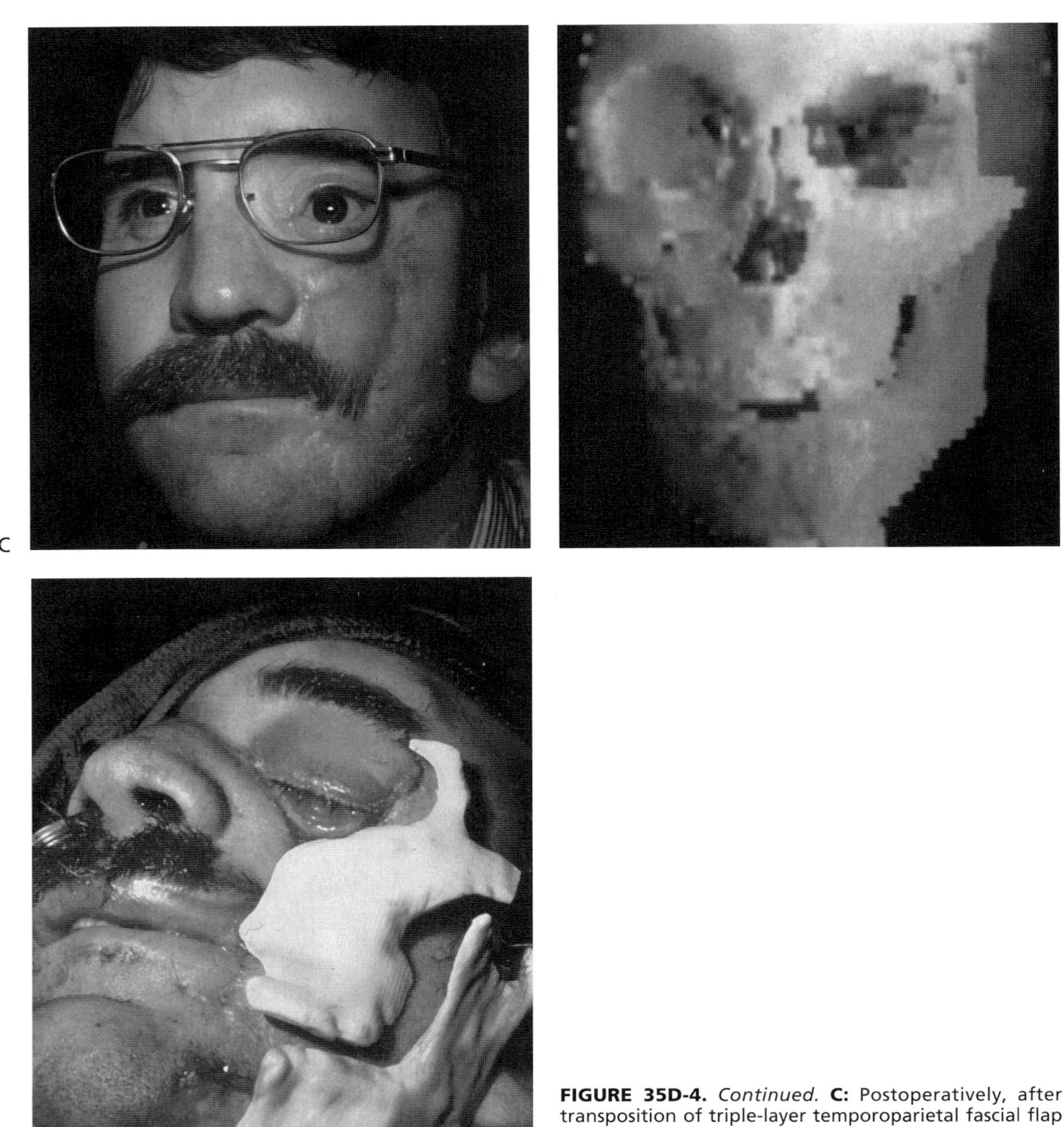

FIGURE 35D-4. *Continued.* **C:** Postoperatively, after transposition of triple-layer temporoparietal fascial flap for reconstruction of cheek, orbit, and beard. Eye prosthesis in place. **D:** Subtraction analysis of orbital and jaw defects. **E:** Computer-generated models of mandibular and zygomatic defects. (From Rose EH, Norris MS. The versatile temporoparietal fascial flap: adaptability to a variety of composite defects. *Plast Reconstr Surg* 1990;85:224, with permission.)

on the screen and project a reasonable expectation of the surgical outcome to the patient. In a step-by-step facial analysis, the surgeon is able to delineate each of the distracting facial elements and develop a plan to correct the myriad of deformities (Figs. 35D-5, 35D-6, and 35D-7). This approach provides the patient with better insight into the complexity of the reconstruction, so that expectations are more realistic, and indirectly involves the patient in the decision-making process.

Each patient at the initial consultation undergoes facial video imaging. A high-resolution digital camcorder (Sony VX3-CCD) captures and transmits the facial image to a capture board (Targa 64). A computer in MS-DOS mode (Intel 80486) is used with Mirror II Aesthetic Software (Canfield

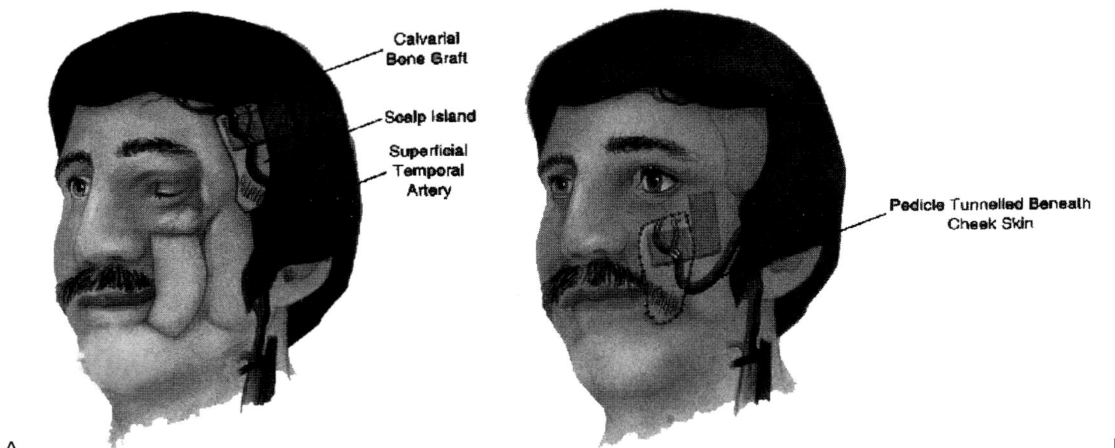

FIGURE 35D-5. A: Design of temporalis fascial flap with L-shaped strut for orbital rim. **B:** Bony contour of orbit restored. Platform provided for prosthetic eye inset into socket. Axial pedicle determined by Doppler auscultation. (From Rose EH, ed. *Aesthetic facial restoration.* Philadelphia: Lippincott–Raven Publishers, 1998:245, with permission.)

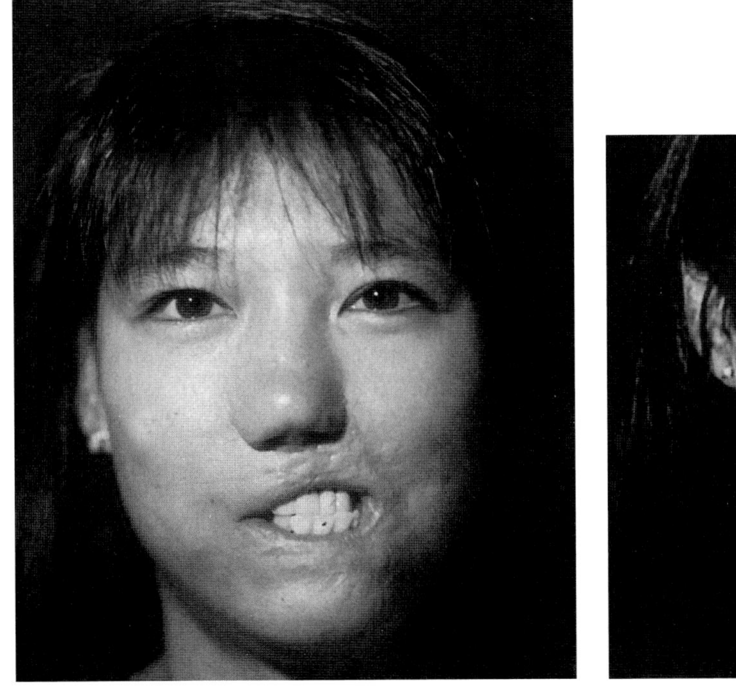

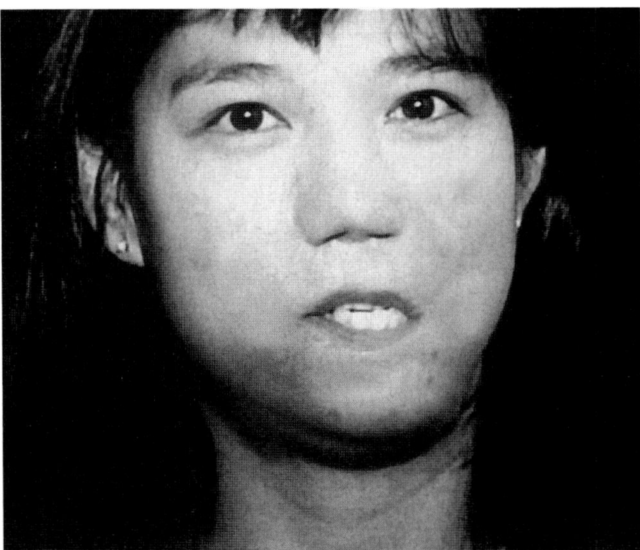

FIGURE 35D-6. Patient 3. A 29-year-old Vietnamese woman sustained a grenade injury to her face as an infant. **A:** Contracted upper lip with insufficient lining. **B:** Video projection of desired surgical results by image modification software. *(continued)*

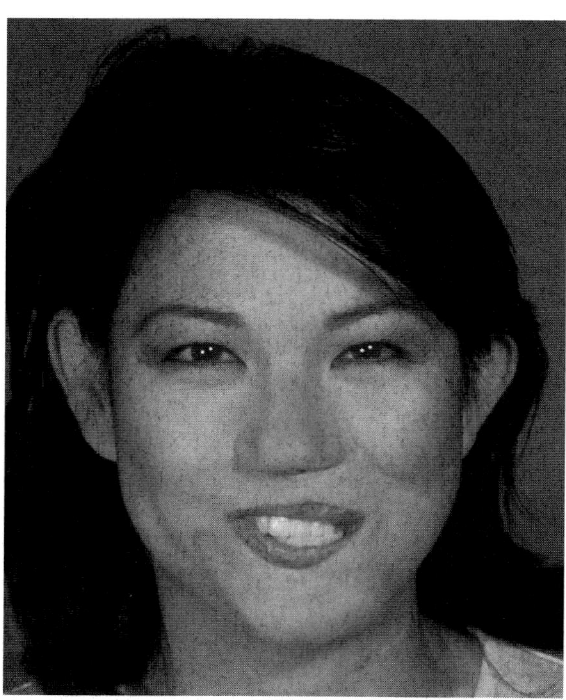

C

FIGURE 35D-6. *Continued.* **C:** Actual surgical outcome. (From Rose EH, Norris MS. The versatile temporoparietal fascial flap: adaptability to a variety of composite defects. *Plast Reconstr Surg* 1990;85:224, with permission.)

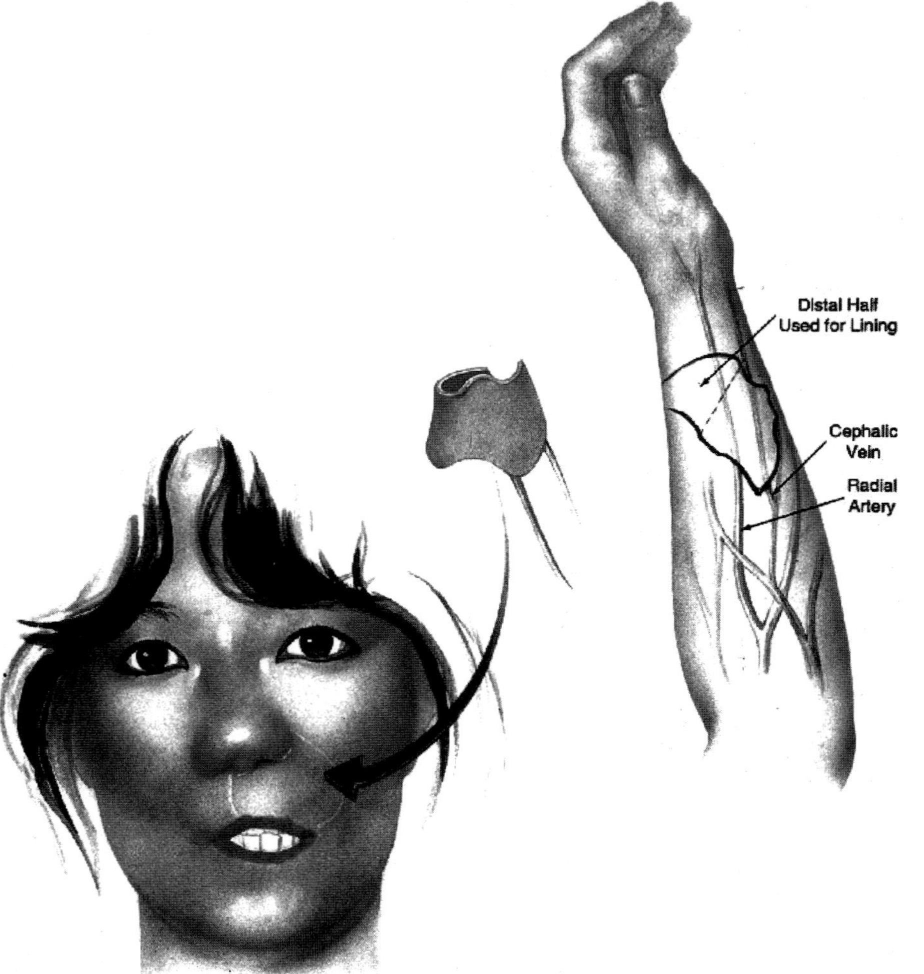

FIGURE 35D-7. Patient 3. **Right:** Design of a prepatterned island defect centered over the radial artery. **Center:** Flap transfer. Distal half is folded into sulcus for mucosal lining. **Left:** Flap inset into upper lip defect. (From Rose EH, ed. *Aesthetic facial restoration.* Philadelphia: Lippincott–Raven Publishers, 1998:170, with permission.)

Medical) to modify the image on the television monitor. Prints of the original and modified images are replicated on a high-resolution Sony video printer. The "shaped" menu allows stretching, cutting, repositioning, rotation, or resizing of facial features. These alteration functions are particularly useful in projecting chin or malar augmentation, nasal tip and base realignment, browlift, and maxillary/mandibular movement. The "copy" tool permits overlay of the facial segment from one image to another, which is particularly useful in the cephalometric overlay of soft tissue. The "draw" menu allows the surgeon to draw freehand lines or shapes, which are particularly helpful in outlining flap design. The "warp" tool visibly shows soft tissue movement in flap advancement or changes in profile (i.e., straighter nasal bridge, submental lipectomy, or flap debulking). The "blend" tool corrects unsightly scars or contour depressions.

Video image prints are used preoperatively for planning and intraoperatively for reference. With a 6-gigabyte hard drive, thousands of pictures can be stored and retrieved individually for postsurgical comparison or collectively according to the database classification. Video images can be converted to 35-mm transparencies for lectures and conferences. In our office, these image storage and retrieval systems have replaced conventional photography and cumbersome slide collection and sorting.

POSTSURGICAL CORRECTIVE MAKEUP

Makeup is an essential component in the overall strategy of aesthetic facial restoration. In the past, too much emphasis has been placed on exact color matches of flaps and grafts, precluding the use of valuable donor resources similar in texture and thickness. During the past decade, with the integration of the services of a professional aesthetician into our reconstructive practice, the focus of our endeavors has been geared to balance and symmetry of facial features. The more advanced formulas of sheer, flesh-colored foundations have made it possible to blend restored facial components into the overall facial integrity. In effect, the contoured tissue transfer serves as a palette onto which the face is painted. In surgical planning, I can concentrate on sculpting the face with the assurance that the aesthetician will be able to complete the facial portrait.

Millard said that "to establish facial form is not enough," and that the goal is also to achieve "a beautiful appearance" (11). As part of our surgical package, a kit of skin care products and custom-matched camouflage makeup is included for postoperative application. A trained aesthetician teaches both our reconstructive and cosmetic patients the art of makeup application as part of the daily ritual. Just as patients who have had facelifts are judged by their made-up appearance (and photographed that way!), reconstructive patients should be assessed by the same standards. The application of camouflage creams beneath the foundation to cover scars and color mismatches becomes as routine as brushing one's teeth or combing one's hair each morning. These tricks enable patients to put their best face forward, and in a world obsessed with appearance, the end justifies the means.

CONCLUSION

Dr. Menick has stated that the "primary function of the face is to look normal." In an era of managed care and cost containment, judgment calls are made by detached administrators weighing the efficacy of the treatment versus the drainage on corporate resources. In an attempt to save money, "simpler operations" performed by in-network providers may end up costing more in the long run because of the need for repeated surgeries and prolonged loss of time from school or work, not to mention the emotional angst to which patients and their families are subjected. Most of our patients are in their teens and 20s (average age in our series is 21.6 years) (4), and each can look forward to *five or six decades of productivity* (in lieu of disability and societal detachment). Overall, the costs of facial microvascular free-tissue transfers at our institution (Mount Sinai Medical Center in New York) compare favorably with those of sophisticated organ transplants (kidneys, lungs, heart), which are generally performed on much older persons (12) and necessitate prolonged pharmacologic antirejection regimens. Commitment to a comprehensive strategy of facial restoration, as outlined, may be more costly in the initial phases of reconstruction, but in the long term, it can provide more definitive outcomes and give the disfigured patient a second chance to enter the mainstream of society.

REFERENCES

1. Auchauer BM. Reconstruction of the burned face. *Clin Plast Surg* 1992;19:623.
2. Feldman SS. Facial resurfacing: the single sheet concept. In: Brent B, ed. *The artistry of plastic surgery.* St. Louis: Mosby, 1987.
3. Rose EH. *Aesthetic facial restoration.* Philadelphia: Lippincott–Raven Publishers, 1997.
4. Rose EH. Restoration of the severely disfigured face in burn victims: a comprehensive strategy. *Plast Reconstr Surg* 1995;96:1573.
5. Lineweaver WC, Buncke HS, Oliva A, et al. Factors associated with clinical microvascular transplant failure: directions for research. Presented at the 58th annual meeting of The American Society for Plastic and Reconstructive Surgeons, San Francisco, 1989.
6. Khouri RF, Shaw WW. Reconstruction of the lower extremity with microvascular free flaps: a ten-year experience with 304 consecutive cases. *J Trauma* 1989;29:1086.
7. Harashina T. Analysis of 200 free flaps. *Br J Plast Surg* 1988;41:33.

8. Rose EH, Norris MS. The versatile temporoparietal fascial flap: adaptability to a variety of composite defects. *Plast Reconstr Surg* 1990;85:224.
9. Rose EH, Norris MS, Rose JM. Application of high tech three-dimensional imaging and computer-generated models in complex facial reconstruction with vascularized bone grafts. *Plast Reconstr Surg* 1993;91:252.
10. Woolson ST, Dev P, Fellingham LL, et al. Three-dimensional imaging of bone from computerized tomography. *Clin Orthop* 1986;202:239.
11. Millard DR Jr. *Principalization of plastic surgery.* Boston: Little, Brown and Company, 1986.
12. Aronoff R. Personal communication. USPHS Division of Organ Transplantation. Telephone 301-443-7577.

36

FACIAL REANIMATION

JULIA K. TERZIS
BERKAN MERSA

Facial reanimation is a challenging area of reconstructive surgery. The goal of facial reanimation is to provide symmetrical, coordinated voluntary and involuntary motion and competent eye and oral sphincters. Etiologic factors include congenital abnormalities, trauma, and tumors and infections, which can affect adjacent structures. Therefore, the surgeon must be familiar with microsurgery, oculoplastic surgery, the reconstruction of deformities of bony structures, the use of alloplastic biomaterials, and facelift and corrective rhinoplasty procedures.

FACTORS AFFECTING OUTCOME

Differential Diagnosis

In the medical literature, about 100 causes of facial paralysis are identified (1). Distinguishing Bell's palsy from other forms of facial paralysis is important because typical Bell's palsy can improve within 3 to 6 months. Additionally, intratemporal and extratemporal facial nerve involvement should be differentiated. Because the intratemporal portion of the facial nerve contains both motor and sensory fibers, involvement at this level is manifested as a decrease in lacrimation, hyperacusia, and taste disturbances on the anterior two-thirds of the tongue. The extratemporal facial nerve contains only motor fibers, and involvement at this level does not affect sensory functions. Another important step in the diagnosis is to determine whether the facial paralysis is complete or incomplete because the choice of surgical strategy for reanimation depends on this determination.

Expectations of the Patient

Patients must be informed before facial reanimation surgery is undertaken that their facial functioning will never be completely normal and that their original facial appearance cannot be restored. Anticipated improvements, donor morbidity, complications, and sequelae should be outlined in detail preoperatively for each stage of the surgery. Patients' expectations may vary depending on the cause of paralysis. The expectations of patients with facial paralysis after elective aesthetic procedures are different from those of patients after traumatic injury, tumor extirpation, Bell's palsy, or developmental mishap. Patients with long-standing facial paralysis are generally pleased with any improvements that follow reanimation surgery, whereas those who have undergone elective aesthetic procedures are likely to be much more critical of the surgical results. Patients with more realistic expectations, regardless of the cause of paralysis, tend to be happier with the results of reanimation surgery.

Capability of the Surgeon

The surgeon should choose the most appropriate treatment for the patient. Current approaches to facial paralysis necessitate the use of microsurgical techniques. Surgeons who are not experienced in microsurgical techniques and are not familiar with facial reanimation should not attempt to perform this type of surgery.

Treatment Plan

No universal recipe for reconstruction is available to fit every patient. Each treatment plan is individualized according to the cultural, socioeconomic, psychologic status, and age of the patient—whether the patient is a child or an adult, and whether the adult patient is mentally young or old. The mental age correlates with the patient's lifestyle, range of activities, and expectations. A combination of these factors will determine how the patient perceives the results of the reconstructive procedure—as favorable or unfavorable.

Cooperation of the Patient

The patient must be informed in detail about the surgical procedure, postoperative regimen, and rehabilitation before beginning treatment. Although the patient may be given

J. K. Terzis: Division of Plastic Surgery and Reconstructive Surgery, Eastern Virginia Medical School; and Department of Plastic Surgery, Sentara Norfolk General Hospital, Norfolk, Virginia

B. Mersa: Department of Surgery, Division of Plastic Surgery, Eastern Virginia Medical School, Norfolk, Virginia

new pathways for facial expression, if they are never used, the result will be unfavorable. The patient must be willing to complete the entire surgical program, including postoperative rehabilitation, to obtain optimal results.

Revisions

All serious facial reanimation surgical procedures, especially those involving free-muscle transfers, require final revisions. Although the segmental innervation of gracilis (2) and latissimus dorsi muscles (3,4) allows the muscles to be sculpted as much as needed, surgeons are unable to predict the ultimate result after free-muscle transplantation. Bulkiness and wrinkles on the cheek skin over the muscle flap always require revision surgery.

Preoperative Evaluation

The surgeon should be a critical evaluator. If the deformity and surgical indications are evaluated incorrectly, the surgeon will fail to choose the best method of repairing the original deformity and the outcome of the treatment will be suboptimal. If more than one method is available to correct a deformity, the advantages and disadvantage of each method must be compared to achieve the best possible result for an individual patient.

MANAGEMENT OF FACIAL PARALYSIS

Diagnosis

History and Clinical Presentation

The first effort should be to differentiate idiopathic Bell's palsy from other causes of paralysis because improvement tends to occur early. The onset is acute and unilateral. Most patients with Bell's palsy describe a viral prodrome. They also may present with pain or paresthesia of the face or neck. The stapes reflex is decreased or absent in almost all patients. The forehead muscles are intact. Other cranial nerves, such as the trigeminal and hypoglossal, may be involved.

It is important to characterize the onset of paralysis. A sudden onset indicates trauma, infection, toxic, vascular, or iatrogenic causes. A slow onset is mostly associated with neoplasm.

A review of the previous medical records is extremely important, especially when facial paralysis follows tumor removal. Information regarding tumor size and location, the operative report of tumor extirpation, the degree of facial nerve involvement, the histologic type of the tumor, previous resection attempts, and the number of previous surgical corrective procedures on the face are necessary to establish a realistic strategy for facial reanimation.

Facial paralysis may be present at birth. Evidence of birth trauma and the use of suction or forceps can be found in the history and medical records. Unilateral or bilateral developmental facial paralysis is also common in children. It may be associated with other anomalies, such as an underdeveloped mandible (especially the vertical segment) or structures of the outer or inner ear. Developmental facial paralysis is usually incomplete and involves mostly the middle and upper face. The lower face typically escapes. Möbius' syndrome is a developmental disorder associated with bilateral facial nerve involvement. Other cranial nerves, especially the sixth, third, fifth, ninth, and twelfth, may be involved. These patients may have other anomalies, such as syndactyly or Poland's syndrome. Surgery for tumors such as cystic hygroma or lymphangioma is another cause of facial paralysis. Medical records of previous surgeries are helpful in these cases to establish the involvement of previously unaffected branches of the facial nerve.

Iatrogenic facial nerve injuries following facial surgery are also very common. During aesthetic facelift procedures, the mandibular branch can be injured (Fig. 36-1). The frontal branch can be injured during temporomandibular joint surgery.

Specialized Testing

1. *Electromyography.* An appropriate neurologic evaluation should be performed with needle electromyography to survey each of the facial muscle targets.
2. *Cranial nerve examination.* Testing the integrity of all cranial nerves is mandatory, especially before a cranial nerve transfer, such as nerve V or XII to nerve VII, is attempted. The blink reflex, corneal reflex, taste, tongue movements, and swallowing should be assessed carefully. The detection of multiple cranial nerve involvement may help to establish the diagnosis and extent of involvement in other syndromes, such as Möbius'. In developmental paralysis, a preoperative neuroophthalmology consultation is also required to rule out amblyopia. An ear, nose, and throat consultation is often necessary to examine the stapedial reflex, or to evaluate facial paralysis that develops after removal of an intratemporal tumor, such as a cholesteatoma.
3. *Radiology.* Bilateral symmetrical polytomography and computed tomography are beneficial to evaluate the facial canal in developmental facial paralysis. Angiography of the donor site (face and neck) is also necessary before a free-muscle transfer is performed, especially if the patient has sustained facial trauma or has previously undergone surgery.
4. *Video and photographic documentation.* Protocols have been established for preoperative photography and video documentation. Photographs and videotapes are obtained at rest and while the patient is talking, smiling, closing the eyes slightly and tightly, lifting the brow, depressing the lower lip, and stretching the neck (for platysma evaluation). The patient is also videotaped for 4 minutes to evaluate the blink reflex. Letting the patient

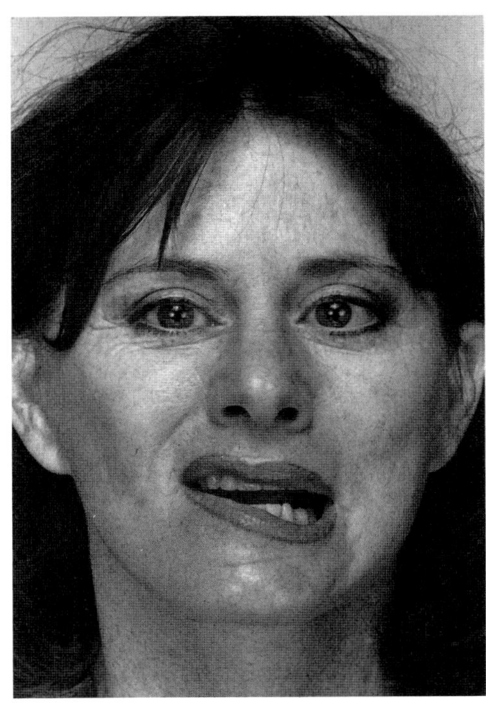

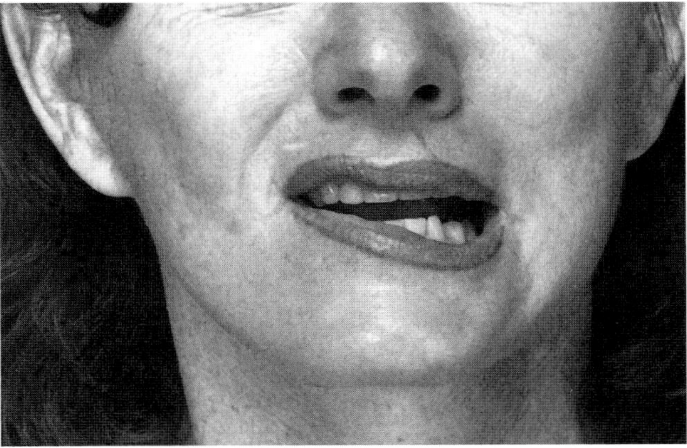

A B

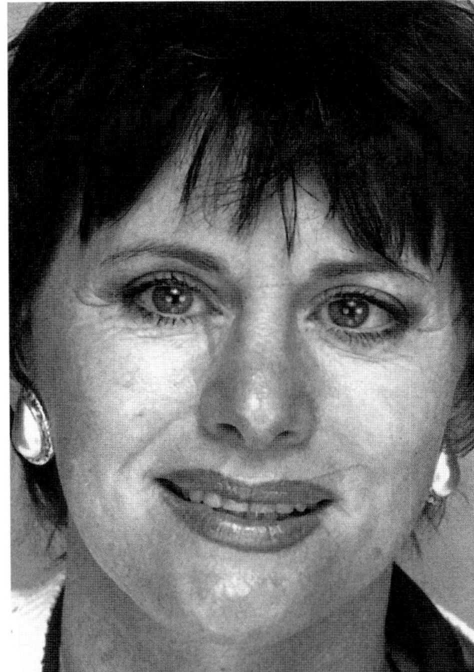

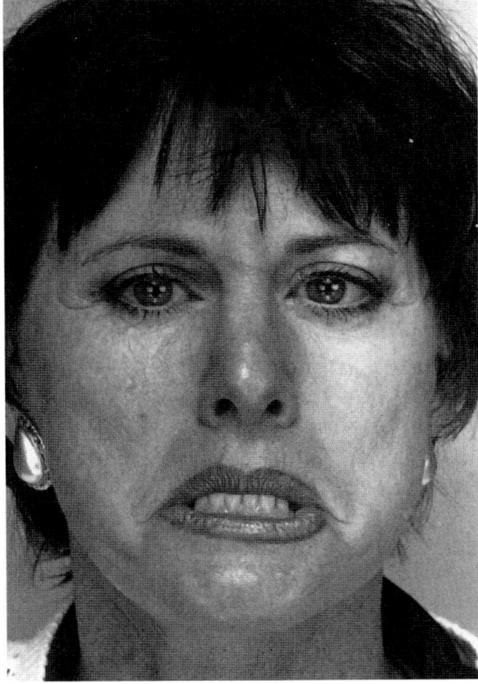

C D

FIGURE 36-1. A,B: A 50-year-old woman with incomplete facial paralysis following a facelift procedure. When her bandages were taken off, a right depressor paralysis was present. Preoperative needle electromyography of the right depressor yielded fibrillations. An exploration was performed 1 month after the facelift surgery. Dense scarring and right mandibular and cervical branch injury were encountered. Reconstruction consisted of facial (VII)-to-facial (VII) nerve transfer, with the buccal branches used as the motor donor. **C:** Patient 1 year after reconstructive surgery. The lower lip is completely symmetrical during smiling. **D:** A nearly full depression of the lower lip has been restored.

watch a funny television show is useful to document spontaneous animation. Measurement and analysis of the direction and extent of movement of the upper and lower lips, nasolabial fold, and nasal base during full smiling are useful in determining how to inset the free muscle in reanimation surgery (5).

Treatment

Treatment strategies differ for acute and chronic cases (Fig. 36-2). In the acute period, because the targets are still present, neural microsurgery (including microneurolysis, direct repair, or ipsilateral nerve grafting) should be performed for target resuscitation. These procedures provide the best result because neither scar nor neuroma has formed. Stimulation of the distal segments of the cut nerve branches, which is possible only in the first 72 hours, makes it easier to identify and match the cut nerve ends. If primary end-to-end repair is not possible, interpositional nerve grafts can be used. If the paralysis has been present longer than 6 months and no ipsilateral donors are available, the surgeon should proceed with cross-facial nerve grafting; however, a "baby-sitter" procedure must also be performed to salvage the muscle targets. If the target atrophy is too advanced, the transfer of a local muscle such as the temporalis or the transfer of a free muscle such as the gracilis or pectoralis minor should be added to the plan as soon as the cross-facial nerve grafts reach the paralyzed side of the face.

Neural Microsurgery Procedures

Nerve Grafting

Traumatic defects and ablative tumor surgery are the main indicators for facial nerve grafting. To avoid the detrimental effect of tension on the suture lines (6), a longer graft than necessary should be harvested because shrinkage of up to 20% will occur (7). The most commonly used nerve grafts for facial nerve grafting are the sural and saphenous nerves. Sural nerve harvesting leaves an anesthetic area over the lateral aspect of the dorsum of the foot and the lateral malleolus, but this area decreases with time. Scarring is also associated with the sural nerve donor site, although it can be minimized with interrupted incisions or perhaps the currently developed endoscopic harvesting techniques (8).

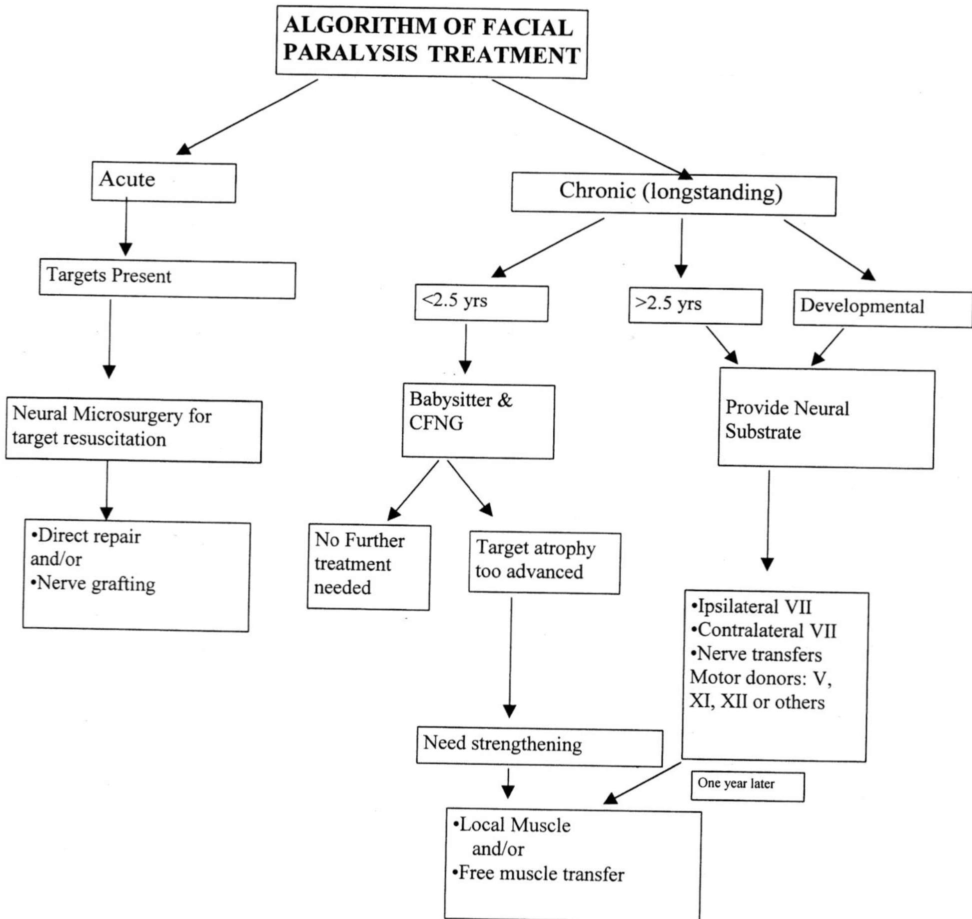

FIGURE 36-2. Algorithm for the treatment of facial paralysis.

The results of reinnervation can be less than anticipated. Possible reasons for failure include disruption of suture lines, use of improper technique to accomplish the nerve coaptations, and atrophy of the reinnervated muscle (6,9).

Cross-facial Nerve Grafting

Cross-facial nerve grafting was first reported by Scaramella (10) and Smith (11), popularized by Anderl and Muhlbauer (12), and subsequently modified and improved (13–15). Modifications relate mainly to the number of cross-facial nerve grafts; the route, location, and methodology of tunneling; and the selection of nerve branches on the nonparalyzed side. The technique used by the senior author (JKT) is as follows: A modified facelift incision is made to explore the nonparalyzed side. A nerve stimulator is used to identify and select the facial nerve branches after electrophysiologic mapping. Two to four sural nerve grafts are preferred. The second stage is usually performed 9 to 12 months later, when a positive Tinel's sign has been observed at the distal end of the cross-facial grafts. At this stage, the distal ends of the cross-facial nerve grafts are coapted with selected branches of the facial nerve on the paralyzed side.

"Baby-sitter" Procedure

The baby-sitter procedure involves a partial hypoglossal transfer to the ipsilateral facial nerve during the first stage of cross-facial nerve grafting to help maintain the bulk and tonus of the facial muscles (16). A 40% splitting of the hypoglossal nerve can be used effectively without damaging the tongue muscles. In a second stage, the cross-facial nerve grafts may be used for coaptation with contralateral facial nerve branches for direct neurotization of the facial muscles, or to supply the muscle transfers (17). If the paralysis has been present for more than 6 months, cross-facial nerve grafting must be supplemented with the baby-sitter procedure because the grafts are relatively weak motor donors.

If the frontozygomatic and cervicofacial branches of the normal facial nerve are carefully selected as motor donors for cross-facial nerve grafting, the uninvolved side of the face should not be impaired. In some cases, mild weakness may develop during the immediate postoperative period, but this weakness resolves typically in 3 months (18). The donor site complications in cross-facial nerve grafting are the same as in other nerve grafting. The anesthetic area on the lower extremity typically is eventually decreased by terminal sprouting from neighboring sensory nerves.

Postoperative care is very important. The motions of the mouth and jaw must be limited to protect the coaptation sites. A dressing of fluffy cotton rolls and elastic bandages is placed around the patient's head to protect the repairs. During the first 24 hours, a plaster of Paris wrap is also utilized and subsequently removed. Antiemetics are given to prevent vomiting in the early postoperative period. The patient takes fluids or a soft diet and speaks only through the teeth for 2 to 3 weeks. In 6 weeks, massage and ultrasound treatment should be started over the coaptation sites to prevent the formation of scars around the nerves and adhesions with the overlapping cheek skin flap. Intensive slow-pulse stimulation of the denervated muscles can be started at this time to prevent further atrophy while the facial fibers are elongating across the face. Facial exercises, biofeedback, and physical therapy are important in restoring coordinated facial movements bilaterally.

Cross-facial nerve grafts are also used to innervate the free-muscle transfers and on occasion to neurotize the orbicularis oculi and depressor muscles directly. The cross-facial nerve grafting procedure is accepted by surgeons who deal with dynamic facial reanimation as the standard first-stage operation.

Neurotization Procedures

The main donor nerves for crossover procedures are the hypoglossal, spinal accessory, and trigeminal nerves. The main advantages of nerve transfers are the following:

1. Ipsilateral donors can be powerful motor nerves to rehabilitate the facial musculature.
2. Because of the short distances involved, denervated muscles can be reinnervated rapidly.

Hypoglossal Nerve

The criteria for use of the hypoglossal nerve for facial paralysis are the following:

1. The extracranial part of the facial nerve should be intact.
2. Some ipsilateral facial musculature should be present.
3. A direct VII-to-VII repair of the facial nerve injury or ipsilateral nerve grafting (VII-graft-VII) is not possible.
4. Facial paralysis is irreversible (19–21).

Patients with denervation of less than 18 months' duration are suitable for this procedure. When the denervation is more prolonged, fibrosis of the facial musculature prevents resuscitation, even if powerful ipsilateral motors are used. If the entire hypoglossal nerve is transferred to the ipsilateral facial nerve, the patient invariably experiences various degrees of tongue atrophy and difficulty in speaking and swallowing (19,21). The other chief complaints of patients who undergo hypoglossal-facial crossover are overactivity and mass movements. Synkinesis and mass movements are seen in almost all patients, especially during talking and eating. Involuntary movements of one portion of the face typically occur while another part of the face moves voluntarily. The most commonly used method to overcome these unpleasant problems is reeducation; physical therapy is used to teach the patient to control facial muscles (22). Other methods attempted are injection of botulinum toxin (23,24), which prevents acetylcholine release at the neuromuscular endplate, magnetic stimulation (25), and selective myectomy (26). Rubin et al. (27) advised a Z-plasty technique to restore tongue function. The aim of this technique is to provide muscular neurotization from the normal side across the midline into the atrophic side.

To avoid the detrimental effects of hypoglossal palsy, the senior author (JKT) in 1984 introduced the baby-sitter procedure (16), in which the hypoglossal nerve is split with a diamond knife and 40% of the proximal motor fibers are used for ipsilateral facial nerve neurotization. This technique is used to stop the denervation clock and maintain the bulk of the denervated facial muscles while the first stage of the cross-facial grafting procedure is simultaneously performed. At the second stage, the distal ends of the cross-facial grafts are coapted with more peripheral branches of the involved facial nerve. The baby-sitter–VII coaptation is not severed. The previously denervated facial musculature now receives motor input from both the baby-sitter nerve and the cross-facial nerve grafts. The baby-sitter nerve serves to maintain the bulk of the facial muscles while the cross-facial motor fibers from the contralateral nerve VII function as the pacemaker (16). The baby-sitter procedure avoids tongue deficit and provides powerful motor donors for rapid muscle rejuvenation.

Spinal Accessory Nerve

Although transfer of the spinal accessory nerve can provide good resting tonus, shoulder disabilities are experienced by almost all patients if the entire accessory nerve is used. Loss of the ability to elevate the abducted arm, increased shoulder pain during activity, and frozen shoulder are the main forms of morbidity associated with this transfer. Transposition of sternocleidomastoid branch of the accessory nerve avoids shoulder paralysis (28,29). The senior author (JKT) uses a partial accessory transfer, which involves 50% of the branch to the sternocleidomastoid and 40% of the branch to the trapezius. After these delicate splitting procedures, paralysis does not develop in the sternocleidomastoid or trapezius muscle.

Trigeminal Nerve

In cases of facial paralysis associated with Möbius' syndrome, the facial nerve is involved bilaterally. The masseter branch of the trigeminal nerve can be used as a motor source for free-muscle transfers instead of a cross-facial nerve graft if it is not involved in the developmental mishap. As with other transfers of chewing muscles, the patient is retrained by biting for smile.

Transposition of Local Muscles

The most commonly used transpositions are those involving the masseter and temporalis muscles (7). The patient must be reeducated after transposition of these muscles; their innervation remains the trigeminal nerve. The main disadvantage of the use of chewing muscles is lack of synchronization with the healthy side of the face. This disadvantage is lessened by placing a cross-facial nerve graft and coapting the cross-facial nerve graft to the motor nerve of these muscles.

Masseter Muscle

The masseter is a very powerful chewing muscle that can be used to reanimate the mouth (30,31). One of the main disadvantages of masseter transposition is lateral and posterior displacement of the muscle because of its deeper location. Involuntary facial movements during eating and talking are also a significant problem for these patients. Therefore, use of the masseter muscle is associated with poor symmetry and coordination.

Temporalis Muscle

The temporalis is the most commonly used muscle for transposition (31–34). It can be used to reanimate both oral and eye sphincters simultaneously, but the results, especially for the eye sphincter, are not satisfactory. If the excursion and length of the muscle are not assessed correctly, lower eyelid ectropion develops. Transposition of this muscle empties the entire temporal fossa and causes a concave deformity. Currently, alloplastic materials that can be reshaped have been used in an attempt to address this problem. Another cosmetic sequela of temporalis transfer is swelling over the zygomatic arch. Other complications are similar to those associated with masseter transposition, such as involuntary facial movements during biting, chewing, and talking and a lack of symmetrical and coordinated facial movement.

Platysma and Digastric Muscles

Depression of the paralyzed lower lip must be included in the overall treatment plan. Although most surgeons focus on smile and eye reanimation, lack of depression of the lower lip leads to an unfavorable aesthetic and functional result. Pedicled platysma and digastric muscles are beneficial for providing depression to the lower lip.

If it is available and not involved, the platysma is the first choice for depressor reanimation of the lower lip because it is innervated by the facial nerve. When the platysma is absent or paralyzed, the digastric muscle can be used. The lower cross-facial nerve graft is usually coapted with the nerve to the anterior belly of the digastric muscle. This arrangement offers the opportunity for coordinated and symmetrical depression. The tension with which the transferred muscle is inset is extremely important. If the muscle is inset with too much tension, a deformity of the lip contour can result (Fig. 36-3). The senior author has had substantial experience with both of these muscles, and overall the morbidity associated with both transfers is minimal.

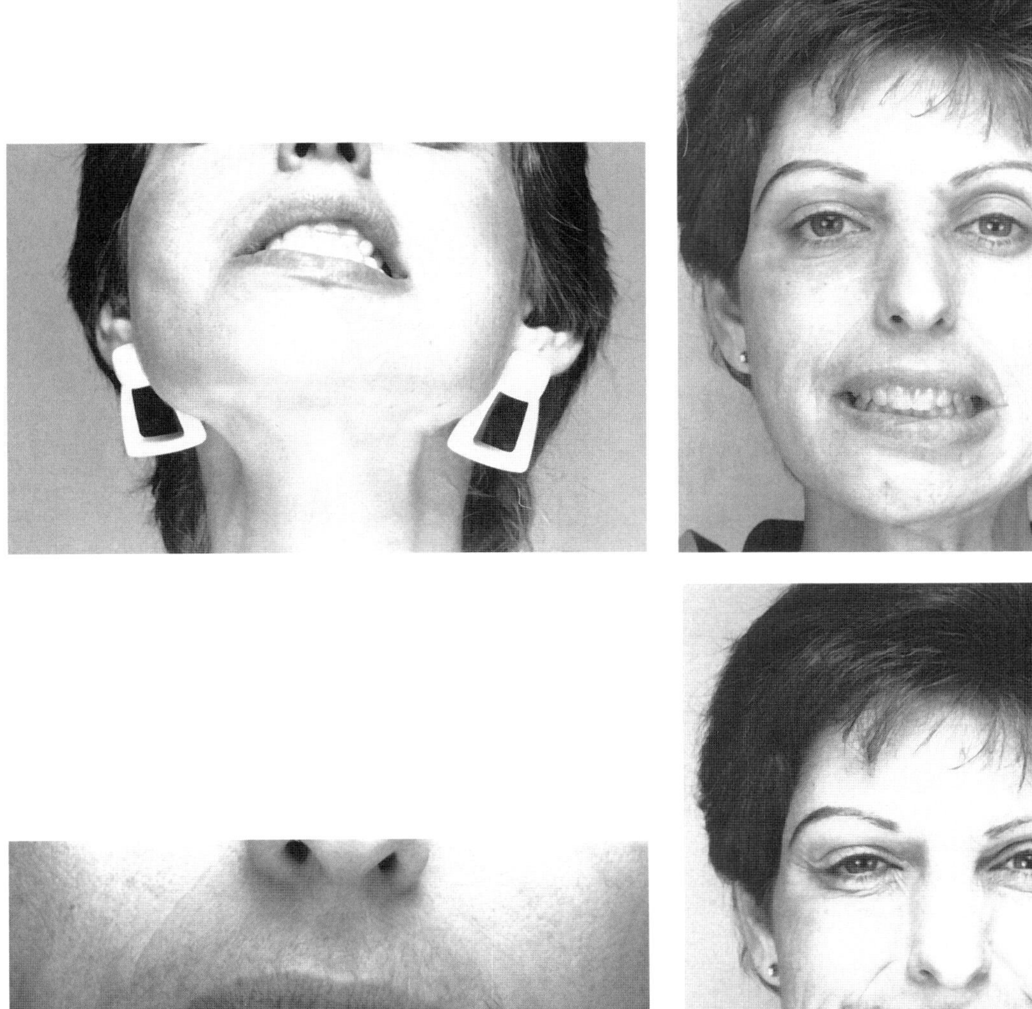

FIGURE 36-3. A: A 34-year-old woman with right-sided facial paralysis after removal of a hemangioma at the age of 7 months. An incomplete paralysis was noted after the surgery. At age 7, a static sling procedure was performed elsewhere to improve her smile. The patient's complaints included an inability to move her lips. In the first stage, four cross-facial nerve grafts were placed. Twelve months after the first stage, a right minitemporalis muscle was transferred to the right modiolus and upper lip. Additionally, a right digastric muscle was microsurgically transferred to the lower lip. **B:** Note the deformity in the right lower lip. **C,D:** The patient after correction of the deformity by advancing and mobilizing the orbicularis oris muscle and resecting a wedge of mucosa from the right lower lip.

Transfer of Free Muscles

Free-muscle transfer is indicated when the facial muscles are absent or their function is substantially diminished. Muscle atrophy should be proved with needle electromyography before surgery. If the ipsilateral facial nerve is available, the nerve of the muscle transplant is coapted directly to it. In the absence of an available ipsilateral facial nerve, cross-facial nerve grafting from the healthy side is preferred. The results with cross-facial nerve grafting are always superior to those obtained with other motor sources because the cross-facial nerve grafts offer the possibility of coordinated facial movement. If the facial nerves are absent bilaterally, ipsilateral hypoglossal, trigeminal, accessory, or other motor nerves may be used as donors for the transplanted muscle.

When the donor muscle is selected, the factors to be considered are the following:

1. The strength, bulk, and excursion of the transplanted muscle should be appropriate for the muscle being substituted.
2. The neurovascular pedicle must be reliable.
3. Donor site morbidity must be minimal.
4. The origin and insertion of the free muscle must fit the requirements of the contralateral face.
5. Two surgical teams should be available for simultaneous donor harvesting and recipient preparation (17,35,36).

When a smile restoration procedure is planned, preoperative measurements and videotapes of the patient are needed to assess the excursion and force vectors. The direction and degree of pull required at the level of the alar base, upper lip, commissure, and nasolabial fold should be considered carefully, and the free-muscle unit placed accordingly (5,36).

Numerous muscles have been used for facial reanimation as free-tissue transfers, including gracilis (37–39), pectoralis minor (36,40,41), rectus abdominis (42), latissimus dorsi (3,4), extensor digitorum brevis (43), and serratus anterior (44). Attempts to reconstruct two functions, eye closure and upper lip elevation, with a single muscle flap usually produce unsatisfactory results except in the case of the pectoralis minor (because of its dual innervation) (40,41).

Gracilis

Gracilis is the first choice for free-muscle transplantation to reanimate the paralyzed face in adults (37–39). Its advantages include easy access, rare anatomical variations of the pedicle, easy shaping and debulking, and appropriate excursion to mimic the zygomaticus major muscle during smiling. Disadvantages include a single direction of pull. Although it is a strong adductor muscle, its absence results in no functional loss. Excess bulk of the muscle is another main disadvantage; however, this is easily prevented by meticulous shaping. It is preferable to debulk the muscle *in situ* and perform meticulous hemostasis at the same time to prevent possible hematoma formation after transfer (36,39). Secondary revision is always needed. During this revisional stage, extreme care must be taken to prevent injury to the supplying cross-facial nerve graft and vascular pedicle. Excessive debulking may downgrade the performance of the muscle, and one can lose the original result. Skin wrinkles resulting from adhesions of the muscle to the overlying skin are one of the most common unfavorable results (Fig. 36-4). This problem can be eliminated by transposing a vascularized, pedicled temporoparietal fascia flap between muscle and skin.

If the pulling force of the free muscle is inadequate, the upper lip, commissure, and nasolabial fold excursion can be strengthened by utilizing a minitemporalis muscle flap, which may provide up to 1 cm of additional excursion to the previously transferred free muscle.

Pectoralis Minor

The main indication for the pectoralis minor free-muscle flap is developmental facial paralysis in young children (36,40,41). The length and width of the muscle at this age are ideal to fit the involved face. Furthermore, the bulk at this age is optimal, and no sculpting is needed before transplantation. One of the main advantage of this muscle is that it can be transplanted as a whole. Because no sculpting is required, the integrity of each muscle fiber remains intact, the risk for hematoma formation is minimal, and downgrading through debulking is totally avoided. Donor site morbidity is minimal. Removal of the muscle causes no functional loss, and the scar is acceptable (41). Dual innervation of the muscle is another important advantage. The upper third is innervated by a branch of the lateral pectoral nerve, and the lower two thirds by the medial pectoral nerve. This arrangement allows independent movement of the upper and lower parts of the muscle. Thus, separate reanimation of the eye and mouth is possible. However, because of its deep position and the short and complex neurovascular pedicle, this muscle flap is difficult for an inexperienced surgeon to harvest. Furthermore, brachial plexus injury is possible if the surgeon is not familiar with the anatomy of the infraclavicular region. The pedicle is also much shorter than that of the gracilis and is variable. If debulking is necessary, it has to be done after the muscle is harvested, which prolongs the ischemia time. If necessary, debulking is performed during the revision stage (Fig. 36-5).

Before the planned free-muscle flap is transferred, the percentage of bulk loss should be estimated. Despite accurate preoperative planning, free muscles usually require revision. An important factor in free-muscle transplantation is related to muscle tension. The tension of the muscle must

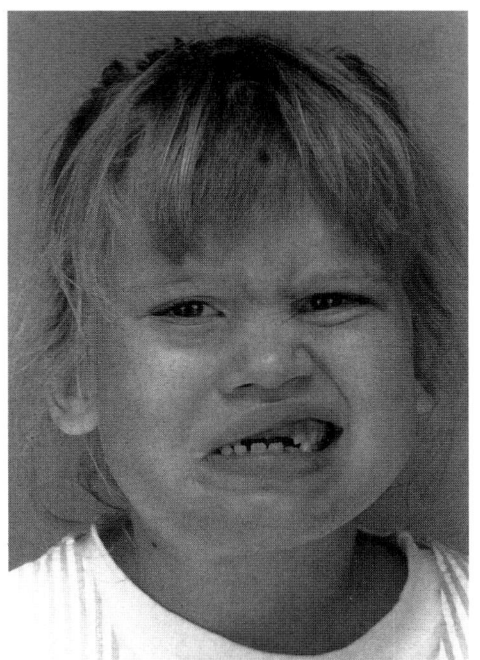
A

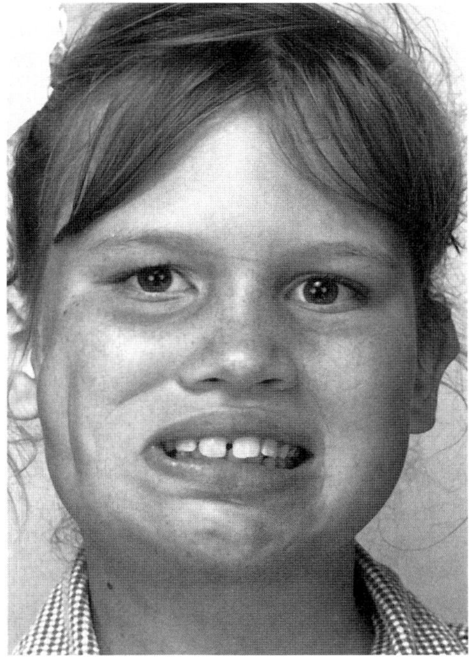
B

FIGURE 36-4. A: A girl, 6 1/2 years old, with unilateral developmental facial paralysis. The medical records stated that vacuum extraction had been attempted twice at delivery. Immediately after birth, a right-sided facial paralysis was noted. Chief complaints of the patient were drooling and an inability to close her eye. The patient underwent the first stage of facial reanimation surgery at age 6 1/2, which consisted of cross-facial nerve grafting. Nine months after the first surgery, a free gracilis muscle was transferred. **B:** About 18 months after the free-muscle transfer, the patient presented with a full-denture symmetrical smile. However, her right cheek displayed several wrinkles that formed only when she smiled. The deformity was corrected with the transfer of a pedicled temporoparietal fascia flap that draped the free muscle.

be marked *in situ* so that it can be reproduced following transfer. The muscle is marked every 1 cm along its longitudinal axis. A rule of thumb in adjusting the tension of the transferred muscle is the following: For facial reanimation, the tension of the muscle should be the same as the tension *in situ,* or slightly less. In contrast, for extremity reconstruction, the tension of the free muscle should be greater than the tension *in situ.* To avoid injury to the transferred muscle unit in the immediate postoperative period, a custom-made external holding device is placed to maintain the position of the commissure; in this way, inadvertent jaw movements (as the patient awakens) do not affect the insetting of the free muscle. The device is anchored with an elastic band attached to a 2-in Ace bandage wrapped around the forehead. During the postoperative period, the patency of the vascular anastomosis is checked every hour with a Doppler flowmeter. The patient is kept on a liquid or soft diet for 2 to 3 weeks and must speak without opening the mouth. After the onset of muscle contraction, patients are trained to perform facial exercises in front of a mirror, so that coordinated animation of both sides of the face can be restored. Additionally, adult patients can be referred to a rehabilitation center for motor biofeedback until the transplanted muscle functions in a coordinated fashion with the contralateral side (22). At 6 weeks, ultrasound therapy and manual massage are carried out to minimize scar formation on the operated side and to help to avoid scar adhesions between the skin envelope and the free-muscle unit.

Terzis and Noah (36) analyzed 100 cases of free-muscle transplantation for facial paralysis. Various factors were correlated with the onset of functional return, including age, sex, and ischemia time in free-flap transplantation. This study showed no correlation between ischemia time (0 to 3 hours) and the onset of muscle contraction. The onset of contraction was slightly earlier in women than in men, and the return of function was earlier in young than in older patients.

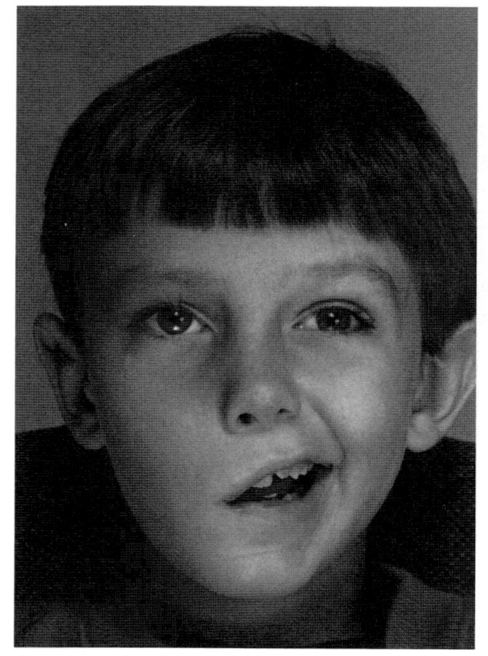

A

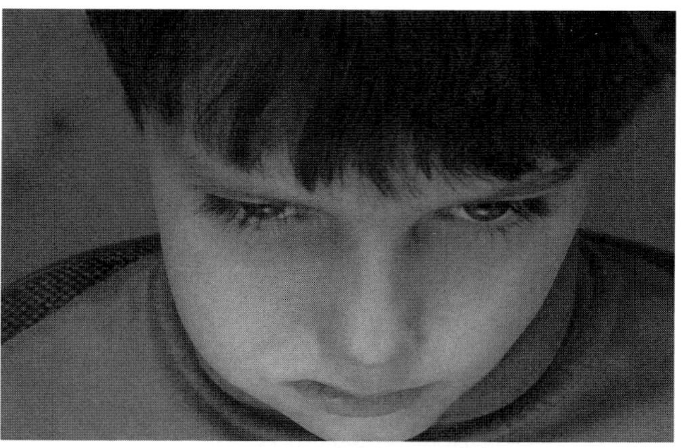

B

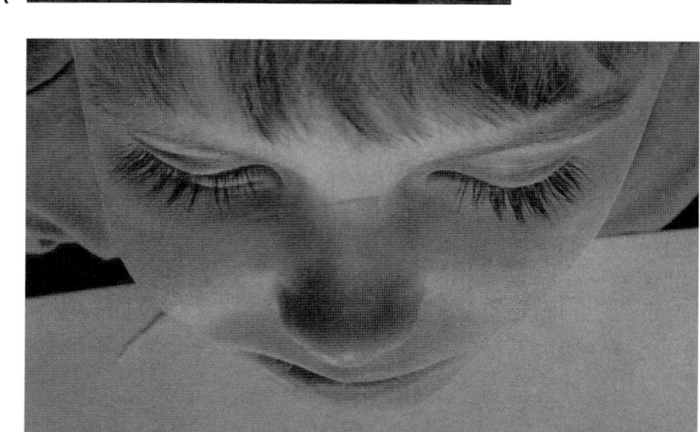

C

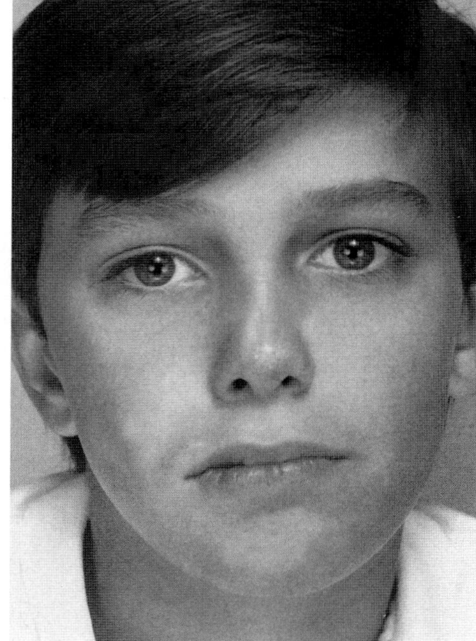

D

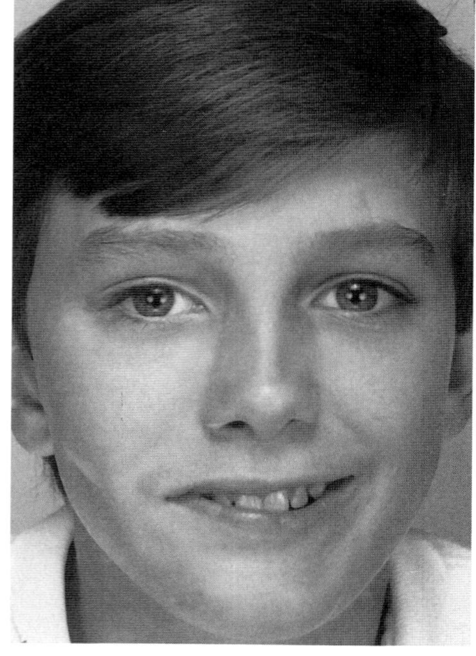

E

FIGURE 36-5. A: A boy, 6 1/2 years old, was born with right-sided developmental facial paralysis. Forceps were used to assist delivery. Facial paralysis was noted immediately after birth. A transmastoid exploration was performed at age 1. The operation notes stated that a mass of soft tissue was encountered between the second genu and the stylomastoid foramen, and that the nerve ended abruptly in this tissue. Biopsy revealed fibrous connective tissue with bony spicules and focal chronic inflammation. The patient underwent cross-facial nerve grafting as a first-stage surgery. One year later, the contralateral pectoralis minor muscle was transferred for smile restoration. **B:** Patient was seen at 9 1/2 years of age with swelling on the right cheek. **C:** A formal reexploration of the right cheek was performed, with debulking of soft tissue. **D:** Two years after revisional surgery, improved contour of the right face is seen in repose. **E:** Patient smiling. Note symmetry and lack of bulk on the right cheek.

UNFAVORABLE RESULTS OF EYE MANAGEMENT PROCEDURES

Denervation of the orbicularis oculi muscle results in insufficient eyelid closure. Gravity pulls the lower eyelid downward when the orbicularis oculi tonus is lost. The ectropion everts the margin of the lower lid and the punctum lacrimalis, so that tear flow and the lacrimal drainage system are disturbed. Constant exposure of cornea gives rise to loss of the tear film, dryness of cornea, conjunctivitis, and keratitis. If the condition progresses, corneal ulceration and blindness can develop.

The age of the patient, presence of the blink reflex and corneal sensation, the degree of lagophthalmos, and the experience of the surgeon are critical factors in determining the method of treatment.

Nonsurgical Methods

In the early period, the following nonsurgical methods protect the eye from the detrimental effects of chronic exposure:

1. Eye glasses or contact lenses
2. Artificial tears and ophthalmic ointments
3. Lid taping
4. Occlusive moisture chambers
5. Scleral shells

When nonsurgical methods become inadequate and lagophthalmos is permanent, surgical treatment should be considered. If the orbicularis oculi muscle is not yet atrophied, cross-facial nerve grafting or direct neurotization of the muscle can relieve the lagophthalmos.

Tarsorrhaphy

Lateral overlapping tarsorrhaphy tightens and shortens the upper and lower eyelids (45). Although it may provide adequate functional results, the cosmetic results are unsatisfactory. The lateral tarsal strip procedure can be used as an alternative to the lateral overlapping technique (46). With this technique, no lid notching is required, baseline tear production is preserved, and the tarsal plate is not sacrificed. Therefore, if additional procedures are contemplated, less morbidity may occur than with the classic overlapping technique. Both of these techniques are commonly used, but neither provides equally sized eyes and coordinated movement. They also limit vision and provide poor corneal protection.

Eye Spring

Eye springs provide good cosmetic and functional results, especially in young patients who do not have a normal blink reflex or in those with an intact corneal reflex and intact trigeminal nerve. The eye spring is inserted through two or three small incisions between the skin and tarsal plate. Extreme care is taken to avoid injury to the globe. Spring breakage and extrusion through the skin have not been very common complications (47). Reduction in tension is a more common complication, but this can be corrected under sedation. If drooping of the lower eyelid is also a problem, specialized upper and lower eyelid springs may be preferable (48,49).

Lid Loading

Gold weight is one of the most useful methods to relieve lagophthalmos (45,50). Different gold weights should be taped to upper eyelid before surgery is performed with the patient in the upright position. Gold evokes a minimal tissue reaction, is easy to carve into the desired shape, and is of a suitable color in partially translucent eyelids because it blends with the skin tone in fair-skinned persons. When the weight is inserted, the pocket must be large enough to anchor to the tarsal plate. Complications listed in the literature are displacement of the implant (Fig. 36-6), implant infection, entropion, inflammatory reaction to gold, poor eyelid contour, corneal ulceration and scarring, asymmetrical closure, residual lagophthalmos, and thickening of eyelid tissue over the prosthesis (51,52). These problems require implant removal and the use of a different reconstructive method.

Minitendon Graft for Lower Eyelid

A minitendon sling to the lower eyelid is the treatment of choice for paralytic ectropion (45). It also helps to decrease lagophthalmos because it raises the lower eyelid. A palmaris longus tendon graft, prepared from the nondominant hand, is utilized for the procedure. A longitudinal split of the tendon is performed before it is transferred to the eye (47). The punctum is canalized to prevent injury. If the lower lid is still lax, symmetry with the normal eye is insufficient, and tearing cannot be controlled, retightening may be necessary. The harvesting of palmaris longus does not leave any functional morbidity. If the graft harvesting is performed with interrupted incisions, donor site scars are acceptable. Some synthetic implants are used instead of tendon graft, but extrusion, migration, failure of the material, inflammatory reactions, and infection are common.

Physiologic Methods of Eye Reanimation

The transplantation of free platysma muscle and the transfer of pedicled contralateral frontalis muscle for eye sphincter substitution have been used in patients with permanent unilateral facial paralysis of long duration (53). Both muscles are innervated by the facial nerve and have a thin, flat belly—features that make them ideal for eye sphincter substitution. Furthermore, the density of innervation in these muscles is comparable with that of the orbicularis oculi mus-

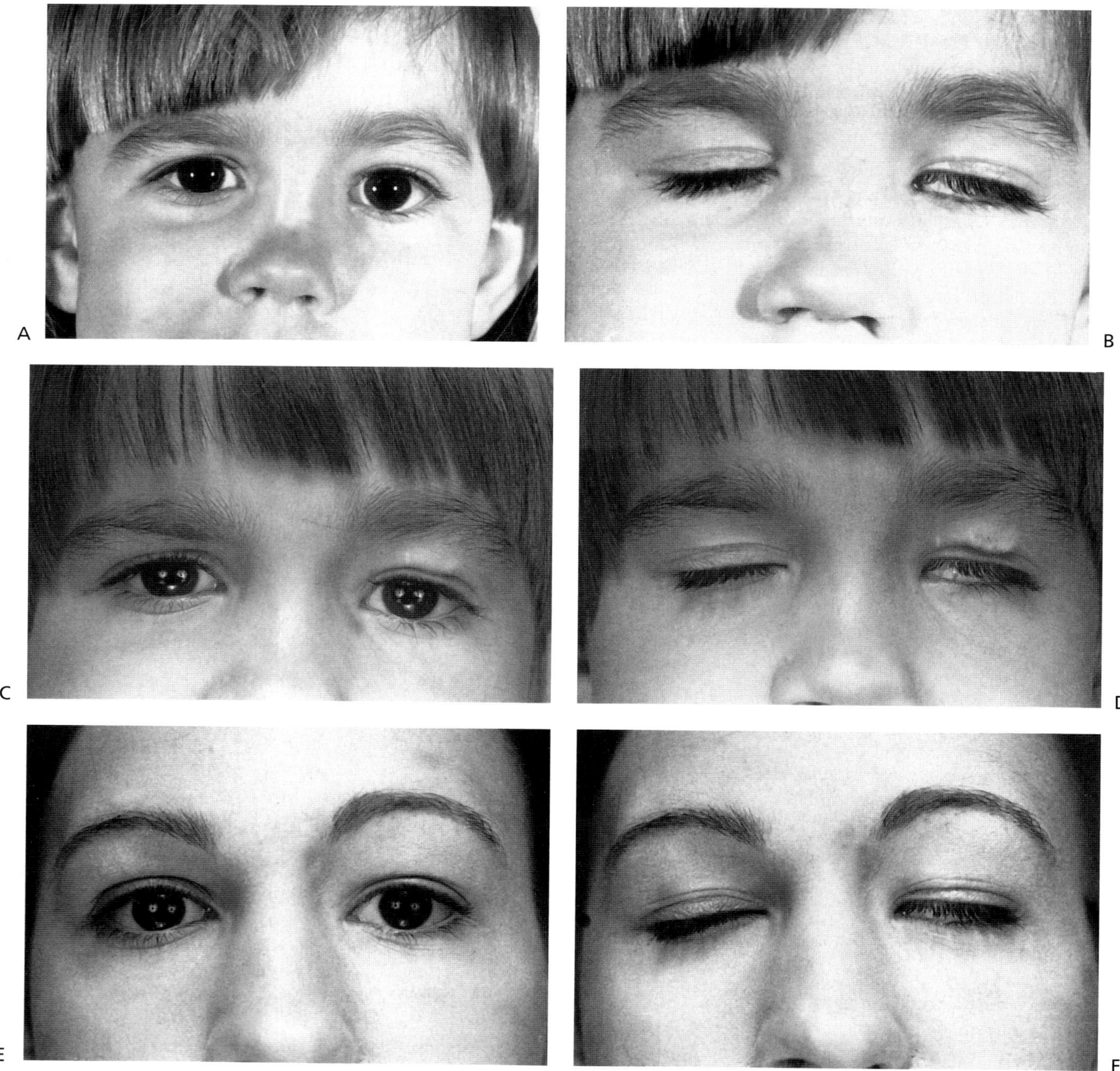

FIGURE 36-6. A,B: A 3-year-old girl with left-sided developmental facial paralysis. Facial paralysis was noted immediately after delivery. At age 3, cross-facial nerve grafting was performed. Patient had a pectoralis minor transfer 10 months later for smile restoration. Seventeen months after the second stage, a gold weight was placed in the left upper eyelid and a minipalmaris tendon graft was performed to improve eye closure. Patient is seen here preoperatively with eyes open (A) and closed (B). **C,D:** Gold weight was displaced at the fourth postoperative month, probably because of manual rubbing by the patient. **E,F:** Patient at 13 years of age, 7 1/2 years after removal of the gold weight and tightening of the minitendon graft to the left lower lid.

cle. These are good alternatives for experienced microsurgeons, especially if other salvage methods fail or the patient is very young. Harvesting of the platysma muscle is accomplished through a submandibular incision, and isolation of the frontalis is carried out through a bicoronal incision, which is hidden in the hair. Elevation of the platysma muscle may interfere with the sensory supply to the overlying skin, but this is transient. Free transfer of the platysma entails all the risks and complications of a vascularized tissue transfer. However, greater freedom in reshaping the muscle is possible. In contrast, transfer of the frontalis muscle carries less vascular risk, but webbing at the medial canthus level invariably requires Z-plasty revision (47,53).

REFERENCES

1. May M, Klein SR. Differential diagnosis of facial nerve palsy. *Otolaryngol Clin North Am* 1991;24:613–645.
2. Manktelow RT, Zuker RM. Muscle transplantation by fascicular territory. *Plast Reconstr Surg* 1984;73:751–757.
3. Mackinnon SE, Dellon AL. Technical considerations of the latissimus dorsi muscle flap: a segmentally innervated muscle transfer for facial reanimation. *Microsurgery* 1988;9:36–45.
4. Dellon AL, Mackinnon SE. Segmentally innervated latissimus dorsi muscle: microsurgical transfer for facial reanimation. *J Reconstr Microsurg* 1985;2:7–12.
5. Paletz JL, Manktelow RT, Chaben R. The shape of a normal smile: implications for facial paralysis reconstruction. *Plast Reconstr Surg* 1994;93:784–789.
6. Terzis JK, Faibisoff B, Williams B. The nerve gap: suture under tension vs. graft. *Plast Reconstr Surg* 1975;56:166–170.
7. Baker DC. Facial paralysis. In: McCarty JG, ed. *Plastic surgery.* Philadelphia: WB Saunders, 1990:2237–2319.
8. Copek L, Clarke HM, Zuker RM. Endoscopic sural nerve harvest in pediatric patients. *Plast Reconstr Surg* 1996;98:884–888.
9. Millesi H. Nerve grafting. In: Terzis JK, ed. *Microreconstruction of nerve injuries.* Philadelphia: WB Saunders, 1987:223–237.
10. Scaramella LF. Preliminary report on facial nerve anastomosis. Read before the Second International Symposium on Facial Nerve Surgery, Osaka, Japan, 1970.
11. Smith JW. A new technique of facial reanimation. In: Hueston JT, ed. *Transactions of the Fifth International Congress of Plastic and Reconstructive Surgery.* Melbourne: Butterworth-Heineman, 1971.
12. Anderl H, Muhlbauer W. Surgery of facial palsy. In: Jackson IT, ed: *Recent advances in plastic surgery.* New York: Churchill Livingstone, 1981:181–199.
13. Fisch U. Facial nerve grafting. *Otolaryngol Clin North Am* 1974;7:517–529.
14. Samii M. Nerves of the head and neck. In: Omer GF, Spinner M, eds. *Management of peripheral nerve problems.* Philadelphia: WB Saunders, 1980:507–547.
15. Lee KK, Terzis JK. Management of acute extratemporal facial nerve palsy. In: Terzis JK, ed. *Microreconstruction of nerve injuries.* Philadelphia: WB Saunders, 1987:587–600.
16. Terzis JK. "Babysitters." An exciting new concept in facial reanimation. Read before the Sixth International Symposium on the Facial Nerve, Rio de Janeiro, Brazil, 1988.
17. Hamilton SLG, Terzis JK, Carraway JT. Surgical anatomy of the facial musculature and muscle transplantation. In: Terzis JK, ed. *Microreconstruction of nerve injuries.* Philadelphia: WB Saunders, 1987:571–586.
18. Cooper TM, McMahon B, Lex C. Cross-facial nerve grafting for facial reanimation: effect on normal hemiface motion. *J Reconstr Microsurg* 1996;12:99–103.
19. Sobol MS, May M. Hypoglossal-facial anastomosis: its role in contemporary facial reanimation. In: Rubin LR, ed. *The paralyzed face.* St. Louis: Mosby, 1991:137–143.
20. Gavron JP, Clemis JD. Hypoglossal-facial anastomosis: a review of forty cases caused by facial nerve injuries in the posterior fossa. *Laryngoscope* 1984;94:1447–1450.
21. Pensak ML, Jackson CG, Glasscock ME. Facial reanimation with the XII-VII anastomosis: analysis of the functional and psychological results. *Otolaryngol Head Neck Surg* 1986;94:305–310.
22. Diels HJD, Combs D. Neuromuscular retraining for facial paralysis. *Clin Otolaryngol* 1997;30:727–743.
23. Mountain RE, Murray JA, Quaba A. Management of facial synkinesis with *Clostridium botulinum* toxin injection. *Clin Otolaryngol* 1992;17:223–224.
24. Smet-Dieleman H, Van de Heyning PH, Tassgnon MJ. Botulinum A toxin injection in patients with facial nerve palsy. *Acta Otorhinolaryngol Belg* 1993;47:359–363.
25. Oge AE, Yazici J, Boyaciyan A, et al. Magnetic stimulation in hemifacial spasm and post-facial palsy synkinesis. *Muscle Nerve* 1993;16:1154–1160.
26. Guerisso JO. Selective myectomy for postparetic facial synkinesis. *Plast Reconstr Surg* 1991;87:459–466.
27. Rubin LR, Mishriki YY, Speace G. Reanimation of the hemiparalytic tongue. *Plast Reconstr Surg* 1984;73:184–194.
28. Poe DS, Scher N, Panje WR. Facial reanimation by XI-VII anastomosis without shoulder paralysis. *Laryngoscope* 1989;99: 1040–1047.
29. Ebersold MJ, Quast LM. Long-term results of spinal accessory nerve-facial nerve anastomosis. *J Neurosurg* 1992;77:51–54.
30. De Castro CP, Zani R. Masseter muscle rotation in the treatment of inferior facial paralysis. *Plast Reconstr Surg* 1973;52:370–373.
31. Baker DC, Conley J. Regional muscle transposition for rehabilitation of the paralyzed face. *Clin Plast Surg* 1979;6:317–331.
32. Rubin LR, Lee GW, Simpson RL. Reanimation of the long-standing partial facial paralysis. *Plast Reconstr Surg* 1986;77: 41–49.
33. Manktelow RT, Laeken NV. Facial paralysis: principles and treatment. In: Georgiade GS, ed. *Plastic, maxillofacial and reconstructive surgery.* Baltimore: William & Wilkins, 1997:507–520.
34. Rubin LR. Reanimation of the partially paralyzed face. In: Rubin LR, ed. *The paralyzed face.* St. Louis: Mosby, 1991:220–227.
35. Terzis JK, Schnarrs RH. Facial nerve reconstruction in salivary gland pathology: a review. *Microsurgery* 1993;14:355–367.
36. Terzis JK, Noah ME. Analysis of 100 cases of free-muscle transplantation for facial paralysis. *Plast Reconstr Surg* 1997;99: 1905–1921.
37. Harii K, Ohmori Y, Torii T. Free gracilis muscle transplantation with microneural anastomosis for the treatment of facial paralysis. *Plast Reconstr Surg* 1976;57:133–143.
38. Sassoon EM, Poole D, Rushworth G. Reanimation for facial palsy using gracilis muscle graft. *Br J Plast Surg* 1991;44: 195–200.
39. Manktelow RT. Free muscle transplantation for facial paralysis. In: Terzis JK, ed. *Microreconstruction of nerve injuries.* Philadelphia: WB Saunders, 1987:607–615.
40. Terzis JK, Manktelow RT. Pectoralis minor: a new concept in facial reanimation. *Plast Surg Forum* 1982;5:106.
41. Terzis JK. Microneurovascular free transfer of pectoralis minor muscle for facial reanimation. In: Strauch B, Vasconez LO, Hall-Findlay EJ, eds. *Grabb's encyclopedia of flaps.* Philadelphia: Lippincott–Raven Publishers, 1998:537–546.
42. Hata Y, Yano K, Matsuka K. Treatment of chronic facial palsy by

transplantation of the neurovascularized free rectus abdominis muscle. *Plast Reconstr Surg* 1990;86:1178–1187.
43. Mayou BJ, Watson JS, Harrison DH. Free microvascular and microneural transfer of the extensor digitorum brevis muscle for the treatment of unilateral facial palsy. *Br J Plast Surg* 1981;34:362–367.
44. Whitney TM, Buncke HJ, Alpert BS, et al. The serratus anterior free muscle flap: experience with 100 consecutive cases. *Plast Reconstr Surg* 1990;86:481–490.
45. Jackson IT. Surgical correction of lagophthalmos. In: Terzis JK, ed. *Microreconstruction of nerve injuries.* Philadelphia: WB Saunders, 1987:617–633
46. Becker FF. Lateral tarsal strip procedure for correction of paralytic ectropion. *Laryngoscope* 1982;92:382–384.
47. Terzis JK. Our experience with eye reanimation microsurgery. *Plast Reconstr Surg* 2001 (*in press*).
48. May M. Gold weight and wire spring implants as alternatives to tarsorrhaphy. *Arch Otolaryngol Head Neck Surg* 1987;113:656–660.
49. May M. Paralyzed eyelids reanimated with a closed-eyelid spring. *Laryngoscope* 1988;98:382–385.
50. Chapman P, Lamberty BGH. Results of upper lid loading in the treatment of lagophthalmos caused by facial palsy. *Br J Plast Surg* 1988;41:369–372.
51. Dinces EA, Mauriello JA, Kwartler JA. Complications of gold weight eyelid implants for treatment of fifth and seventh nerve paralysis. *Laryngoscope* 1997;107:1617–1622.
52. Neuman AR, Weinberg A, Sela M. The correction of seventh nerve palsy lagophthalmos with gold lid load (16 years' experience). *Ann Plast Surg* 1989;22:142–145.
53. Lee KK, Terzis JK. Microsurgical reanimation of the eye sphincter. In: Terzis JK, ed. *Microreconstruction of nerve injuries.* Philadelphia: WB Saunders, 1987:635–650.

Discussion

FACIAL REANIMATION

KIYONORI HARII
HIROTAKA ASATO

Microneurovascular free-muscle transplantation is recognized as a good reconstructive option for treating longstanding or established facial paralysis in which the mimetic muscles of the cheek are severely atrophied or absent. A stronger contraction can be achieved with free-muscle transplantation than with conventional regional transposition of the temporalis or masseter muscle, and therefore a symmetrical balance of the cheeks during smiling, especially in patients with unilateral facial paralysis. However, to obtain optimal results, the contraction of the transplanted muscle should correspond to the involuntary movements of the contralateral facial muscles during smiling. It is still difficult and challenging to restore a natural or nearly natural smile, although many forms of free-muscle transplantation have been developed since the first reports of successful transfers of gracilis muscle (1–3).

In this discussion, we introduce some technical suggestions for avoiding unfavorable results and obtaining better outcomes in free-muscle transplantation performed for smile reconstruction; these are based on our experience with 387 transfers in 375 cases (September 1973 through December 1997).

K. Harii and H. Asato: Department of Plastic and Reconstructive Surgery, Graduate School of Medicine, University of Tokyo, Tokyo, Japan

PREPARATION OF THE RECIPIENT SITE

It is important to observe the normal cheek preoperatively while the patient is smiling and determine the position of the newly created nasolabial fold on the paralyzed side.

1. *Incision and undermining of the recipient cheek.* Through a preauricular facelift incision, the paralyzed cheek is widely raised just above the level of the superficial parotid fascia to accept the subsequent muscle transplant. The level of the undermining should be kept constant, and the undermining should proceed from a point anterior to the parotid gland toward the lips. If the undermining is too superficial, an unnatural tethering or wrinkling may accompany muscle contraction. This is caused by muscle adhering to the skin and may result in a cosmetic problem at the anterior cheek. The undermining should be as wide as possible, wider than the subsequent muscle transplant, and should extend 1 to 2 cm beyond the position of the newly created nasolabial fold. We usually do not incise the nasolabial fold in the primary muscle transplantation to avoid a visible scar at the nasolabial region. However, we often incise here in a secondary revision procedure to shorten or reattach muscle and to create a natural nasolabial fold.

2. *Exposure of the recipient vessels.* Either the superficial temporal or facial vessels are used as the recipient artery and vein. The superficial temporal vessels are traced proximally to

obtain a sizable diameter. When the superficial temporal vein is too small, use of the deep temporal vein is recommended.

A small additional incision, about 2 to 3 cm long, can be placed at the submandibular region when the facial vessels are exposed. In some situations, the superficial thyroid artery and external jugular vein can be used, but the preauricular facelift incision should be extended to the submandibular region. Muscles with a long, vascular stalk, such as the latissimus dorsi, should be chosen as the donor muscle to reach recipient vessels located away from the face.

3. *Creation of the new nasolabial fold.* The lateral portion of the atrophied orbicularis oris muscle and the insertions of the zygomaticus major and minor muscles to the orbicularis oris muscle are exposed in the upper and lower lips to fix the end of the transplanted muscle segment. Several stay sutures (usually three to four stitches) are then placed at the lateral border of the orbicularis oris muscle in the upper and lower lips. When these stay sutures are pulled toward the zygomatic region, the position and shape of the newly created nasolabial fold can be visualized, and the fixation position of one end of the muscle segment is thus correctly determined (Fig. 36D-1).

4. *Pullout suture to secure muscle fixation.* To prevent jaw movements from injuring the muscle fixation and to secure the fixation in the appropriate position during the early postoperative period, a pullout suspension suture of 2-0 or 3-0 monofilament nylon is placed deeply at the corner of the mouth. It is fixed by a small pillow to the skin either behind the ear lobe or in the temporal region. This fixation is simple and can be pulled out about 2 weeks postoperatively, and it may be more comfortable for the patient than the external holding device described in Dr. Terzis' chapter.

5. *Removal of soft tissue over the zygoma.* Another end of the muscle segment is fixed to the zygomatic region, but this produces bulkiness at the zygoma, which frequently requires a secondary debulking operation. To minimize such a problem, a part of the soft tissue over the zygoma should be excised at the position of the muscle attachment (Fig. 36D-2).

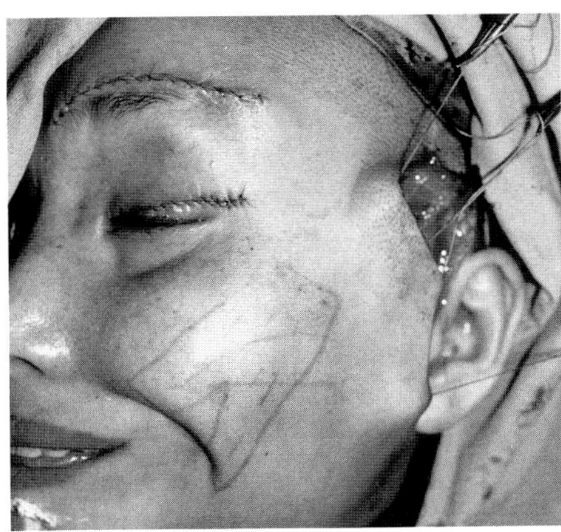

FIGURE 36D-1. The position of the new nasolabial fold is determined by pulling stay sutures toward the zygoma. Stay sutures *(arrows)* are anchored to the lateral portion of the atrophied orbicularis oris muscle.

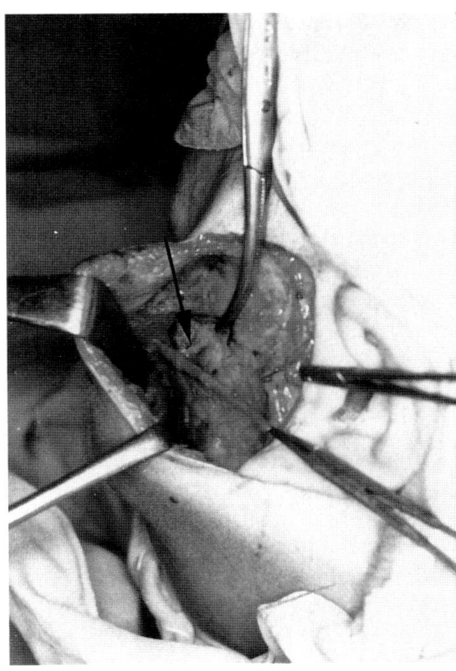

FIGURE 36D-2. A small part of the soft tissue over the zygoma *(arrow)* is removed to prevent bulk after muscle fixation to the zygoma.

This procedure is easy in cases of complete paralysis, but care must be taken in cases of incomplete paralysis not to damage functioning branches of the facial nerve.

SELECTION OF MOTOR SOURCE

Most important is the selection of a motor nerve in the recipient bed to produce a natural or nearly natural smile.

1. *Ipsilateral facial nerve.* In optimal cases, a functioning stump of the facial nerve is available in the recipient cheek. The facial nerve canal in the temporal bone can be opened when the proximal facial nerve trunk is expected to be available.

2. *Motor nerve other than the facial nerve.* Motor nerve branches from other nerves, such as the trigeminal motor nerve and the hypoglossal nerve, can be used if the bilateral facial nerve is not available (e.g., Möbius' syndrome). We prefer to use the hypoglossal nerve (not the main trunk, but a small branch innervating the suprahyoid muscles) as the recipient motor nerve in elderly patients who are unable to undergo a lengthy, two-stage procedure for cross-facial nerve grafting. Muscle contraction recovers early (on average, 6 months postoperatively). Many patients are able to smile voluntarily and are satisfied with the results (4). Problems encountered include muscle contraction that does not correspond to rapid, involuntary movements during smiling and unnatural contraction during biting, chewing, and tongue movements.

3. *Cross-facial nerve graft.* A two-stage method including cross-facial nerve grafting has long been championed, as described in Dr. Terzis' chapter. Many modifications and improvements have been developed (5,6), and satisfactory results have been obtained [180 of 234 patients (77%) undergoing two-stage procedures in our present series were satisfied with the results]. However, a result is not obtained for at least 2 years, although this method can produce a far better smile than other conventional procedures. If axon recovery through a long sural nerve graft crossing the face is disturbed, the result after muscle transplantation can be unfavorable.

SELECTION OF DONOR MUSCLE

Types of Donor Muscles

Muscles with parallel fibers and good excursion are recommended. A donor muscle should also be easy to harvest, and its removal should cause little or no functional morbidity. To date, many muscles have been reported as good candidates (7–9). We have mainly used gracilis (63.8%), latissimus dorsi (31.0%), a combination of latissimus dorsi and serratus anterior (4.4%), and others (0.8%). Short, small muscles, such as the extensor brevis, do not produce a strong contraction because a muscle transplanted to the face markedly loses its original contraction power and excursion.

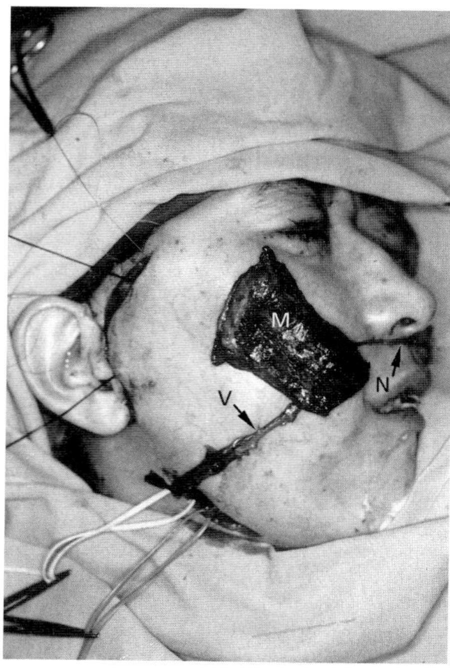

FIGURE 36D-3. A segment of the latissimus dorsi muscle is placed into the cheek pocket. *M,* latissimus dorsi muscle segment; *arrow V,* vascular pedicle hooking up with the facial vessels; *arrow N,* thoracodorsal nerve crossing through the upper lip to the contralateral facial nerve branches.

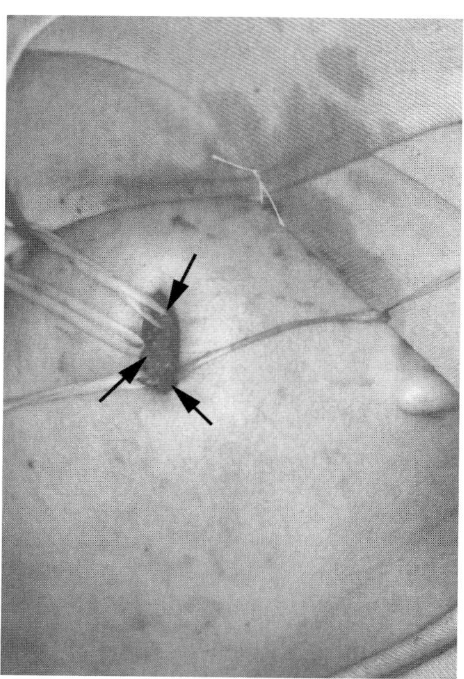

FIGURE 36D-4. Through a small incision, about 1.5 cm long, at the anterior margin of the parotid gland, several (mainly zygomatic and buccal) branches of the intact facial nerve are exposed *(arrows).*

Harvesting a Muscle Segment

A segment of the muscle with appropriate size and thickness (about 3 to 4 cm wide, 8 cm long, and 1.5 cm thick in an adult Asian) should be removed from a large muscle with its neurovascular pedicle. Following complete isolation of the muscle segment with its neurovascular pedicle, the length of the muscle required (8 to 10 cm) is measured and divided by a disposable stapler (10). Thinning and trimming are then carried out *in situ* to secure hemostasis and avoid postoperative hematoma.

One-stage Latissimus Dorsi Muscle Transplantation

To shorten recovery time and obtain a good result, several authors (11,12) use a one-stage method in which the muscle motor nerve is crossed directly over the face and connected with a branch of the contralateral facial nerve.

We use a segment of the latissimus dorsi muscle, from which the thoracodorsal nerve dissected to a length of more than 15 cm can be crossed over the face (13). The thoracodorsal vessels nourishing the muscle segment are usually anastomosed to the facial vessels while the thoracodorsal nerve is crossed through the upper lip to the branches (mainly the zygomatic and buccal branches) of the contralateral facial nerve (Fig. 36D-3). The facial nerve branches are exposed through a small incision placed at the anterior margin of the parotid gland; this leaves a small, invisible scar on the cheek (Fig. 36D-4).

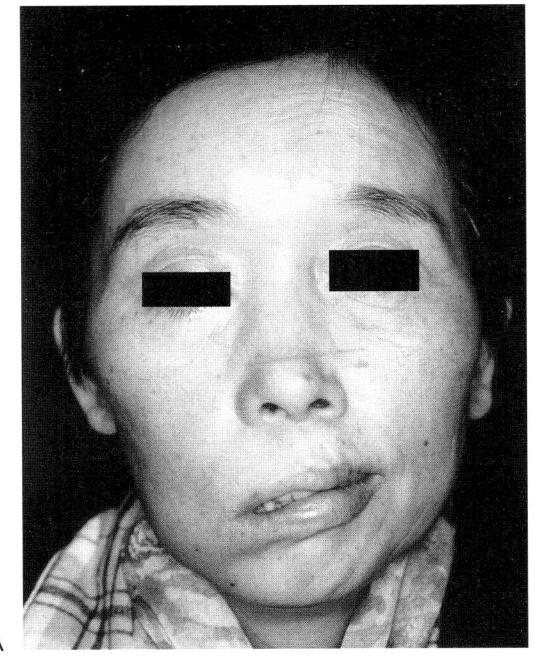

A

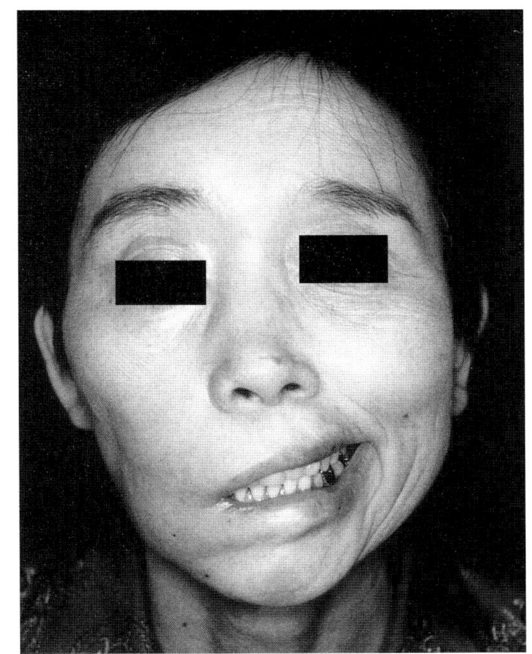

B

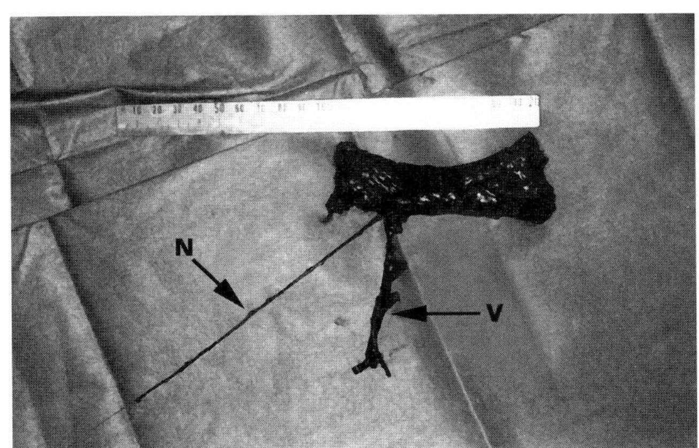

C

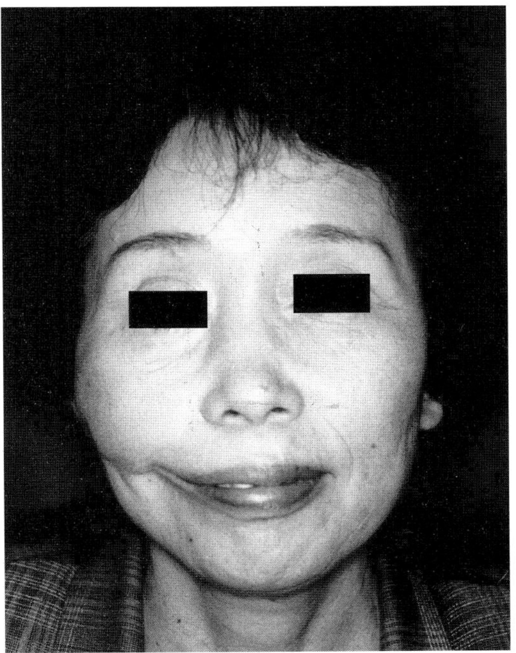

D

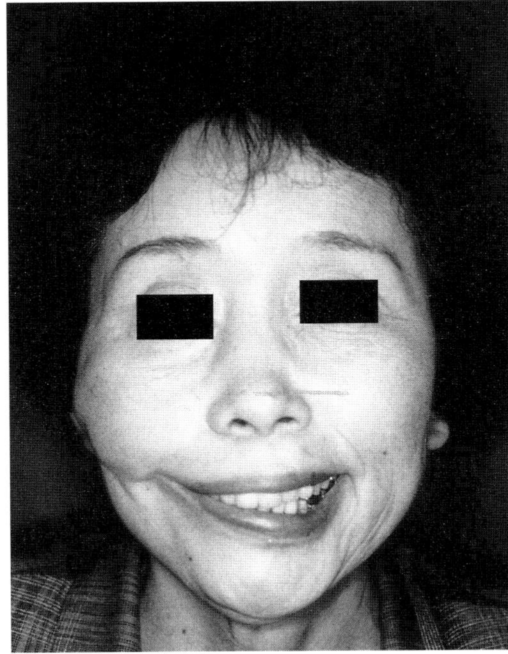

E

FIGURE 36D-5. A 54-year-old woman with right-sided complete paralysis, about 3 years after resection of an acoustic tumor. Her smile was reconstructed by means of a one-stage latissimus dorsi muscle transplantation. **A,B:** Preoperative views. **C:** Isolated latissimus dorsi muscle segment. *Arrow V,* thoracodorsal vessels; *arrow N,* thoracodorsal nerve. **D,E:** In postoperative views at 2 1/2 years, the patient has a good smile without secondary revision.

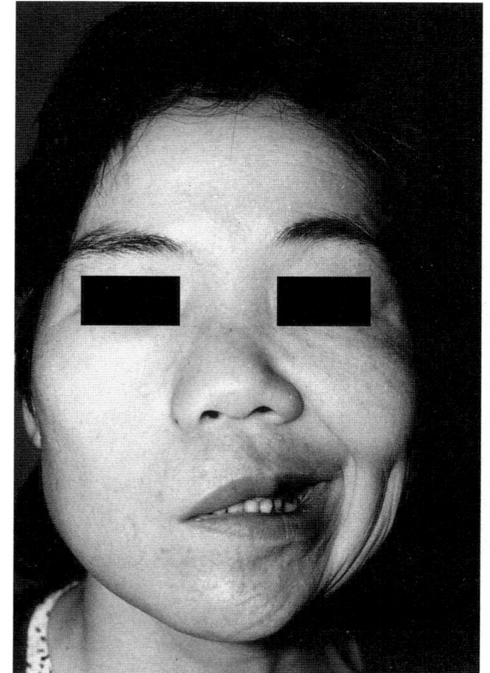

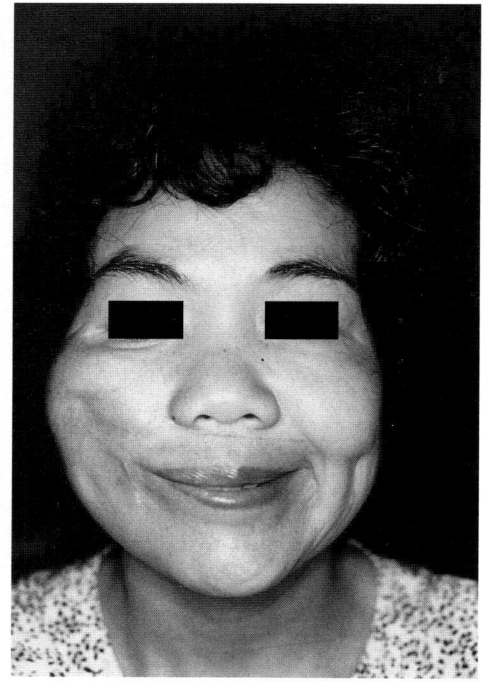

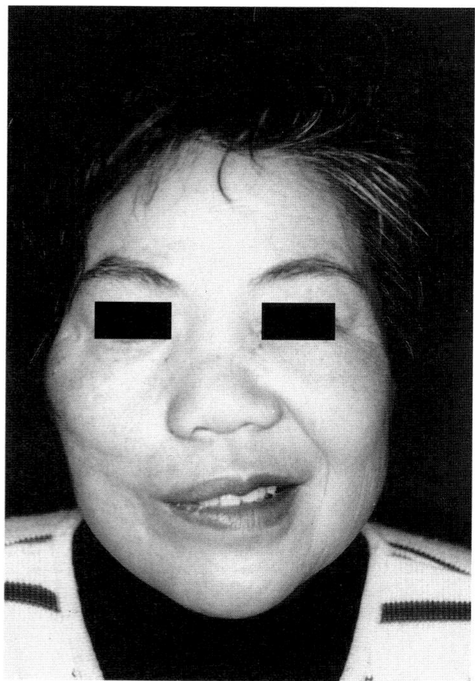

FIGURE 36D-6. A 41-year-old woman with right-sided complete paralysis after acoustic tumor resection was treated with a two-stage reconstruction combining cross-facial nerve grafting and gracilis muscle transplantation. **A:** Preoperative view. **B:** Excessive bulk at the zygoma and excessive contraction of the transplanted gracilis 3 years after gracilis muscle transfer. **C:** Good shape and smile after debulking of the muscle through the nasolabial incision.

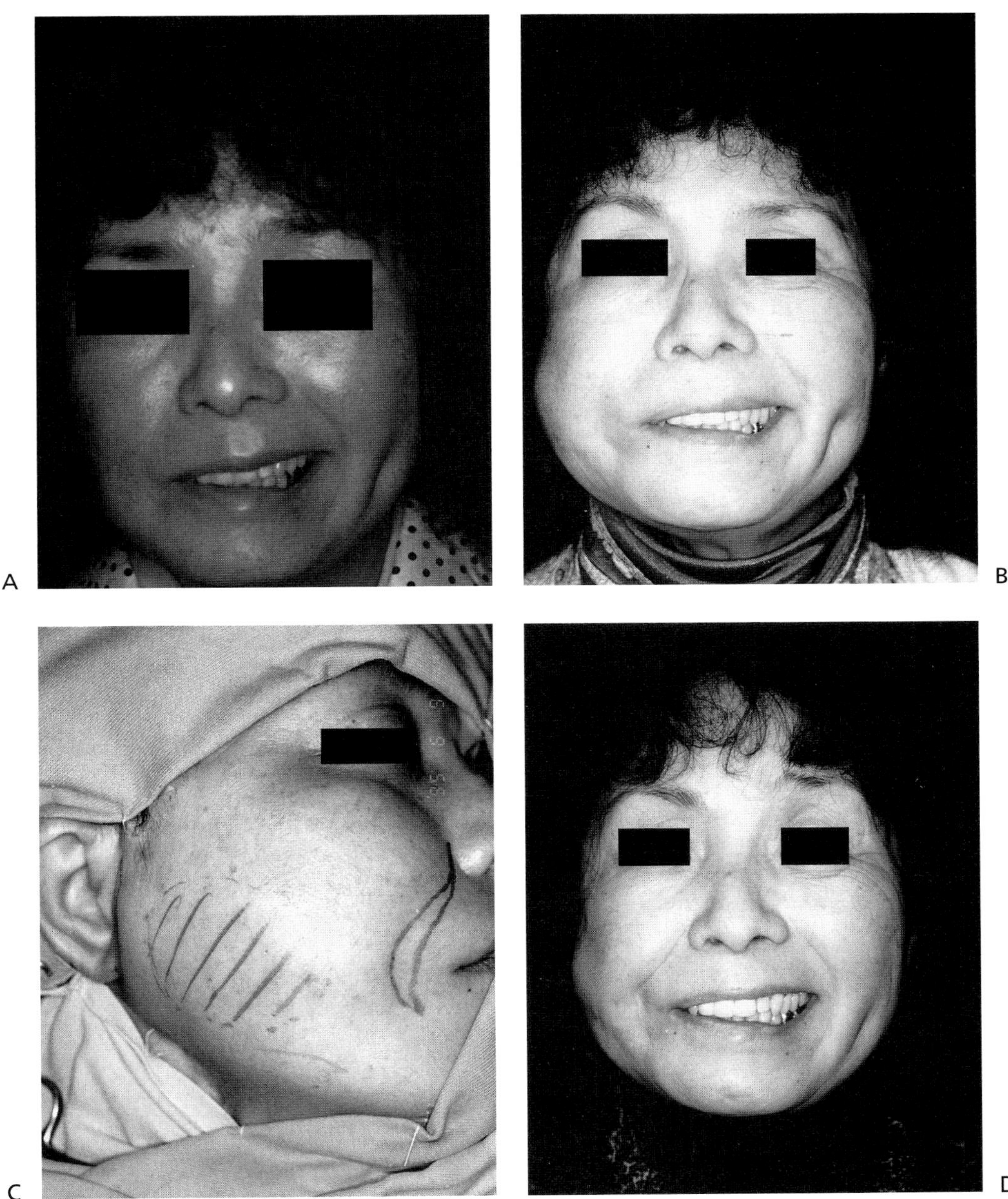

FIGURE 36D-7. A 50-year-old woman with right-sided complete paralysis after surgery for otitis media, performed about 20 years earlier, was treated with a gracilis muscle transfer combined with a cross-facial nerve graft. **A:** Preoperative smile. **B:** Insufficient contraction and bulk at the cheek 2 years after the muscle transfer. **C:** Muscle shortening and debulking carried out through a nasolabial incision. **D:** Stronger contraction of the muscle has been obtained, although slight bulkiness still exists.

Reinnervation of the transplanted muscle occurs significantly faster (average, 7.4 months) than when the two-stage method is used (average, 8.2 months). Because a one-stage latissimus dorsi muscle transplantation can yield satisfactory results [6 of 82 patients (80%) in our present series are satisfied with the results] in comparison with the two-stage method and cross-facial nerve grafting, we now prefer to use it in most cases (Fig. 36D-5).

POSTOPERATIVE CARE

Bulky pressure dressings with suction drainage prevent hematoma formation. Patients are permitted to resume a soft diet 2 weeks postoperatively. Doppler flowmeter is the only available monitor in the immediate postoperative period because the transplanted muscle segment is placed beneath the cheek skin. Denervation potentials at 1 month postoperatively can be used to evaluate muscle survival.

Postoperatively, we do not stimulate the muscle electrically or ultrasonically. Only manual massage of the cheek is recommended beginning 2 months postoperatively.

COMPLICATIONS

Unfavorable results of free-muscle transplantation can be caused by vessel occlusion secondary to thrombosis at anastomotic sites, kinking or torsion of the pedicle, and compression of the pedicle, all of which lead to muscle necrosis. Hematomas frequently compress the muscle or produce a marked fibrosis. In our present series (387 muscle transplants in 375 cases between September 1973 and December 1997), five muscle transplants apparently become necrotic because of thrombosis (artery, two cases; vein, three cases). In addition, seven cases of hematoma, two of temporary salivary fistulas, and three of partial necrosis of the cheek skin developed. Postoperative monitoring with a Doppler flowmeter is mandatory.

UNFAVORABLE RESULTS AND SECONDARY CORRECTION

Bulkiness

Muscle had to be debulked in about 30% of our cases, in which patients complained of asymmetry of the face or excessively strong contraction of the transplanted muscle (Fig. 36D-6). Excessive debulking may reduce the muscle contraction power too much and lead to an unfavorable final outcome. In three cases, complete paralysis after a secondary debulking procedure resulted from accidental nerve damage.

Insufficient Muscle Contraction

When muscle contraction is insufficient, we prefer to shorten the transplanted muscle through an incision at the nasolabial fold (Fig. 36D-7). In 45% of our cases, either muscle shortening or reattachment of the end of the muscle the proper position was required. Suspension of fascia was also carried out in some cases.

Unnatural Movements

Selection of the facial nerve branches on the unaffected side is crucial for a good result. In five of our cases, contraction was sufficient only for eye closure or whistling, and these patients were not able to produce a symmetrical smile. As no effective means to correct this problem is available, selection of the facial nerve branches must be carried out meticulously.

Scar, Unnatural Tethering, and Wrinkles

Because the muscle end is soft and fragile, anchoring sutures to the nasolabial and lip regions may break and slip out of place, causing unnatural tethering of the cheek skin and malposition of the newly created nasolabial fold (Fig. 36D-8). In some cases, wrinkles on the cheek skin become a problem. Undermining deeply to the cheek and solid fixation of the muscle end to the lateral portion of the orbicu-

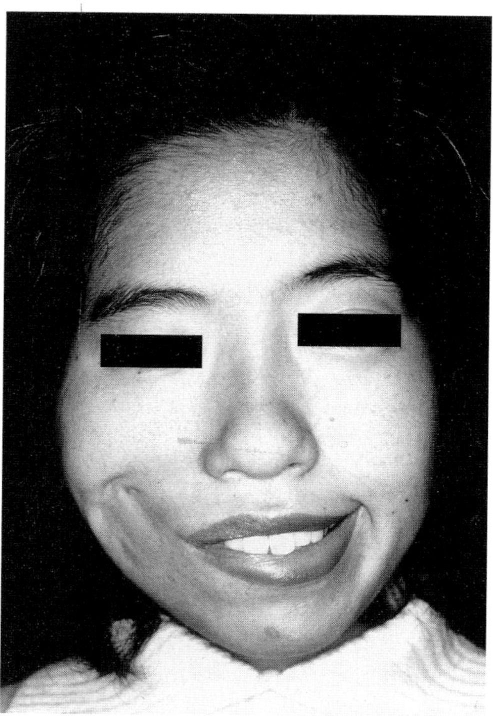

FIGURE 36D-8. Unnatural tethering of the gracilis muscle transplanted to the right cheek requires secondary revision.

laris oris muscle are required to prevent this situation. For correction, removal of the adhesion with placement of a fat graft or transposition of the buccal fat may be effective. Reattachment of the muscle end to the correct position in the nasolabial fold is also advisable.

REFERENCES

1. Harii K, Ohmori K, Torii S. Free gracilis muscle transplantation with microneurovascular anastomoses for the treatment of facial paralysis: a preliminary report. *Plast Reconstr Surg* 1976;57:133–143.
2. O'Brien BMcC, Franklin JD, Morrison WA. Cross-facial nerve grafts and microneurovascular free muscle transfer for long established facial palsy. *Br J Plast Surg* 1980;33:202–215.
3. Harii K. Refined microneurovascular free muscle transplantation for reanimation of paralyzed face. *Microsurgery* 1988;9:169–176.
4. Ueda K, Harii K, Yamada A. Free neurovascular muscle transplantation for the treatment of facial paralysis using the hypoglossal nerve as a recipient motor source. *Plast Reconstr Surg* 1994;94:808–817.
5. O'Brien BMcC, Pederson WC, Khazanchi RK, et al. Results of management of facial palsy with microvascular free-muscle transfer. *Plast Reconstr Surg* 1990;86:12–22.
6. Harii K. Microneurovascular free muscle transplantation. In: Rubin LR, ed. *The paralyzed face.* St. Louis: Mosby, 1991:178–200.
7. Harrison DH. The pectoralis minor vascularized muscle graft for the treatment of unilateral facial palsy. *Plast Reconstr Surg* 1985;75:206–213.
8. Terzis JK. Pectoralis minor: a unique muscle for correction of facial palsy. *Plast Reconstr Surg* 1989;83:767–776.
9. Whitney TM, Buncke HJ, Alpert BS, et al. The serratus anterior free-muscle flaps: experience with 100 consecutive cases. *Plast Reconstr Surg* 1990;86:481–498.
10. Asato H, Harii K, Nakatsuka T, et al. Use of the disposable stapler to ensure proper fixation of a transferred muscle in the treatment of facial paralysis. *J Reconstr Microsurg* 1997;14:199–204.
11. Kumar PAV. Cross-face reanimation of the paralyzed face, with a single stage microneurovascular gracilis transfer without nerve graft: a preliminary report. *Br J Plast Surg* 1995;48:83–88.
12. Koshima I, Moriguchi T, Soeda S, et al. Free rectus femoris muscle transfer for one-stage reconstruction of established facial paralysis. *Plast Reconstr Surg* 1994;94:421–430.
13. Harii K, Asato H, Yoshimura K, et al. One-stage transfer of the latissimus dorsi muscle for reanimation of a paralyzed face: a new alternative. *Plast Reconstr Surg* 1998;102:941–951.

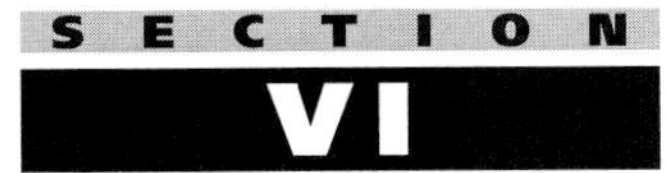

TRUNK

37

BREAST RECONSTRUCTION WITH IMPLANTS AND EXPANDERS

R. JOBE FIX
JORGE I. DE LA TORRE
LUIS O. VÁSCONEZ

The introduction of silicone breast implants in the 1960s had a tremendous impact on the evolution of breast reconstruction (1). At the time, the options for extirpative surgery were either the Halsted radical mastectomy (2) or the Patey modified radical mastectomy (3). Although the Patey mastectomy preserved the pectoralis major muscle, both procedures resulted in significant breast deformity. In early reconstructive efforts, a breast implant alone was used to recreate the breast mound. The result was often quite unsatisfactory because the only available coverage was a thin layer of overlying skin and subcutaneous tissue.

Breast reconstruction with gel-filled silicone prostheses was successful despite a high incidence of capsular contracture (4,5). When they became available, polyurethane implants demonstrated a lower incidence of capsular contracture. As silicone gel implants fell out of favor, saline implants were used more frequently. Severe capsular contracture occurred very commonly (6,7) and produced an unnatural, rounded breast mound rather than the more aesthetically pleasing teardrop shape.

In the late 1970s, the introduction of the latissimus dorsi myocutaneous flap (2) improved the results of breast reconstruction with the silicone implant. The latissimus dorsi muscle, when transposed to the chest, reproduced the anatomy destroyed by mastectomy (8). The latissimus muscle replaced the lost pectoralis major muscle, and the skin island replaced the ellipse of skin removed as part of the mastectomy. The implant that was then inserted and simulated the breast mound.

The introduction of skin expanders by Radovan (9) presented a unique opportunity to expand the remaining skin and muscle and replace the tissue that had been resected. Following adequate expansion, the tissue expander was removed and replaced with a smaller implant. Ideally, proper coverage of the implant was obtained, and the excess skin and muscle re-created the shape of a normal ptotic breast. Unfortunately, achieving symmetry was difficult, and the rate of complications remained high (10,11). Frequently, multiple procedures over a prolonged period of time were required to achieve acceptable results (12).

R. J. Fix, J. I. de la Torre, and L. O. Vásconez: Department of Surgery, Division of Plastic Surgery, University of Alabama at Birmingham, School of Medicine, Birmingham, Alabama

BASIC PRINCIPLES FOR SUCCESSFUL BREAST RECONSTRUCTION

The goals to strive for in breast reconstructive surgery are safety, simplicity, and symmetry. Avoiding complications related to overall patient safety is the fundamental concern with any surgery, but it is particularly important with elective surgery. The safety of the patient is essential and should remain the primary concern in any reconstructive procedure. The simpler an operative technique is, the more reproducible and reliable it will be and the fewer the number of unfavorable results. Of the many techniques currently available for breast reconstruction, few can be described as simple. As with any breast surgery, attention to symmetry is critical. In addition, particular difficulties arise with the use of implants, which must be addressed. The successful reconstruction of an aesthetically pleasing breast depends on preserving or reestablishing breast symmetry. Three elements are essential to recreate a symmetrical breast. These include locating the inframammary fold properly, creating the natural ptotic shape of the breast, and providing projection similar to that of the contralateral breast mound (Figs. 37-1–37-5).

Inframammary Fold

Various definitions and descriptions of the inframammary fold have been presented in the past (13–15). Anatomical

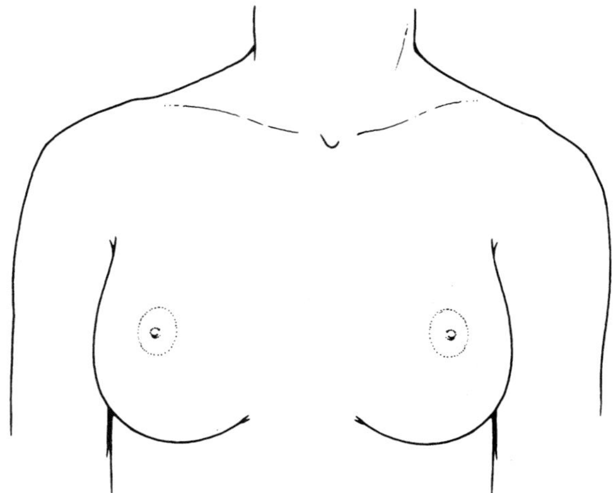

FIGURE 37-1. Normal projection, ptosis, and location of inframammary fold.

and histologic studies indicate the presence of fibrous connections between the dermis and chest wall. Explained simply, the inframammary fold is the lower pole of the normal breast. In a breast reconstructed with a transverse rectus abdominis myocutaneous (TRAM) flap, the inframammary fold represents the lower edge of the TRAM flap. With an implant or expander, the lower pole of the capsule surrounding the implant represents the inframammary fold. This is particularly important because in the majority of the cases, a certain degree of capsular contracture will develop and raise the level of the implant. Therefore, to obtain symmetry with the opposite inframammary fold, the implant must be initially placed at a lower level.

Of clinical importance is the determination by Carlson et al. (16) that little or no breast tissue is present below the normal inframammary fold. Consequently, if the inframammary fold is marked percutaneously before the mastectomy [we use through-and-through silk sutures (Fig. 37-6)], the oncologic surgeon need not extend the dissection beyond that point. In addition, the markings provide a landmark for the reconstructive surgeon. If reconstruction is planned with the use of an implant with or without an expander, it should be placed at least 2 to 3 cm below the preoperative marking of the inframammary fold.

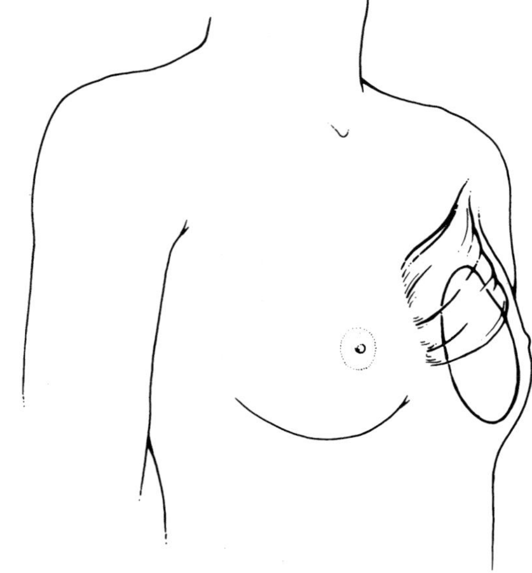

FIGURE 37-3. Inadequate projection and ptosis with partial coverage of submuscular implant.

Projection

Projection can be defined as the transverse diameter over the curved surface of the breast from the midsternal line to the anterior axillary line. The lateral aspect of the breast does

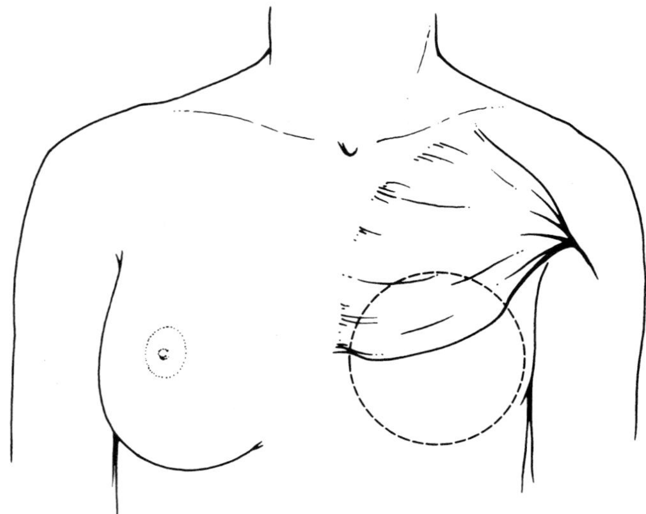

FIGURE 37-2. Location of subpectoral implant.

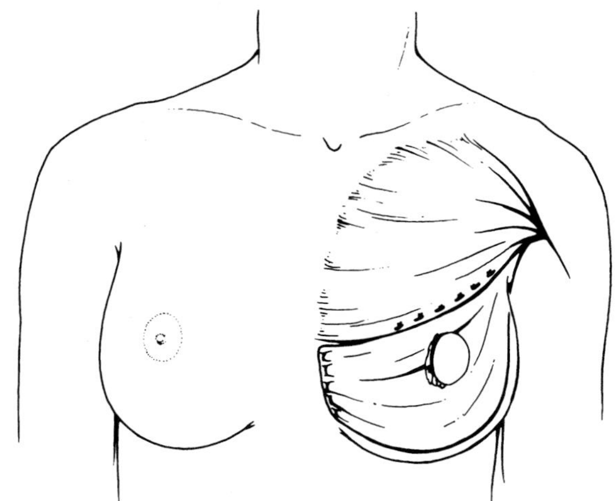

FIGURE 37-4. Location of implant with latissimus dorsi coverage.

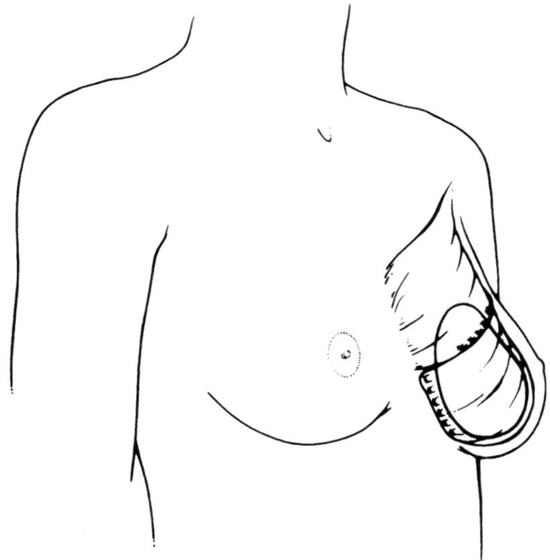

FIGURE 37-5. Complete coverage of implant and skin paddle of latissimus dorsi flap with natural ptosis and projection.

not extend beyond the anterior axillary line. Following mastectomy, the three-dimensional curved surface of the breast becomes a two-dimensional flat surface. Thus, to provide projection, the transverse diameter of the breast must be increased. Tissue can be added in the form of a skin island placed either vertically or obliquely. The transverse diameter can be increased at the expense of the vertical dimension by using either zigzag incisions or, as advocated by Hall-Finley (17), reverse Z-plasties (Fig. 37-7). Although skin expansion can increase the transverse diameter and thus provide projection, overexpansion is limited by subsequent complications, such as excessive thinning of the skin and muscle and unacceptable telangectasia of the overlying skin. In secondary reconstruction, the mastectomy scar must be lengthened to allow development of the skin envelope and permit proper projection.

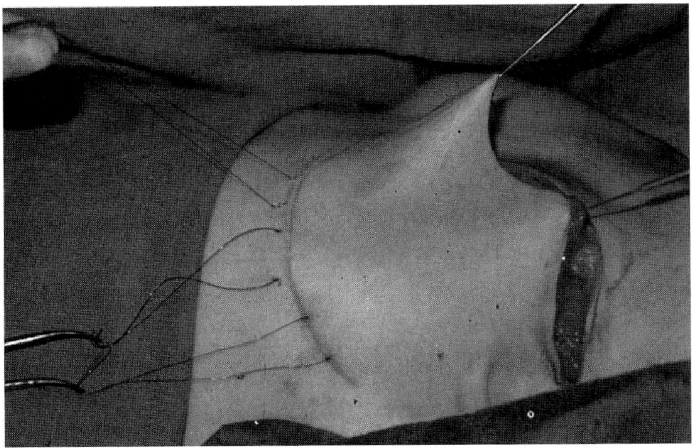

FIGURE 37-6. Preservation of the inframammary fold with temporary sutures.

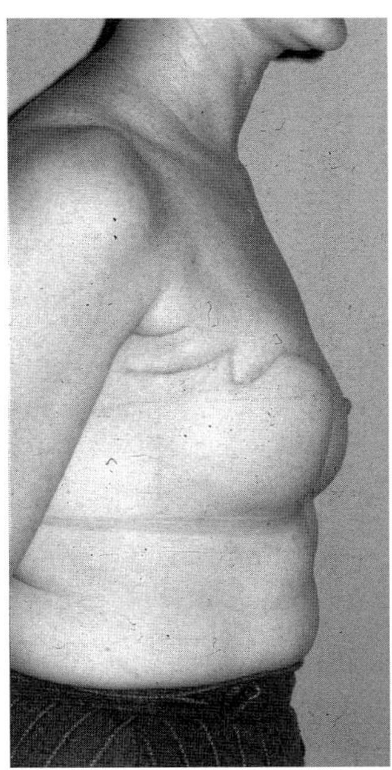

FIGURE 37-7. Z-plasty release of mastectomy scar to increase projection.

Ptosis

Ptosis can be defined as the vertical component of a line drawn over the curved surface of the breast meridian. To develop ptosis, this vertical dimension, which extends from the midclavicle through the nipple to the inframammary fold, must be increased. This can be achieved by stretching the overlying skin or tissue and allowing it to redrape while the position of the inframammary fold is kept fixed. This principle has been made clinically applicable by the ingenious modifications of Pennisi (18) and Ryan (19), in which a portion of the chest skin is deepithelialized and sutured to the intercostal space to create an inframammary fold. Inflation of an expander over a period of time stretches the overlying skin and provides a semblance of ptosis. Two problems were immediately apparent when this procedure was performed. The first was difficulty in determining the proper location of the inframammary fold, particularly in delayed reconstructions. It is very easy to misplace the inframammary fold, usually too high relative to the contralateral fold. The second problem is placing a relatively tenuous suture line in the inframammary fold. Exposure of the implant was not unusual, particularly in thin patients.

COMPLICATIONS OF IMPLANTS AND EXPANDERS

Despite tremendous effort and notwithstanding the extensive clinical knowledge that has been gained during the past two decades, complications in breast reconstruction occur with painful frequency. Frequently, multiple procedures over a prolonged period of time are required to obtain acceptable results (20). The most common complications related to the use of implants include exposure and malposition of the implant, inadequate ptosis, capsular contracture, and infection. Each of these complications is discussed.

Exposure of the Implant

Exposure occurs most often at the site of the mastectomy scar, particularly if the implant is not successfully covered with muscle. Preventing implant exposure is difficult and requires that muscle be placed between the incision and the implant. Two plans of management are available when the implant becomes exposed or even earlier, when the skin edges first become necrotic. The wound can be treated with Betadine and allowed to separate, or the implant can be removed surgically. If the underlying muscle is intact, wound care will be sufficient, and the implant will not be lost. On the other hand, if muscle has retracted and the implant is exposed, it is preferable to remove the implant immediately. Once the wound has reopened, reapproximation should be avoided because invariably this will result in failure. If the reconstruction has been performed without transposition of the latissimus dorsi myocutaneous unit and the implant becomes exposed, it is best to remove the implant, wait several months, and then reconstruct secondarily with the latissimus dorsi myocutaneous unit.

Malposition of the Implant

Malposition usually occurs because the implant has been placed too high at the time of surgery and subsequent capsular contracture elevates the implant further on the chest wall. Once this occurs, it is very difficult to lower the implant by means of nonoperative methods. The operative approach consists of dividing the capsule inferiorly and extending the pocket at least 2 to 3 cm below the desired postoperative level, so that as the capsular contracture reforms, the implant will remain at the proper level.

When the implant has been placed too low and the inframammary line is lower than the contralateral, normal one, manual elevation and taping are often successful in raising it to the proper level. An effective but hazardous approach is percutaneous closure of the excessive inferior pocket. This technique risks puncture of the implant and should be avoided. If taping and nonoperative methods fail, it is preferable to reopen the incision and close the pocket under direct vision. A few nylon sutures are placed at the proper level to promote adherence of the capsule. Removal of the remainder of the capsule is usually not necessary. If, however, the capsule demonstrates significant calcifications, it should be removed.

Inadequate Ptosis and Rounded Reconstruction

The normal inflammatory response of the body is to encapsulate any foreign object, including an implant. As the capsule contracts, the surface area decreases, but the volume remains the same. Therefore, although the implants may have a teardrop or anatomical shape, the body will form a capsule and a spherical shape will result. Currently, experience with the use of *these* biodimensional breast implants is not sufficient for us to make an educated statement regarding their effectiveness. Usually, a certain degree of spherical shape of the reconstructed breast must be accepted. On occasion, in an effort to obtain symmetry, an implant is placed on the contralateral side to create symmetrical fullness in the upper pole.

Capsular Contracture

In almost every case, a certain amount of capsular contracture is expected and occurs. Severe capsular contracture (i.e., Baker class III and class IV) does not occur, as it often does when the latissimus dorsi myocutaneous unit has been transposed; however, it is much more common if reconstruction involves minimal subcutaneous coverage (Fig. 37-8). In a patient who has undergone reconstruction with an expander and without the benefit of the latissimus dorsi myocutaneous unit, the treatment of capsular contracture should include this transposition as a secondary procedure. On the other hand, if an asymptomatic capsular contracture develops in a patient who has received a latissimus dorsi myocutaneous unit, it is preferable not to reoperate. More often than not, open capsulotomies or capsulectomies are followed by the re-formation of thicker capsules.

Infection

Infections occur rarely in patients with implants (21) (Fig. 37-9). When they do, it is best to remove the implant. Although the literature indicates that an implant can be salvaged by continuous irrigation with saline and antibiotic solution, with increased hospitalization cost, this method of

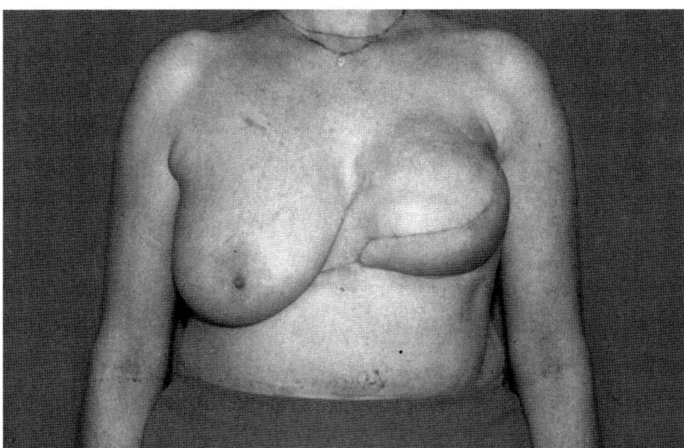

FIGURE 37-8. Capsular contracture resulting in abnormal ptosis and projection and location of the inframammary fold with implant reconstruction.

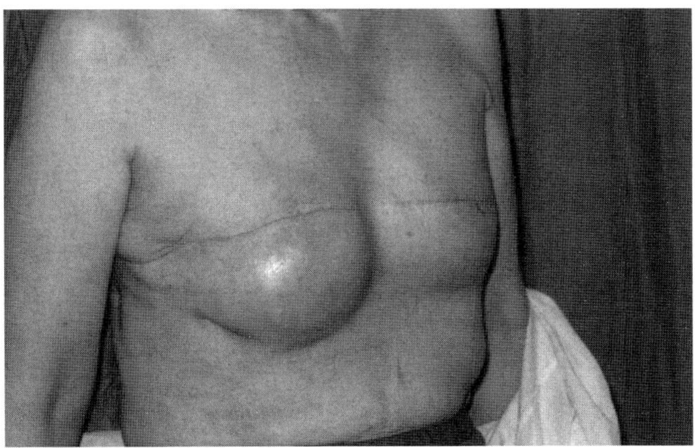

FIGURE 37-9. Characteristic appearance of an infected implant.

treatment is not cost-effective. It is better to remove the implant, support the patient, and wait a minimum of 6 months before undertaking another reconstruction.

REDUCING COMPLICATIONS: SUCCESSFUL USE OF IMPLANTS

Despite the potential complications, the use of implants offers several advantages in breast reconstruction. Undesirable results and complications can be reduced with the proper use and placement of implants and expanders. In addition, as extirpative and reconstructive techniques evolve, it should be possible to obtain better results with fewer problems.

Coverage

The entire circumference of the implant must be covered with sufficiently thick padding, which usually includes muscle (Fig. 37-10). This is essential at the site of the incision or in areas prone to skin necrosis following the skin-sparing mastectomy. Not only does this practice decrease the incidence of extrusion, but it also helps to decrease the development of capsular contracture. We have found the latissimus dorsi myocutaneous flap to be invaluable when implants are used for breast reconstruction.

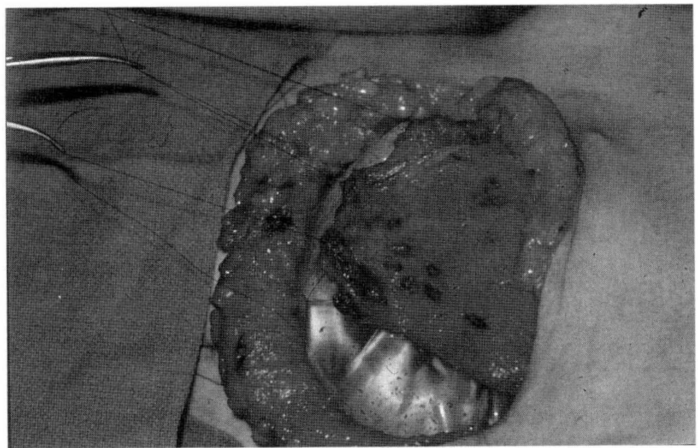

FIGURE 37-10. Muscle coverage of a permanent implant.

Position

The position of the implant must be properly established with regard to the inframammary fold. At surgery, the inferior pole of the implant should be placed 2 to 3 cm below the marked inframammary fold. Even with moderate capsular contracture, the implant will be elevated. It is almost impossible to lower the implant nonoperatively, although it is relatively easy to elevate it 1 or 2 cm with proper taping.

Pocket Size

The pocket must be properly positioned and large enough to accommodate the fully inflated implant. The use of sutures, both medially and laterally, is necessary to define the pocket. Adequate projection and ptosis of the reconstructed breast can then be obtained without the implant slipping laterally into the axilla. When immediate reconstruction is performed, a drain is placed at the axillary level and brought out through a separate incision.

Port Access

Finally, when a permanent implant/expander is used, the injection port must be easily accessible. The port should be placed in the subcutaneous tissue level to aid in localization and inflation. In addition, the port should remain sufficiently remote from the implant to minimize the risk for implant injury. We prefer bringing the port to the inferior midaxillary line or along the costal margin 5 cm below the implant.

CHANGING CONCEPTS: THE SKIN-SPARING MASTECTOMY

Just as the Halsted radical mastectomy was supplanted by the Patey modified mastectomy, the modified mastectomy has been gradually replaced by the skin-sparing mastectomy during the last 10 years. Sufficient data are now available to indicate that the skin-sparing mastectomy performed through a periareolar incision, often without the addition of an axillary incision, is not associated with a greater incidence of local recurrence than the modified mastectomy (22). In our institution, excluding cases that involve skin adherence of the tumor or inflammatory breast carcinoma, the skin-sparing mastectomy is the rule. This has the advantage of simplifying the reconstruction, particularly when it is performed with autologous tissue.

However, the skin-sparing mastectomy does have limitations that must be considered, particularly in respect to breast reconstruction with the use of implants or expanders (23). When a patient undergoes a skin-sparing mastectomy, the breast, nipple, and areola are totally extirpated through a keyhole incision. In patients who have previously undergone a biopsy, the biopsy scar is also excised. To ensure the viability of the skin flaps, the dissection is performed at the subcutaneous level just superficial to the breast tissue itself, so that the subcutaneous vascular plexus is preserved. This plexus becomes apparent during dissection of the flaps. In the proper plane, deep to the plexus, the dissection is relatively avascular; on the other hand, if the flap is too thin, considerable bleeding will be caused by injury to the plexus.

With experience, the oncologic surgeon becomes more adroit and effective at undermining the flaps at the proper subcutaneous level. Nonetheless, it is the responsibility of the plastic surgeon to evaluate the vascular viability of the skin flaps. If the viability of the flaps is of concern, it is best to resect them rather than allow them to necrose in the postoperative period. Even in the hands of the experienced oncologic surgeons in our institution, the incidence of skin necrosis is 14% in patients who have undergone skin-sparing mastectomies.

The advantages of the skin-sparing mastectomy derive from preservation of the inframammary fold and the entire skin envelope. Projection and ptosis are no longer a problem in reconstructive efforts, particularly those performed with autologous tissue (24). The only requirement is to place the correct amount of tissue in the preserved skin envelope and leave a round skin island to simulate the removed nipple and areola. In cases involving a reduction in breast volume and contralateral reduction mammoplasty, or when the nipple and areola are very large, a purse-string suture can be used to decrease the skin envelop and narrow the diameter of the areola while maintaining projection.

On the other hand, skin-sparing mastectomy presents additional problems in patients who undergo reconstruction with implants. In these patients, implant exposure is very common, even when the serratus anterior muscle or the anterior rectus sheath musculofascial flap is used for coverage. Exposure of the implant occurs at the site of the periareolar incision or impending exposure of the implant on the inferior pole, if implant coverage is insufficient. Another complication, which follows an effort to provide total muscle coverage, is placement of the implant too high. With the inevitable capsular contracture, the inframammary fold will appear higher than the contralateral one. Lastly, if the implant is excessively expanded, the soft tissue may thin out considerably, so that telangectasia and translucency of the skin develop. In our series, one or more of these complications occur in at least 50% of the cases. Therefore, we do not perform immediate reconstructions with implants in patients who have undergone skin-sparing mastectomy without transposing the latissimus dorsi myocutaneous flap.

LATISSIMUS DORSI AND IMPLANT RECONSTRUCTION

Use of the latissimus dorsi myocutaneous flap has been shown to be a reliable and reproducible method of breast reconstruction (Fig. 37-11). It provides excellent coverage when either an implant or a permanent expander prosthesis is used. The myocutaneous flap provides such excellent coverage that the second operation, required to replace a temporary expander with a permanent implant, can be safely eliminated. This procedure is suitable for immediate reconstruction following skin-sparing mastectomy or in delayed reconstruction. The unilateral or bilateral transposition of latissimus dorsi myocutaneous flaps for immediate reconstruction in the patient who has undergone a skin-sparing mastectomy has reduced postoperative complications and undesirable results.

Technique for Unilateral Reconstruction

The skin island should be marked preoperatively with the patient standing to place the incision at a level that will be covered by the brassiere (Fig. 37-12). After the skin-sparing mastectomy has been completed, it is essential to pack the pocket with a sponge soaked in Betadine and temporarily close the mastectomy incision with staples. To obtain excellent exposure and decrease the risk for injury to the pedicle, the incision is extended superiorly along the anterior border of the latissimus dorsi muscle, and the skin flaps are elevated superiorly above the tip of the scapula and inferiorly for a distance of about 10 cm. Ideally, the skin island is of sufficient width to re-create the excised areola; however, to reduce donor site morbidity, it is kept narrow enough to permit primary closure without tension.

At the superior border of the latissimus dorsi muscle, just above the tip of the scapula, dissection is started bluntly deep to the latissimus dorsi. It is continued posteriorly to the

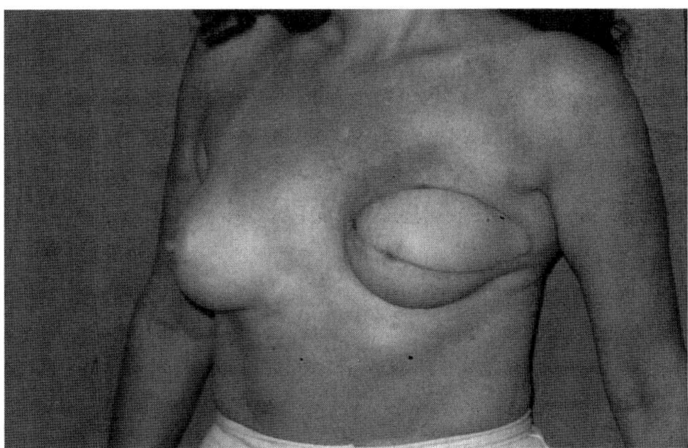

FIGURE 37-11. Good ptosis and projection following latissimus dorsi coverage of an implant.

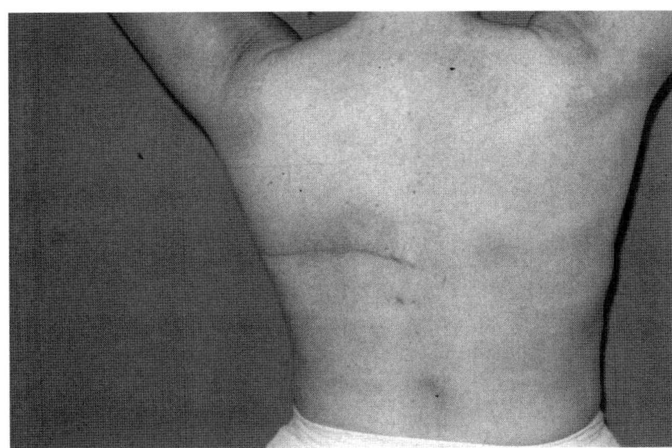

FIGURE 37-12. Minimal donor site morbidity following latissimus dorsi harvest.

fascial origin of the latissimus dorsi, approximately 3 cm from the midline, which is incised caudally 10 cm inferior to the skin island. Cautery is then used to divide the latissimus dorsi muscle and obtain hemostasis. Once the anterior border of latissimus dorsi has been reached, it is dissected either sharply or bluntly. The latissimus dorsi muscle itself is then supported peripherally with four Allis clamps, one in each corner, to visualize, clip, and divide the perforating vessels. It is important to avoid including portions of the serratus anterior muscle.

The dissection then extends along the anterior border of the latissimus dorsi muscle to identify the descending branch of the serratus anterior muscle and the thoracodorsal vessels. Once the pedicle is identified, it is protected as the posterior portion of the muscle is divided toward its insertion on the humerus. It is not necessary to divide the insertion of the latissimus dorsi muscle, but it must be freed sufficiently so that it can be transposed like a pendulum and not be fixed posteriorly like a rotational flap, which will create a bulge along the axillary line.

With the myocutaneous unit dissection complete, a tunnel between the mastectomy scar and the posterior dissection is created to transpose the unit anteriorly. It is critical that the opening be made large enough to transpose the unit, but the pocket must not extend beyond the midaxillary line, or the implant will migrate posteriorly. To accomplish this, particularly when the latissimus dorsi myocutaneous flap is transposed, it is necessary to suture the medial portion of the latissimus muscle to the lateral border of the sternum. Inferiorly, it is sutured to the subcutaneous tissue just below the inframammary fold rather than to the chest wall. Laterally, it is sutured to the pectoralis major muscle and to the chest wall at the midaxillary line to prevent migration of the implant beyond the anterior axillary line.

Once the myocutaneous unit has been transposed anteriorly, the back wound is thoroughly irrigated, hemostasis is checked again, and the wound is closed in layers. Two suction catheters are usually placed in the back and are brought out through separate stab wounds in a dependent portion of the back. The bean bag is deflated, and the patient is placed in the supine position (Fig. 37-13). The contralateral breast should be prepared and draped to check for symmetry. Once the latissimus dorsi myocutaneous unit has been transposed anteriorly, a pocket is created under the pectoralis major muscle. The medial origin of the pectoralis major muscle is partially divided from its lower sternal insertion to approximately 3 o'clock in relation to the nipple. The latissimus dorsi muscle is then sutured medially to the undersurface of the pectoralis major muscle superiorly, medially, and superolaterally, which allows enough room for a large prosthesis to be inserted. It is essential to close the pocket lateral to the midaxillary line with interrupted nylon sutures. The inferior border of the latissimus dorsi muscle is then sutured to the subcutaneous tissue level of the lower skin flap and not to the chest wall, again in an effort to maintain an adequate pocket. The skin island is circumscribed to correspond to the resected areola, and the rest of the skin island is then removed down to the subcutaneous tissue level.

A saline implant is inserted underneath the inferior lateral portion of the latissimus dorsi, where the sutures have been placed but not tied. The sutures are tied and the implant is inflated. Initially, the implant should be overinflated; if tension on the skin is not excessive, the implant can then be inflated to the desired volume. If a permanent implant/expander type of prosthesis has been used, the appropriate filling port connections are made and the portal is placed subcutaneously away from the implant, at the anterior axillary line or along the costal margin.

At this point, the patient is placed in the sitting position to assess symmetry. It is preferable to have the inframammary fold lower than that of the contralateral, normal breast, but it is also important to ensure that the lateral

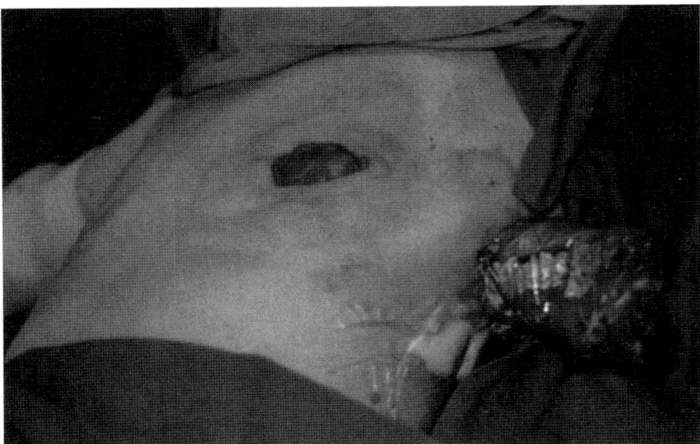

FIGURE 37-13. Latissimus dorsi harvested for bilateral subcutaneous mastectomy reconstruction with an implant.

pocket is not excessive. The wound is closed after a suction catheter has been placed along the axilla and midaxillary line and brought out through another stab wound away from the implant.

Technique of Bilateral Reconstruction for the Latissimus Dorsi Myocutaneous Flap

If bilateral skin-sparing mastectomies are planned, proper coordination between the oncologic and plastic surgeon is essential. It is suggested that the plastic surgeon begin the procedure, harvesting the latissimus dorsi myocutaneous units with the patient in the prone position. Symmetrical skin flap incisions are placed within the brassiere line. The myocutaneous flaps are dissected up into the axilla to allow for a satisfactory transposition. Following dissection, they are placed in sterile plastic bags.

The back wounds are closed in layers and with drains, and then the patient is turned to the supine position, prepared again, and redraped. The oncologic surgeon proceeds with the mastectomies, and then the reconstruction is performed as previously described. Although the operative time is significant, recovery following bilateral breast reconstruction with the use of latissimus dorsi myocutaneous flaps is rapid and straightforward.

REFERENCES

1. Cronin TD, Gerow FJ. Augmentation mammoplasty: a new "natural feel" prosthesis. In: *Transactions of the Third International Congress of Plastic and Reconstructive Surgery.* Amsterdam: Excerpta Medica, 1963.
2. Halsted WS. The results of operations for the cure for cancer of the breast performed at Johns Hopkins Hospital from June 1889 to January 1894. *Johns Hopkins Bull* 1895;4:297.
3. Patey DH. A review of 146 cases of carcinoma of the breast operated upon between 1930 and 1943. *Br J Cancer* 1967;21:260.
4. Moore TS, Farrell LD. Latissimus dorsi myocutaneous flap for breast reconstruction: long-term results. *Plast Reconstr Surg* 1992;89:666.
5. McCraw JB, Maxwell GP. Early and late capsular "deformation" as a cause of unsatisfactory results in latissimus dorsi breast reconstruction. *Clin Plast Surg* 1988;15:717.
6. Jarrett JR, Cutler RG, Teal DF. Aesthetic refinements in prophylactic subcutaneous mastectomy with submuscular reconstruction. *Plast Reconstr Surg* 1982;69:624.
7. Slade CL. Subcutaneous mastectomy: acute complications and long-term follow-up. *Plast Reconstr Surg* 1984;73:84.
8. Bostwick J, Vásconez LO, Jurkiewicz MJ. Breast reconstruction after radical mastectomy. *Plast Reconstr Surg* 1978;61:682.
9. Radovan C. Breast reconstruction after mastectomy using temporary expander. *Plast Reconstr Surg* 1982;69:195.
10. Slavin SA, Colen SR. Sixty consecutive breast reconstructions with the inflatable expander: a critical appraisal. *Plast Reconstr Surg* 1990;86:910.
11. Gibney J. The long-term results of tissue expansion for breast reconstruction. *Clin Plast Surg* 1987;14:509.
12. May JW Jr, Attwood J, Bartlett S. Staged use of soft tissue expansion and lower thoracic advancement flap in breast reconstruction. *Plast Reconstr Surg* 1987;79:272.
13. Maxwell GP, Falcone PA. Eighty-four consecutive breast reconstructions using a textured silicone tissue expander. *Plast Reconstr Surg* 1992;89:1022.
14. Boutros S. The intradermal anatomy of the inframammary fold. *Plast Reconstr Surg* 1998;102:1034.
15. Bayati S. Inframammary crease ligament. *Plast Reconstr Surg* 1995;90:501.
16. Carlson GW, Grossl N, Lewis MM, et al. Preservation of the inframammary fold: what are we leaving behind? *Plast Reconstr Surg* 1996;98:447.
17. Holle J, Pierini A. Breast reconstruction with an external oblique abdominus muscle turnover flap and a bipedicled abdominal skin flap. *Plast Reconstr Surg* 1984;73:469.
18. Pennisi VR. Making a definite inframammary fold under a reconstructed breast. *Plast Reconstr Surg* 1977;60:523.
19. Ryan JJ. A lower thoracic advancement flap in breast reconstruction after mastectomy. *Plast Reconstr Surg* 1982;70:153.
20. May JW Jr, Attwood J, Bartlett S. Staged use of soft tissue expansion and lower thoracic advancement flap in breast reconstruction. *Plast Reconstr Surg* 1987;79:272.
21. Gibney J. The long-term results of tissue expansion for breast reconstruction. *Clin Plast Surg* 1987;14:509.
22. Kroll SS, Shusterman MA, Tadjalli HE, et al. Risk of recurrence after treatment of early breast cancer with skin-sparing mastectomy. *Ann Surg Oncol* 1997;4:193.
23. Carlson GW, Bostwick J III, Styblo TM, et al. Skin-sparing mastectomy. Oncologic and reconstructive considerations. *Ann Surg* 1997;225:570.
24. Hidalgo DA, Borgen PJ, Petrek JA, et al. Immediate reconstruction after complete skin-sparing mastectomy with autologous tissue. *J Am Coll Surg* 1998;187:17.

Discussion

BREAST RECONSTRUCTION WITH IMPLANTS AND EXPANDERS

R. BARRETT NOONE

In discussing how to prevent and correct the complications and unfavorable results of reconstruction with breast implants and expanders after mastectomy, Drs. Fix, de la Torre, and Vasconez make a strong case for use of the latissimus dorsi musculocutaneous unit to cover the breast implant. A better result—namely, an improved inframammary fold, a more pleasing projection, and a greater degree of ptosis—can be achieved with the latissimus dorsi musculocutaneous flap than with an implant alone. It is generally accepted that the goals of safety, simplicity, and symmetry can be attained even more effectively with autogenous tissue reconstruction, specifically reconstruction with the transverse rectus abdominis musculocutaneous (TRAM) flap. Accordingly, in the algorithm I use for evaluating candidates for breast reconstruction, if ptosis is needed to create symmetry with the contralateral breast, and if the patient is otherwise a candidate for autogenous reconstruction, then autogenous reconstruction is the first choice. It is extremely difficult to produce a definitive inframammary fold and a modest to moderate degree of ptosis with implant/expander reconstruction alone unless the latissimus dorsi flap is added.

IMPLANT RECONSTRUCTION

In the patient with a small, nonptotic normal breast, implant or expander reconstruction alone is a first choice and avoids the potential complications of autogenous reconstruction. Therefore, in the usual practice setting, use of the latissimus dorsi flap is most often not necessary.

In many patients, if the healthy breast is small and nonptotic, the contralateral breast can be reconstructed with an implant filled with saline solution or silicone, without any need for soft tissue expansion. An approximation of the implant size can be obtained by weighing the mastectomy specimen in grams and converting the result to milliliters of saline solution. With this type of patient, symmetry can often be achieved without multiple office visits to adjust or expand the implant, and without a second operative procedure. If a breast of reasonable size cannot be created at the time of surgery, and if only a small degree of adjustment is necessary, then the adjustable saline implant is a good choice (Spectrum Adjustable Implant, Mentor Corporation) (1). In a delayed reconstruction, however, or an immediate reconstruction in which some ptosis is needed and a size adjustment of more than 50 to 75 mL might be necessary for the final result, then I proceed with either a two-staged reconstruction (initial expansion followed by replacement with a permanent implant) or a single-staged reconstruction with an expander/implant that has a final composition of 75% saline solution and 25% silicone gel (Becker expander/implant, Mentor Corporation).

In their introduction, the authors refer to the historically significant polyurethane implants, indicating that they demonstrated a lower incidence of capsular contracture. In my experience, this was true for a few years following reconstruction, after which a marked increase in capsular contracture was noted.

INFRAMAMMARY FOLD

In their discussion of how to create a symmetrical breast, the authors correctly devote attention to the inframammary fold. As they state, a distinct fold is particularly difficult to achieve with a nonautogenous reconstruction. It is generally agreed among oncologic and reconstructive surgeons that the resection of breast tissue in a mastectomy does not have to be extended below the inframammary fold. The fold can be clearly marked in most patients and highlighted with full-thickness skin sutures preoperatively, as described by the authors. However, the extent of the dissection during the mastectomy is not the most important factor in determining the position of the inframammary fold postoperatively; it is the placement of the implant. In most instances, it is necessary to provide complete muscle coverage of the implant or expander to prevent exposure in the event of marginal skin necrosis of the mastectomy flaps. Therefore, coverage with the pectoralis major muscle, a portion of the pectoralis minor, the serratus anterior, the external oblique, and the fascia of the rectus abdominis is necessary. For the

R. B. Noone: Division of Surgery, University of Pennsylvania School of Medicine, Philadelphia, Pennsylvania; Division of Plastic Surgery, Main Line Hospitals, Bryn Mawr Hospital, Bryn Mawr, Pennsylvania

inframammary fold to form a definitive crease, a capacious pocket must be developed at the lower pole of the breast reconstruction. To achieve this, it is necessary to release the medial attachment of the rectus abdominis fascia from the fifth and sixth ribs medially. Laterally, the same release is necessary in the anatomical location where the rectus fascia communicates with the external abdominal oblique muscle (2). If care is taken with this portion of the dissection, a larger lower pocket is created for an implant or expander.

In some situations, it may be acceptable to use only skin and subcutaneous tissue rather than a total muscle cover at the lower pole of the implant (3). This arrangement is appropriate in heavy patients, whose skin flaps are protected by a thick layer of adipose tissue superficial to the plane of dissection of the mastectomy. In these patients, the lower border of the superior hemisphere of the usual muscle pocket, consisting of the pectoralis major, pectoralis minor, and serratus anterior, can be sutured to the subcutaneous tissue. The lower portion of the pocket is then not restricted, so that the creation of an inframammary fold and ptosis is facilitated, especially if the expansion technique is used. It must be emphasized that the usually recommended total muscle cover should not be omitted in these cases unless the viability of the mastectomy skin is unquestionably good, as determined by the intravenous fluoroscein-Wood's lamp technique (4). All areas of nonfluorescent tissue must be excised, and the viability of skin flaps with a thickness of more than 1 cm should be ascertained before this technique is attempted. However, in the carefully selected patient, an excellent inframammary fold can be achieved with a modest to moderate degree of ptosis following skin expansion.

PROJECTION

It is very difficult to achieve projection with any type of implant reconstruction unless supplemental tissue is used to increase the transverse diameter. The authors discuss the use of zigzag incisions, or Z-plasties. Although these techniques are beneficial in patients undergoing delayed reconstruction, their usefulness is limited in immediate reconstruction. In the latter case, the degree of projection is usually determined by the ability to develop a large muscle pocket rather than by the ability to limit skin contracture. In the immediate situation, the skin is usually sufficiently loose and abundant that it does not limit the transverse diameter; rather, the problem is the inability first to constrict or later to stretch the muscle pocket.

In regard to the techniques that have been introduced to improve ptosis, I agree with the authors' analysis of the difficulties inherent in the skin advancement, deepithelialization techniques of Pennisi and Ryan. My experience has been similar; it is difficult to position and achieve a symmetrical inframammary fold, and the suture line at the inframammary fold is tenuous.

COMPLICATIONS OF IMPLANTS AND EXPANDERS

In their discussion of the complications of implants and expanders, the authors present a good management plan for the exposed implant. However, in our experience, the incidence of implant exposure is not high, even when necrotic edges on the skin flap must be managed. In our original series of 244 patients who underwent reconstruction immediately, marginal skin necrosis was noted in 21 (9.1%). In the patients in whom skin necrosis developed but who had good muscle cover, the implants could be salvaged, and only eight patients (3.4%) lost their implants (5,6). Of course, if implant exposure is a result of poor muscle cover and skin necrosis intervenes, then implant salvage is not possible, and I agree with the authors' recommendation of immediate implant removal. It is in the secondary reconstruction of the patient with a failed implant that the latissimus dorsi flap is applied to good advantage. In addition to the skin removed during the mastectomy, skin and sometimes muscle must be debrided at the time of implant removal, and the natural processes of contracture and epithelialization that take place during wound healing lead to yet a greater deficiency of skin in the area of the wound. Therefore, secondary reconstruction without the introduction of additional tissue is extremely difficult and produces a result that is far less than ideal.

The authors describe the use of external taping to manipulate the implant position in cases of malposition. I have not found taping to be helpful unless it is done in the operating room at the time of surgery. Once malposition has developed, fibrous contracture is usually evident and cannot be manipulated by taping. I would not favor percutaneous closure of an excessive inferior pocket for two reasons. The first, of course, would be fear of perforating the implant. The second would be that after suture removal, the inferior displacement would be likely to recur because of lack of adherence of the capsule surfaces. When performing an open capsulorrhaphy to close the inferior pocket, I prefer to remove the implant and indicate the correct inframammary fold with transcutaneous sutures or methylene blue marking applied with a Keith needle while the patient is sitting before I excise the capsule from the inferior pocket. I prefer to juxtapose two surfaces of fresh, unscarred tissue at the inframammary fold rather than rely on a capsule-to-capsule sutured closure. Once the internal capsulorrhaphy has been performed and the inframammary fold secured and compared with that on the opposite side, then a decision is made regarding how to manage the rest of the capsule. In many instances, anterior and superior capsulotomy is necessary, but in others, only an inferior hemisphere capsulectomy is needed, so that the posterior surface of the capsule and the superior surface beneath the muscle are preserved. I certainly agree with the authors that in the presence of significant calcifications or leaking gel infiltration of the capsule, that a total capsulectomy should be performed. After inferior internal capsulorrhaphy, external taping for 1 to 2 weeks postoperatively is helpful.

In their discussion of capsular contracture, the authors indicate the necessity of using the latissimus dorsi musculocutaneous unit in treating contracture. Although such a procedure may certainly provide a superior aesthetic result and prevent a second capsular contracture, it would be my preference to perform a capsulectomy as the initial standard treatment for capsular contracture rather than proceed directly to a latissimus dorsi flap. It has not been my experience that a more severe capsular contracture occurs following capsulectomy in more than half of patients. Although capsules do recur, many can be successfully deterred with capsulectomy. It must be recognized that although it is less frequent, capsular contracture does occur with the latissimus dorsi flap (as noted in reference 5 of Chapter 37), and at the same rate as after breast augmentation. I would prefer to introduce additional muscle cover to treat a second capsular contracture rather than a first.

I am in complete agreement with the authors' suggestions to manage infected implants by removing the implants and treating the infection before another reconstruction is attempted. Although the salvage of infected implants with irrigation and systemic antibiotics has been reported, the almost certain capsular contracture around the salvaged implant and the unpleasing aesthetic result are not worth the inconvenience, potential hazards of systemic infection, and expense of attempts at salvage.

SKIN-SPARING MASTECTOMY

The skin-sparing mastectomy has been a major advance toward achieving better aesthetic results after immediate reconstruction with autogenous tissue. It is particularly suited to the rectus abdominis musculocutaneous flap. If an implant is to be used with a skin-sparing mastectomy, the authors correctly recommend the latissimus dorsi flap. However, the decision for or against a skin-sparing mastectomy should be made preoperatively by the oncologic surgeon and plastic surgeon jointly. Skin-sparing mastectomies should not be performed routinely; the use of this technique should be determined according to the reconstruction plan. When implant or expander reconstruction is to be performed in a small-breasted woman without ptosis, it is unwarranted to subject both the patient and the general surgeon to the difficulties of the skin-sparing technique and the added potential for skin necrosis. Excision of the nipple and areola, with preservation of the medial, unscarred skin and tailoring of the skin excision laterally and toward the axilla, can be carried out effectively; this technique obviates the need for a purse string suture around the thin skin flaps remaining after skin-sparing mastectomy and provides a good reuslt with minimal lateral scarring. In a patient with a small nipple and areola who has undergone a well-performed skin-sparing mastectomy, if a total muscle cover is present, I believe a purse string closure can be effective. However, this is an unusual patient, and usually some form of "dog-ear" excision of skin is necessary in implant reconstruction in the absence of a latissimus dorsi flap. I agree with the authors that when any degree of ptosis or projection is desired with a skin-sparing mastectomy, the latissimus dorsi flap should be added.

LATISSIMUS DORSI FLAP

The chapter provides an excellent description of the technique of the latissimus dorsi musculocutaneous flap, which was the mainstay of breast reconstruction in the late 1970s and early 1980s. Although it is often not necessary to divide the insertion of the latissimus dorsi muscle from the humerus, I usually attempt to do this to provide a better arc of rotation and eliminate the posterior axillary fullness that inevitably results from inadequate release of the latissimus insertion.

The authors make a good case for the latissimus dorsi flap to provide optimal results in implant reconstruction. However, they do so without discussing the contraindications to use of the latissimus dorsi, in addition to the disadvantages and complications of the technique. If a skin island is moved with a muscle, the patient obviously will have a back scar. In addition, muscle function is lost, a problem of particular importance to the athletic woman who may want to continue rowing or cross-country skiing, especially after the bilateral procedure. Also, because of a cosmetic excavation deformity of the back, suction lipectomy of the opposite side is occasionally required to achieve symmetry. The inconvenience of patient positioning and the additional length of surgery are not prohibitive; however, care must be taken in positioning the patient to avoid stretching injuries to the brachial plexus. Thoracic outlet syndrome has been reported (7), and a back seroma is a frequent complication in the early postoperative period.

CONCLUSION

In summary, if autogenous tissue reconstruction is contraindicated or not desired by the patient, I recommend a single-stage implant reconstruction for the woman with small, nonptotic breasts and a single-stage Becker expander/implant or two-stage expander/implant reconstruction for modest ptosis. The latissimus dorsi flap is reserved for patients who require a greater degree of ptosis, those with tissue deficiency at either the skin or muscle level, patients undergoing delayed reconstruction after radiation, and patients with recalcitrant capsular contracture after a second capsulectomy.

REFERENCES

1. Noone RB. Adjustable implant reconstruction. In: Spear SL, ed. *The breast: principles and art.* Philadelphia: Lippincott–Raven Publishers, 1998:357–374.
2. Noone RB. Immediate reconstruction after mastectomy. In: Noone RB, ed. *Plastic and reconstructive surgery of the breast.* Philadelphia: BC Decker, 1991:344–371.
3. Dowden RV. Achieving a natural inframammary fold and ptotic effect in the reconstructed breast. *Ann Plast Surg* 1987;19: 524–529.
4. Singer R, Lewis CM, Franklin JD, et al. Fluorescein test for prediction of flap viability during breast reconstructions. *Plast Reconstr Surg* 1978;61:371–375.
5. Costiglione CL, Noone RB, Murphy JB, et al. Complications after immediate breast reconstruction and their management. *Plast Surg Forum* 1987;10:221.
6. Noone RB. Immediate reconstruction after mastectomy. In: Noone RB, ed. *Plastic and reconstructive surgery of the breast.* Philadelphia: BC Decker, 1991:344–371.
7. Rubio PA, Rose FA. Thoracic outlet syndrome caused by a latissimus dorsi flap for breast reconstruction. *Chest* 1990;97:494–495.

38

BREAST RECONSTRUCTION WITH AUTOLOGOUS TISSUE

STEPHEN S. KROLL

The use of autologous tissue for breast reconstruction after mastectomy, especially with transverse rectus abdominis myocutaneous (TRAM) flaps, is becoming increasingly popular with both patients and surgeons (1–4). Autologous tissue has the potential to deliver results of the highest possible quality, providing a feel and consistency very similar to that of a real breast (5,6). Unlike many implant-based reconstructions, autologous tissue reconstructions usually tend to improve with time as tissues soften, pain subsides, and scars fade. Patients who have undergone successful reconstructions with autologous tissues therefore are likely to be very happy with the results and grateful to their surgeons.

Unfortunately, autologous tissue reconstruction is a two-edged sword. Breast reconstruction with TRAM and other autologous flaps can be technically demanding and requires training that, at least in the past, has not been available in all plastic surgery training programs. Flaps do not always survive, and not all results are equally good. When this surgery is performed improperly, donor site complications can leave the patient much worse off than she was previously (7–9). With autologous tissue, the potential gain is greater than it is with implant-based reconstruction, but the risks are greater also.

Complications seen after autologous tissue breast reconstruction include hernias and bulges (9,10), partial or complete flap loss, fat necrosis (11), abdominoplasty flap necrosis (12), umbilical necrosis (12), breast malposition, and keloids. Fortunately, most of these complications can be avoided, at least in the great majority of cases. Unfortunately, even in the best of hands, the incidence of complications is not zero. For this reason, patients should always be warned about complications before the surgery is undertaken and that "this could happen to you." It is a good idea, in general, to promise less than the surgeon can deliver rather than the other way around. Patients are rarely unhappy when they are expecting a difficult time and the recuperation turns out to be easy. If they are promised an easy recovery but complications develop, however, they may well become angry and litigious.

S. S. Kroll: (Deceased) Formerly Department of Plastic Surgery, University of Texas M. D. Anderson Cancer Center, Houston, Texas

PATIENT SELECTION

One of the most important ways to minimize complications is careful patient selection. Not every patient is a candidate for reconstruction with a TRAM flap. Obese patients are at higher risk for complications of all kinds than thin patients are, and in markedly obese patients, the risk is even higher (13–15). Most of my failures in TRAM flap breast reconstruction have been in obese patients (Fig. 38-1). Avoiding TRAM flap reconstruction in very obese patients will therefore eliminate a large number (if not the great majority) of problems and complications. Overly obese patients who desire TRAM flap breast reconstruction should be asked to lose weight before the reconstruction is undertaken if they think that is possible. If the patient believes that she would be unable to lose enough weight to become an acceptable candidate for a TRAM flap, reconstruction with an extended latissimus dorsi flap can be a good alternative (16,17) (Fig. 38-2).

Patients who have a potbelly habitus are also poor candidates for reconstruction with either a TRAM or a Rubens fat pad flap. For one thing, the large amount of intraabdominal fat puts pressure on the abdominal wall repair and increases the risk for bulge or hernia (Fig. 38-3). For another, less subcutaneous fat is available to transfer, and so the size of the breast that can be obtained will be limited. For these reasons, the breasts of patients with a potbelly habitus should be reconstructed with techniques other than TRAM or Rubens flaps. As in obese patients, a latissimus dosi flap can be a good alternative for these patients.

Patients who smoke are usually not good candidates for single-pedicle TRAM flaps (3,13,14) or deep inferior epigastric perforator (DIEP) flaps (18–20). In both these flaps, blood perfusion is less robust than in free TRAM flaps, and partial flap necrosis is a significant risk (Fig. 38-4). Patients who smoke are therefore best offered reconstruction with types of

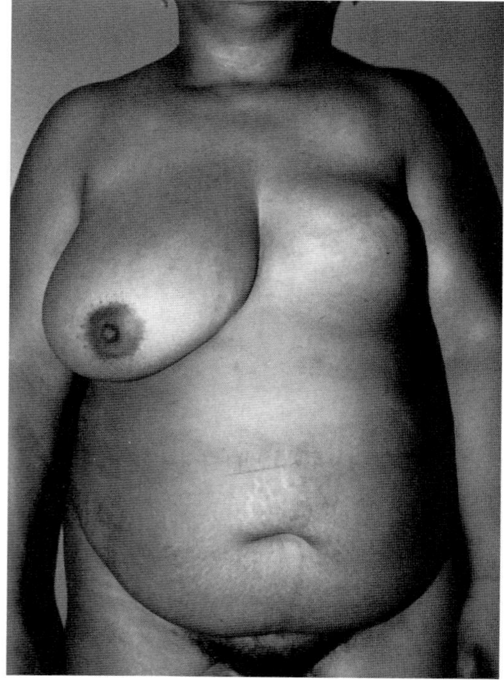

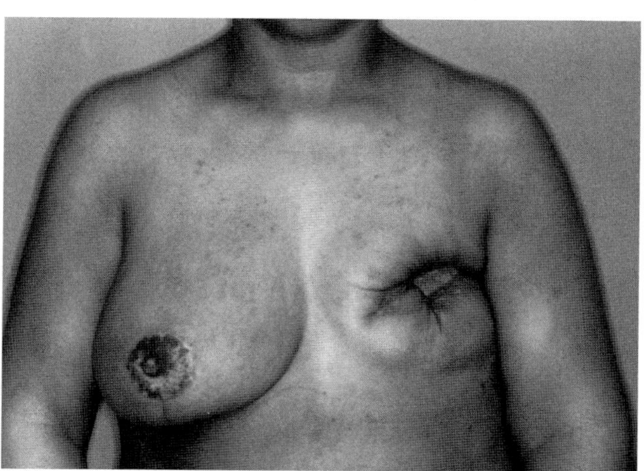

FIGURE 38-1. A: Very obese patient with unsuccessful tissue expander reconstruction of left breast. Because of her obesity, the patient was not a good candidate for a TRAM flap. **B:** After loss of 85% of the flap through late pedicle thrombosis and obstruction, probably caused by traction on the pedicle by the heavy flap.

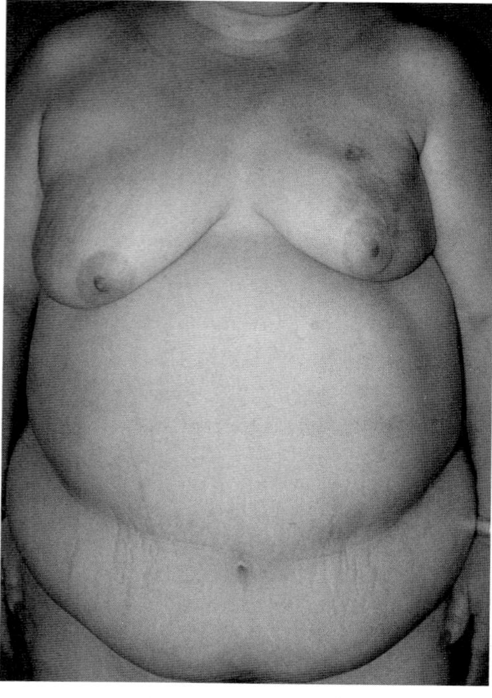

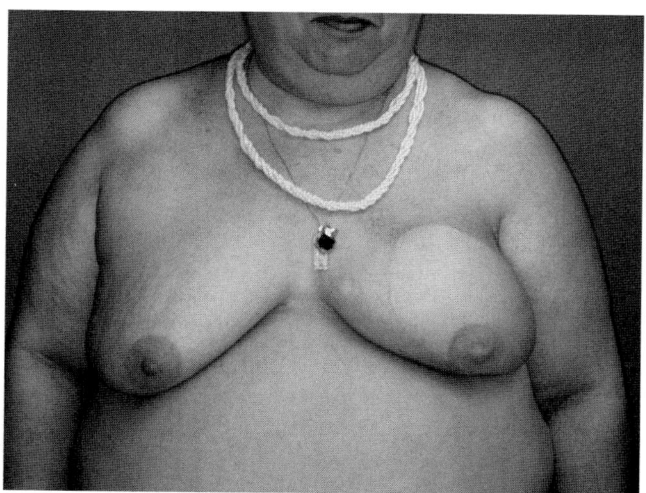

FIGURE 38-2. A: Very obese patient requesting immediate reconstruction of the left breast. **B:** Result of reconstruction with an extended latissimus dorsi flap. (From Kroll SS. *Breast reconstruction with autologous tissue: art and artistry.* New York: Springer-Verlag, 2000:166, with permission.)

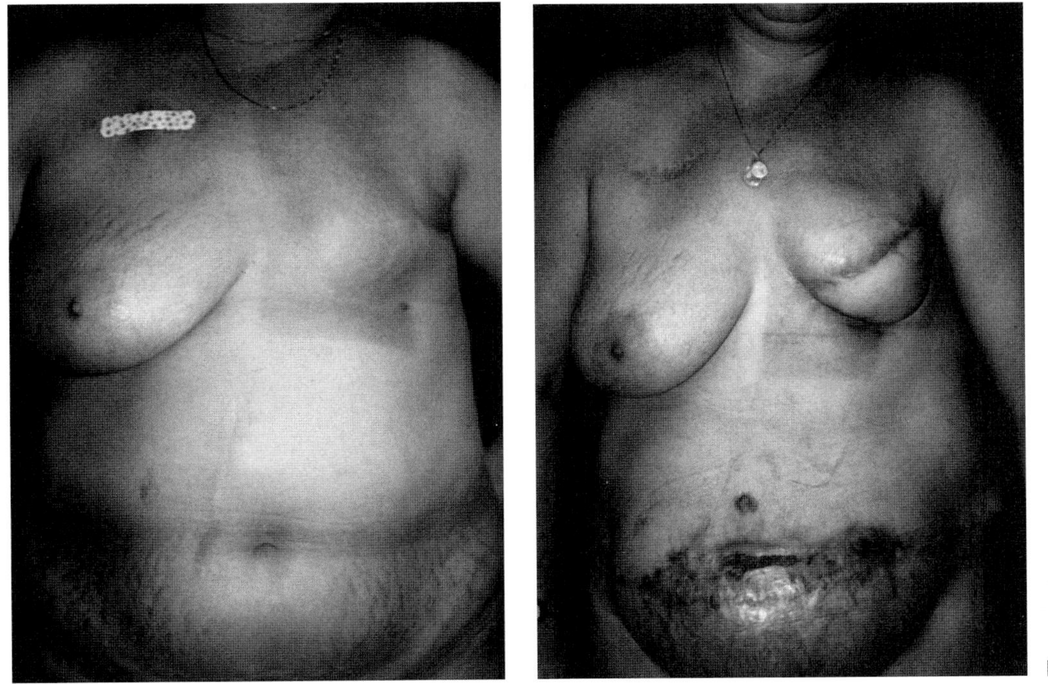

FIGURE 38-3. A: Patient with potbelly habitus who requested breast reconstruction with a TRAM flap. **B:** Patient after double-pedicled TRAM flap reconstruction, with a small, unsatisfactory breast and an abdominal bulge.

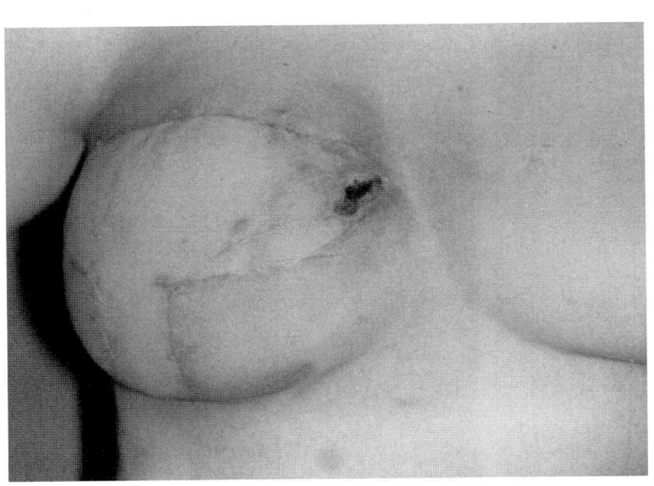

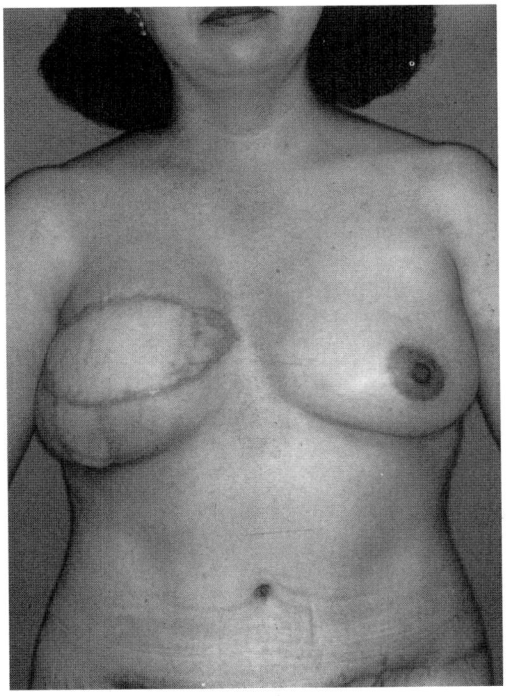

FIGURE 38-4. A: In this patient, who had undergone a delayed reconstruction of the right breast with a DIEP flap, partial flap loss developed medially. **B:** After debridement of the necrotic tissue and reshaping of the breast, the result is improved. (From Kroll SS. *Breast reconstruction with autologous tissue: art and artistry.* New York: Springer-Verlag, 2000:304, with permission.)

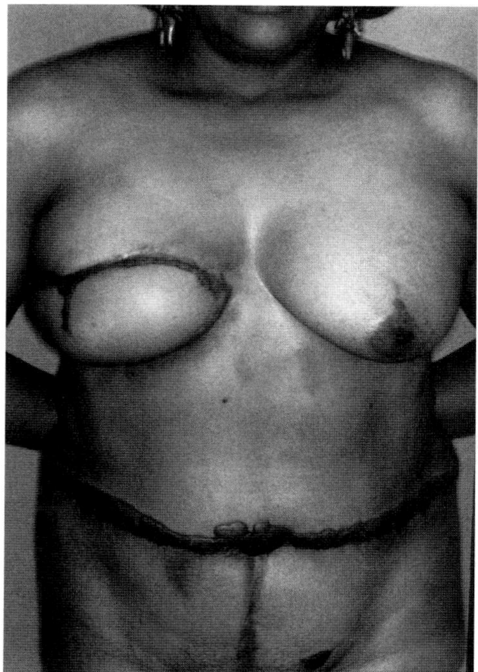

FIGURE 38-5. Patient with keloids following a TRAM flap breast reconstruction. The breast shape is good, but the scars spoil the effect. (From Kroll SS. *Breast reconstruction with autologous tissue: art and artistry.* New York: Springer-Verlag, 2000:156, with permission.)

TRAM flaps that have better than average perfusion (e.g., free, supercharged, or delayed TRAM flaps) unless they can stop smoking for several months before the reconstruction.

Some patients are just not candidates for any breast reconstruction at all. Patients with unrealistic expectations, those who are ambivalent about having the reconstruction, and those who are in poor general health are better off not undergoing reconstruction. Patients who are keloid formers (Fig. 38-5) should be approached only with great caution and perhaps should not be offered reconstruction. Personally, I hesitate to offer TRAM or other complex flaps (but not latissimus dorsi flaps or implant-based reconstruction) to patients who are older than 65, but this is a relative contraindication and can vary depending on the patient's general health.

FLAP SELECTION

For most patients who are candidates for reconstruction with autologous tissue, the best option is some type of TRAM or DIEP flap. This is because the donor site is relatively inconspicuous and because the lower abdominal fatty tissue is soft, pliable, and a good substitute for the missing breast. The DIEP flap is associated with less morbidity than the TRAM flap and is therefore ideal for patients who are suitable candidates. "Suitable candidates" should not smoke, should not require survival of the entire flap to have an adequately sized breast, and should have adequately sized perforators (18–21). Because the perforators ultimately must be assessed in the operating room under direct vision, it is best to tell patients that the final decision to perform a DIEP flap will be made in the operating room. If their vessels are deemed to be unsuitable, a free (or perhaps even pedicled) TRAM flap will be performed instead.

If a TRAM flap is chosen, I generally prefer the free TRAM flap to the pedicled version because less muscle sacrifice is required and the flap blood supply is better. This option is practical in an institution like my own, where adequate equipment, assistance, and nursing care are available, but it may not be practical everywhere. I prefer the free TRAM flap because donor site morbidity is less than with a pedicled flap, and because I believe that the improved flap blood supply makes it possible to attain the best possible aesthetic results. However, it is far better to have a live pedicled TRAM flap than a dead free one, so I advise surgeons to use whichever type of flap they are most comfortable with. Moreover, even in my own practice, I tell patients that the pedicled TRAM flap may be used if I find, in the operating room, that the recipient vessels are unsatisfactory.

If a TRAM flap is not possible because of a previous abdominoplasty or TRAM flap, the next choice is usually either a gluteal flap or an extended latissimus dorsi flap (16,17). Each of these procedures has its own advantages and limitations. The extended latissimus dorsi flap is technically simple, but it leaves a conspicuous donor site scar, and the tissue does not always lend itself to good breast shaping. The gluteal free flaps are technically more difficult than a free TRAM flap, but the donor site scar is usually not objectionable and the quality of the breast that can be obtained is high. At the time of this writing, I prefer the superior gluteal perforator (S-GAP) flap because the donor site morbidity is less than that seen with other gluteal flaps (22,23). The choice between the extended latissimus dorsi and the S-GAP flap for any given patient is usually heavily influenced by the relative amount of fat and skin laxity in the buttock versus the back. In the end, however, it is the patient who makes the decision, guided and supervised by the surgeon.

If neither an extended latissimus dorsi or an S-GAP flap is possible, other options include the Rubens fat pad flap (24) and the inferior gluteal free flap (25,26), and also the use of an implant. All these techniques are useful and capable of achieving good results, but for various reasons they are chosen less often than the methods previously discussed. Fortunately, the overwhelming majority of patients who desire autologous tissue reconstruction are candidates for some type of TRAM (or DIEP) flap.

BULGE AND HERNIA

Unquestionably, the most serious and harmful adverse consequence of a TRAM flap breast reconstruction is an abdominal bulge or hernia that cannot be repaired. Even if the best possible result is obtained in the breast, a patient with a bulge or hernia that cannot be repaired will usually be unhappy and regret having had the surgery. Like most complications, this is easier to prevent than to treat. Prevention of a TRAM flap bulge or hernia begins with the avoidance of unnecessary sacrifice of deep abdominal fascia.

As we all know, with a DIEP flap it is possible to transfer lower abdominal tissues without sacrificing any muscle or fascia. Although hernias can certainly develop after DIEP flaps, they are rare and, more importantly, easy to repair. On the other hand, it can be difficult or impossible to repair a bulge or hernia following a bilateral or double-pedicled conventional TRAM flap in which a wide section of fascia has been removed from each side. However, surgeons need not limit their practice to DIEP flaps to minimize hernias. The amount of fascia that is harvested can be limited in any type of TRAM flap by visualizing the perforators and incising the fascia close to them. When free TRAM flaps are used, because of their usually excellent blood supply, they can be designed to approximate the fascia-sparing qualities of perforator flaps (Fig. 38-6).

Once the flap has been harvested, preferably without excess sacrifice of fascia, the abdominal wall must be repaired correctly. Repair must include the internal oblique fascia, which is stronger than the external oblique layer and therefore essential to the repair (10). In the most inferior part of the abdomen, these two layers often separate, and the internal oblique fascia tends to retract laterally (Fig. 38-7). It is therefore easy not to include it in the suture repair unless it is specifically looked for. The surgeon can ensure that it is included by repairing the abdominal wall in layers or, alternatively, simply by taking care to include the internal oblique with each stitch in a single-layered closure. Either way, the surgeon must be sure to sew it to strong, solid tissue medially. This is done either by including the strong midline fascia in each stitch, or by tugging firmly on the needle after each stitch is placed through more lateral fascia to make sure that the tissue is strong enough to maintain the repair securely. If the needle pulls through, it must be repositioned more medially until it holds.

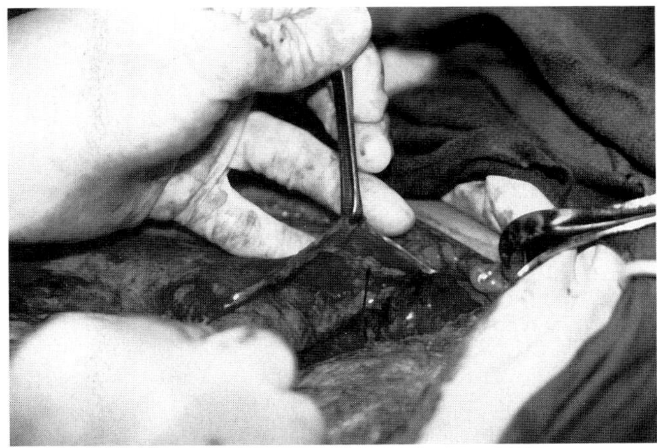

FIGURE 38-7. The internal oblique fascia *(arrow)* tends to separate from the external oblique fascia (held by Allis clamp) and retract laterally in the lower abdomen, so that it is easy to fail to include this layer in the repair.

If excessive amounts of fascia are not sacrificed, synthetic mesh is rarely necessary unless the tissues are of poor quality and will not hold the sutures well. If mesh is used, it should reinforce the fascia rather than replace it (7). Otherwise, if the mesh becomes infected (which is rare but does occur), the patient will have a severe hernia problem when the mesh is removed.

If a bulge or hernia does develop, it must be repaired aggressively (27). True hernias are rare (Fig. 38-8), and their re-

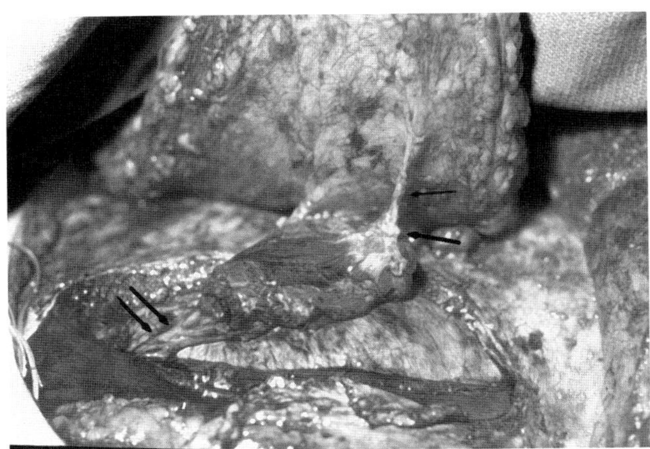

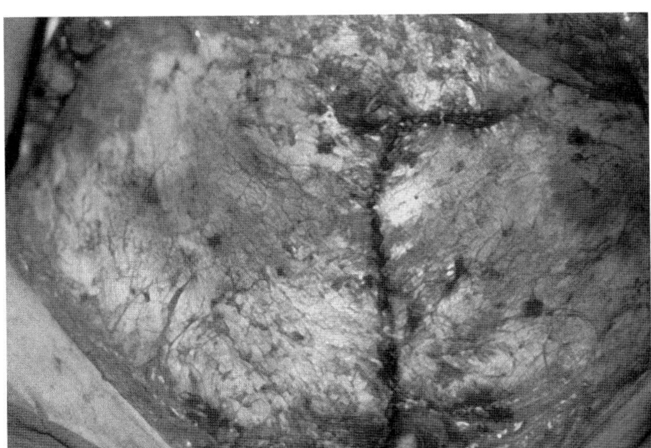

FIGURE 38-6. A: Free TRAM flap with standard muscle and deep inferior epigastric vessels *(double heavy arrows)* harvested but only a small ring of fascia *(single heavy arrow)* harvested around the base of each perforator *(thin arrow)*. **B:** Abdominal wall after closure of the donor defect. Essentially no fascia is missing. (From Kroll SS. *Breast reconstruction with autologous tissue: art and artistry.* New York: Springer-Verlag, 2000:60, with permission.)

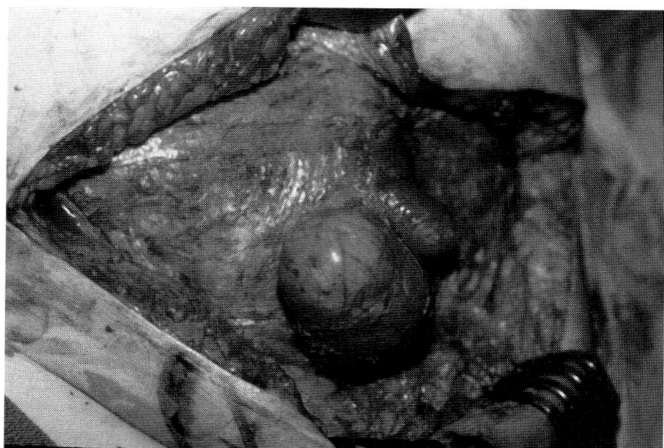

FIGURE 38-8. True hernia after TRAM flap breast reconstruction, with a defect of both internal and external oblique layers. This type of hernia is uncommon. (From Reece GP, Kroll SS. Abdominal wall complications: prevention and treatment. *Clin Plast Surg* 1998;25:235–249, with permission.)

pair is straightforward. Bulges (sometimes called *TRAM hernias*), in which the external oblique fascia remains intact but is stretched out, are more problematic. Simple plication of the bulge is not sufficient. In most cases, the problem is caused by separation of the internal oblique fascia. If the abdomen is entered through a vertical paramedian incision, a shelf caused by retraction of the internal oblique can usually be identified (Fig. 38-9). If this shelf is grasped with Allis clamps, pulled medially, and then sutured to the strong midline fascia, the bulge can usually be successfully repaired.

In the past, I believed the use of reinforcing mesh to be optional in the repair of unilateral TRAM flap bulges. More recently, I have become convinced that it is best to place a layer of mesh over the abdominal wall to reinforce it whenever a bulge or hernia has occurred unless infection is present. One should consider the presence of a bulge or hernia as a possible indicator of weak tissues, so that reinforcement is prudent. The mesh should be placed over a wide area (Fig. 38-10) and sutured under slight tension.

The avoidance of bulges and hernias is one of the most important objectives of any good TRAM flap surgeon. Prevention is usually the best way to manage this problem, and eliminating excessive sacrifice of fascia goes a long way toward achieving this goal. It is for this reason that I personally have abandoned the use of the double-pedicled TRAM flap for reconstruction of a single breast and am using DIEP flaps more and more often (for appropriately selected patients).

ABDOMINOPLASTY FLAP NECROSIS

Blood is supplied to the abdominoplasty flap by lateral perforators that arise from intercostal vessels. If the flap is widely undermined, the central inferior margin of the flap can necrose. If a wide tunnel is then created connecting the abdominoplasty dissection and the breast pockets (as in a bilateral, conventional, pedicled TRAM flap), the risk for necrosis is increased even further and can be significant (Fig. 38-11). This is especially true in patients who smoke.

Abdominoplasty flap necrosis can be minimized by limiting the extent of undermining of the abdominoplasty flap. Personally, I prefer to undermine little more than the area directly overlying the rectus abdominis sheath (Fig. 38-12). In this way, the lateral perforating vessels that supply blood to the abdominoplasty flap are preserved. Visible pleats may be created when the TRAM flap donor site is closed, but these usually disappear with time and, moreover, are far less objectionable than abdominoplasty flap necrosis. Abdominoplasty flap necrosis can also be reduced by using free TRAM flaps, for which a tunnel need not be created. In that way, one of the sources of interruption of the abdominoplasty flap blood supply is eliminated.

COMPLETE FLAP LOSS

Complete loss of a pedicled TRAM flap is rare but does occur. A previous cholecystectomy or congenitally small superior epigastric vessels can both lead to severe flap ischemia and even total loss of the flap. For that reason, I always dissect and include the deep inferior epigastric vessels when I perform a pedicled TRAM flap so that I have the option of "supercharging" the flap by performing an auxiliary microvascular anastomosis to rescue the flap if necessary (28). Often, only a venous anastomosis need be performed to improve flap perfusion sufficiently for survival. Awareness of this fact can be important in cases in which the axillary vein but no convenient recipient artery is available.

If an auxiliary microvascular anastomosis is not possible, the condition of the flap can sometimes be improved by nonmicrovascular auxiliary drainage. If the flap is blue, releasing the end of the deep inferior epigastric vein usually decompresses the flap and restores a healthier pink color. After a few minutes, the vein can be reclamped. Intermittent drainage of this sort will sometimes tide the flap over while venous channels in the muscle pedicle are dilating (Carl Hartrampf Jr., personal communication). If this is not sufficient to resolve the problem, a catheter can be placed in the vein, secured with a tie, and used to drain the flap intermittently during the early postoperative course as necessary (Carl Hartrampf Jr., personal communication). The catheter must be kept open by a heparin lock and the lost blood will have to be replaced, but this is preferable to loss of a flap. When the intermittent drainage is no longer required (as determined by flap color), the catheter is simply withdrawn.

Complete flap loss is always a risk when free TRAM flaps are used, no matter how experienced or skilled the surgeon. The risks can be reduced by having good exposure, making sure the vein is not twisted, and avoiding tension on the pedicle. If the breast is large, I ask the patient to wear a brassiere

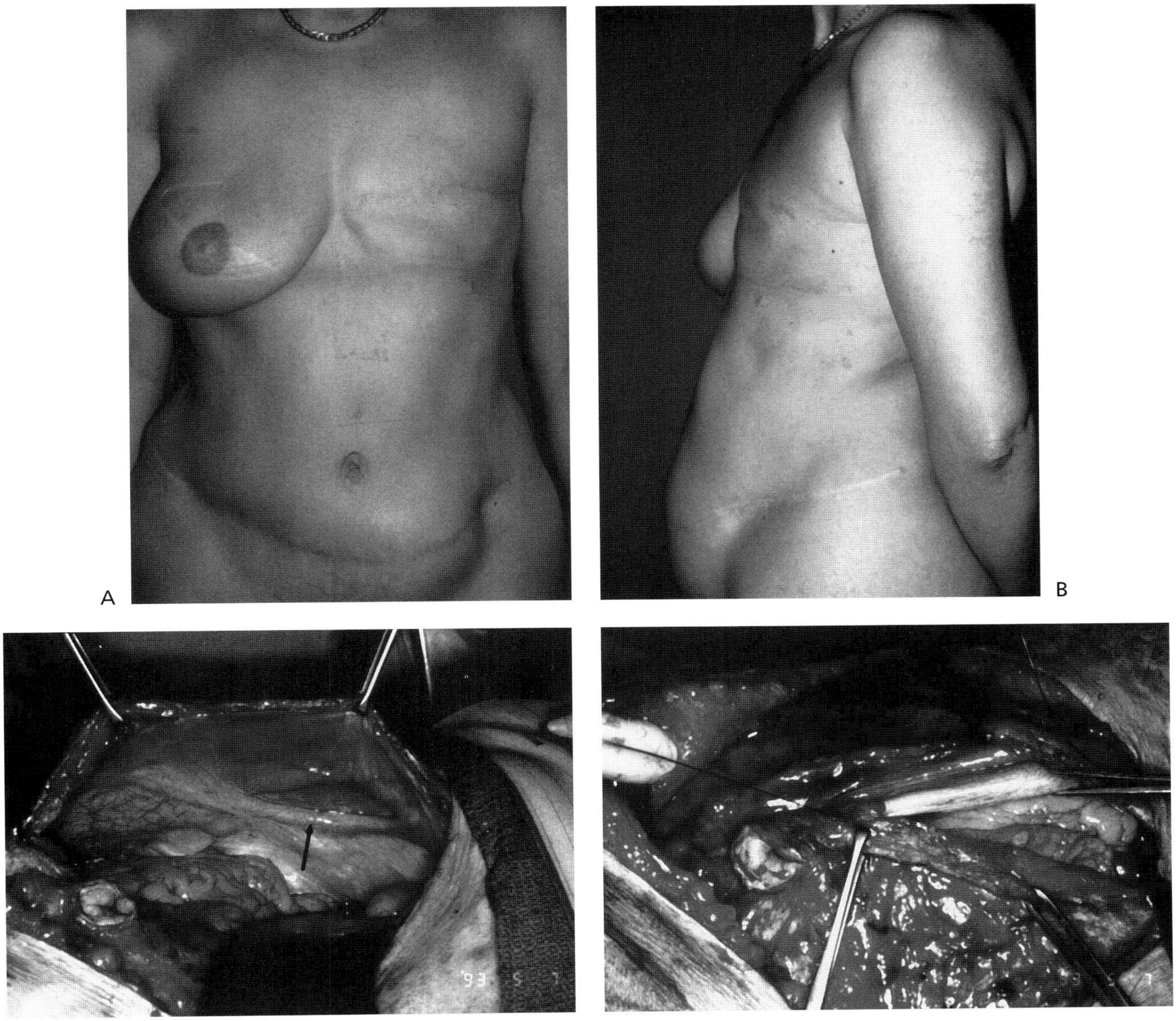

A

B

C

D

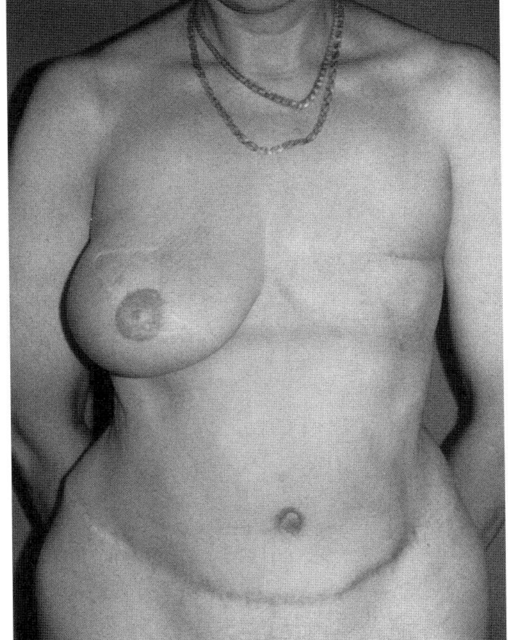

E

FIGURE 38-9. A,B: Patient with left lower abdominal bulge after reconstruction of the right breast with a TRAM flap. The left breast was not reconstructed. **C:** After the abdominal cavity was entered, a shelf consisting of the retracted internal oblique fascia *(arrow)* could be seen and palpated. **D:** This shelf of tissue was grasped with Allis forceps and pulled medially. It was then sutured to the strong midline abdominal fascia with heavy (No. 1) running sutures. **E:** Subsequently, the bulge did not recur. (From Kroll SS, Schusterman MA, Mistry D. The internal oblique repair of abdominal bulges secondary to TRAM flap breast reconstruction. *Plast Reconstr Surg* 1995;96:100, with permission.)

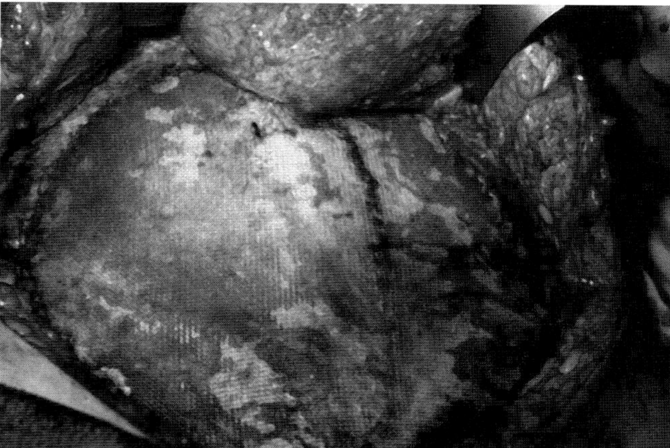

FIGURE 38-10. Mesh used to reinforce the abdominal wall repair. It should cover a wide area and be sutured under mild tension.

night and day for 30 days to support the flap and prevent a combination of gravity and ptosis from pulling on the pedicle. Tension caused by gravity when a patient with a large reconstructed breast is in the upright position is a very real problem with free TRAM flaps, especially when the thoracodorsal vessels have been used as recipients, and was probably the cause of the failure shown in Fig. 38-1. Avoiding the use of free TRAM flaps in very obese patients and having patients with large flaps wear a brassiere will help to prevent this problem.

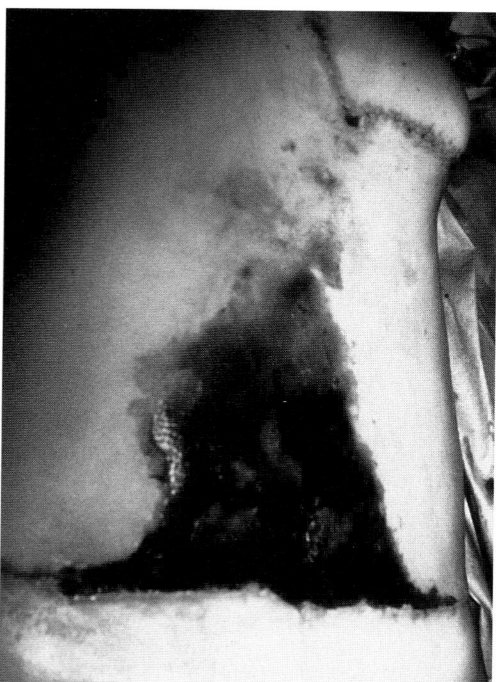

FIGURE 38-11. Patient with a history of smoking who had undergone bilateral conventional TRAM flap breast reconstruction. Extensive abdominoplasty flap necrosis developed. (From Kroll SS. Necrosis of abdominoplasty and other secondary flaps after TRAM flap breast reconstruction. *Plast Reconstr Surg* 1994;94:637 with permission.)

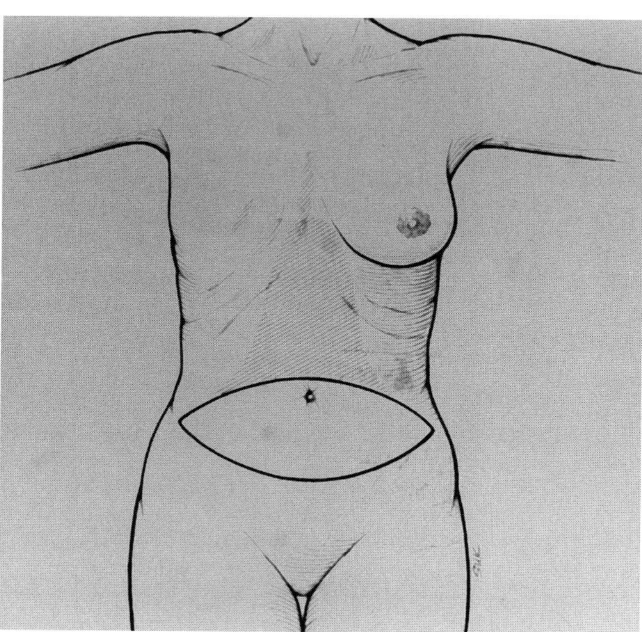

FIGURE 38-12. Schematic showing area that should be undermined when a TRAM flap is created. Further undermining is unnecessary and increases the risk for necrosis. (From Kroll SS. *Breast reconstruction with autologous tissue: art and artistry.* New York: Springer-Verlag, 2000:89, with permission.)

PARTIAL FLAP LOSS

Partial flap loss is a much more common problem in pedicled TRAM flaps than in free TRAM flaps (11,29,30). It also tends to be more severe in pedicled TRAM flaps (Fig. 38-13). The incidence of this problem can be significantly reduced by not performing single-pedicled TRAM flaps in patients who smoke and by "supercharging" pedicled TRAM flaps in which perfusion appears to be poor after transfer to the chest. Delay of the TRAM flap is also said to improve blood circulation and reduce the risk for partial flap loss, but I have no personal experience with that approach.

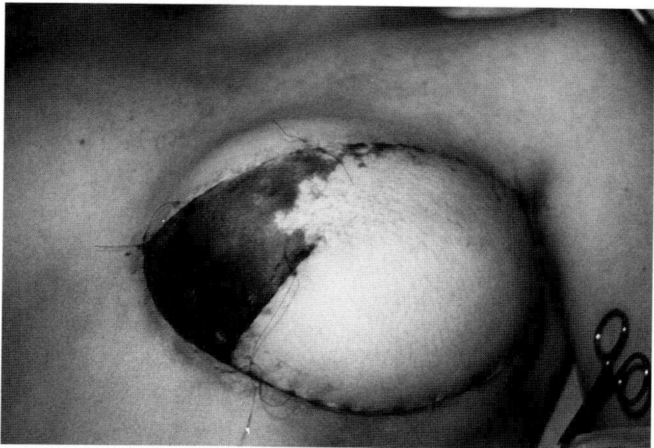

FIGURE 38-13. Patient with partial flap necrosis after pedicled (conventional) TRAM flap procedure.

If part of the flap bleeds only dark (venous) blood after transfer to the chest, it should be debrided back to good tissue that bleeds bright red when incised. If it is not possible to do this without unacceptably reducing the size of the breast, the flap should be "supercharged" or otherwise augmented. Dead or dying tissue should not knowingly be left in place as part of the breast.

If partial flap loss does occur, it should be treated early and aggressively. The best approach is to return the patient to the operating room for early debridement and repair of the defect (31). The best time is usually between the fourth and sixth postoperative days, after the patient has had a chance to recover a bit from the first operation but before the dead tissue has had time to become infected. The presence of fever is not a contraindication to this approach. After debridement of the necrotic tissue, the patient will usually feel better and the fever often disappears.

The defect created by debridement can sometimes be repaired simply by repositioning and reshaping the existing flap. Even if the breast is made smaller, if a good shape is obtained, a satisfactory result with symmetry can ultimately be achieved by reducing the opposite breast. If insufficient tissue remains to create even a small breast, a second flap may be necessary (Fig. 38-14). Provided that the patient is a good

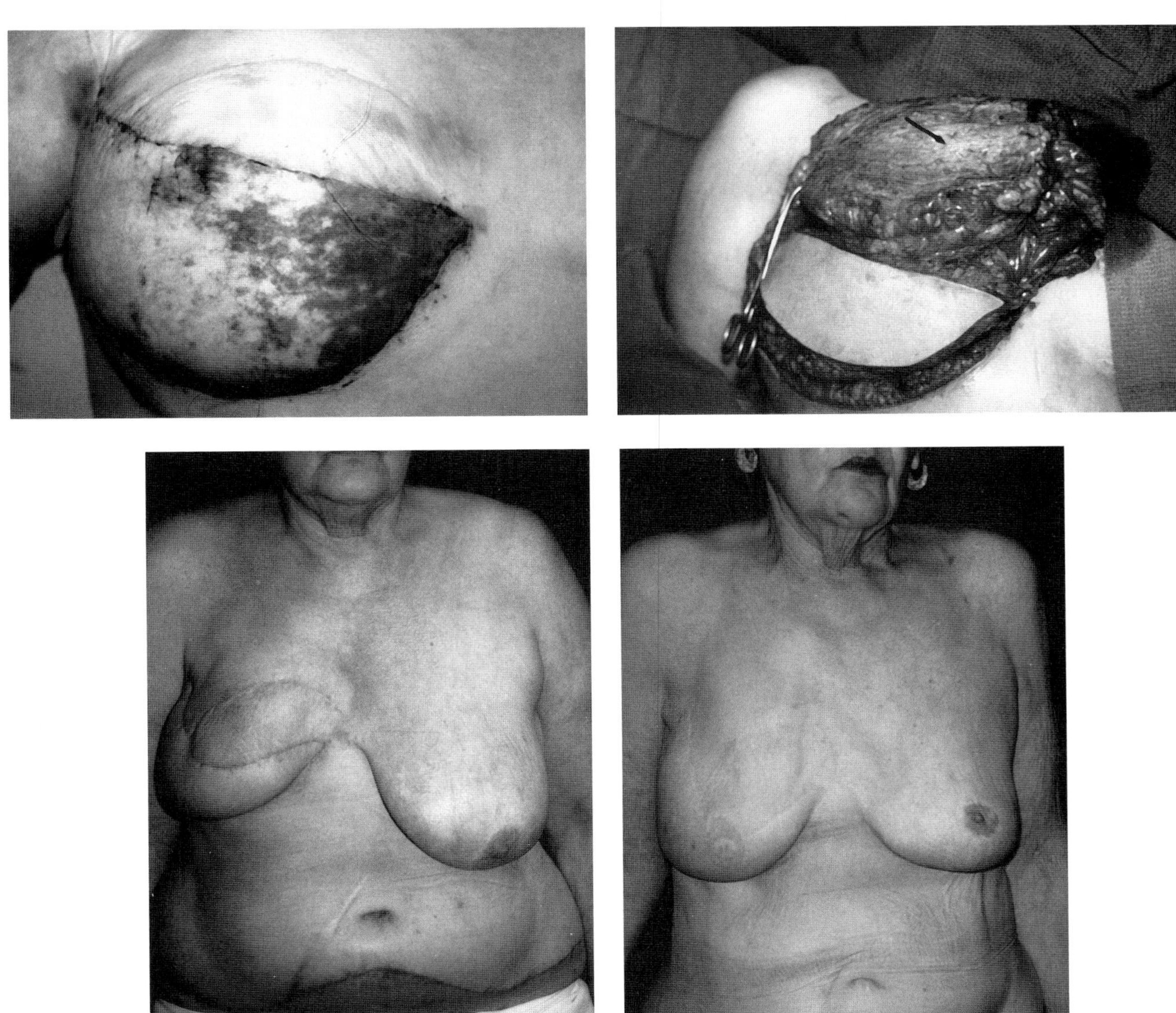

FIGURE 38-14. **A:** Patient with partial flap loss 2 days after creation of a pedicled TRAM flap. **B:** The TRAM flap *(arrow)* was debrided back to living tissue and a latissimus dorsi flap was used to add tissue and cover the deficient breast. **C:** The early result was smaller than the opposite breast but had a reasonable shape. **D:** The final result after reduction of the opposite breast. (From Kroll SS, Freeman P. Striving for excellence in breast reconstruction: the salvage of poor results. *Ann Plast Surg* 1989;22:58, with permission.)

candidate for a second flap and that the surgeon is confident of his or her ability to achieve success, early repair with a second flap is often worthwhile. Although it may seem drastic, there is no better time to perform the second flap procedure than when the patient is already in the hospital, anesthetized, and under the control of the surgeon. Provided that the outcome is successful, the patient will leave the hospital satisfied and content. If she leaves the hospital with a chronic, draining wound, however, neither she nor her surgeon will be happy for long.

MASTECTOMY FLAP NECROSIS

Mastectomy flap necrosis is completely different from TRAM flap necrosis because the volume of dead tissue is small and the underlying TRAM flap is well vascularized. Most cases of mastectomy flap necrosis heal satisfactorily with conservative or even no treatment (Fig. 38-15). Dead tissue should be debrided for hygiene and delayed primary repair performed if possible. If delayed closure is not possible, the wound should be allowed to heal secondarily. Often, the scar can be removed later as part of a breast revision. Split-thickness skin grafting should be avoided because it fixes the defect permanently (instead of allowing it to contract); additionally, texture and color match are poor. If skin grafting is required, a full-thickness graft is preferred.

FAT NECROSIS

The causes of fat necrosis are similar to those of partial flap loss, and prevention is essentially the same. The use of flaps (such as the free TRAM) with the best blood supply will re-

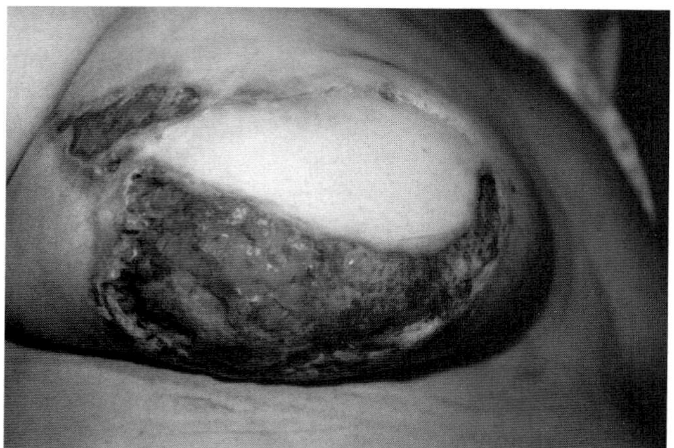
A

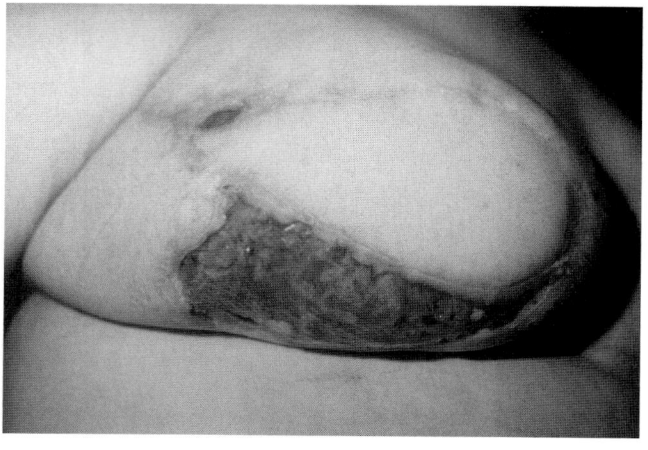
B

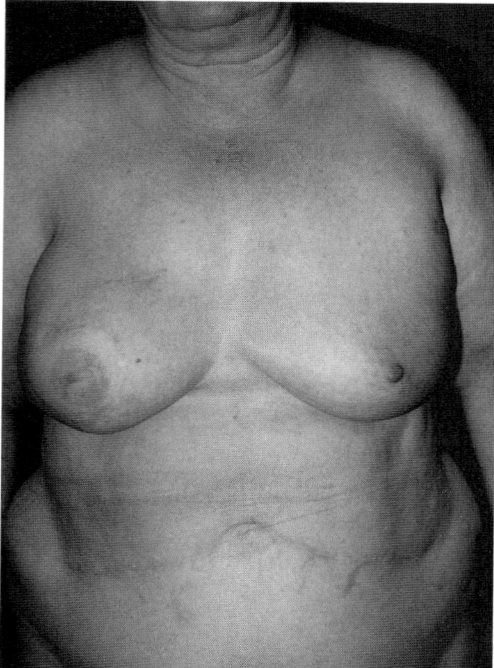
C

FIGURE 38-15. A: Patient with extensive mastectomy flap necrosis after immediate reconstruction with a free TRAM flap. **B:** Four weeks later, the wound is clean and granulating. **C:** After secondary healing and scar revision, the mastectomy flap necrosis has only minimally affected the final result.

duce the incidence of fat necrosis (11), as will careful patient selection. The treatment of fat necrosis, however, differs from that of partial flap loss because ordinarily the diagnosis is not made until several months after the operation, so that aggressive treatment is not possible.

Most cases of fat necrosis resolve spontaneously, with gradual softening of the scar tissue taking place over a period of many months. Needle biopsy may be required to allay fears of recurrent tumor, but usually reassurance and observation are all that is required. Exceptions to this rule arise when the necrotic area is very large (> 4 cm) or the necrosis fails to resolve, in which case the tissue should be excised. Necrotic fat should also be excised if the breast mound is too large and excision of the fat can be combined with breast reshaping to improve breast symmetry (Fig. 38-16). Infections, as always, should be treated with drainage and antibiotics.

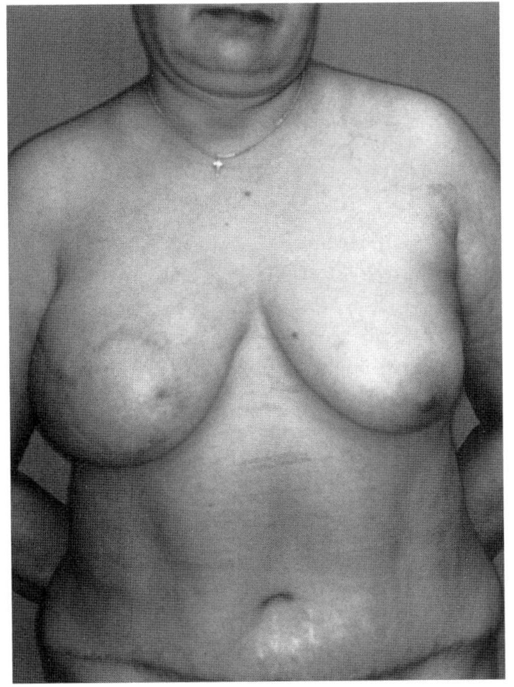
A

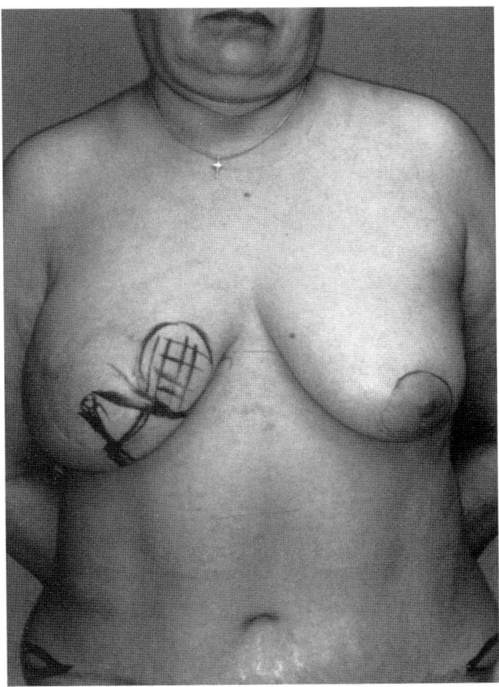
B

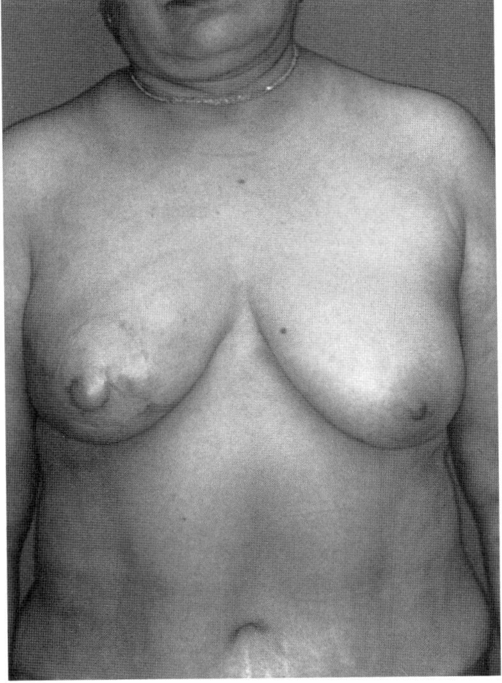
C

FIGURE 38-16. A: Patient with right breast mound reconstruction that is too large. An area of fat necrosis is present medially. **B:** Plan for excision of the fat necrosis *(cross-hatched circle)* and reduction of the breast mound. The part of the flap marked for reduction will be deepithelialized and rotated into the defect created by removal of the necrotic fat. Closer to the nipple, a wraparound flap was made out of excess skin and subcutaneous fat. **C:** Result of the revision, with improved breast symmetry and elimination of the area of fat necrosis.

UMBILICAL NECROSIS

Umbilical necrosis is common, especially in patients who use tobacco (12), but usually of little long-term consequence. Like fat necrosis, it generally heals spontaneously (Fig. 38-17). The usual treatment is drainage, frequent dressing changes, and reassurance. Unless an underlying synthetic mesh becomes infected and must be removed, umbilical necrosis usually resolves without additional surgery within a period of 2 months.

DIEP FLAPS

From the outside, TRAM and DIEP flaps are virtually indistinguishable. From the inside, however, they are quite different (18,19). Surgeons must keep these differences in mind if they are to avoid tissue loss and stay out of trouble (21). Although fewer perforators supply the DIEP flap, so that the blood supply is less robust, the arterial blood flow to the flap is nearly always adequate. It is the venous drainage that most often is inadequate. If, in elevating the flap, the surgeon finds an unusually large *superficial* inferior epigastric vein, the risk for venous insufficiency in the flap is increased (19). The presence of a large superficial vein should be taken as a warning of the possible presence of unusually small perforator veins. When I find a large superficial vein, I strongly consider converting the procedure to a standard free TRAM flap unless I find a large, visible vein in one of the flap perforators.

Even if the superficial inferior epigastric vein is of normal size, I like to find a perforator with a palpable pulse and a vein that I can see (wearing 4.5-magnification loupes) before I commit to performing a DIEP flap. If I cannot find at least one perforator that meets these two criteria (and usually I can), I abandon the plan to perform a DIEP flap and do a free TRAM flap instead.

When the DIEP flap is elevated, good loupe magnification and bipolar electrocautery are essential. Care must be taken to avoid traction on the perforators, which are fragile when dissected away from the protection of the enveloping muscle. I personally prefer to dissect the deep inferior epigastric vessels all the way down to their origins, in this way obtaining both a long pedicle (to help avoid tension) and large-caliber vessels (to make the anastomosis easier). Although the inexperienced DIEP flap surgeon may be tempted to include three or four perforators in every flap, this temptation should usually be resisted. Harvesting too many perforators adds excessive time to the procedure and also requires division of too many of the motor nerve branches that run between the perforators and must be cut to allow extraction of the flap. If only one or two perforators are harvested, few motor nerves need be divided. Moreover, if these divided motor nerves are sufficiently large, they can be repaired after the flap is harvested, so that ultimately all function of the rectus abdominis muscle is restored.

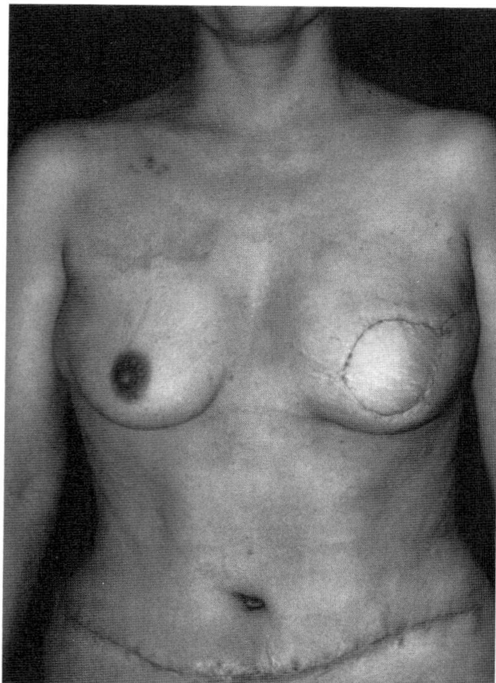
A

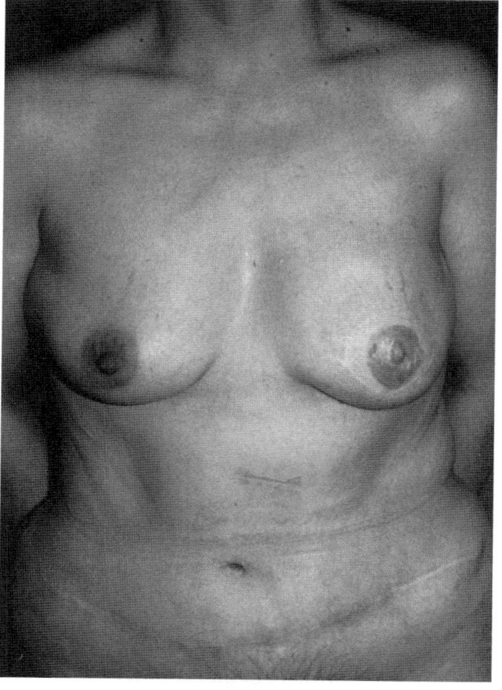
B

FIGURE 38-17. A: Patient with umbilical necrosis after pedicled TRAM flap reconstruction. **B:** Same patient after completion of the reconstruction. The umbilicus healed spontaneously, as is usually the case.

BREAST MALPOSITION

Although the conscientious surgeon always attempts to obtain breast symmetry in every operation, complete success is rarely achieved in the initial surgical procedure. Patients should be told preoperatively that at least one revision will almost certainly be necessary, even when the initial result is fairly good. If the initial result is aesthetically poor, the final result can sometimes still be quite good provided the revisions are successful. The surgeon should therefore not accept a poor result with autologous tissue without at least considering ways to improve the shape, position, and symmetry of the breast.

If the reconstructed breast is just too large, the excess can be sculpted away to leave a remaining breast of the desired size (Fig. 38-18). If the breast has excess tissue laterally but is missing tissue medially, however, the tissue can be shifted by means of an island V-to-Y flap technique (32) instead of merely sculpted away and discarded (Fig. 38-19). Although this approach adds scars to the breast, the improvement in shape is more important and justifies the additional scarring.

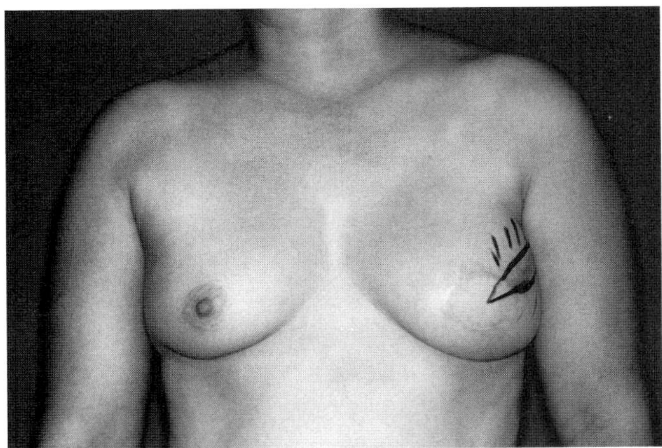
A

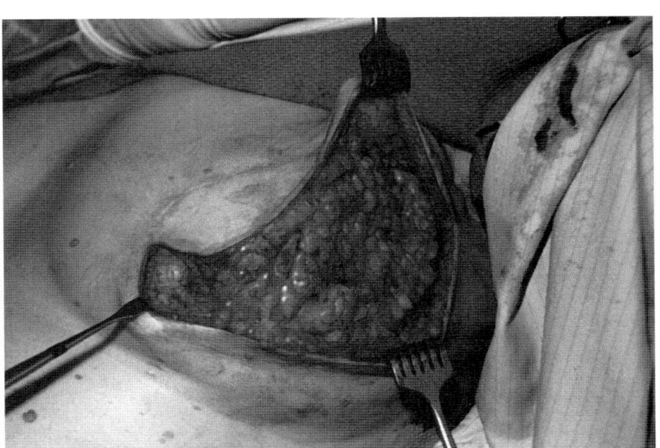
B

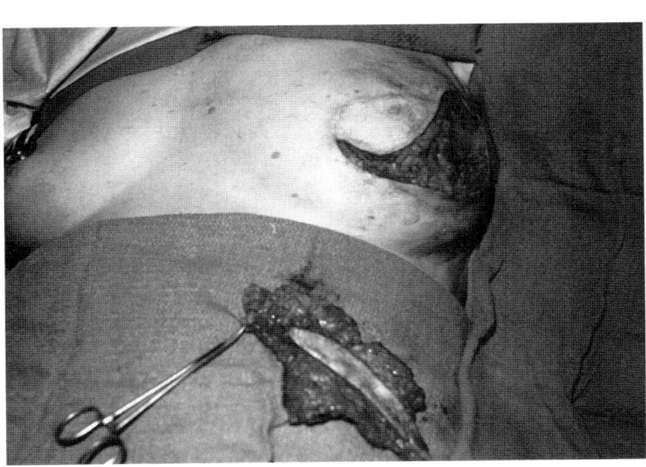
C

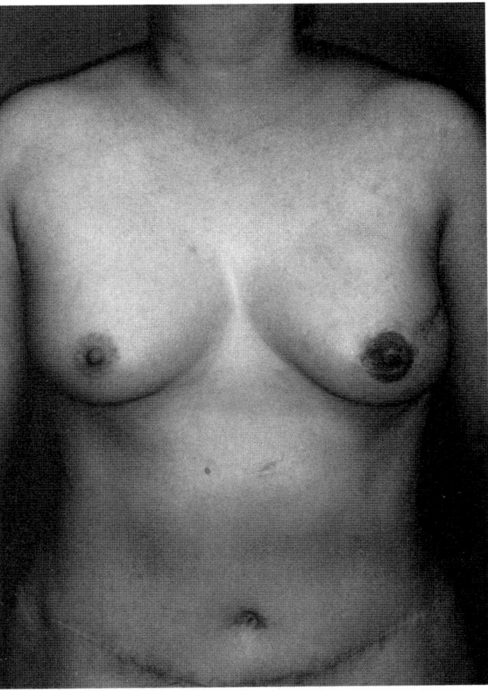
D

FIGURE 38-18. A: Patient with left reconstructed breast mound that is too large laterally. The plan for reduction, with removal of a small ellipse of skin and a wider area of underlying fat, is demonstrated. **B:** Mastectomy flaps were elevated superiorly and inferiorly to expose the lateral underlying breast. **C:** The removed specimen shows how tissue was sculpted widely away from the periphery of the mound, instead of just a wedge being excised. **D:** The result shows a smooth contour and no depressed scar. (From Kroll SS. *Breast reconstruction with autologous tissue: art and artistry.* New York: Springer-Verlag, 2000:296, with permission.)

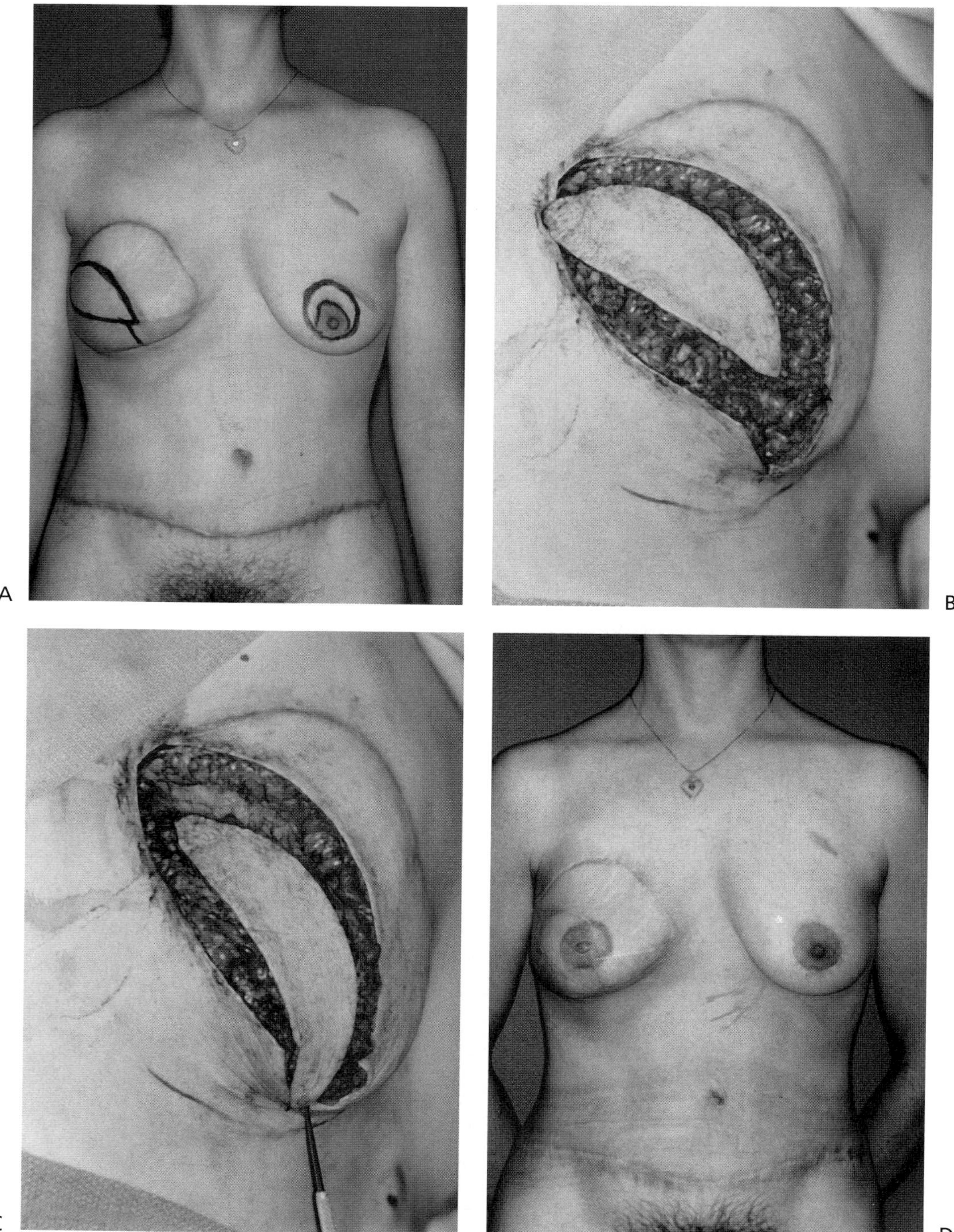

FIGURE 38-19. A: Patient after right breast mound reconstruction. Breast is too full superolaterally and deficient inferomedially. The plan for transfer of tissue from the upper, outer quadrant to the lower, inner quadrant with use of an island V-to-Y flap is depicted. **B:** The flap was elevated on a subcutaneous pedicle. **C:** With advancement of the flap inferiorly, the lower pole was augmented while the excess tissue superolaterally was reduced. **D:** The final result. A crescent mastopexy was also performed on the left breast. (From Kroll SS. *Breast reconstruction with autologous tissue: art and artistry.* New York: Springer-Verlag, 2000:302, with permission.)

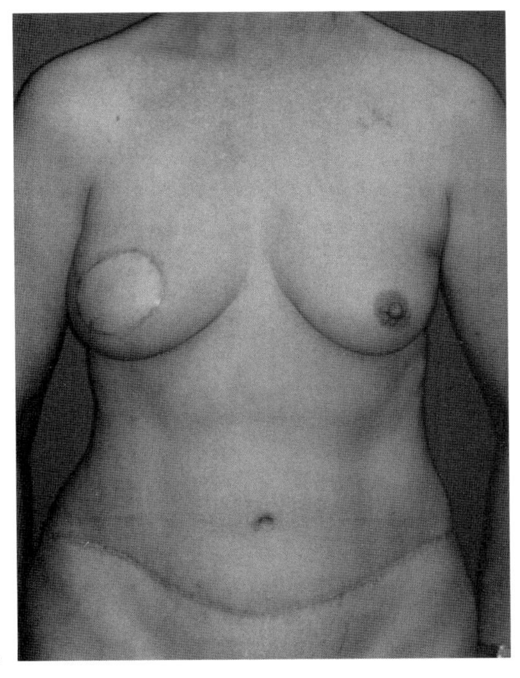

A

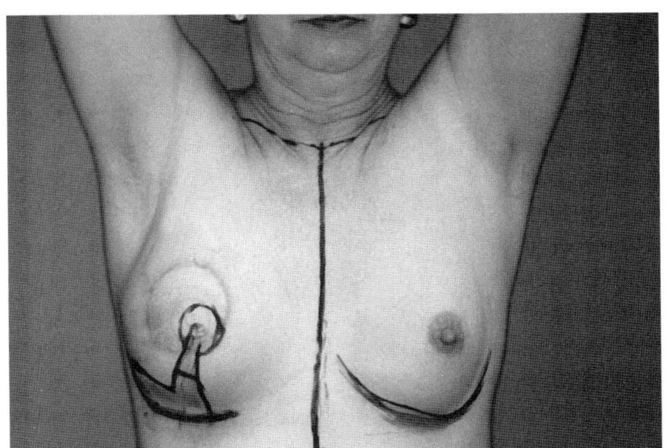

B

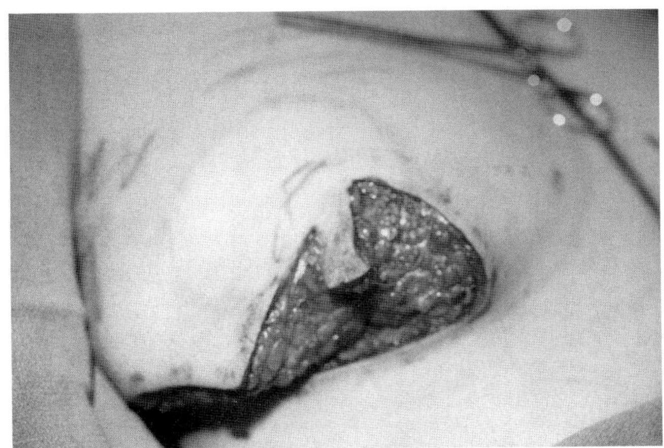

C

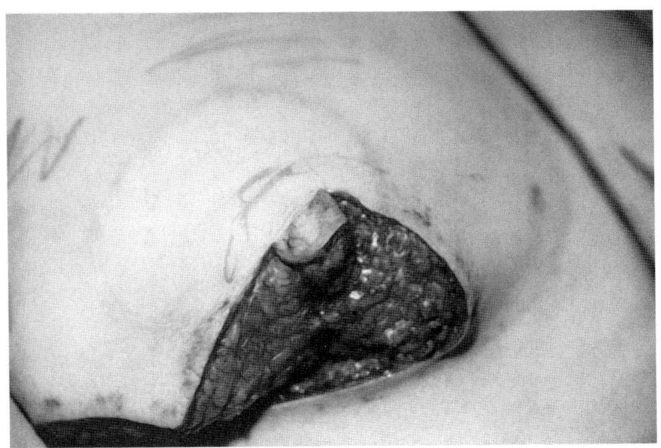

D

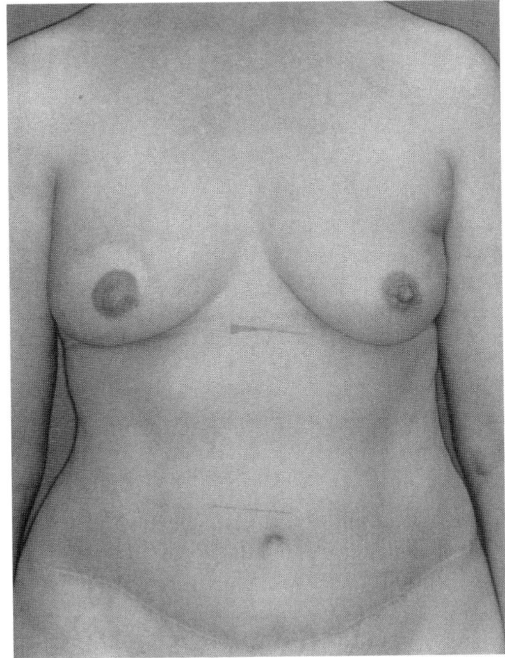

E

FIGURE 38-20. A: Patient with right reconstructed breast mound that is too large. **B:** Plan for revision with use of a J-shaped pattern of breast reduction. **C:** A superiorly based flap of skin and subcutaneous fat was created with tissue that would have been discarded. **D:** The flap was wrapped around on itself to create a nipple. **E:** Final result 1 year later. (From Kroll SS. Integrated breast mound reduction and nipple reconstruction with the wraparound flap. *Plast Reconstr Surg* 1999;104: 687–693, with permission.)

If the breast mound is too low, the inframammary fold can be lifted with reduction mammoplasty techniques. Excess skin can be wrapped around on itself to bank tissue for later use in reconstruction of the nipple (Fig. 38-20). In this way, nipple reconstruction can be accomplished without removal of tissue from the breast mound and subsequent flattening. At the same time, breast shape and projection can be improved by means of techniques similar to those employed in breast reduction and mastopexy (33).

A complete discussion of the revision of autologous tissue breasts is beyond the scope of this chapter, and readers are referred to other publications (32–34) and encouraged to use standard plastic surgical procedures in imaginative ways to improve the results of their reconstructions.

CONCLUSION

Autologous tissue breast reconstruction has the potential to provide excellent results, but it also can lead to severe complications. Fortunately, most of these complications can be prevented by careful patient selection, avoidance of excessive sacrifice of fascia, avoidance of unnecessarily wide undermining, and meticulous repair of the abdominal wall. Most other complications can be successfully managed or resolve spontaneously with time. When properly performed, autologous tissue breast reconstruction can be highly rewarding. No surgeon, however, no matter how good or how experienced, can avoid complications completely. Patients should therefore be informed preoperatively of the risks and indicate a willingness to accept them before the surgery is undertaken.

REFERENCES

1. Hartrampf CR Jr, Scheflan M, Black PW. Breast reconstruction with a transverse abdominal island flap. *Plast Reconstr Surg* 1982;69:216–224.
2. Grotting JC. Immediate breast reconstruction using the free TRAM flap. *Clin Plast Surg* 1994;21:207–221.
3. Hartrampf CR Jr, ed. *Breast reconstruction with living tissue.* New York: Raven Press, 1991.
4. Schusterman MA, Kroll SS, Miller, MJ, et al. The free TRAM flap for breast reconstruction: a single center's experience with 211 consecutive cases. *Ann Plast Surg* 1994;32:234–242.
5. Kroll SS, Baldwin BJ. A comparison of outcomes using three different methods of breast reconstruction. *Plast Reconstr Surg* 1992;90:455–462.
6. Shaw WW, Orringer JS, Ko CY, et al. The spontaneous return of sensibility in breasts reconstructed with autologous tissues. *Plast Reconstr Surg* 1997;99:394–399.
7. Hartrampf CR Jr. Closure of the donor defect for breast reconstruction with rectus abdominis myocutaneous flaps [Discussion]. *Plast Reconstr Surg* 1985;76:563.
8. Hartrampf CR Jr. Abdominal wall competence in transverse abdominal island flap operations. *Ann Plast Surg* 1984;12:139.
9. Mizgala CL, Hartrampf CR Jr, Bennett GK. Assessment of the abdominal wall after pedicled TRAM flap surgery: 5- to 7-year follow-up of 150 consecutive patients. *Plast Reconstr Surg* 1994;93:988–1002.
10. Kroll SS, Marchi M. Comparison of strategies for preventing abdominal-wall weakness after TRAM flap breast reconstruction. *Plast Reconstr Surg* 1992;89:1045–1053.
11. Kroll SS, Gherardini G, Martin JE, et al. Fat necrosis in free and pedicled TRAM flaps. *Plast Reconstr Surg* 1998;102:1502–1507.
12. Kroll SS. Necrosis of abdominoplasty and other secondary flaps after TRAM flap breast reconstruction. *Plast Reconstr Surg* 1994;94:637–643.
13. Hartrampf CR Jr, Bennett GK. Autogenous tissue reconstruction in the mastectomy patient: a critical review of 300 patients. *Ann Surg* 1987;205:508–518.
14. Beasley ME. In: Hartrampf CR, ed. *Breast reconstruction with living tissue.* New York: Raven Press, 1991:161–174.
15. Kroll SS, Netscher DT. Complications of TRAM flap breast reconstruction in obese patients. *Plast Reconstr Surg* 1989;86: 886–892.
16. McCraw JB, Papp C. In: Hartrampf CR Jr, ed. *Breast reconstruction with living tissue.* New York: Raven Press, 1991:211–250.
17. McCraw JB, Papp C, Edwards A, et al. The autogenous latissimus breast reconstruction. *Clin Plast Surg* 1994;21:279–288.
18. Blondeel PN. One hundred free DIEP flap breast reconstructions: a personal experience. *Br J Plast Surg* 1999;52:104–111.
19. Blondeel PN, Van Landuyt K, Monstrey SJ. Surgical-technical aspects of the free DIEP flap for breast reconstruction. *Operative Tech Plast Surg* 1999;6:27–37.
20. Allen RJ, Treece P. Deep inferior epigastric perforator flap for breast reconstruction. *Ann Plast Surg* 1994;32:32–38.
21. Kroll SS. Free TRAM or DIEP flap: which to choose? *Operative Tech Plast Surg* 1999;6:83–85.
22. Allen RJ, Tucker C Jr. Superior gluteal artery perforator free flap for breast reconstruction. *Plast Reconstr Surg* 1995;95: 1207–1212.
23. Blondeel PN. The sensate free superior gluteal artery perforator (S-GAP) flap: a valuable alternative in autologous breast reconstruction. *Br J Plast Surg* 1999;52:185–193.
24. Hartrampf CR Jr, Noel RT, Drazen L, et al. Ruben's fat pad for breast reconstruction: a peri-iliac soft-tissue free flap. *Plast Reconstr Surg* 1994;93:402–407.
25. Codner MA, Nahai F. The gluteal free flap breast reconstruction: making it work. *Clin Plast Surg* 1994;21:289–296.
26. Nahai F. Inferior gluteus maximus musculocutaneous flap for breast reconstruction. *Perspect Plast Surg* 1992;6:65.
27. Kroll SS, Schusterman MA, Mistry D. The internal oblique repair of abdominal bulges secondary to TRAM flap breast reconstruction. *Plast Reconstr Surg* 1995;96:100–104.
28. Beegle PH. In: Hartrampf CR, ed. *Breast reconstruction with living tissue.* New York: Raven Press, 1991:175–182.
29. Schusterman MA, Kroll SS, Weldon ME. Immediate breast reconstruction: why the free TRAM over the conventional TRAM flap? *Plast Reconstr Surg* 1992;90:255–262.
30. Grotting JC, Urist MM, Maddox WA, et al. Conventional TRAM flap versus free microsurgical TRAM flap for immediate breast reconstruction. *Plast Reconstr Surg* 1989;83:842–844.
31. Kroll SS. The early management of flap necrosis in breast reconstruction. *Plast Reconstr Surg* 1991;87:893–901.
32. Kroll SS. The V-to-Y island advancement flap for re-shaping of autologous tissue breast mound reconstructions. *Perspect Plast Surg* 1999.
33. Kroll SS. Integrated breast mound reduction and nipple reconstruction with the wraparound flap. *Plast Reconstr Surg* 1999;104:687–693.
34. Kroll SS. *Breast reconstruction with autologous tissue: art and artistry.* New York: Springer-Verlag, 1999.

Discussion

BREAST RECONSTRUCTION WITH AUTOLOGOUS TISSUE

JACK FISHER

Proper planning and careful patient selection are essential in minimizing the possibility of an unfavorable result in autogenous breast reconstruction. Often, a failed reconstruction does not represent a failure in surgical technique, but rather a failure to select the correct operation for the individual patient. This premise is reiterated when Dr. Kroll states, "One of the most important ways to minimize complications is careful patient selection." Although this statement seems obvious, it is a fundamental issue in reconstructive surgery.

PATIENT SELECTION

In general, I agree with the author that autologous reconstructions tend to require less revisionary surgery, on a long-term basis, than reconstructions based on implants and tissue expanders. However, some of this disparity is not necessarily related to the procedures themselves, but to poor patient selection (1). Higher revision rates in implant-based reconstructions may be a consequence of selecting patients who would have been better candidates for autologous reconstruction as the primary procedure (Fig. 38D-1).

The author points out that breast reconstruction with autologous tissue is a demanding procedure. This is true, but creating an excellent result with an implant-based reconstruction can at times be still more difficult; the use of an implant limits the ways in which the breast mound can be shaped, whereas a breast made of autologous tissue can readily be shaped. As the author describes in his case reports, in several patients, significant improvements were achieved by adjusting the autologous reconstruction through either volume manipulation or skin envelope reduction. Attempts at modification can be more difficult with an implant-based reconstruction. So, as the author points out, although autologous breast reconstruction is associated with greater potential morbidity at the donor site, it may allow more latitude in secondary revisions. First, if the volume is too great, it is relatively easy to reduce most autologous reconstructions. Second, the inframammary fold and skin envelope are more easily readjusted (Fig. 38D-2). Obviously, if the volume or amount of skin is inadequate after autologous reconstruction, then either an implant or other autologous tissue may be required.

As our experience in procedures such as the transverse rectus abdominis myocutaneous (TRAM) flap has increased, we are better able to identify the high-risk patient, especially the patient who is obese. Initially, it was felt that the more fat, the better, until it became apparent that this is true only up to a point. The presence of too much adipose tissue in the lower abdomen can be detrimental, leading to fat necrosis and skin loss. As the author appropriately points out, obese patients are a major source of TRAM flap failures. Carefully evaluating the obese patient can dramatically reduce complications that might require later revisions. The problem then is to define those patients who, because of their weight, are poor candidates.

Another factor that must be taken into consideration, besides the patient's weight, is the contour of the abdomen, specifically the shape or laxity of the abdominal panniculus. A patient who is not excessively obese may, because of a hanging panniculus, be a poor candidate for TRAM flap breast reconstruction. The reason is that the hanging panniculus distracts or distorts the musculocutaneous perforators exiting the fascia, so that identification of the appropriate skin territory is difficult, if not impossible (Fig. 38D-3). It is important to examine these patients in a standing position to determine the relationship of the overlying abdominal skin to the periumbilical or dominant vascular perforators.

I agree with the author that if a patient is obese or unable to lose weight, it is much safer to consider a latissimus dorsi flap breast reconstruction. I also agree with the author that patients who smoke are not good candidates for pedicled TRAM flaps because of their higher rate of complications related to loss of the transferred tissue. However, the author feels that a free TRAM flap is a safer procedure in smokers, and he may be correct in regard to the tissue transferred to the chest. In my experience, complications in smokers are more likely to be related to the abdominal wall donor site—skin necrosis and delayed healing secondary to ischemia.

J. Fisher: Department of Plastic Surgery, Vanderbilt University; Department of Plastic Surgery, Baptist Hospital; Nashville Plastic Surgery, Nashville, Tennessee

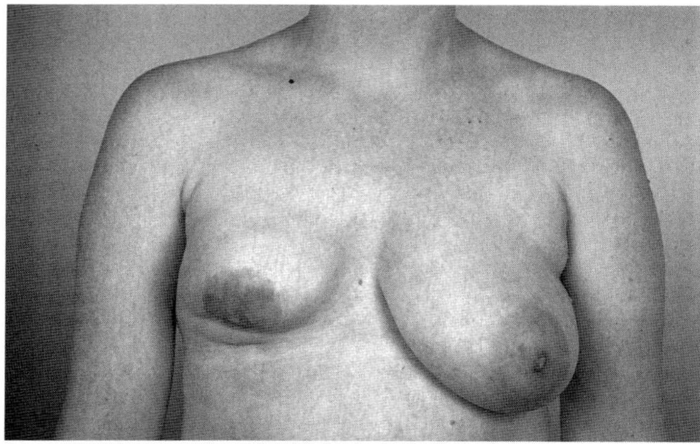

A

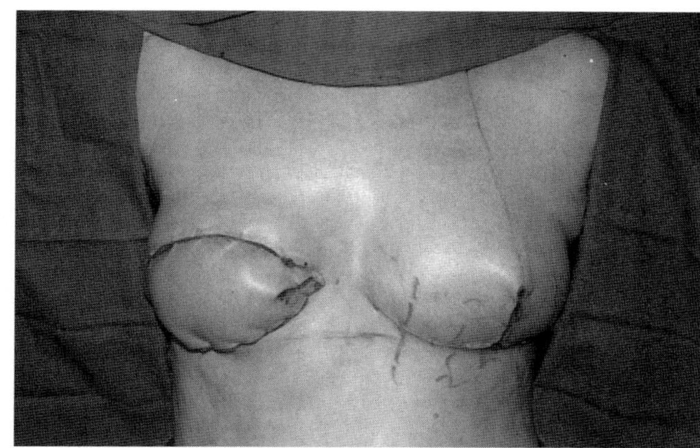

B

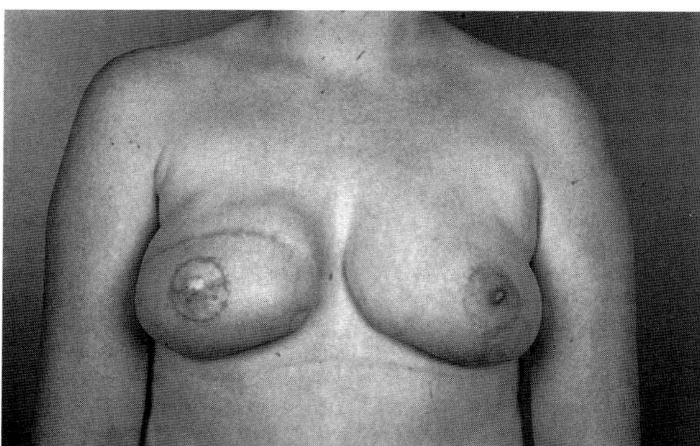

C

FIGURE 38D-1. A: This 30-year-old patient had previously undergone reconstruction with an implant. It was not possible to achieve symmetry with an implant because of inadequate soft tissue and a large contralateral breast. **B:** A pedicled TRAM flap was created, with reduction on the contralateral side. The previous nipple-areolar reconstruction was removed. **C:** Final result after new nipple-areolar reconstruction.

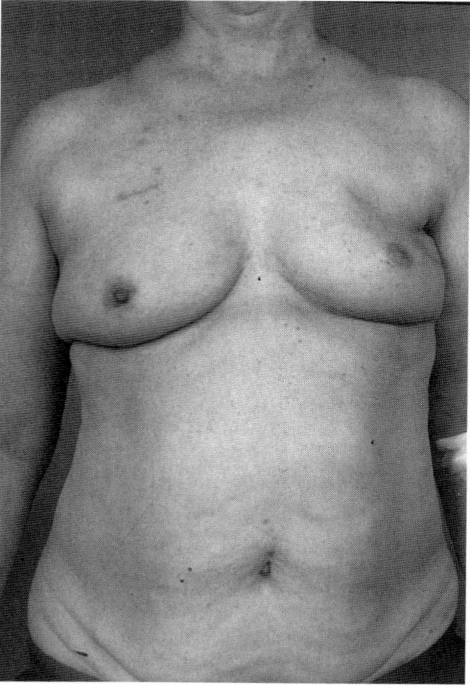

A

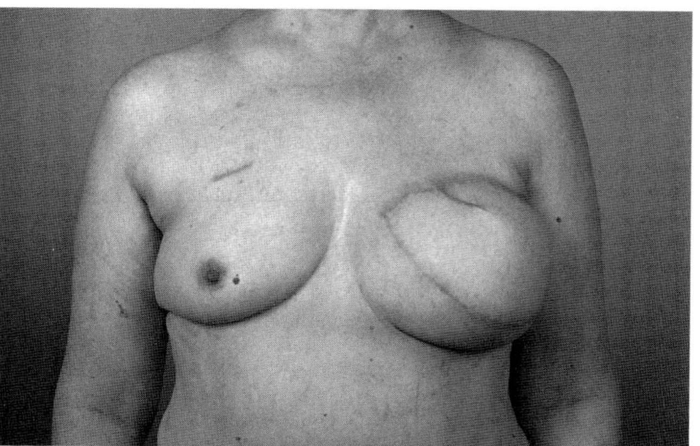

B

FIGURE 38D-2. A: This patient had previously undergone a lumpectomy and radiation treatment. The breast was reconstructed with a double-pedicled TRAM flap. **B:** The inframammary fold is too low and the volume of the reconstruction too great. (*continued*)

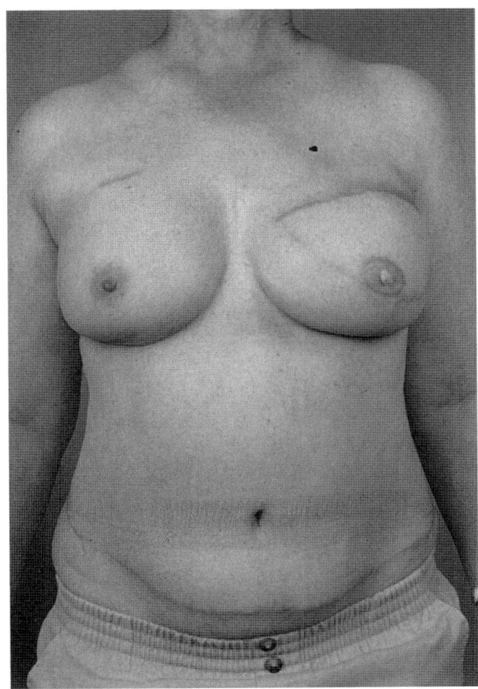

C

FIGURE 38D-2. *Continued.* **C:** With volume reduction of the flap and elevation of the fold, a satisfactory result is obtained. This case demonstrates that it is possible to sculpt or reshape a TRAM flap and modify a misplaced inframammary fold (From Fisher J, Greenberg L. Secondary revision of unsatisfactory breast reconstruction. *Perspect Plast Surg* 2001;14:92, in press).

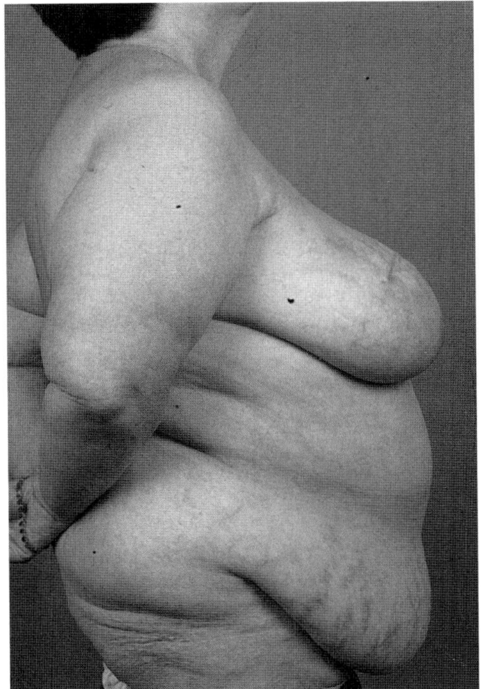

A

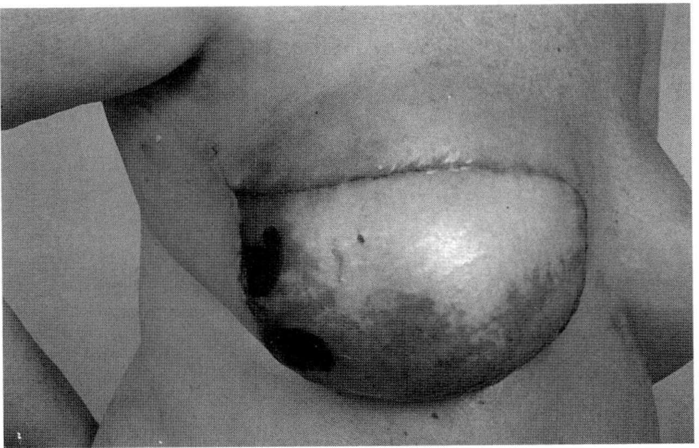

B

FIGURE 38D-3. A: Patient who is a poor candidate for a TRAM flap because of a hanging panniculus, which makes identification of the proper skin territory difficult. **B:** Patient with a single-pedicled TRAM reconstruction in which a hanging panniculus led to incorrect identification of the skin island and subsequent partial flap loss.

One could make the argument that a free flap requires less elevation of the abdominal wall panniculus, so that this potential complication is reduced. The author believes that because a free-tissue transfer can be performed with limited abdominal wall mobilization and without the need for a tunnel, this risk is reduced in a patient who smokes. Abdominal wall problems are probably now of greater significance, on a long-term basis, than any other issue in TRAM reconstructions, whether the flap is placed by microsurgery or as a pedicle.

Finally, in regard to patient selection, Dr. Kroll appropriately points out that some patients may not be candidates at all for a breast reconstruction, and this possibility must be carefully considered, especially when complex cases with multiple comorbidities are assessed.

FLAP SELECTION

Dr. Kroll prefers the free TRAM flap to the pedicled TRAM flap, stating that it has a better blood supply and requires the sacrifice of less muscle. Although this statement may be true in a broad sense, my preference is to use the pedicled TRAM flap. Provided that patients are selected properly and the pedicled TRAM flap is used appropriately, I feel that use of the free TRAM flap offers no specific benefit (2). I do not believe that blood supply is a factor so long as the pedicled TRAM flap is used appropriately and conservatively. It is important that zone 1 be the major source of tissue when pedicled TRAM flaps are created because this is the best-vascularized territory. The assumption that one can perform a pedicled TRAM flap aggressively and cross the midline with a single pedicle or take the entire lateral tissue is mistaken. I agree with the author that the perfusion rate is higher in a free TRAM flap, and that if one crosses the midline or uses the extreme lateral portion, blood flow and viability are greater. So the issue is really not one of which is better or worse, free flap or pedicled flap, but of how to use each safely and appropriately. In regard to donor site morbidity, my personal experience is that with careful muscle dissection and muscle sparing, a pedicled flap has an excellent closure.

The author points out that a team is required to perform numerous free-tissue transfers reliably, and that the pedicle procedure may be more appropriate for some practices than for others. At our institution, where we have no aversion to microsurgery, we prefer the pedicled TRAM flap in most cases. The free-tissue transfer is reserved for patients in whom, because of prior procedures (specifically, subcostal or other abdominal incisions), a pedicled TRAM flap would not be appropriate.

Another important issue is abdominal wall complications. As Dr. Kroll points out, the patient who undergoes a successful reconstruction with a TRAM flap that is followed by an abdominal wall complication does not necessarily view the reconstruction as successful, especially if secondary surgery is required. I have discovered two ways in which to improve abdominal wall contour and reduce morbidity at the abdominal wall donor site. The author mentions the first, and the one I consider most important—that the internal oblique fascia must be included in the abdominal wall repair. It is easy to miss this layer during the surgical closure. The other issue, more subtle, relates to TRAM flaps with a single pedicle. When TRAM flaps first became popular in the early 1980s, they were primarily single-pedicled flaps. After several years of follow-up, it became apparent that bulges had developed in many of the patients with single-pedicled TRAM flaps, not on the side where the procedure had been performed, but on the opposite side. It became apparent that a good fascial closure of the donor site with time placed stress on the contralateral fascial tissues of the lower abdomen. These bulges were not hernias but attenuations of the contralateral fascia. Once this problem was recognized, it was found that imbrication or plication of the contralateral anterior rectus sheath, in conjunction with a good repair of the donor site fascia, reduced the later development of bulges. The author gives a good description of how to repair abdominal wall weakness, depending on etiology, which need not to be repeated here.

I am inclined to disagree with the author's abandonment of the double-pedicled TRAM flap to reconstruct a single breast. Each of us must identify the techniques that yield the best and safest results. In our practice, the double-pedicled TRAM flap is an excellent procedure when more tissue is required for a satisfactory breast reconstruction (Fig. 38D-4). I feel that with proper attention to detail, good fascial abdominal closure, and possibly the use of overlying mesh, the rate of complications at the abdominal donor site in these patients is insignificant. On the other hand, I do agree with Dr. Kroll, in general, that the less tissue sacrificed from the abdomen, the better.

The author describes causes of flap failure, both complete and partial. He states that partial flap loss is greater in pedicled than in free TRAM flaps. Again, the key here is appropriate patient selection and proper execution of the procedure. The single pedicled flap skin must be used without significant deviation across the midline or excessive use of lateral tissues. When these two situations are avoided, I believe the incidence of partial flap loss or fat necrosis is no greater than in a free-tissue transfer. Again, if one wants a large skin island with a single-pedicled blood supply, the free TRAM flap does offer this advantage. It is how the flaps are used, both free and pedicled, that determines the complication rates.

Other problems discussed include umbilical necrosis. I agree with the author that this condition should be treated very conservatively because in most instances it heals with a very acceptable result. This complication can occur in either free or pedicled TRAM flaps.

One of the major benefits of the TRAM reconstruction, free or pedicled, is that it allows one to revise the results of

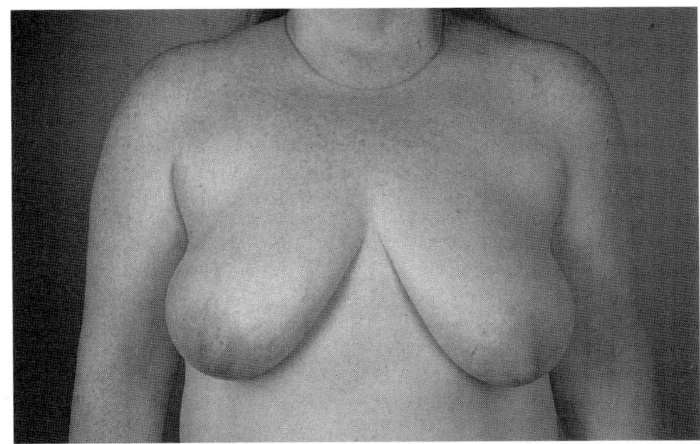

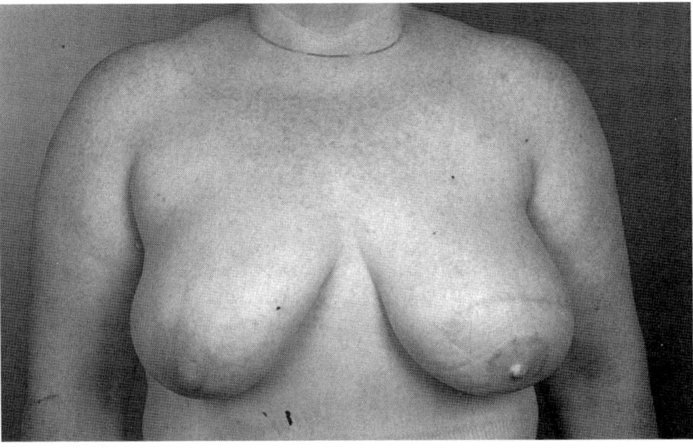

FIGURE 38D-4. A: Preoperative appearance of a patient with a cancer of the left breast. **B:** Patient underwent immediate reconstruction with a double-pedicled TRAM flap. Patient wanted symmetry without a reduction of the remaining breast. A double-pedicled TRAM flap was required to create a symmetrical volume.

the initial operation when the breast mound is less than satisfactory. The autologous reconstruction is like a sculptor's block of clay or granite. A mediocre result can frequently be transformed into an excellent one in a simple secondary procedure. Frequently, the difference between a mediocre and an excellent result is related to the inframammary fold. Creating a fold secondarily can significantly improve the final result. Techniques such as liposuction can be used to adjust the volume and contour of the TRAM flap reconstruction, but they are of limited use in a patient with an implant-based reconstruction.

The author addresses issues related to the sculpting of TRAM flaps. As he points out, the technique is not within the scope of this presentation, but it can be of great benefit in this form of reconstruction.

CONCLUSION

In general, a patient does not care whether an autologous flap transferred for breast reconstruction is free or pedicled. What the patient does care about is what the final breast reconstruction looks like, and whether complications have developed. Dr. Kroll addresses these issues appropriately and makes excellent suggestions regarding how to reduce and correct problems. Surgeons have their own biases and specific ways of performing surgery. The basic principles, however, are always the same— proper patient selection, proper execution of the procedure, and appropriate management of problems when they do occur. In autologous breast reconstruction, the critical portion of the operation is not moving the tissue to the recipient site; rather, it is shaping and contouring the tissue to provide the best result possible for the patient.

REFERENCES

1. Fisher J, Greenberg L. Secondary revision of unsatisfactory breast reconstruction. *Perspect Plast Surg* 2001;14:92 *(in press).*
2. Clungston PA, Gingrass MK, Azurin D, et al. Ipsilateral pedicled TRAM flaps: the safer alternative? *Plast Reconstr Surg* 2000;105:77–82.

39

NIPPLE AND AREOLA RECONSTRUCTION

L. FRANKLYN ELLIOTT

Reconstruction of the nipple and areola continues to be significant in breast reconstruction. The nipple and areola complex completes the breast reconstruction and breast unit in most patients' minds. In some cases with a poor or modest breast mound result, the patient will nonetheless be satisfied with the overall result if a natural nipple and areola complex has been created. It is important, therefore, to understand the seminal importance of nipple and areola reconstruction, and the litany of options that have been suggested over the years to accomplish it. In the earlier decades of breast reconstruction, the nipple and areola were not emphasized as they are today. Breast reconstruction techniques were less than optimal, aesthetic results of nipple and areola reconstruction were modest, and scars were created during the process of reconstruction. However, as both autogenous tissue and implant techniques have improved, the breast mound is made to resemble the opposite side much more closely, and in the case of bilateral reconstruction, the appearance of both mounds is much more natural (Fig. 39-1). For this reason, we tend to be more critical now of the results of nipple and areola reconstruction. Fortunately, the techniques for this procedure have also improved, so that the operation have been simplified and the results are more natural (1).

In an earlier era of nipple and areola reconstruction, tissues were taken from the opposite breast or other parts of the body. Tissue was obtained from the areola of the opposite breast in the case of a large areola or breast reduction. Although this technique can be successful, the indications for using it are limited. When tissues are taken from a nipple of adequate vertical height or adequate horizontal width, very natural results can be produced. These techniques continue to be quite satisfactory in patients who have enough tissue to donate. However, with the availability of modern techniques that do not require grafts, the sharing of tissues from the opposite breast is increasingly questionable in view of the scarring and possible change in sensibility that result.

L. F. Elliott: Atlanta Plastic Surgery; and Department of Plastic Surgery, Emory University, Atlanta, Georgia.

In another chapter in the history of nipple and areola reconstruction, grafts of various sorts were obtained from distant sites on the body. Nipple reconstruction was performed with tissue from distant sites, such as the earlobes, elbows, toes, and labia. The most popular tissues for areolar reconstruction have been labial and perilabial tissues, and also the upper inner thigh. Again, the use of these sites creates scars, and patients are often frightened when the techniques are explained to them. The color, particularly of the areola grafts, cannot be controlled, and pigmentation is often darker than on the opposite side. This is a very difficult situation to correct, and the discrepancy must almost always be corrected by tattooing the opposite side. In addition, the nipple grafts are composite grafts of both skin and fat from the locations mentioned above, and therefore they must receive vascularization from the underlying bed.

The poor "take" of these grafts is well-known in fundamental plastic surgery. Projection and width are limited when these techniques are used, with projections of less than 0.5 cm being common. Over and over again, patients are obviously relieved when they are told that tissue from remote sites will not used to achieve an acceptable and natural nipple and areola reconstruction.

Storage of the nipple and areola has been suggested in the past as an appropriate reconstructive technique. The nipple and areola complex is removed at the time of mastectomy and stored as a graft on some remote, less obvious location. Once the breast reconstruction has been completed, the nipple and areola complex can then be transferred, as a full-thickness graft, back to the appropriate site on the breast mound. Of concern when this technique is used is the possibility of transferring malignant cells, both to the temporary host site and to the breast mound itself. Furthermore, maintenance of projection of the nipple is very unreliable when two transfers are used, as required in this technique. For these reasons, nipple and areola preservation and transfer have fallen out of favor, especially in view of the introduction of local fat flaps and tattooing (2).

The timing of nipple and areola reconstruction remains somewhat controversial. Some surgeons advocate immedi-

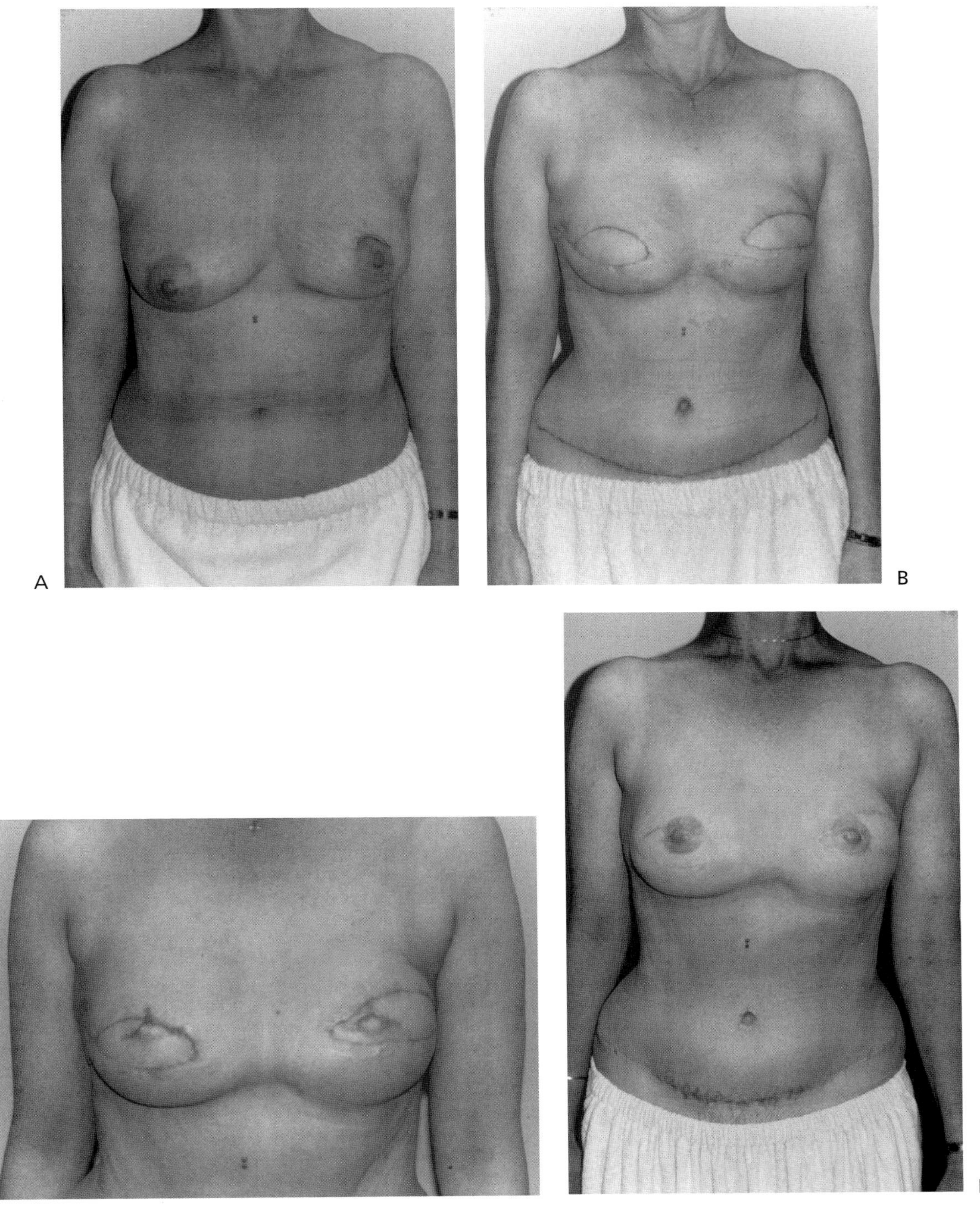

FIGURE 39-1. A 45-year-old patient underwent bilateral mastectomy and bilateral pedicled TRAM flap reconstruction. **A:** Preoperative view. **B:** Four months postoperatively. **C:** One month after bilateral nipple reconstruction. **D.** One year after nipple reconstruction and 10 months after tattooing.

ate nipple and areola reconstruction at the time of autogenous tissue breast reconstruction. Although few surgeons advocate this technique in the instance of a pedicled transverse rectus abdominis myocutaneous (TRAM) flap, it may be reasonable to use it with a free TRAM flap. This is because the free TRAM flap is immediately well vascularized, and perfusion is generally complete from the time of vascular connection. The pedicled TRAM flap, on the other hand, passes through various stages during the first 24 hours as venous outflow adjusts to the reverse flow situation.

Even though immediate nipple and areola complex reconstruction is possible, it should generally be avoided. Positioning the nipple and areola complex on a newly formed breast mound is less reliable than positioning it in the delayed setting. After 2 to 3 months of healing, settling, and resolution of edema and possibly seroma, the breast mound assumes its final position, and a nipple and areola site can be chosen more accurately. Furthermore, a second operation, albeit small, gives the surgeon an opportunity to "tune up" the breast mound and donor site. For these reasons, secondary nipple and areola reconstruction is preferred in most patients.

The patient who has undergone implant/expander breast reconstruction is not a candidate for immediate nipple and areola reconstruction. In this situation, all dimensions of the breast mound change during expansion and in the secondary procedure, in which expanders are exchanged for permanent implants and capsulotomies are performed. Thus, for a patient with an implant/expander reconstruction, nipple and areola reconstruction is carried out at the second operation, or even at a third operation, which would be performed for nipple and areola reconstruction only.

The position of the nipple and areola reconstruction on the breast mound is of paramount importance (3). In the case of symmetrical breast mounds, positioning the reconstruction is relatively straightforward. The location is chosen by measuring from the midline and from the sternal notch to the normal side and then to the reconstructed side. In the case of a bilateral reconstruction with symmetrical breasts, a site at the intersection of the vertical and horizontal meridians of one breast is chosen and transposed to the opposite side. If the breasts are asymmetrical, as when a reconstructed breast is elevated in comparison with a more ptotic, unoperated opposite breast, the choice of position is somewhat problematic. In general, however, it is wise to choose a site for the nipple and areola complex that is appropriate for the breast on which it is being placed. In the case of a ptotic opposite breast, the breast is lifted to a position of symmetry with a brassiere to create symmetry of the breast mounds and the nipple and areola positions while the patient is dressed. It is not appropriate to place the nipple and areola complex more inferiorly on an asymmetrical reconstructed breast mound in an effort to "balance" it with that of the opposite ptotic breast. This option creates symmetry of the nipple and areola complex in the vertical and horizontal planes, but the position is not natural on the reconstructed side relative to the breast mound and does not work as well when a brassiere is worn. Of course, the best option is to elevate the opposite breast, provided the patient consents to this operation. Then, symmetry of both the nipple and areola complexes and the breast mounds can be achieved.

Unfavorable results with nipple and areola reconstruction can be caused by the position of the nipple and areola alone. Sometimes, these cannot be avoided and must be accepted by both patient and surgeon if the patient will not consent to an additional procedure. On the other hand, perfectly reasonable results can be achieved even without symmetry if the proper position of the nipple and areola is chosen on the reconstructed breast, even though it may not match the opposite breast in terms of shape and ptosis. This must be explained in detail to patients preoperatively. They will either acquiesce to a procedure on the opposite breast or accept the asymmetry as a natural result.

Normal areolar tissue is often irregular, discoid, or asymmetric. A careful analysis of the dimensions preoperatively is critical to achieving the most symmetrical and natural result. Graft techniques have been successful in achieving symmetry, but the results are not easily revised and are characterized by scar at the periphery. Tattoo techniques for areolar reconstruction, on the other hand, can be easily revised in the outpatient setting, both in shape and color.

CURRENT TECHNIQUE

A modification of the star flap, popularized by Hartrampf, is my first choice for nipple and areola reconstruction, both in autogenous tissue breast reconstructions and in expander/implant breast reconstructions (Fig. 39-2A–G). It is not surprising that we have moved from grafts to flaps in nipple and areola complex reconstruction, as we have in so many other areas.

The site of the nipple and areola reconstruction is chosen preoperatively with the patient in a sitting position, as described above. The base of the flap is the exact spot at which the nipple will be located when this technique is used. A taller nipple can be achieved by making the central flap longer, and a wider nipple can be achieved by widening the central flap. Both lateral flaps are drawn in a linear curve pattern and are elevated as partial-thickness flaps to the border of the central flap. The central flap contains both underlying fat and, distally, split-thickness skin in a pointed pattern (Fig. 39-2C,D). Once each lateral flap is elevated to the border of the central flap, a deep cut is made through the underlying dermis and fat to recruit an appropriate amount of fat for elevation with the central flap. This deep incision is continued superiorly after the pointed portion of the flap is elevated as a partial-thickness flap. Thus, a three-sided incision through the dermis and underlying fat is made to free the desired amount of underlying fat for the subsequent nipple reconstruction.

The amount of fat to be recruited for the nipple reconstruction is generally about twice as much as one expects to have 1 year later. Thus, the reconstructed nipple is initially twice as large as one expects it to be once final healing occurs. The recruitment of adequate amounts of fat is not a problem, though, when autogenous tissue has been used for the breast reconstruction.

On the other hand, in the case of an implant/expander

breast reconstruction, the tissues beneath the skin consist only of dermis and a very small amount of fat, muscle, and capsule between the skin surface and the underlying implant. The height and width of the reconstructed nipple and areola in this instance are limited. However, additional volume can be recruited by designing all the flaps to include underlying fat and muscle down to the capsule of the underlying implant. Therefore, the bilateral side flaps and the pointed central flap are elevated with underlying fat and muscle. In this manner, additional bulk is recruited for the nipple reconstruction, even when implants have been used.

Once the flaps have been elevated, bleeding is carefully controlled with a needlepoint cautery to reduce damage to adjacent fat. Hematomas, even small ones, will cause subsequent necrosis and loss of nipple height.

While the nipple flap is held out with a single hook (Fig. 39-2E,F), the donor sites are closed to avoid a breast defect in those areas and to lock the nipple flap in an uplifted, projected position. The closures are made with a 3-0 polyglycolic acid suture; the most important sutures are at the base of the nipple flap. Once the sutures have been placed, the nipple flap is maintained in the appropriate position by the sutures alone.

The flap is usually designed to be based inferiorly so that the force of gravity on the flap will maintain it into an erect and elevated position. Superiorly based flaps may be chosen, however, because of scar patterns, but gravity may cause them to tip inferiorly over time.

Once the flap is elevated and the donor sites closed, the bilateral flaps can be sutured to each other along the superior border of the nipple flap with 4-0 polyglycolic acid sutures (Fig. 39-2G,H). The suture at the base of the flap is also tied to the underlying skin closure. Finally, the pointed flap is sutured down to form the nipple tip with a 5-0 catgut suture.

After the nipple reconstruction has been completed, the dressing, which plays a very important functional role, is applied. The nipple is bathed in antibiotic ointment and then covered with a petrolatum gauze. Finally, this inner component is surrounded with gauze pads from which holes are cut out in the center and stacked to the height of the nipple. The dressing is then covered with Medpor tape. We leave the dressings on for 5 to 7 days. Once the dressings are removed, the patient is taught how to apply 4 × 4-in gauze pads with holes cut out of the center, supported by either light tape or a brassiere, for another 2 weeks. Areola reconstruction is performed 2 to 3 months after nipple reconstruction. This allows adequate time for the scars created by the star flap to mature, and for the nipple itself to shrink through scarring. Scarring is an impediment to intradermal tattooing because of the relatively unpredictable retention of instilled pigment in scar tissue. Thus, tattooing is not performed immediately in this method of nipple reconstruction.

Tattooing itself is a simple process in most cases, requiring an outpatient visit of less than 1 hour (4). Occasionally, instillation of a local anesthetic is necessary, especially in patients whose breast reconstruction has been performed more than 3 to 4 months earlier. However, in most cases, the degree of insensibility is sufficient that the tattooing can be performed without any anesthesia.

An intradermal tattooing machine is used, with the pigments chosen carefully to match the opposite side or, in bilateral cases, according to the patient's preference. In general, more pigmentation is added than is necessary because the color of the tattoo will lighten in essentially every case. The blood supply of scar tissue differs from that of normal skin and tissue, so the uptake of dye is not predictable. On the other hand, subsequent tattooing is certainly not difficult. Secondary tattooing procedures can be undertaken as desired by the patient.

Suboptimal results in nipple and areola reconstruction are multifactorial in origin. When a nipple is reconstructed on an autogenous tissue breast mound, nipple height can be lost because of inadequate vascularity of the nipple flap. Scars in the area of the proposed nipple and areola complex reconstruction will affect the planning and orientation of the star flap. Obviously, a scar that represents a deep incision across the base of a planned star flap will result in either failure or inadequate height of the flap. Scars that are not situated across the base but in the footprint of the design may affect the viability of the underlying fat component, and shifting the axis of the design may be warranted. The skin components of the flaps are usually safe even if scarring is present because they are essentially split-thickness grafts.

How the underlying fat on the central flap is handled is very important. Trauma or electrocauterization will diminish the vascularization of the fat and result in significant postoperative atrophy. Therefore, hemostasis must be achieved, but not at the cost of significant fat injury. The precise use of needlepoint cautery is helpful in avoiding this problem.

Occasionally, it is necessary to place an implant behind a TRAM flap to achieve symmetry. This is usually done at a secondary operation, not at the time of primary autogenous tissue transfer. Our experience indicates that reconstruction of the nipple and areola at the time of placement of an implant places undue stress on the nipple flap because the entire autogenous tissue mound has been elevated to create a pocket for the implant. Although the autogenous tissue may be perfectly viable, elevating it from the chest wall and creating a superficial flap are too much for one operation. This practice generally results in an inadequate nipple height and should be avoided.

The nipple reconstruction should be delayed if revisions of the reconstructed breast, either with liposuction or incisions, are necessary near the proposed nipple site. On the other hand, deep liposuction or revisions in remote sites of

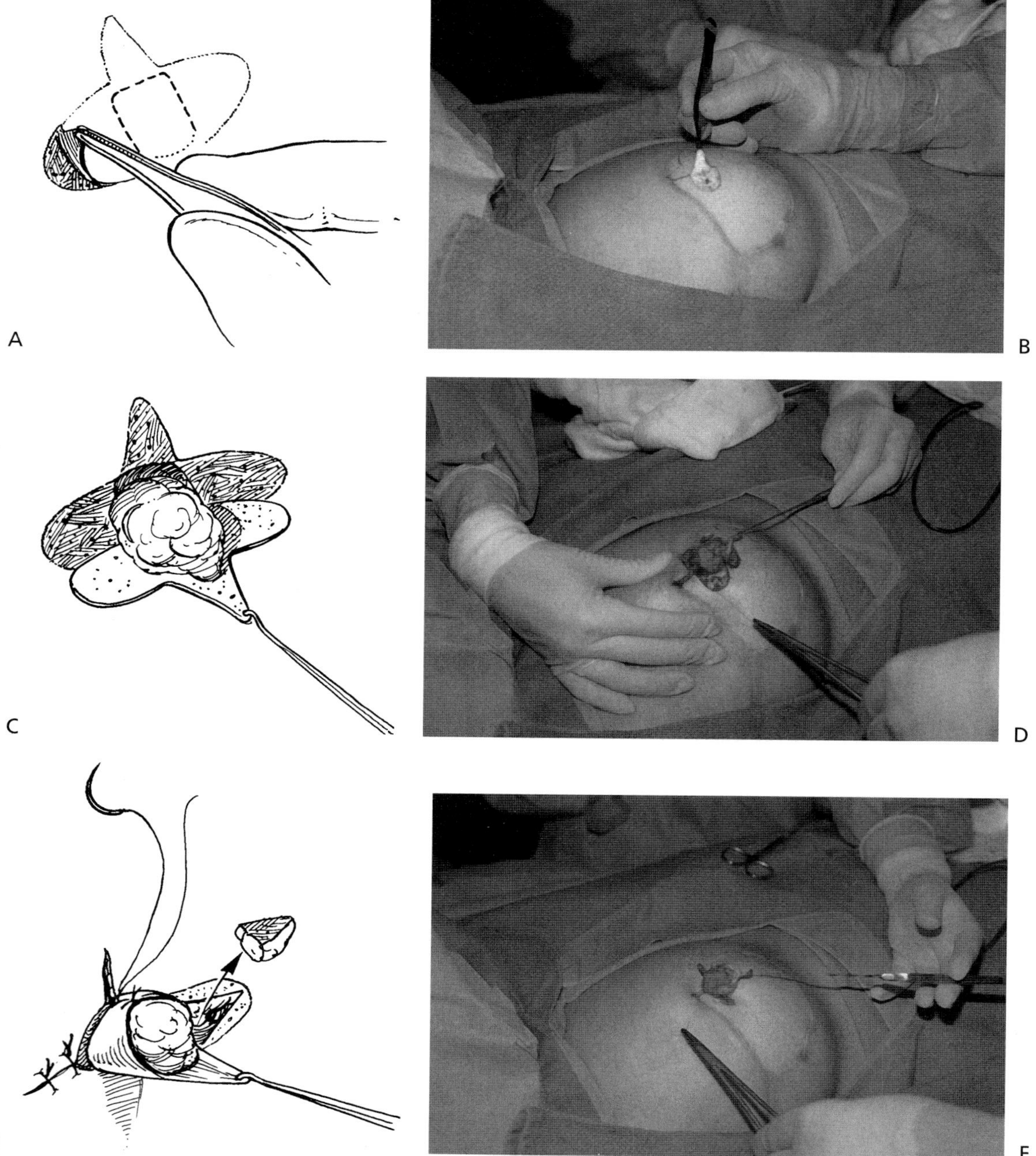

FIGURE 39-2. A: Artist's depiction of design of star flap with partial elevation of partial-thickness lateral flap. **B:** Intraoperative view of A. **C:** Drawing of elevation of star flap with medial, lateral, and superior partial-thickness flaps and central flap with underlying fatty element. **D:** Intraoperative view of C. **E:** Drawing of flap maintained in erect position by closure of partial-thickness defects and suture of medial and lateral flaps superiorly. Note that defects are converted to full thickness before closure to facilitate and flatten the closure. **F:** Intraoperative view of E. (*continued*)

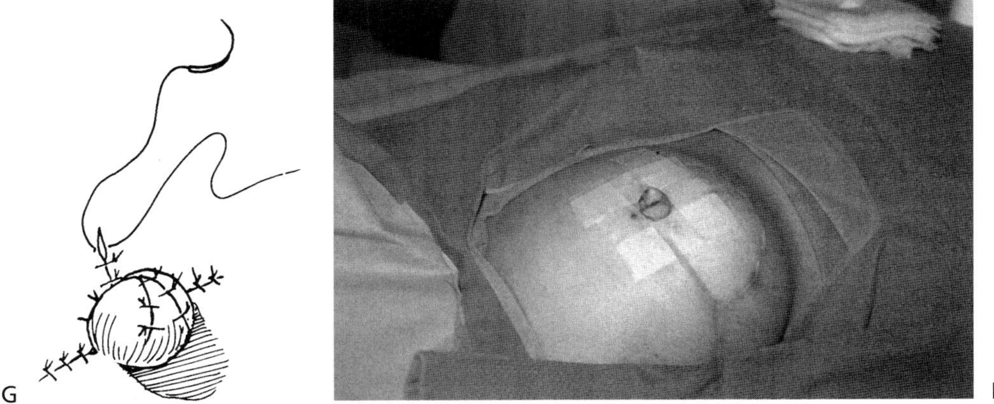

FIGURE 39-2. A: (*Continued*) **G:** Drawing of final kin closures. **H:** Intraoperative view of G.

the breast can be performed at the same time as nipple reconstruction with safety.

Palpable fat necrosis beneath the proposed nipple site after autogenous tissue breast reconstruction poses a significant problem in achieving adequate nipple height and width. In this situation, prior resection of the necrotic fat is essential to achieve a fully viable breast mound before nipple reconstruction is undertaken. Any firmness of the fat used for nipple flap reconstruction will result in significant atrophy of the nipple and generally a need for a secondary procedure.

Secondary nipple reconstructions are occasionally necessary to correct the above-mentioned problems. In these settings, it is almost always best to repeat the star flap reconstruction. Three to six months should pass before a secondary star flap reconstruction is undertaken, but if this amount of time is allowed, a secondary star flap is usually successful. In some cases, scarring of the reconstructed breast in the area of proposed nipple reconstruction is so severe that a star flap is not the best choice. In this situation, we generally use the dermal fat flap based inferiorly and surround this flap with a full-thickness skin graft obtained from another incision site. This technique is technically more demanding because a remote full-thickness skin graft is needed, and we have found that although it is successful in many cases, it is not as reliable as the skate flap, and, of course, a remote site must be used for the skin graft harvest.

In a case of inadequate projection of the nipple over an implant reconstruction, again, a repeated star flap is the best choice. Scarring in the area can actually be helpful in increasing the bulk of the newly created nipple. However, if the scarring is simply too severe for a secondary star flap to be considered, nipple sharing or even grafting from remote sites can be the best option.

Occasionally, the reconstructed nipple is larger than that of the opposite side. It is important to analyze this problem in terms of width versus height. If the nipple is too wide, wedges can be removed from the sides of the nipple reconstruction to make the circumference smaller. If the nipple is too tall in comparison with the opposite nipple, a wedge can be removed from the top of the nipple reconstruction. Either of these minor procedures can be carried out with essentially no discomfort to the patient, and symmetry with the opposite side is achieved.

Sometimes, the nipple is smaller than desired but not completely flattened, and one would like to augment the nipple reconstruction already present. The best procedure in this situation depends on the degree of augmentation needed. If the asymmetry is minor, only a partial addition of flap may be needed from one side or the other. Rotation of a small, adjacent flap of skin and fat will usually suffice. On the other hand, if an enlargement of 50% or more is required, a redo of the star flap is the best choice. It is essential, though, with this technique to make the operative result at least two times the size of the final desired result.

Pitfalls in tattooing are chiefly limited to the lack of persistence of adequate pigmentation. Natural colors can be chosen and combined to achieve a very symmetrical result, and if the result is not exact, additional tattooing methods can be used. However, it is generally not the tint or color of the original tattooing, but rather fading, that is the biggest problem. Although we know of no effective means to prevent this problem, we have found that secondary tattooing is generally a very satisfactory way to deal with it.

In addition, we have noted that certain dye colors tend to fade more than others. For instance, brown, black, tan, and red pigments seem to retain coloration more persistently than most others. On the other hand, we are cautious in using orange pigments because this color may appear unnatural after 6 months to 1 year.

CONCLUSION

In summary, improvements in nipple and areola reconstructive techniques have kept pace with the more significant and better-known improvements in breast reconstruction. Happily, these improvements have led to a simpler approach to nipple and areola reconstruction, for both the surgeon and the patient. Predictable natural results can be achieved in the vast majority of cases without incurring remote scars or painful donor sites. For this reason, nipple and areola reconstruction is increasingly accepted and has become a vital element of successful breast reconstruction.

REFERENCES

1. Arton MA, Eskenazi LB, Hartrampf CR. Nipple reconstruction with local flaps: the star and wrap flaps. *Perspect Plast Surg* 1991;5:178.
2. Hartrampf CR, Culbertson JH. Dermal fat flaps for nipple reconstruction. *Plast Reconstr Surg* 1984;73:982.
3. Little JW. Nipple-areolar reconstruction. In: Spear S, ed. *The breast.* Philadelphia: Lippincott–Raven Publishers, 1998:661–668.
4. Spear SL, Convit R, Little JW. Intradermal tattoo as an adjunct to nipple-areolar reconstruction. *Plast Reconstr Surg* 1989;83:907.

Discussion

NIPPLE AND AREOLA RECONSTRUCTION

J. WILLIAM LITTLE

It is not surprising that I can agree with so many of Frank Elliott's ideas regarding nipple and areola reconstruction. Dr. Elliott represents one of the premier units for breast reconstruction worldwide, one that has contributed greatly to bringing breast reconstruction to its currently high level of safety and effectiveness. I thoroughly agree with his emphasis on the importance of nipple and areola reconstruction in creating a natural appearance in a reconstructed breast. I also agree with the low priority that he places on graft techniques in accomplishing this end. I have abandoned areolar grafting (except to aid in closure of the nipple donor site) since embracing intradermal tattooing as the method of choice in nipple and areola coloration. The only graft site that yields predictable results in nipple reconstruction is the opposite nipple, and use of the opposite nipple as a donor site is associated with problems related to sensitivity and sensation. Furthermore, when the opposite nipple is shared, the final two nipples have less than half the projection of the original nipple. It is far better, I feel, to match the projection of the remaining nipple, a goal that can virtually always be achieved through various reconstructive options available today by local flap. I also agree with his recommendation to delay nipple and areola reconstruction to a second or even third stage, for all the reasons he details. One of the most common and detracting complications of nipple and areola

J. W. Little: Division of Surgery, Georgetown University School of Medicine, Washington, DC

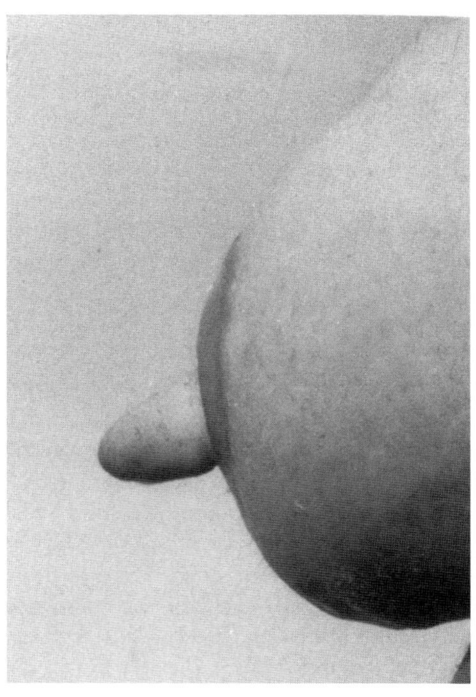

FIGURE 39D-1. Oversized skate nipple from early in the author's experience leaves little doubt about the potential of this design for projection.

reconstruction is malposition, an unfavorable result that is particularly difficult to correct. With respect to coloration, any enthusiasm that remains today for the use of autopigmented grafts from the genital region demonstrates, more than anything else, a limited clinical follow-up, as all such grafts in time lose color and require tattooing. It is far better to tattoo at the onset and avoid unnecessary and regrettable intrusion at these specialized and sensitive donor sites—ultimately to no purpose. With respect to the tattoo adjunct, I agree that coloration should be delayed until after the nipple and areola reconstruction has been performed, and that the initial coloration should be darker than desired. However, I have found that local vasoconstrictors minimize bleeding and hence the amount of hemosiderin pigment embedded with the tattoo pigments; the initial darkening is thus reduced and typically clears in 2 to 6 weeks. I certainly agree that scarred recipient sites make poor tattoo beds. One of Dr. Elliott's recommendations that surprises me, however, is his counsel against nipple reconstruction at the time a mammary implant is placed beneath the soft tissues fol-

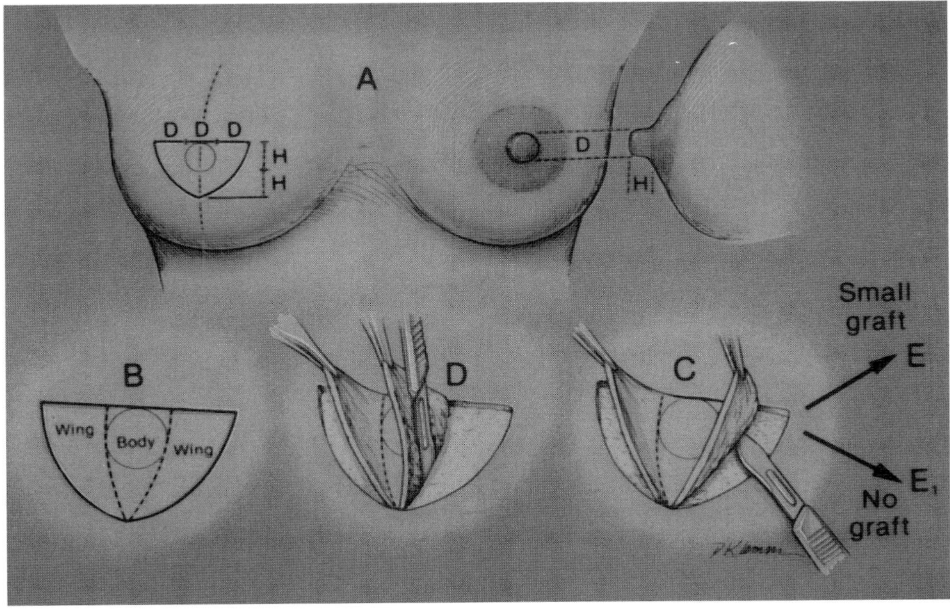

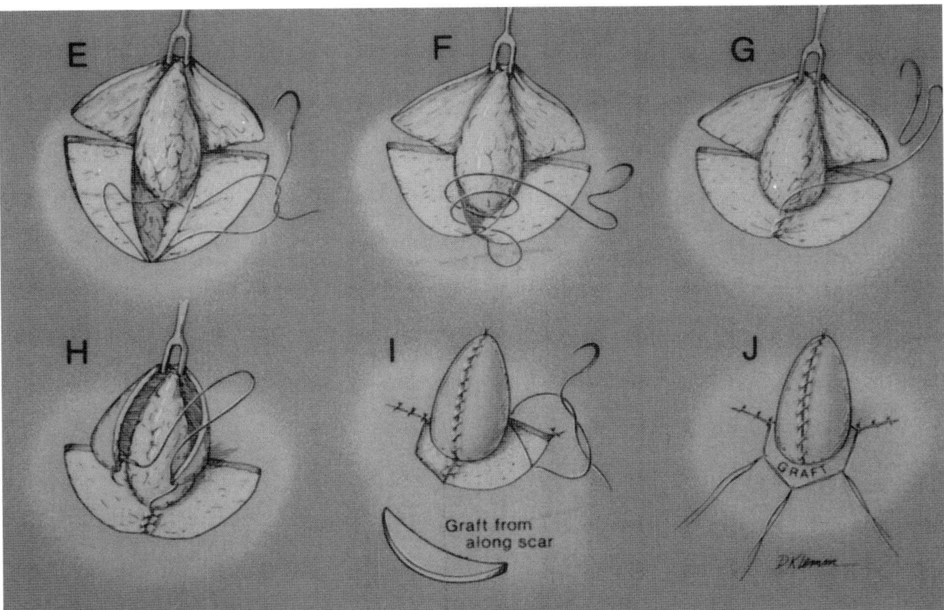

FIGURE 39D-2. Skate flap reconstruction of the nipple with skin graft closure. (Reproduced in part from Little JW. Nipple-areolar reconstruction. In: Cohen J, ed. *Mastery of plastic and reconstructive surgery.* Boston: Little, Brown and Company, 1994:1324–1348, with permission.)

lowing autologous reconstruction. The nipple reconstruction that I favor has a track record of hardiness that would not arouse such concern on my part.

That Dr. Elliott prefers the star flap developed by his colleague and mentor, Carl Hartrampf, is no surprise. It provides an excellent, reliable, and tidy solution to many nipple reconstructions, one that is far easier to execute than its precedent, the dermal-fat flap with wraparound full-thickness graft. And I agree with his advice to create a nipple with twice the dimensions that are ultimately desired. Although the exact ratio may vary from technique to technique (I use the same 2:1 figure), all nipple reconstructions by local flap lose a predictable amount of bulk and projection during the ensuing 4 to 6 months, a fact that must be taken into account at the time of surgical planning.

Dr. Elliott devotes a considerable portion of his discussion to positioning, the primary goal of nipple and areola reconstruction. The surgeon should strive for both a centric relation within the reconstructed breast mound and symmetry with the opposite nipple and areola. He gives little consideration, however, to the goal I consider to be second most important in nipple and areola reconstruction—lasting nipple projection. When nipples of small to moderate size are to be matched, a wide range of options is available with neat designs that allow primary closure of the donor sites. Perhaps the most appealing of these, from a design point of view, is the intricate and inventive star flap. Others include the double-opposing flap and related variants, and the skate flap, closed primarily without skin graft. With respect to nipple projection, the double-opposing and skate flaps have an advantage over the star flap, which is that the full heights of the former designs contribute entirely to nipple projection. This theoretical advantage has been confirmed clinically in a comparative study of late projection after the star and double-opposing designs; a small but significant advantage has been noted with the latter (1).

However, in pursuit of a larger nipple, I find these tidy designs with their closed donor sites inadequate. When the demands of the 2:1 rule are met in pursuit of a large opposite nipple, direct closure of the donor sites becomes counterproductive to the final outcome. Closing wide donor sites under tension at the site of nipple reconstruction produces three untoward effects. First, I have found that the greater the surface tension in the skin surrounding the nipple reconstruction, the greater the loss of nipple projection in the months following reconstruction. Second, the greater the tension in the closure of such sites, the greater the inappropriate flattening of the very portion of the breast silhouette where maximum projection or coning is desirable. Third, the greater the tension in the closure of wide donor sites, the greater the spread of final donor site scars. In this regard, as Dr. Elliott points out, intradermal tattooing of scarred beds is generally unsatisfactory. A clear alternative to closure under tension, of course, is the application of a thinned, full-thickness skin graft from any location, most often along an existing mastectomy or other scar. As the entire height of the skate design contributes to the height of the final nipple, the resulting proportions can be enormous when a graft is used to help close the secondary defect (Fig. 39D-1). As much of the donor site as possible is closed by V-to-Y techniques to either side and direct advancement centrally; a crescent-shaped defect is left that is rarely wider than a centimeter (2) (Fig. 39D-2). So long as the graft lies within the ultimate pigmented pattern of the areola, its presence remains unnoticed. The graft, then, presents a far better bed for intradermal tattoo than the spread scar.

CONCLUSION

Dr. Elliot is to be commended for his well-written chapter on nipple and areola reconstruction and the importance of this technique in achieving an overall favorable outcome in breast reconstruction. His star flap is an excellent technique for the straightforward reconstruction of nipples of small to moderate size, although equally effective alternatives are available. When pursuing a large opposite nipple, however, I prefer a technique in which the full height of the design is used to accomplish nipple projection; donor site closure by skin graft is an alternative to direct closure under tension. Tattoo remains the treatment of choice for reconstruction of the areola and coloration of the new nipple.

REFERENCES

1. Kroll SS, Reece GP, Miller MJ, et al. Comparison of nipple projection with the modified double-opposing tab and star flaps. *Plast Reconstr Surg* 1997;99:1602.
2. Little JW. Nipple-areola reconstruction. In: Spear SL, Little JW, Lippman ME, et al., eds. *Surgery of the breast: principle and art.* Philadelphia: Lippincott–Raven Publishers, 1998:661–669.

40

GYNECOMASTIA SURGERY

GARY J. ROSENBERG

There is no doubt that the condition of gynecomastia has been recognized over the millennia. Figurines of Pharaohs Seti and Tutankhamen displayed in the Cairo museum truly demonstrate gynecomastia. Aristotle was the first to recognize gynecomastia (1–3). The term *gynecomastia* was first used and published by Galen (4). Paulus Aeginata (5) was the first to publish surgical intervention for gynecomastia, in the 7th century AD. It was during the Golden Age of the Moorish Empire that there was an abundance of writings describing gynecomastia. Among this group of writers were Albucasis, Paracelsus, Fabricius ab Aguapendente, and Haly Abbas (1,6).

Medical and surgical treatments of gynecomastia were revisited in the 1800s, paralleling the emergence of modern medicine and surgery. Numerous publications in Europe and the United States documented these emerging techniques (7–11). Thorek (12) described a surgical technique of subcutaneous mastectomy for the treatment of gynecomastia. Four years later, Webster (13) also described subcutaneous mastectomy, which remained the treatment of choice until the early 1980s. Teimourian and Pearlman (14), as well as Courtiss (15), first described combined surgical excision with liposuction. In 1984, I first described suction lipectomy alone as a surgical solution for gynecomastia. This was followed by a series of publications (16–21).

ETIOLOGY AND EVALUATION

Before any surgical intervention, a thorough history, physical examination, and laboratory workup are essential. This is particularly important for the patient with gynecomastia. Studies reviewing thousands of cases, as well as selected autopsies, indicated an instance of gynecomastia between 36% and 65% (22–24). Etiology and workup of gynecomastia, as well as in-depth discussion of the endogenous and exogenous causes, are discussed thoroughly in the literature (25–33). New medications, such as ranitidine (Zantac), cimetidine (Tagamet), and ketoconazole (Nizoral), are constantly being added to the list (21).

The majority of patients can be treated with patience and reassurance, because the majority of cases resolve without treatment. However, with persistent gynecomastia, surgical intervention is indicated.

Azzopardi (34) and McDivitt et al. (35) demonstrated that although breast cancer is rare in males, it does occur and accounts for 1% of all breast cancers. They also state that there is practically an absence of preceding gynecomastia in patients with breast carcinoma. However, patients with Klinefelter syndrome show an association of breast carcinoma and gynecomastia.

CUTTING TECHNIQUES

The majority of cutting techniques are based on the work of Thorek (12) and Webster (13). These, in turn, were based on the works of Albucasis reported centuries earlier (6). The common theme of these techniques is a subcutaneous mastectomy. Any intraareolar and periareolar incisions have been described without skin resection (12,13,36–41). Large gynecomastia and gigantomastia have been treated with subcutaneous mastectomy, with large amounts of skin excision, or simple mastectomy, dating back to the works of Paulus Aeginata (5,42–50).

COMPLICATIONS OF SURGICAL EXCISION TECHNIQUES

As with surgical excision of the female breast, postoperative complications occur, and not rarely. Therefore, the surgeon must pay close attention to meticulous hemostasis to avoid postoperative hemorrhage or hematoma. If hematoma occurs, it must be recognized early and treated aggressively. The incision should be opened and the hematoma evacuated completely (Fig. 40-1). Failure to do so can lead to contour irregularities. The use of suction drainage greatly assists

G. J. Rosenberg: Florida Aesthetic Surgery Center, Delray Beach, Florida

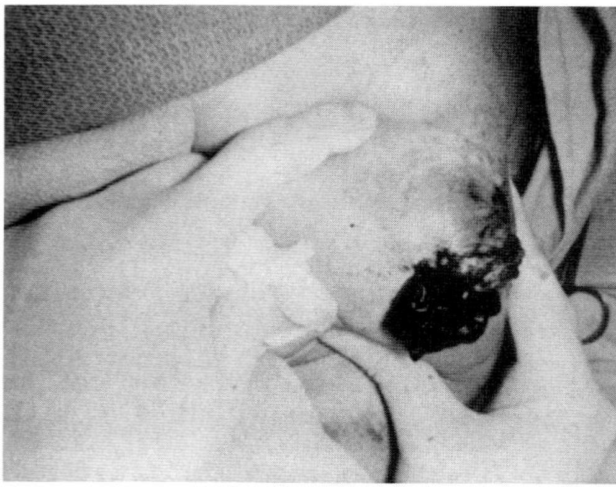

FIGURE 40-1. Evaluation of 6-hour postoperative hematoma.

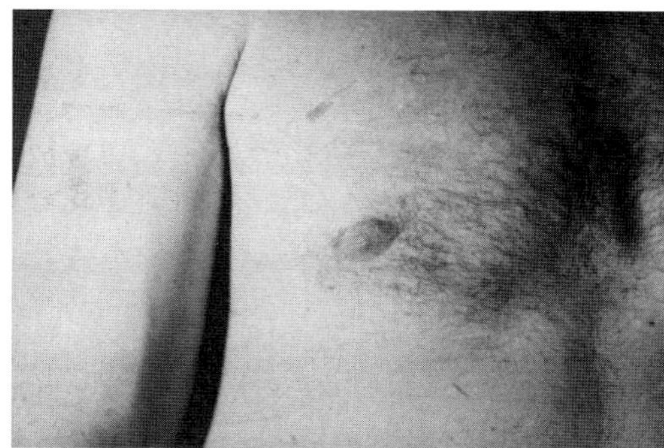

FIGURE 40-3. The areola, which originally was round, has become oval. This can be changed by a small superior skin excision and advancement of the areola.

the surgeon in avoiding hematoma or seroma formation. It can be removed after 24 to 48 hours.

Adherence to proper sterile surgical technique is of utmost importance to avoid postoperative infection. The large dead space created, and the diminished capacity of blood flow to the nipple–areola complex, has an associated risk of infection. One of the two most common postoperative complications of the surgical excision techniques for gynecomastia is saucer deformity (Fig. 40-2) and distortion of the areola (Fig. 40-3). When performing surgical excision, one must leave behind 1 cm of subareolar tissue and carefully bevel the edges of resection to prevent the areola from adhering to the underlying pectoralis muscle. Failure to do so can lead to fibrous attachments of the areola with an obvious saucer deformity. This is a Catch-22, because the immediate subareolar tissue is the point of origin of gynecomastia (21). Aggressive thinning of the subareolar tissue at the time of subcutaneous mastectomy also can lead to slough of the nipple–areola complex.

The other most common complication is hypertrophic scarring (Fig. 40-4). When the surgical incision is confined within the areola, the scars usually go unnoticed and heal without hypertrophy. Incisions that extend onto the breast skin, or skin excision techniques, can lead to hypertrophic scarring. As with breast reduction surgery for the female, meticulous surgical technique and avoidance of tension still can result in hypertrophic scarring.

Secondary surgery performed to correct deformities caused by inappropriately planned excisional surgery is difficult. Distortion of tissue planes, dense fibrosis, and gross skin irregularities make this surgery particularly difficult (Fig. 40-5). Compromise of the blood supply to the nipple–areola complex must be addressed. Nipple tattooing is of great assistance in camouflaging distortion of the areola.

The surgeon must consider inconvenience, down time, and expense to the patient. Time away from work, inability to perform normal daily functions, and time away from leisure activities are of paramount concern to all patients.

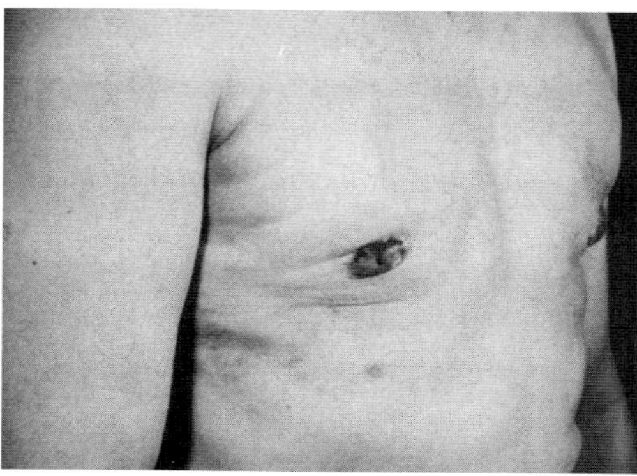

FIGURE 40-2. Saucer-shaped deformity of the breasts after resection for gynecomastia.

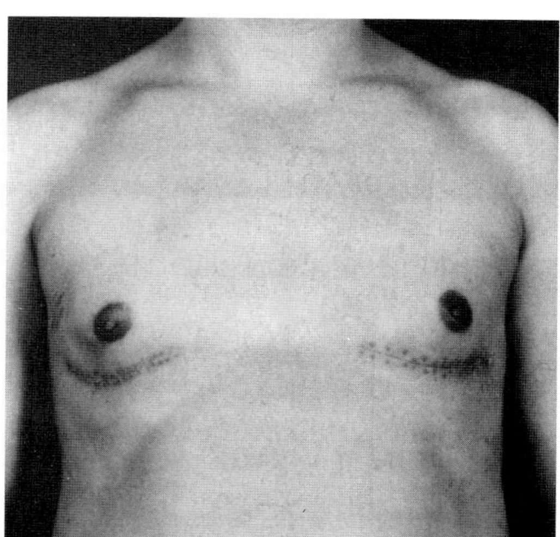

FIGURE 40-4. Gynecomastia resected through inframammary incisions with widely placed mattress suture marks.

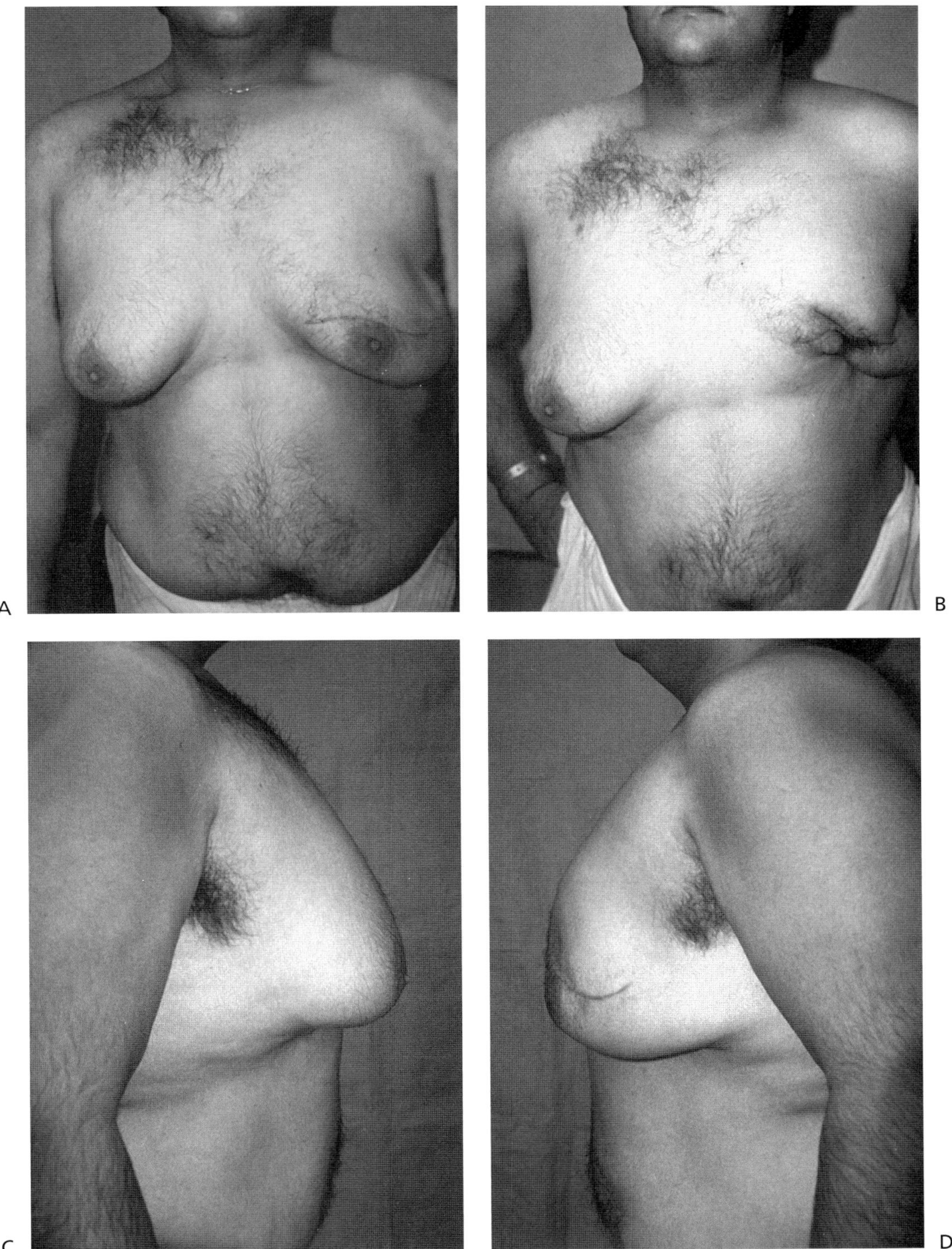

FIGURE 40-5. Post simple mastectomy and nipple grafting and tattooing. Immediate **(A)** and 6-month **(B)** views of a general surgeon's attempt at correction with subcutaneous mastectomy. Only one side was operated on. **C:** Nonoperated right side preoperatively. **D:** Left side after subcutaneous mastectomy (original manifestation). (*continued*)

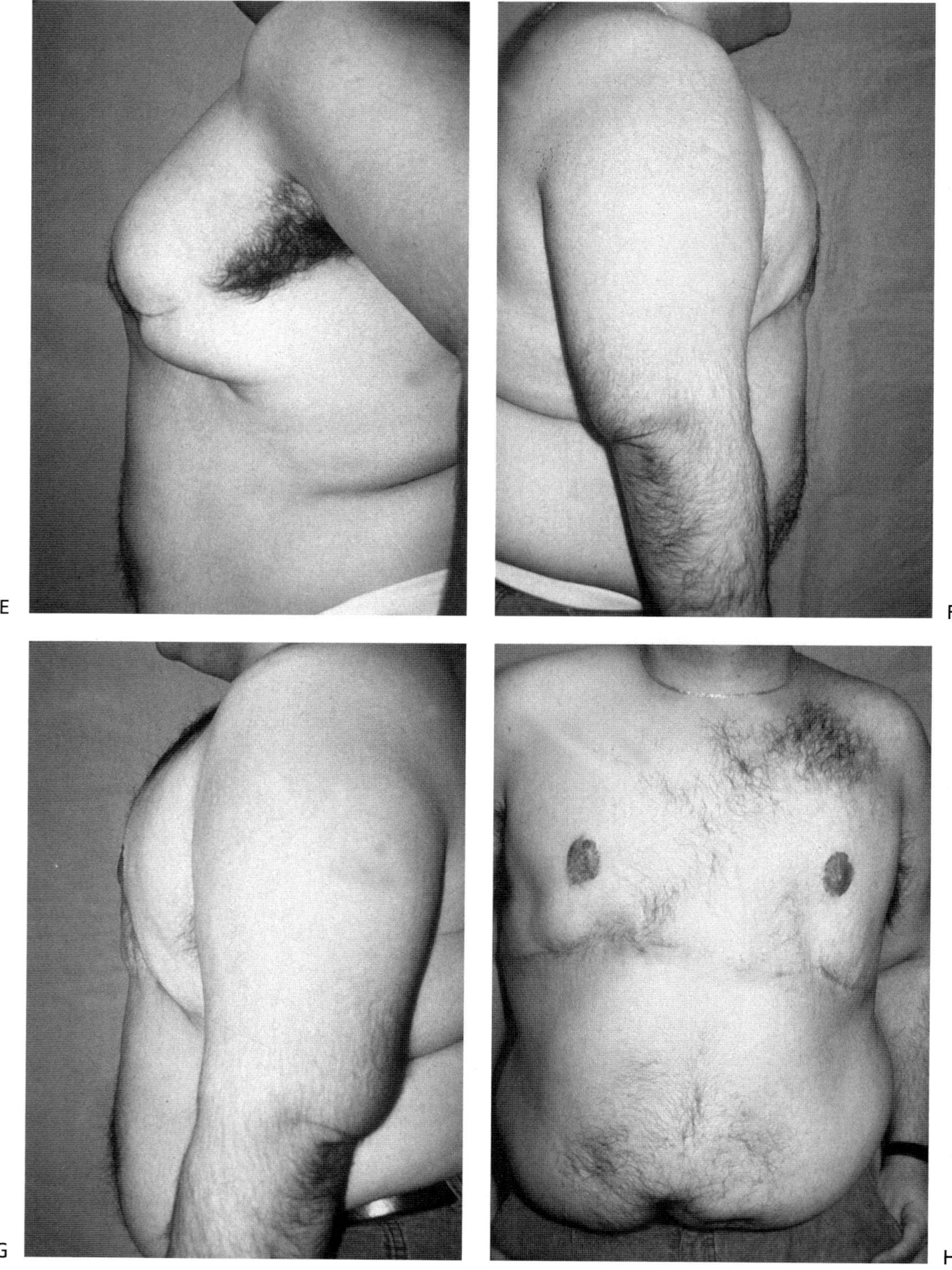

FIGURE 40-5. (Continued) **E:** Left side 6 months later. **F:** Right side after simple mastectomy. **G:** Corrected left side after simple mastectomy. **H:** Front view after simple mastectomy. Scars concealed to create inframammary fold.

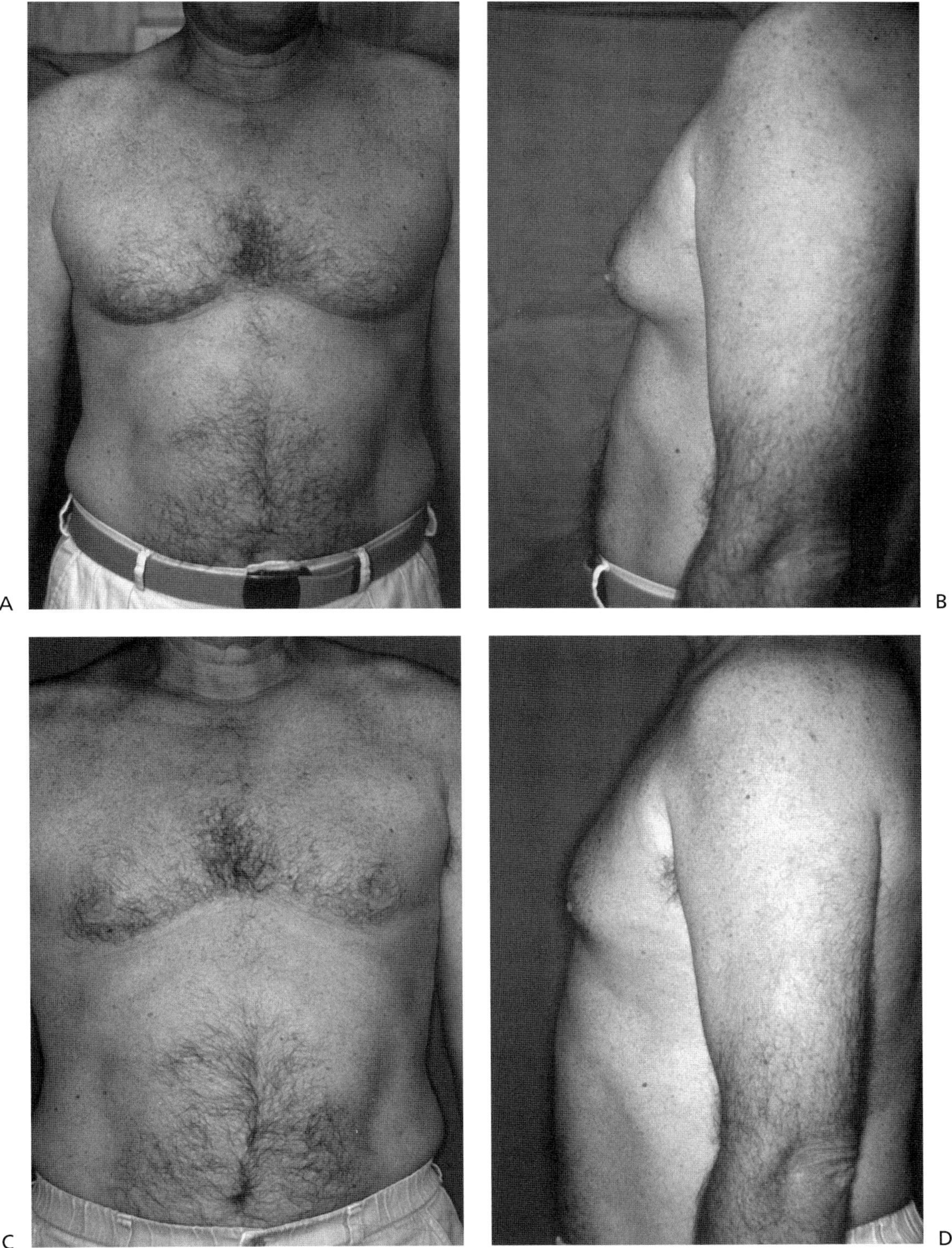

FIGURE 40-6. Preoperative **(A,B)** and 1-year postoperative **(C,D)** views in a 33-year-old man.

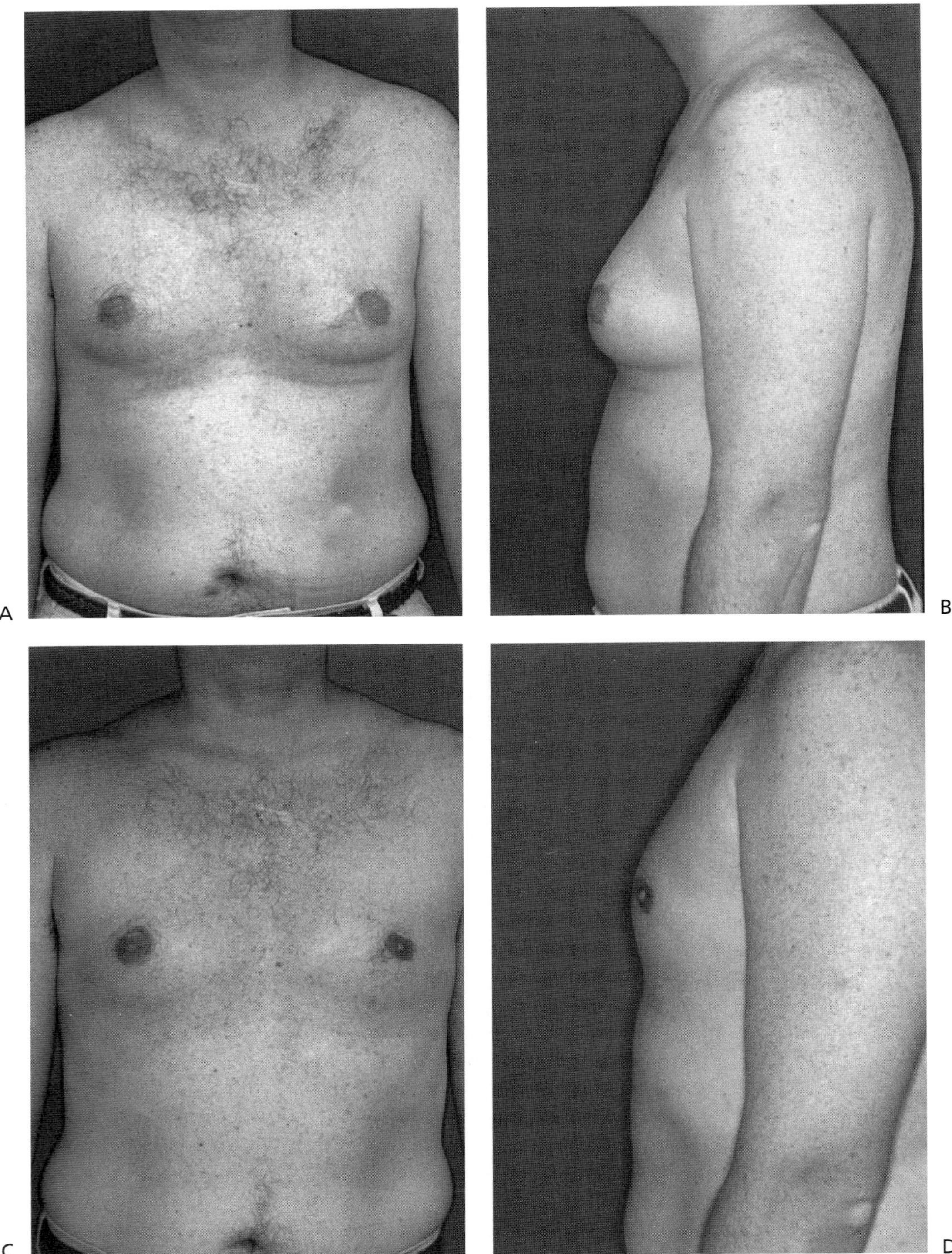

FIGURE 40-7. Preoperative **(A,B)** and 1-year postoperative **(C,D)** views in a 54-year-old man.

LIPOSUCTION

In the 1980s, Teimourian and Pearlman (14) and Courtiss (15) combined sharp excisional techniques with liposuction. I first introduced liposuction alone for treatment of gynecomastia. This technique remained essentially unchanged until the advent of ultrasonic liposuction (internal and external) (16–21). Through a 1-cm superior areolar incision, the parenchymal and glandular tissue is first aspirated using the Rosenberg cannula (18). Periareolar and lateral suctioning is completed to remove the fat. A spatulated cannula is used to remove the immediate subareolar tissue. As previously mentioned, this is the point of origin of the gynecomastia. This step is very important to prevent recurrence. Unlike the surgical excision techniques, the surgeon need not worry about compromise of the blood supply, nipple distortion, saucer deformity, or areolar slough.

Next, the inframammary crease in undermined to allow redraping of the skin. For small or moderate gynecomastia, suction lipectomy is extended to the clavicle, sternum, 2 cm below the inframammary crease, and to the anterior axillary fold. For large gynecomastia, suction lipectomy is extended to the posterior axillary fold and the iliac crest.

The advent of internal, as well as external, ultrasonic lipoplasty greatly facilitated the removal of parenchymal, glandular, and adipose tissue (51–53).

Although I have not seen these complications, the theoretical complications would be those of suction lipectomy performed in other areas of the body, including hemorrhage, infection, hematoma, seroma, fat necrosis, irregularities, waviness, dimpling, crepiness of the skin, or asymmetries.

The most common undesirable result is that of underresection. Although it is inconvenient, it is easy to rectify by a touchup procedure.

Occasionally, an individual nodule of parenchymal or glandular tissue may be left behind. This is easily removed with local anesthesia and direct aspiration. If a small aggregate of fat is left behind, it is treated with direct application of external ultrasound without aspiration.

The use of a compressive garment for 2 weeks after the procedure is of paramount importance in avoiding hematoma, seroma, or improper draping of the skin. All patients are allowed to return to full activities 24 hours after suction lipectomy or treatment with internal ultrasonic or external ultrasonic lipoplasty.

The most difficult problem that I have faced has been the male patient with minimal gynecomastia. Although the results may be good to excellent, patients still may insist that their chest is not perfect. A review of the preoperative photographs often is helpful. However, sometimes it is more useful to plan a minimal procedure under local anesthesia. As with many cosmetic and reconstructive procedures, a frank discussion with the patient, before surgery, of the realistic expectation can avoid this problem.

Minimal discomfort and rapid recovery with return to full activities the day after surgery have made this a popular procedure in my practice. The long-term results and paucity of problems have led to high patient satisfaction (Figs. 40-6–40-7).

REFERENCES

1. Karsner HT. Gynecomastia. *Am J Pathol* 1946;22:235.
2. Kessel FV, et al. Surgical treatment of gynecomastia: an analysis of 275 cases. *Ann Surg* 1963;157:142.
3. Menville JG. Gynecomastia. *Arch Surg* 1933;26:1054.
4. Erdheim S. Über Gynäkomastia. *Arch Surg* 1928;208:181.
5. Aeginata P. *The seven books of Paulus Aeginata,* vol. 2, book 6, section 46. London: London Sydenham Society, 1848. Adams F, translator.
6. Letterman G, Schurter M. Gynecomastia. In: Georgiade NG, ed. *Reconstructive breast surgery.* St. Louis: CV Mosby, 1976: 229–253.
7. Bédor H. Quelques considérations appuyées des faits particulaires sur la gynecomastie sur l'hypertrophie des mamelles chez l'homme. *Gaz mé Paris* 1836;4:689.
8. Foot. Remarks on gynecomastia. *Dublin Q J Med Soc* 1866; 12:451.
9. Gorham J. Extraordinary development of the mammae in the male. *Lancet* 1840;11:637.
10. Hassler. Gynecomastie: Mastite chronique et adénite axillaire polyganglionnaire. *Arch Met Pharm* 1894;23:531.
11. Eve PF. Hypertrophy of the male mamma: removed. *Nashville J Med Surg* 1854;7:454.
12. Thorek M. *Plastic surgery of the breast and abdominal wall.* Springfield, IL: Charles C Thomas, 1942:155.
13. Webster JP. Mastectomy for gynecomastia through a semicircular intra-areolar incision. *Ann Surg* 1946;124:557.
14. Teimourian B, Pearlman R. Surgery for gynecomastia. *Aesthetic Plast Surg* 1983;7:155.
15. Courtiss EH. Gynecomastia: analysis of the 159 patients and current recommendations for treatment. *Plast Reconstr Surg* 1987;79:740.
16. Rosenberg GJ. Gynecomastia: suction lipectomy as a contemporary solution. *Plast Reconstr Surg* 1987;80:379.
17. Rosenberg GJ. Gynecomastia: analysis of 159 patients and current recommendations for treatment [Discussion]. *Plast Reconstr Surg* 1987;79:753.
18. Rosenberg GJ. A new cannula for suction removal of parenchymal tissue of gynecomastia. *Plast Reconstr Surg* 1994;94:548.
19. Rosenberg GJ. Surgical correction for gynecomastia: an update. *Adv Plast Reconstr Surg* 1994;10:285.
20. Rosenberg GJ, Colon GA. Gynecomastia: two perspectives. In: Marchac D, Granick MS, Solomon MP, eds. *Male aesthetic surgery.* Boston: Butterworth-Heinemann, 1996:287.
21. Rosenberg GJ. Gynecomastia. In: Spear SL, ed. *Surgery of the breast: principles and art.* Philadelphia: Lippincott-Raven Publishers, 1998:831.
22. Nydick M, et al. Gynecomastia in adolescent boys. *JAMA* 1961;178:449.
23. Nuttall FQ. Gynecomastia as a physical finding in normal men. *J Clin Endocrinol Metab* 1979;48:338.
24. Williams MJ. Gynecomastia: its incidence, recognition and host characterization in 447 autopsy cases. *Am J Med* 1963;34:103.
25. Letterman G, Schurter M. Gynecomastia. In: Georgiade NG, ed. *Reconstructive breast surgery.* St. Louis: CV Mosby, 1976: 229–253.

26. Letterman G, Schurter M. Gynecomastia. In: Courtiss EH, ed. *Male aesthetic surgery.* St. Louis: CV Mosby, 1982:295.
27. Riefkohl R, McCarty KS. Gynecomastia. In: Georgiade NG, ed. *Aesthetic breast surgery.* Baltimore: Williams & Wilkins, 1983:334.
28. Mahoney CP. Adolescent gynecomastia: differential diagnosis and management. *Pediatr Clin North Am* 1990;37:1389.
29. Kessel FV, et al. Surgical treatment of gynecomastia: an analysis of 275 cases. *Ann Surg* 1963;157:142.
30. Leung AK. Gynecomastia. *Am Fam Physician* 1989;39:215.
31. Lewin ML. Gynecomastia: the hypertrophy of the male breast. *J Clin Endocrinol* 1941;1:511.
32. Beck W, Strabbe P. Endocrinological studies of the hypothalmo-pituitary-gonadal axis during danazol treatment in pubertal boys with marked gynecomastia. *Horm Metab Res* 1982;14:653.
33. Lewis CM. Lipoplasty: treatment of gynecomastia with tamoxifen: a double blind-crossover study. *Metabolism* 1986;53:705.
34. Azzopardi JG. *Problems in breast pathology.* Philadelphia: WB Saunders, 1979;322–324.
35. McDivitt RW, et al. Tumors of the breast. In: *Atlas of tumor pathology, second series, fascicle 2.* Washington, DC: Armed Forces Institute of Pathology, 1968.
36. Letterman G, Schurter M. The surgical correction of gynecomastia. *Am Surg* 1969;35:322.
37. Pitanguy I. Transareolar incision for gynecomastia. *Plast Reconstr Surg* 1966;38:414.
38. Sinder R. Gynecomasty—surgical correction by use of a Z incision in the areola. Paper presented at the First International Congress of the International Society of Aesthetic Plastic Surgery, Rio de Janeiro, February 1972.
39. Barsky AJ, Kahn S, Simon BE. *Principles and practices of plastic surgery,* 2nd ed. New York: McGraw-Hill Book Co., 1964.
40. Simon BE, Hoffman S. Correction of gynecomastia. In: Goldwyn RM, ed. *Plastic and reconstructive surgery of the breast.* Boston: Little, Brown and Company, 1976:305.
41. Simon BE, Hoffman S, Kahn S. Classification and surgical correction of gynecomastia. *Plast Reconstr Surg* 1973;51:48.
42. Menville JG. Gynecomastia. *Arch Surg* 1933;26:1054.
43. Vogt LG. Beitrag zur plastichen Operation der Gynäkomastie. *Chirugie* 1941;13:322.
44. Campos F. Sobre um caso de ginecomastia, bilateral e seu tratamiento cirúrgico. *Arq Cir Clin Exp* 1942;6:703.
45. Maliniac JW. Breast hypertrophy in the male. *J Clin Endocrinol* 1943;3:364.
46. Malbec EF. Ginecomastia: nueva technica operatoria. *J Int Coll Surg* 1946;9:652.
47. Letterman G, Schurter M. Surgical correction of massive gynecomastia. *Plast Reconstr Surg* 1972;49:259.
48. Dufourmentel C, Mouly R. Développement recents de la plastic mammaire par la méthode oblique laterale. *Ann Chir Plast* 1965;10:277.
49. Skoog T. A technique of breast reconstruction. Transposition of the nipple on a cutaneous vascular pedicle. *Acta Chir Scand* 1963;126:453.
50. Skoog T. *Plastic surgery.* Stockholm: Almquist & Wiskell International, 1974.
51. Rosenberg GJ. External ultrasonic lipoplasty: an effective alternative. Presented at the annual meeting of the American Society of Aesthetic Plastic Surgery, Los Angeles, CA, May 1998.
52. Rosenberg GJ, Cabrera RC. External ultrasonic lipoplasty: an effective method of fat removal and skin shrinkage. *Plast Reconstr Surg* 2000;105:785–791.
53. Silberg BN. The use of external ultrasound assist with liposuction. *Aesth Surg J* 1998;18:284.

Discussion

GYNECOMASTIA SURGERY

ROBERT M. GOLDWYN

Dr. Rosenberg has described many of the complications of the surgical treatment of gynecomastia and their prevention. As he mentioned, a thorough history and physical examination can prevent trouble later, e.g., not thinking of the possibility of a cancer, especially if the patient has unilateral or asymmetrical gynecomastia. During the initial consultation, the patient's expectations must be understood. What a young bodybuilder compensating for his gynecomastia may want from the operation may be far different from the expectations of an older male whose gynecomastia has resulted from the hormonal treatment of prostatic cancer. In the latter instance, removing as much breast tissue as possible may be advisable, even at the risk of a slight concavity, in order to prevent regrowth with continuing hormonal therapy. It is important to inform a patient about the possible effect of the procedure on sensation. I had a few patients who rejected the operation because they did not want to impair what was, for them, an important erogenous zone.

R. M. Goldwyn: Department of Surgery, Beth Israel Deaconess Medical Center, Harvard Medical School, Boston, Massachusetts

When the patient is seen initially, he must understand his financial responsibilities. In my state, almost no insurance company will cover the correction of gynecomastia, except when the gynecomastia is a result of the administration of hormones for prostatic cancer. Even then, the bureaucratic battle to gain approval is lengthy. When a complication occurs, the uninsured patient may have the additional expense of the hospital unless the surgeon has his or her own surgical facility. Because I do not have my own operating room, I have the patient sign a form emphasizing his financial responsibilities (Fig. 40D-1). The authorization that I use for the correction of gynecomastia is specific but not inclusive (Fig. 40D-2).

My best results for most patients with gynecomastia have been with combined tumescent liposuction and limited excision. I have not been able to consistently avoid excision, even though Dr. Rosenberg's cannula is extremely helpful. Unlike him, however, I have not yet used ultrasound liposuction, which, according to Dr. Rosenberg and others, is excellent for this problem.

Meticulous hemostasis, if excision is used, is mandatory. This is more difficult when the gynecomastia is corrected through a small periareolar incision. I ask patients to avoid heavy exercise for 2 weeks to prevent bleeding.

Seromas can be exasperating. I used to keep drains in for 5 days. When liposuction is the predominant part of the procedure, I do not resort to drains. Although I have not done a controlled randomized study, my impression is that the incidence of seroma is about the same without drains in that situation.

Dr. Rosenberg wisely notes that it is easier to do more later than to produce a saucer deformity, which is very difficult to remedy. It can be improved but rarely eliminated by waiting at least 4 months, then using fat grafts or local flaps of fat.

Still unsolved is what to do with patients who have severe gynecomastia. Does one make more than a periareolar incision and graft the nipple–areola complex in one stage? My preference is to do the subcutaneous mastectomy through a periareolar incision, allow for tissue shrinkage, and then do a revision as a secondary operation, removing the excess wrinkled skin but still through a periareolar approach. In truth, my results have been acceptable but not notable. In males who are very hairy, an extension of the incision horizontally beyond the areola in both directions is less visible than in less hirsute patients, but one can never predict which patient will have objectionable, prominent scarring.

In cases of severe gynecomastia, Simon and Hoffman (1) have recommended radical excision with grafting and accepting a transverse scar on either side of the nipple–areola complex. In their words, "it is a triumph of hope over experience to expect late shrinkage of the redundant skin."

Murphy et al. (2) also have advocated total mastectomy

ROBERT M. GOLDWYN, M.D.

Because insurance coverage varies with different companies, I understand that I may be responsible for the hospital costs associated with any surgery undertaken to improve a result or to treat a complication. While I understand that Dr. Goldwyn would be willing to forego his fee for additional work if it is not covered by insurance, I understand that he cannot assume responsibility for the hospital charges.

I understand also that it is not his policy to return the original surgical fee in the event that I am displeased with the result and wish to consult another physician/surgeon for evaluation, treatment, or reoperation.

____

Date

____

Signature

____

Witness

FIGURE 40D-1. Form stipulating the patient's responsibility for hospital costs associated with improving a result or treating a complication.

ROBERT M. GOLDWYN, M.D., INC.

—AUTHORIZATION—

CORRECTION OF GYNECOMASTIA

____

Patient's Name

1. I authorize Robert M. Goldwyn, M.D. (the "Doctor") and his assistants to perform upon me (or my.______________________.) the operation known as correction of gynecomastia.
2. The nature and effects of the operation, the risks and complications involved, as well as alternative methods of treatment, have been fully explained to me by the Doctor and I understand them.

   The following points, among others, have been specifically made clear:

   a. The scars are permanent and although they usually are not prominent, they may be.
   b. Although having the breasts made smaller and symmetrical is the surgical objective, perfect symmetry of nipples, areolae, breasts, and chest cannot always be achieved.
   c. Complications after correction of gynecomastia can be those after any surgical procedure.
   d. Bleeding and infection may occur and may require an additional procedure (s) for treatment.
   e. There is the rare possibility that the blood supply to one or both nipples and areolae may become impaired and necrosis (death of tissue) may result. This complication may require later reconstruction.
   f. Swelling and ecchymosis (black and blue marks) take several weeks to disappear; several months are necessary for the breasts and chest to assume their final shape.
   g. While every attempt will be made to make each breast, including nipple and areola, as normal and pleasing in appearance as possible, these objectives cannot always be attained.
   h. Sensation to the breast, including nipple and areola, is usually altered and may be decreased permanently.

FIGURE 40D-2. Authorization form for correction of gynecomastia.

3. I authorize the Doctor to perform any other procedure which he may deem desirable in attempting to improve the condition stated in Paragraph 1. or any unhealthy or unforeseen condition that may be encountered during the operation.
4. I consent to the administration of anesthetics by the Doctor or under the direction of the physician responsible for this service.
5. I understand that the practice of medicine and surgery is not an exact science and that reputable practitioners cannot guarantee results. No guarantee or assurance has been given by the Doctor or anyone else as to the results that may be obtained.
6. I understand that the two sides of the human body are not the same and can never be made the same.
7. For the purpose of advancing medical education, I consent to the admittance of authorized observers to the operating room.
8. I give permission to Robert M. Goldwyn, M.D., Inc. to take still or motion clinical photographs with the understanding that such photographs remain the property of the corporation.
9. I am not known to be allergic to anything except: (list) ____________________

____

I certify that I have read the above authorization, that the explanations referred to therein were made to my satisfaction, and that I fully understand such explanations and the above authorization.

Signed ____

Patient or person authorized to consent for patient

Witness ______________________________ Date ______________

FIGURE 40D-2. (Continued)

and free nipple grafting as the best option. They identified standard nipple distances to aid the surgeon in the placement of the nipple–areola graft.

Beraka (3) prefers the short transfer scar at the level of the nipple to the inframammary scars described by Murphy et al. because he objects to what he considers the residual feminine appearance of the chest wall.

With better conditions for ambulatory surgery, the treatment of gynecomastia is less a problem today than it was a decade ago. However, the outcome can never be guaranteed.

REFERENCES

1. Simon BE, Hoffman S. Correction of gynecomastia. In: Goldwyn RM, ed. *Plastic and reconstructive surgery of the breast.* Boston: Little, Brown and Company, 1976:305–325.
2. Murphy TP, Ehrlichman RJ, Seckel BR. Nipple placement in simple mastectomy with free nipple grafting for severe gynecomastia. *Plast Reconstr Surg* 1994;94:818–823.
3. Beraka GJ. Correction of gynecomastia with an inframammary incision and subsequent scar [Letter]. *Plast Reconstr Surg* 1995;96:1753–1754.

41

CHEST AND ABDOMINAL WALL RECONSTRUCTION

MIMIS N. COHEN

Acquired defects of the trunk, anterior chest wall, back, and abdominal wall are primarily caused by infection, ablative resection of primary or recurrent tumors, complications of surgical procedures, trauma, and radiation. These defects can be superficial, involving only some layers of the soft tissues of the thorax and abdomen, or full thickness, extending to the bony framework and even beyond into the thoracic cavity, mediastinum, spinal cord, and abdominal cavity. In many instances, such defects represent life-threatening conditions, because vital structures such as the heart and great vessels, lungs, spinal cord, or abdominal viscera are exposed. Furthermore, some patients present with poor general health and several significant underlying medical problems that could affect not only the outcome of the reconstructive procedure, but the patients' lives as well. Thus, reconstructive procedures in these areas carry mortality and morbidity rates higher than the rates for the majority of reconstructive procedures performed in other areas of the body.

By far the highest mortality and morbidity are encountered with patients undergoing reconstruction for intrathoracic defects, which include bronchopleural fistula, empyema, heart and great vessel perforation, and esophageal or tracheal fistula. Arnold and Pairolero (1) reported their 10-year experience. In a series of 87 patients, the overall mortality rate was 14.9%, and the complication rate was over 25%. Several complications resulted in intrathoracic sepsis and ultimately, death. On first view, these results might be considered disappointing. The very fact, however, that a significant number of patients in these series were salvaged from a potentially lethal condition fully justifies the use of these reconstructive procedures for the management of intrathoracic catastrophes.

M. N. Cohen: Divisions of Plastic Surgery, the University of Illinois at Chicago and Cook County Hospital, Chicago, Illinois

Given the high risk associated with reconstructive procedures in the trunk, it is imperative for the surgeon to plan each procedure accordingly. Unless it is an absolute emergency, all procedures should be scheduled after hemodynamic stabilization of the patient, control of infection, and improvement of nutritional status. Furthermore, because the margin for error for the reconstructive surgeon dealing with such patients is small, every effort should be made to achieve immediate successful coverage and reconstruction while minimizing the risk of complications.

The purpose of the reconstruction of defects in the trunk is to restore form and function, eradicate local infection, provide stable coverage with well-vascularized tissues, achieve obliteration of all residual cavities, and attain a healed wound (2). The reconstructive techniques for various defects in the trunk have improved significantly over the past years, primarily because of the extensive use of muscles, musculocutaneous flaps, or omentum, as single flaps or in combination. The availability of these flaps enables the surgeon to successfully cover large full-thickness defects of various etiologies, by providing well-vascularized tissues to cover chest wall, back, and abdominal wall defects. It also allows the surgeon to undertake a wide excision of malignant tumors with clear margins and to perform aggressive debridement of devitalized soft tissues, cartilage, and bone. Such debridement is a prerequisite for successful long-term management of defects caused by infection or radiation necrosis.

The advantages of using autogenous tissue for the reconstruction of defects in the trunk are as follows:

- Healthy, well-vascularized flaps with considerable bulk, if needed, are mobilized from areas distant to the defect, the zone of infection, radiation, or tumor and used to obliterate any residual dead space. They provide immediate coverage of all exposed vital structures and reconstruction of the tissue defect. Due to their excellent vascularity, these flaps assist in the elimination of residual local infection and promote wound healing. Therefore, the need for wound care is reduced, hospitalization and convalescence are shortened, and medical costs are decreased.

- Flaps provide stable coverage of bone grafts or synthetic meshes or patches, which contribute to the stability of the chest or abdominal wall. Thus, respiratory functions are improved, paradoxical movement during breathing is reduced or eliminated, and the tone of the abdominal wall is restored as needed.

The disadvantages of using muscle flaps or omentum include the need for additional lengthy procedures for already debilitated individuals, the potential donor site morbidity, and the possible loss of function of a muscle unit. Most of these disadvantages, however, are offset by the significant advantages of using such flaps (3).

PRINCIPLES OF RECONSTRUCTION OF THE TRUNK

With accumulated experience and better understanding of the anatomical and functional requirements of each area, basic reconstructive principles have been established and currently are widely accepted. A variety of flaps are available for the reconstruction. Regardless of the choice of flap, however, the surgeon should adhere to the reconstructive principles in order to achieve consistently good results and minimize the possibility of complications. These principles are summarized in Table 41-1.

TABLE 41-1. BASIC PRINCIPLES FOR RECONSTRUCTION OF VARIOUS DEFECTS OF THE TRUNK

1. Close cooperation between the plastic surgeon and the primary surgeon
2. Timing of reconstruction based on the patient's condition and the requirements of the reconstruction (immediate vs. delayed, early definitive vs staged reconstruction)
3. Complete drainage of any purulent collection; control of infection with local care and appropriate systemic antibiotics
4. Wound preparation and management, as needed
5. Extensive debridement of all devitalized soft tissue, cartilage, and bone
6. Removal of all foreign bodies from the wound
7. Selection of appropriate flap(s) based on reconstructive requirements of the area, size, location, and extent of defect, tissue availability, and surgeon's preference and experience
8. Obliteration of all residual cavities and reinforcement of suture lines, when needed, with muscle flaps
9. Reestablishment of skeletal stability and abdominal fascial continuity
10. Meticulous surgical techniques, hemostasis, judicious placement of drains, and tension-free closure

COOPERATION WITH THE PRIMARY SURGEON

Successful management of patients with complex and sometimes life-threatening defects of the trunk requires close cooperation between the plastic surgeon and the referring primary surgeon. In most instances, a team approach is extremely beneficial, because the talent, knowledge, and expertise of each surgeon is used to address the multiple surgical and systemic problems of each patient.

In some extreme situations, the plastic surgeon will be called upon to manage a surgical emergency in the operating room without previous knowledge of the patient and without having the opportunity to extensively evaluate the patient, understand the reconstructive requirements, and adequately plan for the reconstruction. In all other cases, however, close cooperation, joint evaluation, and extensive planning are necessary to provide successful solutions to very difficult surgical problems and reduce the incidence of complications. For example, when consulted to manage a patient who developed an infected median sternotomy after cardiac surgery, the plastic surgeon should have detailed knowledge about the patency of the internal mammary artery(s), whether one or both arteries were used as bypass conduit(s), and whether the internal mammary artery was injured or ligated during previous debridements. Such knowledge is imperative for planning the appropriate reconstructive procedure and for excluding some flaps or flap designs, such as a turnover pectoralis major muscle flap, from the list of options available for the reconstruction. Furthermore, part of the debridement should be performed by the cardiac surgeon who is familiar with the position of bypass grafts and suture lines on the heart and who will be able to manage rare but potential complications of cardiac bleeding or even rupture of the cardiac wall during the debridement. The presence of the primary specialist not only will result in a more extensive debridement of all necrotic tissues before the reconstruction, but also will enable immediate management of the potential complications of debridement and simultaneous management of complex problems. For all these reasons, the team approach is highly recommended in the management of complex defects of the trunk.

The patient shown in Fig. 41-1 represents successful management of this type of complication through a team approach (4). During the mediastinal debridement, a necrotic area on the right ventricular wall ruptured and led to massive bleeding. Hemostasis was obtained with a Foley

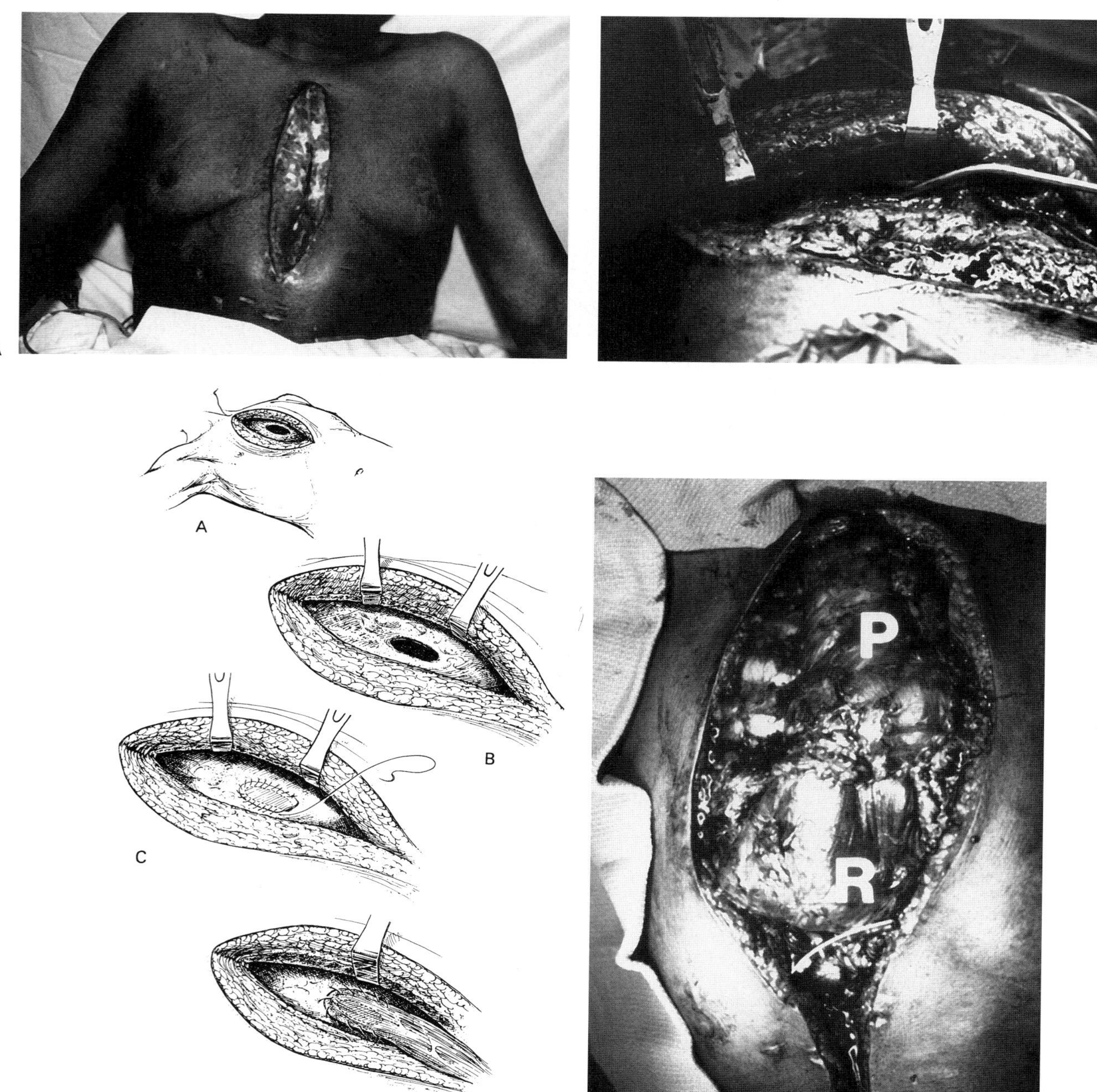

FIGURE 41-1. A: Chest wound 4 weeks after bypass surgery. **B:** Defect of right ventricle (suction tip indicating the defect of the right ventricular free wall). **C:** Cardiac defect was closed with a fascia lata graft and reinforced with a right rectus abdominis muscle flap. (From Cohen M, Marschall MA, Goldfaden D, et al. Repair of right ventricular free wall defect with a pedicled muscle flap. *Ann Thorac Surg* 1987;44:651–652, with permission.) **D:** Turnover pectoralis major muscle was used to fully obliterate the mediastinum. (*continued*)

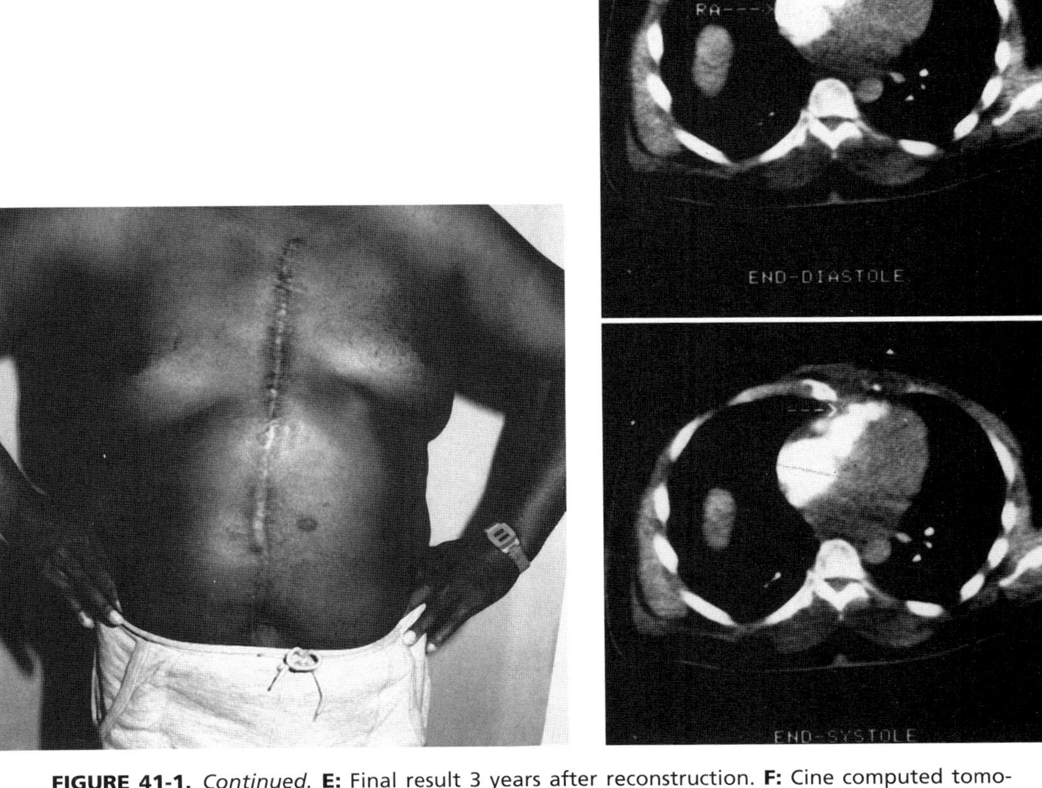

FIGURE 41-1. *Continued.* **E:** Final result 3 years after reconstruction. **F:** Cine computed tomographic scan demonstrating the motion of the right ventricle *(arrow)* without evidence of aneurysm formation and a normal ejection fraction.

catheter and transthoracic mattress sutures that buttressed the ventricular defect against the chest wall. After stabilization, the cardiac and mediastinal wounds were closed simultaneously. The patient was placed on cardiopulmonary bypass, and the cardiac defect was debrided further to healthy myocardium. At that point, the defect measured 6 cm in diameter and could not be closed primarily. To avoid using synthetic material in a heavily contaminated field, a piece of fascia lata was harvested and sutured around the cardiac defect. A right rectus abdominis muscle was harvested and sutured over the patch around the healthy myocardium to further secure the suture line and obliterate the dead space in the lower mediastinum. Finally, the right pectoralis major muscle was mobilized based on perforators of the internal mammary artery to fully obliterate the superior mediastinal cavity. The patient's postoperative course was uneventful. A cine computed tomographic scan obtained several months after the reconstructive procedure demonstrated motion of the right ventricular free wall with normal ejection function and no evidence of pseudoaneurysm around the repaired area.

TIMING OF THE PROCEDURE

Timing of the reconstructive procedure is important to a successful outcome. When dealing with acute infections after cardiac, thoracic, abdominal, or vascular procedures, every effort should be made to drain the purulent collection, debride all necrotic tissues, and administer culture-specific antibiotics systemically as soon as the infection is recognized. A high index of suspicion is necessary to diagnose early an infection and treat it appropriately, even before symptoms and signs of a postoperative infection become clear. Some patients present initially with only vague symptoms and signs, such as low-grade fever, malaise, leukocytosis, pleural effusion, local tenderness, or minimal drainage from the suture line. Significant drainage from the wound, fluctuation, cellulitis, sepsis, ileus, and other signs of infection might be absent in the early stages. Appropriate action should be taken as soon as the diagnosis of an infection is made. Such early intervention and management will reduce the risk for extensive tissue infection and destructive colonization or infection in vascular suture lines, which could result in graft thrombosis, pseudoaneurysms, rupture, and bleeding. Sepsis, such as mediastinitis or peritonitis, which is more difficult to control and might even jeopardize the patient's life, can be prevented with early intervention.

I favor immediate coverage of the debrided wound with appropriate flaps, if the infection is recognized and treated early. If the area is grossly contaminated, there is a large purulent collection, or the patient is unstable due to uncontrolled sepsis or other medical conditions, the wound should be left open after the debridement and drainage of all purulent collections, packed with saline-soaked gauzes, and closed a few days later when the appearance of the wound has improved or when the patient's general condition permits.

Immediate reconstruction is indicated for the majority of defects resulting from tumor extirpation or excision of radionecrotic areas (5,6). On the other hand, patients presenting with complex penetrating injuries to the abdomen or other abdominal catastrophes who require lengthy abdominal procedures and large volumes of resuscitation, which result in significant swelling of the bowel, or patients with significant losses of the anterior abdominal wall caused by various infections might be considered candidates for staged abdominal wall reconstruction (7). Any attempt to

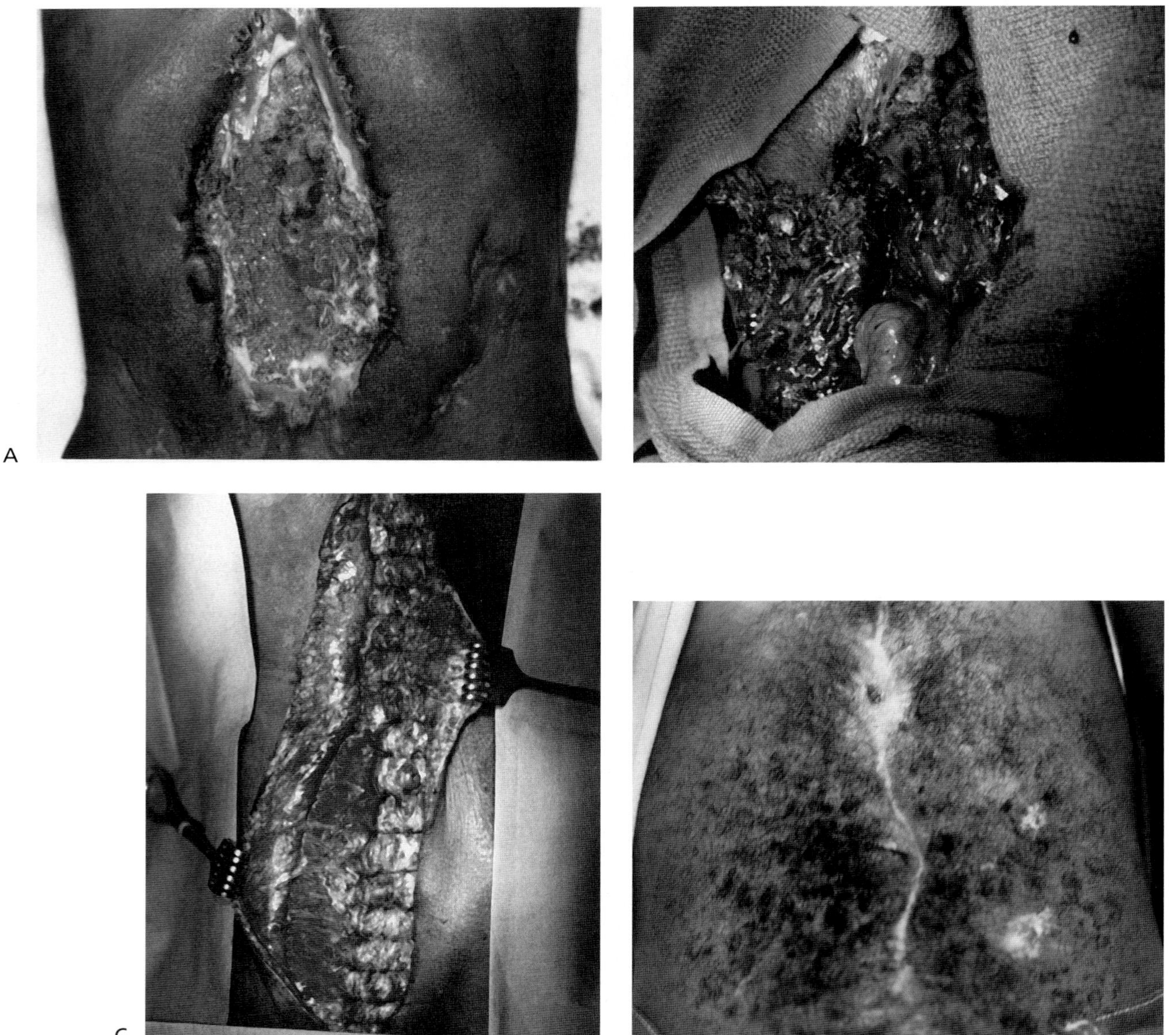

FIGURE 41-2. A: Enteric fistula after temporary closure of the abdomen with a synthetic mesh. **B:** After debridement of the wound and removal of the mesh, the fistula was repaired by the General Surgery Service. **C:** Layered closure was achieved using the component reparation technique. **D:** Final result 9 months after reconstruction.

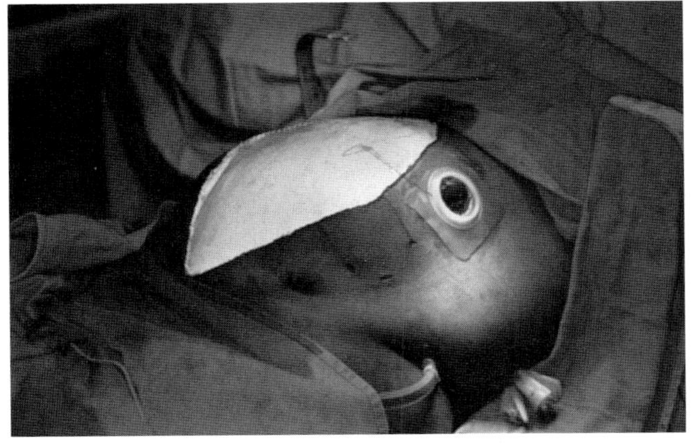
A

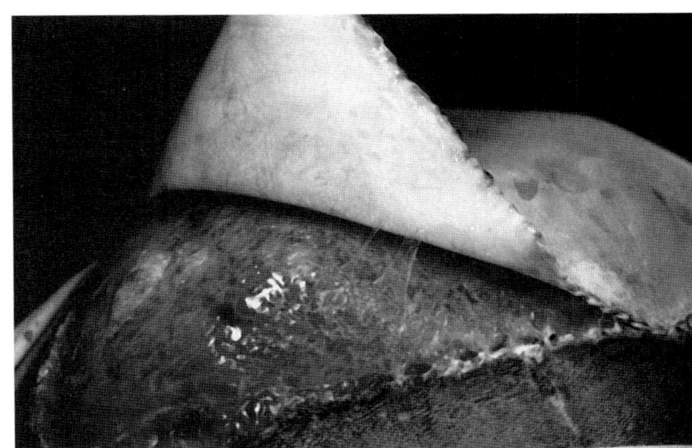
B

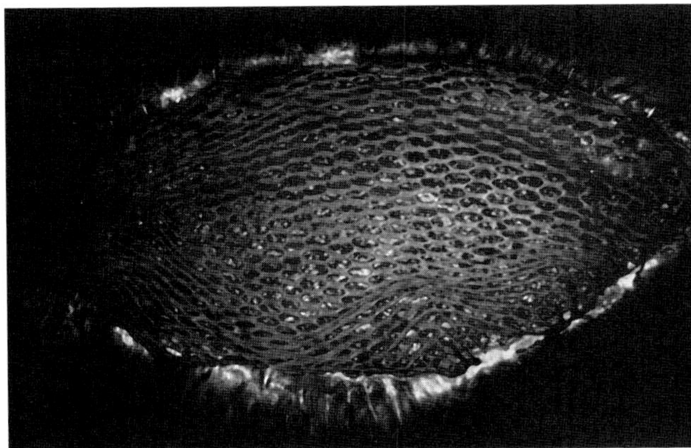
C

FIGURE 41-3. A: Temporary coverage of abdominal wound with Gore-Tex patch at the time of initial intervention. **B:** Removal of the Gore-Tex patch 10 days later reveals a smooth granulating layer over the abdominal viscera. **C:** Due to persistent distension of the bowel and the patient's poor general condition. Split-thickness skin graft was used to provide temporary coverage.

close the abdomen under tension might result in complications ranging from wound dehiscence, infection, and tissue necrosis to the abdominal compartment syndrome, with significant impact to their cardiovascular, respiratory, and renal systems (8). Polypropylene mesh (Marlex or Prolene) has been recommended for temporary coverage of abdominal wounds. Some authors demonstrated subsequent coverage of the granulation tissue over the mesh with split-thickness skin grafts, or local, regional, or distant flaps. The short-term results from coverage of synthetic meshes with split-thickness skin grafts have been reasonably good. The long-term results from this technique, however, have not proved uniformly successful. A high rate of failure with mesh extrusion a few months after the reconstruction has been reported (9). Furthermore, the rate of complications associated with this technique is relatively high and range from infection to enteric fistulae (Fig. 41-2). For these reasons, I favor staged abdominal wall reconstruction when closure of the abdominal cavity or immediate reconstruction is not deemed appropriate (10). The wound initially is covered with saline-soaked gauzes or a Gore-Tex patch to provide coverage and reduce the risk of dryness of the bowel. One week to 10 days later, a split-thickness skin graft is applied directly over the exposed viscera to stabilize the wound and to reduce the risk of infection, rupture of anastomosis, fistulae, and excessive loss of fluids and electrolytes (Fig. 41-3). As soon as the patient's condition permits, the surface of the skin graft can be dermabraded or excised and the abdominal wound closed in layers or, if necessary, with flaps (Fig. 41-4).

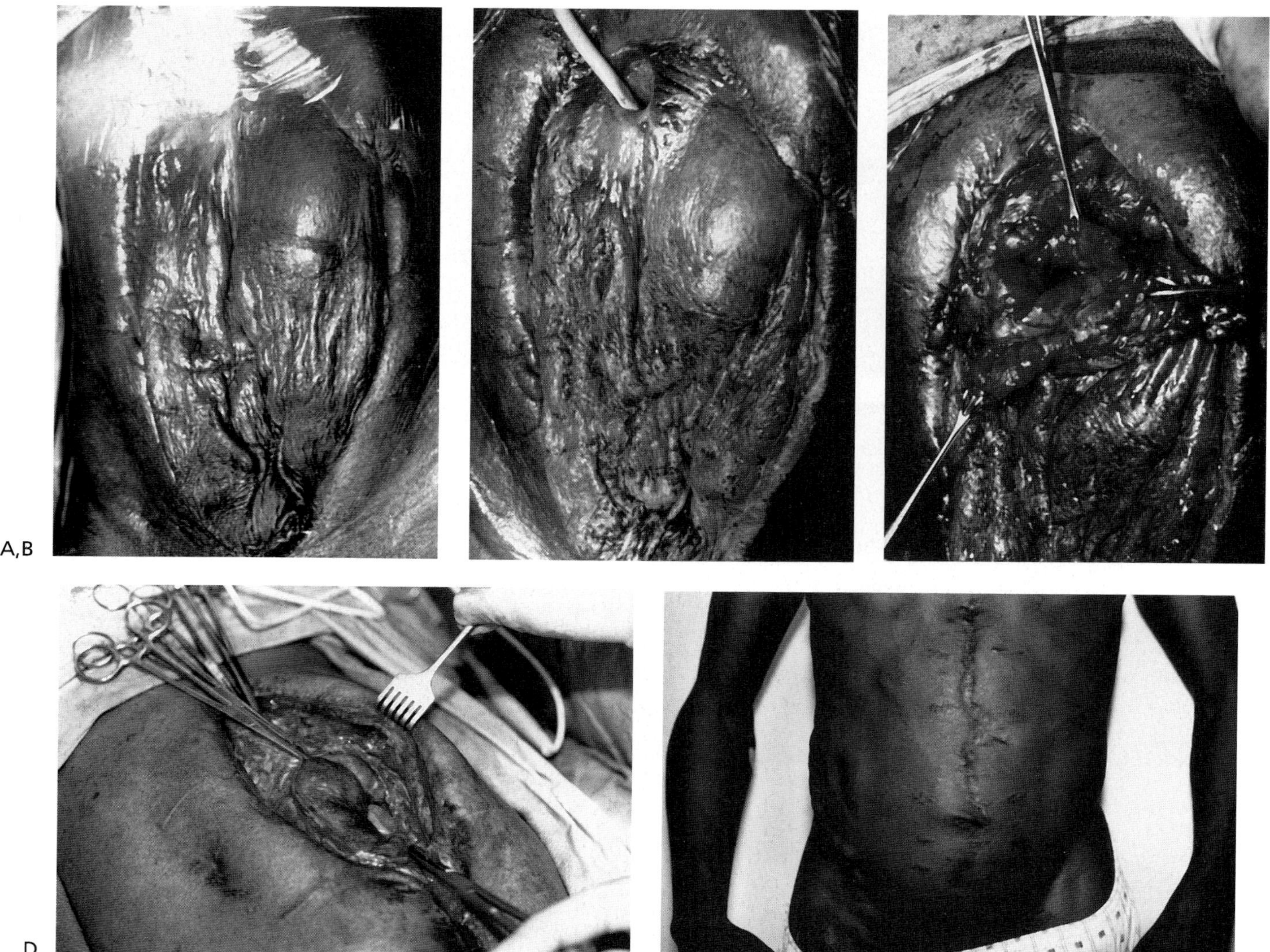

FIGURE 41-4. **A:** Patient 3 months after management of gunshot wound to the abdomen with a split-thickness skin graft over the abdominal viscera. A residual gastric fistula also was present at the time of final reconstruction. **B:** The surface of the skin graft was dermabraded. **C:** The gastric fistula was repaired by the trauma service, and the abdomen was closed in layers using the component separation technique. **D,E:** Final result 16 months after reconstruction. The patient maintains good abdominal tone without evidence of hernia or bulging.

WOUND PREPARATION

Adequate wound preparation is a major prerequisite for successful management of acute or chronic infected wounds. This includes control of infection with local wound care and systemic antibiotics, drainage of all purulent collections and loculations, wide debridement, when possible, of all necrotic soft tissue, bone, and cartilage, and removal of all foreign bodies from the wound. Inadequate control of the infection prior to the reconstruction probably will result in partial or complete failure of the reconstructive procedure, disruption of suture lines, tissue necrosis, partial or complete reexposure of vital structures, and possibly generalized sepsis. These conditions might have significant impact on already debilitated patients and can result in prolonged hospitalization, need for additional wound care, and possibly additional reconstructive procedures to salvage the patients and achieve stable wound coverage (11,12).

Wound infection and dehiscence after a major reconstructive procedure should be managed aggressively, particularly in the presence of additional purulent collection, tissue necrosis, generalized sepsis, or exposure of vital structures. Control of sepsis should include local wound care, drainage of purulent collections, and administration of systemic antibiotics. If such a condition is recognized early, then after debridement and control of infection, some flaps

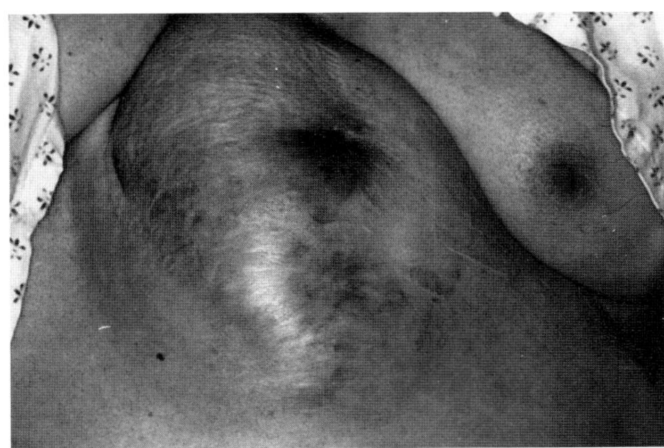
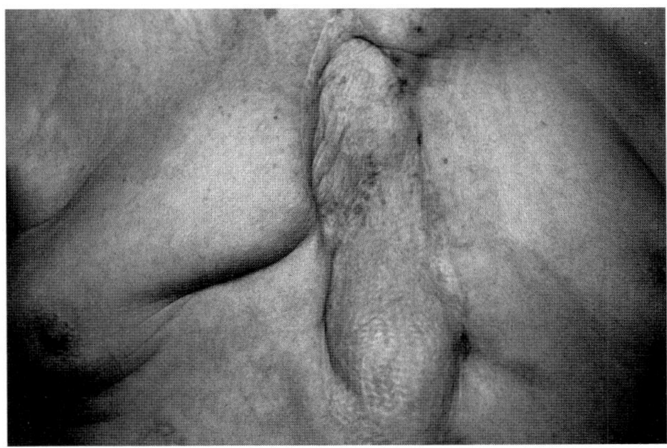

FIGURE 41-5. A: Recurrent infection and purulent collection after debridement and reconstruction of an infected median sternotomy. **B:** Following drainage of the collection and additional debridement, a large residual cavity was created. The previously used pectoralis major muscles could not be mobilized further to provide adequate obliteration of residual cavity. A rectus abdominis musculocutaneous flap was used to provide obliteration and coverage. Final view 1 year after the reconstruction.

can be salvaged and reused to fully obliterate and cover the defect. When this is not possible, additional flaps must be used to achieve full obliteration of residual space, coverage of exposed vital structures, and wound coverage (Fig. 41-5).

In contrast, superficial tissue loss due to persistent local infection can be managed conservatively with wound care and local debridement. Small wounds can be allowed to heal secondarily. Larger wounds will require definitive coverage, when the patient's condition permits, with split-thickness skin grafts or local flaps (Fig. 41-6).

Residual osteomyelitis or costochondritis could result from inadequate debridement or recurrent infection, which could lead to partial or complete disruption of the suture line or persistent draining sinuses over the area of infection. As soon as residual osteomyelitis or costochondritis is diagnosed, a treatment plan should be established. Appropriate systemic antibiotic therapy should be instituted based on wound cultures. Before exploration and definitive surgical treatment, a computerized tomographic scan is recommended to assist in the full evaluation of the extent of the cartilaginous or bony involvement and identification of potential residual locations within the mediastinum or chest. Sinograms could be of some help when dealing with chronic sinuses.

Before the debridement, I like to inject diluted methylene blue and peroxide within the sinus tract. This technique assists in the identification and debridement of all scarred and involved tissues around the sinus. Extensive clinical evaluation during the time of exploration, however, might reveal the presence of additional tissues involved in the infectious process. Radical debridement of all involved costal cartilages and bone is indicated to treat the problem. The subsequent residual cavity shall be obliterated either by readvancement of the previously used muscle flap(s) or with an additional flap (Fig. 41-7).

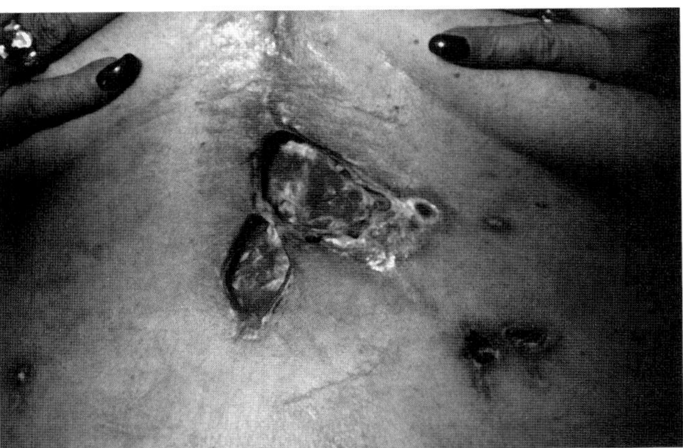
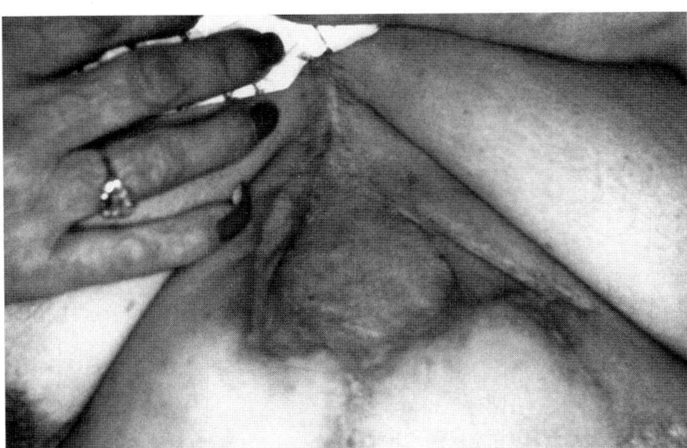

FIGURE 41-6. A: Superficial tissue loss after reconstruction for infected medial sternotomy. **B:** After adequate debridement, a split-thickness skin graft was used to provide stable coverage.

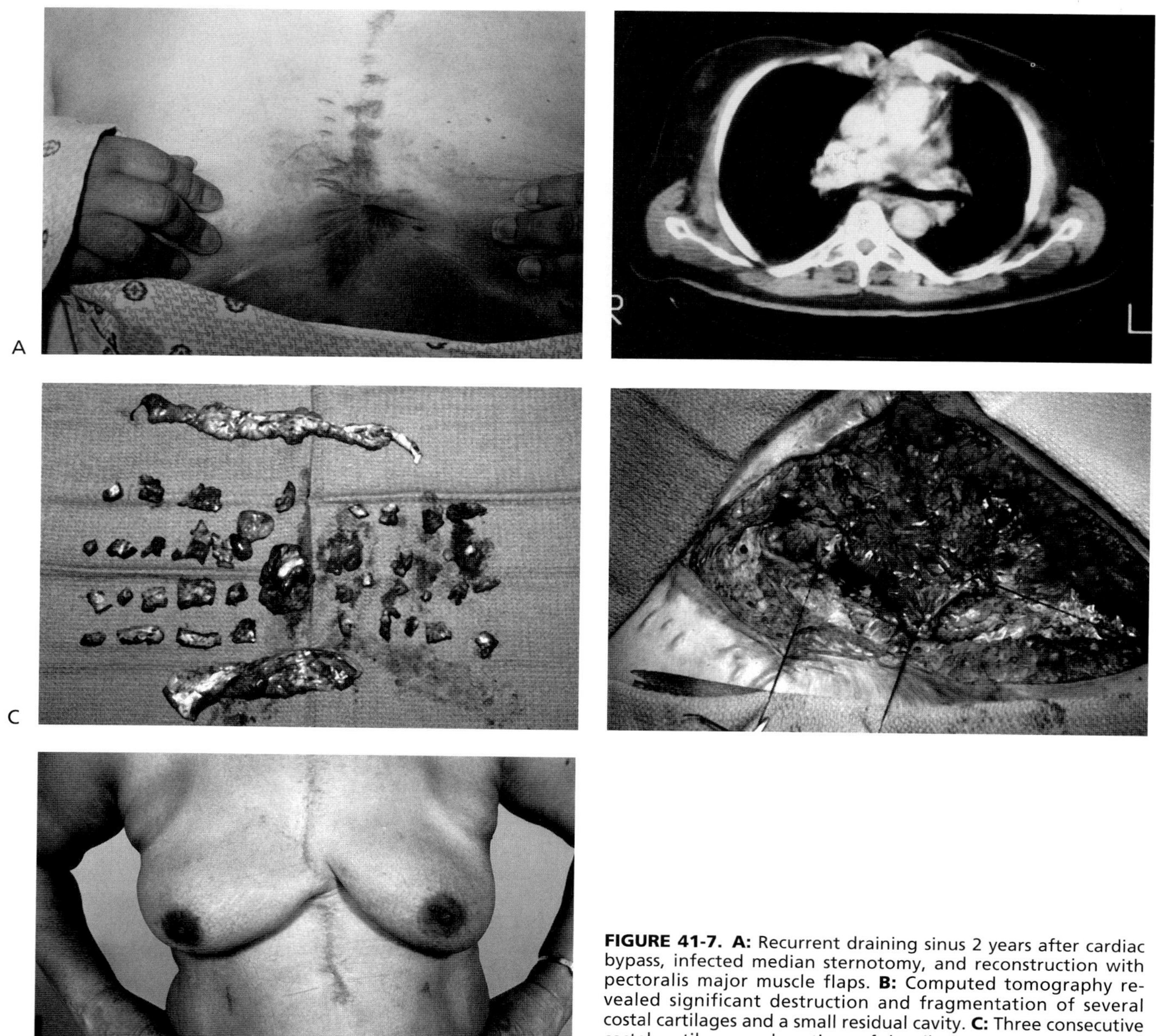

FIGURE 41-7. A: Recurrent draining sinus 2 years after cardiac bypass, infected median sternotomy, and reconstruction with pectoralis major muscle flaps. **B:** Computed tomography revealed significant destruction and fragmentation of several costal cartilages and a small residual cavity. **C:** Three consecutive costal cartilages and portions of the ribs were debrided. **D:** The subsequent defect was covered by readvancing the left pectoralis major muscle flap. **E:** Final result 2 years after reconstruction.

Chronically exposed meshes could be heavily colonized and must be removed or replaced before the definitive reconstructive procedure. The patient shown in Fig. 41-8 had temporary coverage of the abdominal wall using a Marlex mesh after complications of abdominal procedures. Inadequate debridement of the mesh prior to wound coverage with a tensor fascia lata flap resulted in infection, partial loss of the distal portion of the flap, and some mesh exposure. Retrospectively, this patient should have undergone complete removal of the infected mesh prior to the reconstruction.

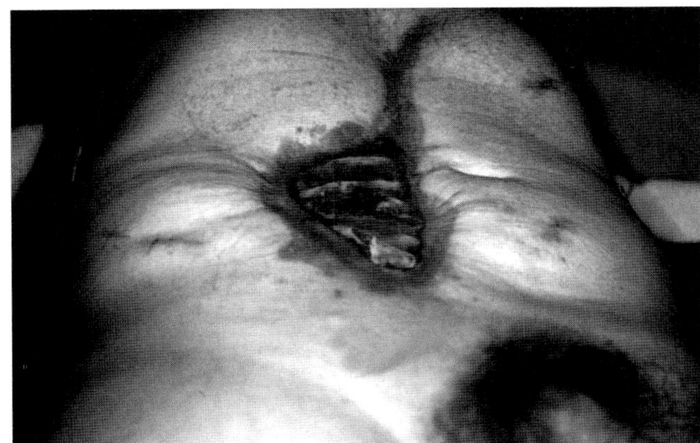

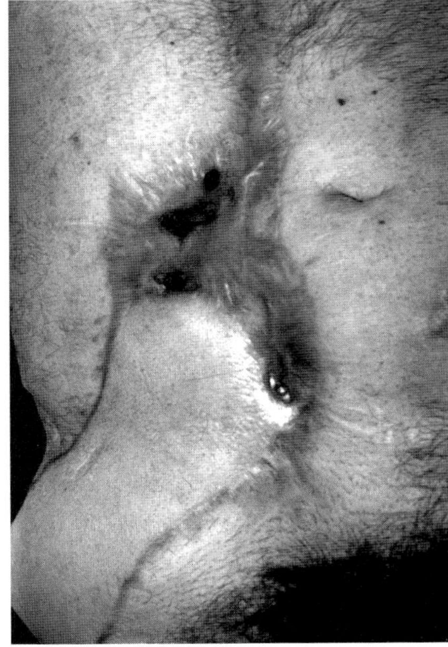

FIGURE 41-8. A: Infected Marlex mesh after multiple abdominal procedures. **B:** The wound was covered with a tensor fascia lata flap. Several weeks after reconstruction, an infection developed around the distal portion of the flap and resulted in partial loss of the flap and small mesh exposure.

PLANNING FLAP SELECTION: SURGICAL TECHNIQUE

Meticulous planning is extremely important before any reconstructive procedure. Planning is even more important for procedures in the chest wall, back, and abdomen because, in many instances, as mentioned earlier, the surgeon is dealing with debilitated patients with complex medical problems. Thus, the margin of error is virtually nonexistent, and every effort should be made to achieve the best possible result in one setting.

Placement of incisions, particularly on the abdominal wall, requires special attention. Most patients present with one or several scars from previous interventions that have deprived the abdominal wall of part of its vascular supply. Every effort should be made to avoid placing incisions parallel or across previous scars, because this practice might jeopardize the vascularity of the involved areas of the abdominal wall and can result in a dehiscence or tissue necrosis.

The patient shown in Fig. 41-9 presents with such a complication. He underwent multiple abdominal procedures through several incisions and was referred with a large ventral hernia and tissue loss between the "railroad track" parallel abdominal wall incisions. The entire bridge of unstable tissue between these scars had to be excised, the hernia was reduced, and the fascial defect was reinforced with a Gore-Tex patch. The overlying skin was closed under no tension after minimal undermining. More than 1 year after the reconstruction, the patient remains well, with a healed, stable abdominal scar and no evidence of recurrence of the ventral hernia.

Several flaps are available for reconstruction of defects in the anterior chest wall, back, and abdomen. Over the last 20 years, specific indications for flap selection have been established based on the location and size of a given defect. Before deciding on the use of a specific flap, the surgeon should thoroughly evaluate the patient, understand the functional and aesthetic requirement of the area, and plan the reconstructive procedure accordingly. Selection of the muscle that will result in the smallest possible functional deficit also is important (13,14).

Scars on the chest wall, abdomen, and lower extremities or across muscles, musculocutaneous units, or their vascular pedicles may preclude the use of some muscles and dictate another flap selection. A history of previous abdominal intervention, particularly for peritonitis, might preclude the use of the greater omentum. The final decision for flap selection should be made at the time of the operation, after complete debridement of the wound and full evaluation of the three-dimensional size of the defect. The surgeon should be familiar with the functional requirements of each anatomic area and plan the reconstruction in such a way to restore, as close as possible, the function of the area along with wound coverage.

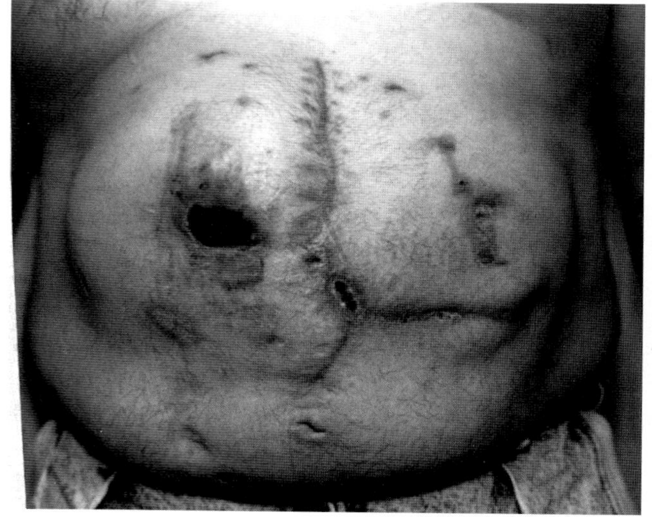

A

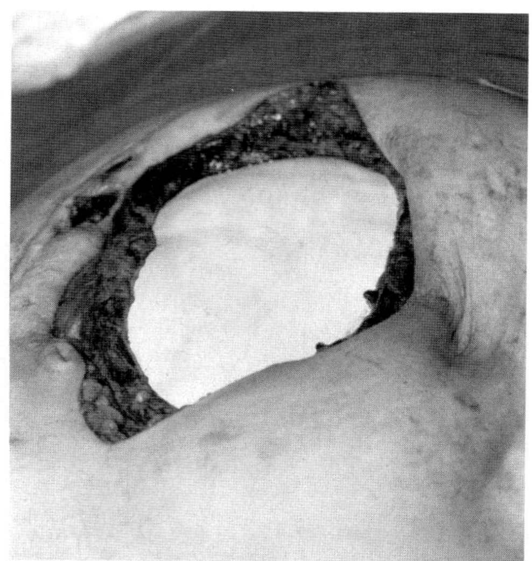

B

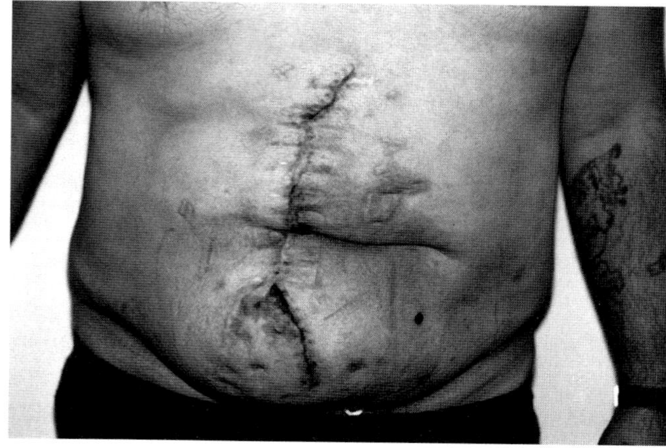

C

FIGURE 41-9. A: Recurrent abdominal wall hernia and tissue loss following multiple abdominal procedures. **B:** After extensive debridement, a Gore-Tex patch was used to provide fascial continuity and stability. **C:** Final result after reconstruction. There is a stable scar and no evidence of ventral hernia recurrence.

In some instances, structural defects of the bony framework of the thorax need to be addressed simultaneously. The decision for bony reconstruction depends not only on the location and size of the defect, but also on the patient's respiratory reserves and the presence or absence of active infection. There is no consensus in the literature regarding the type, location, and size of the skeletal defects that absolutely need to be reconstructed to reestablish bony continuity and stability, prevent paradoxic respiration, and preserve pulmonary and cardiac function (15). As a rule, bone grafts and prosthetic materials are strongly contraindicated in the presence of an active infection (2). For example, bony defects of the manubrium and the sternoclavicular joint following on-block resection of a malignant tumor can be stabilized immediately with bone grafts or synthetic material before soft tissue coverage with muscle flaps is undertaken. Midline defects following sternal debridement for infected median sternotomy, however, should be covered with flaps only; they remain relatively stable because of adhesions within the mediastinum. The location and size of the bony defect also should be taken into consideration before skeletal reconstruction. Acute defects in the lateral thorax over three to four ribs should be stabilized with synthetic material. Defects after resection of radionecrotic tissues do not normally require stabilization due to the presence of adhesions and fibrosis between the lung and the thoracic cavity. Upper and posterior defects usually do not require bony reconstruction, because the scapula and the surrounding soft tissue provide the necessary support (2).

Structural defects of the abdominal wall need to be managed, and the continuity of the abdominal musculofascial system should be taken into consideration and reestablished, when possible. One must understand how the intact musculofascial system of the abdominal wall interacts with the muscles of the back to maintain body balance and participate in various movements of the trunk. One also must understand important body functions such as breathing, defecation, micturition, vomiting, coughing, and childbirth. Detailed knowledge of the vascular anatomy and the innervation of the muscles of the abdominal wall is necessary to design the best possible reconstructive procedure.

When adequate tissues are available for the reconstruction, immediate approximation is recommended. For medium-size abdominal defects without significant tissue loss, the components separation technique as described by Ramirez et al. (16) is suggested. This technique is based on detailed understanding of the various planes between the muscle and fascia of the anterior abdominal wall and the location of the branches of the six lower intercostal nerves between the internal oblique and the transversus abdominis muscles. The rectus abdominis muscle with its overlying fascia are separated from the underlying posterior rectus sheath and mobilized medially along with the attached internal oblique and transversus abdominis muscles. A relaxing incision of the anterior rectus sheath fascia is necessary, along with dissection between the external and internal oblique muscle plane, to achieve adequate mobilization

In my experience, midabdominal defects up to 15 cm in the horizontal dimension can be closed with this technique without tension. Functional reconstruction is achieved along with wound closure. If excess tension is recognized during closure, the surgeon should not hesitate to reinforce the abdominal wall with a synthetic mesh or patch to avoid hernia formation. A synthetic mesh or patch or an autologous fascia lata graft also should be used to reestablish fascial continuity when inadequate musculofascial tissues make closure impossible, as long as adequate skin is available for coverage. If adequate skin is not available, then coverage should be achieved with a pedicled or even a free flap. In most instances, there is no need for structural reinforcement with synthetic material when flaps are used. This decision, however, should be based on the size and location of the defect and the quality of surrounding tissues.

Meticulous surgical techniques of reconstruction include a flap design that can reach the defect without tension or torsion of the vascular pedicle. All dead spaces should be obliterated by the flap. When necessary, a combination of flaps should be used to achieve the reconstructive goals. Before inserting the flap(s), meticulous hemostasis should be carried out in both the recipient and donor sites, and all wounds should be copiously irrigated with an antibiotic solution. Flaps should be inset with multiple absorbable sutures. Appropriate drains should be placed under all areas of dissection in both the recipient and donor sites and in the mediastinum or the thoracic cavities, when indicated.

Total flap necrosis is an extremely rare complication of reconstructive procedures in the trunk. It is attributed primarily to technical errors, accidental division of the pedicle, vascular spasm, torsion during flap inset, or, in some instances, poor perfusion. It is possible to salvage a flap if such condition is recognized early, particularly when perfusion to the flap is disturbed by torsion of the vascular pedicle, spasm, or tension in the suture line. On the other hand, progressive flap loss should be managed aggressively as soon as possible with wound care and a new flap harvesting that will provide stable coverage and assist in the prevention of further complications.

Hematomas and seromas are not uncommon and have been reported in approximately 5% to 20% of cases. Meticulous hemostasis is of cardinal importance in the prevention of hematomas. Small seromas can be treated conservatively with aspiration. Recurrent seromas, particularly in the donor site of the latissimus dorsi muscle, can be difficult to eradicate because a pseudocapsule will form around the seroma within a couple of weeks. Drainage with insertion of a drain should be the first step for treatment of large seromas. Some authors have recommended the use of fibrin glue, talcum powder, or even quilting to obliterate the dead space and prevent seroma formation. In the majority of cases, timely management results in resolution of the problem and does not further affect the length of hospitalization or final outcome.

Donor site anatomy should be normalized, when possible. For instance, defects of the anterior rectus sheath fascia after harvesting of the rectus abdominis musculocutaneous flap should be repaired to reestablish fascial continuity and prevent significant postoperative bulging of the abdominal wall or even a hernia. Finally, overlying skin should be closed under no tension to prevent ischemia and possible tissue necrosis. If primary skin closure without tension cannot be achieved, a split-thickness skin graft should be applied over the raw surfaces to facilitate immediate coverage and timely healing.

OUTCOME OF RECONSTRUCTION OF THORACIC DEFECTS

Accumulated experience and better understanding of the pathophysiology of various conditions, the anatomical and physiologic requirements of each area, and the reconstructive options have enabled us to achieve consistently successful results in the majority of conditions such as infected median sternotomy, chest wall reconstruction after tumor extirpation and excision of radionecrosis, back reconstruction, and abdominal wall reconstruction. (5,6,11,13).

Short-term outcome for reconstructive procedures to correct these conditions has been well described. Unfortunately, there still is a lack of information on the long-term results and the final functional outcome of these procedures. The long-term donor site morbidity is not always clear, and the time frame necessary for the patient to return to preoperative functions is not always defined. Furthermore, functional loss from the use of various muscle units for reconstructive purposes is not well defined. Functional outcomes are supported by subjective references, but little objective data are available (17). Pairolero et al. (18) reported a 37% incidence of pain after transposition of the pectoralis major muscle for infected sternotomy wounds. The pain generally was always present, made worse by activity, and usually not relieved by analgesics or other pain clinic techniques. Ringelman et al. (19) reported a 51% postoperative incidence of pain or discomfort located mainly in the central chest and shoulder. Forty-two percent of patients in this study also noticed abnormal motion of the sternal halves. Presumably, this could have been prevented if more aggressive debridement of the sternum was performed. Mobilization of the pectoralis major did not significantly affect shoulder strength, presumably due to the overlapping function of the shoulder girdle muscle and the associated compensation. There was an 11% incidence of hernia formation and a 42% incidence of abdominal weakness or bulging in patients who had abdominally based flaps. These values are significantly higher than the 2.4% and 0.9% rates reported by Nahai et al. (13).

Return to work was approximately the same (50%) as in studies of patients who underwent uncomplicated coronary artery bypass grafting or cardiac transportation. One-third of the patients reported their inability to resume postoperatively the same activities they had enjoyed preoperatively.

Because some patients suffer from various medical conditions affecting their daily activities, it is difficult to attribute a direct percentage of their disability due to the reconstructive procedure. On the other hand, donor site complications and weakness from loss of muscular units, such as abdominal wall hernias or bulges after use of the rectus abdominis muscle, should always be taken into consideration when selecting a flap for reconstructive purposes. When options are available, preference should be given to the flap(s) that will result in the least functional deficit while having a high possibility from a successful reconstruction.

CONCLUSIONS

Reconstruction of defects in the trunk requires close cooperation between the plastic surgeon and the referring primary surgeon. Some of these patients present with life-threatening emergencies, whereas others suffer from several complex medical conditions. The margin of error is very small, and every effort should be made to plan the reconstructive procedures well and in a timely fashion, adhere to the basic reconstructive principles, and select the appropriate flap(s) that will provide for successful coverage and reconstruction with the least donor site morbidity.

REFERENCES

1. Arnold PG, Pairolero PC. Intrathoracic muscle flaps: a 10-year experience in the management of life-threatening infections. *Plast Reconstr Surg* 1989;84:92–98.
2. Cohen M. Reconstruction of the chest wall. In: Cohen M, ed. *Mastery of plastic and reconstructive surgery.* Boston: Little, Brown and Company, 1994:1248–1267.
3. Cohen M, Marschall MA. Reconstruction for infected and dehisced median sternotomy. *Probl Gen Surg* 1989;6:585–601.
4. Cohen M, Marschall MA, Goldfaden DM, et al. Repair of ventricular free wall defect with pedicled muscle flaps. *Ann Thorac Surg* 1987;44:651–652.
5. Arnold PG, Pairolero PC. Chest wall reconstruction: experience with 100 consecutive patients. *Ann Surg* 1984;199:725–732.
6. Bostwick J III, Hill LH, Nahai F. Repairs in the lower abdomen, groin or perineum with myocutaneous or omental flaps. *Plast Reconstr Surg* 1979;63:186–194.
7. Fabian TC, Croce MA, Prichard EF, et al. Planned ventral hernia. Staged management for acute abdominal wall defects. *Ann Surg* 1994;219:643–653.
8. Eddy V, Nunn G, Morris JA Jr. Abdominal compartment syndrome. The Nashville experience. *Surg Clin North Am* 1997;77:801–812.
9. Voyles CR, Richardson PJ, Bland KI, et al. Emergency abdominal wall reconstruction with polypropylene mesh: short-term benefits versus long-term complications. *Ann Surg* 1981;194:219–223.
10. Cohen M, Ramasastry S. Abdominal wall reconstruction: experience with 218 patients. *Plast Surg Forum* 1999;XXII:160–163.
11. Cohen M, Ramasastry SS. Reconstruction of complex chest wall defects. *Am J Surg* 1996;172:35–40.
12. Core GB, Grotting JC. Reoperative surgery of the abdominal wall. In: Grotting JC, ed. *Reoperative aesthetic and reconstructive plastic surgery, vol. 2.* St. Louis: Quality Medical Publishing, 1995:1325–1375.
13. Nahai F, Rand RPF, Hester RT, et al. Primary treatment of the infected sternotomy wound with muscle flaps. A review of 211 consecutive cases. *Plast Reconstr Surg* 1989;84:434–441.
14. Stahl PS, Koff GS. Preoperative surgery of chest wall. In: Grotting JC, ed. *Preoperative aesthetic and reconstructive plastic surgery, vol. 2.* St. Louis: Quality Medical Publishing, 1995:1207–1279.
15. Gaeber GM, Seyfer AE. Complications of chest wall resection and the management of flail chest. In: Waldhausen JA, Orringer MB, eds. *Complications of cardiothoracic surgery.* St. Louis: Mosby-Year Book, 1991:413–421.
16. Ramirez OM, Ruas E, Dillon AL. Components separation method for closure of abdominal wall defects: an anatomic and clinical study. *Plast Reconstr Surg* 1990;86:519.
17. Fraulin FOG, Gormon L, Zorrilla L, et al. Functional evaluation of the shoulder following latissimus dorsi muscle transfer. *Ann Plast Surg* 1995;35:349–355.
18. Pairolero PC, Arnold PG, Harris JB. Long-term results of pectoralis major muscle transposition for infected sternotomy wounds. *Ann Surg* 1991;213:583–590.
19. Ringelman PR, VanderKolk CA, Cameron P, et al. Long-term results of flap reconstruction in median sternotomy wound infection. *Plast Reconstr Surg* 1994;93:1208–1216.

Discussion

CHEST AND ABDOMINAL WALL RECONSTRUCTION

CRAIG H. JOHNSON
PHILLIP G. ARNOLD

Reconstruction of the human trunk continues to provide unique challenges to the plastic surgeon. Some of the difficulties reside in the unique combination of physiologic function, aesthetic issues, and the structural contribution of the chest wall to the overall upright nature of the human body. The wide variety of etiologies and indications that brings patients to the point of chest wall and abdominal wall reconstruction also contributes greatly to the complexity and detail required to achieve a successful outcome. Toward that end, at our institution we continue to feel that a multispecialty team approach is imperative to the generation of a successful outcome and a safe return of the patient to the best possible overall health. The plastic surgeon works in concert with the thoracic surgeon, together providing the unique set of skills to manage these difficult problems.

CHEST RECONSTRUCTION

The reconstruction of the chest generally can be divided into the chest wall, the sternal region, and the intrathoracic contents. Indications for chest wall reconstruction in our practice are very similar to those cited: trauma, tumor (primary or recurrent), infection, and radiation injury. In our experience, 25% of patients have a combination of these indications (1).

It generally is agreed that the critical first step in the management of chest wall problems is in the initial resection or debridement. It must be thorough and complete. Even the most elegant of reconstructions is doomed to fail in the face of inadequate resection or debridement. Complete eradication is aided by the team approach. The plastic surgeon and thoracic surgeon, together, use a strategy of resecting to the limits of vascularized tissue coverage available.

When the defect encompasses three to four ribs or more, our preferred method of chest wall reconstruction currently uses 2-mm thin Gore-Tex patches. We find the stability that can be achieved when the patch is sewn in a tight circumferential fashion, creating an almost trampoline-like effect, negates the need for rib grafting or methylmethacrylate sandwiches. When covered with vascularized tissue, such as a myocutaneous flap, it provides durable support. We personally have been disappointed with our own experience in the use of the methylmethacrylate construct, including difficulties with infection and a rather challenging surgical task for removal should it become necessary in the postoperative complicated wound. Prolene mesh would be a second choice, but Marlex mesh continues to be looked upon with disfavor due to its fragmentation and stranding in the postoperative complicated wound. Recent reviews at our institution showed that the most common rib resection usually resulted in the loss of four ribs (2). Most of these patients have not undergone reconstruction with skeletal support, but rather have been reconstructed with Gore-Tex patch.

Sternal reconstruction for infection or radiation necrosis continues to be best managed with adherence to the principles of thorough surgical debridement and a prolonged course of dressing changes, followed by transposition of muscle flaps, most often the pectoralis major musculature advanced to midline and based on the thoracoacromial vascular leash as a primary principle of management. Structural stability often is maintained by the fibrosis induced by radiation or the significant scarring induced by infection, such that we find no need for rigid stabilization. We find midline advancement based on the thoracoacromial perfusion most beneficial, as this musculature reconstruction can be divided again in the midline should reentry to the mediastinum be necessary, such as in the case of redo coronary artery bypass (3). Many times the internal mammary perfusion has been used in previous coronary procedures or has been debrided during the course of removal of a very thorough sternectomy so that modifications, such as pectoralis major turnover flaps, are not possible or practical.

We use caution in evaluating the various reports in the literature regarding sternal infection. There is a significant difference between the wound that develops serous sanguinous drainage within the first 5 to 7 days postoperatively, and the wound that has dehisced between 7 and 21 days postoperatively, and the wound that has a draining sinus

C. H. Johnson and P. G. Arnold: Department of Plastic Surgery, Mayo Clinic, Rochester, Minnesota

tract and evidence of frank osteomyelitis on a computed tomographic scan 6 months after surgery.

At our institution, we most often apply omental transposition as our backup, secondary, or rescue plan. However, omentum is a first choice for us in certain circumstances, such as radiation necrosis of the chest wall. This often occurs in the area of the anterior chest wall and, at times, may involve portions of the sternum. The ability to mold and shape the omentum, allowing for contouring, gives the omentum particular aesthetic appeal. We usually wait 48 to 72 hours for final split-thickness skin grafting, to generate a healthy granulation bed, ensuring full skin graft take. We have not found a preponderance of need nor a good solution for the structural reconstruction of the sternum. Patient comments in the postoperative period after sternal reconstruction are generally aesthetic in nature rather than functional or physiologic.

Some of the most life-threatening situations can occur with intrathoracic reconstruction issues, especially as it relates to bronchopleural fistula in the management of the bronchial stump. In the preantibiotic era, bronchopleural fistulas were commonly seen as sequelae of pneumonia. Bronchopleural fistula commonly presents today as a postsurgical complication after pulmonary resection for malignancy. We continue to aggressively use intrathoracic muscle transposition, most commonly the serratus anterior, as a means to buttress radiated bronchial stumps, to reinforce bronchial stump closure after bronchopleural fistula management, and in the obliteration of dead space management when closing the pleural space. We deliver the muscle through a separate second thoracotomy via the resected second rib bed. In our own experience, we have found that there is simply inadequate tissue on the human skeleton to provide enough muscle to transpose in an intrathoracic position such that the entire pleural space can be obliterated. As such, once the pleural cavity has been fully and completely cleaned and the bacterial count has been lowered as best as possible, we use a Clagett-type closure with obliteration of the pleural space using an antibiotic impregnated saline solution. Currently we use Dabs solution (1 L of normal saline, 80 mg gentamicin, 500 mg neomycin, and 1 million units of polymyxin B). Care must be taken to ensure that there is no retained air within the pleural space. A cross-table lateral x-ray in the operating room with subcutaneous tissue and skin closed in watertight fashion generally allows one to be certain of complete obliteration. The results of this method of management have been extremely satisfactory, with primary wound healing obtained in greater than 80% of these very difficult to manage wounds (4). We have yet to see the long-term healed wound or long-term survival of those unfortunate patients who have the lethal combination of radiation and fungal infection. These difficult wounds often end up being treated with long-term chronic dressing changes.

The importance of preserving the latissimus dorsi and serratus anterior musculature in the initial thoracotomy incision cannot be overemphasized. This again shows the need for communication in the team approach between the plastic surgeon and the thoracic surgeon.

ABDOMINAL WALL RECONSTRUCTION

Any discussion of resection of the trunk and reconstruction should include management of the diaphragm. Tumors can certainly involve this structure where it may be necessary to release the diaphragm from its normal attachments in order to manage an abdominal or chest wall tumor. Our current practice uses reattachment of the diaphragm above or below its normal attachment if the resection involves this area. This usually can be done without worrying about the innervation and will maintain separation of the abdominal and thoracic cavity and its respective contents.

Some of the most challenging situations we currently face in reconstruction of the abdominal wall include the massive hernial defects developing after intraabdominal catastrophe and difficulty in closing the wound. These, as stated in the foregoing chapter, are best managed in a staged fashion. Use of separation of components works quite well, but we have been personally impressed that defects beyond 10 to 12 cm are stretching the limits of this methodology. When one needs to achieve more than 5 cm per side (10 cm total), we prefer to add other modalities to our armamentarium. We continue to see good results with the use of intraabdominal tissue expanders. Our initial experience placed these in the subcutaneous plane above the external–internal oblique musculature. Computed tomographic scans demonstrated skin expansion as well as intraabdominal recruitment of musculofascial components, and this observation led to our current practice of placing the tissue expanders in a longitudinal fashion beneath the planes of external and internal oblique. This avascular plane allows for easy placement of the tissue expanders, and inflation with 1 to 2 L of fluid provides ample recruitment to manage even the largest hernia defects, including those in the 25-cm transverse diameter range (5).

In Table 41-1, Dr. Cohen provides an excellent framework for those thinking of embarking down the road of trunk reconstruction management. We would add to this table the inclusion of excellent pulmonary care in the postoperative state, provided ideally by a team that manages these problems, ventilators, and the various parameters of the patient on a 24-hour basis. The patient should be placed in an intensive care unit that is appropriately equipped and staffed to deal with the issues that arise from the management of this physiology. Appropriate "nursing surface" also is mandatory, including a Clinitron bed if necessary or a decubitus mattress so that the wound can be appropriately "pampered" while it is healing. This would include meticulous nursing care, which sometimes is not provided and actually can contribute to further postoperative wound difficulties. These topics alone probably have made some of the greatest difference in our success at Mayo Clinic in the management of these difficult trunk wounds.

It is important to emphasize that muscle flaps do not replace common sense and good surgical judgment. One cannot simply close a questionably contaminated wound "early" with a muscle flap and expect that it will result in primary healing every time. Debridement is of paramount importance in having the responsible surgeons look directly at the wound at the time of dressing change and seems to be the most critical part of the decision as to "when to close." In simplified terms, if the gauze dressing that comes out of the wound is green, purulent, or contaminated, it is not time to close the wound. We often have remarked that we do not know the patients in whom we waited too long before embarking on secondary closure, but we do know the patients in whom we closed too early, as the patient makes this wound very obvious in the short-term postoperative period.

REFERENCES

1. Arnold PG, Johnson CH. Chest wall reconstruction. *Surg Oncol Clin North Am* 1997;6:91–114.
2. Arnold PG, Pairolero PC. Chest wall reconstruction: an account of 500 consecutive patients. *Plast Reconstr Surg* 1996;98:5.
3. Arnold PG, Pairolero PC. Intrathoracic muscle flaps: a ten year experience in the management of life threatening infections. *Plast Reconstr Surg* 1989;84:92.
4. Jacobsen WM, Petty PM, Bite U, et al. Massive abdominal wall hernia reconstruction with expanded external/internal oblique and transversalis musculofascia. *Plast Reconstr Surg* 1997;100:326–335.
5. Pairolero PC, Arnold PG. Thoracic wall defects: surgical management of 205 consecutive patients. *Mayo Clin Proc* 1986;61:557.

VII

HAND

42

CONGENITAL ANOMALIES

JOSEPH UPTON
STEPHEN PAP

An unfavorable result (outcome) in a pediatric patient is difficult to determine for a number of reasons. Babies born with congenital upper limb malformations recognize their present condition as normal and may not fully recognize their differences until they are fully socialized. The remarkable plasticity of the cerebral cortex to reprogram the central computer and the adaptive capacity of the very young allow children to easily compensate for anatomical deficiencies (1). Because there are no standardized methods for evaluation of upper limb function in the newborns and young children, documentation of change is difficult.

The long-term effect of growth is the major difference between children and adults. Although one of the surgical goals in young patients is to release potential contractures and to allow unrestricted growth, the effect of growth and progression of a deformity may not be obvious initially. When significant growth is anticipated, parents must always be advised that additional correction may be needed for their child's limb malformation. For example, the presence of a longitudinal epiphyseal bracket (LEB) along a proximal phalanx in an Apert thumb or a central synpolydactyly (SPD) may not be initially obvious. Continued growth may result in a progressive deformity. Early release of the LEB may not protect the finger or thumb from future angulation or rotational deformity. Unnecessary dissection and partial devascularization of the distal ulna during a centralization procedure may further restrict growth of an already compromised forearm bone. The deforming force of a scar following a syndactyly release or strong muscle tendon units seen with a radial club hand also may set the stage for progressive deformity.

The correct timing for surgery is not always clear with young children. Although it is technically possible to attempt correction of most upper limb malformations shortly after birth, the decision to operate early, if at all, is not easy. Surgery within the neonatal period rarely is indicated. We have encountered two indications for early surgery: (i) decompression of a tight constriction band associated with distal limb vascular insufficiency and edema, and (ii) revascularization and resurfacing of a potentially gangrenous arm associated with cutis aplasia, which is a form of neonatal Volkmann ischemic compression contracture. If the surgeon has any reservations about early surgery, it is best to delay. The ultimate goal is to complete all major (re)constructions before the child enters school at 5 to 6 years of age. Inappropriate early surgery may impair growth, create unnecessary contractures, and alter sensibility, all of which alone or collectively will affect function. As the hand matures, new adaptive patterns may develop and obviate the need for surgical correction. Each child's deformity should be considered individually!

In the past, classification of upper limb malformations has been a nosologic quagmire, primarily because the etiology and mechanisms of malformation are so poorly understood. Surgeons tend to be strict constructionists who want an orderly system for both documentation of the anatomical abnormalities and standardization of therapeutic approaches. In this unique field of surgery, every anomaly can be slightly different, even in those with enantiomorphic or mirror image malformations affecting both upper limbs. At the present time, the system (2) adopted by the American Society for Surgery of the Hand (ASSH) and the Federation of Hand Societies and recently amended by Ogino (3) has provided broad general categories and allowed surgeons to communicate on a more meaningful level. Future classifications based on genetic findings will prove to be very technical and not of obvious value to the clinical surgeon. However, in the future, the congenital hand surgeon will need to be familiar with a basic understanding of molecular genetics (4).

DUPLICATION

Within the hand plate, the existence of extra parts as duplications have been classified as preaxial (radial), central, and postaxial (ulnar). Duplications constitute by far the most

J. Upton: Department of Surgery, Division of Plastic Surgery, Harvard Medical School, and Department of Surgery, Division of Plastic Surgery, Beth Israel Deaconess Medical Center, Boston, Massachusetts

S. Pap: Department of Surgery, University of Massachusetts Medical School, and Department of Surgery, Division of Plastic Surgery, University of Massachusetts Memorial Health Care, Worcester, Massachusetts

common group of congenital upper limb differences and in many Asian series outnumber the combined sum of all other categories (1).

Radial (Postaxial) duplications are the most commonly reported in most published series and usually consist of a digit with a phalanx connected to the fifth finger by a soft tissue bridge. Nubbins that have been tied off in the newborn nursery often do not spontaneously separate (Fig. 42-1A). As adolescents, these patients often come to the hand surgeon for removal of a mass on the ulnar side of the fifth finger, which often has been misdiagnosed as a wart (Figs. 42-1B–C). We know of one infant who exsanguinated from an unrecognized familial coagulopathy following a supernumerary digit ablation in the newborn nursery. We recommend that when these parts are excised in the nursery, the base should be cauterized and the skin sutured with absorbable chromic sutures. More complicated duplications with larger skin bridges should be corrected electively in the operating room. With more complete forms, it is best to obtain radiographs of the duplication, because what may seem to be an obvious duplication of the fifth ray may, in fact, be one of the ring rays.

The potential problems with the treatment of *central duplications* are common, as outlined in the section on syndactyly. Extra parts may exist in the form of widened phalanges with longitudinal epiphyseal brackets (LEBs), transverse phalanges, oblique phalanges, and Y-shaped metacarpals and phalanges with or without conjoined or separate nail matrices. The osseous correction is highly individualized. Intrinsic muscle abnormalities and bizarre extrinsic tendon insertions are the rule, not the exception, in these hands. The long-term functional and aesthetic outcome is *never* normal!

Ulnar (Preaxial) thumb duplications are most common in white and Asian populations. In fact, the presence of a duplicated thumb in an African-American patient warrants a workup for an associated syndromic abnormality (1). These malformations are classified according to their level of duplication within the axial skeleton (5). The complexity of a surgical correction and the potential unfavorable outcome increase with the more proximal levels of duplication. Careful scrutiny of both abnormal soft tissue and skeletal anatomy and comparison to the normal side are advised in all preoperative discussions with the parents of these children.

Type I and II duplications that occur at the distal phalangeal level are the easiest to treat and usually involve ablation of the radial osseous element with preservation of the soft tissue. The retained nail is always smaller than the normal side, and motion of the interphalangeal (IP) joint may be decreased. Unfavorable results usually show a large soft tissue bulge on the radial side of the distal phalanx where the retained soft tissue has not been trimmed.

A

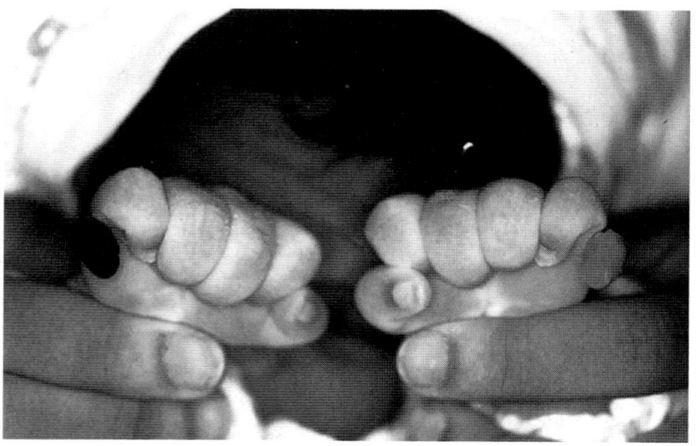

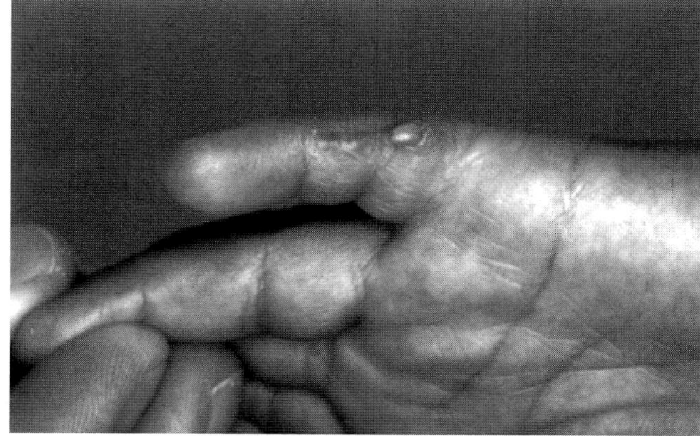

B

C

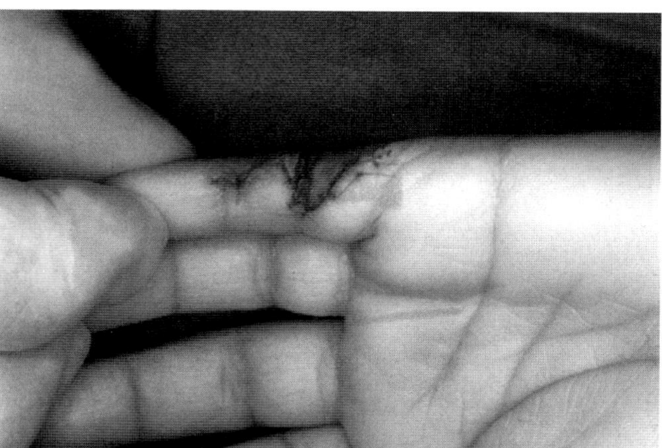

FIGURE 42-1. Duplication. **A:** Despite efforts to tie off these duplicated parts, the one on the left side did not spontaneously separate at 3 weeks. **B,C:** A scar with some underlying cartilage often is left and misdiagnosed as a wart *(top)*. The tissue should be excised and corrected with a Z-plasty.

Type IV duplications occur at the metacarpophalangeal (MP) joint, are the most common variety, and at the time of original correction may present many problems: an offset articular surface, a bifid metacarpal head, thenar intrinsic muscles attached to the radial partner, shared extrinsic flexor and extensor mechanisms, and a deficient first web space. All must be corrected if a maximal functional and aesthetic result is to be achieved. The Z-deformity is seen when the two partners diverge at the proximal phalangeal level and converge toward each other at the distal phalangeal level. Following ablation of one partner (usually the radial), the MP joint deviates in one direction and the IP joint in an opposite direction (Fig. 42-2). Initial correction may require osteotomies of the metacarpal

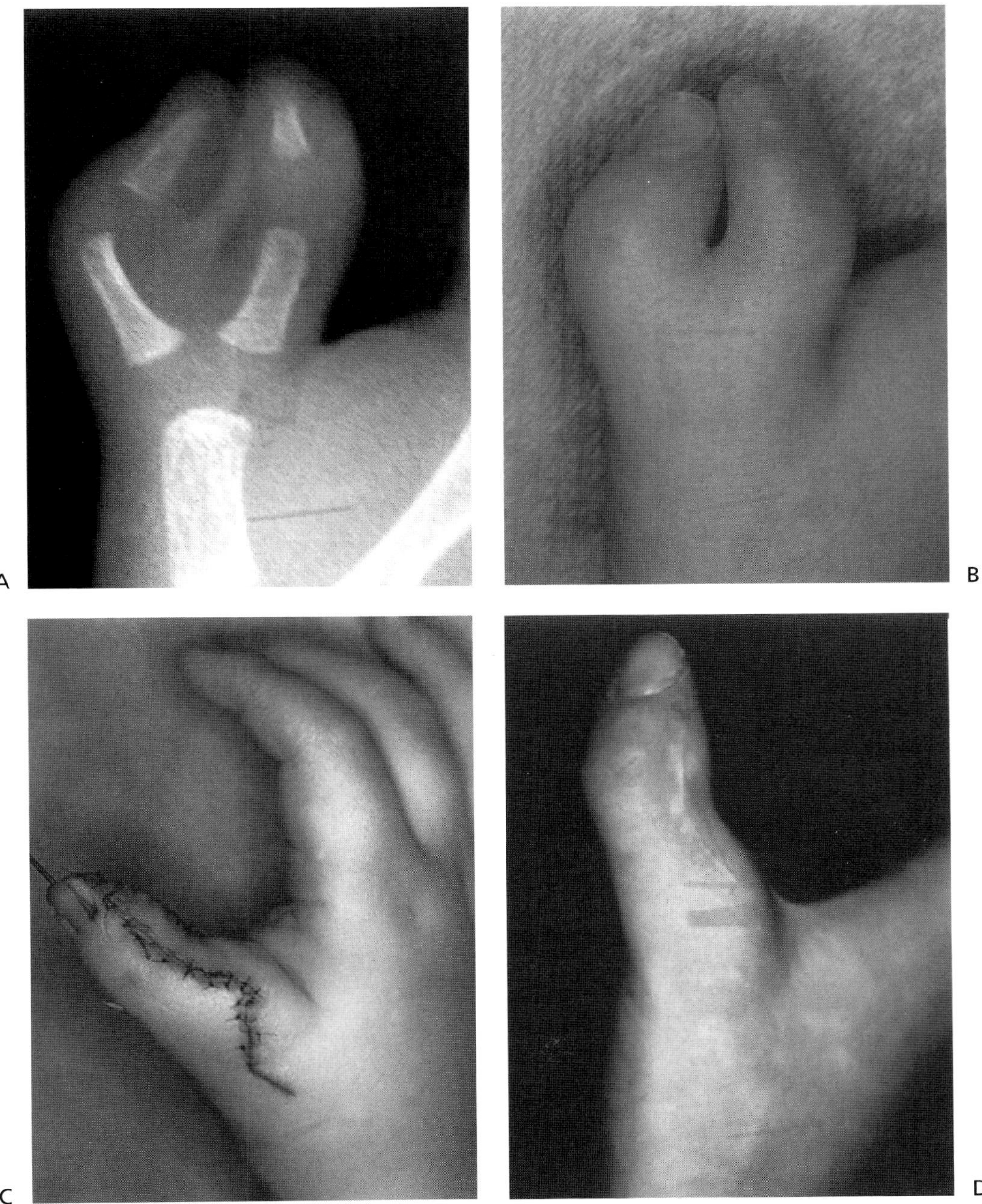

FIGURE 42-2. Duplication. **A,B:** Radiograph and appearance of a type IV duplication demonstrate divergence at the metacarpophalangeal (MP) joint and convergence at the interphalangeal (IP) joint. **C:** The radial thumb was saved with preservation of the ulnar collateral ligament, a phalangeal osteotomy, and centralization of the flexors and extensors. **D:** Twelve years later, the patient presented with recurrent deformity due to abnormal growth. There had been no change in the decreased range of motion at the MP and IP joints.

and/or proximal phalanx to properly align the longitudinal axis of the thumb. Eccentric distal extrinsic tendon insertions also must be centralized. The greatest dilemma with type IV duplication occurs when both duplicates are small and of equal size. We prefer to augment the retained ulnar partner with the radial soft tissue. Others prefer the Bilhaut procedure, in which skeletal and soft tissue elements are combined, leaving a wide thumb with a broad, flat nail marked with a longitudinal ridge and decreased IP joint motion (6).

Type V and VI duplications at the metacarpal level are much less common and have the least favorable outcomes. Because all elements of the thumb (bones, joints, intrinsic and extrinsic muscles, tendons, nail, ligaments and skin) are abnormal, many problems can and do occur. The first metacarpal is short and often positioned in an adducted position with a very deficient first web space, which is masked by a very lax ulnar collateral ligament of the ulnar thumb (Fig. 42-3). All of these problems must be corrected. Incisions are very important. The solution includes an incision much like that utilized for the cleft hand and repositioning of the thumb ray in palmar abduction (7) This transposition often requires a metacarpal osteotomy or a carpometacarpal (CMC) joint transfer. In our experience, persistent laxity of the ulnar collateral ligament at the MP joint level, adherence of the extensor mechanism, and failure to properly define the deficient first web space are the most persistent long-term problems (Fig. 42-3).

A separate category, type VII, is used for triphalangeal thumbs, which constitute slightly less than one-fifth of all preaxial duplications. Many types of configurations are encountered, and no standard type is seen. A whole teratologic sequence of abnormal intermediate phalanges is seen. The seven types described progress from the very small triangular bone to a completely normal phalanx. Often not only duplicate but also triplicate thumbs are present. It is important to reconstruct the best possible thumb from all the available parts (Fig. 42-4). Early excision of the very small extra bones does not always correct the ulnar deviation of the thumb, nor does it increase IP joint motion. Reported results are controversial. In those with more substantial intermediate bones, a partial reduction and fusion of one of the two articulating joints is recommended. There are two surgical caveats: (i) joint with the best motion should be saved; and (ii) excessive shortening must include shortening of the extensor mechanism to prevent a mallet deformity. In this situation, a longer thumb with good motion most often is the best thumb.

A,B

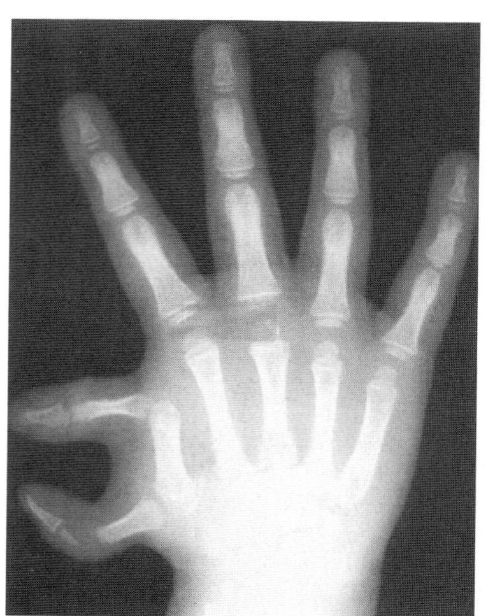

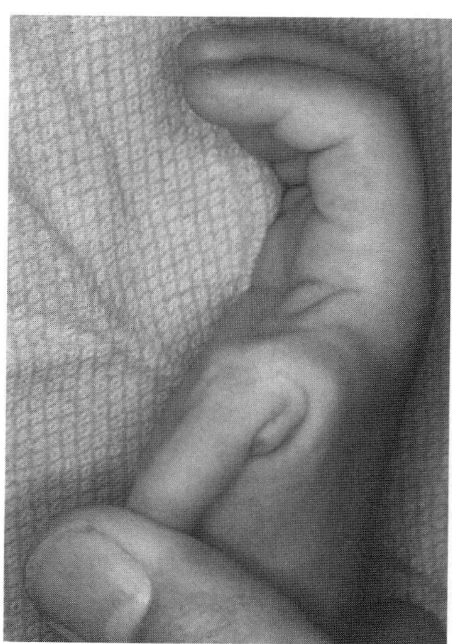

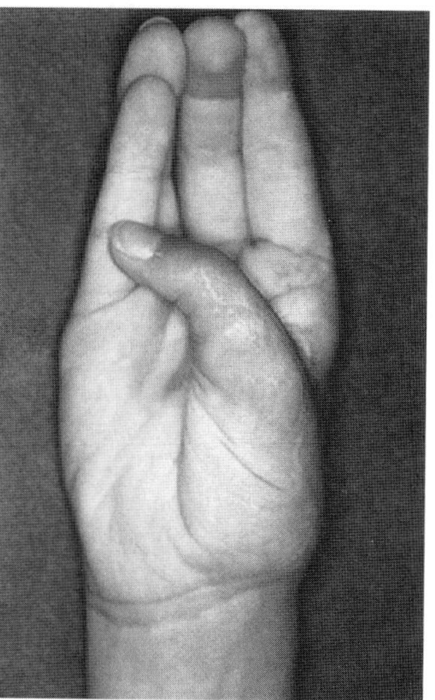

C

FIGURE 42-3. A: Radiograph of a type VI thumbs duplication at the carpometacarpal joint level shows an adducted first ray with a short metacarpal. **B:** Extreme laxity at the metacarpophalangeal joint is common. A secondary tenolysis of the extensor tendon with interposition of silicone sheeting was performed 3 years after initial correction. **C:** Eleven years later, full flexion is still limited by the tight extensor mechanism.

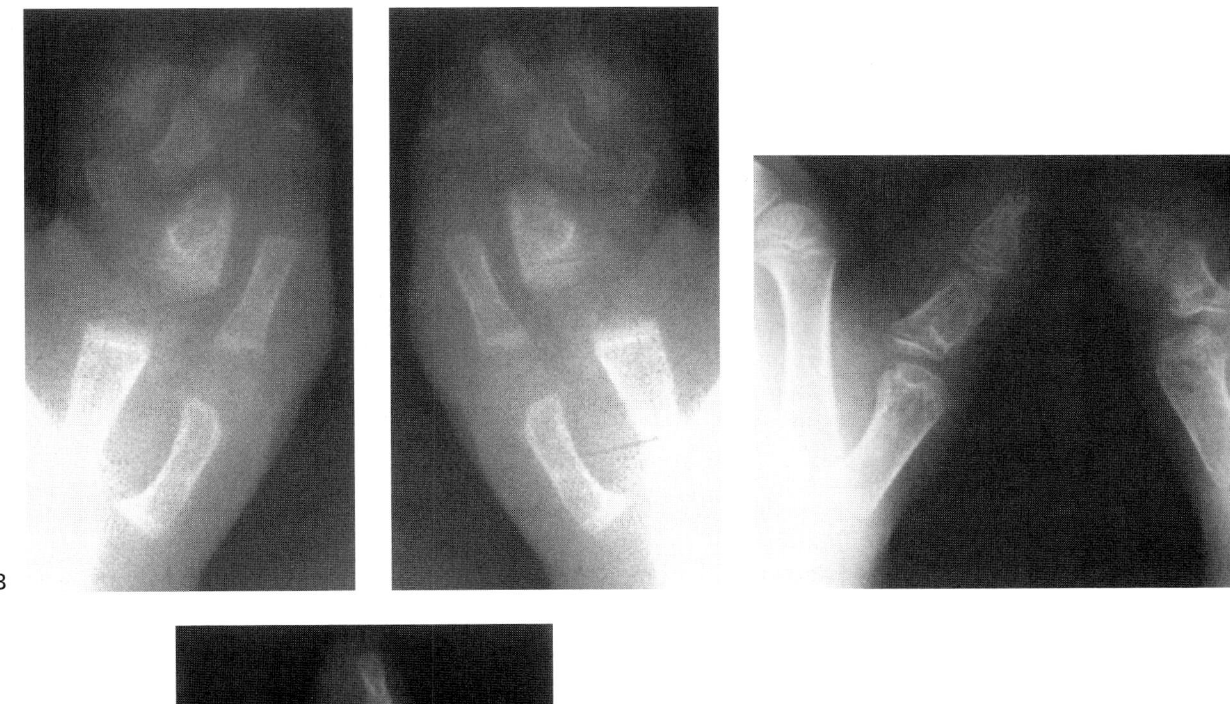

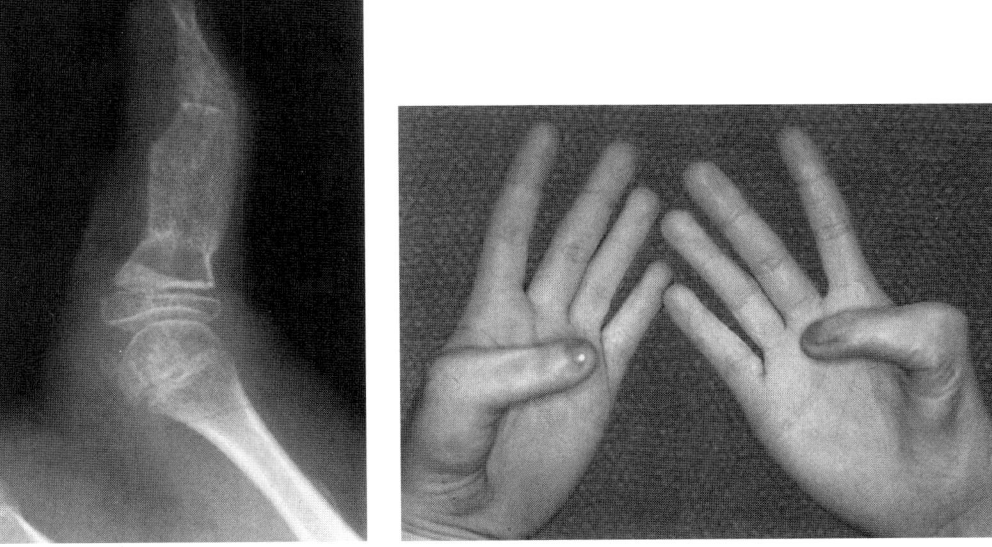

FIGURE 42-4. Duplication. **A,B:** Radiographs of an unusual complex mirror image thumb duplications show a radial biphalangeal thumb and an ulnar partner duplicated at the metacarpophalangeal level (MP) and with a triphalangeal component. **C:** Ten years and four operations later, the patient presented with short thumbs, instability at the interphalangeal (IP) joints, and radial clinodactyly. The left proximal phalanx had grown more than the right proximal phalanx. **D:** Following distraction lengthening, both thumbs were fused at the IP joint. **E:** At age 25 years, the patient demonstrates excellent stability and MP flexion. Note the abnormal nails and hypoplasia of thenar intrinsic muscles.

SYNDACTYLY

Webbed digits occur in isolation or as part of more complex malformations within the Apert hand, synpolydactyly (SPD), typical cleft hand, and the symbrachydactulous hand among others. As a group, they comprise the second most frequent anomaly treated by the upper limb surgeon. Unfavorable outcomes increase predictably from simple to complex forms.

The importance of meticulous surgery, careful hemostasis, and adequate postoperative immobilization following release of routine simple complete and incomplete syndactylies cannot be overemphasized. The permutations of flaps and grafts for the correction of webbing are quite varied. More than 60 methods have been described (1). It is best for the surgeon who frequently operates on these children to stay with one or two methods that he or she finds most acceptable. An incomplete "take" of a full-thickness skin graft or a commissure flaps at the critical palmar base of a web release will, with growth, invariably result in a predictable scar contracture and "web creep" (Fig. 42-5A). Occasionally, an unknown propensity for hypertrophic scarring or keloid formation will become manifest (Fig. 42-5B). Almost as many problems occur with the donor site as with the recipient hand. Grafts harvested within the hair-bearing escutcheon will sprout hair during adolescence (Fig. 42-6). Although utilization of the always abundant preputial skin is a good idea, these grafts tend to become infected and with time develop extreme hyperpigmentation. Incisions not closed within the natural skin creases with widen with time. The ideal donor tissue comes from extra digits or toes, which should not necessarily be sacrificed earlier in life if they can be used later (1).

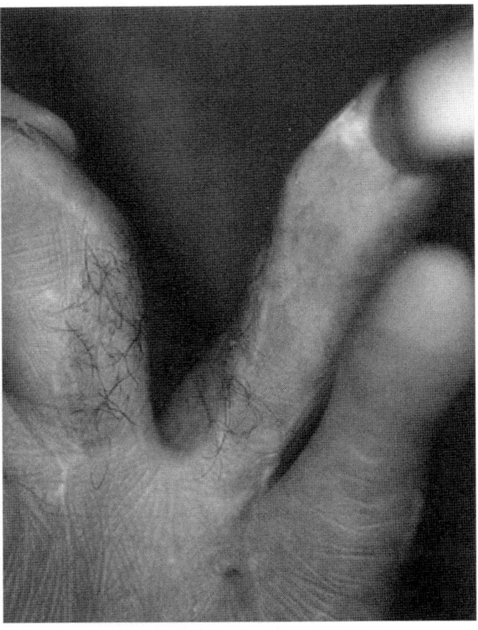

FIGURE 42-6. A very tight interdigital commissure is bordered by hirsute grafts which will contract with additional growth.

Poor or compromised outcomes occur increasingly from the simple to more complex forms of syndactyly. In the Apert hand, conjoined nails and side-to-side union of the

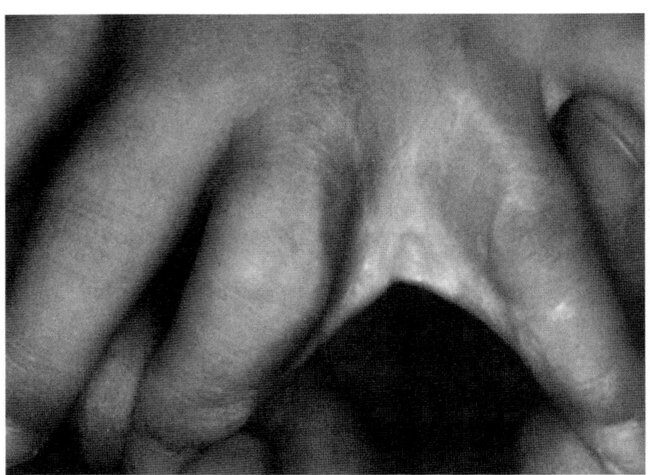

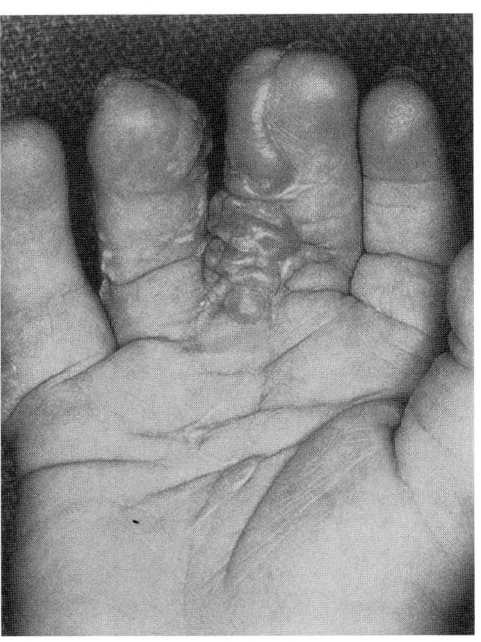

FIGURE 42-5. Syndactyly. **A:** This scar along the palmar border of the web space release resulted from an incomplete graft take. With growth, the commissure has advanced distally. **B:** Keloid scars in a white child are seen at all surgical margins.

A

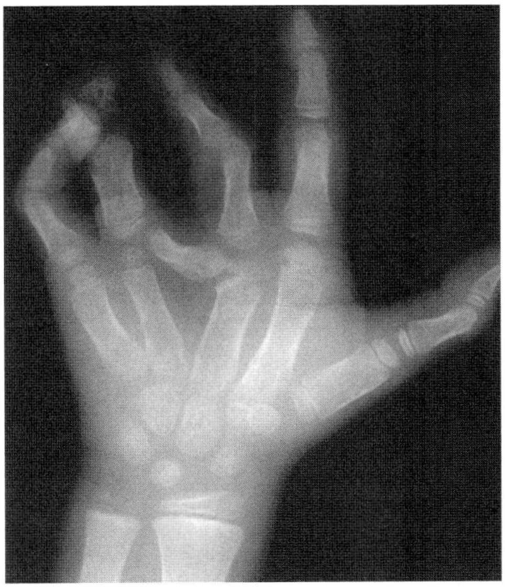

B

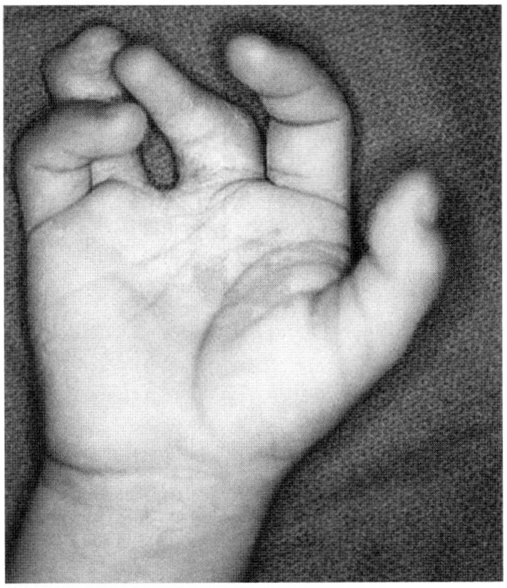

C

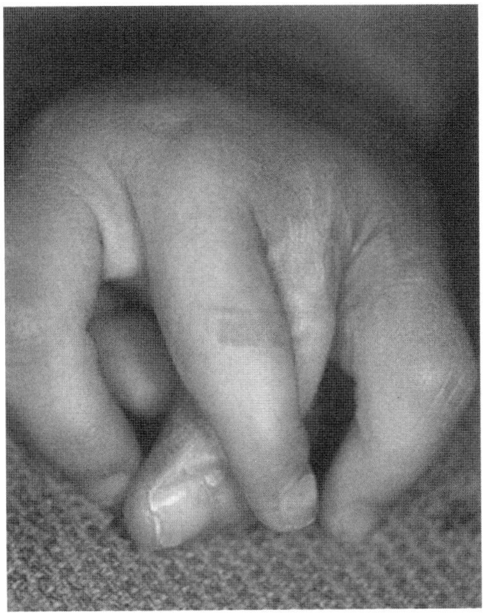

D

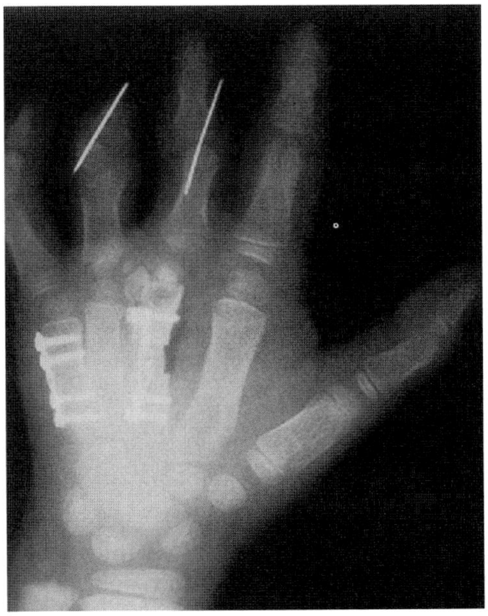

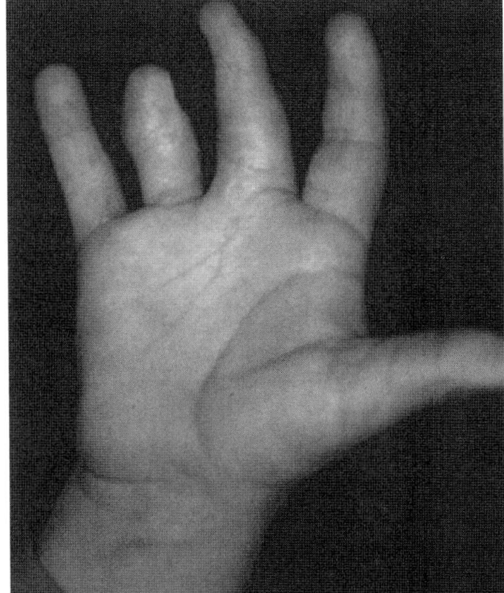

E

FIGURE 42-7. Synpolydactyly. **A,B:** Malrotation and angulation of short central digits are seen in a child 6 years after soft tissue correction of a synpolydactyly involving long and ring rays. The abnormal oblique phalanx between the long and ring metacarpals was saved. **C:** The digits overlap during flexion. **D:** Postoperative radiograph shows a complex osseous correction that included metacarpal lengthening using the extra phalanx as a graft, osteotomy of the fifth metacarpal to correct rotation, osteotomy of the ring proximal phalanx for correction of angulation, and repositioning of the long and ring metacarpal heads for correction of scissoring. **E:** The central digits are straight and have diminished interphalangeal joint motion.

distal phalangeal segments dictate the need for construction of paronychial and eponychial folds, reduction of nail matrices, and reduction of abnormal osseous width. Sometimes nails and phalangeal width are not even considered by the surgeon. With the exception of the distal IP joint of the fifth finger, well-segmented joints represented by lucency on radiographs obtained early in childhood will not move with time. Correction of the thumb radial clinodactyly in Apert children with an opening wedge osteotomy and bone graft harvested from the ring–small metacarpal synostosis is the key to a functional correction. This procedure will create a thumb-to-fifth finger pinch and grasp between a longer and straighter thumb and a mobile fifth ray. The goals for correction of these hands with osseous coalitions must be less stringent than for those with simple syndactyly (1).

Similarly, most patients with SPD will not have predictable IP or MP joint motion, depending on the proximal level of the duplication. In these patients, creation of a digit with (i) MP motion, (ii) no rotation, (iii) no angulation, and (iv) acceptable length and width of a normal finger is realistic. In no other area of hand surgery are poor functional and aesthetic outcomes so predictable. This may account for the paucity of literature on SPD hands. A well-planned, staged correction is critical. For example, in some patients with complex cleft hands and SPD hands, the syndactyly may represent a blessing in disguise. An LEB along a proximal or middle phalanx can be excised and grafted, or a phalanx can be moved into a more useful position before the soft tissue separation has been performed.

Osseous correction at the time of original separation is important. The past dictum of "separate before 7, revise during adolescence" no longer prevails in the surgical treatment of syndactyly (Fig. 42-7). Overzealous correction may, however, result in a vascular compromise and ultimate loss of the digit(s), particularly in SPD hands (8).

RADIAL DYSPLASIA

Preaxial (radial) failure of formation (arrest of development) or radial dysplasia as a group constitutes the third most common group of congenital differences. This failure of formation is longitudinal and includes a wide spectrum of anomalies from the shoulder to the tip of the thumb. Partial or total absence of the radius is the most common forearm deficiency and results in radial club hand posturing. Isolated hypoplasias of the thumb are seen much more frequency and treated. Most are unilateral, with a preference for males. In the syndromic types, it is important to consider three syndromes: TAR (thrombocytopenia and absent radius), Holt-Oram (congenital heart disease plus a radial deficiency), and VACTERL (anomalies of *v*ertebrae, *a*nus, *c*ardiovascular tree, *t*rachea, *e*sophagus, *r*enal system, and *l*imb). Small children with radial ray differences all should be tested for Fanconi anemia, which is not present at birth but may develop during childhood. This is a potentially fatal aplastic anemia that can be confirmed with a diepoxybutane (DEB) test and treated aggressively (9). Children with one of these syndromes may die from an associated malformation during childhood.

Both syndromic and nonsyndromic radial ray defects are comprehensive deformities. All soft tissue and skeletal structures from the shoulder to fingertip can be involved. The anatomical deformities range from minor thenar muscle hypoplasias to complete absence of the radius and a hypoplastic limb and shoulder. Before operating on the forearm, wrist, and hand, it is essential to carefully consider the shoulder and elbow, which position the forearm and hand in space. Adaptive patterns must be recognized, and a planned operation on the wrist or hand should improve function.

Early surgery is advocated for those with moderate and severe deficiencies. The present regimen consists of centralization by 6 to 8 months, pollicization between 12 and 18 months, and all secondary revisions by the time the child enters school between age 5 and 6 years (8). By the time these children reach the adolescent years, their adaptive patterns have been maximized, and further manipulation of their hands and forearms may be meddlesome. Young adults and older people should be evaluated with great scrutiny. Their presentation to the hand surgeon may be indicative of a life crisis more appropriately treated first by a psychiatrist. Those who have been raised in regions of the world where this type of correction was not available may be good candidates. However, they do not tolerate these procedures as easily as young children. Common sense and a thorough evaluation should identify those patients whose present function will not be enhanced by surgery.

The hand surgeon often may focus initially on distal limb deficiencies and ignore the elbow and shoulder. Restoration of elbow flexion is performed before centralization in selected patients. In many children, a passively mobile elbow is present with an absent biceps–brachialis flexor mechanism, which can be replaced effectively with a transfer of the sternoclavicular portion of the pectoralis major muscle. A strip of rectus fascia attached to the muscle is used for fixation into the ulna. The proximal muscle origin can be shifted from the humerus to the acromion. In our hospital, we have seen consistently poor results when the triceps or latissimus dorsi muscles were transferred for elbow flexion. We strongly prefer the pectoral transfer.

For those with radial club hands, centralization of the carpus and hand over the distal ulna is performed within the first year of life, preferably by 6 months of age. Distraction of tight soft tissue structures in severe deformities is preferred over carpectomy or ulnar shortening. The repositioned hand is balanced by the dynamic transfer of functional forearm motors to the dorsal and ulnar portion of the wrist into the extensor carpi ulnaris tendon. With time, those wrists that do have some motion usually drift back into slight flexion and radial deviation. In these patients, it is important to maintain passive correction with night splints. Most surgeons prefer to place the ulna beneath the radial side of the carpus (radialization) (10). In this position, a strong transfer may cause the wrist to dislocate in an ulnar direction. The most common unfavorable outcome following centralization is altered growth that results from partial devascularization of the epiphysis within distal ulna. This phenomenon is difficult to document accurately, because these ulnas are programmed to be short (11). These forearms are always short, and those with the more severe hypoplasias often will request lengthening during their adolescent or young adult years. Lengthening of the ulna is a very effective procedure if performed slowly so that the abnormal muscle tendon units will not be damaged by rapid distraction.

THUMB HYPOPLASIA

Thumb hypoplasias occur in conditions other than radial ray dysplasias and include the constriction ring syndrome, chorionic villus sampling defects, cleft hands, symbrachydactylies, hypoplastic hands, and duplications. Any or all soft tissue and skeletal components of the thumb may be deficient. Not all require treatment, and all cases must be carefully individualized.

The classification system advocated by the Germans (12,13) has been used for years and recently was amended by Manske et al. (14), who made a clear distinction in the type III thumbs between those with (IIIA) and without (IIIB) a CMC joint. In types I and II, differences in all soft tissue and skeletal structures are present and very little, if any, surgery is indicated. The one very effective procedure performed in these hands is a release of the first web space. We prefer the four-flap Z-plasty because it results in a normal, concave configuration between the thumb and index rays, but this procedure should not be used in all cases.

Failure to recognize the need for additional tissue in severe cases will always yield an unfavorable outcome. Many children with type III thumbs simply do not have enough local tissue for creation of a good web space. Tissue can be transferred effectively as fasciocutaneous flaps pedicled on either the dorsal interosseous or radial artery systems. In the hypoplastic mitten hand and the Apert hand, advancement and readvancement of dorsal skin with repeated procedures is quite effective. Distant or local pedicle or island flaps can be avoided. During the correction of type IIIA thumbs, the pollex abductus abnormality often is missed. This anomaly occurs when tight connections between flexor and extensor tendons combine to make both flexors and radial deviators (Fig. 42-8).

Pollicization of the index ray is the treatment of choice for some type IIIA, and all type IIIB, IV, and V thumb deficiencies. The surgeon will be challenged by many families who are intuitively convinced for one reason or another that the type IIIB and IV thumbs should be constructed and not pollicized. The use of videotapes and actual preoperative and postoperative plaster molds of these hands are quite effective during these long consultations. Some parents of children with type IIB thumbs will absolutely insist on a staged reconstruction.

All pollicized thumbs lack both the pinch strength and mobility of the normal thumb. Although palmar abduction can be strengthened with an abductor digiti quinti muscle transfer (Huber transfer), these will never be normal thumbs. With proper incisions and technique, the appearance can be remarkably good. Syndromic patients with a stiff index ray before this surgery will have a very stiff, minimally functional thumb. The most unsatisfactory results

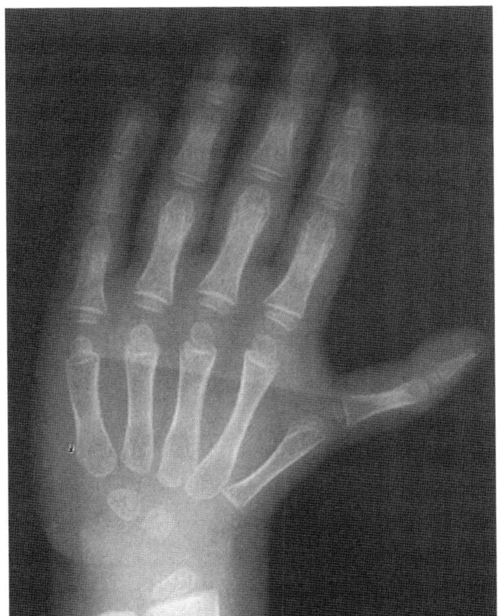

A

FIGURE 42-8. Thumb hypoplasia. **A:** Radiograph of a type IIIA hypoplastic thumb of a 2-year-old child prior to first web release, collateral ligament reconstruction using local tissue, and abductor digiti quinti (AbDQ) transfer. The transfer was attached to the thumb proximal phalanx. *(continued)*

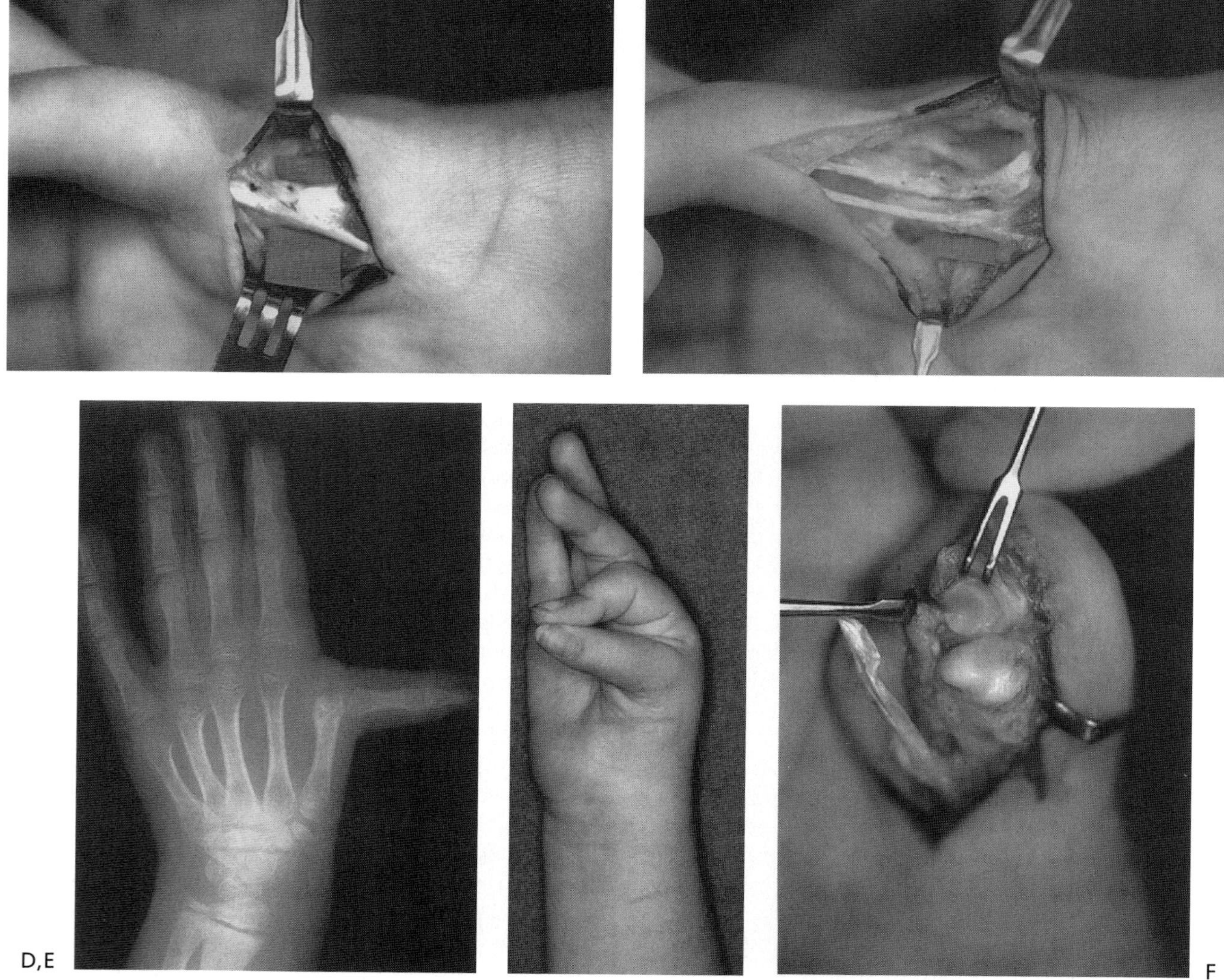

FIGURE 42-8. (Continued) **B,C:** The pollex abductus before and after separation shows the connections between the displaced extensor mechanism and the thumb flexor. **C:** Note the displaced extensor *(top)* and the distal abnormal muscle belly of the thumb flexor (FPL). **D,E:** Fifteen years later, the patient presented with excessive radial deviation, a small web space, and an ineffective pinch. **F:** At the time of metacarpophalangeal arthrodesis, the radial side of the metacarpal head was completed eroded due to the persistent pull of the AbDQ.

are obtained when parents refuse to have a type IIIB or IV floating thumb ablated in lieu of pollicization. The outcome following staged thumb constructions, which can even include a microvascular transfer of the second toe for reconstruction of the CMC joint, will *never* be as good as a well-executed index pollicization (15).

VASCULAR ANOMALIES

The treatment of vascular anomalies remains one of the most challenging and perplexing areas in hand surgery. The classification proposed by Mulliken and Glowacki (16) 19 years ago is now accepted and used clinically worldwide. It separates these anomalies into two broad groups: hemangiomas and malformations. *Hemangiomas* undergo rapid cellular proliferation and eventual complete spontaneous involution within childhood and require very little aggressive surgical treatment in the upper limb. The mechanism(s) of involution is unknown. *Malformations* appear at or shortly after birth, grow with the child, and do not involute. Their natural history and response to treatment are characterized by their cell type. Capillary malformations are confined to the dermis and clinically represent port-wine staining. No surgical treatment is necessary, but these cutaneous birthmarks may be associated with deeper lymphatic, venous, mixed lymphatic venous (CLVM), or high-flow arteriovenous malformations (CAVM) with arteriovenous fistulas (AVFs). Proper treatment of these conditions is contingent on a correct diagnosis.

The diagnosis is made primarily by physical examination, because over 95% of these lesions are easily distinguished by their natural history and appearance. Ultrasound is used to distinguish between hemangiomas and malformations. Magnetic resonance imaging has become the gold standard for the diagnosis and identification of specific types of malformations.

The treatment of most slow-flow malformations is predictable. In the venous malformations (VM) group, the response to single or staged surgical excisions and sclerotherapy is quite good. Although well-localized large malformations with large-caliber channels in the arm and forearm respond well to sclerosis with absolute alcohol, an occasional compartment syndrome may occur due to muscle necrosis and bleeding within the flexor pronator muscle mass (Fig. 42-9). Staged excisions in the hand and wrist regions are predictable (17,18). Lymphatic malformations (LMs) are much more difficult to treat. Those with cutaneous vesicles are prone to develop periodic wildfire β-streptococcal infections, which must be treated aggressively. The rubbery hard, indurated LMs and lymphatic venous malformations (LVMs) often are adherent to all adjacent structures and obliterate normal fascial planes. Although resections of large macrocystic malformations from the chest wall, axilla, arm, and forearm provide dramatic improvement, single or staged excisions on the dorsum of the hand and/or digits are very disappointing. It is impossible to control postoperative edema on the palmar surface of the hand. The residual swelling and scar formation in the wrist and hand make it difficult to maintain active motion of extrinsic tendons and intrinsic muscles. For these children, absolute reconstructive priority should be directed to the thumb and the first web space. In massively involved hands, amputation often is the end result. Results in the mixed LVM or CLVM group are dependent on the amount of macrocystic or microcystic lymphatic component.

In the entire malformation category, alteration in the size of the lesion and subsequent symptoms occur frequently in females during pregnancies and periods of taking antiovulant medication (19). Following delivery and periods of breast-feeding, these malformations do not regress to their prepregnancy size.

Fast-flow arteriovenous malformations (AVMs) contain AVFs and have been categorized into three groups. The first type consists of single or multiple localized aneurysmal lesions with AVFs along the major vessels. The second type is more extensive but still confined primarily to a single axial artery territory within the forearm, hand, or digit. Both

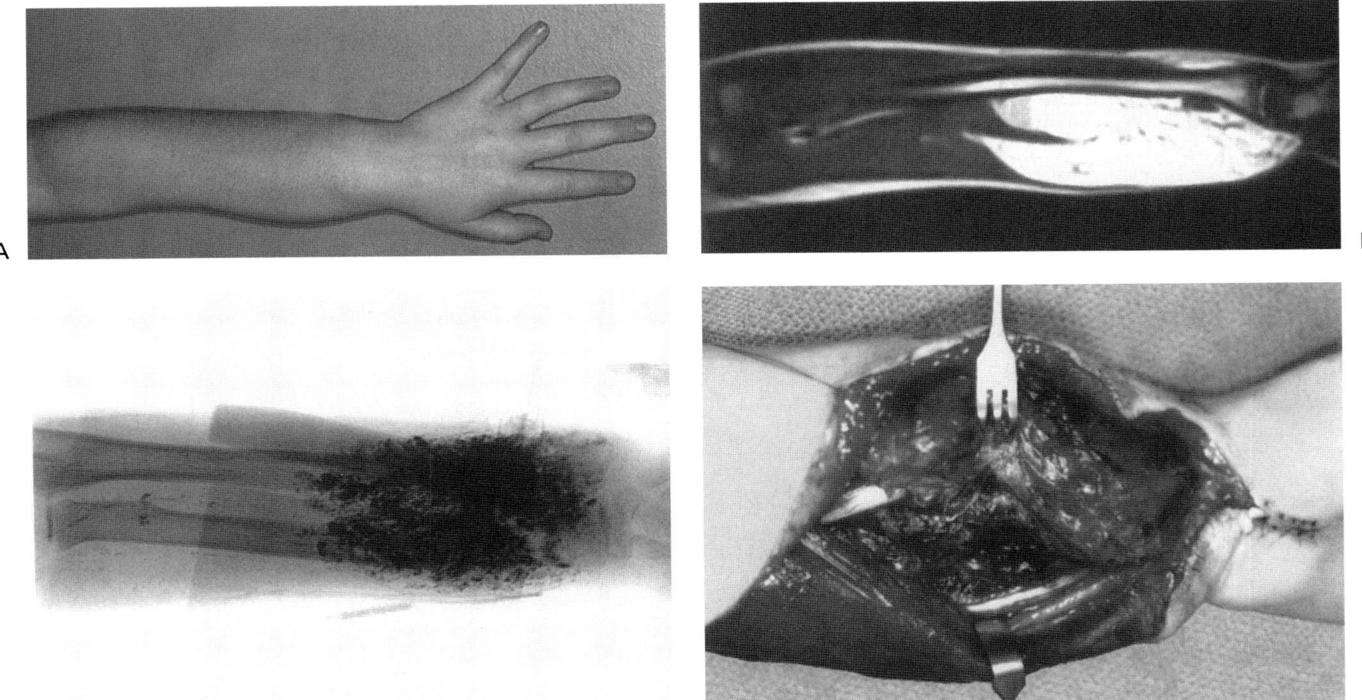

FIGURE 42-9. Vascular malformations. **A,B:** The clinical appearance and magnetic resonance imaging scan of a slow-flow vascular malformation localized to the distal forearm and along the interosseous membrane. **C:** Direct puncture sclerotherapy (needle above) with absolute alcohol was used. **D:** The swelling and bleeding caused a compartment syndrome. Large clots and necrotic tissue are seen along the interosseous membrane.

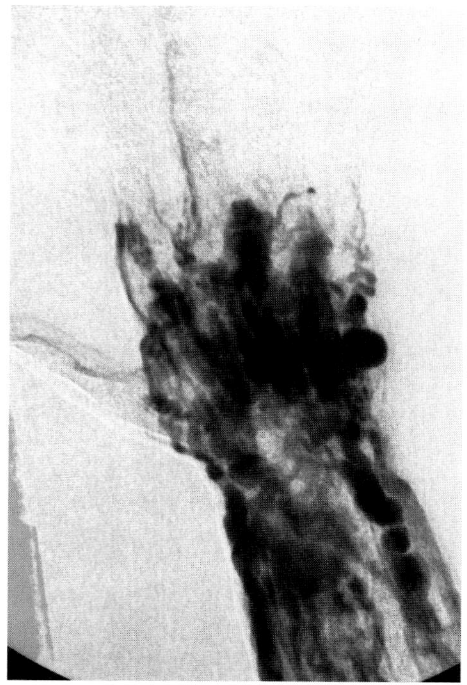

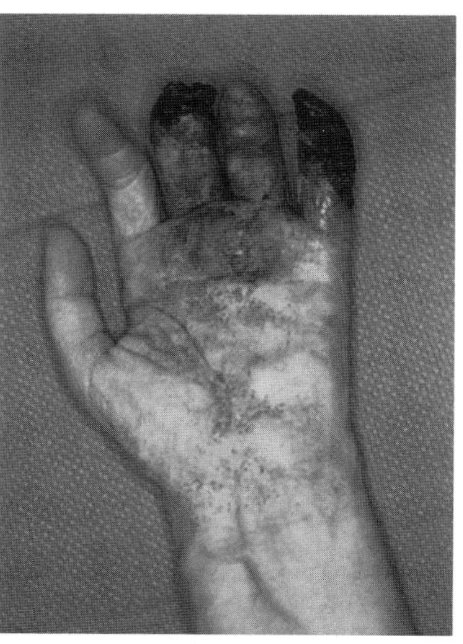

FIGURE 42-10. Vascular malformation following embolization. **A,B:** Radiograph and appearance of a hand following embolization for a fast-flow arteriovenous malformation (AVM) of the forearm and hand. Only the radial digital artery to the long finger has not been occluded. Pain from the digital gangrene was excruciating and necessitated performance of a below elbow (BE) amputation.

types respond well to carefully planned surgery and microsurgical revascularization or resurfacing, if needed (17). The third group presents with diffuse, pulsating, painful, and pernicious lesions with multiple AVFs involving large areas of the extremity. Although some patients manage for a lifetime, most are very symptomatic. Skillful efforts with embolization and even the most heroic surgery often result in amputation (Fig. 42-10). In our group of 33 fast-flow AVF patients, 19 lost a part or all of the upper extremity (19).

CLEFT HAND AND SYMBRACHYDACTYLY

During the past decade, a clear distinction between the typical and atypical cleft hand has been made on nosologic grounds (3). Patients with typical clefts have V-shaped clefts within the central portion of the hand, syndactyly, camptodactyly , bilateral hand and foot involvement, frequently a positive family inheritance, and occasionally the associated ectrodactyly, ectodermal dysplasia, and clefting (EEC) syndrome. Three chromosomal loci have been identified but have not been sequenced. Atypical cleft hands are now preferably called symbrachydactyly and are characterized by a U-shaped cleft, hypoplastic nubbins representing digits, unilateral upper limb and no lower limb involvement, and a negative family history. There are no known genetic abnormalities.

Surgery for the severe cleft hand often is meddlesome due to the child's remarkable adaptive capacities. Flatt's characterization of these hands as "a functional triumph and a social disaster" is quite appropriate (20). In most deep clefts involving the central (long) ray, the *index* finger is located in a "no man's land" between a potentially functional thumb and a normal ring finger. Most incisions for correction create partially ischemic random flaps for reconstruction of the thumb–index web space. It is difficult to move the index ray in an ulnar direction, to shorten it if necessary, and to create a transverse metacarpal ligament. With growth, the index metacarpal becomes longer and tends to position the index ray in more abduction and radial deviation than desired. Incision planning and the position of the transposed index ray are key to this reconstruction (7). In those patients with one or no digits on the hand, the foot must be used as a donor site for thumb or fifth (ulnar) digital construction. These surgeries are the most difficult toe-to-hand transfers imaginable and often present with a potpourri of anomalous structures. Often there is little skeletal support in the hand and limited motors for extrinsic flexion and extension. If the metatarsal head with its growth plate is included in the transfer, the already compromised "lobster claw" foot will become more vulnerable.

The outcome from surgical correction of symbrachydactylies depends on the amount of skeletal and soft tissue available. Often the border rays of the hand (thumb and fifth digit) are the most complete parts of the hand. Both are hypoplastic, and the MP joint of the fifth finger often is flail and joined to a very hypoplastic ring ray in a complete, simple syndactyly. The three central rays are short and webbed together. In extreme deficiencies, they consist of hypoplastic nubbins that retract with carpal motion. Many operations often are needed to both stabilize and provide a flexor mechanism to the thumb, to broaden the cleft during removal of the nubbins or hypoplastic digits. and finally to lengthen and stabilize the deficient fifth finger. Staged flexor reconstruction of the thumb often results in poor functional motion in young children due to limited compliance and restricted motors in the forearm. Efforts to maintain length and MP joint motion of the fifth finger often fail and usually are best treated with an arthrodesis and bone graft with skeletal maturity. A good functional outcome would consist of (i) a mobile radial ray with intact thenar intrinsic muscles, (ii) a central cleft, and (iii) a stable ulnar post.

Many of these hypoplastic hands have a small, mobile, and intact thumb and digits represented only by hypoplastic soft tissue nubbins. Metacarpals are present with or without an intact MP joint. The digits can be augmented with free nonvascularized bone grafts, toe or digit phalangeal transfers, or free vascularized transfers. Free bone grafts tend to resorb, especially when transferred on top of a terminal phalangeal segment (Fig. 42-11). Toe phalangeal transfers with intact periosteum and collateral ligaments are a better alternative but are not completely predictable. Our experience with more than 100 patients treated over a 22-year period has documented survival and normal growth in 40%, survival with poor growth in 40%, and either complete or partial resorption in 20% of all phalangeal transfers. The most favorable factors for acquisition of a blood supply and

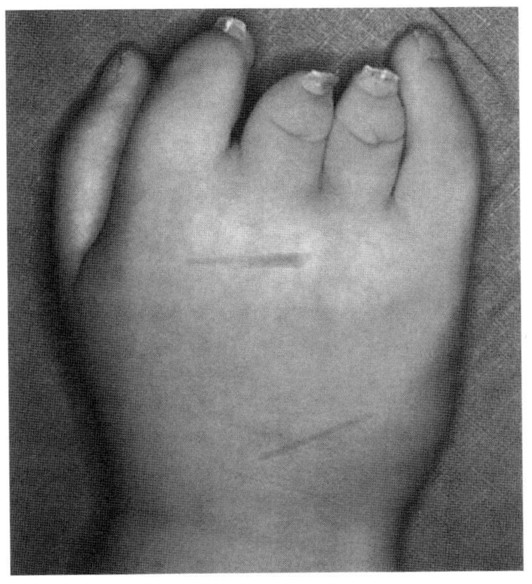
A

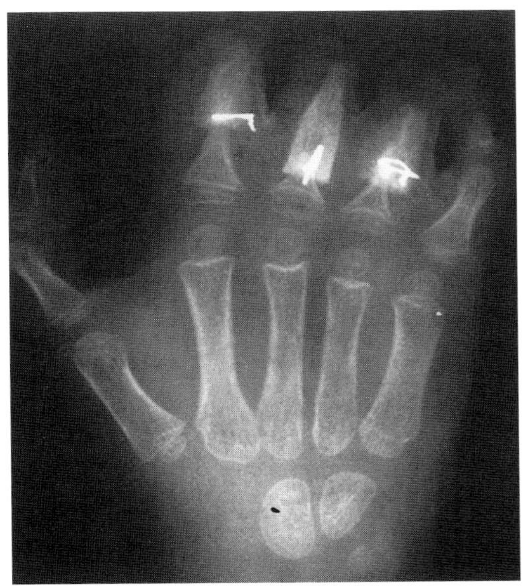
B

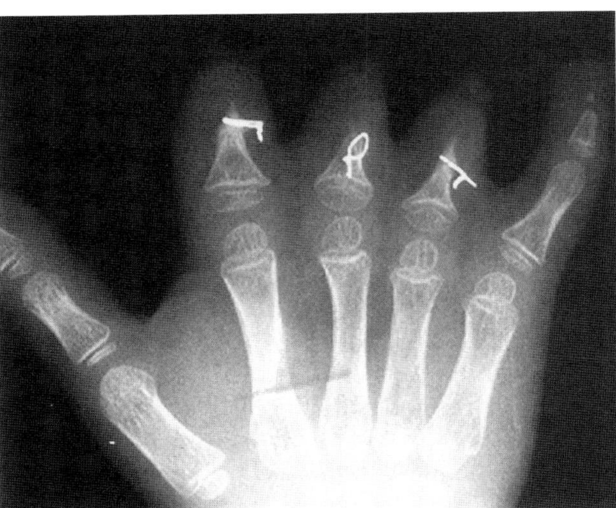
C

FIGURE 42-11. Synbrachydactyly. **A:** initial appearance of a unilateral symbrachydactyly before augmentation with three corticocancellous iliac crest bone grafts. **B:** Radiograph immediately after bone grafting. **C:** Four years later, there is complete resorption of the bone grafts.

normal growth have been (i) the presence of vascularized bone proximal and distal to the implant and (ii) transfer before 2 years of age.

OVERGROWTH

Overgrowth, macrodactyly, or digital gigantism represents a nosologic "black hole" of many different conditions, all of which are very difficult to treat. Dilemmas concerning the best surgical options, poor functional outcomes, and disastrous aesthetic results account for the paucity of reports in the hand literature. At present there is no practical classification of overgrowth anomalies that are seen with vascular malformations, neurofibromatosis, the Proteus syndrome, nerve territory oriented macrodactyly (NTOM), hemihypertrophy, and multiple hereditary exostosis among other conditions. The extent of overgrowth is not predictable in each condition and ranges from minimal to massive. To date, efforts to identify the mechanism of overgrowth have been futile.

The overgrowth seen with vascular anomalies is not related to flow. It occurs with both fast-flow and slow-flow anomalies. Significant hypertrophy in the upper limb is seen with slow-flow VMs and LMs. Often there are associated malformations elsewhere that dictate higher priority for treatment. Staged soft tissue excision combined with epiphysiodesis are the present treatment of choice (17). The mixed LVMs, CLVMs, the Parkes Weber syndrome (complex-combined fast-flow anomalies: CAVM, capillary arteriovenous fistula, [CAVF], capillary lymphatic arteriovenous malformation, [CLAVM]), and the Klippel-Trenaunay anomaly (capillary lymphatico venous malformation [CLVM], skeletal overgrowth) also may demonstrate gross skeletal overgrowth along with a vascular malformation.

The Proteus syndrome is a recently described entity named after the Greek god Proteus, who could change his identity at will to escape detection by other gods. Among the associated malformations are limb overgrowth, hand and digital gigantism, and, in selected children, a cerebriform appearance of the glabrous surfaces on the hands or feet. The genetic mutation responsible for this condition is not known. The metacarpals and phalanges of the hand grow asymmetrically and often have associated cartilaginous masses within the volar plates. Neurovascular structures and tendons appear normal but large. Despite soft tissue reduction, excision of cartilaginous masses, early epiphysiodeses, and corrective osteotomies, it is very difficult to maintain range of motion, as these children selectively neglect the use of the affected portion of their hand. When left uncorrected, these digits and hands can grow to monstrous proportion.

The pediatric hand surgeon struggles most frequently with the NTOM, which may involve one or more digits or the thumb. The options for massive hypertrophy at birth are either to amputate or to perform early radical soft tissue excisions (Fig. 42-12). The latter are often (but not always) futile but do produce straight digits with limited IP motion and decreased sensation. Acceptable aesthetic results are possible. Amputation and transposition of adjacent uninvolved digits often are preferable. The median, ulnar, or digital nerves may be infiltrated with lipomatous tissue, which makes it impossible during dissection to distinguish normal from abnormal fascicular bundles. However, in many hands the nerves are normal and course through abnormally large bundles of fat. Our approach for the past 2 decades has been to preserve the digital artery, including vincular branches to the IP joint system, and to neurolyse the digital nerve, which then is left to reinnervate the skin flap and pulp. One side of a digit at a time is reduced. Despite early aggressive soft tissue excision and early epiphysiodeses, it is still very difficult to control the width of the skeletal segments. During the reduction of infantile gigantic digits, we have amputated the distal phalangeal segment and transferred the nail matrix/nail plate complex to the middle phalanx as a pedicle flap. The results are never optimal, but the nail will survive and grow.

Neurofibromatosis has been separated into specific types with specific inheritance patterns. All types may have an associated extremity overgrowth. The involved digits demonstrate hypertrophy along specific nerve distributions. For example, involvement of the common (or proper) digital nerve to the second web space would clinically result in large index and long digits that deviate away from one another. Often the digits may be joined in a complete syndactyly. The entire median or ulnar nerve territory may be involved. The sausage-shaped nerves are infiltrated with lipomatous deposits and follow a long circuitous course through the hand. During dissection, one may encounter a normal segment of digital nerve, lose it in a hypertrophied mass, and then find it exiting as a normal structure with a more distal dissection. Subcutaneous tissue planes may be grossly infiltrated by plexiform masses of abnormal nerves. Although removal of subcutaneous plexiform masses in the axilla, chest wall, arm, and forearm yields outstanding outcomes, aggressive excisions in the hand and digit usually result in a stiff, oversized digit with poor sensation. Two-point discrimination and light touch are never normal in these children preoperatively. The most unfavorable result in these children is the malignant transformation into neurofibrosarcomas. In the past 21 years, three of our patients with significant upper limb and neck involvement died of their malignancy.

Hemihypertrophy may affect the upper and/or lower extremities. Associated renal or adrenal tumors may be detected with early ultrasound examination. The gross enlargement of the arm and more commonly the forearm is not in the subcutaneous tissue planes but in the muscular layers. The extra muscles seen in the forearm usually are duplicates of wrist and superficial flexor bellies that histologically do not have the normal longitudinal orientation of fibers. The limited excursion of these muscles with longitudinal, transverse, and oblique fibers affects growth results in

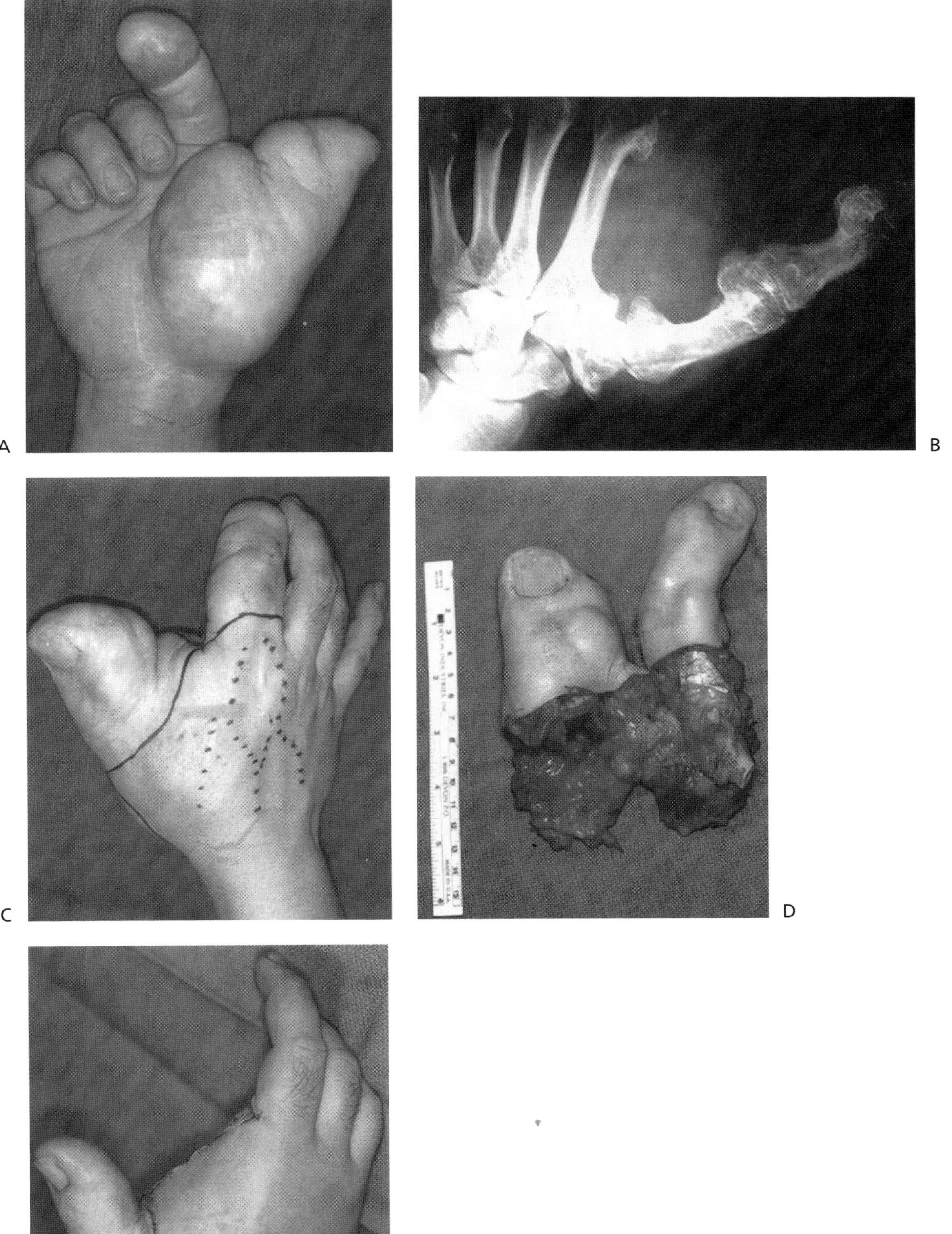

FIGURE 42-12. Overgrowth. **A:** Fifteen previous surgical procedures were unsuccessful in this 30-year-old accountant with nerve territory oriented macrodactyly and massive hypertrophy of soft tissue and skeleton. **B:** The affected skeletal parts show a marked increase in length and width and exostosis at every joint margin. **C,D:** Reconstruction consisted of amputation of the thumb and index rays followed by microvascular great toe transfer **(E)**. Both function and appearance have improved.

MP flexion and ulnar deviation of the wrist and digits. All types of intrinsic muscle duplications may be encountered in the hand. Most of these extra muscles insert into phalanges. Early recognition and release or excision of these abnormal intrinsic or extrinsic muscles will provide better dynamic balance to the hand and minimize secondary skeletal growth deformities. Unfortunately, most are not recognized early. Despite aggressive soft tissue releases, tenotomies, joint releases, muscle excisions, and osteotomies, the final result is always less then optimal in those who present with a grossly enlarged hand with wrist and digital flexion contractures.

CAMPTODACTYLY

Digits with camptodactyly present with proximal IP (PIP) joint flexion contractures in the anteroposterior plane, in contrast to clinodactyly in which the deviation is in a radioulnar plane. Because this condition is present in more than 60 syndromes, the hand surgeon often associates this entity with a genetic condition. Less than half of the patients who are seen have syndromic designations. These PIP flexion contractures often involve multiple digits, are severe and fixed early in childhood, and respond poorly to operative management. Early recognition and aggressive stretching at birth are the treatment of choice. Night splinting alone merely maintains the correction that has been achieved with exercise and stretching. Surgical correction of PIP joint flexion contractures is sequential and starts with longitudinal release of skin that is converted to a Z-plasty. This is followed by incision of the fibrous substrata, flexor sheath, volar plate, accessory collateral ligaments, and finally flexor digitorum superficialis tendon before the joint can be extended to 0 degrees. A full-thickness hypothenar skin graft may be necessary for contractures greater than 70 degrees. Despite excellent wound healing and flap and graft take, secondary contractures will occur with growth, particularly with a noncompliant child. Surgery on a digit with a longstanding contracture of greater than 45 degrees and characteristic radiologic signs (widened middle phalanx, narrowed joint space, and flattened dorsal condyle on a true lateral view) will always yield a very unfavorable outcome (1).

Nonsyndromic flexion contractures of the PIP joint usually involve the fifth finger, may be present at birth, and commonly progress during the adolescent growth spurt, particularly in females. Most are associated with abnormal intrinsic muscle origins and insertions within the hand and tight superficial flexor muscle tendon units. With early diagnosis in the neonate, they can be corrected with stretching and splinting alone. In older children with good passive mobility and contractures of less than 70 degrees, surgery is a reasonable option in the properly selected patient. Similar to those with syndromic involvement, those who present late with the hallmark radiologic signs of a long-standing contracture on a true lateral radiograph have predictably poor results following soft tissue releases. Skeletal realignment with either arthrodesis or osteotomy will provide a more permanent result.

DISTRACTION LENGTHENING

Although the technique of distraction lengthening of long tubular bones has a 90-year history, applications in the upper extremity are not described before Matev's lengthening of the thumb following trauma in 1970 (21). Since 1977, we have used the technique for correction of congenital differences in 94 patients with distraction of 132 skeletal segments. Several important points about the indications, technique, complications, and outcomes should be emphasized.

Indications

These procedures are performed for both aesthetic and functional reasons. Lengthening of the deviated or short thumb at the metacarpal or proximal phalangeal level is the prime functional indication for this procedure. Correction of brachydactylies associated with short metacarpals is performed primarily for appearance. Lengthening of distal phalanges alone is not performed due to poor outcomes and complications. In central complex SPD patients, a metacarpal or phalanx may be lengthened to create a ray of normal length and appearance. The goal in these patients is to create a straight digit free of rotation or angulation and with preservation of MP joint motion. In symbrachydactylies, the goal is to create a post or stable ulnar digit to oppose the mobile thumb with pinch and grip. Lengthening of the forearm in older children and adolescents with longitudinal (usually radial) deficiencies is for aesthetic improvement. More proximal humeral lengthening in those with phocomelia deficiencies is for functional and prosthetic indications. More individualized indications exist in hands in which a skeletal part was transposed for reconstruction of an adjacent ray.

Technique

There are significant differences between lengthening in the hand and wrist compared distraction of long tubular bones in the lower extremity. In the leg, the distraction rarely increases length more than 15%. New bone fills the gaps by spontaneous "callostasis." In the upper extremity, metacarpals and proximal phalanges are rapidly lengthened by 100% or more of their original length and much larger gaps are created. This gap is not always surrounded by well-vascularized skeletal muscle. In the hand and wrist, lengthening is a two-step procedure: (i) application of the distraction apparatus and osteotomy followed by (ii) removal of distractor, bone graft, and rigid internal fixation. The only exception would be the child or young adult who needs a small lengthening at the metacarpal or forearm level where the bone segment is completely surrounded by well-vascularized skeletal muscle. In these patients, external fixation is maintained until solid trabecular bone fills the gap. However, most of these corrections can be achieved during a single procedure. At the digital level, the distraction gap is surrounded by tendon, subcutaneous tissues, and skin. The regenerate bone formed during "callostasis" is not structurally strong and will require some type of rigid support in addition to a bone graft.

Complications

Problems with distraction are directly proportional to the amount of time the external fixation device was left on the patient. Although pediatric patients of all ages protect the external fixation devices from their siblings and friends, problems begin to appear after 6 to 8 weeks of distraction. Pin tract infections, wound breakdown, cellulitis, and skin maceration are most common. Rambunctious children may break the apparatus. After 1 month of lengthening at a rate of 0.5 to 1.0 mm per day, the joints distal to the distraction become very stiff: MP joint for metacarpal and PIP joint for proximal phalangeal lengthening. The second stage must routinely include a release of these joints, if necessary. Intrinsic muscles (dorsal and palmar interossei, thenar and hypothenar musculature) may become fibrotic and create long-term problems. No one has specifically documented the effect of lengthening on the intrinsic musculature of the hand, but we have seen fibrotic muscles with aggressive rapid distraction. Bone exposure may result from excessive distraction at the phalangeal level. Forearm lengthening takes much longer than 6 to 8 weeks and may cause elbow flexion contractures despite conscientious therapy. The lengthening must be slow and the surgeon must be careful not to lose flexor or extensor function of the wrist and hand.

Outcomes

The outcomes of this staged process are predictable but occasionally outcomes are not what the patient and family expected. Careful preoperative counseling is mandatory. There may be a tremendous amount of discomfort and surgery for a minimal gain in length. Humeral distraction is very predictable as long as the radial nerve is not injured during the process. Forearm (radius or ulna) lengthening of greater than 6.0 to 8.0 cm in older children or adolescents commonly develop secondary elbow contractures and persistent wrist and digital flexion. For this reason, the carpus and metacarpal portion of the hand must be stabilized within the external fixation apparatus. These children do well as long as the functioning flexor-pronator musculature is not injured. Surprisingly, there have been no long-term residual nerve-related problems in this entire series. Metacarpal lengthening result in the most predictable and best outcomes, especially when a short metacarpal is extended to the length of its adjacent partner(s). Phalangeal lengthening is the most unpredictable, particularly at the middle and distal level. Patients with the constriction ring syndrome have the worst outcomes because the blood supply to these digits is precarious from birth. Following digital distraction and bone grafting, the surgeon must emphasize to the patients and parents that the digit, although longer, will be narrow and stiff. The appearance is definitely enhanced and sensation should not change. Nails cannot be created without microvascular toe transfers.

In short, distraction lengthening in the hand is a very powerful tool in the properly selected and informed patient and family.

MICROSURGERY

Applications of microsurgery to the treatment of congenital hand differences have evolved slowly during the past decade. The slow progress has been due in part to the erroneous assumptions that pediatric vessels were more prone to spasm, donor site dissections were more difficult, and there were potential growth deficiencies. Although the vessels are smaller and more delicate, the same principles observed in adults apply to these pediatric patients. The most crucial factors include careful preoperative planning, and a meticulous and atraumatic recipient and donor site dissection. Whenever possible, it is essential to convert a micro to a macro operation.

Toe transfers have been the primary indication in congenital hand surgery. The most predictable and best outcomes have been obtained in the constriction ring syndrome and in adactyly patients associated with the chorionic villus sampling syndrome. In both conditions, the proximal anatomy is absolutely normal. Adactylous hands or those with only one border ray benefit most from toe transfers in both syndromic and nonsyndromic patients. The major limitation seen in all of these difficult transfers is a decreased range of motion due to the reduced excursion of the abnormal proximal forearm extrinsic motors (22). The surgeon must always be alert to recognize anomalous anatomy, which becomes the rule instead of the exception in these hands. One example would be the connection of extrinsic flexor and extensor tendons within the palm. The foot in a growing child can be severely compromised by an unnecessary dissection at the metatarsal or tarsal level in order to reach arterial conduits of sufficient size. An open plantar dissection through the first web space is recommended. Judicious use of vein grafts should take precedence over an extensive dissection of the plantar arch. The most devastating failure in all of microsurgery is the loss of an elective toe transfer in a growing child!

The most dramatic and useful applications involve both

soft tissue and skeletal replacement in unusual conditions, such as cutis aplasia congenita, or following severe burns or other traumatic conditions. Contrary to popular belief, the newborn brachial, ulnar, and radial arteries are sufficiently larger than 1.5 mm in size and allow performance of predictable anastomoses under the operating microscope (not loupes). The well-vascularized transferred tissue is programmed to grow at the same rate as it would in its original location. Strict immobilization of the pediatric upper limb is important and usually is related to unfavorable outcomes. Because leech therapy is difficult to maintain in these patients and families, prompt exploration of congested flaps is recommended.

ACKNOWLEDGMENT

The authors thank Mary Beth Ezaki, M.D., for her assistance with several of the figures.

REFERENCES

1. Upton J. Congenital anomalies of the upper limb. In: May J, Littler JW, eds. *Plastic Surgery,* vol. 8. Philadelphia: WB Saunders, 1989:5212–5398.
2. Swanson AA. A classification for congenital limb malformations. *J Hand Surg* 1976:1:8–22.
3. Ogino T. Congenital anomalies of the hand: the Asian perspective. *Clin Orthop* 1966;323:12–21.
4. Witt PW, MacArthur CA. Molecular biology and congenital hand anomalies: from molecules to mutations in man. *Plast Reconstr Surg* 1998;102:2254–2267.
5. Wassel HD. The results for surgery of polydactyly of the thumb: a review. *Clin Orthop* 1969;64:175–181.
6. Bilhaut M. Guerison un pouce bifide par un nouveau procede operatoire. *Congres Francais Chir* 1890;4:576–580.
7. Upton J. The surgical approach to the cleft hand. In: Saffar P, Amadio PC, Foucher G, eds. *Current practice in hand surgery.* London: Martin Dunitz, 1997:421–428.
8. Buck-Gramcko D. Congenital and developmental conditions. In: Bowers WH, ed. *The interphalangeal joints. The hand and upper limb,* vol. 1. Edinburgh: Churchill Livingstone, 1987:194–197.
9. Auerbach AD. Fanconi anemia diagnosis and the diepoxybutane (DEB) test. *Exp Hematol* 1993;21:731–733.
10. Buck-Gramcko D. Radialization as a new treatment for radial club hand. *J Hand Surg* 1985;10:964–968.
11. Lamb DW. Radial club hand: a continuing study of sixty-eight patients with one hundred and seventeen club hands. *J Bone Joint Surg Am* 1977;59(A):1–13.
12. Blauth W. Der hypoplasticher Daumen. *Arch Orthop Unfallchir* 1967;92:225–246.
13. Buck-Gramcko D. Congenital Malformations. In: Nigst H, Buck Gramcko D, Millesi H, eds. *Handchirurgie* (English edition). Stuttgart: G. Thieme Verlag, 1988:12.93–12.107
14. Manske PR, McCarroll HR, James M. Type III-A hypoplastic thumb. *J Hand Surg* 1995;20:246–253.
15. Shibata M, Yoshizu T, Seki T, et al. Reconstruction of a congenital hypoplastic thumb with use of a free vascularized metatarsophalangeal joint. *J Bone Joint Surg Am* 1998;80:1469–1476.
16. Mulliken JB, Glowacki J. Hemangiomas and vascular malformations in infants and children: a classification based on endothelial characteristics. *Plast Reconstr Surg* 1982;69:412–420.
17. Upton J. Vascular anomalies of the upper limb. In: Mulliken JB, Young AE, eds. *Vascular birthmarks.* New York: WB Saunders, 1988:343–380.
18. Upton J, Mulliken JB, Murray JE. Classification and rationale for management of vascular anomalies in the upper extremity. *J Hand Surg Am* 1985;10:970–975.
19. Upton J, Coombes C, Mulliken JB, et al. Vascular malformations of the upper limb: a review of 270 patients. *J Hand Surg* 1999;24: 1019–1035.
20. Flatt AE. *The care of congenital hand anomalies.* St. Louis: Quality Medical Publishing, 1994:337–363.
21. Matev IB. Thumb reconstruction after amputation at the metacarpophalangeal joint by bone lengthening. *J Bone Joint Surg Am* 1970;52:957–965.
22. Kay SP, Wiberg M. Toe to hand transfer in children. Part 1: technical aspects. *J Hand Surg* 1996;21:723–734.

Discussion

RONALD M. ZUKER
MEIR COHEN

Drs. Upton and Pap have put together a very detailed and complete chapter on congenital anomalies of the upper limb. It is an honor to be asked to provide a discussion. The introduction in particular addressed the issues of growth and the unfavorable outcomes that may occur. Timing of surgery also is central to a successful outcome. Early surgery allows for cerebral integration of the new part or function that is provided and avoids the likeliness of developing movements and adaptations that are inef-

R. M. Zuker and M. Cohen: Division of Plastic Surgery, The Hospital for Sick Children, Toronto, Ontario M5G 1X8, Canada.

fectual and difficult, if not impossible, to correct later in life.

Their chapter is extremely clearly written and comprehensive. There are some points that warrant augmentation and some that we feel lend themselves to a more in-depth discussion.

One can never overemphasize the importance of both a detailed history and a complete musculoskeletal examination. It serves to distinguish not only congenital from acquired deformities, but also isolated from syndromic anomalies.

The authors point out that "babies born with congenital upper limb malformations recognize their present condition as normal and may not recognize their differences until they are fully socialized." The same may also be said of the parents. It is not infrequent that the hand surgeon is asked to evaluate a toddler with an obvious congenital hand anomaly (i.e., thumb hypoplasia), first noticed by the parents as late as 2 or 3 years, in association with minor hand trauma. On the other hand, generalized acquired diseases may be confused with isolated hand conditions and even with congenital anomalies. The 2-year-old girl whose hand is shown in Fig. 42D-1 was referred by a hand surgeon for treatment of a soft tissue mass of the third finger diagnosed as a congenital vascular malformation. A complete musculoskeletal examination revealed a tender knee and ankle joints as well.

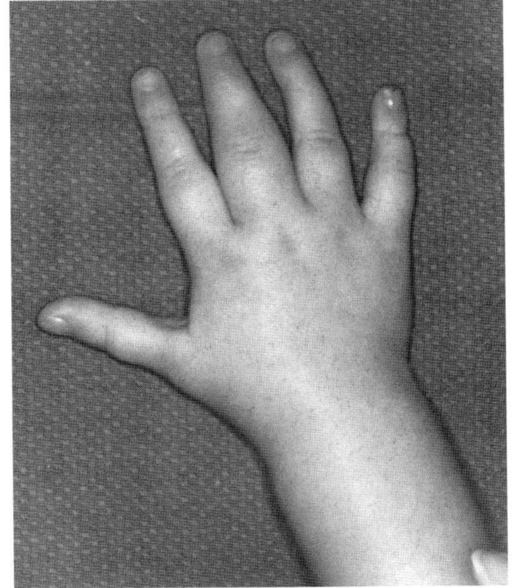

A

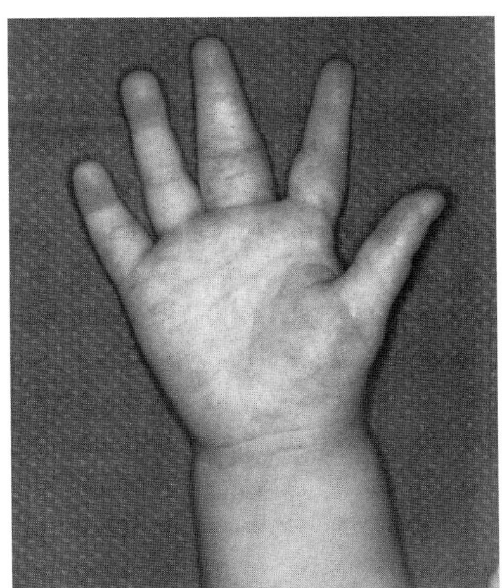

B

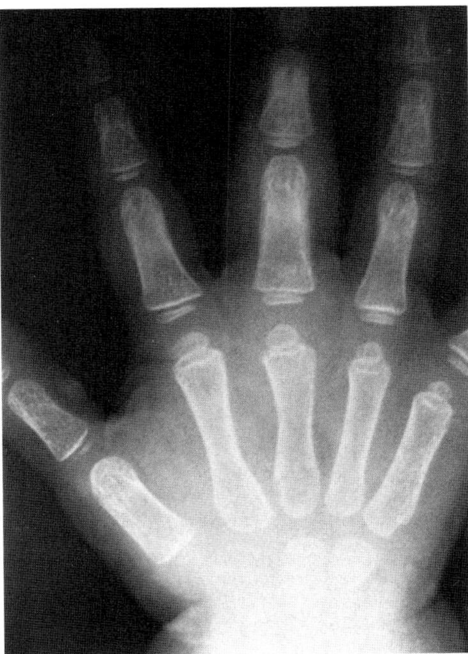

C

FIGURE 42D-1. A: Dorsal view of the hand of a 2-year-old child with diffuse swelling misdiagnosed as a vascular anomaly. **B:** Palmar view. **C:** Radiographic evaluation revealed periosteal reaction of proximal phalanx.

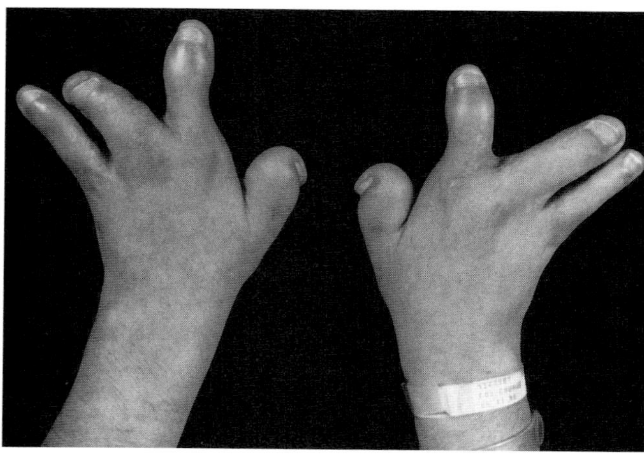

FIGURE 42D-2. Poor result following ray amputation with loss of hand balance and reduced function.

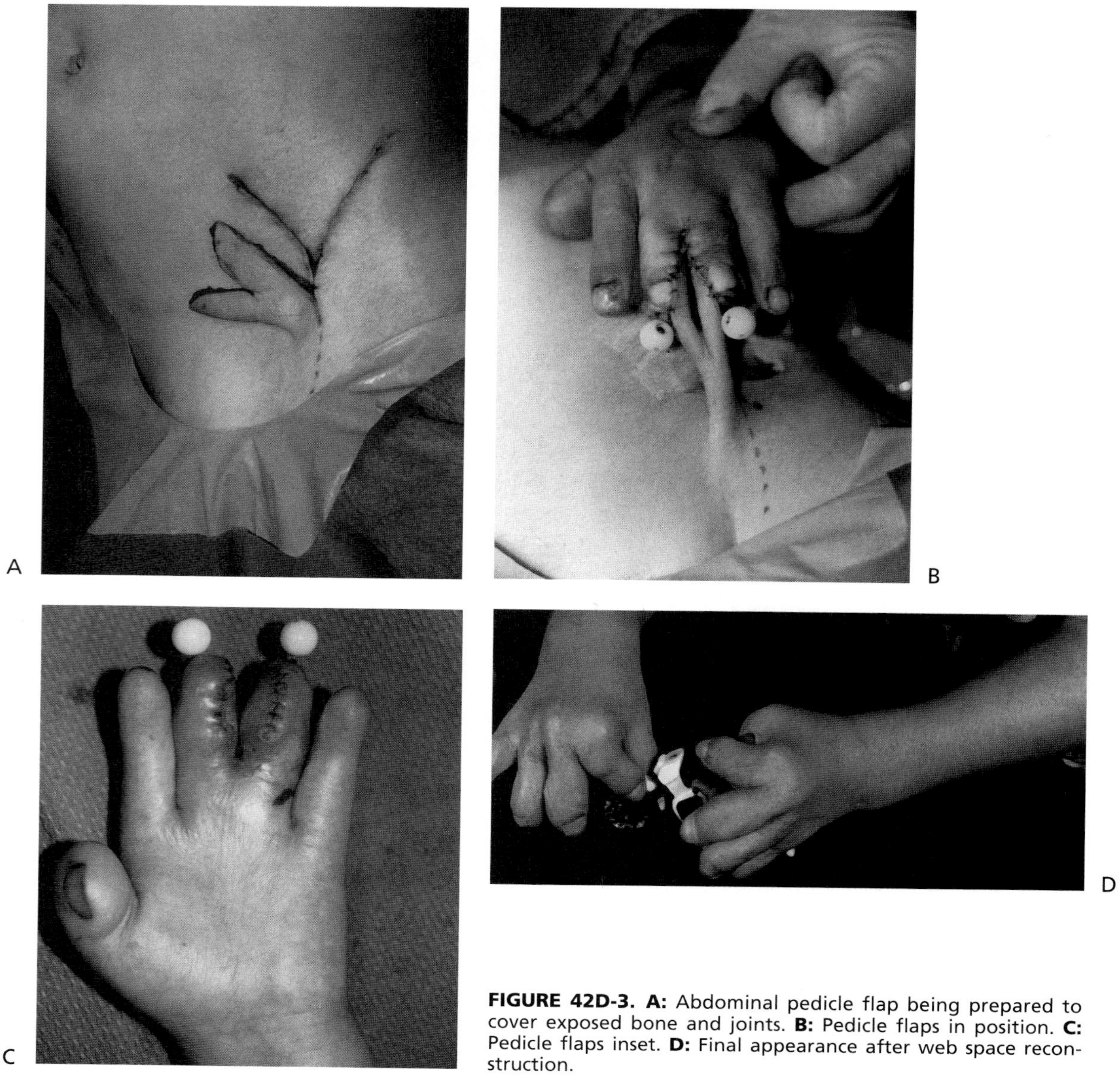

FIGURE 42D-3. A: Abdominal pedicle flap being prepared to cover exposed bone and joints. **B:** Pedicle flaps in position. **C:** Pedicle flaps inset. **D:** Final appearance after web space reconstruction.

The radiograph (Fig. 42D-1C) revealed a significant periosteal reaction on the proximal phalanx. The corrected diagnosis was juvenile rheumatoid arthritis.

Careful history-taking with a detailed review of all systems should always be undertaken when evaluating the child with a complex congenital hand anomaly. A complete whole-body assessment focusing on the musculoskeletal system will reveal the hypoplastic pectoralis major muscle of Poland syndrome, the foot contracture of arthrogryposis multiplex congenita, and the constriction band of the leg in amniotic band syndrome.

With respect to the section on duplication, it is worth commenting on the potential unfavorable result in the common type IV preaxial duplication. Very often there is a redundant segment of the metacarpal head on the radial side. It is tempting to remove this component to obtain a smooth radial contour. However, removal often incorporates a segment of the growth plate of the metacarpal head with potential growth disturbance. The unoperated ulnar side of the metacarpal head will continue to grow, but there will be a deviation toward the operated side where the plate was violated. This progressive deformity can be avoided by leaving the growth plate intact and accepting temporarily the contour irregularity of the oversized redundant metacarpal head. This can be addressed later with a minor contour adjustment when growth is almost complete.

In the syndactyly group, we cannot agree more with the authors' attention to meticulous detail in ensuring the complete survival of the full-thickness skin graft. In fact, in no other area of surgery does an incomplete take of the graft predict an unfavorable result. We have a particular interest in the complex syndactyly of Apert syndrome. Every effort should be made to create a five-digit hand, with separation of the conjoined fingers into four independent entities. Excision of rays all too often further disrupts the already compromised balance of the hand and leads to severe functionally impaired and aesthetically unacceptable results (Fig. 42D-2). Digital separation can be difficult and lead to exposed bone and joints. The use of small abdominal pedicle flaps can be very useful in covering these structures and in providing tissue for assistance in contour restoration. These flaps are appropriately positioned and maintained with secure bandages for 2 weeks until definitive separation and insetting. Final separation, web space creation, and contour adjustment lead to an acceptable, albeit far from perfect, result (Fig. 42D-3).

The section on radial dysplasia is excellent and the results of pollicization exceptional. We agree fully that toe transfers for reconstruction of the hypoplastic thumb are not indicated. They do not look appropriate, do not function well, and are far inferior to a well-planned and well-executed pollicization.

The section of vascular anomalies reflects the wealth of experience and depth of knowledge the authors bring to this subject. Similarly, the sections on the cleft hand reflect the challenge of differentiating a technical success over a practical improvement. One area of congenital hand surgery that commonly leads to an unfavorable result is surgery for overgrowth. This is best left to the hands of experts who have experience dealing with these complex, frustrating problems. Diminution in function, poor aesthetics, and unhappy children are all too often the result of ill-advised intervention.

In the section on camptodactyly, the authors emphasize early detection, stretches, and splinting. In our experience, this almost always is sufficient, and the need for surgical intervention rare. This is fortunate, as the results of surgery usually are abysmal. All too often the child is made worse with a swollen, tender, stiff, and scarred digit. This condition generally is best managed nonoperatively.

Clinodactyly involves digital deviation, but in the lateral plane as opposed to the anterior posterior plane of camptodactyly. Surgery for clinodactyly is mainly for aesthetics, as rarely is it a functional issue. The surgery can, however, lead to significant problems. Wedge osteotomies can be complicated by malunion, nonunion, diminished tendon gliding and can lead to functional impairment. As it is primarily a problem of cosmesis, surgery should not be undertaken without thorough discussion with the child and family.

The last section involves a description of the roles of distraction osteogenesis and microsurgery. These fields continue to evolve and likely will be of significant importance to the pediatric hand surgeon of the future.

In conclusion, an unfavorable result following surgery for congenital anomalies of the upper limb can occur in four situations. First, the wrong operation can be performed, such as an extensive release of a mild camptodactyly. Second, the correct operation could have been performed, but not effectively, such as a significant loss of a full-thickness skin graft in a syndactyly release. Third, the operation could have been performed at the wrong time, such as a growth arrest for overgrowth far beyond the age when it might have been effective. Fourth, the operation may have been performed well, at the correct time, but in the wrong patient who was emotionally or psychologically not able to use the additional unit or the functional adaptation.

Surgery for congenital anomalies of the upper limb must be preceded by a detailed history, a thorough musculoskeletal evaluation that often involves repeat visits, and a well-executed, well-timed procedure on the right patient.

43

BONE AND JOINT INJURIES

NORMAN WEINZWEIG
JEFFREY WEINZWEIG

Care of bone and joint injuries of the hand often is relegated to inexperienced emergency room house officers. Consequently, mistreatment of fractures and dislocations of the metacarpals and phalanges commonly occurs. Ultimately, the hand surgeon is consulted in an attempt to recoup functional losses resulting from no treatment, undertreatment, overtreatment, or inappropriate treatment of these relatively "minor" injuries that can have disastrous consequences.

Proper initial diagnosis and timely appropriate treatment of the tubular bones and small joint injuries of the hand can be simple and straightforward, yet they are often missed by the unwary. The goal in fracture management is not simply bony healing in the correct position, but also minimizing the soft tissue scarring that often results in prolonged disability. In fact, "injury to bone is only one element and often not even the most important element of the injury created by a fracture" (1).

Complications cause significant functional loss and cosmetic deformity that can be avoided by obeying basic principles and techniques (1–8). In certain circumstances, however, the unfavorable result cannot be avoided because of the very nature of the injury (such as a gunshot wound or crush injury that shatters the articular surface, thereby limiting motion) regardless of treatment. Less than optimal results often are obtained whenever bone and soft tissue are disrupted, regardless of the skill and diligence of the surgeon. This chapter will discuss the most commonly encountered problems following bone and joint injuries of the hand, with emphasis on prevention of complications and treatment of established complications.

N. Weinzweig: Divisions of Plastic Surgery and Orthopedic Surgery, University of Illinois at Chicago and Cook County Hospital, Chicago, Illinois
J. Weinzweig: Department of Plastic Surgery, Brown University School of Medicine, Rhode Island Hospital, Providence, Rhode Island

BASIC PRINCIPLES OF FRACTURE MANAGEMENT

First and foremost, treat the patient, *not* the radiograph. Generally, a force of sufficient magnitude to fracture the tubular bones of the hand can cause significant injury to the enveloping soft tissues, flexor and extensor tendons, ligaments, intrinsic muscles, and neurovascular structures (Fig. 43-1). This important factor must be considered in the treatment plan, rehabilitation protocol, and prognosis. In some cases, such as crush or roller injuries, carpal tunnel release and/or fasciotomy for ischemic intrinsic muscles must be performed in timely fashion to avoid devastating complications.

History and Physical Examination

Key to diagnosis and treatment of hand fractures is a thorough history and physical examination. History should include handedness, occupation, avocation, mechanism of injury (crush injury with compartment syndrome), time since injury ("golden period"), and place of injury (home, farm, industry). Physical examination often can provide the diagnosis and should include inspection for open fracture, localized tenderness, swelling, deformity (angulation, rotation, shortening), alignment (fingers should form a gentle arc without overlapping when partially flexed and all nailbeds must point toward the scaphoid), range of motion (ROM; active/passive flexion and extension, intrinsic tightness), and neurovascular status.

Radiographs

The importance of adequate radiographs cannot be overemphasized. Malpractice suits are won by the plaintiff when the treating physician either does not order radiographs for a "minor" injury or "sprain" or obtains inadequate radiographs that fail to demonstrate the extent of bone or joint injury. Radiographs should include three planes: anteroposterior,

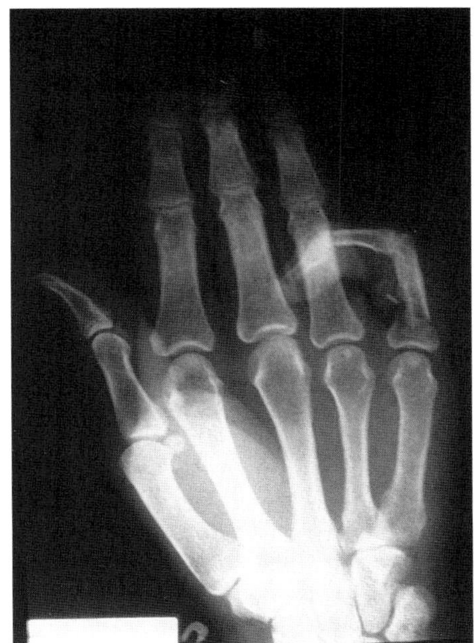

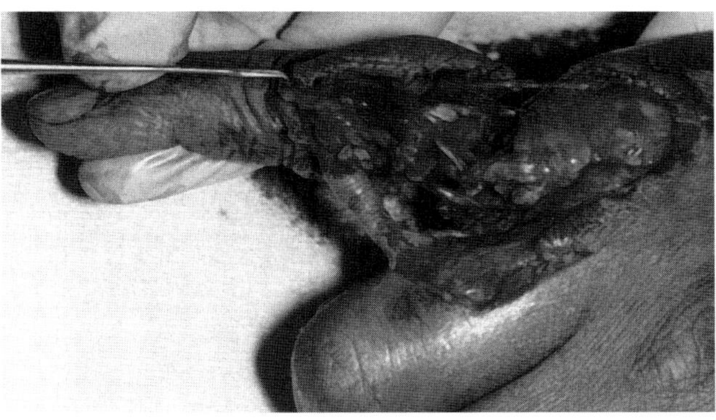

FIGURE 43-1. A: Radiograph demonstrating the extent of bony injury. **B:** The radiograph often does not predict the severity of injury to the surrounding soft tissues, flexor and extensor tendons, ligaments, intrinsic muscles, and neurovascular structures.

lateral, and oblique views of the individual digit. With only two views, one may miss either the fracture or the degree of displacement (Fig. 43-2). The radiology requisition should clearly state that radiographs of the injured digit, *not* the hand, are needed. Lateral radiographs of the hand are taken with the fingers held in full extension and superimposed upon each other. Thus, phalangeal fractures often can be obscured by the overlying silhouettes of the adjacent digits. Postreduction views should be obtained to check the status of reduction in 5 to 7 days. Special views should be obtained when indicated, such as a Brewerton view for clarification of ligament-avulsion injuries of the metacarpal head, a Robert view (true anteroposterior view of thumb metacarpal with hand in maximal pronation) for the first metacarpal-trapezium joint (Bennett or Rolando fracture), and a reverse Robert view for the fifth metacarpal-hamate joint.

Reduction, Retention, and Rehabilitation

The goal of fracture management is the restoration of normal function by achieving the three R's: reduction, retention, and rehabilitation. After accurate fracture reduction, the

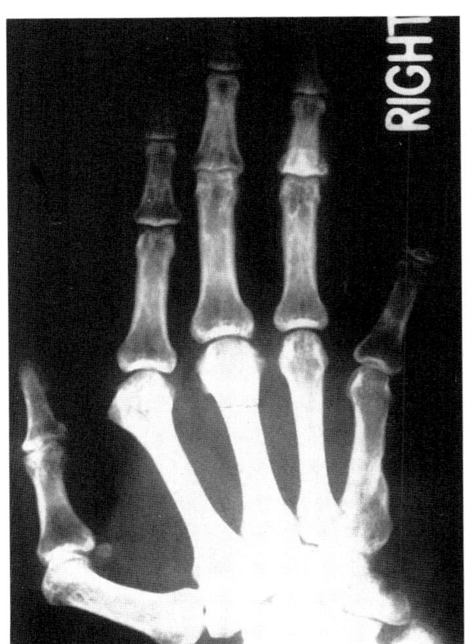

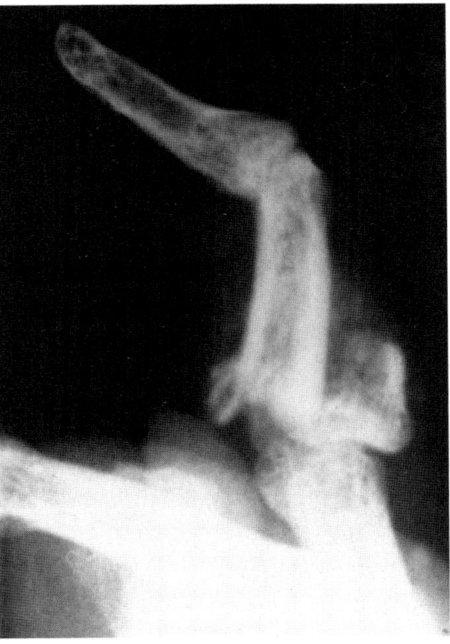

FIGURE 43-2. This patient sustained an open transverse fracture of the base of the middle phalanx of the ring finger. **A:** The fracture is difficult to appreciate on the anteroposterior radiograph. There also is a malunion at the base of the metacarpal of the little finger. **B:** The fracture and degree of displacement of the fragments of the middle phalanx are apparent on the lateral view.

hand should be immobilized in the "intrinsic plus" or "safe position," with the extremity elevated to minimize edema. Proper positioning of the proximal and distal bone fragments during immobilization, appropriate use of internal fixation when indicated, and early motion are mandatory. Inappropriate or prolonged splinting can result in articular and extra-articular changes and the development of joint contracture, deformity, or stiffness (Fig. 43-3). The metacarpophalangeal (MP) joints of the digits should be splinted in maximal or near-maximal flexion. Because the metacarpal head is cam shaped, flexion maintains the collateral ligaments at maximal length. When splinted in extension, the collateral ligaments shorten causing a loss of flexion. The interphalangeal (IP) joints should be splinted in near-maximal extension. Splinting of the IP joints in flexion promotes the development of checkrein ligaments causing volar plate contracture with permanent loss of flexion at the IP joints (9).

The majority of fractures can be treated successfully by nonoperative means (10). This is possible because most fractures are functionally stable before or after closed reduction and will do well with protective splinting and early mobilization. Repeat radiographs should be performed at 5 to 7 days to check the status of the reduction. Unstable fractures cannot be reduced in closed fashion or, if reduced, cannot be held in the reduced position without supplemental fixation. Internal fixation is required to provide stability and allow early mobilization. Initially unstable fractures can be reduced and converted to a stable position by either external immobilization (cast, cast with metal outrigger splint, or anteroposterior plaster splint), closed reduction and percutaneous pin fixation (CRPP), or open reduction and internal fixation (ORIF). Many complications occur because of failure to recognize fractures that are inherently unstable and progress to malunion. Indications for internal fixation include uncontrollable rotation, angulation, or shortening; displaced intra-articular fractures involving more than 15% to 20% of the articular surface; fracture-subluxations of the thumb and little finger carpometacarpal (CMC) joints; unstable fractures that failed closed manipulation, such as spiral fractures of the proximal phalanges or transverse fractures of the metacarpals; metacarpal head fractures; multiple digit fractures; and open fractures (11,12).

Immediate movement of the uninvolved fingers should be permitted to prevent stiffness. An exercise program should be directed toward the specific fracture or dislocation with early mobilization of the injured finger. Always keep in mind that the proximal interphalangeal (PIP) joint is the most important joint in the hand. For nondisplaced fractures treated in closed fashion, motion can be started within 3 weeks, if stable. Midshaft proximal phalangeal fractures require 5 to 7 weeks of immobilization for clinical stability. Midshaft middle phalangeal fractures having a greater ratio of cortical to cancellous bone require 10 to 14 weeks of immobilization (same as a scaphoid fracture). Comminuted fractures with disruption of the periosteum and open fractures can take twice as long as simple and closed fractures to achieve bony union. Failure to immobilize a fracture site for a sufficient period of time can result in loss of reduction with subsequent malunion (Fig. 43-4). Radiologic union lags behind clinical stability and usually is not seen for 3 to 5 months. One of the best criteria for initiation of mobilization is whether or not the fracture site is tender. Fractures that are no longer tender to palpation generally are healed well enough to begin active mobilization.

A,B

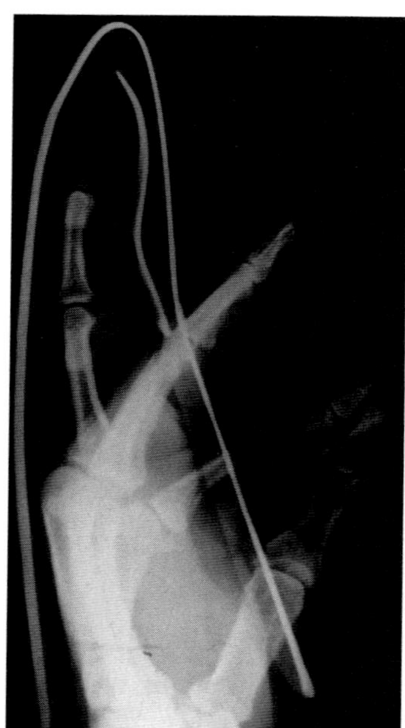

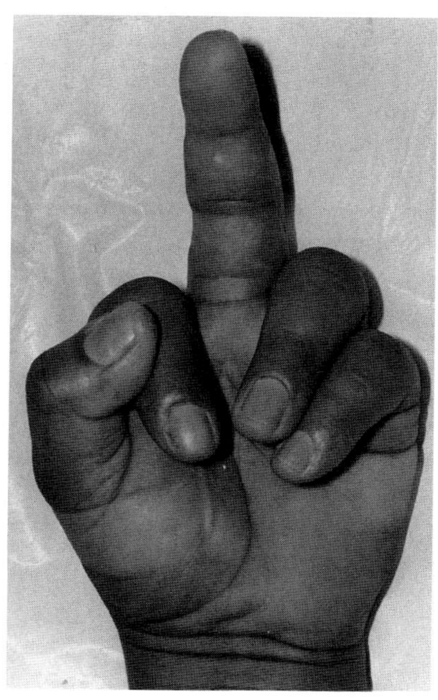

FIGURE 43-3. A: This patient was splinted in metacarpophalangeal (MP) joint extension for 7 weeks following a comminuted intra-articular fracture of the base of the proximal phalanx of the middle finger. **B:** This procedure resulted in stiffness and loss of flexion of the middle finger due to shortening of the collateral ligaments of the MP joint.

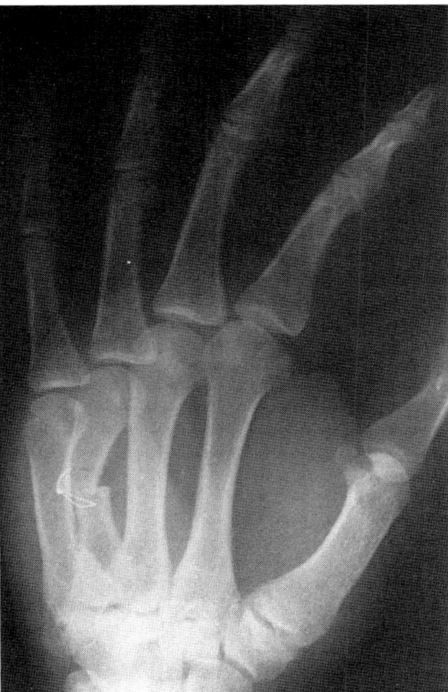

FIGURE 43-4. Premature removal of the oblique Kirschner wire and early mobilization resulted in loss of reduction for this midshaft metacarpal fracture.

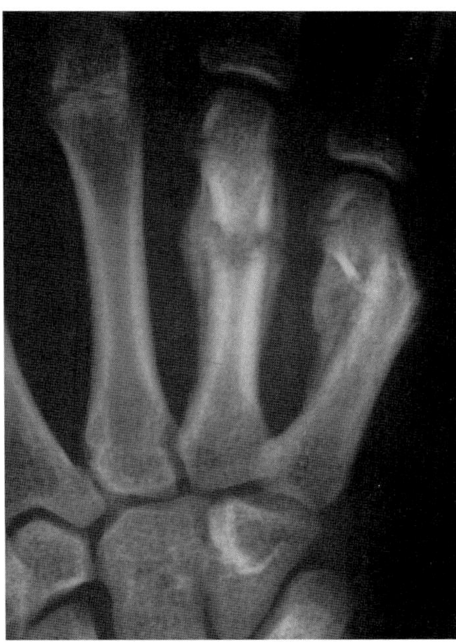

FIGURE 43-5. Malunion resulted from untreated fractures of the metacarpals of the ring and little fingers. Excessive callus formation caused significant tendon adherence that restricted motion.

MALUNIONS

The natural tendency of untreated fractures is to unite, as seen in the fractured bones of animals, primitive tribesmen, and prehistoric skeletons. However, we must ensure that the fractured bones heal or unite in the correct position. Malunion is the most common bony complication of metacarpal and phalangeal fractures (Fig. 43-5). This complication occurs in a variety of predictable patterns based on the biomechanical forces of the injury; the interactive forces of the intrinsic muscles, tendons, and ligaments acting on the fracture site; and the external forces of the applied fixation method(s) resulting in the deformities of *rotation, angulation,* and *shortening*. Remember, all malunions are far more easily prevented than corrected later.

Rotational Deformities

Rotational deformities manifest themselves by overlapping or scissoring of the fingers during flexion, resulting in diminished grip strength and dexterity (Fig. 43-6). These complications are commonly seen after spiral and oblique fractures of the phalanges and metacarpals. Malrotation may be difficult to assess radiographically and often is a clinical diagnosis. This deformity is not obvious when the fingers are extended, although nailbed asymmetry can be appreciated. All fingernails must point toward the scaphoid when making a fist.

No degree of rotational deformity can be accepted, because as little as 5 degrees of rotation in a metacarpal translates into 1.5 cm of digital overlap. Immobilizing the injured finger with an adjacent normal digit and carefully monitoring the planes of the fingernails will help minimize this complication. However, it often is deceptively difficult to control rotation by external immobilization alone. CRPP

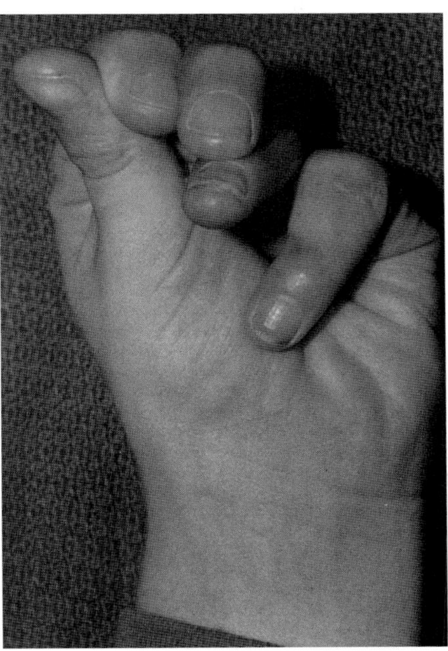

FIGURE 43-6. Rotational deformities are characterized by overlapping or scissoring of adjacent fingers during flexion. Malrotation may be difficult to assess radiographically and is often a clinical diagnosis.

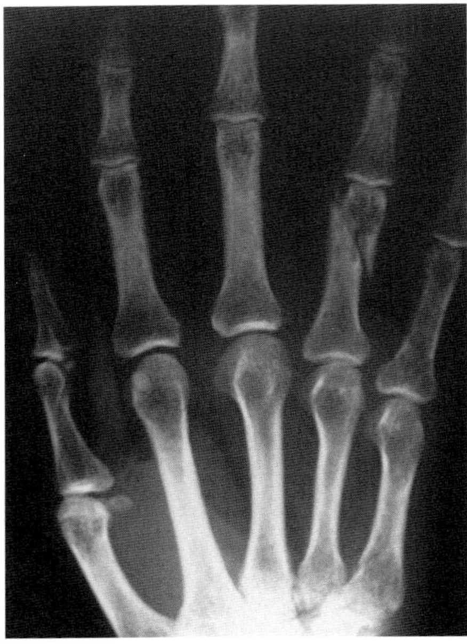

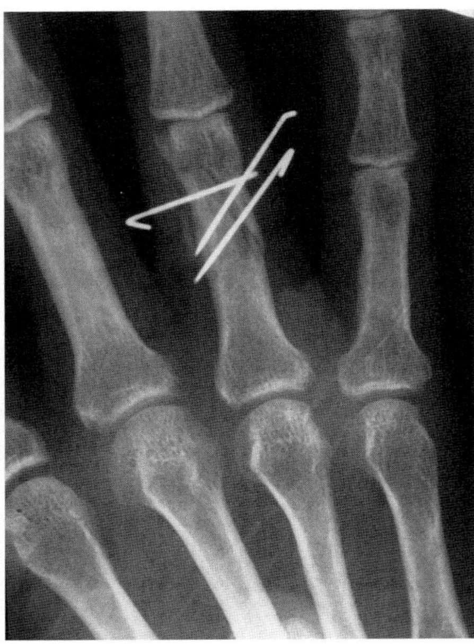

A,B

FIGURE 43-7. A: This patient sustained an oblique fracture of the proximal phalanx of the ring finger. Initial treatment by buddy taping and splint immobilization for 6 weeks resulted in a rotational deformity. **B:** Refracture was performed through the previous fracture site and stable fixation was achieved with Kirschner wires.

or ORIF should be considered, especially for phalangeal fractures (Fig. 43-7). Intraoperatively, the alignment of the fingers can be difficult to assess clinically due to marked edema of the hand and patient uncooperativeness or unconsciousness. In the latter case, the surgeon can compress the muscle bellies along the ulnar aspect of the mid forearm to produce flexion of the fingers (Fig. 43-8). With limited finger flexion, the rotational deformity may not be obvious. Unless significant flexion can be restored, correction of the malunion should not be attempted. However, if there is significant finger flexion and the overlap is obvious, osteotomy should be performed to correct the cosmetic deformity and functional impairment.

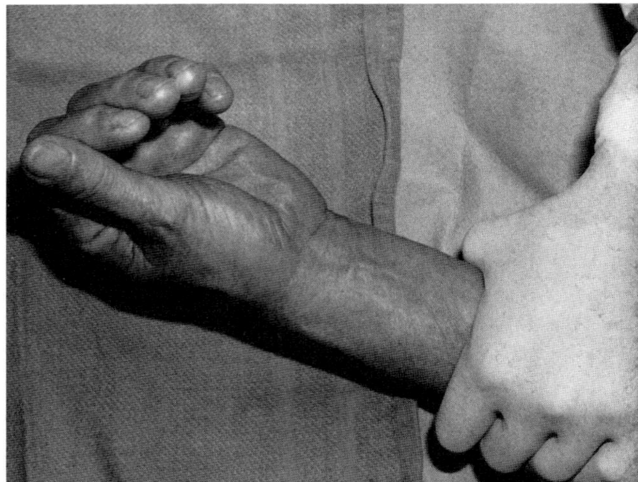

FIGURE 43-8. To assess the alignment of the fingers intraoperatively, compression of the muscle bellies along the ulnar aspect of the mid forearm produces flexion.

Osteotomy can be performed through either the previous fracture site or the base of the metacarpal. Phalangeal deformities can be corrected directly by phalangeal osteotomies; however, this requires considerable dissection about the extensor mechanism that often results in scarring, tendon adherence, and stiffness of the MP and PIP joints with loss of digital motion. Thus, phalangeal osteotomies generally are reserved for simultaneous correction of rotational and angulation deformities. This approach also permits concomitant soft tissue procedures, such as tenolysis or capsulotomy. For a pure malrotation deformity regardless of the site of malunion, most surgeons prefer a transverse osteotomy through the cancellous base of the metacarpal, or Weckesser's technique (13). This technique places the osteotomy outside the fibrous flexor tendon sheath, making it less prone to tendon adhesions. According to Weckesser, correction of up to 25 degrees of malrotation in either direction can be achieved. Gross and Gelberman (14) noted that metacarpal rotation was not equivalent to phalangeal correction. Because the proximal phalanx is not rigidly fixed to the metacarpal, phalangeal correction was approximately 70% of metacarpal rotation. Actual digital correction averaged 18 to 19 degrees in the index, long, and ring fingers and 20 to 30 degrees in the small finger. Another technique is Manktelow's step-cut osteotomy (15); however, this is far more complicated than Weckesser's technique. It requires more dissection and does not offer any significant advantages.

Lateral Angulation Deformities

Lateral angulation usually is caused by either displacement of an articular condyle or actual bone loss at the time of injury, such as following a gunshot wound or crush injury.

The articular condyles are critical in maintaining lateral alignment, and every effort should be made to preserve them, restore them, and maintain their normal position. Although most malunions are fairly amenable to late correction, it is almost impossible to correct PIP joint incongruity due to a malunited condylar fracture of the phalanx. Only anatomical reduction of a condylar fracture should be accepted using either CRPP or ORIF. In the case of actual bone loss, immediate or early bone grafting can be performed if the enveloping soft tissues are adequate. Lateral angulation deformities of the metacarpals are uncommon, because the metacarpals are splinted by the neighboring metacarpals and the strong proximal and distal intermetacarpal ligaments.

For lateral malunions, osteotomy, arthroplasty, and arthrodesis are treatment options. Corrective osteotomy can be performed through either the old fracture site or proximal to the level of deformity. Refracture is indicated if the malunion is a recent one or secondary to a displaced articular condyle. A laterally deviated phalanx can be corrected by a closing or opening wedge osteotomy directly through the site of malunion. A small wedge is removed by carefully measuring a cutout pattern on preoperative films. Alternatively, a closing wedge osteotomy can be performed by a series of progressively smaller burs using the Hall drill, as described by Froimson (16). Regardless of technique, it is desirable to leave periosteum intact at the apex of the osteotomy to provide stability and allow hinging of the bone on this "internal splint." Fixation often can be achieved by a single oblique K-wire. If instability persists, Lister's intraosseous wiring technique can be used (17). Arthroplasty is indicated when the joint surface is damaged and there is painful restricted motion. Implants do not provide lateral stability, and their use is limited to the middle and ring fingers where some lateral support is provided by the adjacent fingers (Fig. 43-9).

Arthrodesis is the treatment of choice for symptomatic angulation deformities of the distal IP joints where stability, not motion, is important. The decision is far more difficult at the PIP joint, where many factors, including the age, sex, occupation, avocation, and digit involved, come into play. When there is painful and restricted movement of the thumb and/or index finger MP joint(s), where lateral stability is important in pinch, arthrodesis is the procedure of choice. The ideal position of PIP joint arthrodesis varies from least flexion in the index finger (20 to 30 degrees) to most flexion in the small finger (35 to 45 degrees).

Dorsal-Volar Angulation Deformities

Dorsal-volar angulation typically is caused by transverse fractures of the metacarpal and phalangeal shafts as result of muscle-tendon imbalance across the fracture site. Metacarpal shaft fractures tend to angulate dorsally due to pull of the intrinsic muscles. In extra-articular fractures of the proximal phalanx, the fragments angulate volarly, with the interossei flexing the proximal fragment and the central slip extending the distal portion. In extra-articular fractures of the middle phalanx, the proximal and distal fragments are displaced by the forces of the central slip, the terminal extensor tendon, and the sublimis insertion. Direction of angulation depends on the location of the fracture with respect to the insertion of the sublimis. Fractures proximal to the sublimis insertion angulate dorsally; fractures distal to the sublimis insertion angulate volarly.

Radiographically, dorsal-volar angulation is less obvious than lateral angulation. In fact, it often is overlooked on anteroposterior radiographs. If lateral views are not performed, the fracture may be missed until bony healing is complete. However, lateral radiographs may be difficult to interpret because overlapping of fingers immobilized in a splint or cast can obscure the fracture. Therefore, lateral views of the injured finger, not the hand, must be specifically requested. Slightly obliqued views (a lateral view with 10 to 15 degrees of pronation for the ring and small fingers and 10 to 15 degrees of supination for the index and long fingers) may be easier to interpret than lateral views because the other fingers are rotated out of the way.

Phalangeal Malunions

Stable, nondisplaced, or impacted proximal and middle phalangeal fractures are treated by temporary protection with a splint followed by buddy taping (dynamic splinting). Remember, an undisplaced fracture requires protection, *not* immobilization. Closed reduction and external immobilization of the forearm, wrist, and injured digit, as well as the adjacent digit(s), usually is adequate. Various traction techniques of external fixation are used for markedly comminuted fractures or for bone loss; however, excessive traction should be avoided because it may prevent bony union. Unstable fractures require internal fixation (18–21).

Established volar angulation of the proximal phalanx often results in a "pseudoclaw" deformity of the finger. If the angulation is greater than 30 degrees, the patient will develop a compensatory flexion deformity of the PIP joint that may result in a fixed contracture. An intact extensor mechanism at the midportion of the proximal phalanx envelops two-thirds of the circumference of the tubular bone and acts as a tension band to transmit compression forces to the volar cortex and distraction forces to the dorsal cortex during active flexion. Therefore, "wounding of the extensor apparatus of the dorsum of the phalanges in association with fracture presents one of the most difficult of all problems of the hand" (19) (Fig. 43-10).

For significant dorsal-volar deformities, corrective osteotomy or refracture at the site of deformity is the only treatment (Fig. 43-11). This is performed via a lateral approach to avoid injury to the extensor mechanism. Froimson (16) prefers a dorsal opening wedge osteotomy at

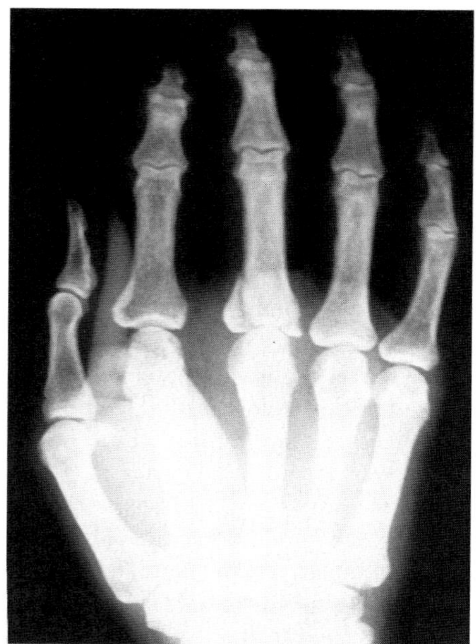

A

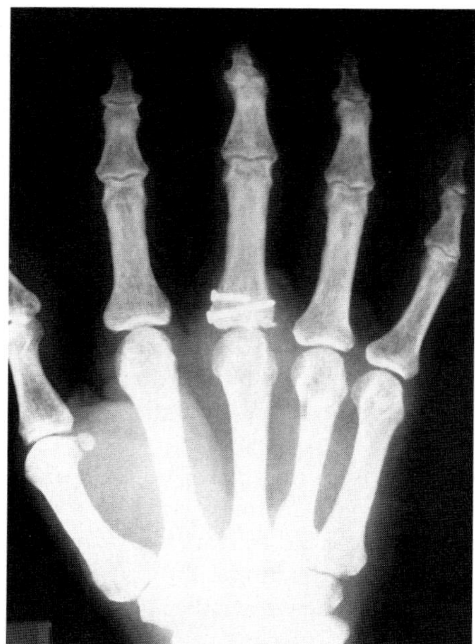

B

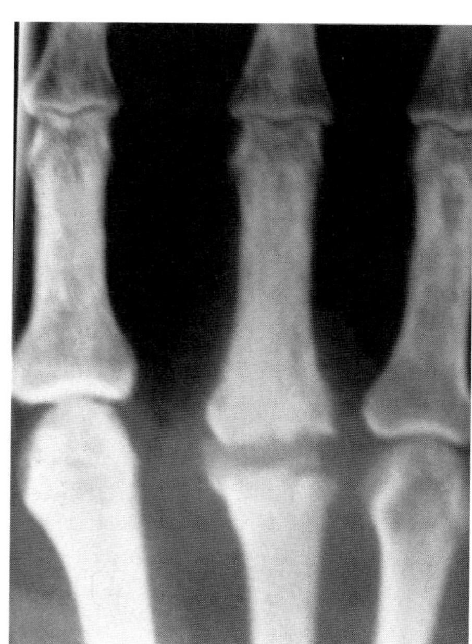

C

FIGURE 43-9. A: This elderly gentleman sustained an intra-articular fracture to the proximal phalanx of the middle finger. **B:** An attempt was made to achieve articular congruity by open reduction and internal fixation using two screws. **C:** Despite an aggressive occupational therapy program, there was residual pain and stiffness of the metacarpophalangeal (MP) joint. Silastic joint arthroplasty of the MP joint was performed to correct this problem.

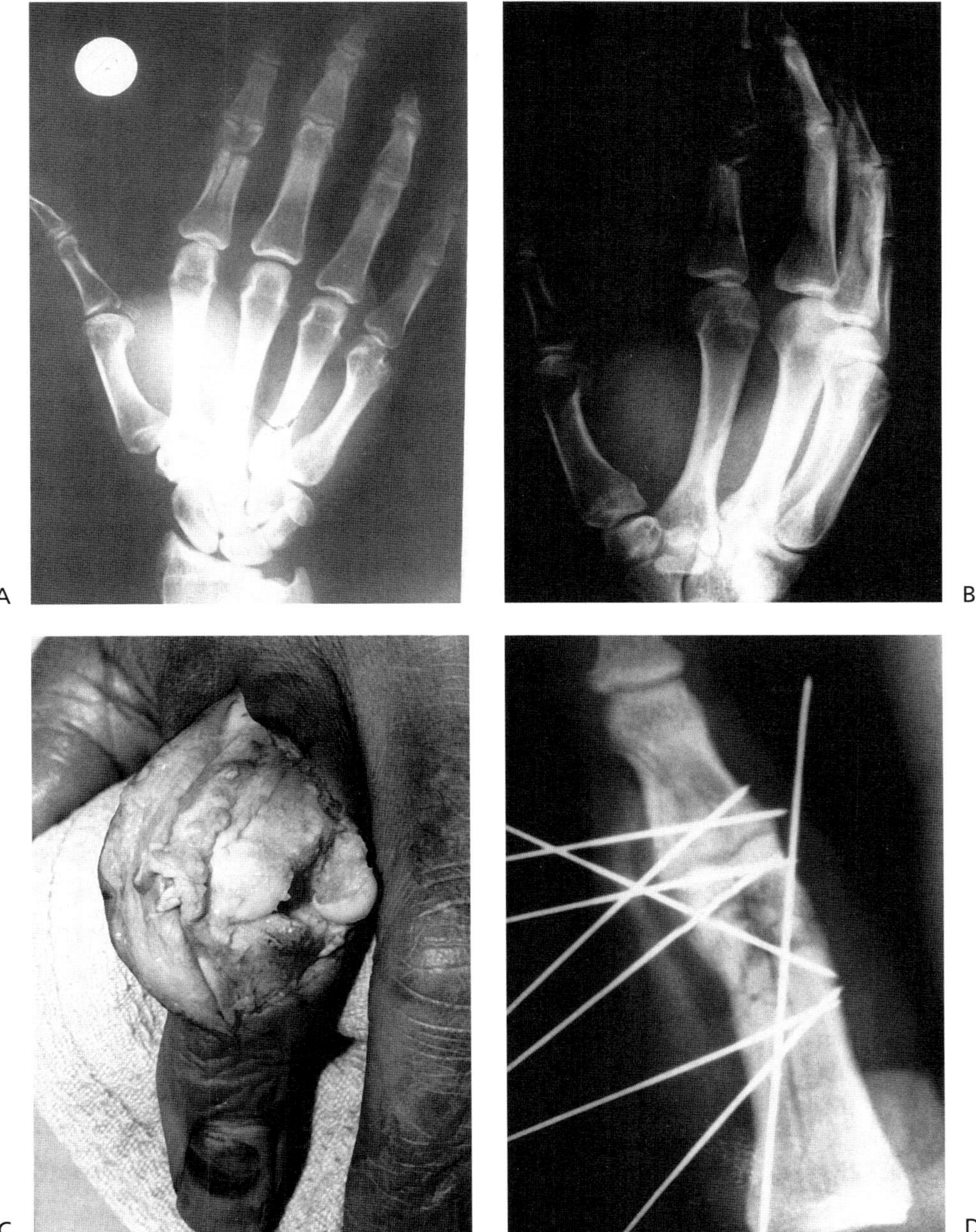

FIGURE 43-10. A,B: This patient sustained severe blunt trauma to his index finger that resulted in markedly comminuted fractures of the proximal and middle phalanges. **C:** Open reduction was performed in an attempt to achieve joint congruity. Note the extensive comminution and disruption of the extensor mechanism. Comminuted fractures with disruption of the periosteum and open fractures take longer to achieve bony union than simple or closed fractures. **D:** Internal fixation was accomplished using Kirschner wires. It is important to maintain internal fixation for a sufficient period of time to achieve clinical stability.

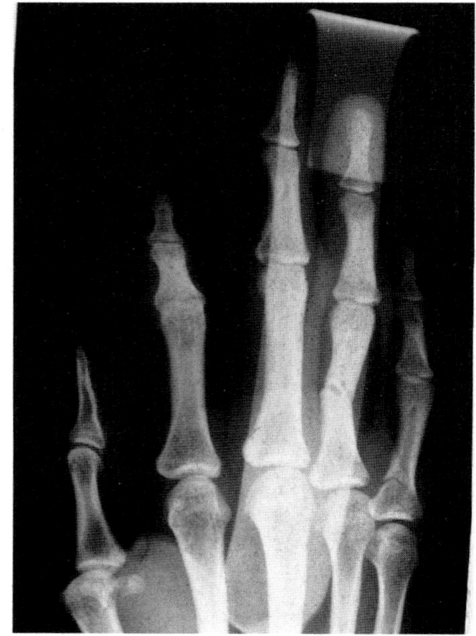

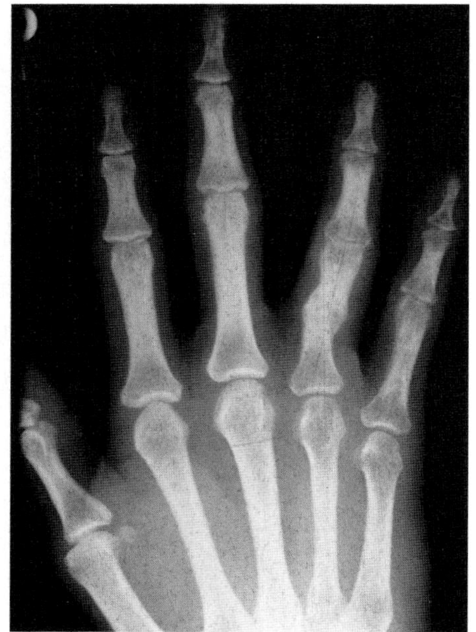

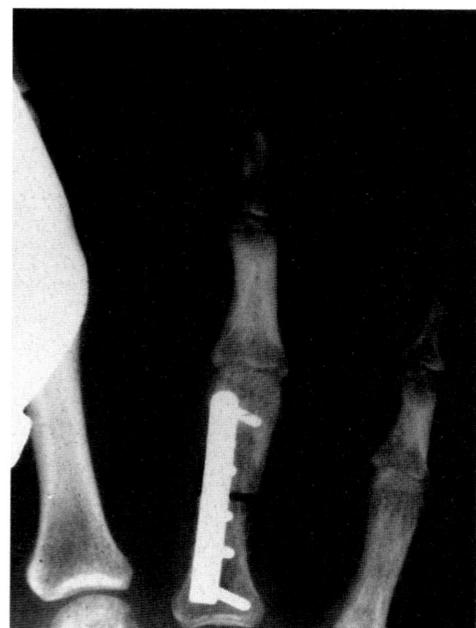

FIGURE 43-11. A: This transverse fracture of mid shaft of the proximal phalanx of the ring finger was treated with a metallic extension splint. No buddy taping or cast immobilization was used. **B:** Malunion of the proximal phalanx with 32 degrees of volar angulation and 15 degrees of ulnar deviation. **C:** An osteotomy was performed through the fracture site to correct the angulation deformities.

the malunion site, which requires a bone graft. Our preferred method is a simpler volar closing wedge osteotomy, which avoids a bone graft; this results in several millimeters of shortening that usually is not problem.

Metacarpal Malunions

Metacarpal neck fractures result in volar cortex comminution and dorsal angulation due to the interosseous muscles exerting a strong volar force. Malunion results in loss of prominence of the metacarpal head dorsally, and a palpable metacarpal head in the palm causing pain on grip. There is controversy over the amount of angulation that should be accepted, ranging from 30 to 70 degrees. Generally, angulation is unacceptable if there is "pseudoclawing" of the finger on digital extension. "Pseudoclawing" is compensatory MP joint hyperextension and PIP joint flexion on attempted extension of the digit. Up to 40 degrees of angulation can be accepted in the mobile ring and little metacarpals. For greater than 40 degrees of angulation, volar comminution, extensor lag, or unacceptable reduction, treat with CRPP. For the fixed index and middle metacarpals, no more than 10 to 15 degrees of angulation is acceptable, because these metacarpals lack compensatory

CMC motion. For the metacarpals, no rotation is acceptable, because as little as 5 degrees of rotation in a metacarpal fracture can cause up to 1.5 cm of digital overlap.

Isolated fractures of the shafts of the index and middle metacarpals tend to be relatively stable due to the splinting effect of the strong proximal and distal intermetacarpal ligaments. These two metacarpals are quite immobile due to the lack of compensatory CMC joint motion; usually they can be treated in closed fashion. However, simultaneous fracture of these bones results in instability with a tendency for malunion; usually internal fixation is necessary. The ring and little fingers are much more mobile, facilitating cupping and opposition of the thumb. This renders them more unstable after fracture, with a greater tendency for unacceptable rotation, scissoring of the fingers, and painful palmar prominence of the metacarpal head. Often, internal fixation is necessary. Plate fixation of the index and little fingers is recommended because these border metacarpals are exposed to uncontrolled external forces.

Transverse fractures of the metacarpal shafts usually are caused by direct blows. The more proximal the fracture, the less angulation that can be tolerated. Oblique and spiral fractures result from torsional forces acting on the finger as a lever arm. Lateral radiographs are mandatory, especially for spiral oblique fractures, to visualize impingement of a spike on the extensor mechanism. Closed reduction and plaster immobilization usually is adequate. Placing a patient in a "clamdigger" or "intrinsic plus" splint prevents contractures. If closed reduction is unsuccessful, perform an ORIF. Remember, immobility is the chief cause of stiffness (12,18).

Shortening

Malunion secondary to shortening most commonly results from metacarpal fractures and usually does not cause either significant cosmetic deformity or functional loss, especially when there is less than 5 mm of shortening. The metacarpal fragments are secured by the strong proximal and distal intermetacarpal ligaments (Fig. 43-12). On the other hand, long spiral and short oblique fractures of the proximal phalanx are inherently unstable. Reduction is impossible to maintain by closed methods. When the proximal phalanx is shortened, it can produce a bony spike distally that can impinge on the base of the middle phalanx volarly, restricting PIP joint flexion. Patients often have no clinical deformity; however, active flexion of the PIP joint is abruptly halted. The volar spike can be appreciated best on lateral radiographs. Formal osteotomy usually is not necessary, because simple excision of the offending spike will correct the problem and allow full flexion. This usually is approached by either a midline or a volar zigzag approach, with the tendon sheath retracted. In the case of significant deformity, corrective osteotomy may be necessary.

A
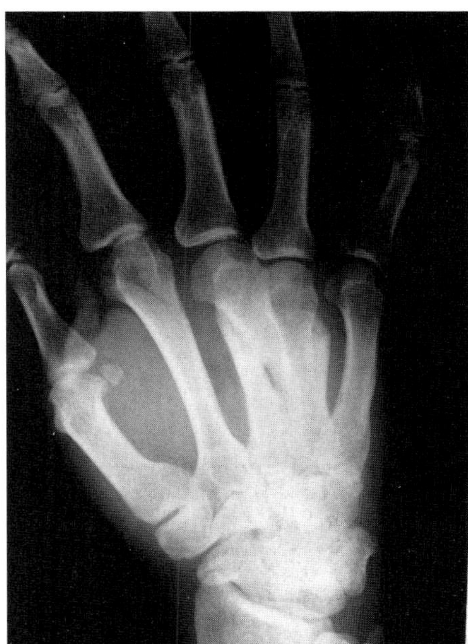

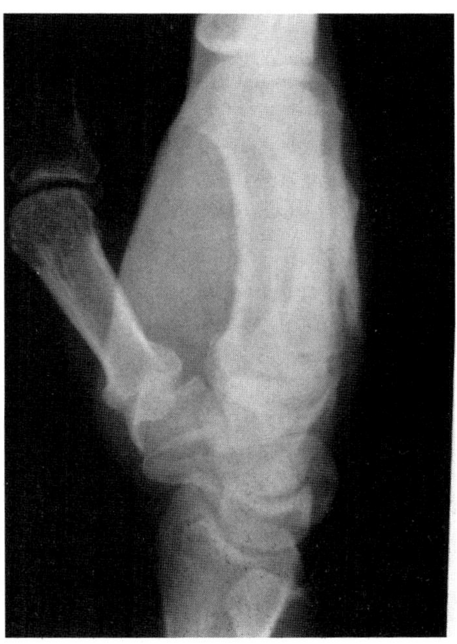
B

FIGURE 43-12. A,B: Malunion secondary to shortening usually occurs after metacarpal fractures. Often, this does not cause significant cosmetic deformity or functional loss, especially when there is less than 5 mm of shortening. ***(continued)***

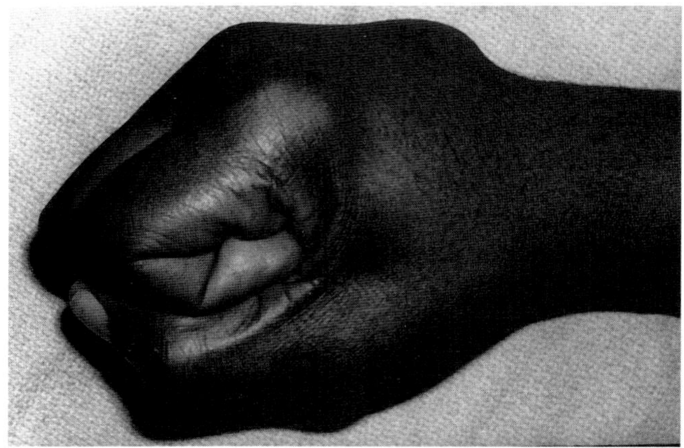

C

FIGURE 43-12. (Continued). **C:** Despite the obvious dorsal deformity, there is little functional disability.

NONUNIONS

Nonunions in the hand are uncommon. They occur following open fracture with segmental bone loss, soft tissue interposition, distraction at the fracture site, premature removal of internal fixation, loss of reduction, or inadequate immobilization. Of all the tubular bones of the hand, nonunion has the greatest propensity to occur in the middle phalanges of the fingers or the proximal phalanx of the thumb. The ratio of cortical to cancellous bone is greatest in the distal part of the middle phalanx, with clinical union taking as long as 3 months. Premature removal of internal fixation may lead to nonunion (Fig. 43-13).

Delayed union is seen quite frequently. One should not be hasty to operate on a nonunion or delayed union, because radiographic union may take 3 to 5 months. Jupiter et al. (3) recommended operative intervention at 4 months after injury to avoid stiffness secondary to additional immobilization. Earlier mobilization in patients who underwent plate fixation resulted in significantly greater total ROM than in the group fixed with Kirschner wires. On the other hand, Wray and Glunk (8) reported satisfactory results in 13 patients treated with K-wires at 3 months after injury. The key was initiation of active motion at 2 to 3 weeks compared with 6 weeks in the series of Jupiter et al.

Treatment of metacarpal nonunion by bone grafting and rigid plate fixation usually produces good results. However, for phalangeal nonunion, no treatment is entirely satisfactory, because bone grafting often will result in union complicated by a stiff finger. For nonunion adjacent to a joint, treatment consists of bone excision, arthroplasty, or arthrodesis.

The term *fibrous malunion* is a misnomer; it is not a true malunion because bone is not solidly united. A fibrous malunion implies a strong fibrous union in a malaligned position. Stress films may be helpful in establishing the diagnosis. In treating these problems, the fracture site usually must be debrided back to fresh bone to facilitate bone grafting and rigid plate fixation.

RESTRICTED DIGITAL MOTION

Restricted digital motion may be secondary to tendon adherence at the fracture site (either flexor or extensor); capsular contracture, especially at the PIP joint; or joint stiffness (9). Contributing factors include crush injury, associated soft tissue and/or joint injury, multiple fractures per finger, or immobilization for longer than 4 weeks. If a patient is unable to flex or extend the digit satisfactorily, one must ascertain whether this is due to tendon adhesions or joint stiffness. In tendon adherence, there is a discrepancy between active and passive joint ROM. In joint stiffness, active and passive ROM are equal.

Tendon Adherence

Fractures do *not* occur as isolated injuries to bone. Physiologic insult to the surrounding structures often has a more significant impact on functional outcome than the fracture itself. Tendon adherence is more likely to occur following crush injuries, but it also can be seen following prolonged or improper immobilization (22). Tendons often become adherent to the fracture callus, especially in the vicinity of the proximal phalanx where the extensor hood encircles almost two-thirds of the tubular bone and the flexor tendons are intimately bound to the volar surface of the phalanx by the A2 pulley. This complication is best prevented by early active ROM exercises during the healing phase. Surgical treatment is undertaken only after maximum passive ROM has been restored with an aggressive occupational therapy program.

Flexor Tendon Adherence

Flexor tendon adherence is characterized by a discrepancy between active and passive PIP joint flexion necessitating flexor tenolysis. Passive flexion is greater than active flexion, assuming there is no joint stiffness or extensor tendon adherence. For persistent flexor tendon adherence with concomitant significant PIP flexion contracture, either the sublimis must be excised or PIP joint arthrodesis performed as a salvage procedure.

Extensor Tendon Adherence

Extensor tendon adherence is characterized by a significant active extensor lag of the PIP joint without any fixed con-

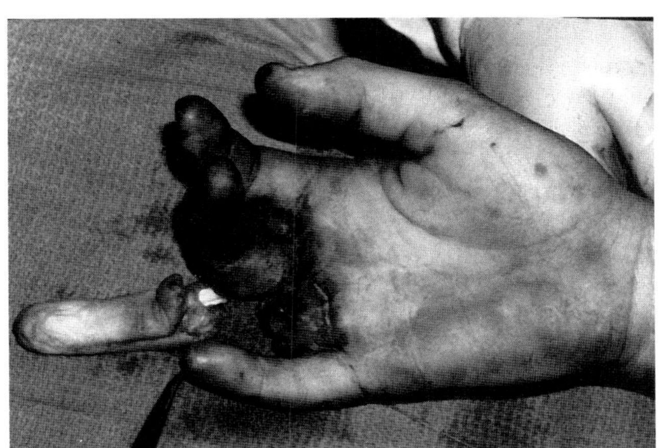
A

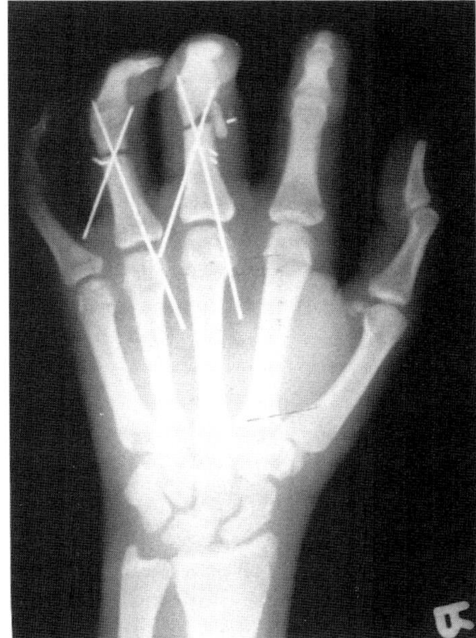
B

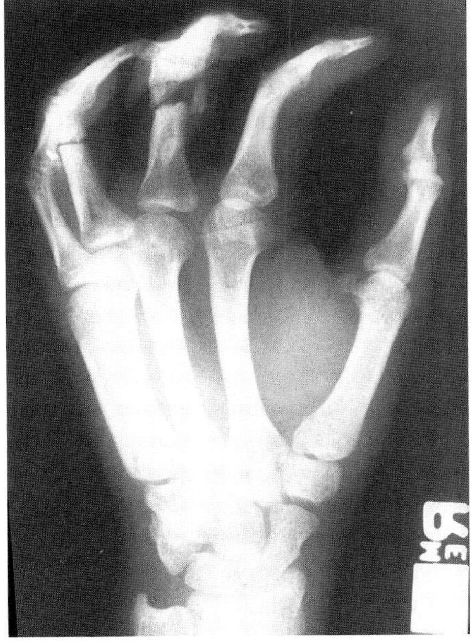
C

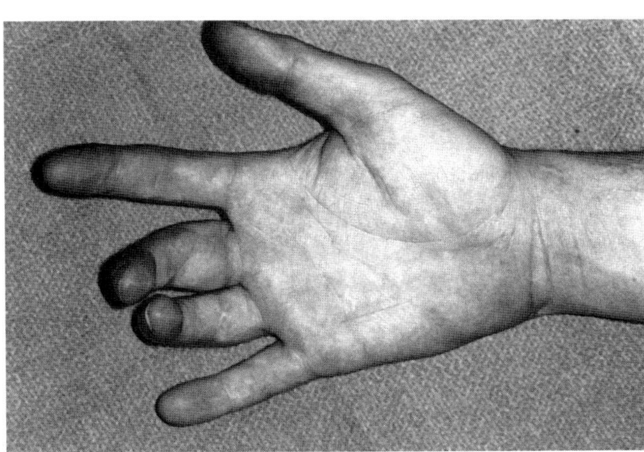
D

FIGURE 43-13. A,B: This patient underwent replantation of his middle and ring fingers. Crossed Kirschner wires were used for fixation of the proximal phalangeal fractures. **C:** The patient developed nonunions due to either distraction at the fracture sites and/or premature removal of internal fixation. There was no evidence of radiographic bony healing even at 1 year. **D:** The nonunions were asymptomatic, but there was significant stiffness and rotational deformity of the fingers.

tracture of that joint. There is limited active and passive PIP joint flexion and limited active but good passive PIP joint extension. Extensor tenolysis can be extremely tedious due to extensive tendon–bone contact that makes it much more difficult to perform than flexor tenolysis. Attempts to restore active PIP joint extension often are disappointing (23). In the case of extreme scarring, Stark et al. (24) recommend the use of inert interpositional materials such as paratenon, polyethylene film, or Silastic sheeting to prevent readherence of the tendons. They noted improved ROM in ten of 15 patients who had combined extensor tenolysis and silicone interposition.

Joint Stiffness

Prolonged joint stiffness usually results from one or a combination of the following: (i) improper position of immobilization, such as a "90-90" position for fractures of the metacarpal neck, (ii) prolonged immobilization, (iii) soft tissue capsular contracture, (iv) intra-articular incongruity, (v) arthrofibrosis, and (vi) an inadequate rehabilitation program. Joint stiffness often is fully correctable by an aggressive therapy program consisting of active and passive ROM exercises combined with dynamic splinting or, if necessary, serial casting. Swelling should be controlled by wrapping the involved digit with a compressive dressing, such as Coban (3M). One should never operate until after an adequate trial of therapy that includes splinting and until the soft tissue induration and edema have subsided. Good patient compliance is mandatory. The most common late residuals are MP extension contracture treated by Curtis' dorsal capsulectomy (25) and PIP flexion contracture treated by Watson's checkrein release (26). Other options for severe refractory PIP joint stiffness include arthrodesis in a functional position and amputation.

Treatment of MP joint stiffness may require both nonsurgical and surgical methods. First, active and passive motion exercises and dynamic splinting are used. Patients with 60 degrees of MP flexion usually regain sufficient additional motion by conservative therapy to obviate surgery; those with 40 degrees or less of MP flexion after a conservative program require surgical release of the shortened collateral ligaments to regain flexion.

PIP joint stiffness in either flexion or extension is common following hand fractures. Conservative therapy such as active and passive motion exercises and dynamic splinting with knuckle benders and reverse knuckle benders are helpful in regaining motion. In the case of limited PIP flexion, the lateral bands of the extensor mechanism have become adherent and cannot glide volarly during flexion; these bands must be mobilized to restore flexion. When the PIP joint is fixed in severe flexion, the accessory collateral ligaments or hypertrophic checkrein ligaments must be released from the lateral margin of the volar plate and the fibrous tendon sheath to facilitate joint extension (26).

SMALL JOINT INJURIES

Small joint injuries of the hand most commonly are complicated by stiffness and pain, with instability and arthrosis seen to a lesser degree. These can be devastating injuries with severe consequences. It is crucial to recognize complications before they develop and to understand the anatomical features of the joints and of a specifically tailored therapy program (7,27).

Articular Fractures of the Phalanges

Condylar fractures include those that are stable without displacement, unicondylar unstable, and bicondylar or comminuted. Unicondylar fractures of the proximal phalanx are common athletic injuries that are missed often, because the athlete can flex the finger quite well. Oblique radiographs are mandatory to visualize the fracture and its displacement. These fractures are inherently unstable, and unrestricted use of the injured finger will result in displacement with angulation and joint incongruity. Displaced unicondylar fractures require ORIF with either Kirschner pins or a lag screw. Often, the extensor tendon insertion is damaged, resulting in a moderate flexion contracture or an extensor lag that can be partially corrected by dynamic extension splinting. Comminuted intraarticular fractures are severe injuries that can have devastating consequences often necessitating arthroplasty or arthrodesis. Schenck (28) reported excellent results using dynamic traction splinting for these cases, with significant remodeling of the articular surfaces at long-term follow-up.

Intraarticular fractures of the middle phalanx can result in volar lateral plateau compression, avulsion of the collateral ligament insertions, and fractures of the dorsal base or volar base.

Volar lateral plate compression is treated by ORIF, bone grafting, and early ROM. Fractures of the dorsal base are treated based on the amount of articular surface involved and the degree of subluxation. If less than 20% of the joint surface is involved without subluxation, an extensor gutter splint is applied. If greater than 20% is involved with subluxation, internal fixation is performed using Kirschner wires and/or a tension band wire or a lag screw if the fragment is at least three times the screw diameter. For comminuted fractures, ORIF with bone grafting and external fixation is performed. For fractures involving the volar base (less than 20% TO 30% of the joint surface) without subluxation, maintain reduction with a dorsal blocking splint that prevents PIP joint extension past the point of stability but allows unrestricted flexion.

Unrecognized Joint Dislocations

Unrecognized joint dislocations occur frequently. These injuries often are diagnosed simply as "sprains," and radiographs usually are not obtained. Trainers, coaches, and misinformed patients often fail to recognize the instability of the reduction and believe that the injured finger will be fine because it is mobile. Thus, diagnosis is delayed, which results in a chronically swollen and painful joint with limited motion. Most dislocations of the PIP and MP joints are dorsal and can be appreciated best by lateral films. Treatment options include late open reduction, arthroplasty, and arthrodesis.

Dorsal Dislocations of the Proximal Interphalangeal Joint

These dislocations are easily reducible but unstable. The patient usually can reduce the dislocation himself or herself, allowing flexion; however, the dislocation recurs on extension due to disruption of the volar plate. Healing of the volar plate is facilitated by application of a dorsal extension block splint maintaining the PIP joint in 20 to 30 degrees of flexion for 3 weeks.

Chronic PIP joint dislocations alter bony contours and degenerative arthritis develops. Treatment involves repair of the volar plate. If the rent is in the membranous portion of the volar plate, multiple fine sutures are used to repair the volar plate. If the thick cartilaginous portion is separated from the middle phalanx, a pullout wire is used to approximate the volar plate to the middle phalanx. Occasionally, one slip of the sublimis tendon can be "tenodesed" for additional volar support. The finger then is splinted in flexion for 3 weeks before gentle exercises are initiated. No attempt is made to restore full flexion for at least 6 weeks, at which time dynamic splinting is begun.

Late open reduction for a joint dislocation that cannot be reduced in closed fashion can result in an excellent functional outcome. Using a dorsolateral approach, the joint is exposed by dividing the collateral ligaments. The volar plate is identified and replaced in its normal anatomical position, making reduction of the joint possible.

Chronic irreducible dislocations of the PIP or MP joints usually are associated with significant soft tissue shortening. Satisfactory reduction cannot be performed without resection of bone. Treatment often involves either arthroplasty or arthrodesis.

Volar Dislocations of the Proximal Interphalangeal Joints

These dislocations are less common and often go unrecognized in the emergency room. Usually, the central slip of the extensor mechanism is avulsed, and one or both collateral ligaments are damaged. Failure to reduce and immobilize the PIP joint in extension will result in a progressive boutonnière deformity. If recognized early, closed reduction and either splinting or CRPP for 6 weeks can be performed. If recognized late, open reduction and repair of the central slip and collateral ligaments will be necessary.

Carpometacarpal Joint Dislocations

The CMC joints form the proximal transverse arch of the hand and demonstrate varying degrees of mobility. The index and middle CMC joints are the most stable, with less than 5 degrees of motion. The ring and little CMC joints are more mobile, allowing 15 to 30 degrees of flexion and extension, respectively. CMC joint dislocations usually result from significant blunt trauma causing concomitant fracture and disruption of the intermetacarpal ligaments. Dislocation is most common on the ulnar aspect of the hand. Clinically, the deformity is masked by marked dorsal edema. Dorsal dislocation of the metacarpals can be visualized best in lateral and oblique radiographs. If recognized early, CRPP for 6 to 8 weeks usually can be performed. Cast immobilization usually is inadequate to maintain the reduction and the joints will redislocate. If recognized late, closed reduction may be impossible so that open reduction is necessary. If the joints are asymptomatic, arthroplasty may be possible; however, if there is significant pain and instability, arthrodesis may be required.

FRACTURES OF THE THUMB METACARPAL

Extra-articular

Extra-articular fractures of the base of the thumb metacarpal are relatively common. These transverse or slightly oblique fractures tend to angulate dorsally due to extension of the proximal fragment by the abductor pollicis longus and flexion of the distal fragment by the flexor pollicis brevis. Splint immobilization alone cannot control these muscle forces and progressive angulation ensues, resulting in malunion. For angulation less than 20 to 30 degrees, compensatory motion at the very mobile CMC joint is satisfactory. However, angulation greater than 30 degrees results in compensatory hyperextension of the MP joint that usually is unacceptable.

Intra-articular

Intra-articular fractures of the thumb metacarpal base must be recognized before they can be treated. A true lateral radiograph (demonstrating superimposition of the MP volar plate sesamoids) must be obtained. A Bennett fracture is an intra-articular fracture-subluxation involving the base of the thumb metacarpal. The strong anterior oblique ligament (volar beak ligament) stabilizes the variable-sized ulnovolar fragment in anatomical position while the metacarpal shaft fragment subluxates radially, proximally, and dorsally. The major deforming forces are the abductor pollicis longus and adductor pollicis. Supination also occurs.

Treatment requires *anatomical* reduction. Any incongruity of the articular surface is considered unacceptable because eventually it will lead to degenerative arthritis with ensuing pain, weakness, and loss of motion (29). Reduction of the fracture-dislocation is easy; retention is difficult. Cast immobilization is insufficient to restore stability. Reduction must be maintained by either CRPP or ORIF with K-wire or screw placement. Longitudinal traction is applied to the thumb metacarpal, which is radially extended, abducted, and pronated with direct pressure over the fracture site. The thumb metacarpal then is stabilized by fixing it to the index metacarpal, the trapezium, or both, using one or two Kirschner wires, between the thumb and index metacarpals, thumb metacarpal to trapezium, thumb metacarpal to ulnovolar fragment, or any combination of the above.

A Rolando fracture is an intra-articular fracture of the base of the thumb metacarpal in T, Y, or comminuted form. Treatment is by closed or open reduction and K-wire or screw placement. For comminuted fractures, treatment options include a thumb spica cast, oblique skeletal traction, limited open reduction, and internal fixation or external fixation.

Failure to achieve anatomical reduction in the fracture-dislocations will inevitably progress to osteoarthritis of the basal joint of the thumb. Eventually, pain, weakness, and loss of motion will mandate arthroplasty or arthrodesis. For the mobile thumb-CMC joint, we prefer to preserve motion of the joint by performing a ligament reconstruction as described by Eaton et al. (30). If significant degenerative disease has occurred, the base of the metacarpal is resected and hemiarthroplasty of the basal joint is performed using either an anchovy of palmaris longus or the proximal stump of the flexor carpi radialis tendon or a Silastic implant. For laborers requiring strong and stable pinch, arthrodesis is performed.

An intra-articular fracture-dislocation involving the base of the little finger metacarpal is analogous to a Bennett fracture of the thumb. The deforming forces are the extensor carpi ulnaris and hypothenar muscles. Anatomical reduction of the mobile CMC joint is necessary.

COMPLICATIONS OF RIGID INTERNAL FIXATION

Rigid internal fixation with plates and screws or lag screws has gained tremendous popularity over the past decade because it facilitates early mobilization of the joints, thus combating stiffness (4,6,31–38). However, aggressive dissection for rigid internal fixation disrupts the soft tissues, causing additional scarring, tendon adhesions, and stiffness. Furthermore, secondary procedures occasionally are necessary for implant removal, plate fracture, or technical failures.

Poor understanding of basic principles and techniques of the Association for the Study of Internal Fixation (ASIF) is responsible for most of the complications of metacarpal and phalangeal fractures seen by the hand surgeon. For example, it is essential to have bone-to-bone contact of the cortices opposite the plate; otherwise, bone grafting is required. Improper choice of fixation frequently occurs. Screw fixation alone is not satisfactory for a transverse fracture; the fracture line must be 2 to 2.5 times the diameter of the bone to consider screws only. Often, too much or too little hardware is used. Precise operative technique with respect to the minifragment set is essential, as the margin for error is very small. Correct use of a tapping device is a very difficult skill to master because the surgeon must "feel" penetration of the opposite cortex; there is no calibration of the threads of the tap. Overpenetration of the tap or drill may damage the flexor tendons, leading to delayed rupture. In phalangeal fractures, a plate should not be used if lesser methods of fixation will suffice.

The literature on rigid plate fixation reports variable functional outcomes. Dabezies and Schutte (31) reported excellent results (greater than 90% of normal) in 27 metacarpal and 25 phalangeal fractures (excluding fractures associated with significant soft tissue injury). Ford et al. (32) reported at least 220 degrees of total active motion in 75% of 26 metacarpal fractures. However, Stern et al. (6) reported less than satisfactory results in 38 fractures following stainless steel plate fixation of metacarpal and phalangeal fractures with 42% complications, mainly stiffness. Complications occurred most commonly with phalangeal fractures (67%). ROM greater than 210 degrees was achieved in 76% of all digits, but in only 56% (five of nine) phalangeal fractures. They concluded that most complications resulted from the severity of the initial fracture, extensive soft tissue dissection to apply the plate, and plate interference with tendon excursion. The prime determinants of outcome probably were not the plates themselves but the circumstances in which they were used. The minicondylar plates had 50% major complications probably because they were used for open, phalangeal, and periarticular fractures (36). Unfortunately, advances in plate design are inadequate to prevent problems associated with plate fixation, such as interference with tendon excursion or soft tissue damage due to addition dissection.

One must not forget that Kirschner wire fixation provides sufficient stability for fracture healing without the need for extensive soft tissue dissection in plate application. Although this does not provide true rigid fixation, the stable fixation allows early protected motion.

INFECTION

Open Fractures

Infected fractures rarely occur in the hand (39). In their series of 204 open digital fractures, Chow et al. (40) reported the incidence of infection to be only 2%. The majority of infected fractures occur following an open fracture with either major soft tissue destruction or vascular compromise. An open fracture of the hand is a true surgical emergency. Commonly caused by low-velocity gunshot wounds, open fractures are converted to clean wounds by early and thorough hydrojet irrigation and debridement. Formal exploration of the entire bullet tract is not necessary; entrance and exit wounds are simply cleansed. All open fractures are cultured; patients are placed on intravenous antibiotics.

Skeletal stability is restored either primarily or as soon as possible (as in case of an extensive open injury with multiple fractures) by either simple immobilization, K-wire fixation, external fixation, or immediate bone grafting (in special cases). The timing of internal fixation depends on the degree of contamination and the extent of soft tissue injury. An external fixator should be considered for severely contaminated wounds or those with significant bone loss; it maintains length by stabilizing the fracture until the infection is eliminated and tissue equilibrium is reached, at which time bone grafting can be performed (Fig. 43-14). Severely comminuted fractures extending onto joint surfaces may obviate any method of fixation, and arthrodesis may be necessary. Soft tissue coverage may be necessary before or at the same time as fracture fixation or bone grafting (41,42).

The role of antibiotics in the management of open phalangeal fractures is still controversial. In a prospective study of 85 patients with open distal phalangeal fractures, Sloan et al. (43) found a 30% infection rate in those not treated with antibiotics compared to only 3% in the treated group. On the other hand, Suprock et al. (44) found a similar incidence of infection in treated and untreated groups in their prospective series of 91 open phalangeal fractures. They concluded that vigorous irrigation and debridement are adequate primary treatment for open phalangeal fractures. They do not recommend antibiotics for routine use in open finger fractures.

Osteomyelitis

Bone infections can become chronic in nature. Treatment of osteomyelitis depends on whether there is bony union of the fracture. Persistent osteomyelitis after union of an infected fracture can be due to the presence of a foreign body, untreated organisms, or a poorly vascularized tissue bed. Treatment involves removal of the foreign body, multiple deep tissue and bone cultures, and provision of well-vascularized soft tissue coverage. Treatment of an infected nonunion is directed at stabilizing the fracture, debriding all infected and nonviable tissue, and using appropriate antibiotics. When the infected nonunion involves a joint, fusion often is indicated, especially if the joint is stiff. If the joint has satisfactory motion, a trial of debridement and stabilizing the fracture while mobilizing the joint is indicated. Following multiple attempts to remove the osteomyelitic bone and antibiotic therapy, the result is often a stiff, useless digit. Amputation at the next proximal level should be considered, especially if the patient wishes an early return to work.

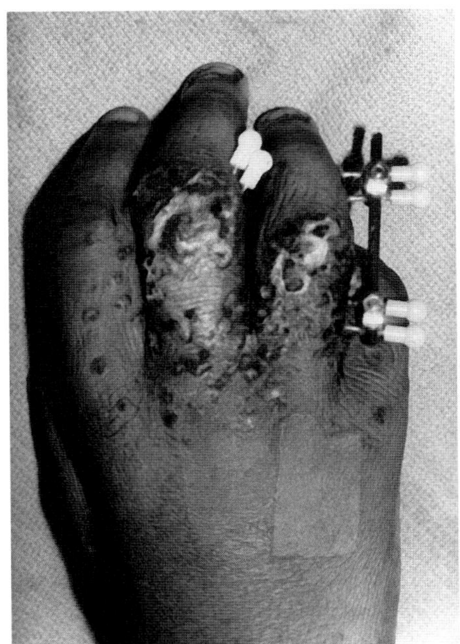
A

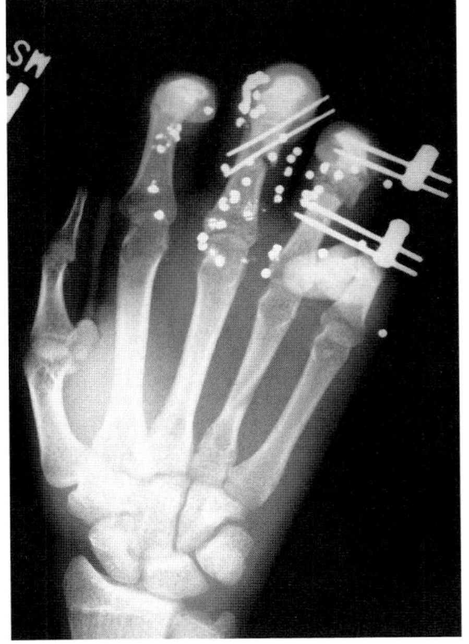

B

FIGURE 43-14. A,B: An external fixator should be considered in severely contaminated wounds or those with significant bone loss. It maintains length by stabilizing the fracture until the infection is eradicated and tissue equilibrium is reached, at which time bone grafting can be performed.

CONCLUSIONS

Long-term disability resulting from inappropriate treatment of bone and joint injuries is tremendous, especially in workmen. The goal is not simply getting bones to heal in correct position but also minimizing soft tissue scarring, which adds further physiologic insult to injury. By obeying basic principles of fracture management and rigid internal fixation, the surgeon can avoid complications.

REFERENCES

1. Eaton RG, Glickel SZ. Fractures and dislocations. In: McFarlane RM, ed. *Unsatisfactory results in hand surgery.* Edinburgh: Churchill Livingstone, 1987:281–300.
2. Green DP. Complications of phalangeal and metacarpal fractures. *Hand Clin* 1986;2:307–328.
3. Jupiter JB, Koniuch MP, Smith RJ. The management of delayed union and nonunion of the metacarpals and phalanges. *J Hand Surg Am* 1985;10:466–475.
4. Page SM, Stern PJ. Complications and range of motion following plate fixation of metacarpal and phalangeal fractures. *J Hand Surg Am* 1998;23:827–832.
5. Seitz WH Jr, Froimson AI. Management of malunited fractures of the metacarpal and phalangeal shafts. *Hand Clin* 1988;4: 529–536.
6. Stern PJ, Wieser MJ, Reilly DG. Complications of plate fixation in the hand skeleton. *Clin Orthop* 1987;214:59–65.
7. Wilson RL, Liechty BW. Complications following small joint injuries. *Hand Clin* 1986;2:329–345.
8. Wray RC Jr, Glunk R. Treatment of delayed union, nonunion, and malunion of phalanges of the hand. *Ann Plast Surg* 1989;22:14–18.
9. Weckesser EC. Rotational osteotomy of the metacarpal for overlapping fingers. *J Bone Joint Surg Am* 1965;47:751–756.
10. Reyes FA, Latta LL. Conservative management of difficult phalangeal fractures. *Clin Orthop* 1983;214:332–336.
11. Belsky MR, Eaton RG, Lane LB. Closed reduction and internal fixation of proximal phalangeal fractures. *J Hand Surg Am* 1984; 9:725–729.
12. Diwaker HN, Stothard J. The role of internal fixation in closed fractures of the proximal phalanges and metacarpals in adults. *J Hand Surg Am* 1986;11:103–108.
13. Watson HK, Weinzweig J. Stiff joints. In: Green DP, Hotchkiss RN, Pederson WC, eds. *Operative hand surgery,* 4th ed. New York: Churchill Livingstone, 1998:552–562.
14. Gross MS, Gelberman RH. Metacarpal rotational osteotomy. *J Hand Surg Am* 1985;10:105–108.
15. Manktelow RT, Mahoney JL. Step osteotomy: a precise rotation osteotomy to correct scissoring deformities of the finger. *Plast Reconstr Surg* 1981;68:571–576.
16. Froimson AI. Osteotomy for digital deformity. *J Hand Surg Am* 1981:6;585–589.
17. Lister GD. Intra-osseous wiring of the digital skeleton. *J Hand Surg Am* 1978;3:427–735.
18. Huffaker WH, Wray RC Jr, Weeks PM. Factors influencing final range of motion in the fingers after fractures of the hand. *Plast Reconstr Surg* 1979;63:82–87.
19. James JIP. Fractures of the proximal and middle phalanges of the of the fingers. *Acta Orthop Scand* 1962;32:401–412.
20. Strickland JW, Steichen JB, Kleinman WB, et al. Phalangeal fractures. *Orthop Rev* 1982;11:39–50.
21. Widgerow AD, Edinburg M, Biddulph SL. An analysis of proximal phalangeal fractures. *J Hand Surg Am* 1987;12:134–139.
22. Shirven T, Trope J. Complications of immobilization. *Hand Clin* 1994;10:53–61.
23. Creighton JJ, Steichen JB. Complications in phalangeal and metacarpal fracture management: results of extensor tenolysis. *Hand Clin* 1994;10:111–116.
24. Stark HH, Boyes JH, Johnson L, et al. The use of paratenon, polyethylene film, or silastic sheeting to prevent restricting adhesions to tendons in the hand. *J Bone Joint Surg* 1977;59A: 908–913.
25. Curtis RM. Capsulectomy of the interphalangeal joints of the fingers. *J Bone Joint Surg Am* 1954;36:1219–1232.
26. Watson HK, Light TR, Johnson TR. Checkrein resection for flexion contracture of the middle joint. *J Hand Surg Am* 1979;4: 67–71.
27. Hastings H II, Carroll C IV. Treatment of closed articular fractures of the metacarpophalangeal and proximal interphalangeal joints. *Hand Clin* 1988;4:503–527.
28. Schenck RR. Dynamic traction and early passive movement for fractures of the proximal interphalangeal joint. *J Hand Surg Am* 1986;11:850–858.
29. Cannon SR, Dowd GSE, Williams DH, et al. A long-term study following Bennett's fracture. *J Hand Surg Am* 1986;11:426–431.
30. Eaton RG, Lane LB, Littler JW, et al. Ligament reconstruction for the painful thumb carpometacarpal joint: a long-term assessment. *J Hand Surg* 1984;9A:692–699.
31. Dabezies EJ, Schutte JP. Fixation of metacarpal and phalangeal fractures with miniature plates and screws. *J Hand Surg Am* 1986; 11A:283–288.
32. Ford DJ, El-Hadidi S, Lunn PG, et al. Fractures of the metacarpals: treatment by A.O. screw and plate fixation. *J Hand Surg Am* 1987;12B:34–37.
33. Green DP, Butler TE. Fractures and dislocations in the hand. In: Rockwood CA, Green DP, Bucholz RW, et al., eds. *Fractures in adults.* Philadelphia: Lippincott-Raven Publishers, 1996: 607–744.
34. Hastings H. Unstable metacarpal and phalangeal fracture treatment with screws and plates. *Clin Orthop* 1987;214:37–52.
35. Heim U, Pfeiffer KM. *Small fragment set manual: internal fixation of small fractures,* 2nd ed. New York: Springer-Verlag, 1982.
36. Ouellette EA, Freeland AE. Use of the minicondylar plate in metacarpal and phalangeal fractures. *Clin Orthop* 1996;327: 38–46.
37. Pun WK, Chow SP, So YC, et al. Unstable phalangeal fractures: treatment by A.O. screw and plate fixation. *J Hand Surg Am* 1991;16A:113–117.
38. Stern PJ. Fractures of the metacarpals and phalanges. In: Green DP, ed. *Operative hand surgery.* New York: Churchill-Livingstone, 1993:695–758.
39. Szabo RM, Spiegel JD. Infected fractures of the hand and wrist. *Hand Clin* 1988;4:477–489.
40. Chow SP, Pun WK, So YC, et al. A prospective study of 245 open digital fractures of the hand. *J Hand Surg Am* 1991;16B:137–140.
41. Duncan RW, Freeland AE, Jabaley ME, et al. Open hand fractures: an analysis of the recovery of active motion and of complications. *J Hand Surg Am* 1993:18A;387–394.
42. Swanson TV, Szabo RM, Anderson DD. Open hand fractures: prognosis and classification. *J Hand Surg Am* 1991;16A:101–107.
43. Sloan JP, Dove AF, Maheson M, et al. Antibiotics in open fractures of the distal phalanx? *J Hand Surg Am* 1987;12B:123–124.
44. Suprock MD, Hood JM, Lubahn JD. Role of antibiotics in open fractures of the finger. *J Hand Surg Am* 1990;15A:761–764.

SUGGESTED READING

Swanson AB. Fractures involving the digits of the hand. *Orthop Clin North Am* 1970;1:261–274.

Discussion

BONE AND JOINT INJURIES

ROBERT R. SCHENCK

The authors have taken us on a whirlwind tour of the kaleidoscope of bone and joint injuries of the hand, covering not only the pathophysiology but also the varied methods of treatment of these often complex problems. Certain refrains are repeated thematically in their encompassing symphony, and it behooves us to pick these out of the score, for in finding them, readers will be able to identify the main axioms and then apply them in their own treatment of bone and joint injuries.

Recurrent themes in this chapter are as follows:

- Limited range of motion and stiffness are related to the severity and complexity of the injury.
- Recognition of the fracture is a *sine qua non* for successful treatment.
- Immobility is the chief cause of stiffness.
- Stability of the fracture and correct angulation and alignment must be achieved.
- Motion is the key to satisfactory results.

Were these truths to be embedded into the thinking pathways of our computer chip brains, the treatment of hand problems would result in fewer complications of treatment and better functional results.

Because the authors' approach is fundamentally sound, thorough in presentation, and accurate in detailing the pathophysiology and treatment methods available, I will not quibble over relatively minor points of emphasis. What this discussion can add is an expansion on the themes of avoiding immobility, promoting motion, and not disturbing fracture position and stability, which are all necessary to obtain the best functional result. As the authors correctly stated, the proximal interphalangeal (PIP) joint *is* the most important joint in the hand. The corollary to this is that it is critical to select the best treatment option for injuries of the PIP joint. Unfortunately, there are a large number of options for treatment of this joint, and whenever multiple options exist, it often indicates that none are perfect. However, in recent years one method has been gaining in ascendancy, that of dynamic traction.

PATHOPHYSIOLOGY OF PROXIMAL INTERPHALANGEAL FRACTURE-DISLOCATIONS

The skeletal system is designed to transmit forces from a proximal structure, through joints, to a more distal point of application. Stability of the PIP joint is created by the bone structural design of the proximal phalangeal bicondylar distal head fitting against the two middle phalangeal fossae, supplemented by the lateral stability provided by the collateral ligaments. Fracture of the volar proximal articulating surface of the middle phalanx creates instability with a tendency for dorsal dislocation of the middle phalanx that is proportionate to the percent of articular surface represented by the fracture fragment(s). Using the Schenck (1) classification system, grade III and IV fractures, those with 21% to 40% and more than 40% middle phalangeal articular surface, respectively, are those that often will result in significant dorsal PIP joint subluxation or dislocation (Fig. 43D-1).

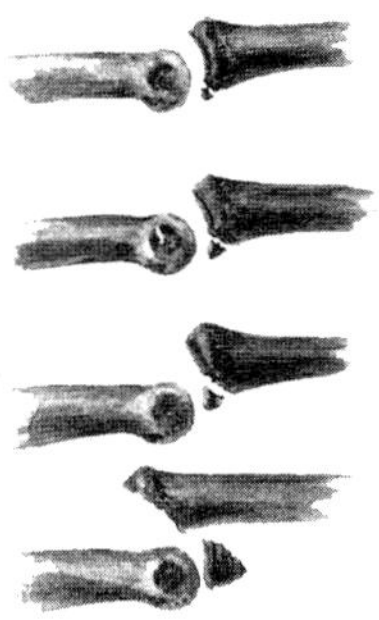

Grade	Fracture	Grade	Dislocation
I	< 10%	A	< 25%
II	11-20%	B	25-50%
III	21-40%	C	> 50%
IV	> 40%	D	Total

FIGURE 43D-1. Proximal interphalangeal joint fractures or dislocations can be classified into four grades of severity, both of the fracture and of the subluxation or dislocation. Four common combinations of fracture and subluxation or dislocation of the proximal interphalangeal joint are shown. (From Schenck RR. Classification of fractures and dislocations of the proximal interphalangeal joint. *Hand Clin* 1994;10:179–185, with permission.)

R. R. Schenck: Departments of Plastic and Orthopaedic Surgery, Rush-Presbyterian–St. Luke's Medical Center, Chicago, Illinois

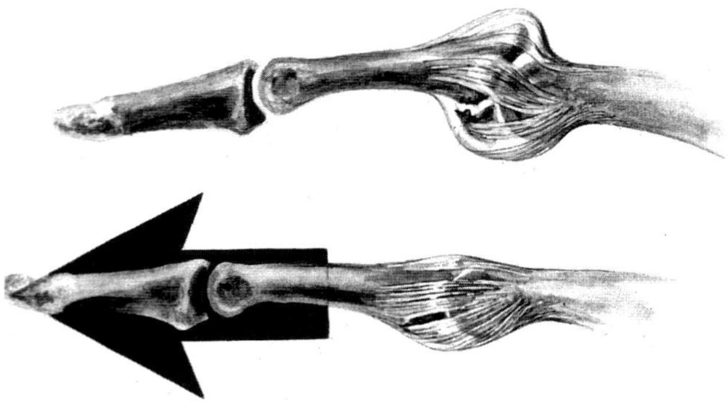

FIGURE 43D-2. In fracture-dislocation of the proximal interphalangeal joint, a distal traction force applied to the distal head of the middle phalanx allows the collateral ligaments and volar plate to reduce the comminuted fragments. Vidal et al. (2) aptly termed this process *ligamentotaxis.* (From Schenck RR. Advances in reconstruction of digital joints. *Clin Plast Surg* 1997; 24:175–189, with permission.)

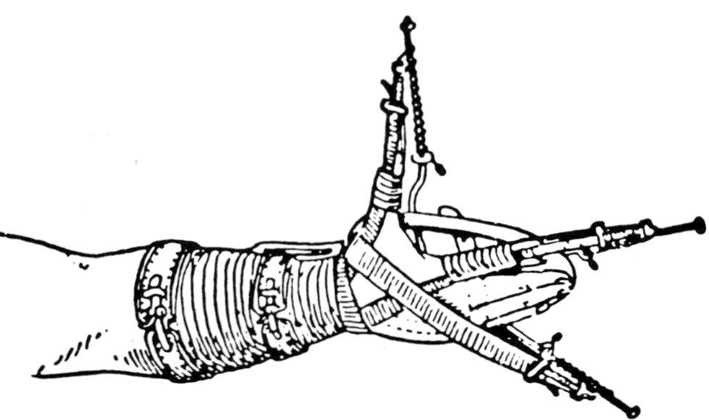

FIGURE 43D-3. Traction was used as a means to treat fractures in the hand for more than a century, as shown in this 1889 drawing by Bardenheuer. Although traction was refined, it gradually fell out of favor soon after World War II and was replaced by the widespread use of Kirschner pins. (From Schenck RR. Advances in reconstruction of digital joints. *Clin Plast Surg* 1997;24:175–189, with permission.)

A

B

C

D

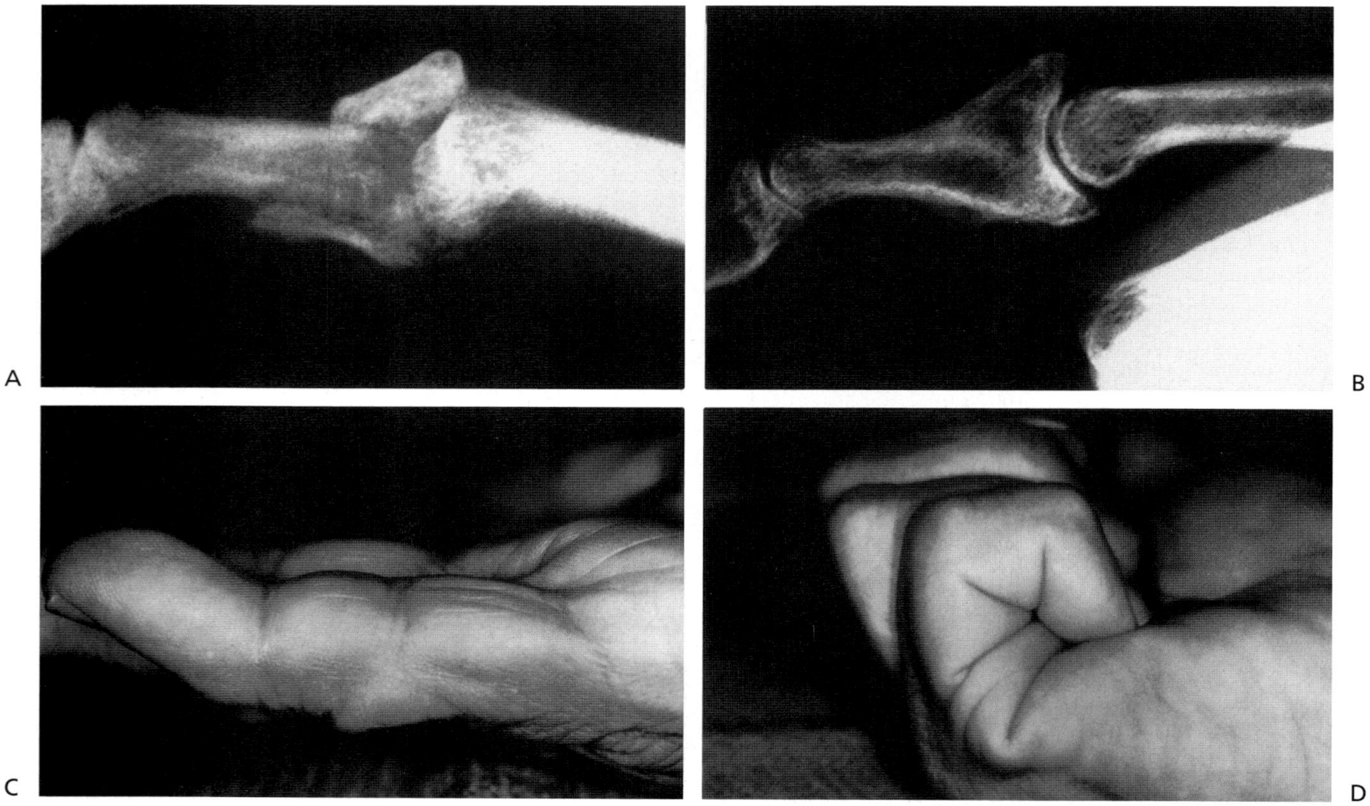

FIGURE 43D-4. A: A 44-year-old man with a severely comminuted intra-articular fracture of the right small finger that, upon surgical exploration, showed internal fixation to be impossible. **B:** Dynamic traction through the distal phalanx was used for 6 weeks. The radiograph taken at 20 years shows the symmetrically preserved joint surfaces appropriate for his age. **C:** The patient lacked full extension by only 5 degrees at the PIP joint. **D:** The proximal interphalangeal joint actively flexed to 85 degrees and the distal interphalangeal joint to 75 degrees without pain or other symptoms. (Modified from Schenck RR. Dynamic traction and early passive movement for fractures of the proximal interphalangeal joint. *J Hand Surg [Am]* 1986;11:850–858, with permission.)

THE DYNAMIC TRACTION METHOD

Dynamic traction can be defined as a method of treating intra-articular fractures of the hand that combines *distal traction* and *movement.* Distal traction reduces fracture-dislocations and realigns joint surfaces through a process that Vidal et al. (2) named *ligamentotaxis* (Fig. 43D-2). Traction was an *old* treatment method (3–5) (Fig. 43D-3) that later was abandoned because of resultant joint stiffness (6). A *newer* method was that of movement (7,8). Movement had been shown by extensive experimental research by Salter et al. (9,10). In 1986, Schenck (11) gave the first report of the use of dynamic traction, a *new* method that combines traction and movement, for treatment of PIP joint injuries. The original series of ten patients ended with an excellent 87 degrees of final range of motion, from 5 degrees in extension to 92 degrees in flexion. The first patient (Fig. 43D-4) of this series was treated with dynamic traction in 1979 for a pilon fracture that was so comminuted that exploration revealed surgery could not help, because of the multiplicity of small fragments of the entire middle phalangeal joint surface. At 5-year follow-up, the up had PIP joint flexion to 85 degrees. The patient has now been followed for 20 years, with maintenance of the same range of motion, preservation of joint space, and no pain. The last patient of the original series was treated in 1984 for a severe (grade IIIC) fracture-dislocation of the PIP joint (Fig. 43D-5). That patient has now been followed for 15 years, again with 110 degrees of motion maintained, no pain, and actual improvement of the articular surface configuration with the passage of time (Fig. 43D-6).

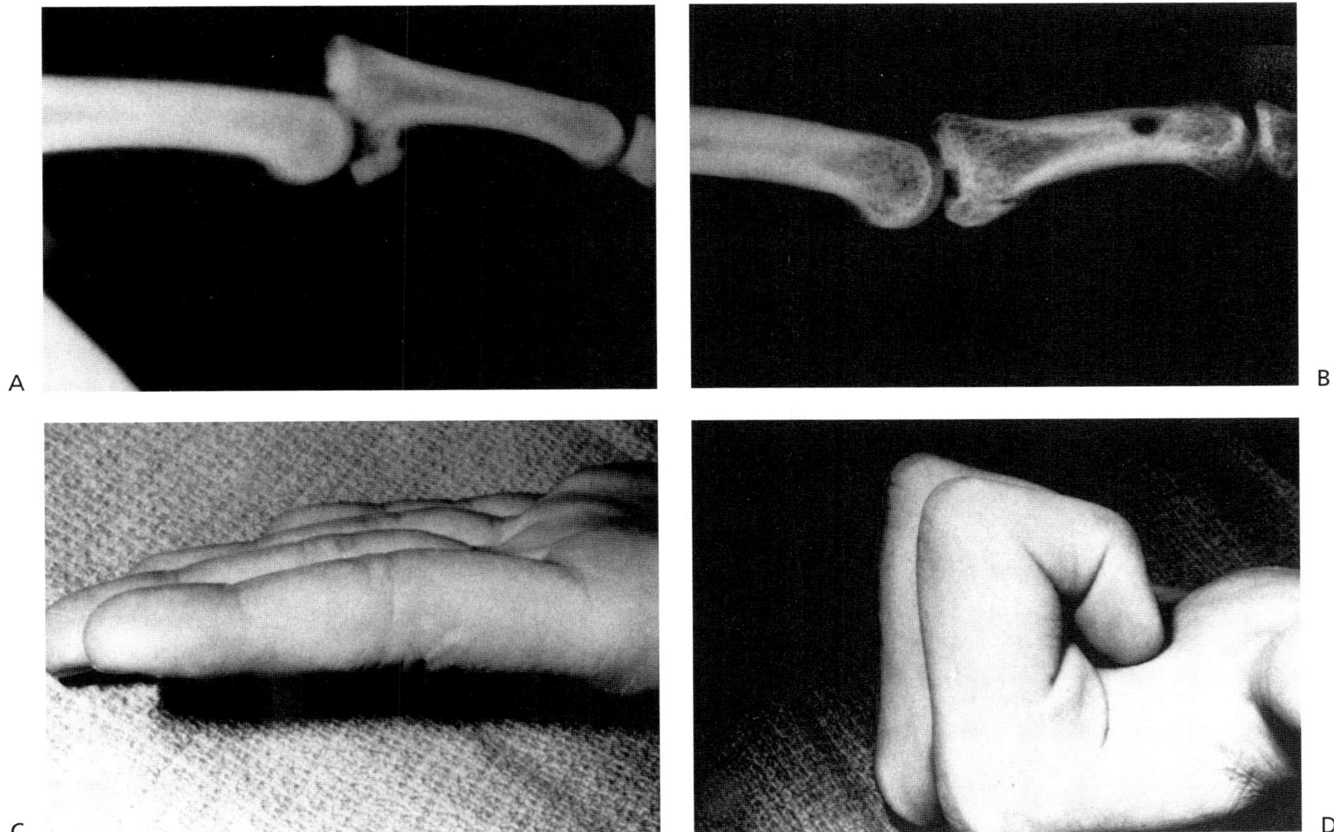

FIGURE 43D-5. A: Severely comminuted fracture-dislocation of the proximal interphalangeal joint of the left index finger of an 18-year-old woman, which resulted from an injury with a 16-inch-diameter softball. **B:** Radiographic follow-up 6 months after injury and treatment with dynamic traction splinting for 7 weeks showed excellent healing of the palmar fragments, with a limited area of depression centrally. **C:** The proximal interphalangeal (PIP) joint had full extension, and the distal interphalangeal (DIP) joint lacked only 5 degrees of extension. **D:** There was 110 degrees of flexion at the PIP joint and 65 degrees at the DIP joint. The patient was otherwise asymptomatic. (From Schenck RR. Dynamic traction and early passive movement for fractures of the proximal interphalangeal joint. *J Hand Surg [Am]* 1986;11:850–858, with permission.)

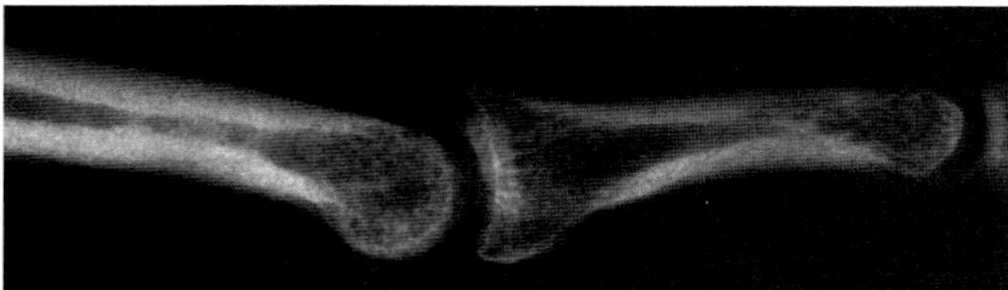

FIGURE 43D-6. Fifteen-year follow-up x-ray of the patient shown in Fig. 43D-5 demonstrating maintenance of articular cartilage space, an amazing restoration of the now near-normal articular configuration, and healing of the previous centrally depressed area. The patient remains with 110 degrees of pain-free motion at the proximal interphalangeal joint and is without other symptoms.

THE DYNAMIC TRACTION SPLINT

Details of construction of the dynamic traction splint were detailed by Kearney and Brown (12), and an example of the splint is shown is shown in Fig. 43D-7. The patient is instructed to keep the splint on at all times, day and night, except when dressing. The moveable component's position is changed by the patient every 10 minutes, alternating between the positions of flexion and extension of the involved joint. The splint usually is worn for 6 weeks, but this can be varied between 4 and 8 weeks, depending on the severity of comminution of the fracture. If available, an office fluoroscopic x-ray machine may be used to monitor progress of healing. Once the splint and the transosseous wire are removed, hand therapy measures can be added to restore the end ranges of motion.

SUMMARY

This chapter outlined the basic principles of fracture treatment. Careful study of the authors' review and application of the principles described will lead to better functional results in the treatment of bone and joint injuries of the hand. The goals of maintenance of fracture reduction and early motion are exemplified by the application of dynamic traction to treat injuries at the PIP joint. Variations of this method, and its underlying principles, can be applied to other fracture locations in the hand.

> To understand motion is to understand life.
>
> Leonardo da Vinci

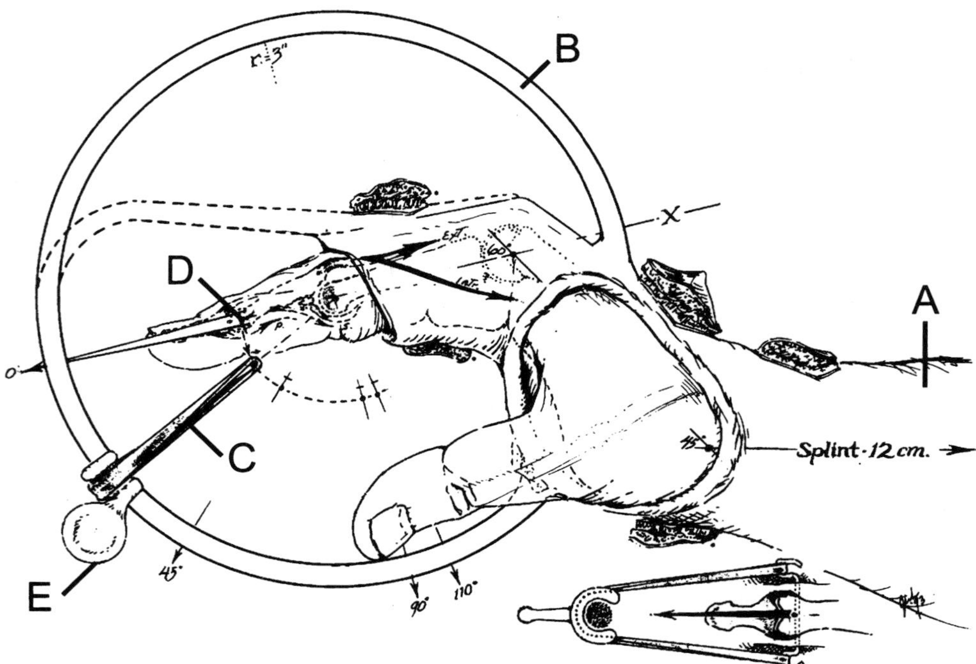

FIGURE 43D-7. Components of the arcuate dynamic traction splint. **A:** Splint base with the wrist at 45 to 60 degrees of extension, and a projection restraining the proximal phalanx with the metacarpophalangeal joint flexed 50 to 60 degrees. **B:** A 6-inch-diameter hoop is mounted on the base splint, with its 3-inch radius centered at the proximal interphalangeal joint, and positioned in line with the digit's motion arc. **C:** Size 19 rubber band(s) provides 300 to 450 g of traction by being attached to the transosseous wire drilled through the distal head of middle phalanx **D**. **E:** The moveable component with tab protects the rubber band from wear and is used to passively move the finger through a flexion/extension arc. (Modified from Schenck RR. Classification of fractures and dislocations of the proximal interphalangeal joint. *Hand Clin* 1994;10:179–185, with permission.)

REFERENCES

1. Schenck RR. Classification of fractures and dislocations of the proximal interphalangeal joint. *Hand Clin* 1994;10:179–185.
2. Vidal J, Buscayret WC, Connes H. Treatment of articular fractures by "ligamentotaxis" with external fixation. In: Brooker AF, Edwards CC, eds. *External fixation: the current state of the art.* Baltimore: Williams & Wilkins, 1979:75.
3. Bardenheuer B. *Die permanente Extensionbehandlung, die subcutanen und complicerten Fracturen und Luxationen extremitaten und ihre.* Stuttgart: Folgen, 1889.
4. Bohler L. *Treatment of fractures,* 4th ed. Baltimore: William Wood, 1939.
5. Bunnell S. Suggestions to improve the early treatment of hand injuries. *US Army Med Serv Bull* 1945;3:81.
6. Cleveland M. *Surgery in World War II: orthopaedic surgery in the European theater of operations.* Washington, DC: Department of the Army, 1956.
7. McElfresh EC, Dobyns JH, O'Brien ETD. Management of fracture-dislocation of the proximal interphalangeal joints by extension block splinting. *J Bone Joint Surg* 1972;54:1705–1711.
8. Dobyns JH, McElfresh EC. Extension block splinting *Hand Clin 1994* 1994;10:229–237.
9. Salter RB, Ogilvie-Harris DJ. The healing of intra-articular fractures with continuous passive motion. In: Cooper R, ed. *AAOS instructional course lectures.* St. Louis: CV Mosby, 1979:102–117.
10. Salter RB, Simmonds DF, Malcolm BW, et al. The biological effect of continuous passive motion on the healing of full-thickness defects in articular cartilage. *J Bone Joint Surg* 1980;62:1232–1251.
11. Schenck RR. Dynamic traction and early passive movement for fractures of the proximal interphalangeal joint. *J Hand Surg [Am]* 1986;11:850—858.
12. Kearney LM, Brown KK. The therapist's management of intra-articular fractures. *Hand Clin* 1994;10:179–185.

SUGGESTED READING

Schenck RR. The dynamic traction method: combining movement and traction for intra-articular fractures of the phalanges. *Hand Clin* 1994;10:187–198.

44

FLEXOR TENDON INJURIES

PROSPER BENHAIM
NEIL FORD JONES

Loss of the normal flexor tendon gliding function remains one of the most problematic sequels of all hand injuries. Such dysfunction can result directly from tendon lacerations or attritional ruptures, or from tendon adhesions that arise secondarily from other related crush injuries, fractures, or systemic disease. Historically, early hand surgeons recognized the significant deficit that arose from zone II flexor tendon lacerations, routinely opting for tendon grafts or two-stage reconstructions for these "no man's land" injuries in preference over the primary or delayed primary repairs that are more commonly performed today. Flexor tendon injuries often become the focus of the patient's life, especially within the context of the prolonged rehabilitation period, the psychological and economic impacts, and the need for secondary surgery that often is required even in the most motivated of patients. In addition, the thousands of flexor tendon injuries that occur each year in the United States account for millions of lost days of work and hundreds of millions of dollars of economic cost. This chapter will cover the spectrum of complications that can occur following flexor tendon repairs, stressing avoidance and therapies designed to correct these complications.

TENDON RUPTURES

Following a primary flexor tendon repair, the incidence of tendon ruptures ranges from 3% to 9% in most series (1–7). Critical evaluation of such studies is difficult, given the wide variety of specific tendon repairs, suture material, suture caliber, zone of laceration, and rehabilitation regimes encountered within the different studies. Nonetheless, some of the larger representative studies are summarized to illustrate the range of results obtained.

In general, postoperative motion programs using either the modified Kleinert active extension/passive flexion protocol (8) or the Duran and Houser controlled passive motion protocol (9) tend to have the lowest rupture rates, although overlap exists with early active flexion protocols. Edinburg et al. (10) reported a 2% rupture rate in 99 flexor tendon repairs in all five of Verdan's zones performed in 36 patients followed by a modified Kleinert postoperative regimen. This is one of the lowest rupture rates reported in a large series in the literature. Gault's retrospective review of 67 patients with 176 flexor tendon repairs performed using a 3-0 or 4-0 Kessler Mason-Allen core suture and 6-0 epitendinous suture technique with a modified Kleinert motion protocol resulted in a 3.4% rupture rate, again one of the lowest rupture rates reported (7). Tonkin and Lister (5) used a similar technique supplemented by a primary sheath repair technique in 31 zone II tendon lacerations and reported a 6% rupture rate. A paradoxical increase in the rupture rate was noted by Strickland and Glogovac (6) when they compared postoperative immobilization (16% rupture) versus controlled passive motion using the modified Duran protocol (4% rupture) in patients with zone II lacerations only. An update of that study noted that the rupture rate in the controlled passive motion group was only slightly higher when both superficialis and profundus tendons were injured and repaired (5%) (4).

Controlled active flexion protocols have been introduced in an attempt to improve the often disappointing range of motion achieved with passive motion programs. Concerns have been raised that active flexion protocols would result in higher rupture rates. The published literature fails to answer this question definitively, although there is a trend toward slightly higher rupture rates. The largest series examining controlled active flexion included 233 patients with 347 individual zone I and II flexor tendon injuries, with a 5.8% rupture rate in fingers and 16.6% in thumbs (1). A nearly identical rupture rate of 5.7% was reported by Kitsis et al. (11) in 130 patients with 339 individual tendon lacerations. A higher rupture rate for flexor pollicis longus repairs also was suggested by Gault (7), who reported a 12.5% rupture rate in 16 flexor pollicis longus repairs when compared to a 4% rupture rate in 100 repairs in the fingers. Small et al. (2) reported a higher rupture rate of 9.4% in 138 zone II flexor

P. Benhaim and N. F. Jones: Division of Plastic and Reconstructive Surgery, Department of Orthopaedic Surgery, University of California, Los Angeles, Los Angeles, California

tendon injuries treated postoperatively with early active flexion that began within 48 hours of surgery. In one of the few prospective studies, Baktir et al. (12) compared the modified Kleinert protocol in 33 patients with an early active flexion protocol in 38 patients. They noted only two ruptures in each group of patients with nearly equivalent rupture rates, postoperative functional outcome, and grip strength. In contradistinction, another prospective, matched-pair study of 52 patients with 92 zone II tendon injuries that compared passive flexion and active extension with active flexion and extension noted a markedly higher tendon rupture rate of 46% in the controlled active flexion group compared with a rate of 7.7% observed in the modified Kleinert treatment group (13). No other study in the literature has documented this high of a rupture rate with early active flexion protocols.

Ruptures usually occur at the tenorrhaphy site, most commonly within the first 2 postoperative weeks. However, delayed ruptures can occur as late as 6 to 10 weeks postoperatively, with the average day of rupture being 38 days in one study of seven treated ruptures (3). If recognized early, the recommended treatment for a rupture is another primary repair, which usually produces a good-to-excellent functional result in an average of 57% to 67% of cases (1–3,7). These results are approximately 10 to 15 percentage points lower than the good-to-excellent results obtained after uncomplicated primary repairs performed in each respective study. The chances of approximately 60% good-to-excellent function after re-repair of the ruptured tendon suggests that an attempt at salvage re-repair of the ruptured tendon is indicated in preference to abandoning the ruptured tendon altogether and proceeding with a two-stage tendon graft reconstruction. Unless a ruptured tendon is attenuated over a long segment, infected, or significantly retracted secondary to an unrecognized rupture or a delayed presentation, the ruptured tendon should be repaired if possible. If the patient is not a candidate for repair of the rupture or two-stage reconstruction, salvage procedures include distal interphalangeal (DIP) joint arthrodesis if the superficialis tendon remains intact or conversion to a superficialis finger by insertion of the distal tendon stump into the middle phalanx in cases where both flexor tendons are involved.

Research over the past 15 years has focused on developing new suture techniques to strengthen the repair, decrease the likelihood of prerupture "gapping" at the tenorrhaphy site, and theoretically allow earlier motion protocols to be performed without an increase in rupture rates. Most ruptures are preceded by the development of "gapping" at the tenorrhaphy site, which can significantly weaken the tendon, increase tendon length, decrease the effective tendon excursion, and act as a nidus for adhesion formation (14–17). The strength of a repair is almost fully dependent on the suture strength and repair technique during the first 3 weeks after the initial repair (18), with an average 50% decrease in strength occurring by 1 week and a 33% decrease at 3 weeks in unstressed immobilized tendons (17,18). Most ruptures occur at the suture knot or through the suture itself (19). Strength also is dependent on the caliber of the suture and the intrinsic properties of the suture material itself. Increasing the suture size from 4-0 to 3-0 improves strength, but it does so at the cost of increasing total suture mass and size of the suture knot (20). Addition of stress to a healing tendon by incorporating early motion into the postoperative rehabilitation program induces more rapid healing, greater tensile strength, and fewer adhesions, but it is highly dependent on having a repair technique that is strong enough to withstand this application of load without allowing significant "gapping" or rupture at the tenorrhaphy site (17,21–23).

The primary focus of most surgeons has been in designing repairs with a greater number of suture strands crossing the repair site to decrease gapping and increase strength while minimizing excess bulk that potentially would limit tendon excursion. Several two-, four-, six-, and eight-strand suture repair techniques have been described, with a general emerging pattern suggesting that the tensile strength of a particular tendon repair is proportional to the number of suture strands crossing the repair site. The standard two-strand techniques, including the common modified Kessler suture, are strong enough for passive motion protocols, but they are mechanically inadequate to withstand early active flexion or light grip, especially in the first 3 weeks after a repair when evaluated by biomechanical testing *in vitro* (17,24–27). In a unique study that compared 20 variables of flexor tendon repair in a cadaver model, Singer et al. (28) examined eight different core suture techniques, four types of suture material, two suture sizes, four epitenon suture techniques, and two distances from the repair site with the Taguchi method of statistical analysis to identify the optimal combination of repair parameters. The strongest repair was the augmented Becker core suture, followed by a four-strand modified Kessler suture technique using 3-0 Mersilene placed 0.75 cm from the tenotomy site, supplemented by a volar epitenon suture. The Becker repair was 7.5 times stronger than a standard 4-0 nylon modified Kessler suture technique (28). An alternate method of increasing core suture repair strength includes the addition of an epitendinous, small-caliber (6-0), inverting suture designed to minimize the unevenness and exposed raw tendon surface at the repair site, producing a smoother contour that improves excursion and reduces adhesion formation. This type of suture can add significant strength, with an estimated 25% to 40% increase in strength over a two-strand repair (17,29,30). The standard running epitendinous suture also has been modified to further increase the overall strength of the repair. Wade et al. (30) reported an overall 89% increase in strength when a horizontal mattress epitendinous suture was added to a core suture repair. A running-locking loop epitendinous suture also has been shown to be 3.8 times stronger than a simple running suture and

1.7 times stronger than a Lembert running suture (31). Silfverskiold et al. (32) introduced an epitendinous 6-0 cross-stitch technique without the use of a core suture that is stronger than a modified Kessler suture. In a study of 46 patients with 55 tendon repairs, this epitendinous cross stitch alone without an additional core suture only had a 3.6% rupture rate even with the use of an early active and passive motion protocol (33).

In one of the largest prospective series of patients repaired with a modified Kessler core suture and a 5-0 polyester Halsted epitendinous suture, Kitsis et al. (11) reported remarkable results in 130 patients with 339 flexor tendon lacerations in 208 individual digits treated with an early active flexion protocol. Results were judged as excellent to good in 92% of cases, fair in 7%, and poor in only 1%, with a rupture rate of 5.7%. Only 87 of the 208 digits had zone II injuries, but even here the incidence of excellent-to-good results was still 89% (11). Although proponents of early active flexion protocols emphasized the importance of using a strong multistrand repair, questions remain about the additional bulk, technical difficulty, and possible vascular strangulation effects of such repairs that may offset some of the advantages afforded by these stronger types of repairs and that may not actually result in lower rupture rates (34). Excellent results have been obtained using only a modified Kessler core suture and early active flexion protocols (2,11,12).

TENDON ADHESIONS

Tendon adhesions remain the most common complication encountered after flexor tendon repairs. The significance of these adhesions is partially dependent on the location of the tendon laceration, with zone II repairs being most susceptible to a poor outcome secondary to adhesions. The presence of the flexor digitorum profundus (FDP) and flexor digitorum superficialis (FDS) tendons within the confines of a relatively tight fibro-osseous tunnel pulley system in zone II magnifies the effect of adhesions (Fig. 44-1A–B). Adhesions may occur between tendon and the surrounding tissues or between the superficialis and profundus tendons. Similarly, zone IV injuries within the carpal tunnel involve multiple tendons that can scar to each other as well as to the inner boundaries of the carpal tunnel, thereby eliminating independent motion of individual fingers. However, tendon repairs in other zones are not immune to adhesions, which can be just as functionally limiting as in zone II and zone IV repairs. The degree of associated soft tissue and bony injuries also greatly affects the formation of adhesions.

Repaired tendons heal by both intratendinous and extratendinous scar tissue formation. The challenge for hand surgeons is to optimize primary intratendinous healing and scarring while minimizing extratendinous scarring. A number of specific intraoperative maneuvers have been routinely incorporated into most surgeons' approach to tenorrhaphy. Recognition of the importance of atraumatic surgical technique, reduction of bulk at the repair site, and adequate soft tissue cover now is well established in providing local conditions that diminish the formation of extratendinous scar and subsequent adhesion formation. The location of the A1, A2, and A4 pulleys relative to the repair site is important with regard to whether the bulk of the repair passes beneath one of these pulleys. This can be determined easily by passive flexion and extension of the digit intraoperatively. For example, a proximal zone II repair that has difficulty gliding beneath the A1 pulley can be converted effectively into a zone III repair by excision of the A1 pulley and, if necessary, even the proximal half of the A2 pulley without incurring a significant risk of bowstringing postoperatively.

Although never studied formally, it is our clinical impression that excellent hemostasis should be obtained after release of the tourniquet before skin closure in order to lessen the risk of postoperative hematoma, which not only jeopardizes the viability of overlying skin flaps but also can increase the risk of adhesions as the blood either organizes or induces an inflammatory reaction as it hemolyzes. Hemostasis is achieved, preferably with a bipolar electrocautery unit to focus more precisely the application of electrocautery energy and again to reduce adhesions that can be generated by large areas of thermally injured tissues. When intact, the vincular blood supply to the flexor tendons should be preserved. Avoiding indiscriminate division of the vincula by either overly aggressive dissection or inadvertent injury should be a high priority.

Numerous researchers investigated the role of tendon sheath repair in improving nutritional supply to the healing tendon and minimizing the development of peritendinous adhesions by restoring a smooth gliding surface. Experimental models demonstrated improved tendon gliding following flexor sheath repair or reconstruction with sheath interposition grafts (35,36), although tendon sheath narrowing following repair also was shown to induce formation of adhesions (36,37). Proponents cite improved range of motion when primary tendon sheath repair is performed (38,39), but none of these studies is controlled, randomized, or even comparative to a cohort of patients not undergoing sheath repair. Other investigators have been unable to demonstrate any benefit of tendon sheath repair, either experimentally or clinically (40,41). Tendon nutrition, as measured by tritiated proline uptake, also was not improved in animal models when comparing sheath excision to sheath incision and repair (42,43).

Research has indicated that local application of aprotinin may inhibit the amount of adhesion formation following tenorrhaphy (44). Aprotinin is a proteinase inhibitor that inhibits trypsin, plasmin, plasma kallikrein, and tissue kallikrein in humans, with its antiplasmin effect reducing fibrin production (45). It is a bioabsorbable gel that can be applied topically on the tendon repair site and is fully reab-

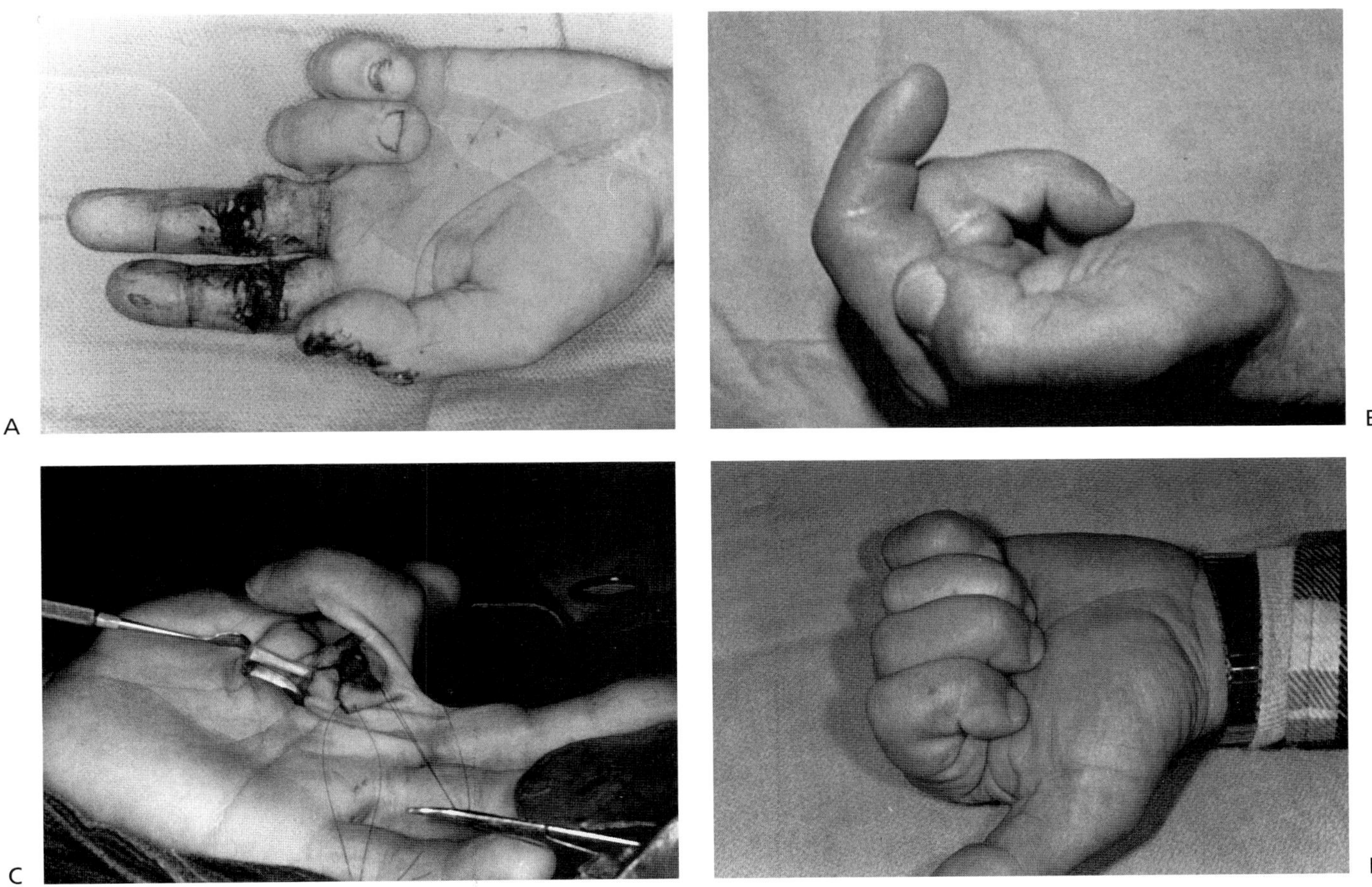

FIGURE 44-1. A: Zone II lacerations of the flexor digitorum superficialis and profundus tendons in both the left index and middle fingers. The resting posture of the hand demonstrates full extension of these fingers, indicating that both of the flexor tendons have been lacerated in each finger. **B:** Postoperatively, near-full active flexion in the middle finger is achieved, but only limited active flexion in the proximal and distal interphalangeal joints of the index finger is possible secondary to adhesions. **C:** Following extensive tenolysis, nearly full flexion in the index finger is obtained when longitudinal traction is applied to the flexor digitorum profundus tendon in the distal palm. **D:** Final result after tenolysis showing full active flexion in both the index and middle fingers.

sorbed by 4 weeks. Komurcu et al. (44) studied the effect of aprotinin in a rabbit model of tendon crush injury and showed a reduction in tendon adhesions with sheath repair and aprotinin application. However, unrestricted early motion was allowed, which is clearly a confounding variable that is quite dissimilar from the protected motion protocols used clinically. The sheath repair also had an independent benefit, calling into question the validity of this study in the context of human flexor tendon repairs (44). Although in clinical use in Europe, no peer-reviewed study has been published to date on the efficacy of aprotinin for flexor tendon repairs in humans. The ultimate utility of such a modality remains unclear.

Although intraoperative techniques have evolved to maximize the strength of the repair and minimize tendon adhesions, many would argue that the dramatic changes in postoperative motion protocols have been largely responsible for decreasing the incidence and severity of postoperative tendon adhesions. The earliest tendon repairs were routinely protected with prolonged periods of immobility. Restricted early motion protocols were suggested as early as 1927, but it was not until 1960 that a passive extension and rubber band passive flexion concept was introduced (46,47). This was later modified by Kleinert to include active extension and rubber band passive flexion. Lister et al. (8) demonstrated that the active contraction of the extensor digitorum communis tendons was accompanied by relaxation of the antagonistic FDP tendons, which had the beneficial effect of minimizing tension on the flexor tendon repair site. The controlled passive motion protocol of Duran and Houser (9) was another significant advance because it highlighted the importance of differential gliding between the superficialis and profundus tendons and suggested that at least 3 to 5 mm of gliding was necessary overall to prevent adhesion formation. Early active flexion protocols are the newest addition, with ongoing studies attempting to characterize more clearly the role for such an approach (1,2,11–13).

FLEXOR TENOLYSIS

Tenolysis frequently is necessary to improve the active range of flexion when significant peritendinous adhesions limit the excursion of the flexor tendon despite an appropriate course of postoperative therapy (Fig. 44-1B). The ideal patient should have stable soft tissue coverage with mature scar remodeling, an adequate neurovascular supply, supple joints with full passive range of motion that will not restrict motion post tenolysis, and a muscle that has sufficient power to move the digit through a full range of motion (48,49). Selection of sufficiently motivated patients also is important. Contraindications to tenolysis include fixed joint contractures, incompletely healed or insufficient soft tissue coverage, unstable or incompletely healed fractures, nonunions, uncooperative patients, and psychiatric problems that preclude a rehabilitative effort. Certain concomitant problems can be addressed at the same time as the flexor tenolysis as long as the corrective maneuver can withstand immediate postoperative motion. Examples include extensor tenolysis for extensor tendon adhesions, intrinsic muscle release for intrinsic tightness, release of checkrein ligaments, and capsulotomy for contractures of the proximal interphalangeal (PIP) or DIP joints (48).

The timing of tenolysis is variable and dependent on the individual circumstances of the specific flexor tendon injury. Tendon adhesions following replantation of a digit in a severely crushed hand will be treated much differently and generally later than an isolated single flexor tendon laceration sustained in a clean simple injury. The primary goal in delaying tenolysis is to allow for softening and maturation of the surrounding soft tissues. A plateau in regaining active flexion also should have been reached in therapy (50). The minimum recommended time for tenolysis is 3 months, although various authors have suggested a period of 6 to 9 months as the preferred time for tenolysis (49,51–53). In a study of 145 zone II flexor tendon injuries, May and Silferskiold (54) noted that 37% of the final DIP joint motion and 9% of the final PIP motion was achieved between 3 and 12 months postoperatively. In addition, of 27 digits judged to have a poor outcome at 3 months, only ten remained in a poor category at the 1-year evaluation, with 17 digits improving significantly between the 3- and 12-month evaluation time points. This indicates that early tenolysis at 3 months may be premature and should be delayed until at least 6 to 12 months after the initial repair (54).

Tenolysis generally is performed under regional anesthesia, although Schneider (50) and Hunter et al. (55) have argued for local anesthetic techniques to allow intraoperative assessment of the effectiveness of "pullthrough" of the flexor tendons. Wide surgical exposure is achieved through either a palmar Bruner or a midlateral incision, often dictated by the configuration of the original wound and incisions used at the initial surgery. Gentle surgical technique is mandatory to avoid injury to the annular pulleys. Specifically, the A2 and A4 pulleys should be preserved to prevent bowstringing of the tendons. A combination of sharp and blunt dissection is used to release the peritendinous and intertendinous adhesions. Dissection should begin in a relatively unscarred portion of the tendon and then proceed into the more scarred regions. Customized instruments have been developed to assist with this often difficult task. Frequent reassessment with longitudinal traction on the proximal tendon is useful to identify any residual adhesions that still require release (Fig. 44-1C). Although as much sheath as possible is conserved, unnecessary bulk from scar tissue should be sharply excised. If extensive adhesions are encountered or if one is unable to define or preserve pulleys, the surgeon should strongly consider abandoning tenolysis and proceeding with placement of a silicone tendon rod as the initial step of a two-stage tendon reconstruction. A similar approach is used if there is significant attenuation of the tendon (50).

The success of tenolysis is partially dependent on the cooperation and motivation of the patient, which greatly influence the patient's ultimate functional recovery (Fig. 44-1). Following tenolysis, motion is begun either immediately or within a few days. Some patients have difficulty performing early motion because of a relatively low pain tolerance. For these patients, the surgeon should consider placement of an indwelling small-bore catheter at the operative site to allow intermittent injections of local anesthetic. Bupivacaine 0.25% or 0.5% may be infused for 2 to 3 days postoperatively to provide local pain relief and allow sufficient early motion to prevent reformation of adhesions. These injections may even be controlled by the patient with a portable unit on an outpatient basis similar to the way that patient-controlled narcotic analgesia is administered in the inpatient setting for postoperative pain control.

Excellent (75% to 100% of normal total active motion) or good (50% to 74% of normal total active motion) results have been achieved following flexor tenolysis in 65% to 67% of patients reviewed in two series (4,56). Foucher et al. (51) reported improvement in 84% of 78 digits undergoing tenolysis, with total active motion improving by 68 degrees from 135 degrees preoperatively to 203 degrees postoperatively. Four digits did not improve and nine digits were worse, losing an average of 25 degrees in total active motion. Tenolysis of flexor pollicis longus repairs resulted in improvement in 78% of thumbs, with a 50-degree increase in total active motion from 65 degrees preoperatively to 115 degrees following tenolysis.

Tenolysis may predispose the tendon to rupture, which can occur anywhere along the tendon. The underlying cause likely is related to devascularization in the tendon segment undergoing tenolysis and the associated nutritional deficit that occurs. The report by Foucher et al. (51) of 78 flexor tenolyses had a very low 2.5% rupture rate, possibly related to a postoperative regimen of immobilization in flexion followed by subsequent passive extension to lyse any early developing adhesions. Although this may have protected against early ruptures, this and other studies clearly demonstrate the efficacy of tenolysis in improving functional range of motion following primary tenorrhaphy with an acceptable level of morbidity.

BOWSTRINGING

The arrangement of the flexor tendons and the overlying tendon sheath in each digit is a well-designed system that maximizes mechanical efficiency by ensuring that the flexor tendons remain in close contact with the underlying metacarpals and phalanges during active flexion. When this relationship is disrupted, the tendon will directly pull between the remaining proximal and distal pulleys, with consequent palmar migration of the tendon on active flexion (Fig. 44-2). This phenomenon of "bowstringing" can significantly reduce the functional outcome following a primary flexor tendon repair, tenolysis, or two-stage tendon reconstruction.

The retinacular system of the flexor tendon sheath consists of five annular and three cruciate ligaments. The thicker annular pulleys are primarily responsible for maintaining the flexor tendons close to the underlying bones, thereby preventing bowstringing during flexion. The thinner cruciate pulleys collapse on flexion, allowing full flexion without buckling of the sheath/tendon construct. The tendon sheath by itself is inadequate to prevent bowstringing. The A2 pulley, located at the proximal portion of the proximal phalanx, and the A4 pulley, located at the middle portion of the middle phalanx, are the two most important pulleys to preserve. In any flexor tendon surgery, windows should be made in the flexor sheath between these two critical pulleys. In the thumb, the oblique pulley is the most important (57–59).

Injuries to the A2 or A4 pulley may occur at the time of the initial injury or iatrogenically at the time of surgical repair or during tenolysis. Loss of integrity of the A2 or A4 pulley results in mechanical inefficiency as the flexor tendon bowstrings across the phalanges and metacarpophalangeal joint. This results in a decrease in total active flexion and relative weakness. Clinical diagnosis usually is obvious, with tendon visibly bowstringing on attempted active flexion. Flexion can be improved by mechanically blocking the bowstringing tendon by compression of the tendon against the underlying bones with the examiner's finger. Conservative therapy with a pulley ring can prevent bowstringing, although most would recommend pulley reconstruction.

There are several techniques for pulley reconstruction. Leaving its distal insertion intact, one slip of the FDS can be used to reconstruct the distal A2 or proximal A4 pulley when a superficialis repair is not planned or if the superficialis remains intact (60,61). Free tendon grafts also may be used, either sutured to the remnants of the missing pulleys (Kleinert) (62) or passed circumferentially around the proximal or middle phalanges (Bunnell loop) (Fig. 44-3) (63,64). Lister (65) has proposed the alternative use of extensor retinaculum from the dorsal wrist, whereas Karev (66) has described a belt-loop technique that uses two parallel strips of volar plate to reconstruct the A1, A3, or A5 pulley (Fig. 44-4A–B) (60). Widstrom et al. (67) evaluated six different techniques for pulley reconstruction in a human cadaver model and examined the efficiency with which tendon excursion is transformed into finger flexion. All pulley reconstructions had at least an 80% mechanical effec-

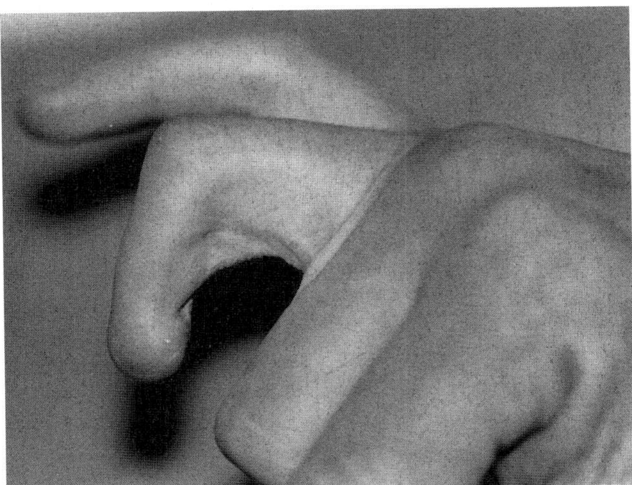

FIGURE 44-2. Example of flexor tendon bowstringing in the ring finger. The initial injury included an extensive crush injury to the volar aspect of the proximal and middle phalanges, as well as a tip amputation of the ring finger distal phalanx. Two prior tenolyses had been attempted.

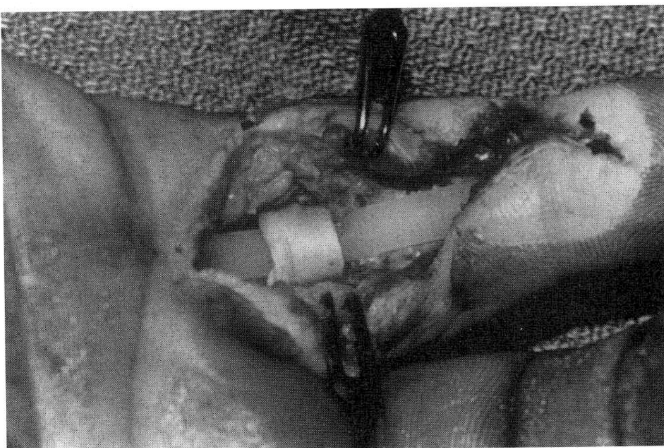

FIGURE 44-3. Reconstruction of an A2 pulley with use of one entire flexor digitorum superficialis tendon wrapped circumferentially around the proximal phalanx (Bunnell loop).

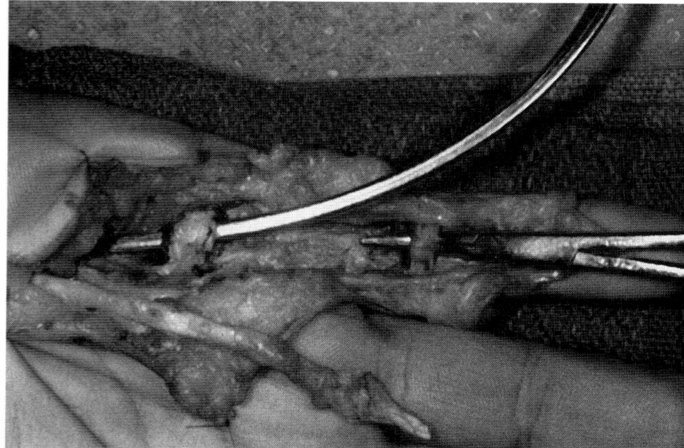

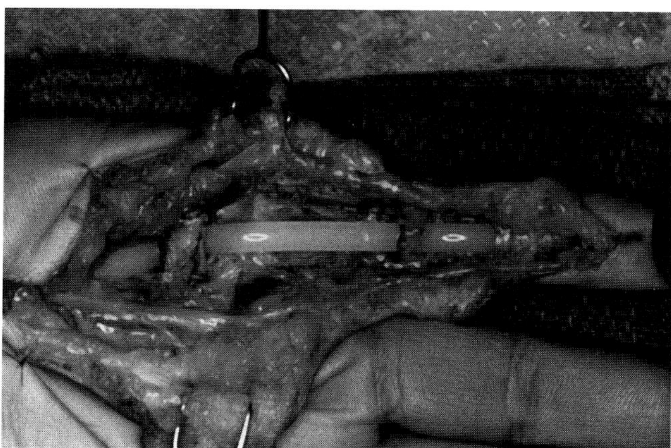

FIGURE 44-4. A: Karev loop reconstruction of flexor tendon sheath pulleys, with use of the metacarpophalangeal joint volar plate to reconstruct an A1 pulley and use of the proximal interphalangeal joint volar plate to reconstruct an A3 pulley. This patient had severe tendon adhesions that could not be treated adequately with tenolysis. **B:** Stage I flexor tendon reconstruction with placement of a silicone rod through the newly created Karev loops.

tiveness when compared to an uninjured normal retinacular system, with the Karev belt-loop procedure producing the most efficient system. The strongest reconstructions were the Karev and Bunnell loop techniques; the weakest was the Kleinert rim technique. (67)

Pulley reconstruction may need to be performed at the first-stage flexor tendon graft procedure concomitant with placement of the silicone tendon rod. The reconstructed pulley should be strong, must not loosen, and should provide a smooth gliding surface. There is disagreement as to the number of pulleys that need to be constructed, with different authors recommending a minimum of two, three, or four pulleys (60,61).

TWO-STAGE FLEXOR TENDON GRAFTING

Two-stage reconstruction of the FDP should be considered in four circumstances:

1. Primary flexor tendon repair is not possible due to segmental injury to the flexor tendon or severe associated soft tissue or bony injuries
2. Tenolysis becomes too extensive to restore digital flexion
3. The tendon bed is severely scarred (Fig. 44-5)
4. Crucial pulleys are missing.

Stage I involves excision of the scarred tendons and placement of a silicone tendon implant (Fig. 44-5B). Pulley reconstruction and capsulotomies of the PIP joint and occasionally the DIP joint may be necessary. The distal end of the implant is secured to the distal phalanx with either a pullout suture with external fixation over a dorsal button, a screw, or a bone anchor. The distal fixation can be augmented with remnants of the FDP insertion if still present. The proximal end of the silicone rod is placed in the distal forearm without fixation to the proximal remnant of the flexor tendon. With passive flexion and active extension of the fingers, the pistoning effect and gliding of the silicone tendon implant induce the formation of a smooth-walled neotenosynovium that will provide a gliding tunnel for the subsequent tendon graft. Stage II, which usually takes place at least 3 months later, involves removal of the implant and replacement with a tendon graft (68–71).

The palmaris longus tendon is the preferred donor tendon for a palm-to-fingertip flexor tendon graft, but it is present in only 85% to 88% of humans (72,73). The palmaris longus often is too short for the more usual distal forearm-to-fingertip graft, especially when the musculotendinous junction is relatively distal. Sometimes the plantaris tendon is more appropriate for a distal forearm-to-fingertip graft, but it is present in only 80% to 94% of patients, and up to 11% of plantaris tendons that are present are too small (2 mm or less diameter) to be used as a graft (73–76). The presence or absence of the palmaris tendon does not predict the presence or absence of the plantaris tendon, with only 2% of 186 cadavers in one study missing both the palmaris longus and plantaris tendons. In the 22 cadavers without both palmaris tendons, 14 still had bilateral plantaris tendons (73). If both the palmaris and plantaris tendons are missing, the donor tendon of choice is the long toe extensor tendon to the second, third, or fourth toe. The fourth toe extensor is preferred if only a single graft is required.

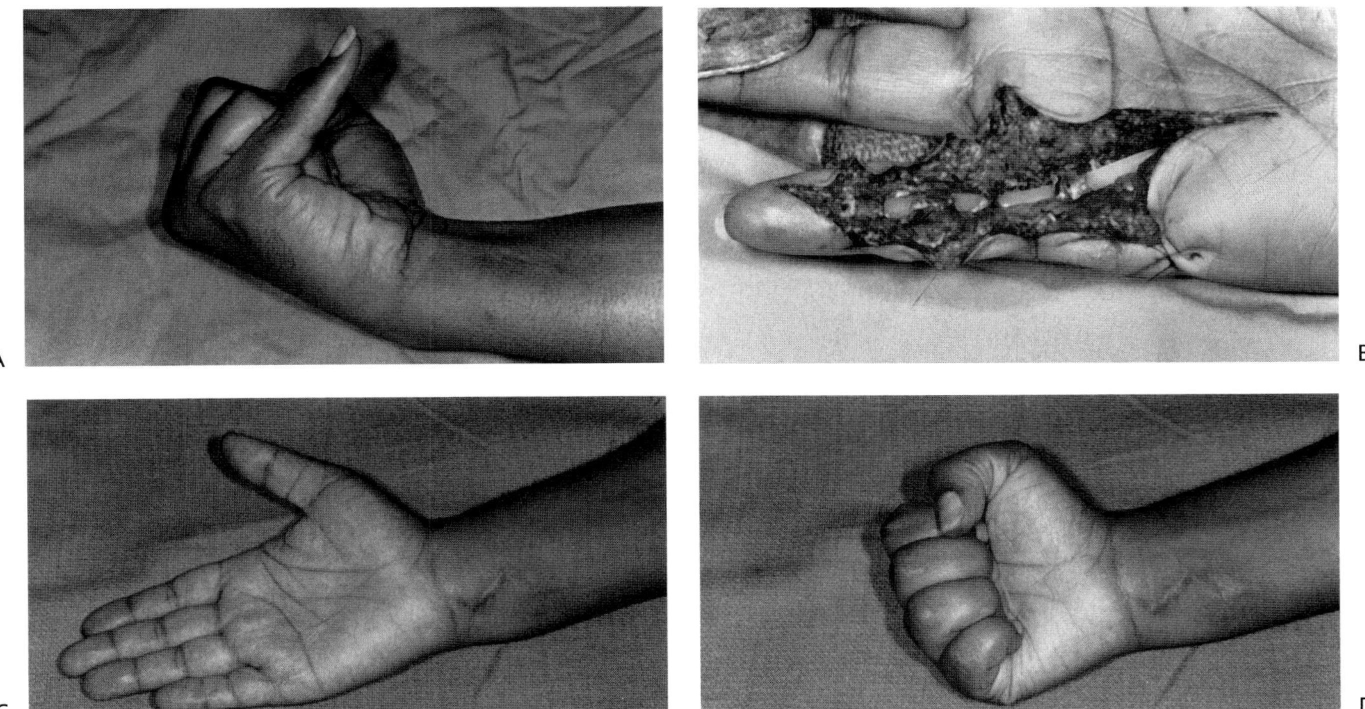

FIGURE 44-5. **A:** This patient had missed lacerations of the small finger flexor digitorum superficialis and profundus tendons 4 months ago. Metacarpophalangeal joint flexion and interphalangeal joint extension are achieved through lumbrical muscle contraction. At 4 months after injury, delayed primary repair of the tendon lacerations is not possible. A two-stage tendon reconstruction will be required. **B:** Intraoperative photograph demonstrating placement of the silicone tendon rod through intact pulleys that were preserved. **C:** Postoperative result following stage II of the tendon reconstruction. Full active extension is demonstrated. **D:** Postoperative result following stage II of the tendon reconstruction. Full active flexion of the small finger is demonstrated.

COMPLICATIONS OF TWO-STAGE FLEXOR TENDON GRAFTING

Complications following stage I have become relatively uncommon as experience with this technique has grown. Synovitis in response to the silicone component of the tendon rod is the most frequently observed complication. Clinical manifestations include inflammation, swelling, pain, stiffness, and thickening of the developing pseudosheath. The most common cause of synovitis is rupture of the distal fixation point of the implant, with subsequent altered motion characteristics on passive flexion of the proximally displaced distal end of the implant. Buckling of the implant can cause synovitis, but this should be prevented at the time of surgery by proper selection of implant size and confirmation of smooth gliding of the implant within the remaining sheath and pulleys. Overly aggressive motion may induce synovitis as well (71,77–79). Treatment involves immobilization of the hand for at least 1 week and administration of antiinflammatory medications.

Differentiating synovitis from the less common infection can be difficult, with synovitis being notable for lack of a systemic response that typically accompanies infection. Infection generally occurs within the first 2 weeks and is characterized by erythema, diffuse swelling, pain, and occasional epitrochlear or axillary adenopathy (Fig. 44-6). Fever and leukocytosis also may be observed. The risk of infection can be reduced at the time of initial placement by the use of

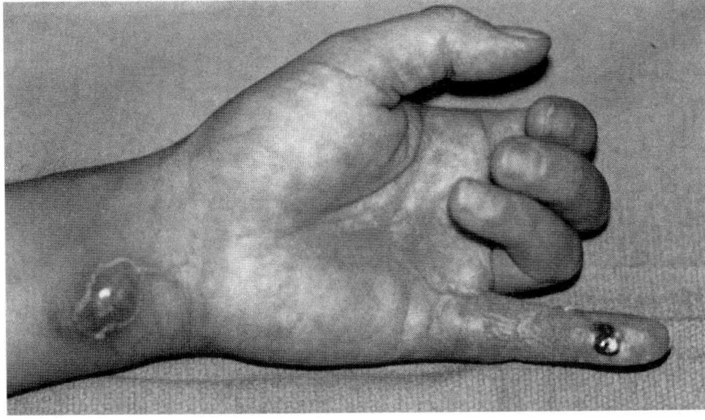

FIGURE 44-6. Infection of a silicone tendon rod. The distal forearm is tender, swollen, and red, symptoms that are all suggestive of an abscess. The distal end of the rod has eroded through the volar aspect of the distal phalanx, and mild seropurulent drainage was observed.

a "no touch" technique that minimizes adherence of glove powder, gauze, or airborne particles to the highly electrostatic tendon implant (71,77–79). Treatment of an infected implant is prompt removal of the implant, irrigation and debridement of any residual fibrinopurulent material, splinting, and antibiotics. After the infection has cleared fully and soft tissue healing has occurred, replacement of a second silicone tendon rod may be repeated, usually 6 months after removal of the infected implant without any significant increase in recurrent infection.

Complications following stage II include formation of peritendinous adhesions, flexion contracture of the PIP or DIP joint, rupture of the tendon graft juncture sites, and incorrect length of the tendon graft. Adhesions occur most commonly at the proximal juncture, but they may occur at any location where nutritional supply is poor, smooth gliding is impaired, or pulleys are constrictive (77). Secondary tenolysis 4 to 6 months later may be required to release such adhesions if they fail to respond to hand therapy interventions. Overall results following 43 two-stage tendon reconstructions were relatively poor, with only 39% of patients achieving a good-to-excellent total active range of motion and 35% with poor results. However, following tenolysis, which was required in 47% of the cases, results improved significantly to 55% good to excellent, 30% fair, and 16% poor (80). Tenolysis was required in only 16% of two-stage reconstructions in a series reported by Amadio et al. (81).

Most early flexion contractures of the PIP or DIP joint respond to night splinting, assuming that an appropriate length tendon graft was used (79). If no progress is made with hand therapy or the contractures are not recognized or treated proactively, tenolysis and/or capsulotomies may be required to improve the range of motion. If the entire native musculotendinous unit and attached tendon graft shorten significantly, a proximal step-lengthening procedure should be considered to salvage the tendon graft reconstruction.

Although the tendon graft may rupture proximally or distally, the typical Pulvertaft weave used proximally prevents most such ruptures. Distal ruptures are more likely and typically occur at the bone–tendon interface. In the largest 10-year experience with 150 two-stage reconstructions, there was a 14.1% rupture rate, with the ruptures occurring almost equally at the proximal (7.4%) and distal (6.7%) tendon graft junctures (71). These ruptures occurred at an average of 12 weeks following surgery (range 2 to 60 weeks. In the series of 43 two-stage reconstructions reported by Strickland (4), the rupture rate was only 7%. In this same series of patients treated by a single surgeon, tenolysis of the tendon grafts had a slightly higher rupture rate of 8% when compared with the 7% rupture rate following the initial tendon graft surgery and greater than the 4% rupture rate following primary tenorrhaphy without grafting (4). A rupture rate of 4% in 101 patients with 130 reconstructions is the lowest reported in a large series, but follow-up was incomplete, with only 89 patients available for long-term evaluation (81). If a tendon graft rupture is recognized early, reattachment should be attempted. If unsuccessful, one can consider conversion to a "superficialis finger," in which the flexor tendon graft attachment is transferred proximally onto the base of the middle phalanx to reconstruct the FDS instead of the FDP (77).

Excessive length of the tendon graft results in inefficient and incomplete active flexion, whereas a short tendon graft produces a flexion posture that prevents full extension. During surgery, the tension should be adjusted after the distal skin incision has been closed, leaving only the proximal incision at the wrist open. If tension has been adjusted correctly, the operated digit should adopt its usual position in the normal cascade of the fingers and should flex and extend appropriately during a tenodesis maneuver.

SINGLE-STAGE (PRIMARY) TENDON GRAFTING

In the acute or subacute injury where primary flexor tendon repair is not possible, one occasionally can consider the use of immediate single-stage flexor tendon grafting. The usual situations for its use are when an attritional rupture has occurred or when an acute repair has been delayed beyond the point when a primary tenorrhaphy on a retracted tendon can be performed without undue tension. Requirements for this technique include full passive range of motion of the finger, intact neurovascular status, intact pulleys, age older than 5 years, and lack of significant scarring of the flexor sheath or inflammation or digital edema. Contraindications include joint contractures, unstable or incompletely healed phalangeal fractures, severe crush injury, impending or actual skin loss that may jeopardize soft tissue coverage, sensory loss, and compromised vascularity (82,83).

The preferred tendon graft from the palm to the distal phalanx is the palmaris longus tendon, although the plantaris or toe extensor tendons are equally acceptable. Tendon sheath and pulleys should be preserved. When both the superficialis and profundus tendons are divided, the superficialis tendon is divided proximally in the mid palm and the distal insertion is preserved to prevent a swan-neck deformity. The distal profundus tendon is divided 1cm proximal to its insertion and the proximal end is trimmed back into zone III in the palm. After the tendon graft is interposed, it is secured distally into the distal phalanx with a pullout suture technique and reinforced with the remaining profundus tendon stump. The proximal juncture is performed with either a Pulvertaft weave or end-to-end suture after the appropriate tension has been adjusted.

If the superficialis tendon remains intact, the surgeon must weigh the risks of FDP reconstruction against the alternatives of DIP joint arthrodesis, tenodesis, or no intervention at all, because most patients will have adequate function if the FDS remains intact. In selected patients who specifically require FDP function (e.g., musician), primary flexor tendon grafting in this situation is performed by passing the tendon graft through Camper's chiasm of the intact superficialis tendon (82,84).

Potential complications are similar to those encountered following primary tenorrhaphy. Tendon adhesions are the most common complication; they may require secondary tenolysis 3 to 6 months following graft placement. Graft ruptures, if recognized early, should be treated with reinsertion. If the tendon graft rupture cannot be salvaged, it may necessitate conversion to a two-stage tendon graft technique. If the FDS distal insertion is missing, PIP joint hyperextension or swan-neck deformity may develop. A lumbrical plus deformity may occur if the tendon graft is too long (see below), whereas a tendon graft that is too short may lead to inability to extend the digit fully. Finally, the surgeon must be cautious in performing a primary tendon graft through an intact superficialis, which may actually make the patient's overall function worse, especially if the FDS is damaged or if additional scar is introduced at Camper's chiasm.

LUMBRICAL PLUS DEFORMITY

Tendon grafts occasionally are used to reconstruct the FDP distal to the origin of the lumbrical muscle from the radial aspect of the FDP. If the interposed tendon graft is too long, the effective length of the profundus tendon is increased and the patient will be unable to completely flex the DIP joint. In an attempt to produce full flexion at the DIP joint, the FDP tendon will contract more proximally than usual, thereby exerting more tension on the attached lumbrical muscle. This results in paradoxical finger extension at the level of the PIP and DIP joints on attempting active flexion, a condition termed the *lumbrical plus deformity* (85,86). A similar situation can arise if a distal FDP avulsion or laceration is not repaired, with consequent proximal migration of the FDP tendon that exerts tension on the lumbrical muscle and produces the lumbrical plus deformity. Such a deformity can be prevented by determination of the appropriate length of an interpositional tendon graft or by early repair of distal FDP avulsions. If a lumbrical plus deformity develops, treatment involves transection of the lumbrical tendon at the level of the radial lateral band of the extensor mechanism at the proximal phalanx. This can be performed easily under local anesthesia (87).

QUADRIGA EFFECT

Unlike the independent FDS musculotendinous units, the FDP tendons arise from a common muscular origin. Several clinical scenarios can produce distal tethering or shortening of a single FDP tendon, including overadvancement of a flexor profundus repair, inadequate length of an interpositional tendon graft, suturing the flexor profundus to the extensor tendon to cover an amputation stump, or significant scarring. These conditions not only produce a flexion posture of the involved finger but also result in weakening of the other three FDP tendons because of their common shared origin. Maximal flexion is achieved in the involved finger before full flexion is reached in the other three digits, thereby limiting complete flexion at the DIP joint of an adjacent finger and producing weak grip. The PIP joints flex but DIP joint flexion is incomplete. This is termed the *quadriga effect* (87,88).

Prevention is dependent on the underlying cause. Distal avulsion of the FDP should be repaired within several days of the injury to minimize the degree of shortening of the proximal musculotendinous unit. Delay in the diagnosis and subsequent repair may require excessive advancement of the shortened musculotendinous unit in order to achieve primary coaptation, resulting in a quadriga effect. Flexor tendon grafts should be carefully adjusted in length to avoid either too tight a reconstruction that may result in a quadriga effect or too loose a reconstruction that may result in a lumbrical plus deformity. In finger amputations, one must avoid the temptation to suture the FDP tendon stump to the extensor tendon at the amputation stump in order to achieve bony coverage. Such a maneuver tethers the FDP distally, creating an instant quadriga effect. FDP tendon adhesions at the amputation stump also may produce the same effect (89).

Treatment of an established quadriga effect is dependent on the underlying cause. Options include adjustment of the length of a flexor tendon graft, release of the distal FDP scar or tenodesis fixation points, or tenolysis of peritendinous or intertendinous adhesions. Salvage procedures include tenotomy of the profundus tendon and conversion to a superficialis finger, DIP joint arthrodesis, or two-stage tendon reconstruction only in special circumstances where FDP function is of critical importance (e.g., for a musician).

SWAN-NECK DEFORMITY

Zone II flexor tendon injuries present the surgeon with the option of repairing the FDP only or repairing both the superficialis and profundus tendons. Advantages of repairing both flexor tendons include increased strength, stabilization of the PIP joint, and provision of a better gliding surface for the FDP tendon. An FDP repair alone reduces the bulk of the repair, minimizes intertendinous adhesion formation, simplifies the repair, minimizes operative time, and introduces the possibility of an FDS-to-FDP tendon transfer in the situation where a segment of FDP tendon is missing or severely damaged. However, if the FDS tendon is not repaired, a swan-neck deformity may develop with hyperextension at the PIP joint and flexion at the DIP joint as a result of tendon imbalance and loss of PIP joint stabilization, especially in patients with normally hyperlax PIP joints.

In most situations, the FDS tendon should be repaired routinely, both to enhance gliding of the FDP tendon and to prevent a swan-neck deformity. If the FDS tendon is intact and only the FDP requires repair, the surgeon occasionally may have to consider dividing one slip of the FDS because of limited excursion of a bulky FDP repair through Camper's chiasm. If the FDS is completely transected and repair is not indicated, the FDS should be sectioned proximal to the chiasm if at all possible for two reasons: (i) the remaining distal portion of the FDS can act as a passive restraint to the PIP joint; and (ii) the long vincular blood supply to the FDP tendon can be maintained through the distal portion of the FDS (57,90). If the FDS tendon is divided distal to the chiasm, the ends of the FDS tendon should be reflected outward and sutured to the periosteum of the proximal phalanx to produce a tenodesis effect across the PIP joint to help prevent a swan-neck deformity (90) .

Treatment options for an established swan-neck deformity include volar plate advancement, sublimis tenodesis, spiral oblique retinacular ligament reconstruction (91), and Littler's ulnar lateral band technique to reproduce the action of the oblique retinacular ligament (92).

INFECTION

The incidence of infection following primary tenorrhaphy is not known and has not been well studied, but it probably is quite low. In a prospective study of 250 simple and complex hand lacerations randomized to treatment with either amoxicillin-clavulanate or no antibiotic therapy, the infection rate was 5% in the antibiotic group and 3.2% in the group not receiving antibiotics (93). In a double-blind randomized prospective study of 87 patients with a variety of open hand injuries reported by Peacock et al. (94), the overall infection rate was only 1.1% without any significant advantage in patients treated with prophylactic antibiotics. A retrospective study of 140 patients with flexor tendon injuries also demonstrated a low infection rate that was not significantly decreased by antibiotic treatment (95). In a review of 150 two-stage flexor tendon grafts, Wehbe et al. (71) reported a 4% infection rate following stage I of the reconstruction and 0.7% following stage II.

Although the excellent vascularity of the hand helps prevent infection, the principles of appropriate wound irrigation and debridement still need to be followed closely in the initial treatment of flexor tendon injuries in order to minimize the risk of infection, especially in heavily contaminated wounds. If an infection develops, treatment is individualized to address the severity and location of the infection. Superficial infections and cellulitis may be treated effectively with elevation, immobilization, and antibiotics. Local debridement also may be necessary. Deep infections may compromise the results of the flexor tendon repair and may require additional surgical drainage.

REFERENCES

1. Elliot D, Moiemen NS, Fleming AF, et al. The rupture rate of acute flexor tendon repairs mobilized by the controlled active motion regimen. *J Hand Surg [Br]* 1994;19:607–612.
2. Small JO, Brennen MD, Colville J. Early active mobilisation following flexor tendon repair in zone 2. *J Hand Surg [Br]* 1989;14:383–391.
3. Allen BN, Frykman GK, Unsell RS, et al. Ruptured flexor tendon tenorrhaphies in zone II: repair and rehabilitation. *J Hand Surg [Am]* 1987;12:18–21.
4. Strickland JW. Results of flexor tendon surgery in zone II. *Hand Clin* 1985;1:167–180.
5. Tonkin M, Lister G. Results of primary tendon repair with closure of the tendon sheath. *Aust N Z J Surg* 1990;60:947–952.
6. Strickland JW, Glogovac SV. Digital function following flexor tendon repair in Zone II: a comparison of immobilization and controlled passive motion techniques. *J Hand Surg [Am]* 1980; 5:537–543.
7. Gault DT. A review of repaired flexor tendons. *J Hand Surg [Br]* 1987;12:321–325.
8. Lister GD, Kleinert HE, Kutz JE, et al. Primary flexor tendon repair followed by immediate controlled mobilization. *J Hand Surg* 1977;2:441–451.
9. Duran RJ, Houser RG. Controlled passive motion following flexor tendon repair in zones 2 and 3. In: *AAOS symposium on tendon surgery in the hand.* St. Louis: CV Mosby, 1975:105–114.
10. Edinburg M, Widgerow AD, Biddulph SL. Early postoperative mobilization of flexor tendon injuries using a modification of the Kleinert technique. *J Hand Surg [Am]* 1987;12:34–38.
11. Kitsis CK, Wade PJ, Krikler SJ, et al. Controlled active motion following primary flexor tendon repair: a prospective study over 9 years. *J Hand Surg [Br]* 1998;23:344–349.
12. Baktir A, Turk CY, Kabak S, et al. Flexor tendon repair in zone 2 followed by early active mobilization. *J Hand Surg [Br]* 1996; 21:624–628.
13. Peck FH, Bucher CA, Watson JS, et al. A comparative study of two methods of controlled mobilization of flexor tendon repairs in zone 2. *J Hand Surg [Br]* 1998;23:41–45.
14. Schneider LH. Suture techniques. In: Schneider LH, ed. *Flexor tendon injuries.* Boston: Little, Brown and Company, 1985: 33–46.
15. Ejeskar A, Irstam L. Elongation in profundus tendon repair. A clinical and radiological study. *Scand J Plast Reconstr Surg* 1981;15:61–68.
16. Seradge H. Elongation of the repair configuration following flexor tendon repair. *J Hand Surg [Am]* 1983;8:182–185.
17. Strickland JW. The Indiana method of flexor tendon repair. *Atlas Hand Clin* 1996;1:77–103.
18. Wagner WF Jr, Carroll CT, Strickland JW, et al. A biomechanical comparison of techniques of flexor tendon repair. *J Hand Surg [Am]* 1994;19:979–983.
19. Trail IA, Powell ES, Noble J. The mechanical strength of various suture techniques. *J Hand Surg [Br]* 1992;17:89–91.
20. Taras JS, Skahen JR, Raphael JS, et al. The double-grasping and cross-stitch for acute flexor tendon repair. *Atlas Hand Clin* 1996;1:13–28.
21. Gelberman RH, Amifl D, Gonsalves M, et al. The influence of protected passive mobilization on the healing of flexor tendons: a biochemical and microangiographic study. *Hand* 1981;13: 120–128.

22. Gelberman RH, Woo SL, Lothringer K, et al. Effects of early intermittent passive mobilization on healing canine flexor tendons. *J Hand Surg [Am]* 1982;7:170–175.
23. Gelberman RH, Vande Berg JS, Lundborg GN, et al. Flexor tendon healing and restoration of the gliding surface. An ultrastructural study in dogs. *J Bone Joint Surg [Am]* 1983;65:70–80.
24. Savage R. In vitro studies of a new method of flexor tendon repair. *J Hand Surg [Br]* 1985;10:135–141.
25. Thurman RT, Trumble TE, Hanel DP, et al. Two-, four-, and six-strand zone II flexor tendon repairs: an in situ biomechanical comparison using a cadaver model. *J Hand Surg [Am]* 1998; 23:261–265.
26. Winters SC, Gelberman RH, Woo SL, et al. The effects of multiple-strand suture methods on the strength and excursion of repaired intrasynovial flexor tendons: a biomechanical study in dogs. *J Hand Surg [Am]* 1998;23:97–104.
27. Schuind F, Garcia-Elias M, Cooney WPD, et al. Flexor tendon forces: in vivo measurements. *J Hand Surg [Am]* 1992;17: 291–298.
28. Singer G, Ebramzadeh E, Jones NF, et al. Use of the Taguchi method for biomechanical comparison of flexor-tendon-repair techniques to allow immediate active flexion. A new method of analysis and optimization of technique to improve the quality of the repair. *J Bone Joint Surg Am* 1998;80:1498–1506.
29. Wade PJ, Muir IF, Hutcheon LL. Primary flexor tendon repair: the mechanical limitations of the modified Kessler technique. *J Hand Surg [Br]* 1986;11:71–76.
30. Wade PJ, Wetherell RG, Amis AA. Flexor tendon repair: significant gain in strength from the Halsted peripheral suture technique. *J Hand Surg [Br]* 1989;14:232–235.
31. Lin GT, An KN, Amadio PC, et al. Biomechanical studies of running suture for flexor tendon repair in dogs. *J Hand Surg [Am]* 1988;13:553–558.
32. Silfverskiold KL, Andersson CH. Two new methods of tendon repair: an in vitro evaluation of tensile strength and gap formation. *J Hand Surg [Am]* 1993;18:58–65.
33. Silfverskiold KL, May EJ. Flexor tendon repair in zone II with a new suture technique and an early mobilization program combining passive and active flexion. *J Hand Surg [Am]* 1994;19: 53–60.
34. Aoki M, Manske PR, Pruitt DL, et al. Work of flexion after tendon repair with various suture methods. A human cadaveric study. *J Hand Surg [Br]* 1995;20:310–313.
35. Tang JB, Ishii S, Usui M, et al. Flexor sheath closure during delayed primary tendon repair. *J Hand Surg [Am]* 1994;19: 636–640.
36. Tang JB, Seiichi I, Masamichi U. Surgical management of the tendon sheath at different repair stages. *Chin Med J (Engl)* 1990; 103:295–303.
37. Tang JB, Shi D, Zhang QG. Biomechanical and histologic evaluation of tendon sheath management. *J Hand Surg [Am]* 1996; 21:900–908.
38. Tonkin MA. Primary flexor tendon repair: surgical techniques based on the anatomy. *World J Surg* 1991;15:452–457.
39. Tang JB, Zhang QG, Ishii S. Autogenous free sheath grafts in reconstruction of injured digital flexor tendon sheath at the delayed primary stage. *J Hand Surg [Br]* 1993;18:31–32.
40. Peterson WW, Manske PR, Kain CC, et al. Effect of flexor sheath integrity on tendon gliding: a biomechanical and histologic study. *J Orthop Res* 1986;4:458–465.
41. Gelberman RH, Woo SL, Amiel D, et al. Influences of flexor sheath continuity and early motion on tendon healing in dogs. *J Hand Surg [Am]* 1990;15:69–77.
42. Peterson WW, Manske PR, Lesker PA. The effect of flexor sheath integrity on nutrient uptake by chicken flexor tendons. *Clin Orthop* 1985;201:259–263.
43. Peterson WW, Manske PR, Lesker PA. The effect of flexor sheath integrity on nutrient uptake by primate flexor tendons. *J Hand Surg [Am]* 1986;11:413–416.
44. Komurcu M, Akkus O, Basbozkurt M, et al. Reduction of restrictive adhesions by local aprotinin application and primary sheath repair in surgically traumatized flexor tendons of the rabbit. *J Hand Surg [Am]* 1997;22:826–832.
45. Wimann B. On the reaction of plasmin or plasmin streptokinase complex with aprotinin or alpha1-antiplasmin. *Thromb Res* 1980;17:143–152.
46. Schneider LH. Postoperative management in flexor tendon repair. In: Schneider LH, ed. *Flexor tendon injuries.* Boston: Little, Brown and Company, 1985:151–160.
47. Young RES, Harmon JS. Repair of tendon injuries in the hand. *Ann Surg* 1960;151:562.
48. Sotereanos DG, Goitz RJ, Mitsionis GJ. Flexor tenolysis. *Atlas Hand Clin* 1996;1:105–120.
49. Fetrow KO. Tenolysis in the hand and wrist. A clinical evaluation of two hundred and twenty flexor and extensor tenolyses. *J Bone Joint Surg [Am]* 1967;49:667–685.
50. Schneider LH. Tenolysis. In: Schneider LH, ed. *Flexor tendon injuries.* Boston: Little, Brown and Company, 1985:111–123.
51. Foucher G, Lenoble E, Ben Youssef K, et al. A post-operative regime after digital flexor tenolysis. A series of 72 patients. *J Hand Surg [Br]* 1993;18:35–40.
52. Strickland JW. Flexor tenolysis. *Hand Clin* 1985;1:121–132.
53. Wray RC, Moucharafieh B, Weeks PM. Experimental study of the optimal time for tenolysis. *Plast Reconstr Surg* 1978;61: 184–189.
54. May EJ, Silfverskiold KL. Rate of recovery after flexor tendon repair in zone II. A prospective longitudinal study of 145 digits. *Scand J Plast Reconstr Surg Hand Surg* 1993;27:89–94.
55. Hunter JM, Schneider LH, Dumont J, et al. A dynamic approach to problems of hand function using local anesthesia supplemented by intravenous fentanyl-droperidol. *Clin Orthop* 1974;104:112–115.
56. Whitaker JH, Strickland JW, Ellis RG. The role of tenolysis in the palm and digit. *J Hand Surg* 1977;2:462–470.
57. Leddy JP. Flexor tendons—acute injuries. In: Green DP, ed. *Operative hand surgery.* New York: Churchill Livingstone, 1993:1823–1851.
58. Doyle JR. Anatomy of the finger flexor tendon sheath and pulley system. *J Hand Surg [Am]* 1988;13:473–484.
59. Lin GT, Amadio PC, An KN, et al. Functional anatomy of the human digital flexor tendon pulley system. *J Hand Surg [Am]* 1989;14:949–956.
60. Schneider LH, Hunter JM. Flexor tendons—late reconstruction. In: Green DP, ed. *Operative hand surgery.* New York: Churchill Livingstone, 1993:1853–1924.
61. Strickland JW. Flexor tendon injuries. Part 4. Staged flexor tendon reconstruction and restoration of the flexor pulley system. *Orthop Rev* 1987;16:39–51.
62. Kleinert HE, Bennett JB. Digital pulley reconstruction employing the always present rim of the previous pulley. *J Hand Surg* 1978;3:297–298.
63. Kleinert HE, Schepel S, Gill T. Flexor tendon injuries. *Surg Clin North Am* 1981;61:267–286.
64. Lin GT, Amadio PC, An KN, et al. Biomechanical analysis of finger flexor pulley reconstruction. *J Hand Surg [Br]* 1989;14:278–282.
65. Lister GD. Reconstruction of pulleys employing extensor retinaculum. *J Hand Surg* 1979;4:461–464.
66. Karev A. The "belt loop" technique for the reconstruction of pulleys in the first stage of flexor tendon grafting. *J Hand Surg [Am]* 1984;9:923–924.
67. Widstrom CJ, Johnson G, Doyle JR, et al. A mechanical study of

six digital pulley reconstruction techniques. *J Hand Surg [Am]* 1989;14:821–825.
68. Hunter JM. Artificial tendons. Early development and application. *Am J Surg* 1965;109:325.
69. Hunter JM, Salisbury RE. Flexor-tendon reconstruction in severely damaged hands. A two-stage procedure using a silicone Dacron reinforced gliding prosthesis prior to tendon grafting. *J Bone Joint Surg [Am]* 1971;53:829–858.
70. Hunter JM. Staged flexor tendon reconstruction. *J Hand Surg [Am]* 1983;8[5 Pt 2]:789–793.
71. Wehbe MA, Mawr B, Hunter JM, et al. Two-stage flexor-tendon reconstruction. Ten-year experience. *J Bone Joint Surg [Am]* 1986;68:752–763.
72. Reimann AF, Daseler EH, Anson BJ, et al. The palmaris longus muscle and tendon. A study of 1,600 extremities. *Anat Rec* 1944;89:495.
73. Vanderhooft E. The frequency of and relationship between the palmaris longus and plantaris tendons. *Am J Orthop* 1996;25:38–41.
74. Daseler EH, Anson BJ. The plantaris muscle. An anatomical study of 750 specimens. *J Bone Joint Surg* 1943;25:822–827.
75. Harvey FJ, Chu G, Harvey PM. Surgical availability of the plantaris tendon. *J Hand Surg [Am]* 1983;8:243–247.
76. Schneider LH. Secondary procedures in flexor tendon surgery. In: Schneider LH, ed. *Flexor tendon injuries.* Boston: Little, Brown and Company, 1985:77–109.
77. Taras JS, Marion M, Culp RW. Staged flexor tendon reconstruction with Hunter implants. *Atlas Hand Clin* 1996;1:129–152.
78. Weinstein SL, Sprague BL, Flatt AE. Evaluation of the two-stage flexor-tendon reconstruction in severely damaged digits. *J Bone Joint Surg [Am]* 1976;58:786–791.
79. Soucacos PN, Beris AE, Malizos KN, et al. Two-stage treatment of flexor tendon ruptures. Silicon rod complications analyzed in 109 digits. *Acta Orthop Scand Suppl* 1997;275:48–51.
80. LaSalle WB, Strickland JW. An evaluation of digital performance following two-stage flexor tendon reconstruction. *J Hand Surg [Am]* 1983;8:263–267.
81. Amadio PC, Wood MB, Cooney WPD, et al. Staged flexor tendon reconstruction in the fingers and hand. *J Hand Surg [Am]* 1988;13:559–562.
82. Strickland JW. Flexor tendon injuries. Part 3. Free tendon grafts. *Orthop Rev* 1987;16:18–26.
83. Tubiana R. Technique of flexor tendon grafts. *Hand* 1969;1:108–114.
84. Stark HH, Zemel NP, Boyes JH, et al. Flexor tendon graft through intact superficialis tendon. *J Hand Surg [Am]* 1977;2:456–461.
85. Parkes A. The "lumbrical plus" finger. *Hand* 1970;2:164–165.
86. Lister G. Pitfalls and complications of flexor tendon surgery. *Hand Clin* 1985;1:133–146.
87. Schneider LH. Acute flexor tendon injuries. In: Schneider LH, ed. *Flexor tendon injuries.* Boston: Little, Brown and Company, 1985:47–75.
88. Verdan CE. Syndrome of the quadriga. *Surg Clin North Am* 1960;40:425.
89. Neu BR, Murray JF, MacKenzie JK. Profundus tendon blockage: quadriga in finger amputations. *J Hand Surg [Am]* 1985;10[6 Pt 1]:878–883.
90. Ariyan S, Cuono CB. Acute hand injuries. In: Goldwyn RM, ed. *The unfavorable result in plastic surgery.* Boston: Little, Brown and Company, 1984:939–965.
91. Thompson JS, Littler JW, Upton J. The spiral oblique retinacular ligament. SORL. *J Hand Surg [Am]* 1978;3:482–487.
92. Burton RI. Extensor tendons—late reconstruction. In: Green DP, ed. *Operative hand surgery.* New York: Churchill Livingstone, 1993:1955–1988.
93. Cassell OC, Ion L. Are antibiotics necessary in the surgical management of upper limb lacerations? *Br J Plast Surg* 1997;50:523–529.
94. Peacock KC, Hanna DP, Kirkpatrick WC, et al. Efficacy of perioperative cefamandole with postoperative cephalexin in the primary outpatient treatment of open wounds of the hand. *J Hand Surg [Am]* 1988;13:960–964.
95. Stone JF, Davidson JS. The role of antibiotics and timing of repair in flexor tendon injuries of the hand. *Ann Plast Surg* 1998;40:7–13.

Discussion

FLEXOR TENDON INJURIES

MARK H. GONZALEZ

The authors provide an outstanding chapter on the complications of flexor tendon surgery based on an exhaustive review of the literature and their own considerable experience.

M. H. Gonzalez: Division of Orthopaedic Surgery, Cook County Hospital, University of Illinois, Chicago, Illinois

Tendon ruptures are a dreaded complication of flexor tendon surgery. Early passive motion has been shown to improve the strength of a tendon repair and in one study has shown a decreased rate of rupture (1–3). In an attempt to further improve range of motion after flexor tendon repair, early active motion has been advocated (4). As the authors state in their chapter, this may show an increased rate of tendon rupture. The literature does not give a definitive answer on the effect of active motion on the rate of tendon rupture, but the rate seems to be slightly increased (5,6). Early motion with stress to the repair has been shown to increase tensile strength, but it may place the tendon at increased risk for gapping at the repair site, which is antecedent to tendon rupture (7).

In an attempt to decrease the risk of gapping, stronger repairs with a greater number of suture strands have been designed (4,5,8). The authors point out that this too is not without a down side. Many of the multistrand repairs are technically difficult, are bulky, and may cause strangulation of the tendon. The work of flexion also may be increased, which decreases tendon gliding (9).

The circumferential stitch first repair with the core stitches placed last has been advocated by Sanders (10). The advantages of the repair are stated to be a less bulky repair, as well as knot placement outside of the repair site. This is thought to increase tendon gliding as well as the strength of the repair because of an increased surface area for tendon healing. Animal studies have shown both a positive and negative effect of having the knots outside the repair site (11–13).

Tendon rupture can be difficult to distinguish from tendon gapping or tendon adhesion. Ultrasound has been used to differentiate the two conditions. Drape et al. (14) perform magnetic resonance imaging when rupture is suspected. Long gapping or frank disruption is treated with re-repair, whereas short gaps with adhesions are treated with tenolysis (14).

A factor often ignored in tendon rupture is patient compliance. In our experience, the most important cause of tendon rupture is patient noncompliance and removal of the splint. Early motion protocols require knowledgeable patient participation. Noncompliant patients and patients with substance addiction or alcoholism are very poor candidates for further surgery.

The treatment plan following tendon rupture must take into account the patient's needs and occupation, and the time after rupture. Based on financial constraints, some patients may opt not to undergo reconstruction for an isolated flexor pollicis longus (FPL) or flexor digitorum superficialis (FDS) rupture. Good results have been reported when repair is done within 14 days of tenorrhaphy rupture (15). A rupture that occurs several weeks after repair may not be reparable, and the patient may be a candidate for a single-stage or two-stage tendon graft. Similarly, a rerupture in the face of wound breakdown and infection is a poor candidate for immediate re-repair and may require a delayed two-stage tendon reconstruction after eradicating the infection and obtaining a stable wound.

The technique of tendon repair after rupture is more challenging than primary repair. The stitch commonly fails at the knot, but pullout of the stitch from the tendon also can occur. Frequently the tendon ends appear mop-like and frayed. Resection of the tendon ends must be judicious and should be avoided, if possible. Resection greater than 1.5 cm for the index finger and 1.0 cm for the other digits can lead to a quadriga effect (16). The core stitch must be extended into the intact portion of the tendon to bypass the frayed end. A braided polyester stitch is preferred because of its superior strength. The addition of a second core stitch as advocated by Strickland (17) is technically simple to do and will greatly increase the strength of the repair. The ends are difficult to oppose, and a meticulous closely spaced circumferential stitch is necessary for strength of repair and to consolidate the frayed ends so as to permit gliding through the pulleys (18).

Two-stage tendon grafting is technically demanding but can give excellent results (19). The pulleys can be reconstructed at the first stage. One complication we have noted after grafting in patients with a hyperextensible proximal interphalangeal joint is a swan-neck deformity due to a lack of FDS function. In such cases, before placing the silicone tendon, a short 2-cm segment of an FDS slip is preserved and sutured to the sheath.

Hunter (20) has attempted to develop a permanent artificial tendon. A permanent artificial tendon has not yet been constructed, but this line of work has led to the development of an active tendon implant to be used in stage I. Advantages of the active tendon implant are thought to be improved gliding and improved maintenance of strength.

In certain instances, an FDS finger is a useful salvage procedure (21). The indications for this procedure include digits with a destroyed or severely scarred distal interphalangeal joint, digits with a severely damaged distal pulley system, and digits with a tendon graft that ruptured at its distal insertion. The tendon graft is tensioned and attached to the middle phalanx.

Rupture of an FDP tenorrhaphy in the presence of an intact FDS tendon may cause limited functional loss. Single-stage tendon grafting through an intact FDS decussation has potential for scarring and further loss of motion (22–24). This procedure is recommended for younger patients with supple joints and a reasonable need for distal interphalangeal function. The tendon graft can be passed either through or around the decussation, depending on which allows freer motion of the graft. Schneider (24) reports that a significant percentage of patients who undergo single-stage grafting through an intact superficialis will require subsequent tenolysis. Two-stage tendon grafting through an intact FDS decussation has been described and should be reserved for cases with a normally functioning FDS and a scarred bed (25) .

Distal interphalangeal joint tenodesis or fusion is a reasonable option, especially if there is normal FDS pull-through and normal proximal interphalangeal flexion.

Rupture of an FPL tenorrhaphy may not be as disabling as rupture of an FDS and FDP repair (26). Loss of interphalangeal joint flexion is not critical, and patients are most disabled by a floppy interphalangeal joint that hyperextends during pinch. Occasionally after rupture, scarring about the interphalangeal joint produces enough stability so that the joint does not hyperextend with pinch, and no further treatment is necessary. Interphalangeal instability during pinch may be treated most simply with an interphalangeal fusion or tenodesis.

If thumb flexion is imperative, options include re-repair, single-stage tendon graft, FDS transfer, or two-stage tendon graft. The single-stage tendon graft or the superficialis transfer should be performed only when there is minimal scarring and intact pulley function (19). Scarring about the tendon bed or incompetent pulleys will require two-stage tendon reconstruction with pulley reconstruction.

The authors discuss the key issues of tendon adhesion. They emphasize the importance of hemostasis and atraumatic surgical technique. The importance of sheath closure in avoiding tendon adhesions has been debated in the literature (27–29). It has been suggested that an intact tendon sheath can improve tendon nutrition and mechanically act as a funnel to allow passage of the tendon repair under a pulley. In a randomized study, Saldana et al. (30) compared the results of flexor tendon repair with and without sheath repair, but they could show no difference between the two techniques.

REFERENCES

1. Feehan LM, Beauchene JG. Early tensile properties of healing chicken flexor tendons: early controlled passive motion versus postoperative immobilization. *J Hand Surg [Am]* 1990;15:63–68.
2. Hitchcock TF, Light TR, Bunch WH, et al. The effect of immediate constrained digital motion on the strength of tendon repairs in chickens. *J Hand Surg [Am]* 1987;12:590–595.
3. Strickland JW, Glogovac SV. Digital function following flexor tendon repair in zone II: a comparison of immobilization and controlled passive motion techniques. *J Hand Surg [Am]* 1980; 5:537–543.
4. Savage R, Risitano G. Flexor tendon repair using a six strand method of repair and early active motion. *J Hand Surg [Br]* 1989; 14:396–399.
5. Thurman RT, Trumble TE, Hanel DP, et al. Two-, four-, and six-strand zone II flexor tendon repairs: an in situ biomechanical comparison using a cadaver model. *J Hand Surg [Am]* 1998; 23:261–265.
6. Elliot D, Moiemen NS, Fleming AF, et al. The rupture rate of acute flexor tendon repairs mobilized by the controlled active motion regimen. *J Hand Surg [Br]* 1994;19:607–612.
7. Kitsis CK, Wade PJ, Krikler SJ, et al. Controlled active motion following primary flexor tendon repair: a prospective study over 9 years. *J Hand Surg [Br]* 1998;23:344–349.
8. Aoki M, Kubota H, Pruitt DL, et al. Biomechanical and histologic characteristics of canine flexor tendon repair using early postoperative mobilization. *J Hand Surg [Am]* 1997;22:107–114.
9. Aoki M, Manske PR, Pruitt DL, et al. Work of flexion after tendon repair with various suture methods. A human cadaveric study. *J Hand Surg [Br]* 1995;20:310–313.
10. Sanders WE. Advantages of "epitenon first" suture placement technique in flexor tendon repair. *Clin Orthop* 1992;280: 198–199.
11. Papandrea R, Seitz WH Jr, Shapiro P, et al. Biomechanical and clinical evaluation of the epitenon-first technique of flexor tendon repair. *J Hand Surg [Am]* 1995;20:261–266.
12. Pruitt DL, Aoki M, Manske PR. Effect of suture knot location on tensile strength after flexor tendon repair. *J Hand Surg [Am]* 1996;21:969–973.
13. Aoki M, Pruitt DL, Kubota H, et al. Effect of suture knots on tensile strength of repaired canine flexor tendons. *J Hand Surg [Br]* 1995;20:72–75.
14. Drape JL, Silbermann-Hoffman O, Houvet P, et al. Complications of flexor tendon repair in the hand: MR imaging assessment. *Radiology* 1996;198:219–224.
15. Allen BN, Frykman GK, Unsell RS, et al. Ruptured flexor tendon tenorrhaphies in zone II: repair and rehabilitation. *J Hand Surg [Am]* 1987;12:18–21.
16. Malerich MM, Baird RA, McMaster W, et al. Permissible limits of flexor digitorum profundus tendon advancement—an anatomic study. *J Hand Surg [Am]* 1987;12:30–33.
17. Strickland JW. Flexor tendon injuries: II. Operative technique. *J Am Acad Orthop Surg* 1995;3:55–62.
18. Wade PJ, Wetherell RG, Amis AA. Flexor tendon repair: significant gain in strength from the Halsted peripheral suture technique. *J Hand Surg [Br]* 1989;14:232-5—23.
19. Schneider LH. Flexor tendons: late reconstruction. In: Green DP, Hotchkiss RN, Pederson WC, eds. *Green's operative hand surgery,* 4th ed. New York: Churchill Livingstone, 1999: 1898–1949.
20. Hunter JM. Tendon salvage and the active tendon implant: a perspective. *Hand Clin* 1985;1:181–186.
21. Schneider LH, Hunter JM, Fietti VG. The flexor superficialis finger: a salvage procedure. In: Hunter JM, Schneider LH, Mackin EJ, eds. *Flexor tendon surgery in the hand.* St. Louis: CV Mosby, 1986:312–318.
22. Jaffe S,Weckesser E. Profundus tendon grafting with the sublimis intact: the end result of 30 patients. *J Bone Joint Surg Am* 1967;49A:1298–1308.
23. Stark HH, Zemel NP, Boyes JH et al. Flexor tendon grafting through intact superficialis tendon. *J Hand Surg* 1977;2: 456–461.
24. Schneider LH. Treatment of isolated flexor digitorum profundus injuries by tendon grafting. In: Hunter JM, Schneider LH, Mackin EJ, eds. *Flexor tendon surgery in the hand.* St. Louis: CV Mosby, 1986:518–525.
25. Wehbe MA. Staged tendon reconstruction: technique and rationale. In: Hunter JM, Schneider LH, Mackin EJ, eds. *Flexor tendon surgery in the hand.* St. Louis: CV Mosby, 1986, pp. 260–264.
26. Kilgore ES Jr, Newmeyer WL, Graham WP 3d, et al. The dubiousness of grafting the dispensable flexor pollicis longus. *Am J Surg* 1976;132:292–296.
27. Peterson WW, Manske PR, Lesker PA. The effect of flexor sheath integrity on nutrient uptake by chicken flexor tendons. *Clin Orthop* 1985;201:259–263.
28. Peterson WW, Manske PR, Kain CC, et al. Effect of flexor sheath integrity on tendon gliding: a biomechanical and histologic study. *J Orthop Res* 1986;4:458–465.
29. Tonkin M, Lister G. Results of primary tendon repair with closure of the tendon sheath. *Aust N Z J Surg* 1990;60:947–952.
30. Saldana MJ, Ho PK, Lichtman DM, et al. Flexor tendon repair and rehabilitation in zone II open sheath technique versus closed sheath technique. *J Hand Surg [Am]* 1987;12:1110–1114.

45

EXTENSOR TENDON INJURIES

DAVID NETSCHER

The balance between the extensor and flexor tendon systems and between the extrinsic and intrinsic systems is delicate. Thorough knowledge and understanding of extensor tendon anatomy and mechanics are essential to prevent disturbance of this balance when treating extensor tendon injuries.

Extensor tendon anatomy is classified by zone. Each zone has features peculiar to its location, and each has its own requirements for management of injury. The nature of the injury, its location, its specific manner of treatment, and the rehabilitation protocol individually and collectively influence outcome.

General complications include tendon adhesions and finger stiffness, rupture of the tendon repair, and joint contracture. Specific complications relate to the site of injury and may include chronic mallet, boutonnière, swan-neck deformities, and joint infection. This chapter outlines relevant anatomy, describe the zones of tendon injury, discuss site-specific treatment recommendations and avoidance of complications, evaluate postoperative rehabilitation protocols, and discuss treatment of both the general and specific complications.

ANATOMY OF EXTENSOR TENDONS AND EXTENSOR PHYSIOLOGY

Finger flexion and extension are synchronized movements, and the extensor mechanism cannot function without the balance of the flexor antagonists (1). The wrist extensors, the extensor carpi radialis longus, the extensor carpi radialis brevis, and the extensor carpi ulnaris (ECU), act synergistically with the flexor digitorum profundus (FDP) and flexor digitorum superficialis (FDS). The wrist is stabilized in extension and the finger extensors are relaxed, countering any extension tenodesis effect and allowing a more powerful flexion grasp. Grip strength is decreased markedly with paralysis or injury to the extensors. Similarly, finger extension is enhanced with slight wrist flexion.

Over the proximal phalanx, the extensor hood is joined by tendons of the intrinsic muscles to form a broad expanse, covering about two-thirds of the circumference of the phalanx. The lateral bands represent a continuation of the more volar fibers of the intrinsic tendons together with a portion of the central extensor tendon, which fans out over the dorsum of the proximal phalanx. The more central fibers insert into the base of the middle phalanx as the central slip. Fibers from the intrinsic tendon also swing inward and contribute to the central slip, interdigitating with those fibers from the central extensor tendon, which fan toward the lateral band (Fig. 45-1). The fibers of each system are not attached to each other at the point of crossing; the crossing angle changes with proximal phalangeal joint motion from approximately 30 degrees in full extension to 90 degrees in full flexion (2,3). This arrangement provides the extensor mechanism at this level elastic properties from nonelastic components. During proximal interphalangeal (PIP) joint flexion, the tendon mesh opens and allows volar migration of the lateral bands, increasing their effective length to permit distal interphalangeal (DIP) joint flexion. This subtle balance between the relative tensions of the central slip and the lateral bands is upset, for example, in a boutonnière deformity.

The triangular ligament and retinacular ligaments also play their parts in this precisely balanced system. The triangular ligament lies just distal to the PIP joint in the midline, connecting the medial edges of the lateral bands and preventing their separation during PIP joint flexion. At the level of the PIP joint, the transverse retinacular ligaments attach to the volar edge of the lateral bands and prevent their dorsal migration. The oblique retinacular ligament passively affects DIP extension: as the PIP joint extends, the oblique retinacular ligament tightens passively and results in DIP extension (Fig. 45-2).

The lumbrical muscles act synergistically with the muscles that both extend and flex the fingers, assisting both the FDS and FDP with metacarpophalangeal (MP) joint flexion and the extensor digitorum communis (EDC) and interosseous muscles with interphalangeal (IP) joint exten-

D. Netscher: Division of Plastic Surgery, Baylor College of Medicine, and the Plastic Surgery Service, Department of Veterans Affairs, Medical Center, Houston, Texas

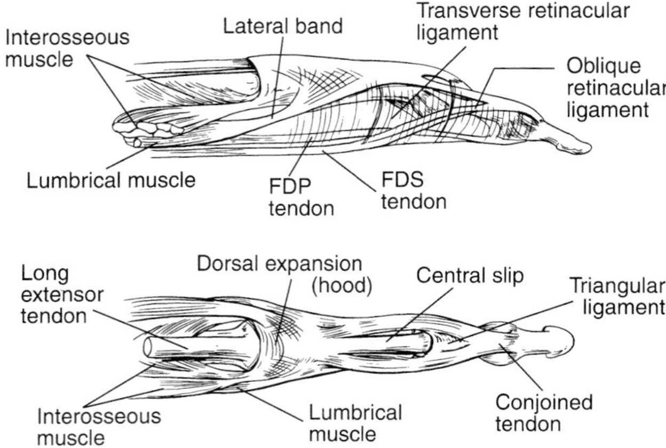

FIGURE 45-1. Anatomy of the extensor mechanism on the finger.

sion. Electromyographic studies demonstrated that the lumbricals continuously flex the MP joint throughout full active finger extension (4), preventing MP joint hyperextension and allowing IP joint extension. Without the lumbricals, the fingers would assume a hooked position, as often occurs with ulnar nerve palsy, with hyperextension of the MP joints and flexion of the IP joints.

Electromyographic studies determined that the EDC is the primary extensor at the MP joints (5). The force of the EDC is transmitted to the proximal phalanx through the sagittal bands' lasso effect on the volar plate. Flexor tenodesis affects MP joint extension; full flexion of the IP joints diminishes the tenodesis effect, allowing the MP joint to achieve greater extension than when the IP joints are held straight.

The thumb extensor system differs from that of the fingers. The dorsal hood for the thumb is somewhat similar to that of a finger in that its primary central component is the extensor pollicis longus (EPL) tendon, which extends the MP joint through the sagittal bands. The extensor pollicis brevis (EPB) and, occasionally, the adductor muscle contribute to the thumb's dorsal hood. The abductor pollicis longus (APL) tendon inserts at the base of the first metacarpal, the EPB inserts at the base of the proximal phalanx, and the EPL inserts at the base of the distal phalanx. The MP joint of the thumb is extended by the EPB, which also assists with carpometacarpal (CMC) extension and, occasionally, with IP extension. The IP joint is extended primarily by the EPL. The thumb has no lumbrical or interosseous muscles; the abductor pollicis brevis, adductor pollicis, and, occasionally, opponens pollicis muscles assist, through the dorsal expansion, in extension of the thumb's IP joint (6).

The extensor tendons enter the hand from the forearm through a series of six canals, five of which are fibro-osseous and one of which is fibrous (the fifth dorsal compartment contains the extensor digiti minimi [EDM]). The first compartment contains the APL and EPB; the second contains the radial wrist extensor; and the third contains the EPL, which angles around the Lister tubercle. The fourth compartment contains the EDC to the fingers, as well as the extensor indicis proprius (EIP). The fifth compartment contains the EDM, and the sixth contains the ECU. The communis tendons are joined distally near the MP joints by fibrous interconnections called juncturae tendinum, which usually are found only between the communis tendons and usually are three in number. The EDM and EIP are each capable of independent extension and are positioned to the ulnar side of the adjacent communis tendons (7). It is impor-

A

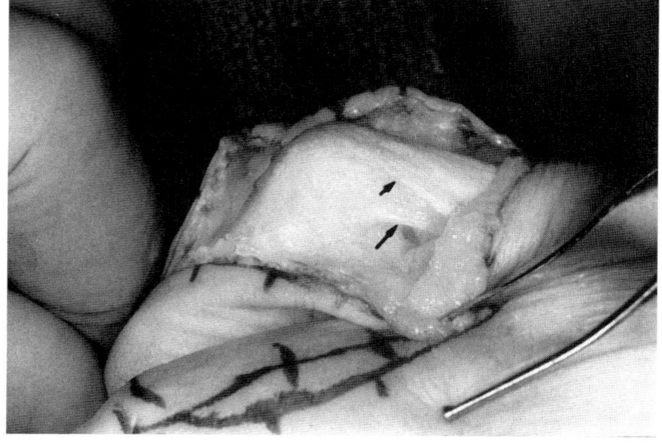

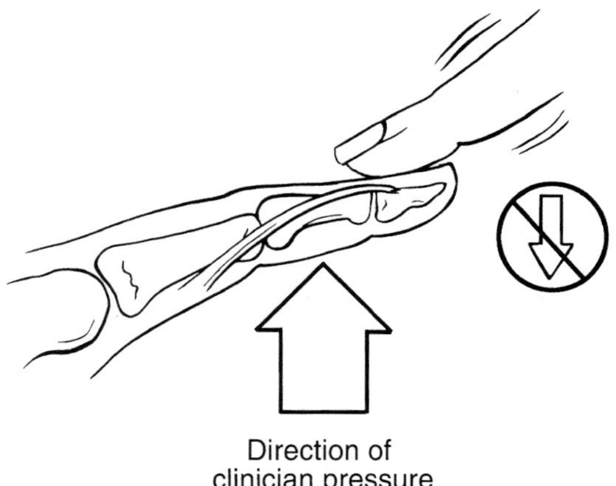

B

FIGURE 45-2. A: Operative photograph showing lateral band of the extensor mechanism *(small arrow)* and oblique retinacular ligament *(large arrow)* passing from flexor sheath proximally to the dorsal extensor mechanism distally. **B:** The oblique retinacular ligament results in a tenodesis effect between the proximal interphalangeal (PIP) and distal interphalangeal (DIP) joints. PIP extension tightens the ligament, which then extends the DIP joint. (It is more difficult for the palpating examiner's finger to passively flex the DIP joint).

tant to note that independent extension of the index finger is not lost following transfer of the EIP (8). Because of the juncturae interconnections, laceration of the middle finger communis tendon proximal to the juncturae may result in only incomplete extension loss of the middle finger (9). The EIP and EDM have no juncturae connections. The EIP muscle can be bifid and send a tendon slip to either side of the EDC of the index finger or may send a single slip to the middle finger where it will lie ulnar to that tendon. The EDM tendon usually is bifid and receives a contribution from the EDC in 80% of hands. The EDM is located on the ulnar side of the little finger extensor tendons. Occasionally, the EDM tendon sends a slip to the ring finger and may even receive a slip from the ECU tendon. The EDC to the little finger is present less than 50% of the time and, when absent, is almost always replaced by a junctura tendinum from the ring finger to the extensor aponeurosis of the little finger (10). A junctura tendinum also has been reported to occur sometimes between the index EDC and the EPL (11).

The forearm contains two layers of extensor muscles. The superficial layer is composed of five muscles, and the deep layer consists of four shorter muscles. Three muscles are found above the elbow in the superficial layer. Starting proximally and following the radial nerve innervation sequence, the extensor carpi radialis longus originates on the lateral humeral condyle and inserts distally at the base of the second metacarpal, the extensor carpi radialis brevis inserts at the base of the third metacarpal, and the EDC originates on the distal humerus and travels with the extensor carpi muscles. The two other muscles in the superficial layer, the EDM and the ECU, originate below the elbow joint. The deep muscles originate in mid forearm, primarily from the interosseous membrane, and cross the forearm obliquely toward the radial aspect of the wrist. The proximal to distal sequence of deep extensor muscles of the forearm consists of the APL, which inserts at the base of the first metacarpal, the EPB and EPL, and the EIP.

ZONES OF EXTENSOR TENDON INJURY AND INJURY EVALUATION

To facilitate understanding and treatment of tendon injuries, international agreement on the anatomical nomenclature for the flexor and extensor zones of the hand was reached in June 1980 at the First Congress of the International Federation of Societies for Surgery of the Hand in Rotterdam (12). The extensor tendon system is divided into nine zones (Fig. 45-3).

Fingers

Zone I	***Over the DIP joints***
Zone I	Over the middle phalanx
Zone III	Over the apex of the PIP joint
Zone IV	Over the proximal phalanx
Zone V	Over the apex of the MP joint
Zone VI	Over the dorsum of the hand
Zone VII	Under the extensor tendon retinaculum
Zone VIII	Distal forearm
Zone IX	Mid and proximal forearm

Thumb

Zone T-1	***Over the IP joint***
Zone T-2	Over the proximal phalanx
Zone T-3	Over the MP joint
Zone T-4	Over the first metacarpal
Zone T-5	Between the CMC joint and radial styloid
Zone T-6	Under the extensor tendon retinaculum
Zone T-7	Distal forearm
Zone T-8	Mid and proximal forearm

The management of injuries to the extensor mechanism demands the same skill and knowledge needed in the care of flexor tendon injuries. Injuries to the relatively exposed and superficially located extensor tendons are common. The dorsal aspect of the hand and wrist is covered with a thin layer of supple skin with minimal subcutaneous tissue. The tendon is thin in the distal finger joint and, with sufficient force, may be subject to closed rupture. Penetrating wounds that disrupt the tendon also may enter a neighboring joint. The degree of joint contamination must be evaluated and considered in the treatment plan.

Simple loss of continuity due to laceration of the extensor mechanism in the hand and fingers usually is not associated with immediate tendon end retraction because of the multiple soft tissue attachments and interconnections (13). The extensor mechanism of the hand is extrasynovial, except at the wrist where the tendons are covered with a synovial sheath. Paratenon surrounds the extensor tendons over the dorsum of the hand; tendons covered with paratenon do not

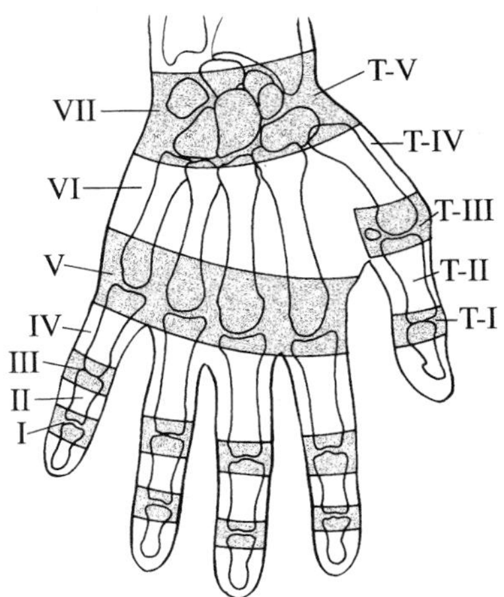

FIGURE 45-3. Zones of extensor tendon injury.

separate widely when lacerated (14). Whereas divided extensor tendons usually retract only on the dorsum of the wrist, the EPL often is devoid of junctura connections and is more likely to retract from the hand into the forearm when lacerated. Because most injured extensor tendon ends do not retract, tendon injuries, especially in the fingers, often may be treated successfully by splinting alone. Gap formation in the hand and fingers following laceration usually is due to unopposed flexion of the joints rather than to tendon retraction (14).

Evaluation of the injury and the patient begins in the emergency room, and wound assessment is completed frequently by exploration of the wound in the operating room. Radiographs are a mandatory part of the initial assessment, because they not only reveal obvious fractures but also may show foreign bodies and unexpected avulsion fractures (Fig. 45-4). Accurate evaluation prevents the overlooking of associated injuries that may, if left untreated, jeopardize good results. The surgical focus should be on avoiding complications that might interfere with the smooth gliding and integrated action of the tendons, including adhesions, attenuation and rupture, joint and soft tissue contractures, and secondary deformities due to alteration of the synergistic balance between flexors and extensors.

Complications may arise from various sources.

1. *Contaminated and crush injuries.* Open wounds may be tidy or untidy (ragged wounds with devitalized tissue, bacteria, and foreign bodies). A treatment delay of more than 6 to 8 hours effectively converts a relatively clean wound into a potentially infected one. Wood chips and sawdust are intensely irritating to tissues and can cause dense tendon adhesions. Heavily contaminated agricultural injuries, such as those caused by cornpickers, chain saws, and power lawn mowers, may cause multiple tearing wounds with extensive devitalization and contaminated particles forced deep into the tissues (15). The mainstay of treatment is adequate debridement and extensive wound irrigation. All foreign material and devitalized tissue must be meticulously removed, and release of the surgical tourniquet allows further assessment of nonviable and ischemic tissue. Wounds may be left partially open for drainage. In heavily contaminated wounds, a mix of aerobic and anaerobic gram-negative organisms may be resistant to many antibiotics.

Crushing injuries often involve the dorsum of the hand. Approximation of the ends of shredded extensor tendons may result in considerable regeneration and restoration of extensor function. A good case can be made for insertion of a silicone rod beneath a skin flap for future tendon graft or

A

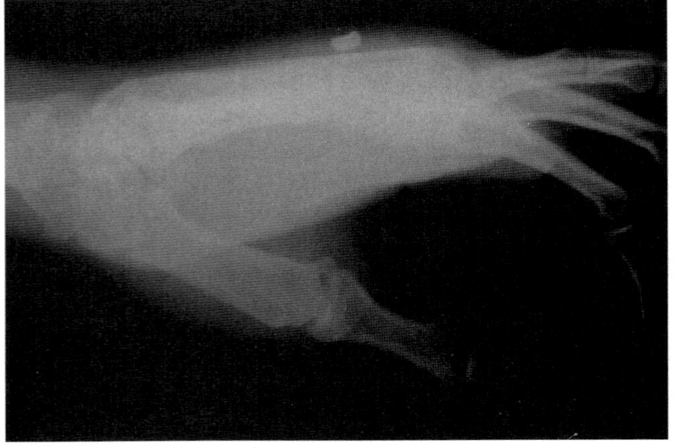

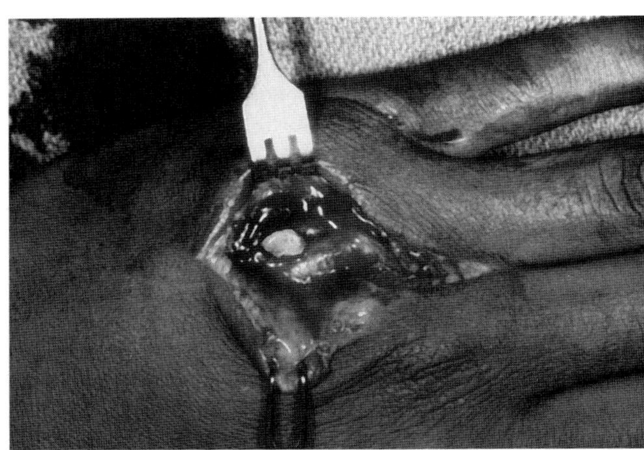

B

C

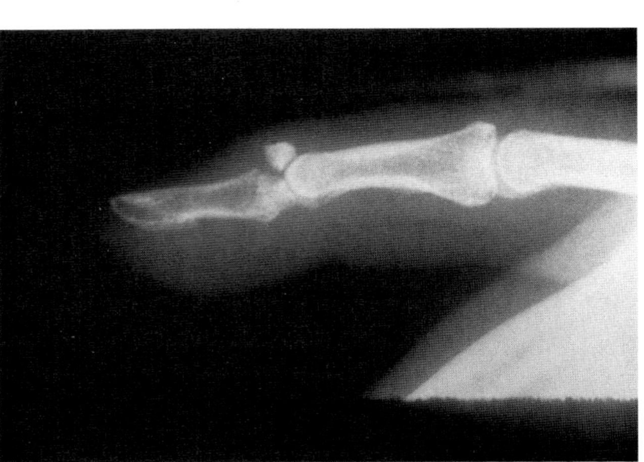

FIGURE 45-4. A: Radiograph of a patient with a seemingly innocuous small wound over the dorsum of the ring finger metacarpophalangeal joint revealed a radiopaque foreign object. **B:** On surgical exploration, the object was confirmed to be a tooth embedded within the joint after a so-called fight-bite injury. **C:** Radiograph of a finger after a closed "jamming" injury shows a dorsal avulsion distal phalangeal fracture.

transfer when the tendon has been avulsed. Crushing injuries are likely to be associated with metacarpal fractures, the reduction and fixation of which may interfere with extensor tendon gliding and sometimes require subsequent tenolysis.

2. *Human and animal bites.* Although dog and cat bites may produce a septic arthritis (Fig. 45-5), the contaminating organisms usually are not as virulent as those associated with human bites, *Eikenella corrodens,* and anaerobic gram-positive bacteria. *Pasturella multocida* is usually the infecting organism in dog and cat bites and responds to penicillin or a cephalosporin. The extensor surface of the MP joint is the most common site for a human bite injury; the tooth, or teeth, penetrates the extensor expansion and dorsal capsule at the joint and may strip off a small piece of articular cartilage. These wounds initially appear innocuous and may be neglected. A patient with such a wound rarely wishes to admit to having struck his flexed knuckles against someone's teeth. In its contaminated environment, the injured tendon retracts over the joint, and full-blown infection with septic arthritis may rapidly establish itself. The wound should be surgically enlarged and explored without delay and left open. The most suitable antibiotics are a combination of intravenous penicillin and a cephalosporin.

3. *Associated neurovascular injuries.* Lacerations on the dorsum of the forearm and wrist may divide the superficial radial nerve or ulnar sensory nerves. Microneural repair of the involved nerve prevents subsequent painful neuromas. In the more proximal forearm, the multiple branches of the posterior interosseous nerve may be divided among the extensor muscle bellies. This region marks the so-called filum terminale of the posterior interosseous nerve; repair of that nerve structure may be difficult and confusing in the mass of hematoma and lacerated muscle bellies (16).

4. *Problems with skin cover and scars.* Exposed tendons should always be covered with soft tissue to prevent desiccation and loss of viability. A wound sutured under tension to give tendon coverage is apt to break down, exposing the ten-

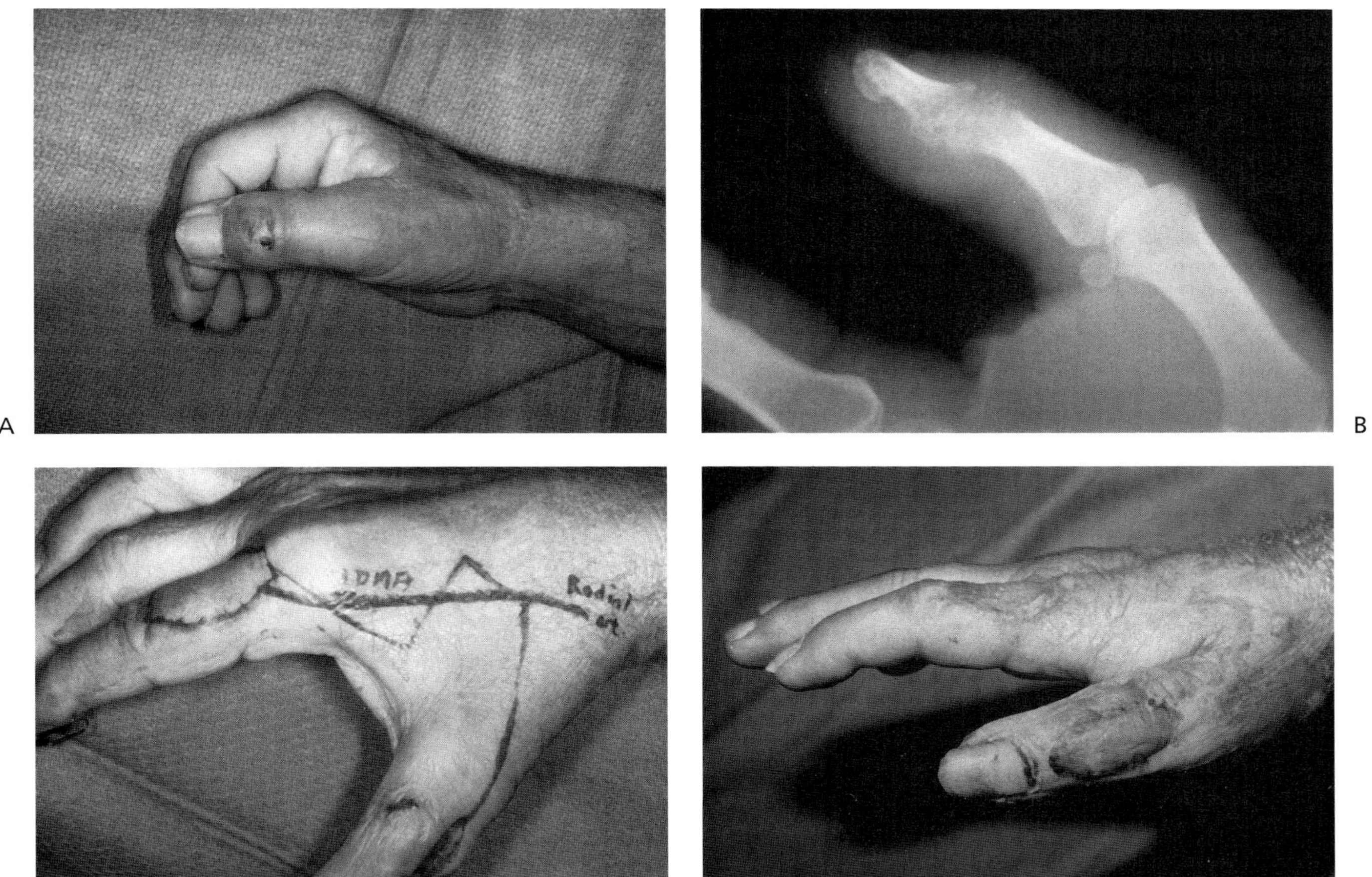

FIGURE 45-5. A: This patient had a single penetrating cat-tooth injury to the dorsum of the thumb interphalangeal joint and presented some days later with pain and swelling. **B:** Radiograph shows osteomyelitis and an associated septic arthritis of that joint. **C,D:** After debridement of soft tissue, extensor tendon, bone, and an appropriate duration of antibiotics and wound care, bone grafting interphalangeal joint arthrodesis was completed with soft tissue coverage provided by means of a first dorsal metacarpal artery flap.

don and resulting in contracture. Tension across a wound also impedes capillary refill and may contribute to postoperative edema and limit or preclude early motion.

Degloving and crushing injuries are common in the dorsum of the hand. Small skin defects may be covered with local rotational or transposition flaps. A cross-finger (16) or homodigital flap may be used to cover exposed finger joints and tendons (Fig. 45-6). A larger defect may require a more distant flap that may be raised as a tubed pedicle groin flap (17). Neurovascular free flaps are the procedure of choice of the experienced and confident surgeon.

5. *Hematoma.* Breakdown products of red blood cells cause irritation and stimulate formation of dense adhesions. Hematoma in subcutaneous tissue, in addition to being an excellent bacteria culture medium, causes necrosis of overlying skin flaps, a response thought to be chemical rather than totally mechanical in nature (18). Once surgical wound debridement is complete, the tourniquet is deflated. At least

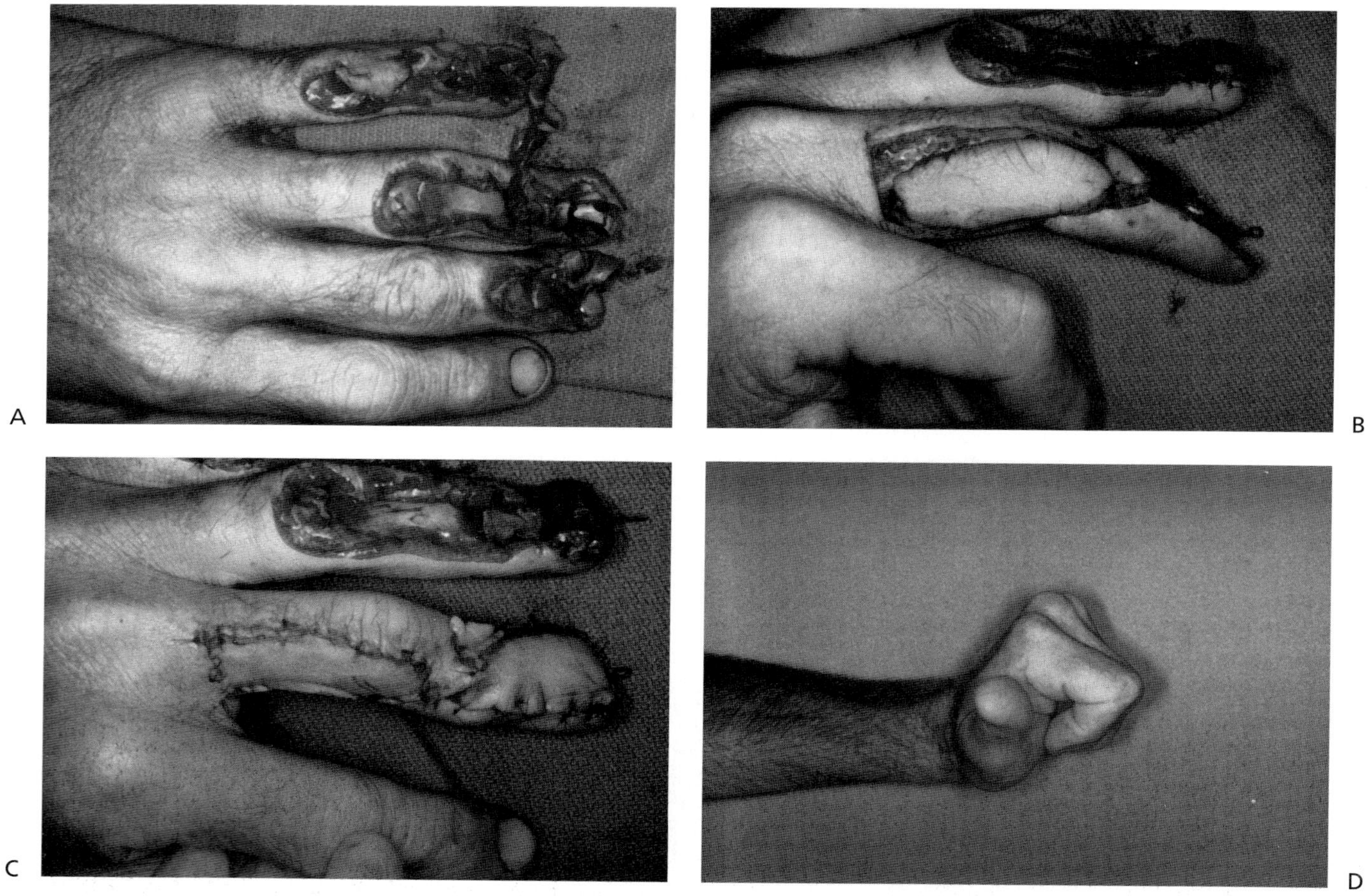

A

B

C

D

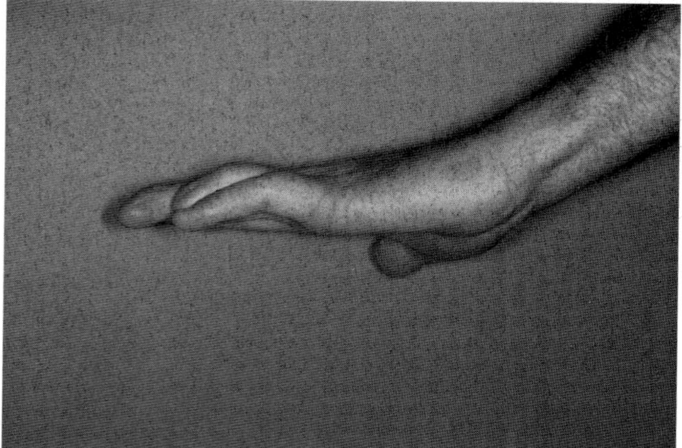

E

FIGURE 45-6. A: Planing injury of dorsum of the fingers resulted in denuding of soft tissue down to bone devoid of periosteum and exposure of joints. **B,C:** After debridement, immediate reconstruction with tendon grafts was made possible because adequate soft tissue coverage could be obtained by homodigital distally based turnover flap. **D,E:** Subsequent tenolysis was required. This second procedure was made feasible by having good-quality dorsal soft tissue coverage. The patient had a good functional result noted 8 months after the initial injury.

10 minutes should be allowed to elapse for reactive hyperemia to subside, and then meticulous hemostasis should be accomplished.

6. *Complications resulting from failure to recognize a tendon injury.* Extensor tendon injuries often are missed for the following reasons:

A. They may be associated with closed injuries, and pain and swelling may mask injury to the extensor mechanism (closed mallet and boutonnière deformities).

B. Interconnecting juncturae tendinum may maintain MP joint extension if the tendon is divided proximal to the juncturae. Some extensor lag usually is present in this case.

C. Both the index and middle fingers have dual extensor tendons; only one of these may be ruptured on either finger. The EDM often is a double tendon.

D. Complete laceration of the extensor tendon at the MP joint may not be detected because hood expansion provides some extension.

E. The intrinsic thenar muscles have an extending action at the thumb IP joint and may mask division of the EPL.

It is important to recognize and treat these injuries with appropriate repair and splinting, because extensor lag and deformity will occur with the passage of time.

7. *Complications arising from surgical technique of tendon repair.* Prerequisites for tendon repair are aseptic conditions with good lighting, good instruments, adequate anesthesia, appropriate magnification, and delicate handling of tendon ends. Failure to produce a smooth repair may result in adhesion formation, tendon locking, or tendon rupture. The flat extensor tendons should be repaired with a figure-of-8 stitch or with a central core suture that avoids the concertina effect that a lateral core suture has on a flat tendon.

Even a perfectly repaired, cleanly cut tendon will be weak for a lengthy period of time as the collagen matures. If a repaired tendon is not protected, stretching and scar attenuation may occur. A clinical sign of stretching of the repair is the patient's inability to fully extend the fingers, with an extension lag. Postrepair tendon stretching also encourages adhesion formation as collagen fills the gap caused by the stretching. Frank rupture may occur; when it occurs early, it usually is due to the suture giving way. This complication almost always can be avoided by having good surgical technique and postoperative management.

The ideal suture material has not been found. Monofilament nylon and proline sutures stretch and fray and are notorious for unraveling of the knot, a major cause of tendon separation (19). Both are too bulky for suitable repair of extensor tendon injuries. A coated 4-0 or 5-0 gauge polyester, requiring at least five square throws for a secure knot, is probably the best suture material for extensor tendon repair.

Total active range of motion and grip strength are accepted indicators of hand function after flexor tendon injuries. Extensor tendon injuries, however, both reduce range of flexion because of the extensor tenodesis effect and cause extension lag. Based on these factors, a total active range of motion rating system for extensor tendon injuries is as follows (20):

Excellent	Full flexion and extension
Good	10 degrees or less of extension lost, 20 degrees or less of flexion lost
Fair	11 to 45 degrees of extension lost, 21 to 45 degrees of flexion lost
Poor	45 degrees or more of both extension and flexion lost

Using this grading system, a retrospective study of 101 digits revealed that 60% of all fingers with extensor tendon injury had an associated injury, such as fracture, dislocation, or joint capsule or flexor tendon injury, which resulted in good-to-excellent results in 35% of cases, in contrast to 64% with good-to-excellent results in patients without associated injuries (20). The same study found that distal zone injuries (I through IV) healed less favorably than proximal zone injuries (V through VIII).

GENERAL PRINCIPLES OF POSTOPERATIVE MANAGEMENT AND SPLINTING

Postoperative management of extensor tendon injuries has evolved over the past 20 years, from immobilization for 4 to 6 weeks to controlled passive motion and now to protected active motion. The more traditional forms of immobilization may be useful in children and uncooperative patients. Early mobilization (before 10 days) reduces the postoperative adhesions (21) common in extensor tendon injuries, particularly in crush-type injuries. An active mobilization program allows the patient to achieve the necessary amount of tendon excursion. Dynamic splinting is useful in promoting a healed gliding surface in flexor tendon injuries and now has been advocated in early motion for finger extensor tendon injuries in zones V, VI, and VII, and in thumb extensor injuries involving zones T-4 and T-5. Depending on which finger is involved in the injury, 27.3 to 40.9 degrees of MP joint flexion produces 5 mm of EDC sliding. The EPL of the thumb will slide 5 mm with 60 degrees of IP joint flexion. A 5-mm slide causes no repair site disruption and limits adhesion formation (22,23).

Typically 3 to 5 days postoperatively, the hand is positioned in a splint with the wrist at 45 degrees of extension and the MP and IP joints supported at 0 degrees in an elastic extension outrigger device. Positioning of a palmar blocking splint limits MP flexion to that which results in 5-mm extensor tendon excursion (Fig. 45-7). The patient actively flexes the MP joints, allowing dynamic traction on the outrigger device to passively return the digital joints to 0 degrees.

In zone T-4 and T-5 thumb injuries, the EPL is splinted with the wrist extended and CMC joint in neutral position.

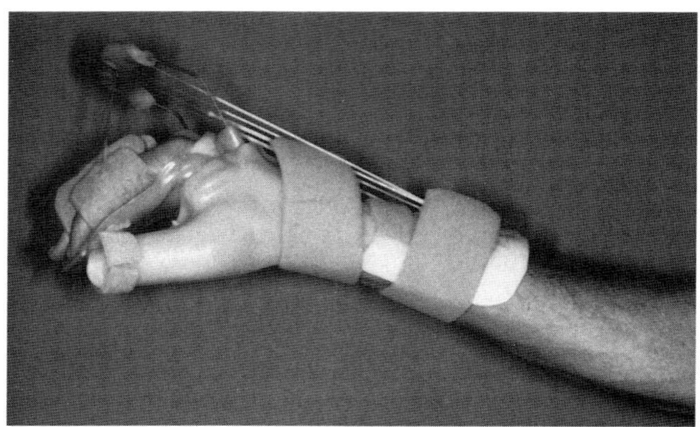

FIGURE 45-7. Extension outrigger splint initially may be fabricated with a palmar blocking platform. This palmar block subsequently is removed to allow unrestricted finger flexion. (Courtesy of Dorit H. Aaron, MA, OTR, CHT, FAOTA, and staff of the Houston Hand Fellowship Program, Houston, TX.)

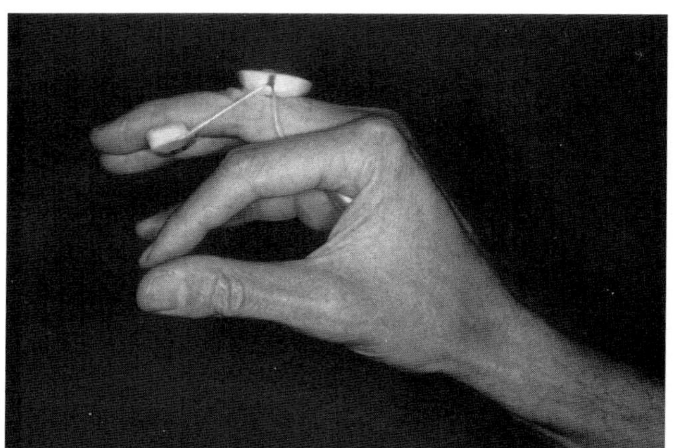

A

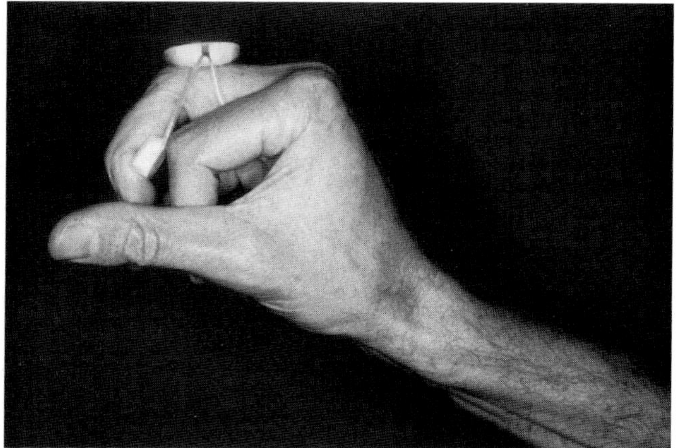

B

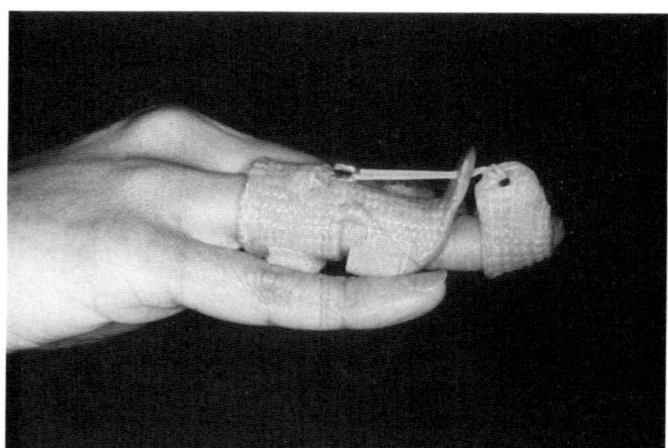

C

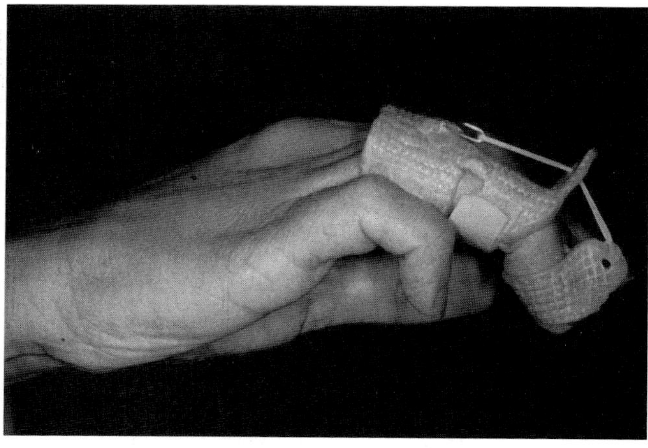

D

Central tendon adhesions

Attenuation

E

FIGURE 45-8. A–D: Examples of dynamic splints that can be used when extensor tendon injuries have occurred over the dorsum of the finger. (Courtesy of Dorit H. Aaron, MA, OTR, CHT, FAOTA, and staff of the Houston Hand Fellowship Program, Houston, TX). **E:** If extensor tendon adhesions are allowed to develop through immobilization, then late mobilization will cause attenuation of a repaired central slip.

Dynamic traction is maintained with the MP joint at 0 degrees but allowing 60 degrees of active flexion. After 4 weeks, active motion is started with the wrist supported in extension. After 7 weeks, resistance and functional electrical stimulation are considered safe modalities.

Efficacy of dynamic splinting of extensor tendon injuries in zones II through IV is less well documented (Fig. 45-8). Some advocate early active short arc motion for repaired extensor tendon injuries in zones III and IV (21). A study of long-term results of extensor tendon repair reported that intradigital extensor tendon injuries that are treated only with immobilization had high percentages of fair and poor results compared with those of more proximal, similarly treated injuries and that injuries in zones III and IV had higher percentages of resultant extensor lag (35%) and loss of flexion (71%) than similar injuries in other extensor tendon zones (24).

Any possibility of adhesion formation or shortening of the extensor tendon on the dorsum of the digit must be minimized if a reasonable result is to be obtained. Postinjury tendon-to-bone adherence in zone IV and nongliding because of periosteum–tendon proximity may, with a late mobilization program, cause gaping or attenuation of the repaired central slip because the more proximal segment is bound by adhesions. Increased resistance in zone IV will increase internal tendon tension in zone III, which may exceed the tensile strength of the repair. Poor results following immobilization programs have resulted in a search for alternative mobilization regimens.

The mean moment arm for an extensor tendon of the PIP joint of the middle finger is calculated to be 7.5mm (25). Central slip excursion when the PIP joint is moved through angular rotation of 57.29 degrees equals the moment arm of the tendon (7.5 mm). To obtain the physiologic excursion necessary for an early motion program (3 to 5 mm recommended excursion) (26,27), the joint must be moved through 28.65 degrees. Force analysis shows that the resistance applied to the central slip with an upward motion of 30 degrees of flexion to 0 degrees of extension against gravity is 291 gm (28,29). A mattress suture gapes 2 mm at the 488 g mark and fails at 840 g; a figure-of-8 suture gapes at 587 g and fails at 690 g.

The short arc motion (30,28) protocol for zones III and IV consists of a Thermaplast finger splint that maintains the IP joints at 0 degrees and allows unrestricted motion at the MP joints and wrist. A second Thermaplast splint to the injured finger is used hourly, allowing 30 degrees of active flexion at the PIP joint and 20 to 25 degrees of flexion at the DIP joint, returning to 0 degrees of extension. The wrist is positioned at 30 degrees of flexion and the MP joint at 0 degrees during this active short arc motion. Thus, the PIP joint is actively flexed and extended in a controlled range (30). An alternative protocol is the splinting of the PIP joint in extension at night, with the application of a Capner splint during the day. The dynamic extension splint allows active PIP joint flexion but protects the central slip from stretching by synergistic muscle action and relaxation (31).

TREATMENT OF EXTENSOR TENDON INJURIES AT SPECIFIC ZONES

Zone I (Over the Distal Interphalangeal Joint)

Loss of continuity of the conjoined lateral bands at the distal joint of the finger results in a mallet deformity. Active extension is lost, although full passive extension usually is present. The PIP joint may be hyperextended due to unopposed central slip tension and palmar plate laxity. Open injuries in this zone may be due to either sharp or crushing lacerations, but closed injuries are more common. The usual mechanism of injury is a sudden, acute, forceful flexion of the extended digit that results in rupture of the extensor tendon or avulsion of the tendon with or without a small fragment of bone from the distal insertion. Forced hyperextension of the distal joint may result in a fracture at the dorsal base of the distal phalanx. The relative avascularity of the extensor tendon at the DIP joint probably explains its tendency to rupture in this area and explains, as well, the poor results after primary repair (32). Mallet deformities are classified as follows (33):

Type I	Closed or blunt trauma with loss of tendon continuity with or without a small avulsion fracture
Type II	Laceration at or just proximal to the DIP joint with loss of tendon continuity
Type III	Deep abrasion with loss of skin, subcutaneous tissue, and tendon substance
Type IV	(a) Transepiphyseal plate fracture in children; (b) hyperflexion injury with fracture of 20% to 50% of the articular surface; (c) hyperextension injury with fracture of the articular surface (usually greater than 50%) and volar subluxation of the distal phalanx.

Closed tendon ruptures respond to prolonged splinting of the DIP joint in extension (14). Prolonged splinting is required for all mallet deformities, and ulceration of skin over the dorsum of the DIP joint is a potential complication. The dorsal skin of a hyperextended IP joint normally will blanch. After acute injury, this area is compromised further by edema and by direct application of a dorsal splint (Fig. 45-9). Dorsal ulceration may be prevented by the use of a volar splint initially with the DIP joint in neutral position, followed by the application of a dorsal hyperextension splint when the edema has subsided. If full-thickness necrosis of skin results from ill-advised splinting, immediate treatment includes wound care and dressings if the area is small and superficial or a split-thickness skin graft if the defect is large. Exposure of the joint or underlying tendon urgently re-

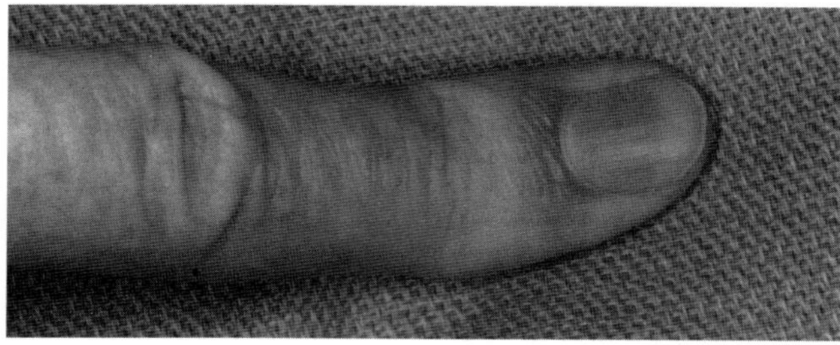
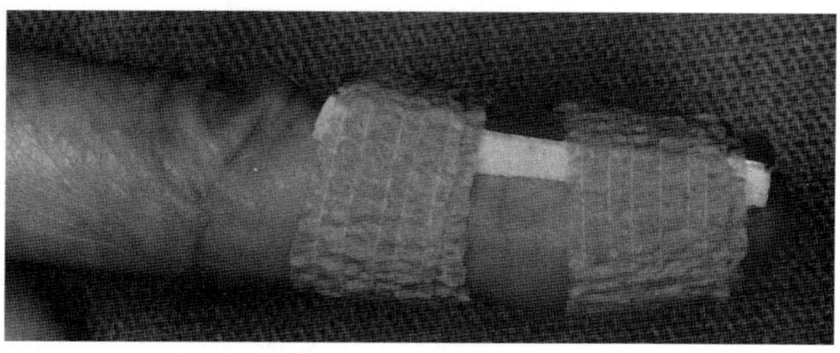

FIGURE 45-9. A: Hyperextension at the distal interphalangeal joint results in dorsal skin blanching. **B:** Dorsal padded aluminum splint for treatment of closed mallet injury.

quires flap coverage, i.e., a reversed cross-finger subcutaneous flap (16).

Excellent-to-good results can be anticipated in approximately 80% of closed zone I injuries when early treatment is provided. The extended position of the DIP joint must be maintained continuously for at least 6 weeks for the splint to be effective. This is followed by 2 weeks of night splinting and a progressive weaning away from the splinting program. Operative repair not only is unnecessary for closed injury but probably is contraindicated.

Open type II wounds may be treated by suture repair of the friable tendon ends or by DIP joint immobilization with a finger splint and additional transarticular Kirschner pin support. The pin is removed after 4 weeks, but splinting continues. Gentle active motion begins at 6 weeks.

Soft tissue reconstruction with a local flap is the treatment of choice for type III wounds in which tendon and soft tissue loss has occurred. Type III injuries may be caused by a grinding tool or due to an avulsive scrape against a roughened surface. Either immediate or later tendon reconstruction, with a minitendon graft, may be necessary (Fig. 45-10).

Operative treatment has, in the past, been recommended for type IV mallet finger injuries with fracture fragments involving more than one-third of the articular surface, particularly when volar subluxation is present at the distal phalanx. Various surgical approaches, including fixation of the DIP joint in extension with a 0.028-inch diameter Kirschner wire and the placement of a pullout stainless steel wire over a button, have been advocated for reduction of the intra-articular fragment. At least one study, however, has reflected the belief that restoration of joint congruity does not influence the end result, because the articular surface usually remodels to produce a near-normal, painless joint (34). We have abandoned open reduction and internal fixation, even with volar subluxation of the distal phalanx, and recommend external splinting alone.

Mallet finger deformity can recur unless DIP joint splinting and hyperextension are maintained for at least 6 weeks because the pull of the profundus tendon always stretches extensor tendon repair at this level. Even after 6 weeks, the splint should be worn during heavy work. At the first sign of extension lag, continuous splinting is resumed. Although splinting for more than 4 weeks after recurrence is unlikely to help any further, nonoperative splinting, even in delayed presentation of mallet finger, sometimes is successful and should always attempted. Failure of nonoperative splinting for a significant residual deformity is an indication for surgery. Surgical procedures for chronic mallet deformity are as follows:

A. The terminal tendon is mobilized and advanced for insertion into the distal phalanx with nonabsorbable suture placed through a drill hole in the dorsum of the terminal phalanx.

B. When the tendon is intact with an elongated scar, a tuck can be taken and the tendon overlapped and secured with nonabsorbable suture.

C. A minitendon graft from an accessible tendon (i.e., the palmaris longus) can bridge the defect between the end of the tendon when the tendon ends are too friable to hold sutures by securing it to bone by a drill hole and weaving into the proximal tendon (35).

In all cases of repaired chronic mallet deformity, a longitudinal Kirschner wire holds the joint in extension for 6 weeks. Once the pin is removed, the splint is worn part time and at night. It is worn continuously if there is any tendency to further deformity. Late cases of mallet deformity with painful arthritis are best treated by arthrodesis at approximately 15 degrees of flexion.

Swan-neck deformity, usually seen as a late result of chronic mallet deformity, is a classic manifestation of the dynamic imbalance between the extrinsic and intrinsic extensor mechanisms. Coexistent volar plate laxity allows PIP joint hyperextension. Relative lengthening of the distal extensor mechanism occurring secondary to disruption at the DIP joint allows dorsal migration of the lateral bands at the PIP joint and further accentuates this deformity. The powerful FDP becomes an unopposed deforming force at the DIP joint. Reconstructive techniques involve correction of the flexed posture at the DIP joint and of the hyperextended posture at the PIP joint by a tendon graft that mimics the

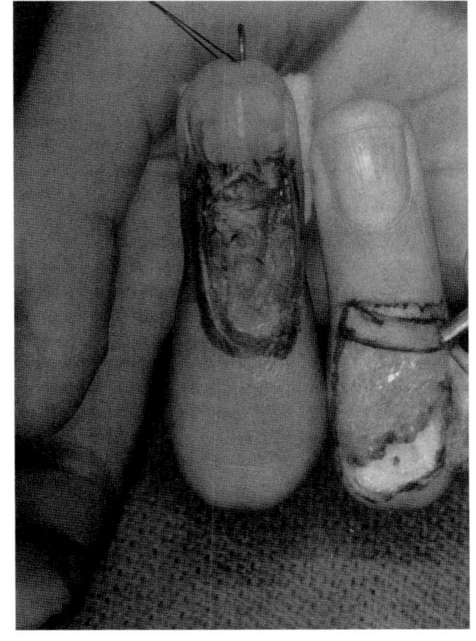

A

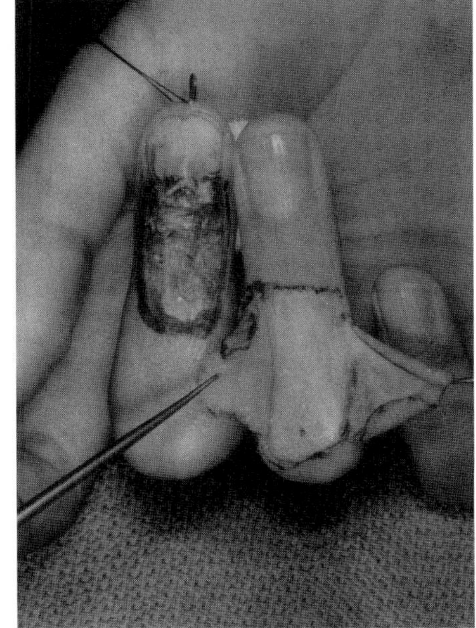

B

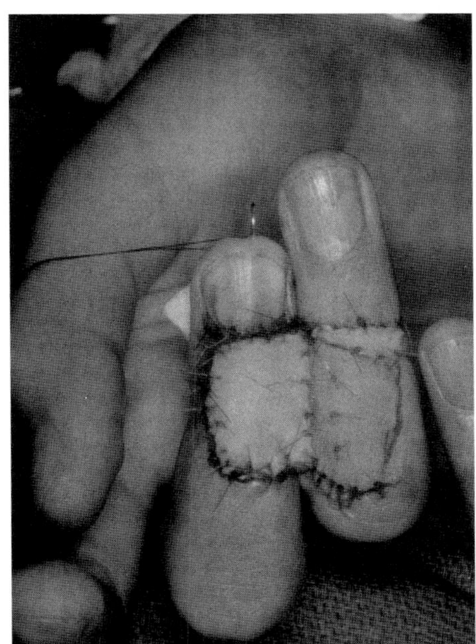

C

FIGURE 45-10. A–C: A child scraped the dorsum of the distal interphalangeal joint on concrete while roller blading. After placement of a mini-tendon graft, soft tissue reconstruction of dorsal skin and eponychial fold is done with a reverse cross-finger flap. A portion of donor skin is retained on the subcutaneous flap to provide deep surface lining to the eponychium, and a full-thickness skin graft is placed over the flap at the recipient area.

dynamic function of the oblique retinacular ligament (spiral oblique retinacular ligament reconstruction) (Fig. 45-11) (36). Tension on the graft is adjusted so that the PIP joint rests in 20 degrees of flexion and the distal joint is at full extension. A protective transarticular Kirschner pin across the PIP joint is removed at 4 weeks. The digit then is supported with a dorsal splint. Active PIP joint flexion is instituted, although the 20 degrees of extension block is maintained and gradually straightened over the next 6 to 10 weeks. A minimal flexion contracture probably will persist at the PIP joint.

Zone II (Over the Middle Phalanx)

Partial lacerations of less than 50% of the tendon can be treated by skin wound closure and active motion in 7 to 10 days. Complete lacerations require suturing followed by a short period of static splinting of the fully extended IP joint.

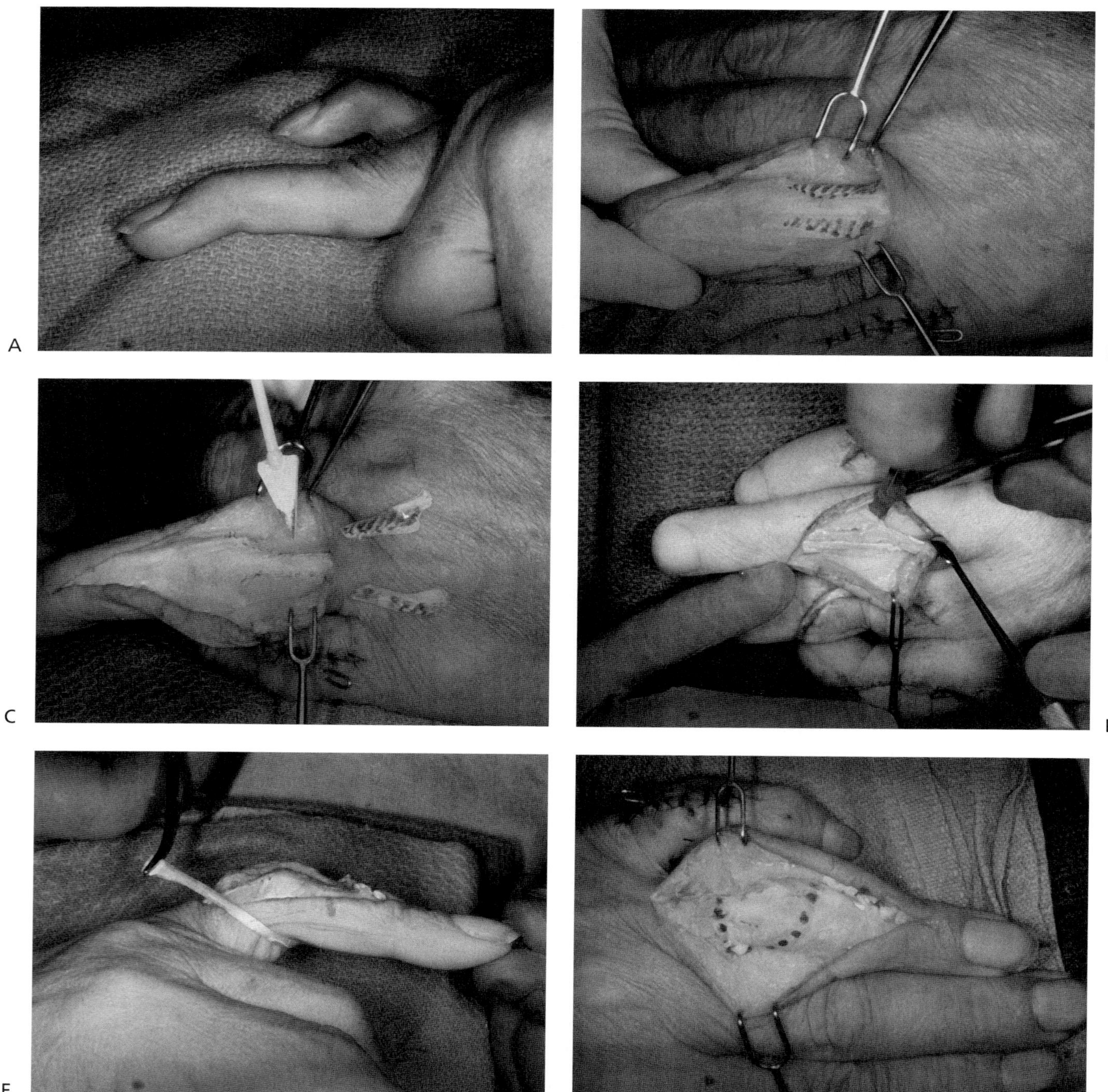

FIGURE 45-11. A: Swan-neck deformity with intrinsic tightness. **B:** Portion of extensor mechanism containing lateral bands is marked out to be excised. **C:** Excised "wing tendons" of distal intrinsic release to include the lateral bands and oblique fibers of the extensor mechanism. **D:** Dorsal proximal interphalangeal joint capsulotomy is done deep to the extensor mechanism to restore passive flexion. **E,F:** A free tendon graft for spiral oblique retinacular ligament (SORL) reconstruction is sutured distally into the dorsal extensor mechanism and passes volar to the flexor tendon sheath and then emerges through a transverse drill hole in the shaft of the proximal phalanx.

Short arc range of motion, as already described, then is instituted.

Zone III (Over the Apex of the Proximal Interphalangeal Joint)

Acute traumatic boutonnière deformity is caused by division of the extensor mechanism central slip at PIP joint level (37). The lateral bands migrate volarly, stretch the triangular ligament (38), and begin to act as joint flexors with volar migration to the axis of rotation of the PIP joint (3). DIP joint hyperextension follows secondary to shortening of the oblique retinacular fibers and lateral bands. MP joint hyperextension eventually occurs because of the increased but distorting pull of the finger extensors.

Boutonnière deformity resulting from open wounds over the dorsum of the IP joint can be prevented by repair of the central slip of the extensor mechanism and corrective postoperative splinting (Fig. 45-12). The severity of closed PIP joint injuries often is not appreciated at the time of injury. If the joint is heavily bruised and a boutonnière deformity is suspected, the finger should be splinted for a few weeks until the surgeon can be certain that no deformity is present. The rare volar dislocation of the base of the middle phalanx is an injury usually associated with central slip disruption and should be immediately reduced and splinted.

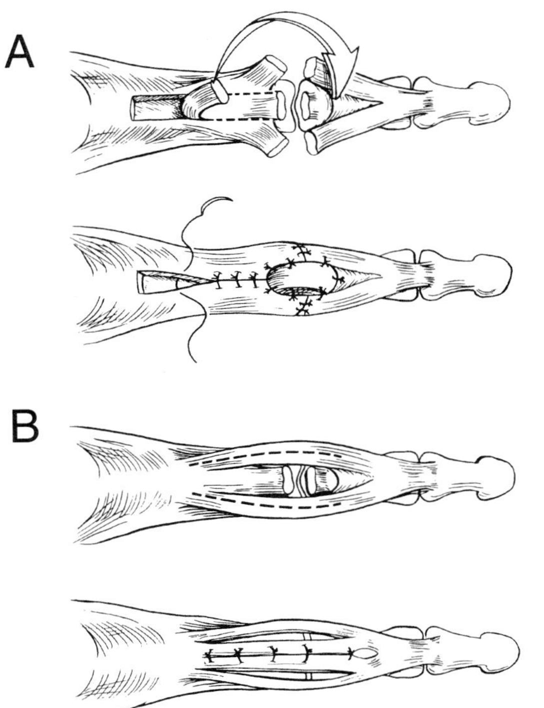

FIGURE 45-12. In an acute open boutonnière deformity, the central slip may be deficient and alternative methods for reconstruction exist.

Occasionally, a small avulsion fracture at the central slip may be seen with these volar dislocations. If the fragment is large, open reduction and fixation are necessary. Closed boutonnière deformities of recent origin usually respond well to splinting of the PIP joint in extension and encouraging DIP joint flexion (Fig. 45-13) (39). A dynamic PIP flexion splint is worn during the day and a static splint at night. The dynamic splint allows active PIP joint flexion but protects the central slip from stretching by synergistic muscle action and relaxation.

Surgical correction of chronic boutonnière deformity is exacting, and full extension of the PIP joint is difficult to achieve although it may be much improved. Curtis et al. (40) described a stepwise approach to the correction of a mobile boutonnière deformity that involves an initial release of the transverse retinacular fibers so that the lateral bands can once again migrate dorsally (Fig. 45-14). Extensor tenolysis follows, and subsequent incremental reconstruction reinforces the central slip mechanism with or without a distal Fowler release. The Fowler release involves a tenotomy of the lateral bands distal to the triangular ligament that allows proximal migration of the extensor apparatus with correction of DIP joint hyperextension and improvement of PIP joint flexion (41). Several operations to reinforce the central slip mechanism over the dorsum of the PIP joint have been described, ranging from use of one or both of the lateral bands for central slip reconstruction, to plication of the attenuated central slip, to use of small tendon or fascial grafts (Fig. 45-14).

Delay in treatment of a mobile boutonnière deformity often results in a fixed flexion PIP deformity. Passive serial splinting or use of a joint jack to overcome some of the contracture is necessary initially (Fig. 45-14). The transverse retinacular ligaments become secondarily contracted and must be divided during correction of the deformity. The oblique retinacular ligaments also tighten secondarily and contribute to DIP hyperextension, so they also require division. The presence of secondary joint changes may necessitate PIP joint arthrodesis.

Zone IV (Over the Proximal Phalanx of Finger and Thumb)

Injuries at zone IV are similar to zone II injuries in that lacerations in this location may be only partial because of tendon width and the underlying curvature of the osseous phalanx. Complete lacerations of the central tendon must be repaired to prevent relative tendon lengthening and a resulting imbalance between central slip and lateral bands. The PIP joint must be maintained in full extension following repair. An isolated laceration to the lateral band must be repaired and protected motion begun immediately. Lacerations to the thumb must distinguish between EPB and EPL tendon injuries; each tendon should be repaired when transected.

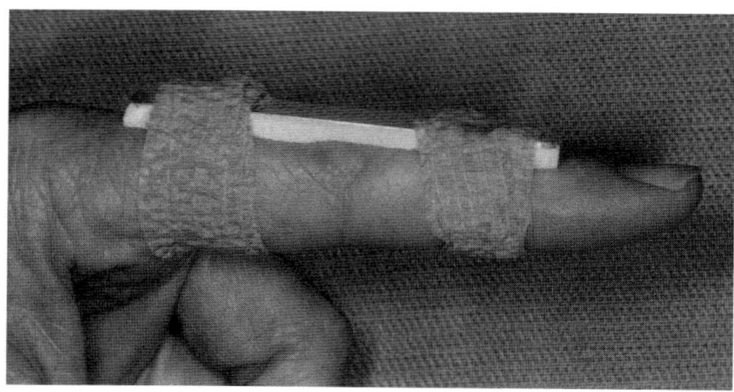

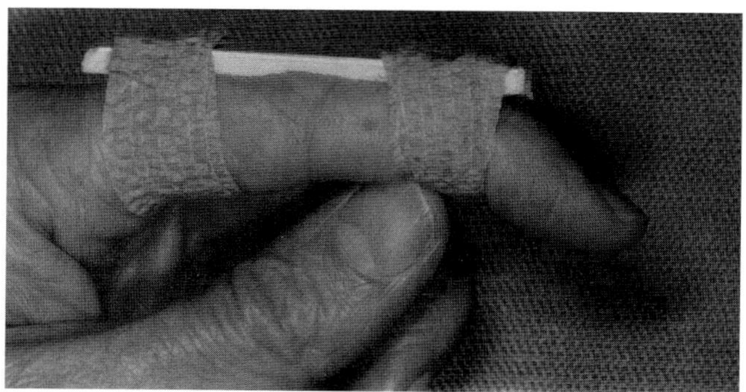

A B

FIGURE 45-13. A,B: Extension splinting of the proximal interphalangeal joint for closed boutonnière deformity enables flexion at the distal interphalangeal joint.

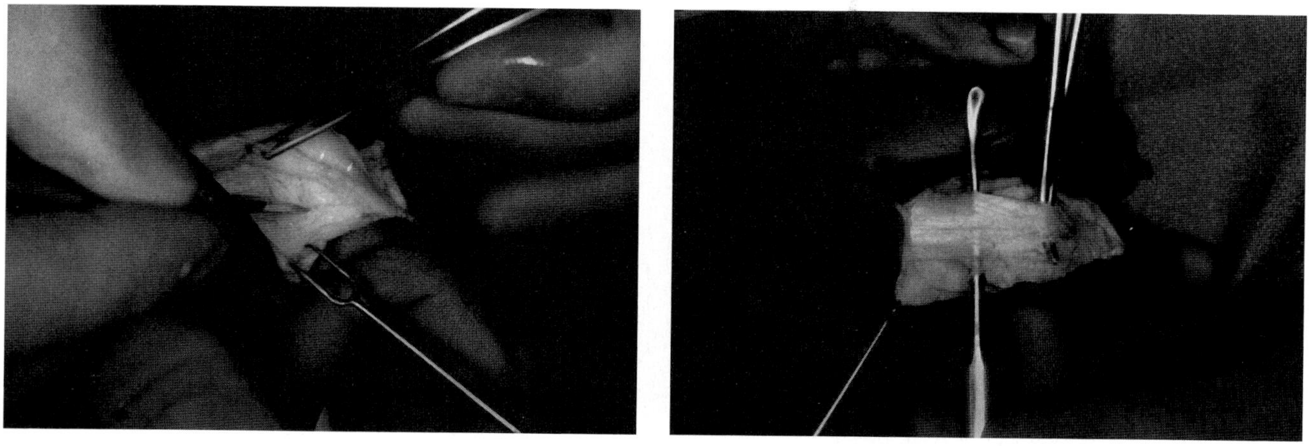

A B

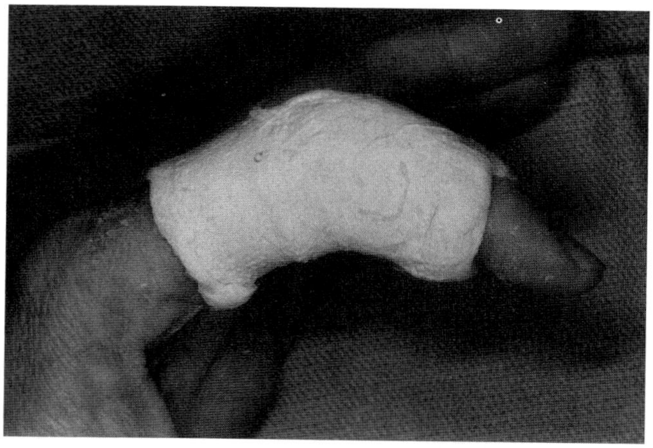

C 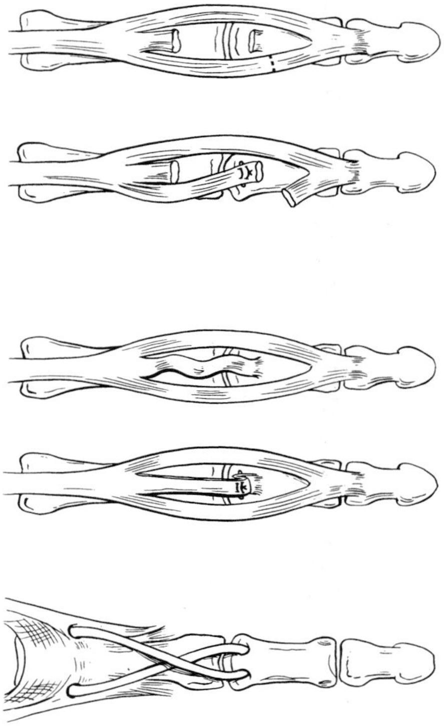 D

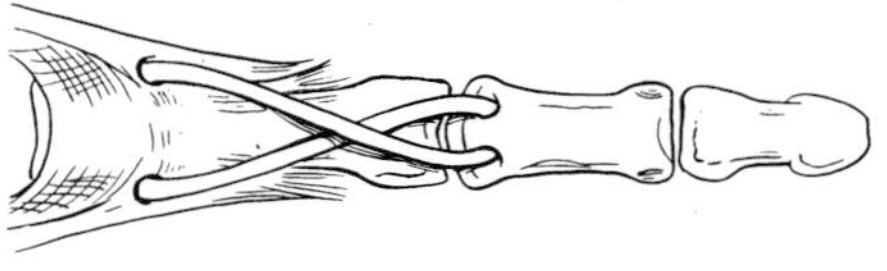

FIGURE 45-14. A: When surgically treating a chronic boutonnière deformity, sharp division of the transverse retinacular fibers enables the lateral bands *(arrow)* to be repositioned dorsally. **B:** Extensor tenolysis will permit improved tendon gliding, which is a prerequisite before reconstructing the central tendon. **C:** Proximal interphalangeal joint flexion contractures may require preliminary serial splinting to overcome that deformity before embarking on surgical repair. **D:** Numerous alternative methods for reconstruction of the central slip include using local tissues from the lateral band or plicating redundant tissue, but occasionally a free tendon graft is required that secures into bone distally and into the extension expansion proximally.

Zone V (Over the Metacarpophalangeal Joints)

A penetrating injury over the MP joint extensor surface should carry a high index of suspicion for originating from a human bite. Radiographs should be taken and appropriate wound exploration and irrigation performed. Administration of parenteral antibiotics is necessary. The hand should be splinted with the wrist in approximately 45 degrees of extension and the MP joint flexed at approximately 20 degrees, allowing the soft tissues, including the capsule and the extensor hood, to find their own positions over the joint. Even complete lacerations at this level are seldom associated with significant tendon retraction. Formal tendon repair, undesirable in a contaminated wound, may not be required with judicious splinting. Skin closure can be carried out in a delayed primary manner.

Lacerations involving the sagittal bands at this level must be repaired so that the extensor tendon will remain centralized over the dorsum of the joint. Failure to repair this type of injury may result in subluxation of the extensor tendon and associated loss of extension.

Traumatic dislocation of the extensor tendon may occur at the MP joint following laceration of the sagittal bands of the extensor hood or following a closed injury involving either forceful flexion or extension of the finger. The middle finger is most commonly involved in forceful extension injuries without laceration; the lesion occurs secondary to a tear of the sagittal band and oblique fibers of the extensor hood and usually occurs on the radial side. Ulnar dislocation of the extensor tendon then occurs and is associated with incomplete finger extension and ulnar deviation of the involved digit. Fresh injuries are repaired with figure-of-8 nonabsorbable sutures. An injury more than a few weeks old may require alternative methods of repair, such as passage of a retrograde slip of the central extensor tendon around the lumbrical, reinforcing the side on which the tear occurred, or reinforcement with a proximally detached junctura (Fig. 45-15) (42).

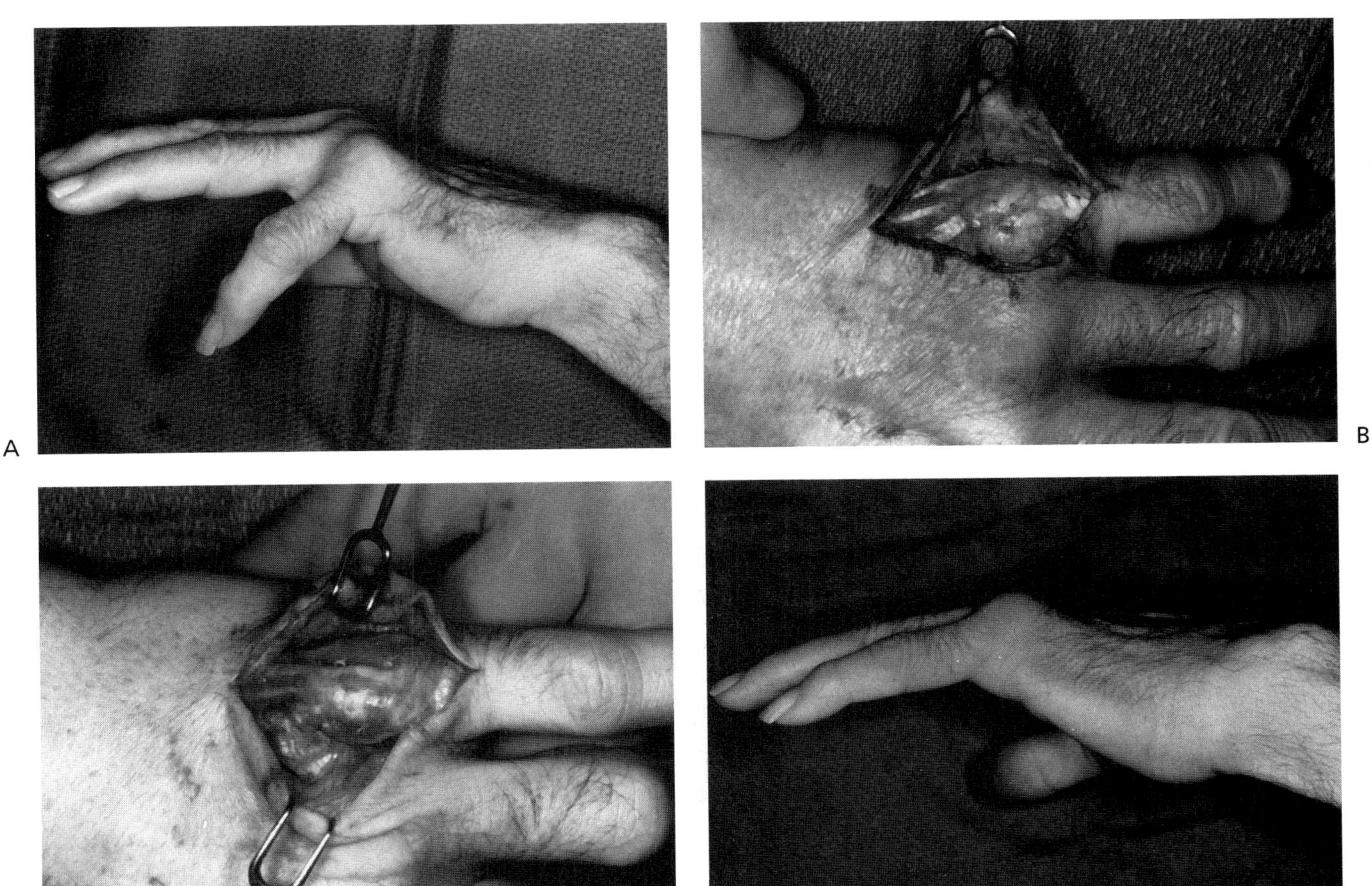

FIGURE 45-15. A: Patient with inability to extend his little finger due to sagittal band rupture. **B:** The radial sagittal band is found to be attenuated and the extensor tendons are subluxed in an ulnar direction. (*continued*)

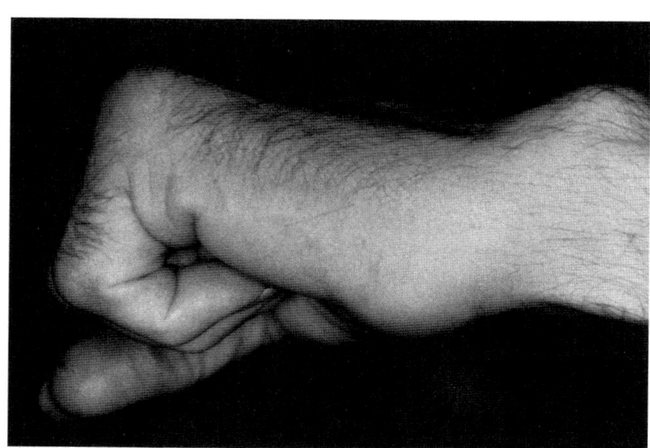

E

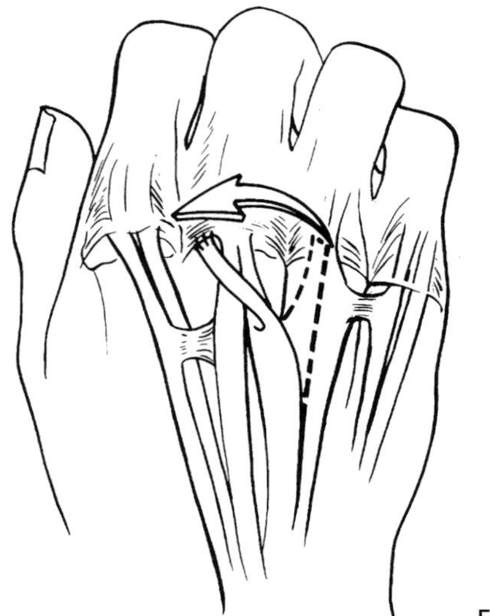

F

FIGURE 45-15. (Continued) **C:** Correction is achieved by centralizing the extensor tendons using horizontal mattress reefing sutures that, after postoperative therapy, restored excelling finger function **(D–F)**. When insufficient sagittal band tissue remains for repair, then a junctura may be used for the reconstruction.

Zones VI and VII (Over the Metacarpals and Wrist)

Extensor tendons at the levels of the metacarpal and wrist are substantial enough to accept a variety of core sutures. Dynamic splinting postoperatively generally ensures excellent results for these injuries. In zone VI, the tendon may retract proximal to the extensor retinaculum, an event particularly likely to occur with a laceration of the EPL. If the extensor tendon has retracted proximally, the proximal stump should be retrieved and threaded back through its appropriate fibro-osseous canal to the distal stump. With extensor injuries at wrist level, the traumatic opening in the retinaculum may be extended to facilitate tendon repair. Portions of the retinaculum either proximal or distal to the suture line should be preserved to prevent bowstringing.

Traumatic disruption of the compartment containing the ECU results in ulnar subluxation of this tendon during pronation. A new compartment can be fashioned from a portion of extensor retinaculum (43).

Zone VIII (Distal Forearm)

Injuries at the muscle–tendon junction in the distal forearm may be difficult to manage. Although the distal tendon will accept and hold sutures well, the proximal muscle belly does not. A search, however, within the lacerated muscle belly will locate the intramuscular origin of the tendon, which is more likely to hold a 4-0 core suture. Repair of the surrounding perimysium with a running suture reduces the risk of mass adhesions. If the tendon is not repaired within 4 weeks of injury, muscle contracture occurs and retraction becomes permanent. Secondary repair may require a mini-tendon graft or tendon transfer.

Zone IX (Mid and Proximal Forearm)

A demonstrated loss of function in the proximal forearm on clinical examination may be due to muscle or nerve injury, or both. Preoperative diagnosis may not be possible because the muscle may be hemorrhagic and the muscle planes difficult to identify immediately after injury. Identification is aided by evacuation of the hematoma, irrigation, and gentle sponging of cut muscle ends. If a nerve injury is identified, the appropriate nerve branches must be traced out to their insertions. Penetrating wounds often injure the nerve near its entrance to the muscle belly, and repair may be complicated by retraction of the distal nerve stump into the muscle belly. If the injury involves muscle only, the muscle belly is repaired with multiple figure-of-8 polyglactin sutures. In extensive muscle defects involving two or more muscles, free tendon grafts restore muscle continuity (44). With repair of injuries to muscles arising at or above the lateral epicondyle, the wrist must be supported in 45 degrees of extension and the elbow immobilized at 90 degrees of flexion.

LATE COMPLICATIONS OF EXTENSOR TENDON INJURIES

Joint Contractures

Extension contractures and dorsocapsular adhesions at the MP joints may occur secondary to prolonged extension splinting of these joints. Inability to passively flex the MP joints may be due to either extrinsic tendon adhesions or dorsocapsular contracture. If the extrinsic extensor tendon is adherent to the metacarpal, the limitation of excursion distal to that point will restrict or preclude simultaneous flexion of the MP and PIP joints (45). Extensor tendon adhesions and joint capsular contractures sometimes occur simultaneously. Failure of surgical tenolysis to restore full passive and active motion calls for additional joint release and possible incremental collateral ligament release (46). MP capsulotomy elevates the extensor mechanism; the capsule is transversely incised from beneath at the level of the joint. Although the opening of a portion of the sagittal bands may be necessary, complete release leads to extensor tendon subluxation and should be avoided. Progressive incremental release of the collateral ligament from its dorsal to volar aspect may be required.

Extensor Tendon Adhesion and Extrinsic Extensor Tendon Tightness

The decision for operative intervention for extensor tendon adhesions, as with joint contractures, is delayed for a minimum of 4 months after the original repair and is made only when progress with hand therapy is at a standstill. Tenolysis is the procedure of choice if the condition and length of the extensor tendon are reasonable and the problem is one of adherence and scarring at the tendon. However, if the problem is inadequate tendon length or scarring of a long segment of tendon proximal to the juncturae tendinum, a Littler extrinsic tendon release may be preferred (47). Extrinsic tightness following complete tenolysis or the presence of extensive scarring proximal to the juncturae tendinum requires an extrinsic extensor tendon release. This procedure separates the intrinsic and extrinsic extensor tendon systems and, thus, separates the dual extrinsic–intrinsic extensor control at the PIP joint (Fig. 45-16). Extrinsic extensor tendon release is contraindicated in a patient with weak intrinsic function. The sagittal bands at the MP joint and the central tendon insertion at the base of the middle phalanx must be preserved carefully; the extrinsic extensor extends the MP joint only and relies on the intrinsic system to extend the PIP joint. The central portion of the extensor mechanism is excised over the proximal phalangeal shaft and the distal extent of the tendon resection carried 5 to 8 mm proximal to the PIP joint to avoid disturbing the confluence of the lateral bands and the insertion of the extensor mechanism onto the middle phalanx. Extending the tendon excision too far distally may cause a boutonnière deformity.

We prefer curvilinear longitudinal skin incisions for extensor tenolysis and/or extrinsic extensor tendon release. The entire skin incision does not necessarily have to be sutured closed, but a generous flap remains for extensor tendon coverage. The skin incision may be left open proximally and distally to avoid added tightness over the dorsum of the finger. Immediate motion is instituted postoperatively under the supervision of a hand therapist.

Intrinsic Extensor Tendon Tightness

Both extrinsic and intrinsic extensor tendon tightness may ensue following crushing injuries, and both are associated with limitation of PIP joint flexion. With intrinsic tightness, passive placement of the MP joint in full extension limits active and passive PIP joint flexion (Fig. 45-17) (48). If therapy does not completely correct the problem, surgery is indicated. This procedure, along with the surgery for extrinsic extensor tendon tightness, eliminates dual control of PIP joint extension by excision of the "wing tendons" (49). Intrinsic PIP joint extension is eliminated, leaving extrinsic tendons to extend the PIP joint (Fig. 45-16B). When intrinsic tightness is associated with swan-neck deformity, the

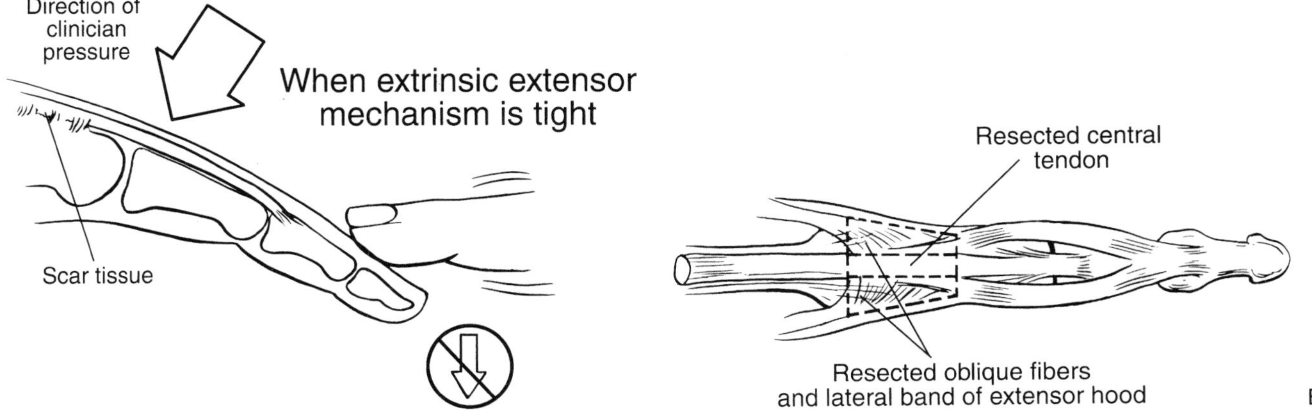

FIGURE 45-16. A: Extrinsic extensor tendon adhesions and tightness are demonstrated by greater difficulty in passive flexion of the finger at the interphalangeal joints when the metacarpophalangeal joint is in a flexed position. **B:** Extrinsic release resects the central tendon proximal to its insertion into the middle phalanx.

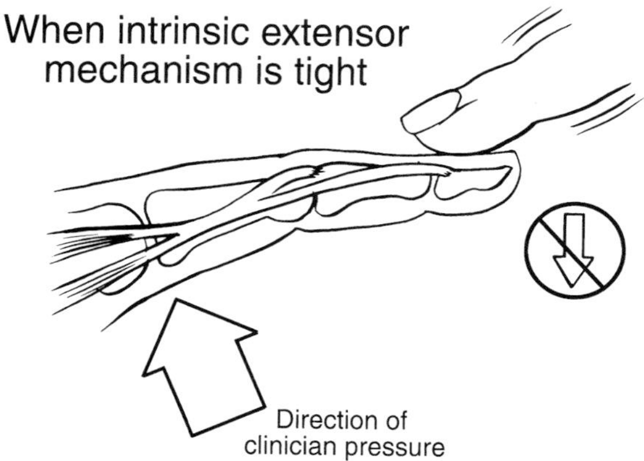

FIGURE 45-17. Intrinsic tightness is demonstrated by the finding that passive flexion of the interphalangeal joints is made more difficult when the metacarpophalangeal joint is positioned in extension.

intrinsic release is carried out as described, followed by a procedure to correct volar plate laxity of the PIP joint.

Extensor Tendon Ruptures

Acute rupture following primary tendon repair may be reconstructed once the tendon ends are freshened. Postoperative dynamic splinting similar to that following primary repair yields a result comparable to that of primary repair. Delayed diagnosis of tendon rupture may require either a tendon grafting procedure or tendon transfers. Rupture of the EPL tendon probably should be repaired in a delayed manner with EIP transfer from the index finger directly through a subcutaneous tunnel into the extensor tendon expansion distal to the MP joint of the thumb (Fig. 45-18). Multiple extensor tendon ruptures on the dorsum of the hand may be treated by side-to-side suturing to adjacent

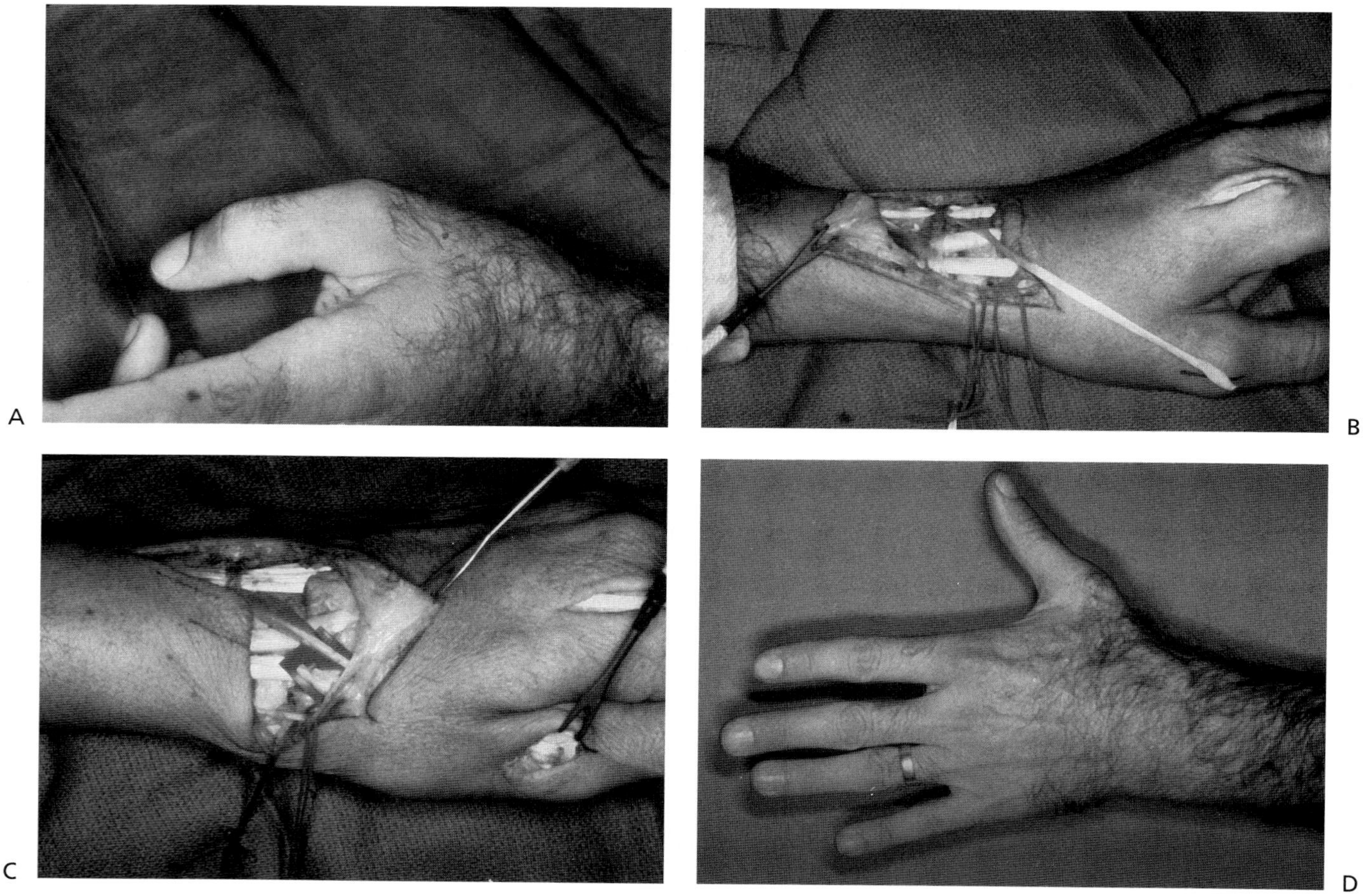

A B C D

FIGURE 45-18. A: Delayed rupture of the previously repaired extensor pollicis longus tendon is noted by the inability to extend the thumb at both metacarpophalangeal and interphalangeal joints. **B,C:** The extensor indicis proprius is transferred to the extensor mechanism, inserting it distal to the metacarpophalangeal joint of the thumb. **D:** Full active thumb extension has been restored

tendons. The repair site should be placed well distal to the extensor retinaculum and, whenever possible, should be away from areas of previous scar. Two tendons may be sutured into the adjacent remaining tendons; three or more tendon ruptures are best treated by means of a formal tendon transfer. My preferred method of tendon transfer is initially to set the tension of the adjacent tendons to each other in a side-to-side manner and then to transfer the FDS tendon of the ring or middle finger directly into the conjoined tendons either through the interosseous membrane or around the radial side of the forearm.

SUMMARY

Treatment of the later complications of extensor mechanism injuries can be quite difficult. Once the delicate balance between the extrinsic and intrinsic systems is disturbed, restoration of fully coordinated hand function is a formidable task. Early recognition and appropriate treatment will prevent some of the untoward late sequelae of extensor tendon injuries.

REFERENCES

1. Thompson ST, Wehbe MA. Extensor physiology in the hand and wrist. *Hand Clin* 1995;11:367–371.
2. Schultz RJ, Furlong J, Storace A. Detailed anatomy of the extensor mechanism at the proximal aspect of the finger. *J Hand Surg* 1981;6:493–498.
3. Zancolli E. *Structural and dynamic angles of hand surgery,* 2nd ed. Philadelphia: JB Lippincott, 1979.
4. Landsmeer J, Long C. The mechanism of finger control, base of electromyograms and location analysis. *Acta Anat* 1965;60:333.
5. Kendal FP, McCreary EK. *Muscle testing and function,* 3rd ed. Baltimore: Williams & Wilkins, 1983.
6. Tubiana R. Architecture and function of the hand. In: Tubiana R, ed. *The hand, vol. 1.* Philadelphia: WB Saunders, 1981:71.
7. Long C, Brown ME. Electromyographic kinesiology of the hand: muscles moving the long finger. *Arch Med* 1964;43:1701.
8. Moore JR, Weiland AJ, Valdata L. Independent index extension after extensor indices proprius transfer. *J Hand Surg* 1987;12A:232–236.
9. Nichols HM. *Manual of hand and injuries,* 2nd ed. Chicago: Yearbook Medical Publishers, 1960:180–181.
10. Godwin Y, Ellis H. Distribution of extensor tendons on the dorsum of the hand. *Clin Anat* 1992;5:394–403.
11. Steichen JB, Petersen DP. Junctura tendinum between extensor digitorum communis and extensor pollicis longus. *J Hand Surg* 1984;9A:674–676.
12. Weber E. Synovial nutrition. In: *Proceedings of the First Congress of the International Federation of Societies for Surgery of the Hand.* Rotterdam: IFSSH, 1980.
13. Kaplan EB. Anatomy, injuries, and treatment of the extensor apparatus of the hand and fingers. *Clin Orthop* 1959;13:24–41.
14. McFarlane RN, Hampole MK. Treatment of extensor tendon injuries of the hand. *Can J Surg* 1973;16:366–375.
15. Beatty MR, Zook EG, Russell RC, et al. Grain auger injuries: the replacement of the corn picker injury? *Plast Reconstr Surg* 1982;69:96–102.
16. Atasoy E. Reversed cross-finger subcutaneous flap. *J Hand Surg* 1982;7:481–483.
17. McGregor IA, Jackson IT. The groin flap. *Br J Plast Surg* 1972;25:3–16.
18. Mulliken JB, Healy NA, Murray JF. An experimental study of hematoma and flap necrosis. *Surg Forum* 1977;28:531–533.
19. Pennington DG. The locking loop tendon suture. *Plast Reconstr Surg* 1979;63:648–652.
20. Newport ML, Blair WF, Steyers CM. Long-term results of extensor tendon repair. *J Hand Surg* 1990;15A:961–966.
21. Evans RB. Immediate active short arc motion following extensor tendon repair. *Hand Clin* 1995;11:483–512.
22. Evans RB, Burkhalter WE. A study of the dynamic anatomy of extensor tendons and implications for treatment. *J Hand Surg* 1986;11A:774–779.
23. Hung LK, Chan A, Chang J, et al. Early controlled active mobilization as dynamic splintage for treatment of extensor tendon injuries. *J Hand Surg* 1990;15A:251–257.
24. Newport ML, Shukla A. Electrophysiologic basis of dynamic extensor splinting. *J Hand Surg* 1992;17A:272–277.
25. Brand PW, Hollister A. *Clinical mechanics of the hand,* 2nd ed. St. Louis: Mosby-Year Book, 1993.
26. Duran RJ, Houser RG. Controlled passive motion following flexor tendon repair in zones II and III. In: *The American Academy of Orthopedic Surgeons: Symposium on Tendon Surgery in the Hand.* St. Louis: CV Mosby, 1975:105.
27. Gelberman RH, Botte MJ, Spiegelman JJ, et al. The excursion and deformation of repaired flexor tendons treated with protected early motion. *J Hand Surg* 1986;11A:106–110.
28. Evans RB, Thompson DE. An analysis of factors that support early active short arc motion of the repaired central slip. *J Hand Ther* 1992;5:187–201.
29. Newport ML, Williams D. Biomechanical characteristics of extensor tendon suture techniques. *J Hand Surg* 1992;17A: 1117–1123.
30. Evans RB. Early active short arc motion for the repaired central slip. *J Hand Surg* 1994;19A:991–997.
31. O'Dwyer FG, Quinton DN. Early mobilization of acute middle slip injuries. *J Hand Surg* 1990;15B:404–406.
32. Warren RA, Kay NRM, Norris SH. The microvascular anatomy of the distal digital extensor tendon. *J Hand Surg* 1988;13B: 161–163.
33. Doyle JR. Extensor tendon injuries. In: *Hand surgery update.* Rosemont, IL: American Academy of Orthopedic Surgeons, 1994:769.
34. Wehbe MA, Schneider LH. Mallet fractures. *J Bone Joint Surg* 1984;66A:658–669.
35. Nichols MH. Repair of extensor tendon insertions in the fingers. *J Bone Joint Surg* 1951;33A:836–841.
36. Thompson JS, Littler JW, Upton J. The spiral oblique retinacula ligament SORL. *J Hand Surg* 1978;3:482–487.
37. Doyle JR, Blythe W. Anatomy of the flexor tendon sheath and pulleys of the thumb. *J Hand Surg* 1977;2:149–152.
38. Harris C, Rutledge GL. The functional anatomy of the extensor mechanism of the finger. *J Bone Joint Surg* 1972;54A:713–726.
39. Boyes JH. *Bunnell's surgery of the hand,* 5th ed. Philadelphia: JB Lippincott, 1970.
40. Curtis RM, Reid RL, Povost JM. A staged technique for the repair of the traumatic boutonniere deformity. *J Hand Surg* 1983; 8:167–171.
41. Fowler SB. Extensor apparatus of the digits. Proceedings of the British Orthopaedic Association. *J Bone Joint Surg* 1949;31B: 477.

42. Carroll C, Moore JR, Weiland AJ. Post-traumatic ulnar subluxation of the extensor tendons: a reconstructive technique. *J Hand Surg* 1987;12A:227–231.
43. Burkhart SS, Wood MB, Linscheid RL. Post-traumatic recurrent subluxation of the extensor carpi ulnaris tendon. *J Hand Surg* 1982;7:1–3.
44. Botte MV, Gelberman RH, Smith DB, et al. Repair of severe muscle belly lacerations using a tendon graft. *J Hand Surg* 1987;12A:406–412.
45. Burton RI. Extensor tendons: late reconstruction. In: Green DP, ed. *Operative hand surgery.* New York: Churchill Livingstone, 1988:2107.
46. Guelmi K, Sokolow C, Mitz V. Dorsal tenolysis and arthrolysis of the proximal interphalangeal joint, 19 cases. *Ann Chir Main Memb Super* 1992;11:307.
47. Littler JW. Principles of reconstructive surgery of the hand. In: Converse JM, ed. *Reconstructive plastic surgery.* Philadelphia: WB Saunders, 1964:1612–1632.
48. Eaton RG. The extensor mechanism of the fingers. *Bull Hosp Joint Dis* 1969;30:39–47.
49. Finochietto R. Retraction de Volkmann de los musculos intrinsecos de la mans. De La Sociedad de Cirugia de Buenos Aires. Tomo IV, 1920.

Discussion

EXTENSOR TENDON INJURIES

WILLIAM P. GRAHAM III
DONALD R. MACKAY

The author provides a brief lucid description of the extensor mechanism and its physiology, recognizing the intricate interactions and contributions of the dual extrinsic and intrinsic components. Using the international classification for levels of tendon injuries permits discussion of the significance of injuries at different levels with respect to prognosis, treatment, and potential sequelae.

The mechanism of injury and the appreciation of the importance of tidy versus untidy injuries are cited. Emphasis is placed on the avoidance of chronicity and the risk this poses relative to the ease of ultimate correction. The importance of specific hand therapy with dynamic splinting is acknowledged, along with the importance of the role of the therapist and the specificity of the postoperative prescriptions. However, discussion of the pitfalls of unsupervised or overexuberant therapy and their consequences is lacking.

In discussing contaminated and crushing injuries, the author advises consideration of primary placement of silicone rod to create space for later tendon grafting. Caution must be observed when placing such a foreign body in a wound of this nature due to its basic "untidy" character. A more conservative approach involves delayed insertion of such a rod(s) once early healing has proceeded without complications.

W. P. Graham and D. R. Mackay: Section of Plastic and Reconstructive Surgery, Department of Surgery, Penn State Geisinger Health System, Hershey, Pennsylvania

The loose, pliable dorsal skin is prone to avulsion and often must be replaced. The classic groin flap of MacGregor and Jackson (1) has stood the test of time and is within the armamentarium of every hand surgeon. Today, free flaps, with and without innervation, and reverse radial forearm flaps are more the procedure of choice for the competent surgeon. They are fast becoming the standard to which one may be expected to adhere.

Restoration of a thin, gliding, pliable cover is essential for appropriate extensor tendon excursion. Even with minor loss of paratenon and some underlying tendon injury, a split-thickness skin graft allows excellent tendon excursion and early return to functionality.

With regard to type III mallet deformities, the author proposes immediate or late reconstruction when arthrodesis may be an expedient and reasonable consideration. With type IV injuries and open acute distal tendon lacerations, the new microanchors provide secure fixation to the bone and obviate the need for a pullout suture. Temporary internal splinting with a small Kirschner wire is important. By placing the wire obliquely, it is easier to seat the anchor in the distal phalanx. Since adopting this technique, we no longer rely on a pullout wire and believe that we have produced less trauma and hence less cicatrix resulting in a more favorable outcome.

For the patient with the chronic mallet deformity that has progressed to a recurvatum of the proximal interphalangeal joint (PIP), reconstruction of the spiral oblique retinacular ligament is not always feasible, especially if the distal joint is ankylosed. In such cases, an arthrodesis of the distal joint in a more favorable attitude and a judicious release of the central extensor slip at the middle phalanx permit return of flexion in the mobile PIP joint.

In his discussion of zone III injuries of the closed variety, the author recommends a dynamic PIP flexion splint. We believe the splint should be of the dynamic extensor type, which limits flexion and restores the relaxed digit to the fully extended attitude.

Curtis et al. (2), in discussing their stepwise approach to the chronic boutonnière deformity (zone III), point out that surgical release of an unyielding volar capsular contracture of the PIP joint must be done first, followed by a second procedure to deal with the boutonnière deformity. They stress that full passive extension must be achieved presurgically. Furthermore, as described by the author, a modified Fowler tenotomy of the lateral bands at the middle phalanx is done by step-cutting them and resuturing to prevent the occurrence of a mallet deformity (3).

The author appropriately notes the need to preserve portions of the extensor retinaculum to prevent bowstringing in zone VI and VII injuries. As in the performance of synovectomies for treatment of the rheumatoid patient, the extensor retinaculum can be split transversely and a portion transferred beneath the tenorrhaphy site to avoid triggering or postoperative adhesions. This keeps the traumatized and repaired segment of the tendon free of the restricting extensor compartments.

When treatment of zone VIII injuries has been delayed, tendon transfers often prove more effective than trying to repair the disrupted tendon with a short intercalated graft. Adjusting the tension of these small grafts more often than not results in too tight a reconstruction or an extensor lag.

The more proximal the muscle injury, the more important is the immobilization of the elbow and the positioning of the wrist. The author's citation of the work by Botte et al. (3) on tendon grafting muscle lacerations bears reinforcing, as it is a frequently overlooked adjunct to the repair of these high forearm injuries. Up to three grafts are used in each divided muscle.

The author cites the typical complications that follow extensor tendon and dorsal hand injuries. The site of the extensor tendon adherence often can be defined preoperatively by careful physical examination, as noted in the text. When adherence of the extensor mechanism precludes full flexion with tethering of the digit, an extensor plus state exists (3).

The greater the degree of trauma associated with the hand injury (especially with fractures), the greater are the risks to the volar structures (joint capsule, volar plate, and flexor tendons). When a combination of adherence of the extensor mechanism dorsally and tendon adhesions within the flexor sheath occurs, then any surgical procedure must be planned to evaluate the patient, permitting active motion of the digits after the completion of the extensor release. A good anesthetic combination is intravenous regional block supplemented with an intermetacarpal or sensory wrist block. As with all tenolyses, active assisted motion and dynamic elastic traction are started in the immediate postoperative period. Joint releases and tenolyses can be augmented with local instillation of dilute steroid solution (5 mg/mL triamcinolone).

Extensor tendon ruptures following acute repair are unavoidable at times, especially with early motion, even when the patient is appropriately instructed and splinted. The author suggests the use of a superficialis transfer to power multiple ruptured extensor communis tendons. He suggests bringing this through the interosseous membrane, which often proves to be restrictive and precludes adequate excursion. Because the superficialis is not synergistic with the digital extension, a more appropriate choice might utilize the flexor carpi ulnaris, prolonging it with a tendon graft as needed for treatment of this problem.

The critical balance of the intricate extensor mechanism cannot be overemphasized. The delicate relationship of the intrinsic and extrinsic elements with the profound effects of even minor changes in the amplitude of glide often is overlooked.

REFERENCES

1. MacGregor IA, Jackson IT. The groin flap. *Br J Plast Surg* 1972;25:3–16.
2. Curtis RM, Reid RL, Probost JM. A staged technique for the repair of the traumatic boutonniere deformity. *J Hand Sur [Am]* 1983;8:67–171.
3. Botte MV, Gelberman RH, Smith TB, et al. Repair of severe muscle belly lacerations using a tendon graft. *J Hand Surg* 1987;12A:406–412.

SUGGESTED READINGS

Dolphin JA. Extensor tenotomy for chronic boutonniere deformity of the finger. *J Bone Joint Surg Am* 1965;47:161–164.

Kilgour ES Jr, Graham WP, Newmeyer L, et al. The extensor plus finger. *J Hand Surg* 1975;7:159–165.

46

NERVE INJURIES

SALEH M. SHENAQ
ALDONA JEDRYSIAK

In the field of peripheral nerve surgery, the considerable number of unfavorable results remains a significant problem. Despite the advent of microsurgical techniques, predictable and complete recovery remains an elusive goal. As we enter the 21st century, we are working to overcome these deficiencies, which lie not as much in our surgical skill, but in our ability to manipulate the molecular environment. We have been striving to perfect our operative intervention to facilitate nerve regeneration, but the key to better results may be more biologic than surgical. This chapter will discuss the current concepts in treatment of nerve injury, illustrating its pathophysiology, diagnosis, and common pitfalls in management.

PATHOPHYSIOLOGY

Anatomy

Peripheral nerve anatomy is comprised of the cell body and axon, Schwann cells, connective tissue stroma, microcirculation, and sensory and motor end-organs (1). The two basic nerve fibers are *type A* and *type C,* which are myelinated rapidly conducting fibers and unmyelinated slow conducting fibers of the sympathetic system, respectively. Schwann cells surround each myelinated nerve fiber individually, whereas unmyelinated nerve fibers are enveloped by Schwann cells in groups (2). *Type A* fibers are subdivided according to size into the largest $A\alpha$ fibers for proprioception, $A\beta$ fibers for touch sensation, $A\gamma$ fibers for muscle stretch receptors, and smallest $A\delta$ fibers for fast pain sensation. *Type C* fibers carry dull pain sensation and temperature (3).

The cross section of a nerve is partitioned into well-defined layers. Endoneurium, a layer of loosely packed collagen, cushions each axon and its Schwann cell sheath, protecting it against stretch and elongation (1). An average of 10,000 axons group to form a fascicle, which is surrounded by the perineurium, a compact connective tissue layer composed of collagen and elastin that provides most of the tensile strength of the nerve. Internal epineurium, a loose connective tissue stroma, envelops the fascicles along with the microcirculation. The final layer is the external epineurium, which serves to bind the contents of the nerve trunk together.

Nerves can be described as monofascicular, oligofascicular (few), or polyfascicular (many) according to their fascicular content. The proportion of the internal cytoskeleton in the cross section of a nerve can range from 20% to 80%, depending on the number of fascicles present. The ratio of connective tissue to the amount of neural tissue is much higher in a polyfascicular nerve, where a larger surface area needs to be covered. The more fascicles present, the more stroma is required to ensheathe them and the greater the tensile strength. Generally, the proximal nerve trunk has a greater number of fascicles than the distal portion and, therefore, is more resistant to stretch (3).

The mesoneurium extends from the epineurium to the surrounding tissues and allows the nerve to glide around joints during movement. It also carries the extrinsic blood supply (4). The intrinsic blood supply is located within the epineurium and transverses both the perineurium and endoneurium to provide the dominant blood supply to the nerve.

Classification/Grading of Peripheral Nerve Injury

In his pioneering work, Seddon (5) proposed a simple yet clinically applicable system for grading nerve injuries, based on the amount of destruction of the structural components.

Neuropraxia occurs when the Schwann cell sheath is disrupted but the axon remains intact. It is considered the mildest type of injury. Compression, ischemia, or demyelinating toxins can cause a loss of the insulating sheath, resulting in a lack of conductivity at the site of injury. Because the axons remain intact, stimulation distal to this point still elicits a response. Conduction is restored when remyelination occurs, usually hours to 3 months after injury (2).

S. M. Shenaq and A. Jedrysiak: Division of Plastic Surgery, Baylor College of Medicine, Houston, Texas

Axonotmesis involves injury to the Schwann cell myelin sheath as well as the underlying axon. This is a more severe type of injury because the distal part of the nerve undergoes wallerian degeneration. Therefore, stimulation of the nerve more than 72 hours after injury does not elicit a response. The surrounding endoneurium continues to serves as a guide for regenerating axons, and recovery can be followed by an advancing Tinel sign.

Neurotmesis constitutes injury of all the anatomical components, the myelin sheath, the axons, and the surrounding connective tissue. This total nerve disruption makes regeneration impossible and surgical intervention necessary.

Sunderland (6) expanded this classification into five grades as follows: grades I and II correspond to neuropraxia and axonotmesis, respectively; and grades III to V correspond to increasing severity of neurotmesis. More specifically, grade III depicts injury of the axon, endoneurium, and basal lamina of Schwann cells. The recovery typically will be indicated by an advancing Tinel sign but will be incomplete because the axons are required to grow through some degree of scar tissue. Grade IV injury frequently is caused by traction where disruption of the endoneurium and perineurium occurs, but continuity is preserved by scar. Grade V is total discontinuity of all structures and usually is caused by a laceration. Mackinnon and Dellon (7) added grade VI, or neuroma-in-continuity, which describes a common situation where combinations of nerve injury grades are present. Surgical intervention typically is indicated in grades IV to VI.

Nerve Regeneration

Despite the advances made in the past two decades, the pathophysiology of nerve degeneration and regeneration is still poorly understood. Following axotomy, the survival of the two portions of the nerve depends on the connection and communication between the two segments. Neuronal cell death can occur in the proximal segment, an event that depends on the age of the cell and proximity of the injury. Early nerve repair can prevent cell death because the degenerating nerve stump provides a neurotropic stimulus. When the stimulus is perceived, the nucleus increases in size, accelerating the production of structural proteins (8). At this point, the nerve metabolism shifts from maintaining conductivity to rebuilding structural components.

Distally, the nerve undergoes wallerian degeneration, where the axon deteriorates and macrophages and Schwann cells then perform the breakdown of myelin. Several weeks are required for the cleaning process, and hollow endoneurial tubes are left behind. These become filled with Schwann cells, which generate trophic stimuli to initiate new axonal growth. The regenerating axons send several amebic sprouts, which comprise a growth cone, along the endoneurial tubes at an average rate of 1 to 2 mm/day (9), Over time, the new axons become myelinated and enlarge after they reach their end-organ target. The axons unsuccessful at this task eventually degenerate, resulting in the number of axons in a nerve fascicle to decrease.

Schwann cells are the rate-limiting factor in axonal regeneration; in their absence, regeneration ceases. In tissue culture, neurons survive and produce axons only in the presence of Schwann cells or a nerve growth factor. Similarly, specialized fibroblasts found in epineural and perineural tissue are essential for nerve regeneration by producing collagen for endoneural tube formation. The collagen production process requires a negative feedback mechanism to keep it in check; otherwise, fibroblast activity will not facilitate nerve regeneration but will impede it by forming a scar. The amount of "extra" collagen formed is directly proportional to tension on the repair, the amount of soft tissue damage, and the amount of foreign body present. Some authors advocate resecting a strip of epineurium 2 to 3 mm wide at each end to decrease scar formation at the repair site (10).

The motor axons are in a race for time to reach the muscle end-organs before they atrophy. After 12 months, muscle fibrosis and scarring markedly impair functional recovery; after 18 months, muscle atrophy is complete. Normal muscle is composed of a mixture of type I and II fibers. Conversion to one type is seen after reinnervation, therefore demonstrating that muscle type is nerve dependent. Accordingly, evidence of reinnervation may be obtained by performing a muscle biopsy and finding discrete groups of either type I or II fibers (1).

Sensory receptors do not undergo significant end-organ atrophy, and recovery of sensation is possible years after injury. Sensory modalities do not return uniformly; pain along with sweat gland function returns first, followed by cold then warm sensation, with soft touch being the last to return.

Neurotrophism is the ability to influence the direction of nerve regeneration. Neurotropism is the ability to influence maturation of the nerve. Studies have shown that growing axons will preferentially grow toward distal nerve stumps rather than toward muscle or tendon (11). This is due to a nerve growth factor known to be present in the distal nerve stump (12), which provides neurotrophic support and prevents neuronal death after axonal degeneration. Similarly, a purified acidic fibroblast growth factor placed in a collagen-filled nerve guide has been shown to increase the number of myelinated axons crossing a 5-mm nerve gap distance (13). Perhaps in the future, a neurotrophic analogue infiltrated around the repair site can enhance post-lesion repair by increasing the number of outgrowing axons.

TYPES OF NERVE INJURY

Pathology of Peripheral Nerve Injury

It is necessary to differentiate between the diverse mechanisms of nerve injury in order to make the correct diagnosis and provide the best type of operative intervention. For simplification, the various mechanisms can be globally divided into two categories, according to the vector of the force acting on the nerve. The force vector direction is longitudinal in the case of traction and cross-sectional in the case of pressure. Most injury mechanisms are a combination of these forces.

Effect of Traction

Traction exposes the peripheral nerve to tension, which causes straightening and stretching of the nerve fibers and their fascicles. Nerves have a slightly undulating course and can tolerate 8% stretch without any perceptible changes (14). The amount of resting tension is determined by the perineural and epineural structures and provides cushioning for the fascicles, as seen by nerve shortening after a laceration (2). Therefore, a nerve with many fascicles that contains a large amount of perineural tissue is considered more resistant to stretch than a monofascicular nerve.

As progressive elongation occurs, the diameter of the nerve fiber decreases, which causes pressure deformation of the endoneural contents. This results in ischemia and disturbances of conductivity of the nerve. The elastic limit is approached at 15% stretch, at which point breaking of the fascicles usually occurs. However, substantial stretch can be tolerated if this force is exerted in small increments over a long period of time.

Effect of Pressure

The characteristics of injuries caused by pressure are dependent on the magnitude of the force and the size of the area over which it is exerted. Sharp injuries, where a large amount of force is exerted over a small and narrow area, typically result in nerve transection. Blunt pressure causes direct mechanical damage and ischemia that indirectly increase the severity of the injury. The susceptibility of nerves to acute and chronic compressive forces is a function of their internal anatomy and location.

Mechanisms of Peripheral Nerve Injury

Blunt trauma delivers forces that stretch and compress the nerve, frequently causing a neuroma-in-continuity. Depending on the magnitude of the force, the nerve may undergo total disruption or avulsion, which reduces the chances for a favorable outcome. Sharp lacerations frequently cause a grade V or VI injury, but they are associated with the best prognosis because they offer the greatest opportunity for primary nerve repair. Missile injuries are less likely to sever a nerve, but they produce devastating soft tissue damage due to pronounced cavitation effects. Because nerves frequently run in neurovascular bundles, trauma to vascular structures can result in profound damage with a large amount of subsequent scarring. Ischemia is an integral part of compressive injury, which affects the largest motor fibers first, spares the small sympathetic nerve fibers, and frequently produces hyperesthesia.

Thermal nerve injury can range from grade I to IV, depending on the severity of the surrounding soft tissue damage. The low conduction resistance of nerves makes them especially susceptible to severe injury in electrical burns, where a large amount of current can pass through and cause extensive damage to nerves and muscles. After the injury, necrosis ensues and the nerve is replaced by scar. The surrounding tissue scar can worsen the injury by causing compression of the nerve.

There are several potential types of iatrogenic injury. The most common are compression and traction injury during operative positioning or during cast immobilization. Another common type is injection injury that occurs when an agent is injected close to a nerve. Its severity depends on both the nature of the agent injected and the proximity of the needle to the nerve. An intraneural injection leads to nerve inflammation and edema, and an intrafascicular injection can quickly lead to necrosis. Nerve injury caused directly by retractors, electrocautery, or transection may occur without notice. The best outcome occurs when it is immediately recognized and repaired; therefore, careful attention when dissecting around vital structures cannot be overemphasized. Iatrogenic damage due to ionizing radiation induces extensive fibrosis of the surrounding tissues with compromise of the blood supply and ensuing intraneural damage. Other causes of nerve damage can result from compression in entrapment syndromes or due to a mass effect of a growing tumor. Systemic diseases, such as diabetes mellitus, gout, systemic amyloidosis, and hypothyroidism, also can have an indirect influence on peripheral nerve injury.

CLINICAL EVALUATION

A thorough history and physical examination are essential when treating a nerve injury, not only to form a diagnosis, but also to establish a baseline that can be used in the future to assess recovery and prognosis. The mechanism of injury, timing of onset, signs, and symptoms must be clearly documented. Muscle evaluation should proceed in a stepwise fashion, using a widely accepted grading system such as the British Medical Research Council (MRC) Motor Grading. A sensory examination that includes two-point discrimination should be performed. It is not possible to differentiate between axonotmesis and neurotmesis for 3 weeks after injury because the electrical conductivity may persist during this time. After 3 weeks of careful observation, a baseline electromyogram and nerve conduction velocities of both affected and unaffected extremities should be performed, and repeated after 3 months at 4- to 6-week intervals. If no recovery is demonstrated or if recovery plateaus, axonotmesis or neurotmesis is presumed and operative exploration and repair are indicated.

PRINCIPLES AND TECHNIQUE

Ideal Nerve Repair and Results

The ideal nerve repair should provide optimal conditions for the axons to cross the site of repair and grow along the endoneurial tubes to reach the corresponding end-organ before it undergoes degeneration (15). Unfortunately, this ideal is not possible for several reasons. The growing axon is stimulated by a global neurotropic stimulus, but there is no specific way for it to reach the end-organ that it innervated before transection. In the best of circumstances, sensory axons reach appropriate sensory organs and motor axons reach appropriate synergistic muscles. As well, out of all the growing axons, only a fraction of them will be successful at reaching the end-organ.

Principles of Nerve Repair

In an open injury, exploration of the nerve is indicated. If a clean cut is found, immediate repair should be undertaken. In case of significant soft tissue damage, it is advisable to perform a delayed primary or early secondary repair because it is difficult to establish immediately how much of the nerve is damaged. A period of 3 to 4 weeks allows time for fibrosis of the nonviable nerve segment and gross identification for excision (16).

Techniques of Nerve Repair

Neurolysis

Scar surrounding a nerve is detrimental to its conductive function. Ischemia can result from the scar's chronic strangulation effect on the microcirculation. Any tethering attachments to surrounding structures put traction on the nerve and obstruct its ability to glide when the extremity is in motion. This is significant because the length difference between nerve and arm in flexed position is 20% (17). Although external neurolysis is beneficial, overzealous dissection from surrounding tissues can result in increased vascular compromise. This is an explanation for the poor results obtained when a large gap is overcome by extensive mobilization (18). Internal neurolysis is controversial because, even when it is performed with great precision, some fascicles are transected, leading to small neuroma formation. The microcirculation is disrupted, and fibrosis may recur (17).

Neurorrhaphy

Neurorrhaphy, or end-to-end repair, should be performed in a stepwise fashion (17). Preparation for the repair starts by resection of the proximal and distal nerve stumps. The two ends can be approximated using a tension-relieving suture to overcome the retraction of the mesoneurium (19). Recent studies showed that local neurotrophic factors are the main contributors to the correct alignment of axons, and loose approximation is preferred over tight closure with a large amount of suture. Local fibrin contributes to coaptation, and if there is a small amount of tension on the repair, a minimum number of sutures should be used. To prevent scar formation at the repair site, a 2-mm strip of epineurium can be removed. There are several guidelines to keep in mind when aligning the two severed ends. The location of the dorsal blood vessel, the mesoneurium, and the external shape of nerve are useful in determining the correct orientation. Anatomical internal topographic maps that are available for various peripheral nerves facilitate fascicular identification (20). Histologic staining can differentiate motor from sensory nerves, because acetylcholinesterase and choline transferase are limited to motor fibers, whereas carbonic anhydrase is unique to the sensory fibers. This method has become clinically applicable, because the incubation time for the carbonic anhydrase has decreased from 24 hours to 1 hour (21).

The amount of dissection performed near the site of repair should be just enough to overcome a small nerve gap. At no time should the repair be performed under tension, as this increases the amount of fibrosis and impairs vascular perfusion. Another important consideration is minimizing the amount of suture material used. Monofilament suture ranging from 8-0 to 10-0 have been advocated, but 9-0 nylon is best because its breakage point correlates with excess tension on the nerve repair and indicates the need for a nerve graft.

Controversy remains about the preferred method for nerve repair. Epineural repair has been a preferred method because it involves less operative difficulty and time while providing a strong, dependable repair. Its disadvantages are the misleading external appearance that conceals distortion of the internal architecture and the presence of dead space (18).

Fascicular repair appears theoretically attractive but is best used for injuries where several large fascicles are present. When nerve loss occurs, the rapidly changing cross-sectional fascicular patterns do not correspond, and this mismatch leaves some fascicles unrepaired and the suture line crowded. This type of repair is only possible for larger fascicles, and any mismatch in the size of the fascicles compromises the result.

However, neither epineural nor fascicular repairs have shown any conclusive advantage in studies. Therefore, a compromise between epineural and fascicular techniques frequently is made to "group fascicular repair," which optimizes the fascicular apposition.

Other methods of coaptation include welding with the CO_2 laser, using coupling devices, and fibrin glue. The milliwatt carbon dioxide laser has not found popularity, largely due to thermal damage and lack of repair strength (22). Similarly, fibrin glue is not recommended for primary nerve repair. It is mostly used for nerve grafting, which is completely tension free.

Nerve Grafts

In the last two decades, the importance of minimizing tension at the suture line has been shown. Nerve guides were implemented to provide a structural bridge for axonal regeneration and improve outcomes. Despite the disadvantages of two suture lines and donor site scars, a nerve repair with a graft that is tension free was found to be superior to primary repair under tension (23,24).

Gaps are produced in three different ways. Small gaps are created by retraction of the stumps after the nerve is severed and are reversible for a short time after the injury. With time, nerve elasticity decreases, scar tissue forms, and the force required to approximate the severed ends increases. In cases where ragged nerve edges are trimmed by a few millimeters, the gap can be repaired primarily if done soon after the injury. True loss of substance occurs in some injuries where a segment of nerve is damaged and needs to be excised. In these cases, the gap distance is comprised of the loss of length due to elastic recoil of the connective tissue elements plus the actual loss of nerve tissue. The stress strain curve rises sharply after 5% stretch, creating a critical gap distance beyond which primary approximation is not possible or requires an unacceptable amount of tension (25,26). Maneuvers such as nerve mobilization, limb flexion, and nerve transposition are insufficient, and a nerve graft frequently is required. The amount of scar that needs to be excised can be evaluated grossly, microscopically, or histochemically. Determination of nerve viability is difficult based purely on the appearance of the nerve, and it has not been shown to correlate with function (3). A classification scheme for description of nerve grafts has been developed distinguished by four criteria: (i) origin of graft, (ii) mechanical aspects, (iii) donor nerves, and (iv) circulation (17). The most commonly used donor nerve is the sural nerve, a large and purely sensory nerve that innervates the lateral aspect of the foot. It provides the longest graft length, up to 40 cm in adults. Other possible donor nerves include the medial and lateral antebrachial cutaneous nerves, the terminal branch of the posterior interosseous nerve, and the tibial nerve. Once the donor nerve is harvested, it is divided into interpositional nerve grafts with lengths longer than the gap to provide for elongation during movement. Given the minimal tension on nerve grafts, some authors prefer using fibrin alone for coaptation to decrease the operative time. Studies have shown that there is no difference between fibrin and sutures in tension-free repairs (27). The main disadvantages of nerve grafts are their inherent limitations in length and thickness, as well as the donor neurologic deficits (28). Moreover, the functional result when a nerve graft is used decreases as its length increases. This has led to the development of vascularized nerve grafts, where donor sites described include the sural nerve as well as the ulnar nerve in brachial plexus reconstruction. In cases of amputated parts, harvesting a vascularized nerve graft also should be considered.

Nerve Guides

The idea of using conduits to facilitate axonal regeneration dates back to the beginnings of peripheral nerve surgery, when suture was used as a nerve guide (29). In cases where primary repair is not possible, a cylindrical tube, not necessarily nerve tissue, can be used to bridge the gap and guide the regenerating axons (17). Tubulization also serves to protect the site of repair and decrease scar formation by reducing the number of invading fibroblasts. Nerve guides also provide a local microenvironment where neurotrophic and neurotropic factors promote the migration of regenerating nerve sprouts. These conduits are advantageous for small gaps because a donor site nerve defect is avoided. Many materials have been tried for this purpose, including bone, tendon, Gore-Tex, Millipore (30), collagen (31), Surgicel (32), Silastic tubes (33), silicone, and others (34) with variable success. Only collagen and vein conduits have proved functional in nerve gaps measuring less than 3 cm. Vein grafts are useful because their tissue structure is similar to nerves, specifically their inner endothelial cells, outer fibroblast, and collagen layers. Other advantages include ease of harvest, abundant supply, and ability to permit diffusion of nutrients into the luminal space (35) .Other conduits, such as polyglycolic acid, have been used clinically, with results superior to those of nerve graft (36). A pseudosynovial vascularized sheath was used to bridge a 3-cm nerve gap and revealed no difference when compared to sural nerve graft at 1 year (37).

Allografts

Allografts are useful in severe injuries that require large amounts of nerve graft. To date, there has been little success with fresh nerve grafts, but encouraging results have been reported with pretreated grafts. The main problems are related to graft preservation and immunologic suppression rejection phenomena (38). The required part of the allograft is the connective tissue scaffold; therefore, pretreatment with radiation or freeze drying to eliminate the cellular component decreases immunologic activity. Short-term immunosuppression typically is necessary because only the connective tissue scaffold is required (36).

Intraoperative Electrodiagnostic Testing

Intraoperative electrophysiologic assessment of nerve action potentials is useful in making surgical decisions. The presence or absence of nerve action potentials across a lesion determines the need for simple neurolysis or resection of the damaged nerve segment with interpositional nerve grafting. Often, a normal-appearing nerve will not be functional, and this technique has helped greatly in improving surgical outcomes.

POSTOPERATIVE CARE AND REHABILITATION

The extremity should be immobilized for 3 to 4 weeks after nerve repair, followed by 1 week of night splinting. Massage and electrical stimulation are implemented to prevent denervated muscle from atrophying. Muscles that are starting to function should be splinted intermittently to avoid fatigue and fibrillation (10).

Intensive physiotherapy after a period of immobilization with passive joint movement is crucial to avoid stiffness. Edema should be treated with elevation and elastic bandages to avoid secondary diffuse fibrosis. The skin is protected to avoid lesions and burns due to insensibility. Postoperative motor and sensory reeducation maximize the surgical result. The patient is given various shaped objects with different surfaces and is asked to identify them with eyes open and then closed to correlate visual and sensory input.

RESULTS

Factors Affecting Results

Several factors affect the prognosis and timing for recovery:

1. Proximity of the lesion to the parent body cell
2. Distance between the lesion and the end-organ
3. Amount of retrograde degeneration and involution of the proximal segment
4. Complexity of the nerve
5. Degree of axonal disruption.

Many obstacles stand in the way of achieving a good result in nerve repair. Axons require stimulation to grow, and as they regenerate through the site of repair they encounter some degree of scarring. The amount of scarring is dependent on the mechanism of injury and the amount of traction present at the repair site. Regeneration proceeds very slowly through scar, if at all. Additionally, the amount of variation in the cross-sectional pattern makes it difficult to assure correct anatomical alignment of the neural tubules that serve to guide the axons in regeneration. The axons also may propagate outside of the neural tubules and remain functionally useless.

Regeneration is an unpredictable chance event that is dependent on both biologic and technical factors. Patient age, the mechanism and severity of injury, and the degree of surrounding fibrosis are unchangeable biologic variables that influence the number of axons that will be successful at crossing the repair site. Fortunately, technical factors can be modified to optimize the nerve repair. Identifying correctly the type of nerve injury and choosing the best operative intervention are paramount. The timing of the repair and deciding from among neurolysis, neurorrhaphy, and nerve grafting also are critical. In primary repair, the extent of correct apposition of nerve fibers and avoiding tension greatly enhance the final outcome.

SUMMARY OF ESSENTIALS IN NERVE REPAIR

1. Understanding anatomy (both normal and abnormal)
2. Accurate and detailed clinical assessment
3. Timing of repair according to the mechanism of injury
4. Clean bed for nerve repair
5. Sound microsurgical technique
6. Tension-free repair
7. Appropriate technique of nerve repair
8. Immobilization
9. Physical therapy
10. Rehabilitation.

FUTURE

As with any complex tissue, "regeneration" after nerve injury is slow and incomplete. It is important to consider that repair of a transected nerve, even if performed with impeccable microsurgical skill, is unlikely to result in complete return of motor or sensory function.

Our future progress depends on laboratory investigative studies to find advances in biochemistry, immunology, and genetics. Complete success requires the ability to manipulate the axonal microenvironment as an adjunct to continual improvement in microsurgical techniques.

REFERENCES

1. Mitchell JR, Osterman AL. Physiology of nerve repair: a research update. *Hand Clin* 1991;7:481–490.
2. Gerald GA, Goodkin R, Kliot M. Evaluation and surgical management of peripheral nerve problems. *Neurosurgery* 1999;44:825–839.
3. Ehni BL. Treatment of traumatic peripheral nerve injury. *Am Fam Phys* 43:897–905.
4. Smyth JW. Factors influencing nerve repair. *Arch Surg* 1993;93:335–341.
5. Seddon HJ. Three types of nerve injury. *Brain* 1943;66:237–288.
6. Sunderland S. A classification of peripheral nerve injuries producing loss of function. *Brain* 1951;74:491—516.
7. Mackinnon SE, Dellon AL. Nerve repair and nerve grafts. In: *Surgery of the peripheral nerve.* New York: Thieme, 1988:89–129.
8. Watchmaker GP, Mackinnon SE. Advances in peripheral nerve repair. *Clin Plast Surg* 1997;24:63–72.

9. Holmquist B, Kanje M, Kerns JM. A mathematical model for regeneration rate and initial delay following surgical repair of peripheral nerves. *J Neurosci Methods* 1993;48:27–33.
10. Brunelli G, Monini L, Brunelli F. Problems in nerve lesions surgery. *Microsurgery* 1985;6:187–198.
11. Mackinnon SE, Dellon AL, Lundborg G, et al. A study of neurotropism in the primate model. *J Hand Surg* 1986;11:888–894.
12. Richardson P, Ebendal T. Nerve growth activities in the rat peripheral nerve fascicle. *Brain Res* 1982;246:57.
13. Cordeiro PG, Seckel BR, Lipton SA, et al. Acidic fibroblast growth factor enhances peripheral nerve regeneration in vivo. *Plast Reconstr Surg* 1989;83:1013.
14. Peripheral nerve lesions: diagnosis and therapy.
15. Millesi H. Peripheral nerve injuries: nerve sutures and nerve grafting. 25–37.
16. Ducker TB, Kauffman C. Metabolic factors in surgery of peripheral nerves. *Clin Neurosurg* 1977;24:406.
17. Millesi H. Progress in peripheral nerve reconstruction. *World J Surg* 1990;14:733–747.
18. Smith JW. Peripheral nerve surgery: retrospective and contemporary techniques. *Clin Plast Surg* 1986;13:249—254.
19. Tsuge K, Ikuta M, Sakaue M. A new technique for nerve suture. *Plast Reconstr Surg* 1975;56:496.
20. Sunderland S. The intraneural topography of radial, median, and ulnar nerves. *Brain* 1945;68:243.
21. Terzis JK. The use of carbonic anhydrase in the sensory motor differentiation of peripheral nerve trunks: possible histochemical aid to nerve repair Presented at Symp Sur le Plexus Brachial, Lausanne, Switzerland, December 3–4, 1984.
22. Terris DJ, Fee WE. Current issues in nerve repair. *Arch Otolaryngol Head Neck Surg* 1993;119:725–730.
23. Millesi H, Meissel G. Consequences of tension at the suture site. In: Gorio A, Millesi H, Mingrino S. eds. *Posttraumatic peripheral nerve regeneration.* New York: Raven Press, 1981:81.
24. Hentz VR, Rosen JM, Xiao SJ, McGill KC, Abraham G. The nerve gap dilemma: a comparison of nerves repaired end to end under tension with nerve grafts in a primate model. *J Hand Surg* 1993;18:417–425.
25. De Medinaceli L, Prayon M, Merie M. Percentage of nerve injuries in which primary repair can be achieved by end-to-end approximation: review of 2,181 nerve lesions. *Microsurgery* 1993;14:244–246.
26. Miyamoto Y, Watari S, Tsuge K. Experimental studies on the effects of tension on intraneural microcirculation in suture of peripheral nerves. *Plast Reconstr Surg* 1979;63:398.
27. Daverio PJ, Krupp S. Sutureless nerve anastomosis. Transactions 8th Congress Plastic and Reconstructive Surgery, June 26–July 1, 1983.
28. Seddon HJ. Nerve grafting. *J Bone Joint Surg* 1963;45A: 447–461.
29. Vanlair C. De la regeneration des nerfs peripheriques par la procede de la suture tubulair. *CR Acad Sci (Paris)* 65:99-101, 1882.
30. Campbell JB, Bassett AL, Husby JT, et al. Microfilter sheathing in peripheral nerve surgery. *J Trauma* 1961;1:139.
31. Kline DG, Hayes GJ. The use of resorbable wrapper for peripheral nerve repair. Experimental studies in chimpanzees. *J Neurosurg* 1964;21:737.
32. Gabrielson GS, Stenstoeam S. A contribution of peripheral nerve suture. *Plast Reconstr Surg* 1966;8:68.
33. Lehman RA, Hayes GJ. Regeneration in peripheral nerves. *Brain* 1967;90:285.
34. Collin W. Nerve regeneration through collagen tubes. *J Dent Res* 1984;63:987.
35. Suematsu N. Tubulation for peripheral nerve gap: its history and possibility. *Microsurgery* 1989;10:71–74.
36. MacKinnon SE, Dellon AL. *Surgery of the peripheral nerve.* New York: Thieme, 1988.
37. Dellon AL, MacKinnon SE. An alternative the classical nerve graft in management of the short nerve gap. *Plast Reconstr Surg* 1988;82:849.
38. Sunderland S. *Nerve and nerve injuries.* New York: Churchill Livingstone, 1978.

Discussion

NERVE INJURIES

A. LEE DELLON

The chapter on nerve injuries by Shenaq and Jedrysiak is a scholarly discussion of the *treatment* of traditional nerve injuries. The chapter clearly outlines the basic neuroanatomy of the peripheral nerve, reviews the classic staging and understanding of the pathophysiology of peripheral nerve injury, and describes the modern concepts of microsurgical nerve repair and nerve grafting. Although the chapter describes what to do with the most common problems encountered with the peripheral nerve, i.e., nerve compression and nerve division after trauma, it does *not* address the problem of preventing nerve injury or the treatment of the injured nerve when it presents as a complication of plastic surgery.

In my personal practice of plastic surgery, the treatment of peripheral nerve injuries comprises about 80% of my patient population. About half of these patients had been op-

A. L. Dellon: Department of Plastic Surgery and Neurosurgery, Johns Hopkins University, Baltimore, Maryland

Dr. Dellon has a proprietary interest in the Pressure-Specified Sensory Device™ and in the Neurotube™.

TABLE 46D-1. UNFAVORABLE RESULTS DUE TO NERVE INJURY: CUTANEOUS NEUROMA

Region of Nerve Injury	Initial Surgical Procedure	Nerve Involved
Face	Facelift	Greater auricular
	Browlift	Supraorbital
Neck	Flap or neck dissection	Cervical plexus
Chest	Breast reconstruction	Intercostal
Hand	Carpal tunnel decompression	Palmar br. median
Forearm	de Quervain release or ganglion excision	Radial sensory and/or lateral antebrachial
Elbow	Tennis elbow release	Posterior cutaneous nerve of forearm
	Ulnar nerve decompression	Medial antebrachial
Groin	Flap or hernia repair	Ileoinguinal
Abdomen	Abdominoplasty	Ileohypogastric
Knee	Flap or orthopedic surgery	Infrapatellar branch of saphenous nerve
Ankle	Flap	Sural, calcaneal
	Tarsal tunnel decompression	Saphenous
Foot	Toe transfer	Peroneal, superficial/deep
Hip	Harvesting bone graft	Lateral femoral

TABLE 46D-2. UNFAVORABLE RESULTS DUE TO NERVE INJURY: STRETCH/TRACTION

Region of Nerve Injury	Initial Surgical Procedure	Nerve Involved
Face	Facelift	Infraorbital
	Browlift	Supraorbital
	Mandibular lengthening	Inferior alveolar
Neck	Flap	Cervical plexus, spinal accessory
Hand	Limb lengthening	Digital
Forearm	Limb lengthening	Radial sensory
Groin/hip	Flap	Lateral femoral cutaneous
Abdomen	Reconstruction	Lateral femoral cutaneous
Knee	Flap	Common peroneal

TABLE 46D-3. UNFAVORABLE RESULTS DUE TO NERVE INJURY: MISDIAGNOSIS

Original "Misdiagnosis"	Correct Diagnosis	Nerve Involved
Recurrent carpal tunnel syndrome	Radial sensory nerve entrapment	Radial sensory
Recurrent carpal tunnel syndrome	Pronator syndrome	Proximal median
Recurrent tennis elbow	Radial tunnel syndrome	Radial nerve
Temporal mandibular joint dysfunction	Thoracic outlet syndrome	Brachial plexus
Poor result of nerve repair	Neuroma-in-continuity	Any nerve

erated on by someone who made them worse. Many of these patients had a complication that could have been avoided. All of these patients have a complication that requires treatment. The patient's presenting complaints are pain, numbness, or loss of motor function. The unfavorable results due to a nerve injury usually can be related to (i) a cutaneous neuroma in the surgical incision, (ii) placing traction on a major nerve, (iii) cutting a major sensory or motor nerve, or (iv) failure to appreciate a second existing diagnosis when the patient returns to the original treating physician with "persisting" complaints (Tables 46D-1–46D-3.)

CUTANEOUS NEUROMA

Prevention

Cutaneous neuroma *should* be a preventable complication of surgery. The prevention comes from knowledge of regional anatomy as described in the textbooks. However, realization that there is extensive variability in the anatomical distribution of cutaneous nerves means that even the most knowledgeable surgeon may have this complication.

An unfortunate situation is exemplified by the patient who presents with pain at the site of a venipuncture from an intravenous line or preoperative blood work. The patient, awake at the time, feels the nerve injury as a lightening-like bolt of pain in the distribution of the cutaneous nerve and instantly reports the event. The patient typically is in pain at the venipuncture site. Often this patient will become litigious. The diagnosis and treatment of this problem generalizes into the prevention and treatment of pain from any surgical incision. I tell the patient that there was no way this particular nerve injury could have been prevented due to the wide variability of the cutaneous nerves and the blood vessels. I have testified that this is not grounds for a malpractice action against either the hospital or the phlebotomist. The treatment is a program of desensitization with a therapist, warming the site of pain and massaging in a steroid cream, or both. If the pain persists for 6 months, it is reasonable to explore the wound to see if the nerve is still intact but adherent to the vein, or whether there is a neuroma.

This same approach applies to the prevention and treatment of all the situations listed in Table 46D-1. Knowledge of the anatomy of the cutaneous nerves should allow the plastic surgeon to avoid the greater auricular nerve during a facelift, the supraorbital nerve during a browlift, the cutaneous nerves over the dorsoradial aspect of the forearm during an extensor tendon release for de Quervain tenosynovitis, or ganglion excision (1,2). The known course of the palmar cutaneous branch of the median nerve should permit an incision for carpal tunnel decompression that will result in a pain-free scar at that site (3). It is helpful if the surgeon wears loupes during the dissection.

If the cutaneous nerve is identified during the surgery but the nerve still becomes either partly divided or severely stretched so that the surgeon is concerned that a painful neuroma will develop and cause postoperative pain, a decision must be made as to whether to repair the nerve or to complete its division and relocate the proximal end of the nerve into an area that will not be subject to movement or pressure. This decision should be made based on (i) the degree of preoperative discussion the surgeon had with the patient regarding the potential risks of the procedure, which may have included a discussion of postoperative numbness or dysesthesias in the skin around the incision; (ii) the area that will become anesthetic if the nerve is divided; and (iii) the willingness of the patient to endure the paresthesias and probable dysesthesias during neural regeneration if the nerve is repaired. For example, if the nerve is the medial antebrachial cutaneous nerve and it is injured doing an anterior transposition of the ulnar nerve (4), or if one of its small branches crosses the incision and is clearly severely stretched or torn during retraction, it may be most appropriate to dissect this divided nerve proximally and relocate that end into the triceps muscle, accepting an area of numbness about the scar. In contrast, if the nerve is the supraorbital nerve and it is divided during an endoscopic browlift, it may be more appropriate to make a new incision over the eyebrow and repair the nerve. This choice can be made because the resultant area of numbness usually is unacceptably disturbing to patients, and there is a chance of a painful neuroma in the eyebrow, which also is usually unacceptable to patients.

During abdominoplasty (5) or groin flap procedures, little can be done to prevent injury to the cutaneous nerves. This is because they often are within 1 to 2 cm from the usual anatomical description, and the location from which they go within the abdominal wall musculature to the skin also is variable. It is remarkable that there are not more painful neuromas of the abdomen and groin.

Treatment

The program for neuroma treatment is outlined in Table 46D-4 (6). Every patient must have 6 months of desensitization. This treatment should be started by the surgeon, who instructs the patient on application of heat to the scar, followed by twice daily 5-minute massages with a steroid-containing cream, such as 0.1% betamethasone. If no progress is made within 3 to 6 weeks, referral to a therapist is appropriate for a structured program of desensitization with fluidotherapy, different grades of materials, and vibration. This is a form of sensory reeducation for type C and Aδ fibers (7). To this may be added ultrasound massage with steroid iontophoresis. If the scar remains painful, intrascar injection of steroid should be attempted. Dexamethasone, which is water soluble, is the ideal steroid to inject because it will not cause damage even if it is inadvertently injected into the nerve. If this aggressive nonsurgical approach does not relieve the pain by 6 months, then neuroma resection is appropriate.

Before resecting a neuroma that is believed to be the source of the patient's pain, it is critical to block this nerve with a local anesthetic. This demonstrates not only that the nerve imputed to be the source of pain is, in fact, the source of pain, but also that the patient is willing to accept the skin area that will become anesthetic as an anesthetic area of his or her body. It is critical that in areas such as the forearm, where it is known that more than one cutaneous nerve can be involved in the pain mechanism, that the first block be done proximal to the neuroma pain area, in which the two nerves overlap (2,8,9). For example, in the dorsoradial forearm, the lateral antebrachial cutaneous nerve should be blocked first in the volar forearm. After determining the extent of pain relief from this first block, the second block can be placed more distally in the dorsoradial forearm, realizing that this will block both the lateral antebrachial cutaneous

TABLE 46D-4. TREATMENT OF THE PAINFUL NEUROMA

- I. Nonoperative (first 6 months)
  - A. Steroid cream massage by patient into painful scar
  - B. Refer to a therapist
    - 1. Desensitization
    - 2. Ultrasound with scar massage
  - C. Steroid injection into scar, repeat A and B
- II. Operative (after 6 months of pain not relieved by I above)
  - A. Identify correctly the nerve that is the source of the pain
    - 1. Use known anatomy
    - 2. Use differential nerve blocks
  - B. Intraoperatively
    - 1. Resect the neuroma
    - 2. Implant the proximal nerve end into muscle

nerve and the radial sensory nerve. A second area in which this potential for choosing the "wrong" nerve or not enough "right" nerves to resect is the dorsum of the foot. In this region, the saphenous nerve and the superficial and deep peroneal nerves, medially, and superficial peroneal nerve and the sural nerve, laterally, can overlap; all can be involved in the pain mechanism (10–12). Because the sensory nuclei of the peripheral nerve fibers that are transmitting the pain message reside in the dorsal root ganglion, no known treatment to the distal end of the divided nerve can prevent neural regeneration. At the time of neuroma resection, it is critical to place the proximal end of the divided nerve into an area where it will be free from pressure and movement. This almost always dictates that the nerve be translocated away from joints and tendons and that it be placed deeply. It has been demonstrated that a divided sensory nerve placed into normally innervated muscle will not form a classic end-bulb neuroma (13). Instead, the nerve sprouts, encounters no nerve growth factor from the divided distal stump's Schwann cells, encounters no denervated sensory end-organs awaiting reinnervation, and stops regenerating. The nerve must be placed loosely into the muscle and the adjacent joints taken through a full range of motion, demonstrating the nerve will not pull out of the muscle (14,15). The nerve does not need to be sutured into the muscle. If a stitch is used, it should be placed only through the epineurium. If the stitch is placed through the nerve itself, a new nerve injury will be produced.

PLACING TRACTION ON THE NERVE

Prevention

Wound closure must be done under sufficient tension to accomplish the purpose of the surgery. Usually, we attempt to close wounds with minimal tension to ensure that the scar will form under the most favorable circumstances and that the circulation to the skin will not be compromised. However, there are circumstances where tension not only is unavoidable but is the desired outcome. In facial rejuvenation surgery, the reshaped skin must be placed under some degree of tension; in flap closure of soft tissue defects, the flap's distal edge often is under tension. If cutaneous nerves that are pulled tightly by this flap tension, the patient may experience postoperative pain or paresthesias in the distribution of these nerves.

Given that tension will be required in certain wound closures, what can the surgeon do? In general, a nerve can be stretched about 15% acutely before it stops functioning. Most often, this is sufficient for the skin to stretch without drawing a cutaneous nerve out of position. The surgeon in facelift procedures must attempt to leave the greater auricular nerve on the sternocleidomastoid muscle so that it is not redraped or stretched with the facial skin flap. If the supraorbital nerve is viewed to be under tension in the browlift, either the degree of lift must be reduced or an attempt must be made to loosen the nerve within the supraorbital notch.

When flaps are draped in relationship to major nerves, such as the peroneal nerve at the knee or the ulnar nerve at the elbow, the flap rotation must be done such that tension on the nerve is avoided. If it is clear that this will be a problem, then the peroneal nerve can be decompressed as it crosses the fibular neck by incising the peroneus longus fascia (14,16). There may be a wide fibrous band deep to the peroneus longus muscle as well, and this should evaluated. For the ulnar nerve at the elbow, a submuscular transposition may be necessary (17,18). The plastic surgeon involved in limb lengthening or mandibular distraction must be aware that stretching of the peripheral nerve will result in pain. In the literature on lower extremity limb lengthening, up to 30% of patients required decompression of the peroneal or tibial nerves. Monitoring the cutaneous pressure threshold of the lip, thumb, dorsum of the foot, or plantar aspect of the big toe can identify when nerve dysfunction is beginning. The rate of distraction can be slowed accordingly. The device that performs this function, the Pressure-Specified Sensory Device™ (Sensory Management Services, LLC, Baltimore, MD), can be used to monitor any peripheral nerve function (7,19). The limb lengthening group at Kernan's Hospital, University of Maryland, has reduced their nerve decompressions to zero during this last year as the result of monitoring each patient with this type of quantitative sensory testing (A. Bhave, J. Herzenberg, D. Paley, presentation at the 1999 American Society for Peripheral Nerve Meeting).

Treatment

If the patient has postoperative pain that seems to be related to traction on a nerve, the decision must be made whether to follow this situation and hope that, with time, the normal stretch/relaxation curve will reduce the tension, or to approach the problem surgically. The nonoperative approach to follow is identical to that described in Table 46D-4, with appropriate regional modifications.

If the pain does not diminish sufficiently or disappear by 6 months and there is no concern about diminished motor function, then the nerve may be approached surgically as described in Table 46D-4 for cutaneous neuroma. If critical function is lost and exploration of the nerve reveals a severe stretch/traction injury with no electrical activity that will pass across this segment of the nerve, then this region should be excised and a nerve graft reconstruction done (20). If the nerve has critical sensory or motor function, decompression of the nerve is appropriate. An example relates to anterolateral thigh pain following an abdominal or groin procedure. The lateral femoral cutaneous nerve has sufficient variability that the nerve can be expected to be located adjacent to the anterior superior iliac crest and within the inguinal ligament in at least one-third of patients (21). The physical examination will have a positive Tinel sign at this area, or at least pressure in this area will cause pain on the affected side but not on the contralateral side. Neurolysis of the lateral femoral cutaneous nerve from the internal oblique to the thigh fascia is the indicated treatment (22). Another example is the patient who awakens from cardiac bypass surgery with an ulnar or median nerve compression, or the patient who awakens from a total hip or knee arthroplasty with peroneal nerve palsy. Because sensory function will return before motor function, quantitative sensory testing using the Pressure-Specified Sensory Device, measuring one-point moving, one-point static, two-point moving and then two-point static touch, will identify a nerve regeneration pattern (7). If this pattern is present, then recovery of motor function can be predicted. If this pattern is not present, then the nerve should be decompressed (A.L. Dellon, presentation at the 1998 American Society for Peripheral Nerve Meeting).

CUTTING A MAJOR SENSORY OR MOTOR NERVE

Prevention

Knowledge of anatomy should prevent the occurrence of this complication. Sometimes because of a new technology such as the endoscope, a major nerve, such as the median or ulnar nerve, is cut. Sometimes because of previous surgery in the area, the major nerve is not where the surgeon thought it would be. For this latter situation, the surgeon should be using loupe magnification and intraoperative electrical stimulation. The anesthesiologist should be instructed not to use paralytic agents after induction of anesthesia.

Treatment

The divided nerve should be repaired using microsurgical technique as soon as the complication is recognized. If the surgeon is aware that the nerve has been divided at the time it was divided, then the nerve should be divided at that time. This occurrence should be recorded in the operative notes and the patient notified that the event occurred. Appropriate postoperative rehabilitation for the specific repaired nerve should be instituted (7).

MISDIAGNOSIS OF RECURRENT CARPAL TUNNEL SYNDROME

Prevention

In my experience, the most common area for this problem is related to carpal tunnel syndrome. Carpal tunnel decompression is a very common procedure in the United States. This implies that a number of patients will be back to see their doctor with "recurrent" or "persistent" symptoms. In my experience, the only carpal tunnel syndromes that have recurred have been related to recurrent tenosynovitis, such as occurs in patients with rheumatoid arthritis, or in patients who fell and caused direct trauma to the carpal tunnel. This surgery usually is so successful that the plastic surgeon should immediately consider a diagnosis other than recurrent or persistent carpal tunnel syndrome as the correct diagnosis. The two most common "other diagnoses" are entrapment of the radial sensory (23) nerve and pronator syndrome. The best way to identify these syndromes is not with traditional electrodiagnostic studies, which, in my experience, have a false-negative rate greater than 75% for these diagnoses.

The pronator syndrome can be identified by manual muscle testing, looking for anomalous relationships between the pronator teres, lacertus fibrosis, and flexor superficialis with the median nerve, which travels between or beneath potentially fibrous arcades (24). Quantitative sensory testing with the Pressure-Specified Sensory Device over the thenar eminence also can identify the pronator syndrome (D. Rosenberg, J. Connolly, A.L. Dellon, presentation of the 2000 American Society for Surgery of the Hand Meeting). This is because the palmar cutaneous branch of the median nerve, which innervates this area, arises from the median nerve proximal to the carpal tunnel, and proximal median nerve compression can cause dysfunction of this skin area.

Radial sensory nerve entrapment can be identified by a positive Tinel sign in the forearm, usually located adjacent to where the brachioradialis tendon inserts into the radius. It also can be identified by a positive stretch/traction sign along the course of the radial sensory nerve (the same physical examination as a positive Finkelstein sign) or by worsening of the patient's symptoms with forearm pronation (14,23). It can be documented with quantitative sensory testing that demonstrates an elevated cutaneous pressure threshold over the dorsoradial aspect of the hand (7).

Treatment

Clearly, if the pronator syndrome or radial sensory nerve entrapment is identified in the patient who returns to the physician with complaints of "recurrent carpal tunnel syndrome," then these nerve compressions should be treated rather than reoperating on the median nerve at the wrist. The technique for these decompressions has been described elsewhere (14).

MISDIAGNOSIS: POOR RESULT AFTER NERVE REPAIR

Prevention

The reason I consider a poor result after a nerve repair to be a misdiagnosis is because the correct diagnosis is a "neuroma-in-continuity." Many explanations have been given for a poor result after nerve repair, such as the patient's age, the delay between nerve injury and the repair, the location of the nerve injury, and an avulsion injury instead of a clean laceration (25). However, the most likely reason a nerve repair gives a poor result is because the two ends of the nerve that were joined still contained injured nerve segments. The most neglected technique in peripheral nerve surgery is resection of damaged nerve tissue (26). Resection of this damaged nerve tissue is the best way to prevent a poor result from a nerve repair.

Why is this misdiagnosis not routinely prevented? Most nerve repairs are done within a few days of the nerve injury; therefore, the surgeon cannot know, even when he or she examines the injured nerve with magnification, how much of that nerve will produce scar tissue. Experimental studies demonstrated that it is usually 3 weeks after the injury before the surgeon can examine the nerve and resect it appropriately to remove all the damaged tissue (27,28). If the injury was made with a thin knife, probably a few millimeters of resection is sufficient. If the injury was made with a ¼-inch saw blade, perhaps 1 cm needs to be resected. If the injury involved an avulsion, the true extent cannot be estimated. In this case, the surgeon doing the primary repair, not wanting to do a primary nerve graft to replace the needed neural tissue, which can only be approximated, does not resect enough tissue. The result is neural regeneration into an area of tension that produces a painful neuroma-in-continuity with poor distal regeneration—a poor result.

Today this problem can be prevented by resecting the length of tissue expected to be damaged based on the mechanism of injury. The defect to be reconstructed primarily does not need to be an autologous nerve graft. For almost 2 decades there has been a search for a bioabsorbable nerve guide that could be placed between the two ends of a nerve. This would facilitate regeneration and then the tube would be resorbed, leaving an intact nerve between the two divided ends. Clinical work with such a tube was first reported in 1990 in a small series of patients (14,29,30). In March 1999, the United States Food and Drug Administration approved the Neurotube™ (NeuroRegen, LLC, Bel Air, MD) for use. This is a bioabsorbable conduit made of polyglycolic acid. The results of a randomized prospective study comparing the use of this tube to a primary nerve repair was presented to the American Association of Plastic Surgery at its 1999 meeting. This study demonstrated that the Neurotube gave statistically significantly more patients excellent results and statistically significantly more patients a lower (better) two-point discrimination than did the primary repair of a divided digital nerve (31). The Neurotube is permitted for nerve defects up to 3 cm. Use of this device will permit sufficient resection of injured nerve at the time of primary repair, such that most of the poor results of nerve repair hopefully can be prevented.

Treatment

Treatment of the poor result of nerve repair is resection of the neuroma-in-continuity. The nerve reconstruction can be achieved with a traditional interposition interfascicular autologous nerve graft or, if the resultant nerve defect is smaller than 3 cm, with one or more Neurotubes. The results of the prospective randomized peripheral nerve study also demonstrated that for nerve defects larger than 7 mm, the Neurotube gave statistically significantly more patients excellent results and statistically significantly more patients a lower (better) two-point discrimination than did a nerve graft of the defect (31). In addition to achieving superior results for the nerve reconstruction, the Neurotube permits nerve reconstruction without the need to create a nerve graft donor site or a new nerve deficit with its own potential to become a source of pain.

REFERENCES

1. Dellon AL, Mackinnon SE. Susceptibility of the superficial sensory branch of the radial nerve to form painful neuromas. *J Hand Surg* 1984;9B:42–45.
2. Saplys R, Mackinnon SE, Dellon AL. The relationship between nerve entrapment versus neuroma complications and the misdiagnosis of deQuervain's disease. *Contemp Orthop* 1987; 15:51–57
3. Naff N, Dellon AL, Mackinnon SE. The anatomic course of the palmar cutaneous branch of the median nerve, including a description of its own unique tunnel. *J Hand Surg* 1993;18B: 316–317.
4. Dellon AL, Mackinnon SE. Injury to the medial antebrachial cutaneous nerve during cubital tunnel surgery. *J Hand Surg* 1985;10B:33–36.
5. Liszka TG, Dellon AL, Manson PN. Iliohypogastric nerve entrapment following abdominoplasty. *Plast Reconstr Surg* 1994; 93:181–184.
6. Mackinnon SE, Dellon AL. Algorithm for neuroma management. *Contemp Orthop* 1986;13:15–27.
7. Dellon AL. *Somatosensory testing and rehabilitation.* Bethesda, MD: American Occupational Therapy Association, 1997.
8. Mackinnon SE, Dellon AL. Overlap of lateral antebrachial cutaneous nerve and superficial sensory branch of the radial nerve. *J Hand Surg* 1985;10A:522–526.
9. Mackinnon SE, Dellon AL. Results of treatment of recurrent dorsoradial wrist neuromas. *Ann Plast Surg* 1987;19:54–61.
10. Coert JH, Dellon AL. Clinical implications of the surgical anatomy of the sural nerve. *Plast Reconstr Surg* 1994;94:850–855.
11. Aszmann OC, Ebmer JM, Dellon AL. The cutaneous innervation of the medial ankle: an anatomic study of the saphenous, sural and tibial nerve and their clinical significance. *Foot Ankle* 1998;19:753–756.
12. Dellon AL, Aszmann OC. Treatment of dorsal foot neuromas by translocation of nerves into anterolateral compartment. *Foot Ankle* 1998;19:300–303.
13. Dellon AL, Mackinnon SE. Treatment of the painful neuroma by neuroma resection and muscle implantation. *Plast Reconstr Surg* 1986;77:427–436.
14. Mackinnon SE, Dellon AL. *Surgery of the Peripheral Nerve.* New York: Thieme, 1988.
15. Evans GRD, Dellon AL. Implantation of the palmar cutaneous branch of the median nerve into the pronator quadratus

for treatment of painful neuroma. *J Hand Surg* 1994;19A: 203–206.
16. Mont MA, Dellon AL, Chen F, et al. Operative treatment of peroneal nerve palsy. *J Bone Joint Surg* 1996;78A:863–869.
17. Dellon AL. Operative technique for submuscular transposition of the ulnar nerve. *Contemp Orthop* 1988;16:17–24.
18. Dellon AL: Techniques for successful management of ulnar nerve entrapment at the elbow. *Neurosurg Clin North Am* 1991;2: 57–73.
19. Dellon AL. Management of peripheral nerve problems with quantitative sensory testing in the upper and lower extremity. *Hand Clin* 1999;15:697–715.
20. Campbell J, Dellon AL. Traction injury to the spinal accessory nerve. *J Neurosurg* 1990;72:500–502.
20. Aszmann OC, Dellon ES, Dellon AL. The anatomic course of the lateral femoral cutaneous nerve and its susceptibility to compression and injury. *Plast Reconstr Surg* 1997;100:600–604.
22. Nahabedian MY, Dellon AL. Meralgia paresthetica: etiology, diagnosis and outcome of surgical management. *Ann Plast Surg* 1995;35:590–594.
23. Dellon AL, Mackinnon SE. Radial sensory nerve entrapment in the forearm. *J Hand Surg* 1986;11A:199–205.
24. Dellon AL, Mackinnon SE. Musculoaponeurotic variations along the course of the median nerve in the proximal forearm. *J Hand Surg* 1987;12B:359–363.
25. Dellon AL. Sensory recovery in replanted digits and transplanted toes. *J Reconstr Microsurg* 1986;2:123–129.
26. Dellon AL. Resection: nerve repair's most neglected technique. *Plast Surg Tech* 1995;1:191–199.
27. Zachary LS, Dellon AL. Progression of the zone of injury in experimental nerve injuries. *Microsurgery* 1987;8:182–185.
28. Zachary LS, Dellon AL, Seiler WA IV. Relationship of intraneural damage in the rat sciatic nerve to the mechanism of injury. *J Reconstr Microsurg* 1989;5:137–140.
29. Mackinnon SE, Dellon AL. Clinical nerve reconstruction with a bioabsorbable polyglycolic acid tube. *Plast Reconstr Surg* 1990; 85:419–424.
30. Crawley WA, Dellon AL. Inferior alveolar nerve reconstruction with a polyglycolic acid, bioabsorbable nerve conduit: a case report. *Plast Reconstr Surg* 1992;90:300–302.
31. Weber RA, Breidenbach WC, Brown RE, Jabaley ME, Mass DP. A randomized study of polyglycolic acid conduits for digital nerve reconstruction in humans. *Plast Reconstr Surg* 2000; 106:1036–1045.

47

REPLANTATION, REVASCULARIZATION AND TOE-TO-HAND TRANSPLANTS

HARRY J. BUNCKE
GREGORY M. BUNCKE
GABRIEL M. KIND
RUDOLF F. BUNTIC

REVASCULARIZATION

Microvascular transplantation of the large toe to replace the thumb, or the second toe to replace single or multiple digits, is now a common form of reconstruction. Although toe transplantation can be one of the most rewarding procedures in upper extremity reconstruction, it is one of the most technically demanding microsurgical transplants. Both harvesting of the flap and inset of the toe on the hand are fraught with operative nuances and hazards that can lead to less than favorable results. In addition to surgical factors, postoperative monitoring, splinting, and therapy are important elements of the reconstruction that can improve outcome or adversely affect results if neglected. Anticipating potential problems, accurate monitoring, and early action when difficulties are encountered can help the surgeon avoid unfavorable results and greatly improve both patient and surgeon satisfaction for the procedure (1).

GREAT TOE TRANSPLANTATION

Flap Loss

Of course, the most unfavorable result is the total loss of the transplant. Fortunately, this is a rare occurrence (Fig. 47-1). Meticulous preoperative planning and careful attention to microsurgery principles are essential to avoiding flap failure. Bone synostosis or joint reconstruction and skin flaps all can be planned preoperatively using clay models of the anticipated transplant. The position of the vascular pedicle, tendon, nerve, and vessel repairs can be prepared for before surgery. This is particularly important with multiple toe transplants, because the vascular pedicles may dictate that the toes be removed from the right or the left foot. Preliminary transplants of skin, muscle, or bone may be needed to prepare the platform for the elective toe transplant.

Even with excellent planning and technique, failure does occur. In our experience with 129 great toe transplants, only four failed entirely, with a survival rate of 96.9%. Similar results can be expected with single and multiple transplants of the lesser toes. Only 3.9% have been lost in our experience with 130 second toe transplants.

Complete failure may require amputation with closure of the surgical stump, but occasionally a failing large toe transplant can be partially salvaged, covering the proximal phalanx with a tubed pedicle to preserve function and length. Tubed pedicles and bone grafts were the only method available for thumb reconstruction before the era of microsurgery and still can be valuable tools. A neurovascular island transfer from the ring finger can follow a tube flap to provide sensation on the volar surface of the lost distal transplant (Fig. 47-1B–F).

Tendon adhesions, joint ankylosis, and poor sensation, alone or in combination, can produce an unsatisfactory result. Fortunately, all of these problems can be corrected or partially corrected by secondary surgeries, which are not uncommon with toe transplants. More than 30% of our patient with great toe-to-thumb transplants require secondary operations. There are measures that can be taken during the initial procedure that help to minimize these problems or help the surgeon prepare for future reconstruction (2,3).

H. J. Buncke, G. M. Buncke, G. M. Kind, and R. F. Buntic: The Buncke Clinic, San Francisco, California

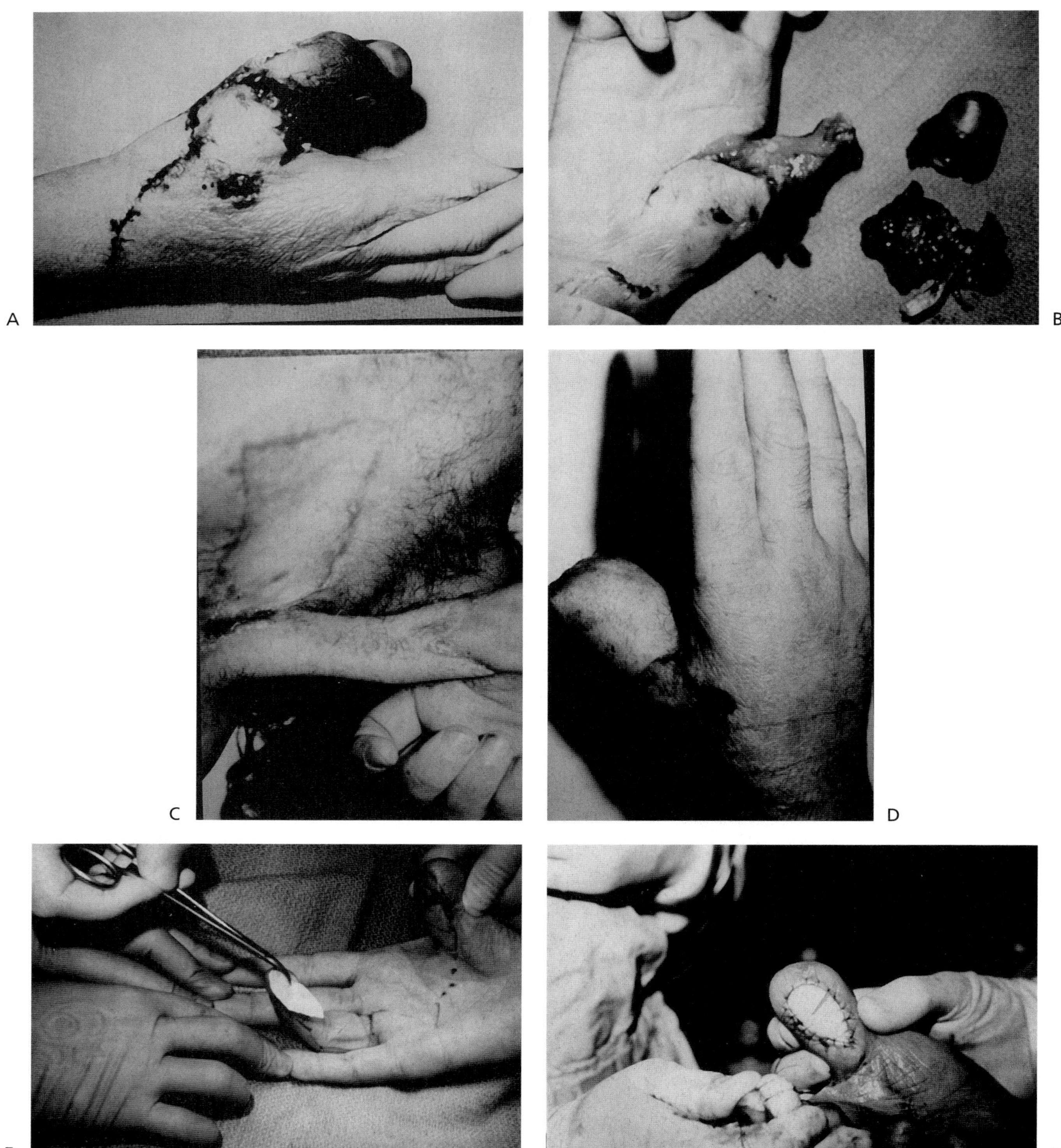

FIGURE 47-1. A: Failed great toe transplant. **B:** The necrotic tissue was debrided to viable proximal phalanx. **C,D:** An abdominal tube pedicle was formed to cover the open wound. **E,F:** A neurovascular island flap from the ring finger was designed and inset onto the reconstructed thumb to provide sensation.

Failure of Function

Osteosynthesis

A surviving transplant does not necessarily predict good function. Poor function may be related to a number of problems, including an improper anatomical position. The toe must be pronated into appropriate opposition with an adequate web space to permit grasping of large objects. Although intraoperative x-ray films can be helpful, we have found fluoroscopy more valuable. The portable Fluoroscan (Fluoroscan Imaging Systems, Northbrook, IL) machine gives multiple views of an osteosynthesis site, so that small angulation in any plane can be seen and corrected. Similar to hand fractures, angulation or rotation of the bone can be magnified markedly when thumb flexion and opposition are achieved. After bone fixation is performed, the thumb must be manually manipulated by the surgeon: adduction, abduction, opposition, flexion, and extension are tested to assure normal thumb orientation. Considerable time is spent correctly aligning the toe. Rushing through the positioning of the transplant and bone fixation are not necessary, because the toe can tolerate several hours of warm ischemia quite easily. If the position is incorrect, then immediate consideration should be given to repositioning the toe if possible, because often this can be more difficult to do later. After microvascular repairs are performed, any correction of bone malalignment can result in arterial or venous injury and should be avoided.

Bone fixation can be achieved with K-wires, screws, or plates. Bone contact needs to be solid to decrease the chance of nonunion. A single four-cortical screw fixation of the native thumb proximal phalanx embedded into the toe proximal phalanx is an excellent choice when anatomy allows. It requires minimal subperiosteal dissection and leaves joints free for early motion.

After adequate fixation is achieved, the flexor tendon is repaired, followed by microsurgical arterial repair. The hand is repositioned for the venous and extensor tendon repair, and finally the nerve repairs and skin closure.

Tendon Rupture

Rupture of the flexor and extensor tendons is uncommon. Sound intraoperative repairs are necessary to lessen the chance of rupture. The flexor tendon is repaired with a Pulvertaft-type weave if adequate tendon is available to perform the repair in the wrist. Harvesting the flexor hallucis tendon at the ankle allows repair at the wrist level, where tendon glide will be superior to that achieved in zone II (Fig. 47-2). If a tendon ruptures in zone II or III in the postoperative period, repair may be difficult and may endanger vessel or nerve anastomoses. If repair must be done in the hand or flexor sheath, then a standard type of flexor tendon repair is performed, often with epitendinous suturing.

Adequate tendon usually is available to perform extensor tendon repair with a Pulvertaft weave; therefore, extensor rupture is unlikely in this setting.

A neutral position usually is required to balance flexor and extensor tendon tension and to optimally position blood vessels and avoid kinking.

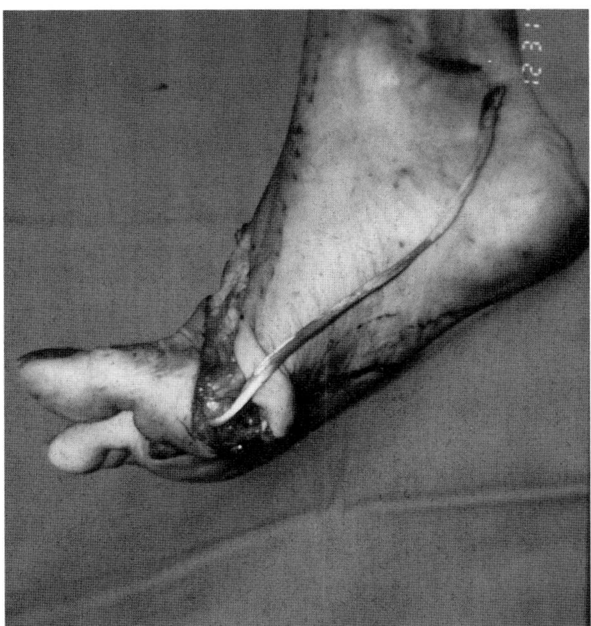
A

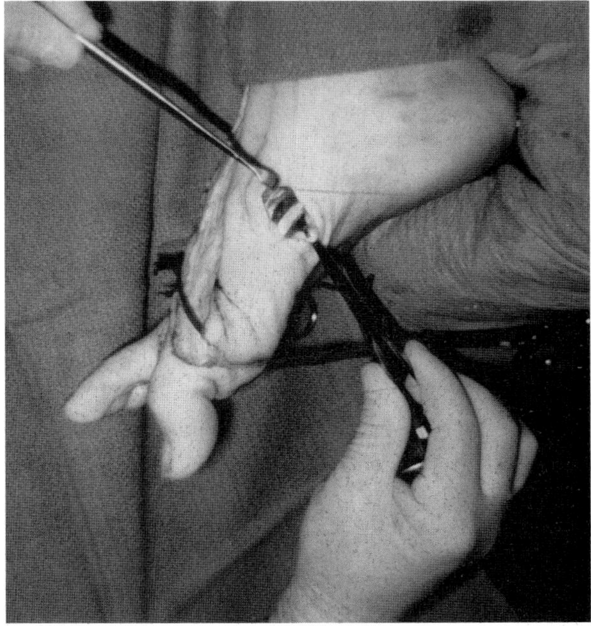
B

FIGURE 47-2. Additional length on the great toe flexor tendon can be achieved by a stair step incision on the medial plantar surface **(A)** or just posterior to the medial malleolus **(B)**.

Tendon Adhesion

Tendon adhesion to some degree is inevitable, because transected and repaired tendons will scar in the healing process. However, steps can be taken to minimize the extent of adhesion and later to lyse adhesions, if necessary. As mentioned previously, a long flexor tendon is harvested with the toe so that tendon repair is not performed in zone II. If flexor tendon adhesion becomes a problem, flexor tenolysis is performed in the wrist within 2 to 4 months of the initial operation to facilitate tendon glide. If tenolysis is performed near the inflow artery, as often is necessary, injury to the digital artery may result in arterial insufficiency even if many months have passed. Microsurgical arterial repair is indicated in this circumstance and necessitates postoperative splinting and immobilization. Tendon adhesion will recur in this case. We have not had the misfortune of losing a toe at this stage of the reconstruction.

Loss of passive interphalangeal (IP) or metacarpophalangeal (MP) flexion due to extensor tendon adhesion is common and needs further surgical treatment if it is unresponsive to hand therapy. If passive range of motion is restricted at these joints, extensor tenolysis and dorsal capsulotomy, sometimes with excision of the dorsal collateral ligaments, can significantly improve passive range of motion. This usually is carried out before flexor tenolysis is performed. Simultaneous flexor and extensor tenolysis are avoided to minimize edema and resulting stiffness.

Poor Joint Motion

The toe metatarsophalangeal joint is an extension joint and flexes poorly. Using this joint is avoided if possible, but it may be needed if the first metacarpal is missing. The IP joints can become stiff and are affected by prolonged immobilization and extensor tendon adhesion. Intrinsic joint stiffness can be affected by patient age or lack of use. Plate fixation during the osteosynthesis, with early motion and therapy, can help minimize stiffness and result in more supple joint motion. If this fails, secondary surgery may be required to tenolyse the extensor tendon and release the dorsal joint capsule or dorsal collateral ligaments to improve range of motion of joints.

On rare occasions, joints in the transplant must be replaced with Silastic or other types of prostheses. Patient age and potential demand on the hand are considered when investigating this option.

Even when good joint and tendon motion is present, full function can be compromised by a tight first web space,

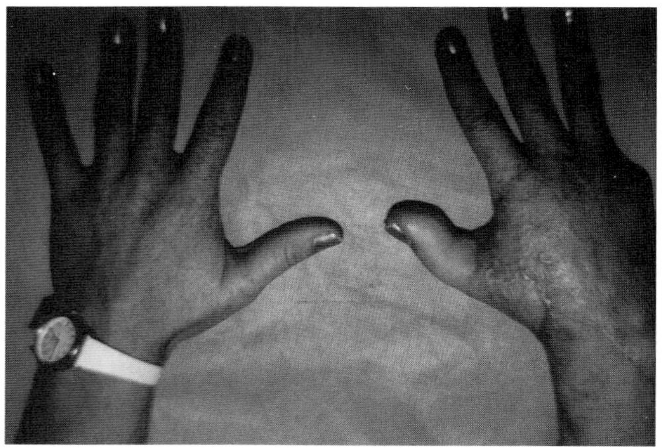

A

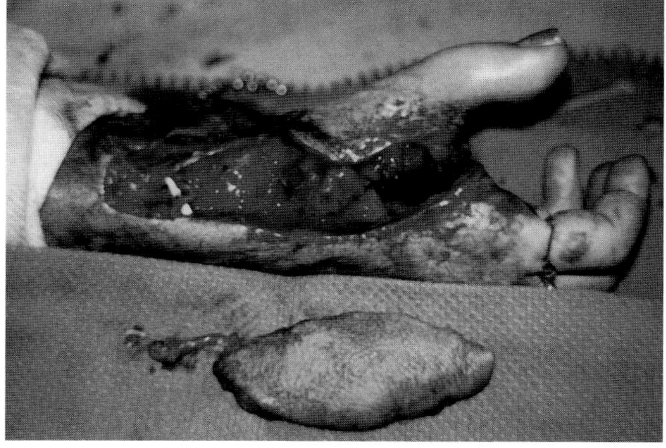

B

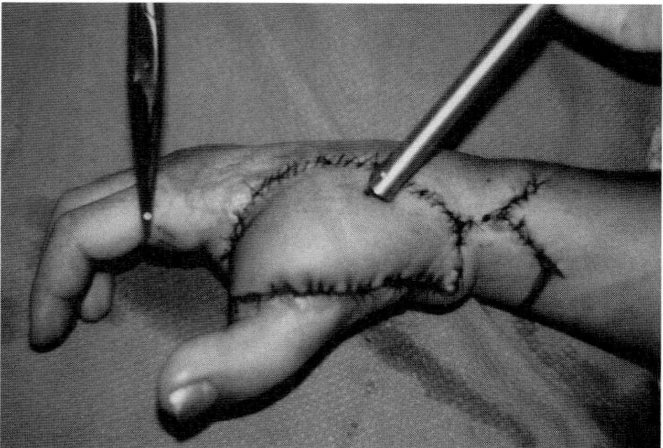

C

FIGURE 47-3. A 30-year-old woman developed a first web space contracture after a crush injury and great toe to thumb reconstruction. A lateral arm flap from the opposite arm was used to widen the first web space and fill the web with supple tissue.

which fortunately can be corrected with an additional microvascular transplant. In our hands, the lateral arm flap is the best choice (Fig. 47-3).

Poor Sensation

Most transplants regain useful sensation, with 5 to 6 mm of two-point discrimination, or at least protective sensation. Absence of sensation return can be a frustrating problem, because return of feeling is the most important factor in making the transplanted digit useful to the patient. The initial underlying reason for toe transplantation may play a role in the poor outcome. Sharp amputation injuries where clearly normal nerves are repaired to the transplanted toe should, in the majority of cases, develop good sensation. However, when the underlying diagnosis was a crush or avulsion injury, the proximal nerve may have been more severely affected. Proximal nerve can be resected to "snails eyes," where healthy nerve ends are sprouting. If this requires resection of proximal nerve to the point where nerve grafting is necessary, this is more desirable than finding later that the toe does not develop sensation. The foot has ample nerve graft available in the toe harvest wound: both the terminal deep peroneal nerve and terminal branches of the superficial peroneal are available and are good choices as donors. Using this approach, only in a small percentage of cases are secondary neurolyses and nerve grafts required. When the digital nerves have been avulsed from the median nerve back to the wrist, primary repair may not be possible, even with long nerve grafts. In this instance, the radial digital nerve can be anastomosed to the dorsal radial sensory nerve and the ulnar digital nerve to one-half of the ulnar digital nerve to the index.

CONSIDERATIONS IN SECOND TOE TRANSPLANTATION

Second or third toe transplantation has unique aspects differentiating this procedure from great toe transplantation. In Asia, the second toe is more commonly used to reconstruct the thumb, because the large toe is needed to wear zori slippers. In the United States, second toe transplants usually are used to reconstruct the index through small fingers. In second toe transplantation, all the pitfalls of great toe to thumb reconstruction can be seen and have been discussed earlier. However, using a second toe in thumb and finger reconstruction differs considerably from great toe transplantation and requires attention to several unique aspects of this procedure (4).

Flap Loss

The failure rate for our second toe transplants has been 3.9%. All the elements of flap harvesting and careful technique required in a microsurgical procedure are especially applicable to this difficult procedure. A tubed pedicle or cross-finger flap can be used to salvage length in a failed second toe, which then can be used to hold a prosthesis.

Second Toe for Thumb Reconstruction, Appearance, and Flexion Contracture

Choosing a second toe transplant for thumb reconstruction has many disadvantages that lead to unfavorable results inherent in the toe anatomy itself. These are a trade-off for saving the great toe and must be considered with each patient's needs specifically in mind.

Aesthetically, the second toe is less pleasing (Fig. 47-4). It does not resemble the thumb to the extent that a great toe does: the nail is smaller, the distal phalanx is not as prominent with less volar pulp volume, and the second toe has two IP joints rather than one. The toe also has a tendency to develop a flexion contracture. The appearance of this can be quite bizarre and limits thumb function to a greater degree than a single IP flexion contracture. To avoid an early postoperative flexed position and later contracture, care must be taken not to repair the extensor tendon with too much laxity. Rather, tension by the extensor pollicis longus tendon needs to be maintained on the reconstructed thumb. The toe also is K-wired with a single wire to keep the proximal and distal IP joints in full extension. This can cause some joint stiffness that is better than flexion contractures.

Anatomical Position and Osteosynthesis

The positioning of the second toe transplant when reconstructing the index through small fingers is less complex than thumb reconstruction. One need only consider flexion and extension of the MP and IP joints, rather than the variable positioning of the thumb saddle joint and need for opposition. Nevertheless, poor anatomical position is easy to

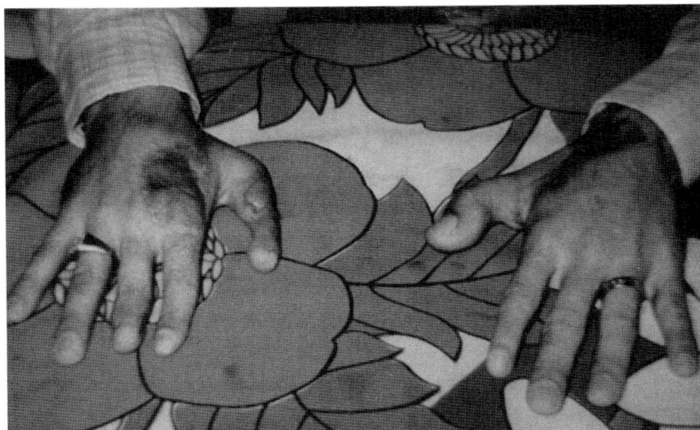

FIGURE 47-4. Patient who had a second toe transplant to the right thumb and a great toe transplant to the left thumb after bilateral thumb amputations. The great toe is both cosmetically more appealing but also more like a true thumb in function.

achieve and requires great care to avoid. Similar to hand fractures, angulation or rotation of the bone can be magnified markedly when flexion is achieved. The transplanted toe is checked in flexion and extension to ensure normal anatomical position, and only after adequate fixation is achieved are the tendons repaired, followed by microsurgical repair.

Bone fixation can be achieved with K-wires, screws, or plates. Four-cortical screw fixation is more difficult to achieve in a second toe transplant, and we favor K-wires and plating. The IP joints often are pinned in extension to minimize tension on the tendon repairs and to prevent flexion contracture. If the extensor tendons are not balanced appropriately, an extensor lag of the IP joints can result. After checking the position in flexion and extension and using fluoroscopy to ensure adequate bone alignment and hardware placement, tendon and vessel repair can proceed with all the considerations noted for great toe transplants.

Unfavorable results, such as loss of transplant, tendon rupture, poor joint motion, and poor sensory recovery, are treated similarly in second toe transplants as in great toes.

DONOR SITE DIFFICULTY

Donor site complications and problems can lead to an unfavorable result. The most common difficulty is delay in healing over the first metatarsal head. This usually is caused by taking too much skin with the toe transplant or trying to preserve the entire first metatarsal head (Fig. 47-5). Because most of the weight is transferred to the lateral four metatarsal heads after removal of the large toe, the first metatarsal head can be shaved down considerably in its dorsal and tibial sides to reduce bulk and permit closure without tension.

Wound complications from the second toe harvest site are fewer in number because skin flaps created in the donor dissection are smaller. Adequate proximal resection of the second metatarsal must be performed to minimize wound tension at closure. Much of the remaining tension can be removed by approximating the deep transverse metatarsal ligament with the heads of the first and third metatarsals. When there is little tension, complications are minimized in the routine postoperative patient.

Patients with vascular complications in the transplanted toe requiring heparin tend to have more difficulty with delayed healing in the foot. Hemorrhage into the donor wound with resultant edema and ecchymosis generally is greater, requiring longer-term foot elevation and delayed rehabilitation.

Neuroma pain on the plantar surface of the donor area can occur. This usually results when the plantar nerves are not transected far enough back from the metatarsal heads and the neuroma of healing becomes trapped in the weight-bearing area. Treatment consists of secondary mobilization and proximal transposition of the excised neuroma stump. Painful neuromas of the terminal branches of the superficial peroneal nerve can be a problem and are treated in a similar fashion.

Hypertrophic and unstable scars can develop, particularly after prolonged secondary healing. These usually are re-

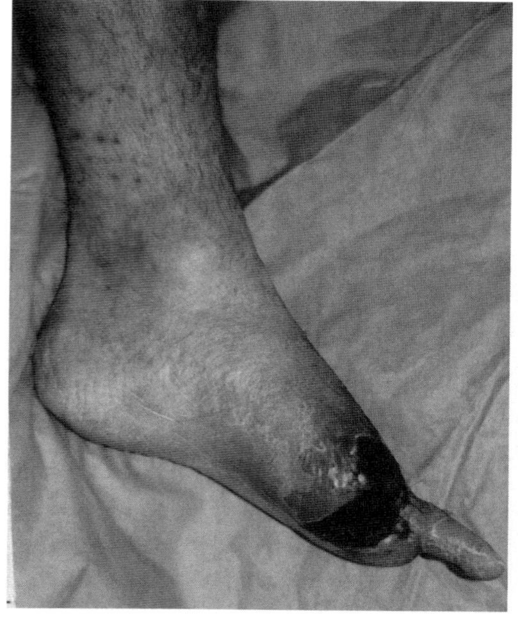

A

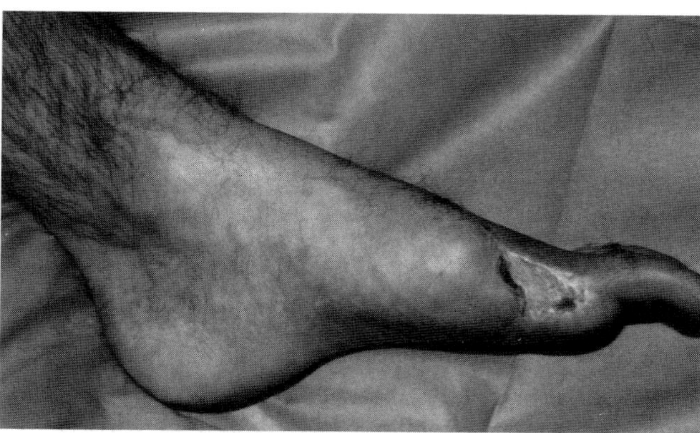

B

FIGURE 47-5. A 34-year-old man developed necrosis of the skin flap raised at the donor site of a great toe transplant. After shortening the first metacarpal, the donor site was closed and skin grafted.

vised with scar excision and skin grafts and, in rare instances, with a second microvascular skin flap or muscle flap.

OTHER FACTORS

One of the rarest unfavorable results occurs when a patient fails to use the transplant, despite a good anatomical position and acceptable function of the tendons, joints, and nerves. This may occur because of poor patient compliance, lack of patient understanding of the overall goals of the operation, or other personal gain factors of which the patient is not consciously aware or perhaps does not reveal. Self-mutilation and Munchausen syndrome are the ultimate unfavorable results after toe transplantation procedures.

At its best, reconstruction of the thumb, or single or multiple digits by toe transplant, is an excellent procedure that restores function to an otherwise compromised hand. There are some centers that believe the large toe is too great a sacrifice in terms of foot function, and second toes are preferred. In our experience with careful postoperative gait analysis, loss of the large toe is not a severe handicap. Most patients live a perfectly normal existence, participating in a wide variety of sports and physical activities. With careful planning and compulsive attention to detail, results of toe transplantation can be excellent.

REPLANTATION

The successful replantation of an amputated part is a dramatic demonstration of a "miracle" of modern medicine. Such a procedure involves the repair of every structure of the involved part. Depending on the mechanism of injury, the trauma can extend a great distance from both sides of the amputation site. A successful result from a replantation involves not just the restoration of blood flow to the part, but also the successful healing and return to function of all involved structures.

The most obvious unfavorable result following replantation is the early postoperative failure of the part to survive. Preoperative evaluation of both the amputated part and the patient is mandatory to decrease the likelihood of postoperative complications. Frequently other injuries are missed in the excitement of dealing with an amputated part (5). A careful history is mandatory to elucidate any significant medical history. Concurrent significant medical issues, peripheral vascular disease, hypercoagulopathy, and significant associated trauma are all relative contraindications to replantation. Furthermore, a careful description of the mechanism of injury itself may provide significant details that would affect intraoperative decision making. An amputated digit that appears to be relatively clean cut may have a significant crush or avulsion component. Such information is extremely useful during the preoperative discussion with the patient.

Thorough examination of the amputated part and the wound itself should be performed in the emergency room. We routinely discuss with the patient any possibilities other than replantation and amputation. For instance, local or tube pedicle flaps may be used to preserve the length of a digit in the setting of a nonreplantable digit with associated tissue loss. This is especially true for thumb amputations, in which length preservation is very important.

Once a replantation has been performed, the most common postoperative complication is vascular insufficiency. The importance of adequate microvascular debridement and replacement with vein grafts has long been recognized (6). Currently, most cases of postoperative vascular insufficiency are due to venous congestion, although loss of arterial inflow is not uncommon. If a replanted part becomes pale and cool with minimal bleeding following pinprick, arterial insufficiency can be presumed. Release of a constrictive dressing can be followed by the removal of several sutures. In a child especially, arterial insufficiency can be the result of vascular spasm. Application of topical agents, such as papaverine or lidocaine, can be done at the bedside after the removal of several sutures. A stellate or brachial block should be considered, if not already done. A decreased hematocrit may contribute to arterial spasm and should be corrected. If these interventions fail to restore arterial inflow, reexploration should be done if the replanted part is to be salvaged.

A replanted part that appears slightly swollen, with a slight purple tinge, has rapid capillary refill, and briskly bleeds dark red blood when poked with a needle can be presumed to have venous congestion. If this occurs in the early postoperative period and is not resolved with the release of constrictive dressings or sutures, then the best solution generally is reexploration. However, frequently a part will be replanted that will be found at the time of replantation to have few if any veins to repair. Reexploration in such cases will prove fruitless, and relief of venous congestion must be performed by some mechanical means. In the case of digital replantation, this is most commonly done by the removal of the distal two-thirds of the nail followed by medicinal leech therapy (Fig. 47-6) (7,8). Other replanted parts that frequently have poor venous outflow include acral parts, such as ears, lips, and noses. Leech therapy has been shown to help the survival of such parts, especially if instituted promptly after recognition of venous congestion (9–12). Once leech therapy is begun, patients should have antibiotic coverage to include *Aeromonas hydrophila* (13); we routinely use cefotaxime (Claforan). Using this antibiotic, we have not seen *Aeromonas* infection with leech use in our institution.

Heparin infusion is started at the time of the recognition of venous congestion. The heparin is titrated to the amount of bleeding from the replanted part, with the partial thromboplastin time (PTT) checked daily and kept at or below 1.5 times normal. Generally, the success of such therapy is re-

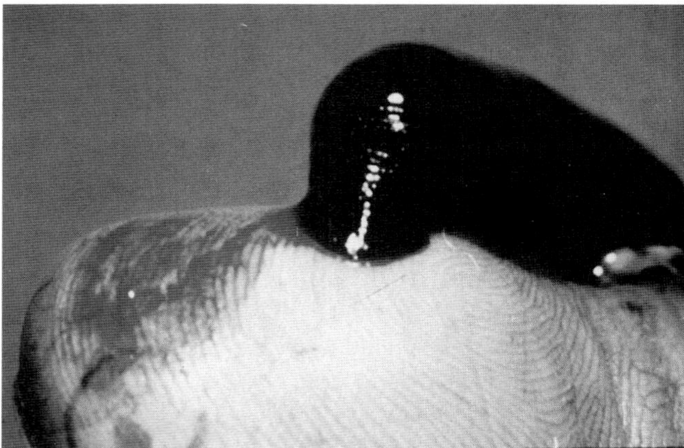

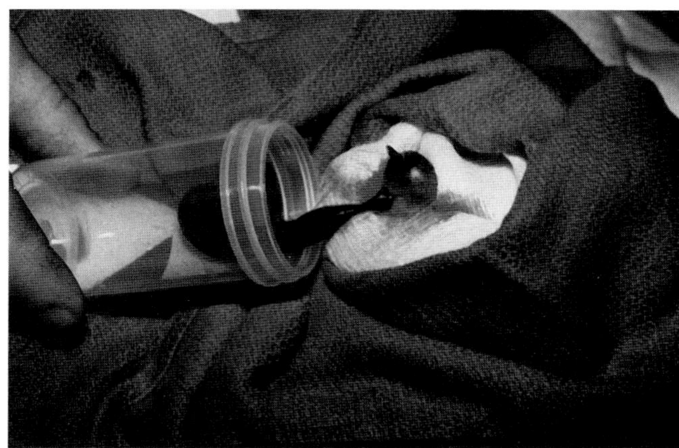

FIGURE 47-6. A,B: Medicinal leech therapy to a replanted digit.

lated to the degree of congestion present and the time at which it begins. Transient venous congestion occurring several days after replantation usually is overcome by such methods. However, as previously noted, venous congestion beginning in the early postoperative period is much more difficult to overcome and usually will requires a significant amount of blood loss before the amputated part develops a new intrinsic venous outflow system. The use of more than one anticoagulant increases the incidence of blood transfusion following digital replantation from 2% to 53% (14).

We have found the use of surface fluorometry to be the best postoperative monitoring system for replanted digits (15,16) and other parts with a cutaneous component (10). The fluorometer gives an objective reading of tissue perfusion and differentiates between arterial and venous insufficiency. Many other monitoring systems have been described and have been used with varying degrees of success (17–19).

The difficulty of digital replantation is reflected in the survival rates in reported series. Early large series demonstrated survival rates of approximately 80% (20–27), and more recent reports continue to have survival rates from 70% to 90% (28–30). This has occurred while the survival rates for microvascular transplantation of composite tissue has increased to 96% (31). One explanation is that although global microvascular skills have improved, the indications for replantation have widened and a greater number of severely traumatized digits are undergoing attempted replantation. In any event, any surgeon performing replantation must be able to deal with a failed replant. The management of such situations depends on the amount and location of tissue loss.

Loss of the border digits usually is adequately treated with amputation and closure. Loss of the long or ring fingers results in a significant deficit in grip, and consideration should be given to ray amputation (Figs. 47-7–47-9). In the case of multiple digital amputation where not all of the dig-

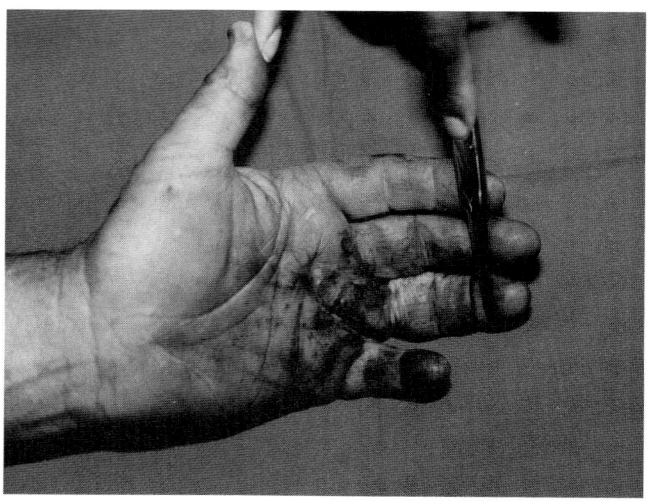

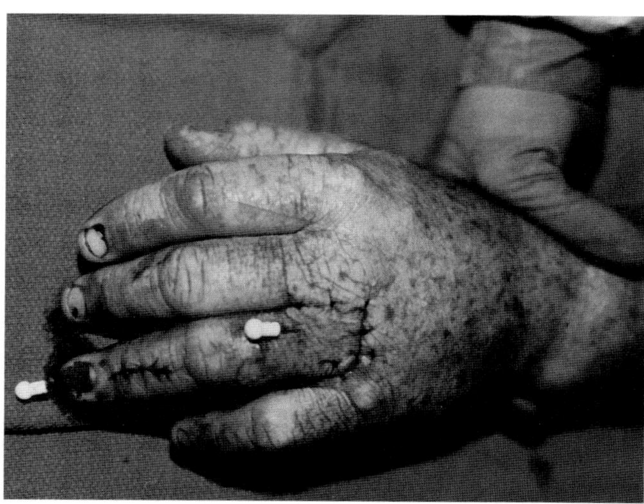

FIGURE 47-7. Preoperative **(A)** and postoperative **(B)** appearance of a ring finger following roller injury.

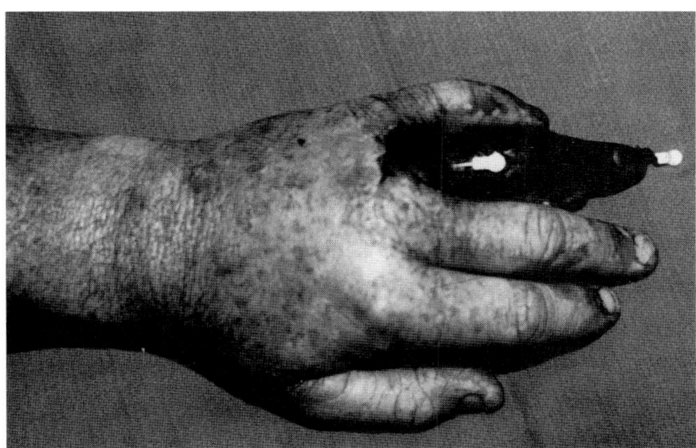

FIGURE 47-8. Five days later, there is complete necrosis of the replant.

its are replantable, transpositional digital replantation is favored over replantation of a border digit (32,33). This can significantly increase the function of the involved hand. Digital prostheses can be of great psychological benefit in selected patients and in our opinion should be offered to nearly all patients with missing digits (Fig. 47-10) (34). These digital prostheses lack motion and sensation, and they do not contribute to the overall function of the hand. There are useful orthotic devices that improve function for patients with thumb or multidigit loss. Great toe transplantation can provide a functional replacement for the thumb that is sensate, has IP joint motion, and renders exceptional cosmetic results (6). Second toes have been used for single digit replacement, but do not offer the degree of functional and cosmetic results obtained by great toe reconstruction of the thumb (Fig. 47-4). Generally, second toe reconstruction of digital loss is reserved for injuries that result in the loss of multiple digits.

An amputated digit, by definition, has disruption of every structure with loss of blood supply to the distal part. All repaired structures in a replanted part therefore must heal in the face of relative reduction of blood flow, and also are healing in a wound in which all neighboring structures have been transected and repaired. In such a setting, it is no surprise that there is a significant complication rate of healing tendons, bone, and nerves.

The rate of nonunion of a replanted digit depends on the zone and mechanism of injury. In our experience, crush injuries result in the highest rate of malunion as well as most of the other postoperative complications. For extra-articular zone II injuries, 15% of the replanted digits treated in our practice undergo a secondary operation to achieve bony union. At the time of the secondary procedure, the fibrous nonunion is removed, exposing healthy bone, and the fracture is secured with plate and screws. Cancellous bone grafting is used when indicated.

All replanted digits will be stiff to some extent following replantation because of the requisite immobilization, multiple structures involved, and tissue and joint swelling. The majority of digits amputated in zone I and successfully replanted will be able to overcome these obstacles through dedicated hand therapy. Approximately 15% of digits replanted in zone I will continue to have inadequate range of motion following a course of hand therapy and will undergo tenolysis with or without joint capsule release.

In contrast, the vast majority of digits in zone II that undergo successful replantation will continue to have significant limitations of motion due to tendon adhesions and joint contracture and will require secondary operations (25,26,35–38). The classic surgical approach to the stiff finger involves the dorsal release of involved structures followed by a check of the flexor side of the digit with flexor tenolysis performed if necessary. Our experience has been

A

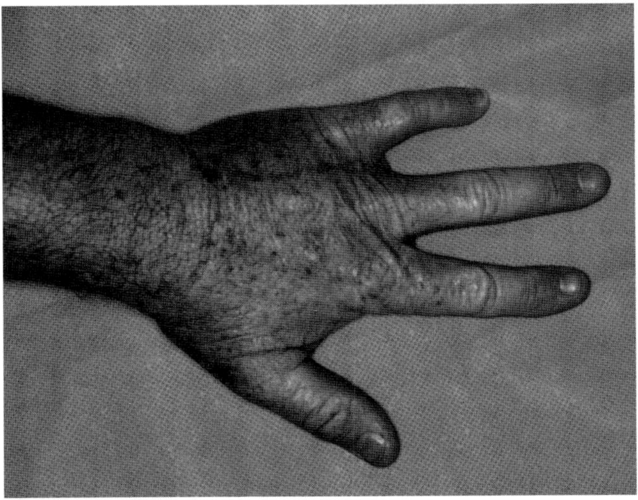

B

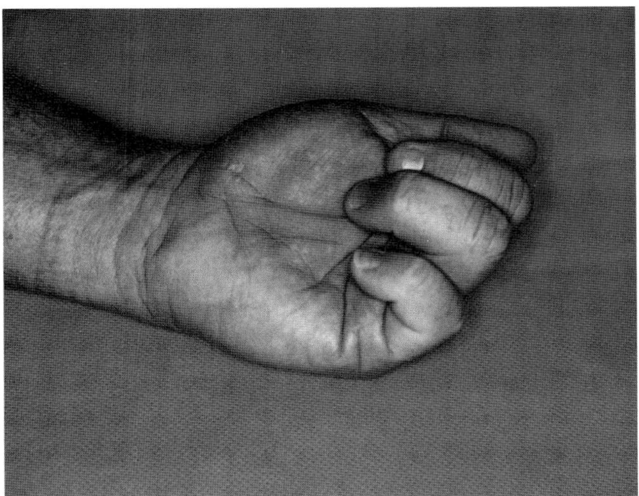

FIGURE 47-9. A,B: Three months after ray amputation.

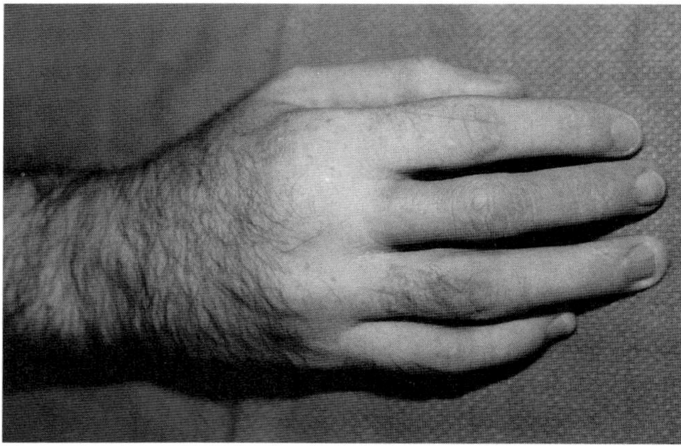

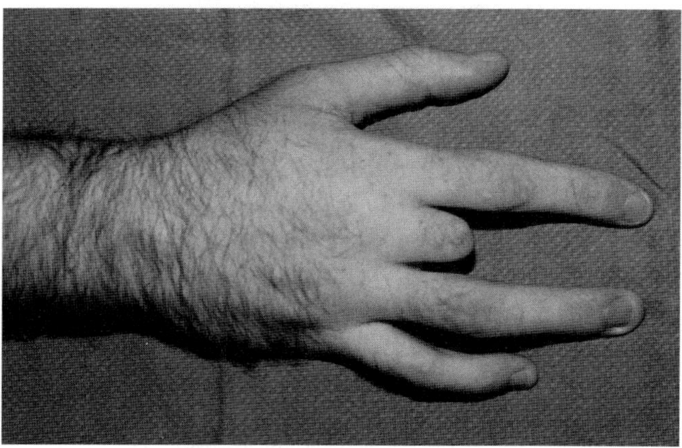

FIGURE 47-10. Right long finger loss, with **(A)** and without **(B)** prosthesis.

that such an approach is tolerated poorly by the replanted digit. Simultaneous dorsal and volar approaches result in a significant amount of swelling and minimal gains from the combined tenolysis procedures. We began to stage such tenolysis procedures, beginning with a dorsal approach followed approximately 6 weeks later by a volar approach if needed. Our protocol is as follows. Once bony union is established and gains in hand therapy have plateaued, patients with an inadequate passive range of motion undergo extensor tenolysis. The decision to perform joint capsulotomy is made at the time of operation. If range of motion is incomplete after complete extensor tenolysis, then joint capsule release is performed. Postoperatively the patient is returned to hand therapy and followed closely. Once the dorsal wound is completely healed and further gains in passive range of motion have plateaued, if active range of motion remains significantly less than passive range of motion, flexor tenolysis is performed (Figs. 47-11–47-16) (39).

Tendon rupture is always a concern during postoperative rehabilitation, especially following tenolysis. We carefully assess the condition of the tendon at the time of surgery. Those tendons that do not appear to have healed completely or are frayed are enrolled in a "frayed tendon" protocol (40). This is a carefully supervised course of hand therapy that involves primarily place-and-hold techniques for several weeks. This allows for less load to be placed on the tendon in the weeks after surgery. Using this technique, we have a very low rate of tendon rupture, currently 1% to 2%. Nonetheless, tendon rupture can occur, especially in poorly compliant patients (Fig. 47-17).

Joint contracture is a significant problem following replantation. It occurs more commonly in amputations caused by crush trauma and in sharp amputations that occur near joints. Replantations that occur through a joint usually cause significant articular trauma and are best treated with arthrodesis at the time of replantation. Late joint degeneration also occurs and again is more common in crushed fingers and in those with trauma in or near the joint

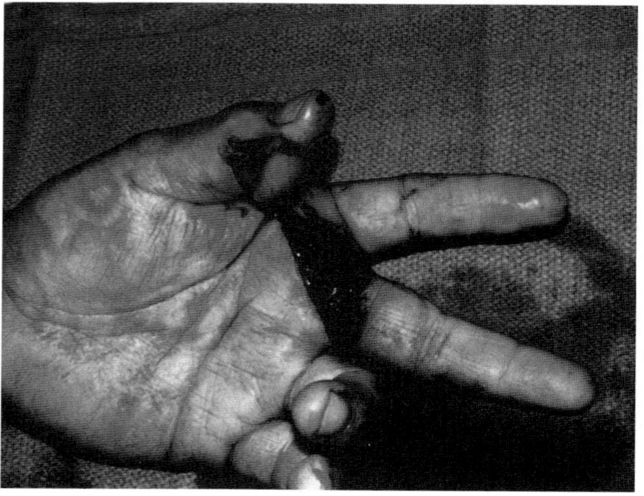

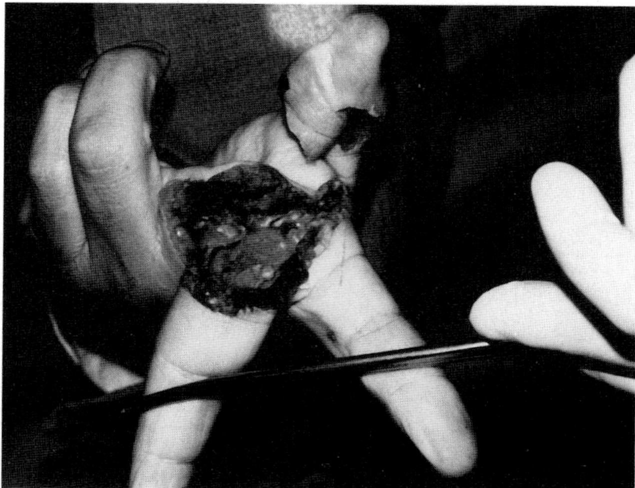

FIGURE 47-11. A,B: Table saw injury to the right hand of a 47-year-old man.

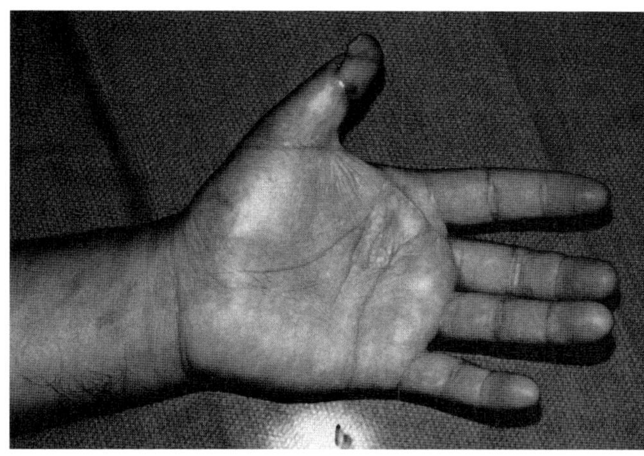
A

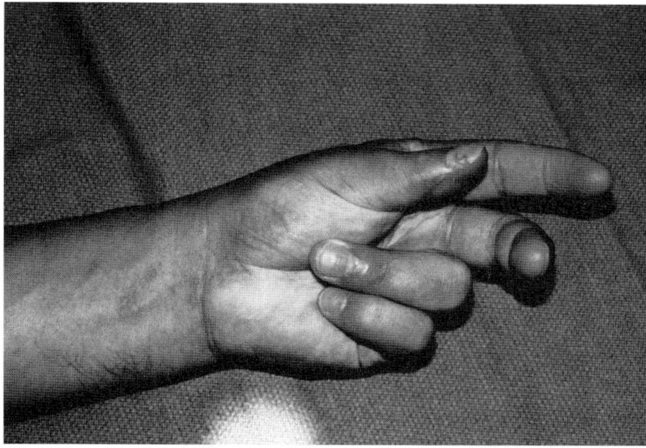
B

FIGURE 47-12. A,B: Appearance and range of motion 3 months later.

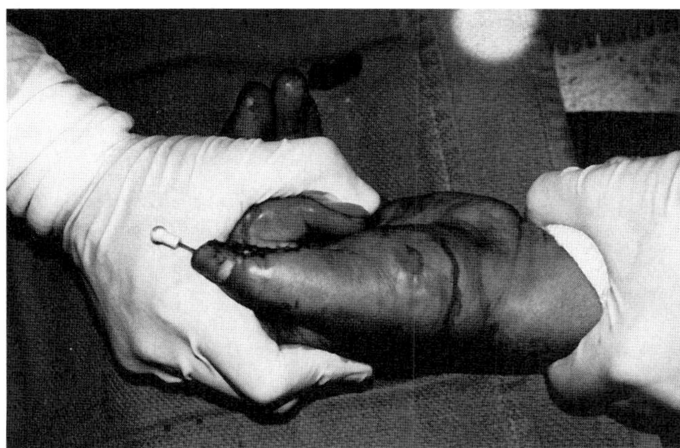

FIGURE 47-13. Intraoperative view at the time of extensor tenolysis and metacarpophalangeal joint capsulotomy.

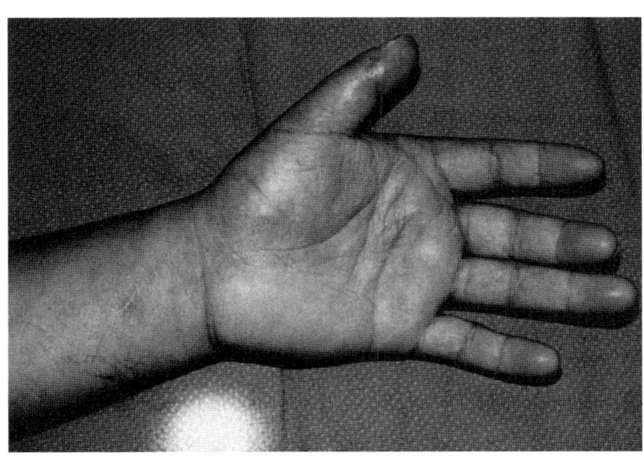
A

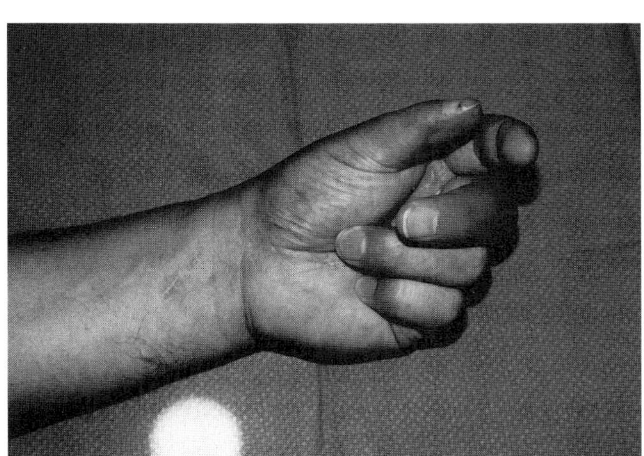
B

FIGURE 47-14. A,B: Appearance and range of motion 2 months later at the time of flexor tenolysis.

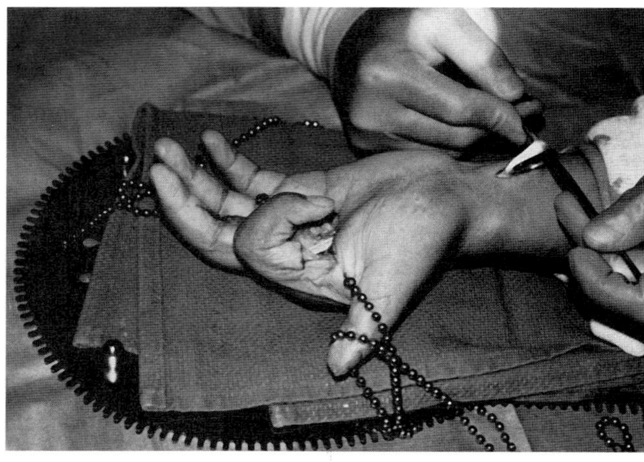

FIGURE 47-15. Intraoperative view of flexor tenolysis.

A

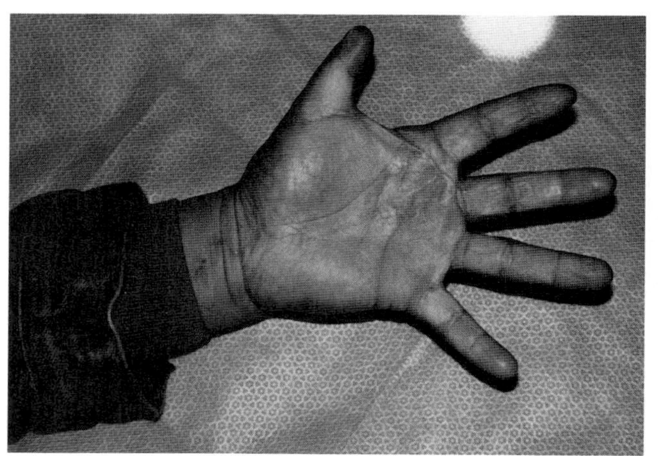

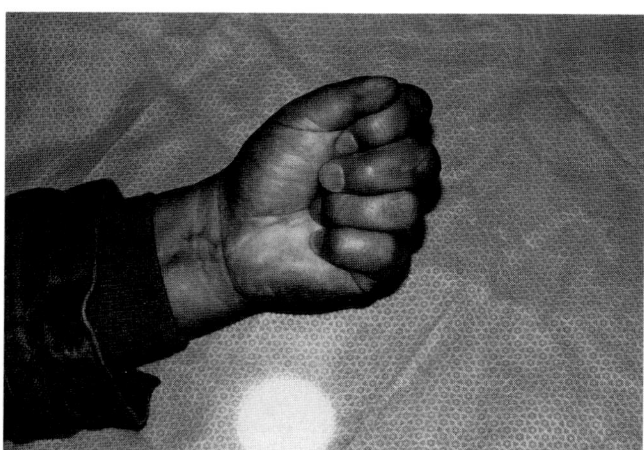

B

C

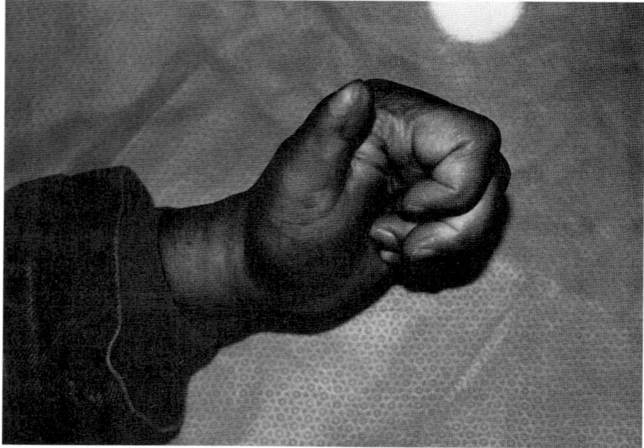

FIGURE 47-16. A–C: Final appearance and range of motion 9 months after injury.

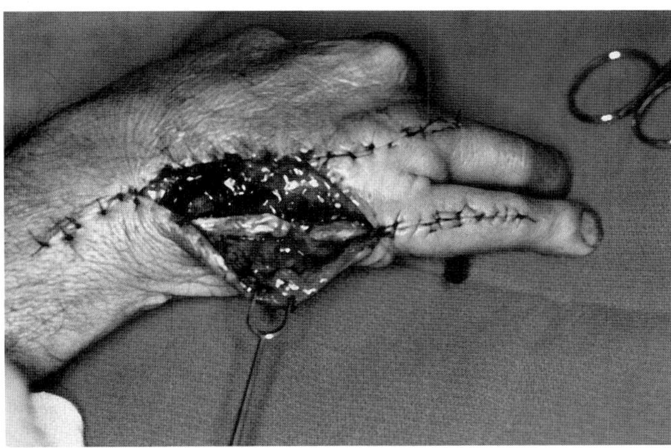

FIGURE 47-17. Extensor tendon rupture 5 days after extensor tenolysis. Patient had worn a "joint jack"-type device overnight, which maintained the finger in complete composite flexion. He removed the device and actively extended the finger, resulting in rupture.

itself. Proximal IP joints with significant degenerative joint disease may be treated by Silastic arthroplasty (41). However, many replanted digits with significant trauma near the proximal IP joint have lost a significant amount of the collateral ligaments and stabilizing structures of the joint capsule. This makes Silastic arthroplasty much less stable, especially in the border digits. We recently began to use a two-piece proximal IP joint replacement system that seems to offer sufficient stability to use in such salvage situations (42).

Digital function and use following replantation have been shown to depend to a large degree on the extent of digital nerve regeneration. Most replanted digits demonstrate significant nerve regeneration, with the worst results in crushed digits (43). Care must be taken at the time of digital nerve repair to debride all traumatized nerve tissue. If this results in a nerve gap, later nerve grafting or primary nerve grafting with a venous conduit is preferable to repair under tension or inadequate debridement (44,45).

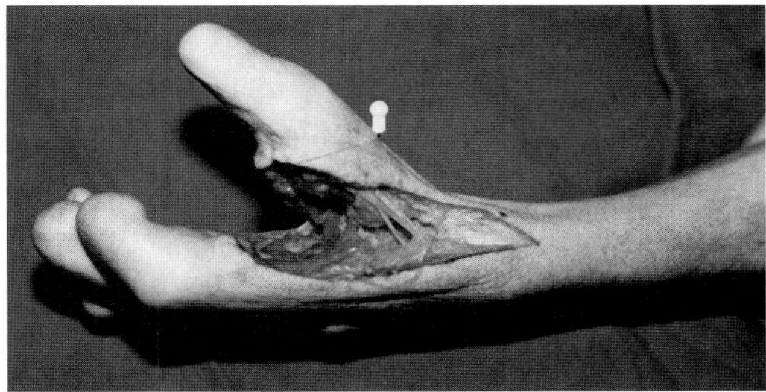

FIGURE 47-19. Intraoperative view showing first web space release.

Soft tissue contracture of the first web space is common after thumb replantation. This can be due as much to contracture of the powerful intrinsic adductors of the thumb as to tissue loss or scarring. An attempt should be made in any thumb replantation to splint the thumb in abduction. We typically secure the thumb in abduction with K-wires to maintain the first web space. Despite such internal and external splinting, some patients will develop first web space contracture. In thumb replantation patients, this can usually be treated by scar release and Z-plasty or some other tissue rearrangement, with the occasional need for full-thickness skin grafts. In patients with more severe hand trauma, web space contracture can be severe. After web space and adductor release, we typically use a lateral arm microvascular transplant for tissue replacement and wound coverage (Figs. 47-18–47-21).

Replantation of digits is by far the most common replantation procedure performed. Replantation of larger structures introduces a whole new set of potential problems (46,47). Patients with major limb loss are more frequently victims of significant trauma and need to be approached as in any major trauma situation. Compartment release should be performed on any part replanted that has an intact muscle compartment. Thus, a replanted hand should have com-

A

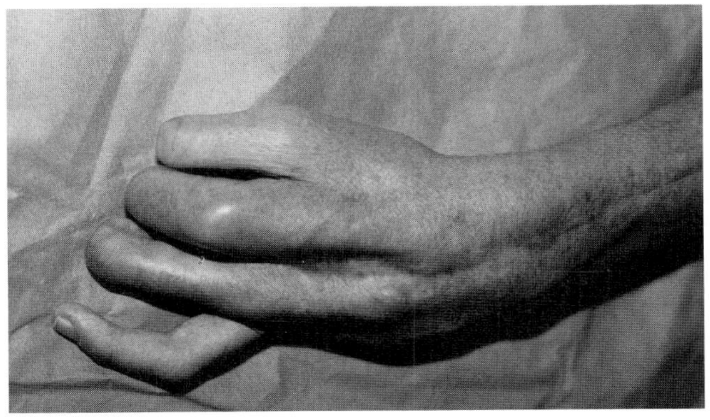

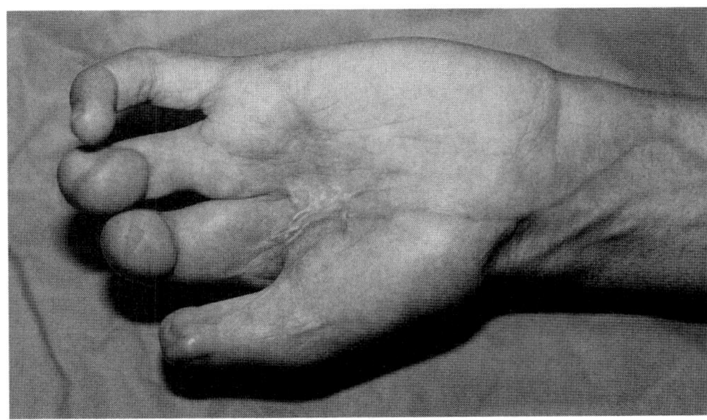

B

FIGURE 47-18. A,B: Contracted first web space following a blast injury.

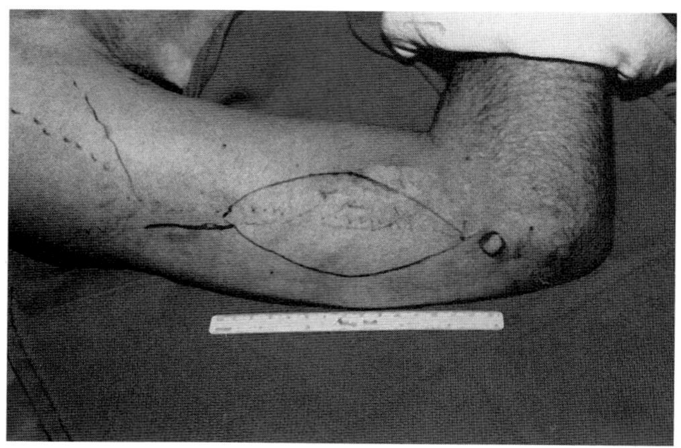

A

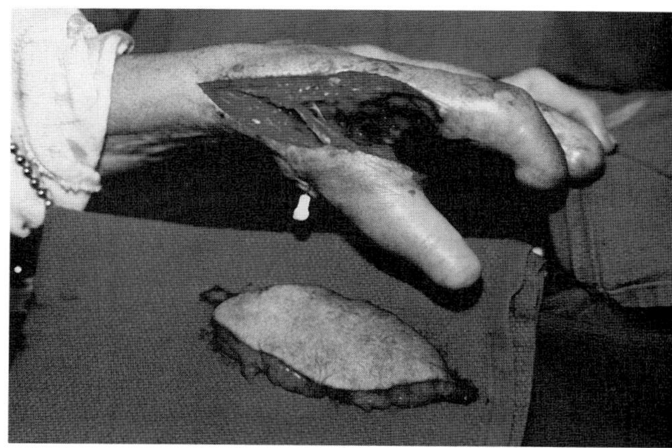

B

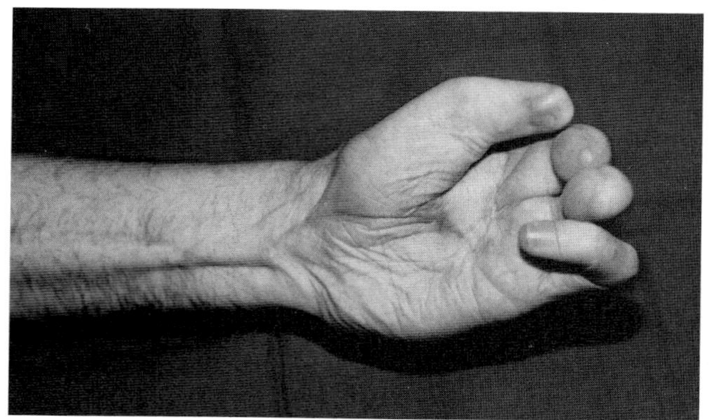

C

FIGURE 47-20. A,B: Lateral arm flap was harvested. **C:** Immediate result after flap inset.

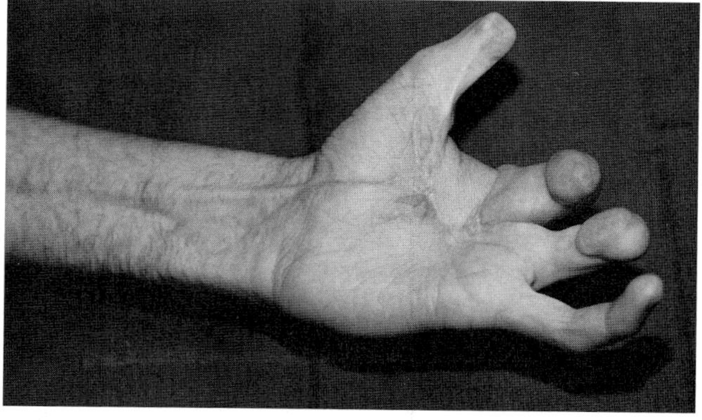

A

B

FIGURE 47-21. A,B: Appearance 5 months later, showing functional web space.

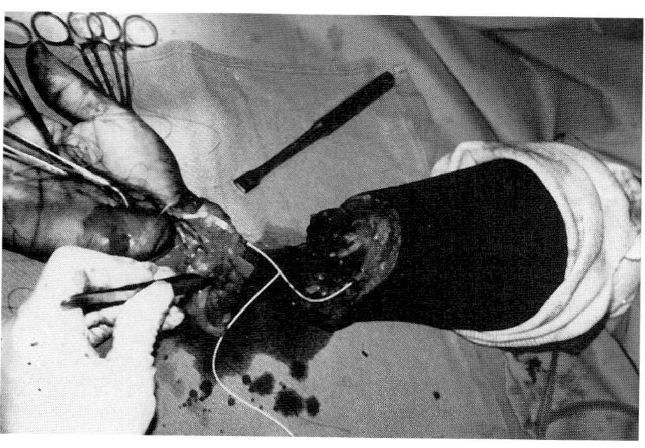

FIGURE 47-22. Amputated right hand perfused via a pediatric T-tube during replantation.

partment release of all of the intrinsic compartments of the hand. This usually can be easily done during the tagging process before revascularization. Typically, we revascularize larger parts through Silastic shunts while the bony fixation is being performed. This cuts down greatly on the ischemia time and allows for washout of metabolic byproducts. Deaths have been reported following replantation of large body parts when such by-products are allowed to recirculate (48,49). The shunts that we use are pediatric T-tubes. The extra limb of the T-tube is helpful in that blood can be drawn easily and heparin can be given to flush out the shunt periodically (Fig. 47-22). If bony fixation is taking an excessively long time, these shunts can also be placed on the venous side of the circulation.

CONCLUSIONS

Replantation procedures are technically demanding and are associated with a high rate of postoperative complications. As in most areas of surgery, careful attention to detail will result in improvements in outcome. A successful replantation offers a chance at reconstruction unmatched by any other means and is significantly rewarding to both patient and surgeon. Early reports of replantation emphasized survival, and although this is still a significant surgical accomplishment, it is recognized that the restoration of function of a replanted part is the ultimate goal. Despite the relatively high rates of postoperative complications, many reports attest to the functional and psychological benefits of replantation of digits and larger more proximal replantations (50–52). Hopefully, further experience with these difficult procedures will result in more successes and less unfavorable results.

REFERENCES

1. Buncke HJ, ed: *Microsurgery: transplantation-replantation. An atlas text.* Philadelphia: Lea & Febiger, 1991:6–88.
2. Buncke HJ, Valauri FA, Buncke GM. Great toe-to-hand transfer. In: Meyer V, ed. *Microsurgical procedures: the hand and upper limb.* New York: Churchill Livingstone, 1991;8:84.
3. Wei FC, Chen HC, Chuang DC, et al. Aesthetic refinements in toe-to-hand transfer surgery. *Plast Reconstr Surg* 1996;98:485.
4. Yim KK, Wei FC. Secondary procedures to improve function after toe-to-hand transfers. *Br J Plast Surg* 1995;48:487.
5. Partington MT, Lineaweaver WC, O'Hara M, et al. Unrecognized injuries in patients referred for emergency microsurgery. *J Trauma* 1993;34:238.
6. Alpert BS, Buncke HJ, Brownstein J. Replacement of damaged arteries and veins with vein grafts when replanting crushed, amputated fingers. *Plast Reconstr Surg* 1978;61:17.
7. Gordon L, Leitner DW, Buncke HJ, et al. Partial nail plate removal after digital replantation as an alternative method of venous drainage. *J Hand Surg* 1985;10:360.
8. Lineaweaver WC, O'Hara M, Stridde B, et al. Clinical leech use in a microsurgical unit: the San Francisco experience. *Blood Coagul Fibrinolysis* 1991;2:189.
9. Kind GM, Buncke GM, Placik OJ, et al. Total ear replantation. *Plast Reconstr Surg* 1997;99:1858.
10. Anthony JP, Lineaweaver WC, Davis JW, et al. Quantitative fluorometric effects of leeching on a replanted ear. *Microsurgery* 1989;10:167.
11. Walton RL, Beahm EK, Brown RE, et al. Microsurgical replantation of the lip: a multi-institutional experience. *Plast Reconstr Surg* 1998;102:358.
12. Yao JM, Yan S, Xu JH, et al. Replantation of amputated nose by microvascular anastomosis. *Plast Reconstr Surg* 1998;102:171.
13. Lineaweaver WC, Hill MK, Buncke GM, et al. Aeromonas hydrophila infections following use of medicinal leeches in replantation and flap surgery. *Ann Plast Surg* 1992;29:238.
14. Furnas HJ, Lineaweaver WC, Buncke HJ. Blood loss associated with anticoagulation in patients with replanted digits. *J Hand Surg* 1992;17:226.
15. Silverman DG, LaRossa DD, Barlow CH, et al. Quantification of tissue fluorescein delivery and prediction of flap viability with the fiberoptic dermo-fluorometer. *Plast Reconstr Surg* 19890;66:545.
16. Graham B, Walton RL, Elings VB, et al. Surface quantification of injected fluorescein as a predictor of flap viability. *Plast Reconstr Surg* 1983;77:826.
17. Stirrat CR, Seaber AV, Urbaniak JR, et al. Temperature monitoring in digital replantation. *J Hand Surg* 1978;3:342–347.
18. Powers EW, Frayer WF. Laser Doppler measurement of blood flow in microcirculation. *Plast Reconstr Surg* 1978;61:250.
19. Hovius SE, van Adrichem LN, Mulder HD, et al. Comparison of laser Doppler flowmetry and thermometry in the postoperative monitoring of replantations. *J Hand Surg Am* 1995;20:88–93.
20. Lendvay PG. Replacement of the amputated digit. *Br J Plast Surg* 1973;26:398.
21. Biemer E. Replantation of fingers and limb parts. Technique and results. *Chirurgie* 1977;48:353–359.
22. Kleinert HE, Juhala CA, Tsai TM, et al. Digital replantation: selection, technique and results. *Orthop Clin North Am* 1977;8:309.
23. Morrison WA, O'Brien BM, MacLeod AM. Evaluation of digital replantation: a review of 100 cases. *Orthop Clin North Am* 1977;8:295.
24. MacLeod AM, O'Brien BM, Morrison WA. Digital replantation: clinical experiences. *Clin Orthop* 1978;133:26.
25. Morrison WA, O'Brien BM, MacLeod AM. Digital replantation and revascularization: a long term review of 100 cases. *Hand* 1978;10:125.
26. Weiland AJ, Villarreal-Rios A, Kleinert HE, et al. Replantation of digits and hands: analysis of surgical techniques and functional results in 71 patients with 86 replantations. *J Hand Surg Am* 1977;2:1.
27. Tamai S. Twenty years experience of limb replantation: review of 293 upper extremity replants. *J Hand Surg Am* 1982;7:549.
28. Holmberg J, Arner M. Sixty five thumb amputations. A retrospective analysis of factors influencing survival. *Scand J Plast Reconstr Surg Hand Surg* 1994;28:45–48.
29. Zumiotti A, Ferreira MC. Replantation of digits: factors influencing survival and functional results. *Microsurgery* 1994;15:18.
30. Patradul A, Ngarmukos C, Parkpian V. Distal digital replantations and revascularizations: 237 digits in 192 patients. *Br J Hand Surg* 1998;23:578.
31. Khouri R. Practice patterns and outcome data in a prospective survey of 495 microvascular free flaps. Presented at the 11th annual meeting of the American Society for Reconstructive Microsurgery, Tucson, Arizona, January 16, 1996.
32. Ross EH, Buncke HJ. Selective finger transposition and primary metacarpal ray resection in multidigit amputations of the hand. *J Hand Surg Am* 1983;8:178.

33. Chiu HY, Lu SY, Lin TW, et al. Transpositional digital replantation. *J Trauma* 1985;25:440.
34. Pereira BP, Kour A-K, Leow E-L, et al. Benefits and use of digital prostheses. *J Hand Surg Am* 1996;21:222.
35. Urbaniak JR, Roth JH, Nunley JA, et al. The results of replantation after amputation of a single finger. *J Bone Joint Surg* 1985;67:611.
36. Jupiter JB, Pess GM, Bour CJ. Results of flexor tendon tenolysis after replantation in the hand. *J Hand Surg Am* 1989;14:35.
37. Tark KC, Kim YW, Lee YH, et al. Replantation and revascularization of hands: clinical analysis and functional results of 261 cases. *J Hand Surg Am* 1989;14:17.
38. Chiu HY, Shieh SJ, Hsu HY. Multivariate analysis of factors influencing the functional recovery after finger replantation or revascularization. *Microsurgery* 1995;16:713.
39. Kind GM, Buntic RF, Buncke GM, et al. The role of tenolysis following digital replantation and revascularization. Presented at the 67th Annual Scientific Meeting of ASPRS/PSEF/ASMS, Boston, Massachusetts, October 3–7, 1998.
40. Cannon NM. Enhancing flexor tendon glide through tenolysis . . . and hand therapy. *J Hand Ther* 1989;April-June:122–137.
41. Hage JJ, Yoe EPD, Zevering JP, et al. Proximal interphalangeal joint silicone arthroplasty for posttraumatic arthritis. *J Hand Surg Am* 1999;24A:73–77.
42. Linscheid RL, Murray PM, Vidal M-A, et al. Development of a surface replacement arthroplasty for proximal interphalangeal joints. *J Hand Surg Am* 1997;22:286.
43. Dellon AL. Sensory recovery in replanted digits and transplanted toes: a review. *J Reconstr Microsurg* 1986;2:123–129.
44. Yamano Y, Namba Y, Hino Y, et al. Digital nerve grafts in replanted digits. *Hand* 1982;14:255.
45. Chiu DTW, Strauch B. A prospective clinical evaluation of autogenous vein grafts used as a nerve conduit for distal sensory nerve defects of 3 cm or less. *Plast Reconstr Surg* 1990;86:928–934.
46. Kutz JE, Jupiter JB, Tsai TM. Lower limb replantation: a report of nine cases. *Foot Ankle* 1983;3:197.
47. Gayle LB, Lineaweaver WC, Buncke GM, et al. Lower extremity replantation. *Clin Plast Surg* 1991;18:437.
48. Rosen HM, Slivjak MJ, McBrearty FX. The role of perfusion washout in limb revascularization procedures. *Plast Reconstr Surg* 1987;80:595.
49. Dell PC, Seaber AV, Urbaniak JR. The effect of systemic acidosis on perfusion of replanted extremities. *J Hand Surg Am* 1980; 5:433.
50. Merle M, Dautel G. Advances in digital replantation. *Clin Plast Surg* 1997;24:87–105.
51. Cheng GL, Pan DD, Zhang NP, et al. Digital replantation in children: a long-term follow-up study. *J Hand Surg Am* 1998; 23A:635–646.
52. Graham B, Adins P, Tsai TM, et al. Major replantation versus revision amputation and prosthetic fitting in the upper extremity: a late functional outcomes study. *J Hand Surg Am* 1998;23A: 783–791.

Discussion

REPLANTATION, REVASCULARIZATION AND TOE-TO-HAND TRANSPLANTS

FU-CHAN WEI
VIVEK JAIN

TOE-TO-HAND TRANSPLANTS

This chapter provides a comprehensive and in-depth review of the possible unfavorable results in toe-to-hand transplantation. It provides useful and strategic tips for their prevention and management. Toe-to-hand transplantation is as rewarding a procedure as it is technically demanding. It requires a dedicated team approach, beginning from patient selection, meticulous preoperative planning, careful toe harvesting and insetting, precise microsurgical anastomosis of vessels and nerves, intense postoperative monitoring, and splinting and hand therapy. We have performed more than 1,400 toe-to-hand transplantations for thumb as well as finger reconstruction, and our overall success rate has been 97%.

Great Toe Transplantation

Preoperative planning of the vascular pedicle, nerve, and tendons of the recipient site should be made in toe trans-

F.-C. Wei and V. Jain: Department of Plastic and Reconstructive Surgery, Chang Gung Memorial Hospital, College of Medicine, Chang Gung University, Taipei, Taiwan

plantation. The type of toe transplants must be considered, balancing the reconstructive goal with potential donor site morbidity (1).

Precise microanastomosis is the key to prevent flap loss; therefore, a proper healthy recipient vessel that is out of the zone of injury and has good spurting should be selected. Proper digital artery, common digital artery, superficial and deep arch, or, if necessary, ulnar or radial artery can be used. For veins, good lumen and wall thickness matching to the donor vein should be selected. Flow insufficiency or repeated spasms immediately after the microanastomosis may be due to imperfect anastomosis, microthrombi at the anastomosis site, or anastomosis at the zone of injury. Redo of anastomosis with direct repair or even with a vein graft should be considered.

Failure of Function

Osteosynthesis

We agree that the toe should be pronated into the appropriate opposition with an adequate web space without any angulation. Good bone contact and stability, which can be obtained by many methods of fixation, permit early movements and union.

We use intraosseous wiring, which is simple, quick, and reproducible, requires minimal soft tissue exposure, and needs only small bony segments (5 mm) so that skeletal length and joints can be preserved (Fig. 47D-1) (2). This provides enough stability to permit passive mobilization in the immediate postoperative period. Any residual angulation or malrotation can be corrected by appropriate splinting, because it is not a rigid fixation. The incidence of nonunion is only 1.5% (2).

In toe-to-thumb transplantation, the position assumes importance only when thenar function is limited. When it is adequate, the new thumb usually can perform pulp-to-pulp, pulp-to-tip, and pulp-to-side grips without difficulty.

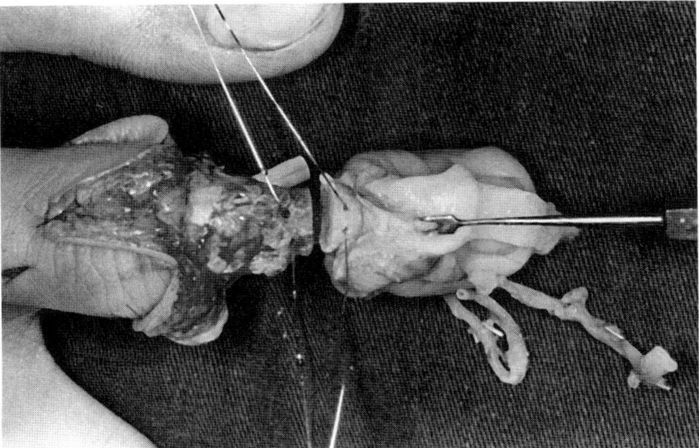

FIGURE 47D-1. Intraosseous wiring used for osteosynthesis of the transplanted toe.

Tendon Rupture

We harvest flexor hallucis longus at the midfoot level and not at ankle because it increases the operative exposure at both the donor as well as recipient site and, in our experience, does not contribute to the results.

The flexor tendon is repaired using a modified Kessler technique and extensor tendon with the Pulvertaft interweaving technique. For the site of flexor tendon repair, whenever possible we prefer the proximal phalanx, or in palm at least 2 cm from the Al pulley in the thumb. In distal finger reconstruction with toe transfer, flexor digitorum superficialis insertion is preserved and the tendon is repaired distal to this, if possible (Fig. 47D-2). If not, then it is repaired in the palm at least 2 cm from the Al pulley. In toe transfer to proximal finger, the repair is performed in the middle or proximal palm away from the Al pulley or more proximally in the wrist away from the carpal tunnel.

The extensor tendon usually does not retract much; therefore, it requires only minimum elevation for repair.

Rupture of flexor tendons occurs in a few patients despite early postoperative rehabilitation programs (3).

Tendon Adhesion

We agree that steps must be taken to minimize adhesions, which to some extent are inevitable, and to lyse them if necessary.

Stable osteosynthesis permits immediate/early mobilization, and postoperative intensive supervised progressive hand therapy (3) constitutes a main part of our postoperative regimen. This helps prevent joint stiffness and tendon adhesions, and it improves coordination and dexterity of the reconstructed hand. We agree that adhesions unresponsive to hand therapy should be managed by tenolysis of extensor followed by flexor. The incidence of secondary procedures involving tendons, bone, and joints in our series was 9%, 1.5%, and 2.3%, respectively (4).

Tendon adhesion usually is limited to the site of repair. Because a minimal amount of extensor tendon is elevated, extensor adhesion was very rare in our series.

Poor Joint Motion

If the first metacarpal is short or missing, rather than including the first metatarsal and first metatarsophalangeal joint, we prefer to reconstruct metacarpal length using bone graft from the iliac crest or amputated part. None of our great toes were taken proximal to the metatarsophalangeal joint (5). We preserve the first metatarsophalangeal joint for two main reasons: (i) it maintains the weight-bearing area of the foot, and (ii) flexion is limited because it is an extension joint.

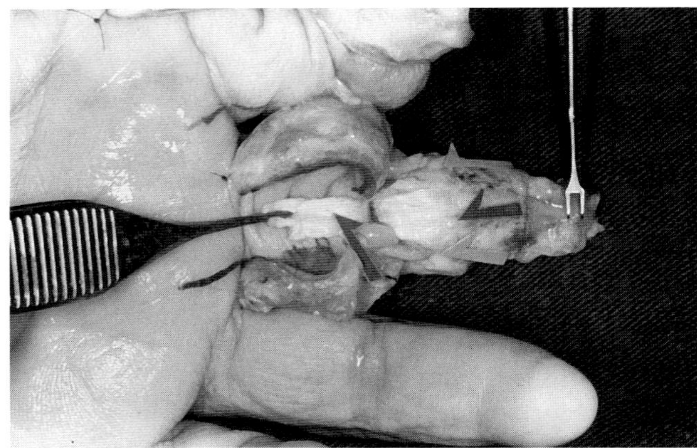

A

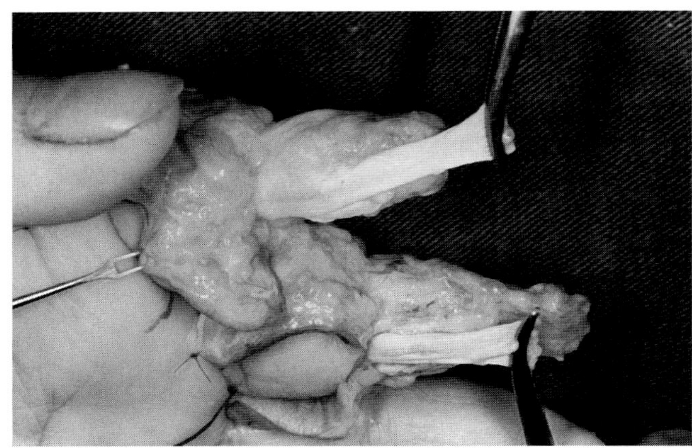

B

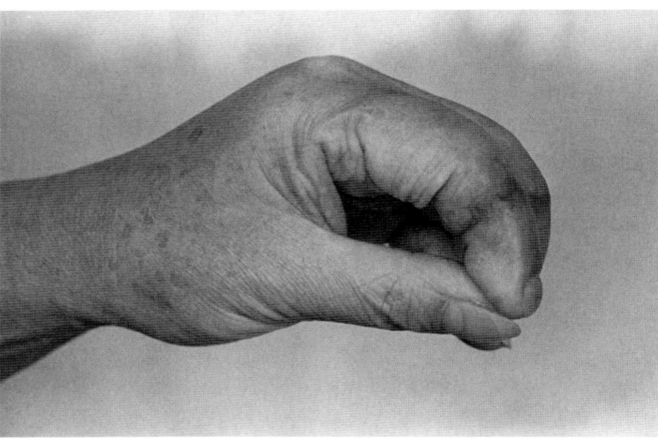

C

FIGURE 47D-2. Repair of flexor digitorum profundus distal to insertion of the intact flexor digitorum superficialis. **A:** Flexor digitorum superficialis insertion and flexor digitorum profundus reflected back. **B:** Adequate excursion of flexor digitorum profundus. **C:** Final result.

Stable bony fixation and dedicated postoperative therapy usually prevent poor joint motion, which is evidenced by only 2.3% of the patients in our series requiring a secondary procedure for joint stiffness (4). We agree that the tight first web space should be released of all contracted soft tissues and reconstructed with either ipsilateral free lateral arm flap or pedicled groin flap before toe transfer.

Poor Sensation

We agree that most toe transplants regain useful sensation with two-point discrimination less than 15 mm, despite the large discrepancy in numbers of myelinated nerve fibers between the fingers and the toe.

Sensory reeducation, both early and late, helps better interpretation of peripheral impulses by using higher cortical functions such as memory, concentration, and learning (6).

Early sensory reeducation focuses on perception of touch submodalities (7). Late-phase sensory reeducation focuses on size, shape, and object recognition. In a study of the effect of delayed sensory reeducation (33 months after toe transplantation), sensory improvement averaged 7 mm in static discrimination and 6 mm in moving two-point discrimination (8).

Considerations in Second Toe Transplantation

Flap Loss

We agree that meticulous preoperative planning, careful technique, and vigilant postoperative monitoring help reduce transplant failure. In case of flap failure, the first choice is another toe transfer if conditions are suitable and patient is agreeable.

Skeletonization of the failed toe transplant and covering with a skin tube with or without additional innervated flap reconstruction is another alternative, but the results usually are inferior.

Appearance and Flexion Contracture

We agree that the second toe usually is slender and less pleasing and does not resemble the thumb as the great toe does. Use of the second toe is indicated for patients who want their great toe preserved; when the size of the second toe is comparable to the thumb; when suboptimal function and appearance of the reconstructed thumb are acceptable, as in old age or with a nondominant hand; in transmetacarpal thumb amputation so that the length and the metacarpophalangeal joint can be reconstructed with the metatarsophalangeal joint (9); and in children (5).

The tendency to claw can be prevented by releasing the extensor digitorum longus attachment from the metatarsophalangeal joint, suturing the extensor digitorum brevis to the extensor hood or interosseous tendon, tight extensor repair, pinning interphalangeal joints in extension for 6 weeks, and nighttime extension splints for at least 1 year (9).

Persisting claw deformity can be corrected by distal interphalangeal joint arthrodesis.

Anatomical Position and Osteosynthesis

We agree that positioning of the toe transplant is crucial for finger and thumb reconstruction. Any angulation or malrotation must be checked and corrected.

Osteosynthesis can be achieved using various devices. We prefer intraosseous wiring, as it is easy, fast, and reproducible, it requires minimal soft tissue dissection, and it preserves skeletal length as well as the joint because it requires only a few millimeters of bone on either side.

Donor Site Problems

The great toe makes a better thumb functionally and cosmetically, but the donor site of the great toe is worse than that of second toe. Therefore, in great toe transplantation, we always harvest distal to the metatarsophalangeal joint, preserving 1 cm of the proximal phalanx because it improves the appearance and maintains important pushoff during gait. If the first metacarpal is deficient, we reconstruct it before toe transfer by bone graft from the ileum or the amputated part. If necessary, we use a pedicled groin flap, which will save more skin in the donor foot and allow closure without tension (5).

To prevent delayed wound healing of the donor site, the wound should be closed meticulously without any tension. Sutures should be removed in 3 to 4 weeks, and weight bearing on this wound should be avoided until sound healing has occurred.

Shortening of the first metatarsal transfers the load laterally and causes lateral metatarsalgia, which should be avoided. We agree that there are fewer complications from second toe harvest sites. Suturing of the deep transverse metatarsal ligament with heads of the first and third metacarpals reduces tension. It is not necessary to resect metatarsal proximally for wound closure, but skin is trimmed to narrow the new web for better cosmesis.

Neuromas can be prevented by proximal resection of the nerves and by burying the nerve ends in the muscles.

We agree with the authors that careful planning and attention to detail lead to excellent results. The success rate in most centers is already over 95%, and the information in this chapter will go a long way to further improving the results of this modern surgery.

REPLANTATION

Replantation leading to successful healing and return to function is a miracle of modern medicine. An accurate history of the mechanism of injury, preoperative evaluation of the patient in entirety and of the amputated part, and any associated medical conditions play important roles in preoperative planning.

Vascular Insufficiency

We agree that adequate debridement of the artery and vein should be done to ensure normal anatomy and blood flow; if necessary, interposition vein grafts should be used (10). In avulsion injuries, a digital artery from the neighboring normal digit can be used to provide successful flow to the injured finger (11).

Release of dressing and sutures, topical lidocaine, papaverine, and ganglion block are helpful. We have a low threshold for reexploration for arterial/venous insufficiency. Removal of the nail and use of leeches can help in cases of venous congestion, and care should be taken to prevent complications (12). We prefer not to use leeches, because of the associated incidence of hepatitis C. In addition, it is difficult to control leeches in any one body part. Medicinal leeches should be used with caution, as the injected volume can further jeopardize vascular flow.

Titrated heparin infusion can relieve venous congestion, although it may lead to excess blood loss, especially if it is used with other anticoagulants such as low-molecular-weight dextran (13).

Alternative techniques to improve venous outflow include arteriovenous shunting and pinpricks (14), silicone shunts (15), and pharmaceutical leeches (16), which have been used with success.

Monitoring

A wide variety of monitoring techniques can be used, including surface fluorometry, thermometry, and laser Doppler flowmetry. We agree that surface fluorometry is a good technique. In our center, we have a dedicated microsurgical intensive care unit where patients are continuously monitored in the postoperative period. We believe this helps in early identification of potential vascular insufficiency and that, combined with our low threshold for reexploration, helps to improve the success rate.

Survival Rates

We agree that the survival rates of replantation are lower than those of free-tissue transfers. This probably is due to multiple factors, including wider indications for replantation, more extensive trauma than is being visualized, attempts to salvage more serious crush and avulsion injuries, and more emphasis given to planned free flaps. The results in the elderly can be good; hence, age is no longer a contraindication to replantation (17).

Transpositional digital replantation preserves greater hand function and reduces the need for secondary reconstructive procedures. It is indicated for multiple digits and severe crush injuries, and for injuries distal to zone V (18). Thumb reconstruction can be performed using various techniques that provide a mobile, sensate, and cosmetically acceptable thumb (19).

In severely injured hands, multiple toe transfers along with free composite tissue transfers can be used for reconstruction (20). Nonunion and malunion are more common with crush injuries, especially in zone II, and are managed by secondary surgery with bone grafting if indicated.

Stable osteosynthesis with dedicated hand therapy helps increase range of motion. In indicated cases, extensor tenolysis and, if necessary, arthrolysis can be used, especially in zone II. Flexor tenolysis can be undertaken at the second stage, if necessary. Joint contracture in periarticular amputations, especially crush injuries, can be managed by primary fusion or secondary joint replacement (21).

Digital sensibility returns quicker with sharp amputations than in crush or avulsion injuries (22). During primary repair, emphasis is on proper debridement and repair without tension, and primary nerve grafting, if necessary (23).

First web space contracture is best prevented by splinting; established contractures are best managed by release and reconstruction with free lateral arm flap. Major limb replantation should include compartment release as part of the debridement. Larger parts should be revascularized using Silastic shunts to reduce ischemia time and allow washout of metabolic by-products to prevent serious complications (15). Replantations are technically demanding, and success should be evaluated by restoration of function.

REFERENCES

1. El-Ganunal TA, Wei FC, Ma HS, et al. Biomechanical analysis of foot function following transfer of combined second and third toes from the same foot. *J Hand Surg (submitted).*
2. Yim KK, Wei FC. Intraosseous wiring in toe-to-hand transplantation. *Ann Plast Surg* 1995;35;66–69.
3. Yim KK, Wei FC. Secondary procedures to improve function after toe-to-hand transfer. *Br J Plast Surg* 1995;48:487–491.
4. Wei FC, Cossens B, Lanos D, et al. Multiple microsurgical toe tohand transfer in reconstruction of mutilated hand. *Ann Hand Surg* 1992;11:177.
5. Wei FC, Chen HC, Chuang CC, et al. Microsurgical thumb reconstruction with toe transfer: selection of various techniques. *Plast Reconstr Surg* 1994;93:345–351.
6. Wilson MC. Sensory re-education. In: Gelberroan RH, ed. *Operative nerve surgery and reconstruction.* 1st ed. Philadelphia: JB Lippincott, 1991:827.
7. Dellon AL, Curtis RM, Egderton MT. Evaluating recovery of the sensation in hand following nerve injury. *John Hopkins Med J* 1972;30:225.
8. Wei FC, Ma HS. Delayed sensory re-education after toe-to-hand transfer. *Microsurgery* 161995;:583-5—85.
8. Wei FC, Tarek AEG. Toe-to-hand transfer current concepts, techniques and research. *Clin Plast Surg* 1996;23:103–116.
10. Bernard SA, Buncke HJ, Brownstein M. Replacement of damaged arteries and veins with vein grafts when replanting crushed amputated fingers. *Plast Reconstr Surg* 1978;61:17–22.
11. Cheng SL, Chuang DC, Wei FC, et al. Successful replantation of an avulsed middle finger. *Ann Plast Surg* 1998;41:662–666.
12. Lineaweaver WC, Hill MK, Buncke GM, et al. *Aeromonas hydrophila* infection following use of medicinal leeches in replantation and flap surgery. *Ann Plast Surg* 1992;29:238–244.
13. Fumass HJ, Lineaweaver WC, Buncke HJ. Blood loss associated with anticoagulation in patients with replanted digits. *J Hand Surg* 1992;17:226.
14. Jeng SF, Wei FC, Noordhoff MS. Replantation of amputated facial tissue with microvascular anastomosis. *Microsurgery* 1994;15:327–333.
15. Chen SH, Chang YL, Ho WP, et al. Simultaneous bilateral forearm revascularization. *Plast Reconstr Surg* 1991;87:346–353.
16. Jeng SF, Wei FC, Noordhoff MS. Successful replantation of a bitten off vermilion of lower lip by microvascular anastomosis case report. *J Trauma Injury Infection Crit Care* 1992;33: 914–916.
17. Wei FC, Epstein MD, Chen HC, et al. Microsurgical reconstruction of distal digits following mutilating hand injuries: result in 121 patients. *Br J Plast Surg* 1993;46:181–6.
18. Chiu HY, Lu SY, Lin TW, et al. Transpositional digital reimplantation. *J Trauma* 1995;25:440.
19. Wei FC, Chen HC, Chuang CC, et al. Microsurgical thumb reconstruction with toe transfer: selection of various techniques. *Plast Reconstr Surg* 1994;93:345.
20. Wei FC, Seah CC, Chen HC, et al. Functional and aesthetic reconstruction of a mutilated hand using multiple toe transfer and iliac osteocutaneous flap: a case report. *Microsurgery* 1993;1: 388–390.
21. Hage JJ, Yoe EPD, Zevering JP, et al. Proximal interphalangeal joint silicone arthroplasty for post traumatic arthritis. *J Hand Surg* 1999;24A:73—77.
22. Tark TT, Kim YW, Lee YH, et al. Replantation and revascularisation of hands: clinical analysis and functional results of 261 cases. *J Hand Surg* 1989;14A:17–27.
23. Dellon AL. Sensory recovery in replanted digits and transplanted toes: a review. *J Reconstr Microsurg* 1986;2:123–129.

48

THUMB RECONSTRUCTION

ROSA L. DELL'OCA
VINCENT R. HENTZ

A deficient thumb, caused by trauma or developmental mishap, presents a great challenge, because restoration of normal function and appearance is difficult to achieve. Given surgical limitations and patient's desires, the definition of "unsuccessful" varies widely. For the surgeon, an unfavorable result arises from an error of omission, poor preoperative planning, failure to anticipate potential problems or commission, faulty technique, or misguided postoperative management. For the patient, the result is unfavorable when expectations are not met, regardless of whether or not there were errors of either omission or commission. Alternatively, "success" is gauged in two realms, that which the surgeon aspires to and achieves and that which the patient hopes for and gains. It is imperative that all parties involved have realistic expectations of the outcome from surgical or nonsurgical treatment. An appropriate plan develops through careful consideration of the patient's occupation and functional demands, psyche, age, motivation, and commitment to postoperative therapy. Each individual case must be evaluated on its own merits and shortcomings, for, in the final analysis, as Gaul (1) suggested, "the owner of the hand is the only one who really knows how to evaluate the results."

Function is of the utmost importance, but aesthetic considerations occasionally may be of equal concern. Requisites for satisfactory thumb reconstruction can be categorized into three primary areas: structure, sensibility, and posture. Pollex is derived from the Latin term *polleo,* which implies strength. The importance of length, strength, stability, and free lateral movement of the thumb was eloquently stated by Sir Charles Bell (2) in the frequently quoted Fourth Bridgewater Treatise. These considerations may well be viewed as comprising the structure of the thumb. Second, sensate but pain-free skin coverage is an absolute requirement for protection and stereognosis, and to ensure use. Finally, the posture of the thumb concerns its attitude and mobility with respect to the remaining four fingers. These three areas of consideration assume variable importance depending on the level and magnitude of the thumb deficit. Accordingly, efforts at surgical reconstruction must focus on the particular areas of deficiency peculiar to the individual case.

Just as the priorities in posttraumatic thumb reconstruction vary with the level of amputation, the potential causes of an unfavorable result differ according to the particular level of deficit. We will discuss the most commonly accepted advantages and shortcomings of specific reconstructive procedures as they relate to the five levels of injury to the thumb as illustrated in Fig. 48-1. Rather than completely describe the operative techniques, we will focus on key steps of the procedures and on certain principles that, when adhered to, diminish the risk of an unfavorable result.

LEVEL OF AMPUTATION AND ITS RELATIONSHIP TO THE UNFAVORABLE RESULT

Level I

Level I includes the distal two-thirds of the terminal phalanx, the nail structures, and the volar tactile surface to the level of the interphalangeal joint flexion crease. The priorities of restoration at this injury level focus less on maintaining or restoring length and more on maintaining the aesthetic, tactile, and dorsal skin-stabilizing contributions of the nail and replacing the durable, sensate pulp. As terminal hypesthesia presents less of a problem than an irritable tender neuroma or unstable skin coverage, the time-honored commandment that the thumb should never be shortened solely to facilitate skin closure might be overemphasized (3). If shortening the bone by several millimeters leads to a sensate tip without oppositional loss in length (4), then this is an acceptable sacrifice. However, the distal phalanx supports and defines the nail plate. Phalangeal shortening where less than 30% to 40% remains beneath the nail matrix results in a volarly curved nail's having the appearance of a parrot's beak. Furthermore, distal phalangeal irregular-

R. L. Dell'Oca and V. R. Hentz: Division of Hand Surgery, Stanford University Medical School, Palo Alto, California

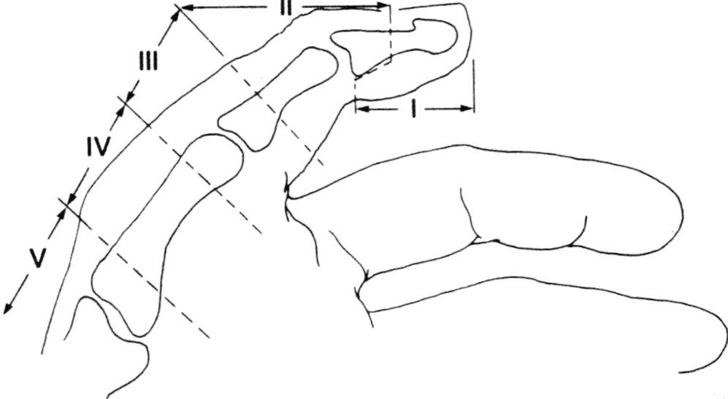

FIGURE 48-1. Levels of traumatic loss of the thumb. **I:** Distal half of terminal phalanx, nail plate and matrix, and volar soft tissue of entire terminal segment. **II:** Through proximal phalanx leaving intact metacarpophalangeal (MCP) joint. **III:** Proximal to or through MCP joint with nearly entire metacarpal and intrinsic musculature left intact. **IV:** Between proximal and distal thirds of metacarpal with significant loss of thenar muscular cone but preservation of trapeziometacarpal joint. **V:** Loss through or proximal to trapeziometacarpal joint . (From Hentz VR, Littler JW, Pellegrini VD. Thumb reconstruction. In: McFarlane RM, ed. Unsatisfactory results in hand surgery. Edinburgh: Churchill Livingstone, 1987:113–143, with permission.)

ities or incomplete repairs in the germinal matrix produce a grooved nail. In sum, the most important reconstructive goal is stable sensate durable pulp and tip coverage. Correspondingly, unfavorable outcomes are related to factors such as poor choice of donor tissue and technical errors that compromise ultimate sensation. The next dilemma centers on the extent and status of the remaining nail, the condition of the distal phalanx, and the needs and desires of the patient to determine whether the team embarks on nail remnant preservation and, if necessary, the tedious process of bone lengthening or proceeds to complete germinal matrix ablation to avoid a problematic nail remnant. This decision also must consider that although earlier procedures for late reconstruction of the injured nail and supporting matrix were technically complex with often unsatisfactory results and frequent residual deformity (5), the more recently described microvascular wraparound great toe flap (4) or transfer of a partial great toe distal phalanx (6), although also technically demanding, has improved on the results for nail reconstruction, albeit at a high expense to the donor site.

Level II

Level II injuries include loss of the terminal joint with shortening of the proximal phalanx to the junction of the proximal and middle thirds. As in level I injuries, for the more distally located level II injuries, function is minimally affected, again leaving durable and sensible skin coverage as the primary concern during reconstruction. Unfavorable results occur for the same reasons noted for level I. For more proximally located level II injuries, structure is moderately compromised due to skeletal shortening; however, restoration of length at the expense of lesser quality skin coverage is not a profitable trade-off. Although not an absolute necessity with this modest deficit in thumb length, phalangealization, distraction lengthening, osteoplastic procedures, and even microsurgical tissue transfers provide a functional and esthetic remedy. These last procedures address both the structural (length) deficit and the loss of sensation. However, as the complexity of the reconstruction increases and as more reconstructive goals are added to the operative plan, so do the opportunities for complications leading to an unfavorable outcome.

Level III

The most common level of traumatic amputation lies within the zone extending from the base of the proximal phalanx to the metacarpal neck, which is level III. Although sparing most of the thenar cone of muscles, shortening to this degree results in significant loss of function, especially with concomitant injury to the soft tissues of the first web space and ensuing contracture. Beginning at this level of loss and in a more absolute sense for level IV and V amputations, provisions for reconstructive thumb substitution become paramount. Occasionally, with sparing of the web space and preservation of good thumb–index breadth, adequate function may remain or may be augmented with phalangization (Fig. 48-2). Usually, however, restoring function necessi-

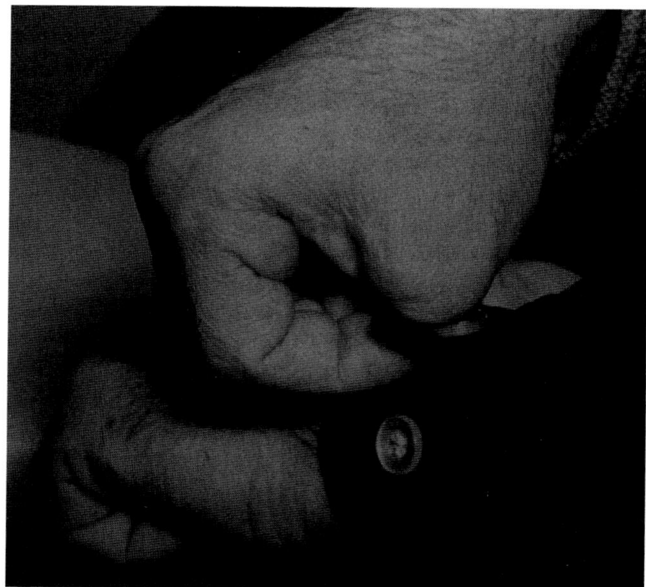

FIGURE 48-2. Loss of some portion of the thumb is, in itself, insufficient indication for reconstruction. If the remaining digits have normal function and the web remains soft, the residual thumb stump may possess substantial thumb-like function. (From Hentz VR, Littler JW, Pellegrini VD. Thumb reconstruction. In: McFarlane RM, ed. Unsatisfactory results in hand surgery. Edinburgh: Churchill Livingstone, 1987:113–143, with permission.)

tates the addition of real length by using such techniques as distraction lengthening, osteoplastic reconstruction pollicization, or microvascular tissue transfer.

Level IV

Level IV injuries involve the proximal and middle thirds of the thumb metacarpal and are associated with significant loss of intrinsic muscle control of the basal joint. They represent a major challenge for thumb reconstruction. Specific priorities of restoration at this level include adding length and stabilizing the trapeziometacarpal joint either by fusion or with multiple tendon transfers. As the available length of the remaining metacarpal diminishes, so does the ability of osteoplastic methods to reconstruct the thumb, leaving digital pollicization or some type of microvascular replacement by toe transfer as the better option. At this level, more than two-thirds of cases involve injury to another digit that provides a great candidate for transfer.

Level V

Injuries at level V involve loss of the unique trapeziometacarpal joint along with its associated governing intrinsic musculature. They closely resemble the congenital deficiencies, and similarly the benchmark treatment remains pollicization. Following in the hierarchy of reconstruction, microvascular toe transfers followed by osteoplastic reconstruction and bone lengthening all face the difficulty of reproducing the basal joint. Some argue that the trapeziometacarpal articulation is too difficult to reproduce and, therefore, the proximal phalanx of the transposed digit or the bone graft should be fused to the trapezium or the remainder of the carpus. In any event, the more essential functional attribute of the basal joint system of the thumb is stability rather than mobility. The only caveat is that, in fusing the proximal phalanx to the carpus, a modest degree of extension in the plane of the palm must be provided so that the fingers are free to close unobstructed by the newly created thumb (7).

AVOIDING UNFAVORABLE OUTCOMES IN RECONSTRUCTION

Skin Coverage

For essentially all level I and for many level II injuries, the principal reconstructive challenge is to provide durable sensate skin cover for the prime contact surface of the thumb, pulp, and tip areas. The same need for durable and sensate skin cover exists for amputations at more proximal levels, in addition to other reconstructive needs such as basal joint stability, acquisition of necessary length, positional requirements, and those of movement and strength.

A detailed discussion of the numerous methods for management of the thumb tip injury (level I) is not within the scope of this text. However, application of general principles will help to avoid the specific complications and minimize the shortcomings peculiar to each technique. Digital nerves should be shortened proximal to the level of existing skin to avoid formation of an irritable neuroma in an area vulnerable to unbuffered repetitive trauma. Split- and full-thickness skin graft coverage provide simple, efficient, and economical coverage with the least additional bulk to the tip, but usually requires later revision with a more stable, sensate replacement, except in children (8). Healing by secondary intention provides a well-contoured sensate tip with adequate bulk; however, it usually necessitates bony shortening. Although lateral (Cutler) or volar (Atasoy) V-Y advancement flaps provide mobilization of several millimeters of sensate skin of adequate bulk, further elevation to the distal palmar crease (9) with metacarpal and interphalangeal flexion of up to 45 degrees allows 1 to 2 cm of advancement without persistent interphalangeal flexion contracture if adequate physical therapy follows (10). This requires skin grafting proximally, unless more extensive volar advancement flaps are created with mobilization to the proximal flexion crease (Figs. 48-3–48-4) or a V-Y incision is extended into thenar eminence. Extension of the tip of the V to a line drawn from the radial border of the middle finger to the wrist (11) permits coverage of a defect extending from the interphalangeal joint to the tip with bone exposure from nail fold to tip, but there is a higher risk of persistent interphalangeal joint flexion contracture. Flexion contracture may be infrequent, but the loss of normal hyperextension occurs in more than one-third of cases compared to the contralateral thumb (12).

As homodigital flaps are appropriate for defects up to 2.5 cm or 50% of the pulp (level I injuries), heterodigital flaps are more appropriate for level II injuries. Sensory innervated cross-finger flaps harvested from the radial innervated area of the index finger, such as the kite or flag flap (13), are complex procedures requiring surgical assault on an otherwise normal digit (1), with a higher rate of complications for resurfacing to injuries at level I. Overstretching the radial nerve to cover distal (level I) defects may result in neuroma and hypesthesia and may only ultimately return sensation to the digit at a protective level or worse in the form of double sensitivity (14). Furthermore mobilization of the radial sensory branches risks irritation of these temperamental nerves and may invite a reflex sympathetic dystrophy. The position and duration of immobilization may jeopardize the integrity of the thumb web in an already injured digit and as with other flap procedures, contracture following immobilization is more pronounced in patients of increasing age over 40.

The greater utility of heterodigital flaps is in the reconstruction of more severely injured thumbs (level II and beyond). At level II, if local flaps are not available to provide satisfactory coverage of the amputation stump, then more

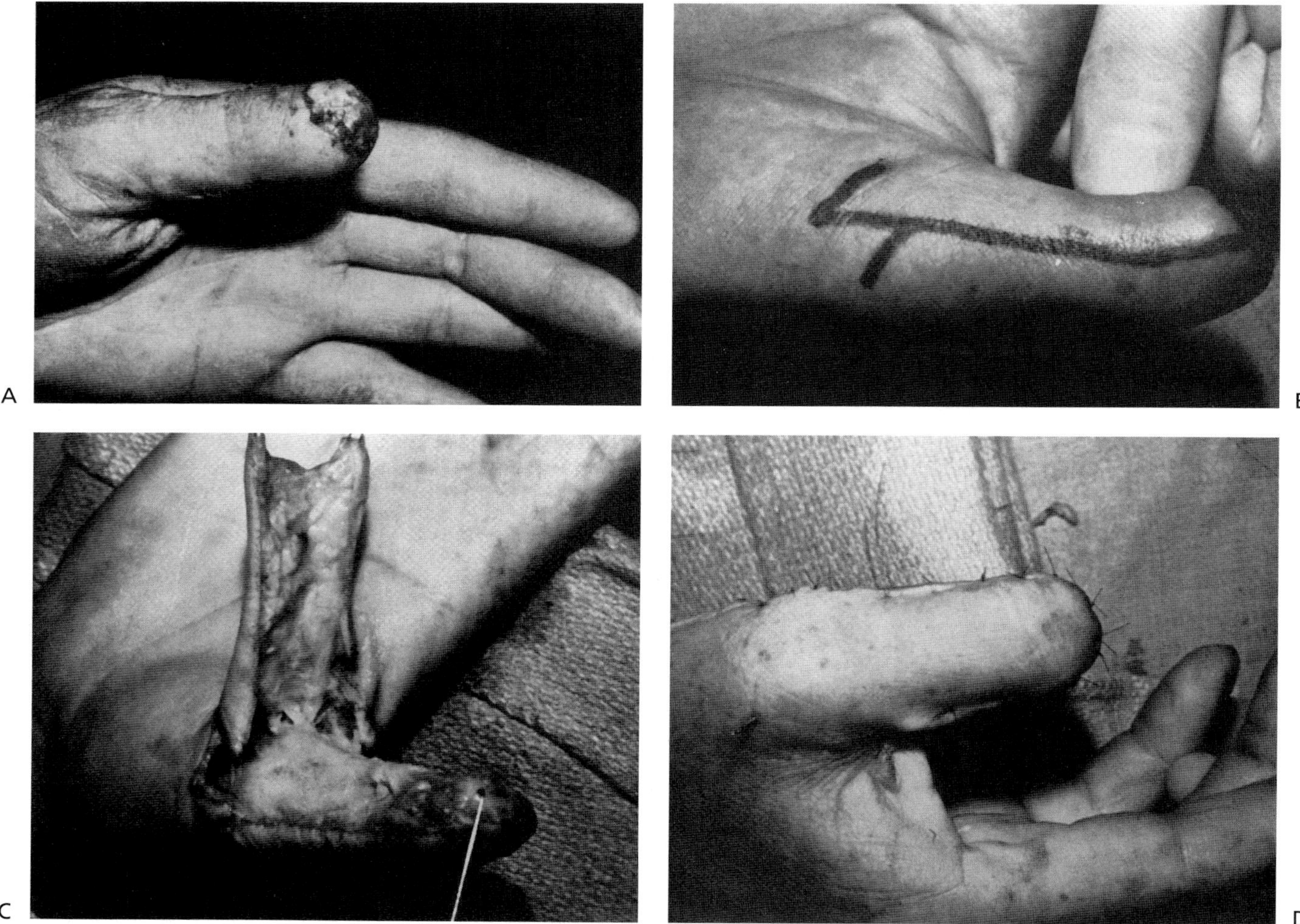

FIGURE 48-3. A–D: The volar soft tissue can be advanced distally 1 to 1.5 cm. A small Z-plasty on either side at the proximal end of the incision provides for additional advancement. (From Hentz VR, Littler JW, Pellegrini VD. Thumb reconstruction. In: McFarlane RM, ed. Unsatisfactory results in hand surgery. Edinburgh: Churchill Livingstone, 1987:113–143, with permission.)

creative and complex soft tissue rearrangement is required with its attendant risks and complications. With the decreased demand for pedicle length, so diminishes the risks of radial sensory flaps. Although they provide coverage as determined by the dimensions between the midlateral lines and as distal as the interphalangeal joint of the index finger, two-point discrimination is limited to 10 to 15 mm (1). This theme pervades the use of most local sensory flaps, including the dorsal web rotation flap described by McFarlane and Stromberg (15), which is based distally on the palmar skin of the intact commissure, providing good-quality coverage with satisfactory fixation of the skin while preserving the web space during the required period of immobilization. Recent improvements of these cutaneous flaps include extension by including fascia of the first dorsal interosseous muscle (16), expansion by creating a second web space bilobed island flap to resurface both volar and dorsal defects (17), and permutation by using the middle or ring finger (14).

The standard neurovascular island pedicle based on a proper digital nerve to an adjacent finger improves on two-point discrimination, attaining static two-point discrimination of 5 to 15 mm (average 9 mm) and moving two-point discrimination of 3 to 12 mm (average 7.4 mm). It also provides adequate-quality skin of good color and texture approximating the contralateral thumb. This improved sensation comes at the price of "double sensitivity" secondary to insufficient cortical reorientation (4,18). In a study of 17 patients, 35.5 % had referral to the thumb and the index finger and 5.8 % to the index finger alone (18). To laborers, this represents a significant handicap, which can be ameliorated by incising the donor nerve and annealing it to the ulnar digital nerve of the thumb (Fig. 48-5). In the same study of 13 patients, this allowed 100% sensory perception from the thumb within a

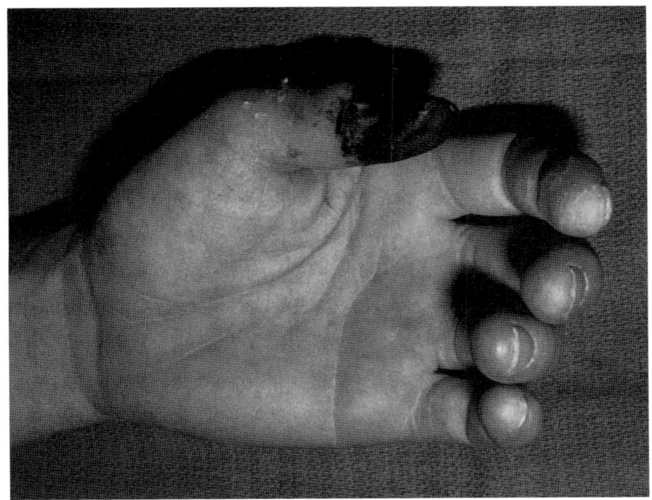

A

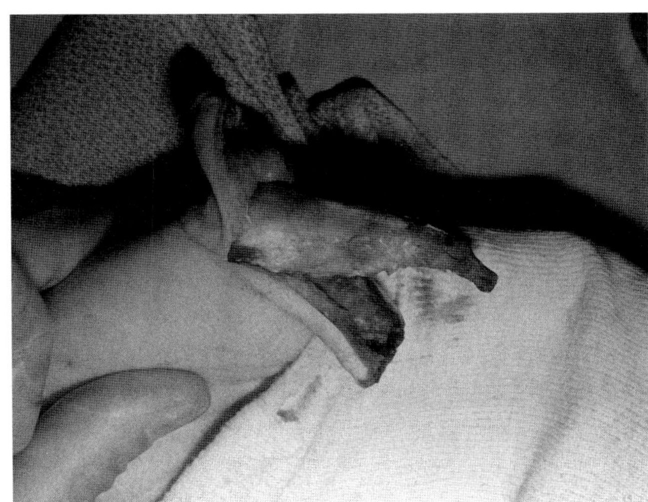

B

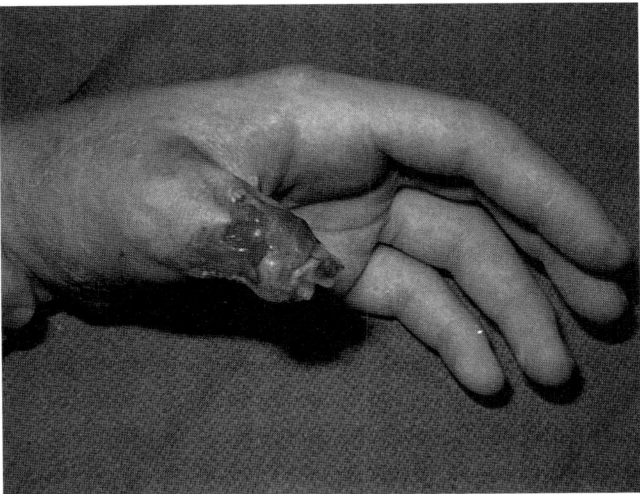

C

FIGURE 48-4. A–C: Volar soft tissues remain well nourished when advanced on the neurovascular bundles. It is not feasible to combine a volar advancement with a similar advancement of the dorsal soft tissues without risk of necrosis of the dorsal flap. (From Hentz VR, Littler JW, Pellegrini VD. Thumb reconstruction. In: McFarlane RM, ed. Unsatisfactory results in hand surgery. Edinburgh: Churchill Livingstone, 1987:113–143, with permission.)

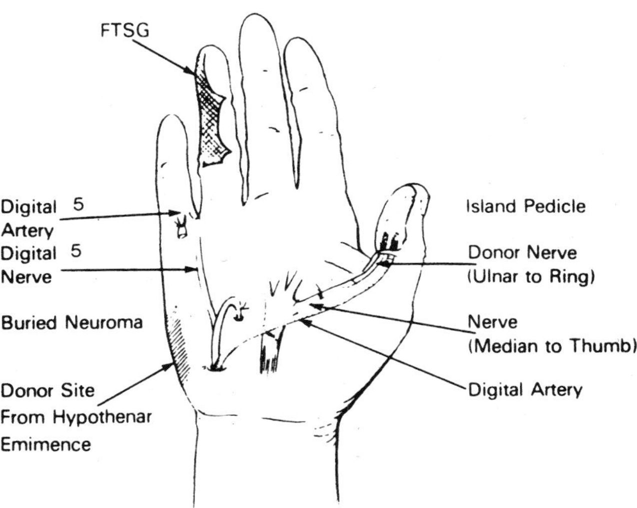

FIGURE 48-5. Need for cortical reorientation can be avoided by suture of the proper digital nerve of the neurovascular island to the stump of one of the digital nerves to the thumb. However, sensibility then is dependent on the quality of the neural repair and axonal regeneration. (From Hentz VR, Littler JW, Pellegrini VD. Thumb reconstruction. In: McFarlane RM, ed. Unsatisfactory results in hand surgery. Edinburgh: Churchill Livingstone, 1987:113–143, with permission.)

few months; however, both static and moving two-point discrimination suffered, with values 6 to 15 mm (average 10.1 mm) and 4 to 15 mm (average 8.4 mm), respectively. This may be an acceptable compromise in light of follow-up studies demonstrating absent two-point discrimination in up to 80% of island pedicle flaps transposed on intact nerves despite preservation of sharp/dull discrimination (19). Therefore, in the very young, who remain adept at cortical reorientation, and the very old, who have limited sensory recovery after nerve repair, the conventional Littler (18) method is appropriate. For patients dependent on manual dexterity, the Foucher modification (20) of "debranchment and rebranchment" is an important option to be considered. Neuroma formation is a preventable complication of this procedure; it can be avoided by correctly burying the donor nerve deep within the interosseous muscle. Digital neurovascular island pedicle transfer should not be routinely used as a primary or emergency procedure because it requires a more complex and extensive dissection. Although prone to hyperesthesia (50%), cold intolerance, and progressive deterioration in sensibility, these issues abate at this level secondary to decreased traction on the pedicle (19). Decreasing overstretching by raising the flap from the terminal phalanx with a cuff of donor tissue around the pedicle further ensures against these risks (21). However, arguments can be made to harvest the skin from the proximal and middle segments to preserve sensibility in the donor fingertip or better yet transfer skin from an already injured digit (22). Unfortunately, proximal and middle phalangeal skin is less well innervated, and transection of terminal nerves may lead to dysesthesias in the donor fingertip.

An important caveat concerns the use of this procedure in thumbs afflicted with causalgic pain, especially those resulting from avulsion injuries (23). The procedure has not alleviated symptoms in this situation, nor has the theoretical advantage of providing additional circulation to the injured thumb provided any improvement in cold intolerance. Therefore, although neurovascular island pedicle skin transfer from an adjacent digit provides very functional and durable skin coverage, many of the anticipated benefits from preserving the integrity of artery and nerve have not been realized in subtotal thumb reconstruction.

Regional Reversed (Retrograde) Pedicle Flaps for Thumb Reconstruction

As a consequence of the search for new donor sites for microvascular free-tissue transfers, the vascular anatomy of the upper limb was reappraised recently. These studies led to the development of a number of unique island pedicle flaps that can be harvested from the injured limb in a retrograde fashion and based on one of the major longitudinal forearm vessels.

The first flap described was the radial forearm flap. The radial forearm flap provides thin skin coverage at the sacrifice of the radial artery, which possibly adds to regional vascular insufficiency as well as leaves an unsightly donor site. A retrograde flap based on the ulnar artery has been described. Its transfer is associated with the same potential vascular deficit as for the reversed radial artery flap. A variation based on the dorsal ulnar artery can be harvested without compromising the ulnar artery. These flaps are most useful in restoring skin cover about the first web space. The reverse posterior interosseous flap provides the same type of coverage as the radial artery flap without sacrificing either of the major vessels to the hand.

Distant Pedicle Flaps for Skin Coverage

Another alternative for skin coverage is to use distant pedicle flaps with their attendant risks and complications. The traditional groin flap offers satisfactory skin coverage at the expense of a bulky and mobile subcutaneous layer, poor sensibility, and dependency leading to edema and significant stiffness of the hand and inefficiency of the frequent need to delay division. The infraclavicular pedicle flap eliminates the significant disadvantage of dependency, stiffness, and bulkiness when it can be used in men. A visible unsightly scar usually precludes its use in the women (24).

A final issue related to skin integrity is web space contracture. This can be corrected with pedicle skin flaps such as dorsal rotation flaps, radial or posterior interosseous artery flaps, distant flaps (25), or cross-arm flaps (26).

Structural and Postural Restoration

For the more proximal injuries (levels II to V), the second issue after adequate skin coverage is whether or not structural lengthening is required or desired and the most appropriate method to meet this need.

Phalangization

Deepening of the thumb web space, otherwise known as phalangization, not only creates an illusion of increased length but also may truly augment hand breadth, allowing a firmer grasp of larger objects. Preservation of the adductor function of pinch and grip (27) defines the geometric limitations of enlarging the web space in a manner consistent with Littler's (28) tetrahedral configuration in contrast to a simple cleft or commissure. In the absence of soft tissue contracture and with preservation of pliable web space musculature, a traditional Z-plasty often will suffice to broaden the web space. Note, however, that the cleft produced by a standard 60-degree Z-plasty can be minimized with better distribution of tension with a four-flap Z-plasty.

Severe contracture as discussed earlier necessitates recruitment of additional skin, preferably from local flaps, analogous to a syndactyly release (Fig. 48-6). Unfortunately, subcutaneous tissue of distant flaps retains the phenotypic characteristic of the site of origin and may all too well reflect

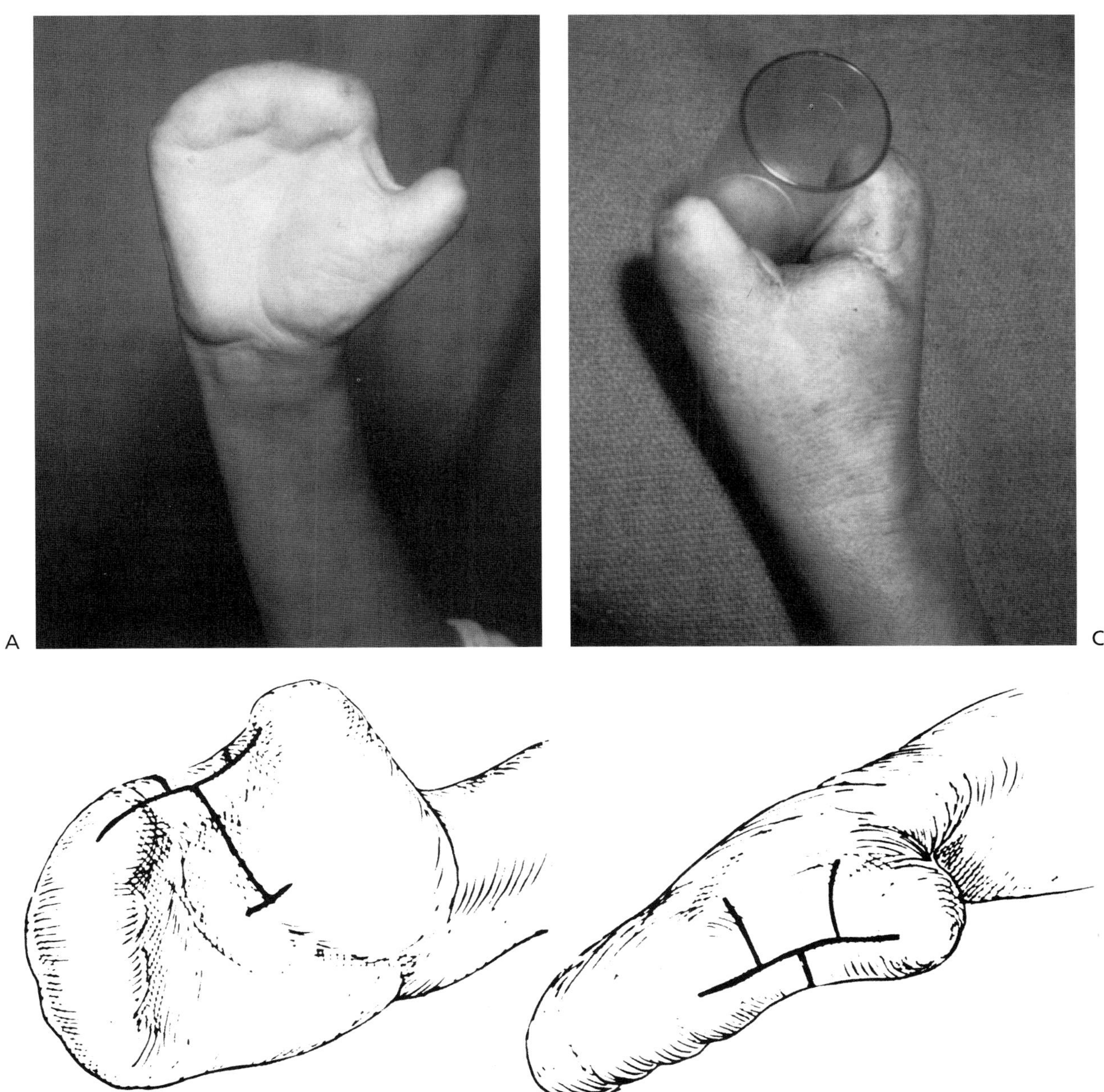

FIGURE 48-6. A–C: The remaining thumb skeleton can assume an appearance of greater length by deepening the first web space. Rearrangement of the soft tissue much like that for release of syndactyly, rather than a standard Z-plasty, is advocated. This results in an increased ability to grasp objects of greater diameter. (From Hentz VR, Littler JW, Pellegrini VD. Thumb reconstruction. In: McFarlane RM, ed. Unsatisfactory results in hand surgery. Edinburgh: Churchill Livingstone, 1987:113–143, with permission.)

changes in body weight (Fig. 48-7). Proximal adductor origin release as described by Matev (29) maintains functional continuity but does not allow for significant deepening and contributes little to the phalangization of an already shortened thumb amputation. Systematic division of the first dorsal interosseous muscle followed by the leading edge of the adductor usually is sufficient; however, extreme contracture requiring complete release of the adductor may be fraught with significant flexion-adduction weakness. This situation can be avoided by recession of the adductor with more proximal reattachment to the shaft of the metacarpal (30). Resection of a useless index ray (27) or pollicization of a damaged index finger may further enlarge the web space.

Even more extreme cases may require trapeziometacarpal capsulotomy or even trapezial excision, to afford sufficient thumb metacarpal abduction to provide a functional web

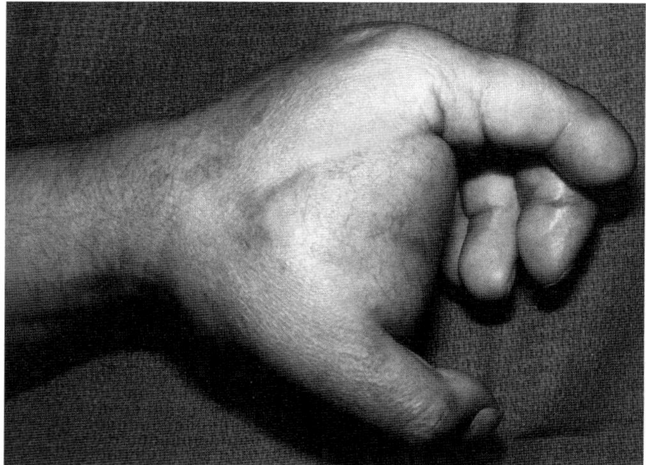

A

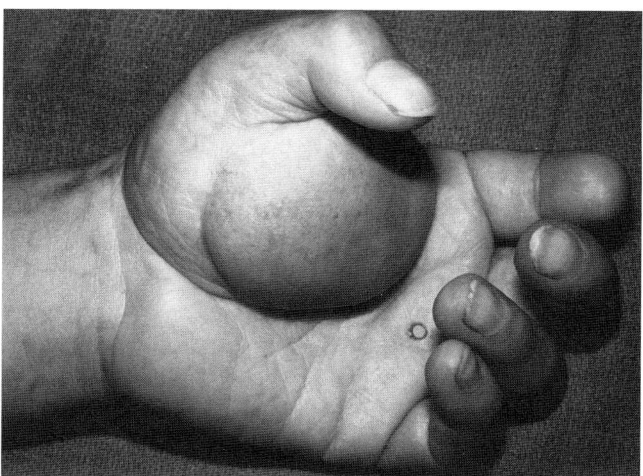

B

FIGURE 48-7. A,B: The choice of distant flaps for coverage of defects or as an element in osteoplastic pollicization must take into account future changes in patient body weight. The abdominal flap retains the fat storage capabilities of the donor site. In this case, marked weight gain is reflected in the development of a bulky flap that interferes with function. (From Hentz VR, Littler JW, Pellegrini VD. Thumb reconstruction. In: McFarlane RM, ed. Unsatisfactory results in hand surgery. Edinburgh: Churchill Livingstone, 1987:113–143, with permission.)

space. Dissection at this level demands careful attention to the superficial radial artery and its branch, the princeps pollicis, to maintain adequate circulation to the thumb.

Finally, treatment of recurrent contractures may require prolonged splinting for up to 6 months postoperatively, along with tendon transfer to augment poorly functioning thenar musculature. This procedure is most appropriate for level II injuries.

Distraction Osteogenesis

Although first described for metacarpal lengthening, distraction osteogenesis has been applied to phalangeal lengthening for congenital and traumatic thumb insufficiencies (29). It provides for better more precise functional grip but does not improve pulp pinch (31).

Previous advocates of this technique advocated bone grafting the defect created by the elongation process. Seitz and Dobyns (32) promote healing by callotasis (regenerate bone) as structurally adequate, physiologically sound, and comfortable for the patient. Given a metacarpal of length that is near normal (two-thirds) or 3 cm, and good skin coverage, distraction lengthening (29) affords elongation of up to 1 mm per day, resulting in an increase of 50% to 100% (2 to 4.5 cm, average 3.5 cm) over 2 to 4 months. New bone organizes into a trabecular network by approximately 2 months after surgery and into lamellar bone by 4 months, with central, normal hematopoietic marrow (32). Requiring 30 days for distraction anticipates the necessary two-fold for children and three-fold for adults (32) additional isometric distraction to allow intramembranous ossification within the gap of connective tissue. Complications range from common benign pin-track infections to significant deleterious compromise in skin and bone vascularity. Proceeding slowly with the initial distraction process and after gain of 50% in length avoids ischemia and thus the likelihood of infection and skin slough. Matev (29) recommends lengthening 0.7 to 0.75 mm per day beginning 3 to 4 days after surgery. Seitz and Dobyns support this and lengthens their patients 1 mm per day (rhythmic lengthening of 0.25 mm four times per day) beginning 5 days postoperatively in a child and 7 days in an adult. This allows adequate callus formation while preventing premature consolidation.

The most common complication is pin-site problems. Pin-track infections respond well to oral antibiotics and debridement. They can be prevented by meticulous pin-site care and stable fixation where the use of four pins has been found to be the most important variable in stability (33). Distal skin slough requires creative skin flap acrobatics. Adequate surgical soft tissue exposure and careful traction pin placement prevent soft tissue injury, whether vascular, neurologic, or tendinous. Distal sensibility transiently diminishes during lengthening but returns to the normal preoperative level at the conclusion of the distraction process (31).

As mentioned, adults take longer to achieve mature bone. Although ossification can be accelerated by bone growth electrostimulation with a noninvasive electromagnetic or semi-invasive needle bone stimulation during the second half, Matev (29) recommends bone grafting for patients older than 20 years with a gap larger than 3 cm. He suggests that the long-term lack of trophic disorders is attributable to this interposition type of bone lengthening. Another potential pitfall, fracture of the graft, can be avoided by adequate protection of the bone graft with a plaster splint for 25 days while the graft undergoes incorporation and maturation. Manktelow and Wainwright (34) assert that a step osteotomy eliminates the need for a bone graft. Notice that children frequently do not require bone grafting to consolidate the gap produced during lengthening due to active periosteal new bone formation.

Aside from poor skeletal fixation, failure of bone regeneration may result from osseous devascularization secondary to inadequate preservation and closure of the periosteum, or from heat necrosis with the use of a power saw instead of an osteotome to make the osteotomy or corticotomy. Device stability and integrity can be jeopardized by bending the pins to force the fit at the time of device placement, which makes the pins weaker and prone to failure. Rotational or angular deformity may result with premature removal of the distraction device before achieving solid consolidation along the full length and width. Reapplication of the device until the deformity is corrected, with immobilization until complete consolidation is present on radiographs, ameliorates this complication.

Ramsundar et al. (35) claim that rotational and angular deformities can be prevented by using Ikuta's phalangeal compression-distraction-fixation device. Like Ilizarow's device it provides distraction. It functions as a compression device by steadying the bone graft and providing good bony contact to allow filling of the defect. As a fixation device, it maintains stability to prevent angulation and malrotation.

Finally, and most importantly, nonpliable soft tissue coverage presents the greatest resistance to lengthening and may result in flexion deformity of the proximal phalangeal remnant at the metacarpophalangeal joint or, less commonly, radial subluxation of the trapeziometacarpal joint. Prevention of joint complications such as luxation requires recognition of ligamentous injuries rendering the joint unstable, where tension forces transmitted across the joint during the distraction process can result in luxation or malalignment. Even with stable joints, however, inadequate rehabilitation or poor pin or device position may result in a stiff adjacent joint. In addition to the previous guidelines, congenital cases require special attention to placement of the Kirschner (K-)wires 5 mm away from growth plate. Furthermore, metacarpal and phalangeal lengthening can be repeated at 1- to 2-year intervals in children. Unfortunately, this results in a thin digit without interphalangeal movement, so its use requires strong indications (36). Hierner et al. (36) recommend starting at age 5 years, because this procedure tolerates few errors and requires strict compliance.

Osteoplastic Pollicization

Osteoplastic reconstruction had its beginnings in Gillies' "cocked-hat flap," where stable skin coverage allowed raising a volar-based skin flap that would accommodate a bone graft. Although this procedure provided 1- to 1.5-cm increase in length, observations suggest that it compromised sensation. Although some claim that normal two-point discrimination persisted (37), others found sensation was equal to or worse than the dorsal skin over the metacarpal because repositioning of the skin required division of cutaneous nerves. Occasionally, wound breakdown and bone resorption resulted in a sensitive nonfunctional tip. Furthermore, tissue rearrangement decreased web depth and compromised cosmesis.

Gillies' cocked-hat procedure fell from favor because of these complications and the overall lack of sufficient functional gain. The procedure was modified in a number of ways to provide a more substantial thumb replacement for level III and IV injuries. This led to the multiple staged procedure of attachment and subsequent division of a nonsensate tubed pedicle flap and installation of bone graft at the time of attachment, between attachment and division (37), or at division of the pedicle (Fig. 48-8). The complicating issues of attaching the hand to the end of a tubed pedicle flap for a prolonged period of time was discussed earlier. The insensate pedicle flaps spurred the incorporation of a neurovascular island flap, which also added the risk of another procedure and the problem of cortical reorientation. Furthermore, each bone graft donor site had its inherent problems, and none was resistant to bone absorption.

Bone graft donor sites have included rib, clavicle, anteromedial region of tibia, and iliac crest. The osteogenic potential of the iliac crest and the need for cast protection of the leg following tibial graft harvest to avoid pathologic stress fracture appear to make the pelvis a more favorable graft (Fig. 48-9). Few surgeons have continued use of the tibia as the preferred donor site. However, the inherent curvature of the ilium presents unique problems as well.

Other sources of osteoplastic pollicization include the radial forearm osteocutaneous graft (38) with neurovascular island flap, which can be complicated by radius fractures and donor site problems, and the dorsalis pedis free flap plus iliac crest bone graft.

Proper graft position within the tubed flap and its angle of attachment to the recipient bone should restore the normal flexion arc to the thumb. This may be accomplished by either proper orientation of the natural curvature of the graft or creation of a greenstick fracture at the appropriate level (Fig. 48-10). The graft should be 1 to 2 cm shorter than that required to restore normal length to the injured thumb to compensate for the loss of dexterity with the equivalent of fused metacarpophalangeal and interphalangeal joints. Normal length without normal flexibility and control frequently results in less than optimal function (39). Given the relative avascularity of the graft and that bone resorption requires a blood supply, the more likely reason for resorption may be a manifestation of disuse atrophy secondary to suboptimal sensibility in the overlying skin or hypersensitivity at the very tip of the bone graft. The vascularized wraparound flap offers a solution for a one-stage procedure that provides

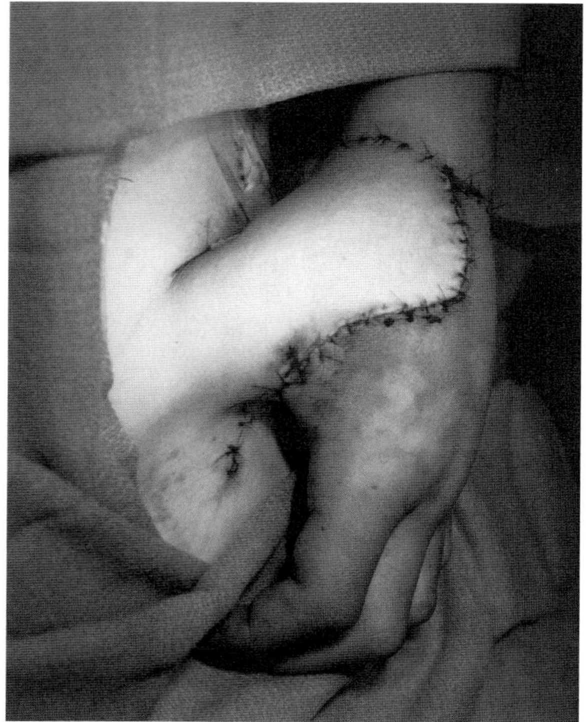
A

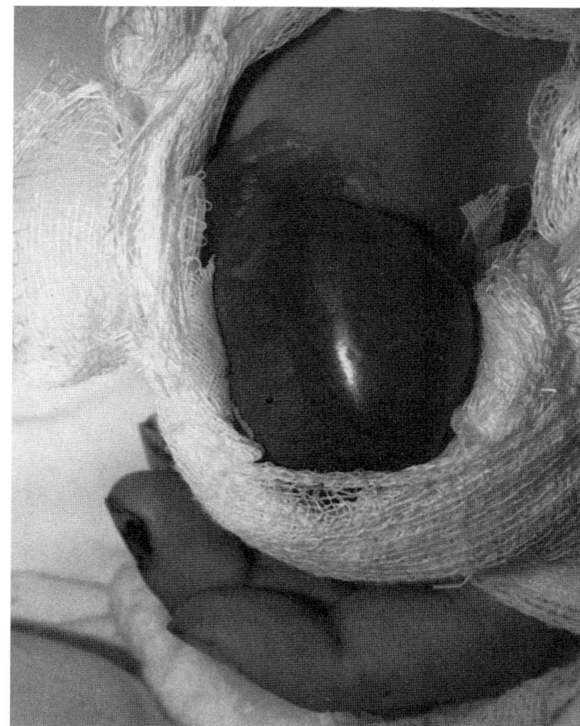
B

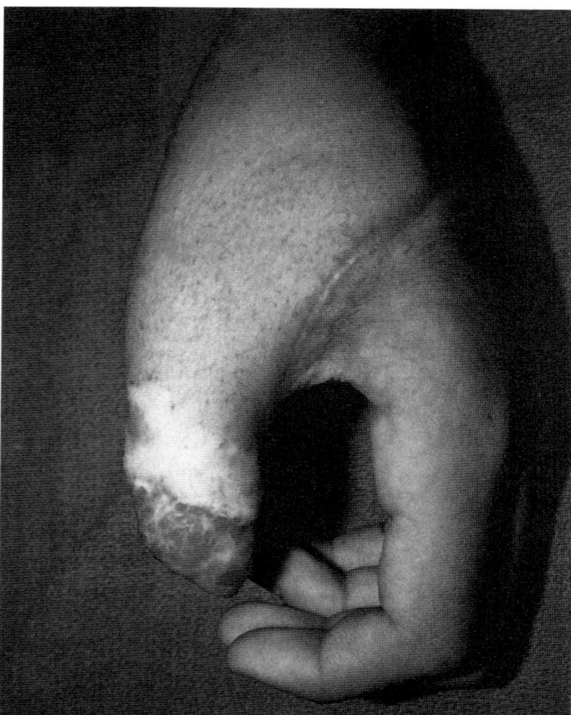
C

FIGURE 48-8. A–C: The multiple stages required for osteoplastic pollicization allow numerous opportunities for development of complications leading to an unfavorable result. In this case, a very long groin flap was used to cover the remaining skeleton after an avulsion injury. There was no means to temporarily occlude the pedicle to determine if revascularization of the flap via newly formed recipient site vessels was adequate to nourish all the flap. Following division of the flap, the distal soft tissue suffered from ischemia with subsequent loss of some length of the flap. (From Hentz VR, Littler JW, Pellegrini VD. Thumb reconstruction. In: McFarlane RM, ed. Unsatisfactory results in hand surgery. Edinburgh: Churchill Livingstone, 1987:113–143, with permission.)

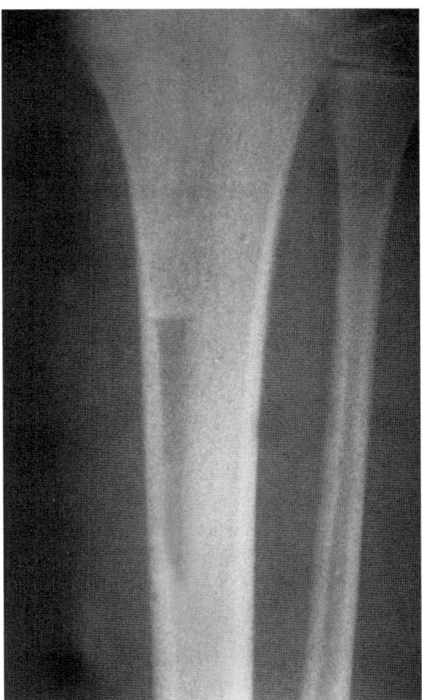

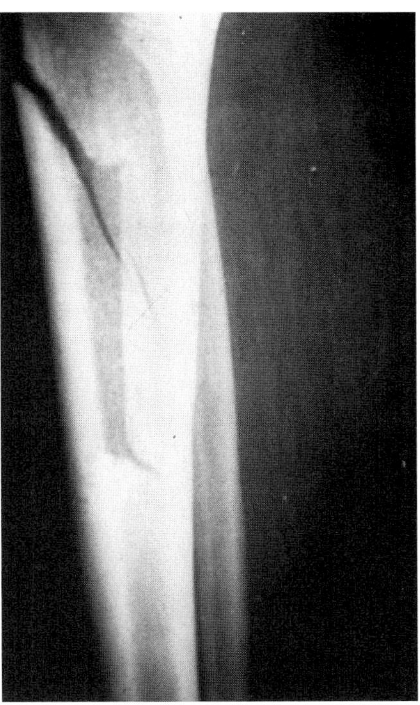

FIGURE 48-9. A,B: Attention to detail must extend to the postoperative period. Harvesting of a bone graft, e.g., from the anterior surface of the tibia, focuses stresses transmitted through the tibia with weight bearing (stress risers). A period of 6 weeks of no weight bearing or protected ambulation in an orthosis is necessary to avoid a potential pathologic tibial fracture. (From Hentz VR, Littler JW, Pellegrini VD. Thumb reconstruction. In: McFarlane RM, ed. Unsatisfactory results in hand surgery. Edinburgh: Churchill Livingstone, 1987:113–143, with permission.)

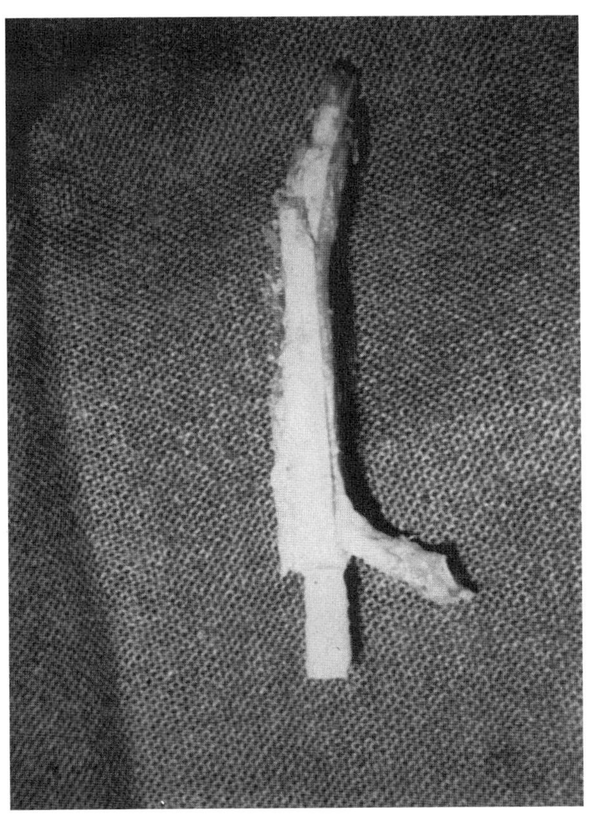

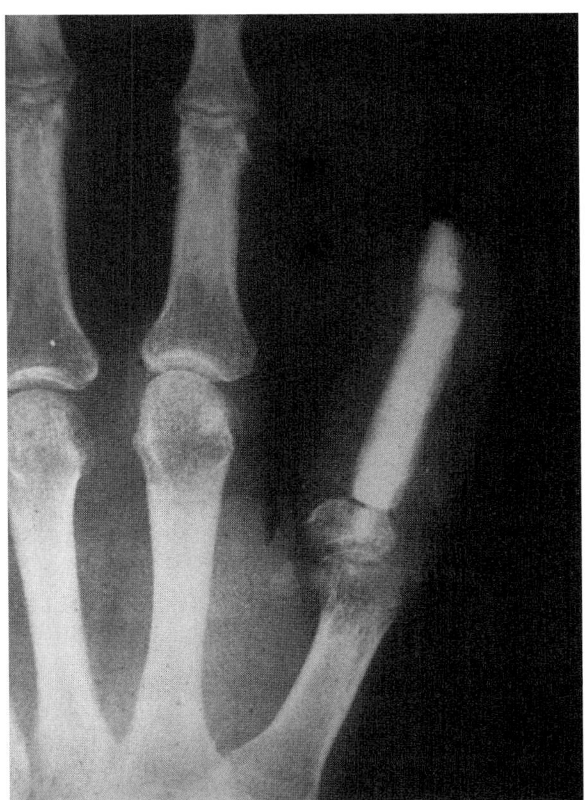

FIGURE 48-10. A,B: Various refinements in osteoplastic techniques have been suggested, including fracturing the bone graft to restore a semblance of terminal flexion. Commonly, in accord with the Wolff law, the terminal fracture remodels over time. (*continued*)

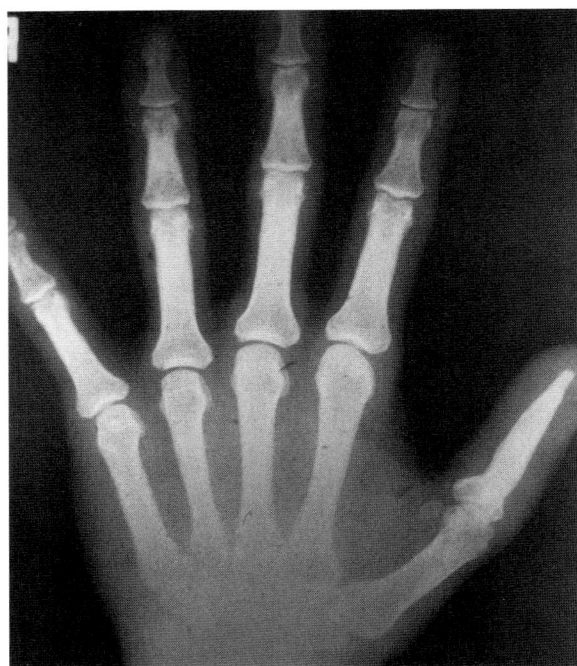

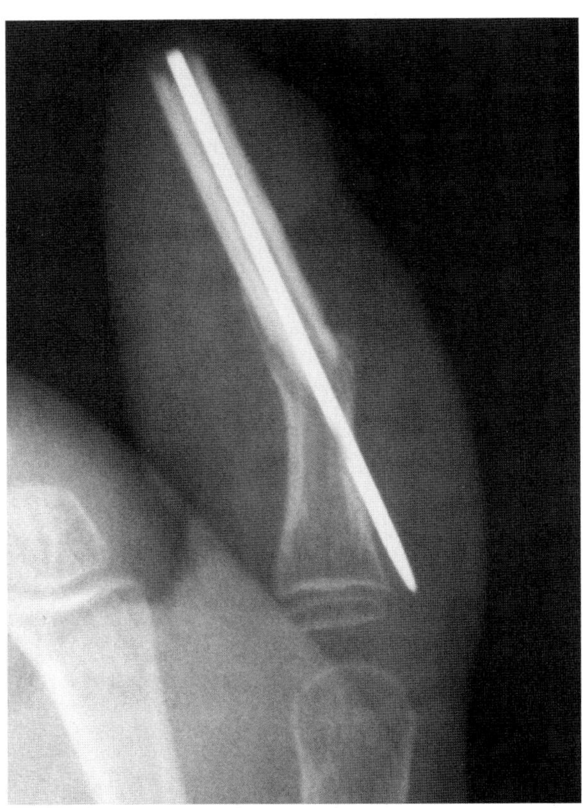

FIGURE 48-10. (Continued) **C,D:** This occurs to a lesser degree when the bone graft itself is mechanically fixed to the recipient site in some flexion. (From Hentz VR, Littler JW, Pellegrini VD. Thumb reconstruction. In: McFarlane RM, ed. Unsatisfactory results in hand surgery. Edinburgh: Churchill Livingstone, 1987:113–143, with permission.)

sensate coverage and prevents bone resorption. Tendons are transferred, allowing function and therefore limiting resorption. The best results with this approach are obtained with nearly complete preservation of the metacarpal and the surrounding thenar muscular core to control the critical trapeziometacarpal articulation (Fig. 48-11).

With less than one-half to one-third of the normal length of the metacarpal intact (level IV), the abnormal proportions of the reconstructed thumb and loss of intrinsic control of the basal joint result in less than satisfactory results from osteoplastic thumb reconstruction.

Pollicization

Pollicization of a normal digit from a full complement of four normal fingers represents a more facile approach to thumb reconstruction, with the significant advantages of providing normal immediate sensibility (28,40) and faster recovery to normal function without the risk of microsurgical loss (Fig. 48-12) (7). The development of microsurgical free transfer of toe to thumb has intensified the controversy about sacrifice of a normal finger for reconstruction of level III injury (41). Much less debatable is the pollicization of an injured digit, seen frequently with traumatic damage to the thumb (28). This represents the ultimate in "conservation of tissues": adding length, sensibility, and function to the thumb position while affording an opportunity for web reconstruction if the index or long fingers are transferred. Any of the four fingers can be used, depending on the degree of injury; however, the proximity and functional independence of the index finger and the ease with which the long finger spontaneously assumes its place and function make the index finger the easiest and most successful transfer (7,28,42). For the three ulnar digits, skin flaps and more complex palmar incisions, which may hinder grip, are required. The vascular pedicle is more susceptible to mechanical kinking or compression beneath intact skin bridges. Preservation of a dorsal vein is extremely difficult when transposing the long finger and impossible when pollicizing the ring or little fingers. Furthermore, the third metacarpal remains, as does the origin of the adductor pollicis.

Pollicization of the other digits produces an obvious void. In the case of the long finger, it may lead to rotation and overriding of the adjacent index and ring fingers. This may be decreased by transferring the index finger onto the third metacarpal (7). If the index finger is not available, the next best option is the ring finger, because it is shorter than the long finger and, as discussed, the adductor pollicis in-

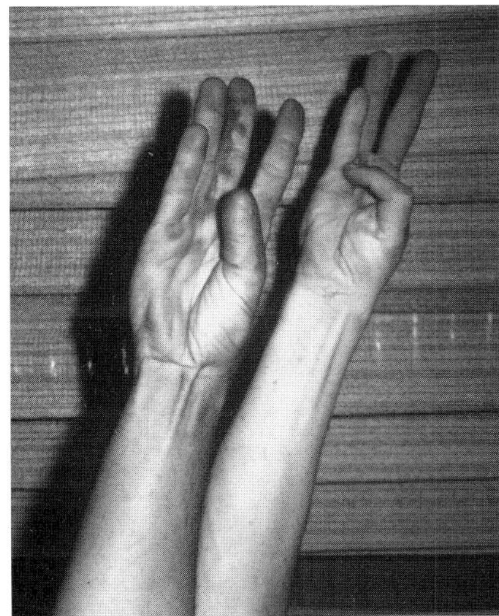
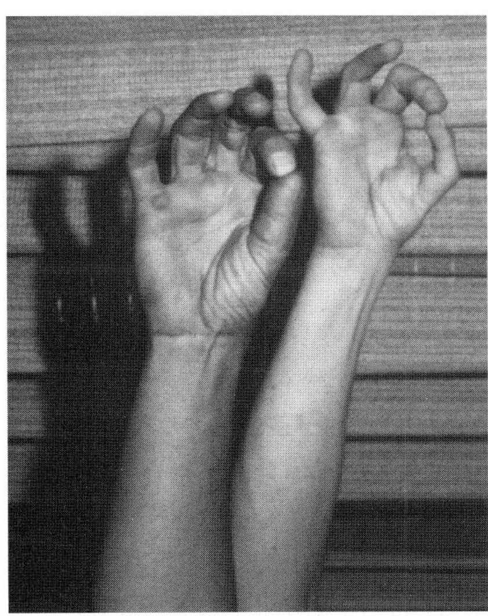
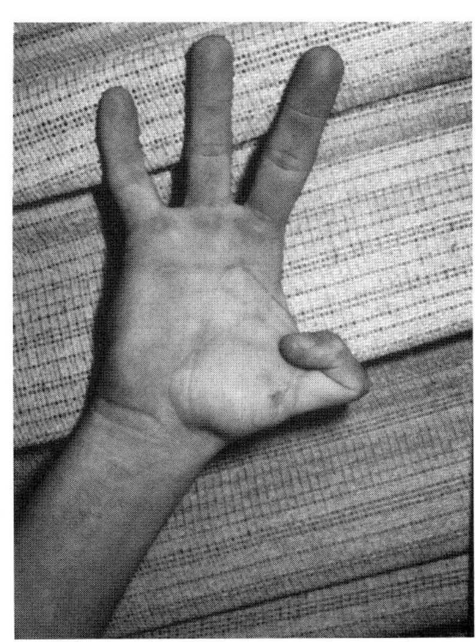

A, B C

FIGURE 48-11. A–C: Appearance of an osteoplastic reconstruction compared to the result after index pollicization. (From Hentz VR, Littler JW, Pellegrini VD. Thumb reconstruction. In: McFarlane RM, ed. Unsatisfactory results in hand surgery. Edinburgh: Churchill Livingstone, 1987:113–143, with permission.)

serts on the third metacarpal and the long finger naturally substitutes for the index finger. Finally, the importance of cupping and providing ulnar support of the hand, as well as the difficulties associated with transferring the hypothenar intrinsic muscles to the ring finger, make the little finger a poor candidate for pollicization.

Abnormal vascular anatomy resulting from the original injury should be delineated by preoperative arteriography. Severely damaged and scarred skin covering the web space and thumb should be excised and replaced by either local flaps during the pollicization or a distant flap in a separate preliminary procedure. Problems and complications contributing to an unsatisfactory result following pollicization can be divided into three general categories: skin incision and web reconstruction, vascular compromise, and management of the skeleton.

Skin Incision and Web Reconstruction

The need to excise unsatisfactory skin overlying the thumb and web space, to interrupt scar constricting the thumb base and provide for satisfactory configuration and coverage of the reconstructed web space, dictates the proper design of skin incisions about the thumb and the need for local or possibly distant flaps. As discussed earlier, interdigitating dorsal and volar web flaps (28) or varying combinations of Z-plasties (42) aid in reconstructing the web space, which should remain at the level of the metacarpophalangeal joint of the reconstructed thumb that corresponds to the PIP joint of the transposed index finger. This necessitates longitudinal incisions to that level on the index ray to allow for positioning of the web and to add skin for coverage of the reconstructed intrinsic musculature. The tendency toward more proximal placement of the web results in a grotesque thumb substitute with an overlying slender profile and illusion of excessive length.

Vascular Compromise

With adequate preparation and meticulous technique, this most devastating complication becomes an infrequent occurrence. Despite preoperative arteriography to determine the condition and number of intact recipient vessels, dissection should begin in the palm to verify neurovascular integrity. Inclusion of perivascular fat with the pedicle preserves small venous channels accompanying the digital arteries. Even better, raising a 1.5-cm strip of skin with the pedicle adds stability and incorporates precious veins (7).

Pollicization of a digit, other than the index finger, requires a palmar incision, which precludes the use of a dorsal vein (7). The pedicle is routed through a plane superficial to the flexor tendons with particular care to avoid graft contortion, constriction by old scars, positioning beneath tight skin bridges, and excessive rotation that might compromise vascular flow to the digit. Brunelli and Brunelli (7) make a V incision in the palm to ensure that vital nerves and vessels are not cut while manipulating the pedicle under tight skin bridges. Once the tourniquet is released, anything other than brisk return of circulation must be investigated immediately and the source discovered and rectified. Surgical delay is possible as a salvage maneuver but seldom is necessary (43). Postoperative vascular insufficiency is avoided by elevation, releasing constricting dressings, and using sympathetic blockade to reduce vasospasm.

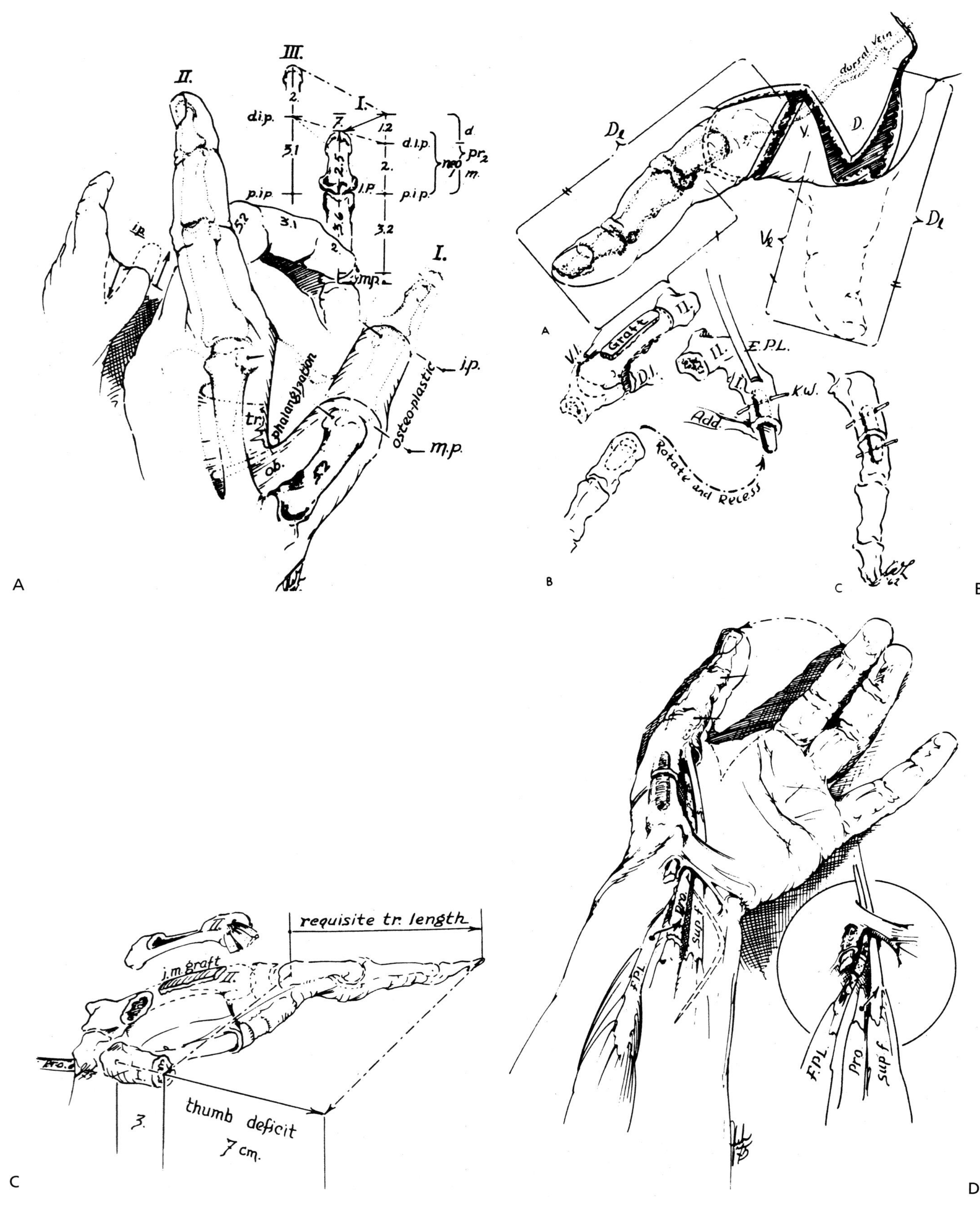
III.
II.
I.
d.i.p.
p.ip.
i.p.
mp.
I.P.
d.i.p.
p.i.p.
neo
pr2
phalangization
osteo-plastic
i.p.
m.p.
tr.
ob.
A
dorsal vein
D1
D.
V.
V2
D1
Graft
II.
V.I.
D.I.
II.
E.P.L.
K.W.
Add.
Rotate and Recess
A
B
C
B
requisite tr. length
j.m.graft
II.
I.
3.
thumb deficit
7 cm.
C
F.P.L.
Pro.
sup f.
F.P.L.
Pro.
sup f.
D

Management of the Skeleton

Skeletal management encompasses both posture and stability of the reconstructed thumb. Posture implies both length and attitude of the thumb relative to the remaining digits. Comparative radiography of the injured and normal thumbs helps to determine the appropriate length; however, from both a cosmetic and functional standpoint, it is better to err on the side of a shorter rather than a longer reconstructed thumb. This requires shortening of either the distal phalanx or the metacarpal. Shortening the metacarpal results in an apparition that is much thinner than the normal thumb, with the following attendant disadvantages: redundant length of the tendons necessitating shortening; the presence of the profundus and superficialis flexor tendons as opposed to a single long flexor in the thumb; and the difficulty of suturing the intrinsic muscles of the thumb (adductor, abductor pollicis brevis, and opponens) onto the tendons of the intrinsic muscles of the index finger (7). By sacrificing the nail with shortening of the metacarpal, there are none of these problems and the resulting thumb better mimics the dimensions of the normal thumb, although without the nail.

With regard to posture, as a condyloid articulation, the thumb metacarpophalangeal joint allows pronation along the thumb's longitudinal axis of 15 to 20 degrees. As the ginglymoid proximal interphalangeal joint cannot mimic this motion, the pollicized segment should be rotated an additional 15 to 20 degrees relative to the thumb metacarpal. In addition, the thumb interphalangeal joint pronates 10 to 15 degrees in flexion, whereas the index terminal joint rotates into supination. Therefore, overall the pollicized segment requires 120 to 140 degrees of rotation (pronation) relative to its original position (42). A good intraoperative guide is to allow the reconstructed thumb tip to oppose the ring finger. Elasticity of the soft tissues tends to neutralize this positioning, making overrotation a rare occurrence.

Secondary procedures such as opposition transfer of the dispensable superficial flexor of the pollicized digit may be required to improve functional rotation of the basal joint even where one half of the metacarpal and the accompanying intrinsic musculature remain intact. Secondary adjustment of flexor tendon tone or transfer of flexor pollicis longus to the reconstructed thumb may be desired for enhanced functional independence and active flexion.

Although instability of the bony juncture between thumb metacarpal and transferred segment is infrequent, joint instability remains a difficult problem. Either placing a free intramedullary graft or designing a spike (tooth) from the proximal phalanx (7) of the transposed digit to fit into the thumb metacarpal remnant with K-wires achieves union. The availability of small but sturdy plating systems makes this a more practical approach than in the past. Hyperextension instability of one or both of the transposed interphalangeal joints is a frequent reminder of the complexity and delicate balance of the intrinsic and extrinsic musculature (Figs. 48-11C, 48-13). Powerful metacarpophalangeal joint flexion is lost with amputation of the sesamoids and detachment of the proximal phalangeal insertion of the flexor pollicis brevis, adductor pollicis, and abductor pollicis brevis. The loss of extrinsic flexor tone following recession of the pollicized digit along with transfer and readjustment of the extensor tendons aggravates the tendency toward interphalangeal joint hyperextension. The two slips of the superficial flexor insertion on the middle phalanx of the pollicized index finger can be used to reinsert the adductor pollicis and flexor pollicis brevis on their respective ulnar and radial sides and restore strong metacarpophalangeal flexion, although at the expense of intrinsic extensor tone to the terminal joint (12). In a similar fashion, the first dorsal and first volar interosseous muscle can be reattached to the lateral bands of the extensor mechanism of the transposed digit at the level of the former proximal interphalangeal joint, functioning primarily to extend the terminal two segments. Alternatively, one of the interosseous muscles can be attached to the former superficialis insertion on the middle phalanx to provide for strong flexion of the newly created metacarpophalangeal joint. Littler has suggested shortening and transferring the index superficial flexor to the pollicized proximal or middle phalangeal segments of the reconstructed thumb to enhance pinch. In the adaptation of Brunelli and Brunelli, the distal phalanx is amputated, leaving the first volar interosseous, first dorsal interosseous, and first lumbrical muscles available to be sutured to the adductor pollicis, opponens, and abductor pollicis brevis, respectively. To prevent hyperextension, the ac-

FIGURE 48-12. A–D: Littler's depiction of thumb reconstruction with emphasis on pollicization. Phalangization achieves "relative" lengthening, osteoplastic reconstruction ideally restores thumb length to the interphalangeal joint level, and pollicization most closely restores a mobile thumb of nearly normal size. Sequential skeletal dimensions are best approximated by long finger pollicization, but overall thumb length is equally well replaced by proper deployment of the index digit **(A)**. Preoperative measurement of volar and dorsal skin lengths adds precision in thumb reconstruction **(B)**. Interdigital dorsal and volar web flaps and recession-abduction-pronation of the transposed part are critical steps in the technique. An intramedullary bone graft fixed by transverse wires is fused to restore an average skeletal length of 10 to 11 cm **(C)**. Secondary suture of the flexor pollicis longus to the profundus tendon of the neothumb enhances independence of function and affords an opportunity to increase flexor tone **(D)**. (From Hentz VR, Littler JW, Pellegrini VD. Thumb reconstruction. In: McFarlane RM, ed. Unsatisfactory results in hand surgery. Edinburgh: Churchill Livingstone, 1987:113–143, with permission.)

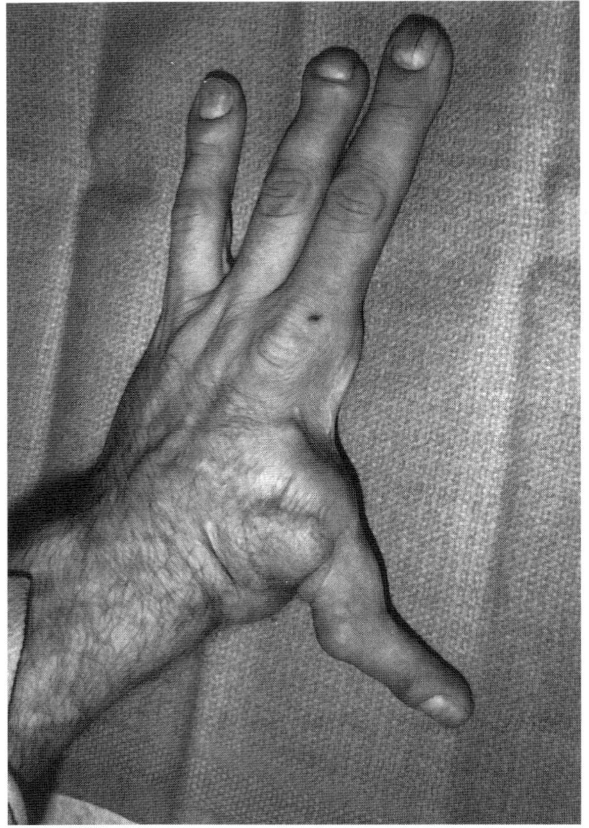
A

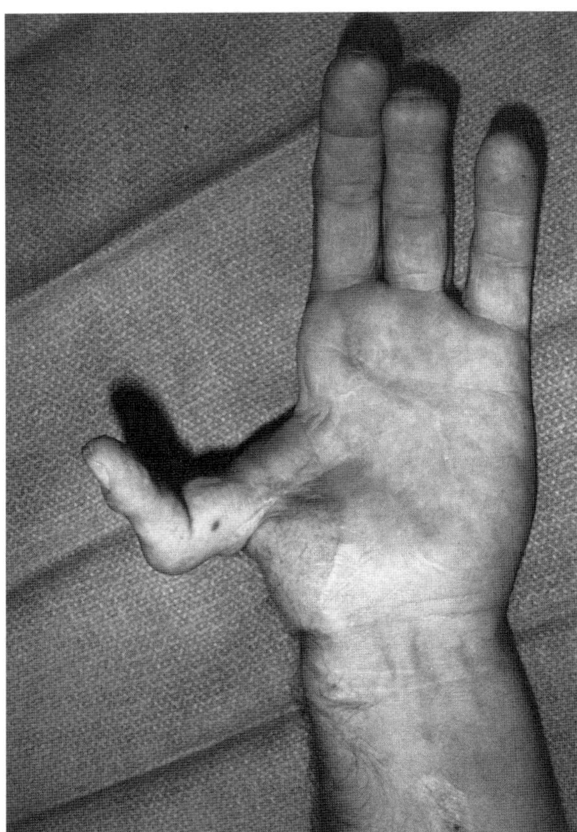
B

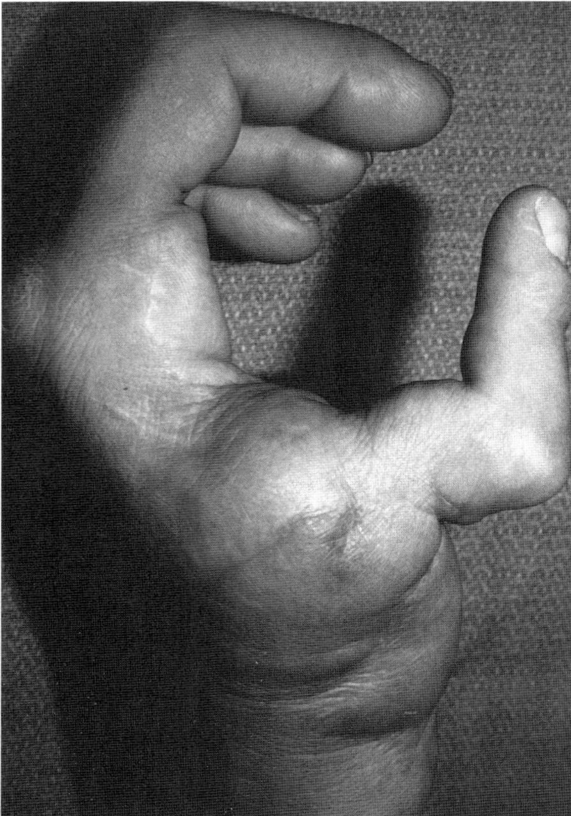
C

FIGURE 48-13. A–C: Dynamic stabilization of the transferred metacarpophalangeal joint into the carpometacarpal joint position is very difficult to achieve. When the basal joint has been destroyed and the index digit is to be transferred , it seems best to fuse the base of the proximal phalanx to the remaining radial carpal element or base of the second metacarpal. (From Hentz VR, Littler JW, Pellegrini VD. Thumb reconstruction. In: McFarlane RM, ed. Unsatisfactory results in hand surgery. Edinburgh: Churchill Livingstone, 1987:113–143, with permission.)

tion of the extensors on the proximal phalanx is weakened by severing the dorsal hood longitudinally. The A1 pulley may be released, and a third transfixing K-wire is used to keep the metacarpophalangeal joint in 25 degrees of flexion for 35 days. Basically, an additional loss in function occurs when a digit other than the index finger is used, causing tendons to cross (7). Interestingly, unlike nerve transposition, tendon transposition is associated with rapid corticalization. This makes the old practice of reattaching transposed tendons to thumb tendons obsolete and prevents subsequent adhesions (7). Amputating the distal phalanx allows easier adaptation of tendon function without the need to fine tune tendon length. For amputations at the level of the trapeziometacarpal joint, the technique is modified by preserving the distal phalanx and implanting the head of the second metacarpal on the trapezium or in its place if it is lacking, such as in congenital malformations.

Voluntary movement is begun the next day. Advantages of transfer without the distal phalanx include a comparably sized thumb; the ability to adjust length by removing as much metacarpal as necessary; the possibility of suturing the tendons of the first dorsal interosseous and lumbrical to the abductor pollicis brevis and opponens and that of the first volar interosseous to the adductor pollicis; the possibility of transferring the first on the second dorsal interosseous muscle, which allows the long finger the ability to be strongly abducted; achieving normal tension of the extrinsic flexor and extensor tendons; and a thumb with two phalanges. Fusion of the new metacarpophalangeal joint serves to simplify and stabilize the system (28).

Index finger pollicization offers a potentially excellent functional reconstruction for injuries at the midmetacarpal level. In addition to restoration of length, it provides normal sensibility, independence of motion, and potential for stability that characterize the normally functioning thumb. However, because of the complexity of the digit being imitated, satisfactory functional restitution will not be achieved by a single operative procedure in all cases. Secondary procedures directed at specific functional deficits may be necessary and were indicated in 80% of cases in one series of thumb reconstruction by pollicization of a previously injured digit (44).

Other Refinements

To avoid the numbness of neuromas caused by cutting the branch for the long finger, Brunelli (7) suggests separating the fascicles to the long finger.

CONSIDERATIONS IN CONGENITAL ANOMALIES

Just when the choice between thumb reconstruction and thumb salvage seems fairly straightforward, a young Asian boy presented with a Blauth type 4 thumb anomaly, and the parents became tearful at the thought of its removal in favor of reconstruction. Unfortunately, reconstructing a type 4 deficiency by shifting it palmarly and proximally, inserting some type of bony support (autogenous corticocancellous iliac crest bone, free fibula, or microvascular transfer of the second tarsometatarsal joint), and providing skin coverage (dorsal hand flap) result in a functionally limited reconstruction (limited tendon excursion and poor joint mechanics) and limit potential for pollicization due to skin damage (45).

It frequently is difficult to decide when a structurally deficient thumb with less than a normal complement of skeletal components is salvageable by staged reconstruction. If the abnormal thumb significantly varies from normal size, it is best to ablate that member and proceed with pollicization of the next most radial digit. Conservation of tissues still can be used to a limited extent to create the illusion of a thenar eminence by subcutaneous burial of these nonfunctional remnants.

To have a more successful outcome with regard to congenital problems, one must initially consider developmental issues apart from the thumb that affect the entire well-being of the child and secondarily affect the success of the procedure. Associated congenital anomalies, such as thrombocytopenia and myocardial septal defects, are considered along with the normal cardiopulmonary development, which is more stable at 12 months. Waiting 1 year allows maturation of the vascular system, such that involution of the endosteal circulation allows more effective use of a tourniquet to provide a bloodless field and the friable veins and arteries of infancy have attained a more substantial thickness. Given that a child demonstrates bimanual grasp between 9 to 12 months, Strickland and Kleinman (45) advocate intervention at 1 year. They are flanked by some of the greatest authorities, where Littler (40) prefers 2 to 4 years, and Flatt (46) prefers 6 to 12 months.

In pollicization for the congenitally absent thumb, the surgical principles are identical to those for posttraumatic thumb reconstruction, with several notable exceptions.

Without scar tissue requiring excision and more available skin coverage for web space construction, the design of skin incisions focuses on interrupting what would otherwise be a circumferential incision at the base of the pollicized digit, placing the volar incision to simulate a thenar crease, and preventing incisions through the potential web space.

There is some controversy centered around the timing and the need to shorten extensor and flexor tendons. Caroll (47) and Buck-Gramcko (48) shorten the extensor tendons (extension indicus proprius and extensor digitorum communis). Littler (40) shortens the flexor digitorum superficialis (FDS) secondarily. Strickland and Kleinman (45) found that tone returned spontaneously in their 50 cases, which parallels the findings of Buck-Gramcko, and therefore they see no need to shorten the FDS. Finally, some authors shorten neither tendon (49). Most agree that shorten-

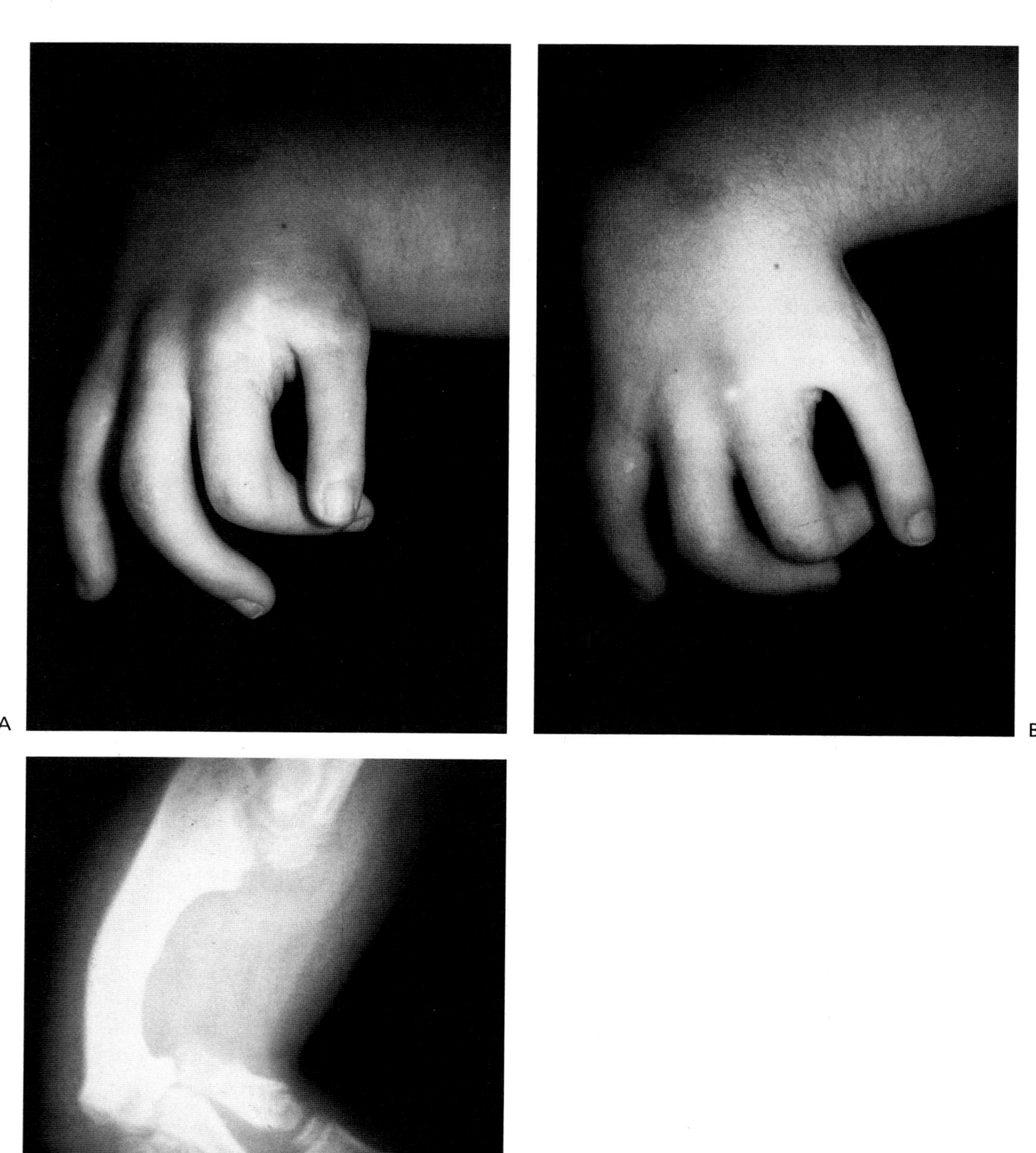

FIGURE 48-14. A–C: Insufficient abduction and rotation along with continued epiphyseal growth of the transposed metacarpal head have reduced this pollicized index finger to minimal functional value. (From Hentz VR, Littler JW, Pellegrini VD. Thumb reconstruction. In: McFarlane RM, ed. Unsatisfactory results in hand surgery. Edinburgh: Churchill Livingstone, 1987:113–143, with permission.)

ing the extensors to the length that the metacarpal is shortened is necessary, whereas shortening of the extensors may not be necessary.

On a more aesthetic level, absence of a true thenar cone frequently gives the false impression of excessive length because of the slender appearance of the pollicized digit. This can be avoided by adequate distal advancement of the abductor indicis and first volar interosseous muscles to the level of the proximal interphalangeal joint by attachment to the respective lateral bands, correct placement of the leading edge of web skin at this same level, and preservation of tissues from a nonfunctional thumb to provide bulk in simulation of a thenar eminence.

Vascular compromise may be related to unanticipated anomalous structures. Malformation of the vascular arches occurs most frequently on the preaxial side of the extremity, with anomalous intermingling of the digital artery and nerve occurring in 15% to 20% of cases and an absent radial digital vessel to the index ray in the four-fingered hand in up to 25% of cases. With the relative predictability of anomalous structures and increased risk of the use of contrast media in young children, arteriography seldom is indicated. To define the blood supply of the pertinent digit, dissection begins in the palm, with extreme care taken to identify and isolate these structures. To ensure sufficient venous outflow, Littler encourages use of both neurovascular bundles, which requires fascicular dissection and one dorsal vein. Other principles include measures to decrease arterial spasm and to prevent tight skin closure. This might include having the surgeons at the beginning of the learning curve take down the tourniquet after the neurovascular dissection before going on to the carpometacarpal joint reconstruction, because the novice usually requires 4 hours while the experienced surgeon requires 2 hours.

Imitation of the absent trapeziometacarpal joint requires strategic positioning of the pollicized digit. Placement volar to its former metacarpal provides for satisfactory opposition. Positioning the digit in 40 degrees of palmar abduction by palmar rotation of the metacarpal head prevents hyperextension at the reconstructed basal joint. The plasticity and growth potential of the infant skeleton, and further adjustment of the digit into 15 degrees of extension and 120 degrees of pronation, allow a crude approximation of this unique articular relationship.

Both Hentz and Littler (50) and Buck-Gramcko (48) emphasize the need for complete epiphyseal arrest of the transposed index metacarpal head to avoid late overgrowth of the new trapezium and subsequent deformity (Fig. 48-14).

There are differing opinions regarding the advisability of primary opponensplasty, most frequently using the flexor superficialis tendon from the pollicized digit, when available (12). As secondary procedures frequently are necessary to increase power and independence, it seems prudent to delay opponensplasty until a specific functional deficit is identified. This allows tendon transfer to be conducted in a more attentive manner rather than at the conclusion of an already long and arduous pollicization. This avoids additional surgery in those patients in whom it is unnecessary and affords the additional benefit of increased cooperation during postoperative retraining in the older child. When the superficial flexor tendon is not available for transfer from the pollicized digit, shift of the abductor digiti minimi (Huber transfer) can provide augmentation of opposition while adding bulk to the thenar eminence. Littler performs shortening of the FDS in the distal forearm and transfer of flexor pollicis longus to flexor digitorum profundus as secondary procedures. Other deficiencies also can be addressed.

With respect to dissection in children, attention must be given to the anomalous neural ring around the common digital artery (51).

Despite adequate skin for the web space, the design of incisions is challenging to prevent scar contractures. Unfortunately, Gosset's (52) palmar-based transposition flap to cover the web space still produced contractures, as did Caroll's (47). Littler (40) designed better skin incisions to prevent web space scarring. In spite of carefully planned skin flaps, redundancy of the proximal flap occurs on dorsoradial side of web space and must be trimmed. The skin flaps accommodate the muscle, and the incisions determine how far the lateral bands can be mobilized from the central tendon and how far the dorsal interosseous and volar interosseous can be advanced (48). Finally, the first web space should be placed at the level of the proximal interphalangeal joint of the index finger (49).

Evolving methods to better meet the well-defined goals of thumb reconstruction (skin coverage, skeletal stability, and function) turned toward microsurgical transfers (53). As with all of the other procedures intent on rebuilding the amputated thumb after surgically successful but functionally disastrous results, these transfers were reengineered many times to become "more successful" and finally rivaled other means while limiting donor site morbidity. Now they fall into a spectrum of procedures that address the necessary requirements at the different levels of amputation or skin loss.

REFERENCES

1. Gaul JS. Radial innervated cross finger flap from index to provide sensory pulp to injured thumb. *J Bone Joint Surg Am* 1969; 51:1257–1263.
2. Bell C. *The hand. Its mechanics and vital endowment as evincing design,* 3rd ed. London: WB Pickering, 1932:162.
3. Bruner J. Salvage of the "all but amputated" thumb. *Plast Reconstr Surg* 1954;14:244–248.
4. Morrison WA. Thumb reconstruction: a review and philosophy of management. *J Hand Surg [Br]* 1992;17:4;383–390.
5. McCash CR. Free nail grafting. *Br J Plast Surg* 1965;8:19–33.
6. Foucher G, Chabaud M. The bipolar lengthening technique: a modified partial toe transfer for thumb reconstruction. *Plast Reconstr Surg* 1998;102:1981–1987.

7. Brunelli GA, Brunelli GR. Reconstruction of traumatic absence of the thumb in the adult by pollicization. *Hand Clin* 1992;8: 41–55.
8. Ward JW, Penslar, JM, Parry SW. Pollicization for thumb reconstruction in severe pediatric hand burns. *Plast Reconstr Surg* 1985;76:6:927–932.
9. Moberg E. Aspects of sensation in reconstructive surgery of the upper limb. *J Bone Joint Surg Am* 1964;46:817–825.
10. Posner MA, Smith RJ. The advancement pedicle flap for thumb injuries. *J Bone Joint Surg Am* 1971;53:1618–1621.
11. Elliot D, Wilson Y. V-Y advancement of the entire volar soft tissue of the thumb in distal reconstruction. *J Hand Surg [Br]* 1993;18:3:399–402.
12. Kelleher JC. Pollicization. In: Goldwyn RM, ed. *The unfavorable result in plastic surgery. Avoidance and treatment.* Boston: Little, Brown and Company, 1972:475–488.
13. Rivet D, Noel X, Martin D, et al. Thumb flaps. In: Gilbert A, Masquelet AC, Hentz VR. eds. *Pedicle flaps of the upper limb,* 2nd ed. London: Martin Dunitz Ltd., 1992:181–210.
14. Hynes DE. Neurovascular pedicle and advancement flaps for palmar thumb defects. *Hand Clin* 1997;13:2:207–216.
15. McFarlane RM, Stromberg WB. Resurfacing of the thumb following major skin loss. *J Bone Joint Surg Am* 1962;44: 1365–1374.
16. El-Khatib HA. Clinical experiences with the extended first dorsal metacarpal artery island flap for thumb reconstruction. *J Hand Surg [Am]* 1998;23:4:647–652.
17. Yao JM, Song JL, Xu JH. The second web bilobed island flap for thumb reconstruction. *Br J Plast Surg* 1996;49:2:103–106.
18. Adani R, Squarzina PB, Castagnetti C, et al. A comparative study of the heterodigital neurovascular island flap in thumb reconstruction, with and without nerve reconnection. *J Hand Surg [Br]* 1994;19:5:552–559.
19. Murray JF, Ord JV, Gavelin GE. The neurovascular island pedicle flap. An assessment of late results in sixteen cases. *J Bone Joint Surg Am* 1967;49:1285–1297.
20. Foucher G, Braun FM, Merle M, et al. La technique du “débranchment-rebranchment” du lambeau en ilot pedicule. *Ann Chir* 1981;35:301–303.
21. Markley JM Jr. The preservation of close two-point discrimination in the interdigital transfer of neurovascular island flaps. *Plast Reconstr Surg* 1977;59:6:812–816.
22. Murray JF. The missing thumb. In: *Symposium on frequent hand problems in plastic and reconstructive surgery,* vol. 9. St. Louis: CV Mosby, 1974:214–222.
23. Tubiana R, Duparc J. Restoration of sensibility in the hand by neurovascular skin island transfer. *J Bone Joint Surg Br* 1961;43:474–480.
24. Chase RA. An alternate to pollicisation in subtotal thumb reconstruction. *Plast Reconstr Surg* 1969;44:421–430.
25. Brown P. Adduction-flexion contracture of the thumb. Correction with dorsal rotation flap and release of contracture. *Clin Orthop* 1972;88:161–168.
26. Reid DAC, McGrouther DA. The contracted thumb web. In: *Surgery of the thumb.* Cambridge: Butterworth and Co., 1986: 139–146.
27. Brown H, Welling R, Sigman R, et al. Phalangizing the first metacarpal. *Plast Reconstr Surg* 1970;45:294–297.
28. Littler JW. Reconstruction of the thumb in traumatic loss. In: Converse JM, ed. *Reconstructive plastic surgery,* 2nd ed. Philadelphia: WB Saunders, 1977:3350–3367.
29. Matev IB. The bone-lengthening method in hand reconstruction: twenty years experience. *J Hand Surg [Am]* 1989;14[2 Pt 2]: 376–378.
30. Tubiana R, Roux JP. Phalangisation of the first and fifth metacarpals. Indications, operative technique and results. *J Bone Joint Surg Am* 1974;56:447–457.
31. Pollack HJ. Reconstruction of the traumatically amputated thumb by continuous Matev distraction. Experiences and results in 48 cases. *Handchir Mikrochir Plast Chir* 1994;26: 6:291–297.
32. Seitz WH Jr, Dobyns JH. Digital lengthening with emphasis on distraction osteogenesis in the upper limb. *Hand Clin* 1993;9:4:699–706.
33. Stuchin SA, Kummer FJ. Stiffness of small-bone external fixation methods: an experimental study. *J Hand Surg [Am]* 1984; 9:718–724.
34. Manktelow RT, Wainright DF. A technique of distraction osteosynthesis in the hand. *J Hand Surg [Am]* 1984;9:858–62.
35. Ramsundar RK, Chifumi F, Kaoru Y, et al. Experience with Ikuta’s phalangeal compression-distraction-fixation device. *J Hand Surg [Am]* 1988;13:4:515–521.
36. Hierner R, Wilhelm K, Brehl B. Callus distraction for lengthening of mid hand and finger stumps in congenital hand abnormalities—personal results and review of the literature. *Handchir Mikrochir Plast Chir* 1998;30:196–202; discussion 203–205.
37. Gillies H, Millard DR. *The principles and art of plastic surgery,* vol. 2. Boston: Little, Brown and Company, 1957:484–488.
38. Matev IB. The osteocutaneous pedicle forearm flap. *J Hand Surg [Br]* 1985;10:179–182.
39. Flatt AE. An indication for shortening of the thumb. Description of technique and brief report of five cases. *J Bone Joint Surg Am* 1964;46:1534–1539.
40. Littler JW. The neurovascular pedicle method of digital transposition for reconstruction of the thumb. *Plast Reconstr Surg* 1953;12:303–319.
41. Lister GD, Kalisman M, Tsai TM. Reconstruction of the hand with microvascular toe to hand transfers: experience with 54 toe transfers. *Plast Reconstr Surg* 1983;71:372.
42. Burton RI, Littler JW. Thumb reconstruction. In: Evart CM, ed. *Surgery of the musculoskeletal system,* vol. 2, 1st ed. New York: Churchill Livingstone, 1983:501–519.
43. Bowe JJ. Thumb construction by index transposition. *Plast Reconstr Surg* 1963;32:414–424.
44. Harkins R, Rafferty J. Digital transposition in the injured hand. *J Bone Joint Surg Am* 1972;54:1064–1069.
45. Strickland JW, Kleinman WB. Thumb reconstruction. In: Green D, ed. *Operative hand surgery.* New York: Churchill Livingstone, 1993:2043–2156.
46. Flatt AE. *The care of congenital hand anomalies.* St. Louis: CV Mosby, 1977:79.
47. Caroll RE. Pollicization. In: Green DP, ed. *Operative hand surgery,* 2nd ed. New York: Churchill Livingstone, 1988: 2263–2280.
48. Buck-Gramcko D. Pollicisation of the index finger. Method and results in aplasia and hypoplasia of the thumb. *J Bone Joint Surg Am* 1971;53:1605–1617.
49. Zancolli E. Transplantation of the index finger in congenital absence of the thumb. *J Bone Joint Surg Am* 1960;42:658–666.
50. Hentz VR, Littler JW. The surgical management of congenital hand anomalies. In: Converse J, ed. *Reconstructive plastic surgery,* vol. 6, 2nd ed. Philadelphia: WB Saunders, 1977:3306–3349.
51. Edgarton MT, Snyder GB, Webb WL. Surgical treatment of congenital thumb deformities (including psychological impact of correction). *J Bone Joint Surg Am* 1965;47:1453–1474.
52. Gosset J. La pollicixation de l’index (technique chirurgicale). *J Chir (Paris)* 1949;65:403.
53. Wei FC, Chen HC, Chuang CC, et al. Microsurgical thumb reconstruction with toe transfer: selection of various techniques. *Plast Reconstr Surg* 1994;93:2:345–351.

Discussion

THUMB RECONSTRUCTION

FU-CHAN WEI
VIVEK JAIN

The authors have presented an excellent overview of various techniques for thumb reconstruction and management of possible unfavorable results.

We agree with most of their comments and would like to emphasize that microsurgical transfer of various foot tissues provides the best thumb reconstruction at all levels. With technical refinements, these procedures have become less complicated and have acceptable donor site morbidity.

A deficient thumb is a challenge to reconstruct. The criteria for reconstruction are to provide a thumb with adequate sensation and of sufficient length to oppose remaining digits; stability of the thumb's moving parts to allow strong pinch; and freedom from pain (1).

A realistic plan should be made considering the patient's occupation, functional demands, age, psychology, motivation, and commitment to postoperative therapy. Functional as well as aesthetic considerations are important, and selection of a technique requires balancing the patient's functional needs, appearance of the reconstructed thumb, and donor site cosmesis.

LEVEL OF AMPUTATION AND ITS RELATION TO UNFAVORABLE RESULT

Level I

The aim is to obtain stable sensate and durable pulp and nail that allow manipulation of fine objects (2). Glabrous skin flaps from the pulp of toes and web space provide matching skin. Great toe wraparound flap (3), partial distal great toe (4), or, if size matches, distal second toe (5) can be used if nail reconstruction is necessary.

Level II

Although function is not seriously affected, various forms of microsurgical toe transfer remain our preference for reconstruction, as they provide better function as well as appearance compared to procedures such as phalangization, lengthening, or any of the osteoplastic procedures. (Fig. 48D-1).

Level III

This most common amputation results in significant loss of function. Procedures such as distraction lengthening or osteoplastic reconstruction not only are lengthy, but they result in less optimal function and cosmesis due to lack of sensation, mobility, and nail (4).

Pollicization may be indicated when four fingers are present, but toe transfer remains our first choice (Fig. 48D-2).

In multiple digit amputation, simultaneous multiple toe transfer provides possible one-stage total reconstruction (6).

Level IV

With loss of the metacarpophalangeal joint and injury to intrinsic muscles, length as well as the joints must be reconstructed. In isolated thumb injuries, pollicization provides optimal motor and sensory function. A damaged finger can also be pollicized (6,7).

When multiple digits are involved or pollicization is not possible, great toe transfer is an useful option. The great toe can be harvested distal to the base of proximal phalanx. The inadequate metacarpal length is augmented with bone graft taken from the ileum or the amputated part, either before or at the time of toe transfer (5).

If the patient prefers to preserve the great toe, second toe with transmetatarsal transfer to restore length and reconstruct joint mobility can be used (Fig. 48D-3) (2).

Level V

The approach to reconstruction is similar to that of level IV. Pollicization remains the treatment of choice. When multiple digits are involved or pollicization is not possible, transmetatarsal second toe with metatarsal transfer or great toe transfer with bone graft augmentation of the metacarpal length can be considered. These toes are transferred to the thumb position as a semipost (Fig. 48D-4).

F.-C. Wei and V. Jain: Department of Plastic and Reconstructive Surgery, Chang Gung Memorial Hospital, College of Medicine, Chang Gung University, Taipei, Taiwan

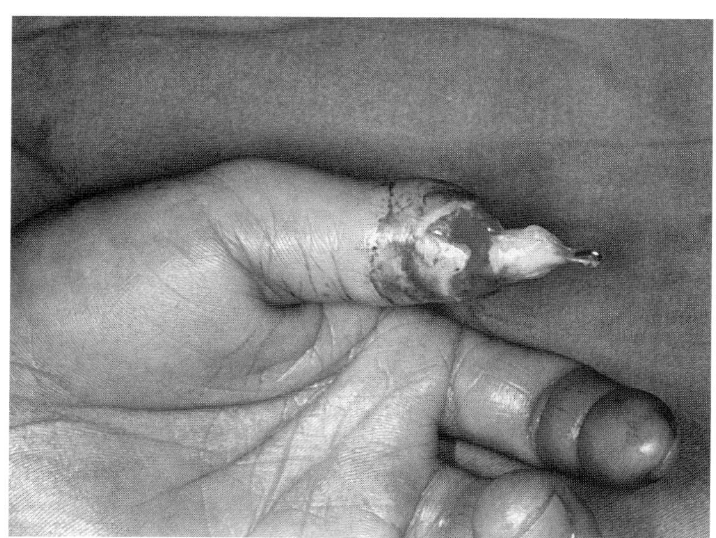
A

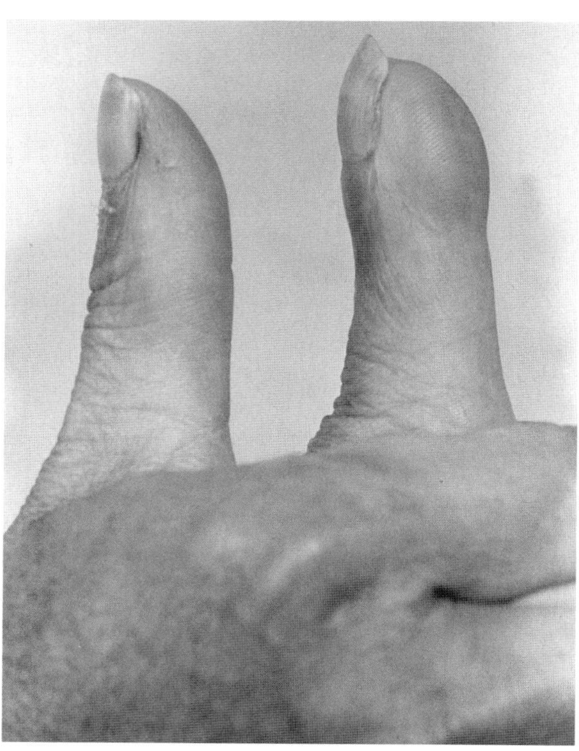
B

FIGURE 48D-1. Thumb amputation at level II reconstructed with a modified great toe wraparound flap including the distal phalanx. **A:** Before reconstruction. **B:** After reconstruction.

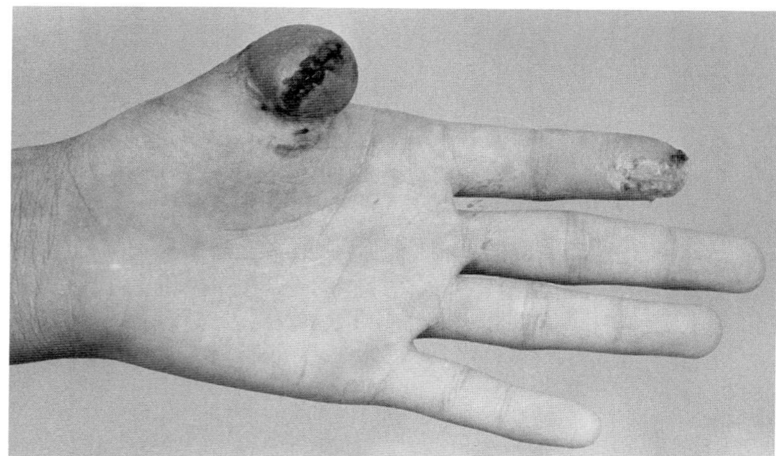
A

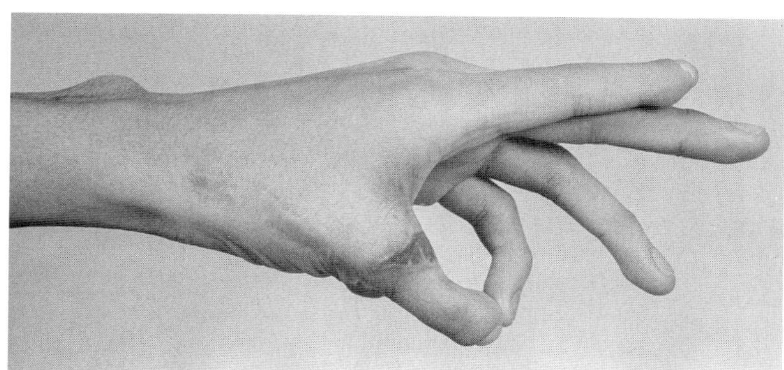
B

FIGURE 48D-2. Thumb amputation at level III reconstructed with a second toe. **A:** Before reconstruction. **B:** After reconstruction.

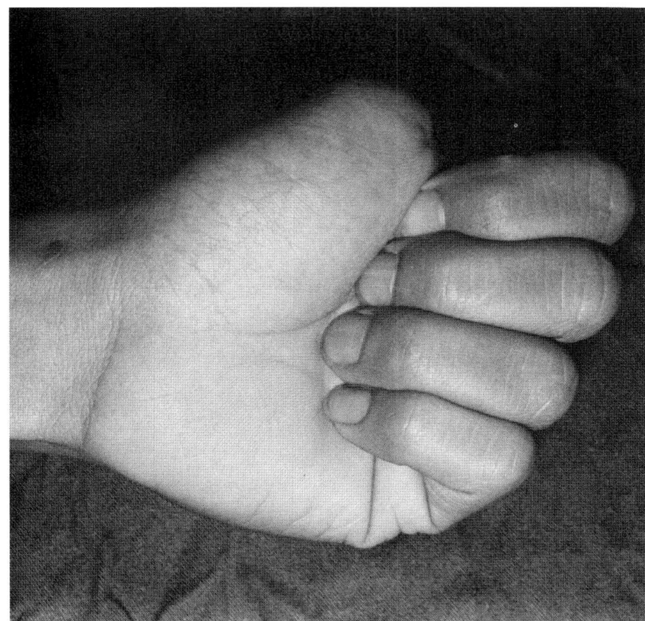
A

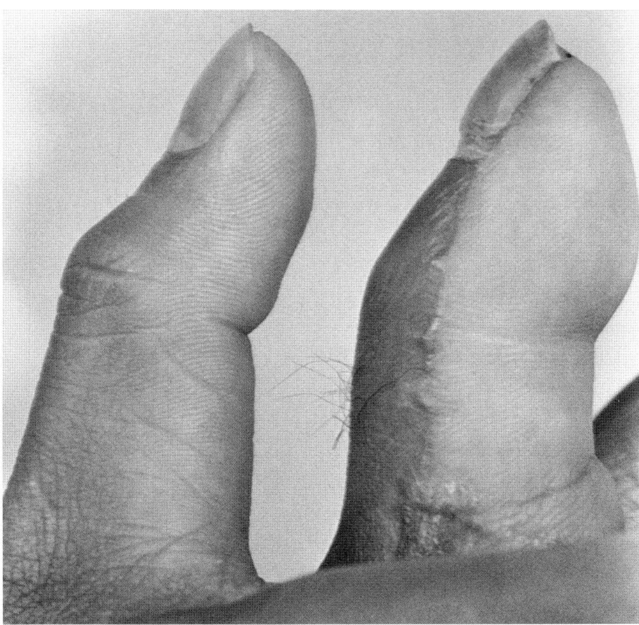
B

FIGURE 48D-3. Thumb amputation at level IV reconstructed with a pedicled groin flap and trimmed great toe. **A:** Before reconstruction. **B:** After complete reconstruction.

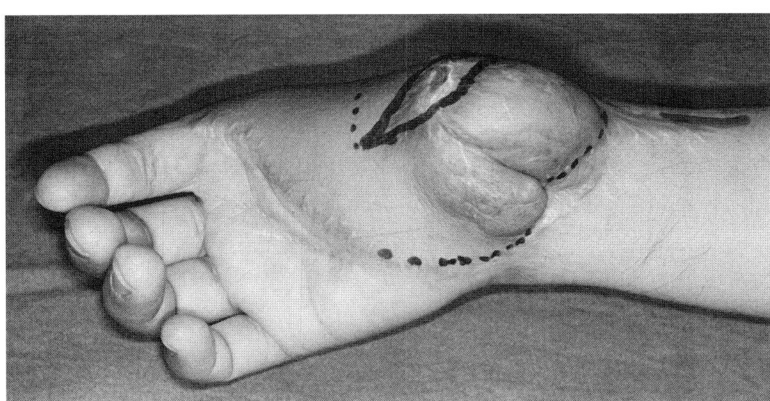
A

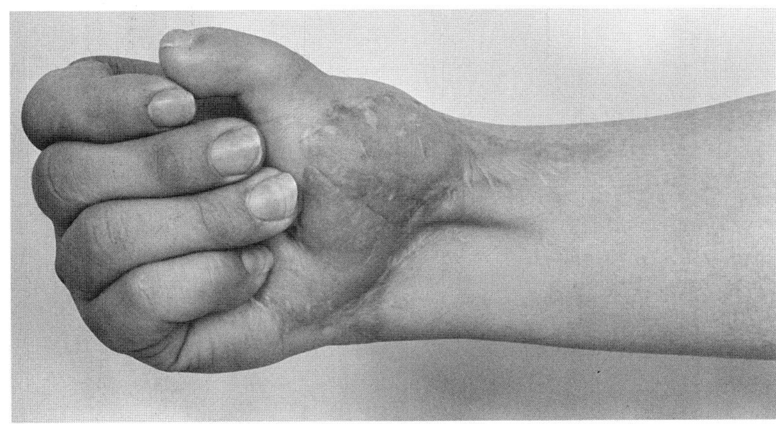
B

FIGURE 48D-4. Thumb amputation at level V reconstructed with a second toe and vascularized iliac bone graft for metacarpal length augmentation. **A:** Before reconstruction. **B:** After vascularized iliac bone grafting and second toe transplantation.

AVOIDING UNFAVORABLE OUTCOMES IN RECONSTRUCTION

Skin Coverage

Sensate and durable skin cover is required over the thumb tip and pulp. Microsurgical transfer of the glabrous skin of the feet and toes provides the perfect match. For the more proximal palmar side and dorsum of the thumb, free flaps are better options because local flaps may induce scarring to already injured tissues and can hamper later reconstructive procedures.

We prefer free ipsilateral lateral arm flap, especially for web space reconstruction. It can be performed under tourniquet, provides adequate sensate skin, and permits primary closure of the donor site if the flap width is smaller than 4 to 5 cm (Fig. 48D-5). However, conventional techniques still play some role. Neurovascular island pedicle flap provides quality skin with sensation (8). Distal elevation of these flaps provides pedicle of adequate length to avoid traction (9).

Retrograde pedicled flaps, such as the dorsal ulnar artery flap and reverse posterior interosseous flaps, can provide coverage without sacrificing a major vessel to the hand. Distant pedicled flaps provide adequate coverage only suitable for the dorsum of the hand and the thumb. Less skin is harvested from the foot during subsequent toe transfer.

DISTRACTION OSTEOGENESIS

Distraction osteogenesis (10,11) provides good length with preservation of sensation and functional grip. However, it is a long, multistage procedure that does not provide a nail or mobility (12) and does not improve pulp pinch (13). It may require secondary bone grafting in adult patients (12).

Osteoplastic reconstruction using various described techniques provide length but require multiple operative procedures, create a stiff and bulky thumb without a nail, lack proper sensation, and result in skin instability at the tip, trophic ulceration, and cold intolerance (14–16). An island flap (17) may be required to improve sensibility and has in-

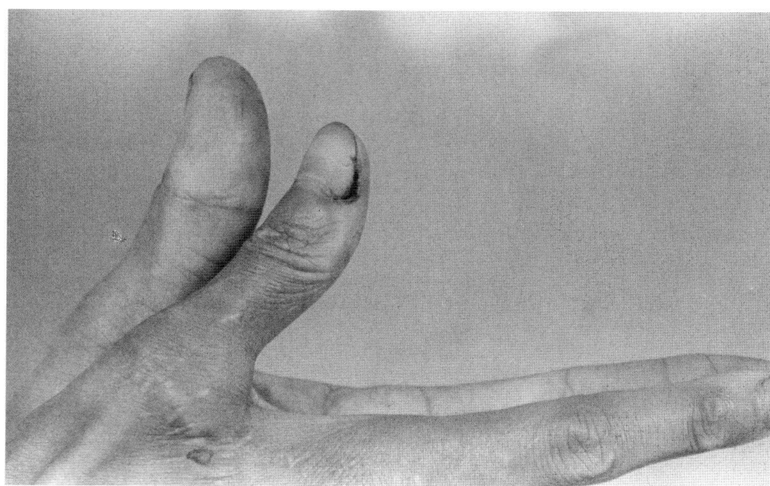

A

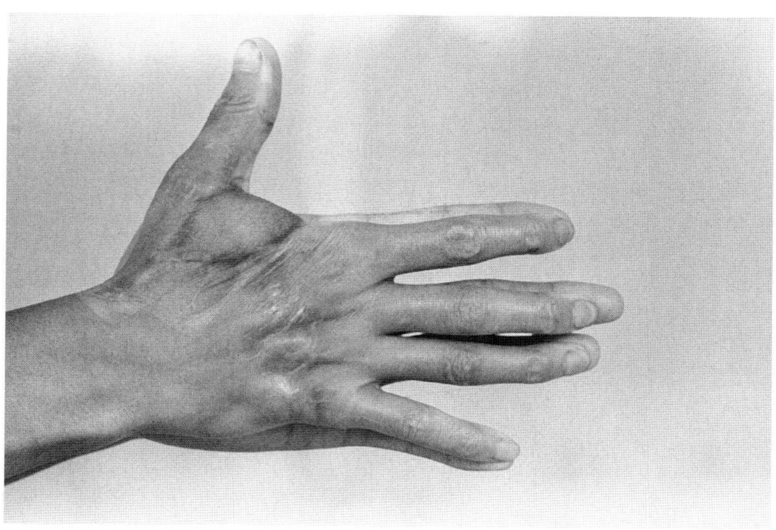

B

FIGURE 48D-5. First web space contracture released and reconstructed with an ipsilateral free lateral arm flap. **A:** Before reconstruction. **B:** After reconstruction.

herent complications, such as web space contracture, graft resorption, and donor site morbidity.

POLLICIZATION

For amputations proximal to metacarpophalangeal joints, pollicization is one choice for thumb reconstruction, provided the other fingers are intact (6). A damaged digit also can be used (7,18).

Pollicization is safe and quick to perform, leads to quick recovery to better sensory and independent motor function, and provides stable thumb reconstruction without the risks associated with microsurgical reconstructions. Toe transfer remains our preference because of its better functional and cosmetic results.

The index finger is the digit of choice for several reasons: its pollicization is the easiest and safest; it does not require crossover of vessels, nerves, or tendons; dorsal veins can be preserved; good web space can be formed after easy removal of the second metacarpal; the long finger covers its place and function spontaneously; there are no scars in the palm; and it is cosmetically better than other digits (6). Secondary procedures, such as opponensplasty or transfer of flexor pollicis longus to the thumb, transfer of adductor pollicis and flexor pollicis brevis to the superficialis tendon at middle phalanx, and insertion of first dorsal and volar interossei to the lateral bands of the extensor mechanism enhance function (19).

CONGENITAL ANOMALIES

We believe the age for surgical intervention should be at least 1 year, when the vascular system has matured and attained reasonable size and thickness that make identification and dissection easier. Associated congenital anomalies should be investigated. Pollicization remains one choice, along with distraction lengthening in indicated cases. Dissection should begin in the palm to identify and deal with any vascular malformations. Both neurovascular bundles should be used, as suggested by Littler. The recipient site is prepared first in toe transfer in cases of floating thumb and ring amputation thumb. As in adults, the web space should be placed at the level of the proximal interphalangeal joint of the index finger (20). Secondary procedures such as opponensplasty are best done at a later stage, balancing the needs and availability.

REFERENCES

1. Littler JW. On making a thumb: one hundred years of surgical effort. *J Hand Surg* 1976;1:35.
2. Wei FC, El-Gammal TA. Toe-to-hand transfer: current concepts, techniques and research. *Clin Plast Surg* 1996;23:103.
3. Morrison WA. Thumb reconstruction: a review and philosophy of management. *J Hand Surg* 1992;17B;383–390.
4. Foucher G, Chaboud M. The bipolar lengthening technique: a modified partial toe transfer for thumb reconstruction. *Plast Reconstr Surg* 1998;102:1981–1987.
5. Wei FC, Chen HC, Chuang CC, et al. Microsurgical thumb reconstruction with toe transfer: selection of various techniques. *Plast Reconstr Surg* 1994;93:345.
6. Brunelli GA, Brunelli GR. Reconstruction of the traumatic absence of the thumb in the adult by pollicization. *Hand Clin* 1992;8:41–55.
7. Cheng MH, Cheng SL, Tung TC, et al. A case report of pollicization of traumatised index finger for reconstruction of traumatic amputation of thumb. *J Surg Assoc Rep China* 1997; 30:134–139.
8. Adani R, Squarzina PB, Castagnetti G, et al. A comparative study of heterodigital neurovascular island flap in thumb reconstruction with and without nerve connection. *J Hand Surg* 1994; 19B:552–559.
9. Markley JM Jr. The preservation of close two point discrimination in the interdigital transfer of neurovascular island flaps. *Plast Reconstr Surg* 1977;59:812–816.
10. Matev I. Thumb reconstruction in children through metacarpal lengthening. *Plast Reconstr Surg* 65:482, 1980.
11. Matev I. The bone lengthening method in hand reconstruction: twenty years experience. *J Hand Surg* 1989;14A:376–378.
12. Foucher G, Hultgren T, Merle M, et al. L'allongroent digital selon Matev. A propos de vingt cas. *Ann Chir Main* 1988;7:210.
13. Pollock HJ. Reconstruction of the traumatically amputated thumb by continuous Matev distraction. Experience and result in 48 cases. *Handchir Mikrochir Plast Chir* 1994;26:291–297.
14. Gillis H, Millard DR. *The principle and art of plastic surgery.* Boston: Little Brown and Company, 1957:484–488.
15. Biemer E, Stock W. Total thumb reconstruction: one stage reconstruction osteocutaneous forearm island flap. *Br J Plast Surg* 1983;36:52.
16. Masquelet AC, Penteado CV. The posterior interosseous flap. *Ann Chir Main* 1987;6:131.
17. Littler JW. The neurovascular pedicle method of digital transposition for reconstruction of the thumb. *Plast Reconstr Surg* 1963;12:303.
18. Littler JW. Reconstruction of the thumb in traumatic loss. In: Converse JM, ed. *Reconstructive plastic surgery,* 2nd ed. Philadelphia: WB Saunders 1977:3350–3367.
19. Kellehar JC. Pollicization. In: Goldwyn RM, ed. *The unfavorable result in plastic surgery. Avoidance and treatment.* Boston: Little Brown and Company, 1972:475–488.
20. Zancolli E. Transplantation of the index finger in congenital absence of the thumb. *J Bone Joint Surg* 1960;42A:658–666.

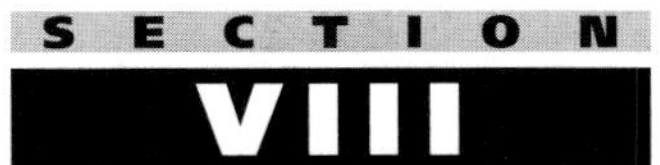

LOWER EXTREMITY

49

RECONSTRUCTION FOR LOWER EXTREMITY TRAUMA

GEOFFREY G. HALLOCK

Accidents are not just a leading cause of death in young people. Equally devastating is the fact that more than 400,000 Americans yearly become disabled from trauma (1). Additional morbidity from loss of limb or dysfunction can only be estimated. The history of our specialty has recorded an intense involvement in the care of traumatic defects (Table 49-1) and a responsibility not only to preserve limbs, but to maximize their function. This group is unique, as most are young and healthy and have few risk factors that would limit reconstructive options. Unfortunately, their normal lifestyle has been disrupted by what is, at the least, an urgent situation requiring prompt decision making, often irreversible, with sequelae that frequently cannot meet unrealistic expectations.

ROLE OF PRIMARY AMPUTATION

Despite technical achievements in trauma management, limb revascularization, microneurovascular surgery, skeletal fixation, and critical care medicine, paradoxically these advances can lead to extraordinarily expensive economic, psychological, or even lethal costs by an attempt at limb salvage, which would be the ultimate undesirable result (2). Before embarking on the lengthy course of multiple operative interventions needed to salvage most lower extremity injuries, assessment by a team of trauma, orthopaedic, vascular, *and* plastic surgeons should decide if primary amputation would be preferable. This should not be considered a failure of treatment, but rather a valid reconstructive option.

Numerous predictive indices, such as AIS (Amputation Index Score), MESI (Mangled Extremity Syndrome Index), PSI (Predictive Salvage Index), LSI (Limb Salvage Index), and MESS (Mangled Extremity Severity Score), are based on objective criteria that assess the initial magnitude of soft tissue, nerve, vessel, bone, and associated injuries (2,3). Unfortunately, although some scores can foretell successful limb viability, none has any predictive utility to avoid a futile salvage effort that may be a functional failure (2). Personality, motivation, and socioeconomic status are strong influences on outcome that are virtually impossible to evaluate in the acute setting (4).

Interestingly, in a prospective study using standardized generic and specific outcome questionnaires, patients who had primary amputations had functional outcome scores less than those with successful limb salvage, yet *all* of these patients had scores lower than many with serious medical illnesses, such as cancer or cardiac disease. This proves that lower extremity trauma is a serious lifestyle-threatening disease that perhaps has been underestimated in its severity (3). Despite these negative aspects, most patients having limb salvage would again choose that option, and few would have accepted a primary amputation, which makes the latter choice even more difficult (3).

The surgeon's clinical impression still is of paramount importance. If the usual criteria deem an attempt to save the limb worthwhile, then that is what should be done. Guidelines for primary amputation are useful (Table 49-2), but they cannot be arbitrary (3–7). Relative factors require flexibility and foresight. The requisite rehabilitation always is difficult, where again the socioeconomic status, degree of family support, and level of education necessary to obtain the optimal result are factors above and beyond the extent of the physical injury (4,8).

REPLANTATION

As a general rule, replantation of the completely or near-amputated lower limb is contraindicated. Unlike the upper extremity where joint fusion in positions of function and retention of fine motor movements alone may be valuable, the lower extremity must be strong enough to support the weight of the body, and muscle contraction is needed for walking and to resist the sequela of dependent edema (9). Fused joints and lack of motor function will hinder stand-

G. G. Hallock: Division of Plastic Surgery, Lehigh Valley Hospital, Allentown, Pennsylvania

TABLE 49-1. FREQUENCY OF FLAP SELECTION BY ETIOLOGY OF DEFECT

	Local		Free		Total
	Muscle	Fascia	Muscle	Fascia	
Cancer	18	11	13	11	53
Iatrogenic	74	16	3	2	95
Trauma					
Initial	35	38	32	15	120
Secondary[a]	12	42	27	21	102
Vascular	6	15	14	4	39
Other	23	28	2	1	54
Total	168	150	91	54	463

Data based on author's total experience over the years 1988 to 1998.
[a]Delayed reconstruction of a traumatic defect or for complications of the initial management.

ing and restrict mobility. Whereas upper limb prosthetic devices cannot yet restore significant hand function, lower limb prostheses often provide a superior option for the different demands of ambulation (10,11).

This is not to say that lower limb replantation cannot be performed successfully. The ideal candidate is the very young, healthy patient with a guillotine-type amputation at a very distal level (4,12). Unfortunately, the nature of lower extremity trauma is more severe than that of the upper extremity (10,12). Extreme contamination, crush, multilevel injury, warm ischemia time exceeding 12 hours, and requirement for severe bone shortening mitigate against even attempting such a feat (4,10,12).

Nevertheless, before a limb is discarded, the salvage of uninjured portions should be considered. Retention of maximum limb length and functioning joints is a reasonable axiom, because this will minimize energy dissipation during ambulation (4). Rather than rely on a delayed tissue transfer to accomplish this, a salvage replantation can avoid altogether the morbidity of a donor site (11,13). For example, the glabrous sole of a foot can provide durable stump coverage (11), and an intact ankle joint can be rotated to simulate a missing knee joint (13). Cross replantation after a bilateral injury can make at least a single useful limb (14). Often, salvaged parts can be sensate and even transferred without microsurgical expertise if their neurovascular status remains intact (13)!

TABLE 49-2. INDICATIONS FOR PRIMARY LOWER LIMB AMPUTATION

Absolute
1. Total leg amputation in an adult
2. Sciatic nerve transection in an adult
3. Irretrievable devascularization

Relative
1. Life-threatening multisystem trauma
2. Insensate plantar foot from any source
3. Crushed foot or degloved plantar surface
4. Widespread leg crush injury, with defunctionalization
5. Extensive bone loss
6. Multiple joint disruption
7. Multilevel injury.
8. Elderly (age >55 years), especially with history of diabetes or advanced peripheral vascular disease
9. Rehabilitation concerns

Data from references 4, 9, 29, 30, and 32.

APPROACH TO LIMB SALVAGE

Unlike wound coverage for other diseases, lower extremity trauma imposes some unique constraints. The timing of restoration of cutaneous coverage, an evolving size or zone of injury, the risk of exposure of underlying vital structures, and a requirement for composite tissues cannot be predetermined.

Timing of Closure

The timing of definitive wound closure depends on the severity and interrelated mechanism of injury; but, most importantly, the overall medical status of the patient must always take precedence (15). Byrd et al. (16) classified tibial fractures according to the energy expended by the mechanism of injury and concomitant soft tissue injury, which directly affects the approach to wound closure (Table 49-3). Godina (17) extended the principle of primary wound management and advocated early closure of all traumatic wounds. This concept, when applied in the acute period before bacterial colonization of the wound, dramatically reduced the incidence of flap failure, rate of infection, bone healing time, number of operations, and length of hospital stay, and it now is probably the consensus approach (8,16).

Yaremchuk (7) proposed that treatment of the severely injured lower extremity be done in four distinct phases:

1. Emergency evaluation, orthopaedic stabilization, and debridement of obviously devitalized tissues

TABLE 49-3. CLASSIFICATION OF OPEN TIBIAL FRACTURES ACCORDING TO BYRD ET AL. (16)

Type I	Low-energy forces causing a spiral or oblique fracture pattern with skin lacerations <2 cm and a relatively clean wound
Type II	Moderate-energy forces causing a comminuted or displaced fracture pattern with skin lacerations >2 cm and moderate adjacent skin and muscle contusion but without devitalized muscle
Type III	High-energy forces causing a significantly displaced fracture pattern with severe comminution, segmental fracture, or bone defect with extensive associated skin loss and devitalized muscle
Type IV	Fracture pattern as in type III but with extreme energy forces as in high-velocity gunshot or shotgun wounds, a history of crush or degloving, or associated vascular injury requiring repair

2. Wound management with serial debridement
3. Soft tissue coverage
4. Delayed bone reconstruction.

Emergency coverage of the wound within the first 24 hours after injury or at the time of the first operative procedure as Godina (17) proposed is *not* essential, except in the most unusual circumstances (e.g., an exposed vascular graft). It may even be detrimental in high-energy wounds where serial radical debridement ensures removal of all devitalized tissues that may not be totally obvious at the initial presentation (7,9,15). The zone of injury invariably is larger than that grossly obvious (Fig. 49-1). Meticulous local wound care can extend the acute period up to 15 days, as shown by Francel et al. (9), with results no different than those of Godina.

Method of Closure

Only when the wound milieu has stabilized should coverage be considered. Closure should never be attempted if unresolved infection or necrotic material is retained, as sepsis will be inevitable. Arteriography can be a helpful adjunct before closure to assess collateral circulation to the foot, perforators to potential local flaps, characteristics of recipient vessels, and congenital anomalies (7,15). The selection process depends on defect location, mechanism of injury, degree of contamination, and presence of any injuries to underlying structures (9).

General

Whenever primary closure or a skin graft is not feasible, standard vascularized flap options for the lower limb should be the initial consideration, if they are not precluded by the trauma itself (Fig. 49-2) (18,19). Their proven reliability is reflected by my experience over the past decade (Table 49-4). The thigh rarely needs flap coverage, as a skin graft often suffices (20). The gastrocnemius muscles are the best local flap for the knee and proximal one-third of the leg. The soleus muscle is the first choice for the mid-third of the leg and sometimes can reach the upper part of the lower third of the leg. Whenever possible, a hemisoleus flap can be used for function preservation. A microsurgical transfer is the best option for the distal leg and foot, as well as significant Byrd type IV injuries throughout the lower limb where the viability or loss of function created by use of a local flap of any type would be circumspect (Fig. 49-1) (16,19). Flap delay or distant-pedicled flaps are tertiary maneuvers valuable only if the first attempt at closure is unsatisfactory or other options are unavailable (8,21).

Foot

Coverage of the foot represents a special challenge. Again, location as well as the magnitude of the injury are important considerations (22). Of all foot regions, the plantar weight-bearing surface is the most unique, as this glabrous, relatively rigid cushion is essential for shock absorption. It is virtually irreplaceable, so that after a plantar avulsion injury, for example, replantation or revascularization whenever feasible is always indicated (23). Local flaps can be used in all regions, but plantar sensation should be maintained and local circulation uninterrupted. Sufficient local tissues must be available. Intrinsic foot muscles often are too small or irrevocably involved by the trauma itself (15,18). Therefore, in high-energy wounds, a free flap more often than not becomes an essential option, as corroborated by this series (Table 49-4). The free flap of choice must allow contouring acceptable for use of normal footwear. The method of resurfacing the sole remains controversial. In a series of muscle or skin flaps used for this purpose, Potparic and Rajacic (24) noted "no significant difference was found in the incidence of complications and functional outcome between fasciocutaneous and skin-grafted muscle flaps. There was no significant difference between reinnervated and non-innervated

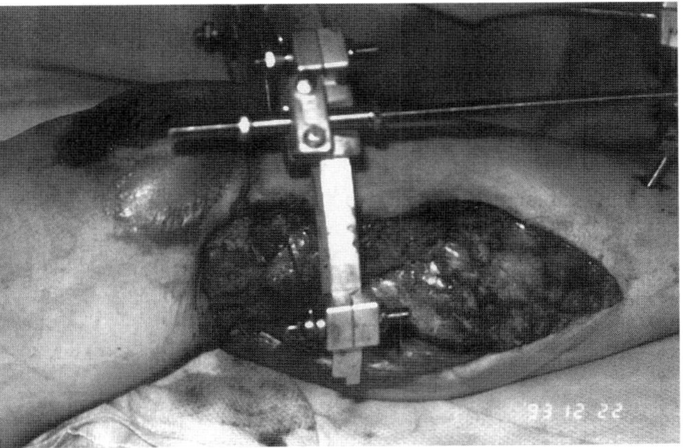
A

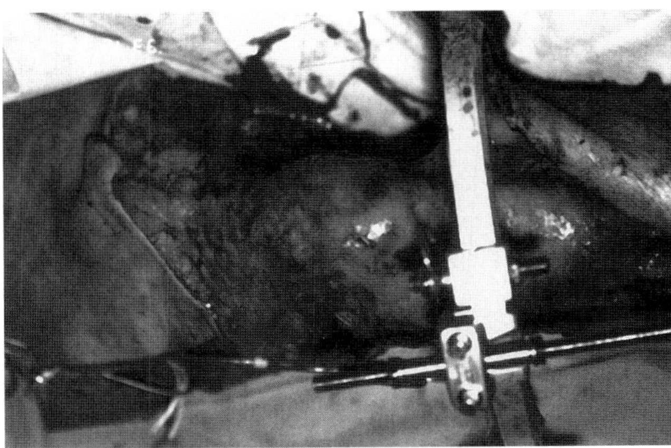
B

FIGURE 49-1. A: Bumper crush injury with open proximal left tibia fracture. **B:** Extensive circumferential zone of injury is more obvious after wide debridement (Byrd type IV injury). *(continued)*

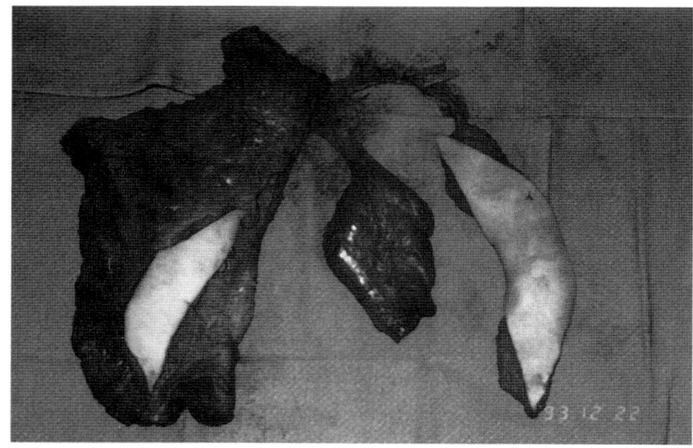
C

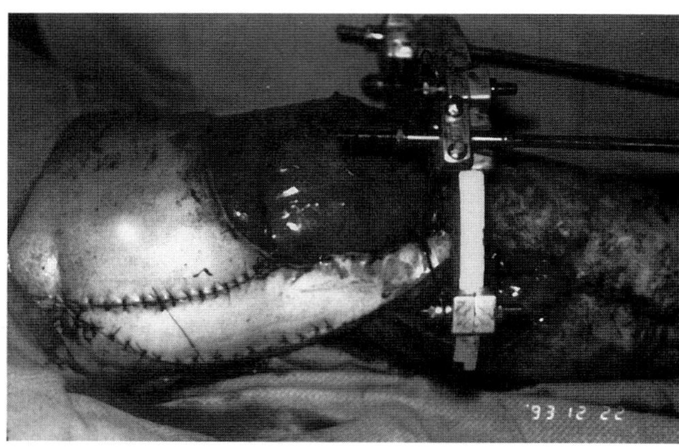
D

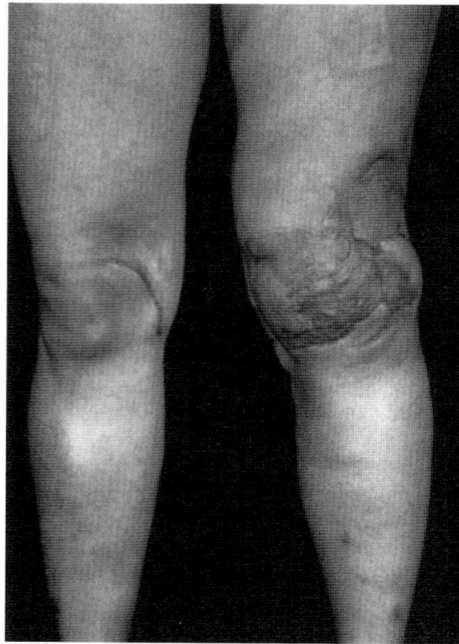
E

FIGURE 49-1. (*Continued*) **C:** Coverage planned via microsurgical transfer of a combined latissimus dorsi musculocutaneous, serratus anterior muscle, and scapular fasciocutaneous flap **(left to right)**, joined only by a common subscapular vascular pedicle (**above,** center in microclamps). **D:** End-to-side microanastomoses were performed to the superficial femoral artery and vein. The scapular flap was designed to prevent tension after closure of the medial thigh recipient vessel site that could compress the vascular pedicle. The serratus anterior muscle covered the patella, and the latissimus dorsi flap was wrapped around the rest of the upper leg. **E:** Normal ambulation was accomplished by this well-motivated woman. Traditional local muscle or even skin flap options would have been too small to close this large defect, even if available. (From Hallock GG. Permutations of combined free flaps using the subscapular system. *J Reconstr Microsurg* 1997;13:47–54, with permission.)

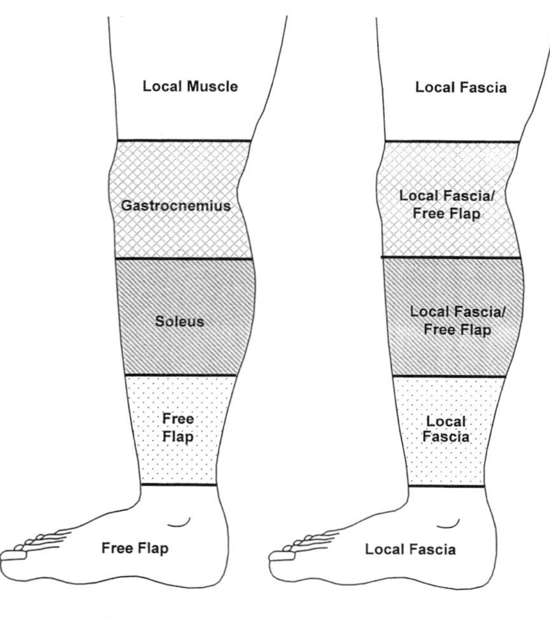

FIGURE 49-2. Standard protocol for initial flap selection of the lower limb by region **(left)** and secondary alternatives dependent on the magnitude of injury or availability **(right)**.

TABLE 49-4. FREQUENCY OF FLAP TYPES USED IN ACUTE LOWER EXTREMITY TRAUMA BASED ON LOCATION AND SEVERITY OF INJURY[a]

		Local			Free		
		Muscle	Fascia	Total	Muscle	Fascia	Total
	II	—	—	—	—	—	—
Thigh	III	2	—	2	—	—	—
	IV	2	—	2	—	—	—
	II	6	1	7	—	—	—
Upper one-third	III	4	1	5	—	—	—
leg and knee	IV	1	1	2	5	2	7
	II	10	3	13	—	—	—
Mid-leg	III	4	3	7	1	—	1
	IV	—	—	—	4	—	4
	II	4	5	9	—	—	—
Distal leg	III	—	1	1	2	—	2
	IV	—	—	—	—	1	1
	II	1	5	6	3	1	4
Foot	III	—	2	2	4	—	4
	IV	—	2	2	8	1	9
Total		34	24	58	27	5	32

[a]Types II, III, and IV injury as defined by Byrd et al. (16), see Table 49-3.

flaps. Neither type of flap should be considered permanent in the presence of peripheral neuropathy." Although cutaneous sensation within the flap may not be necessary to prevent breakdown, deep pressure sensation must be present (25). Ulcerations in these flaps are common and probably related to the deep bony anatomy where mechanical stresses may be concentrated at areas of bony prominence (Fig. 49-3) (25). If foot reconstruction is to be successful, foot sensibility must be replaced by meticulous foot care requiring constant visual observation and common sense (12,21).

Bone Reconstruction

Although bone grafting can be performed at the time of soft tissue coverage, since this is a contaminated milieu at best, it is preferable to wait at least 4 to 6 weeks after the wound is closed to minimize the risk of infection (7,15,16). Except when an autogenous vascularized graft is needed, usually this becomes the domain of the orthopaedist, and our advice is no longer needed. Closed methods to fill segmental bone gaps include vascularized bone grafts or distraction osteogenesis, and bypass techniques involve posterolateral corticocancellous grafts or fibula-pro-tibia (26). The latter require an intact ipsilateral fibula, which therefore should not be violated if at all possible during the preliminary stages of limb salvage, as this is an important secondary option for an intertibiofibular synostosis (8).

Special Considerations

Fascial Flaps

Skin flaps *if* augmented by circulation from the fascial plexus as reintroduced by Ponten *do* have a role in lower extremity coverage, which is a change in concept from the last edition of this book where the advice was to avoid them (21). Simple to elevate, they are most pertinent for small or moderate defects to avoid the loss of marginally expendable local muscles or the morbidity of a comparably more extensive dissection (6,20). Because local muscles are conspicuous by their absence about the distal leg and ankle, fascial flaps may provide the only alternative to complex microsurgical transfers and are especially valuable if such technical capabilities are not available or if mitigating medical problems coexist (27,28).

Many oppose the use of fascial flaps, as the rigidity imposed by the fascia or subcutaneous fat prevents their conforming to fill dead space, whereas muscles are more malleable (15,20,29). Circulation to the skin always is compromised in the obese patient. Most importantly, the trauma itself can deglove the perforators to the fascial plexus, or lacerations and/or prior scars present at the pedicle of the flap can result in devascularization (Fig. 49-4). Muscle always has precedence in the contaminated wound, as its superior vascularity enhances the immunologic response to the wound (30).

The ultimate detriment of the fasciocutaneous flap is a skin graft if needed at the donor site. There is no debate that this is a significant *cosmetic* disadvantage similar to that of the musculocutaneous flap (28). However, from a functional and wound-healing standpoint only, there is no superiority of the muscle flap versus the fascial flap with regard to the donor site, as each has intrinsic limitations that fortunately are uncommon (28).

Distal-Based Flaps

A proximal-based cutaneous flap not only has antegrade inflow and orthograde venous outflow, but it can be sensate.

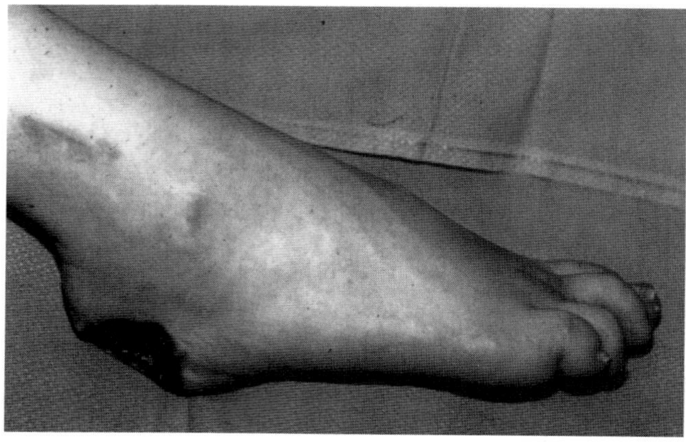

A

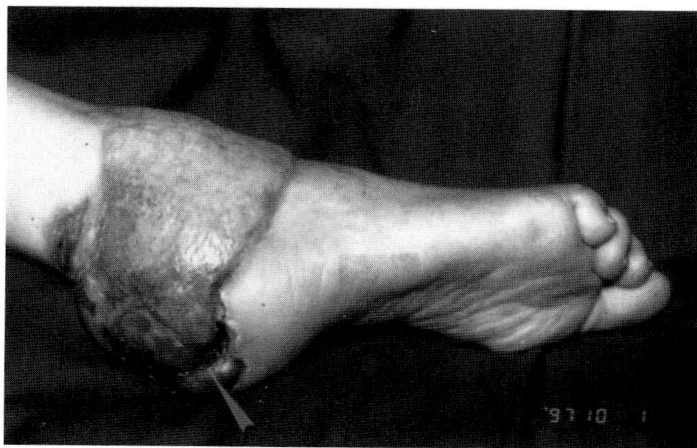

B

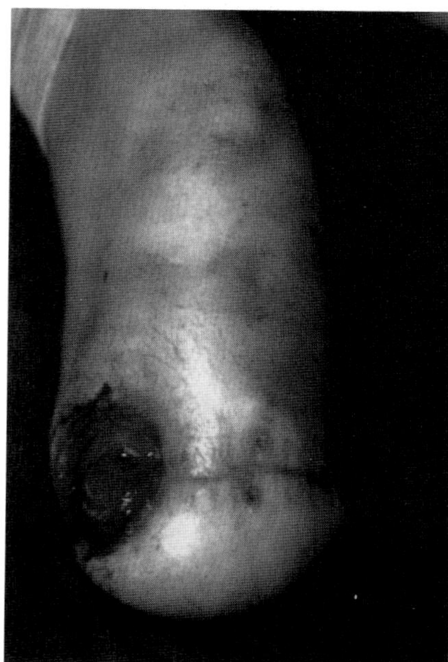

C

FIGURE 49-3. A: Exposed calcaneus after minor trauma resulted in infection in a diabetic with plantar neuropathy. **B:** The skin grafted gracilis free muscle flap survived, but full-thickness ulceration following noncompliant ambulation occurred rapidly *(arrow)*. **C:** Problem ultimately solved by a below-knee amputation that incidentally developed a stump ulcer. More thorough psychosocial evaluation could have predicted the need for primary amputation initially.

However, at the ankle level, the deep fascia blends with the extensor retinaculum such that this orientation risks exposure of tendons at the donor site (20). This can be avoided by basing the flap distally, using proximal skin territories to cover distal defects, and leaving a healthy bed for skin grafting if needed (27). These local flaps are relatively simple to elevate, are taken from the injured extremity, can avoid inclusion of a source vessel to the foot, and could obviate the need for a microsurgical transfer (27). Unfortunately, outflow can be compromised and venous congestion leading to flap death is an omnipresent risk (Fig. 49-5).

Distal-based muscle flaps are possible. The soleus muscle was the most frequently used in the past, but was abandoned due to the high rate of complications presumably due to injury to distal minor pedicles (1,9,18,19). Because of the uncertainties imposed by an often indeterminate zone of injury from significant leg trauma, a microsurgical transfer can predictably be more reliable than any distal-based flap (Table 49-4.)

Microsurgery

General technical aspects of microsurgery are discussed in Chapter 14, but some points are specifically germane to the lower extremity. Although the International Microvascular Research Group (IMRG) states that the rate of free-flap failure is not related to the location of the recipient site or the etiology of the defect (31), my experience is to the contrary. Traumatic lower extremity wounds have been the most difficult to cover successfully with free flaps, probably because these are the most complex wounds. Proper debridement may be the crucial element, not the microsurgery itself (17).

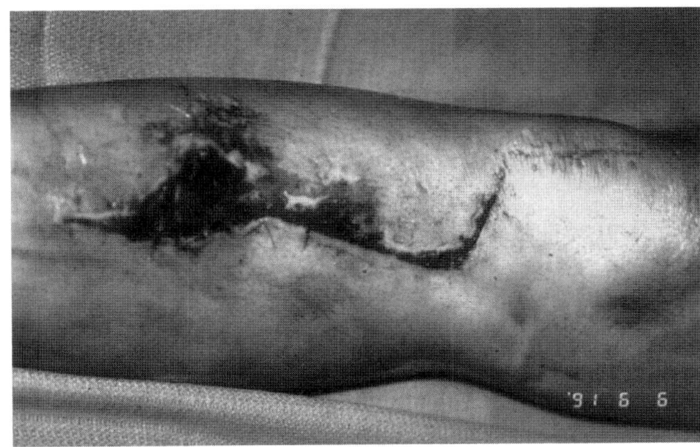

A

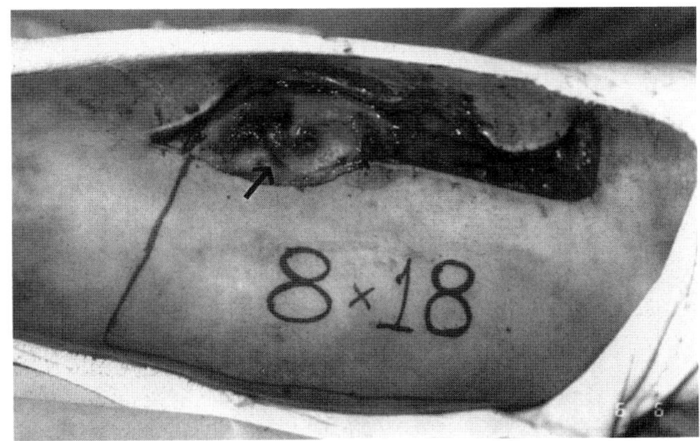

B

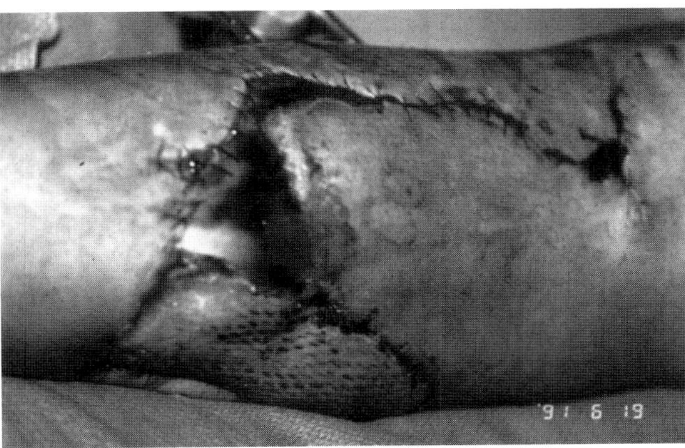

C

FIGURE 49-4. A: Closed mid-tibia fracture after a motorcycle accident was treated by open reduction, with skin necrosis ensuing (patella on **right**). **B:** After appropriate debridement, the fracture became exposed *(arrow)*. A proximal-based medial local Ponten-type fasciocutaneous flap was proposed for coverage. **C:** Necrosis of the distal portion of the flap resulted in failure to cover the fracture site, which ultimately healed after using a soleus muscle flap. Disruption of the fascial plexus by the degloving component of this injury was obviously more than appreciated, and a muscle flap should have been the primary choice. Note the appearance of the skin graft needed to cover the fascia flap donor site.

Early free-tissue transfers maximize the chance of success for many reasons. The recipient vessels adjacent to the wound are still pliable. In time, the zone of injury that *does* extend beyond the limits of nonviable tissue as a response to injury and edema (32) results in their vessel fibrosis and friability, leading to unavoidable injuries and irreversible vasospasm (17). If this occurs, vein grafts to more proximal vessels become mandatory. Even the IMRG observed that the use of vein grafts in general increased the risk of flap failure 2.9-fold (31). A delay in transfer can cause failure because of other unusual events, including venous hypertension from unsuspected deep vein thrombosis (29) or the development of a hypercoaguable state, presumably from cytokines released by the trauma that do not reach a maximum level until about 2 weeks after injury (33).

Whenever possible, inflow should be reestablished by an end-to-side anastomosis. This preserves all collateral flow to the foot. A positive spurt test must always be observed from the recipient artery *before* dividing the free-flap pedicle (32). For outflow, deep veins are used preferentially from a logistical standpoint because they are adjacent to the artery. End-to-end anastomoses usually are used. Two venous anastomoses are always performed, if possible, as this lowers the rate of failure (31).

Tension-free coverage of the microanastomoses is essential and must be planned beforehand. Edema of the leg accumulating during these lengthy procedures can make reclosure of the recipient site difficult. Sometimes a companion flap can be taken with the coverage flap or a local flap raised just to prevent compression of the pedicle (Fig. 49-1.) (34). Monitoring during insetting and in the postoperative period can be challenging, especially for flaps without a cutaneous component. A laser Doppler using a muscle probe normally is accurate, but there is no foolproof system. If for any reason there is any suspicion of anastomotic thrombosis, reexploration as soon as possible is indicated (35). Other maneuvers usually are futile. Microsurgery always carries a risk of total failure that can introduce a myriad of new problems; therefore, this tool demands a total commitment if a high success rate is to be expected (35).

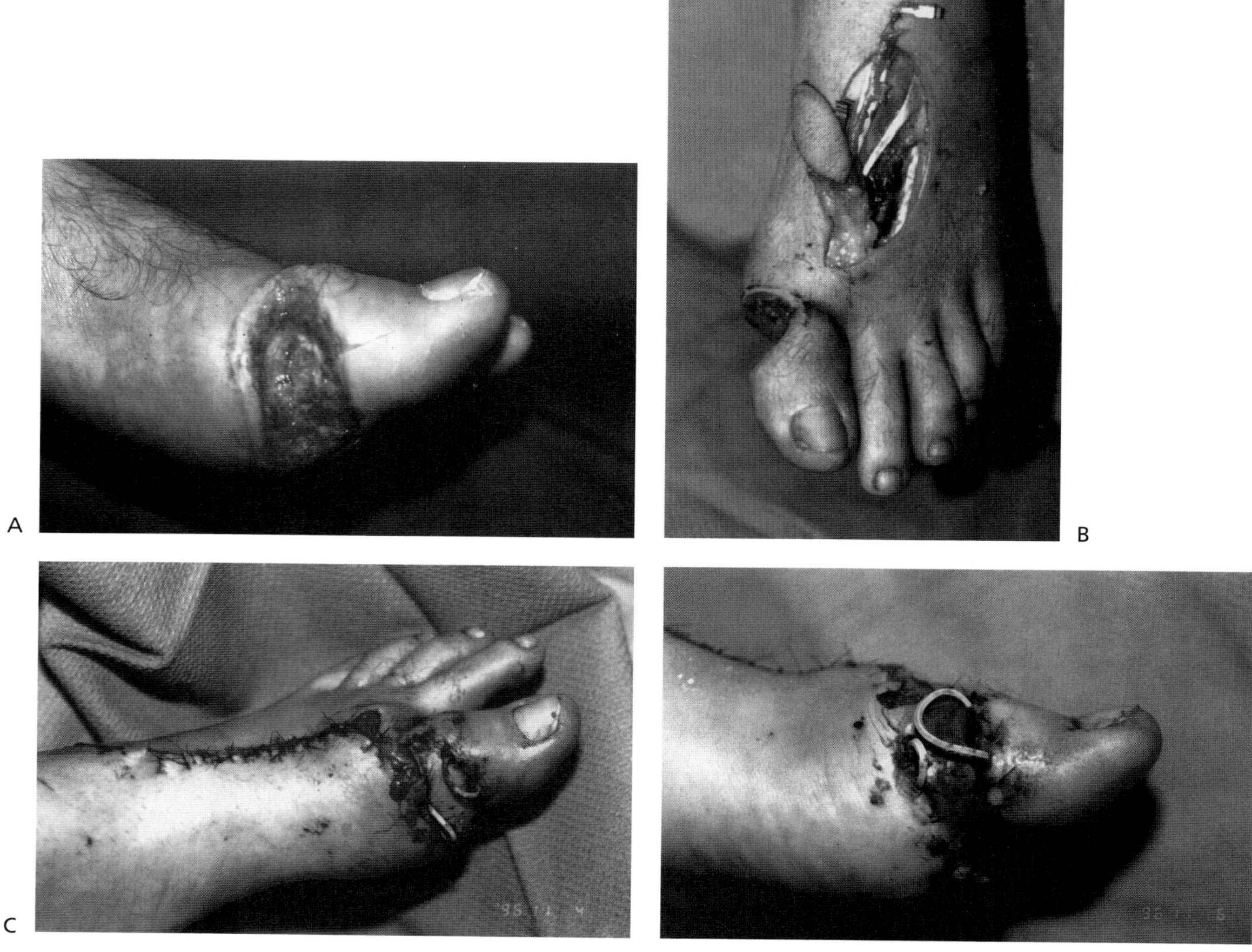

FIGURE 49-5. **A:** Self-inflicted gunshot wound through the metatarsophalangeal joint of the medial left great toe. **B:** Distal-based dorsalis pedis flap designed to rely on reverse flow from the distal communicating branch at the first web space via the first dorsal metatarsal artery, with retention of greater saphenous branches for orthograde venous outflow. **C:** An initially "pink" flap filled the defect, and primary donor site closure was achieved. **D:** Progressive venous congestion resulted in eventual total flap necrosis.

CONCLUSIONS

Traumatic injuries of the lower extremity can be life shattering. A complete return to normalcy is an unrealistic expectation. In one series after lower limb salvage by free flaps, only 28% returned to work of any kind (9). None returned after 2 years of disability, as they lost financial incentives and developed other means of support (9). Primary amputation could hasten the return to a more productive lifestyle. At this time, which patients would benefit more by a protracted attempt at limb salvage cannot be predicted accurately by any objective criteria. Each case must be judged independently by surgeons well versed in this dilemma.

Early wound closure within the acute phase after injury diminishes the risks of failure and onset of complications. Timing is critical, but adequate debridement is paramount. Soft tissue coverage of the lower limb should follow standard protocols, unless the trauma has compromised potential solutions. For the most significant injuries regardless of defect location, microsurgical tissue transfer can maximize both appearance and remaining limb function. Fascial flaps and distal-based skin flaps have a minor role with limited but important indications. Muscle flaps are more versatile, because they adhere more precisely to the wound contour, overcome contamination, and can enhance osteogenesis. Skeletal restoration usually is the last phase of lower limb salvage and should await satisfactory soft tissue healing.

The traumatic lower extremity wound can be the most

complex and challenging of all reconstructive endeavors. Limb survival alone is meaningless if function cannot simultaneously be restored, an outcome that is too often elusive.

ACKNOWLEDGMENTS

Microsurgery assistance was provided by David C. Rice, B.S., Director, Advanced Clinical Technologies Department. Graphics are courtesy of Carol Varma, Medical Illustrationist. Both are with The Lehigh Valley Hospital, Allentown, Pennsylvania.

REFERENCES

1. Flint LM, Flint CB. Evolution, design, and implementation of trauma systems. In: Zuidema GD, Rutherford RB, Ballinger WF, eds. *Management of trauma,* 4th ed. Philadelphia: WB Saunders, 1985:787–800.
2. Bonanni F, Rhodes M, Lucke JF. The futility of predictive scoring of mangled lower extremities. *J Trauma* 1993;34:99–104.
3. Dagum AB, Best AK, Schemitsch EH, et al. Salvage after lower extremity trauma: are the outcomes worth the means? *Plast Reconstr Surg (in press).*
4. Walton RL, Rothkopf DM. Judgment and approach for management of severe lower extremity injuries. *Clin Plast Surg* 1991;18:525–543.
5. Burgess AR. Emergency evaluation. In: Yaremchuk MJ, Burgess AR, Brumback RJ, eds. *Lower extremity salvage and reconstruction.* New York: Elsevier Science, 1989:31–40.
6. Shaw AD, Ghosh SJ, Quaba AA. The island posterior calf fasciocutaneous flap: an alternative to the gastrocnemius muscle for cover of knee and tibial defects. *Plast Reconstr Surg* 1998; 101:1529–1536.
7. Yaremchuk MJ. Acute management of severe soft-tissue damage accompanying open fractures of the lower extremity. *Clin Plast Surg* 1986;13:621–629.
8. Swartz WM, Mears DC. Management of difficult lower extremity fractures and nonunions. *Clin Plast Surg* 1986;13:633–644.
9. Francel TJ, Vander Kolk CA, Hoopes JE, et al. Microvascular soft-tissue transplantation for reconstruction of acute open tibial fractures: timing of coverage and long-term functional results. *Plast Reconstr Surg* 1992;89:478–487.
10. Chen ZW, Yu HL. Lower-limb replantation. In: Urbaniak JR, ed. *Microsurgery for major limb reconstruction.* St. Louis: Mosby, 1987:67–73.
11. Jupiter JB, Tsai TM, Kleinert HE. Salvage replantation of lower limb amputations. *Plast Reconstr Surg* 1982;69:1–8.
12. Gayle LB, Lineaweaver WC, Buncke GM, et al. Lower extremity replantation. *Clin Plast Surg* 1991;18:437–447.
13. Zeng Bing-Fang, Chen Yum-Feng, Zhang Zhong-run, et al. Emergency rotationplasty of ankle to knee. *Plast Reconstr Surg* 1998;101: 1608–1615.
14. Wang D, Yin YS, Gao FG, et al. Cross-replantation of lower extremities in multilimbed amputation: case report and literature review in China. *J Trauma* 1995;38:947–951.
15. Yaremchuk MJ. Flap reconstruction of the open tibial fracture. In: Yaremchuk MJ, Burgess AR, Brumback RJ, eds. *Lower extremity salvage and reconstruction.* New York: Elsevier Science, 1989:159–180.
16. Byrd HS, Spicer TE, Cierney G. Management of open tibial fractures. *Plast Reconstr Surg* 1985;76:719–728.
17. Godina M. Early microsurgical reconstruction of complex trauma of the extremities. *Plast Reconstr Surg* 1986;78:285–292.
18. Mathes SJ, Nahai F. Muscle and musculocutaneous flaps. In: Goldwyn RM, ed. *The unfavorable result in plastic surgery: avoidance and treatment,* vol. 1, 2nd ed. Boston: Little, Brown and Company, 1984:91–122.
19. Yaremchuk MJ, Manson PN. Local and free flap donor sites for lower-extremity reconstruction. In: Yaremchuk MJ, Burgess AR, Brumback RJ, eds. *Lower extremity salvage and reconstruction.* New York: Elsevier Science, 1989:117–157.
20. Lamberty BGH. Use of fasciocutaneous flaps in lower extremity reconstruction. *Perspect Plast Surg* 1990;4:146–162.
21. McGregor IA, Watson JD. Skin flaps. In: Goldwyn, RM, ed. *The unfavorable result in plastic surgery: avoidance and treatment,* vol. 1, 2nd ed. Boston: Little, Brown and Company, 1984:79–89.
22. Hidalgo DA, Shaw WW. Reconstruction of foot injuries. *Clin Plast Surg* 1986;13:663–680.
23. Hidalgo DA. Lower extremity avulsion injuries. *Clin Plast Surg* 1986;13:701–710.
24. Potparic Z, Rajacic N. Long-term results of weight-bearing foot reconstruction with non-innervated and reinnervated free flaps. *Br J Plast Surg* 1997;50:176–181.
25. May JW Jr, Rohrich RJ. Foot reconstruction using free microvascular muscle flaps with skin grafts. *Clin Plast Surg* 1986;13:681–689.
26. Alonso JE, Regazzoni P. Bridging bone gaps with the Ilizarov technique: biologic principles. *Clin Plast Surg* 1991;18:497–504.
27. Fix RJ, Vasconez LO. Fasciocutaneous flaps in reconstruction of the lower extremity. *Clin Plast Surg* 1991;18:571–582.
28. Hallock GG. Relative donor-site morbidity of muscle and fascial flaps. *Plast Reconstr Surg* 1993;92:70–76.
29. Yaremchuk MJ, Brumback RJ, Manson PN, et al. Acute and definitive management of traumatic osteocutaneous defects of the lower extremity. *Plast Reconstr Surg* 1987;80:1–12.
30. Calderon W, Chang N, Mathes SJ. Comparison of the effect of bacterial inoculation in musculocutaneous and fasciocutaneous flaps. *Plast Reconstr Surg* 1986;77:785–793.
31. Khouri RK, Cooley BC, Kunselman AR, et al., International Microvascular Research Group. A prospective study of microvascular free-flap surgery and outcome. *Plast Reconstr Surg* 1998; 102:711–721.
32. Isenberg JS, Sherman R. Zone of injury: a valid concept in microvascular reconstruction of the traumatized lower limb? *Ann Plast Surg* 1996;36:270–272.
33. Choe EI, Kasabian AK, Kolker AR, et al. Thrombocytosis after major lower extremity trauma: mechanism and possible role in free flap failure. *Ann Plast Surg* 1996;36:489–494.
34. Hallock GG. Methods for providing vascularized tissue protection of microanastomoses. *Ann Plast Surg* 1991;27:305–311.
35. Daniel RK. The unfavorable result in elective microvascular reconstructive surgery: a method of pre- and postoperative analysis (comments). In: Goldwyn RM, ed. *The unfavorable result in plastic surgery: avoidance and treatment,* vol. 1, 2nd ed. Boston: Little, Brown and Company, 1984:138–141.

Discussion

RECONSTRUCTION FOR LOWER EXTREMITY TRAUMA

THOMAS R. STEVENSON

Lower extremity trauma is primarily a young working man's disease. Whether physical labor or recreational risk taking causes the injury, the results are often a lifetime of pain and impairment. As such, the disease affects the individual and society. A rapid and complete recovery is in everyone's best interests.

The patient with a serious lower limb injury faces choices. Decisions he makes will affect his life forever. In his chapter, Dr. Hallock makes recommendations for guiding the patient through this process. Dr. Hallock's suggestions are founded on the literature and his own extensive experience. My discussion of his excellent chapter is based solely on subjective opinion and personal variation in technical preferences.

Should a damaged limb be salvaged? The patient always wants limb preservation (1). The plastic surgeon's responsibility is to educate and recommend to the patient a sound treatment plan. Certainly, total leg amputation and irretrievable devascularization are *absolute* indications for amputation. Dr. Hallock further states that sciatic nerve transection in an adult mandates amputation. Unless associated injuries are very significant, the patient will resist this plan. Are there *relative* indications for amputation? Yes, sometimes limb salvage is possible but ill advised. Dr. Hallock's list of *relative* indications for amputation helps guide both surgeon and patient when amputation is likely the best solution.

If attempted limb salvage is chosen, operative timing becomes important. Rapid wound closure has its advantages. Bacteria contaminate all traumatic wounds. Early reconstruction can prevent extensive colonization and the subsequent natural selection of antibiotic-resistant bacterial strains. Early reconstruction may favor better functional recovery and increase the likelihood of return to work, but delayed reconstruction has its advantages as well. Foremost is the opportunity to determine the extent of injury. It is difficult to identify all devitalized tissue in the acute wound. Over time, poorly vascularized structures declare themselves through lack of tissue adherence, desiccation, discoloration, or absent granulation. Serial debridement prepares the wound for treatment. When wound closure is delayed, other noncontiguous injuries are identified and either stabilized or resolved. Delaying treatment gives the patient and his family time to "come to terms" with the injury. In summary, I agree with Dr. Hallock and Yaremchuk et al. (2)—the wound should not be closed immediately nor should wound closure be delayed beyond 2 weeks.

Many factors contribute to the selection of a reconstructive plan. The most important of these are the location of the defect and injuries to associated deeper structures. Although "mechanism of injury and degree of contamination" are considerations, they are of lesser importance. In the clean, well-vascularized, tension-free wound, primary or delayed primary wound closure is done. If tension prevents primary wound closure, the wound should be skin grafted.

When bone, tendon, or reconstructed neurovascular elements are exposed, a flap is indicated. The more robust and dependable fasciocutaneous flaps have replaced random skin flaps. Most fasciocutaneous flaps can be either proximally or distally based. I agree with the comment that proximally based flaps are more reliable. Bipedicle fasciocutaneous flaps, although more difficult to elevate and transpose, are my preference because of better vascularity. Imanishi et al. (3) and Nakajima et al. (4) described variations of fasciocutaneous flaps they term venoadipofascial (VAF), neuroadipofascial (NAF), and venoneuroadipofascial (V-NAF) pedicled fasciocutaneous flaps. These flaps can cover distal limb and foot defects without the need for free-tissue transfer.

Lower extremity muscles are available for transposition. A muscle flap is indicated when the wound has a deep contour deformity or when exposed medullary cavity of bone is present. Chronic osteomyelitis should be treated operatively by extensive debridement and coverage with a well-vascularized muscle flap.

Microvascular free-tissue transfer can provide coverage of a difficult wound using well-vascularized tissue. Absence of an available local flap is an indication for a free flap. I usually obtain a preoperative arteriogram of the damaged limb and, when possible, an ultrasound study to determine the patency of veins proximal to the injury. The parascapular

T. R. Stevenson: Division of Plastic Surgery, University of California, Davis, School of Medicine, Sacramento, California

fasciocutaneous free flap is my preference for soft tissue coverage *except* for defects of the plantar surface of the foot. The latissimus dorsi and rectus abdominis muscle flaps are my favorite choices for free-muscle flaps. I give a slight preference to the latissimus dorsi because its donor site is less symptomatic in the active patient. I choose a free-muscle flap to fill deep wounds or when bone medullary cavity is exposed *and* local muscle is unavailable. Dr. Hallock and I both prefer end-to-side arterial anastomoses. In contrast to Dr. Hallock, I like to transpose the saphenous as a recipient vein, rather than use a concomitant vein adjacent to the posterior or anterior tibial artery. I fully agree that closing skin tightly over microvascular anastomoses is risky. Instead of raising a local flap, I usually either advance the free flap over the anastomotic site or apply a split-thickness skin graft directly on the vessels. Hourly postoperative Doppler arterial checks monitor vessel patency. I raise the muscle flap with a 4 × 6-cm lenticular skin island. Pallor or mottling of this island gives an early indication of an arterial or venous clot.

If a flap (local or free) is needed, the appropriate one is selected based on wound location and size. A wound of the proximal one-third of the leg is covered with a fasciocutaneous or muscle flap. The fasciocutaneous flap can be unipedicle based proximally or distally, or bipedicle. If muscle is needed, I use the medial or lateral gastrocnemius muscle for larger defects and the tibialis anterior muscle for smaller ones. To close a wound of the middle one-third of the leg, I select the soleus muscle or, for a small wound, the tibialis anterior. I find elevation of the hemisoleus flap to be difficult and usually transpose the entire soleus muscle. If the wound is so large that it requires both the medial gastrocnemius and soleus muscles, I use a free flap instead. Harvesting both gastrocnemius and soleus is too debilitating. Free-tissue transfer is my choice for a distal one-third leg wound. Distally based muscle flaps are unreliable in this region. An exposed metal plate, in any location, should be covered with a flap. Bone grafting should be delayed, preferably until the soft tissues have healed.

The foot wound deserves special attention. Large avulsed or amputated portions of skin ideally are replanted or revascularized, but this is rarely possible. A defect of the dorsal foot is treated with a skin graft, local fasciocutaneous flap, dorsalis pedis flap, extensor digitorum brevis flap, or free flap. On the plantar surface of the foot, a wound on the non-weight-bearing portion can be skin grafted. As alternatives for the weight-bearing forefoot, I consider a local transposition flap, free flap, or transmetatarsal amputation. I prefer to skin graft a wound involving one-third or less of the plantar heal. If two-thirds of the plantar heel is missing, I transpose a local fasciocutaneous flap. I use free-tissue transfer for a wound of the entire plantar heel and prefer a muscle graft with split-thickness skin graft. Notwithstanding the report by Potporic and Rajacic (5), I find the free fasciocutaneous flap less durable on the plantar surface of the foot. The proximally or distally based sural nerve V-NAF is my choice for a difficult wound of the posterior heel.

Recovery of function first depends on a properly planned and successful operation. Also important are postoperative physical therapy, orthotics and prosthetics where indicated, and patient compliance. Combining these elements provides the best chance for the patient to be ambulatory, pain free, and employed.

REFERENCES

1. Dagum AB, Best AK, Schemitsch EH, et al. Salvage after severe lower-extremity trauma: are the outcomes worth the means? *Plast Reconstr Surg* 1999;103:1212–1220.
2. Yaremchuk MJ, Brumback RJ, Manson PN, et al. Acute and definitive management of traumatic osteocutaneous defects of the lower extremity. *Plast Reconstr Surg* 1987;80:1–12.
3. Imanishi N, Nakajima H, Fukuzumi S, et al. Venous drainage of the distally based lesser saphenous-sural veno-neuroadipofascial pedicled fasciocutaneous flap: a radiographic perfusion study. *Plast Reconstr Surg* 1999;103:494–498.
4. Nakajima H, Imanishi N, Fukuzumi S, et al. Accompanying arteries of the lesser saphenous vein and sural nerve: anatomic study and its clinical applications. *Plast Reconstr Surg* 1999;103:104–120.
5. Potparic Z, Rajacic N. Long-term results of weight-bearing foot reconstruction with non-innervated and reinnervated free flaps. *Br J Plast Surg* 1997;50:176–181.

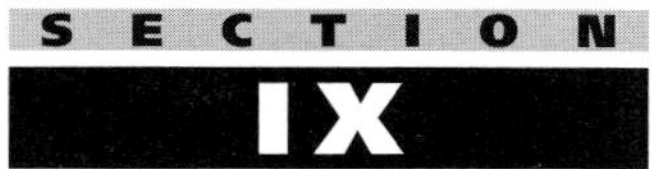

COSMETIC SURGERY

50

BLEPHAROPLASTY

STANLEY A. KLATSKY
NICHOLAS ILIFF
PAUL N. MANSON

The eyes are more eloquent than the tongue.
Japanese proverb (1)

The eyes are one of the most expressive features of the face, capable of displaying physical health as well as changes of emotion. Castanares (2) emphasized that "the eyes are a prime element of youthfulness and beauty, and the most expressive feature of the face." Aging changes and signs of systemic disease often are first noticed in the periorbital area. It is no wonder then that blepharoplasty is one of the most frequently performed aesthetic surgical procedures.

The apparent simplicity of the procedure, the likelihood of success, and the potential remuneration attract trained and untrained practitioners from diverse surgical specialties. The level of patient satisfaction that appears to accompany blepharoplasty operations is as much related to satisfaction with the doctor–patient relationship as it is to satisfaction with the results. These operations should not propagate complacency, however, for blepharoplasty is a technically demanding procedure that is highly complex, and the complexities and patient disappointment with the postoperative appearance easily yield unsatisfactory results (3,4).

The variety of procedures available for improvement of periorbital aging changes makes the choice a complicated decision and one that is open to considerable interpretation. Incisions can be made with scalpel or laser (5), fat can be resected (2) or preserved, and incisions can be made on cutaneous (6–8) or conjunctival (9,10) surfaces. The periorbital skin can be peeled, the canthus can be tucked (11), or the cheek can be augmented (12) or lifted (13,14) simultaneously. The brow can be lifted (15,16), as can the face.

According to Lowery and Bartley (10), the ideal blepharoplasty has three goals:

1. Enhance the appearance of the eyelids and related soft tissue
2. Reestablish proper eyelid function
3. Maintain the integrity of the visual system.

They emphasized that these goals are best achieved by first completing a comprehensive preoperative evaluation, with thoughtful consideration of associated conditions. An operative plan then is developed that is pursued with meticulous surgical technique and a thorough knowledge of management of complications. Prudent selection of patients and careful attention to detail are criteria that produce satisfactory results.

Patient satisfaction from cosmetic eyelid surgery involves several perspectives:

1. Anatomical or surgical result
2. Personal satisfaction of the patient
3. Reaction of patients, friends, relatives, and associates.

All of these aspects, in combination, contribute to patient satisfaction; however, the contribution of each is not necessarily predictable. The most important aspect is perception of what will make the eyelid more attractive in a particular patient, preoperatively confirming with them that these changes are, in fact, what they desire. In pursuit of this goal, we have found preoperative computer imaging to be helpful in predicting patient satisfaction. Unfortunately, this exercise involves considerable experience (10).

Complications following blepharoplasty procedures are infrequent; however, when they arise, they usually result from

1. Inaccurate or incomplete appraisal of the deformity (misdiagnosis) or of the patient's *perception* of the deformity
2. Iatrogenic errors (surgical misjudgment, technical errors)
3. Random postoperative complications (infection, hematoma, etc.).

S. A. Klatsky, N. Iliff, and P. N. Manson: Division of Plastic Surgery, the Johns Hopkins Medical Hospital, Baltimore, Maryland

Complications can be minimized by careful preoperative evaluation consisting of the following steps:

1. Documentation of the patients perception of the deformity
2. Assessment of the anatomical deformity
3. Evaluation of the psychological profile of the patient
4. Selection of the appropriate surgical technique.

PREOPERATIVE EVALUATION

Comprehensive preoperative evaluation of the patient must begin by delineating the patient's perception of the deformity, that is, what features concern the patient and what steps he or she feels might be taken to improve the appearance. The patient's goals and feelings are explored. This evaluation consists of an assessment of the patient's concerns and goals, the surgeon's evaluation of the anatomical defects to be corrected, and a thorough discussion with the patient of reasonable expectations, surgical procedures to be used, and possible complications. Many surgeons emphasize the importance of first allowing the patient to specifically point out all his or her areas of concern. These concerns should be noted carefully and each discussed in detail. Common misconceptions on the part of the patient include the inability of eyelid procedures alone to eliminate fine wrinkles or crow's-feet, improve skin pigmentation changes, eliminate secondary bags or festoons, modify the position of the brows, or achieve facial rejuvenation such as ptosis of the malar fat pads.

Complete ocular and periocular examination must include an evaluation of the visual system and should include visual acuity, fundus evaluation, and screening for glaucoma, corneal lubrication problems, and common ocular diseases. Many surgeons prefer that an ophthalmologist perform these examinations, providing a "second opinion" (10).

The surgeon's anatomical evaluation must be detailed and systematic. It should begin by evaluating the features of the forehead, the position of the brows, and the effect of elevation of the brows on the eyelid deformity. Deep forehead wrinkles may indicate overly active frontalis action, perhaps a subconscious attempt by the patient to improve ptosis or heaviness of the lids. Brow hooding produces a heavy skin fold in the lateral aspect of the upper lid, but it really is caused by brow ptosis and is eliminated by a browlift. Both soft tissue and bone must be assessed separately in the brow prominence evaluation. Brow ptosis accentuates eyelid excess skin, after creating a "minor ptosis" by weight of the tissue. Merely lifting the brow improves eyelid position. Poor aesthetic results will be obtained if the brow position is uncorrected, as one overexcises eyelid skin in an attempt to compensate. One of the most common mistakes in blepharoplasty is to underestimate the effect of brow position in patients who request lid procedures.

Castanares (2) classified eyelid deformity into several categories:

1. Skin deformities

   A. Blepharochalasis: generally young patients subject to recurrent attacks of edema with thin, atrophic skin (Fig. 50-1)

   B. Dermatochalasis: loose hypertrophic skin generally accompanied by some degree of brow ptosis (Fig. 50-2)

2. Protrusion of orbital fat (Fig. 50-3)
3. Orbicularis hypertrophy (Fig. 50-4)
4. Brow ptosis (Fig. 50-5).

The surgeon's preoperative evaluation should include each anatomical component of eyelid deformity (17):

1. Skin
2. Orbicularis muscle
3. Orbital fat
4. Lacrimal glands
5. Supraorbital rim
6. Brow ptosis.

This classification is particularly useful, because it separates the usual components of eyelid deformity into areas that can be managed by individual variations in surgical technique (18).

A 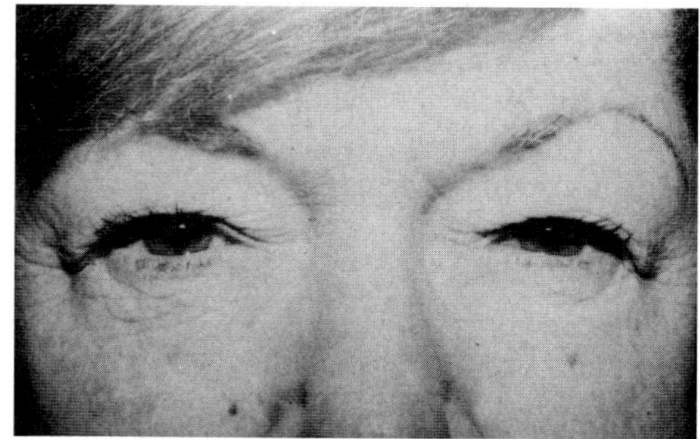

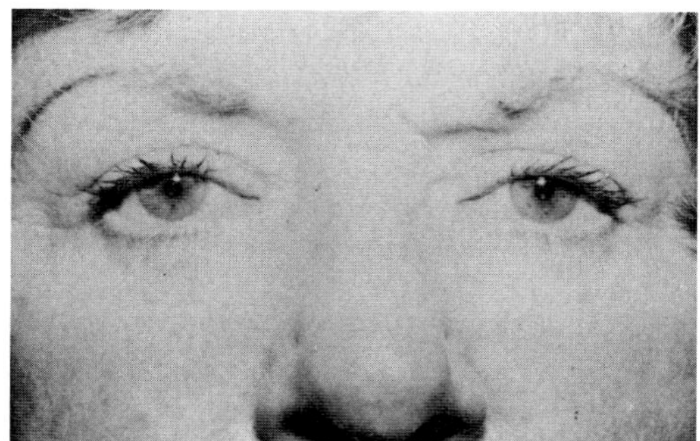 B

FIGURE 50-1. A 55-year-old patient with blepharochalasis and fat excess. **A:** Preoperative. **B:** Postoperative upper and lower lid blepharoplasty.

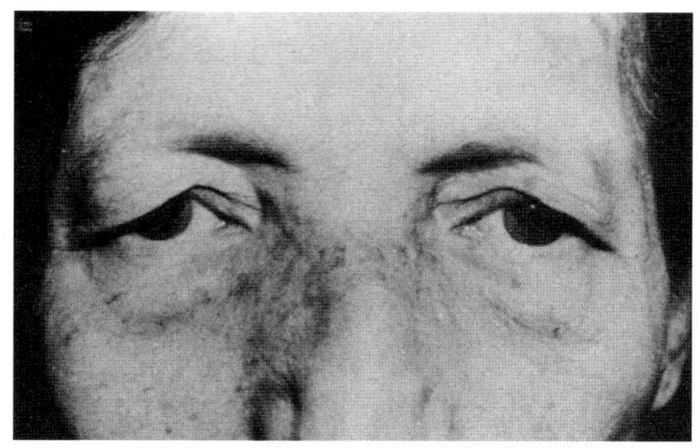
A

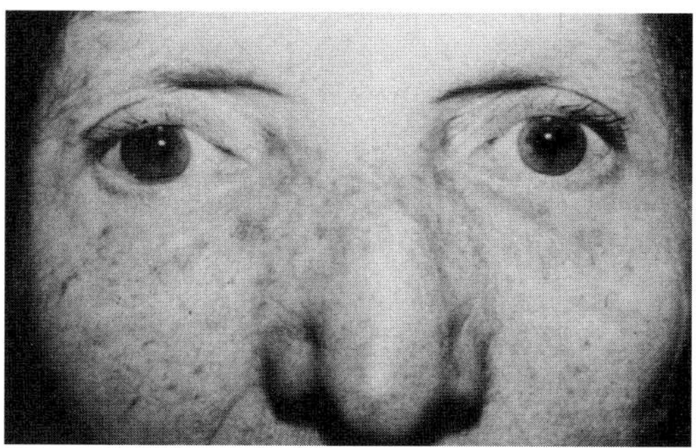
B

FIGURE 50-2. True dermatochalasis. **A:** Preoperative. **B:** Postoperative upper and lower lid blepharoplasty.

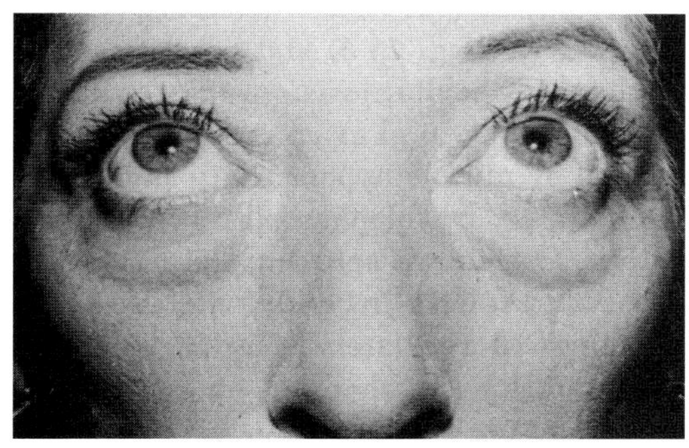

FIGURE 50-3. Upward gaze emphasizes excess fat distribution.

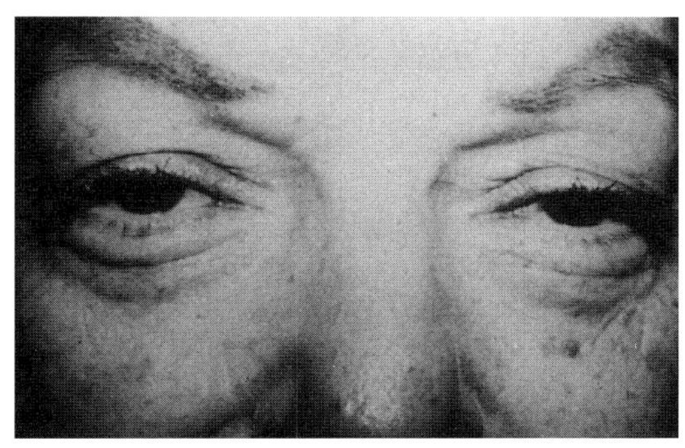
A

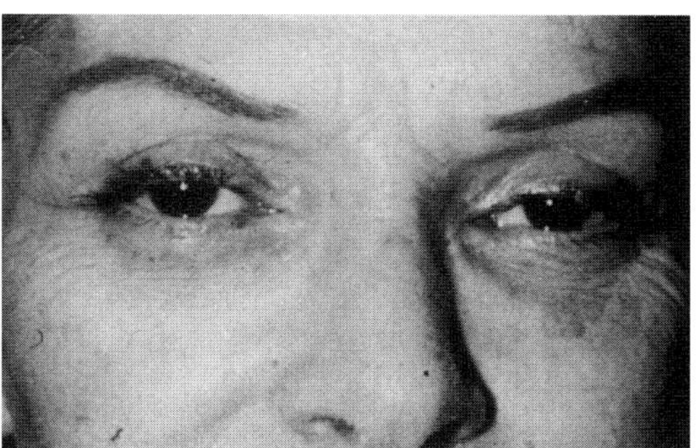
B

FIGURE 50-4. A 55-year-old female patient showing marked orbicularis hypertrophy. **A:** Preoperative. **B:** Postoperative upper and lower blepharoplasty by separate skin and muscle flap technique.

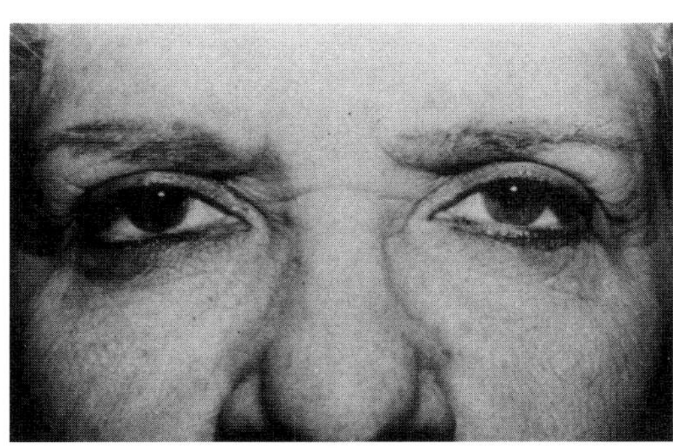
A

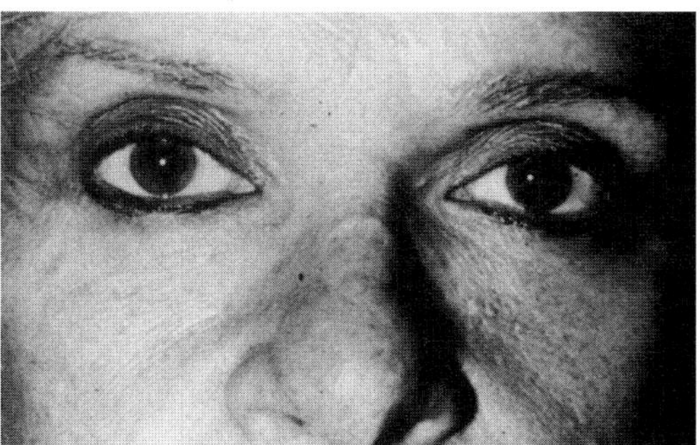
B

FIGURE 50-5. A 58-year-old patient with marked brow ptosis. **A:** Preoperative. **B:** Postoperative correction by coronal browlift.

Skin

Periorbital skin evaluation should include observation of the following:

1. Lid fold. The position of the lid fold or dermatolevator attachment should be noted in millimeters from the lid margin. Many believe that this attachment results from the fascia of the orbicularis muscle sending fibers to the skin (19). This attachment can be assessed by having the patient look down and observing the distance from the ciliary margin to the lid fold (20). Ideally, this should be 10 to 12 mm in whites.
2. Asymmetry. The appearance of eyes generally is reasonably symmetrical; however, one must note any unilateral variation, which may be due to lid or brow ptosis, or bone abnormality. Asymmetrical distances should be compared, with the same tension applied to the eyelid skin.
3. Skin excess. The quantity of excess skin should be measured above the medial and lateral canthi and at the midpupillary line. The reasons for unilateral discrepancies should be carefully considered. The effect of different brow positions on the apparent amount of upper lid skin excess should be noted and pointed out to the patient. A facelift or browlift at the time of blepharoplasty can be discussed as appropriate.
4. Skin wrinkles. Fine skin wrinkling usually is not helped by blepharoplasty techniques alone; in particular, lower lid blepharoplasty should never be considered as a technique to improve skin wrinkling. Ancillary procedures (such as laser treatment or chemical peel) (21,22) may produce improvement in skin wrinkling and perhaps in pigmentation (5).
5. Eyelid elasticity. Eyelid elasticity can be evaluated by observation; palpation; and lid distraction, such as the millimeters of distraction, which the lid may be, retracted from the globe; or the time it takes for the lid to snap back against the globe.
6. Pigmentation and telangiectasia. Skin pigmentation and telangiectasia sometimes are worsened by surgery and generally are not improved by surgery. Patients should be forewarned, and they should avoid sun exposure and sunsensitizing drugs such as tetracycline.

Orbicularis Muscle Abnormalities

Hypertrophic orbicularis (21,23) or excess orbicularis (festoons) must be identified (24). The squint and pinch tests are helpful in the diagnosis (Fig. 50-6). Static abnormalities (festoons) represent sagging muscle and excess skin. Dynamic abnormalities (such as deep crease lines and crow's-feet produced by muscle hyperactivity) are not eliminated by blepharoplasty procedures alone and require muscle resection (25). Facelifts, browlifts, and orbicularis splitting and suspension procedures have all addressed crow's-feet in the lateral canthal area. Several procedures exist to improve festoons: lid or muscle suspension, resection of excess muscle and wide skin undermining by simultaneous facelift (deep plane techniques) (13,14), and eyelid resuspension procedures (11). Specific procedures address orbicularis excess (such as separate skin and muscle flaps) and resection of areas of orbicularis hypertrophy.

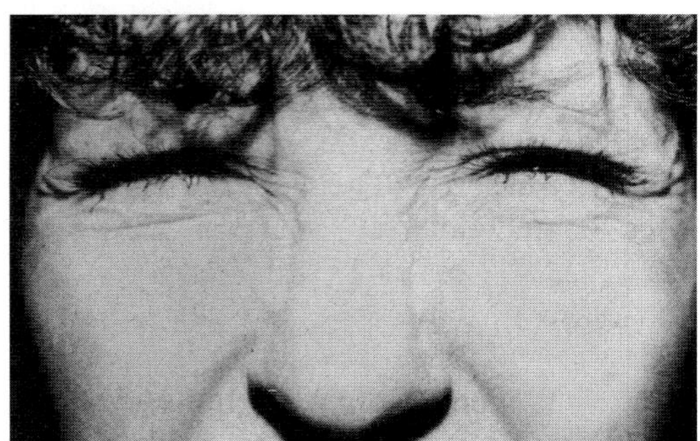

FIGURE 50-6. The squinch test.

Orbital Fat

1. Excess. Palpation and observation of the fat compartments on upward and downward gaze will assist in the identification of excess fat. The upper lid has two extramuscular fat compartments (26) beneath the orbital septum: one compartment located medially and a central extramuscular compartment that extends to the lacrimal gland. The medial compartment is located medially to the end of the upper eyelid incision and communicates with deep (intramuscular cone) orbital fat. The middle compartment is a sausage-shaped fat compartment, which overlies the levator muscle, and represents true extramuscular cone fat. Laterally the lacrimal gland should not be confused with excess fat. May et al. (27) commented on the significance of the upper lateral fat compartment between the orbicularis muscle and the orbital septum, in the lateral brow area. they called this

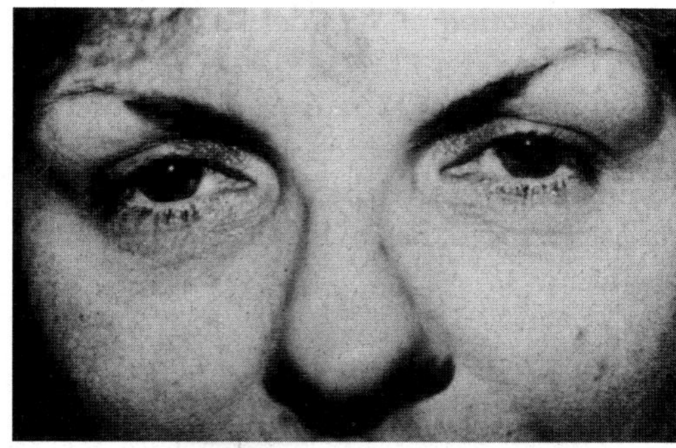

FIGURE 50-7. Brow deformity created by a prominent superior orbital rim.

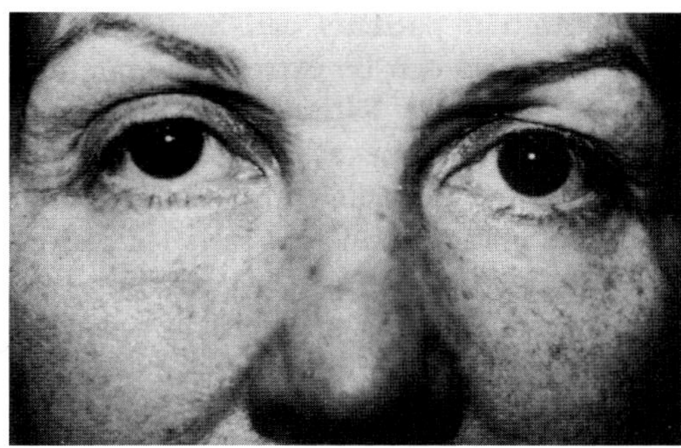

FIGURE 50-8. Prominent left lower orbital rim. Diagnosis is made by palpation.

area *ROOF* (retro-orbicularis orbital fat). Aaiche and Ramirez (28) described a *SOOF* (supra-orbicularis orbita fat) fat compartment in the lower lid.

Lower orbital fat is located in three compartments, with the lateral two compartments separated by Clifford's ligament. Opinion is divided about whether the orbital septum (29) is weak, thus contributing to a true hernia, and whether the problem should be corrected by fat resection, fat preservation (13,14,30,31), ligament tightening with septal repair (32), fat draping, or cautery of the septum.

2. Deficiency. Fat deficiency produces a hollow eye. A hollow upper lid and a high lid crease often accompany ptosis. A prominent lower orbital rim in a hollow-eyed patient may appear as a bulge simulating excess fat.

Lacrimal Gland

Ptosis of the lacrimal gland may masquerade as orbital fat protrusion in the lateral portion of the upper eyelid (33). Diseases of the lacrimal gland, such as tumors and inflammation, may produce excessive prominence of the gland.

Bone

Prominent supraorbital rims or infraorbital rims (34) may masquerade as fat protrusion. Only palpation will differentiate the conditions. Astute observation and examination prevent mistaken identification (Figs. 50-7–50-8).

PSYCHOLOGICAL EVALUATION OF THE BLEPHAROPLASTY PATIENT

The emotional satisfaction of the patient is the principal goal of aesthetic surgery procedures. If this goal cannot be achieved reasonably and predictably, it is valueless to proceed despite the surgeon's expectations, and the surgical procedure should be deferred or canceled. Each patient seeking cosmetic blepharoplasty should have a specific, psychological evaluation by the surgeon as well as a precise anatomical diagnosis of the deformity and a plan for surgery. The psychological evaluation is performed during careful history taking, at which time the surgeon becomes aware of the patient's motivation, expectations, family support, and current life events. The patient's emotional reaction to the deformity should be evaluated in the perspective of the anatomical deformity (sometimes there is an exaggerated response to a minimal deformity). Excessively particular or demanding patients are more likely to be dissatisfied after surgery.

Four factors characterize patients who are good psychological candidates for surgery (35–37):

1. Internal motivation
2. Supportive family, friends, and associates
3. Development of a strong doctor–patient relationship
4. Absence of significant psychopathology.

It is important that the plastic surgeon attempt to recognize those patients who may be prone to dissatisfaction prior to surgery and those with whom preoperative rapport, based on trust and confidence, cannot be established. Zide (38), in a whimsical report, identified four types of troublesome patients. The article by MacGregor (39) should be required reading for all plastic surgeons. A carefully performed history and preoperative consultation are paramount to the identification of patients with overly demanding or excessively particular personalities who have unsatisfactory or unrealistic expectations.

Danger signals for possible patient dissatisfaction (35–39) include external motivations, unrealistic or exalted expectations, surgery during the time of emotional crises or illnesses, and an excessively critical or disapproving spouse or lover. The patient who criticizes other surgeons often presents with excessive praise for the consulting surgeon. Those patients having secondary surgical procedures usually are never as satisfied, especially if the primary surgery was accompanied by a complication. A higher level of patient dissatisfaction usually accompanies revision surgery, and surgeons may inherit someone else's problems and problem patients. Some plastic surgeons refuse to perform secondary procedures on patients initially treated by others, because their dissatisfaction can seldom be completely resolved.

The schizoid, paranoid, neurotic, aloof, self-sacrificing, and overly dramatizing patient should be approached with more caution (40). Overly fastidious (and especially particular) patients are difficult to manage, but they also may be extremely grateful if things go well (21). Patients who wish to have multiple procedures done at the same time, those who have multiple complaints, and those with unfocused goals are more difficult to manage and are less satisfied following aesthetic procedures. Patients who present with photographs of what they wish to look like, patients in the middle of changing social or psychological states, and patients undergoing psychiatric care should be evaluated more carefully before being accepted as candidates for surgery. In general, males exhibit a higher incidence of psychopathology than females (41).

Patients must have good psychological insight into the limitations and possible complications of any surgical procedure to be used. It is particularly helpful to confirm a confident approach of the patient toward the operation. It is common for all postoperative patients to experience a mild transient depression, and this can be expected to be more extensive in patients who are depressed preoperatively. Most blepharoplasty procedures are intended to be restorative, rather than creative (40), but creativity is increasingly necessary to achieve the most pleasing aesthetic results. In general, creative procedures are more prone to dissatisfaction than are restorative procedures. Preoperative imaging in these situations may detect possible dissatisfaction with the proposed change. Many blepharoplasty patients will display mild depression on psychological evaluation; however, they usually have little significant psychopathology. Their expectations from surgery usually are realistic, and they usually have normal relationships with other individuals (40,41).

Psychiatric consultation is helpful to confirm the surgeon's impressions or to arrive at a complex treatment plan. However, the ultimate responsibility for patient selection rests with the surgeon. The patient's emotional status must be clarified completely and the necessary supportive factors identified before surgical care is initiated. Those patients requiring psychiatric referral should not be summarily dismissed (3,41); however, surgeons should offer to see the patient again after psychiatric evaluation, and decisions about surgery should be postponed until all of the factors are known.

OCULAR EXAMINATION

A complete ocular examination is a desirable part of every evaluation and should be accomplished before elective periocular surgery (10). A history should be taken to identify preexisting ocular or skin diseases and to determine their relationship with the proposed surgical techniques. Thyroid disorders, dry eye conditions, skin diseases, and risk factors such as high myopia, maxillary hypoplasia, facial motor nerve or sensory abnormalities, history of amblyopia, shallow orbits with prominent eyes, diabetes, allergies, bleeding tendencies and hypertension should be identified.

Determination of visual acuity and the need for correction are important to avoid confusing postoperative visual impairment with preexisting visual loss. An examination should be conducted to determine any evidence of diplopia or amblyopia. Visual field examinations are important when assessing a patient for functional indications for blepharoplasty, such as superior visual field loss. Applanation tension and fundus examinations are essential to demonstrate evidence of asymptomatic ocular disease, which may adversely affect the result of surgery. Lacrimal function and tear-film adequacy should be assessed. Photographic documentation is recommended, both for preoperative planning and for intraoperative execution. Photographs serve as a record, which can be used for review if the patient questions the postoperative result. Preoperative imaging also is desirable when performed in experienced hands.

SELECTION OF SURGICAL TECHNIQUE

Every surgeon should master a basic blepharoplasty technique, which he or she can modify to accommodate special considerations (42–51) Our basic blepharoplastic technique is as follows.

Upper Lid Blepharoplasty

Marking

Careful marking is one of the most important steps in blepharoplasty. In the upper eyelid, the lower incision is generally 10 to 12 mm above the lash line centrally, with the skin on slight tension. The low points of the incision are generally 5 to 7 mm above the medial and lateral canthal areas. Care is taken to mark the lids equally, under equal tension (52). If an asymmetry is to be corrected, this is accounted for in the markings. The forceps "pinch test" and the vertical sitting position confirm the amount of the skin that can be excised safely before infiltration of anesthesia. Sufficient skin is grasped with the forceps such that the lid margin just begins to open, indicating the amount of skin that can be resected without creating lagophthalmos. Some individuals minimize or eliminate the use of local anesthesia, believing that the injection itself causes tissue distortion that impairs assessment of the degree of skin excess. Others avoid local anesthesia because of vasoconstriction, believing the local anesthesia may have an undesirable effect on end arterial circulation by producing ischemic optic nerve injury resulting in blindness. Vasoconstrictors also might cause rebound or secondary bleeding after the epinephrine effect wears off.

Skin Excision

Skin excision is confined to the marked area. The medial incision should not extend onto nasal skin to prevent contractures. Abundant medial skin excess generally is managed with a properly designed elliptical resection. In some cases, a W or V-Y excision technique is required (52).

Orbicularis Excision

Excision of redundant orbicularis can be completed as a separate step or performed with the skin excision. Caution should be used when excising orbicularis inferiorly in the upper lid, as the orbicularis fascia may be adherent to the orbital septum and levator at the level of the inferior incision. Levator injury has been reported (26)

Orbital Septum

The orbital septum is opened widely. This maneuver permits complete inspection of the fat compartments as well as the lacrimal gland. No part of the orbital septum is resected.

Fat Resection

There are two upper lid fat compartments separated by the superior oblique tendon: the central (sausage-shaped) compartment overlies the levator, and the medial compartment is accessed by blunt spreading in the medial incision. The medial compartment contains lighter-colored, more fibrous fat with prominent blood vessels and branches of the supratrochlear and infratrochlear nerves. A third thinner fat pad is not truly orbital fat but is located under the orbicularis, *anterior* to the orbital septum over the superolateral aspect of the superior orbital rim (ROOF) (27). It sometimes contributes to a prominence in the lateral brow (supraorbital) region. The exact amount of orbital fat to resected is evaluated with light global pressure.

Fat Preservation

Fat preservation (creating a hernia in the orbital septum and draping the fat over the orbital rim) has been advocated in the lower lid (30,31,53) to avoid the late sunken appearance produced by fat resection. In the upper lid, less fat should be resected to avoid an overresected appearance.

Lacrimal Gland Ptosis

A prominent lacrimal gland should not be resected (33,54). The ptotic gland can be sutured or anchored behind the orbital rim to provide suspension. In the case of an enlarged lacrimal gland, a biopsy should be considered (Fig. 50-9).

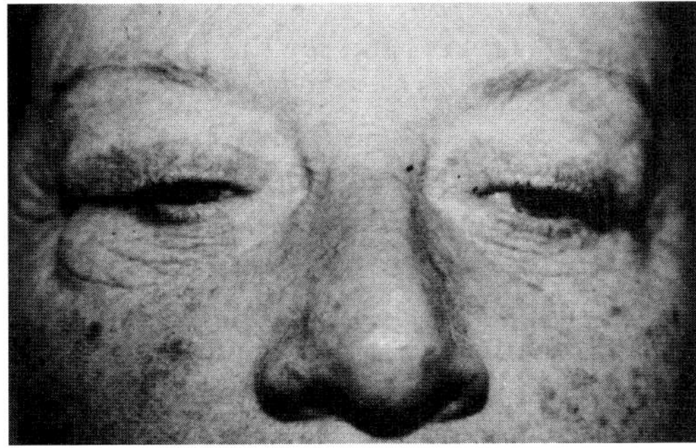

FIGURE 50-9. Blepharoplasty performed elsewhere with residual ptosis of the lacrimal gland and retained excess fat.

Internal Brow Suspension

Upper lid excision is performed more precisely if the brow elevation precedes the upper lid blepharoplasty. The browlift can be performed by either endoscopic or open techniques and includes corrugator resection. In internal brow-pexies, the orbicularis or its fascia is tacked to the frontal bone periosteum or orbital rim through the blepharoplasty incision. This may produce limited elevation and suspension of the brow (15,16).

Anchoring the orbicularis to the supraorbital periosteum, tacking the orbicularis fascia to the frontal periosteum, and resecting the corrugator through the upper lid incision can be included. To avoid a hollow in the area of the corrugator resection, fat from the blepharoplasty can be placed into this area.

Lower Lid Blepharoplasty

Marking

The cutaneous incision is located 2 to3 mm below the lash margin on the skin. It should begin just lateral to the lacrimal punctum and extend horizontally beyond the lateral canthus to the extent necessary for even skin resection.

Undermining techniques may involve the skin alone, a skin-muscle composite flap (21,43,55,56), or simultaneous skin and muscle flaps (23) The skin-muscle flap was popularized because there was less ecchymosis and it was technically easier. The procedure is accompanied by less lower lid ectropion, but less correction of skin tension is achieved. Independent skin and muscle flaps permit the most precise independent resection of skin and muscle excess. Interestingly, some surgeons have found little difference when the results of skin and skin-muscle flaps were compared. Loeb (30,55), Spira (57), and others believe that scleral show is worsened by damage to the pretarsal orbicularis muscle. Therefore, some surgeons step the muscle dissection and avoid elevating the pretarsal muscle component, believing that it has a strong stabilizing influence on lower lid position (Fig. 50-10).

Transconjunctival Blepharoplasty

The transconjunctival lower eyelid blepharoplasty was first described long ago in the French literature; only recently has it become very popular. Potentially, transconjunctival lower eyelid blepharoplasty minimizes some of the complications of the transcutaneous approach, such as scleral show and ectropion. Transconjunctival blepharoplasty has been less popular because of less familiarity of surgeons with the transconjunctival approach and because of the persistent notion among surgeons that lower eyelid wrinkles may be improved by lower lid skin excisions. Transconjunctival blepharoplasty begins with topical and infiltrative local anesthesia. The anesthetic agent must be injected subconjuncti-

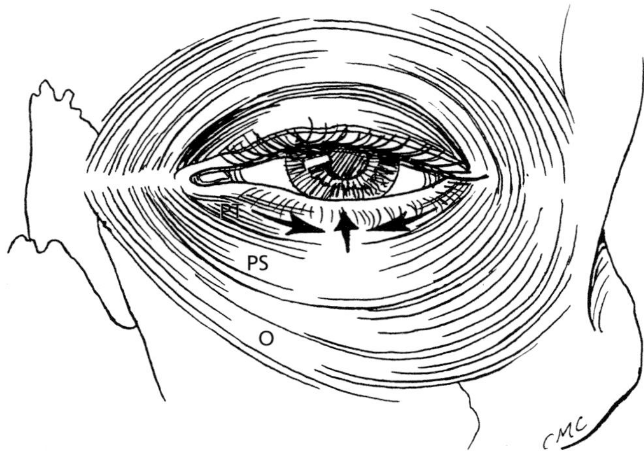

FIGURE 50-10. The function of the pretarsal orbicularis muscle is to pull the lower lid upward by contraction. If this muscle is denervated, the lid tends to droop or sag.

vally. One drop of topical anesthetic is placed on the conjunctiva. The needle is passed through the conjunctival fornix and directed slightly posterior to the inferior orbital rim. A Desmarres lower lid retractor is used to provide exposure, and a lid plate is placed over the globe to protect the cornea. Gentle palpation of the globe underneath the lid plate prolapses the orbital fat, and the area for cutting cautery is identified. The conjunctiva and lower lid retractors are incised directly over the fat, and the fat is exposed. Fat from all three lower fat compartments is teased, separating it from structures such as the inferior oblique, and resected with the cautery. Following the initial resection, the lower lid margin is replaced superiorly, and any residual fat to be resected is determined by inspection. Refinement of fat excision is completed. The conjunctival and lower lid retractors are approximated with a 6-0 plain gut suture with the knot inverted. The major complication of lower eyelid transconjunctival blepharoplasty is underresection of fat, which in some series has been seen in up to 10% of patients. Residual skin redundancy and skin wrinkling are common. Skin wrinkling is easily aggravated by excess fat resection and is managed with laser treatment, peels, or further skin excision.

Lower Lid Fat Resection (Transcutaneous Approach)

The orbital septum is opened from the medial canthus to the lateral edge of the middle compartment. A separate septal incision is made over the lateral fat compartment, which avoids transecting the arcuate ligament of Clifford, which supports the lower lid. The inferior oblique muscle separates the medial from the middle compartment of lower orbital fat (3,38,58). The muscle should be visualized and protected, especially in transconjunctival blepharoplasties. Transconjunctival blepharoplasty has become popular in recent years, presumably because of the reduced frequency of lower lid positional abnormalities (9,59,60). It was described in 1924, but only recently has the procedure been commonly used as a management technique.

Management of Orbicularis Excess

Management techniques for orbicularis excess include resection, plication, and suspension. Punctate cautery (limited destruction) also has been described (61).

Skin Resection

The resection of excess lower lid skin should be accomplished only after careful redraping. Some authors recommend opening the mouth and having the patient look upward to ensure careful redraping to prevent excess skin resection, as the skin must not be tented away from the orbicularis muscle (62). If the skin is tented away from the muscle, ectropion will occur as the skin secondarily becomes adherent to the muscle.

Segmental flaps (dividing the skin vertically until the lid margin is visualized at several points) are suggested to increase the accuracy of skin resection, splitting the skin at the canthus and then proceeding to middle lid areas. Repositioning the eyelid margin over the inferior surface of the cornea (as well as applying light global pressure) are two maneuvers that assist lower lid redraping of the eyelid skin into the depths of the sulcus created by fat resection.

Suturing

Generally, subcuticular suturing is used from the medial to the lateral canthus with interrupted suturing lateral to the lateral canthus.

The following aids are useful in blepharoplasty surgery:

- Lint-free sponges, which help to avoid the formation of small granulomas secondary to foreign body reaction. In the absence of lint-free sponges, washed sponges are used.
- Two to three power loop magnification assists visualization of the delicate planes to be followed in precise surgical dissection.
- Bipolar cautery generates less heat and produces less tissue necrosis. The current is not conducted along orbital structures to the posterior orbit, a mechanism that some believe contributes to possible optic nerve damage.
- Some recommend closing the eyelid incisions only after all four lids are done, to allow late bleeding points to be identified. Local anesthesia with vasoconstrictors masks bleeding, and some believe it creates distracting edema that complicates the perception of how much extra skin is present.

Postoperative Care

The head should be elevated to minimize swelling. Light occlusive dressings for 8 to 24 hours are recommended by some surgeons to prevent edema. Most surgeons prefer to avoid postoperative dressings so that visual function can be monitored. Dressings should never be applied to deliver a pressure greater than 20 mm, as a tight dressing may cause increased intraocular pressure. Intraocular pressures over 50 mm have been documented if a tight dressing is applied incorrectly. Dressings may mask the occurrence of postoperative hematoma and visual deficit. When in a dressing, the patient may not realize he or she cannot see properly if the eye is closed. Additionally, some patients suffer from claustrophobia and do not tolerate the absence of vision. Any dressing should be removed at the first complaint of significant pain, with immediate inspection of the wounds and assessment of visual acuity.

Many surgeons commonly use iced saline, gel, or witch hazel compresses for 48 hours. They provide local wound comfort and reduce postoperative swelling and ecchymosis. Alternating warm and cool compresses are used after 48 hours and hasten the resolution of bruising. Hot compresses are avoided because they may contribute to skin damage in anesthetic lid skin.

SPECIFIC COMPLICATIONS OF BLEPHAROPLASTY

Frequency of Complications

The most common significant complaints observed in our practice are undercorrection, asymmetry, and apparent insufficient resection of skin or fat. One of the most troublesome complaints is the unsatisfactory change in appearance, with smaller eyes, hollowness, shortening of the palpebral fissure, rounding of the palpebral aperture, and scleral show. The most common complaints seen by our colleague specializing in oculoplastic surgery with a large tertiary referral practice are lagophthalmos, dry eye, scleral show, and ectropion (6–8,10,47,63–76).

Patient Dissatisfaction

Patients who have sustained a surgical complication should be followed closely and supported emotionally. Patients may be dissatisfied despite having what appears to be an adequate surgical result (39). Some patients' expectations exceed what can be provided by a well-executed surgical procedure, whereas others fear excessive correction (35). Despite having been carefully told what to expect from surgery, some patients are disappointed that more was not achieved. A perplexing source of dissatisfaction is a negative change in the appearance of the eyes—a postoperative look. This problem usually presents after generous fat resection and consists of slight scleral show, horizontal narrowing of the palpable fissure, and a slightly enophthalmic appearance (Fig. 50-11). Many patients also complain of a sad look. Although most patients adapt to a result that does not reach their level of expectation, those who remain unhappy either become increasingly difficult to manage or pursue litigation.

Keratoconjunctivitis Sicca

1. Dry eye syndrome (33,77–80) as a postoperative sequela usually is produced by operations performed when existing tear lubrication is marginal or deficient.
2. Increased corneal and conjunctival exposure following surgery produces more surface of the eye exposed to the air, which increases evaporation.
3. Incomplete eyelid closure exacerbates evaporation.
4. Reduced rapidity or efficiency of eyelid blink is common in postoperative lids because of edema, scarring, and muscle damage from incisions, so that the tear film is not spread evenly.
5. Reduced orbicularis oculi muscle tone is present from edema, incisions, and partial denervation.

A reduction in the volume of tear secretion is a normal component of aging (77). This reduction coincides with the appearance of aging changes around the eye. Diseases such as hypothyroid states, diabetes, and collagen diseases may produce generalized dry or atrophic mucous membranes causing tear deficiency. Diabetic patients are sensitive to tear deficiency. Eye lubrication is dependent on tear production and the mechanical role of eyelid function. Blepharoplasty procedures change the requirements for lacrimal secretion and the mechanics of tear distribution. They alter eyelid function and thus may precipitate a dry eye syndrome (77,78). Although they do not cause deficiencies of lubrication (which generally are due to underlying conditions), they may make them symptomatic earlier.

Most satisfactory blepharoplasties produce an increased area of corneal and conjunctival surface exposed to the air.

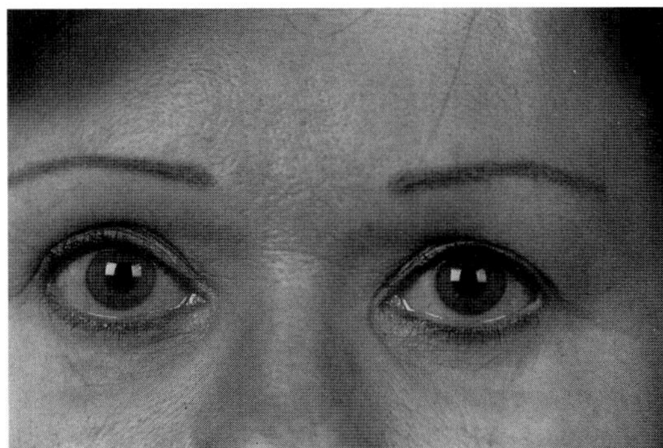

FIGURE 50-11. Sadness and lifelessness of the eyes produced by blepharoplasty. The postoperative appearance shows that the eye looks smaller, the palpebral fissure is slightly shortened, and the lower lid is slightly retracted, especially in the lateral third. All of these changes create a sadder, less vibrant appearance.

The eye is more open or exposed. In patients with marginal lacrimal function, the lacrimal system cannot compensate when forced to protect an increased ocular surface area. Punctate corneal erosions or keratoconjunctivitis sicca are produced. At the extreme, the cornea is damaged and cicatricial replacement leads to visual impairment. Corneal exposure may be produced by incomplete closure of the lids postoperatively or by lids that function slower and do not distribute the tears evenly over the surface of the globe.

Symptoms of Dry Eye or Keratoconjunctivitis Sicca

Dry eye symptoms that may be present preoperatively include conjunctival injection or irritability, itching, soreness, burning, or foreign body sensation, as well as increased mucoid secretion, crusting, and conjunctival injection (Fig. 50-12). Postoperatively, these symptoms persist and may be accompanied by subjective tightness and photophobia. Although the Schirmer test has been reported to be useful in

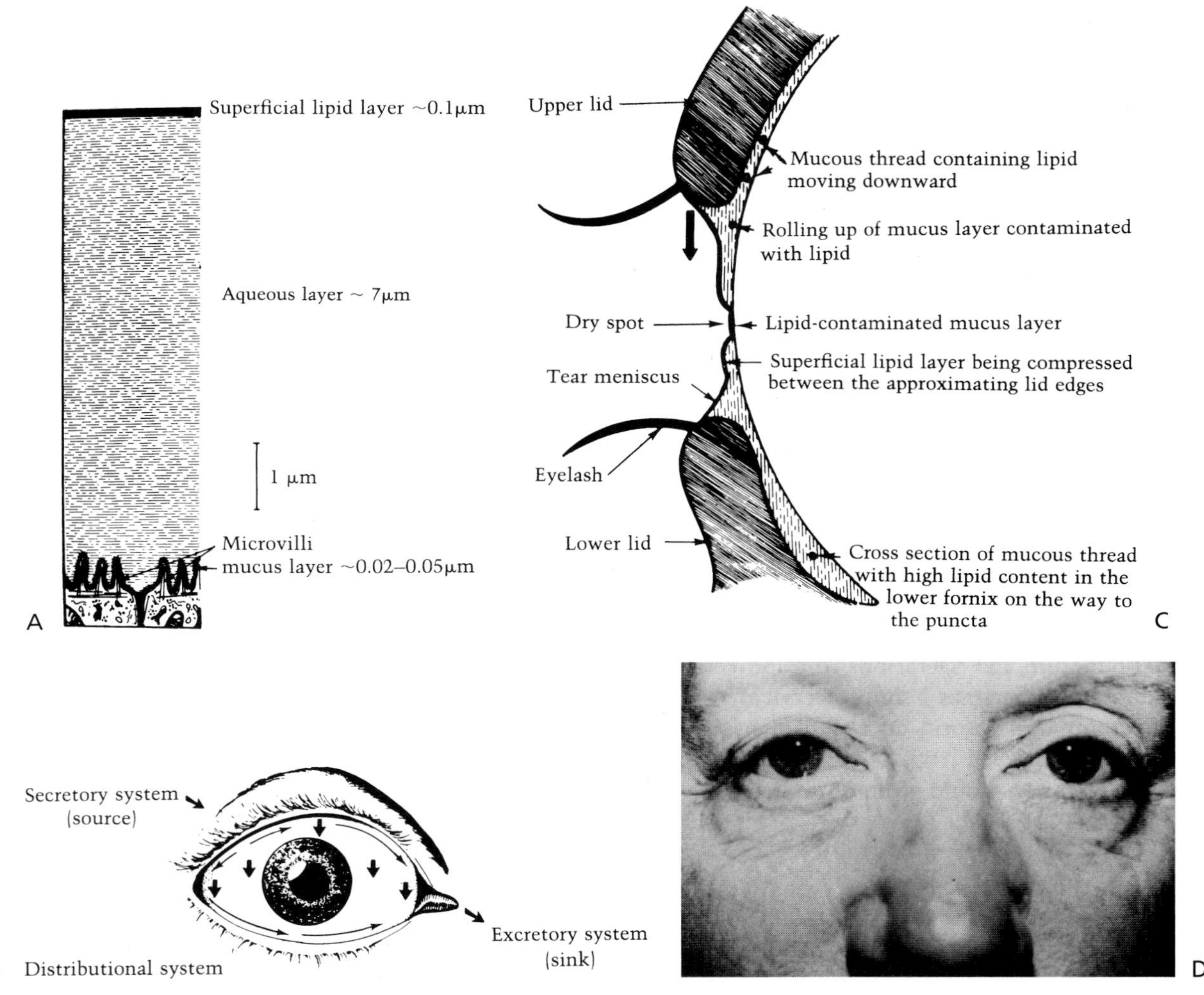

FIGURE 50-12. Three-layer corneal tear film. **A:** Structure and composition of the tear film. The superficial lipid layer consists mainly of waxy and cholesteryl esters and some polar lipids. The aqueous layer contains inorganic salts, glucose, urea, and surface active biopolymer proteins and glycoproteins. The mucous layer is a hydrated layer of mucoproteins rich in sialomucin. **B:** Dynamics of the lacrimal system. The secretory system contains the meibomian glands and the glands of Zeis and Moll, which supply the lipids; the main and accessory lacrimal glands, which supply the aqueous tear layer; and the goblet cells, crypts of Henley, and glands of Manz, which supply the ocular surfactant. The distributional system is composed of the lids and adjacent tear meniscus for tear-film formation and maintenance. The excretory system contains the lacrimal canaliculi and sac, and the nasolacrimal duct. **C:** Tentative mechanism for removal of lipid contaminated mucous layer. **D:** Dry eye. Conjunctival irritation and crusting are seen.

confirming the diagnosis, other tests probably are better. The Schirmer test consists of measuring (on Whatman No. 41 filter paper) the amount of secretion absorbed onto the paper in a 5-minute period. The edge of the paper strip should be bent and placed over the lower eyelid at the junction of the middle and lateral thirds. Less than 10 mm of wetting is considered hyposecretion; less than 15 mm of wetting is considered borderline.

There are actually two Schirmer tests. Schirmer anesthetized is a test of *basic tear secretion,* which consists of measuring the secretion after anesthetizing the cornea. This test represents baseline lacrimal gland secretion. Schirmer without anesthesia is a test of *basic and reflex* secretors. This test consists of measuring the secretion *without* corneal anesthesia and thus includes the main lacrimal gland output.

The measurement of basic secretion theoretically is the most important test, because this represents the level of *basal* lubrication. However, most practitioners accept the Schirmer test without anesthesia as the clinical screening procedure. A Schirmer test may give a false-positive impression of basal protection and inaccurately predict a dry eye syndrome after blepharoplasty. The results of this test on a given patient on a given day may vary; therefore, it is necessary to perform several tests for confirmation if the values are low. Other tests can be used, such as tear lysozyme content and tear electrophoresis; however, staining of the cornea may be observed with a slit lamp following fluorescence or Congo red application, and the presence of minute filamentous ulcerations precisely indicate the presence of keratoconjunctivitis sicca. Low Schirmer tests and positive rose bengal staining may be seen in 2% to 25% of patients in the 40- to 60-year age group.

The decision to perform cosmetic blepharoplasty in patients with marginal tear secretion should be considered carefully (80,81). If surgery is decided, the procedure, especially on the lower lid, should be conservative to prevent decompensation in the patient with marginal lacrimal function. Patients with symptomatic keratoconjunctivitis sicca should be evaluated thoroughly and counseled before surgery. Any lagophthalmos or ectropion should be avoided, and lax lower lids should be tightened with appropriate lid-tightening procedures. Postoperative use of bland lubricants and artificial tears is helpful to prevent corneal irritation.

The value of a routine Schirmer test in blepharoplasty screening is open to considerable question. McKinney and Zukowski (81) analyzed 146 patients undergoing elective blepharoplasty by assessing tear-film breakup time and the Schirmer tests 1 and 2. The tests were evaluated in conjunction with ocular history, orbital and periorbital anatomy, and the Bell phenomenon to determine the value (if any) of identifying patients at risk who developed a post-blepharoplasty dry eye complication. One hundred six patients had test results that were within normal limits, and two of these patients complained postoperatively of a transient gritty or burning sensation. Forty patients had abnormal results in one, two, or all three tests, and 5% postoperatively reported a transient gritty sensations. These four symptomatic patients preoperatively *all* had a dry eye history and abnormal periorbital anatomy. When analyzed alone, however, an abnormal tear-film breakup or abnormal Schirmer test result alone was not a good predictor of post-blepharoplasty dry eye complications. McKinney and Zukowski (81) emphasized that an abnormal preoperative ocular history and abnormal orbital and periorbital anatomy (prominent eyes, scleral show, weak eyelid elasticity, and maxillary hypoplasia) proved to be the best predictors for the possible development of post-blepharoplasty dry eye complications.

Corneal desiccation with normal tear volumes has been documented and is due in part to premature tear-film breakup. Patients compensate for abnormal tear-film breakup by more frequent blinking and increased reflex tear production. Blinking and complete lid closure are expected to be impaired in the immediate post-blepharoplasty period.

McKinney and Zukowski (81) stated that patients with consistently decreased tear-film breakup times were found on biopsy to have decreased or absent conjunctival goblet cells. For this reason, they believed that a tear-film breakup test should be obtained in conjunction with Schirmer test 1, and that it probably is the most useful test for predicting dry eye complications. In determining whether to perform staged upper and lower lid procedures or a more conservative skin excision, McKinney and Zukowski (81) were guided by abnormalities in the following five categories:

1. Preoperative ocular history
2. Orbital and periorbital anatomy
3. Bell phenomenon
4. Schirmer test 1
5. Tear-film breakup test.

These authors believe that patients with abnormalities in one of the preceding categories deserve consideration for a more conservative excision of skin and muscle. If there are abnormalities in two or more of the categories, then consideration should be given to a staged upper and lower lid procedures. They also suggest that contact lens wearers frequently have abnormal Schirmer and tear-film breakup tests. Determining dry eye condition is difficult in this group, especially if the patient is astigmatic.

Lacrimal Gland Resection

Some authors reported that lacrimal glands may be partially resected with impunity; others indicate that those having lacrimal gland resection often will develop dry eye syndromes (33,77). Lacrimal gland resection may be avoided by the "tucking procedure," where the gland is replaced behind the orbital rim and anchored with several permanent sutures (33,82).

Treatment of Dry Eye Syndrome

Treatment of dry eye syndrome consists of lubrication of the cornea and conjunctival surfaces with wetting agents whose viscosity influences the rate of evaporation (26,77). Medications of high viscosity (such as ointments) will last longer, but they will blur vision (72). Treatment of dry eye syndrome includes topical lubricants such as polyvinyl pyrrolidine, polyvinyl alcohol, methylcellulose, petroleum gels or eye drops of 1% or 2% polyvinyl pyrrolidine, mucopolysaccharide, or mucolytic agents such as acetylcysteine. Nighttime taping and patching, protective scleral and soft contact lenses, occlusion of the lacrimal punctum, and operations to improve lower lid position sometimes are helpful. Cervical sympathectomy and parotid duct transplantation into the conjunctival sac have been described, although their application appear limited.

Ectropion and Scleral Show

Scleral show and ectropion may be either temporary or permanent. Scleral show implies a retraction of the lid without distraction of the lid margin from the globe, whereas ectropion implies distraction of the lid margin from the globe. Early postoperative ectropion and scleral show are common, with the latter exceeding the former in frequency. Scleral show usually is maximal in the phase of maximal wound retraction, about 3 to 6 weeks after the operation. Usually it is present in the lateral portion of the lower eyelid and is due to a combination of edema, muscular hypotonicity, wound contraction, and partial denervation of the orbicularis oculi muscle. Early scleral show and ectropion usually subside over a period of weeks. Warm compresses, massage, orbicularis oculi exercises, and resolution of wound induration improve eyelid position. Conservative management is indicated for most cases (Fig. 50-13). If ectropion is observed at the time of surgery following skin closure, the skin segment should be immediately replaced as a graft. Rarely, surgeons save (refrigerate) resected lower lid skin in cases where the judgment regarding skin resection is critical (dry eye or lax lower lid) so that, if ectropion is noted, the skin can be replaced as a graft within a 48-hour period. Persistent ectropion should be treated with lid support, orbicularis muscle (squinting) exercises, gentle upward eyelid massage, warm compresses, and corneal protection with drops or more viscous lubricants, until the ectropion has resolved (Fig. 50-14). Rarely, skin grafting is appropriate. Skin grafting should be performed early if the cornea cannot be protected (Fig. 50-15). Otherwise, one can wait until it is clear that there will be no further improvement with conservative therapy. This may require 3 to 6 months.

Mechanisms of Ectropion and Scleral Show

Scleral show and ectropion represent an imbalance between lower lid elasticity and canthal support versus the gravitational weight produced by the weight of the lower eyelid and cheek tissues (31,81,83–87). Lateral lower eyelid malposition is the first stage of ectropion, which then progresses to scleral show. Inferior descent of the lateral third (5) of the lower eyelid is the most common long-term complication following transcutaneous lower lid blepharoplasty. The malposition usually includes rounding of the lateral canthal angle and slight retraction of the lateral portion of the lower eyelid (Fig. 50-14). The condition may progress to frank scleral show or ectropion in the presence of wound contraction. As the problem becomes more extensive, lid function is compromised and may be associated with conjunctival edema, irritation, chemosis, tearing, and exposure keratitis. Multiple factors contribute to scleral show and ectropion, including lower eyelid laxity, skin shortage, scarring within the middle lamella, a negative vector (Fig. 50-16) produced by the prominent globe and the recessed inferior orbital rim, and loss of elasticity within lower eyelid tissues. Some middle lamella scarring (which reduces the vertical height of the lid) exists after any lower eyelid blepharoplasty (Fig. 50-17). It is maintained that transconjunctival blepharoplasties cre-

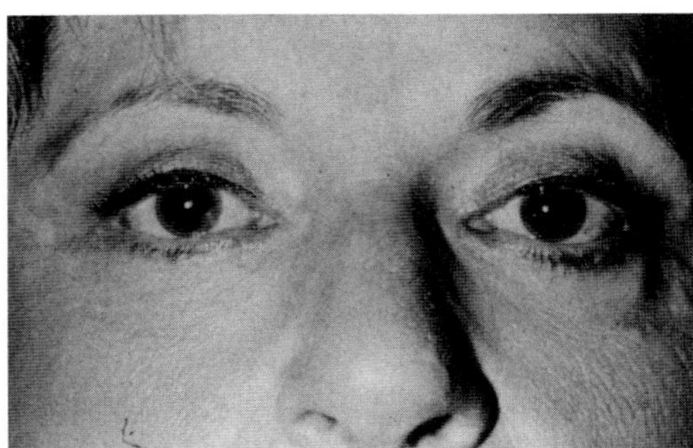

FIGURE 50-13. Lower lid induration and increased scleral show 2 weeks postoperatively.

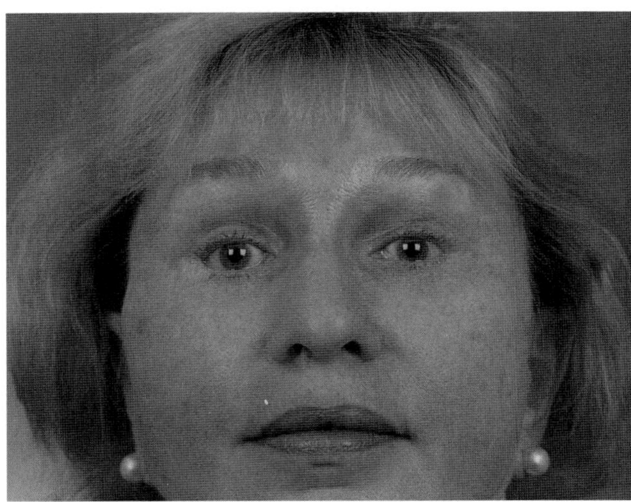

FIGURE 50-14. Ectropion that did not resolve.

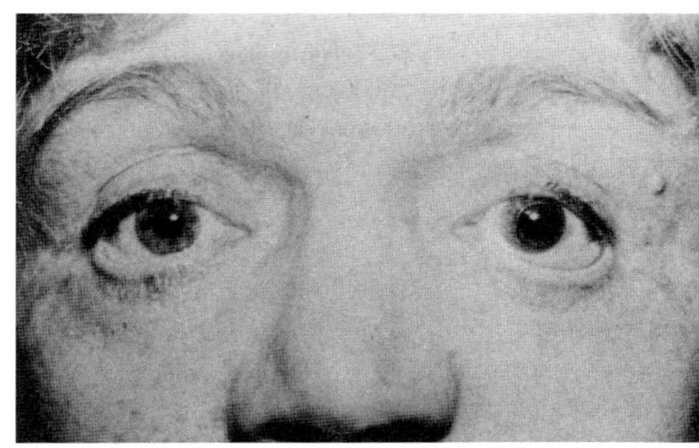
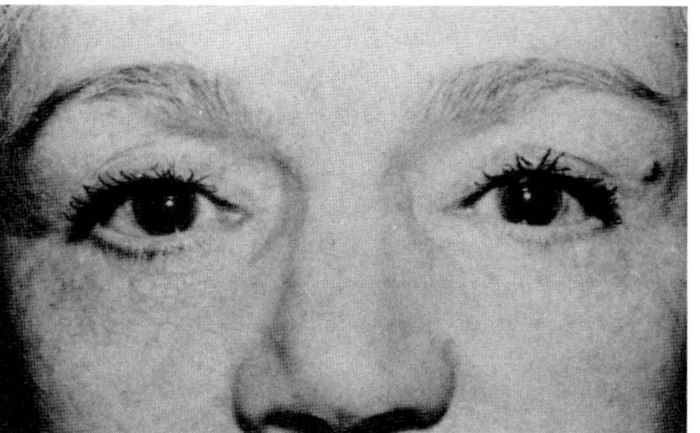

FIGURE 50-15. A 55-year-old patient with severe ectropion following blepharoplasty performed elsewhere. **A:** Preoperative. **B:** Postoperative correction with full-thickness retroauricular grafts.

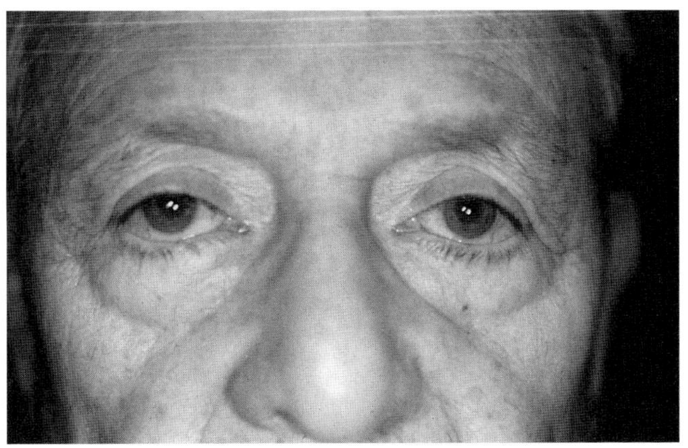
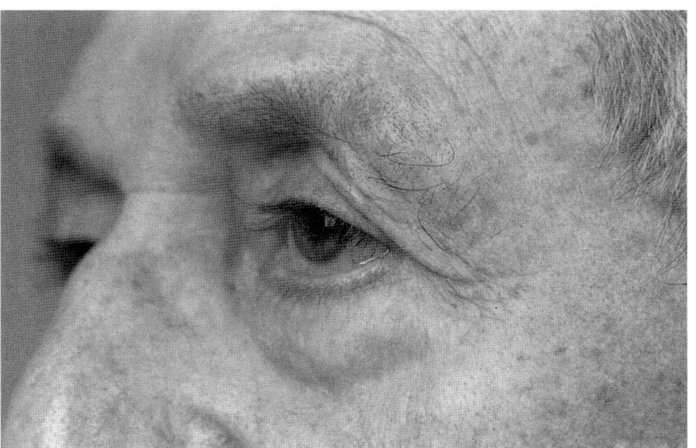

FIGURE 50-16. A,B: Patient with a "negative vector." Prominent globes and a recessed maxilla produce postural changes prone to ectropion.

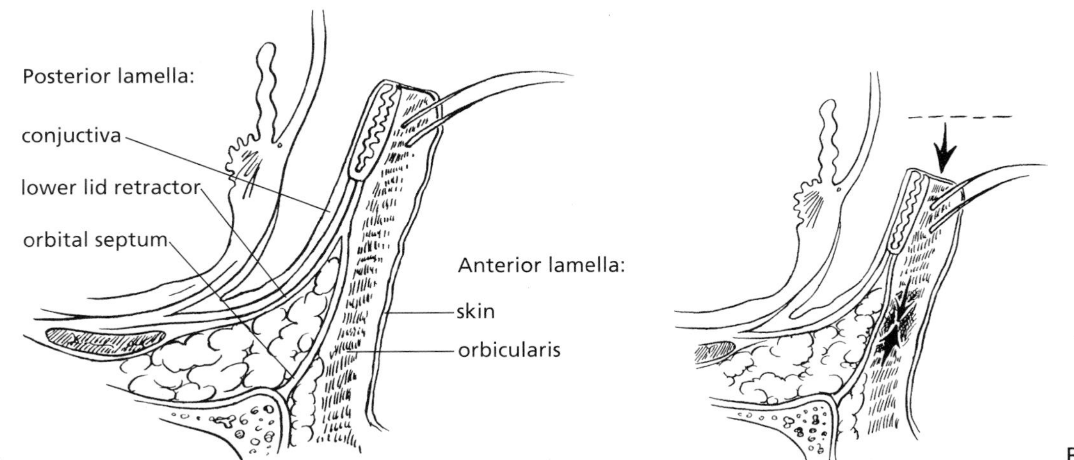

FIGURE 50-17. A: Lamella of the lid. **B:** Anterior lamella scarring reduces the vertical height of the lid and exists to a small extent after any lower eyelid blepharoplasty. Transcutaneous blepharoplasties produce more scarring transconjunctival blepharoplasties.

ate less scarring than do transcutaneous blepharoplasties. Ectropion usually is associated with irritative symptoms, such as xerophthalmia, photophobia, conjunctivitis, and foreign body sensation. Lagophthalmos may result in exposure keratitis and corneal ulceration.

Mechanisms of ectropion (87,88) include the following:

1. Excess skin resection. (Fig. 50-18)
2. Excess muscle resection
3. Suture infolding of the orbital septum or a vertical contracture of the septum that produces shortening of the lid
4. Scar fixation of lower lid structures to the inferior orbital rim
5. Paresis, displacement, or folding of the orbicularis muscle
6. Gravitational drag of the cheek on the lid
7. Contracture within the orbicularis muscle
8. Excessive removal of orbital fat
9. Postoperative hematoma.

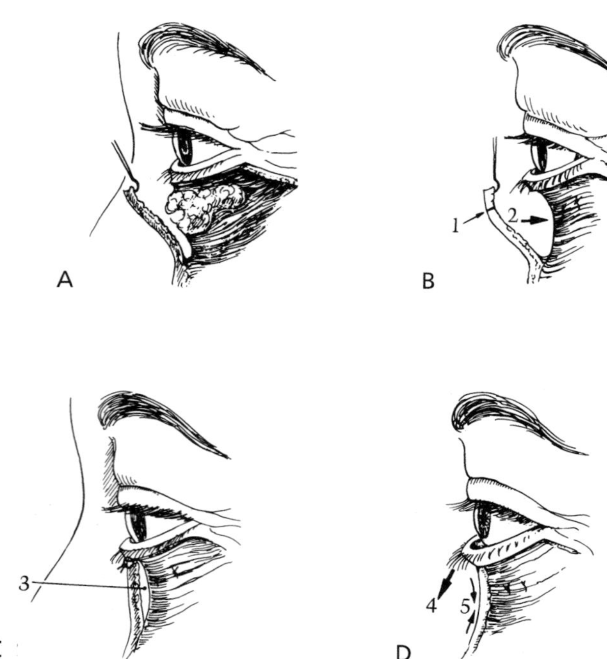

FIGURE 50-18. Contour of lid after fat resection. [Diagram adapted after Rees TD (62).] One of the pitfalls is found in the patient with large fat bags in the lower lids but with virtually no excess skin. The bulging fat stretches the skin tight, and removal of the fat may produce a slight concavity *(B2)*. Apparent skin is excised in such patients. Instead, the skin is looked upon as a full-thickness skin graft *(A)* and is draped over every contour of the wound exactly as a graft would be applied. Bridging over pockets or concavities creates a dead space *(B2,C3)*, where fluid or blood may accumulate. Subsequent contracture of the flap *(D5)* can cause ectropion *(D4)*. The surgeon must always be cognizant of the fact that when the patient is under anesthesia (even local anesthesia), the lower eyelid is relaxed and tends to sag. Failure to take this into account may result in too much skin excision, producing ectropion.

Lower lid retraction has been classified as follows (Fig. 50-19):

Grade 1: Lateral rounding of the lower eyelid
Grade 2: Retraction of the entire lower lid
Grade 3: Moderate retraction with pooling of tears in the inferior cul-de-sac
Grade 4: Lower lid eversion and exposure of the palpebral conjunctiva.

Eyelid ectropion is believed to have an incidence of 1%, whereas lower lid malposition has been recorded to occur in 15% to 20% of patients with transcutaneous lower eyelid blepharoplasty. Edgerton (87) recognized eight causes for postoperative ectropion:

1. Suturing of the orbital septum
2. Scar fixation of the lower lid to the orbital rim
3. Paresis or displacement of the orbicularis muscle
4. Excess gravitational pull from the lower lid and cheek
5. Upward angulation of the orbicularis oculi
6. Faulty wound closure
7. Excessive orbital fat removal
8. Postoperative hematoma resulting in necrosis and contraction.

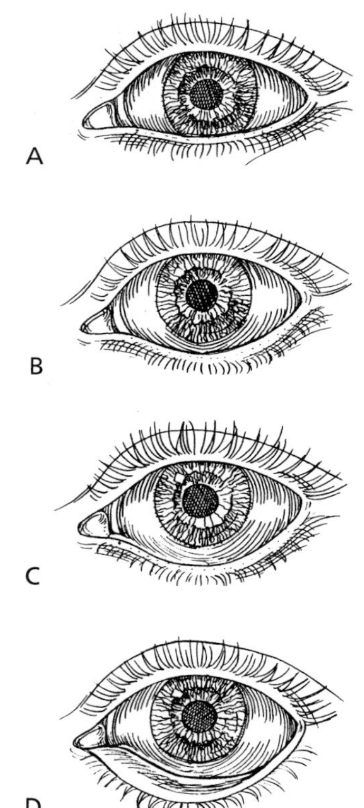

FIGURE 50-19. Lower eyelid retraction is classified as follows. Grade 1: lateral rounding of the lower eyelid. Grade 2: Retraction of the entire lower lid. Grade 3: Moderate retraction with pooling of tears in the inferior cul-de-sac. Grade 4: Lower lid eversion and exposure of the palpebral conjunctiva.

Several authors imply that inflammation and improper dressing placement may produce abnormal adherence of the internal layers of the lower lid and force the lower lid into a downward position (62,87). Studies have shown that lower lid malposition is more common when the amount of lower lid skin resection exceeds 3 mm. Almost all patients with lower lid malpositions can be shown to have preoperative laxity. Carraway and Mallow (84) listed 11 causes of postblepharoplasty ectropion and relate the position of the lower eyelid to a balance of forces between the tarsus and canthal ligaments pulling upward, the pretarsal orbicularis oculi muscle fibers contracting to push the lid upward (Fig. 50-10), and the cicatricial forces involving dissection of the skin, orbital septum, and capsulopalpebral fascia pulling the lid inferiorly. Their causes of postblepharoplasty ectropion are as follows:

1. Excessive skin, fat, and muscle removal
2. Scar contracture
3. Damage to the orbicularis oculi muscle
4. Contracture of the orbital septum
5. Lid edema
6. Hematoma
7. Lax lid margin
8. Proptosis
9. Unilateral high myopia
10. Elongated eyeball
11. Lax canthal support.

Lid hypotonicity with general loss of tone and elasticity of the tissues of the lid margin, the tarsal plate, the canthal ligaments, and the orbicularis muscle, and stretching of the lateral canthal ligament contribute to reduced elasticity (89). The lid snap test, or pulling the lid away from the globe and allowing it to retract, demonstrates the weak lower eyelid (Fig. 50-20). More than 8 mm distraction, delayed retraction, or no retraction is a warning signal. Horizontal shortening of the lower eyelid by wedge tarsectomy, lateral canthopexy, and orbicularis plication sutures have been suggested as prophylactic techniques in these patients. Patients skeletally predisposed to ectropion are those with malar hypoplasia, shallow orbits, and large globes (Fig. 50-16). Even minimal skin or aggressive fat excision in these patients leads to lower eyelid bowing underneath the globe, scleral show, and ectropion (Fig. 50-18). A secondary blepharoplasty patient is at "high risk" for ectropion, as previous surgery may have compromised orbicularis muscle tone. Conservative transcutaneous lower lid blepharoplasty is believed to require preservation of a muscle strip of about 8 mm of pretarsal orbicularis muscle left attached to the tarsus. Beneath the preserved pretarsal muscle, a skin-muscle flap is developed to the lower orbital rim. Some surgeons support the lid for 24 hours with a Frost suture, a suture through the central lower lid margin taped to the forehead, to encourage superior draping on the lid. In high-risk cases, a one-stitch temporary intermarginal tarsorrhaphy can be used.

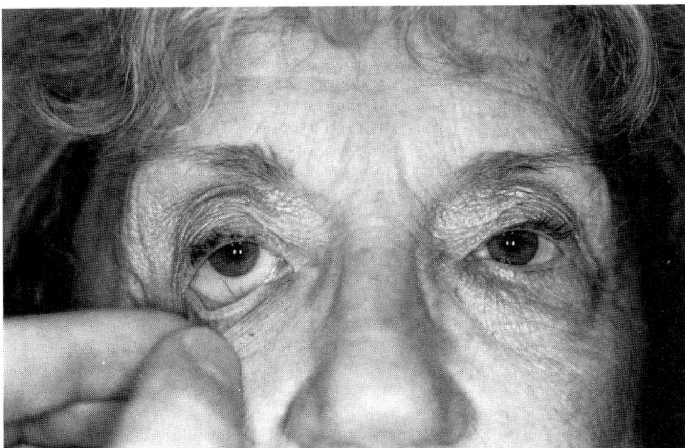

FIGURE 50-20. The lid snap test. Pulling the lid away from the globe and allowing the lid to retract demonstrates the weak lower eyelid. More than 8 mm of distraction, delayed retraction, or no retraction (the lid simply hangs in a distracted position) is a warning signal for a lid predisposed to ectropion.

Light cool dressings reduce postoperative hematoma and edema. Head elevation and a low-salt, alcohol-free diet also help to reduce edema. Removal of sutures at 3 days improves patient comfort and reduces lid reaction. Many surgeons advocate massage of the lower lid, with the patient using his or her finger on the lower lid, pushing it up rather firmly to milk edema out of the lid, holding it there for 10 seconds (the 10-10-10 rule: massage 10 seconds, 10 times a day, for 10 days). Established ectropion can be treated by wedge tarsectomy or tarsal strip procedure or lateral canthal and orbicularis suspension. Some patients require skin grafting to evert the lid margin. Patel et al. (86) believe that lower eyelid retraction involves middle lamella scarring; therefore, they use a hard palate mucosal graft to lengthen and stiffen the middle lamella, much in the manner that the tarsus supports the vertical height of the lower lid. They recommend hard palate mucosa grafts as a spacer with a lateral canthal tightening, using a transconjunctival incision, permitting access for release of lower lid scarring of the retractors and septum, adding the graft. It is their belief that most patients do not demonstrate a true deficiency of anterior lamella (skin and orbicularis muscle), but that their problem relates to middle lamella scarring.

Friedman (90) has attributed the production of ectropion to the ratio of pre- and postclosure tension on the skin incision. The wound tension was measured with a dynamometer at the beginning and at the end of skin resection, and ratios that exceeded a factor of four were necessary to produce ectropion. The study emphasized the relationship between the elasticity of a particular eyelid and the tension that could be tolerated by that eyelid. Ectropion in a given patient was produced by excessive tension as it relates to the elasticity of that particular eyelid. Interestingly, tissue expansion in experimental animals that had ectropion failed to correct the ectropion after several weeks, even when initially it was satisfactory.

Patients with reduced eyelid elasticity should have conservative skin resection, with consideration given to a surgical procedure designed to increase lower lid support, such as muscle plication (91), muscle suspension (91), dermal canthal support (92), tarsal plate resection (21,93), or lateral canthal elevation (61,93).

Precautions that can be taken to prevent overresection include the use of light global pressure at the time of skin redraping, inferior displacement of the cheek produced by finger pressure, or having the patient open the mouth and gaze upward (21,88,94). These movements assist the redraping of the lid relative to placing skin and muscle layers in the depths of the wound created by the fat resection. Muscle and skin must be redraped properly in the depths of the wound to prevent tenting of the skin over the orbicularis that would result in subsequent contracture (Fig. 50-18). Upper lid ectropion is rare, but it may require skin grafts (Fig. 50-21).

Epiphora

Epiphora is produced by hypersecretion or improper processing of tears. Improper processing of tears may be produced by anesthetic injections, paralysis of the orbicularis, injury to the lacrimal punctum at the medial extent of the lower lid incision, ectropion that displaces the punctum away from the globe and the tear lake, and lagophthalmus. Corneal irritation may produce a reflex hypersecretion of tears, making it impossible for the lower lid to manage the volume of tears. Epiphora usually is temporary and resolves within several days to several weeks, unless some anatomical abnormality exists. Blepharoplasty procedures often produce a reflex hypersecretion of the lacrimal glands; thus, the amount of lacrimal secretion produced may be in excess of what the lacrimal system can handle, particularly in view of orbicularis hypotonicity. A specialized portion of the orbicularis muscle exists medial to the lacrimal punctum in the lower lid, which empties the canaliculus. It is important that the lower eyelid incision not extend into this medial orbicularis muscle, as it can injure the area. Corneal abrasions also cause a reflex hypersecretion of tears.

Skin Slough

Skin slough in the lower lid is uncommon and was observed most frequently when skin-only flaps were popular (Fig. 50-22). It usually occurred 3 to 4 mm below the cilia in the lateral portion of the lower eyelid, and often a hematoma was present. Black-and-blue discoloration accompanied by superficial blistering is an early sign of incipient necrosis or slough. Hematomas should be evacuated promptly, and skin slough should be treated conservatively, always allowing the eschar to separate spontaneously. The defect beneath the eschar will spontaneously reepithelialize, and a much smaller deformity than would have been originally anticipated usually is present. The resulting ectropion, if significant, can be treated as previously described. Often it does not require surgical treatment, as it resolves spontaneously.

Ptosis

Preoperative ptosis may have congenital, traumatic, neurogenic, or myogenic causes (95). Mild ptosis noted postoperatively probably is due to edema and thickening in the upper eyelid. Mild ptosis noticed preoperatively (Fig. 50-23) usually contributes to more apparent ptosis noticed postoperatively but might be more difficult to observe in the presence of excessive skin and fat. With regard to ptosis, mild degrees of facial asymmetry and orbital dystopia may be noticed frequently if they looked for. Generally, repair of significant ptosis should accompany upper lid blepharoplasty (Fig. 50-23) (96,97).

Postoperative ptosis may be produced by injury to the levator muscle or its fascia (95,98). The levator fibers attach to the tarsal plate and orbicularis and are close to the skin. Care should be taken when simultaneously resecting skin and orbicularis that these structures are not simultaneously resected. Early ptosis usually is due to the weight of edema

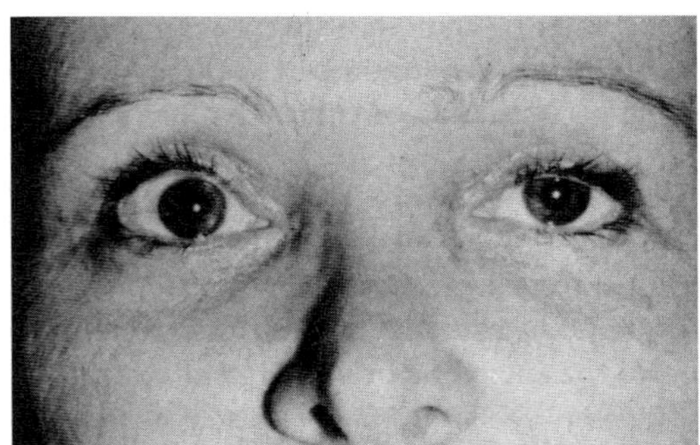

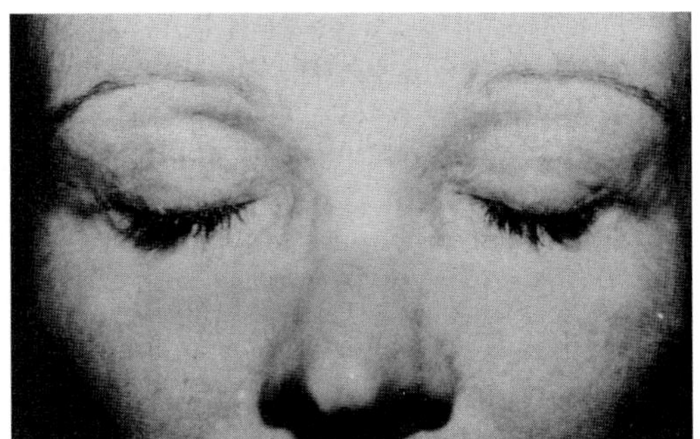

FIGURE 50-21. A: Blepharoplasty performed elsewhere with asymmetry, levator adhesion, right upper lid ectropion, and increased scleral show. **B:** View with the lids closed showing adhesions and cysts in scar, left upper lid.

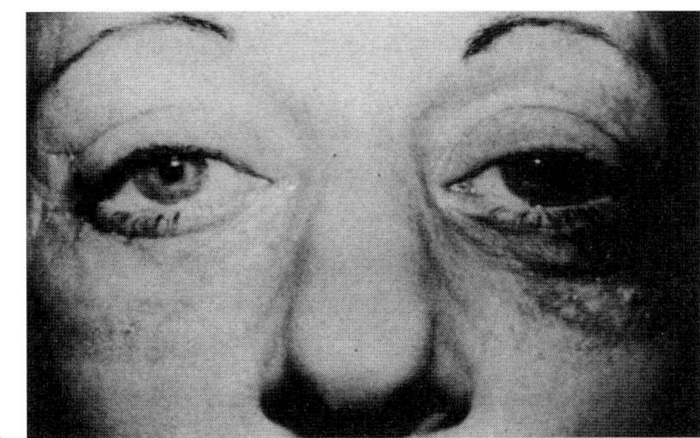
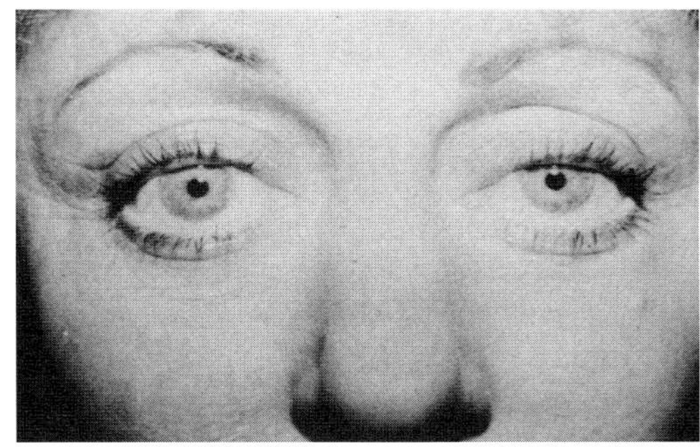

FIGURE 50-22. A: Blepharoplasty 5 days postoperatively with hematoma and slough. **B:** Blepharoplasty 3 months postoperatively. The slough was treated conservatively without surgery.

or hypotonicity of the muscle and frequently accompanies supratarsal fixation techniques, taking 6 to 8 weeks to resolve. Levator injuries may consist of direct transection, hematoma, injuries produced by supratarsal fixation, or those due to septal adhesion. It is important that the aponeurotic extension of the levator muscle be protected (the levator becomes aponeurotic distal to the Whitnall ligament and inserts onto the anterior face of the tarsus; it also sends fibers anteriorly into the orbicularis muscle and subcutaneous tissues). The highest level of these attachments defines the upper eyelid crease.

Direct mechanisms of levator injury include sharp dissection or transection of the levator muscle. Frequently, the aging eyelid displays an attenuated aponeurotic portion, which may be disrupted more easily by either blunt or sharp manipulation. Direct injury to the levator aponeurosis usually occurs at the lower half of the skin muscle excision. At this location, the levator is merging with the septum; therefore, the levator muscle is more vulnerable to injury (Fig. 50-24) in orbicularis resections. Usually, septal incisions are performed more superiorly, because the preaponeurotic fat pad is thickest there and location of the incision in this area helps to protect against direct levator injury.

Eyelid crease enhancement by supratarsal fixation involves approximating the dermis to the levator aponeurosis. In high supratarsal fixations, the unyielding medial and lateral canthal retinaculi maintain traction on the underlying levator aponeurosis. Release of the fixation sutures, if performed early, may relieve this mechanism of ptosis; however, there may be transient impairment of levator muscle excursion. Usually, this mechanism of ptosis resolves spontaneously. Septal levator adhesions may produce ptosis by joining the orbital septum to the levator tendon. Ptosis occurs only if the abnormal junction is made on the levator superior to the point at which the original level of the septum was present. This leads to a mechanical restriction of levator function. Disruption of this adhesion should improve the condition. In general, transient ptosis resolves by 3 months postoperatively. If ptosis exists after this time and shows no improvement, mild or segmental ptosis may be corrected by levator aponeurosis resection. Severe ptosis generally results from extensive injury to the levator aponeurosis, and surgical treatment may necessitate upper eyelid reexploration and identification of damaged aponeurotic fibers and their repair.

Most postoperative ptosis is related to postoperative edema. Occasionally, ptosis may be due to injury to the levator mechanism or its adjacent structures (95). Ptosis noted after blepharoplasty is either acquired or was missed during the preoperative evaluation. A heavy brow may produce ptosis by impinging on the eyelid. Lifting the brow should be performed and its effect on ptosis noted. Acquired ptosis has been classically defined as neurogenic, myogenic, traumatic, or mechanical. Differentiation between congenital and acquired ptosis is of obvious significance. The determi-

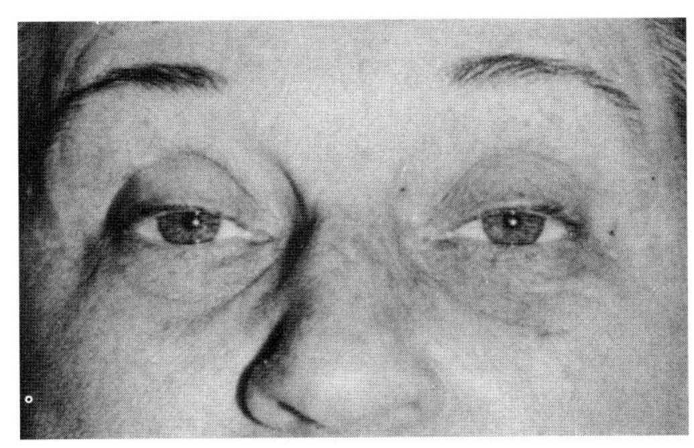
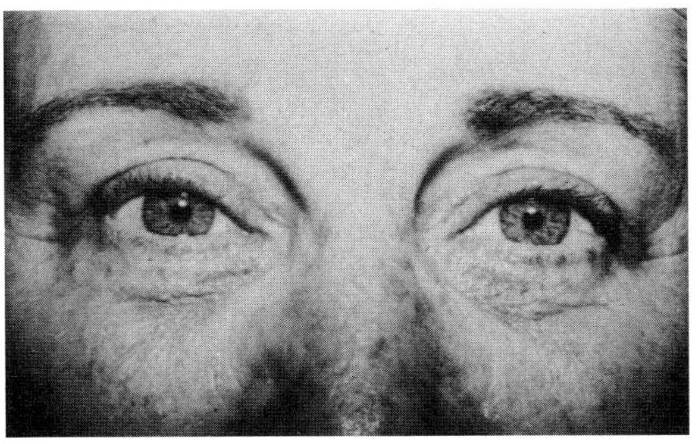

FIGURE 50-23. Ptosis of the upper lids. **A:** Preoperative. Note patient's elevated brows in an attempt to compensate for lid ptosis. **B:** Postoperative correction by levator suspension.

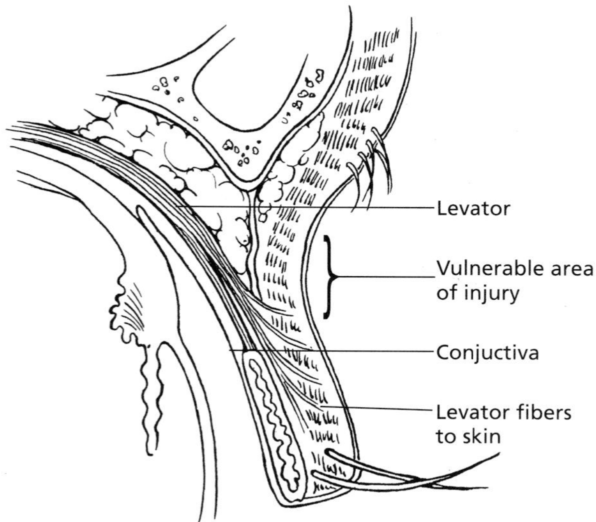

FIGURE 50-24. Levator injury generally occurs in the lower half of the skin-muscle excision in the upper lid. At this location, the levator is merging with the orbital septum, is adherent to the orbicularis oculi muscle, and is more vulnerable to injury in orbicularis resections.

nation must identify the amount of functioning levator muscle present, which determines the procedure to use in its correction. Ptosis after blepharoplasty is considered posttraumatic or involutional if it is associated with an abnormality or defect in the levator aponeurosis. Any increase in length of the aponeurosis allows an inferior descent of the lid margin. Unilateral segmental (partial) injury would create a shift of the tarsal plate medially or laterally. Injuries of the levator aponeurosis may include rarefaction, dehiscence, or disinsertion. Rarefaction refers to thinning of an otherwise intact aponeurotic layer. A dehiscence refers to an anatomical defect in the aponeurosis with intact tissue on each side. Disinsertion refers to disruption of the aponeurosis at its attachment to the superior border of the tarsus, with a migration of its edge superiorly. This appears as a white line on exploration. In all of these types of cases, integrity of the levator muscle is assumed to be present, which exists above the superior transverse Whitnall ligament. Aponeurotic repair completes the surgical reconstruction.

Edema or hematoma in the retroseptal space impairs levator function. Hematomas may result in fibrosis, which may limit the motion of the upper lid. Adhesions between the orbital septum and the levator may limit excursion, resulting in ptosis.

The evaluation of ptosis must establish three data items: the degree of ptosis, the number of millimeters of function of the levator, and the fact that the cornea is being properly protected. Ptosis is quantified in millimeters by noting the position of the upper lid relative to the superior limbus of the cornea in primary gaze. The displacement from normal is noted in millimeters. Any asymmetry should raise concern, but it is seen frequently in the immediate postoperative period. Mild injury is defined as within 2 mm of normal, whereas moderate injury or severe injury is defined as between 2 and 4 mm and greater than 4 mm severe injury, respectively. Levator function is assessed by first immobilizing the brow and noting the excursion of the upper eyelid as the eye travels from down to up gaze. Poor excursion is less than 5 mm; fair is 6 to 8 mm; and, good is greater than 10 mm. The cornea should be examined by slit lamp to be sure that it is being properly lubricated.

Ptosis caused by edema should be treated with warm and cool compresses, and repetitive blinking exercises, which increase circulation and force edema from the lids. Ptosis that lasts more than 4 months postoperatively can be considered for operative correction. Levator advancement or repair of a dehiscence is the preferred procedure.

Asymmetry

Small asymmetries are routine and should be documented preoperatively on physical examination and by preoperative photographs. Generally, significant ptosis or asymmetry should be discussed preoperatively with the patient, emphasizing differences. Patients often notice asymmetry postoperatively, especially in the size of the eyes. The palpebral fissures may be of unequal length and the lids or lid creases of unequal height. Blepharoplasty, through circumferential scarring, may produce a slight scar contracture, rounding the appearance of the eyes and shortening the palpebral fissure. Orbital dystopia and cheek asymmetry are common preoperative conditions. Postoperative asymmetries may be produced by edema, unequal skin excision, malposition of incisions, or supratarsal fixation.

Wound Separation

Wound separation develops most frequently in the lateral portion of the blepharoplasty incisions and is due to tension. Resuturing should be considered. One should be careful when suturing a blepharoplasty incision to avoid any skin eversion or inversion, which leads to incomplete or delayed healing and uneven or wide scarring.

Suture Abscesses

Suture abscesses or milia occur if sutures are retained for an excessive length of time (more than 3 or 4 days). Subcuticular sutures minimize these problems. Drainage of the cysts or abscesses, warm compresses, and topical antibiotics can be used at the discretion of the physician.

Orbital Cellulitis

Orbital cellulitis is a rare condition that has resulted in blindness (99). Fortunately, significant infections are rare in elective periorbital surgery because of the clean nature of the operations and the excellent vascularity in the head and neck area.

Chronic Blepharitis

Chronic blepharitis is a common condition seen in eyelid margins with advancing age and can be aggravated by blepharoplasty. The condition is divided into squamous and ulcerative types. Treatment consists of hygiene and topical and systemic antibiotics to keep the eyelids clean and reduce colonization. A preoperative regimen normally consists of several months of preoperative lid hygiene.

Numbness

Upper eyelid numbness following blepharoplasties usually is temporary (100). Patients often comment about eyelid numbness observed after application of makeup. Extensive temporary numbness in the upper lid or portions of the forehead can be produced by injury to the supratrochlear, infratrochlear, or supraorbital nerves during upper lid fat resection. Care should be exercised, when excising fat, to tease the more dense fibrous structures, which may include the infratrochlear or supratrochlear nerve, away from the fat (Fig. 50-25). Clamping or cauterizing fat should be clearly visualized to avoid damage to adjacent structures.

Loss of Eyelashes

Eyelash loss is produced by direct damage to hair follicles from incisions, dissection, or cautery. The most common cause is incisions that are made too close to the lid margin and violate the hair follicles. It is important to mark the patient before the injection of anesthetic agent so that placement of the incision may be properly positioned.

Edema

Preoperative edema or thickening in the tissues should prompt medical evaluation to exclude thyroid malfunction. Eyelid edema and aging changes, festoons, or secondary bags noticed in the periorbital area may be due to thyroid abnormality. In one series, 4% of patients with blepharoplasty had thyroid abnormalities (101). Of interest, all were being followed by internists without identification of the thyroid problem. The onset of hypothyroid symptoms is slow and, therefore, may be mistaken for aging changes. Following thyroid replacement therapy, the periorbital symptoms may improve to a variable extent, and the may or may not require blepharoplasty.

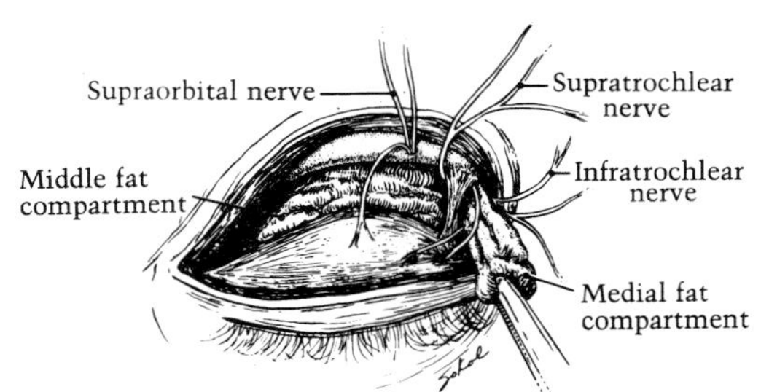

FIGURE 50-25. Supratrochlear, infratrochlear, and supraorbital nerves in medial compartment fat resection.

Conjunctival Edema

Conjunctival edema generally is due to wide dissections, hematoma, or reactions. Extensive edema precipitates conjunctival prolapse, which may be irritating and concerning. Conjunctival prolapse should be managed by a regimen of warm compresses, diuretics, lid support, orbicularis exercises, and eyelid patching with ointment. Steroid ointments are recommended, but glaucoma must be excluded. Rarely, the redundant conjunctiva must be resected.

Induration

Induration is produced by subcutaneous scarring, tissue necrosis, or fibrosis from discrete hematoma. Traumatized muscle is a frequent cause. Fat necrosis occasionally presents as small areas of induration. Sometimes the nodules are painful and generally occur in the lower eyelid. Common sponges shed lint, which causes foreign body reaction. The use of washed or lint-free sponges is recommended. Compresses and local massage are helpful, and minute doses of steroids can be injected intralesionally to hasten resolution (0.1 to 0.2 mL of triamcinolone, 10 mg/mL) Spontaneous resolution is preferred, as steroids may produce subcutaneous atrophy or hypopigmentation. Discrete hematoma should be drained or aspirated as soon as it is noted. Diffuse hematomas are managed with warm compresses, and the residual of diffuse hematoma, hyperpigmentation, may be managed by application of bleaching creams. Hyperpigmentation may persist for months in black, Indian, and other Asian patients.

Muscle Induration/Hematoma

A small intramuscular hematoma may be excised at the time of its generation. Occasionally, excision of a fibrotic area may be indicated for chronic areas of scarring that do not regress following hematoma formation. Although some inject hematomas with steroids, it is not our recommended practice. Discrete hematomas should be drained or aspirated. Diffuse hematomas (ecchymoses) cannot be drained and should be treated conservatively with compresses, massage, and avoidance of sun exposure.

Skeletonized Appearance and Enophthalmos

Patients with deep-set eyes and prominent bony orbital rims are predisposed to a skeletonized appearance following excessive fat resection. Actual enophthalmos may be produced by resection of intramuscular cone fat, but it is our experience that extramuscular fat excision does not produce enophthalmos. Fat resection must be done with caution in all patients and should be limited to that which prolapses beyond the orbital rim on light global pressure. Adherence to this general criterion of fat resection will produce more balanced results than aggressive fat resection. Current procedures advocate redraping the fat over the lower orbital rim; this eliminates the groove between the eyelid and cheek and avoids fat resection (30,53). Other surgeons replace the fat into the orbit, tighten the canthus, and reinforce the orbital septum with a conjunctival flap. Current emphasis is on less aggressive resection of upper lid fat to give a fuller lid and brow. The recent literature has emphasized that excess fat resections become more skeletonized with time. The skeletonized appearance is difficult to correct. In the hands of most surgeons, free fat transplantation has been disappointing (30,31,85), as have augmentation procedures. A condition of trapped orbital fat presenting as a hollow appearance following blepharoplasty has been described (102,103).

Entropion

Entropion is produced by damage to the ciliary margins of the eyelid, leading to inversion and angulation of the upper border of the tarsal plate. Entropion may be produced by incisions that are too close to the ciliary margins or by contracture in the internal lamella of the eyelid (Fig. 50-26). Entropion also may be produced by spasm of the upper portion of the orbicularis muscle, where the lashes turn inward toward the conjunctiva producing severe irritation and tearing. A variety of procedures can be used to treat entropion. Such procedures involve increasing tension on the lower muscular layers or denervation of the pretarsal orbicularis, which is tight or spastic in some patients (76). Techniques for correction vary from release of contracture in the internal lamella to strengthening the mid lamella of the lid by grafting, muscle resection or retraction, muscle denervation, or creating a balancing scar with the ⅓ three-suture technique (76).

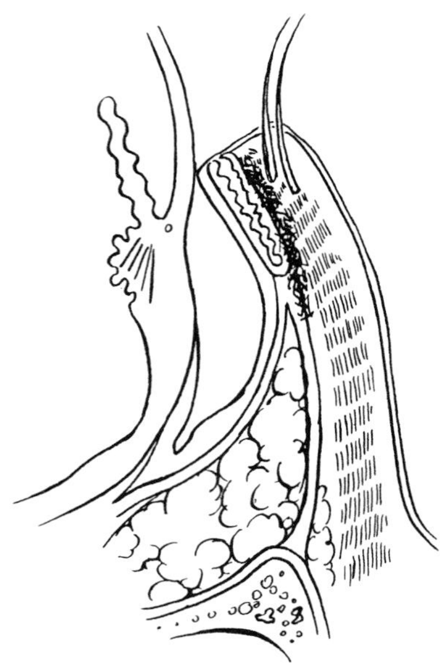

FIGURE 50-26. Entropion can be produced by incisions that are too close to the ciliary margins or by contracture of the internal lamella of the eyelid.

Corneal Abrasions

Corneal abrasion is produced by trauma to the cornea during surgery. Instruments, sutures, and sponges all are capable of producing injury in surgery. Postoperatively dressings, foreign bodies, and desiccation during sleep in patients unable to completely close their eyes because of excessive resection of skin are conditions that cause corneal injury. Protection of the cornea during surgery is accomplished with scleral shields, balanced ocular irrigation, ointment, and a Frost traction suture during lower lid blepharoplasty. If it is the surgeon's custom to set the upper eyelids open, one must be careful to constantly protect the cornea. Corneal abrasion is suspected when there is pain, tearing, and photophobia. The diagnosis is confirmed with fluorescein staining techniques or slit-lamp examination. Treatment consists of the application of a bland ointment with or without patching the eye for 24 to 48 hours. Ophthalmologic consultation is indicated if symptoms do not promptly subside with patching and lubrication. Corneal infection and conjunctivitis are uncommon, but they are serious and may produce corneal scarring by advancing inflammation. Steroid-containing ointments should be used only when glaucoma or bacterial or herpetic infection has been excluded. Bland lubricating ointments are recommended.

Lagophthalmos

Lagophthalmos (inability to close the eyelids) usually is due to excessive skin resection (Fig. 50-27) or damage to the orbicularis muscle or seventh cranial nerve. It rarely can be produced by vertical shortening of the orbital septum, reactions to local anesthetics, postoperative induration from hematoma or infection, or supratarsal fixation. Lagophthalmos requires corneal protection. Generally, the causes are self-limiting and resolve with time; however, a tarsorrhaphy should be accomplished if corneal protection cannot be maintained.

Dermatologic Complications

Increased telangiectasia and pigmentation occasionally are seen following surgery. The conditions usually are present to

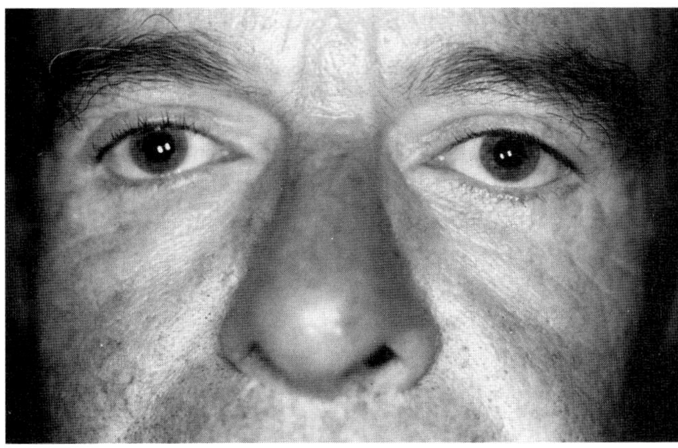

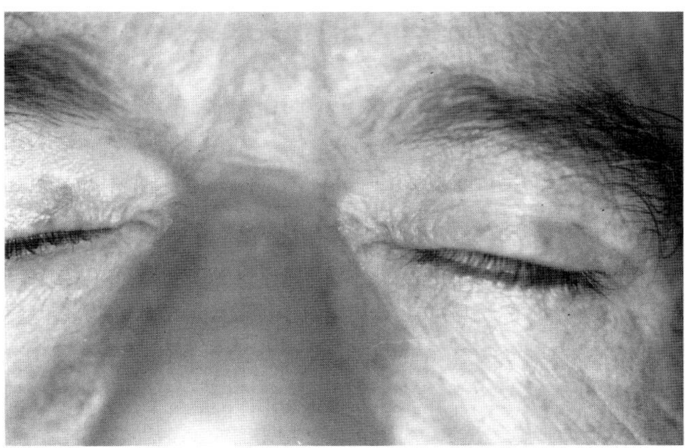

FIGURE 50-27. A,B: Lagophthalmos (inability to close the eyelid) due to excessive skin resection.

some degree before surgery and, in that regard, may be called to the patient's attention. There seems to be an increased tendency in patients with capillary fragility and a history of excessive bruising to develop telangiectasia. Patients who have excessive bruising or hematomas, especially when predisposed by increased skin pigmentation preoperatively, may have excessive hemosiderin deposition. It is important to mention increased pigmentation preoperatively (Fig. 50-28), pointing out to the patient that it may be more conspicuous postoperatively and is aggravated by ecchymosis and sun exposure. Sun-sensitizing antibiotics, such as tetracycline-containing drugs, should be avoided. Resolution of hyperpigmentation may occur slowly, sometimes taking 1 year. Pigmentation may be improved by the use of cutaneous bleaching creams, such as hydroquinone (Eldoquin, Melanex). Sunscreens are recommended.

Hypertrophic Scars and Web Scars

Black and Asian patients are more prone to develop hypertrophic scars, but true hypertrophic scars confined to the eyelid skin are very unusual. To our knowledge, a true keloid occurring in the eyelid has not been described. One is encouraged in eyelid surgery to confine the incisions to eyelid skin, which may be identified by its fine texture and slightly crinkled appearance. Extension of incisions beyond the orbital or eyelid skin margin, beyond the canthus or into cheek, brow, or nasal skin, should be avoided, as they are more conspicuous and produce poorer scars. Extension of incisions onto the nasal skin especially should be avoided to prevent prominent scars and webbing. Hypertrophic or web scars usually respond to nonsurgical treatment (pressure, massage, and judicious steroid injections.) Z-plasty rarely is needed and may produce a more conspicuous pattern of cutaneous scarring.

Inclusion Cysts and Milia

Inclusion cysts and milia commonly occur in areas of suture trauma. Small white nodules may appear and disappear spontaneously, but when they persist, they should be treated by incision, unroofing with the tip of a No. 11 blade and gently extruding the cyst material.

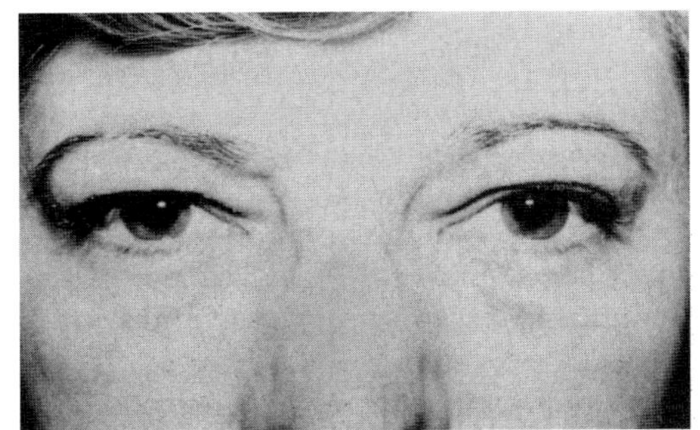

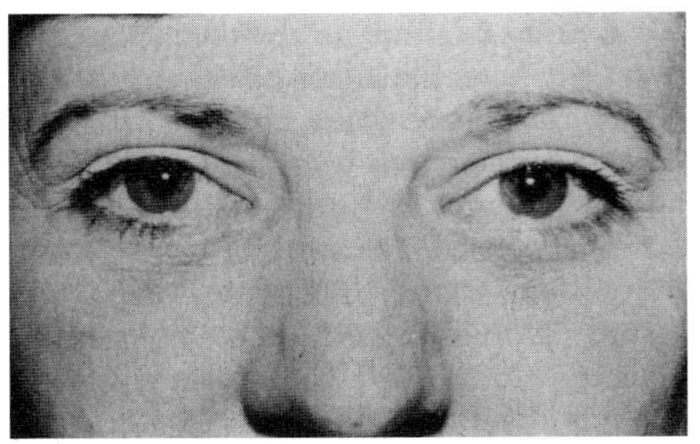

FIGURE 50-28. Increased pigmentation is not changed by a blepharoplasty and can be worsened by hematoma with hemosiderin deposition. **A:** Preoperative pigmentation. **B:** Postoperative pigmentation.

Epithelial Tunnels

Epithelial tunnels are produced by suture retention over an excessive length of time. Generally, it takes more than 4 to 5 days for epithelialization along the suture to occur, producing the tunnel. Such areas may be treated by marsupialization of the tracts or excision of the tunnel edge. Subcuticular closure eliminates the need for early suture removal and minimizes the formation of epithelial tunnels.

Skin Wrinkling

Skin wrinkling occurring after blepharoplasty may be due to release of skin tension after resolution of edema and is increased after excessive fat resection. Skin wrinkling may be more apparent following blepharoplasty in the lower lid. The only treatment possible is reduction in the amount of skin or increase in tension on the lower eyelid, which may produce a lowered eyelid position. Generally, postoperative treatment consists of judicious laser or peel treatment, with consideration for canthal tightening.

Ecchymosis and Hematoma

Ecchymosis and hematoma generally are noticed in the skin of the periorbital region. However, retrobulbar hematomas may occur and are treated by urgent decompression of the incisions and lateral canthotomy. They are discussed in the section on optic nerve injury (p. 871).

Generalized Bruising and Ecchymosis

Generalized bruising and ecchymosis may be due to postoperative nausea and vomiting, excessive physical activity, prolonged clotting or bleeding time due to coagulopathy, or drugs modifying coagulation (aspirin, nonsteroidal medication, clofibrate [Atromid-S], hypertension, and increased capillary fragility). Drugs modifying coagulation should be discontinued 2 to 3 weeks postoperatively, depending their mechanism and length of action.

Acute Periorbital Hematomas

Acute hematomas may occur immediately after injection and are controlled by precise digital pressure. If a small hematoma exists within the muscle, it may be possible to excise the muscle segment or evacuate the hematoma during the course of the blepharoplasty.

Localized Periorbital Hematoma

Localized hematomas noticed in the postoperative period should be evacuated once they have slightly liquefied or may be formally explored and removed. Such procedures often can be accomplished in the office without the need to return the patient to the operating room. Diffuse periorbital ecchymoses resorb slowly over a 2-week period. Resorption can be assisted by warm compresses, and increased scarring is expected.

Subscleral Hematomas

Subscleral hematomas are produced by leakage of blood beyond the tenon capsule. When they occur, the appearance of red eyes often is frightening and alarming to the patient. The patient should be reassured regarding the usual uncomplicated but time-consuming resolution. Frequent application of warm compresses may hasten resorption, but subscleral hematomas often require several weeks for resolution.

Retrobulbar Hematoma

Retrobulbar hematoma is a dramatic bleeding event that has been related to transient visual disturbances (104–106). A consistent relationship between retrobulbar hematoma and permanent visual loss has been difficult to establish (107–109). The most concerning aspect of the condition is that it has been the most consistent feature in cases of visual loss, as has been fat resection, (58,104,110–112). The symptoms of retrobulbar hemorrhage include mydriasis, ecchymosis, proptosis, and pain. Pain is the predominant symptom and alerts the physician to urgently perform a careful visual examination to assess visual acuity and intraocular pressure. The eye may be proptotic and the periorbital tissue congested and firm to palpation. If the eye becomes hard and protrudes between the eyelids, this is an absolute emergency that requires immediate decompression. Decompression should be completed before any other maneuvers are accomplished. The conjunctival capillaries can be injected, and extraocular movements may be limited. Visual loss may or may not occur. Schiøtz tonometry may reveal elevated pressure, sometimes exceeding 115 (normal pressure is 10). Therapy may be based on the degree of proptosis, the presence of central retinal artery circulation, the intraocular pressure, and degree of visual loss. Rees (21,113) observed four retrobulbar hematomas in 15,000 blepharoplasties, a frequency of 0.04%. Each resolved under careful observation without permanent visual impairment. In his cases, it was not necessary to use any aggressive treatment, such as decompression or anterior chamber paracentesis.

Numerous experiments suggested that the visual loss accompanying retrobulbar hemorrhage is transient (104). To simulate the conditions of a retrobulbar hematoma, injection of blood into the posterior closed space of the orbit under excessive pressure has been performed in animals. Transient and resolving (but not permanent) visual loss was produced. The proposed mechanism for visual loss is related to increased intraocular pressure involving either compromise of the circulation through the central retinal artery and veins draining the retina or optic nerve ischemia. Glaucoma and optic nerve ischemia have been postulated as reflex sequelae produced by excessive hemorrhage, which contribute to visual loss. Anterior chamber paracentesis in experimental animals has reversed central retinal artery occlusion (114).

Retrobulbar hematoma usually accompanies a deep or blind injection into the fat compartments or bleeding in the fat that retracts back into the deep orbit. The infraorbital artery may be damaged by a deep injection. For this reason, it is recommended that fat be injected superficially under direct vision after opening the orbital septum completely. Strong traction on orbital fat should be avoided, and vessels in the fat should be electrocoagulated before their retraction back into the orbit. Strong traction on fat has been postulated to avulse veins deep within the orbit, producing hemorrhage. Coagulation of blood vessels in the stump of the orbital fat should be complete. Some individuals have postulated extension of thrombosis along vessels extending distant to the site of application of cautery current, and this progressive thrombosis has been suggested as a mechanism of optic nerve ischemia. Bipolar cautery conceptually would limit the conduction of electrical current along vessels or nerves to a deep orbital location.

If retrobulbar hemorrhage occurs, the pressure within the orbit may rapidly approach systolic pressure (14). When the arterial bleeding vessel is tamponaded, a reflex spasm may occur in the central retinal artery. This triggers a new increase in blood pressure that is accompanied by further arterial bleeding. The increased pressure within the orbit may produce interference with venous drainage of the optic nerve or acute glaucoma by interfering with resorption of fluid through the canal of Schlemm. Fluid resorption is reduced by iris prolapse secondary to increased pressure. Increases in intraocular pressure may produce a reflex diminution of blood flow in the central retinal artery. Experimentally, diminished arterial flow and decreased retinal perfusion have been shown to occur if the intraocular pressure exceeds 30 mm Hg. When the pressure is over 80 to 100, blood flow to the retina ceases. The normal intraocular pressure is 15 mm Hg (44), varies with respiration and pulse, and has a diurnal variation. The amount of vitreous material is relatively static; however, the amount of aqueous fluid varies (105). Aqueous fluid is secreted in the posterior chamber and travels through ports into the anterior chamber, where it is absorbed by the canal of Schlemm. It is produced at the rate of 3 to 4 μL/min, and thereafter 0.3 to 0.mL of this fluid is present in the intraocular cavity.

It was shown experimentally that occlusion of the central retinal artery for more than 2 hours must be present before any permanent ischemic damage occurs. It is important to realize that most retrobulbar hemorrhages are self-limiting and temporary diminution of vision may occur, but visual loss almost always resolves, even without treatment (115). This was the situation occurring in experimental animals.

Treatment of retrobulbar hematoma that does not respond to observation should include opening the incisions, expressing hematoma, and carefully exploring the wound. Deep exploration is not practical. If vision is not restored and a clinically effective decompression is not achieved promptly, a lateral canthotomy should be performed by dividing the lateral canthal tendon. Vision usually is restored within a few minutes to within several hours. The patient should be observed continuously. Mannitol 20% can be given intravenously at a dose of 2 g/kg. The first dose of 12.5 g can be given over 3 to 4 minutes, with the rest given more slowly. A lowering of blood pressure occurs during diuresis. The patient also can be given acetazolamide (Diamox) 500 mg intravenously; thereafter the drug can be continued at the rate of 250 mg every 6 hours. The patient can be given 95% oxygen and 5% carbon dioxide to breathe, which is believed to improve circulation to the brain, retina, and associated organs. Visual acuity and central retinal artery circulation should be monitored throughout the course of treatment. If the globe becomes proptotic, an intermarginal suture will protect the cornea. Globe massage and anterior chamber paracentesis are controversial. Globe massage has been recommended by some authors and can be performed. Anterior chamber paracentesis is *not* believed to be helpful in most cases; the procedure is fraught with complications. Anterior chamber paracentesis may cause lens prolapse and profuse intraocular bleeding. It should be performed only by an experienced anterior segment ophthalmologist and only after all other treatments have been unsuccessful.

Visual Loss and Blindness Accompanying Blepharoplasty

Visual disturbances and blindness (104) may have been present preoperatively and not diagnosed. They also may be coincident with the blepharoplasty, and they may or may not be causally related to the blepharoplasty procedure. The value of a carefully performed preoperative history and physical examination is never to be underestimated. The incidence of visual disturbances resulting in permanent visual loss following blepharoplasty has been estimated to be 0.04% (104), but many have questioned the validity of the methods used in this study. There have been approximately 75 cases of visual loss reported in the literature, but it is not known how accurately the reported cases reflect the true incidence. A precise cause-and-effect relationship has been difficult to establish, but there must be a variety of mechanisms (58,94,104,105,106–110,112).

Preexisting visual disturbances easily go unrecognized by the patient. They also can be missed by the surgeon; thus, the surgeon can be blamed for the preexisting disturbance first noted in the postoperative period. It is normal for patients with amblyopia to have a moderate visual deficit in the affected eye. Such losses of visual acuity should be documented and pointed out to the patient. The following ophthalmologic tests are recommended preoperatively at the discretion of the surgeon: (i) visual acuity; (ii) evaluation of ocular lubrication (see section on dry eye); (iii) evaluation of extraocular movement and levator function; (iv) evidence of accommodation and light reflex; (v) resting level of the eyelids; (vi) tonometry; (vii) evaluation of Bell phenomenon; (viii) funduscopic examination; and (ix) brief general medical evaluation, including measurement of blood pressure.

Common visual disturbances existing preoperatively include amblyopia ex anopsia, glaucoma, and cataract.

Amblyopia is present in 2% of the population and may be responsible for dramatically reduced unilateral visual acuity.

Chronic simple glaucoma is present in 0.09% of the population. The incidence increases when patient age is greater than 50 years. Glaucoma is diagnosed by measurement of intraocular pressure.

Decreased unilateral vision or field spot is diagnosed by confrontation fields.

The eye, like any organ, may be affected by degenerative diseases, such as diabetes, central nervous system demyelinating diseases, and atherosclerosis. Slow visual loss can be produced without dramatic symptoms. Optic atrophy may be a consequence of several neurologic diseases and may be surprisingly asymptomatic. Ophthalmologic consultation should be obtained if visual disturbances are suspected by visual examination or field testing. The decision to perform aesthetic blepharoplasty in the presence of a single eye with good vision should be considered very carefully and discussed explicitly with the patient preoperatively.

In a survey of 16,000 surgeons, DeMere (104) noted that fewer than 15% of patients undergoing blepharoplasty performed by a nonophthalmologist had sufficient preoperative visual screening examinations. One of the best defenses against postoperative complaints is the well-documented preoperative history and physical examination.

Acute Visual Disturbances

Acute visual disturbances resulting in diminished or absent vision have been postulated to be caused by (i) idiopathic events occurring spontaneously; (ii) optic neuritis or atrophy, such as that accompanying central nervous system demyelinating disease, multiple sclerosis, and toxic ambiopia; (iii) thrombosis of the central retinal artery or veins (spontaneous vascular occlusive disease associated with hypertension); (iv) retrobulbar hematoma; and (v) indirect optic nerve injury (104).

Glaucoma

Acute glaucoma may be precipitated by surgery (116). Glaucoma can be diagnosed by a careful preoperative history and measurement of the intraocular pressure. Patients with glaucoma have a history of pain around the eye, headaches, nausea, vomiting, ocular irritation, and conjunctival injection. They may or may not have visual loss, visual field defect, blurring, or rainbow rings. Guyton and Ledford (116) reported a case of angle closure glaucoma following combined blepharoplasty and ectropion repair. Pupil dilatation (from whatever source) may precipitate an angle closure attack in any patient with a shallow anterior chamber or other predisposing factors. Angle closure glaucoma may be a postoperative complication of numerous ophthalmic procedures, such as panretinal photocoagulation, cataract extraction, keratoplasty, and scleral buckling. Patients may be examined with a slit lamp to determine the likelihood of an angle closure before undergoing surgical procedures where pupillary dilatation is a possible side effect. Angle closure glaucoma should be included in the differential diagnosis of acute pain following eyelid or orbital surgery. In this regard, treatable angle closure may mimic retrobulbar hemorrhage and thus be missed.

Double Vision

Visual disturbances, consisting of diplopia or double vision, usually are caused by surgical injury to the inferior oblique or superior oblique muscles (Fig. 50-29) (99,117,118) during fat resection (Fig. 50-28) (119,120). In the lower lid, the muscle is in the field of the lower lid blepharoplasty, whether done transcutaneously or through a conjunctival approach. It is important to carefully tease the fat away from other structures and to visualize and protect muscular structures during fat resection and cauterization.

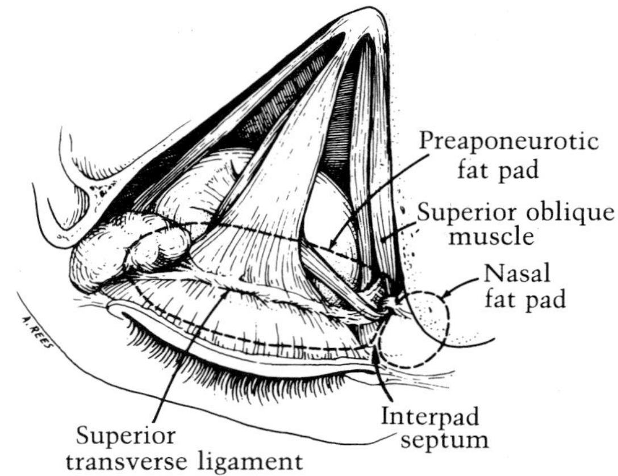

FIGURE 50-29. Extraocular muscles and their relationship to fat resection. The superior oblique muscle can be injured in upper lid blepharoplasty. The superior oblique muscle and its adjacent structure are shown.

Visual Loss from Central Retinal Artery Occlusion

Blindness following blepharoplasty in most cases is associated with retrobulbar hematoma. Several individuals documented the association of blindness with central retinal artery occlusion (105). The mechanism of occlusion is believed to begin with vasoconstriction; some individuals recommend avoiding the injection of vasoconstrictors deep within the orbit. However, in most cases of blindness, central retinal artery occlusion has not been reported. Most authors believe that increased intraorbital pressure is a major factor, whether it is a result of orbital hemorrhage or edema or of operative manipulation. Hepler et al. (121) believed that sudden or complete loss of vision following blepharoplasty was caused by orbital hemorrhage, acute angle closure glaucoma, or optic nerve ischemia, possibly due to orbital manipulation or reduced perfusion pressure of secondary systemic hypotension from operative medications. In all of the reported cases of visual loss following blepharoplasty, fat resection was performed. Additional causes for orbital hemorrhage include eyelid neovascularization secondary to retinal detachment repairs, rebound vasodilatation from epinephrine-constricted vessels escaping cautery during surgery, excessive traction on orbital fat during excision, inadequate hemostasis of excised fat, bleeding diatheses, and arteriosclerosis. The usual mechanism of visual loss is increased intraorbital pressure, which may produce a central retinal artery or vein occlusion, but more commonly causes direct reduction of perfusion pressure for the optic nerve with subsequent occlusion of its vascular supply (Fig. 50-30). Total vascular insufficiency for 60 or 120 minutes produces permanent visual loss.

Systemic antibiotics should be started after opening of the surgical wounds and evacuation of hematoma. The wound should be closed only after drainage has ceased. During the acute treatment phase, the patient should be monitored carefully in terms of visual acuity, pupillary response, funduscopy, and confrontation visual fields to assess the response to therapy.

Blindness is a realistic but rare complication of blepharoplasty. Rest, general sedation, and control of elevated blood pressure are indicated. Some avoid the use of epinephrine because the blood vessels to the retina and optic nerve are end artery vessels. Those individuals believe it is wise not to use a vasoconstricting substance around these vessels as it would in other sites supplied by endarteries, such as the fingers. Most surgeons, however, use vasoconstriction in the anterior orbit. Others relate the possibility of bleeding to the rebound congestion that occurs following the vasoconstrictive effects.

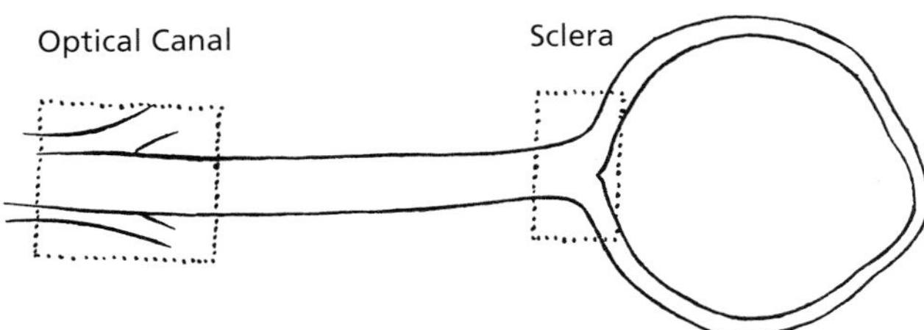

FIGURE 50-30. Areas of vulnerability in the circulation to the optic nerve.

SPECIFIC PROBLEMS IN BLEPHAROPLASTY

Medical Conditions

Medical conditions, such as thyroid (Fig. 50-31) or renal disease, and allergic states, may masquerade as orbital aging changes (100,101,117,122). Appropriate medical evaluation and treatment should be confirmed in these patients before performing surgery. It is emphasized that many patients with orbital aging changes have been followed by internists without identification of the medical problem.

Lateral Canthal Rhytides and Crow's-Feet

Orbicularis division and suspension procedures have been advocated for treatment of lateral canthal rhytides (Fig. 50-32) (61). The youthful eye generally exhibits little scleral show, and the palpebral fissures slant slightly upward toward the lateral canthal area. Division of the orbicularis, accomplished through a temporal rhytidectomy approach, with elevation and suspension of the orbicularis oculi muscle may smooth the lateral periorbital area (61). Simple undermining, separating the skin from the orbicularis, improves canthal rhytides, as does performing the temporal portion of a cervicofacial rhytidectomy. Some surgeons advocate denervation in the lateral portion of the orbicularis, which also may inhibit recurrence of the deep rhytides in this area. Lagophthalmos is a possibility with excessive denervation. Complications resulting from this procedure include hematoma (61), a slight depression just lateral to the canthus (where the orbicularis was previously situated), exaggerated correction (oriental appearance), and facial nerve paralysis (frontal and zygomatic branches) producing lagophthalmus. Hematoma was the most common postoperative complication observed (121). An exuberant blood supply is encountered during dissection beneath the lateral orbicularis. Meticulous hemostasis and a carefully applied facelift dressing will minimize the occurrence of hematoma.

Xanthelasma

The removal of xanthelasma deposits (123,124) can be performed with blepharoplasty procedures if they occur in a

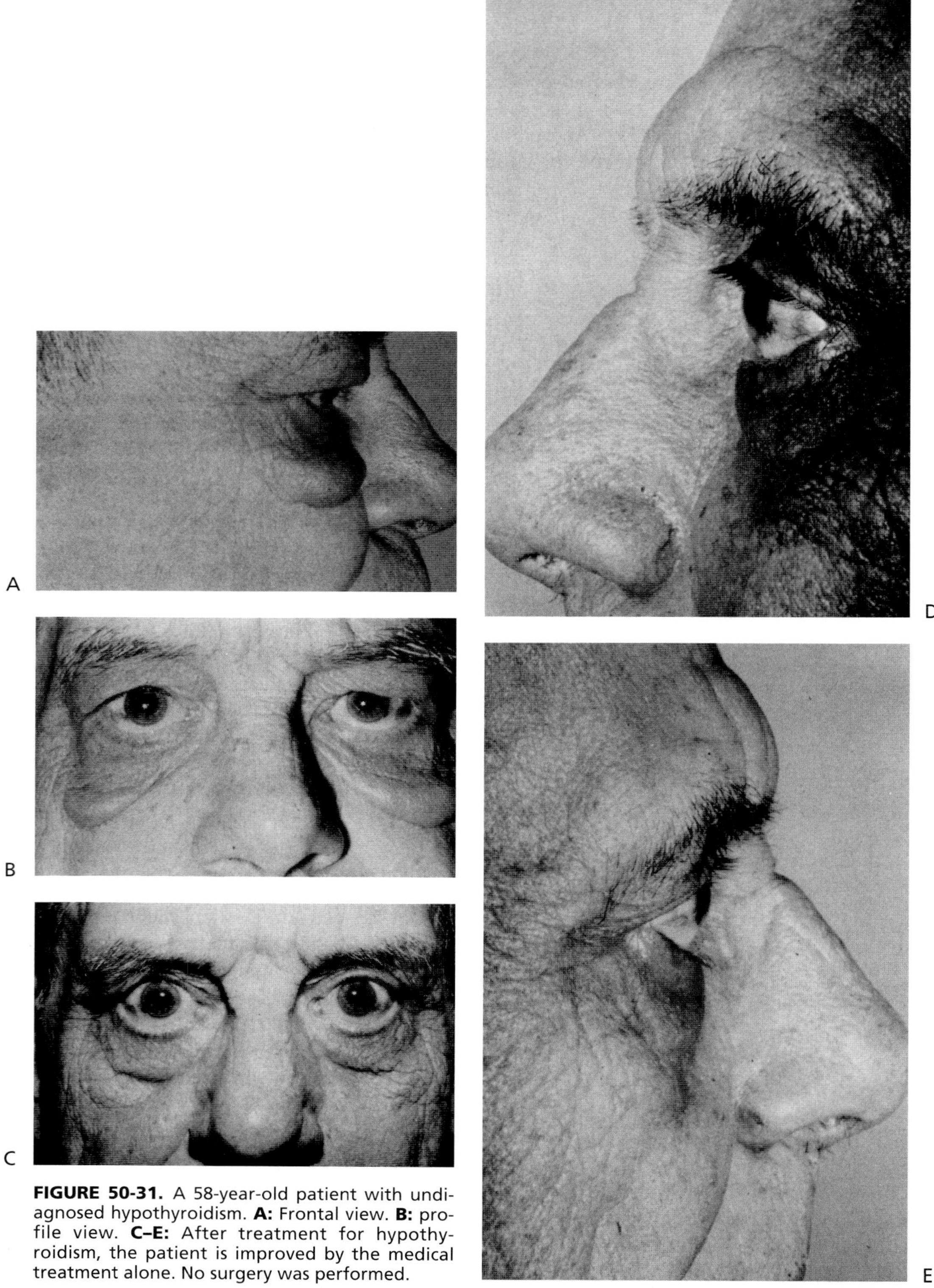

FIGURE 50-31. A 58-year-old patient with undiagnosed hypothyroidism. **A:** Frontal view. **B:** profile view. **C–E:** After treatment for hypothyroidism, the patient is improved by the medical treatment alone. No surgery was performed.

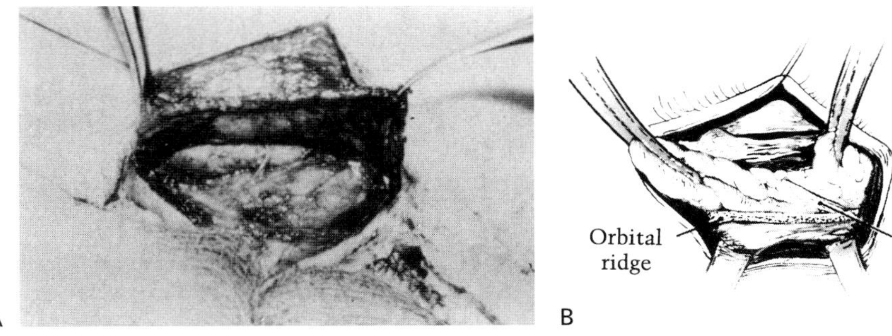

FIGURE 50-32. **A:** Separate skin and muscle flap dissection. **B:** Separate skin and muscle flaps. The location of the inferior oblique is seen.

pattern that is compatible with the incisions planned for blepharoplasty. Imaginative incisional variations sometimes must be used, and skin grafts may be necessary in some cases. The recurrence rate of xanthelasma is 40% and may increase to 80% if all four eyelids are involved. In patients with recurrent xanthelasma, the incidence of recurrence may approach 60% for a single eyelid. The presence of a lipid abnormality does not necessarily affect the incidence of xanthelasma or its occurrence.

Hypertrophic Orbicularis Oculi Muscle

Hypertrophic orbicularis muscle is best handled by resection of excess orbicularis and areas of muscle hypertrophy (21,23,56).

Festoons and Secondary Bags

Festoons were characterized by Furnas (24) as upper lid, brow, lower lid, pretarsal, orbital, preseptal, and jugal (Fig.

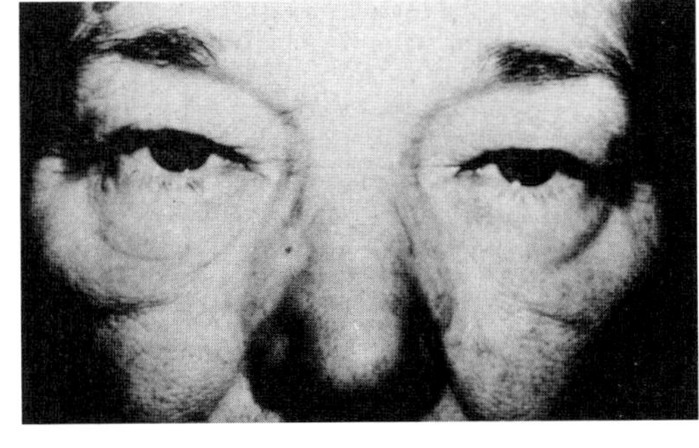

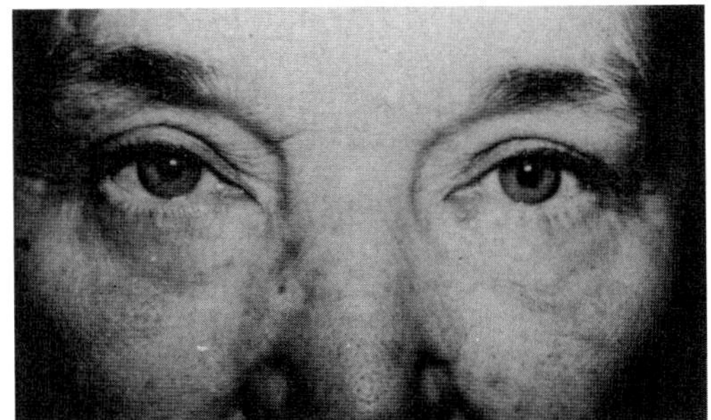

FIGURE 50-33. A 62-year-old patient with dermachalasis, fat herniation, and secondary bags. **A:** Preoperative. **B:** Postoperative blepharoplasty with separate skin and muscle flaps.

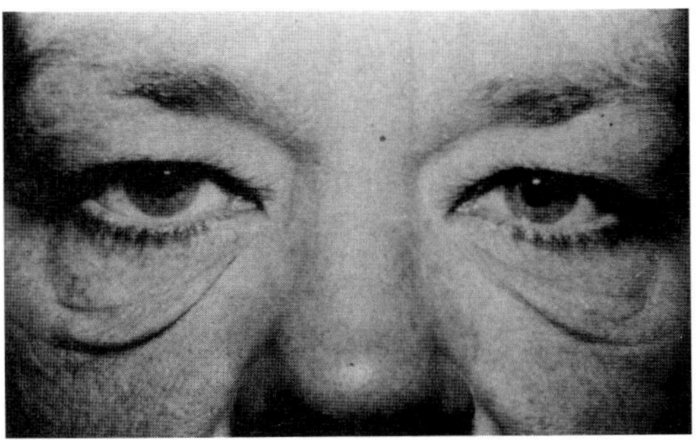

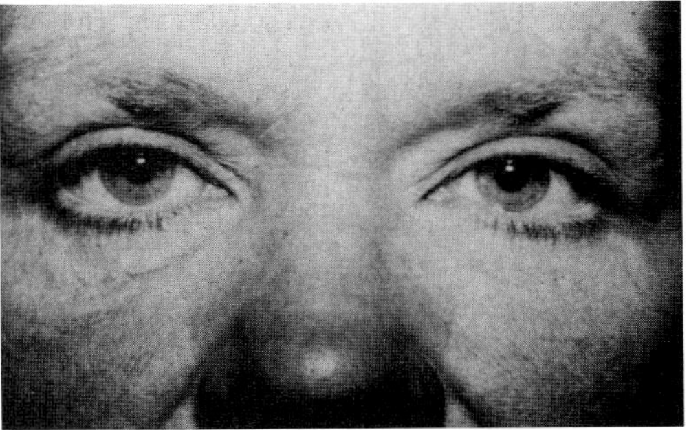

FIGURE 50-34. A 55-year-old patient with upper lid blepharochalasis and lower lid festoons. **A:** Preoperative. **B:** Postoperative upper and lower blepharoplasty with separate skin and muscle flaps.

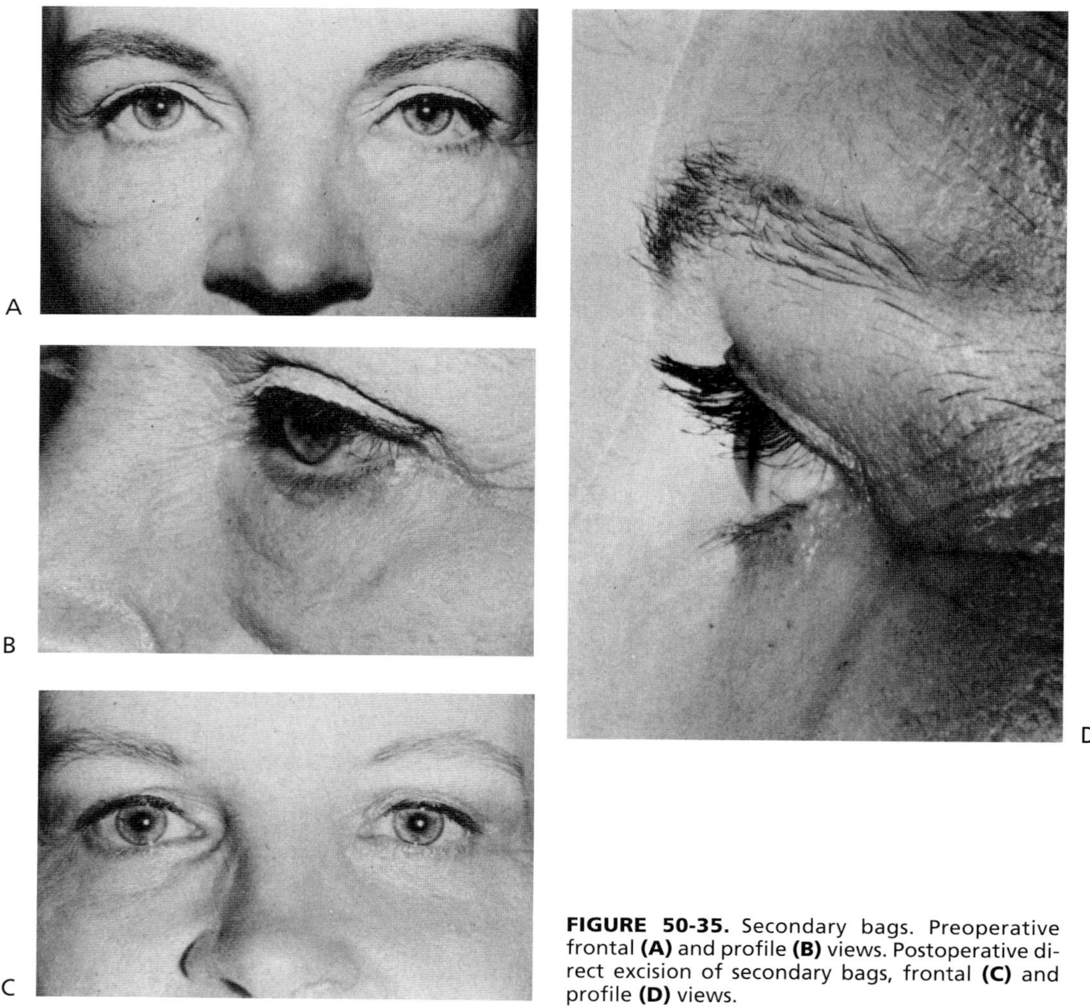

FIGURE 50-35. Secondary bags. Preoperative frontal **(A)** and profile **(B)** views. Postoperative direct excision of secondary bags, frontal **(C)** and profile **(D)** views.

50-33). They may contain only muscle, or muscle and fat (Fig. 50-31). Festoons are further characterized preoperatively by the squinch test or pinch test (24). Festoons are best managed by wide skin undermining, separate skin and muscle flap combinations (23), fat resection, and temporal and cervicofacial rhytidectomy (Figs. 50-32–50-35). Some surgeons believe they are best managed by direct excision if one can accept the cutaneous scar. The challenge is to create adequate tension without producing an eyelid eversion or ectropion. Therefore, subtotal correction is the usual result of more conservative procedures. Care must be taken to improve or correct canthal weakness and accompanying lid elasticity.

Atonic Lower Lids

Atonic lower lids, lowered eyelid elasticity, and reduced skin tone are observed more commonly in patients older than 35 years. These phenomena appear to be more common in men (Fig. 50-36). Abnormal lid laxity can be confirmed by two diagnostic maneuvers: (i) the lid is able to be distracted more than 8 mm from the globe; and (ii) the lid is abnormally slow to return to its usual resting position after inferior distraction (lid snap-back test). Sometimes the lid stands away from the globe until the next blink. Patients with abnormal lid laxity need a lid-tightening procedure concomitant with their blepharoplasty. Lid tightening may be accompanied by canthoplasty, resection of the lateral portion of the lid, or tightening of the pretarsal orbicularis muscle (13,14). "Blepharocanthoplasties" (125) and "dermal canthal suspension" have been suggested (92), as have canthopexies (11).

Supratarsal Fixation

The complications of supratarsal fixation (Fig. 50-37) (20,21,117,126–128) include ptosis that may last 4 to 6

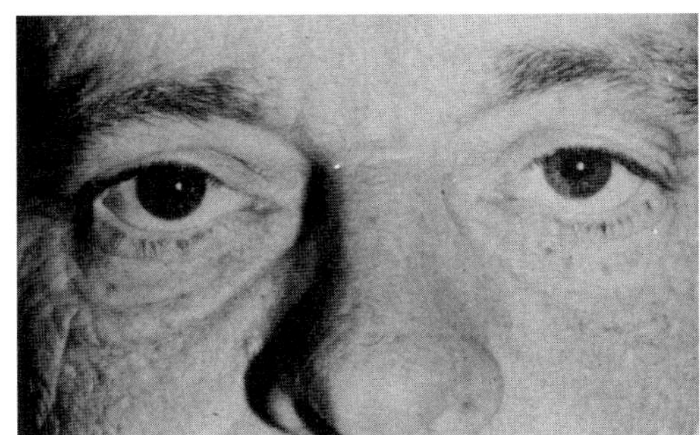

A

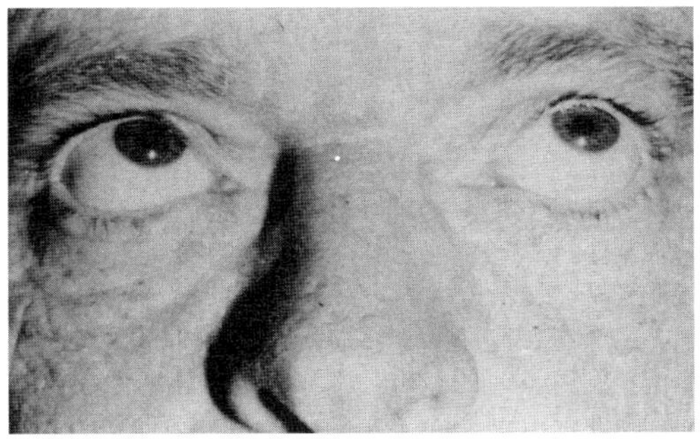

B

FIGURE 50-36. A: A 54-year-old man with lax lower lids, poor tissue turgor, and increased scleral show. **B:** Lax lower lids, looking up, with increased scleral show.

weeks, temporary edema that may last months, and uneven fixation. Many surgeons believe that a well-defined lid crease may be obtained by dermotarsal adhesion following block resection of a strip of orbicularis muscle and skin to expose the tarsal plate (42,80,129). Other surgeons prefer supratarsal fixation to achieve a more predictable result.

Infratarsal Fixation

Infratarsal fixation was described by Sheen (130) and Rees (131), using a technique to recreate the infratarsal crease. Other authors have not described it. Care must be taken in lower lid crease reconstruction to avoid ectropion.

Thyrotoxicosis

Exophthalmos often precedes other symptoms of thyrotoxicosis; therefore, thyroid function screening should be performed in any patient with periorbital edema or prominent eyes (Fig. 50-38). Standard blepharoplasty techniques accentuate the prominent eye deformity by removing the skin and fat that partially mask global prominence. Scleral show, ectropion, and dry eye are likely to be more frequent in patients with exophthalmos who have undergone blepharoplasty procedures. Lateral canthorrhaphy, selective levator myotomy, scleral grafting, and resection of the Müller muscle have been advocated to reduce the deformity of thyrotoxicosis (117,122, 132–139).

Lengthening and Shortening of the Palpebral Fissure

Although various methods for lengthening and shortening the palpebral fissure have been described, their use may cause substantial scarring and deformity; therefore, these techniques should be approached with caution.

CONCLUSIONS

Blepharoplasty is a deceptively simple procedure fraught with subjective and objective complications. Complications

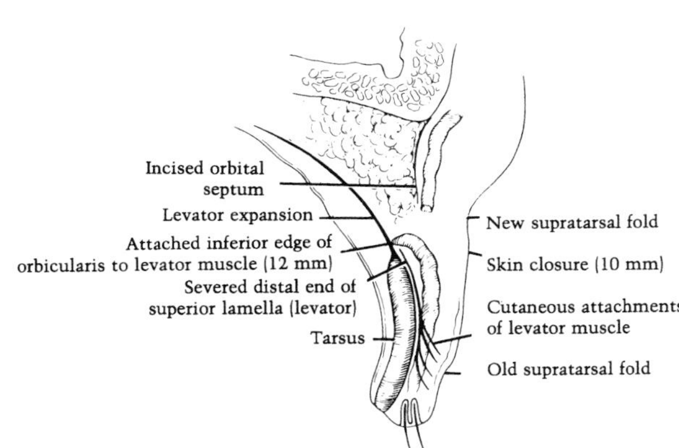

FIGURE 50-37. Supratarsal fixation.

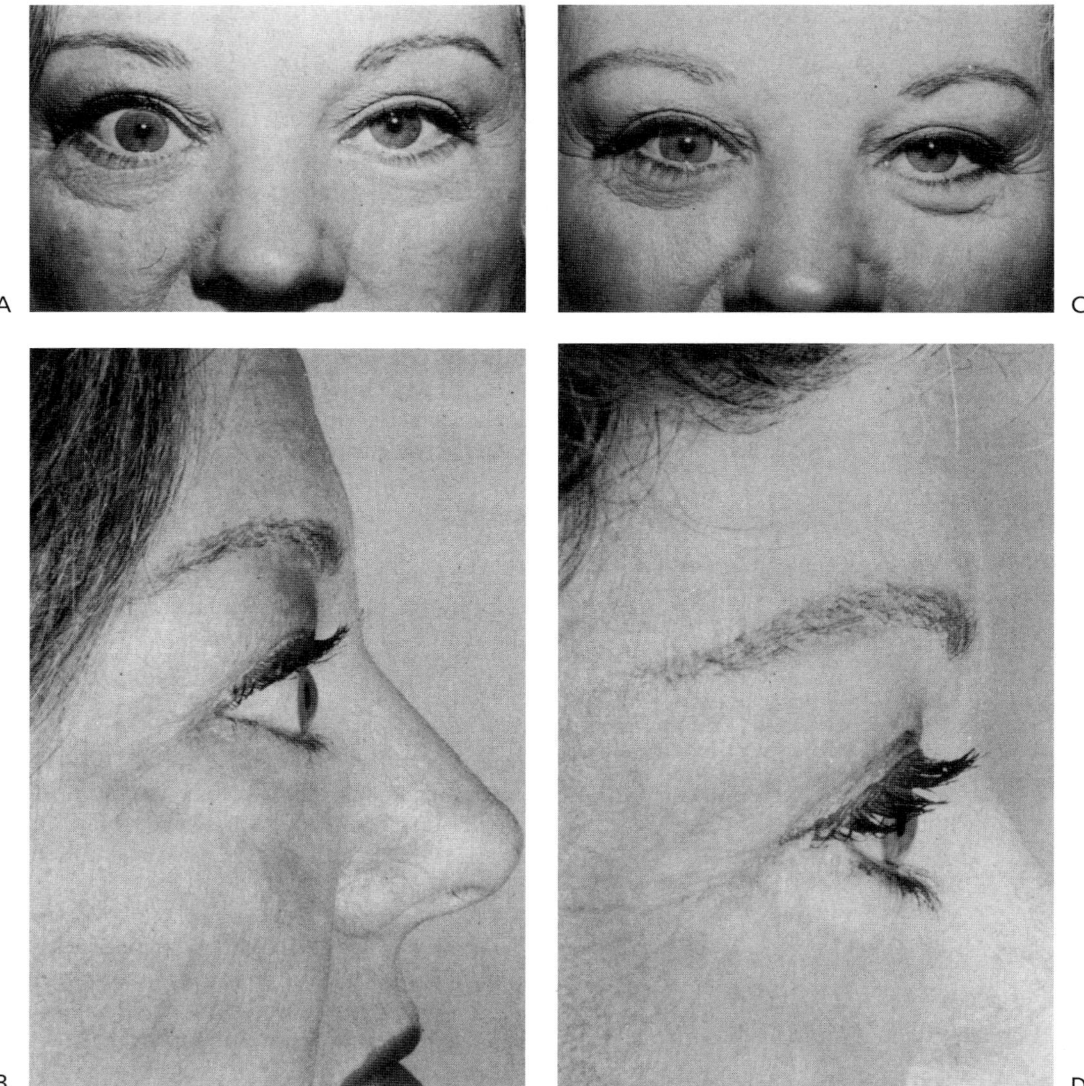

FIGURE 50-38. A 54-year-old patient with treated hypothyroidism and unilateral exophthalmos right eye. Preoperative frontal **(A)** and profile **(B)** views. Postoperative correction with lateral canthoplasty, frontal **(C)** and profile **(D)** views.

can be minimized by a thorough knowledge of anatomy, the literature, an eye for beauty, and an uncompromising insistence on perfection.

REFERENCES

1. Hiraga Y. The double eyelid operation and augmentation rhinoplasty in the oriental patient. *Clin Plast Surg* 1980; 7:533.
2. Castanares S. Classification of baggy eyelid deformity. *Plast Reconstr Surg* 1977;59:629.
3. Berry EP, Berenson M. Evaluating patient satisfaction with the face lift, eyelid operation, or both. *Aesthetic Plast Surg* 1971; 1:131.
4. Berry EP. Planning and evaluating blepharoplasty. *Plast Reconstr Surg* 1974;54:257.
5. Trelles MA, Baker SS, Ting J, et al. Carbon dioxide laser transconjunctival lower lid blepharoplasty complications. *Ann Plast Surg* 1996;37:465–468.
6. Popp JC. Complications of blepharoplasty and their management. *J Dermatol Surg Oncol* 1992;18:1122–1126.
7. Seiff SR. Complications of upper and lower blepharoplasty. *Int Ophthalmol Clin* 1992;32:67–77.
8. Lisman RD, Hyde K, Smith B. Complications of blepharoplasty. *Clin Plast Surg* 1988;15:309–335.
9. Palmer FR, Rice DH, Churukian MM. Transconjunctival blepharoplasty. Complications and their avoidance: a retrospective analysis and review of the literature. *Arch Otolaryngol Head Neck Surg* 1993;119:993–999.

10. Lowry JC, Bartley GB. Complications of blepharoplasty. *Surv Ophthalmol* 1994;38:327–350.
11. Giat PM, Jelks GW, Jelks EB. Evolution of the inferior retinacular techniques and indications. *Plast Reconstr Surg* 1997; 100:1396–1405.
12. May JW, Zenn MR, Zingarelli P. Subciliary malar augmentation and cheek advancement: a 6-year study in 22 patients undergoing blepharoplasty. *Plast Reconstr Surg* 1995;96: 1553–1559.
13. Byrd HB, Salomon A. Endoscopic midface rejuvenation. *Op Tech Plast Reconstr Surg* 5:138–145, 1998.
14. Hamra S. Periorbital rejuvenation in composite rhytidectomy. *Op Tech Plast Reconstr Surg* 1998;5:155–163.
15. Dingham RD, Peled I, Izenberg D. Forehead and brow lifts and their relationship to blepharoplasty. *Ann Plast Surg* 1979;2:32.
16. Ramirez OM. Endoscopic assisted biplanar forehead lift. *Plast Reconstr Surg* 1995;9:323–333.
17. Beard C. Cosmetic blepharoplasty: anatomic considerations. *Trans Am Acad Ophthalmol Otolaryngol* 1969;73:1141.
18. Beard C, Quickert MH. *Anatomy of the orbit,* 2nd ed. Birmingham: Aesculapius Publishing Company, 1977.
19. Kuwabara I, Cogan D, Johnson CC. Structure of the muscles of the upper eyelid. *Arch Ophthalmol* 1975;93:1189.
20. Sheen JH. Supratarsal fixation in upper blepharoplasty. In: Goulian D, Courtiss EH, eds. *Symposium of surgery of the aging face.* St. Louis: Mosby, 1978:129.
21. Rees TD. *Aesthetic plastic surgery.* Philadelphia: WB Saunders, 1981:470–524.
22. Wood RW Jr. Blepharoplasty—surgical versus chemical. *Aesthetic Plast Surg* 1980;4:295.
23. Klatsky SA, Manson PN. Separate skin and muscle flaps in lower lid blepharoplasty. *Plast Reconstr Surg* 1981;67:151.
24. Furnas DW. Festoons of orbicularis muscle as a cause of baggy eyelids. *Plast Reconstr Surg* 1978;61:531.
25. Loeb R. The necessity for partial resection of the orbicularis oculi muscle in blepharoplasties in some young patients. *Plast Reconstr Surg* 1977;60:178.
26. Owsley JQ Jr. Resection of prominent lateral fat pad during upper lid blepharoplasty. *Plast Reconstr Surg* 1980;65:4.
27. May JW, Fearon J, Zingarelli P. Retro orbicularis oculus fat (ROOF) resection in aesthetic blepharoplasty: a six year study in 63 patients. *Plast Reconstr Surg* 1990;86:682.
28. Aaiche AE, Ramirez O. The sub orbicularis oculi fat pad: an anatomical and clinical study. *Plast Reconstr Surg* 1995; 95:37–42.
29. Putterman AM, Urist MJ. Baggy eyelids–a true hernia. *Ann Ophthalmol* 1973;5:1029.
30. Loeb R. Fat pad sliding and fat grafting for leveling lid depressions. *Clin Plast Surg* 1981;8:757.
31. Loeb R. Scleral show. *Aesthetic Plast Surg* 1988;12:165–170.
32. Loeb R. Improvements in blepharoplasty: creating a fat surface for the lower lid. In: *Transactions of the Seventh International Congress of Plastic and Reconstructive Surgery.* Rio de Janiero: Cartgraft, 1979:390–393.
33. Castanares S. Prolapse of the lacrimal gland: findings and management during blepharoplasty. *Aesthetic Plast Surg* 1979;3:111.
34. Marchac D. Relationship of the orbit to the upper eyelids. *Clin Plast Surg* 1981;8:717.
35. Bernstein NR. Emotional reactions in patients after elective cosmetic surgery. In: Goldwyn RM, ed. *Long-term results in plastic and reconstructive surgery.* Boston: Little, Brown and Company, 1980:6–17.
36. Goldwyn RM. *The patient and the plastic surgeon.* Boston: Little, Brown and Company, 1981.
37. Goldwyn RM. The dissatisfied patient. In: Goulian D, Courtiss EH, eds. *Symposium on surgery of the aging face.* St. Louis: Mosby, 1978:81.
38. Zide B. Four patients you love to hate. *Plast Reconstr Surg* 1998;102:1729–1732.
39. MacGregor FC. Patient dissatisfaction with the results of technically satisfactory surgery. *Aesthetic Plast Surg* 1981;5:27.
40. Goin JM, Goin MK. Face lift. In: *Changing the body: psychological effects of plastic surgery.* Baltimore: Williams & Wilkins, 1981.
41. Edgerton MT, Langman M. Psychiatric considerations. In: Courtiss EH, ed. *Male aesthetic surgery.* St. Louis: Mosby, 1982:17.
42. Baker TJ, Gordon HL, Mosienko P. Upper lid blepharoplasty. *Plast Reconstr Surg* 1977;60:692.
43. Beare R. Surgical treatment of senile changes in the eyelids. The McIndoe Beare technique. In: Smith HJ, Converse JM, eds. *Proceedings of the Second International Symposium on Plastic and Reconstructive Surgery of the Eye and Adnexa.* St. Louis: Mosby, 1967.
44. Boo-Chai K. Plastic construction of the superior palpebral fold. *Plast Reconstr Surg* 1964;31:556.
45. Callahan A. *Surgery of the eye: Diseases.* Springfield, IL: Charles C Thomas Publisher, 1956.
46. Castanares S. Correction of the baggy eyelids deformity produced by herniation of the orbital fat. In: Smith J, Converse JM, eds. *Proceedings of the Second International Symposium of Plastic and Reconstructive Surgery of the Eye and Adnexa.* St. Louis: Mosby, 1967:346–353.
47. Colloquium on blepharoplasty. *Ann Plast Surg* 1978;1:66.
48. Converse JM. The Converse technique of the corrective eyelid plastic operation. In: Converse JM, ed. *Reconstructive plastic surgery.* Philadelphia: WB Saunders, 1964:1333–1336.
49. Courtiss EH. Selection of alternatives in cosmetic blepharoplasty. *Clin Plast Surg* 1981;8:739.
50. Guy CL, Converse JM, Morello DC. Esthetic surgery for the aging face. In: Converse JM, ed. *Reconstructive plastic surgery,* 2nd ed. Philadelphia: WB Saunders, 1977:1868–1929.
51. Guy CL, Everett DN. Upper and lower blepharoplasty: standard technique. *Clin Plast Surg* 1981;8:663.
52. Courtiss EH, Webster RC, White MF. Use of double W-plasty in upper blepharoplasty. *Plast Reconstr Surg* 1974;53:25.
53. Hamra ST. Arcus marginalis release and orbital fat preservation in midface rejuvenation *Plast Reconstr Surg* 1995;96:354–362.
54. Smith B. Herniated lacrimal glands and the technique of suspension. In: Proceedings of the Third International Symposium on Orbital Disorders, Amsterdam, 1977.
55. Loeb R. Aesthetic blepharoplasties based on the degree of wrinkling. *Plast Reconstr Surg* 1971;47:33.
56. Rees TD, Tabbal N. Lower lid blepharoplasty. *Clin Plast Surg* 1981;8:643.
57. Spira M. Lower blepharoplasty—a clinical study. *Plast Reconstr Surg* 1977;59:35.
58. Gilbert SE. Transconjunctival blepharoplasty with chemexfoliation. *Ann Plast Surg* 1996;37:24–29.
59. Hugo NE, Stone E. Anatomy for blepharoplasty. *Plast Reconstr Surg* 1974;53:381.
60. Tomlinson FB, Hovey LM. Transconjunctival lower lid blepharoplasty for removal of fat. *Plast Reconstr Surg* 1975;56:314.
61. Su CT, Morgan RF, Mason PN, et al. Technique of division and suspension of the orbicularis oculi muscle. *Clin Plast Surg* 1981;8:673.
62. Rees TD. Complications following blepharoplasty. In: *Symposium on Plastic Surgery in the Orbital Region.* St. Louis: Mosby, 1976:455–459.

63. Baylis HI, Goldberg RA, Kerivan KM, et al. Blepharoplasty and periorbital surgery. *Dermatol Clin* 1997;15:635–647.
64. Lyon DB, Raphtis CS. Management of complications of blepharoplasty. *Int Ophthalmol Clin* 1997;37:205–216.
65. Kikkawa DO, Kim JW. Lower-eyelid blepharoplasty. *Int Ophthalmol Clin* 1997;37:163–178.
66. Millman AL, Williams JD, Romo T, et al. Septal-myocutaneous flap technique for lower lid blepharoplasty. *Ophthalmic Plast Reconstr Surg* 1997;13:84.
67. Alt TH. Blepharoplasty. *Dermatol Clin* 1995;13:389–430.
68. Murakami CS, Plant RL. Complications of blepharoplasty surgery. *Facial Plast Surg* 1994;10:214–224.
69. Castanares S. Eyelid plasty. In: Goldwyn RM, ed. *The unfavorable result in plastic surgery: avoidance and treatment.* Boston: Little, Brown and Company, 1972.
70. Hartman E, Morax PV, Vergez A. Complications visuelles graves de la chirurgie des poches palpebrales. *Ann Ocul* 1962;195:142.
71. Rees TD. Blepharoplasty. In: Courtiss EH, ed. *Aesthetic surgery. Trouble-how to avoid it and how to treat it.* St. Louis: Mosby, 1978.
72. Rees TD. Blepharoplasty: postoperative considerations and complications. In: *Aesthetic plastic surgery.* Philadelphia: WB Saunders, 1980.
73. Rees TD, Dupuis C. Cosmetic blepharoplasty in the older age group. *Ophthalmol Surg* 1970;1:30.
74. Smith B. Postsurgical complications of cosmetic blepharoplasty. *Trans Am Acad Ophthalmol* 1969;73:1162.
75. Stasior OG. Complications of ophthalmic plastic and reconstructive surgery. *Trans Am Acad Ophthalmol Otolaryngol* 1976;81:550.
76. Iliff CE, Iliff WJ, Iliff NT. *Oculoplastic surgery.* Philadelphia: WB Saunders, 1979:20.
77. Holly FJ, Lemp MA. The preocular tear film and dry eye syndrome. *Int Ophthalmol Clin* 1973;13:1.
78. Jelks GW, McCord CD Jr. Dry eye syndrome and other tear film abnormalities. *Clin Plast Surg* 1981;8:803.
79. Rees TD. The dry eye complication after blepharoplasty. *Plast Reconstr Surg* 1975;56:375.
80. Rees TD. Blepharoplasty and the dry eye syndrome: guidelines for surgery. *Plast Reconstr Surg* 1981;68:249.
81. McKinney P, Zukowski ML. The value of tear film breakup and Schirmer's tests in preoperative blepharoplasty evaluation. *Plast Reconstr Surg* 1989;84:572–576; discussion 577.
82. Smith B, Petrelli R. Herniation of the lacrimal glands. *Trans Am Acad Ophthalmol Otolaryngol* 1977;84:988.
83. McCord CD Jr, Ellis DS. The correction of lower lid malposition following lower lid blepharoplasty. *Plast Reconstr Surg* 1993;92:1068–1072.
84. Carraway JH, Mellow CG. The prevention and treatment of lower lid ectropion following blepharoplasty [see Comments]. *Plast Reconstr Surg* 1990;85:971–981.
85. Tenzel RR. Complications of blepharoplasty. Orbital hematoma, ectropion, and scleral show. *Clin Plast Surg* 1981;8:797–802.
86. Patel BC, Patipa M, Anderson RL, et al. Management of post-blepharoplasty lower eyelid retraction with hard palate grafts and lateral tarsal strip. *Plast Reconstr Surg* 1997;99:1251–1260.
87. Edgerton MT. Causes and prevention of lower lid ectropion following blepharoplasty. *Plast Reconstr Surg* 1972;49:367.
88. Rees TD. Correction of ectropion resulting from blepharoplasty. *Plast Reconstr Surg* 1972;50:1.
89. Gonzales-Ulloa M, Stevens EF. Senile eyelid esthetic correction. In: Smith J, Converse JM, eds. *Proceedings of the Second International Symposium on Plastic and Reconstructive Surgery of the Eye and Adnexa.* St. Louis: Mosby, 1967:354–361.
90. Friedman WH. Ectropion after blepharoplasty. *Arch Otolaryngol* 1979;105:455.
91. Adamson JE, McCraw JB, Carraway JH. Use of a muscle flap in a lower blepharoplasty. *Plast Reconstr Surg* 1979;63:359.
92. Edgerton MT, Wolfort FG. The dermal flap canthal lift for lower eyelid support. *Plast Reconstr Surg* 1969;43:42.
93. Soll DB. *Management of complications in ophthalmic plastic surgery.* Birmingham: Aesculapius Publishing Company, 1976.
94. Rees TD. Technical considerations in blepharoplasty. In: *Transactions of the Fourth International Congress of Plastic and Reconstructive Surgery.* Amsterdam: Excerpta Medica Foundation, 1969:1084.
95. Wolfort FG, Poblete JV. Ptosis after blepharoplasty. *Ann Plast Surg* 1995;43:264–266; discussion 266–267.
96. Zide B. Anatomy of the eyelids. *Plast Surg* 1981;8:623.
97. Mustarde JC. Problems and possibilities in ptosis surgery. *Plast Reconstr Surg* 1975;56:381.
98. Baylis HI, Sutcliffe T, Fett DR. Levator injury during blepharoplasty. *Arch Ophthalmol* 1984 Apr;102(4):570–1570,
99. Morgan SC. Orbital cellulitis and blindness following a blepharoplasty. *Plast Reconstr Surg* 1979;64:823.
100. Klatsky SA, Manson PN. Numbness after blepharoplasty. *Plast Reconstr Surg* 1981;67:20.
101. Klatsky J, Manson PN. Thyroid disorders masquerading as aging changes. *Ann Plast Surg* 1992;28:420–426.
102. Soll DB. Correction of superior lid sulcus with subperiosteal implants. *Arch Ophthalmol* 1971;85:188.
103. Goldman B, Friedhofer H, Anger M, et al. Surgical indications for sunken eyelids. *Aesthetic Plast Surg* 1981;5:123.
104. DeMere M. Blindness and eyelid surgery. *Aesthetic Plast Surg* 1978;2:41.
105. Hartley JH, Lester JC, Schatten WE. Acute retrobulbar hemorrhage during elective blepharoplasty. *Plast Reconstr Surg* 1973;52:8; discussion 12.
106. Hayreh SS, Kolder HE, Weingeist TA. Central retinal artery occlusion and retinal tolerance time. *Ophthalmology* 1980;87:75.
107. Goldberg RA, Marmor MF, Shorr N, et al. Blindness following blepharoplasty: two case reports, and a discussion of management. *Ophthalmic Surg* 1990;21:85–89.
108. Callahan MA. Prevention of blindness after blepharoplasty. *Ophthalmology* 1983;90:1047–1051.
109. Waller RR. Is blindness a realistic complication in blepharoplasty procedure? *Ophthalmology* 1978;85:730–735.
110. Huang TT, Horowitz B, Lewis ST. Retrobulbar hemorrhage. *Plast Reconstr Surg* 1977;59:39.
111. Moser MH, DiPirro E, McCoy FJ. Sudden blindness following blepharoplasty. *Plast Reconstr Surg* 1973;51:364.
112. Stasior OG. Blindness associated with cosmetic blepharoplasty. *Clin Plast Surg* 1981;8:793.
113. Rees TD. Prevention of post-blepharoplasty complications. In: Goulian D, Courtiss EH, eds. *Symposium on surgery of the aging face.* St. Louis: Mosby, 1978.
114. Becker W, Talley AR, Logan SE, et al. Effect of anterior chamber paracentesis on decreased retinal circulation due to retrobulbar hematoma in dogs. *Plast Reconstr Surg* 1989;83:421–428.
115. Hayreh SS, Weingeist TA. Experimental occlusion of the central retinal artery of the retina: I. Ophthalmologic and fluorescein fundus angiographic findings. *Br J Ophthalmol* 1980; 64:896.
116. Guyton JL, Ledford JK. Angle closure glaucoma following a combined blepharoplasty and ectropion repair. *Ophthalmic Plast Reconstr Surg* 1992;8:176.
117. Tenzel R. Upper lid complications of blepharoplasty. In: Aston A, Hornblass A, Meltzer M, et al. *Third International Eye Plastic Symposium.* Baltimore: Williams & Wilkins, 1982.

118. Wesley RE, Pollard ZF, McCord CD Jr. Superior oblique paresis after blepharoplasty. *Plast Reconstr Surg* 1980;66:283.
119. Mariey RD, Nelson LB, Flanagan JC, et al. Ocular motility disturbances following cosmetic blepharoplasty. *Arch Ophthalmol* 1986;104:542–549.
120. Hayworth RS, Lisman RD, Muchnick RS, et al. Diplopia following blepharoplasty. *Ann Ophthalmol* 1984.
121. Hepler RS, Sugimura GI, Straatsma BR. On the occurrence of blindness in association with blepharoplasty. *Plast Reconstr Surg* 1976;57:233–235.
122. Smith, F. Multiple excision and Z-plasties in surface reconstruction. *Plast Reconstr Surg* 1946;1:170.
123. Anderson RL, Edwards JJ. Bilateral visual loss after blepharoplasty. *Ann Plast Surg* 1980;5:288.
124. Francois J. *Heredity in ophthalmology.* St. Louis: Mosby, 1961:272–275.
125. Hinderer VT. Blepharocanthoplasty and eyebrow lift. *Plast Reconstr Surg* 1975;56:402.
126. Flowers RS. Anchor blepharoplasty. In: *Transactions of the International Congress of Plastic Surgeons.* Paris: Masson et Cie, 1976:471–472.
127. Flowers RS. Anchor blepharoplasty. Presented at the Third International Symposium of the Eye and Adnexa, New York, 1980; also personal communication.
128. Putterman AM, Urist MJ. Reconstruction of the upper eyelid crease and fold. *Arch Ophthalmol* 1976;94:1941.
129. Spira M. Supratarsal fixation versus orbicularis muscle excision: a comparative study. Presented at the Fourteenth Annual Meeting of the American Society for Aesthetic Plastic Surgeons, 1981.
130. Sheen JH. Tarsal fixation in lower blepharoplasty. *Plast Reconstr Surg* 1978;62:24.
131. Rees TD. The voice of polite dissent: tarsal fixation in lower blepharoplasty (J.H. Sheen). *Plast Reconstr Surg* 1978; 62:295.
132. Goldstein I. Recession of the levator muscle for lagophthalmos in exophthalmos goiter. *Arch Ophthalmol* 1934;1:389.
133. Wortsman J, Wavak P. Palpebral redundancy from hypothyroidism. *Plast Reconstr Surg* 1980;66:1.
134. Grove AS Jr. Upper eyelid retractions and Graves' disease. In: Symposium on Surgical Management of Thyroid Ophthalmopathy. Proceedings of the Annual Meeting of the American Academy of Ophthalmology, Chicago, Illinois, 1980.
135. Moran RE, Letterman GS, Shuster MA. The surgical correction of the exophthalmos. *Plast Reconstr Surg* 1972;49:595.
136. Putterman AM. Surgical treatment of dysthyroid eyelid retraction and orbital fat hernia. *Otolaryngol Clin North Am* 1980;13:39.
137. Smith B, Lisman RD. Cosmetic correction of eyelid deformities associated with exophthalmos. *Clin Plast Surg* 1981; 8:777.
138. Smith B, O'Bear M. Tarsal grafting to elevate the lower lid margin. *Am J Ophthalmol* 1965;59:1088.
139. Castanares S. Blepharoplasty in exophthalmos. *Plast Reconstr Surg* 1971;47:215.

Discussion

BLEPHAROPLASTY

MARK A. CODNER
CHARLES R. DAY

The authors are to be congratulated on a comprehensive and well-written chapter on avoiding an unfavorable result following blepharoplasty. The goal of blepharoplasty, as pointed out by the authors, is to enhance the appearance of the eyes by restoring a more youthful appearance of the eyelids and periorbital region. Improvement in appearance must be accomplished while simultaneously minimizing complications associated with blepharoplasty. Reducing the risk of complications begins with the preoperative assessment. A focus of our research has been the identification of high-risk patients through objective assessment of specific anatomical findings and disease processes that may involve the periorbital region. These findings have been used to define an algorithm for blepharoplasty, canthoplasty, and transpalpebral periorbital surgery (1). The focus of this discussion is to elaborate on the surgical decision-making process associated with high-risk orbital morphology, in order to minimize complications and patient dissatisfaction.

M. A. Codner and C. R. Day: PACES Plastic Surgery and Recovery Center, Atlanta, Georgia

HIGH-RISK PATIENTS

A summary of the distinct groups of patients who are associated with increased risk following blepharoplasty includes systemic disease processes that affect the orbit and periorbital region; local functional and anatomical disorders; and orbital morphology that is associated with postoperative lid malposition (2). Preoperative screening examination should include identification of patients with thyroid eye disease, dry eye syndrome, benign essential blepharospasm, and local immune disorders such as rosacea and pemphigoid. Because this group of patients has an increased risk following blepharoplasty, intervention should be limited to conservative procedures or avoidance of surgery all together.

In addition to this group of patients, specific orbital morphologic findings have been associated with increased risk of complications (3,4). Patients with brow and upper lid ptosis, eye prominence, lower lid laxity, and malar hypoplasia are at increased risk for unsatisfactory results following blepharoplasty. Preoperative assessment begins with an evaluation of the upper lid and brow. An unstable brow demonstrates significant mobility during superior and inferior displacement, with a resting position below the superior orbital rim. Lack of brow stability may result in an unsatisfactory upper eyelid crease following blepharoplasty. Brow descent will cause early recurrence of redundant upper lid skin with visible lateral hooding. In addition, unilateral brow ptosis may be the underlying cause of an asymmetrical upper lid fold and requires recognition and correction prior to blepharoplasty (Fig. 50D-1). Correction should be performed prior to upper blepharoplasty with techniques including open coronal approach, endoscopic-assisted browlift, or transpalpebral internal browpexy.

In addition to brow ptosis, recognition and management of upper lid ptosis should be emphasized before upper blepharoplasty. Acquired ptosis commonly is subclinical and may be recognized only after surgery by the appearance of a high lid crease and droopy eyelid (Fig. 50D-2). Furthermore, the upper blepharoplasty crease incision may actually contribute to dehiscence of the levator aponeurosis, resulting in worsening of the ptosis after blepharoplasty (Fig. 50D-3). Recognition and correction of ptosis with bilateral tarsolevator advancement should be performed to avoid these complications. In addition, supratarsal fixation of the lid crease to the levator aponeurosis should be performed in all cases to prevent post-blepharoplasty ptosis (5).

Upper lid laxity should be evaluated and may demonstrate patients with the "floppy upper lid syndrome"(6). This most commonly is associated with larger burly males and represents a small group of patients who may have functional lid closure complications after surgery. To avoid an overriding upper eyelid, horizontal upper lid tightening should be considered. Surgical options include lateral canthal tightening, canthal repositioning, and horizontal lid

A
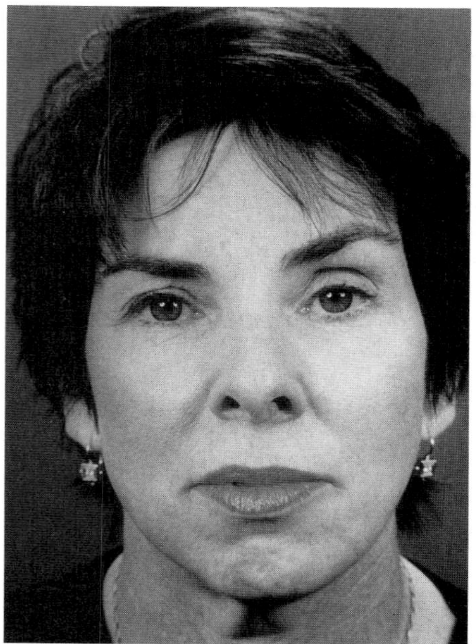
B
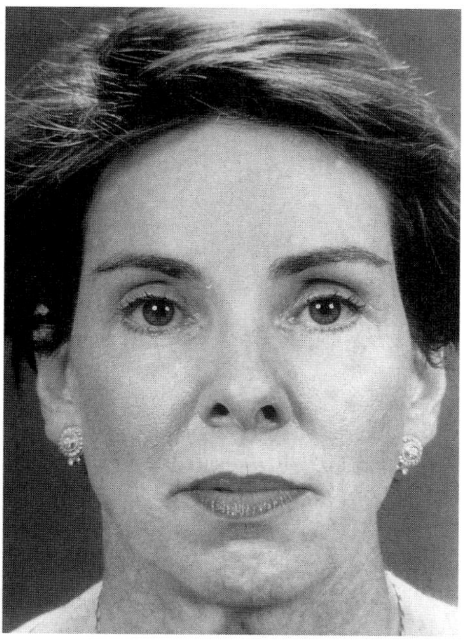

FIGURE 50D-1. A: Patient with significant right unilateral brow ptosis prior to surgery. **B:** Six months after endoscopic brow lift with right unilateral fixation, upper and lower blepharoplasty.

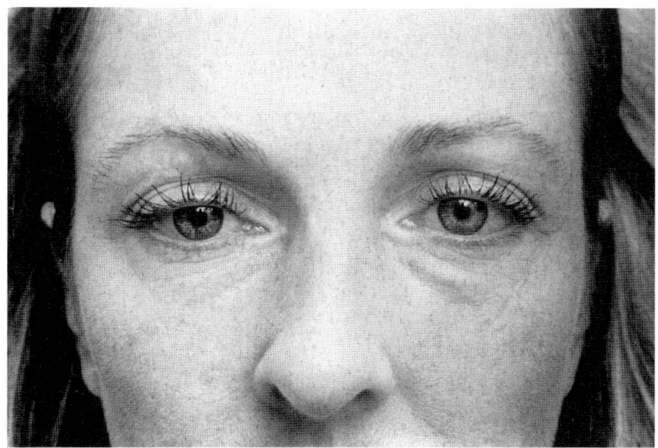

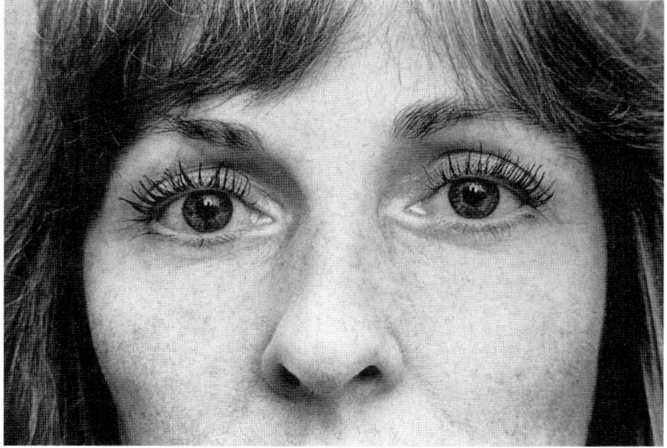

FIGURE 50D-2. A: Patient with acquired right unilateral upper eyelid ptosis. **B:** One year after upper and lower blepharoplasty with right tarsolevator advancement.

shortening depending on the degree of laxity (Fig. 50D-4).

As emphasized by the authors, lower lid malposition represents the most common complication following blepharoplasty (7). Although causes of lid retraction often are multifactorial, including overresection of skin, hematoma formation with foreshortening of the septum, and lid descent from excessive edema, the majority of complications are associated with inadequate recognition or management of eye prominence and tarsoligamentous laxity. Conventional preoperative analysis of tarsoligamentous laxity includes the lid snap-back and lid distraction tests. To provide more objective criteria for lid laxity, intraoperative lid distraction with caliper measurements has been used (8). Anterior lid distraction greater than 6 mm from the globe and lateral lid distraction greater than 3 mm over the lateral orbital rim are considered reliable indications of significant lid laxity (Fig. 50D-5). Preoperative vector analysis has been used as a preoperative determination of eye prominence. The relationship of the globe to the inferior orbital rim is the fundamental basis for vector analysis (4). In addition to this test, use of the Hertel exophthalmometer can provide an objective measurement of globe position in relation to the lateral orbital rim (Fig. 50D-6). Patients with a Hertel greater than 20 mm have been found to have significant eye prominence, which is associated with increased risk for lid malposition following lower blepharoplasty. Patients with a Hertel less than 17 mm have deep-set eye morphology that generally is associated with significant lower lid laxity, representing a second risk factor for lid malposition. In addition to these tests, morphologic findings of preoperative scleral show, lateral canthal descent or phimosis, and malar hypoplasia are indicative of a subgroup of patients who may be at increased risk for lower lid complications following blepharoplasty (Fig. 50D-7). To reduce the risk of lid malposition in this high-risk group of patients, lateral canthal support should be performed in all cases.

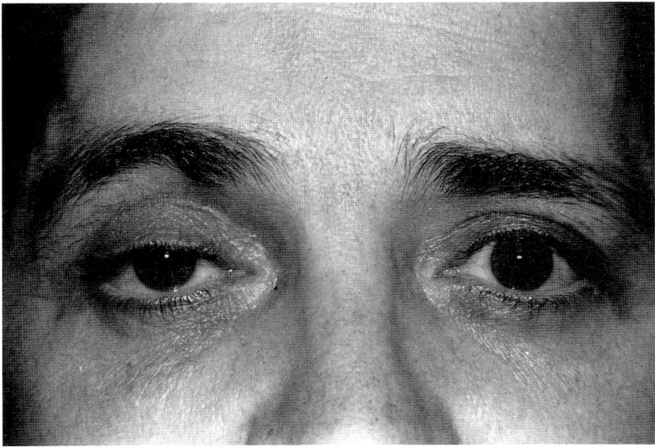

FIGURE 50D-3. Patient with right upper lid ptosis that occurred following upper blepharoplasty.

The two options most commonly used for lateral canthal support are (i) lateral canthoplasty, which requires lateral canthotomy; and (ii) lateral canthopexy, which does not require canthotomy, but produces a lesser degree of horizontal tightening. These techniques are favored over more traditional methods such as the Kuhnt-Szymanowski procedure and tarsal strip, which have been associated with visible notching and narrowing of the palpebral aperture (9,10).

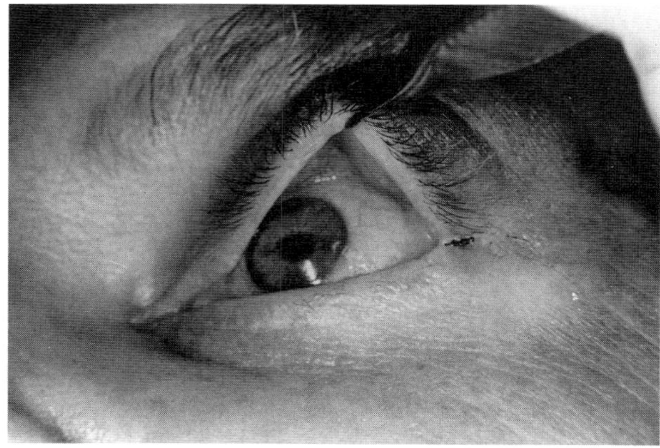
A

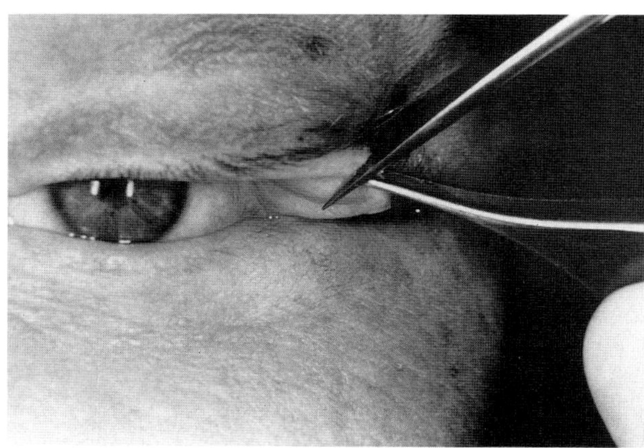
B

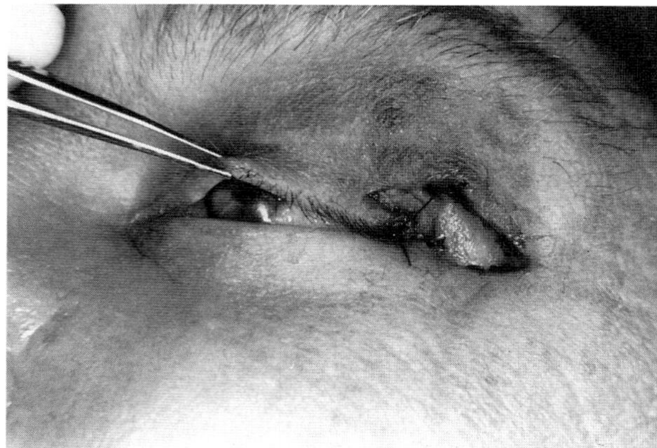
C

FIGURE 50D-4. **A:** Intraoperative examination demonstrating "floppy upper lid syndrome." **B:** Horizontal lid resection of the lateral aspect of the tarsal plate. **C:** Lateral canthoplasty of the upper lid was performed to correct the laxity.

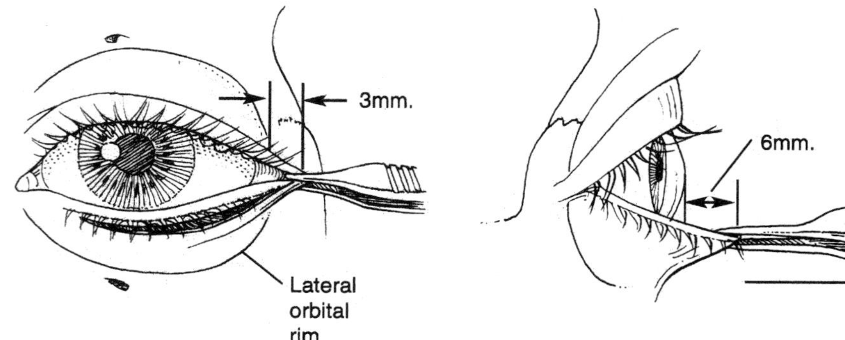

FIGURE 50D-5. Lateral and anterior lid distraction demonstrating measurements used to define significant lid laxity.

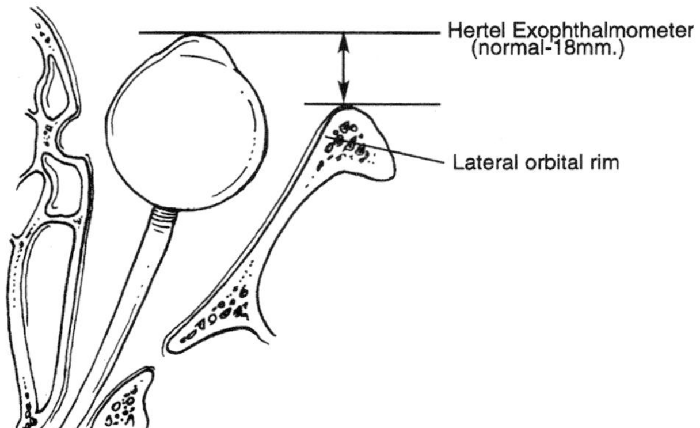

FIGURE 50D-6. Hertel exophthalmometer is used to define the degree of eye prominence compared to the lateral orbital rim.

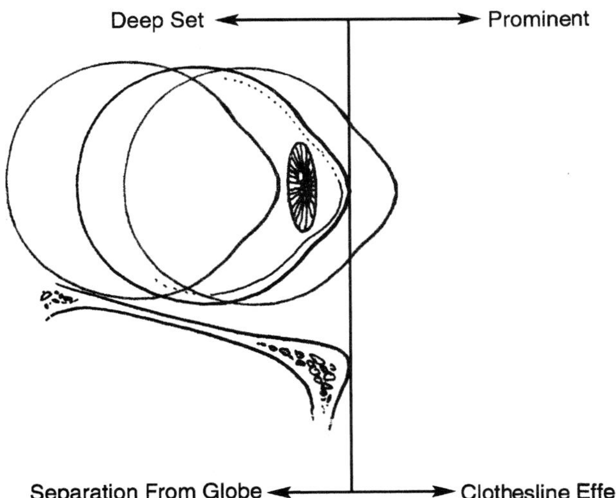

FIGURE 50D-7. Diagram demonstrating the relationship between vector analysis and globe position with the risk of complications associated with excessive lateral canthal tightening.

LOWER BLEPHAROPLASTY TECHNIQUE

An infraciliary lower lid blepharoplasty incision is made from the lateral canthal angle directed laterally in a prominent line. The initial incision lateral to the canthus is kept within the confines of the orbital rim. The medial extension is made with scissors beveling away from the lash margin to preserve at least 4 mm of pretarsal orbicularis muscle. Needle tip electrocautery is used to elevate the skin-muscle flap to the level of the infraorbital rim. Following exposure of the septum, the periosteal origin of the orbitomalar ligament is divided, which exposes the suborbicularis oculi fat (SOOF) (Fig. 50D-8). Release of the orbitomalar ligament is required to elevate the SOOF (11). The suborbicularis dissection is carried laterally and superiorly along the lateral orbital rim to create a bipedicled myocutaneous flap of orbicularis and orbital skin between the upper and lower lid

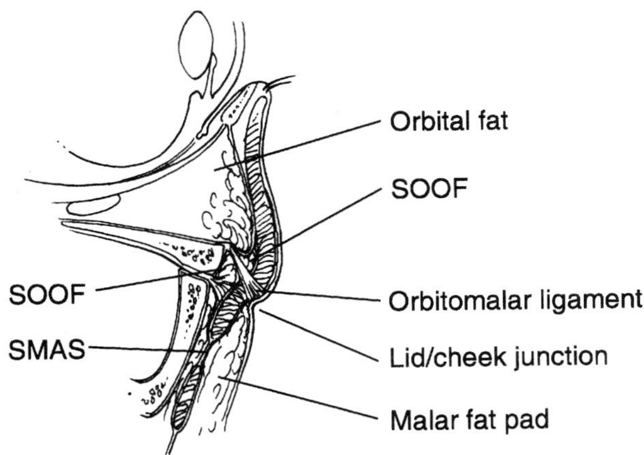

FIGURE 50D-8. Cross-sectional anatomy of the orbital rim demonstrating the orbitomalar ligament.

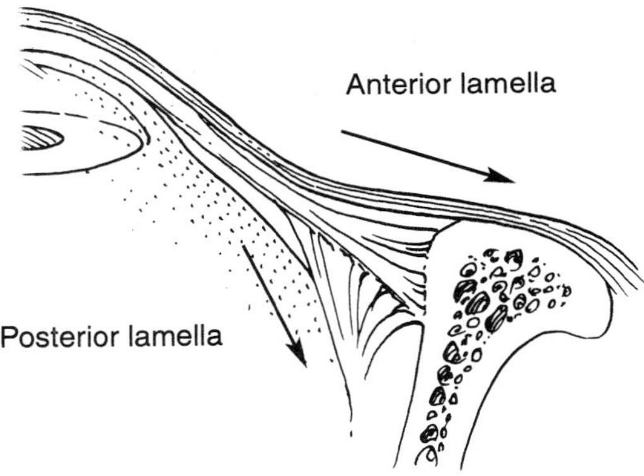

FIGURE 50D-9. Anatomy of the lateral orbital rim demonstrating the anterior and posterior components of the lateral canthus.

incisions. A distance of at least 10 mm should be maintained between the lateral extension of the upper and lower blepharoplasty incisions. Conservative removal of fat and arcus marginalis release with fat transposition are performed most commonly (12,13).

The underlying principle governing performance of canthal tightening is reestablishment of lower eyelid stability through fixation of the tarsoligamentous sling and orbicularis to the lateral orbital rim at separate points corresponding to the two vectors of the normal lateral canthal anatomy (Fig. 50D-9). The tarsoligamentous sling is sutured to the inner aspect of the lateral orbital rim for posterior lamellar support and to insure approximation of the lid margin to the globe. The orbicularis is sutured to the anterior aspect of the orbital rim along the lateral orbital raphe for anterior lamellar support (14). A lateral canthopexy is adequate for lid support in patients who have mild lid laxity, minimal eye prominence, and a lateral canthal position that is superior to the medial canthus (Fig. 50D-10). A transcanthal can-

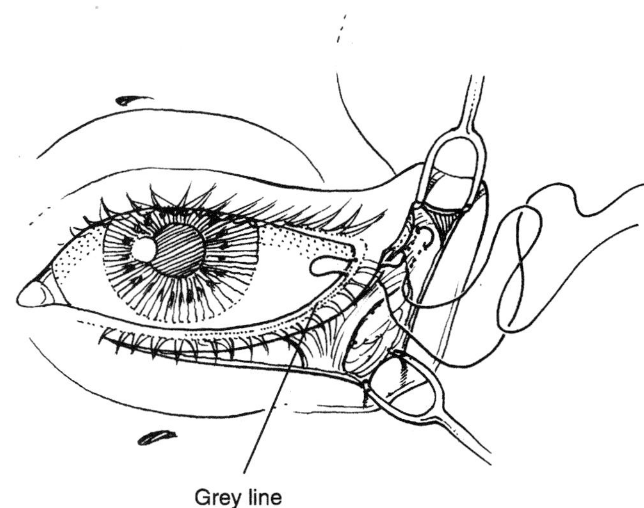

FIGURE 50D-10. Lateral canthopexy used to suture the lateral retinaculum and tarsal plate to the periosteum of the lateral orbital rim.

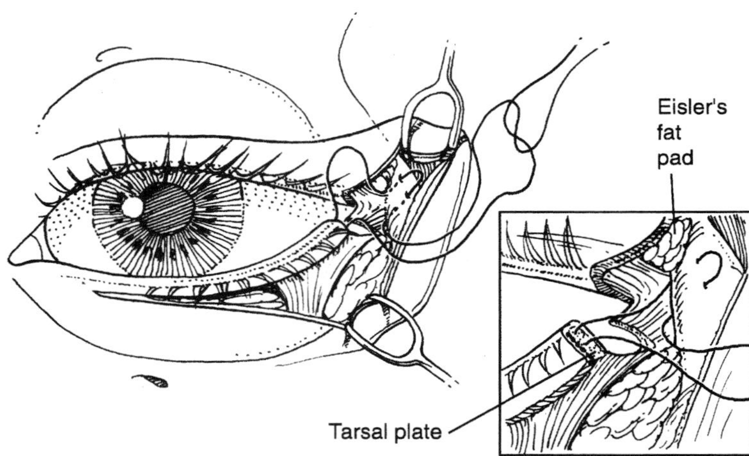

FIGURE 50D-11. Lateral canthoplasty performed by suturing the cut edge of the tarsal plate to the lateral orbital rim at the level of the Eisler fat pad.

thopexy is used most commonly by suturing the tarsal plate and lateral retinaculum to the periosteum of the lateral orbital rim with 4-0 Prolene (8,12).

Lateral canthoplasty is recommended for patients who are at increased risk for lid malposition, including significant lower lid laxity, significant eye prominence, and a lateral canthal position that is inferior to the medial canthus. Canthotomy through the inferior limb of the lateral canthal tendon is performed, preserving the tendon to the upper lid (Fig. 50D-11). Cantholysis should divide the capsulopalpebral fascia and conjunctiva below the lid margin and the inferior arcade. Following release of the lower lid, lid redundancy is managed by full-thickness resection.

Suture fixation of the lower lid is performed using a 4-0 Prolene mattress suture to the periosteum of the inner lateral orbital rim. The suture is placed through the tarsal plate, entering at the inferior margin and exiting through the superior margin. The suture is placed inside the lateral orbital rim at the level of the pupil. Vertical alignment of the mattress suture is required to avoid complications of lash rotation. The goal of lateral canthoplasty is correction of lid laxity while maintaining lid position and shape similar to the preoperative appearance. Overcorrection with supraplacement and loosening of the lid are required for patient with significant eye prominence and for correction of scleral show (Fig. 50D-12). Primary spacer with AlloDerm or ear cartilage should be considered for patients with marked prominence or for a history of Graves ophthalmopathy (15). Following lateral canthoplasty, it is critical to reconstruct the lateral canthal angle with 6-0 nylon alignment suture to avoid webbing of the lateral commissure. The suture is placed to approximate the gray line of the upper and lower lid in a "vest-over-pants" fashion.

The lower blepharoplasty is completed by conservative excision of excess skin and muscle. Suturing the skin-muscle flap to the periosteum along the lateral orbital raphe, using a three-point quilting suture, restores the anterior vector of the lateral canthus. Suspension of the orbicularis is an important part of lower lid support (14). This tension serves to redistribute the lower lid soft tissue while adding lower lid

A 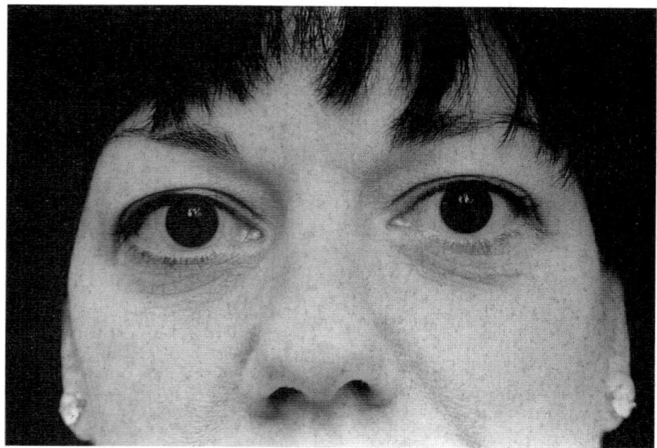

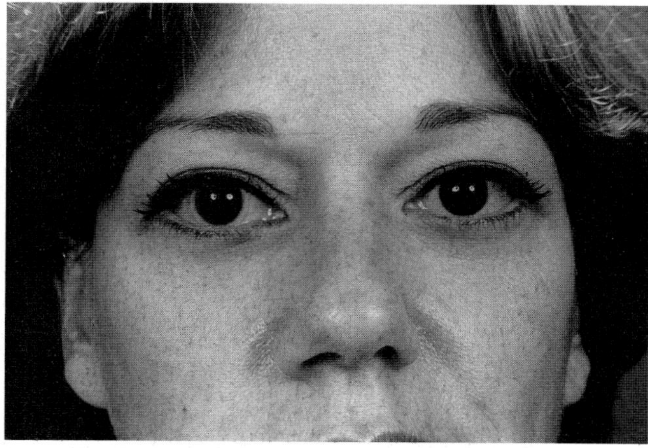 B

FIGURE 50D-12. A: Preoperative appearance of a patient with significant eye prominence, preoperative scleral show, and a Hertel measurement of 20 mm. **B:** Patient 6 months after lower blepharoplasty with lateral canthoplasty and improvement of lid position.

support using a "hammock" of orbicularis, thereby rejuvenating the contours of the lower eyelid. After completion of the lateral canthoplasty and orbicularis suspension, conservative resection is performed so that a tensionless skin closure is obtained. The incision then is closed with a simple running 7-0 silk suture, taking care to incorporate skin and muscle in the closure to minimize visible scar formation.

Just as preoperative evaluation of the upper lid should include evaluation of the brow and position of the retro-orbicularis fat, evaluation of the lower lid should include assessment of the midface with attention to the position of the suborbicularis oculi fat and malar fat pad. To provide an objective determination, a classification system of midfacial aging has been described (16). This classification can assist in surgical planning by emphasizing the procedures needed to correct progressive facial changes of aging.

Type I midfacial aging represents the earliest changes that only involve the lower eyelid, with pseudoherniation of orbital fat and minimal skin and muscle excess (Fig. 50D-13). Type II aging involves the upper midface with minimal descent of the lid–cheek junction and SOOF. As aging progresses, the midface demonstrates significant descent of the lid–cheek junction, with deepening of the nasolabial fold, characteristic of type III midfacial aging. Type IV aging represents more advanced midfacial aging, with the development of the tear-trough deformity and malar bags with significant descent of the malar fat pad. Classification of aging by this method emphasizes the relationship between the midface and lower eyelid. With advanced changes related to aging, the midface and lower eyelid should be managed as a single aesthetic unit.

A discussion of blepharoplasty would not be complete without mention of the options available to improve the midface through the lower blepharoplasty incision (12,16–18). Patients with mild degrees of midfacial aging classified as types I and II are candidates for more conservative techniques, which include limited dissection above the periosteum. Release of the orbitomalar ligament and eleva-

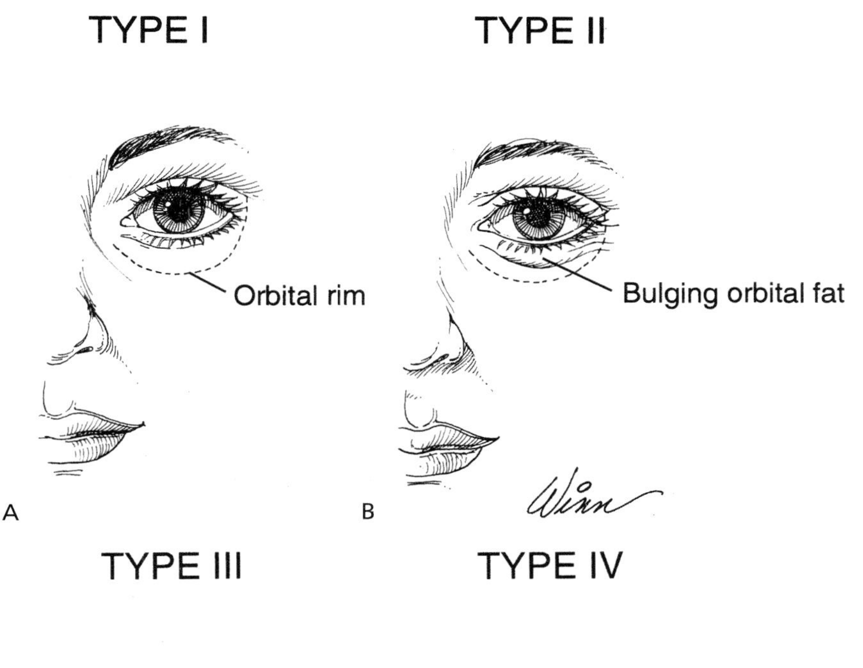

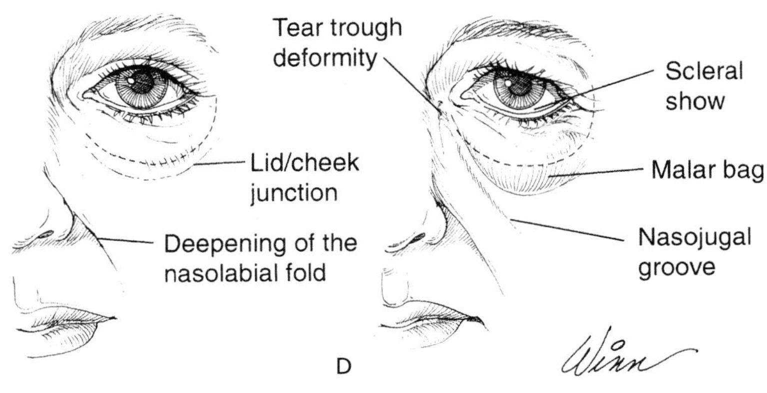

FIGURE 50D-13. A: Type I midfacial aging with minimal pseudoherniation of lower lid fat. **B:** Type II midfacial aging is characterized by bulging lower lid fat and minimal descent of the lid–cheek junction. **C:** Type III midfacial aging demonstrates significant descent of the lid–cheek junction with deepening of the nasolabial folds. **D:** Type IV midfacial aging with advanced signs of aging, including the development of the tear-trough deformity and malar bags.

tion of the SOOF is a safe and effective technique used to camouflage the infraorbital rim. Patients with more advanced midfacial aging, such as types III and IV, require a more aggressive approach. Subperiosteal dissection and release of the midface are necessary to elevate the malar fat pad and restore a more youthful anatomical contour. Recent modifications to reduce the incidence of complications of lid malposition associated with the procedure include postoperative fixation through the lateral aspect of the upper blepharoplasty incision and more limited lower lid incisions to preserve orbicularis innervation (16,19). Overall, the technique should be considered more technically demanding, with an increased risk of complications compared with standard lower lid blepharoplasty; however, the results have been satisfactory with a high level of patient satisfaction.

CONCLUSION

The authors have provided a comprehensive summary of blepharoplasty with an emphasis on useful ways to recognize potential problems before they occur. Although avoiding complications through recognition of high-risk patients is often the best way to minimize risk, complications inevitably will occur following blepharoplasty. Management of these complications may be as simple as patient reassurance with conservative measures or may include surgical revision. This chapter provided a framework for the appreciation of potential technical failure and the formation of a sound surgical approach that may reliably ensure a favorable outcome.

REFERENCES

1. Fagien S. Algorithm for canthoplasty: the lateral retinacular suspension: a simplified suture canthopexy. *Plast Reconstr Surg* 1999;103:2042–2058.
2. McCord CE, Shore JW. Avoidance of complication in lower lid blepharoplasty. *Ophthalmology* 1983;90:1039–1046.
3. Rees TD, LaTrenta GS. The role of Schirmer's test and orbital morphology in predicting dry eye syndrome after blepharoplasty. *Plast Reconstr Surg* 1988;82:619–625.
4. Jelks GW, Jelks EB. The influence of orbital and eyelid anatomy on the palpebral aperture. *Clin Plast Surg* 1991;18:183–195.
5. Wolfort KG, Pobleter JV. Ptosis after blepharoplasty. *Ann Plast Surg* 1995;43:264–267.
6. Dutton JJ. Surgical management of floppy eyelid syndrome. *Am J Ophthalmol* 1985;99:557–560.
7. Carraway JH, Mellow CG. The prevention and treatment of lower lid ectropion following blepharoplasty. *Plast Reconstr Surg* 1990;85:971–981.
8. Codner MA, McCord CD, Hester TR. The lateral canthoplasty. *Op Tech Plast Reconstr Surg* 1998;5:90–98.
9. Smith B, Cherubini TS. Modification of Kuhnt-Szymanowski ectropion repair. In: Smith BC, ed. *Oculoplastic surgery: a compendium of principles and techniques.* St. Louis: Mosby-Year Book, 1970.
10. Anderson RL, Gordy DD. The tarsal strip procedure. *Arch Ophthalmol* 1979;97:2192-–2196.
11. Kikkawa DO, Bradkley NL, Dortzbach RK. Relations of the superficial musculoaponeurotic system to the orbit and characterization of the orbitomalar ligament. *Ophthalmol Plast Reconstr Surg* 1996;12:77–88.
12. Hamra ST. The zygo-orbicular dissection in composite rhytidectomy: an ideal midface plane. *Plast Reconstr Surg* 1998;102: 1646–1657.
13. Hamra ST. Arcus marginalis release and orbital fat preservation in midface rejuvenation. *Plast Reconstr Surg* 1995;96:354–362.
14. McCord CD, Codner MA, Hester RT. Redraping the inferior orbicularis arc. *Plast Reconstr Surg* 1998;102:2471–2479.
15. Schorr NS. "Madame Butterfly" procedure: total lower eyelid reconstruction in here layers utilizing a hard palate graft. Management of the unhappy post-blepharoplasty patient with round eye and scleral show. *Int J Aesthetic Restor Surg* 1995;3:3–26.
16. Hester TR, Codner MA, McCord CD, et al. Evolution of technique of the direct transblepharoplasty approach for the correction of lower lid and midfacial aging: maximizing results and minimizing complications in a 5-year experience. *Plast Reconstr Surg* 2000;105:393–406.
17. Paul MD. The periosteal hinge flap in the subperiosteal cheeklift. *Op Tech Plast Reconstr Surg* 1998;5:145–154.
18. Gunter JP, Hackney FL. A simplified trans-blepharoplasty cheek lift. *Plast Reconstr Surg* 1999;103:2029–2041.
19. Hester TR, Grover S. Avoiding complication of transblepharoplasty lower-lid and midface rejuvenation. *Aesthetic Surg J* 2000;20:61–67.

51

BROWLIFT AND FACELIFT

TRACY M. BAKER
THOMAS J. BAKER
JAMES M. STUZIN

This chapter represents the ideas of three surgeons who deal primarily with patients undergoing aesthetic surgery of the face and brow. It is based on their combined experience in treating more than 10,000 cases during the preceding 40 years. Specific cases, extensive footnotes, and long reference lists are not included. Rather, the authors present their thoughts and observations regarding the treatment and prevention of complications in facelift and browlift surgery.

Unfavorable results in plastic surgery can be broadly categorized into two distinct groups. The first comprises *true surgical complications*—hematoma, infection, hypertrophic scar, slough, and others. Although careful preoperative measures can minimize these events, they inevitably develop in a small percentage of patients. The second category is best described as unfavorable results caused by by *errors of aesthetic judgment*—hairline shifts, poorly placed scars, lines of misdirection in cervical and facial flaps, earlobe and tragal distortions, and overcorrections. These results can in most instances be prevented by careful planning and execution. Only through the most critical analysis of our own work can we fully come to understand and eliminate this latter group.

TRUE COMPLICATIONS OF SURGERY

Complications occur during surgery despite the most heroic efforts to prevent them. This section deals with these inevitable outcomes and the best measures to lower their incidence. Patients in whom unfavorable results develop should be seen *frequently.* Frequent visits reassure the patient, make it possible to deal with problems appropriately, and, it is hoped, prevent legal action. Complications are psychologically difficult for both patient and surgeon. Open and honest discussions during which patients can express their feelings and desires allow them to understand their problem and maintain good relationships with the physician and staff.

Hematoma is the most common true complication following facelift (Fig. 51-1). Avoidable underlying causative factors should be identified and eliminated, and the history and physical examination should reveal most of these. Hypertensive patients should comply with their medication regimens, and their blood pressure should be well controlled. Patients may not be aware of underlying bleeding disorders. Known disorders, a history of easy bruising and bleeding, abnormal laboratory values, and a prolonged bleeding time should all be evaluated thoroughly before surgery. Many patients will not list over-the-counter drugs as "medications" and may unknowingly be taking a preparation that can prolong the bleeding time. A list of commonly taken medications containing aspirin is given to every patient, and preparations on this list are avoided for a minimum of 2 weeks before surgery.

Two perioperative factors of importance that should be controlled are blood pressure and nausea. All patients undergoing facelift in our facility receive 0.1 to 0.3 mg of clonidine (Catapres) orally when they arrive on the morning of surgery. This centrally-acting alpha agonist maintains the systolic blood pressure at 90 to 100 mm Hg throughout the procedure and for several hours in the recovery room. Dissection is facilitated because of the drier field, and postoperative hematomas have been all but eliminated. No cases of "rebound" hypertension causing hematoma have been seen. Nausea and vomiting may follow surgery and contribute to high venous pressures in the head and neck (Valsalva's maneuver). Nausea should be aggressively controlled by any of several excellent medications available. We have found intravenous ondansetron (Zofran) particularly useful in controlling symptoms in patients with a severe history of postoperative nausea and in cases refractory to other medications.

Hematomas should be evacuated as soon as possible. Small collections of less than 2 cm^3 discovered early after they form can be aspirated with a needle if still in liquid

T. M. Baker: Department of Plastic Surgery, University of Miami School of Medicine, Miami, and Department of Plastic Surgery, Mercy Hospital, Miami, Florida

T. J. Baker: Department of Plastic Surgery, University of Miami School of Medicine, Miami, and Department of Plastic Surgery, Mercy Hospital, Miami, Florida

J. M. Stuzin: Plastic Surgery Associates, Miami, Florida

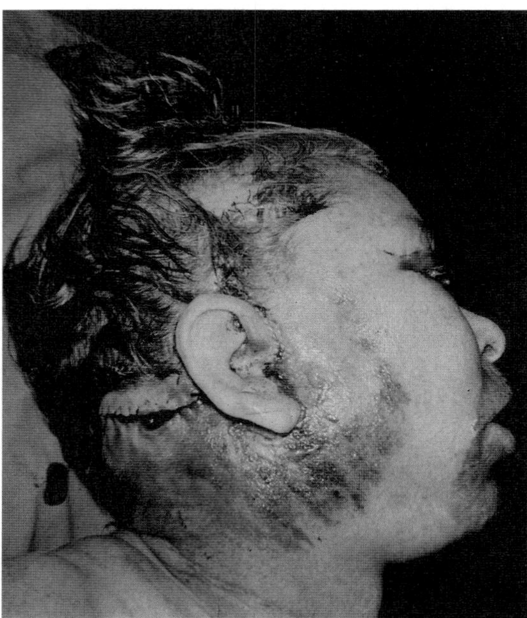

FIGURE 51-1. Hematoma is one of the most common true surgical complications after facelift. In this instance, deleterious effects on the overlying flaps resulted from delayed recognition.

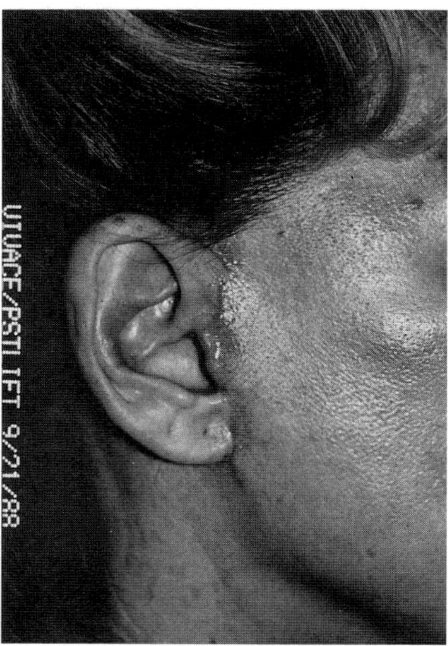

FIGURE 51-2. Tragal infections are commonly caused by gram-negative organisms from the external auditory canal. These infections can prove resistant to treatment, and longer periods of antibiotics may be required.

form. Larger or organized collections should be explored and evacuated. If tense or expanding collections are discovered in the recovery room, when exploration will be delayed, release of the suture lines to relieve tension on the flaps until they are drained may be required. Frequently, the source of bleeding cannot be found at the time of exploration. Because breakdown products of hemoglobin have deleterious effects on local tissues and healing, the proper treatment of all hematomas is warranted.

Infection following rhytidectomy can be an aggressive, tissue-destroying event (Fig. 51-3A). The overwhelming majority of infections in patients undergoing facelift are caused by bacteria from the skin, ear canals, mouth, or nasal passages. *Staphylococcus* and *Streptococcus* organisms cause the vast majority of infections, but *Pseudomonas* and a host of emerging pathogens also contribute significantly. Most infections present at 3 to 5 days after surgery as localized erythema, swelling, and fluctuance. Symptoms of fever, malaise, and associated pain often lag behind the clinical findings. With frequent examinations and clinical awareness, these problems can often be diagnosed early in their course.

Patients undergoing rhytidectomy should receive one dose of intravenous antibiotics before the incision and one to two doses afterward. The antibiotic agent should be targeted to the pathogens most likely to be encountered. Antibiotics given beyond this time period have not been effective in the prevention of infection and may in fact select for resistant bacteria should infection arise. Patients with closed-system drains left in place longer than 24 hours may be considered candidates for oral antibiotic therapy during this time.

Bacterial infections involving the tragus are commonly caused by gram-negative organisms. Clinical infection usually begins several days after surgery and presents as tenderness and erythema in the region of the tragal body (Fig. 51-2). Long-term antibiotic therapy may be required to eradicate these persistent infections fully. Prevention is aimed at preserving the perichondrium with a thin layer of soft tissue coverage over the tragus during elevation of the facial flap.

Treatment of infections associated with facelift procedures should be directed toward wide drainage, generous irrigation, and culture- and sensitivity-specific antibiotic therapy. Some wounds may require debridement, as in cases of significant tissue destruction. When infection is under control, wounds can either be left to heal by secondary intention or closed secondarily if no tissue loss has occurred (Fig. 51-3B,C). Scars can then be revised when appropriate. Hyperbaric oxygen therapy should be considered when available in more severe infections; however, its efficacy has yet to be demonstrated clearly.

Slough may occur as a result of any of several factors with a single basis: compromise of cervicofacial flap circulation (Fig. 51-4). The two most heralded causative factors in slough remain *tension* and *smoking*. Skin tension results from either poor planning or careless execution of the operation. Tension provides no beneficial addition to a rhytidectomy and serves only to distort the normal anatomy, widen scars, and cause tissue loss. Tension should be placed on any of several deep structures (submucosal aponeurotic system, periosteum, and galea) and avoided in the skin. Smoking and the presence of nicotine in the microcirculation of a flap

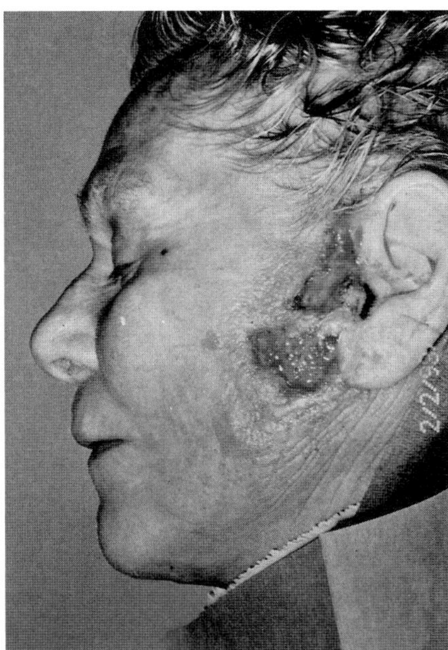
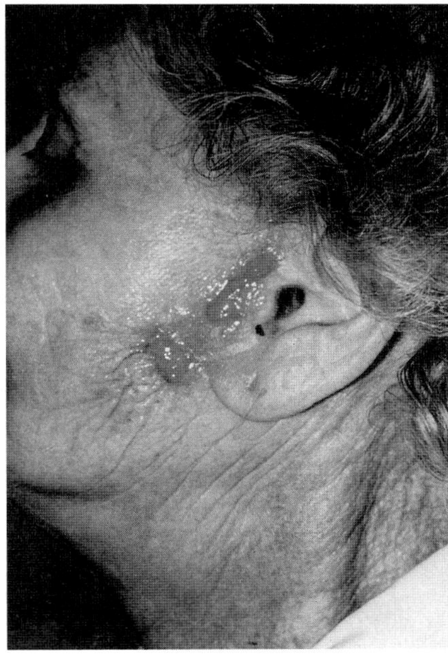
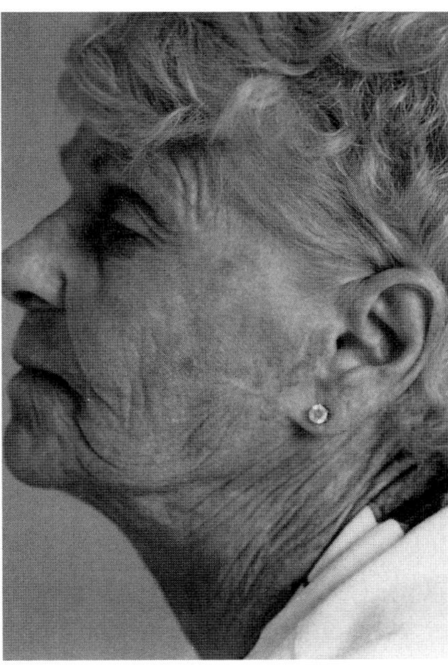

A, B C

FIGURE 51-3. A: *Pseudomonas* infection presenting on the fifth postoperative day after a facelift without any systemic signs. Significant tissue destruction occurred despite early recognition and treatment. The subcutaneous extension of the process is evident several centimeters beyond the edge of the wound inferiorly. **B,C:** After the infection was brought under control, the wound was allowed to heal by secondary intention. Part B shows a clean contracting wound at 4 weeks following surgery. Part C shows the final appearance at 18 months. Small scar revisions at this point can render even these significant defects quite acceptable.

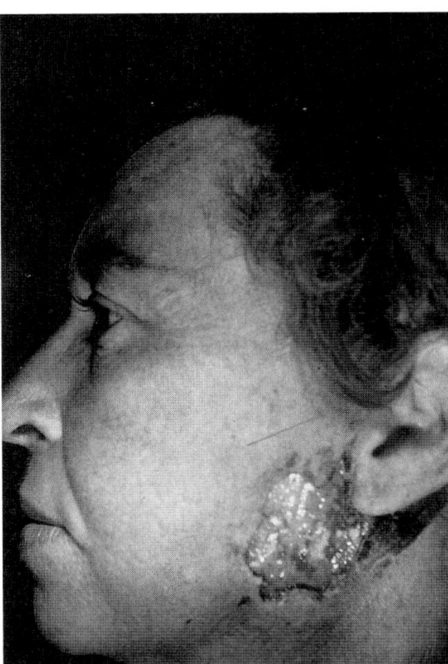

FIGURE 51-4. Slough after facelift is three times more likely in smokers. Other significant factors include flap tension, infection, and unrecognized hematoma. (From Baker TJ, Gordon HL. *Surgical rejuvenation of the face.* St. Louis: Mosby, 1986:217, with permission.)

are known factors in reducing flap survival. Nicotine has a thrombogenic effect, mediated in part by the stimulation of thromboxane A_2. Postauricular slough is three times more common in smokers. Patients should discontinue all nicotine (including transdermal patch preparations) for a minimum of 2 weeks before surgery and for several weeks thereafter. Measuring the urinary nicotine levels can easily detect noncompliance the day before surgery. In patients unable or unwilling to quit smoking, skin flaps should be undermined more conservatively, and patients should be made aware of the increased risks of surgery.

Inadequately treated hematoma and infection result in the destruction of overlying tissues and masquerade as "slough" (Fig. 51-1). Similarly, inappropriately placed "pressure dressings" may congest or strangle the blood supply of a flap. Improper positioning of a patient, with the scapulae flat on the mattress and two pillows under the head, can acutely flex the cervical spine and produce a linear strangulation at the cervical crease anteriorly (Fig. 51-5). The head should be elevated with the neck in the neutral position or in slight extension; the elevation should be behind the torso and shoulders.

The treatment of slough begins with early recognition and elimination of any of the causative factors outlined above. Flaps exhibiting venous congestion may benefit from the topical application of nitroglycerin paste. This vasodilator has significant cardiac and systemic hemodynamic effects and should be used with some caution. The circulation

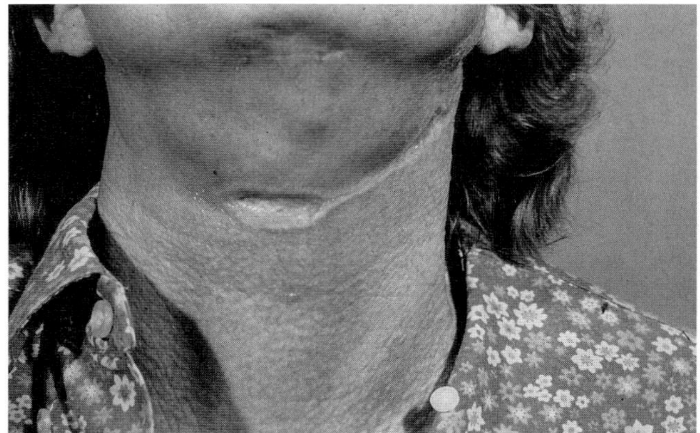

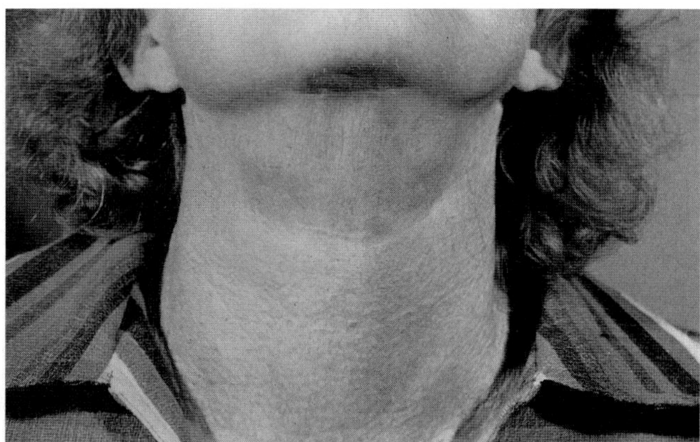

FIGURE 51-5. A,B: Acute flexion of the cervical spine in an attempt to "elevate" the head may result in ischemia and slough of the anterior cervical crease. Appearance at 8 months after healing by secondary intention. Proper elevation includes support of the entire back and shoulders to produce flexion at the waist with a neutral or slightly extended cervical spine.

in flaps exhibiting early ischemia may improve with hyperbaric oxygen. Clean dry eschar should not be debrided, but any necrotic regions exhibiting secondary infection should be adequately removed. The wounds should be allowed to heal completely by secondary intention and revisions performed when appropriate (Figs. 51-3 and 51-5). Skin grafts to larger defects, although at times they may be tempting, should be avoided because they routinely produce inferior aesthetic results (Fig. 51-6).

ERRORS IN PATIENT SELECTION

The relationship between patient and plastic surgeon is unlike any other in medicine. Aesthetic surgery of the face treats the spirit as well as the physical changes of aging. The relationship is personal and intimate. Patients entrust us with the awesome responsibility of performing *elective* surgery. The physical changes imparted by our scalpels on the emotional being, both good and bad, will finalize the

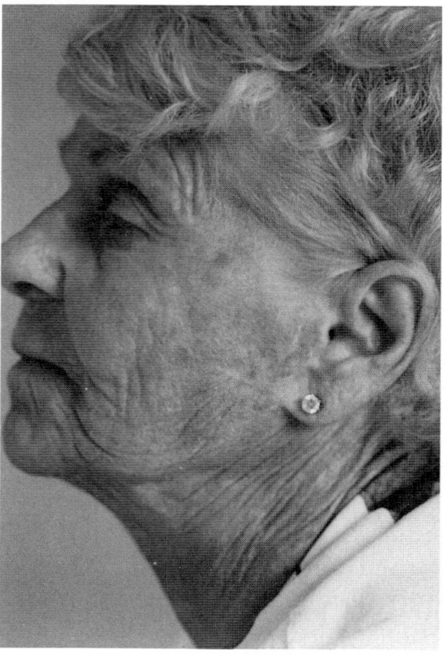

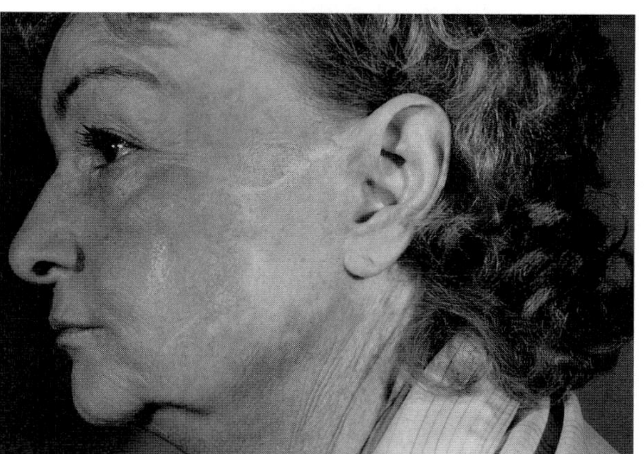

FIGURE 51-6. Compare the final aesthetic results of similar sloughs treated by different methods. **A:** The appearance of a wound allowed to heal by secondary intention. **B:** A similar wound treated by split-thickness skin grafting. However tempting a large, clean, granulating wound may appear, skin grafts routinely produce poor color and texture matches in the face.

permanent bond between surgeon and patient. Before these lifelong relationships are established, each and every one must be carefully considered.

It is sometimes difficult for a surgeon simply to say no to a prospective patient. After all, it is quite flattering to have patients select you as their surgeon. It is financially rewarding and, it is hoped, what we truly enjoy doing. Additionally, saying no sets up a potentially confrontational situation—the patient wants an explanation for the refusal. Surgeons may not want to be seen as weak or unable to deliver the product they were trained to produce. In any event, the initial consultation should be a screening process for both patient and surgeon. Indeed, a patient may see several surgeons and choose one. Likewise, the surgeon needs to evaluate potential patients in the same manner.

The motivation for the proposed procedure must be well founded. The dress and demeanor of the patient should be proper. Questions should be appropriate. The patient should be listening to the surgeon's portion of the dialogue. Depression, severe anxiety, anger, inappropriate emotions, and unrealistic expectations are red flags. Overly flattering patients who may have undergo multiple previous surgeries and who harbor ill feelings toward the previous surgeon(s) can likewise be trouble. Be alert for signs of alcoholism and other substance abuse.

Patients who present overweight need to be counseled regarding the increased risks and limitations of surgery. These patients tend to be sedentary and are at higher risk for cardiac, circulatory, and pulmonary events. Programs modifying eating habits and lifestyle make patients feel better and reduce complications. Additionally, most procedures are anatomically designed for the neck and the face containing normal amounts of fat. Surgical candidates presenting with frank obesity are counseled, and surgery is made contingent on appropriate weight loss.

Preexisting medical conditions are usually not in themselves criteria for exclusion from surgery. The American Society of Anesthesiologists has organized a useful classification to grade a patient's medical status for surgery (Table 51-1). Asthma, insulin-dependent diabetes, hypertension, and other mild to moderate medical problems (PS-2) should be appropriately evaluated and controlled by the patient's physician. Those with more severe problems or multiple medical risk factors should be excluded from surgery (PS-3 or higher). Patients over the age of 65 and younger patients with existing problems should undergo appropriate testing and clearance from their own physicians. "Medical clearance," however, should not supersede the surgeon's own judgment. The final decision and responsibility regarding whether or not to operate rests solely with the plastic surgeon.

TABLE 51-1. CLASSIFICATION OF PHYSICAL STATUS

PS-1	Normal, healthy person
PS-2	Mild systemic disease that results in no functional limitations (hypertension, diabetes, extreme age)
PS-3	Severe systemic disease resulting in functional limitations (angina, previous myocardial infarction, severe pulmonary disease)
PS-4	Severe systemic disease producing a constant threat to life (congestive heart failure, unstable angina, hepatic dysfunction)
PS-5	Moribund patient who will not survive without operation (ruptured abdominal aortic aneurysm)
PS-6	Brain dead, scheduled for organ donation

From the American Society of Anesthesiologists. New classification of physical status. *Anesthesiology* 1963:24:111, with permission.

One of the most common events leading to dissatisfaction in the postoperative period is the failure to detect and point out to the patient preexisting conditions and asymmetries (Fig. 51-7). The patient may be dissatisfied despite an excellent aesthetic result. Resuspension of the brow may reveal an underlying ptosis of the upper lid. Tightening of the cervical skin may reveal ptosis of the submaxillary gland(s). Most faces have a vertically "long side" and "short side." Clinical signs of aging are usually more advanced on the short side—more brow ptosis, more malar and jowl fat descent, and heavier nasolabial folds. Despite independent vectoring, these features can persist postoperatively, when patients are evaluating themselves with a more critical eye. Preoperative evaluations tend to enlighten the patient, whereas postoperative discussions are perceived as excuses. Asymmetries should be thoroughly discussed and documented at the time of consultation to educate the patient and minimize any disappointments.

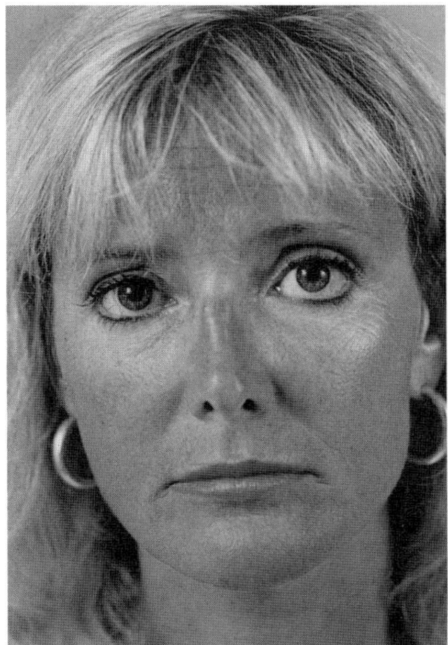

FIGURE 51-7. Note the asymmetries in this attractive 42-year-old woman. The left side of her face is larger than the right, with a broader malar region, a larger and higher orbit, more pretarsal skin show, and an elevated eyebrow. Preexisting asymmetries should be noted and discussed with the patient to avoid postoperative misunderstandings.

ERRORS OF AESTHETIC JUDGMENT

The most common unfavorable results in aesthetic surgery of the face and brow are the consequence of errors of aesthetic judgment. Plastic surgeons and the general public see such patients everyday. In fact, the painfully visible errors of aesthetic judgment may be one of the largest single factors deterring new patients from considering surgery. The distorted, pulled, and overcorrected look is etched in almost every person's memory (Fig. 51-8). Two independent movements in the field of plastic surgery are beginning to minimize these problems. The first is an improved knowledge of surgical anatomy. No longer do we rely solely on the skin to vector all the aging layers of the face. Now that the skin is no longer the vehicle of restoration, we can reposition muscle, fascia, and fat separately and more naturally. The second factor is a general movement away from the purely technical execution of surgery toward a greater awareness of what we are creating aesthetically. This is reflected in the content of the journal articles and courses offered during the last decade. We must first know the normal beautiful if we are to restore or create it surgically.

The remaining sections of this chapter are organized according to anatomy. Errors of aesthetic judgment are discussed with the complications particular to a specific location. Here, the lines here between errors of aesthetic judgment and true complications are not so clear. For example, a hypertrophic scar can happen anywhere but may be more common if undue tension is placed on the skin. The two groups of complications are considered together to facilitate discussion.

THE BROW

The debate between endoscopic versus open approaches to the brow rages on. As we become technically more facile with endoscopic procedures and as our ability to fix the elevated soft tissues in place with accuracy improves, the endoscope will eclipse the open approach in all but the most aged cases. In experienced, well-trained hands, the endoscopic approach has fewer inherent complications. It avoids an ear-to-ear incision across the top the head and so minimizes the associated scar. Similarly, the innervation by the first division of the trigeminal nerve is not interrupted between the incision and the top of the head. Alopecia and even slough along the scar of an open browlift should be minimized. Endoscopic browlift can be considered in both men and women a with thinning or receding hairline. Both procedures increase the vertical height of the forehead. Regardless of the surgeon's approach, it is ultimately the aesthetic result that determines the success of the procedure.

The brow is perhaps the area where errors of aesthetic judgment are most obvious. Figure 51-9 demonstrates the characteristics of a beautiful youthful brow in a 25-year-old woman. The most common error seen in surgery of the

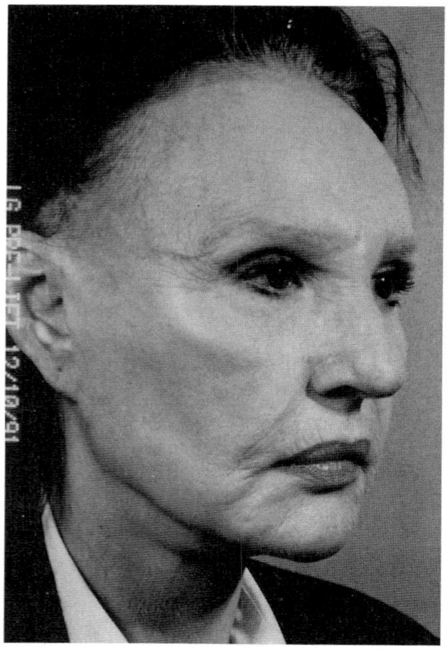

FIGURE 51-8. Errors of aesthetic judgment produce a distorted and operated appearance. This patient demonstrates many of the errors we seek to avoid. Raised frontal hairline, loss of the temporal and sideburn hair, distorted tragus, pulled earlobes, exaggerated distance between the lateral canthus and hairline, and loss of the normal facial contours all contribute to a bizarre appearance.

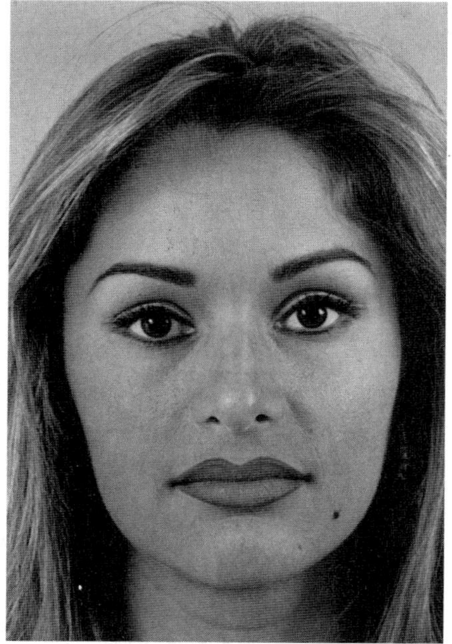

FIGURE 51-9. The aesthetically pleasing youthful female brow. Note the course of the eyebrow, beginning medially at the level of the orbital rim and arching above the rim as it progresses laterally. The peak of the arch is ideally at the junction of the medial two thirds with the lateral one third. The lid sulci are clean and sharp with pretarsal symmetry.

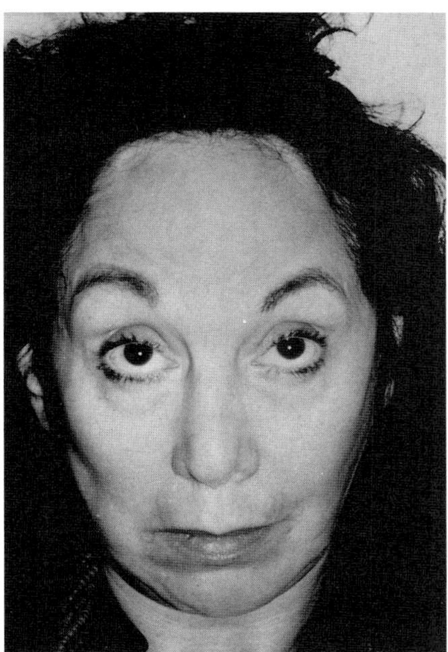

FIGURE 51-10. Excessive release and correction of the brow produce an exaggerated elevation with lateral splaying of the interbrow distance. Additionally, excessive resection of the frontalis muscle in this patient produced an unnatural adherence of the skin to the calvarium. (From Baker TJ, Gordon HL. *Surgical rejuvenation of the face,* 2nd ed. St. Louis: Mosby, 1996:568, with permission.)

brow is overcorrection. Often, the location of the entire brow is too high, particularly medially, where it may splay apart and rest well above the level of the orbital rim (Fig. 51-10). This imparts a look of surprise and is the look many patients envisage when they are apprehensive about a browlift. Care should be taken to maintain the attachments between the bone and overlying soft tissues in the region of the medial brow and glabella. Total release should be avoided in this region when the corrugator and procerus muscles are manipulated.

A hairline incision at the junction of the cutaneous forehead skin and hair-bearing scalp may be an option in some patients with vertically long foreheads. This type of incision should be carefully chosen and discussed with the patient. Designed and executed well in the appropriately selected patient, it can be a rewarding procedure that leaves an indiscernible scar (Fig. 51-11A). The incision should be individually designed for each patient and should meander through the fine hairs along the junction of the scalp and forehead junction. As the incision is extended toward the ear, it can be designed to move posteriorly into the scalp to join the standard facelift incision, or it can be continued as a complete anterior hairline incision. This choice depends on the patient's and surgeon's preference, the distance from the lateral canthus to the temporal hairline, and many other factors. A long horizontal distance from the lateral canthus to the temporal hairline is a classic stigma of browlift and facelift that can be avoided in selected patients with a complete anterior hairline incision. Hairline scars tend to be more visible in patients with a ruddy or dark complexion. Poorly designed incisions can alter hairline contours in bizarre fashions (Fig. 51-11B).

Muscle resections and divisions are a part of all procedures designed to rejuvenate the brow. The removal of large powerful corrugator muscles may leave a visible depression. Fat or fascia grafting of these defects at the time of browlift can help eliminate problems. Weakening of the frontalis muscle by horizontal divisions through the galea and muscle tissue can result in transverse forehead lines. Complete resection of the frontalis muscle will cause a large visible depression and a very unaesthetic adherence of the remaining soft tissues to the calvarium (Fig. 51-10).

Excessive tension in the closure of the standard open browlift may manifest itself as a tension-related hyper-

A

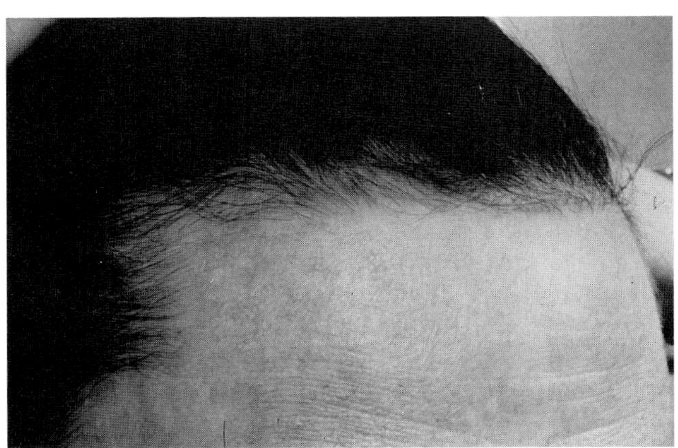

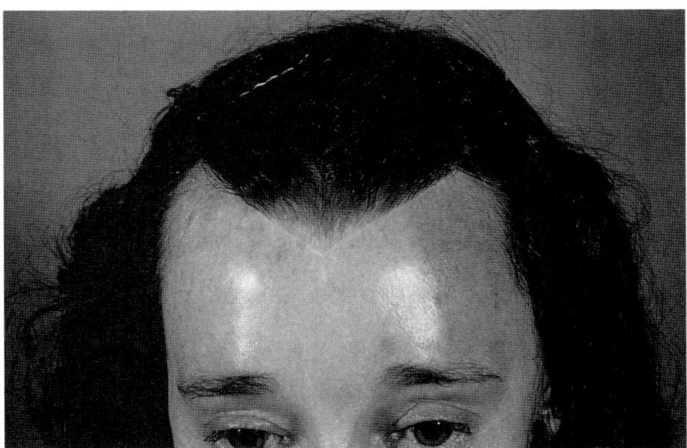

B

FIGURE 51-11. A: A well-designed and executed hairline incision meanders and is hidden within the fine hairs of the anterior hairline. In properly selected patients, this incision can minimize forehead lengthening. **B:** A poorly designed straight-line incision has produced a contrived and unnatural anterior hairline.

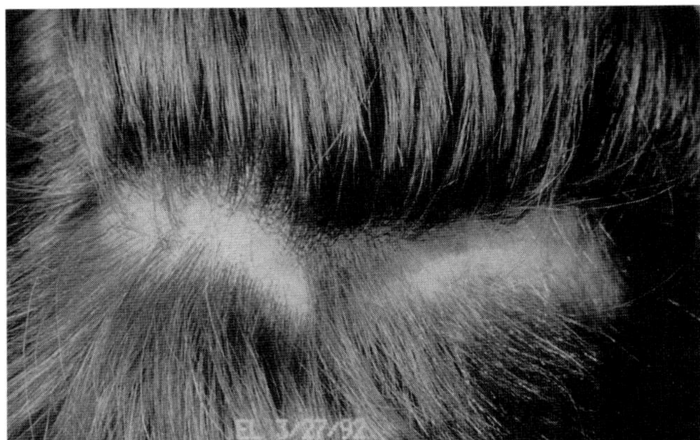

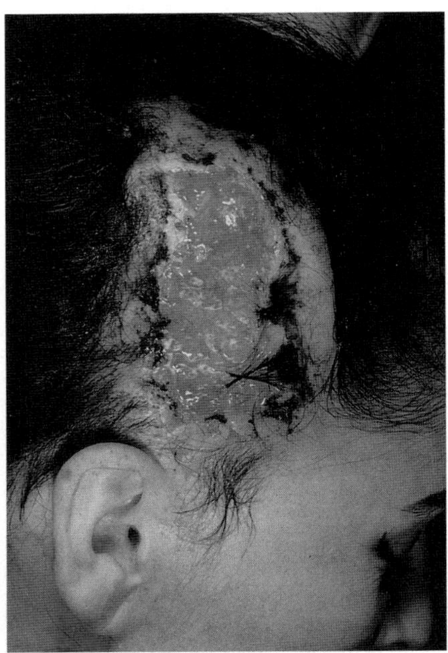

FIGURE 51-12. A: Typical appearance of tension-related alopecia. Transferring the tension load to the galea below the level of the follicle can minimize these events. **B:** A larger scalp slough secondary to infection.

trophic scar, tension-related alopecia, or at the worst, formal scalp slough (Fig. 51-12). Tension on the closure may be minimized by better release of the soft tissues in the lateral orbit and distributing the tension along the closure of the galea in a two-layered fashion. In most modern endoscopic techniques, skin tension is circumvented by the use of suture fixation between the galea and some form of bone anchor. The two most popular methods remain the outer-table cortical bone tunnel and the fixation of Gore-Tex tabs the outer table with titanium microscrews. Although certainly fraught with their own problems, these techniques minimize the tension-related complications seen with the traditional open browlift.

THE FACE

Accurately designed incisions are essential to producing natural results in a facelift procedure. Visible scars and the structures they distort can render a facelift painfully obvious to even a casual observer. During flap redraping and closure, excessive tension can cause migration and distortion even with properly planned incisions.

A telltale stigma of the retrotragal incision is distortion of the tragus (Fig. 51-13A). Here, a flap that was cut too short has produced tension and anterior movement with flattening during scar maturation. The natural sulcus anterior to the tragus is obliterated, and one can look directly into the ear canal. If a retrotragal incision is chosen, it must be executed in such a way that the natural anatomy is not distorted and the principal reason for its use defeated. The tragus should be visualized as a vertically oriented rectangle. The facelift incision should proceed inferiorly as it emerges from the temporal hair and form a curve parallel to the helical rim as it approaches the superior edge of the tragus. The width of the helix in the upper portion of the ear should be maintained by the incision as it descends. At the superior edge of the tragus, the incision should turn 90 degrees posteriorly for several millimeters to define this upper border. At the superoposterior edge of the helix, the incision makes a second 90-degree turn inferiorly to run along the posterior edge. The third side of the tragal rectangle is formed by another 90-degree turn anteriorly along its most caudal extent. Here, the incision makes a last 90-degree turn inferiorly within the crease between the lobe and the face. It should be noted that the flap should be trimmed to fit in a similar fashion without any tension. A redundancy of several millimeters of skin flap over the tragus produces the most natural results. The fat of the facial skin flap overlying the sulcus anterior to the tragus should be removed to re-create this natural recess (Fig. 51-13B). Pretragal incisions should be considered if careful preservation of this important structure is not feasible. Male patients may do better with pretragal incisions, so that beard growth on this important landmark is avoided.

Anterior and inferior migration of the earlobe is produced when the cervicofacial flap is cut too short (Fig. 51-14). Tension in this area serves no function other than to produce distortion. Excessive skin tension in this region causes flattening of the normal contours of the buccal recess. One to two millimeters of facial skin should be preserved

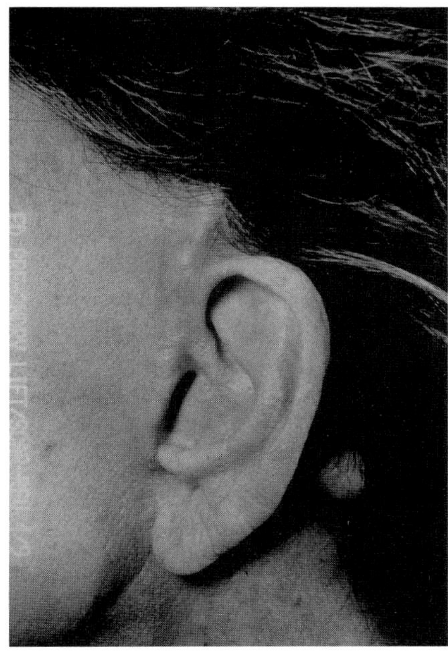

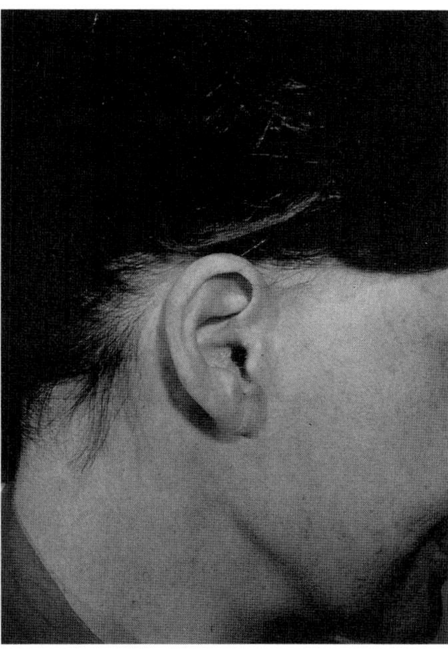

A, B

FIGURE 51-13. A: The common stigma of distortion following retrotragal incisions. Note the flattening and anterior displacement with loss of the pretragal sulcus. **B:** A well-designed retrotragal incision preserving the natural landmarks of the region.

along the caudal border of the earlobe incision to maintain a "detached" earlobe. The lobe normally has an independent axis of −15 degrees (posterior) relative to the axis of the main portion of the ear (Fig. 51-13B). The lobe should be inset as a separate structure to preserve this orientation.

Hairline shifts may occur anywhere that flaps are advanced to bring non–hair-bearing skin into a position previously occupied by hair-bearing skin (Figs. 51-2, 51-8, 51-11B, 51-13A). Care should be taken in planning incisions and flap movement before surgery. The most common and distressing hairline shifts are those within the temple. Here, the natural sideburn becomes obliterated by the advancement of the non–hair-bearing facial skin. This scenario makes it impossible for a female patient to wear her hair pulled back. These situations should be anticipated, and the surgeon should alter the pattern of incisions accordingly. The use of anterior temporal hairline incisions and small triangular darts below the sideburns can eliminate this problem in most instances. Hairline step-offs are produced where incisions cross hair-bearing and non–hair-bearing skin segments. Step-offs along the postauricular hairline can be prevented by proper alignment during advancement and closure of the flap.

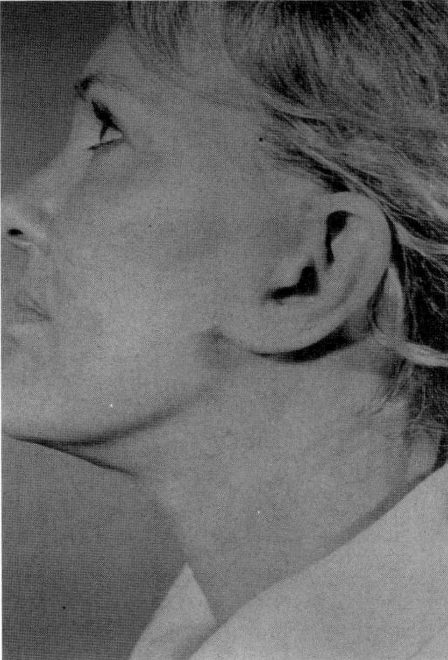

FIGURE 51-14. Earlobe distortion is produced when the cervicofacial flap is trimmed too short. The cheek is in effect hung on the ear. The creation of the "pixie ear" deformity distorts the normal −15-degree axis of the lobe relative to the body of the ear. Correction of this problem poses a difficult surgical challenge.

Hypertrophic scars may occur anywhere along the facelift incision but form most commonly in the postauricular portions of the wound (Fig. 51-13A). It is here that the tension is greatest. Additionally, flexion, extension, and rotation of the cervical spine exaggerate the tension. These forces are at times strong enough to force the scar to migrate well beyond the location of the original incision. Hypertrophic scar formation also depends on skin type. As the melanin content of the skin increases, so does its propensity toward unfavorable scarring. Facelift techniques designed to distribute most of the tension toward the deeper structures (superficial musculoaponeurotic system [SMAS] and platysma) allow the surgeon to redrape and inset the cervicofacial flap without these adverse forces. The SMAS-platysma cervical hammock, rather than the skin, is used as the vehicle to tighten the anterior neck laxity. Once established, hypertrophic scars may be treated by the intralesional injection of steroids at 6- to 8-week intervals. Scar revisions are reserved for those patients who do not respond to steroids.

An injury to the motor branch of the facial nerve is perhaps the most feared and untreatable complication arising in surgery of the face and brow (Fig. 51-15A,B). As surgical techniques in facial rejuvenation become more sophisticated, we are becoming more familiar with the facial nerve. Surgeons unfamiliar with the nuances and variability of its anatomy should spend considerable time observing procedures and perhaps even dissecting in the laboratory before attempting new techniques. Nerve injury is prevented by a knowledge of its *three-dimensional anatomy.* The routine skin flap elevation in any facelift proceeds over the course of all branches of the facial nerve and the great auricular nerve. Thus, knowledge of the two-dimensional course of the nerve within the face is of limited value. Knowing where within the layers of the face the nerve courses guides the surgeon through safe dissections. The anatomy within the face may be thought of as a series of concentric layers. The main branches of the facial nerve are protected proximally by the parotid gland. As they emerge from the anterior edge of the gland, they become more vulnerable to injury. The parotid-masseteric fascia is a thin, semitransparent glistening layer covering the branches of the facial nerve as they emerge from the edge of the parotid gland. Maintaining the integrity of this deep fascia is important, as all the branches of the facial nerve within the cheek lie deep to this layer.

Divisions of large branches of the facial nerve discovered at the time of surgery should be repaired immediately under magnification. Because of numerous cross communications between the branches of the facial nerve, many distal injuries to small segments will, over time, improve clinically. With frontal branch injuries, botulinum toxin injections to the innervated side of the forehead can improve symmetry until healing occurs. Injuries to the great auricular nerve produce numbness in the pinna and can be quite distressing to the patient. These nerves should be repaired if possible. Established neuromas of the great auricular nerve need to be explored and excised, and the ends should be buried separately in the sternocleidomastoid muscle. The spinal accessory nerve (eleventh cranial nerve) may be injured in the posterior triangle of the neck during elevation of the flap (Fig. 51-15C). The nerve exits the jugular foramen at the cranial base and perforates the fibers of the posterior portion of the sternocleidomastoid muscle. From here, it traverses the posterior cervical triangle just beneath the cervical fascia to the underside of the trapezius muscle. Dissection should be above the level of the cervical fascia to protect the nerve throughout its entire course.

Injuries to the integrity of the parotid gland may result in the accumulation of parotid fluid beneath the flap (Fig. 51-16). Significant accumulations may drain through the incision as a parotid "fistula." The cause of these problems is injury to the gland during dissection. Techniques that el-

A, B

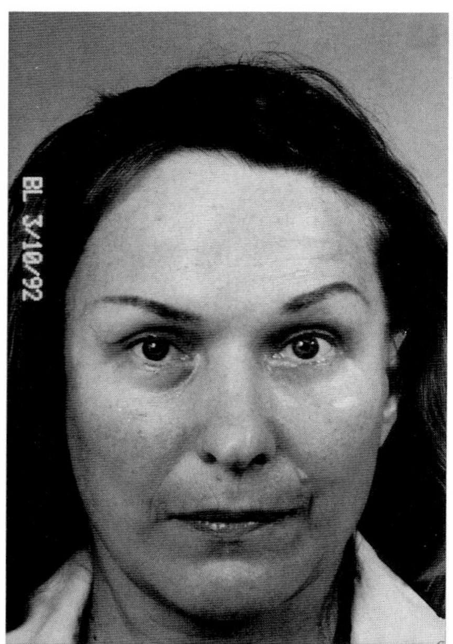

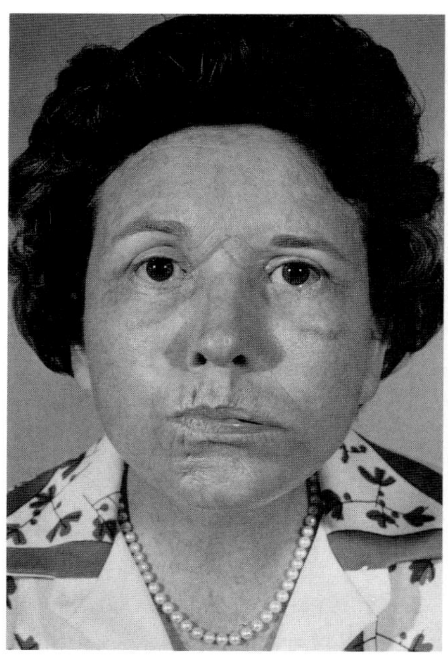

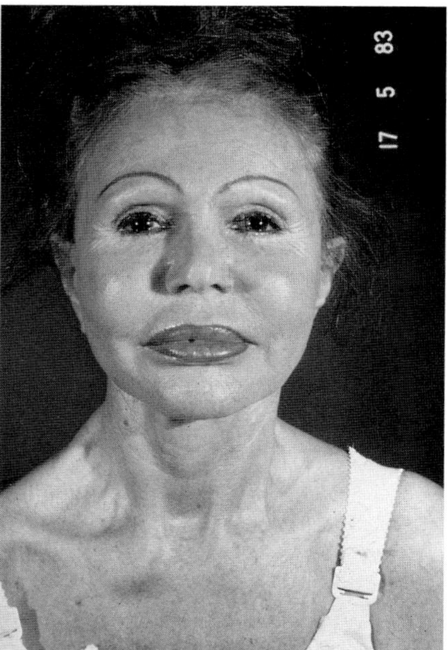

C

FIGURE 51-15. A: Appearance of an injury to the right frontal branch of the facial nerve. Note the absence of forehead rhytids on the affected side. **B:** A more proximal injury to multiple branches of the nerve. **C:** Appearance following injury to the left spinal accessory nerve (cranial nerve XI). Note the loss of mass of the left trapezius muscle. The eleventh cranial nerve can be injured in the posterior triangle of the neck where it lies immediately beneath the cervical fascia. (Part C from Baker TJ, Gordon HL. *Surgical rejuvenation of the face.* St. Louis: Mosby, 1986:211, with permission.)

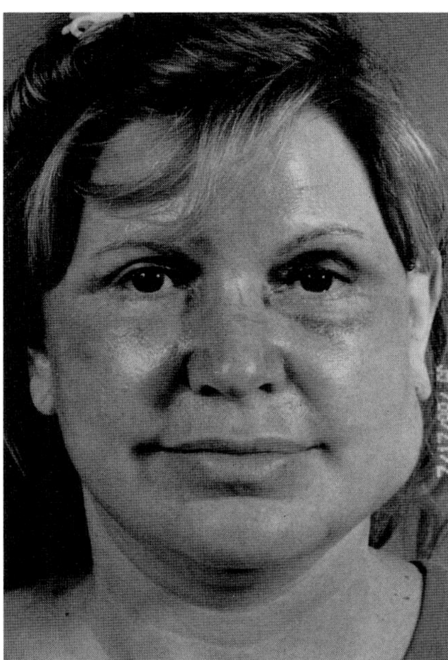

FIGURE 51-16. Appearance 1 week after surgery of a patient with a left parotid cyst. After aspiration of straw-colored fluid with a high amylase content, the cyst collapsed and did not recur.

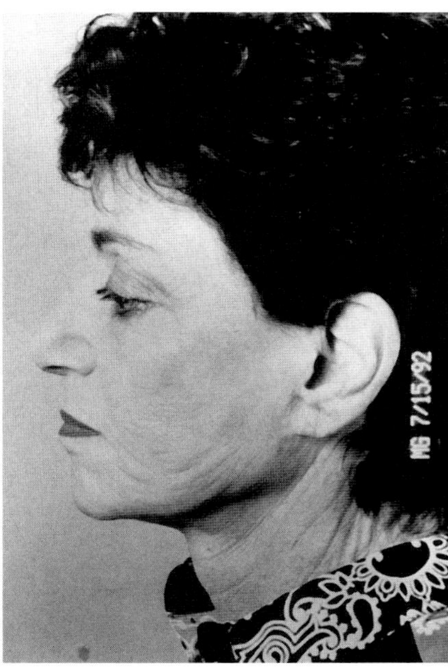

FIGURE 51-17. Lines of misdirection may become evident when the skin is used as the primary vehicle of restoration. Note that despite significant distortion in the lines of skin in the face, the jowl remains redundant.

evate the SMAS are more likely to violate the parenchyma of the gland. Small collections present within a few days and can be aspirated with a needle on two or three separate occasions. Reaccumulations or communication with the outside as a fistula warrants insertion of a closed-system suction drain until the defect seals itself and the drainage diminishes. Two to four weeks may be required for closure of the parotid leak. The origin of the fluid is established by a high amylase content. Injuries to the parotid duct are rare. The presentation is more dramatic and is usually manifested as fistulous drainage to the outside. Sialogram confirms the diagnosis. Consultation with an otorhinolaryngologist is generally required to reestablish the course of the duct surgically.

The creation of a distorted, operated look is perhaps the quintessential error of aesthetic judgment (Figs. 51-8, 51-17). Lines of misdirection in the facial skin are created by overly zealous undermining and subsequent advancement and rotation of the skin flap. More natural appearances can be created by placing the tension and the more superior vectors of movement within the deeper layers of the face and allowing the skin to redrape in a more horizontal vector. Even the most elegantly performed facelift entails some degree of facial change. This distortion increases proportionally with secondary and tertiary procedures. Patients are undergoing their first facelift earlier, and life expectancy continues to increase. Inevitably, a larger percentage of patients will have multiple facelifts. More than ever, we must strive to avoid the stigmata of surgical distortion.

THE NECK

The proper restoration of contour within the neck is an integral part of a successful facelift. Skin, fat, and muscle must be individually considered and addressed. All modern facelift techniques address cervical laxity with a submental incision. Generally speaking, some form of edge-to-edge plication of the platysma muscle along the midline is performed. Transverse platysmal myotomies relieve tension along the midline, allow the repaired muscle to elongate slightly, and reestablish the cervicomental angle. In patients with short, tight platysmal bands, mytomies also make it possible to avoid converting two paramedian platysmal bands into a single midline band.

Long transverse or complete platysmal myotomies may make it possible to visualize the anterior belly of the digastric muscle (Fig. 51-18). Division of the anterior belly eliminates this problem.

The direct excision of redundant skin in the anterior neck should be discouraged. Inasmuch as most facelift techniques can correct even the most severe laxity, the scars resulting from direct excision are not warranted (Fig. 51-19). In addition, most necks require some form of platysmal tightening for optimal results, so that a posterior approach is required.

Ptosis of the submandibular gland may become more evident when the overlying soft tissues are tightened. The gland is subject to the same factors of aging as the overlying skin and platysma, and it should be examined and any

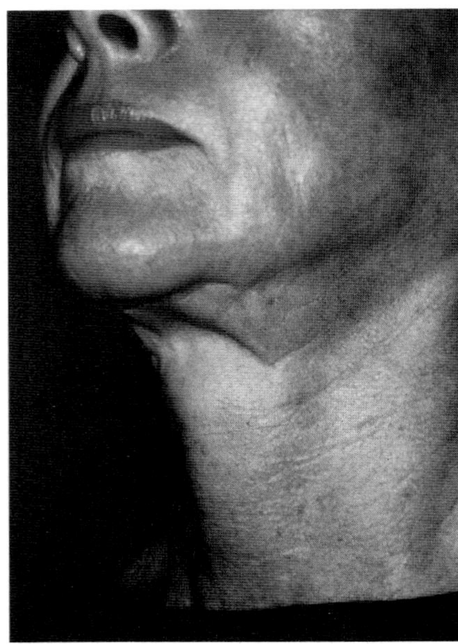

FIGURE 51-18. Complete division of the platysma muscle may create a gap that results in visibility of the anterior belly of the digastric muscle.

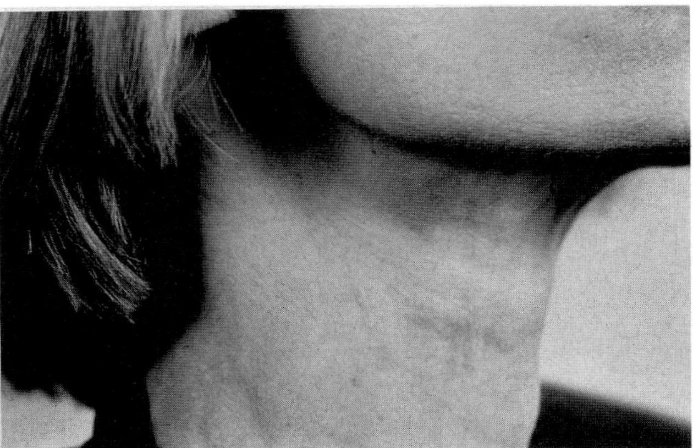

FIGURE 51-20. Excessive resection of the cervical fat produces a harsh, skeletonized appearance. Fat preserved within the neck gives a softer, more youthful look.

problems discussed with the patient before surgery. Correction is difficult and is limited to suture-assisted reefing of the overlying platysma. Direct excision of the gland is usually best avoided.

Fat is an important structure in the youthful neck. If properly proportioned, it softens and feminizes the visible contours within the neck. Overly aggressive suctioning and direct excision of cervical fat leave the neck appearing barren, harsh, and skeletonized (Fig. 51-20). Care should be taken during elevation of the cervical skin flap to preserve a uniform, healthy layer on the undersurface. Excess fat may then be cautiously and conservatively excised under direct vision.

Extensive platysmal work or small unrecognized collections within the neck may organize as regions of significant induration (Fig. 51-21). These areas become evident within

A

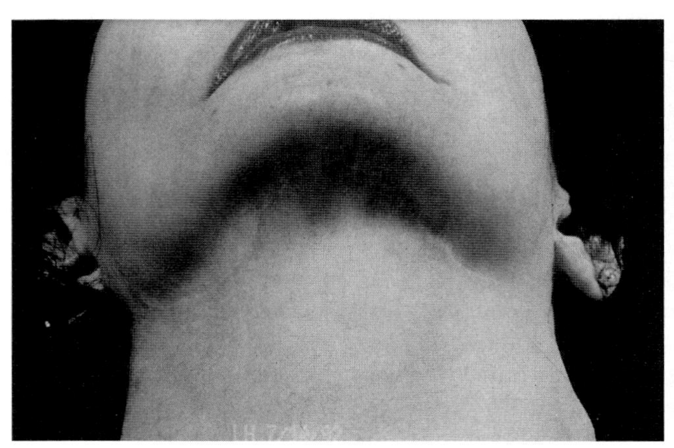

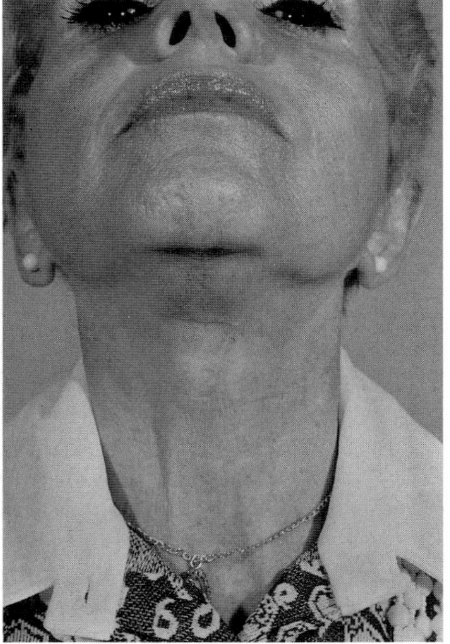

B

FIGURE 51-19. A,B: Two different but equally unacceptable approaches to direct excision of excess cervical skin. These incisions routinely produce poor scars in highly visible locations. Standard facelift incisions can produce equal or superior results in contour without such conspicuous scars. (Part A from Baker TJ, Gordon HL, Stuzin JM. *Surgical rejuvenation of the face,* 2nd ed. St. Louis: Mosby, 1996:326, with permission.)

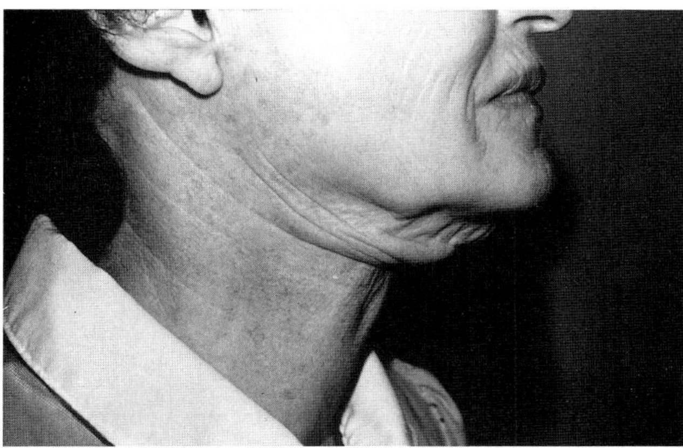

FIGURE 51-21. Seromas may organize and form palpable or even visible indurated masses, particularly in the submental region. Ultrasound treatments delivered via a small paddle directly into the affected area (8 to 10 W/cm^2) significantly speed the resolution of these problems.

the few weeks following surgery and sometimes require several weeks to months to resolve. Transcutaneous ultrasound therapy (8 to 10 W/cm^2) for 15 minutes two to three times each week dramatically speeds resolution.

CONCLUSION

Despite our most diligent efforts, a small percentage of patients undergoing browlift or facelift experience a true surgical complication. It is our awesome responsibility to take all the necessary precautions to limit these events. Most of the unfavorable outcomes resulting from errors of judgment can be prevented by thorough planning and surgical execution. Only through the continued evaluation of our own work can we take the next step forward toward better results. Plastic surgery has no "measuring stick" by which the quality of a result can be evaluated objectively. The desired result is what is aesthetically pleasing. It is our responsibility as aesthetic surgeons to "raise the bar" and continue to challenge ourselves by expanding the possibilities.

SUGGESTED READING

Baker TJ, Gordon HL, Stuzin JM. *Surgical rejuvenation of the face,* 2nd ed. St. Louis: Mosby, 1996.

Baker TM, Stuzin JM, Baker TJ, et al. What's new in aesthetic surgery? *Clin Plast Surg* 1996;23:3–16.

Byrd HS. The extended browlift. *Clin Plast Surg* 1997;24:233–246.

Chang LD. Cigarette smoking, plastic surgery, and microsurgery. *J Reconstr Microsurg* 1996;12:467–474.

Connell BF. The forehead lift: techniques to avoid complications and produce optimal results. *Aesthetic Plast Surg* 1989;13:217–237.

Connell BF. The significance of digastric muscle contouring for rejuvenation of the submental area of the face. *Plast Reconstr Surg* 1997;99:1586–1590.

Ellenbogen R. Avoiding visual tipoffs to face lift surgery. A troubleshooting guide. *Clin Plast Surg* 1992;19:447–454.

Gunter JP. Aesthetic analysis of the eyebrows. *Plast Reconstr Surg* 1997;99:1808–1816.

Guyuron B. Secondary rhytidectomy. *Plast Reconstr Surg* 1997;100:1281–1284.

Guyuron B. Refinements in endoscopic forehead rejuvenation. *Clin Plast Surg* 1997;100:154–160.

Knize DM. Limited incision foreheadplasty. *Plast Reconstr Surg* 1999;103:271–284; discussion, 285–290.

Marten TJ. Facelift planning and technique. *Clin Plast Surg* 1997;24:269–308.

Stuzin JM, Baker TJ, Gordon HL. The relationship of the superficial and deep facial fascia: relevance to rhytidectomy and aging. *Plast Reconstr Surg* 1992;89:441.

Stuzin JM, Baker TJ, Gordon HL, et al. Extended SMAS dissection as an approach to midface rejuvenation. *Clin Plast Surg* 1995;22:295–311.

Wolfort FG, Baker TM, Kanter WR. Aesthetic goals in blepharoplasty. In: Wolfort FG, Kanter WR, eds. *Aesthetic blepharoplasty.* Boston: Little, Brown and Company, 1994.

Discussion

BROWLIFT AND FACELIFT

RAFAEL DE LA PLAZA

I would first like to say that the authors, Tracy M. Baker, Thomas J. Baker, and James M. Stuzin, have presented an excellent review of unfavorable results in browlift and facelift surgery based on their unequaled experience of 10,000 cases treated during the last 40 years. The differences in age between the authors, and the fact that one of them is an accredited anatomist as well as a surgeon, provide a broad view of the evolution of this area of surgery and lend great credibility to their opinions and advice. I am honored to have been invited to comment on this chapter, and at the same time challenged owing to the professional status of these three surgeons. Nevertheless, I accept the challenge with pleasure. I would like to add some personal thoughts and, if possible, supplement their discussion in ways that might be useful to the reader.

COMPLICATIONS

Complications are the bane of our profession, and no surgeon can avoid them entirely. The word *complication* has a negative connotation, but complications do not necessarily lead to an unfavorable result. If anything positive can be said about complications, it is that they are a source of learning, provided the surgeon objectively analyzes the possible causes and does not adopt the attitude that the patient or sheer chance is to blame. In my opinion, *unfavorable results* and *complications* are imprecise terms commonly used in medical jargon that can cause confusion when surgical technique and ability are assessed. In a strict sense and within the field of surgery, we can define complications as conditions that occur during an operation or the postoperative period. Such conditions can interfere with the expected outcome of a surgical procedure and the well-being of the patient. On occasion, the cause cannot be determined. Alternatively, the cause can be an unforeseen event, such as an attack of coughing, an unexpected rise of blood pressure, or trauma, or a pathologic process that was not detected during the preoperative study. Examples include allergic reactions, hematoma, infections, hypertrophic scars, or even keloids.

Rafael de la Plaza: Centro de Quemados y Cirugia Plastica Cruj Roja, Universidad Compluteuse, Madrid, Spain

I agree with the authors that the most frequent complication in facelift surgery is the formation of a hematoma. Among the causes of hematomas are certain coagulopathies that are not detected by routine preoperative tests. Patients with such conditions may have no history of abnormal bleeding or hematoma if they have not previously sustained any significant trauma or undergone surgery. Clinically, during the operation, we may notice more bleeding than usual. In the immediate postoperative period, blood accumulates under the undermined areas and in the nearby tissues. Extension into the neck can create respiratory problems through compression. Unlike ordinary hematomas, which are usually unilateral, hematomas after facelift are often bilateral, and the ecchymosis extends over nearly the entire face and neck. Surgical exploration does not generally reveal the presence of significant bleeding from vessels, only subtle oozing and infiltration of the tissues. When this type of coagulopathy is suspected, a hematologist should be contacted immediately and treatment begun with cryoprecipitates, fresh plasma, or DDAVP (deamino-8-D-arginine vasopressin) to supply the patient with the needed coagulation factors. During my professional career, I have encountered three cases with this type of pathology—one after a rhinoplasty, another after breast augmentation, and the third after a facelift. Although therapeutic action was rapidly undertaken, all these cases caused me enormous stress, considerably delayed the patients' recuperation, and jeopardized the final result. Fortunately, coagulopathies, which can be either hereditary (generally varieties of von Willebrand's disease) or acquired, are not very frequent. During the preoperative study, it is advisable to measure the bleeding time with an Ivy test, which is much more precise than the classic prick in the earlobe.

Another suggested cause of hematoma is the use of anesthesia with controlled hypotension, which is thought to cause frequent rebound effects. My observation is that controlled hypotension does not cause rebound effects in the way that vasoconstrictors do. The arterial blood pressure is raised or lowered by the anesthetist as requested by the surgeon according to the phase of the operation and within the appropriate limits for each patient. The systolic blood pressure is raised periodically to 90 or 100 mm Hg for hemostasis, and at the end of the operation, the anesthesiologist raises the pressure slowly to the level appropriate for the individual patient. Some surgeons favor the use of a compressive dressing, as I do, both in cases with controlled hypotension and in those managed with infiltration of vasoconstrictive agents.

ERRORS

Apart from complications in a strict sense, many other factors can lead to unfavorable results, as described by the authors. I would, however, use a slightly different classification:

- Errors committed by the surgeon during the operation
- Errors in the postoperative period
- Errors in patient selection
- Errors in aesthetic judgment and the undesirable effects of surgical manipulation of tissues

I will comment briefly on each of these.

Errors Committed by the Surgeon during the Operation

The authors have discussed most of these errors, and so I will simply list them:

1. Injuries to nerves or other anatomical structures (e.g., Stensen duct, lacrimal duct, large vessels)
2. Very superficial undermining of the skin with risk for ischemia
3. Closure under excessive tension and consequent ischemia
4. Infection resulting from lack of adherence to the principles of sterile technique
5. Asymmetries
6. Excessive or unevenly placed compressive bandages

Errors in the Postoperative Period

The surgeon, ancillary staff, or patient may make errors in the postoperative period. To prevent them, it is essential that the surgeon provide precise written instructions to the ancillary staff and patient regarding such matters as general positioning of the body and neck, medication, hygiene and asepsis, and the application of ice.

Errors in Patient Selection

I totally agree with the authors' recommendations regarding this important area. The plastic surgeon must elicit the reasons for a consultation within a 20- to 30-minute period. Within that period, the surgeon must evaluate the medical, mental, and social status of the patient, any medications being taken, and possible addictions, and then, taking all these factors into account plus the results of preoperative tests, suggest the correct treatment. The possibility of medicolegal action impels us to be cautious. If even the slightest doubt exists, we should, as the authors suggest, consult the patient's primary care physician and, if the patient has been or is under psychiatric care, the psychiatrist. The opinion of these colleagues regarding the possible benefits of surgery to the patient, the best timing, medication during the preoperative and postoperative phases, and follow-up will be invaluable when the decision is made whether to operate. They can also indicate what psychological control will be necessary postoperatively. When in doubt, I advise patients to postpone their decision, return once or twice more for consultation, and invite them, if they have come alone, to bring along a friend or relative. This practice allows me to get to know them better and appreciate the kind of support they will receive during the postoperative period.

It is essential to know what medications the patient is taking, particularly those that might interfere with hemostasis. It is not only medications containing aspirin that must be considered. Many patients regularly take medications that they forget about or do not think necessary to mention, such as peripheral vasodilators and vitamin E. These substances can cause problems with bleeding, particularly vitamin E at high doses, which is often recommended by dermatologists and other health care professionals. Furthermore, natural medicines are becoming more and more popular; for example, some patients take two or three cloves of garlic or a garlic concentrate capsule daily. It has been shown that the antiinflammatory and analgesic properties of garlic, which also increase the peripheral circulation, can be attributed to an active substance that is very similar to acetylsalicylic acid. I routinely ask patients to stop taking these products 3 weeks before surgery.

Errors in Aesthetic Judgment and Undesirable Effects of the Surgical Manipulation of Tissues

The authors correctly state that the most common unfavorable results in aesthetic surgery of the face and brow are caused by errors of aesthetic judgment. However, equally or even more important is what I refer to as the *undesirable effects of the surgical manipulation of tissues* (1). Obviously, the unfavorable results in both cases are caused by the manipulation of tissues, so what is the difference? In the first case, the cause is technical or mechanical; excessive or inadequate traction of the tissues, performed voluntarily by the surgeon based on erroneous aesthetic criteria, results in overcorrection or distortion of the face. In the second case, the unfavorable result is a consequence of the technique itself and the cause is anatomical—malpositioning, lengthening, sectioning, excising, denervating, and transposing muscles. Such practices can result in serious disturbances in facial expression for which the surgeon alone is responsible, having chosen an inappropriate technique even if it was performed well. We must be cautious when manipulating the muscles and very careful to reestablish the equilibrium between agonistic and antagonistic forces.

We must remember that the great majority of the patients simply want facial rejuvenation. As the authors rightly say, surgery must be directed toward correctly repositioning the tissues to recapture the appearance the patient had 8 or 10 years ago, without altering the normal appearance or expression. For this and other reasons, it is best to choose techniques that damage the tissues as little as possible, techniques I call *physiological* (1,2).

We therefore stress the importance of an extensive preoperative evaluation during the first consultation, which is not only static but also dynamic. The evaluation should be documented with photographs for comparison and a better analysis of the postoperative results.

I also have a few comments to make regarding the anatomical areas considered by the authors.

THE BROW

The techniques of the classic bicoronal incision and the endoscopic forehead lift are evaluated correctly. Loss of sensitivity in the scalp behind the line of the bicoronal incision, with the typical sequence of anesthesia, hypesthesia, and paresthesia, is an excellent example of the undesirable effects inherent in the technique itself that causes patients to complain for several months postoperatively. With the endoscopic technique, of course, these problems are minimized, as is alopecia, which is also unusual in the bicoronal technique when subgaleal or subperiosteal planes are followed and no tension is created in the suture line.

Of the two other alternative approaches to the browlift, one is through an incision in each temporal region, which is very useful when we do not have to manipulate the corrugators, the procerus muscles, or both. The other is through minimal incisions without endoscopy, plus the incision used in upper blepharoplasty when we must perform an upper lid blepharoplasty. The endoscopic technique requires costly equipment and prolonged training if complications are to be avoided and adequate results obtained, whereas the two techniques mentioned above can be performed without special instruments or simply with a simple cold light retractor.

THE FACE

When a pretragal incision is used, in addition to calculating the resection to avoid tension in the suture, we should thin the flap to reproduce the small preauricular depression and insert three transcutaneous-transcartilagenous stitches with a 4-0 to 5-0 monofilament suture. Two of these stitches start from the interior of the tragus, penetrate the skin, cartilage, and dermis of the flap, and return to the interior of the concha, where they are tied. The third stitch starts from the interior of the crus helicis and penetrates the skin and cartilage. Then, after taking the dermis of the flap, it returns, like the others, to be tied in the interior of the crus (Fig. 51D-1). These stitches provide an excellent adaptation of the skin edges and free the suture line from all tension, so that the cutaneous stitches can be removed on the fourth or fifth day. The three stitches described above should be maintained until the tenth day.

To avoid widening and posterior and inferior migration of the retroauricular scars, it is very useful to take three or four mattress stitches passing through the raw depth of the fold (Fig. 51D-2). These stitches not only prevent widening and migration of the scar but also act to suspend the retroauricular flap, which is completed with a small, triangular, deepithelized flap in the horizontal area of the first.

To prevent nerve injury, the authors correctly emphasize the importance of three-dimensional anatomy. However, some of the techniques designed in the last few years violate the principles of anatomical safety underlying the prevention of nerve injuries. For example, we cannot establish a continuous plane of dissection between the preauricular and

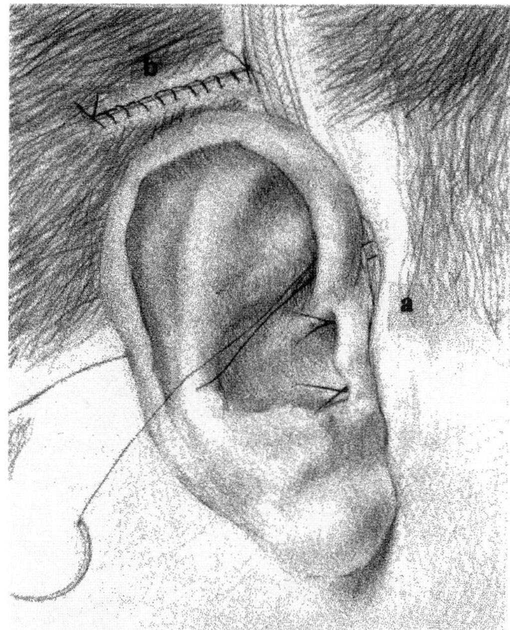

FIGURE 51D-1. a: Transcutaneous-transcartilaginous stitches to relieve tension in the pretragal incision. **b:** I frequently perform a triangular excision of the scalp above the ear to avoid the dropping of the same and to even the length of the sutured edges of the temporal incision.

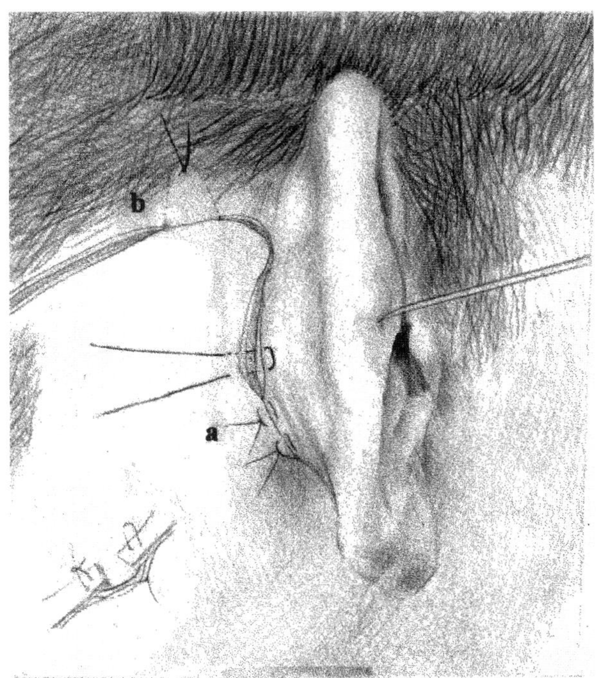

FIGURE 51D-2. a: Mattress stitches passing through the depth of the retroauricular fold to prevent widening and caudal migration of the scar. **b:** Small, triangular, deepithelized flap.

suborbicularis areas without interfering with the innervation of the orbicularis oculi muscle. The innervation of this muscle is from multiple branches that form a plexus shortly after or even before the zygomatic branch of the facial nerve emerges from the parotid gland. Any dissection plane chosen starting from the preauricular incision [superficial subcutaneous, deep subcutaneous, sub-SMAS (submuscular)] on its way to the suborbicularis oculi plane will cross this plexus. Injury to these branches can cause dystonia and dysfunction of the lids. This does not occur when a continuous sub-SMAS (supraperiosteal) plane is followed through the temporal incisions (2).

THE NECK

The authors discuss unfavorable results in the neck extensively and analyze causes and prevention. I wish to add three points:

1. The neck is where perhaps asymmetries are most frequent. These can originate in the platysma, fat, submandibular glands, or the skin itself. Asymmetries should be documented statically and dynamically during the preoperative study, and patients should be informed that they cannot always be completely corrected.
2. Muscles in general and particularly the platysma do not relax with age, except when pathologic conditions are present; on the contrary, they become fibrous, shorter, or even hypertrophic (1). They can also become displaced caudally, so that the face loses its oval shape at the horizontal contour of the mandible. The rules to be followed in surgery of the platysma are based on this information. I agree with almost everything the authors say, except in regard to posterior traction of the platysma.
3. In cases of great cutaneous laxity, traction on the cervical flap upward and backward, as is usual, can give rise to a noticeably receding, uneven hairline. It can also create the appearance of oblique cutaneous folds because of insufficient correction of cervical laxity. This unfavorable result can be avoided or corrected by making incisions on the hairline. This practice allows for ample skin resections and consequently makes it possible to tighten the skin. On the other hand, as we are usually treating older patients, the scars are generally of good quality and easily hidden by the hair.

REFERENCES

1. De la Plaza R, de la Cruz L. Can some facial rejuvenation techniques cause iatrogeny? *Aesthetic Plast Surg* 1994;18:205.
2. De la Plaza R, de la Cruz L. Lifting of the upper two-thirds of the face: supraperiosteal–sub-SMAS versus subperiosteal approach. The quest for physiological surgery. *Plast Reconstr Surg* 1998; 102:2178.

52

SUBPERIOSTEAL FACELIFT

OSCAR M. RAMIREZ

An unfavorable result is any outcome of a surgical procedure that either the patient or the surgeon finds unsatisfactory. An unfavorable result can be gross medical negligence, a complication, an unsatisfactory aesthetic or functional outcome, or expected morbidity that can be either temporary or permanent.

This chapter describes various expected and unexpected complications, and some undesirable although expected forms of morbidity. Methods to avoid or minimize complications and surgical morbidity are also discussed.

SUBPERIOSTEAL APPROACH TO FACELIFT SURGERY

The subperiosteal approach to facelift surgery has been designed to rejuvenate the central oval of the face, including the frontal forehead, brows, glabella, periorbital soft tissues, tear troughs, nasolabial folds, marionette lines, corners of the mouth, and, to a lesser extent, jowls. A more aggressive approach during the subperiosteal facelift can also improve the orbital rims and change the shape of the eyelid socket, chin, and mandible (Fig. 52-1). The subcutaneous repositioning and redraping of excess skin via a cervicofacial rhytidectomy is a complementary technique that improves the lower nasolabial fold, jaw line, jowls, and neck.

Based on my extensive experience, I believe that a combination of these two planes of dissection—subperiosteal for the central oval and subcutaneous for the peripheral semicircle—is the safest way to provide a comprehensive, balanced, total facial rejuvenation (Fig. 52-2). However, like any other technique, this approach has gone through an unavoidable learning curve. Before the unfavorable results of the subperiosteal facelift are described, it is necessary to summarize the evolution of this technique because the rate of complications and unfavorable results is different for each stage of its development.

O. M. Ramirez: Plastic & Aesthetic Surgical Center of Maryland, Lutherville, Maryland

The subperiosteal facelift evolved through six stages:

1. Early development of Tessier's technique, popularized by Psillakis, Krastinova-Lolov, and others (1–4)
2. Period of the extended subperiosteal facelift with use of the temporal fascia suspension flap (5–8)
3. Early development of the endoscopic approach with use of a limited subciliary incision for the midface (9–11)
4. Development of multiplanar subperiosteal-*supra*-periosteal techniques (12)
5. Use of the "open" full blepharoplasty incision to approach the midface combined with a routine canthopexy (13,14)
6. Refinement of endoscopic techniques with avoidance of incisions in the lower eyelid (15–17)

A brief description of each technique enables one to understand the actual and potential complications of each variation.

1. *First stage.* Tessier and his followers approached the forehead through a coronal incision (1). Initially, the dissection was performed at the subgaleal layer. Then, the dissection was changed to the subperiosteal plane 2 cm above the orbital rim to enter the periorbita and in some instances the orbit itself. The transition from the subgaleal plane in the temporal area to the subperiosteal plane in the midface was accomplished with an incision in the periosteum directly on the superior border of the zygomatic arch. The midface was degloved at the subperiosteal plane. Canthopexy was performed almost routinely (2). Cheek augmentation was carried out occasionally with the use of bone harvested from the parietal area. Midface suspension was provided by the tension of the scalp closure after the necessary trimming of the scalp was performed. To overcome this weak point, Psillakis (3) used "fibroadipose" tissue suspension in the cheek area and Krastinova-Lolov (4) used deliberate canthoplasty and bone grafting in the cheek.
2. *Second stage.* To elevate the cheek more effectively and treat the nasolabial fold more reliably, the "extended" subperiosteal facelift initially used the intermediate and deep temporal fascia with an intervening layer of fat (in-

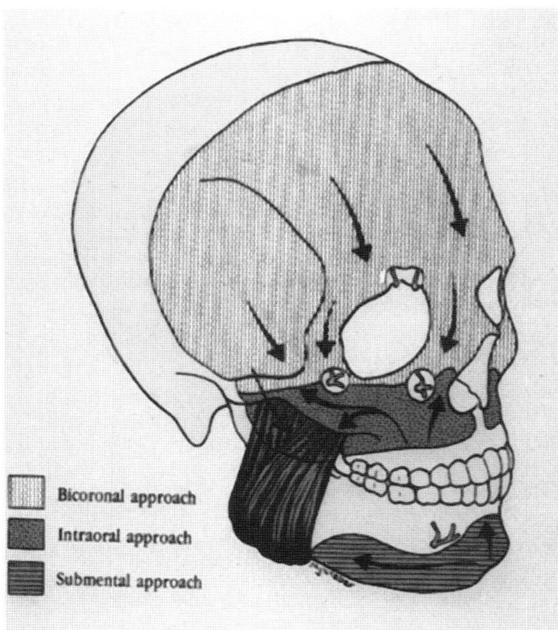

FIGURE 52-1. The traditional subperiosteal facelift is approached through a bicoronal incision for the upper face, an oral sulcus incision for the midface, and a submental incision for the mandible. This aggressive subperiosteal dissection significantly rejuvenates the central oval of the face in a plane that is very safe.

termediate fat pad) as a safer access to the zygomatic arch and a more effective means of suspension (5,6). Because temporal atrophy developed in some thin patients, the suspension was changed to include only the intermediate temporal fascia (7,8) (Fig. 52-3).

3. *Third stage.* When the endoforehead was extended to the midface, the initial access for the midface was via a limited lower blepharoplasty incision. The zygomatic periosteum was dissected in a retrograde fashion, and its connection with the temporal area was made easier and safer. The entire midface was dissected through the same blepharoplasty access. The suspension of the midface was changed to the suborbicularis oculi fat (SOOF) (Fig. 52-4). Canthopexy was performed selectively (9–11).
4. *Fourth stage.* This was a mixed technique in terms of planes of dissection in the midface. The temporal region was dissected at the subgaleal layer, the zygomatic arch at the subperiosteal plane, and the superior, lateral, and inferior orbital rim at the *supra*periosteal plane. From here, the dissection on the midface proceeded above the zygomaticus major muscle in the subcutaneous plane to the nasolabial fold (12).
5. *Fifth stage.* The endoscopic approach to the midface was converted to an "open" approach with the use of a full blepharoplasty incision to dissect the midface (13). The midface was suspended partly with the SOOF and partly with the orbicularis oculi, and the canthus was used to suspend the cheek and improve the tear trough. Others used exclusively periosteum for suspension (14). The zygomatic arch was not dissected, and the excess skin in the upper malar and temple areas was addressed by excising the scalp in the temporal area. The length of the temporal incision was about 6 cm or more.
6. *Sixth stage.* Because of the high rate of complications with the lower eyelid incision, the subperiosteal dissection of the midface was performed endoscopically, with few or no incisions made in key areas of the orbicularis oculi muscle. Three variations have been described. Each

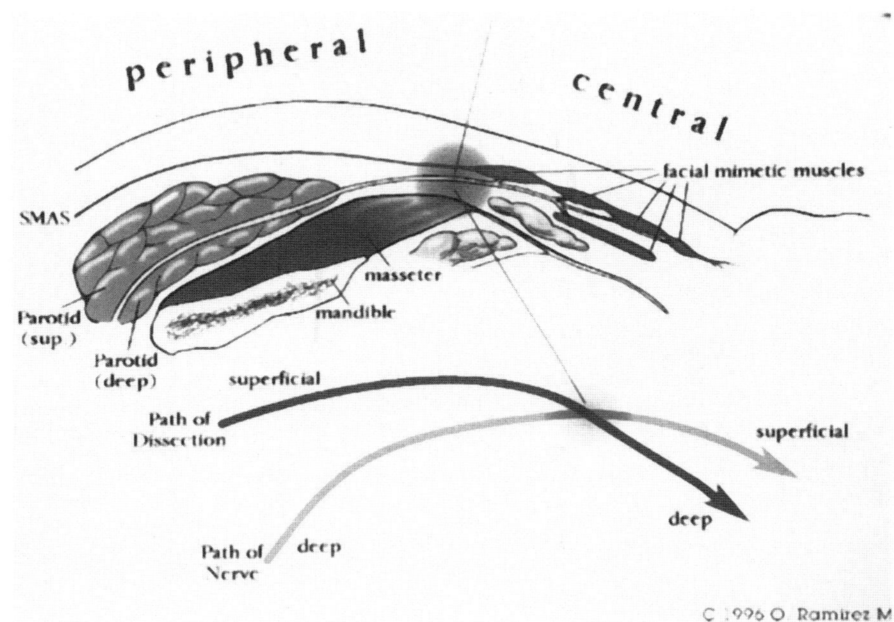

FIGURE 52-2. Subperiosteal facelift for the central oval and subcutaneous rhytidectomy for the peripheral semicircle of the face are the safest combination for a total facial rejuvenation. Intermediate-plane techniques tend to go from a superficial plane at the periphery to a deep plane at the center, whereas the branches of the facial nerve travel from a deep to a superficial plane. At the areas of potential decussation, the branches of the facial nerve can be injured.

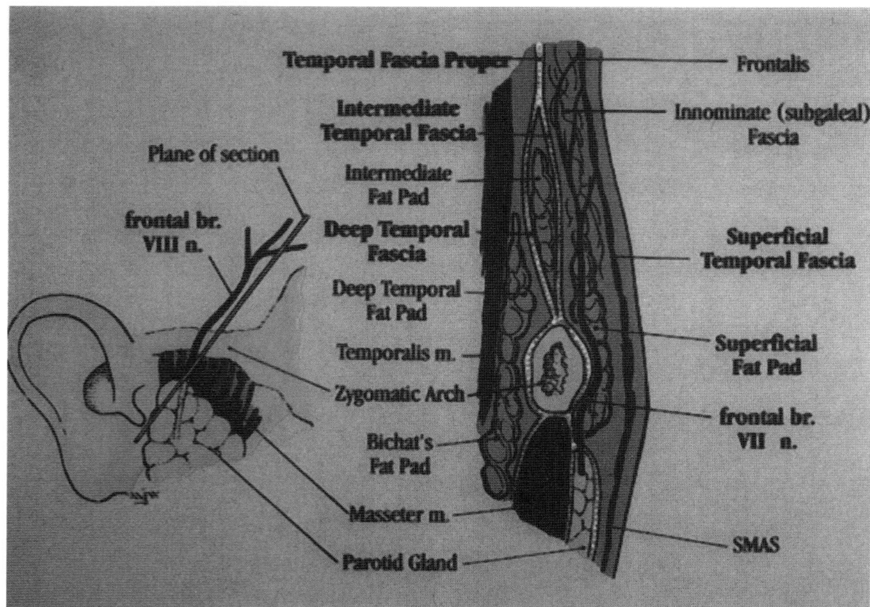

FIGURE 52-3. A thorough knowledge of the temporal anatomy, the relationship of the temporal fascia and fat pads, and the path of the frontal branch as it crosses from the midface to the frontal areas is critical in the approach to the zygomatic arch. This is performed at the subperiosteal plane, with the dissection started underneath the intermediate temporal fascia and continued inferiorly underneath the masseter fascia. The rest of the midface dissection, which is in the subperiosteal plane, is performed through the intraoral sulcus incision. (Reprinted from Ramirez OM. Endofacelift: subperiosteal approach. In: Ramirez OM, Daniel RK, eds. *Endoscopic plastic surgery.* New York: Springer-Verlag, 1996:109–126, with permission.)

can be adapted according to aesthetic need and the ability of the surgeon (15–18).

The first variant is a *crow's foot incision* with or without lateral canthotomy. This is an endoscope-dependent operation performed via 1.5-cm incision (18). The excess fat pads of the eyes are managed with the aid of the endoscope. The entire midface and half to two-thirds of the zygomatic arch are elevated at the subperiosteal plane. The dissection is extended to elevate the fascia of the masseter muscle for 2 to 3 cm inferiorly.

The second variation is performed via *orbicularis-sparing windows.* This is also an endoscope-dependent operation. The skin is elevated off the orbicularis oculi muscle for 1 to 1.5 cm. Two windows, one for the endoscope and another for the periosteal elevator, are made in the most inferior portion of the exposed orbicularis oculi muscle. These are created by blunt separation of muscle fibers without transection. The rest of the surgery is the same as in the basic endoscopic operation.

The third variation is a *no-touch orbicularis midfacelift.* This technique avoids all incisions in the periorbital area. The midface is approached with a combination of slit, temporal, and intraoral incisions.

The advantage of these three variations of stage 6 is that innervation and integrity of the orbicularis oculi muscle are maintained and the critical connections between the preseptal and pretarsal parts, where the innervation for the latter travels, are fully maintained (19).

As one might infer from the array of subperiosteal techniques for the midface, the rates of complications and unfa-

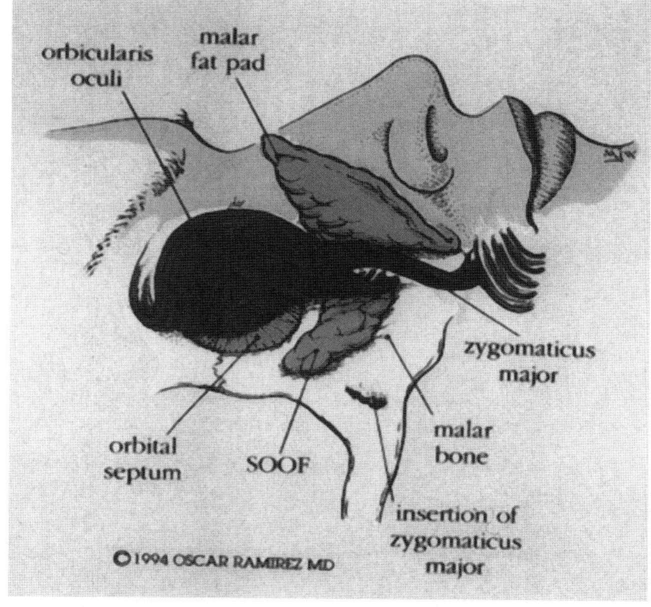

FIGURE 52-4. With the development of endoscopic approaches to the midface, the suborbicularis oculi fat *(SOOF)* pad/periosteum are critical for suspending the midface. From a mechanical and logistical point of view, it is more effective for lifting the cheek. Judicious and precise application of the suture suspensions to this structure is important to avoid potential complications. (Reprinted from Ramirez OM. The subperiosteal approach for the correction of the deep nasolabial fold and the central third of the face. *Clin Plast Surg* 1995;22:341–356, with permission.)

vorable results are different for each technique. Because I have pioneered and taught some of these techniques, I have been asked by other surgeons and self-referred patients to correct complications and unsatisfactory results following all types of facial rejuvenation surgery, including subperiosteal open and endoscopic variations. I have also had my own complications.

COMPLICATIONS OF OPEN FOREHEAD LIFT

Because the browlift/forehead lift is an intrinsic component of the subperiosteal facelift, the related complications are described in this chapter. These include scarring, alopecia, numbness in the forehead, itching, recurrent brow ptosis, brow asymmetry, excessive brow elevation, and hairline elevation. Some frontal nerve injuries can also be included, but the complication rate is completely different in comparison with the rate of nerve injury after the combined forehead lift and midfacelift.

Scarring

The coronal incision has an average length of 32 cm. When the subgaleal approach is used, the rate of scarring of the suture line, manifested by widening and depression of the scar, is almost 100%. This was our observation early in our experience. After we changed the technique to the so-called anchor subperiosteal forehead lift, the rate of widening and depression of the suture line was significantly decreased to less than 3% (20). Although this change in the technique prolongs the operative time by about 30 minutes, the results and the decreased rate of scarring are worth the extra time and effort.

Alopecia

Diffuse alopecia is rare (0.3%); however, alopecia at the suture line is more common. Alopecia is considered to be any loss of hair away from the incision line or an incision that is visible for more than 10 mm (Fig. 52-5). With the subgaleal approach, this complication is about 30%. With the anchor subperiosteal lift, it has decreased to 3%. Alopecia can be prevented by taking the following steps:

1. Bevel the incision to keep the hair follicles in the remaining flap.
2. Suture the scalp under minimal tension.
3. Include the periosteum and galea in the anterior flap and anchor them to the posterior flap.
4. Avoid excessive excision of the scalp and temporal areas.
5. Close the skin with wide skin staples, which are gentler and less constricting to the flap edges and hair follicles. Alternatively, the skin layer can be closed with epidermal 5-0 Prolene sutures without including the hair follicles in the bites.
6. Remove the staples or sutures after a minimum of 1 week.

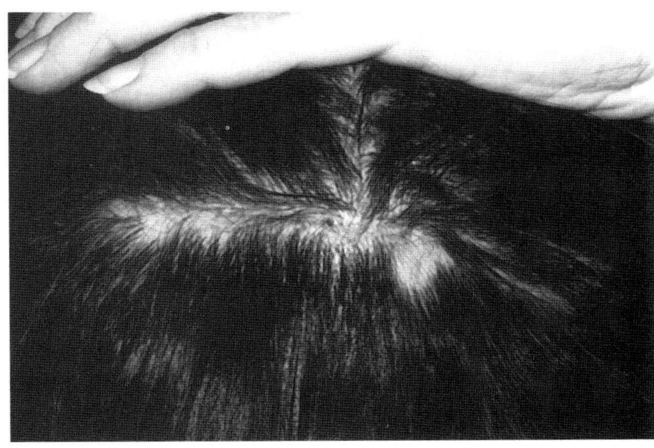

FIGURE 52-5. Alopecia along the suture line of the coronal incision is a frequent complication of the forehead lift and facelift with use of the open technique. It can be avoided with deep anchoring of the periosteal galeal layer, as described by Ramirez (20). (Reprinted from Ramirez OM. The anchor subperiosteal forehead lift. *Plast Reconstr Surg* 1995;95:993–1003, with permission.)

Alopecia and wide scars are usually treated with excision and advancement of the forehead 1 year after surgery. If the scalp is revised before that time, significant tension will be created, and the chance of recurrence will be great.

Numbness in the Forehead

Temporary numbness in the forehead following an open subperiosteal forehead lift occurs almost invariably. Long-term numbness distal to the incision, particularly when coronal incisions are made low, occurs in more than 50% of cases. However, permanent numbness in the forehead itself is rare, occurring in patchy areas in about 3% of cases. It is caused by the transection of small accessory nerves that travel through the frontal cortex to innervate segments of the frontal scalp. In the temple, routine sacrifice of the zygomaticotemporal nerve has produced permanent numbness in about 3% of cases. Prolonged temporary numbness lasting up to about 1 year occurs in about 90% of patients. Prolonged numbness in diffuse areas innervated by the supraorbital and supratrochlear nerves is not uncommon and is related to excessive tension in the frontal scalp. The condition disappears within 3 to 6 months.

Scalp Itching

When the open approach is used, scalp itching occurs in 50% of cases. This is related to transection of the branches of the supraorbital and supratrochlear nerves within the scalp incision, particularly the deep branch of the supraorbital nerve, which has a fairly extensive course and innervates the parietal scalp. Itching can be prevented by placing the coronal incisions as far posteriorly as possible. Itching is more severe when the precapillary incision is used.

Recurrent Brow Ptosis and Brow Asymmetry

Brow ptosis recurs in about 0.6% of patients and is related to insufficient dissection, particularly at the level of the hooding areas. We have noted brow asymmetry in 0.8% of cases; however, minor asymmetry is more common, probably in the range of 5%. None of the patients with minor asymmetry requested surgical correction.

Excessive Brow Elevation

Although in postoperative photographs the brow position often appears much too high, we have had complaints from only 0.2% of our patients, and none of the patients requested surgical correction. Although the opinions of surgeons may differ in regard to an attractive brow position, this probably represents an aesthetic judgment more than an undesirable sequela or complication.

Hairline Elevation

Measurements of hairline elevation vary. However, only 1% of patients expressed any concerns, and none requested surgical correction.

COMPLICATIONS OF OPEN FACELIFT

A series of complications are inherent to the combination of a forehead lift with a midfacelift or a temporal lift with a midfacelift. These include frontal nerve injury, massive swelling, lateral canthal asymmetry, transient numbness of the upper lip, paresis of the zygomaticus and/or buccal nerve branches, patient dissatisfaction, and rare complications.

Frontal Nerve Injury

Frontal nerve injury is probably one of the reasons why acceptance of the subperiosteal facelift into the surgical armamentarium was delayed. The rate of nerve injury has decreased as the operation has been modified to make it safer. Psillakis (3) described a complication rate of 20% (3). When we used the same technique in our initial series, we had a complication rate of 11%. Although all the nerve injuries were temporary, with a return to normal function seen within 1 to 6 months, still they were a difficult problem to accept in an aesthetic operation (5). In our combined series of 545 patients, the rate of temporary frontal nerve paresis was 6.5%, and the rate of permanent injury was 2% (21). My personal rate of nerve complications after use of the "extended" open approach was less than 1% (22). The rate of complications is higher in the combined forehead lift and midfacelift than in the pure forehead lift because of the anatomical configuration of the frontal nerve as it crosses the zygomatic arch. Although it is very unusual for a surgeon to transect the frontal branch of the facial nerve when proceeding with the dissection from the subgaleal plane to the superior border of the zygomatic arch to begin the subperiosteal dissection, probably the traction of the nondominant hand of the surgeon produces a temporary neurapraxia. Furthermore, exposure of the three fascicles of the frontal branch after it crosses the zygomatic arch make it vulnerable to injury by either the scissors or the periosteal elevator. When the "extended approach" is used, the main fascicles of the frontal branch are protected by the intermediate temporal fascia with or without the intermediate temporal fat pad for a length of about 3 cm. The relative rigidity of this fas-

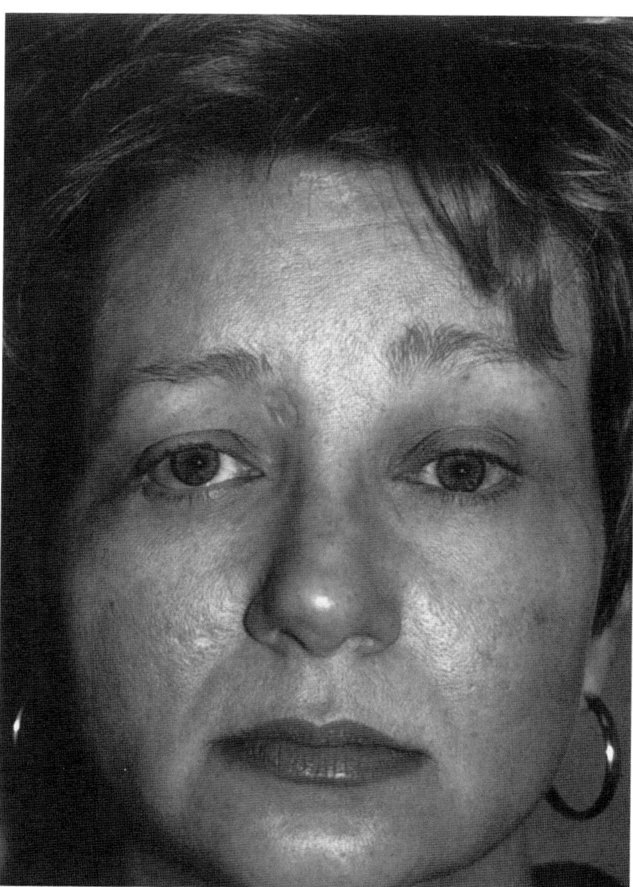

FIGURE 52-6. Frontal nerve injury was a frequent complication of the open subperiosteal facelift. With the newer techniques, it has been almost completely eliminated. However, I occasionally see a patient with this problem who underwent surgery somewhere else.

cia while the flap is placed under tension for the midface dissection keeps the nerve from being overstretched. This is perhaps why the rate of nerve injury is very small with the "extended" subperiosteal variation (Fig. 52-6).

*Supra*periosteal techniques that dissect the zygomatic arch over the periosteum probably have a higher rate of frontal nerve injury. The only explanation of the low rate of this complication by proponents of the technique is that dissection is performed only along the anterior third of the zygomatic arch. Unfortunately, this practice restricts effective vertical lifting of the midface.

Massive Swelling

Massive swelling is more likely to occur when a midfacelift is combined with a forehead lift or vice versa. The chance of massive swelling is greater with a subperiosteal bicoronal lift than with a standard facelift. The rate of severe swelling is 8% (Figs. 7 and 8); for moderate to mild swelling it is about 70%, and for minimal swelling it is 12%. The risk for postoperative swelling is greater when the subperiosteal bicoronal forehead/midfacelift and standard rhytidectomy are combined than when the procedures are staged separately. The addition of excision of the buccal fat pad during the surgery also increases the chances of massive midface edema (17). The addition of eyelid surgery in the same operative setting increases periorbital edema significantly, and the likelihood of significant chemosis is greater.

Methods to minimize massive swelling are the use of gentle, nontraumatic techniques and meticulous hemostasis. The pace of the surgery also tends to influence the degree of edema. If the surgery is quick rather than prolonged and the bandages and ice compresses are applied early after surgery, the degree of edema tends to be less. For these reasons, adding an ancillary procedure to a subperiosteal facelift increases postoperative edema beyond what is contributed by the ancillary operation. The application of small drains under the undermined flaps tends to decrease swelling. Although we have used steroids for many years, we have

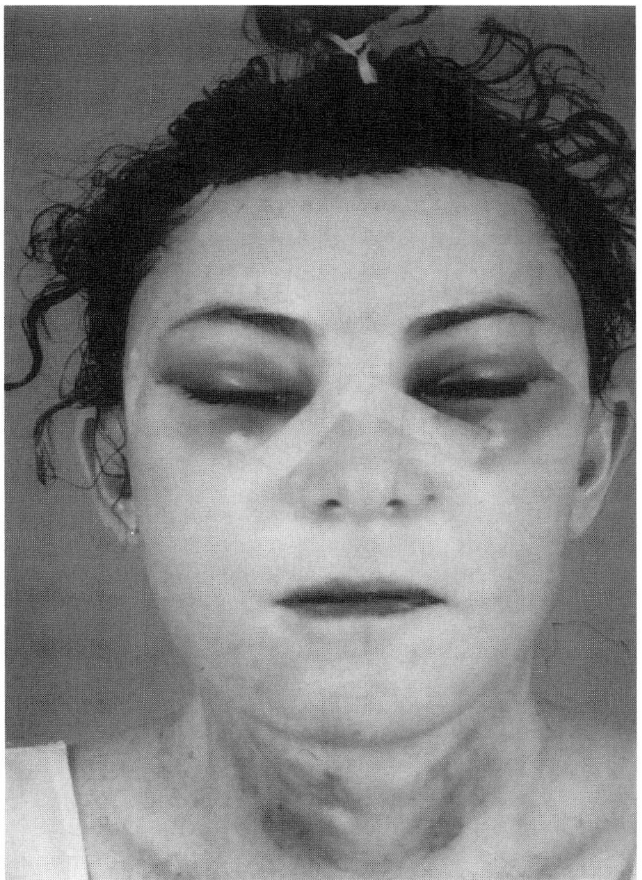

FIGURE 52-7. Anteroposterior view of a female patient after an open subperiosteal approach through a bicoronal incision combined with a lower eyelid blepharoplasty and a subcutaneous cervicofacial rhytidectomy. Note the massive swelling of the face on postoperative day 2. (Courtesy of Mark Zukowski, M.D.)

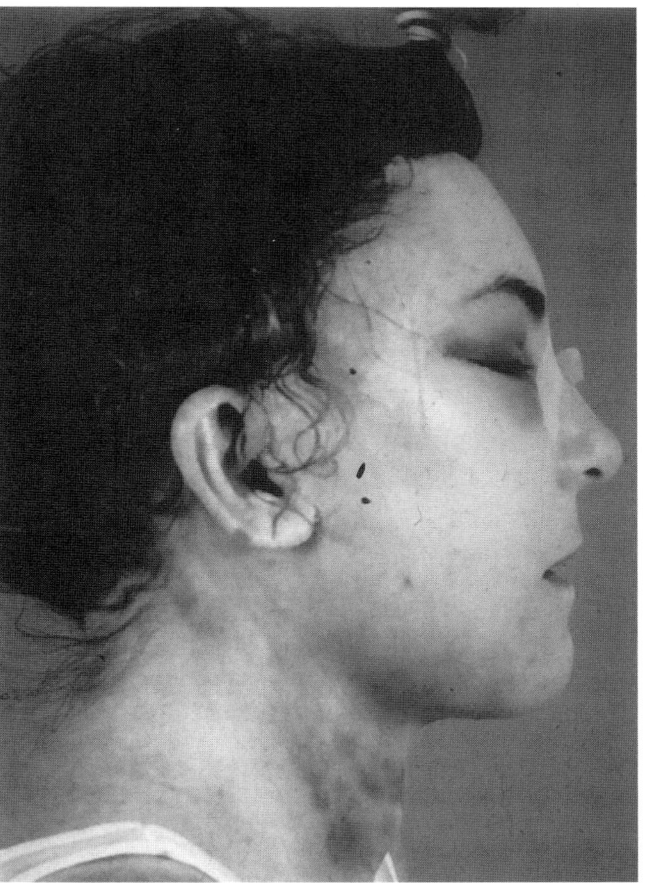

FIGURE 52-8. Lateral view of the same patient. Note the massive facial edema. (Courtesy of Mark Zukowski, M.D.)

abandoned their routine use because short, double-blinded studies at our center did not demonstrate any significant benefit. The way the bandages are applied may also influence the degree of edema. It is necessary to apply tape support to the forehead and central oval of the face and a relatively loose conforming bandage to the neck and peripheral semicircle of the face because with the opposite arrangement, the peripheral bandage tends to act as a tourniquet and increases edema in the central oval of the face.

Lateral Canthal Asymmetry

Asymmetry of the lateral angle of the eyes is a relatively rare event, contrary to popular belief. The eyelid slant should be changed only after a thorough discussion to determine the patient's desires and the surgeon's objectives. I do not recommend placing a direct suture into the lateral canthal area and pulling superiorly unless it is absolutely necessary. In the experience of surgeons performing routine canthopexy, the rate of secondary operations to correct asymmetries is 5% to 20%. I do not perform routine canthopexy/canthoplasty. I use the temporomasseter flap to control the lifting of the cheeks and lower eyelids. The repositioning of the entire orbicularis oculi around the periorbital area produces the effect of a canthopexy, with pleasant, almond-shaped eyes. If this effect is not desired, then a back-cut of the temporomasseter flap near the canthal tendon will prevent it. Excessive slanting of the lateral eyelid raphe discovered early in the postoperative period is corrected by massage in the opposite direction, which usually is sufficient to correct minor asymmetries. If asymmetry is the result of a canthoplasty, then a surgical revision may be necessary to correct the deformity; in this circumstance, massage alone is not helpful.

Transient Numbness of the Upper Lip

Transient numbness of the upper lift is a consequence of contusion, stretching, or bleeding around the infraorbital nerve. This nerve is protected by the following measures:

1. Using the intraoral approach, which permits better control and visualization.
2. Identifying and shielding the nerve during the dissection.
3. Placing a finger on the skin over the infraorbital foramina during the intraoral dissection. The sharp periosteal levator may still scratch the nerve in the underlying cheek envelope. For this reason, the elevators must be kept flat against the bone.

Further causes of numbness of the upper lip are hematoma, seroma, infection, or inflammation of the undermined cheek region. If it is recognized early, it should be treated promptly.

Neurapraxia of the Zygomaticus and Buccal Nerve Branches

This is a rare event, probably related to nerve stretching during the subperiosteal midface dissection or trauma caused by the hypodermic needle during injection. The local anesthetic solution can also produce temporary neurapraxia. For this reason, we recommend using a small-gauge needle and small syringes for injection. Application of a nerve stimulator quickly relieves this condition. We have not seen permanent neuropraxia in this nerve.

THE DISSATISFIED PATIENT

It is not uncommon for a patient to be dissatisfied after an aesthetic procedure. However, dissatisfaction following a subperiosteal lift is not as frequent as people might believe. If the patient and surgeon have communicated effectively regarding their objectives, there should be no reason for dissatisfaction. In most cases, dissatisfaction is caused by undercorrection rather than overcorrection. Forehead lift is not the sole purpose of the operation. The subperiosteal lift should eliminate or diminish crow's-feet, raise the lateral canthus, flatten the skin of the lower eyelid without an external incision, raise the soft tissues of the cheek to a higher position on the cheekbone, and flatten the upper half of the nasolabial fold. When indicated, prominent forehead bossing can be remodeled to improve deep-set eyes and a protruding supraorbital rim. Additionally, the zygomatic, malar, and submalar areas can be augmented.

A common cause of dissatisfaction following surgery is insufficient elevation of the soft tissues resulting from inadequate dissection or unrealistic expectations of the patient. Experienced surgeons can elevate 2 to 3 cm around the cheek areas. Novice surgeons find it difficult to mobilize the flaps and try to compensate with excessive tension of the undermined flaps. The soft tissues should be repositioned without significant tension. Total familiarity with the anatomy to understand and treat the attachments that can hinder the elevation is critical. Only after complete dissection can an unrestricted soft tissue lift to the desired position be obtained.

The subperiosteal approach via the coronal incision is an excellent method to improve the soft tissues up to the level of the upper lip. Mechanically, lifting of the midface is transmitted less and less as the distance from the point of traction increases. For this reason, lower cheek sagging can be eliminated and the lower face and jowl improved in early aging. However, when the patient presents with significant perioral sagging or excess skin and a large jowl, a concomitant subcutaneous rhytidectomy is an excellent added modality to improve these areas and the lower nasolabial fold. This lateral vector of pull also further improves the already undermined areas of the subperiosteal plane (malar and maxillary areas). Conversely, if no subperiosteal undermining is performed, the subcutaneous traction will do very little to remodel these areas. The bidirectional pull produced by the temporomasseter flap and the periauricular skin flap maximizes the effectiveness of the subperiosteal dissection.

The patient usually comes to the consultation requesting eyelid surgery and overall improvement around the eyes and cheeks, particularly the tear troughs and nasolabial folds. These areas can be approached effectively and safely with a subperiosteal facelift.

RARE COMPLICATIONS

Upper Eyelid Ptosis

Upper eyelid ptosis is caused by contusion or laceration of the levator mechanism during intraorbital dissection. It can be avoided through absolute control of the tip of the periosteal elevators at all times. We have not seen this complication in our series; however, we had an opportunity to review a case performed somewhere else. It should be possible to eliminate the complication altogether by not entering the orbital cavity, as we suggested early in our experience.

Ectropion

Ectropion may result when a standard lower blepharoplasty is performed at the same operative setting as the subperiosteal facelift. The "sandwich" dissection of simultaneous subperiosteal and muscle skin flap is significant and should be undertaken only with caution. If a lower blepharoplasty is indicated, it should be carried out with either a minimal skin-only excision or a transconjunctival lower blepharoplasty to remove the fat pad without touching the skin. The excess skin can be corrected with either chemical peel or the new laser technology.

During vertical lifting of the cheek, a significant amount of skin is recruited for excision. Surgeons should avoid excessive skin excision because this can cause significant ectropion.

Dry Eye Syndrome

This extremely rare complication may be caused by inflammation around the minor zygomaticofacial nerve. This nerve exits through the pinpoint foramen and middle malar eminence and carries sympathetic and parasympathetic fibers to the lacrimal glands before emerging as a purely sensory branch. Any inflammation around the nerve can produce retrograde inflammation of the sympathetic and parasympathetic fibers previously mentioned. The symptoms usually subside and disappear as the swelling, inflammation, or infection resolves.

Diplopia

Intraorbital swelling can cause diplopia in the immediate postoperative period. It is usually minimal and resolves within a week or so. The reason why I do not recommend entering the orbital cavity to remodel the brow or resect the fat pad of the eyelid is because the chances of injuring an extraocular muscle are increased, particularly if the eyelid surgery is performed at the end of the operation, when the tissues are already swollen.

Hematoma

This is a rare complication following a subperiosteal dissection. The nonexpansible subperiosteal component does not allow a hematoma to form. I have seen only one case of hematoma, related to a postoperative hypertensive crisis. In this case, drainage of the hematoma had to be delayed until the hypertensive crisis was controlled, which took a couple days. We were able to delay drainage of the hematoma because the subcutaneous dissection was minimal and most of the hematoma was under the periosteum. The patient recovered without any sequelae. Minor hematomas can be drained in the office or at the bedside through small incisions in the ear, mouth, or temporal fossa.

Infection

Infection also is a rare event and has occurred in only one of our patients. It was related to a hole on the anterior wall of the maxillary sinus that had been caused by a prior traumatic event. Treatment was with broad-spectrum antibiotics and drainage of the abscess (Fig. 52-9). Despite use of the intraoral incision, the incidence of infection is extremely low, probably because of the excellent vascularity of the thick flaps, the lack of dead space, and the atraumatic technique. To avoid infection, we routinely give the patient broad-spectrum antibiotics, and we cleanse frequently with Betadine solution during the intraoral manipulation.

Temporary Asymmetrical Smile

This is an unusual complication that may be caused by detachment of the zygomaticus muscle. Swelling and interstitial hematoma around this muscle can produce a temporary decrease in function, which usually lasts 2 to 3 weeks and improves gradually without treatment.

Oriental Look

The subperiosteal lift of the upper face, particularly if combined with a midfacelift, imparts an oriental appearance to the eyelid raphe. The slanting of the lateral canthal area usually lasts for about 1 month to 6 weeks. Upward pulling of

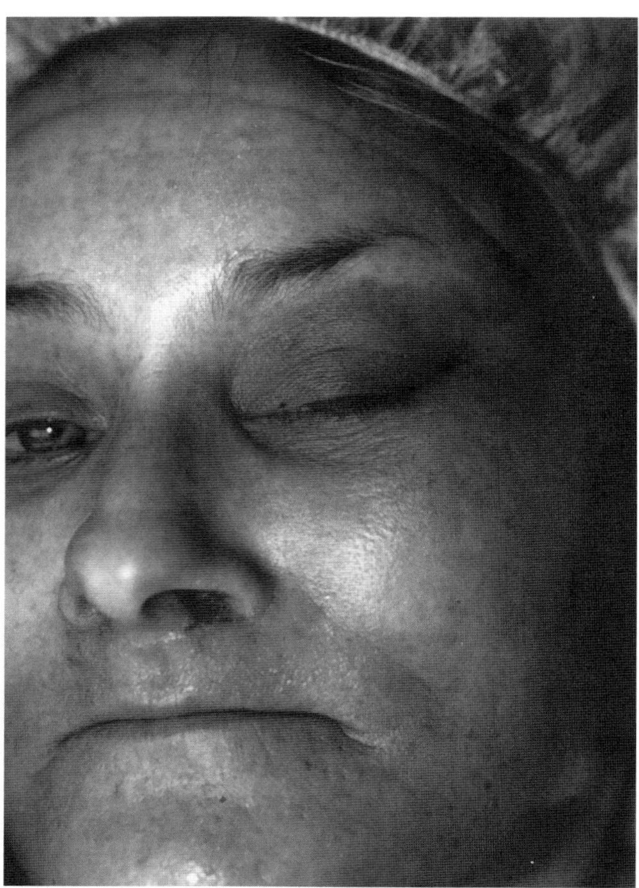

FIGURE 52-9. Despite the use of the intraoral incision to access the midface, infection is a rare occurrence. It should be treated promptly with drainage, irrigation, and antibiotics.

the temporomasseter fascia following the intraorbital detachment of the lateral canthal ligament brings the lateral angle of the eye to a higher position. If during surgery the slanting is judged to be too great, a back-cut in the temporal fascia will relieve the problem. Minimal slanting is desirable and should be left to resolve spontaneously, which usually takes about 4 weeks. In general, patients consider almond-shaped eyes beautiful and aesthetically pleasing.

Depression of the Temporal Fossa

In the first cases in which the extended subperiosteal concept was used, both layers of the tempora fascia were included in the flap, and depression of the temporal fossa was noted fairly often, particularly in thin patients (4%). Shortly after we recognized this sequela, we changed our approach to include only the intermediate temporal fascia in the temporomasseter flap, and thereby eliminated this complication. The treatment for the condition is to inject fat superficially and deep in the temporal fossa (Fig. 52-10).

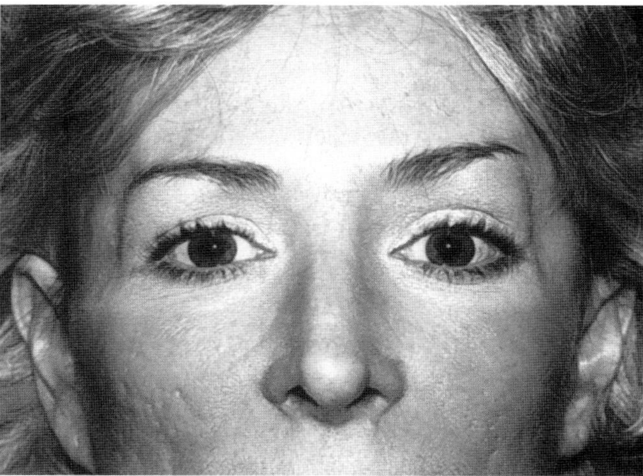

FIGURE 52-10. At first, when both layers of the temporal fascia were used for suspension in the second-stage subperiosteal facelift, temporal atrophy developed in quite a few patients. For this reason, the deep temporal fascia and part of the intermediate fat pad are left undisturbed in the open subperiosteal facelift.

HOW CHANGES IN TECHNIQUE CAN AFFECT THE RATE OF UNFAVORABLE RESULTS IN THE SUBPERIOSTEAL FACELIFT

The complications described are essentially limited to first-stage and second-stage subperiosteal facelifts. Each of the other stages has its unique complications, or lack thereof, and these are technique-dependent. They are also related to the anatomical locations of incisions and the planes of dissection.

Third Stage

During the early development of the endoscopic approach, we used external "tied-over" dressings for the temporary suspension of the advanced brow and forehead (Fig. 52-11). This practice produced about a 5% rate of diffuse alopecia, and it took between 4 to 6 months for the hair to grow back completely (Fig. 52-12). The alopecia was probably related to the pressure of the dressing; hair follicles were sandwiched between the dressing and the swollen galea/pericranium. I very quickly changed the method of fixation to temporary percutaneous screw fixation, which was initially applied at the same paramedian scalp ports for the endoforehead. The screw was applied to the outer cortex, and the scalp was suspended with skin staples. The galea/pericranium was not closed. Two localized problems ensued. One was the development of suture line depression, and the other was localized alopecia around the screw and staples interface. Probably the entrapment of many hair follicles between the screw and the staples caused the alopecia. For this reason, the technique was subsequently modified (23).

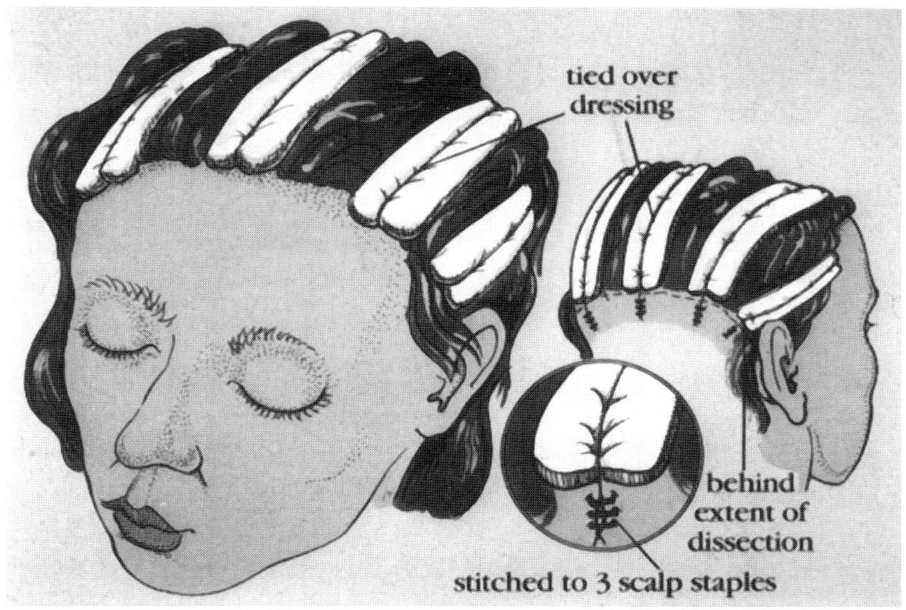

FIGURE 52-11. "Tied-over" dressing suspension originally used in the endoscopic approach to the forehead lift. (Reprinted from Daniel RK, Ramirez OM. Endoscopic-assisted aesthetic surgery. *Aesthetic Surgery Magazine* 1994;14:14–20.)

During the initial endoscopic technique, the midface was approached via a limited subciliary incision. Although it was not routinely performed, many patients required canthopexy to prevent postoperative ectropion. A conservative blepharoplasty was also performed. With the use of this technique, ectropion did not occur. We have seen a few cases of late scleral show.

The midface was suspended with the SOOF rather than the temporomasseter flap. This provided, from a logistical point of view, a better anchoring point that was closer to the problem areas (tear trough and nasolabial folds). Cheek elevation was significantly improved and the other problems corrected. Many surgeons found it difficult to elevate the cheek mound or distribute redundant, thick soft tissues of the cheek around the superolateral malar areas and the zygomatic arch. Surgeons unable to perform a good dissection and an unrestricted upper cheek lift compensated by creating excessive traction on the SOOF, which produced a limited cheek elevation and dimpling and depressions along the traction points (Figs. 13,14). In some cases, dimpling produced a trapdoor swelling on the lower eyelid. Other surgeons converted the endoscope-dependent subciliary approach to an "open" full blepharoplasty incision. They also limited the dissection around the zygomatic arch and did not connect the malar with the temporal pockets. This change in technique required a routine canthopexy in every patient and excisional scalp surgery with a subcutaneous dissection from the temple toward the zygomatic arch to redrape the excess skin in this area.

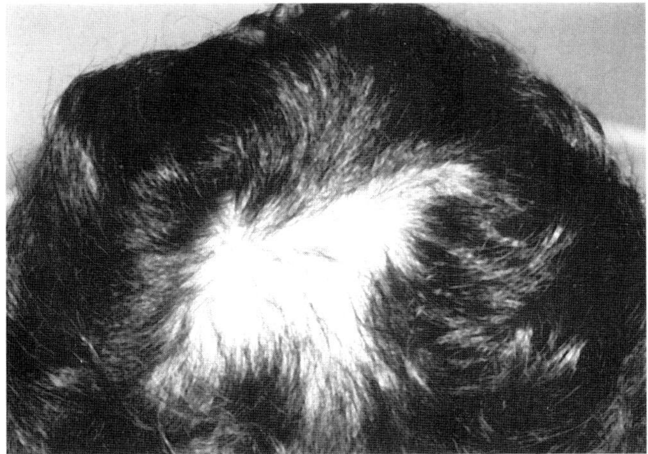

FIGURE 52-12. Diffuse alopecia, seen in 5% of patients in whom the "tied over" dressing suspension is used. This complication is more frequent when the scalp dissection is performed at the subgaleal layer.

Fourth Stage

The fourth stage is a multiplanar procedure in which the temporal subgaleal dissection is changed to a subperiosteal dissection along the zygomatic arch to protect the frontal branch of the facial nerve. The dissection is changed to a *supra*periosteal plane around the orbital rim. The zygomatic-cutaneous ligament is released along the medial origin of the masseter muscle fascia to mobilize the malar pad. The suborbicularis preperiosteal plane is continued over the in-

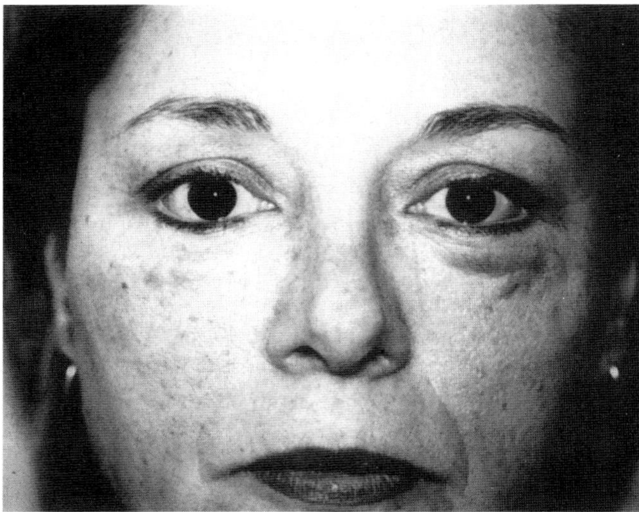

FIGURE 52-13. This patient had a suborbicularis oculi fat *(SOOF)* suspension performed elsewhere. Observe the dimpling, discoloration of the cheek and tear troughs, and chronic edema of the lower eyelid.

fraorbital rim to the infraorbital nerve. The dissection in this technique finishes at this point; however, it can be carried down over the zygomaticus major muscle in a subcutaneous plane to the nasolabial fold. In other words, the suborbicularis dissection changes plane again to the *supra*zygomaticus major muscle plane to reach an even more superficial plane in the malar soft tissues. This dissection obviously passes through the interface between the zygomaticus major muscle and orbicularis oculi muscle, in which the motor branches to the lower orbicularis are located (Fig. 52-15), so that these nerves are placed at significant risk. Other proponents of the supraperiosteal technique, in which they change from a suborbicularis oculi to a *supra*zygomaticus plane, place the motor branches to the orbicularis oculi and the zygomaticus major muscles at significant risk for injury. This produces early paralysis of the muscles, and during the process of recovery and neurotization, significant troublesome synkinesis develops (Fig. 52-16).

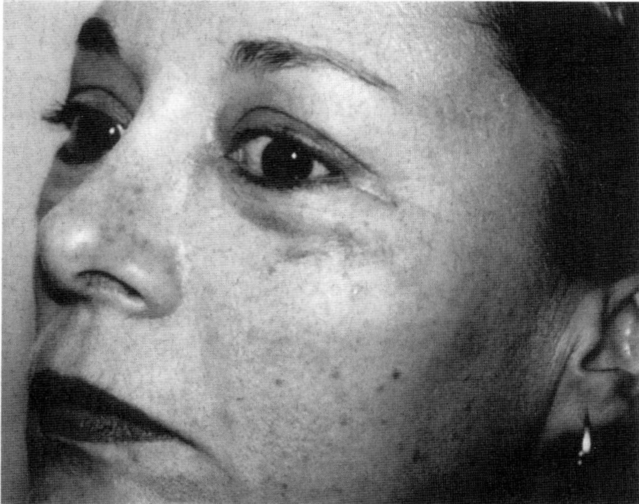

FIGURE 52-14. The three-fourths view shows some of the distortion produced by the "too superficial" application of the suture suspension to the suborbicularis oculi fat *(SOOF)*. Actually, the orbicularis oculi muscle has been grasped in the suture.

Fifth Stage

As was mentioned, some surgeons converted the endoscopic subciliary approach to the midface to an *open* full blepharoplasty incision without use of the endoscope. This required a significantly longer incision, traction on the divided orbicularis oculi muscle, and a routine canthopexy for additional suspension and sometimes horizontal shortening of the lower eyelid whether it was required or not. An array complications was created that would be unacceptable to most physicians (24). The most common complications were ectropion, scleral show, canthal malposition, asymmetry, and orbicularis oculi paralysis or paresis. Less obvious complications were flattening of the tarsal area and vertical external tilt of the ciliary margin. Other complications were related to the incision in the temporal area, such as alopecia and widening of the scar.

Ectropion, scleral show, and flattening of the tarsal area are caused by denervation of the pretarsal muscle. The first two can also be as a consequence of vertical shortening of the external lamella or cicatricial contracture. More severe ectropion and orbicularis oculi paralysis/paresis can be caused by stretching or transection of the motor branches to the orbicularis oculi muscle. Patients have been referred to me with all these problems. Some of these complications also developed in my own patients when this technique was used (Fig. 52-17). For this reason, I have abandoned it completely and would not recommend it.

Sixth Stage

This is the stage of refinements and reappraisal. As was mentioned, the sixth stage comprises three variations. The aim of each is to preserve the integrity, function, and innervation of the orbicularis oculi muscle, particularly the pretarsal portion. The preservation of muscle integrity avoids temporary or permanent paralysis/paresis, which in turn prevents ectropion, scleral show, and flattening of the pretarsal muscle.

The way I most often handle the midface is through the temporal slit incision and the intraoral incision (Fig. 52-18). This is an endoscopic procedure that precludes the use of incisions or tunnels through the orbicularis oculi muscle. The plane of dissection is subperiosteal around the zygomatic arch and the midface, and underneath the intermediate temporal fascia in the temporal area to avoid injuring the frontal branch of the facial nerve. Also, to facilitate the upward movement of the cheek, the subperiosteal dissection on the

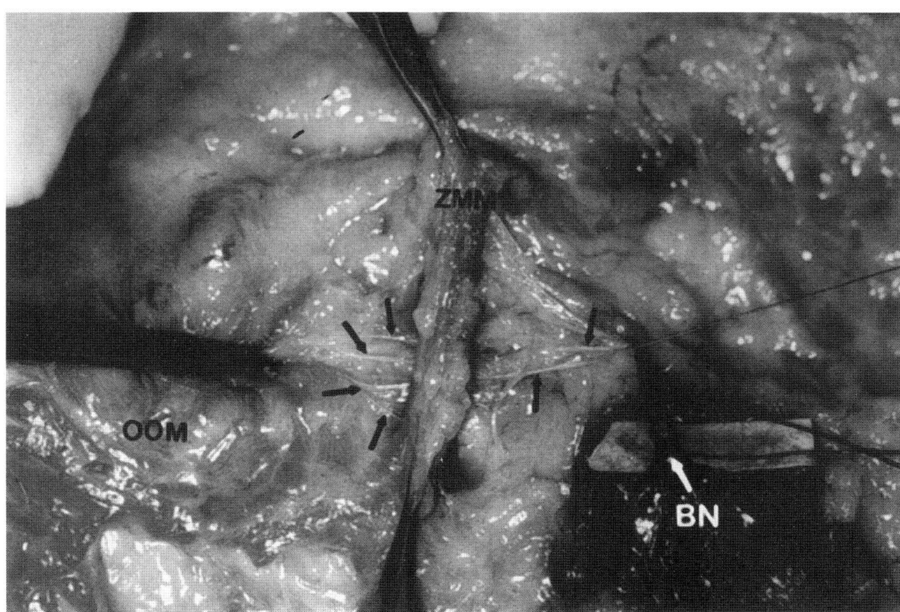

FIGURE 52-15. *Arrows* show the multiple fascicles of the zygomaticus nerve branching to the zygomaticus major muscle *(ZMM)* and coursing underneath the orbicularis oculi muscle *(OOM)*. Multilayer techniques that approach the suprazygomatic plane from underneath the orbicularis oculi muscle can easily injure these nerves. *BN,* buccal nerve.

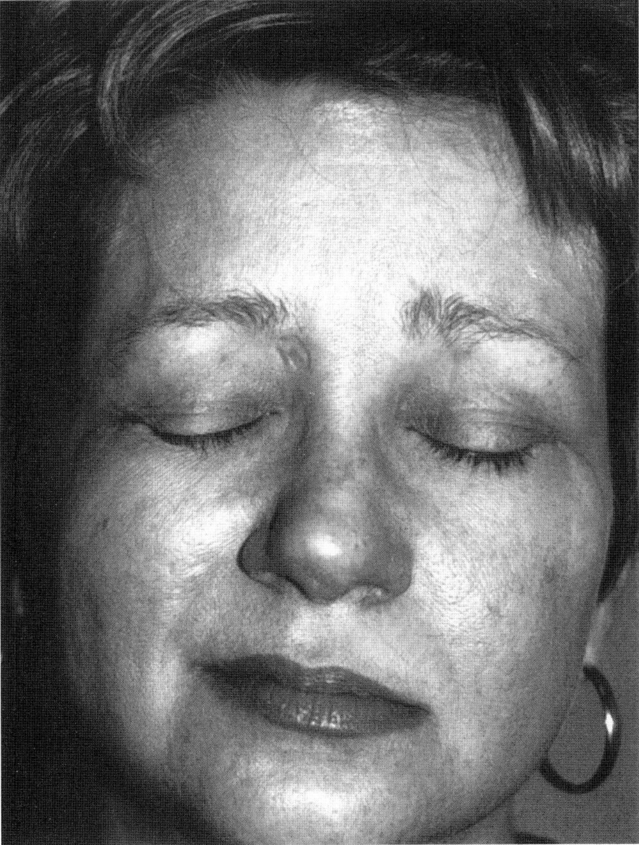

FIGURE 52-16. Planned or unplanned dissection in the intermediate layers of the face can injure the branches of the zygomaticus nerve to the orbicularis oculi muscle. In this patient, neurotization of the branches of the zygomaticus major muscle to the orbicularis oculi muscle has produced a troublesome synkinesis. The eyelids are closed to show the significant contracture of the zygomaticus major and levator anguli oris muscles. The patient also has blepharospasm secondary to the nerve injury.

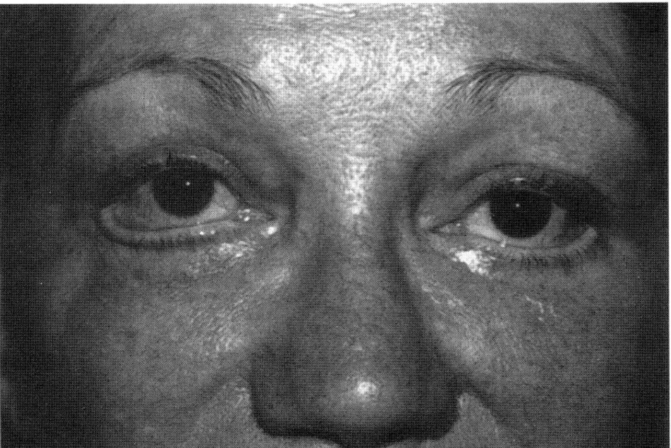

FIGURE 52-17. Lower eyelid ectropion, or scleral show, is a common complication after an "open" subperiosteal cheek lift. The patient's condition on the left is a consequence of the technique and on the right of the technique plus blunt trama to the cheek, with development of a hematoma in the early postoperative course. Any scarring over the already paralyzed pretarsal muscle will be a further factor in the development of ectropion.

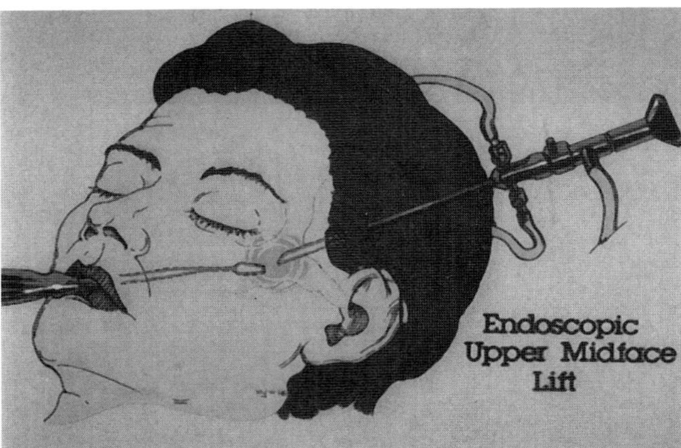

FIGURE 52-18. The safest and least traumatic way to approach the midface is with the combination of a temporal slit incision and an upper oral sulcus incision. The orbicularis oculi muscle is left undisturbed.

zygomatic arch is extended inferiorly, with elevation of the fascia of the masseter muscle. This plane of dissection is not different from our original description of the endoscopic midfacelift (10). By performing the surgery this way, we avoid all the problems seen in stage 5. Because the elevation of the SOOF over the inferior orbital rim diminishes or erases the tear trough deformity, the bulging or excess orbital fat pad becomes less noticeable. Therefore, the rate of orbital defatting has decreased to less than 10% in our series. The skin of the lower eyelid is handled with carbon dioxide laser resurfacing, 35% trichloracetic acid peel, or a cutaneous blepharoplasty with the pinch technique or wide skin undermining and redraping. The last technique is reserved for cases of excessive crepiness or crow's-feet. The orbicularis oculi is left intact. Elevation of the skin and suspension of the orbicularis oculi (without transection) to the lateral orbital rim recruits more muscle over the pretarsal area and re-creates the beautiful pretarsal bulge of youthful eyes. If excessive intraorbital fat is present, it can be reduced via a transconjunctival approach or through small windows in the orbicularis oculi muscle. With this technique, the incidence of ectropion or scleral show has been practically zero.

CONCLUSION

Based on experience with nearly all the stages of the subperiosteal facelift described herein, the best combination in terms of safety and effectiveness to obtain a total facial rejuvenation appears to be the following (Fig. 52-19):

1. Forehead. Endoscopic approach via five slit incisions. Stability is obtained with suspension of superficial temporal fascia to temporal fascia proper and with the application of screws via a percutaneous stab wound incision in the frontal scalp.

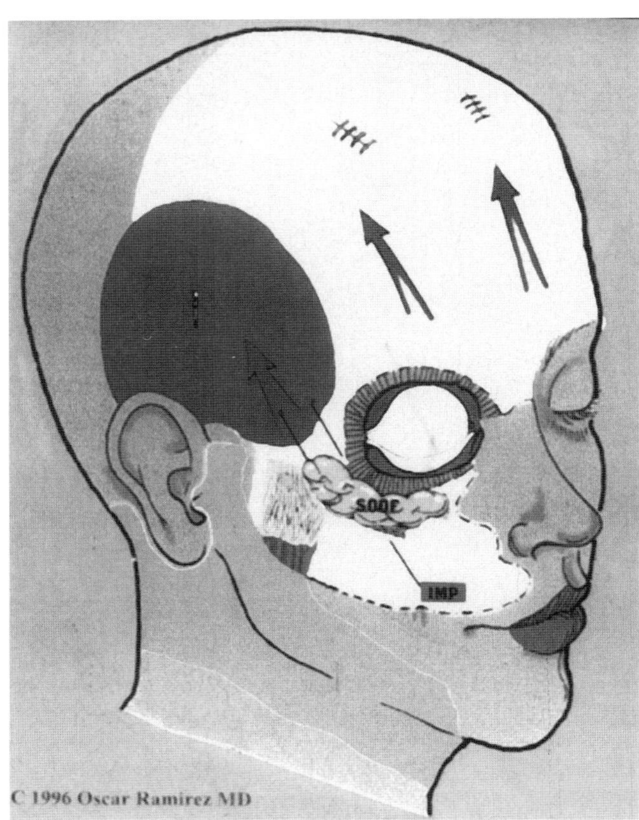

FIGURE 52-19. The best combination for total facial rejuvenation is an endoscopic forehead lift, endoscopic midfacelift, and subcutaneous cervicofacial rhytidectomy. The superior extent of the preauricular incision is limited. (Modified from Ramirez OM. High-tech facelift. *Aesthetic Plast Surg* 1998;22:318–328, with permission.)

2. Midface. Endoscopic approach via temporal slit incision and intraoral incisions. Stability is obtained with suspension of the SOOF, imbrication of the lower malar periosteum, and augmentation of the cheek with Bichat's fat pad.
3. Eyelids. Transconjunctival lipectomy (< 5%) and "skin-only" blepharoplasty or carbon dioxide laser resurfacing. The orbicularis oculi muscle is maintained intact, and no excision or incision of the muscle is performed.
4. Lower face and neck. These are approached via cutaneous cervicofacial rhytidectomy. The upper extent of the incision is at the level of the roof of the helix. Guerrerosantos-Giampapa suture suspension is routinely used for better definition of the neck. Mentopexy is frequently performed.

A brief description of the subperiosteal facelift has been presented. The development of subperiosteal facelift techniques in six stages has been outlined so that the reader will have a better understanding of the potential complications of each of these techniques. The complications of the forehead lift and facelift have been described for and quantified for stages 1 and 2. The actual and potential complications of stages 3 through 5 have been outlined. Our most recent modifications (stage 6) to decrease the rate of complications has been briefly described. The most important factor in understanding and avoiding complications during a subperiosteal facelift is an in-depth knowledge of surgical facial anatomy.

REFERENCES

1. Tessier P. Le lifting facial sous-perioste. *Ann Chir Plast* 1989;34:193.
2. Santana PM. Metodologia craneomaxilofacial en ritidoplastias. *Cirugia Plastica Ibero-Latinoamericana* 1984;10:322.
3. Psillakis JM. Subperiosteal approach as an improved concept for correction of the aging face. *Plast Reconstr Surg* 1988;82:383.
4. Krastinova-Lolov D. Le lifting facial sous-perioste. *Ann Chir Plast* 1989;34:199–211.
5. Ramirez OM, Maillard GF, Musolas A. The extended subperiosteal facelift: a definitive soft tissue remodeling for facial rejuvenation. *Plast Reconstr Surg* 1991;88:227–236.
6. Ramirez OM. The subperiosteal rhytidectomy: the third generation facelift. *Ann Plast Surg* 1992;28:218.
7. Ramirez OM, Fuente del Campo A. Facial rejuvenation: subperiosteal brow and facelift. In: Riley SR, ed. *Instructional courses,* vol 6. St. Louis: Mosby, 1993:41–54.
8. Maillard GF, de St Cyr C, Scheflan M. The subperiosteal bicoronal approach to total facelifting: the DMAS deep musculoaponeurotic system. *Aesth Plast Surg* 1991;15:285–291.
9. Ramirez OM. Endoscopic techniques in facial rejuvenation. An overview. *Aesthetic Plast Surg* 1994;18:141.
10. Ramirez OM. Endoscopic full facelift. *Aesth Plast Surg* 1994;18: 363–371.
11. Ramirez OM. Endoscopic forehead and facelift: step-by-step operative techniques. *Plast Reconstr Surg* 1995;2:129–136.
12. Byrd S. The deep temporal lift. *Plast Reconstr Surg* 1996;97: 928–937.
13. Hester TR, Codner MA, McCord CD. The "centrofacial" approach for correction of facial aging using the transblepharoplasty subperiosteal cheek lift. *Aesth Surg J* 1996;16:51–58.
14. Paul MD. An approach for correcting midface aging with a periosteal hinge flap. *Aesthetic Surg J* 1997;17:61–63.
15. Ramirez OM. Fourth-generation subperiosteal approach to the midface: the tridimensional functional cheek lift. *Aesth Surg J* 1998;18:133–135.
16. Ramirez OM. High-tech facelift. *Aesthetic Plast Surg* 1998;22: 318–328.
17. Ramirez OM. Buccal fat pad pedicle flap for midface augmentation. *Ann Plast Surg* 1999;43:109–118.
18. Ramirez OM, Pozner JN. Subperiosteal minimally invasive laser rhytidectomy—the SMILE facelift. *Aesthetic Plast Surg* 1996; 20:463–470.
19. Ramirez OM, Santamarina R. Spatial orientation of the motor innervation to the lower orbicularis oculi muscle. *Aesth Surg J* 2000;20:107–113.
20. Ramirez OM. The anchor subperiosteal forehead lift. *Plast Reconstr Surg* 1995;95:993.
21. Schefflan M, Maillard GF, Cornette de St Cyr B, et al. Subperiosteal facelifting: complications and the dissatisfied patient. *Aesth Plast Surg* 1996;20:33–36.
22. Ramirez OM. Subperiosteal endoscopic techniques in facial rejuvenation. In: Guyuron B, ed. *Aesthetic surgery.* vol. 5. St. Louis, MO: Mosby, 2000:2609–2630.
23. Ramirez OM. Facelift: an plastic surgeon's perspective. In: Romo T, Millman AL, eds. *Aesthetic facial plastic surgery.* New York: Thieme Medical Publishers, Inc., 2000:187–206.
24. Hurwitz DJ, Raskin EM. Reducing eyelid retraction following subperiosteal facelift. *Aesth Surg J* 1997;17:149–156.

Discussion

SUBPERIOSTEAL FACELIFT

GASTON-F. MAILLARD
LAURENCE GAREY

Facial rejuvenation is one of the most fascinating subjects for the cosmetic plastic surgeon. Only after years of experience can the practitioner aspire to attract the attention of clients in this exclusive domain.

G. F. Maillard: Department of Plastic Surgery, University of Lausanne, Lausanne, Switzerland
L. Garey: Department of Anatomy, Division of Medicine, UAE University, Al Ain, United Arab Emirates

Since the first efforts of Madame Noël in Paris at the beginning of the 20th century simply to retension the skin around the ear under local anesthesia, we have witnessed striking technical advances in various aspects of the field.

Even if a number of surgeons are opposed to subperiosteal dissection, it has to be recognized that Paul Tessier in Paris opened a new field with his craniomaxillofacial surgery, a true "spin-off" for cosmetic surgery. In 1969, as a young resident in plastic surgery, I had the opportunity to watch and assist Tessier in his operations. His surgery was conceptually different from that of the "soft tissue" surgeons whom I had encountered earlier in my training (Clodius, Dufourmentel, Meyer, Millard, Mouly). Tessier followed the same principles applied in orthopaedics: diagnosis of the deformity, precise measurement, then subperiosteal dissection and complete degloving of the face with correction of the underlying skeleton. This was followed by replacement of the facial "mask" (the facial soft tissues) on the skeleton. He called this essentially orthopedic procedure *"orthomorphic" surgery.*

During my training and at the beginning of my academic and hospital career, I had the occasion to undertake a considerable amount of orbital surgery. Indeed, the subject of my "aggregation" thesis at the Faculty of Medicine in Lausanne was plastic surgery of the bony orbit (1). So, early in my independent career, beginning in 1976, it seemed quite logical to apply the concepts of my mentor, Tessier, to cosmetic surgery. My familiarity with subperiosteal dissection explains why I found it quite normal to perform frontal facelifts in the subperiosteal rather than in the subgaleal plane.

As I mastered the technique, I soon began to discover its disadvantages:

1. If no intraoral dissection is performed inferiorly to superiorly, the facial mask does not rise but remains fixed at the midface level.
2. If one exerts traction on a poorly mobilized facial mask through the coronal incision, problems of tension on the branches of the facial nerve can develop, with all the well-known sequelae.

In 1988, I published a first article on an exceptional case of subperiosteal facelift to correct a severe Romberg deformity (2).

My practice of reducing zygomatic fractures by means of Gillies' technique—introducing a subperiosteal elevator through the temporalis aponeurosis deep to the zygomatic arch—gave me the idea of dissecting beneath the deep temporal fascia to protect the frontal branch of the facial nerve. If the periosteum of the zygomatic arch is dissected from above, one inevitably approaches the insertions of the zygomaticus major and minor muscles, so that they are at risk of being torn. Such injury causes subsequent dyskinesia of these important muscles of facial expression. Therefore, initial intraoral dissection is indispensable. This is performed by making an incision in the canine fossa, then totally dissecting the maxillary and malar areas, as in a Caldwell-Luc operation or a maxillary osteotomy by an intraoral approach. Care is taken to free the bony origin of the zygomatic muscles. After this, one approaches this dissection from above, through the deep temporal fascia.

In 1989, Tessier himself and his student Darina Krastinova-Lolov described the subperiosteal facelift at the SOFCEP (Société Française de Chirurgiens Esthétiques Plasticiens) conference in Paris, dedicated to Tessier (3,4). At the ISAPS (International Society of Aesthetic Plastic Surgeons) conference in Zurich in 1989, I described the technique of deep fixation, and Oscar Ramirez presented the same technique during the same session (5,6). The chairman of the session was James Smith of New York, who took us to task energetically, claiming that it was useless and dangerous to attempt such a major dissection for a simple rejuvenation in which skin traction would suffice! However, the co-chairman, Fernando Ortiz-Monasterio, expressed a completely different opinion, concluding that this seemed to be the first statement of a potentially useful idea, and that it should be followed with interest. Next day, Ramirez and I worked together on our notes. Later, we worked in the dissecting room, and finally in the operating theater. We decided to publish our common findings. We agreed on almost all points. The temporoperiosteal flap protected the frontal branch of the facial nerve and permitted a solid vertical suspension of the face. Because of the hazards of the mail and the fax machine, some important correspondence was lost between Baltimore and Lausanne. This poor communication during a period of some months led to my collaborating with Cornette de St.-Cyr in Paris and Scheflan in Tel Aviv, both with a broad surgical experience (7). We adopted the expression *deep musculoaponeurotic system* (DMAS) in our article, as opposed to the older concept of SMAS (superficial musculoaponeurotic system). Then Ramirez and I reestablished contact, and we decided that our article, too, was virtually ready for submission (8). We gradually incorporated the anterior and superficial fibers of the masseter in our flap to be sure of suspending the deep surface by a very solid and almost inextensible flap. Ramirez later adopted the term *temporomasseter flap* rather than DMAS. He had the extremely good idea of organizing several international symposia on deep facelifting, with practical sessions at the Maryland Institute of Anatomy. We had an unique opportunity to undertake extremely detailed anatomical dissections in a perfect technical and academic environment. During the 1993 symposium, Nicanor Isse spoke to us for the first time about endoscopic dissection. Ramirez was quick to jump aboard this moving train, and by the next year, he had converted almost entirely to endoscopic subperiosteal facelift.

In his chapter, it is interesting to review all the stages of Ramirez' development from 1989 to 1999. It appears that his learning curve was quite difficult. It is comforting to note that he has gradually abandoned risky solutions, so that the ultimate outcome is practically Tessier's original method with or without suspension by a DMAS or deep temporomasseter flap, but accomplished by an endoscopic approach.

Such an evolution seems quite logical. Tessier himself teased his young trainees somewhat by saying that the masklift, or subperiosteal facelift, was a very simple technique, and that they had transformed his single-layered method into a *mille-feuilles.* It is perhaps noteworthy that this well-known Parisian pastry, made of alternating layers of thin flaky pastry and vanilla cream, is also known as a Napoleon!

In my opinion, dissection of the face through the lower eyelid should be banned, for it is dangerous. Edema often forms that resorbs only very slowly. I have seen several complications of such midfacelifts through a primary lower lid approach. We should remember that the masklift, or subperiosteal facelift, is in itself a simple technique. The principle is to dissect completely and widely so that the whole facial mask can be lifted to the desired position and fixed without too much tension, which might drag the mask down again. One of the fundamental aspects of either the "open" or the endoscopic masklift is the toning of the orbital septum and the orbicularis oculi muscle. This is achieved without interrupting the continuity of the muscle and produces an appreciable rejuvenating effect, even before the soft cheek and nasolabial fold are suspended.

Therefore, in my opinion, only two techniques are possible today. The first, the *open masklift via a coronal approach,* has the following disadvantages:

1. Some hair loss, and occasional visible scars requiring secondary correction on the scalp
2. Hyposensitivity of the scalp
3. Pruritus of the scalp during the reinnervation phase

This really remains the best technique, permitting a proper surgical exposure and many possible variations in terms of addition or removal of skeletal elements (9).

The other approach is the *endoscopic forehead and midfacelift* of Isse and Ramirez, which is in fact the same dissection except that the approach is endoscopic, without any fancy variations. It should be said that the results are often more modest in terms of tissue mobilization and deep fixation. The technique must be chosen after frank and open discussion with the patient to allow the advantages and disadvantages of the two techniques to be weighed.

1. If a patient refuses a scalp incision, an endoscopic subperiosteal facelift is the only choice, as it leaves only a few small scars in the scalp (although they too can cause minor local problems, such as small patches of alopecia).
2. If enlargement of the forehead is clearly indicated, if the scalp is of good quality and the hair dense enough, and if the patient will accept a hairline scar, one can perform the classic open technique, but with resection of scalp restricted to the central pat and nearly eliminated at the side.
3. A variation is the frontal lift with an incision in front of the hairline. This is the choice when the patient already had a high forehead and a reduction of the extent of this hairless skin is desired. If the scar is wavy, as described by Connell (10), it is quite acceptable. This technique, called the *precapillary forehead lift,* by itself it gives a good rejuvenating effect.
4. Yet another variation, a combination of open and closed techniques, emphasizes the advantages of both without their disadvantages. It is strictly cutaneous and in front of the hairline; the frontalis muscle, galea, and periosteum are left intact, so that the twigs of the frontal branch of the trigeminal nerve are preserved (11).

CONCLUSION

Subperiosteal facelift is a controversial subject. As with any newly introduced approach, a certain amount of time must elapse before, in the light of experience, one can reach some sort of consensus on the specific indications for the technique. In the light of modern developments based on the concept of the SMAS (12), it is out of the question to consider subperiosteal dissection as a new panacea. Nevertheless, precise indications for the use of these deep approaches have been defined:

1. Antimongoloid position of the eyelids
2. Scleral show resulting from a short lower eyelid
3. A "sad look"
4. Patient's desire to have almond-shaped eyes ("star eyes")
5. Orthomorphic rejuvenation or correction of the midface (e.g., onlay grafts, bony corrections)

A major difference between the SMAS lift and the DMAS lift is that traction in the former is obliquely anteroposterior, whereas in the latter it is purely vertical. To avoid any misunderstanding, it should be made clear that although subperiosteal dissection allows lifting of the facial mask in a deeper plane than that of the SMAS, a subcutaneous cervicofacial facelift remains indispensable to achieve proper draping of the skin, just as retensioning of the platysma remains necessary in the neck (11).

In the long term, an important difference becomes apparent; the results are much more stable and durable than with the classic techniques (13) (Figs. 52D-1 through 52D-8).

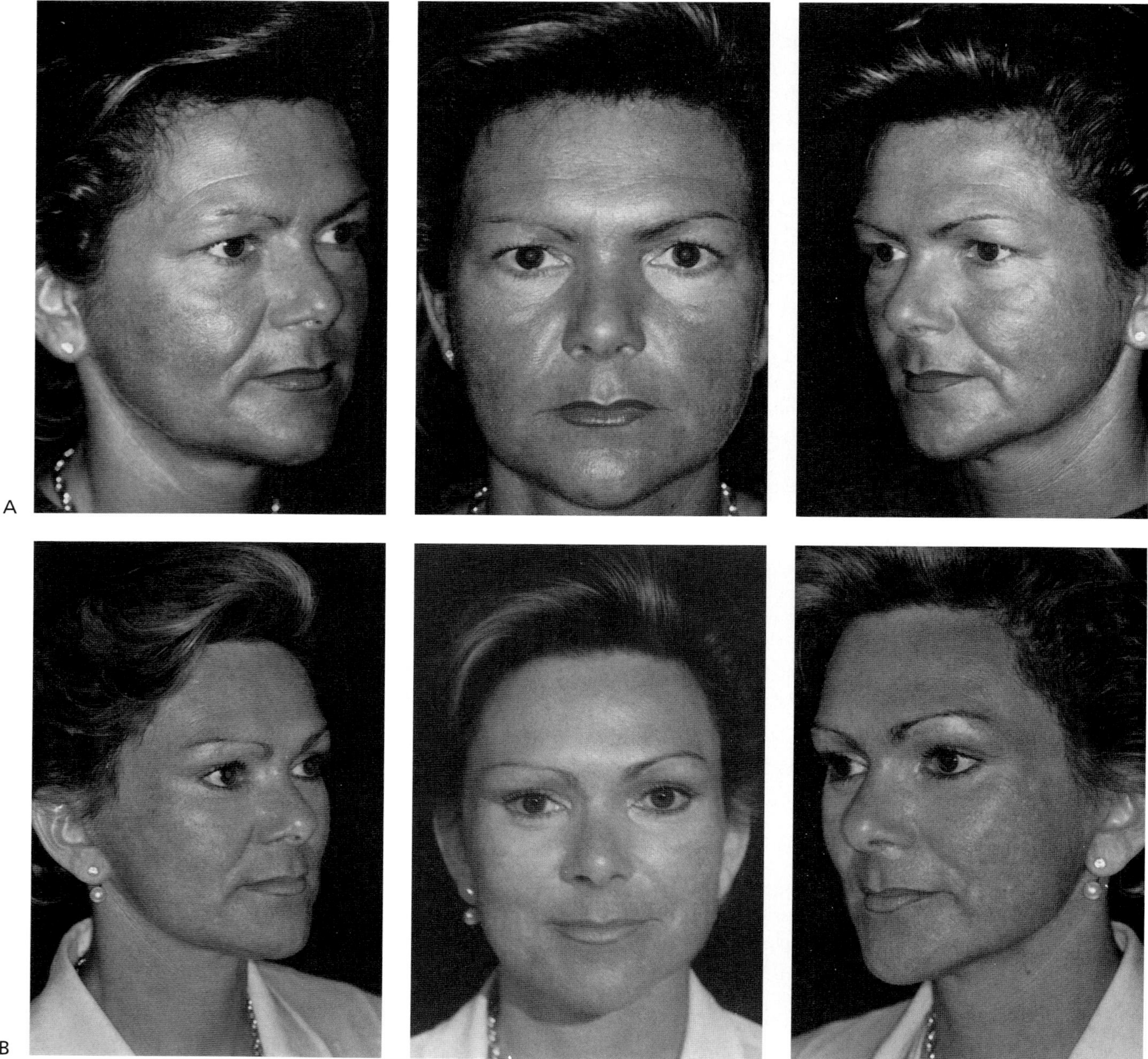

FIGURE 52D-1. Patient **(A)** before and **(B)** after deep musculoaponeurotic system *(DMAS)*-extended subperiosteal facelift.

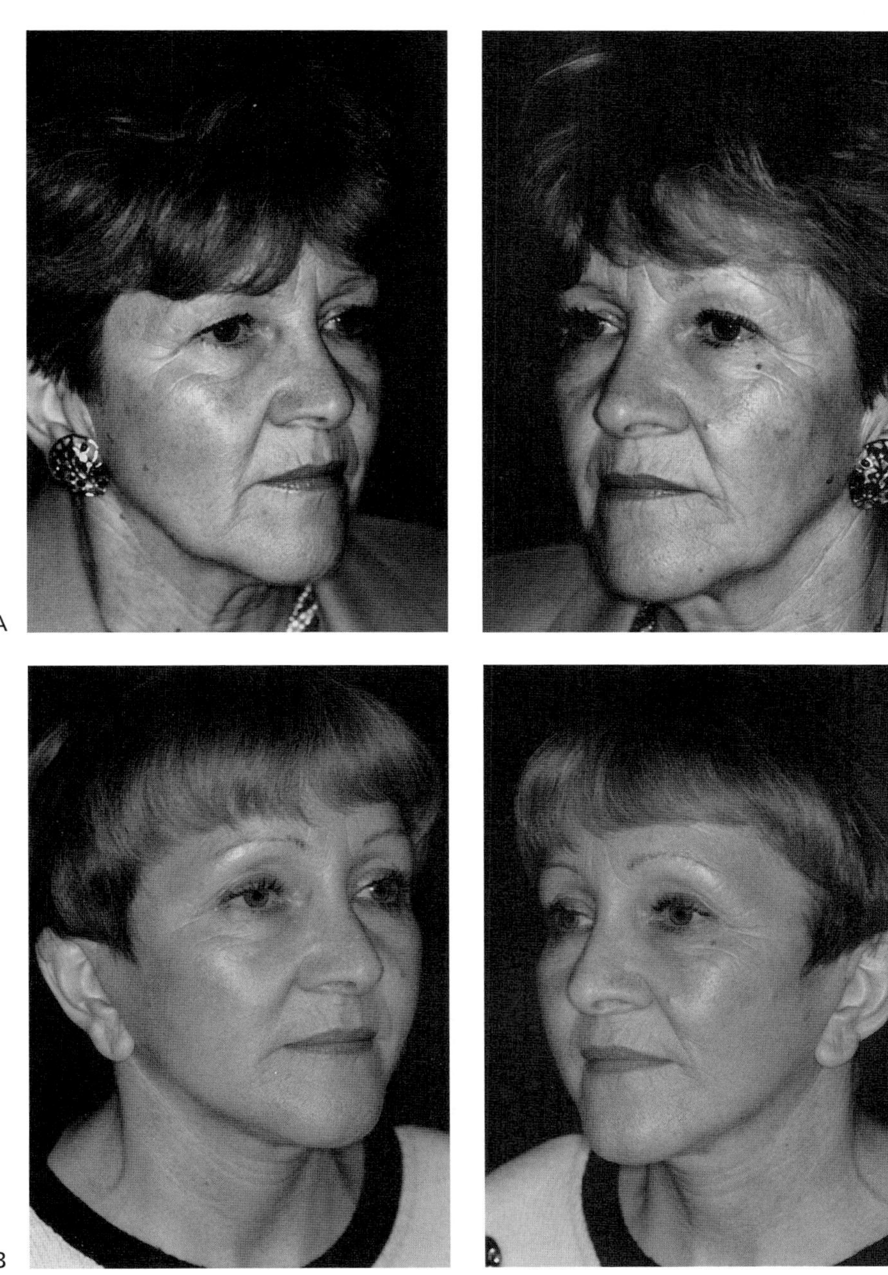

FIGURE 52D-2. Patient **(A)** before and **(B)** after deep musculoaponeurotic system *(DMAS)*-extended subperiosteal facelift.

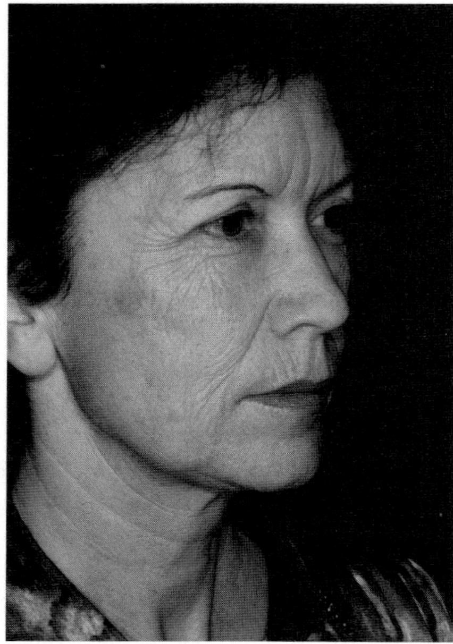
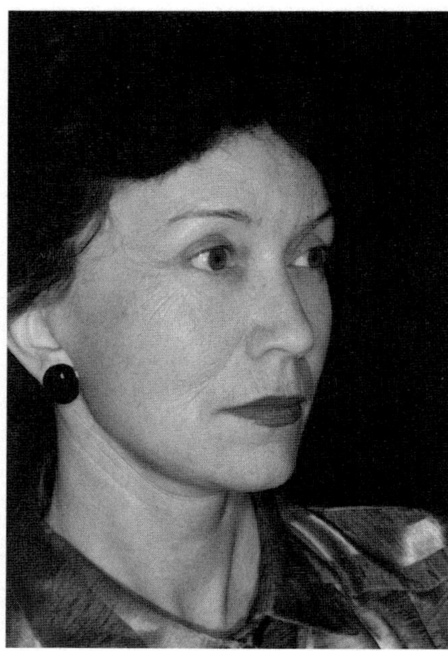

A,B

FIGURE 52D-3. Patient **(A)** before and **(B)** after deep musculoaponeurotic system *(DMAS)*-extended subperiosteal facelift.

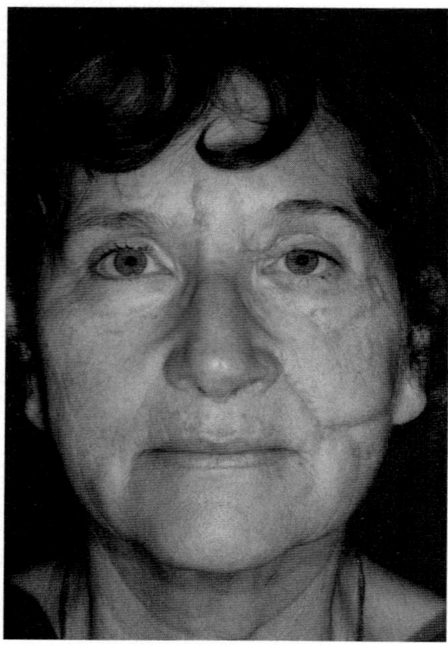
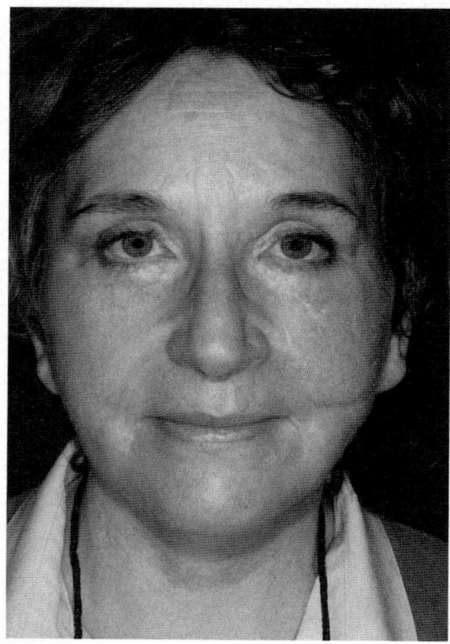

A,B

FIGURE 52D-4. Patient **(A)** before and **(B)** after deep musculoaponeurotic system *(DMAS)*-extended subperiosteal facelift.

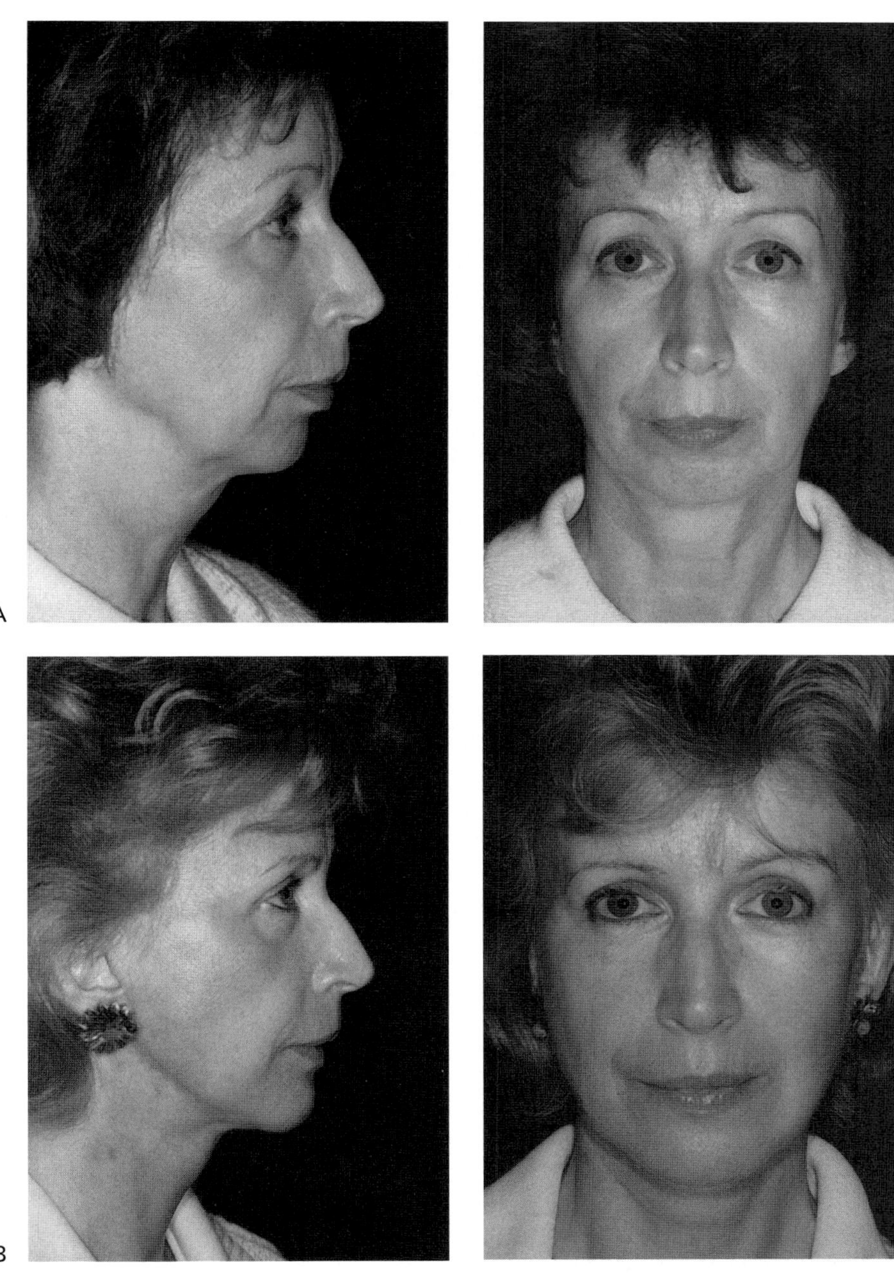

FIGURE 52D-5. Patient **(A)** before and **(B)** after deep musculoaponeurotic system *(DMAS)*-extended subperiosteal facelift.

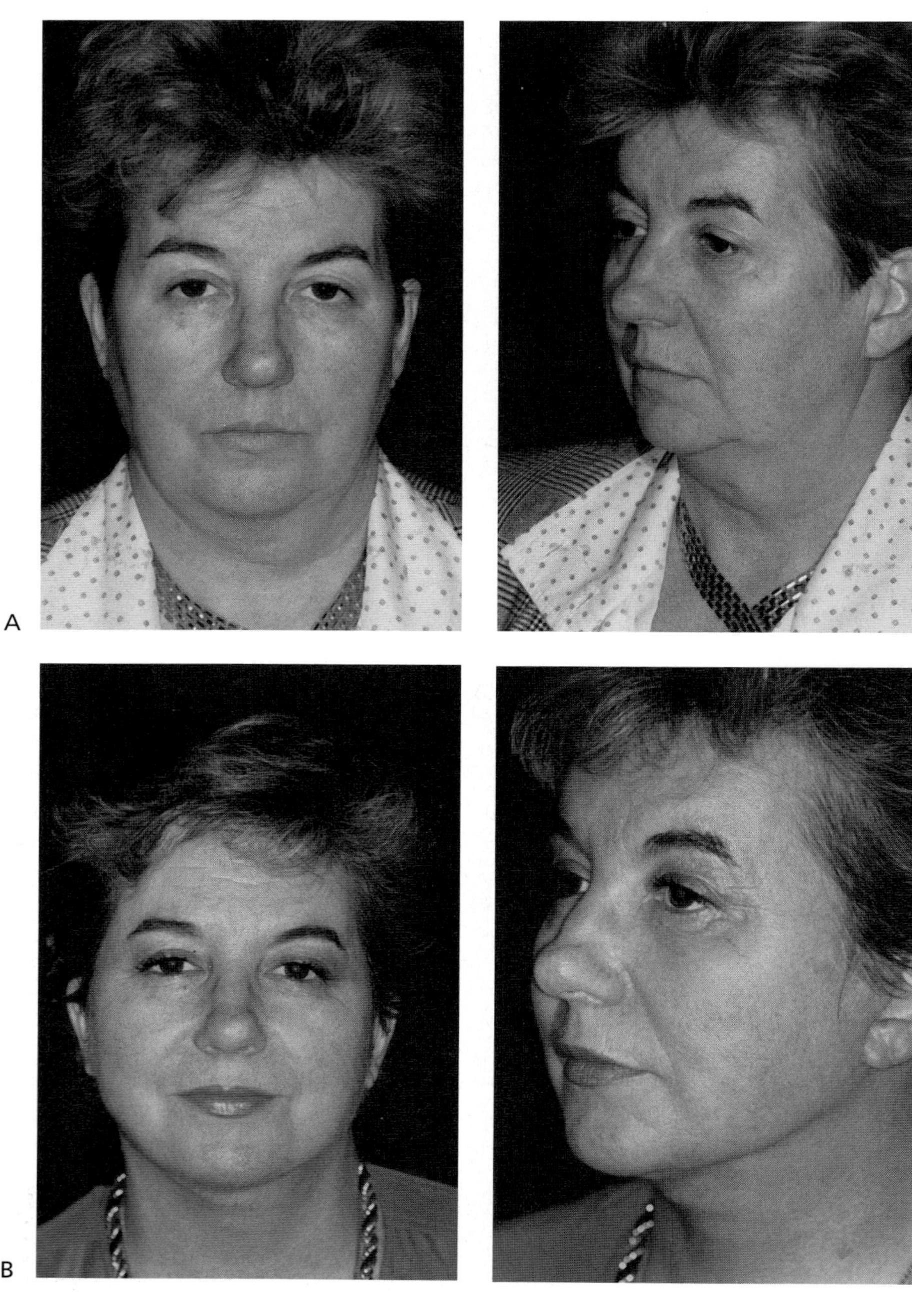

FIGURE 52D-6. Patient **(A)** before and **(B)** after deep musculoaponeurotic system *(DMAS)*-extended subperiosteal facelift.

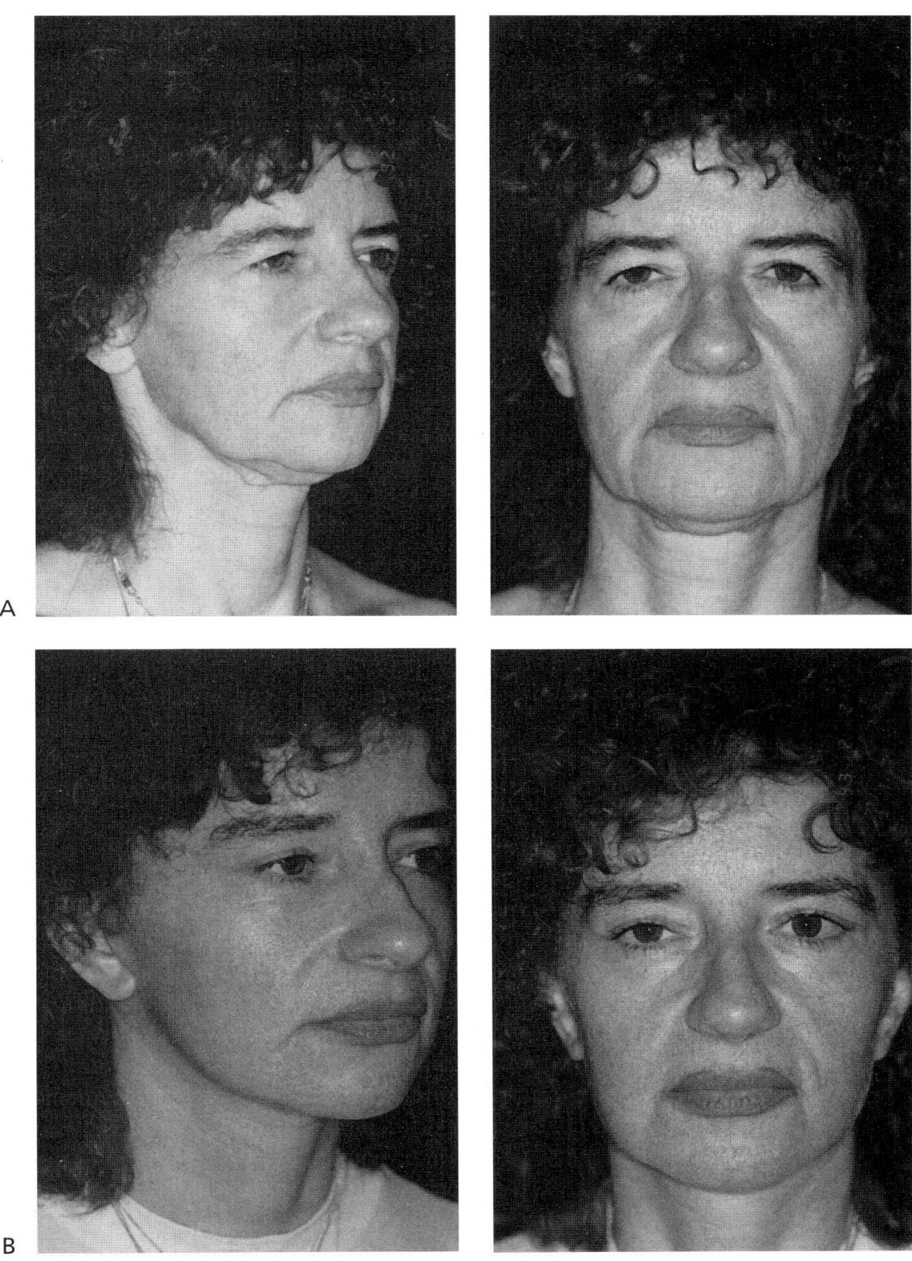

FIGURE 52D-7. Patient **(A)** before and **(B)** after deep musculoaponeurotic system *(DMAS)*-extended subperiosteal facelift.

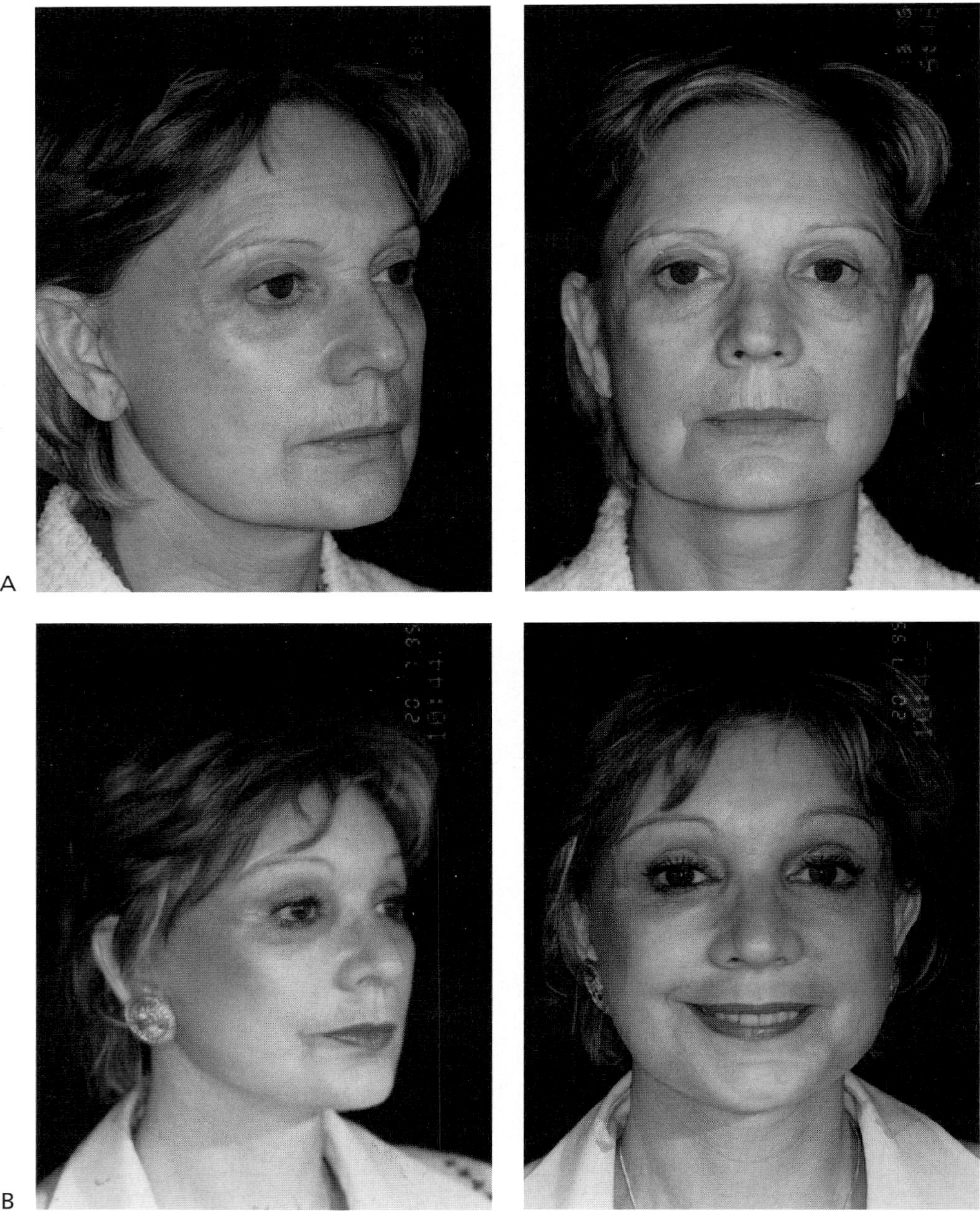

FIGURE 52D-8. Patient **(A)** before and **(B)** after deep musculoaponeurotic system *(DMAS)*-extended subperiosteal facelift.

REFERENCES

1. Maillard GF. *Chirurgie plastique de l'orbite osseuse. Monographie.* Basel, Switzerland: Schwabe Verlag, 1977.
2. Maillard G-F. Case report: subperiosteal facelift and correction of facial skeleton for severe Romberg fat atrophy. *Eur J Plast Surg* 1988;11:136–137.
3. Tessier P. Le lifting facial sous-périosté. *Ann Chir Plast Esthet* 1989;34:193–197.
4. Krastinova-Lolov D. Le lifting facial sous-périosté. *Ann Chir Plast Esthet* 1989;34:199–211.
5. Maillard G.F. *Le lifting facial sous-périosté.* Communication at the International Society for Aesthetic Plastic Surgery Congress, Zürich, 1989.
6. Ramirez O. *Le lifting facial sous-périosté.* Communication at the International Society for Aesthetic Plastic Surgery Congress, Zürich, 1989.
7. Maillard GF, Cornette de St-Cyr B, Scheflan M. The subpe-

riosteal bicoronal approach to total face lifting: the DMAS—deep musculoaponeurotic system. *Aesthetic Plast Surg* 1991;15: 285–291.
8. Ramirez O, Maillard G-F, Musolas A. The extended subperiosteal face lift: a definitive soft-tissue remodeling for facial rejuvenation. *Plast Reconstr Surg* 1991;88:227–236.
9. Hamra ST. Composite rhytidectomy. *Plast Reconstr Surg* 1992;90:1–13.
10. Connell BF. Deep-layer techniques in cervicofacial rejuvenations. In: Psillakis JM, ed. *Deep facelifting techniques.* New York: Thieme Medical Publishers, 1994:161–190.
11. Maillard G-F. The DMAS ("deep musculoaponeurotic system") flap. Extended subperiosteal facelift. Ideas and innovations. *Plast Reconstr Surg* 2000;105:1188–1195.
12. Maillard G-F, Ramirez O, Cornette de St Cyr B, et al. El rejuvenecimiento facial. *Cirugia Plastica Ibero-Latinoamericana* 1996;12:9–20.
13. Maillard G-F. Discussion: facelift without preauricular scars by Antonio Fuente Del Campo. *Plast Reconstr Surg* 1993;92: 654–661.

53

CLOSED RHINOPLASTY

MARK B. CONSTANTIAN

As any surgeon knows who has performed the operation even once, rhinoplasty is exceedingly difficult. The very fact that surgeons calculate and publish their nasal surgery revision rates (a practice that is uncommon in other aesthetic procedures) distinguishes the diminutive "nose job" as an operation that can accomplish harm as well as good, and create favorable or highly unfavorable results.

Why is this so? Is it because the surgeon does not have good, binocular vision through small incisions? Is it because the nasal anatomy is complex and the margin of error narrow? Or is it, as one surgeon told me, that the nose is an idiosyncratic organ, ungoverned by the usual biological laws? It is my intention in this chapter to outline the reasons why I believe rhinoplasty is so difficult; to describe the causes, originating in surgeon–patient interaction and in the operating room, that most commonly produce the unfavorable result; and to provide a framework for avoiding complications or undesired sequelae and correcting them if they occur.

FALLACIES OF THE TRADITIONAL RHINOPLASTY MODEL

Reduction rhinoplasty is an inherently odd operation; the traditional model itself is probably the chief reason that rhinoplasty is so difficult. Many patients and surgeons consider all preoperative noses to be too large; it follows therefore that the successful rhinoplasty should always be a reduction operation. However, rhinoplasty is almost unique when compared with other reduction operations. In breast reduction, for example, skin and underlying support (breast parenchyma) are reduced proportionally, whereas traditional rhinoplasty teaching prescribes skeletal reduction alone; the skeletal reduction presumably produces soft tissue contraction appropriate to the patient's aesthetic goals.

As logical as this model may sound, nature conspires to undo it. Nasal skin does not contract alone. The reduced postoperative skeleton also "contracts" wherever postoperative structural interdependencies have been disturbed but not rebalanced, (e.g., yielding middle vault collapse or alar notching). The soft tissues contract wherever underlying skeletal support has been reduced, but according to their own vectors of contraction, which may or may not follow skeletal shape. An aesthetic operation designed so that the surgeon has the least control over the surface most responsible for the quality of the postoperative result is at best a trying format.

What has confused surgeons in the past is the simple fact that reduction rhinoplasty does sometimes work. The thin-skinned nose that requires only modest dorsal and tip reduction is ideal for a pure reduction strategy; this is the nasal type most commonly shown by authors who espouse a pure reduction model. In clinical practice, however, few such salutary circumstances occur. Much more common is the nose with a high dorsum (in which hump reduction will impair internal valvular support); the nose with poor tip projection (in which reduction alone will provide neither a straight bridge nor optimal tip contour); or the preoperatively unbalanced nose (e.g., one with a low root and high dorsum, or a low dorsum and a large nasal base). The surgeon should be wary of a pure reduction strategy because it does not solve most rhinoplasty problems.

The Two False Assumptions of a Traditional Rhinoplasty Model

Two assumptions underlie the logic of "skeletal reduction, soft tissue contraction," neither of which may be valid in many clinical situations.

Assumption No. 1

The nasal soft tissue cover has an infinite ability to contract to the shape of the underlying skeleton. If the nose is being reduced, the entire surgical result depends on the validity of this assumption. To a limited degree (depending on the quality, thickness, and distribution of the preoperative skin sleeve), nasal skin will shrink, but not necessarily to the

M. B. Constantian: Department of Surgery, Dartmouth Medical School, Hanover, New Hampshire

shape of the underlying skeleton (which may be contracting itself; see below). The vectors of skin sleeve contraction are related to, but independent of, bridge and tip shape: caudal and medial over the bony and upper cartilaginous vaults, posterior over the maxillary arch, cephalad at the caudal septum and alar rims, posterior and concentric at the tip lobule (1). The "end stage" of these vectors is the classical shape of supratip deformity: low dorsum; collapsed middle third (accompanying internal valvular incompetence); high supratip; round, undifferentiated tip lobule; arching alar rims (usually accompanying external valvular incompetence); sharp subnasale; and retrusive upper lip (Fig. 53-1). Indeed, if assumption No. 1 were always true, supratip deformity would never occur, and augmentation would not correct it.

Assumption No. 2

Surgical alterations of the nasal skeleton produce purely regional changes. The classical application of assumption No. 2 is a preoperative plan in which the surgeon will resect all nasal skeleton anterior to a straight line drawn from the nasal root to the tip. Underlying this strategy is the assumption that dorsal reduction affects only bridge height. In fact,

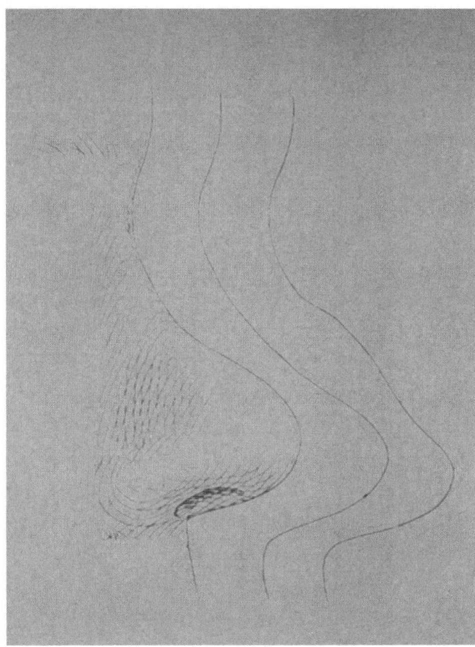

FIGURE 53-1. The vectors of soft tissue contraction following reduction rhinoplasty. The preoperative outline *(left)* may appear to drape to the reduced framework intraoperatively *(center line)*, but if the skeletal structures have been reduced beyond the ability of the soft tissues to coapt, the skin sleeve contracts in a predictable pattern that leads to the classic supratip deformity *(right-hand line)*. See text for details. (From Constantian MB. A model for planning rhinoplasty. *Plast Reconstr Surg* 1987;79: 472–481, with permission.)

however, bridge reduction affects nasal width and nasal length, apparent nasal base size, middle vault support, alar rim contour, and columellar position (2,3). Similarly, alar cartilage reduction can affect tip support and projection, nasal length, alar rim contour, and external valvular support (4). These structural interdependencies are predictable and important in preoperative planning and in interpreting intraoperative nasal appearance, postoperative success, and secondary deformities.

Structural interdependencies in the nose are "global," not regional, and understanding these interrelationships the surgeon may control the postoperative result. Useful to me here is the model of a dynamic nasal equilibrium (1), in which the preoperative nasal shape represents a balance between soft tissues and their underlying support. Skeletal reduction disrupts this equilibrium, the disequilibrated nose cannot and does not remain the same, and change occurs until the nose reestablishes its new equilibrium. Consequently, the degree of disequilibrium at the conclusion of a rhinoplasty determines the amount of postoperative change; the greater the disequilibrium, the greater the postoperative surprise. Therefore, the surgeon who controls the postoperative equilibrium controls the postoperative result; usually, this means maintaining skeletal support where soft tissue contraction is particularly undesirable or unpredictable—in the nasal tip (to control contour) and the middle third (to control internal valvular support). Conversely, soft tissue contraction is safer (and more predictable) over the bony vault, where the skin is thinner and the underlying skeletal shape is simpler. Rhinoplasty is difficult partly because the reduction model is insufficiently complex, because a smaller nose is not always an achievable surgical goal, because many traditional presumptions about nasal structure do not account for the interdependencies that exist, and because rhinoplasty, unlike many surgical procedures that can be pictured and followed step by step in atlases, is a feedback operation that cannot be easily premeasured and premarked; rather, it requires constant readjustments by the surgeon. Rhinoplasty is a uniquely interactive operation, and an effective rhinoplasty model must respect the biological principles on which it is based.

CONSTRUCTING A SURGICAL PLAN

Although this chapter is not a discussion of routine rhinoplasty, the surgeon trying to understand unfavorable results must appreciate not only the surgical strategies that may have preceded them, but also how to avoid them primarily. In trying to solve these problems myself, I have used three aesthetic parameters for the past 20 years to plan primary and secondary rhinoplasties (5). Their simplicity lies entirely in a reliance on soft tissue assessments, which therefore apply whether or not the skeleton influences surface contours.

Skin Thickness and Distribution

Although it may be intuitively obvious that skin thickness affects a rhinoplasty plan, so also does skin distribution; the preoperative large nasal base does not contract to become a small nasal base, but rather a distorted large nasal base (6,7). Because preoperative skin distribution is relatively fixed, skin quality affects both reduction and augmentation. Thicker skin requires *more,* not less, skeletal support (8); the surgeon must therefore be conservative in skeletal reduction and will need more substantial grafts to produce a given postoperative result. Thinner skin may allow greater reductions but requires softer, more carefully tailored grafts to avoid surface irregularities or distortions.

Tip Lobular Contour

Because the nasal base (lower nasal third), with its alar lobules, tip lobule, nostrils, facets, and columella, has a more complex topography than the pyramidal bony and upper cartilaginous vaults, and because the soft tissues of the lower third are thicker, it follows that the surgeon should select first those maneuvers that provide the best nasal base contours.

Ideal tip aesthetics (Fig. 53-2, left) require a defined point of greatest projection, a flat supratip, and a tip lobular mass that falls below the level of greatest projection. The poorly shaped tip lobule (Fig. 53-2, right) has the opposite characteristics—a poorly defined, low point of greatest tip projection, a convex supratip, and a tip lobular mass that lies cephalic to the point of greatest projection. Simple alar cartilage reduction cannot raise the level of the alar dome peaks nor increase tip lobular mass; rather, it produces a smaller replica of the same preoperative tip (Fig. 53-3). To create an aesthetic lobule from the poorly shaped configuration just described, the surgeon must raise the level of greatest projection while increasing the lobular mass caudal to this point. In my practice, the most effective reconstructive technique toward this end is autogenous cartilage grafting (9,10).

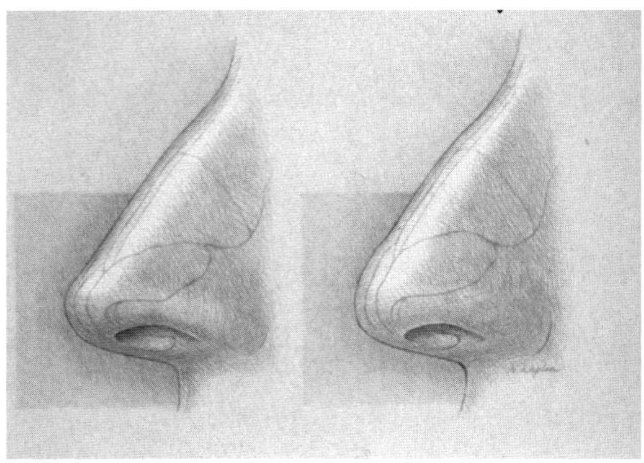

FIGURE 53-2. "Good" and "bad" tip aesthetics. In the well-shaped tip lobule *(left),* the supratip is flat, tip projection is greatest at a discrete point, and the mass of the tip lobule is caudal to this point; in the poorly shaped lobule *(right),* the opposite contours are present. (From Constantian MB. Experience with a three-point method for planning rhinoplasty. *Ann Plast Surg* 1993;30:1–12, with permission.)

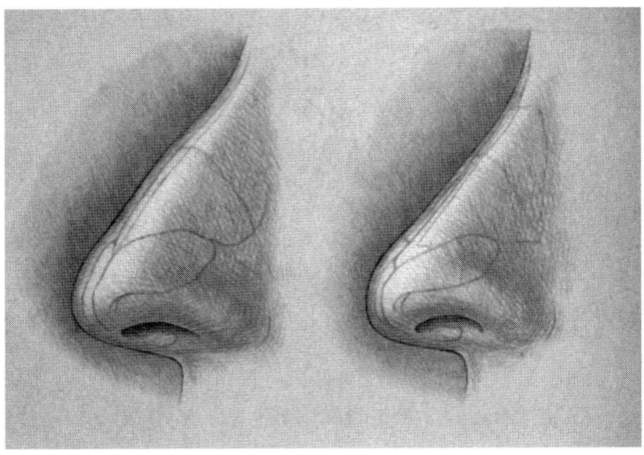

FIGURE 53-3. Reduction of a poorly shaped tip lobule *(left)* does not produce a well-shaped lobule, but rather a smaller version of the same preoperative tip *(right).* (From Constantian MB. Experience with a three-point method for planning rhinoplasty. *Ann Plast Surg* 1993;30:1–12, with permission.)

Balance between Nasal Base Size and Bridge Height

Before the surgeon can select a preferred operative strategy, he or she must first consider the effect of dorsal reduction or augmentation on the apparent size of the preoperative nasal base (5,11). This critical balance most profoundly affects the nasal profile, about which patients usually have the strongest views despite the fact that it is the angle from which they least often see themselves. In general, the higher the dorsum, the smaller the nasal base appears (6,7) (Figs. 4 and 5). This powerful illusion has its most important practical application in the patient who believes that the preoperative nasal base is too large; if the patient also has a convex dorsum, bridge reduction will make a large nasal base appear larger. Optimal balance is necessary for postoperative aesthetics. The patient's goals may be better achieved by a change in balance than in size, a paradoxical effect that most patients, and even many surgeons, have to see to believe.

FOUR COMMON ANATOMICAL PROBLEMS THAT CREATE UNFAVORABLE RESULTS

Although secondary rhinoplasty deformities may seem to come in a limitless variety, four anatomical problems, easy to diagnose preoperatively, particularly predispose to bad outcomes unless recognized and corrected in the operative plan.

Low Nasal Root

The traps posed by this particular entity have not been properly appreciated by many surgeons (Figs. 4 and 5). Skeptics who originally viewed the low root as simply another indication for cartilage grafting have missed the importance of the observation (11).

The nasal root (or radix) ideally begins at the level of the upper lash margin. When the radix begins lower, nasal length (from root to subnasale or tip) is shorter, and the nasal base (subnasale to the most projecting point of the tip), appears larger. The position of the root should influence the operative plan in two circumstances: (a) the patient with a low root, high dorsum, and large nasal base (Fig. 53-4), in whom

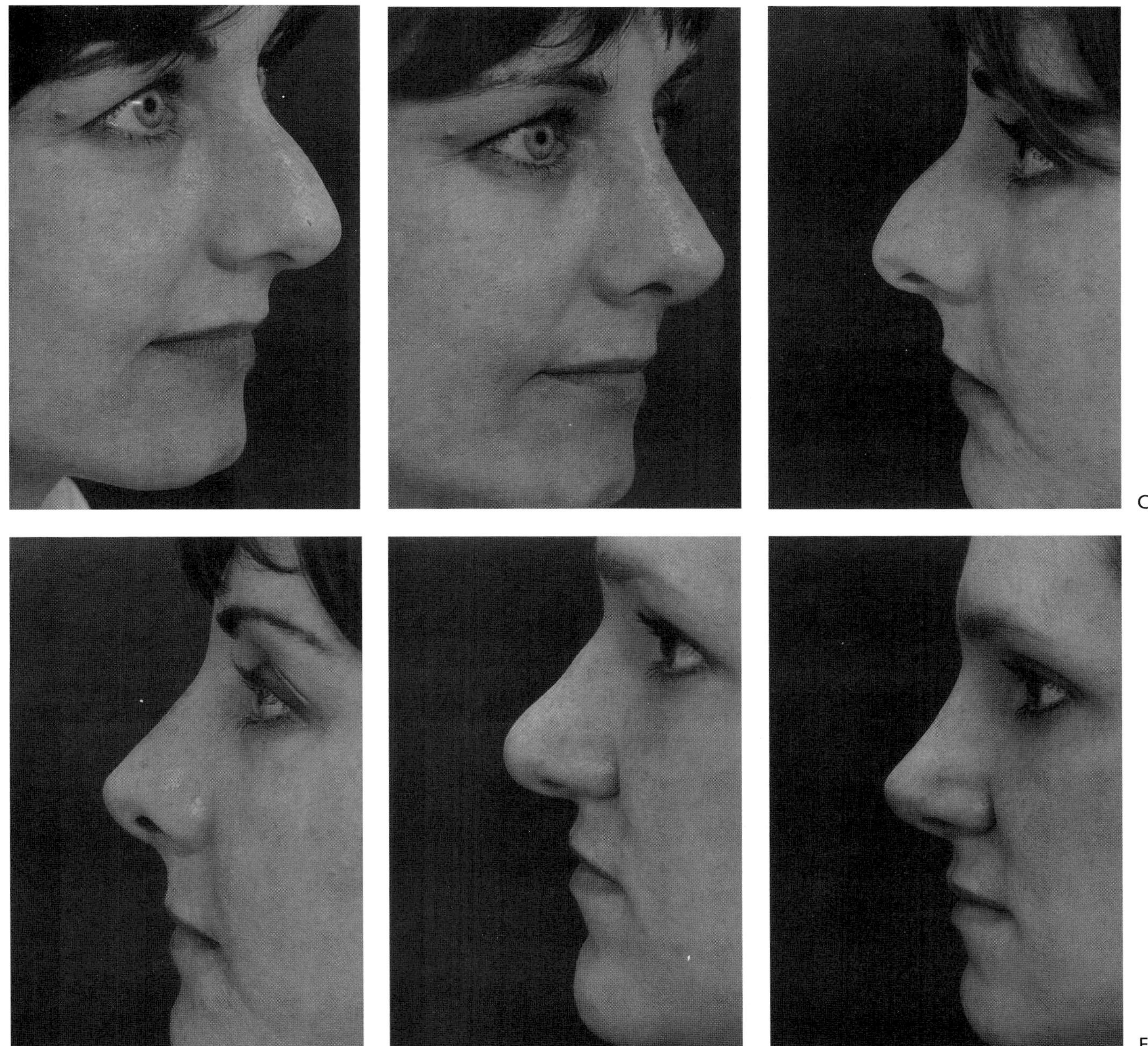

FIGURE 53-4. A–D: Low radix. In this patient, the preoperative nasal root begins near the lower lash margin; to avoid the increase in apparent nasal base size that would occur with a substantial dorsal resection (and to minimize the degree of contraction required in these thick soft tissues), the dorsal convexity was reduced moderately and the nasal root was raised with layered, crushed cartilage grafts. **E,F:** Low dorsum. When the root and dorsum are low, the nasal base appears large; by raising the entire dorsum, the surgeon can decrease the apparent size of the nasal base. The illusion is so powerful that this nasal base appears smaller after surgery even though it is actually larger (from tip grafting).

dorsal reduction will make the nasal base appear undesirably larger; (b) the patient in whom the entire dorsum is low relative to the nasal base (Fig. 53-5). In both cases, the patient often complains most about nasal base size ("The tip of my nose sticks out too far," or "The bottom of my nose is too big"). The surgeon has two choices—either reduce the nasal tip sufficiently to balance the upper nose, or reduce the tip less (or not at all) and raise the dorsum, segmentally (Fig. 53-4) or entirely (Fig. 53-5), to balance the nasal base. Variations of the latter option are generally safer because they require less contraction of thicker tip tissues and are therefore less likely to cause distortion.

Tip with Inadequate Projection

In our discussion of "good" and "bad" tip lobular shapes, I have not mentioned "adequate" or "inadequate" tip projection, terms that are used commonly by nasal surgeons without uniform consensus about their meaning. In my mind, "adequate tip support" describes alar cartilages that can support the tip lobule to the level of the supratip septum. When the alar cartilages are not sufficient to do so, the tip seems to "hang" from the septal angle and is "inadequately projecting" (Fig. 53-6). Tip projection depends less on the size of the nasal base (which is also the product of skin sleeve vol-

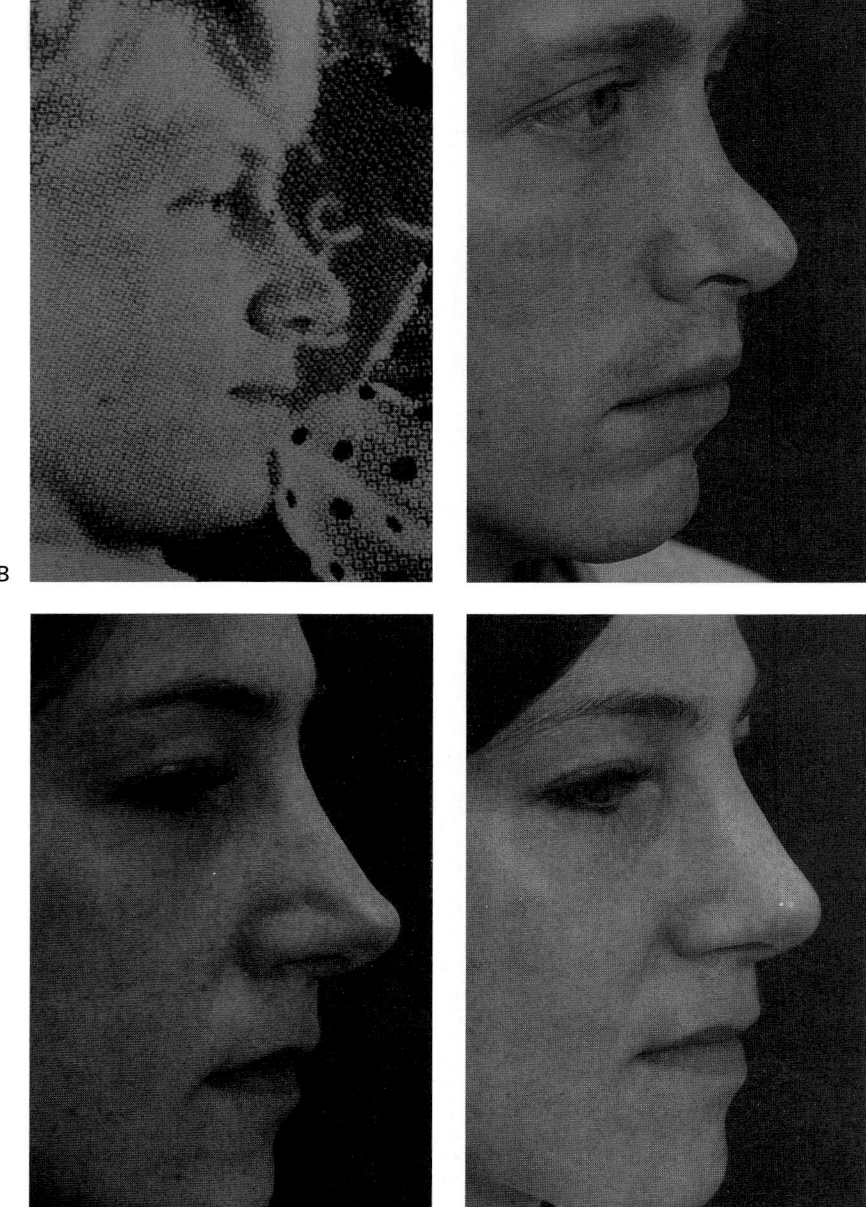

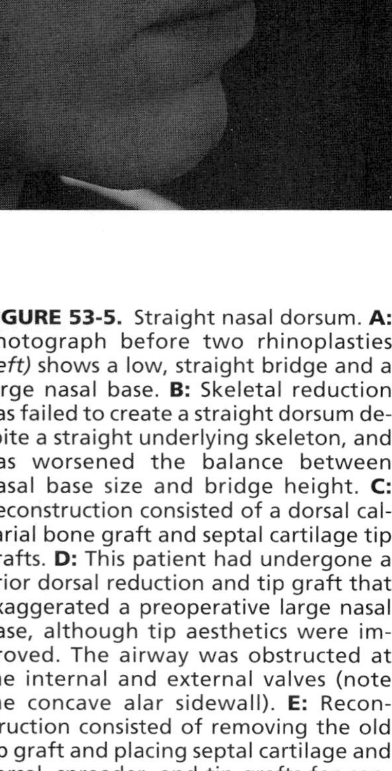

A,B

C

D,E

FIGURE 53-5. Straight nasal dorsum. **A:** Photograph before two rhinoplasties *(left)* shows a low, straight bridge and a large nasal base. **B:** Skeletal reduction has failed to create a straight dorsum despite a straight underlying skeleton, and has worsened the balance between nasal base size and bridge height. **C:** Reconstruction consisted of a dorsal calvarial bone graft and septal cartilage tip grafts. **D:** This patient had undergone a prior dorsal reduction and tip graft that exaggerated a preoperative large nasal base, although tip aesthetics were improved. The airway was obstructed at the internal and external valves (note the concave alar sidewall). **E:** Reconstruction consisted of removing the old tip graft and placing septal cartilage and dorsal, spreader, and tip grafts for contour and support. At 18 months postoperatively, mean nasal air flow had increased more than 15 times over preoperative values.

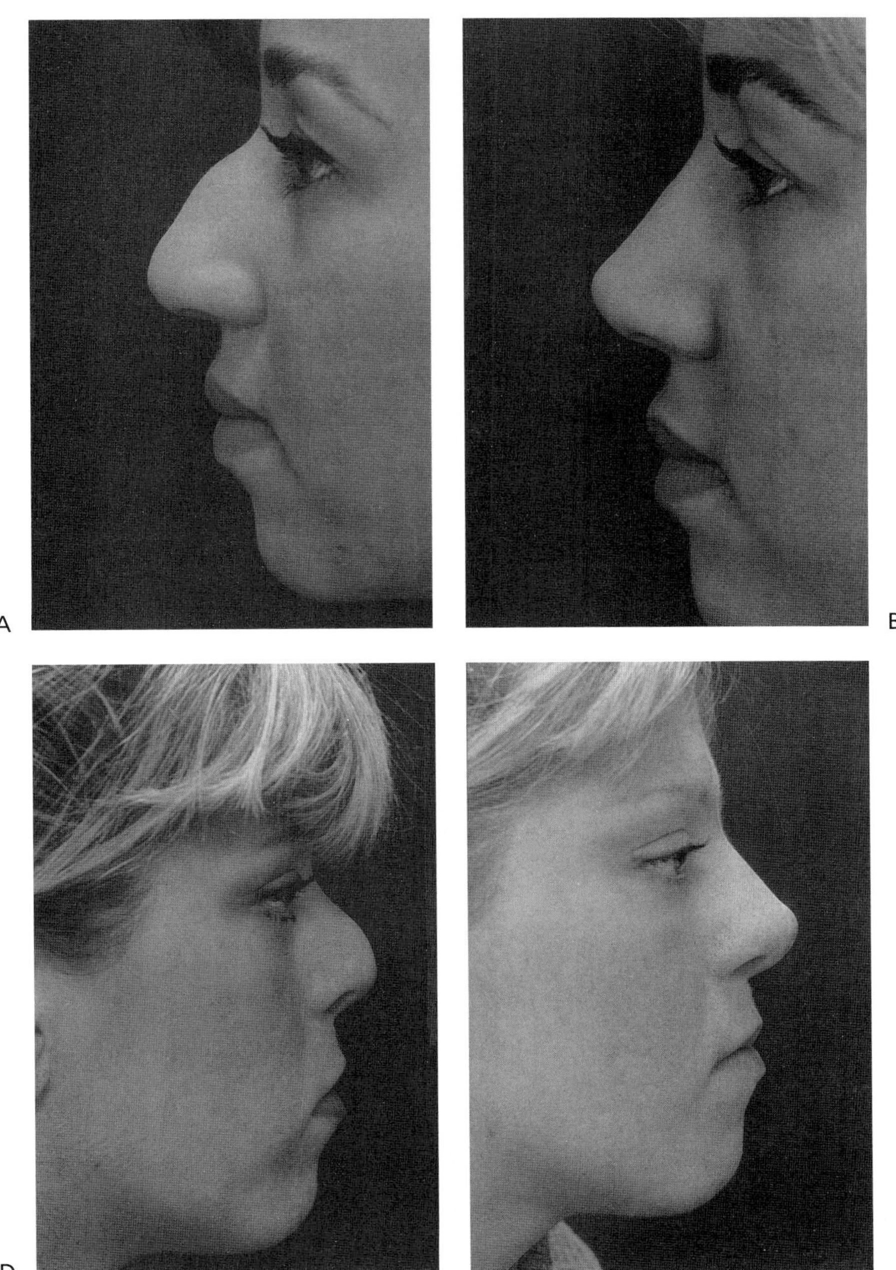

FIGURE 53-6. A–D: Inadequate tip projection. In both patients, the alar cartilages were not sufficiently strong to support the tip to the level of the supratip septum. Reconstruction involved some dorsal reduction and the use of radix and tip grafts.

ume and distribution) than on intrinsic alar cartilage strength. If the preoperative tip does not project to the level of the supratip septum, the surgeon must employ some "tip-strengthening" method (sutures, struts, or grafts) to create a straight postoperative bridge. Inadequate tip projection cannot be rendered adequate by reducing the dorsum; no matter how much the bridge is reduced, an inadequately projecting tip, by definition, cannot support itself sufficiently to create a straight profile (Fig. 53-3).

Related to the inadequately projecting tip is the tip with intrinsic strength that supports the tip lobule only to the level of the supratip septum. Here, the surgeon should be aware that any reduction of alar cartilage strength may create inadequate tip projection; the realistic alternatives are to modify the alar cartilages minimally or not at all (when they are well shaped), or to augment tip support when the alar cartilages require modification for aesthetic reasons.

Narrow Middle Vault

Identified some years ago by Sheen in his seminal paper introducing "spreader grafts" (3), the width and stability of the upper cartilaginous vault has received appropriately increasing attention as a common site of preoperative and postoperative airway obstruction (Fig. 53-7). Although descriptions of valvular collapse had appeared earlier in the rhinoplasty literature (12–14), the missing puzzle piece had been the link between resection of the cartilaginous dorsum and postoperative collapse of the middle nasal third, a phenomenon recognized by other authors but erroneously attributed to avulsion of the upper lateral cartilages from the nasal bones during surgery.

In a recent careful anatomical study (15), cadaver measurements indicated a mean width of 5.5 mm at the septal and upper lateral cartilage confluence 10 mm distal to the caudal bony arch. Posterior to the confluence is a broadened area of septum ("confluence height") that averaged 1.2 mm at the same distance from the nasal bones. The critical anatomical fact to remember is that the width and stability of the upper cartilaginous vault (containing the internal nasal valve) depend not only on the width of the bony vault, but also on the height and width of the middle vault roof.

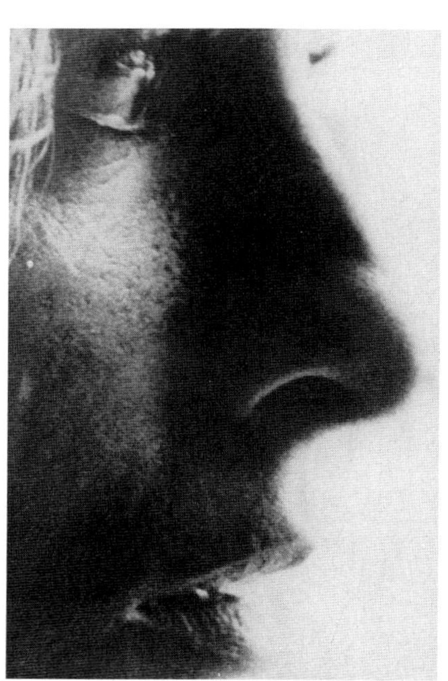

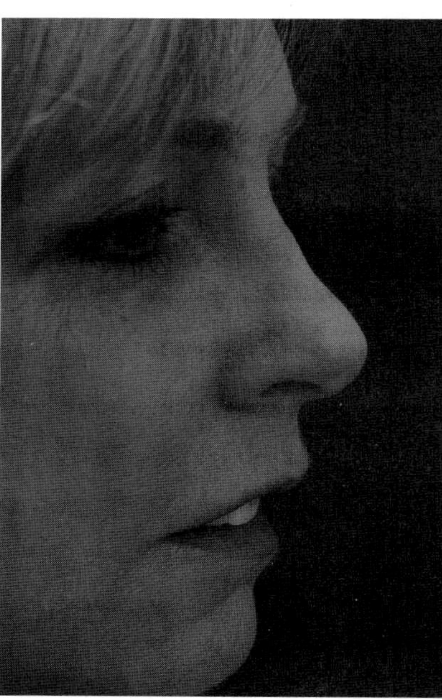

A,B

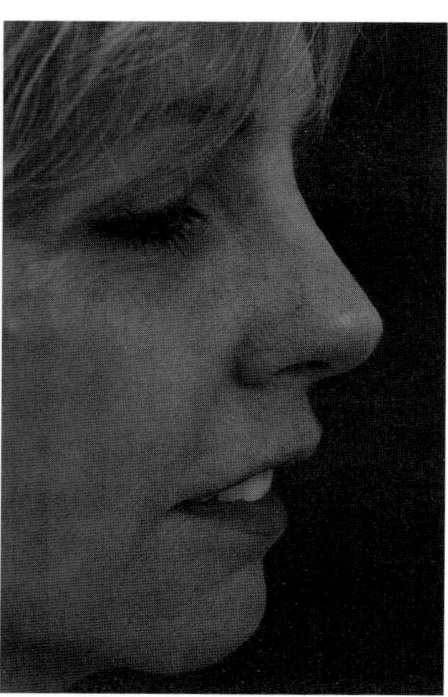

C

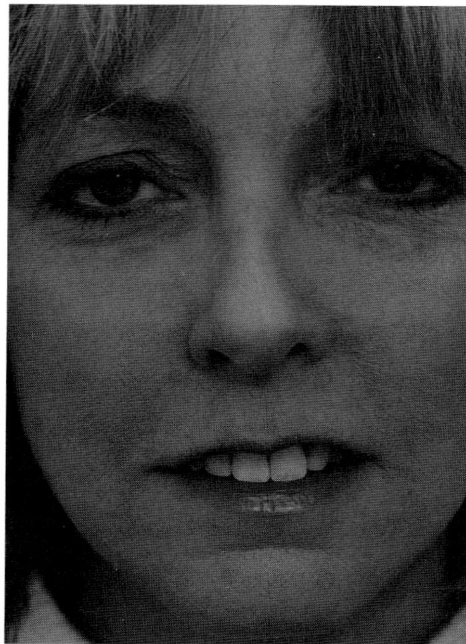

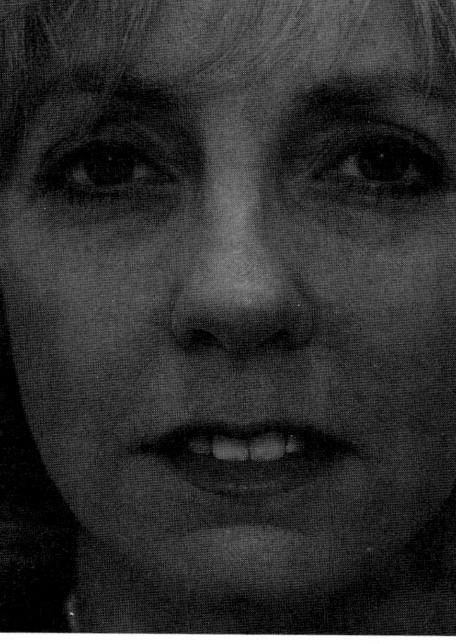

D,E

FIGURE 53-7. A: Narrow preoperative middle vault. A photograph taken before this patient's initial rhinoplasty shows a concave middle third at risk for an increase in airway obstruction following resection of the middle vault roof (see text). **B,D:** Following rhinoplasty, the middle third has become narrower and the airway is obstructed at the internal valve *(right).* **C,E:** Valvular reconstruction was carried out with spreader, dorsal, and tip grafts; air flow increased 28 times over preoperative values following this single operative procedure. **D,E:** Preoperative and postoperative frontal views.

Resection of even 2 mm of middle vault roof during hump removal removes the stabilizing confluence that braces the upper lateral cartilages, which, now unsupported, fall medially and produce the characteristic "inverted V" deformity (3) and varying degrees of associated airway obstruction. An external discontinuity may or may not be visible, depending on overlying soft tissue thickness. It is important for the surgeon to recognize the narrow middle third preoperatively (particularly if a dorsal resection is planned) and to use spreader or dorsal grafts to correct instability that was present preoperatively *or that was created by the surgeon during hump removal* (3,16). The importance of properly supported internal valves cannot be underestimated; rhinomanometric measurements (first reported in 170 patients in what is now a 375 patient study group) have indicated that correction of internal valvular incompetence, with or without septoplasty, at least doubles mean nasal air flow in most patients (16).

Alar Cartilage Malposition

The alar cartilage lateral crura, after leaving the lateral genua, most commonly parallel the anterior third of the alar rims and then diverge from them at 30- to 45-degree angles. In some patients, however, the lateral crura diverge from the rims at greater angles and may even parallel the anterior septum; occasionally, the superior margins of the two lateral crura meet in the midline (17). This anatomical variation

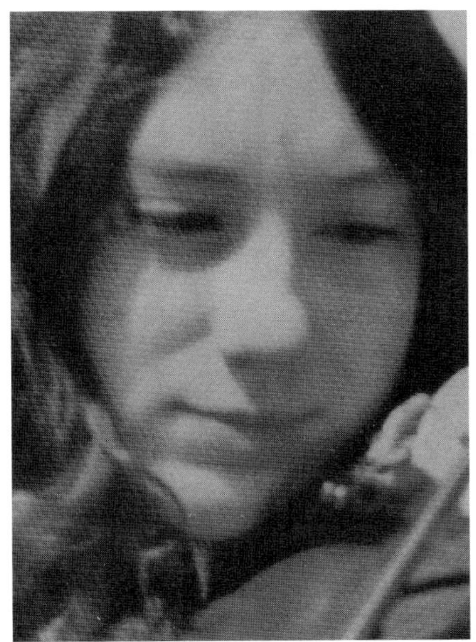
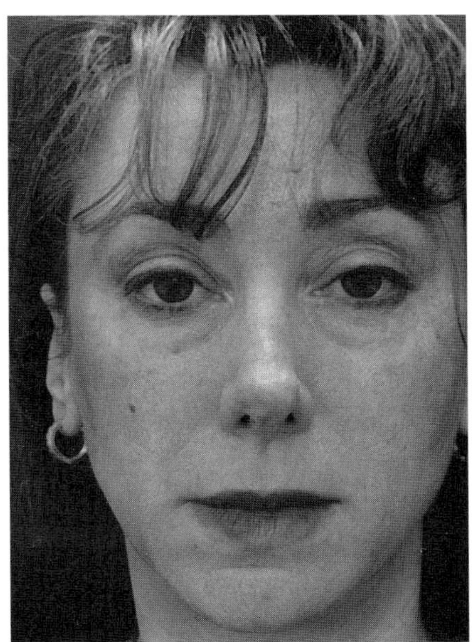
A,B

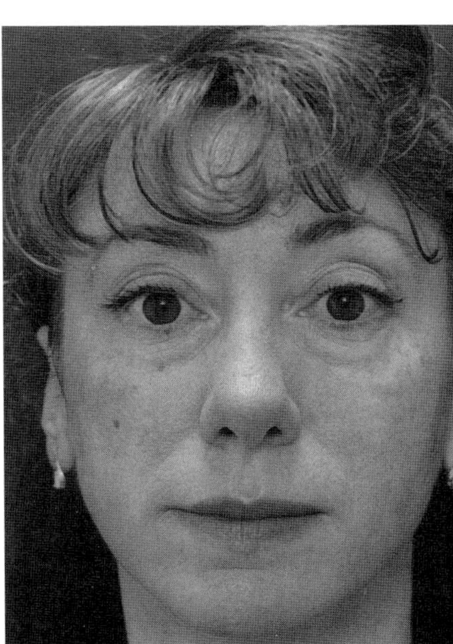
C

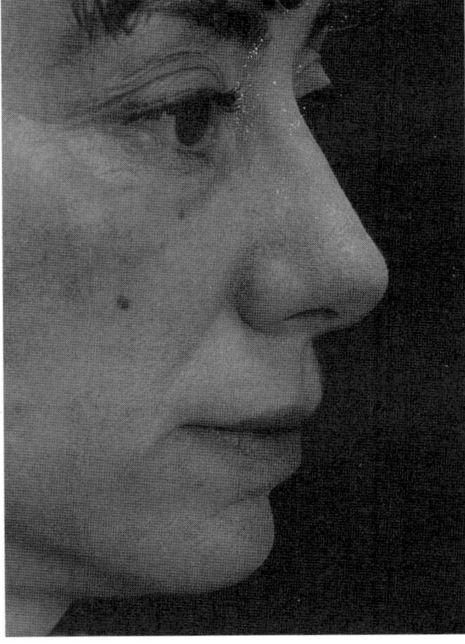
D,E

FIGURE 53-8. Alar cartilage malposition. **A:** A preoperative photograph shows the characteristic lateral wall convexity and "parentheses"; the middle vault is narrow. **B,D:** Following dorsal and tip reduction, the patient's middle third has become narrower, airway obstruction has increased, and the alar cartilage stumps have become knuckled and visible. This type of tip configuration, in which the domes appear amputated at the lateral genua, is characteristic of an unrecognized and operated alar cartilage malposition. **C,E:** Postoperative views following removal of the deformed alar cartilages and placement of spreader, dorsal, tip, and lateral wall septal grafts show smoother contours and an increase in nasal balance. Air flow increased 2.3 times over preoperative values.

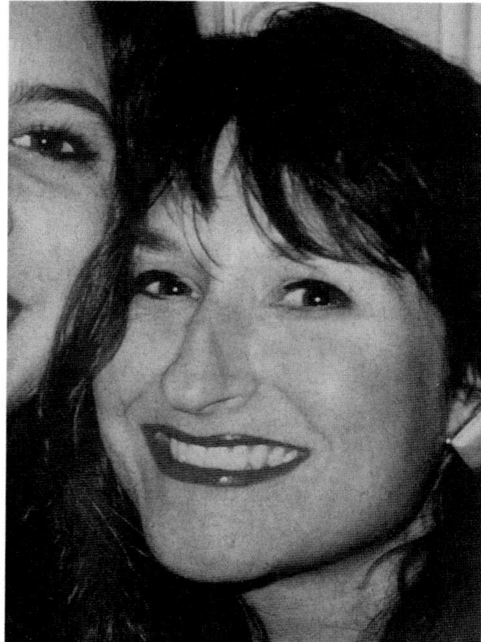
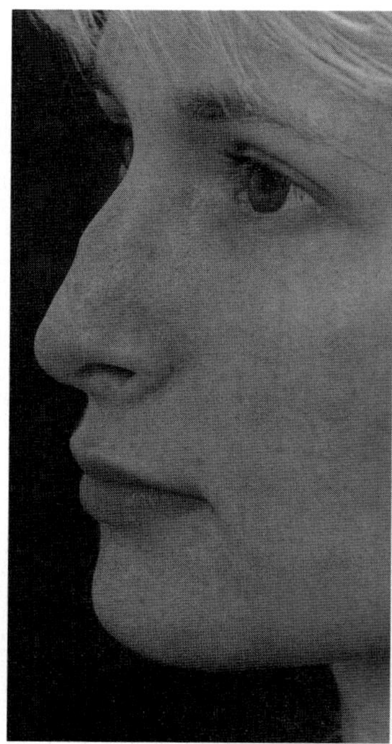
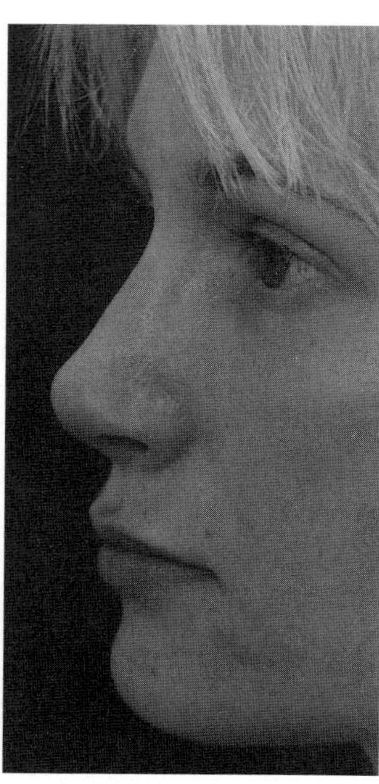

A,B C

FIGURE 53-9. Alar cartilage malposition. **A:** Preoperative views show a characteristic lateral crural deformity with parentheses and tip distortion. **B:** Following dorsal and tip reductions, the airway has become obstructed because of incompetence at the internal and external valves. Note the flat alar sidewall and the new alar rim retraction. **C:** Following dorsal, tip, and spreader grafts and composite skin/conchal cartilage grafts to support and lower the alar rims (9), alar rim contour has improved, tip support is now adequate, and air flow has increased 9.6 times over preoperative values.

has three critical ramifications: (a) *Malposition creates a round or "boxy" tip lobule* with strong lateral "parentheses" that reflect the caudal edges of the underlying alar cartilages; (b) *The abnormal position of the lateral crura places them at risk for an intracartilaginous alar cartilage technique.* Surgeons who favor an incision that splits a normally positioned lateral crus can inadvertently transect the lateral crus in the case of cephalic rotation. Believing that only the cephalic edge of the lateral crus is being resected, the surgeon may remove the entire lateral crus instead. The deformity created is consistent and recognizable (Fig. 53-8). In a recent survey of 20 consecutive secondary patients before a symposium lecture, 70% had tip deformities directly related to failure to recognize an alar cartilage malposition. (c) *The malpositioned lateral crura provide inadequate alar rim support and commonly produce external valvular incompetence.* Less recognized than the internal valve, the external nasal valve is formed by the lateral crus spanning the anterior alar rim and its investing soft tissue cover (4). In a consecutive series of 21 patients with external valvular incompetence, 50% had alar cartilage malposition (18). Preoperative failure to recognize the malpositioned lateral crus often yields new postoperative functional and aesthetic problems. The lateral crus should be relocated or the alar rim splinted to support the external valve and correct the aesthetic deformity (17) (Fig. 53-9).

AVOIDING THE UNFAVORABLE RESULT

Preoperative Diagnosis: Interview

General Remarks

Surgeons frequently remark on how difficult rhinoplasty is for them, forgetting sometimes how difficult it is for their patients. Those surgeons who have seen secondary rhinoplasty candidates devastated by the result of one or more previous operations immediately recognize the importance of a safe and biologically sound surgical plan and particularly an accurate understanding on the part of both patient and surgeon of the aesthetic goals and the realities of the situation (i.e., what is possible and what is not).

Making matters more difficult are the common misconceptions that patients have about their nasal deformities and therefore about the appropriate surgical plan. Because patients so commonly believe that all preoperative noses are too large (and that the only appropriate solution is reduction), a certain amount of education by the surgeon is necessary. The "big" or "wide" nose, the "fat tip," and the "flaring nostrils" are all pleas for reduction. Many patients without airway obstruction do not appreciate the importance of maintaining nasal function, and most do not realize that an improperly performed rhinoplasty can jeopardize the airway (16).

The surgeon must therefore guide the patient to understand that every rhinoplasty is a compromise between the patient's preferred aesthetic goals and the limitations that the preoperative skeleton and soft tissues impose. The priorities, in order of importance, are safety, function, and aesthetics. It is also wise to remember that many preoperative noses already have some desirable features; patient and surgeon should be careful not to destroy them.

In my experience, primary and secondary rhinoplasty patients differ in three cardinal ways. First, the previously scarred and contracted soft tissues are less tolerant of aggressive dissection, multiple incisions, and tight dressings. Secondly, donor sites may have already been consumed, so that the use of more difficult (distorted septum or concha), painful (costal), or frightening (calvarial) donor sites becomes necessary (19). Finally, the patient's morale is less tolerant. Having already invested money, time, discomfort, and emotion in one or more procedures that have not produced satisfactory results, the last thing secondary rhinoplasty patients need is further disappointment. The surgeon should be careful to construct a plan that is based on a clear understanding with the patient of what is possible, and that is founded on sound surgical and biological principles that maximize the airway and respect the patient's aesthetic goals.

Patient History

In as much detail as possible, I try to elicit the patient's operative goals, and, if they are numerous, help prioritize them. Is the major issue bridge height, tip projection, nasal length, asymmetry, or airway? How long has the sense of deformity existed? The latter question is more important in older than in younger patients: a patient in her 60s who has disliked her nasal shape for 40 years may tolerate a larger configurational change than one troubled for only 5 years who may be recognizing only recent signs of aging.

Unless the patient is under 12 years of age (when cosmetic rhinoplasty is rarely a concern), I first interview and examine the patient alone before involving a parent, spouse, or significant other to join us for a discussion of the operative plan (with the patient's permission). Although some family members (particularly protective parents or spouses) do not like this policy until it is explained to them, I think that it is important to establish an individual relationship with patients and listen to their concerns and complaints without the influence of other family members. Not surprisingly, it is usually the family members who object most strongly to this policy who should be excluded from the initial consultation; their presence is invariably distracting to the patient, and my questions directed to the patient, like some odd ventriloquist act, more commonly elicit responses from the parent or spouse instead. If, after an adequate explanation, the patient's family will not permit this policy (which does happen on occasion), I consider this a danger sign that should not be overlooked.

Unique to history taking in the secondary patient is a careful chronology of prior operations, which may be particularly difficult to obtain from patients who are still frustrated and angry about one or more unsuccessful outcomes. Nevertheless, the surgeon should gather as much information as possible about nasal appearance before and after each operation, what the prior surgeon intended to achieve, and how successful the outcome was (to the patient and to the operating surgeon), functionally and aesthetically. If an airway obstruction was part of the original complaint, was it corrected? If not, how soon did the obstruction appear, and after which procedure? What problems was the surgeon trying to correct with revisionary surgeries, and how successful were they? Did prior surgeons plan operations that the patient did not undergo?

In this regard, it is helpful when patients bring preoperative photographs (some will do it automatically), not only so that I can see what the surgeon was trying to correct and how the current deformities may have occurred, but also to place the original objectives in the perspective of the patient's current goals. For the beginning surgeon, a comparison of preoperative photographs with outcomes is invaluable, and teaches an enormous amount about the consistency and variability of nasal skeletal and soft tissue responses to surgical intervention.

Patient's Functional and Aesthetic Complaints

The surgeon should inquire about the airway first to avoid becoming distracted by aesthetic considerations, about which the patient is usually much more interested. I routinely ask questions about periodic or cylic airway obstruction; which airway is worse; any history of nasal trauma; seasonal allergies obstructing the airway; clear rhinitis; episodes of suppurative sinusitis requiring antibiotics; snoring, epistaxis, sinus headache, and what remedies the patient has previously tried, successfully or unsuccessfully. Not infrequently, many secondary patients with poor airways chronically self-medicate with steroid or vasoconstrictive sprays that should be eliminated before surgery. Also important are the patient's work environment and history of tobacco or alcohol use (both of which can cause nasal congestion) and, more important now than in previous years, cocaine use. Finally, I specifically inquire about features that the patient does not want changed and whether or not a change in ethnic appearance is desired.

Specific aesthetics. Some patients are more articulate than others about the changes they want. In this regard, I have found it helpful to ask patients to bring photographs from magazines or elsewhere that illustrate what type of tip and bridge configuration they would ideally prefer. The same words may indicate different things; the patient who requests a "straight" bridge line may mean a slightly concave bridge with a tip that is retroussé, a bridge that forms a straight line from root to tip, or a convex bridge. From these photos I also gather information about tip shape and preferred nasal length. One of the things that patients fear most is the overshortened, upturned nose produced by an aggressive rhinoplasty, yet some patients do want a shorter nose, an important planning decision for patients with large nasal bases, in whom shortening will produce a beneficial illusion (6,7).

Intranasal Examination

I make a habit of examining the internal nose first, so that this most critical functional area is not forgotten in discussing the surface. Patients are always grateful to be able to breathe easily, even when an inadequate airway was not one of the preoperative complaints; patients who breathe poorly (and even mouth breathe during the entire interview) may be unaware of how bad their airways are. More importantly, the surgeon must avoid unintentionally decreasing nasal function postoperatively.

I first wipe the intranasal mucosa gently with 4% pontocaine so that I can examine the internal structures without causing the patient discomfort. Without manipulating the airway, I then ask the patient to breathe deeply with the mouth closed and observe any areas of collapse or asymmetry in the nasal sidewalls. The surgeon who makes a habit of observing his or her patients breathe will be surprised at the number who have sidewall collapse on inspiration at internal or external valves. It is important to determine why this valvular incompetence exists (prior surgery, intrinsic cartilage weakness, or alar cartilage malposition) (4,16).

If sidewall collapse occurs, I occlude one nostril and ask the patient to compare flow through the unobstructed airway with and without support at the area of collapse by a cotton-tipped applicator. In patients with valvular incompetence, the increase in airway size is usually obvious and gratifying. The surgeon may frequently observe a straight septum accompanied by valvular collapse in patients with substantial airway obstruction. In these patients, septoplasty may be indicated to harvest grafts but by itself will not open the airway; the surgeon must place appropriate valvular grafts. Reconstruction of the internal and external valves can triple or quadruple air flow in most rhinoplasty patients, even when septoplasty is not simultaneously performed (4,16,18).

Next, I palpate the septum for substance, contour, and mucosal cover (looking for sequelae of allergy, injury, or perforation). I try to assess whether a "high" (i.e., toward the anterior edge) septal deviation exists; because hump removal can unmask a high septal curvature, the surgeon should be prepared to camouflage or correct the septal deflection with unilateral or asymmetrical thick spreader grafts.

Finally, I assess turbinate size. In my experience, obstructing turbinates are a relatively infrequent cause of postoperative airway obstruction (Table 53-1). Because turbinates warm and humidify inspired air, I avoid turbinectomy (even partial turbinectomy) except in strongly atopic patients, in whom some turbinate resection may be necessary. Most of the time, with adequate septal correction and valvular support, crushing and out-fracture of the turbinates or no turbinate treatment, is all that is necessary.

External Examination

Next, I palpate the external nose to assess cartilage size and substance (remembering alar cartilage malposition, as previously discussed), bony vault length, the firmness of the sidewalls (another assessment of valvular support), and soft tissue thickness. Tip lobular contour is considered, as is the balance between nasal base size and bridge height (see "Constructing a Surgical Plan"). With the patient holding a mirror, I then inquire about each nasal area, whether or not the patient has already mentioned it—width, length, bridge contour, tip shape, nostril size, columellar and upper lip position, and any asymmetries.

My own aesthetic standards are simple. On frontal view, the upper nose should be narrower than the lower nose; symmetrical, divergent lines should connect the two. On oblique view, no regional discontinuities should be apparent, the supratip should be flat, and the tip lobular mass should fall below the level of the peaks of the alar cartilage domes. On lateral and oblique views, the balance between nasal base size and bridge height should be appropriate, neither area dominating. The airways should be patent and stable during forced inspiration. Beyond these basics, the particular details depend on the patient's wishes, preoperative nasal structure, ethnic background, and the peculiarities of the existing skeletal framework and soft tissue cover (overall size, scars, trauma, or operations). For the surgeon who wishes to pursue the discipline of rhinoplasty to its limits, the operation offers, as much or more than any other aesthetic procedure, the possibility of individualizing the details of an aesthetic goal. In this regard, there is no better advice than Osler's admonition to "listen to your patient."

TABLE 53-1. IATROGENIC CAUSES OF AIRWAY OBSTRUCTION[a]

Internal valvular incompetence
External valvular incompetence
Inadvertent loss of tip support
Excessive alar wedge resection
Resection of lining
Excessive shortening
Uncorrected septal obstruction
Excessive narrowing of bony vault
Inadequate turbinate resection

[a] In descending order of frequency.

Forming an Operative Plan

The foregoing aesthetic criteria may seem impossibly simple, particularly in the perspective of countless careful elaborations of nasal proportions based on cephalometrics, classic facial proportions, and numerous calibrated angles. The difficulty in attaining these laudable goals lies in the nature of the medium—the strictures imposed by skin sleeve thickness, volume, and distribution, and the limitations of predictable soft tissue contraction. For example, in a patient with a small face and a large nose, in whom a 4- to 5-mm dorsal resection and proportional tip reduction might be aesthetically desirable in terms of classic facial balance, what is the surgeon to do with all that extra skin? Although patient and surgeon may share the same goals of proper balance and "a nose that fits the face," the real latitude that the surgeon has is much more limited than often realized.

The three parameters that I have found most practical in forming an operative strategy have been discussed earlier, here and elsewhere (5).

Setting Surgical Goals with the Patient

Because a practical rhinoplasty strategy may differ from what the patient imagines or what has been previously tried (e.g., augmentation in a case of supratip deformity), the patient must understand the logic of the surgeon's plan and prefer it to other reasonable alternatives. I am specific about what I propose down to the last graft; not only does this candor place patient and surgeon on the same side of the problem, but it also ensures that minor postoperative irregularities or palpable grafts are more likely to be tolerated by the patient, who has understood and consented to the necessity of each surgical maneuver beforehand. I explain what I will reduce, what I will not modify, and why augmentation is necessary for valvular incompetence, contour, or balance. The discussion of grafts is always more difficult with primary than with secondary patients; the latter, who have already seen the effects of reduction, disequilibrium, and contraction on their nasal configurations and airways are much easier to convince.

I am specific about my choice of donor sites, particularly if more than one possibility exists, and I let the patient decide, as much as possible, how complicated the reconstruction should be. In this way, the more extensive procedure will be better tolerated, and the lesser procedure, even when postoperative imperfections occur, may still be quite acceptable to the patient, who took part in the decision beforehand.

Discussing Potential Complications and Revisions

Patient and surgeon alike must remember that revisions may be necessary, almost predictable in some difficult configurations if the best possible result is desired. Often, such revisions are minor, consisting of modest contour changes or additional augmentations. Nevertheless, the patient must understand preoperatively that some results cannot be predicted and must not mistake the uncontrollable for the uncontrolled.

Some patients attach great importance to a surgeon's revision rates, just as other patients always want "second opinions" (which may or may not be more correct than the first one). I explain to patients that revision rates, even in the most skilled hands, can never be zero because patient and surgeon can control only some aspects of the outcome. Particularly for a patient who has had a prior unhappy surgical experience and has (correctly or not) attributed it to surgical error, the reasons for potential revisions must be clear. Without exaggerating the difficulty of the problem, I try to explain the peculiarities of the patient's situation (difficult anatomy, prior trauma, airway problems, asymmetries, prior scars, unavailable donor sites) and that this operation, just like the previous ones, is an intervention to change nature. I cannot predict the outcome with certainty because I do not know how "cooperative" the soft tissues will be, how difficult the dissection will be, or how "plastic" and suitable the donor material will prove. In some patients, septal cartilage is abundant, adequately thick, and easily fashioned into solid or crushed grafts; in other cases, the same donor site may yield brittle, calcified, irregular pieces that are of inadequate quantity and unsuitable for crushing or other modification (19). The same unknowns exist, with some variation, for conchal, rib, and calvarial donor sites. Unless the surgeon plans to employ alloplastics in the nose (which I do not recommend), the suitability of building materials is always unknown before surgery. This type of discussion is one that most patients readily understand; an adequate preoperative discussion of the uncertainties of surgery will make patients more tolerant of imperfections postoperatively and more understanding if revisions are needed.

My own revision rates for primary and secondary rhinoplasty, in a recent prospective 5-year series (9), were 12% and 15%, respectively, although revision rates steadily decreased during the observation period (particularly for tip grafting, as experience with a new method was gained). Although these figures are both higher and lower than others reported in the literature, revision rates are most meaningful in terms of a particular patient and surgeon; just as some surgeons revise very few rhinoplasties even when improvement might be obtained, some patients will not permit a revision even when it is needed.

Finally, with regard to further revisions, the patient must understand preoperatively that no revision will be considered until the end of the first postoperative year. Resolution of swelling and stabilization of the final appearance take at least that long in the primary nose and longer in the secondary nose; during that time irregularities, asymmetries, or poor contours that initially appear to require revision may improve sufficiently without surgery. Even in situations in which patient and surgeon are convinced that revision will be needed (e.g., tip asymmetry or inadequate support), nothing should be done until healing is complete and an accurate assessment can be made of what should be done; in this setting, revision success will be inevitably higher. The surgeon should control every possible variable.

Who should perform the revision? To some degree, the nature and type of revision and the identity of the surgeon depend on the same factors as in the prior rhinoplasty. The surgeon's model and proposed solution should be clear, and the patient's goals reasonable. Patient and surgeon must understand each other explicitly; each operation may be geometrically more difficult than the last one.

RELATIONSHIP BETWEEN PATIENT AND SURGEON

Ideally, the surgeon–patient relationship during aesthetic surgery should be even more favorable than in many other medical encounters. We have all learned to tolerate the intoxicated or abusive emergency department patient, or the frightened and demanding patient stricken with cancer. In those circumstances, often the best that the surgeon can expect is cooperation with the treatment plan. Although it is always optimal (and probably better for the healing process) when patient and physician like each other, it is not always necessary in those situations.

The same cannot be said for aesthetic surgery, where the risks and complications are just as real as in nonelective procedures and where the emotional turmoil for patient and family may be just as great. In aesthetic surgery, a passable surgical outcome without complications is not the only goal; patients want good outcomes, perfect outcomes, from procedures that change their appearance and that have profound ramifications for that complex part of the psyche that we call "body image." To undertake an aesthetic operation when the patient and surgeon do not understand or (for lack of a better word) "like" each other, is, I think, risky for both parties.

The Body Dysmorphic Patient

"Difficult patients", from the surgeon's standpoint, encompass the intensely anxious, those with unreasonable objectives, and those who are argumentative or unusually demanding of the surgeon's and staff's time. A particular subcategory of patients seeking cosmetic surgery who should be recognized preoperatively are those with body dysmorphic disorder (BDD), previously termed *dysmorphophobia.* The literature on this topic is continually expanding, much of it written by Katharine A. Phillips, M.D., a psychiatrist at Brown University. The topic is a large one but important to the present discussion because, across all cultures, the physical feature most commonly creating emotional distress is the nose (45% of cases) (20,21).

Three criteria must be satisfied for a diagnosis of BDD: (a) The patient must be preoccupied with some imagined defect in appearance; if a slight but real deformity is present, the patient's concern must be markedly excessive. (b) The preoccupation must cause clinically significant distress or impairment in social, occupational, or other important areas of functioning. (c) The preoccupation must not be better defined by another mental disorder (22,23).

For a comprehensive review of this important topic, the reader is referred to a summary of the current literature (23). For our discussion, the following points are pertinent: Among patients with BDD, 72% seek surgery, 48% have thought of suicide, and 27% have a suicide plan. The sex ratio does not appear to differ for BDD; more women than men may have mild BDD, but as many men as women have more severe BDD. Men with BDD are as likely as women to undergo aesthetic surgery. Unfortunately for patient and surgeon, surgical and even other medical treatments are generally not successful in BDD patients and may even worsen their symptoms. In one study, two-thirds of the patients who had undergone surgery reported no improvement or a worsening of their symptoms (23–25). Unfortunately, even when BDD patients are pleased with the surgical result, they often start to obsess about another body area. Rarely, a BDD patient may become violent toward the treating surgeon (23).

In an 18-month period, I performed surgery on three such patients without making the diagnosis beforehand, despite several lengthy preoperative consultations. The diagnostic difficulty for the surgeon is that many patients who have had unfavorable results are understandably apprehensive about further surgery, anxious about every detail of the proposed procedure, and worried about complications. Some are depressed because of their deformities and the financial losses they have incurred, and not all have understanding and support from their families. The BDD patient may share many of the same characteristics, but whereas the first group will feel better after a successful operation, even a spectacular result will disequilibrate the latter. One of my patients abandoned her teaching position at a university and became a recluse for 6 months; another man became unable to work and lost his business.

No simple diagnostic tests are available for these patients, but if BDD is suspected, evaluation by a psychiatrist knowledgeable and interested in this disorder is mandatory. One valuable indicator may be the patient's level of insight about the degree of distress that the deformity is causing. During a 12-month period, two of my patients reequilibrated and returned to their prior occupations; both still seek revisionary surgery. I was unsuccessful in persuading either to obtain psychiatric treatment. The third patient has improved over the last 2 years but still seeks further nasal surgery. The surgeon treating secondary deformities and trying to understand dissatisfied patients should be conversant with BDD so that it is not missed before surgery.

SPECIFICS OF THE OPERATION AND POTENTIAL COMPLICATIONS

Complications Referable to Rhinoplasty

Iatrogenic Airway Obstruction

More common than many of the other complications addressed in this section is a postoperative decrease in airway size, which is particularly troublesome if the airway was not obstructed before surgery. Although attributed by some authors to the narrowing effects of osteotomy, much more common causes are increased (or new) internal valvular incompetence from resection of the middle vault roof (3), or external valvular incompetence created by alar cartilage resection (particularly in cases of malposition) (4,16–18). As discussed above, these complications can be avoided entirely by a thorough preoperative evaluation and the maintenance or creation of valvular competence.

Less commonly, new airway obstruction may be caused by an inadvertent loss of tip support (through septal collapse or excessive dorsal or alar cartilage reduction); excessive alar wedge resection (which can be treated by composite grafts or local flaps) (26); resection of the nasal lining (which should never be performed); overshortening (which will misdirect the air stream); an uncorrected septal obstruction (occurring in fewer than 30% of the secondary patients that I see); an overly narrowed bony vault; or inadequate turbinate resection (27) (Table 53-1).

A decrease in airway size should never be the obligatory exchange for an improvement in nasal appearance; the airway function of virtually all rhinoplasty patients can be maintained or improved if the surgeon remembers the principles of airway structure and basic wound healing.

Incisions

Surgeons have strong opinions about the placement of rhinoplasty incisions, even the invisible ones of the closed approach. The intercartilaginous incision has been indicted (usually by surgeons who prefer the intracartilaginous approach) as the cause of "scarring at the nasal valve." Assuming that no mucosa has been resected, an angular incision that traverses three planes should not create a contracture. Perhaps the surgeons drawing this conclusion are not observing the mucosal wound alone, but what was performed through it instead—resection of the cartilaginous dorsum with medial collapse of the middle third (carrying the mucosa with it). If valvular support is maintained, the intercartilaginous incision is predictably safe.

Other surgeons caution that the transfixing incision invariably reduces tip support. This may be true intraoperatively, but it is hard to understand how the incision itself, once repaired, can decrease tip support. Although some authors have described ligamentous attachments between the caudal cartilaginous septum and its membranous component, their existence has been disputed, and they are not obvious intraoperatively. Any postoperative loss of tip support is more likely to occur not because of the transfixing incision, but because of what was performed through the incision (e.g., alar cartilage or bridge resection). If the surgeon requires the transfixing incision for caudal septal or septal angle access, it should be used.

Circulatory Problems

Circulatory complications occur more commonly after open than after closed rhinoplasty, particularly when cautery has been liberally employed to control columellar bleeding or when excessive retraction has been used. During primary rhinoplasty, the surgeon can make intercartilaginous and intracartilaginous incisions with or without alar incisions (for wedge resections) without fear of circulatory compromise *so long as* the incisions are not made longer than is necessary and packing and dressings are not placed too tightly.

The same is less true in secondary rhinoplasty, in which the surgeon must be more frugal with incision placement. Each nasal area should be approached thoughtfully and incisions planned to minimize the amount of dissection (which not only benefits the circulation but decreases morbidity and assists in graft placement and fixation) (19,27). Soft tissue necrosis can occur in the secondary and tertiary nose if the dissection has been too aggressive, incisions have been too numerous, dressings and packing too tight, or if too many nasal operations have been performed in close succession (Fig. 53-10). The scarring illustrated in Fig. 53-10 is avoidable and cannot be repaired after it occurs. Necrosis in the supratip skin can follow excessive dressing pressure placed to prevent supratip deformity. Supratip deformity

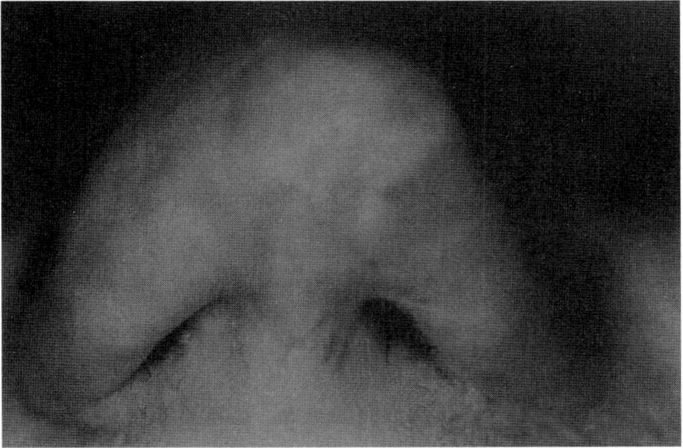

FIGURE 53-10. Scarring and soft tissue loss from repeated nasal surgeries in quick succession.

cannot be prevented, nor a "supratip break" achieved, by pressure on the supratip skin; rather, tip and supratip contours are the result of adequate skeletal support in the bridge and tip (28). I place dressings only firmly enough to immobilize grafts and control postoperative swelling. They need not be tight.

Skeletal Problems

Irregularities and asymmetries occur in any modified skeletal structure, but some points should be noted about their interpretation. Irregularities at the caudal edge of the bony vault are often not the result of inadequate reduction but rather of middle vault collapse, which causes the caudal end of the bony arch to stand out in relief. Further bony vault reduction is not an effective cure; rather, the surgeon must support the middle third.

A palpable or visible low point may appear at the midpoint of the nasal bridge, either intraoperatively or postoperatively. This "middorsal notch" has been interpreted by some surgeons and patients as the result of an untidy resection of the cartilaginous dorsum. More commonly, the middorsal notch is a soft tissue phenomenon that occurs where the thinner, upper nasal skin begins to thicken in its transition to the supratip skin; the middorsal notch represents the cephalic end of a supratip deformity and indicates dorsal overresection. It should be treated by augmentation (29).

Finally, a new frontal asymmetry may develop when dorsal resection has uncovered a high septal deviation (see "Intranasal Examination"). If observed at the time of surgery, a high septal deviation can be camouflaged by onlay grafts or unequally thick spreader grafts (3,16).

Infection

In the absence of other complications, infection is uncommon following rhinoplasty and septal procedures (30). Many surgeons use antibiotics while postoperative packing is in place. Toxic shock syndrome and septic involvement of the cavernous sinus are extremely rare but have been reported (31,32). Minor graft infections also occur on occasion, more often in areas of tissue compromise or where conchal cartilage grafts have been used. Sheen and Sheen (33) have described a technique for irrigation with antibiotic solution that may salvage the graft.

Hemorrhage

Most patients, particularly those who have undergone septal or turbinate surgery, have scant to moderate bleeding for the first 48 to 72 hours postoperatively; after this time, bleeding should subside and ordinarily does not resume. Approximately 3% of patients, however, will rebleed, classically between the sixth and tenth postoperative days. The bleeding patient is always terrified. The surgeon's major task is to calm the anxious patient and elicit cooperation: as occurs in upper gastrointestinal hemorrhage, the calmed patient often stops bleeding. Previously placed packs should be removed, the airway suctioned of clots, and the site of bleeding identified; bleeding frequently ceases spontaneously after the removal of old blood and clots. At other times, reinsertion of a smaller pack (soaked in phenylephrine HCl) is necessary. Less frequently, placement of a posterior pack is required; the surgeon should be familiar and comfortable with its use before the occasion arises.

Rhinitis

In patients without a history of preoperative rhinitis, persistent, clear postoperative nasal drainage should be rare (although it occasionally occurs for a few weeks following surgery when the airway has been dramatically improved). Iatrogenic rhinitis most commonly follows excessive turbinectomy. Proponents of turbinectomy minimize this complication, but it is unquestionably a real and exceedingly difficult entity for which I know of no consistently effective treatment.

Septal Perforation

Small perforations occur occasionally after difficult septoplasty but can be minimized by cautious dissection, repair of any tears in the mucoperichondrial flaps, and placement of silicone splints on each side of the septal partition while the packing is in place. The symptomatic perforation can cause rhinitis, pain, or whistling; more troublesome are crusting and epistaxis, which usually reflect an area of exposed septal cartilage or bone. Even if the perforation cannot be repaired, these latter symptoms can be ameliorated or cured if the surgeon removes areas of exposed septal skeleton and repairs the mucoperichondrium around the perforation to create a uniform, stable surface.

Even when perforations are asymptomatic and I have caused them, I tell the patient that a perforation exists; the alternative will be surprise and anger if the information comes instead from another physician.

Lacrimal Injury

In a series reported in 1968 (34), the incidence of lacrimal obstruction in a group of 27 patients was 78%. Orbital floor injury following nasal osteotomy has also been reported. I have seen one patient in consultation with persistent epiphora 2 years following rhinoplasty, presumably resulting from lacrimal duct injury. These types of problems should be exceedingly rare; the surgeon must know the position of the osteotome at all times and control the fracture line precisely.

Red Nose

The cutaneous manifestations of prior underlying surgery (with its natural circulatory readjustment) vary; in many cases, they never develop, and in others, they occur after the first procedure. Frequently, discoloration decreases as the months progress, but when it persists, the patient should be forewarned that another operation may worsen the condition. Fortunately, laser treatment is often effective (35).

Pink Tip

Nontender tip discoloration, usually occurring early in the postoperative period, is less likely to signal infection than ischemia. I have most frequently seen it in my own patients when a scarred, tight tip lobule has been expanded by multiple grafts. Even when the wound is not closed under tension, internal pressures caused by grafts, packing, and taping may render even a carefully placed dressing too tight. It is wise to check secondary rhinoplasty patients 24 to 48 hours after surgery and split or remove the dressing if the tip color is not perfectly normal. Even at 24 hours, graft position will not be lost by removing the tape; much more is jeopardized if a tight dressing remains too long.

Septal Collapse

This dreaded complication (Fig. 53-11) affects not only nasal aesthetics but the airway. Because bridge contour, nasal length, nasal base support, middle vault support, and the position of the upper lip are affected, the required reconstruction is complex. It is important to maintain a minimum 15-mm dorsal strut during septoplasty, and to obtain a history of prior nasal trauma that will alert the surgeon to septal fractures that may have created permanent areas of instability. In this regard, for the surgeon who prefers "open septoplasty" (i.e., through an open rhinoplasty incision), the dissection should still leave an intact dorsal strut with attached mucoperichondrium. To begin the dissection at the anterior septal edge and proceed posteriorly jeopardizes septal support and can result in collapse if old (unhealed) fracture lines are present.

Other Complications

Intracranial injury, meningitis, and permanent anosmia have been reported but are infrequent; the reader is referred to the literature for more information.

COMPLICATIONS CAUSED BY CARTILAGE GRAFTS

Septal Cartilage

The most "plastic" of the donor materials used in nasal reconstruction, septal grafts may nonetheless become visible or show postoperative irregularities. The surgeon can mini-

A,B

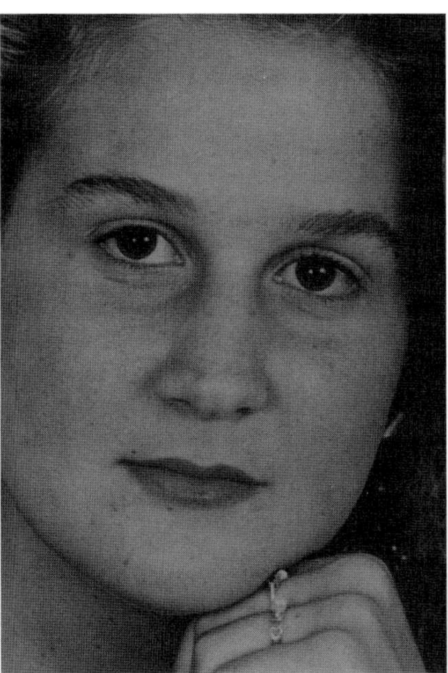

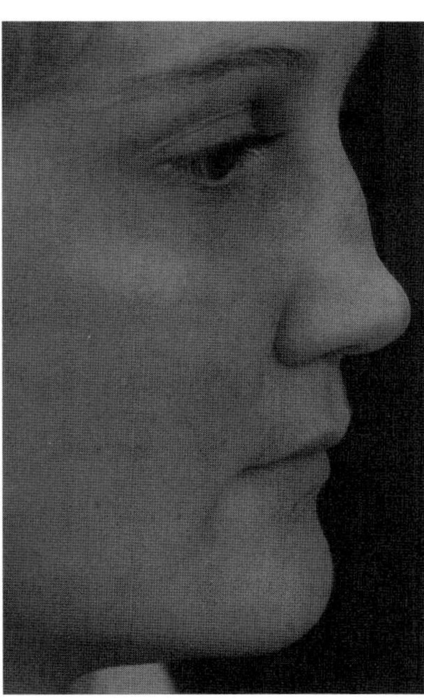

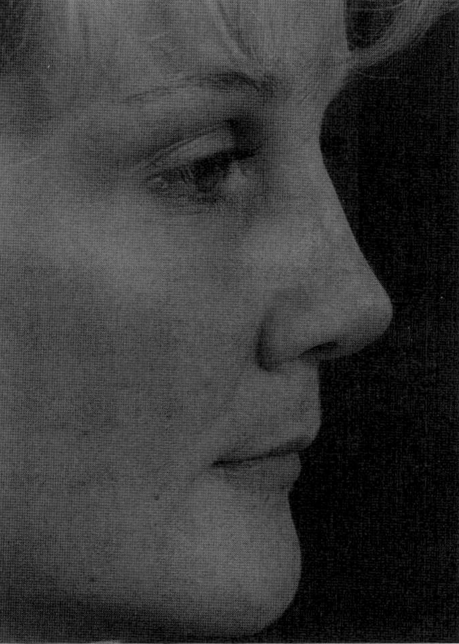

C

FIGURE 53-11. Septal collapse. The functional and aesthetic consequences of septal collapse are consistent; bony vault height apparently increases, internal valvular support (and middle vault width) decreases, the nose lengthens, the columella becomes retracted, the soft tissue maxillary arch falls posteriorly (from loss of caudal septal support), and the subnasale sharpens. Because septal cartilage is unavailable, reconstruction requires the use of other donor sites (in this case costal and rib cartilage). **A:** Preoperative view before septal surgery. **B:** Postoperative view following septoplasty, before reconstruction. **C:** One-year postoperative view.

mize these types of problems by suiting the substance of the graft to its soft tissue cover. Under thick skin, more substantial (and less perfectly regular) grafts are unlikely to be noticeable; beneath thin skin, the surgeon must contour grafts more carefully (9–11,19). Septal cartilage is ideal for dorsal, tip, spreader, lateral wall, or columellar grafts. When the cartilage is used as a solid piece, the edges can be beveled by light scraping with a No. 15 blade; alternatively, the cartilage may be crushed so that it becomes pliable or lacy. In general, the more aggressively septal cartilage is crushed, the more it absorbs postoperatively.

To avoid palpability or visibility, upper dorsal or radix grafts should be crushed, not too wide, and layered to conform to the defect (11). Multiple tip grafts, the consistency of which should suit the soft tissue cover (crushed under thin skin, firmer under thick skin), will contour the tip lobule more naturally than single grafts (9,10).

Conchal Cartilage

Unmodified cartilage harvested from the conchal floor (preserving the posterior wall to avoid deforming the donor ear) forms an excellent dorsal graft for a deep, asymmetrical defect beneath a thick soft tissue cover. The method of trimming, rolling, and fixing the graft has been described by Sheen and Sheen (11). For shorter, shallower defects, or where the soft tissue cover is thinner, ear cartilage is not ideal but can be used as a compromise solution (e.g., for the patient with no available septal cartilage who needs a 1- or 2-mm elevation of a short dorsal defect). Because of its rubbery consistency and thickness, however, single pieces of unmodified conchal cartilage will flatten and deform as the overlying soft tissues heal; unlike septal cartilage, full-thickness conchal cartilage shatters when crushed. In such "compromise" situations, or when thinner grafts are needed, conchal cartilage can be split tangentially and carefully crushed to yield suitable grafts (19).

Calvarial Grafts

Outer-table calvarial bone grafts are well suited for the reconstruction of long, shallow (2 to 3 mm), symmetrical dorsal defects beneath thin soft tissue covers. These grafts must be harvested with exceeding care, as intracranial injuries and subdural hematomas (resulting from vibrations of the mallet and osteotome) have been described. The recipient defect should be cleared of soft tissue and the bony vault roughened to receive the calvarial graft. The bone graft itself should be contoured but not excessively thinned to avoid resorption. Although some surgeons have had mixed success with this donor site, I have used it frequently with only two (of approximately 90) cases of partial absorption (in the supratip). The grafts must be harvested under low speed and with an electric bur to avoid overheating the osteocytes (36).

Costal Cartilage

Costal cartilage is notorious for warping postoperatively, which has dscouraged many surgeons from its use. Nevertheless, when conchal grafts are too short or calvarial grafts too thin, costal cartilage creates an excellent dorsal reconstruction, and slices of costal cartilage (either unmodified or crushed) can fill the maxillary arch, lateral nasal walls, columella, or tip. Two principles help to avoid postoperative distortions: (a) The surgeon should use the smallest rib needed (usually the ninth or 10th), so that less disruption of internal stresses occurs during modification; and (b) the surgeon should consider insertion of a threaded, longitudinal K-wire as an internal splint (37).

CONCLUSION

Rhinoplasty deserves its reputation as difficult surgery, not only because of the limited access and technical precision required, but also because rhinoplasty differs from many other plastic surgical operations. Simple structural modifications may have effects beyond their immediate areas (2,3,7,11). Skin sleeve volume is limited in its contractility, and the skin contracts in ways that are related to, but independent of, skeletal modifications (1). Certain anatomical problems, such as narrow middle vault (3), low root (11), inadequately projecting tip (10), and cephalic malposition of the alar cartilages (17), predispose to unsatisfactory outcomes. The operation itself cannot easily be premeasured and premarked but is an interactive procedure in which the surgeon must make readjustments and decisions based on intraoperative appearance. Furthermore, despite the fact that most patients want smaller noses, the parameter most critical to aesthetic success is nasal balance, not volume. Finally, as is so true in all aesthetic procedures, the relationship between patient and surgeon is paramount, not only because perfection is difficult and elusive, but because rhinoplasty creates a change in facial appearance.

Nonetheless, despite its idiosyncracies and paradoxes, nasal surgery remains a fascinating endeavor for the dedicated surgeon, and an immensely rewarding one for his or her patients.

REFERENCES

1. Constantian MB. A model for planning rhinoplasty. *Plast Reconstr Surg* 1987;79:472–481.
2. Constantian MB. Distant effects of dorsal and tip grafting in rhinoplasty. *Plast Reconstr Surg* 1992;90:405–418.
3. Sheen JH. Spreader graft: the method of reconstructing the roof of the middle nasal vault following rhinoplasty. *Plast Reconstr Surg* 1984;73:230–237.
4. Constantian MB. The incompetent external nasal valve: pathophysiology and treatment in primary and secondary rhinoplasty. *Plast Reconstr Surg* 1994;93:919–931.
5. Constantian MB. Experience with a three-point method for planning rhinoplasty. *Ann Plast Surg* 1993;30:1–12.

6. Constantian MB. An alternate strategy for reducing the large nasal base. *Plast Reconstr Surg* 1989;83:41–52.
7. Sheen JH, Sheen AP. *Aesthetic rhinoplasty,* 2nd ed. St. Louis: Mosby, 1987:118–120.
8. Sheen JH, Sheen AP. *Aesthetic rhinoplasty,* 2nd ed. St. Louis: Mosby, 1987:1032–1044.
9. Constantian MB. Elaboration of an alternative, cartilage-sparing tip graft technique: experience in 405 cases. *Plast Reconstr Surg* 1999;103:237–253.
10. Sheen JH. Tip graft: a 20-year retrospective. *Plast Reconstr Surg* 1993;91:48–63.
11. Sheen JH, Sheen AP. *Aesthetic rhinoplasty,* 2nd ed. St. Louis: Mosby, 1987:383–403.
12. Fomon S, Gilbert JG, Caron AL, et al. Collapsed ala: pathologic physiology and management. *Arch Otolaryngol* 1950;51: 465–484.
13. Kern EB. Evaluation of nasal breathing: an objective method. In: Rees TD, ed. *Rhinoplasty: problems and controversies.* St. Louis: Mosby, 1986:195–202.
14. Sulsenti G, Palma P. A new technique for functional surgery of the nasal valve area. *Rhinology* 1989;10[Suppl]:1–19.
15. Teller DC. Anatomy of a rhinoplasty: emphasis on the middle third of the nose. *Otolaryngol Head Neck Surg* 1997;13:241–252.
16. Constantian MB, Clardy RB. The relative importance of septal and nasal valvular surgery in correcting airway obstruction in primary and secondary rhinoplasty. *Plast Reconstr Surg* 1996;98: 38–54.
17. Sheen JH, Sheen AP. *Aesthetic rhinoplasty,* 2nd ed. St. Louis: Mosby, 1987:988–1012.
18. Constantian MB. Functional effects of alar cartilage malposition. *Ann Plast Surg* 1993;30:487–499.
19. Constantian MB. Rhinoplasty in the graft-depleted patient. *Operative Techniques in Plastic and Reconstructive Surgery* 1995;2:67–81.
20. Denis PB, Denis M, Gomes A. Psychosocial consequences of nasal aesthetic and functional surgery: a controlled prospective study in an ENT setting. *Rhinology* 1998;36:32–36.
21. Phillips KA. *The broken mirror: understanding and treating body dysmorphic disorder.* New York: Oxford University Press, 1996:185.
22. Phillips KA. Body dysmorphic disorder: the distress of imagined ugliness. *Am J Psychiatry* 1991;148:1138–1149.
23. Phillips KA. *The broken mirror: understanding and treating body dysmorphic disorder.* New York: Oxford University Press, 1996.
24. Hollander E, Cohen LJ, Simeon D. Body dysmorphic disorder. *Psych Ann* 1993;23:359–364.
25. Jerome L. Body dysmorphic disorder: a controlled study of patients requesting cosmetic rhinoplasty. *Am J Psychiatry* 1992;149:577.
26. Constantian MB. An alar base flap to correct nostril and vestibular stenosis and alar base malposition in rhinoplasty. *Plast Reconstr Surg* 1998;101:1666–1674.
27. Constantian MB. Closed Rhinoplasty: current techniques, theory, and applications. In: Mathers SM, Hertz VR, eds. Plastic Surgery. 2nd ed. Baltimore: Lippincott, Williams and Wilkins, *(in press).*
28. Constantian MB. The septal angle: a cardinal point in rhinoplasty. *Plast Reconstr Surg* 1990;85:187–195.
29. Constantian MB. The middorsal notch: an intraoperative guide to overresection in secondary rhinoplasty. *Plast Reconstr Surg* 1993;91:477–484.
30. Slavin SA, Rees TD, Guy CL, et al. An investigation of bacteremia during rhinoplasty. *Plast Reconstr Surg* 1983;71:196–198.
31. Casaubon J, Dion MA, Labrisseau A. Septic cavernous sinus thrombosis after rhinoplasty. *Plast Reconstr Surg* 1977;59: 119–123.
32. Toback J, Fayerman JW. Toxic shock syndrome following septorhinoplasty. *Arch Otolaryngol* 1983;109:627–629.
33. Sheen JH, Sheen AP. *Aesthetic rhinoplasty,* 2nd ed. St. Louis: Mosby, 1987:568–578.
34. Flowers RS, Anderson R. Injury to the lacrimal apparatus during rhinoplasty. *Plast Reconstr Surg* 1968;42:577–581.
35. Noe JM, Finley J, Rosen S, et al. Postrhinoplasty "red nose": differential diagnosis and treatment by laser. *Plast Reconstr Surg* 1981;67:661–664.
36. Sheen JH, Sheen AP. *Aesthetic rhinoplasty,* 2nd ed. St. Louis: Mosby, 1987:808–826.
37. Gunter JP, Clark CP, Friedman RM. Internal stabilization of autogenous rib cartilage grafts in rhinoplasty: a barrier to cartilage warping. *Plast Reconstr Surg* 1997;100:161–169.

SUGGESTED READING

Aiach G, Levignac J. *La rhinoplastie esthétique.* Paris: Masson, 1989.
Brady KT, Austin L, Lydiard RB. Body dysmorphic disorder: the relationship to obsessive-compulsive disorder. *J Nerv Ment Dis* 1990;178:538–540.
Gruber RP, Peck GC. *Rhinoplasty: state of the art.* St. Louis: Mosby, 1993.
McKinney P, Cunningham BL. *Rhinoplasty.* New York: Churchill Livingstone, 1989.
Millard DR Jr. *A rhinoplasty tetralogy.* Boston: Little, Brown and Company, 1996.
Phillips KA. An open study of buspirone augmentation of serotonin-reuptake inhibitors in body dysmorphic disorder. *Psychopharmacol Bull* 1996;32:175–180.
Phillips KA, Nirenberg AA, Brendel G, et al. Prevalent and clinical features of body dysmorphic disorder in atypical major depression. *J Nerv Ment Dis* 1996;184:125–129.
Rees TD, La Trenta GS. *Aesthetic plastic surgery.* Philadelphia: WB Saunders, 1994.
Sheen JH, Sheen AP. *Aesthetic rhinoplasty,* 2nd ed. St. Louis: Mosby, 1987:428–431.

Discussion

CLOSED RHINOPLASTY

PETER McKINNEY

Read it, cogitate, and read again. Like rhinoplasty itself, this chapter takes time to absorb because it contains so many pearls of wisdom and so much invaluable information. Herein, the essence of rhinoplasty is distilled into a manageable unit, and this remarkably well-written piece should be required reading for any resident who plans to undertake the rhinoplasty voyage. Because of the infinite complexities and unexplained factors involved in rhinoplasty (evidenced by numerous books devoted to the subject), the operation requires a lifetime of study. Some confusion is created because the nasal terms are used differently among authors. It is almost as if one has to speak several dialects to understand the meaning of the rhinoplasty literature. However, this author sidesteps the trap by defining his terms; for example, some would call the nasal base the lobule and others the tip. We use the author's terms in this discussion.

The fact that Dr. Constantian, unlike many authors, emphasizes rearrangement of the nasal skeletal units (cartilages and bone), rather than just removal, provides a valuable focus. The anatomy differs so much between people (and even between opposite sides in the same person) that a customized approach is necessary for each and every patient. Thus, Dr. Constantian maintains that reduction rhinoplasty, the "standard" approach, will always fail in a certain number of cases. An emphasis on equilibrium in the nose is important because changes in one area bring about alterations in another. For example, raising the dorsum by itself makes the vault look thinner and the nasal base smaller. Surgeons who take pride in a 20-minute rhinoplasty will find that most of their patients' noses will look like the result of a 20-minute rhinoplasty after a few years. I have performed thousands of rhinoplasties and I have found that as knowledge of the operation and the possible tissue rearrangements increase, the operation has become much longer than it was 35 years ago. The additional time is used mainly for cartilage grafting. Primary rhinoplasties that used to take 45 minutes today take 1.5 hours, and some secondary rhinoplasties require up to 3 hours.

One of the author's most valuable contributions is his emphasis on the "skin sleeve." This organ does not have an infinite ability to contract, and indeed contracts concentrically at the base and linearly in the vault—hence the principle of filling the skin sleeve to balance the nose. This is a very difficult concept for patients to accept, but if the radix is low and the base overprojecting, the base can be set back only so far because skin contractility is limited. Raising the radix will rebalance the nose by making the nasal base appear less projected, and less tissue will have to be removed.

Nasal obstruction can be caused by malfunction of the internal or external valve. Dr. Constantian documents this fact with rhinomanometry. It is a concept that has not been emphasized enough. With the use of spreader grafts for the internal valve and onlay support for the external valve, the airway can be improved to a greater degree than with septoplasty or turbinectomy alone. However, insurance companies continue to distort this phenomenon; there is no Current Procedural Terminology (CPT) code for spreader graft, as there is for septoplasty and turbinectomy. Most surgeons do not examine valve function well enough. Forced inspiration, with and without occlusion of one nostril, can provide a great deal of information about nasal patency. The function of the small muscles of the nose should also be evaluated because they may be compromised in a primary rhinoplasty. These muscles (elevators, depressors, compressors, and dilators) can be damaged if the dissection is too superficial to the alar cartilage, either because the dissection is in the wrong plane or because tissues are mistakenly removed to "defat the nasal tip." Fat may be found between the intermediate crura but rarely laterally. Some of these muscles are important for stabilizing and widening the nasal aperture during forced inspiration. If they do not function well after a rhinoplasty, the lateral walls require stabilization with a strut because the dynamic stabilizer has been lost (Fig. 53D-1).

Patients with body dysmorphic disorder (BDD) are seen more often than we realize. (BDD does develop occasionally as a temporary self-limiting phenomenon in the immediate postoperative period secondary to facial distortion from swelling.) Dr. Constantian notes that 72% of patients with BDD seek surgery. A long, repetitious consultation in which the patient does not hear what is wanted—is invariably a red flag. Caution and anxiety are understandable to a point, es-

P. McKinney: Department of Plastic Surgery, Northwestern University Medical School; and Department of Plastic Surgery, Rush Medical College, Chicago, Illinois

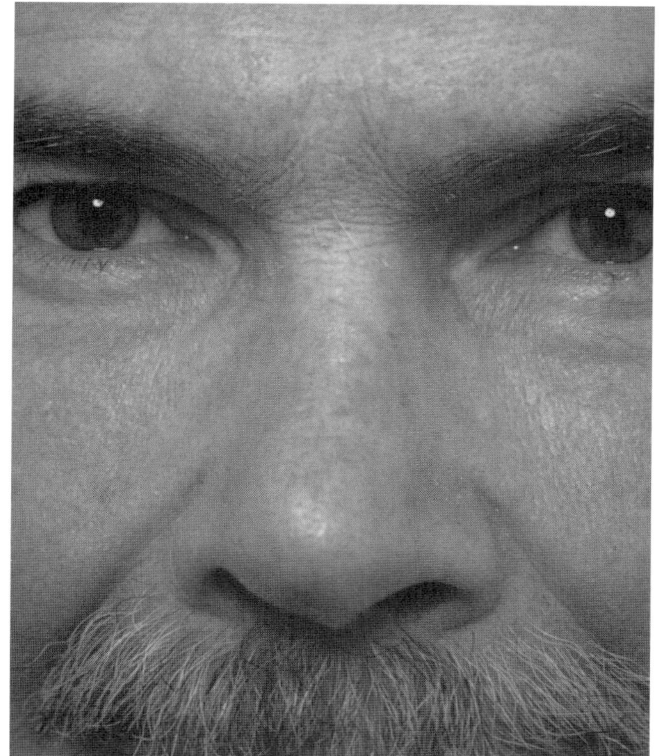
A

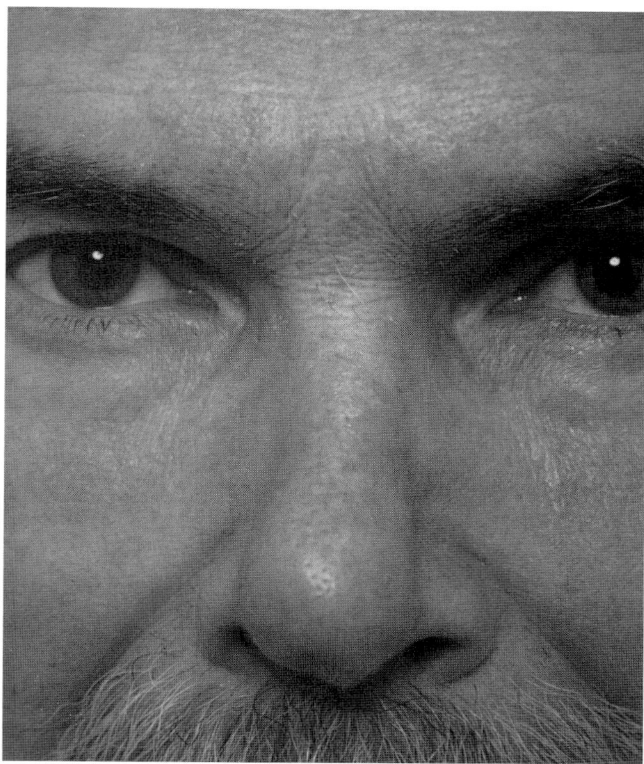
B

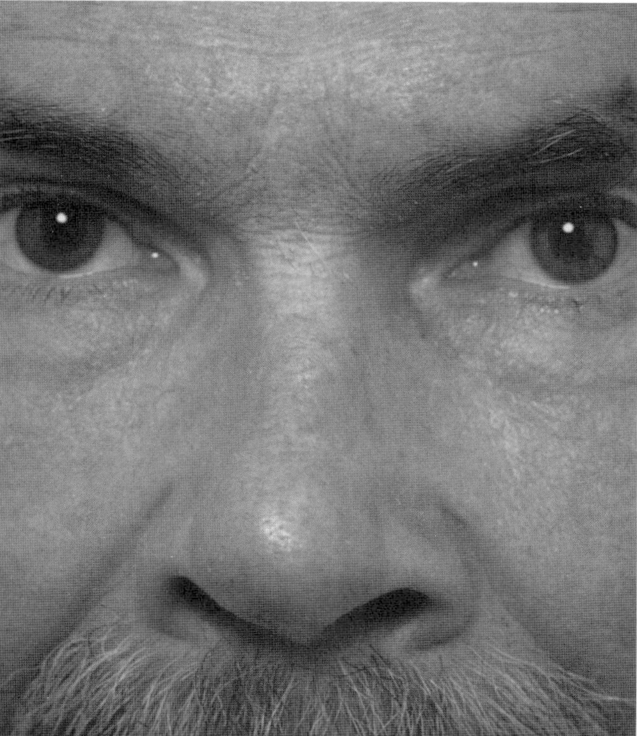
C

FIGURE 53D-1. The small muscles of the nose stabilize the valves during forced inspiration. **A:** Normal inspiration. **B:** Forced inspiration—note the collapse on the left. **C:** Forced inspiration with dilation and stabilization by the small muscles of the nasal base. The left side has been stabilized by the small muscles.

pecially if the patient has previously undergone surgery. However, exaggerated anxiety over a slight imperfection may represent a psychiatric phenomenon of wanting to remain ill, with the imperfection used as an excuse for perceived failure in life. We concur with the author that this type of patient does not readily accept a psychiatric referral. Dr. Gorney was onto BDD when he plotted the defect-to-anxiety ratio (see Chapter 5). (A high level of anxiety and a minimal defect meant potential trouble.) The cheerful, outgoing patient does well, accepting rare failures as something that can be expected and then going on with life. If only we had a waiting room full of those!

Dr. Constantian also discusses alar cartilage malposition, with which most of us are familiar. We would like to add iatrogenic malposition to this discussion. Since the advent of the open procedures and vector suturing, we have seen two patients with malposition of the lower lateral cartilage. In these cases, the placement of interdomal sutures caused an inward rotation of the alar cartilage and a shift of the long axis to a more vertical orientation. In both these patients, the nose was more bulbous after the initial surgery, which was documented photographically. To rectify the problem, the long axis was rotated horizontally in a secondary surgery.

We do disagree with the author about some minor points. When Dr. Constantian states that the nasal lining should never be resected, he is probably referring to the region of the internal valve, and with that we fully agree. However, resection of the nasal lining may be indicated in the ventral caudal septum, lateral wall of the ala, and the septum itself (1,2). Resection of the membranous septum (along with some cartilage) may be necessary to shorten the nose, especially in the older patient. Sometimes, the removal of membrane alone raises the lobule. Resection of the vestibular lining is rare but is useful in the lateral wall to raise the ala in certain patients. Finally, after repair of a severely buckled septum, it may be necessary to resect lining on one

A

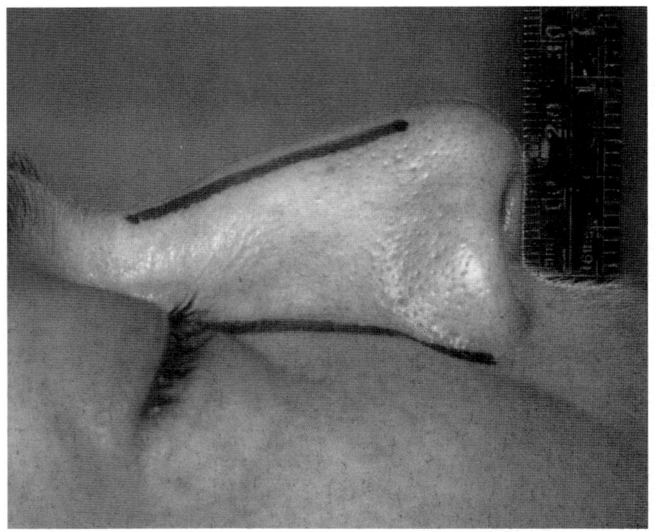

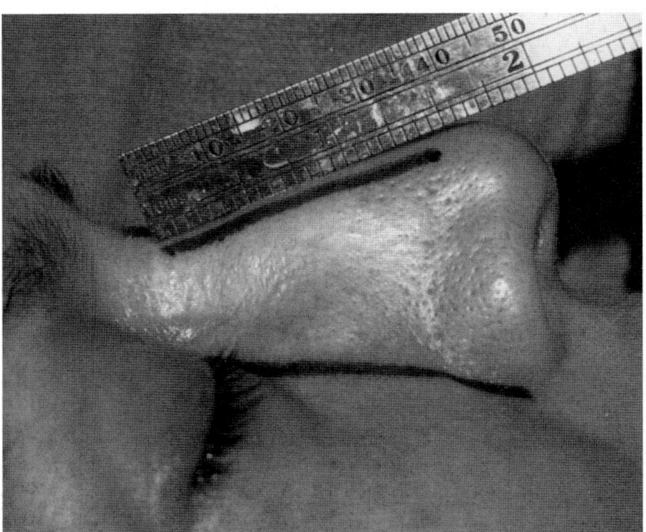

B

C

FIGURE 53D-2. Measuring the nasal base projection from the columella-labial angle to the intersection of the projection line provides convenient relationships for an "aesthetic nose." **A:** The average measurement for base projection is 2.5 cm. **B:** The length of an aesthetic dorsum from the radix to the intersection is 5 cm. **C:** If a line is drawn from the medial canthus to the alar groove, an aesthetic height at the rhinion measures 2.5 cm.

side; otherwise, the redundant membrane can flap back and forth with changes of intranasal pressure.

We also differ with the author's statement that incisions in the region of the internal valve do not cause webbing and so are not a cause of internal valve obstruction. We do see webbing and feel it occurs because the retractor pulls the lining forward. If an incision is made right at the valve, when the tension is decreased the membrane tends to move cephalad, and the scar then webs across the apex of the valve (2).

Another difference of opinion concerns the definition of nasal projection. Dr. Constantian defines projection relative to the septal angle, and indeed this is a useful guideline because with a good result, the tip projection point will be ventral to the septal angle, so that a supratip break will be present. However, the septal angle can change with dorsal resection as the nasal base projection from the facial place becomes smaller. Other authors define projection in absolute terms as the distance from the alar groove to the tip-defining point. We find it more helpful to define nasal tip projection as the distance from the soft tissue of the nasal labio angle to the dorsal line. This is normally about 2.5 cm, or half the length of the dorsum (5 cm). If a line is drawn from the medial canthus to the alar groove just at the rhinion, a distance of 2.5 cm from this line to the maximum height of the dorsum is aesthetic (Fig. 53D-2).

Finally, the observation that a middorsal notch represents the cephalic edge of a supratip deformity is a bit confusing. We would expect a smooth transition of skin rather than an abrupt one, and would attribute this feature to excessive resection of the nasal dorsum.

CONCLUSION

Dr. Constantian has condensed many valuable points into a single chapter on rhinoplasty that is well worth reading and rereading. The concepts of skin sleeve, malrotation, valvular obstruction, rearrangement, nasal balance, and BDD are the foundation of modern rhinoplasty.

REFERENCES

1. McKinney P, Stalnecker ML. The hanging ala. *Plast Reconstr Surg* 1984;73:427.
2. McKinney P, Cunningham BL. *Rhinoplasty.* New York: Churchill Livingstone, 1989:53,115,172.

54

OPEN RHINOPLASTY

RONALD P. GRUBER
GILBERT AIACH

The subject of complications following rhinoplasty has been extensively reviewed (1–3). This chapter considers the complications of rhinoplasty, with an emphasis on those related to the open technique. The open approach to the septum is not discussed because airway problems associated with the septum and turbinate are covered in another chapter.

COMPLICATION VERSUS UNFAVORABLE RESULT

It is important to separate complications from unfavorable results. Although the two terms overlap to a certain extent, it is generally agreed that a complication is an unexpected sequela (and theoretically preventable), whereas an unfavorable result is an expected sequela of surgery (and theoretically not preventable). In surgery other than rhinoplasty, the clearest example of an unfavorable result is capsular contracture following augmentation mammaplasty. A surgeon can do very little to prevent this complication and, as a general rule, cannot be held responsible for it. For that reason, it is considered an unfavorable result. In contrast, whether or not a sponge is left in the breast is very much under the surgeon's control, and this problem is best considered a complication. In rhinoplasty surgery, problems related to the ultimate aesthetic appearance, such as a supratip deformity, generally fall into the category of unfavorable results. This particular problem is less likely to arise when the surgeon is more experienced, but the fact is that no plastic surgeon has complete control over the ultimate architectural outcome of surgery of the nose.

R. P. Gruber: Department of Plastic and Reconstruction Surgery, Stanford University, Stanford, California; and Department of Surgery, Summit Hospital, Oakland, California

G. Aiach: Plastic Surgery Department, Centre Hospitalier Universitaire Henri Mondor, Paris, France

CLOSED VERSUS OPEN APPROACH

This chapter focuses primarily on complications. To focus on unfavorable results (aesthetic problems), a complete treatise on secondary rhinoplasty would be required. However, significant differences between aesthetic outcomes of the open and closed approach are discussed. The open technique is a suitable method to treat many complications and undesirable results, whereas others are best managed with the closed technique.

PREOPERATIVE PHASE

When rhinoplasty is being considered, the history and physical must focus on the desires and expectations of the patient. What is the patient seeking? Can it be achieved? Can most of it be achieved? Will the patient be happy with what is achieved? At least two visits with the patient help the surgeon to understand the patient and allow the patient to understand the limitations of the operation and the surgeon. Male patients are typically more difficult to deal with. Many of them are very demanding. They tend to want to control the situation and are often unforgiving if the ultimate result is not to their liking. For these reasons, video imaging can be extremely helpful. The surgeon should try to create a realistic image of the anticipated outcome. A patient who does not express satisfaction with video images is probably not a good candidate for surgery.

Informed Consent

Because the results of aesthetic rhinoplasty are more unpredictable than those of most other aesthetic operations, informed consent is critical. *Every patient should be told that a touch-up or corrective procedure may be necessary.* A specific issue of informed consent with the open approach is that unless the patient is not concerned about details of the technique, the nature of the incision and the scar that is likely to follow should be discussed. Most patients will agree to an open rhinoplasty and the associated scar if it is explained that the open approach generally produces the best results. However, there will always be a few patients who are not willing to accept that risk. These patients should be given the option of a closed rhinoplasty. Some patients will ask why it is necessary to have a columellar scar when their friends do not. Performing an open rhinoplasty on such a patient creates a potential problem in the event the scar is not all but invisible.

Planning the Operation

Once the decision is made to perform a rhinoplasty, a detailed plan is essential. Unlike many aesthetic operations, rhinoplasty involves a series of steps or maneuvers. Often, they must be coordinated. For example, osteotomies are typically performed toward the end of the operation because the associated swelling and bleeding can obscure components of the overall aesthetic appearance. Writing down the steps to be performed ahead of time is preferable to using an extemporaneous approach. Finally, the timing of the rhinoplasty is important. Ideally, a year should elapse before any touch-up or corrective procedures are performed. Patients often find it difficult to wait that long and put pressure on the surgeon to act sooner. If surgery is to be performed earlier, it is reasonable to do so when the tissues of the nose feel soft and pliable, which indicates that another procedure will be tolerated with a minimum of postoperative nasal swelling and induration.

INTRAOPERATIVE PHASE

Hypertension

The complications of any type of rhinoplasty can begin intraoperatively (4). Hypertension both during and after surgery is an occasional problem. Often, it is caused by a preexisting condition, but in other cases, it is simply due a consequence of anxiety or the epinephrine used with the local anesthetic. Hypertension poses a problem during surgery because it is difficult to operate in a blood-filled field and to manage a patient who is coughing up aspirated blood. It also poses a problem postoperatively in terms of epistaxis, swelling, and ecchymosis. Ideally, the systolic pressure should be kept below 130 mm Hg.

Prevention begins by keeping the patient normotensive before the commencement of surgery and certainly during the surgery. A number of agents are available to reduce pressure (4). Usually, 5 mL of hydralazine (Apresoline) is given first. Because hydralazine takes up to 45 minutes to take effect, chlorpromazine (Thorazine) is sometimes used when the pressure is high and must be reduced in a relatively short period of time. An intravenous push of 2.5 mg of chlorpromazine is given every 5 minutes to a maximum dose of approximately 25 mg, or until the blood pressure has reached a satisfactory level. Chlorpromazine does produce a considerable degree of drowsiness and prolongs the recovery time, but this is a worthwhile exchange for the problems associated with uncontrolled hypertension.

Surgeons who use ketamine should keep in mind that this drug is potentially dangerous when given during (but not at the beginning of) head and neck surgery (5). Bleeding during surgery can cause problems of aspiration. For that reason and because the nose is generally easy to anesthetize, we almost never use ketamine for nasal surgery.

Effects of Cocaine

A serious potential problem with local anesthesia comes from the use of cocaine. It is well-known that the cardiac arrhythmias associated with cocaine are idiosyncratic and not always dose-dependent. These arrhythmias are also more difficult to treat than arrhythmias with other causes. Consequently, one of us (RPG) no longer uses cocaine. Local anesthesia is easily established by direct injection of lidocaine with epinephrine. If the mucoperichondrium of the dorsal septum, the inferior turbinate, and the mucosa of the medial side of the nasal bone are injected, satisfactory anesthesia is obtained for septoplasty and osteotomies. If necessary, cotton soaked in 4% lidocaine with epinephrine is applied topically to the internal airway.

Soft Tissue Perforations

An occasional intraoperative complication is nasal skin perforation by an operative instrument (Fig. 54-1), especially in secondary rhinoplasty, when the skin is intimately adherent to the underlying cartilaginous framework. Skin perforation is best prevented by hyperinflation of the tissues (Fig. 54-2). At the beginning of the case (whether general or local anesthesia is used), the nose should be hyperinflated with local anesthetic. This practice not only improves hemostasis but also facilitates dissection and minimizes skin perforation.

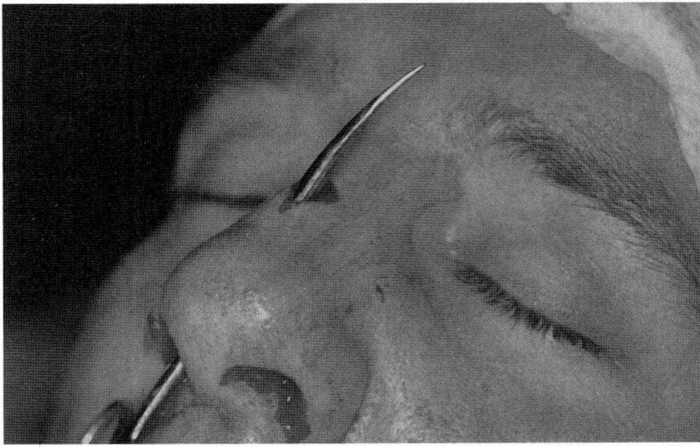

FIGURE 54-1. The dorsal nasal skin of this patient was perforated during the course of dissection.

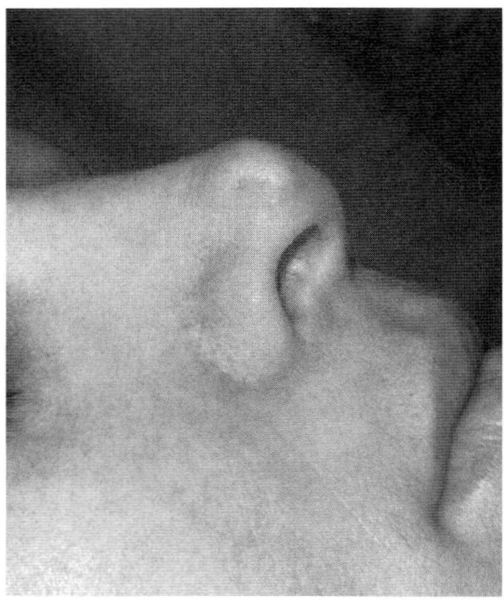

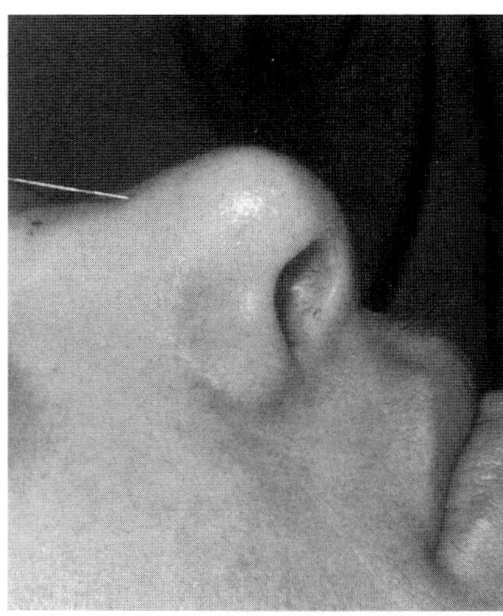

A,B

FIGURE 54-2. Before surgery of the nose is begun **(A)**, the tissues are hyperinflated with local anesthesia **(B)**.

The nose must occasionally be reinfiltrated with local anesthetic (or saline solution) during the course of the operation, particularly the septum and vestibular skin, which do not hold anesthetic very well. The vestibular skin is infiltrated immediately before any manipulation of the domes or lower lateral cartilages. The septum is infiltrated immediately before mucoperichondrial elevation, for the same reason.

EARLY POSTOPERATIVE PHASE

Unaesthetic Result Immediately after Surgery

On occasion, the appearance of the nose may be quite unaesthetic immediately after surgery, when the splint is still in place (Fig. 54-3). The most common problem at this time is that the nose has an obtuse columellar angle. When the splint is removed, the obtuse angle is even more obvious. Both the patient and the surgeon are immediately aware that the nose is unaesthetic and can be quite concerned. The problem is as likely to occur with the open as with the closed approach.

The cause of the problem may be edema or hematoma of the anterior nasal spine. Another likely cause is that an aesthetic error in sculpting has been made. The angle of the septum may have been made too obtuse. Alternatively, if tip cartilages have been sutured to the caudal septum, the sutures at the level of the septal angle may be too tight and cause the anterior aspect of the tip to retract. Many sculpting errors are not apparent until the splint has been removed. Patients undergo surgery in the supine position, so that it is difficult to judge what the nose will look like on the face when the patient is upright.

One way to prevent this problem is to tilt the table upward during surgery to get a better idea of the aesthetic result. Even a Polaroid picture (Fig. 54-4) taken during surgery gives the surgeon a better perspective of the patient's appearance. One of us (RPG) likes to use a video camera

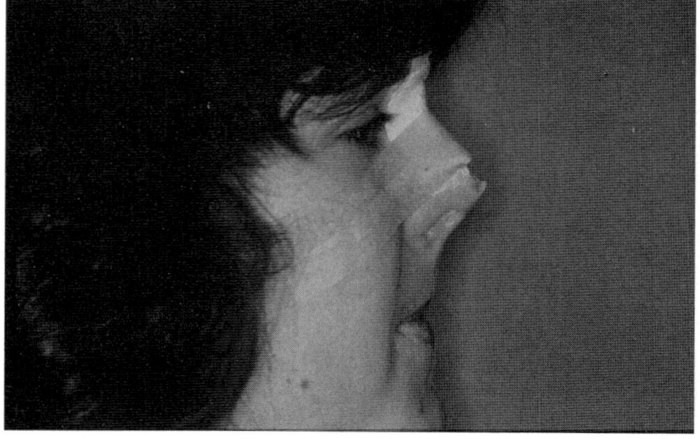

A

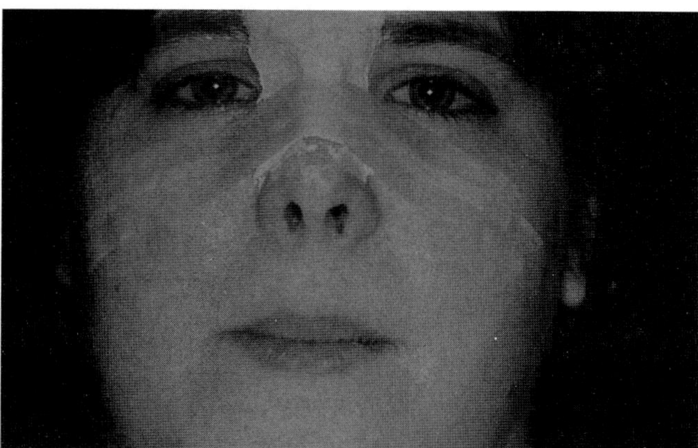

B

FIGURE 54-3. An unaesthetic result may be apparent in the immediate postoperative period. It is better to treat it immediately than to wait months in the hope that the problem will correct itself. **A:** Lateral. **B:** Frontal.

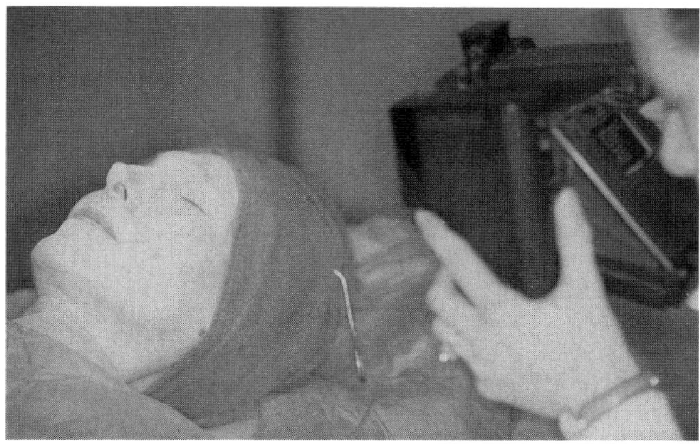

FIGURE 54-4. Because the patient is supine during surgery, it is often difficult to appreciate what the nose looks like relative to the rest of the face. A Polaroid picture provides another perspective (two-dimensional) of the nose.

during surgery to obtain a continuous, two-dimensional profile view of the patient—a perspective different from the three-dimensional view.

This situation should be managed by returning to the operating room and correcting the problem right away. Waiting several months and hoping for a resolution of the problem forces the patient to live with the problem. The patient can easily become unhappy, if not hostile, during this period of watchful waiting. It is just as easy to tell the patient that an immediate adjustment is necessary to get the best possible result. The adjustment can be performed by removing and replacing sutures, probably without cutting the tissues again. We have gone back as late as 12 days following surgery to make a surgical adjustment of this type. Edema and induration are not significantly increased by this practice.

Epistaxis

Unexpected bleeding following elective nasal surgery has been reviewed in detail (6). Epistaxis usually occurs in the first 24 to 48 hours following rhinoplasty. Mild epistaxis is occasionally seen immediately after the removal of packing, which is one of the reasons why we do not use packing unless it is absolutely necessary. The site of bleeding is frequently the caudal edge of the septum. The anterior nasal spine is another potential area of bleeding. The overall incidence of epistaxis is less than 2%.

Prevention begins by keeping the patient off aspirin for at least 10 days before surgery, in addition to the numerous other products on the market (notably nonsteroidal antiinflammatory drugs and ketorolac tromethamine) that affect platelet adhesion. Ideally, all patients should be evaluated for a possible family history of bleeding (e.g., von Willebrand's disease). Careful hemostasis during surgery is an obvious factor. This is easier to obtain in open rhinoplasty simply because the blood vessels along the dorsum of the septum are visualized after the hump is removed. Also, two vessels of the dorsal skin (branches of the lateral nasal artery) can be seen during open rhinoplasty and coagulants administered therein. These vessels often do not bleed until the end of the case, when the effect of epinephrine has worn off. *A distinct advantage of the open approach over the closed is that it is easier to obtain hemostasis and prevent epistaxis.*

Epistaxis is treated as follows: After some sedation, the patient receives local anesthesia to the base of the nose, columella, and portions of the septum. Digital compression of the nares is then applied. More often than not, these measures will resolve the matter. If not, a search for the bleeding vessel may be necessary. While active measures are taken to stop the bleeding, the patient should be reevaluated for the cause of the epistaxis, and a bleeding panel may be required to determine whether the patient has a bleeding diathesis. Epistaxis associated with turbinectomy and septal surgery is discussed in another chapter.

Hematoma

Hematoma is an infrequent complication of rhinoplasty, but it is probably more common than appreciated. The entrapment of a small quantity of blood under the nasal skin, even if it is only 1 to 2 mL, can cause pain if not swelling. The patient's discomfort is out of proportion to what is expected for a rhinoplasty. Small hematomas can be tolerated under the skin of the nose in terms of skin survival, but they are manifested later as an unsatisfactory aesthetic result. Hematomas cause persistent edema and thickening of the subcutaneous tissues for many months, some of which will be permanent. Another site where small hematomas occur is along the lateral osteotomy line and near the radix where the nasal bones are fractured. These hematomas are often not appreciated until the splint is removed, when some redness and swelling are noted, especially in the region of the radix, causing an obliteration of the frontonasal angle.

If the hematoma is large, the treatment involves a return to the operating room for evacuation. If the vessel is not found, the subcutaneous space is irrigated with a thrombin solution or packed with Avitene to stop the bleeding that occurs after hematoma evacuation. If the swelling is along the lateral nasal bone where the osteotomy was performed, the hematoma is suctioned through the canal through which the osteotome was passed. Figure 54-5 shows a patient in whom a small hematoma was seen at the time the splint was removed on postoperative day 6. It was immediately evacuated with a syringe and needle rather than allowed to become a source of problems.

Infection

Infection is a very uncommon complication following rhinoplasty (Fig. 54-6). Nonetheless, subcutaneous infec-

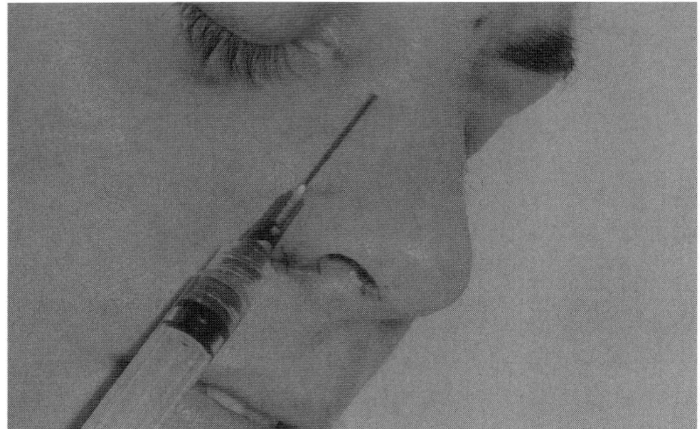

FIGURE 54-5. Occasionally, a small hematoma is seen at the time of splint removal. Unlike simple edema, it is usually quite tender to palpation. It often resolves after simple aspiration.

tions, infectious rhinitis, and even sinusitis can result. In part, this may be because up to 25% of patients are silent carriers of *Staphylococcus aureus.* Packing in the nose is certainly a potential cause of infection if left in place too long. If nothing else, a foul odor may develop the packing is left in place too long. Therefore, if packing must be used, it is left in for no more than 3 days. Early removal also prevents toxic shock syndrome, which is discussed in detail elsewhere (7,8).

Although many feel that antibiotics do not prevent infection, we favor prophylactic antibiotics, such as 250 mg of cephalosporin orally three times daily started the day before surgery and continued postoperatively for a few days. All cartilage grafts are soaked in a bacitracin solution before they are placed in the nose. Infection is treated with drainage and appropriate antibiotics as dictated by the results of culture.

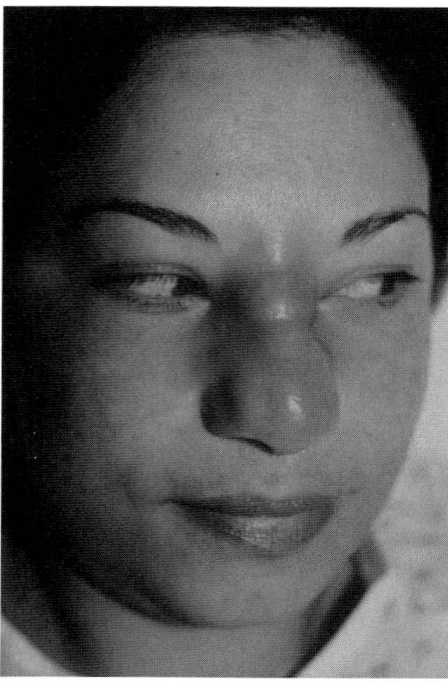

FIGURE 54-6. Although rare, infection does occur following rhinoplasty. When it develops immediately, culture and sensitivity and, if possible, drainage should be performed.

Skin Necrosis after the Open Approach

Major Necrosis

Flap necrosis is a rare but major potential complication in open rhinoplasty (Fig. 54-7). Several potential causes of this problem are the following:

1. Smoking
2. Poor circulation of the nasal skin because of prior trauma or the presence of surgical scars
3. Defatting of the flap such that the dermal circulation is damaged
4. Extensive excisions of the alar base

To avoid flap necrosis, patients are asked to stop smoking 10 days before surgery. *The skin flap is never defatted other than to trim away any soft tissue that is hanging from the dorsal skin like a stalactite.* If the patient has surgical scars on the nose or tip, or has atrophic or discolored skin, the open approach is deferred. Finally, extensive excisions of the alar base are not performed at the time of an open rhinoplasty.

Although any excision of the alar base would seem to carry a great risk for flap necrosis, this has not occurred in the author's experience. There certainly appears to be a potential for interference with the circulation, particularly if the ala is completely detached from the face. Rohrich et al. (9) nicely demonstrated the circulation in the nasal skin and how branches of the lateral nasal artery near the upper alar area contribute significantly to blood flow in the nasal tip. To avoid interfering with the circulation in the open approach, the alar base excision should be conservative. If an extensive resection of tissue is required, it should be deferred for months if necessary, until a time when the viability of the columellar flap is certain. At that time, under local anesthesia, an alar base excision can always be performed as an office procedure.

Sometimes, poor technique with a lack of respect for the tissues leads to soft tissue necrosis. The patient in Fig. 54-8 sustained not only damage to the flap but also to the columella itself, so that a substantial amount of columellar tissue was lost.

The treatment of necrosis is exceedingly difficult and beyond the scope of this chapter. In general, the management involves conservative wound care. The nose has a remarkable ability to heal without too much scarring (Fig. 54-9). The surgeon will most likely want to wait at least a year before deciding what, if any, corrective measure can be implemented. *Intercepting the healing process of the nose early by excision of the wound and grafting or flap rotation is likely to cause further distortion, scarring, and color mismatching.*

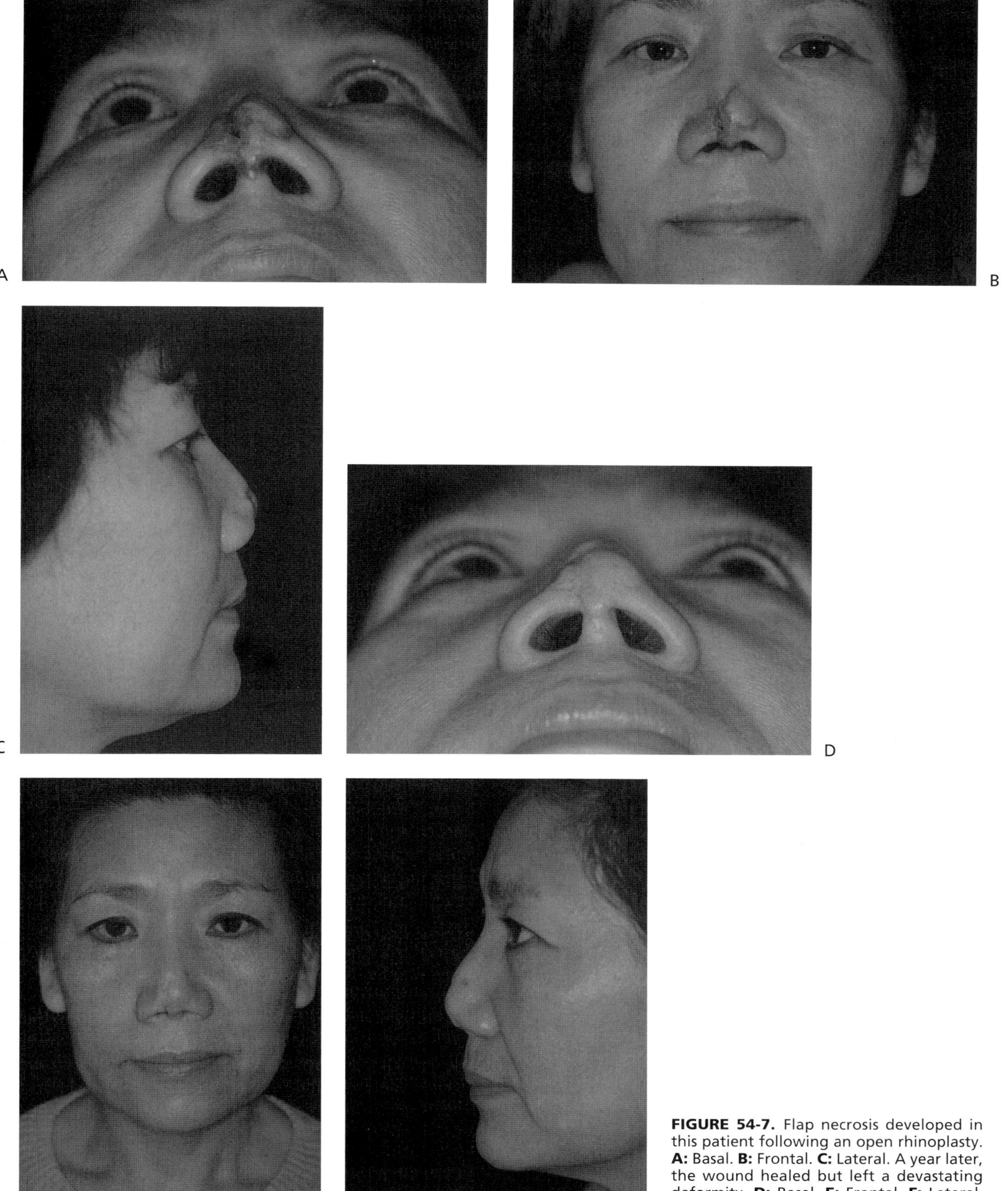

FIGURE 54-7. Flap necrosis developed in this patient following an open rhinoplasty. **A:** Basal. **B:** Frontal. **C:** Lateral. A year later, the wound healed but left a devastating deformity. **D:** Basal. **E:** Frontal. **F:** Lateral. These problems are often a consequence of defatting the flap.

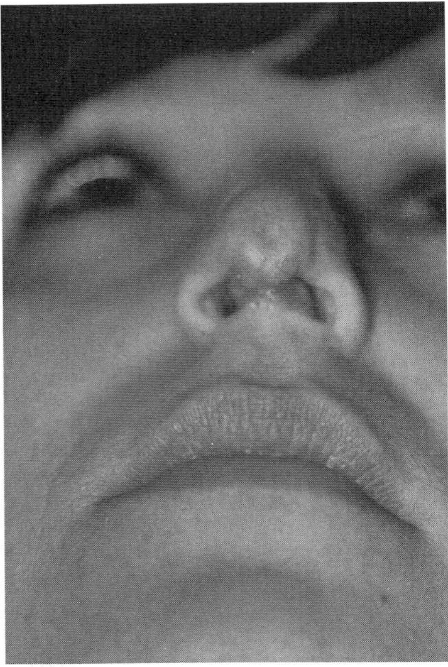
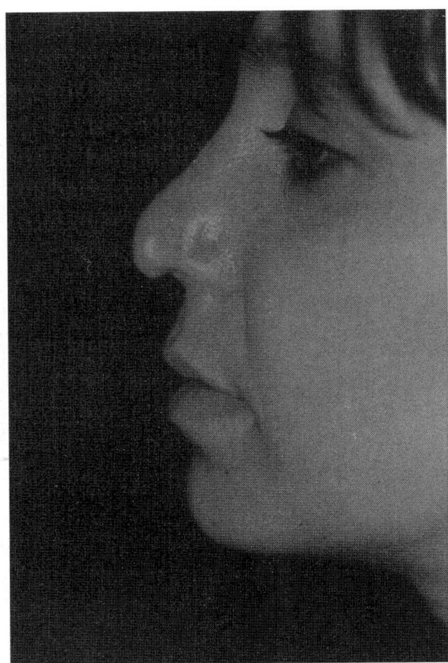

A,B

FIGURE 54-8. Although rare, tissue necrosis can be seen in the columellar area following an open approach. **A:** Basal. **B:** Lateral.

Cyanosis

Occasionally, one may see a slight bluish discoloration of the columellar portion of the nasal flap on the first postoperative day following an open approach (Fig. 54-10). This is usually caused by the tight placement of tape around the tip of the nose. For this reason, patients should be seen on the first day after surgery for an evaluation of the circulation in and around the region of the columella, and release of the tape if necessary. Minor discoloration may be the consequence of minor trauma to the flap during the rhinoplasty. To minimize trauma to the columella flap, it is suggested that the flap not be folded on itself for long periods of time. It is also helpful to unfurl the columella flap when the dorsum is rasped or when scissors are used to resect the dorsum (Fig. 54-11).

Edema and Steroid Atrophy

Edema

Although our initial impression was that edema (and subsequent fibrosis) is not increased after the open approach, our opinion has changed. The extra dissection of the tip and col-

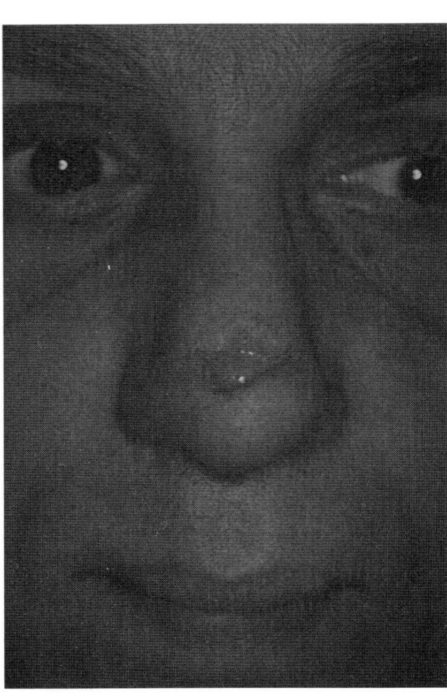
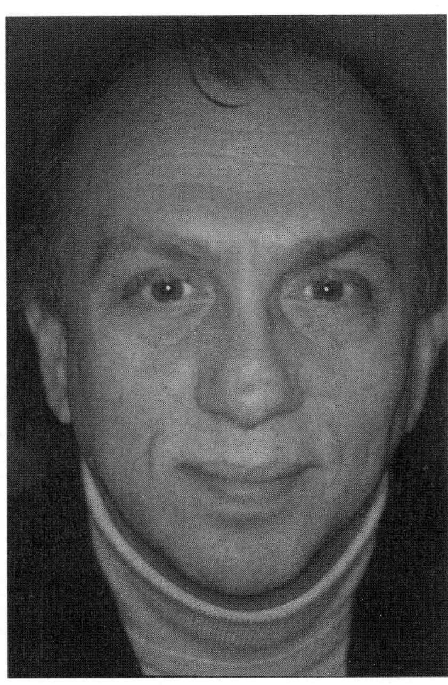

A,B

FIGURE 54-9. Despite skin necrosis **(A)**, the nasal skin has a remarkable ability to heal **(B)**. For this reason, conservative treatment should be given every chance to work before surgical treatments such as grafts or local flaps are considered.

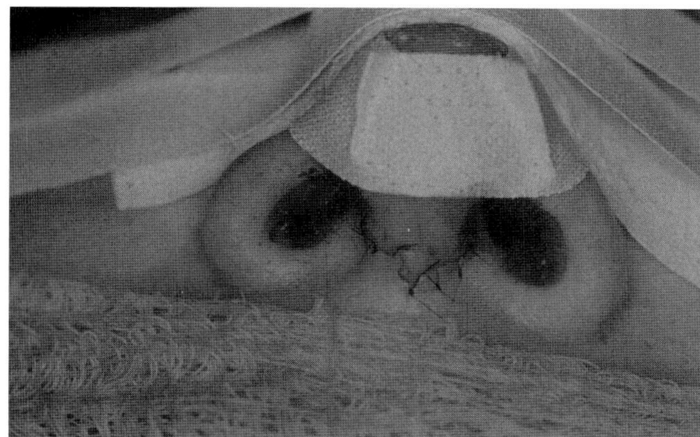

FIGURE 54-10. Occasionally after an open approach, the skin flap may appear mildly blue or cyanotic. If this problem is seen on the first day postoperatively, the tape surrounding the nasal tip should be released.

umella, with interruption of the veins and lymphatics in the columella, probably increases the edema that a patient experiences postoperatively. Figure 54-12 shows a very thick-skinned patient 1 1/2 years following an open rhinoplasty. Postoperatively, severe edema developed; it did not subside and was eventually replaced by fibrosis. Very thick-skinned patients (requiring reduction rhinoplasty) are better candidates for the closed approach. The exception to this rule is the patient whose anatomical structural problems are not amenable to the closed approach. *In the very thick-skinned patient, the surgeon needs to weigh the benefits of increased visibility and better sculpting against the possibility of increased edema and subsequent fibrosis.* The risk for edema and fibrosis is not always offset by the benefit of better sculpting.

If edema persists after 4 to 6 weeks, it is treated with the judicious use of corticosteroids. Triamcinolone (Kenalog-10) is injected into such areas as the supratip or lower lateral cartilage (Fig. 54-13). Because some patients are unusually

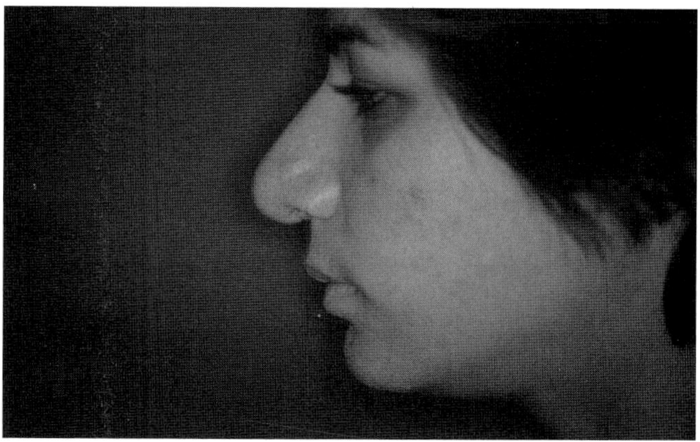

A

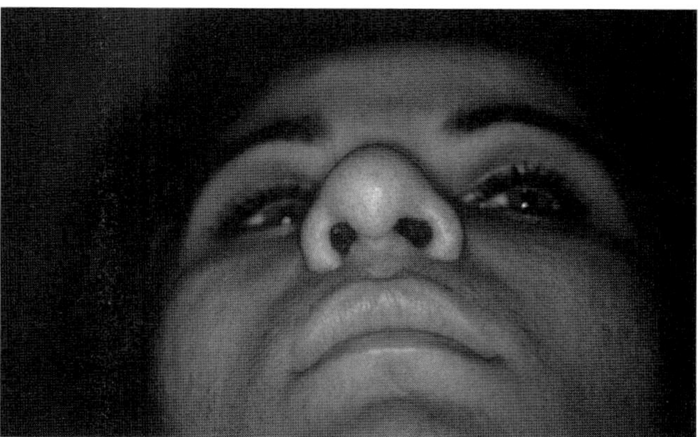

B

FIGURE 54-12. Patient with very thick skin 1 1/2 years after open rhinoplasty. She has a rounded, poorly defined nasal tip. Because of postoperative edema and subsequent fibrosis, a thick-skinned patient is a less suitable candidate for the open approach. **A:** Lateral. **B:** Basal.

sensitive to corticosteroids, a very small initial dose is used. With a No. 27 or No. 30 needle, 0.25 mL (1.25 mg) of triamcinolone and an equal volume of lidocaine are mixed. Slightly less than 0.25 mL (about 1 mg of triamcinolone) is

A

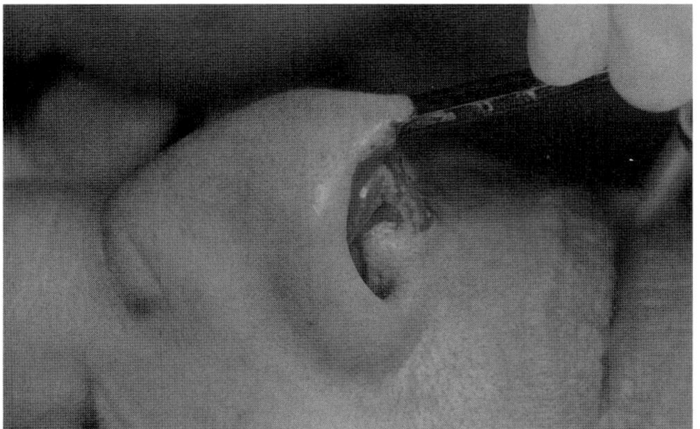

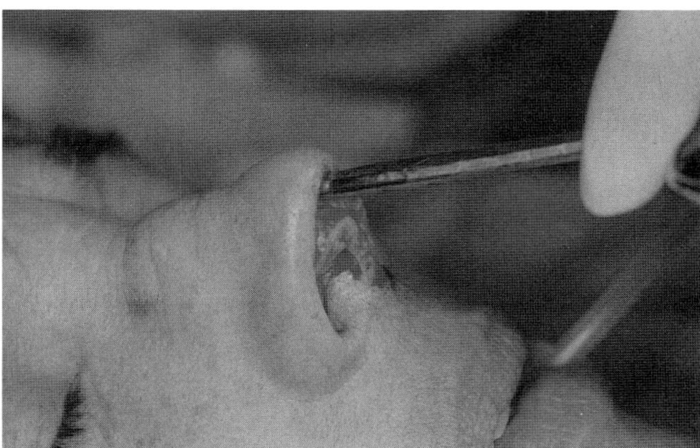

B

FIGURE 54-11. Trauma to the nasal skin flap **(A)** in the open approach is minimized by unfurling the flap **(B)** when the scissors are used or the dorsum is rasped.

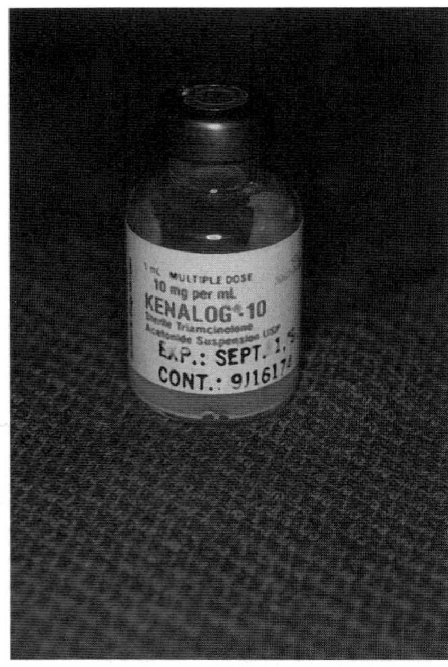

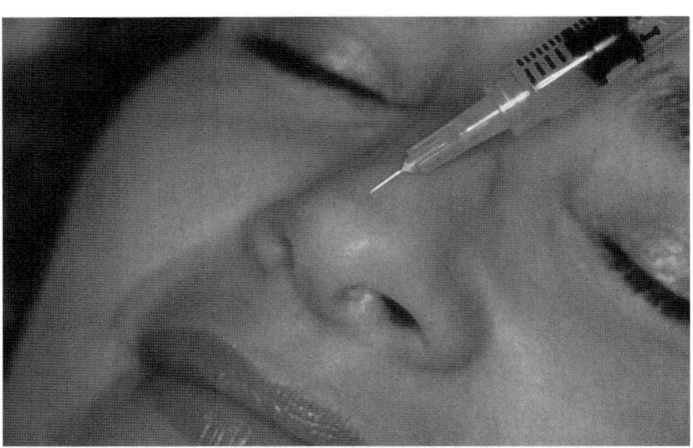

A B

FIGURE 54-13. Early postoperative edema can be treated to some extent with the judicious use of triamcinolone **(A)**. An initial dose of 1 mg is given **(B)**, and the dose is repeated every 2 to 3 weeks as needed.

injected into the thickened area. Care is taken to avoid a wheal in the skin. The injection is repeated at 2- to 3-week intervals and the dose increased as needed. Patient's responses to triamcinolone vary strikingly. Some patients require hardly any before a significant change in the soft tissues is noted, whereas the response of others to several injections over many months is minimal.

Steroid Atrophy

Corticosteroid injection is not without its own potential problems. It is difficult to predict how much of the corticosteroid should be given, and how often. The same problem is encountered in the treatment of hypertrophic scars. Experience is an excellent teacher. After a primary rhinoplasty, the patient in Fig. 54-14 had significant edema in the

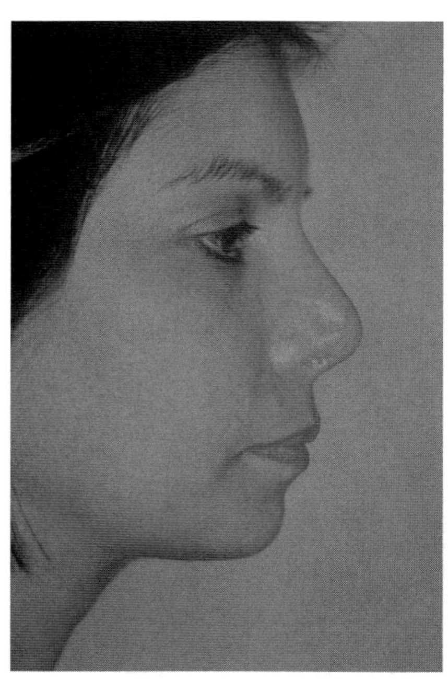

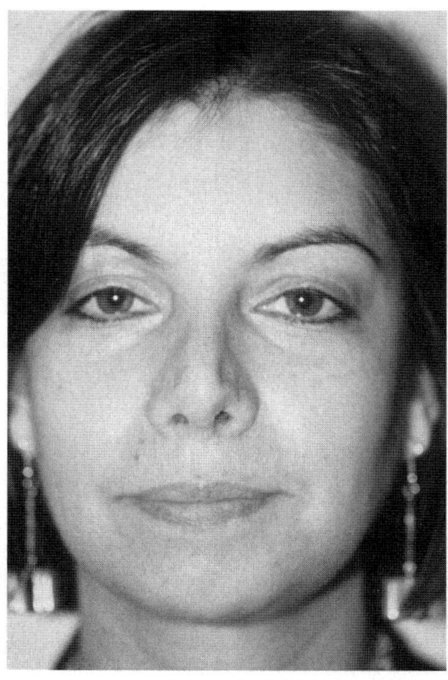

A,B

FIGURE 54-14. The use of corticosteroids for edema can cause steroid atrophy, as in this patient. Therefore, the initial dose should be small and the patient's sensitivity observed. **A:** Lateral. **B:** Frontal.

region of the lateral crura. The patient was given 2 mg of injectable triamcinolone, after which a very marked atrophy of the soft tissues developed that improved only slightly with time.

Steroid atrophy can, of course, be prevented by avoiding the use of corticosteroids altogether. However, many patients do benefit from the judicious use of corticosteroids. A better approach is simply to minimize the first dose (to approximately 1 mg) and wait 3 to 4 weeks to observe the response. Many patients in whom some apparent atrophy does develop show a rebound phenomenon during which the steroid-induced depression improves.

LATE POSTOPERATIVE PHASE

Columellar Scar after a Primary Open Approach

The complication that most concerns those who do not perform open rhinoplasties is the columellar scar. The nature of the scar depends on the type of incision. At least five types of incisions have been used for open rhinoplasty (Fig. 54-15): (a) a chevron type, (b) a slightly curved incision, (c) a stair-step incision, (d) a V-shaped incision, and (e) an incision at the junction of the columella and lip in patients with a short columella. In all cases, the potential for scarring

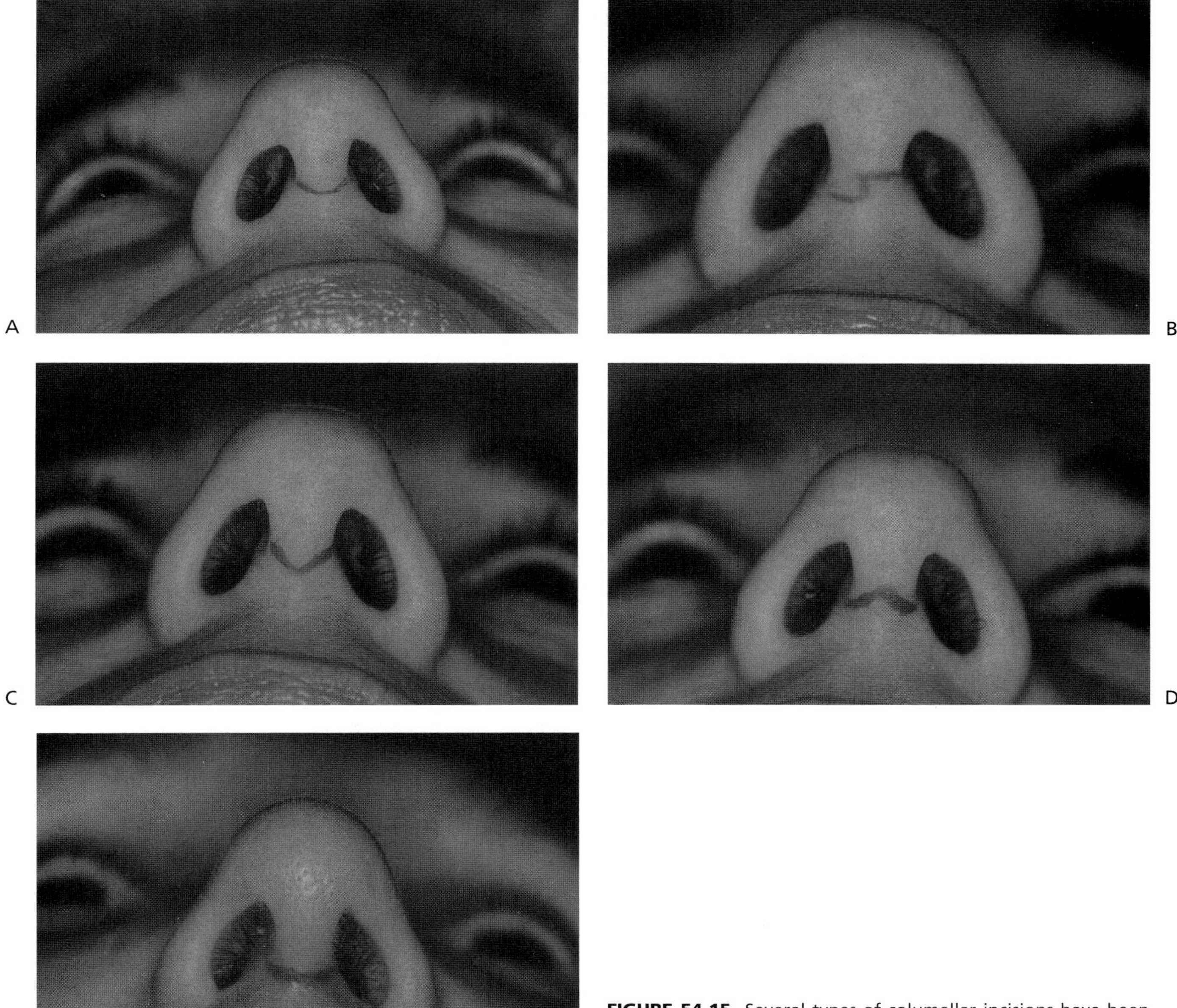

FIGURE 54-15. Several types of columellar incisions have been used over the years to minimize the problem of a visible columellar scar. **A:** Curved. **B:** Stair-step. **C:** Chevron. **D:** Inverted chevron. **E:** Incision at the junction of the columella and lip.

is present although not great. In our experience, a scar that is not satisfactory to the patient develops in approximately 1% of cases and requires some form of treatment. Usually, the problem will be mild retraction; it is not likely to be hypertrophy or widening. Occasionally, thickening of the soft tissue immediately anterior to the scar creates the effect of a hanging columella. This effect (convexity of the columella) is caused by a small degree of fibrosis and edema and is aggravated by the depressed scar. Occasionally, however, a very severe problem develops from this phenomenon (Fig. 54-16). The most common one is notching of the scar at the lateral aspect of the columella. Sometimes, a small degree of hyperpigmentation will be noticeable within the scar (Fig. 54-17).

The problem of scarring can be minimized by the correct choice of incision. *The stair-step incision (popularized by Gunter) seems to give the best overall result.* In the event that a significant notch of the lateral columella is present, it can be camouflaged (on profile view) by the unscarred portion of the other side of the columella (i.e., the stair-step incision breaks up the scar and makes it less apparent on profile view) (Fig. 54-18). In addition, meticulous technique (under magnification) during the repair greatly enhances the final result. A deep layer of absorbable sutures is not necessary. A few 5-0 nylon sutures that slightly evert the closure are more than satisfactory.

If a significant scar develops even though the best measures have been taken to prevent it, the treatment depends on the type of incision employed. The depressed scar *per se* is treated with excision. Additional measures to treat the convexity within the columella itself can be exceptionally difficult. However, if it develops, it is treated much like a hanging columella. A resection of a portion of the caudal septum followed by a repair with semiabsorbable or nonabsorbable sutures will be beneficial. In the case of a chevron incision or a curvilinear one, a small A-plasty sometimes effectively breaks up the depression and improves the results dramatically.

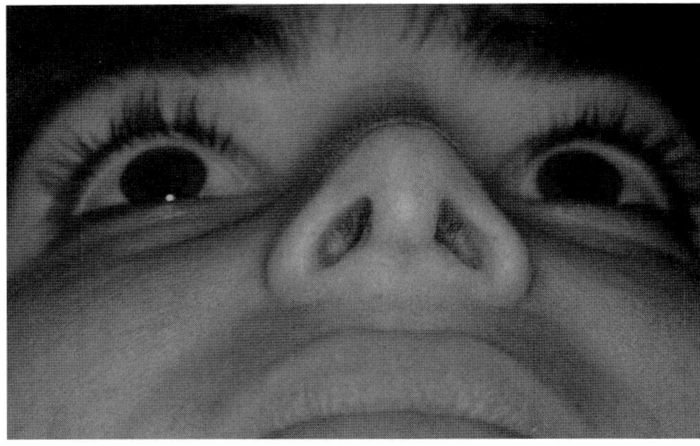

FIGURE 54-17. This patient, who underwent an open rhinoplasty, exhibits hyperpigmentation in the area of the columellar scar.

Columellar Scar after a Secondary Open Approach

Secondary open rhinoplasty following a primary open rhinoplasty can carry its own set of problems (10). In par-

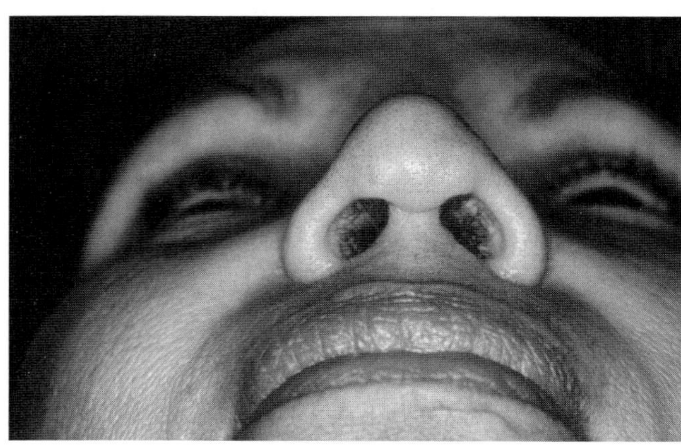

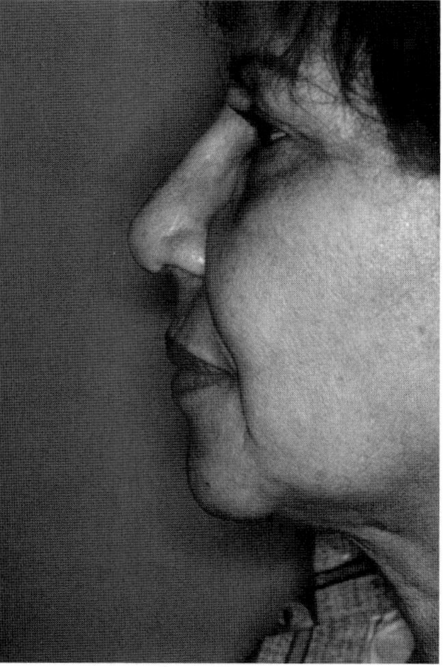

A B

FIGURE 54-16. This patient, who underwent open rhinoplasty, has an unsightly scar that has contracted. **A:** Basal. **B:** Lateral.

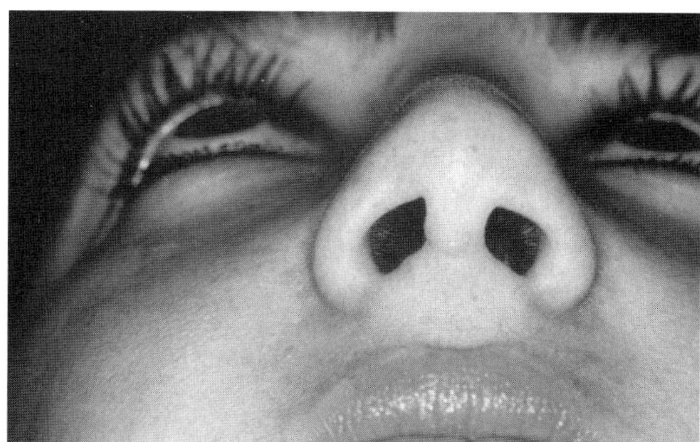
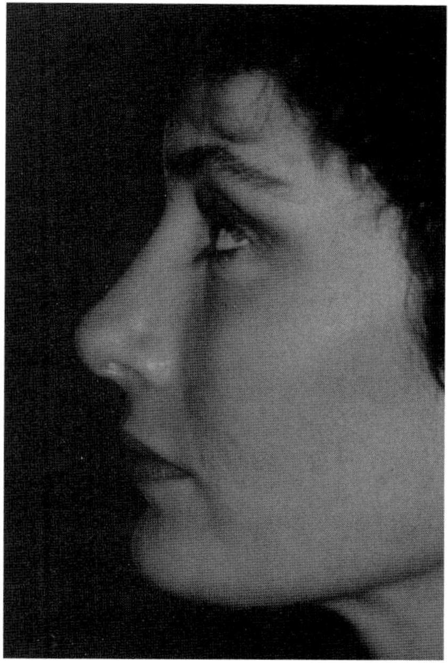

FIGURE 54-18. An advantage of the stair-step incision is that any notching that develops on the lateral columella, as seen from the basal view **(A)**, is not very noticeable in the profile view **(B)**.

ticular, the most difficult scar of the columella is the one following a second open rhinoplasty. Opening the nose for a second time may aggravate any mild depression that already exists. In the patient in Fig. 54-19, a chevron incision was made at the waist of the columella during the first open rhinoplasty. She required a secondary revision of the tip,

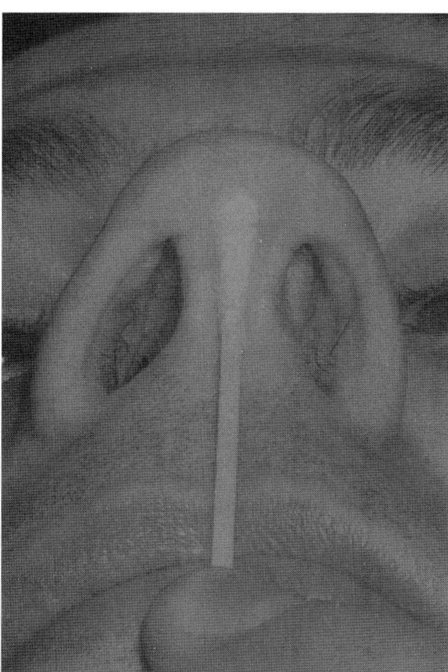

FIGURE 54-19. This patient has a prominent scar in the vestibule where a "rim" incision was made. The caudal septum also impinges on the vestibule. The combination of these two problems contributes to significant airway obstruction.

and so the old incision was reopened. The depressed scar following the second procedure was much more marked than the one following the first procedure (which was relatively unnoticeable).

Prevention of this problem is twofold: (a) Avoid an open rhinoplasty in those patients who already have a columellar scar unless it is necessary to obtain precise control over the cartilaginous framework. This is especially true if the tissues are not soft. (b) Excise the primary columellar scar completely, perform whatever secondary procedures are necessary in the nose, and close the nose with interrupted sutures. Attempt to evert the edges when possible. Scar resection should not prevent closure of the wound or cause a foreshortening of the columella. Should the columellar scar reappear despite these efforts, treatment of the depressed scar and convex columella is similar to that used after a first open rhinoplasty.

Vestibular Scarring

Vestibular scarring can detract from the patient's appearance and cause airway obstruction. A common problem is thickening of the vestibular skin along the location of a "rim" incision bordering the caudal aspect of the lower lateral cartilage (Fig. 54-19). If the rim incision has not been suture-repaired properly, the caudal edge of the lower lateral cartilage can collapse. A thickening then develops along the rim incision that is usually a combination of scar and cartilage that is actually hanging. The same phenomenon can occur on the cephalic side of the lower lateral cartilage, where the "intercartilaginous" incision is usually made. The intercartilaginous incision is not ordinarily repaired because of its remoteness. However, if for some reason the cephalic edge of the lower lateral cartilage does not abut the caudal edge of the upper lateral cartilage reasonably well, a thickening of both scar and cartilage will develop here and can contribute to airway obstruction.

Scar along the area of the transfixion incision can also pose a problem. The transfixion wound can contract and leave a vertical band that is bothersome to the patient, although not likely to obstruct the airway. A scar band contracture is most distressing when it occurs in the area of the dome where an intercartilaginous (or intracartilaginous) incision is made in conjunction with a transfixion incision. It also occurs in the area of the dome where the rim incision rises to the dome and then sweeps down the lateral edge of the columellar rim. This scar, if fully contracted, can impede the airway significantly. It can even cause an external deformity if the dome is pinched.

Vestibular and rim scars are prevented with carefully located incisions and meticulous suture technique. Even so, these problems can still occur simply because the dome is a very small zone in which even a little scar band contracture can have a profound effect in terms of distortion. Packing the vestibule for the first day helps maintain the cartilages in their proper position and prevents blood from accumulating beneath the tissues. However, packing is distressing to patients. A better alternative that has served us well is the use of a "peanut pack" (Fig. 54-20). At the conclusion of vestibular incision repair, a peanut gauze (soaked in antibiotic ointment) is placed in the dome of each vestibule. The peanut gauze is just the right size to press the lower lateral cartilage up against the nasal skin and maintain the integrity of the dome. The two peanut packs are actually sutured to each other before they are placed in the vestibules to prevent inadvertent aspiration by the patient.

Treatment can be difficult. One of us (GA) excises the thickening and advances the mucoperichondrium (or vestibular skin) to close the wound. The other author (RPG) often solves the problem by trimming the edge of the lower lateral cartilage or repositioning it.

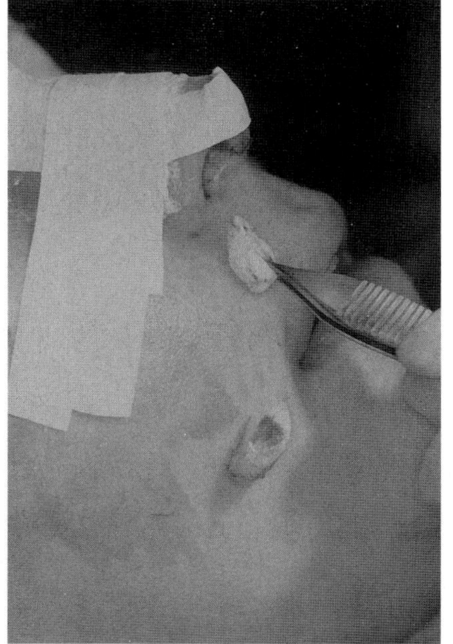

B

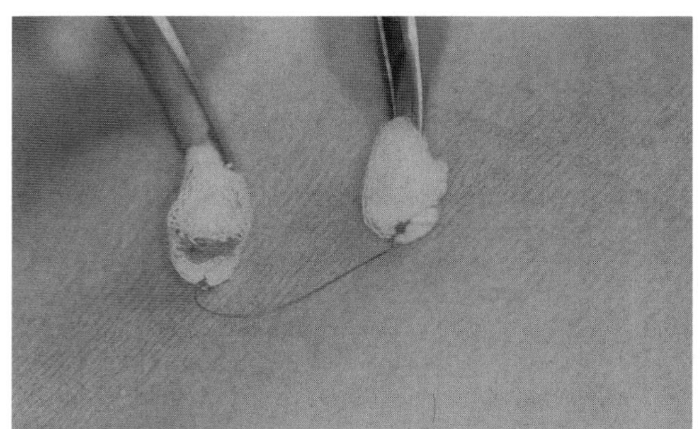

A

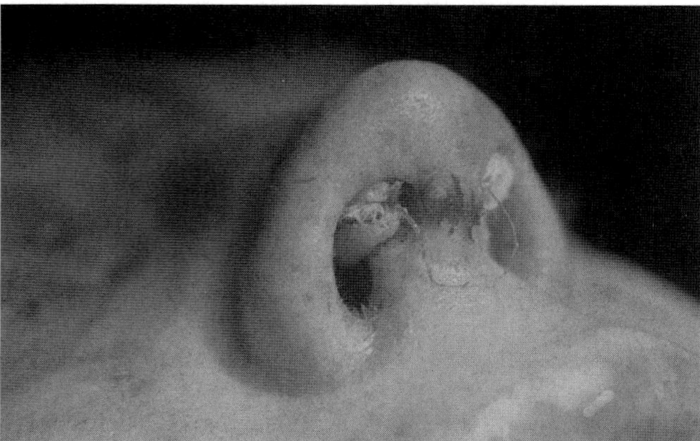

C

FIGURE 54-20. Vestibular scarring and tip cartilage malpositioning can be minimized by the use of a "peanut pack." Two peanut gauzes sutured to each other **(A)** are placed in the area of the vestibular dome and removed on postoperative day 1. **B:** Lateral. **C:** Basal.

Late Skin Problems

Late skin problems include erythema and telangiectasia (Fig. 54-21). These are related to interference with the circulation of the skin and are exacerbated by repeated or extensive surgery and undermining of the skin over the dorsum. Sometimes, postoperative telangiectasia is merely an exacerbation of preoperative telangiectasia. Therefore, it behooves the surgeon to notice the extent of telangiectasia before surgery, point it out to the patient during the consultation, and let the patient know that this problem may be aggravated postoperatively. Telangiectasia is probably more likely to develop with the open approach but do not offset the enormous benefits of the open approach.

Prevention should be aimed at minimizing the amount of surgical dissection. Unfortunately, undermining is frequently necessary to accomplish the major goals of the rhinoplasty. Treatment involves avoiding alcohol and spicy foods, which tend to flare the condition. A more definitive treatment is the use of cautery or argon laser to obliterate the vessels. One or more sessions with the Bovi often suffices (Fig. 54-22). If the problem is diffuse erythema, such treatment will not be effective.

Actual scarring of the nasal skin can be caused by rough handling of the tissues, inadvertent perforation of the skin, or multiple operations. Prevention must be directed toward better surgical technique and the avoidance of multiple procedures. Once the scar occurs, it may be difficult to eradicate. Surgical excision of the scar often leaves another scar that may be no less noticeable than the first.

Implant Complications

Implant exposure is an occasional problem in augmentation rhinoplasty (11) and is why most plastic surgeons avoid the use of alloplastic materials. Implants are more likely to erode

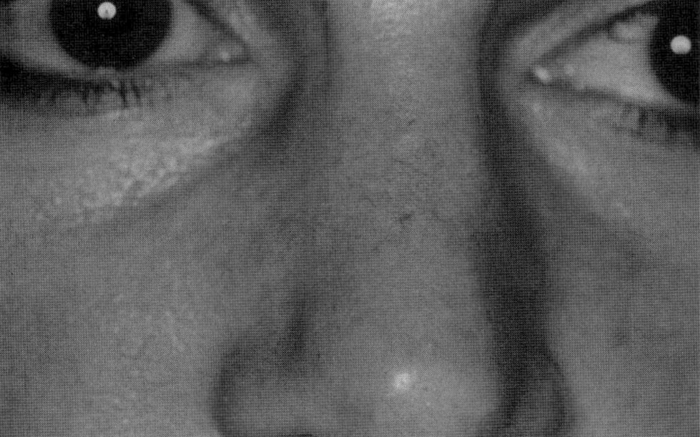

FIGURE 54-21. This patient exhibits telangiectasia and erythema following rhinoplasty. The magnitude of these problems is proportional to the extent of skin undermining, and therefore they are probably more likely to develop after the open than after the closed approach.

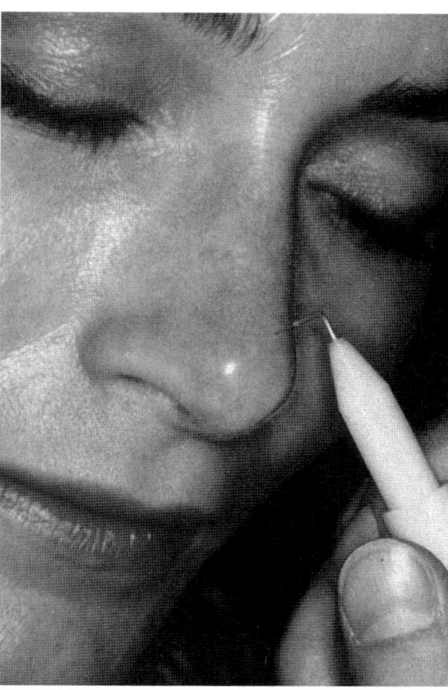

FIGURE 54-22. Treatment of telangiectasia is often but not always accomplished with the use of a Bovi.

in the area of the membranous septum and radix, where the tissues are meager. Even if they do not erode, implants can cause the skin to become so thin (just as in the case of large breast implant) that the implant can be felt or seen through it.

Gore-Tex was originally thought to be a material that might avert the problems associated with silicone. However, perhaps one should not anticipate any significant difference between one type of alloplastic material and another in terms of rejection and infection (12). The best means of prevention is simply to avoid using alloplastic material. If it is to be used at all in the nose, it is probably best confined to the region of the dorsum and supratip, where the skin is thickest.

In Fig. 54-23, one sees a patient who previously received an L-shaped silicone implant during an aesthetic augmentation rhinoplasty. Unfortunately, it became exposed within the vestibule. Because of the threat of ultimate implant loss and infection, early intervention was undertaken and the implant was replaced with a cartilaginous graft taken from the septum. At 13 months postoperatively, one can see that the cartilage graft provides a similar aesthetic result without the risk for silicone exposure.

Allograft/AlloDerm Rejection and Absorption

Allograft

The use of cartilage allografts (homografts) carries with it a potential for rejection (13). Although allografted cartilage is

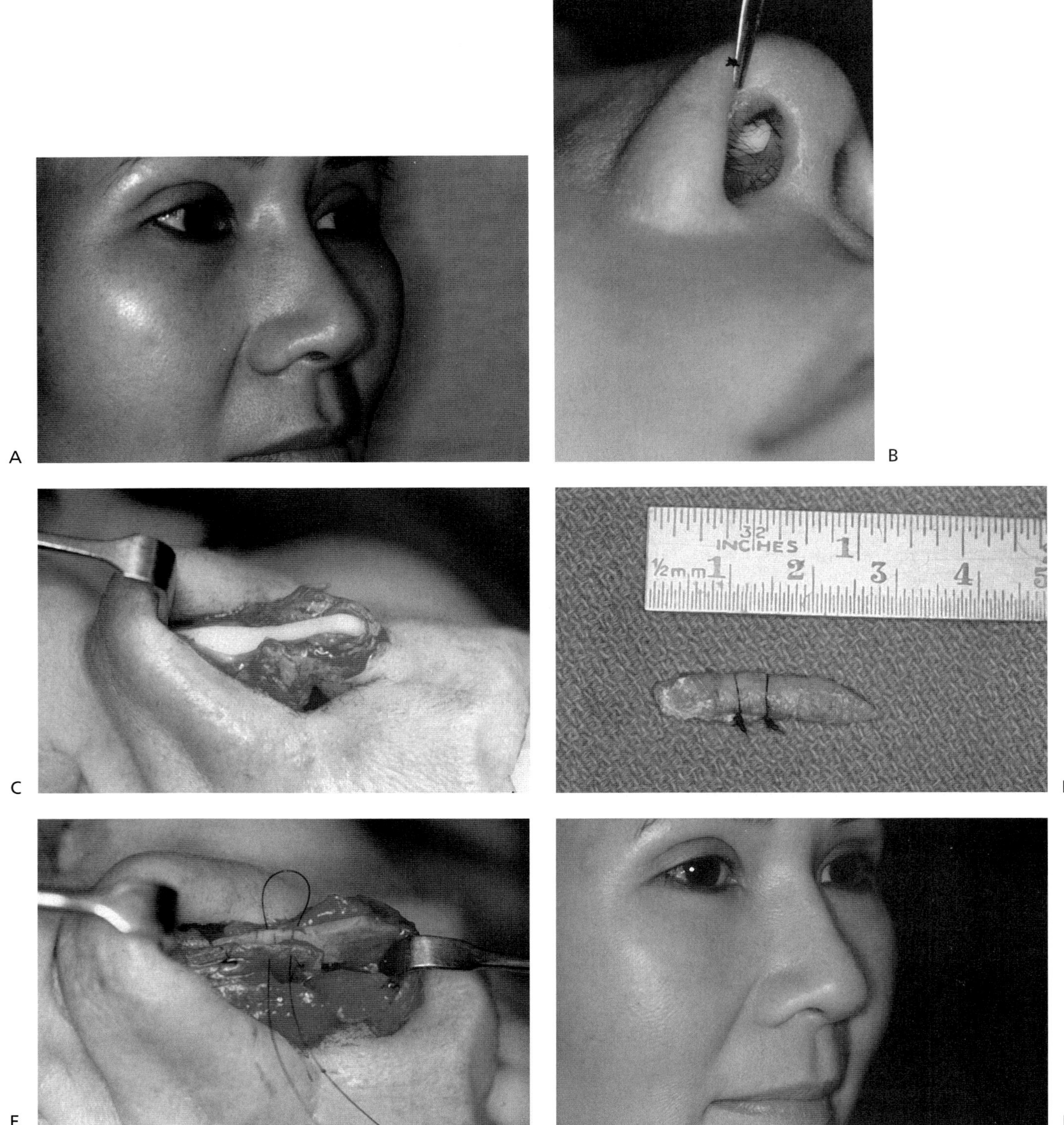

FIGURE 54-23. This patient received a silicone implant **(A)** that subsequently became exposed in the vestibulum **(B)**. Immediate removal **(C)** and replacement with cartilage graft **(D,E)** restored the nasal shape. The patient is seen 13 months postoperatively **(F)**.

generally thought of as being immunologically privileged, the fact remains that some allografts are absorbed, and some even become infected. Simple avoidance of banked cartilage will prevent this unfavorable result. If the use of allografts is confined to small, noncritical areas, such as the dorsum, any absorption that does occur will be less of a problem in terms of secondary correction. Treatment involves the removal of an exposed or infected allograft and replacement with autogenous tissue after the infection has cleared.

AlloDerm

In recent years, banked dermis (AlloDerm) has become available and is popular. AlloDerm is free of cellular material and is said to be immunologically inert. On the other hand, absorption has been seen. Thus, if it is used to augment the nose, it will probably present similar advantages and disadvantages as allografted cartilage. Time will tell.

Complications at the Ear Donor Site

Complications can also develop at the donor site. The ear is a potential problem area because of technique and the inherent tendency of cartilage to warp. Often, the entire concha (cymba and cavum) must be taken for a graft. Although no major deformity of the ear may develop, the ear will occasionally flatten as a result of the concha excision. The patient in Fig. 54-24 illustrates this problem. Prevention involves leaving those parts of the concha that cause the ear to project from the head. The vertical component of the concha cymba as it joins the antihelical rim should not be completely removed. At least 6 mm of the concha cavum is preserved because it keeps the antihelix away from the head.

A discussion of methods to treat the collapse of various portions of the ear is beyond the scope of this chapter. However, it should be stated that if the collapse is apparent at the time of surgery, that is the time to initiate treatment. If too much cartilage is removed, it should simply be returned and sutured. Hoping that the ear will assume a normal shape after too much cartilage has been removed is wishful thinking.

An excellent approach to removing conchal cartilage is by an anterior incision. On occasion, however, the scar in the anterior concha can become hypertrophic (Fig. 54-24). To a large extent, this problem can be avoided by meticulous closure of the donor site and packing the concha. A more definitive way to avoid this problem is to use a posterior approach. Once the surgeon becomes familiar with the anatomy from the posterior approach, it is quite easy to harvest cartilage in this way. The posterior approach is a particularly convenient method when removal of the entire concha cymba is desired. The treatment of scars of the ear, whether anterior or posterior, is the same as for any unsatisfactory scar.

Psychological Problems

The Difficult Patient

As in all types of aesthetic surgery, certain patients are difficult to please. Some, who have preexisting psychological

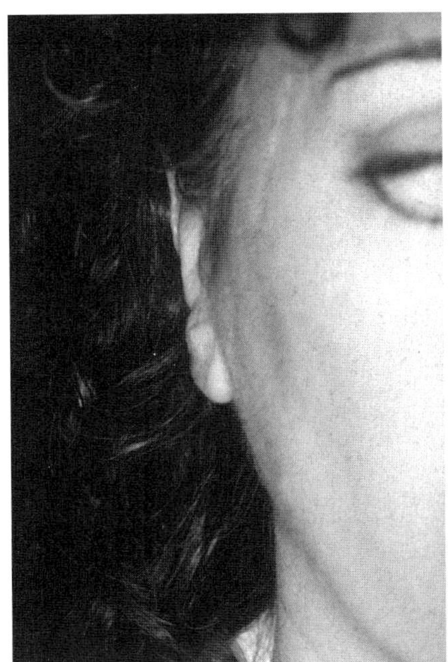
A

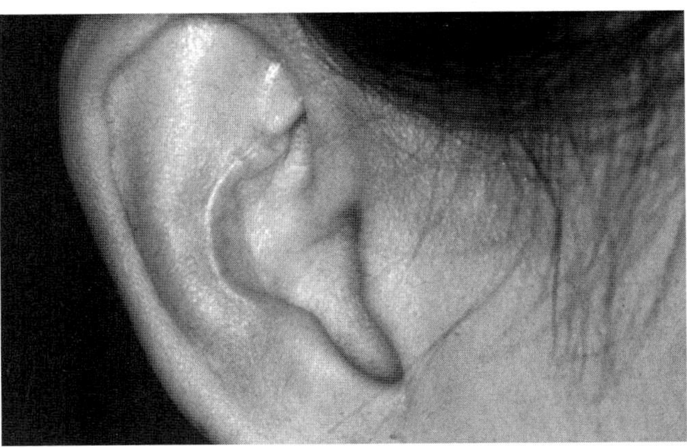
B

FIGURE 54-24. This patient had cartilage removed from the ear but was left with a flat ear **(A)**. The problem is prevented by leaving at least 6 mm of the part of the concha that is perpendicular to the head. If the concha is removed by way of an anterior incision, there is a small chance that the scar will be noticeable or hypertrophic **(B)**.

problems, may not be pleased by even the finest rhinoplasty result. Others simply have expectations that exceed the surgeon's abilities. McKinney and Cook (14) analyzed 200 patients and noted a greater dissatisfaction with postoperative results in female patients than in male patients. Patients in the fifth decade or older and patients not referred by another physician were more likely to be dissatisfied. On the other hand, numerous articles have been written about the difficult male rhinoplasty patient (15,16).

Prevention involves avoiding surgery in this type of patient. The diagram of Gorney (17) separates the most ideal from the least ideal patient. Those who have a minor deformity but a major complaint are at one end of the spectrum, whereas those with a major deformity but a minor complaint are at the other end. Careful preoperative consultation is the best way to detect this type of patient. At the very least, obtaining informed consent is imperative.

Sometimes, patients do not know what they really want. Figure 54-25 shows a female patient who requested a Caucasian-type nose. Drawings of her anticipated postoperative result were superimposed on preoperative photographs. The patient seemed satisfied with the drawings, and there appeared to be no problem with communication. At surgery (through an open technique), a cartilage graft was applied to the dorsum, the tip cartilages were narrowed, and lateral osteotomies were performed. In the early postoperative period, the patient was quite satisfied, but friends and family commented that she did not look as "black" as formerly. She asked that the cartilaginous graft be removed, which was done.

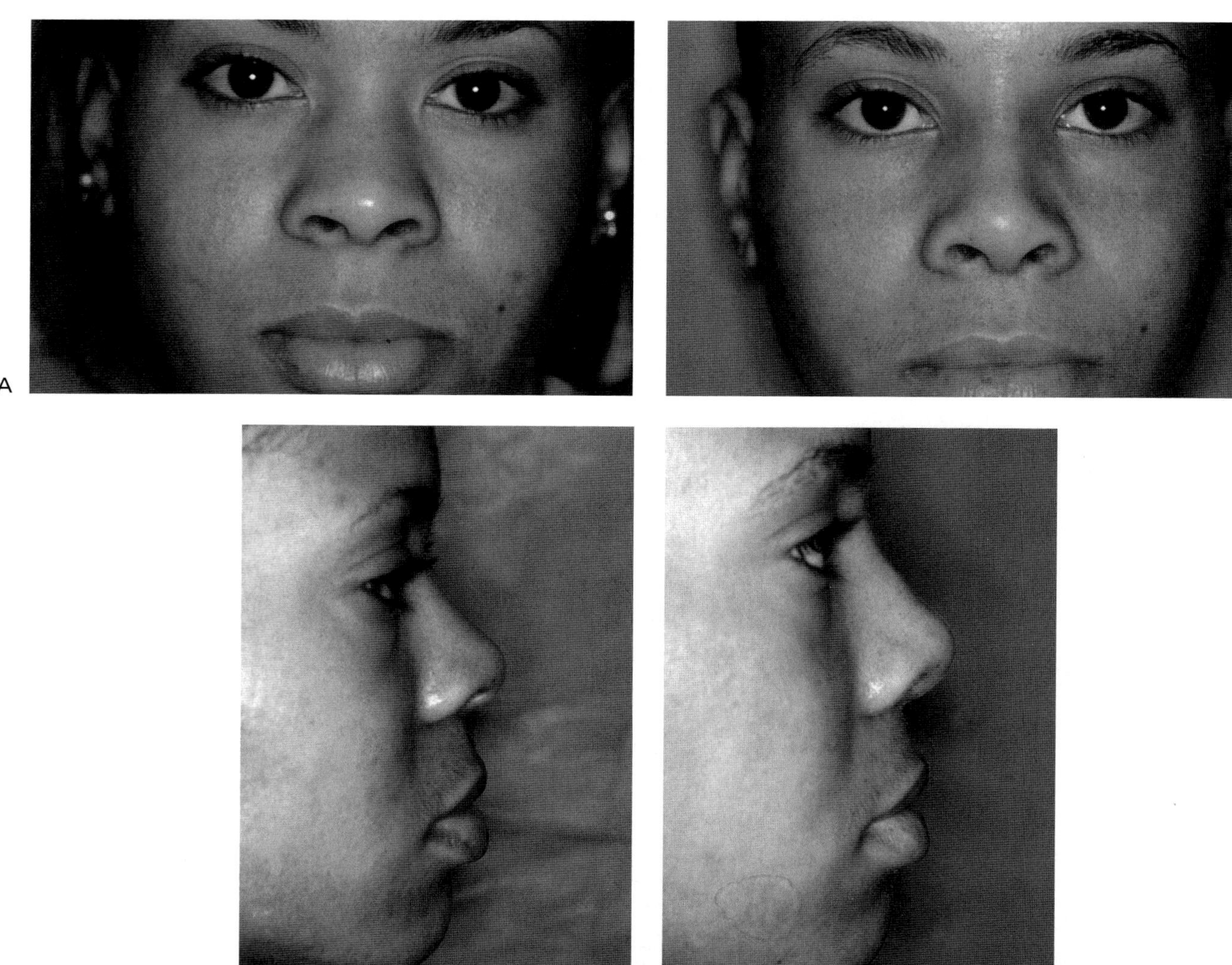

FIGURE 54-25. This patient wanted a more Caucasian nose. **A:** Frontal, preoperative. **B:** Frontal, postoperative. **C:** Lateral, preoperative. **D:** Lateral, postoperative. Alar base excision, radix/dorsal grafting, and dome narrowing with sutures were performed. (*continued*)

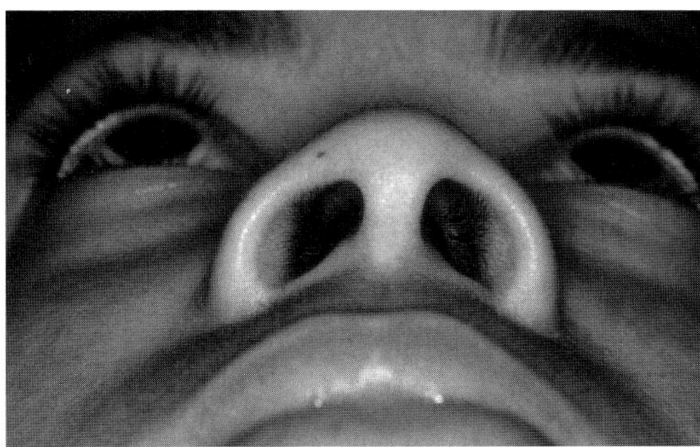
E

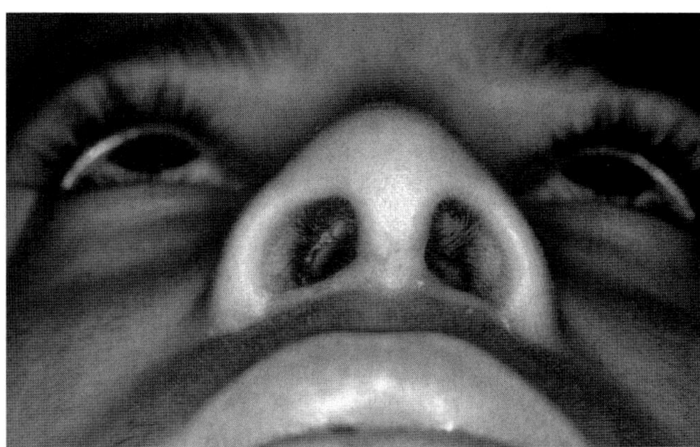
F

FIGURE 54-25. *Continued.* **E:** Basal, preoperative. **F:** Basal, postoperative. Postoperatively, the patient felt that she had lost some of her ethnic identity. As in this case, patients are not always sure of what they want.

Treating the difficult patient requires patience and tolerance. The patient's symptoms should not be dismissed and cannot be ignored because the patient may become hostile and litigious. The patient should be reassured that everything that can be done will be done to give the best result possible. This may mean a secondary procedure at the appropriate time. It also means obtaining a second opinion for the patient before it is requested. A second opinion from a colleague reassures the patient that everything possible is being done and often provides the surgeon with some alternatives that had not been considered.

Role of Video Imaging

The video imager is a tool that can both work for or against the plastic surgeon in detecting potential problems. It can work against the plastic surgeon if the imaged result is offered as an implied result. It can work for the plastic surgeon if it is used to demonstrate to the patient that "this is the best you should expect." We have occasionally encountered patients who did not like the imaged result, which indicated that they were not good candidates for cosmetic surgery. Without the video imager, it would not have been as easy to tell how perfectionistic these patients were.

True Psychological Problems and Body Dysmorphia Syndrome

A large group of patients have mild psychological problems and take or formerly took medications such as Prozac. The behavior of this group may be perfectly normal, and in fact they may be good candidates for aesthetic rhinoplasty.

Patients with true psychological problems are less frequent but pose a different and more significant problem. Some patients hope to relieve their depression by indulging in aesthetic surgery. Others are manic and have a temporary urge to undergo an aesthetic procedure. These patients are not good candidates for surgery. Finally, a small group of patients suffer from dysmorphia. The dysmorphic patient has the potential to hound the surgeon (physically, mentally, or both) whether or not the aesthetic result is satisfactory (18). The dysmorphic patient is invariably a poor candidate for surgery.

The problems associated with psychologically disturbed patients are prevented by making the diagnosis preoperatively, which is not always an easy task. Even after two consultations with a patient, it is not always possible to detect major psychological illness. If the patient happens to have a therapist, a discussion with that person is very helpful. The therapist can suggest whether or not surgery is contraindicated. If a significant psychological disorder is diagnosed after the surgery has been performed, a psychiatrist or therapist should be involved.

ARCHITECTURAL AND ANATOMIC PROBLEMS

Crooked Nose

Unrecognized Crooked Septum

After a primary rhinoplasty, a crooked nose will sometimes be revealed that was not apparent preoperatively. A deviation of the dorsal septum can be camouflaged by a large dorsal hump or lower lateral cartilages, and sometimes the septum is inadvertently scored or malpositioned during submucous resection. The patient in Fig. 54-26 underwent

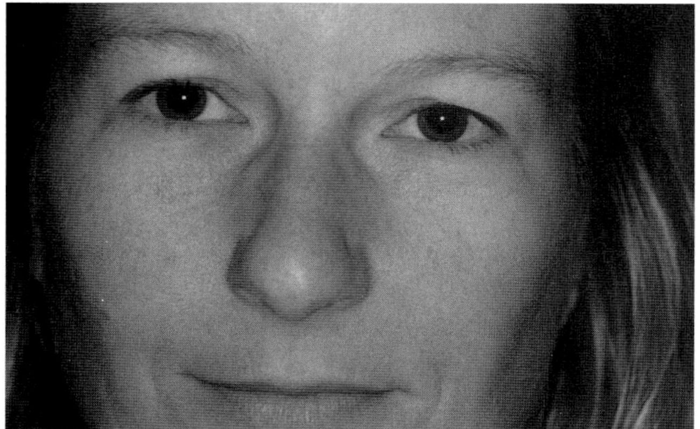

A

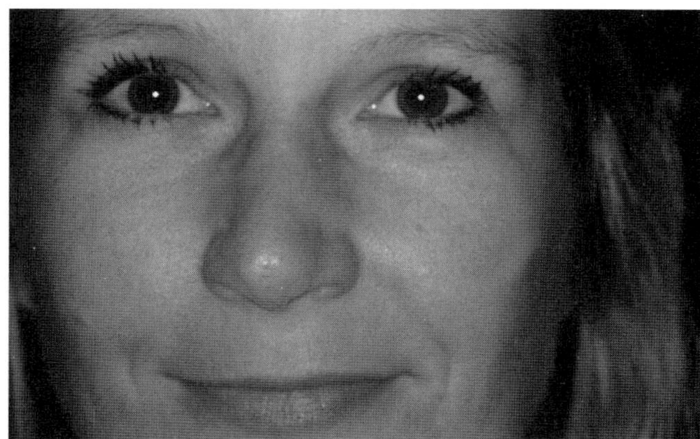

B

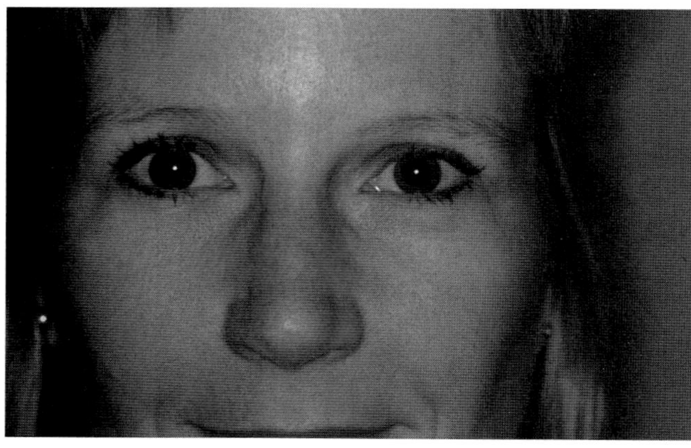

C

FIGURE 54-26. This patient had a broad nose and tip **(A)**. After a rhinoplasty was performed, a crooked nose became apparent **(B)** that had not been noticed preoperatively because it was hidden by the hump. A secondary open approach was used to straighten the nose **(C)**.

a primary rhinoplasty. The slight deviation of the nose to the right side was not readily apparent preoperatively because it was camouflaged by the overall increased width of the nose. However, following rhinoplasty, when the nose was thinned, the deviation was more apparent.

The potential for this complication should be recognized if it is to be prevented. The septum should be straightened intraoperatively, or the dorsal septum should be camouflaged with cartilage. Correction at the time of surgery is easier with the open approach because the direction of the dorsal septum is so easy to see—particularly from the head of the operating table. In this case, prevention was not undertaken. Treatment involved a return to surgery 6 months later to correct the crooked septum. After elevation of the mucoperichondrium bilaterally, the septum was scored vertically on the concave side and released from the vomerine ridge, which allowed it to swing back toward the midline. To secure the septum in the midline position, a suture was passed from the buccal sulcus to the caudal septum and back to the buccal sulcus.

"Recurrent" Crooked Nose

After a crooked nose has been corrected, "recurrence" is sometimes seen. This may be caused by continuous warping of the septal cartilage with time, or other factors may be responsible. It is quite possible that the nose was never straightened completely at the primary procedure. Even if the septum is scored and released fully from the vomerine ridge, such that it now acts like a hinged door, minor retained forces in the cartilage can cause the septum to return to its original position. In addition, malpositioned upper lateral cartilages may force the septum to one side or the other by impinging on its dorsal aspect.

If these problems are detected at the time of the original procedure, the "recurrent" crooked nose can be prevented. The caudal septum can be sutured to the anterior nasal spine or secured to the frenulum, as described above. A batten graft or spreader graft can be attached on one side of the septum. Alternatively, the medial aspect of the upper lateral cartilage can be trimmed where it is impinging on the dorsal septum. As always, the open approach makes it much easier to executive these maneuvers.

Dorsal Problems

Open Roof Deformity

The dorsum is a seemingly mundane part of the nose in comparison with the more complex tip. Nevertheless, numerous potential problems occur there. In the open roof deformity (Fig. 54-27), a gap is visible between the lateral

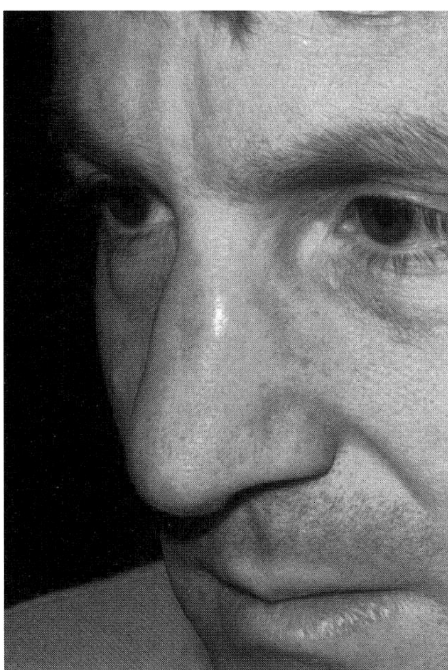

FIGURE 54-27. This patient has an open roof deformity. At the time the hump was removed, an osteotomy was not performed.

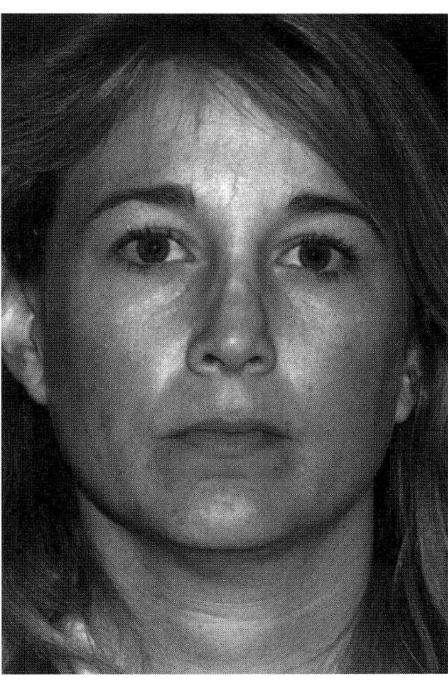

FIGURE 54-28. This patient with thin nasal skin exhibits surface irregularities resulting from dorsal grafts. The open approach has the distinct advantage of avoiding this problem because much of the dorsum and radix can be visualized to note any potential cartilage irregularities.

nasal bones, and the dorsum appears to have a flat top. It is usually caused by a failure to bring the nasal bone sidewalls together. Small open roofs may fill with scar tissue and not be noticeable. Larger ones may not.

Prevention involves ascertaining the size of the open roof at the time of rhinoplasty and deciding if the roof is large enough to warrant closure. The open approach makes it much easier to appreciate the magnitude of the open roof deformity at the time of rhinoplasty because the gap can be visualized. Closure usually involves a lateral and possibly a medial osteotomy. It may sometimes be possible to apply autogenous material (cartilage in the grooves) or a dorsal graft to cover the roof. The open approach also makes it easy to see after a lateral osteotomy has been performed whether the nasal bones have truly migrated medially to close the roof or whether they are failing to close the roof completely because a piece of upper lateral cartilage is obstructing the closure. If the open roof appears postoperatively, a later correction will of necessity involve any of the above maneuvers.

Surface Irregularities

Surface irregularities (Fig. 54-28) are a common problem with both the closed and open approaches. When a graft is applied to the dorsum, radix, or tip, part of the graft may be visible through the skin, particularly if the skin is thin. When small pieces of cartilage grafts are applied to the nose to supplement the larger grafts, they may also cause surface irregularities, particularly where the skin is thin, such as in the radix. Surface irregularities are more likely to occur when small pieces of ear cartilage are used, as opposed to septal cartilage. Although they may feel smooth beneath the skin during surgery, when local anesthesia is distending the skin, small cartilage grafts may feel quite irregular later when healing is complete. The grafts also have the potential to migrate.

Prevention requires good sculpting and immobilization of the grafts with sutures when possible. Providing an exact pocket for the graft is another means of preventing the problem—a task that can be more formidable than good sculpting. Although surface irregularities do occur in the open approach, they are less frequent, simply because one can visualize the architectural framework before the skin is redraped. The treatment of surface irregularities involves either (a) removal of the irregularity by rasping or excising it; (b) removing, reshaping, and replacing the cartilage; or (c) replacing the irregular cartilage with soft tissue, such as dermis.

Inverted V Deformity

The inverted V deformity (Fig. 54-29) is caused by a collapse of the upper lateral cartilage with obliteration of the internal nasal valve. This is more likely to occur in the patient with short nasal bones after a hump reduction. Prevention involves spreader grafts of cartilage between the upper lateral cartilage and the dorsal septum. These grafts not only prevent an aesthetic deformity but also can improve the airway dramatically.

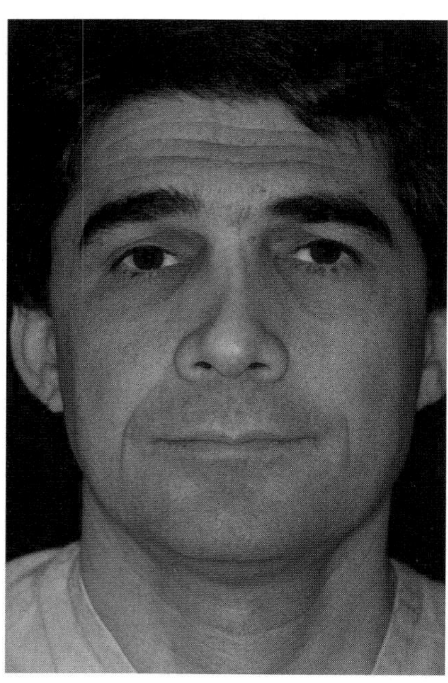

FIGURE 54-29. This patient exhibits an inverted V deformity.

Another method to prevent the inverted V deformity is to develop a "spreader flap" (Fig. 54-30). The upper lateral cartilage is utilized rather than discarded with the hump (Oneal, personal communication). The entire cartilaginous hump is not removed; instead, the upper lateral cartilages are separated away from the septum. Only the hump of the septum is removed. The dorsal edge of the upper lateral cartilage is scored and folded on itself. A small amount of mucoperichondrium is elevated off the dorsal edge of the septum to allow the spreader flap to sit flush up against the dorsal edge of the septum. The width of the spreader flap can be adjusted with absorbable sutures, and it can be sutured directly to the dorsal septum as needed.

If the inverted V deformity is not recognized at the time of surgery, treatment involves the use of spreader grafts, much as has been described above. As in other aspects of rhinoplasty, the open approach has the distinct advantage of allowing visualization of the dorsum and enabling the precise placement of spreader grafts with a corresponding adjustment in the width of the dorsum.

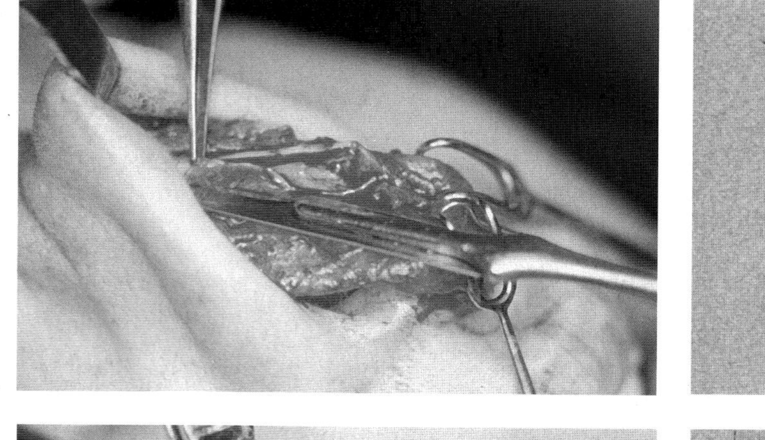

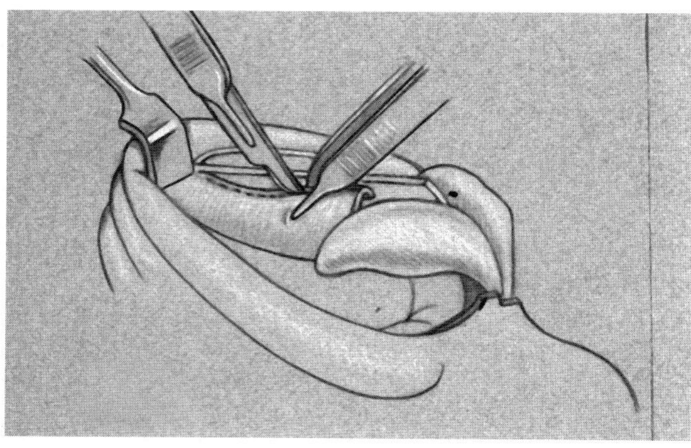

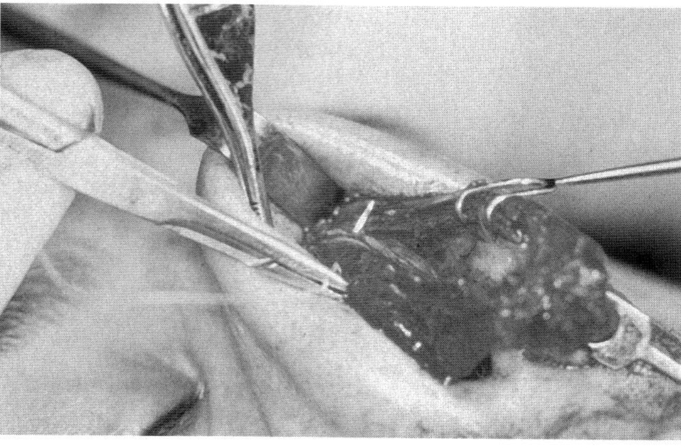

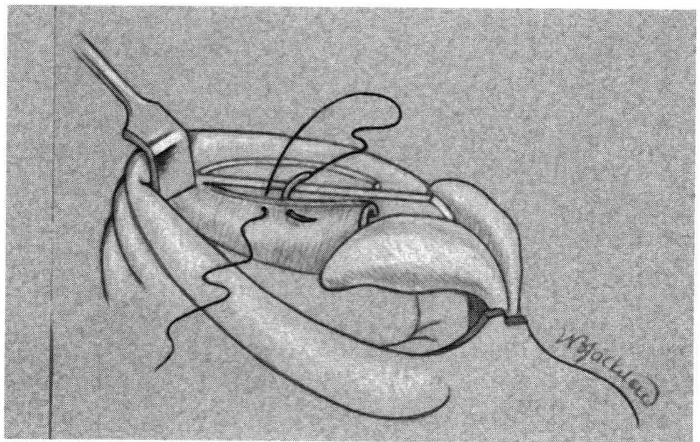

FIGURE 54-30. The inverted V deformity can be prevented by the use of a spreader flap. The upper lateral cartilage is separated away from the septum, and the septal hump is trimmed. The cephalic edge of the upper lateral cartilage is scored **(A,B)**, folded on itself, sutured **(C,D)**, and set against the dorsal edge of the septum. **A,C:** Intraoperative. **B,D:** Schematic.

Supratip Deformity (Polly Beak)

A true "polly beak" deformity is not seen very often nowadays (Fig. 54-31). This is a very pronounced dorsal convex fullness in the supratip area. It is usually caused by overresection of cartilage (dorsal septum, dome, or lower lateral cartilages), after which the skin in the area contracts into a sphere of scar tissue. It is more likely to occur in a reduction rhinoplasty because the skin may not be able to accommodate the smaller anatomical framework. The pathologic mechanics, prevention, and treatment of this problem have been nicely outlined by Sheen (19). As he points out, prevention is a matter of avoiding the tendency to overresect the nasal cartilages in an attempt to make them smaller. The nasal skin requires a substantial framework beneath it—one that prevents the skin from contracting into a polly beak. The width of the lower lateral cartilages should be at least

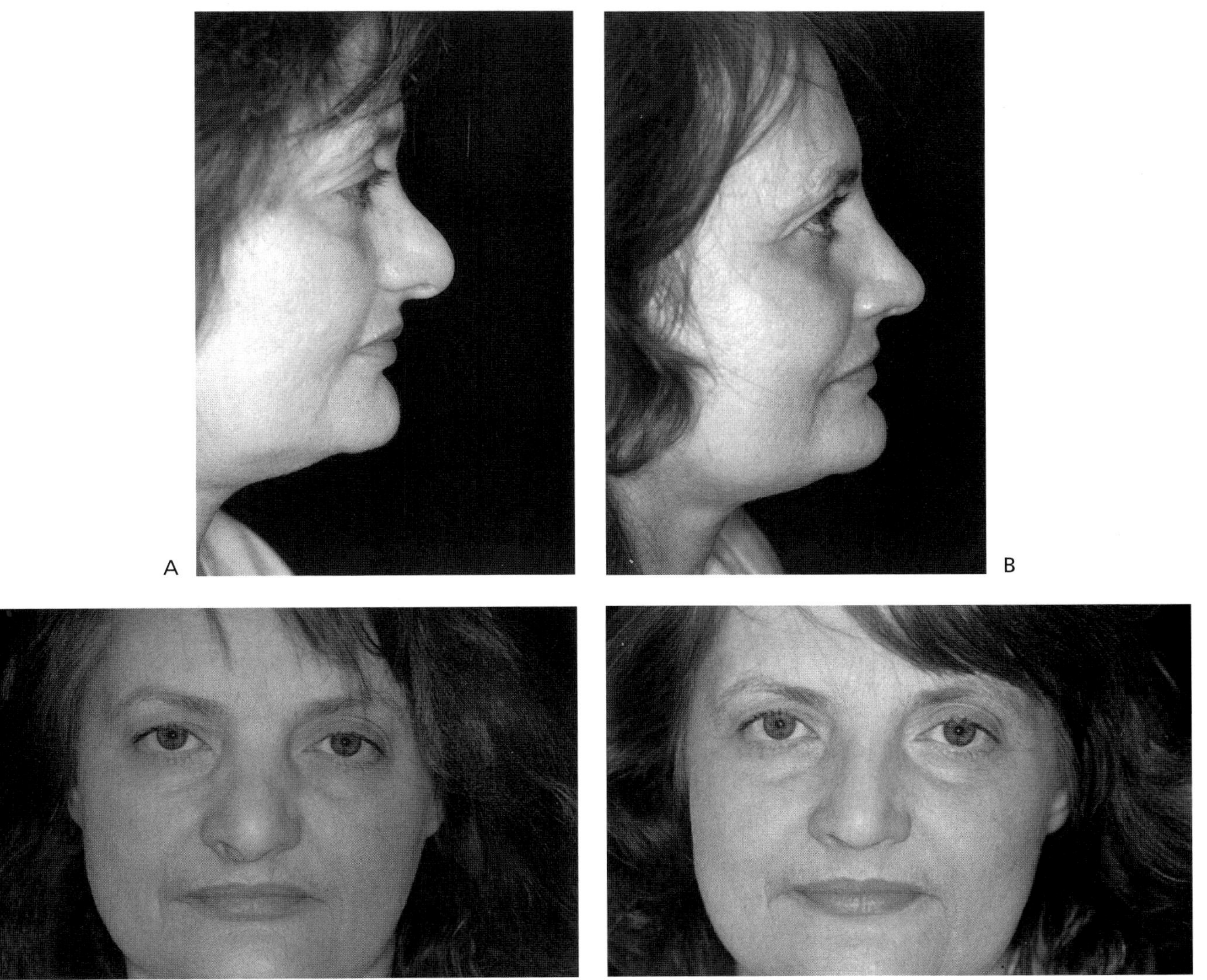

FIGURE 54-31. This patient has a polly beak deformity. Too much cartilaginous tissue was removed from the tip cartilages. **A:** Lateral, preoperatively, **B:** Lateral, 15 months postoperatively. **C:** Frontal, preoperatively. **D:** Frontal, 15 months postoperatively. She also has a radix deficiency. In an open approach, the dorsum was reconstructed with cartilage grafts. *(continued)*

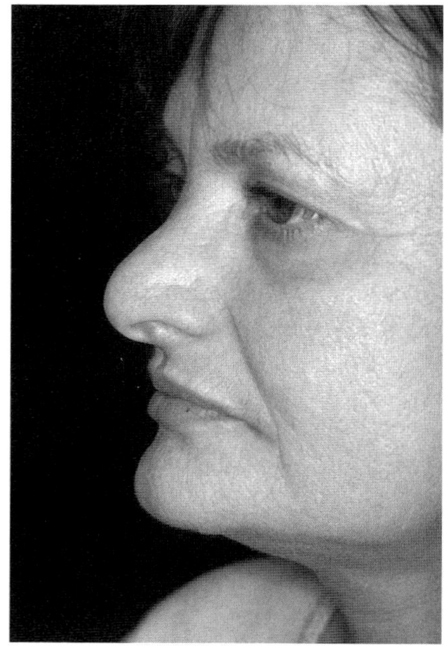
E

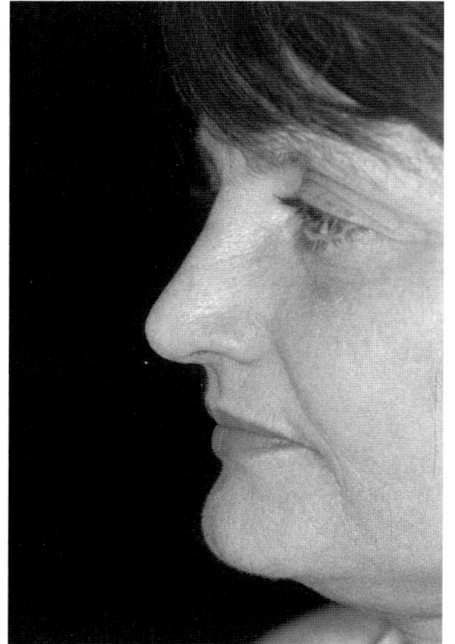
F

FIGURE 54-31. *Continued.* **E:** Oblique, preoperatively. **F:** Oblique, 15 months postoperatively.

5 mm if possible. The tip cartilages need not be more than 6 to 8 mm above the dorsal septum to accommodate the skin thickness in this region. It is generally a good idea in reduction rhinoplasty to keep the nose on the large side of what is normal or aesthetic. By minimizing the extent of reduction, problems of skin accommodation, such as the polly beak, are reduced.

When a nose is treated that already has a full supratip, further resection of the tissues is usually contraindicated. Instead, cartilaginous material in the form of grafts is required to provide a framework on which the skin can drape. The patient in Fig. 54-31 underwent correction by the open approach. She received (a) sutures to reshape and strengthen the dome, (b) a radix graft, (c) a small trim of the distal dorsal septum, and (d) a tip graft.

Alar Collapse

Alar collapse, which occurs particularly during inspiration, is caused by a loss of the architectural shape or integrity of the lower lateral cartilages and dome area. The problem, which is both functional and aesthetic, is prevented by not overresecting the cephalic aspect of the lower lateral cartilage. In an attempt to make the nose thinner, the surgeon is naturally tempted to remove more and more of the lower lateral cartilage. When too much cartilage is removed, collapse is inevitable. As a general rule, it is best to leave a 4- to 5-mm width to the lower lateral cartilage and a 4- to 5-mm width to the dome. With the open approach, it is easy to see the lower lateral cartilage and tip cartilages and so avoid this complication. If the closed approach is used, the cartilage delivery technique (with a "rim" incision) helps the surgeon visualize the cartilages before they are sculpted.

The techniques for management are reviewed elsewhere. One of the best treatments involves the use of cartilage struts deep to the lower lateral cartilage to restore the integrity of that structure (20). The patient in Fig. 54-32, with alar collapse, was treated with cartilage struts to the lower lateral cartilage area and also a spreader graft to strengthen and maintain the proper distance between the tip cartilages.

Complications of Osteotomy

Collapse of the Nasal Bone

Osteotomies are a potential source of several complications. The most significant one is complete collapse of one or both nasal bones (Fig. 54-33). This is caused in part by a disruption of the periosteal attachments on the deep side of the nasal bones, which ordinarily help hold the nasal bones in place, and in part by the absence of bony attachments to the adjacent maxilla or frontal bone, which leaves an island of nasal bone devoid of support.

The nasal bone normally falls medially whenever a lateral osteotomy is made. It falls still further medially and may even collapse if multiple attempts are made to fracture the bone. Each blow of the hammer has the potential to rupture the attachments and force the nasal bone medially. A dull osteotome makes multiple blows necessary. Also, overly wide osteotomes are more likely to disrupt periosteal attachments.

Prevention involves a careful, decisive, and preferably

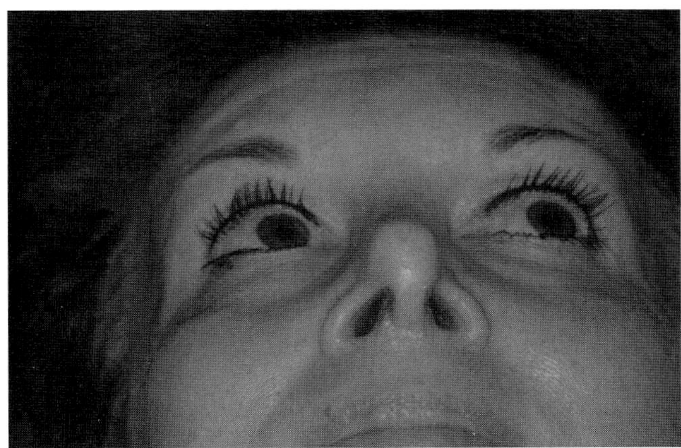

A

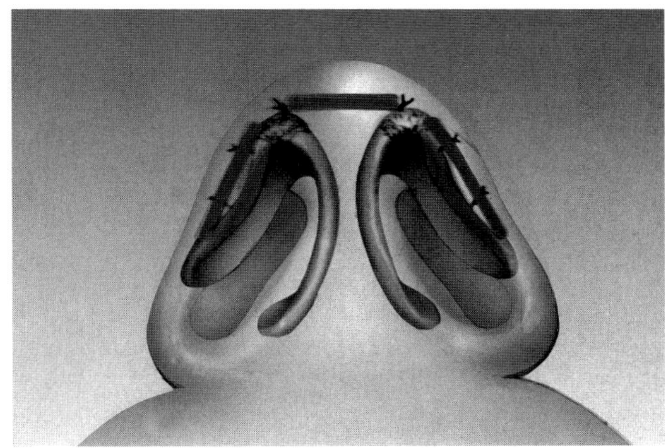

B

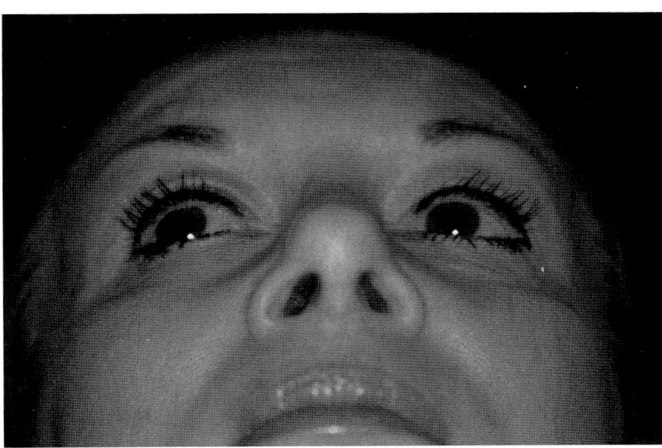

C

FIGURE 54-32. Alar collapse developed in this patient because too much cartilage from the lateral crura was removed **(A)**. At surgery, struts of cartilage graft were used to reinforce the straightness and strength of the lateral crura. In addition, a spreader graft was used to maintain the normal separation between the tip cartilages **(B)**. Postoperatively, alar collapse is no longer seen **(C)**.

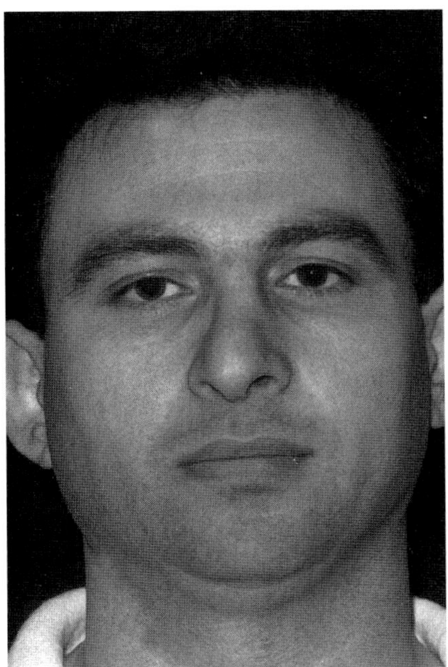

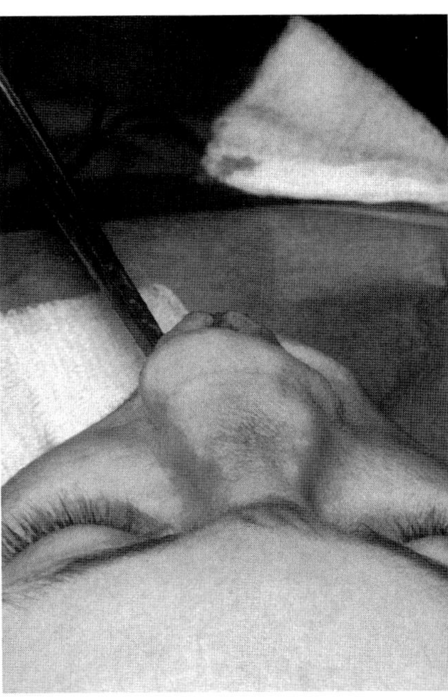

A,B

FIGURE 54-33. This patient exhibits collapse of the right nasal bone **(A)**. Prevention is facilitated by performing both a medial and lateral osteotomy. The nasal bone is first out-fractured to obtain a greenstick effect **(B)**. Then the nasal bone is manually and gently moved medially.

single cut of the bone made by driving an osteotome from the pyriform fossa up to the root of the nasal bone. A medial osteotomy and out-fracturing of the nasal bone (Fig. 54-33) are ways to avoid collapse with a lateral osteotomy. A medial osteotomy is made first, followed by a lateral osteotomy. The nasal bone is then out-fractured (not in-fractured) with the aid of an osteotome. Almost always, the nasal bone will greenstick into an abducted position. At this point, the finger or thumb is used gently to move the nasal bone medially until it reaches the desired position.

Damage to the underlying periosteum (and collapse of the bone) is also less likely if a lateral nasal osteotomy is performed via an external skin approach, in which a very small osteotome is used to perform multiple fractures along the course of the nasal bone. This is an excellent technique but in our opinion makes it more difficult to manipulate the slant of the nasal bone.

If collapse has occurred and is noted at surgery, an osteotome is used to manipulate the lateral nasal bone (provided it is still one fragment) until its posterior edge overlaps the medial edge of the maxilla. If collapse is a late postoperative finding, correction is easiest with onlay grafts of cartilage. Refracturing the bone and trying to get it to remain in a more lateral position is extremely difficult, even when the nose is packed postoperatively.

Stair-step Deformity

A stair-step deformity is another potential problem following osteotomy. It develops when a lateral osteotomy is not flush (not sufficiently posterior) with the maxilla. This problem can be prevented by making a concerted effort to keep the osteotome flush with the maxilla at the level of the pyriform fossa when the osteotomy is performed. One should keep in mind, however, that these low-to-low and low-to-high osteotomies do move the inferior turbinate medially and have the potential to obstruct the airway partially (21). If the stair-step deformity is noted at the time of surgery, the osteotomy is simply repeated at a more posterior level (Rudolph Meyer, personal communication). A late stair-step deformity is treated more easily by applying a cartilage graft to the area of depression rather than by trying to perform an osteotomy and reset the bone.

Saddle Nose Deformity

One of the classic anatomical complications is saddle nose deformity (22) (Fig. 54-34). If this is not recognized at the time of surgery, or if the structural integrity of the septum fails postoperatively, then a depression of the nose will be quite evident. The cause of the problem is usually overresection of the septum, which leads to a loss of integrity of the septum and eventual collapse. The deformity can also occur without significant septal resection if the cartilaginous septum is separated from the vomer. If the septum is contoured to an L-shaped strut, a collapse may occur if the attachment of the vertical component of the L-shaped strut to the area of the anterior nasal spine is lost.

Prevention is aimed first toward identifying the problem. In the closed approach, it is a good idea simply to press on the dorsal nose to see if the integrity of the septum is sufficient (Fig. 54-35). Prevention is also aimed at cautious and conservative resection of the septum. When a central resection of the septum is performed and an L-shaped structure is left, care must be taken to leave a width of at least 1 to 1.5 cm for the vertical and horizontal components of the L-shaped septum that remains. *Prevention of the saddle nose deformity is facilitated by the open approach because the septum is sculpted under direct vision.*

If the problem is discovered at surgery, the open approach allows a relatively easy correction. After the skin of the dorsum is retracted, the mucoperichondrium of both sides of the septum is elevated (if it has not already been elevated for the septal surgery). The entire dorsal septum is inspected (Fig. 54-35), including the junction of the dorsal cartilaginous septum with the bony septum. Direct repair

A

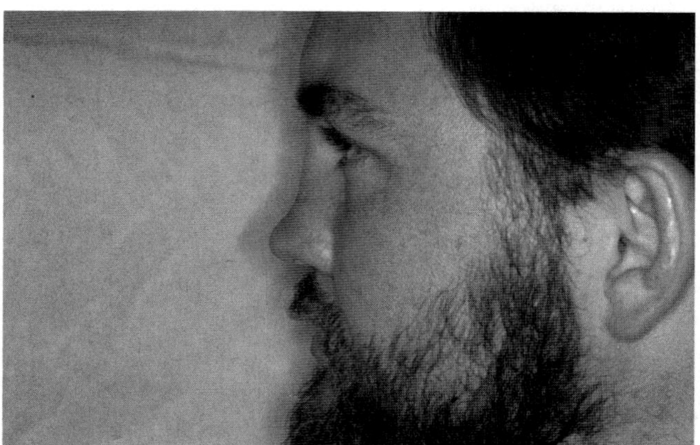

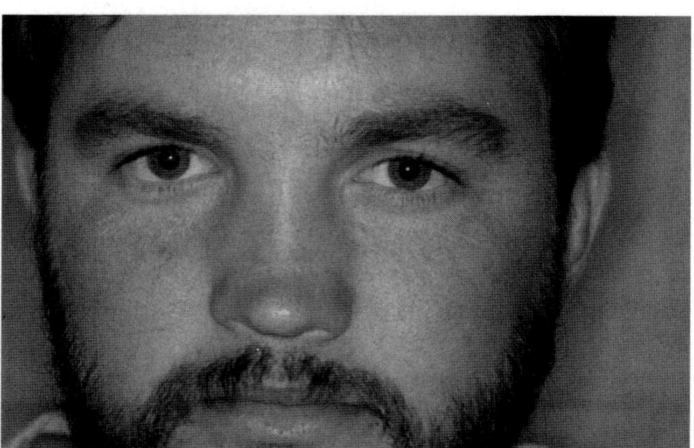

B

FIGURE 54-34. This patient has a saddle nose deformity. The integrity and strength of the cartilaginous septum were lost at the initial rhinoplasty. **A:** Lateral. **B:** Frontal.

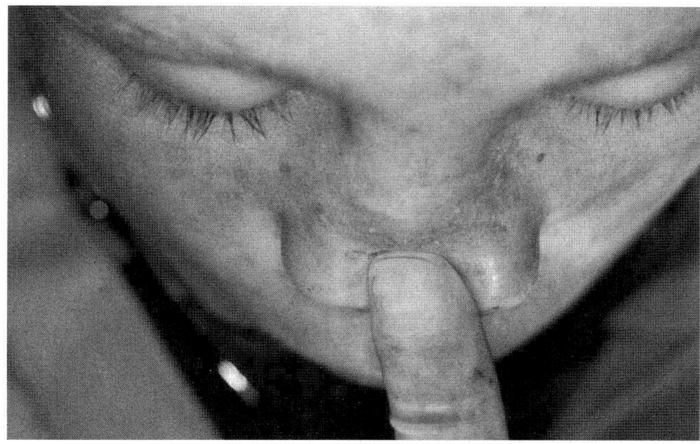

A

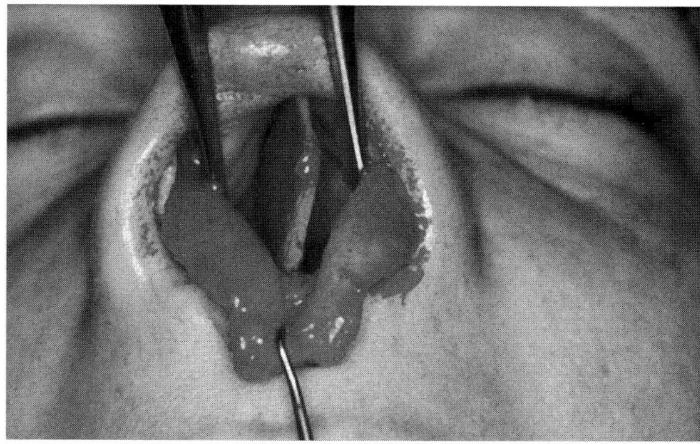

B

FIGURE 54-35. In the closed approach, the integrity and strength of the septum are not always apparent because it cannot be visualized. By manually pressing on the dorsum, however, the integrity is readily verified **(A)**. In the open approach, structural deficiencies of the dorsal septum and its attachment to the bony septum are readily corrected with sutures **(B)**.

with 4-0 nylon sutures restores the integrity of the junction if that in fact is the cause of the saddle nose problem.

If the problem is a collapse of the vertical component of the L-shaped septum following septoplasty, direct exposure of the vertical component is obtained by elevating the mucoperichondrium from both sides of the septum. Reinforcing the septum with cartilage batten grafts and anchoring the caudal septum to the anterior nasal spine area via the buccal sulcus will stabilize the vertical component. Late treatment involves a cartilage graft to the dorsum, and possibly a reconstruction of the horizontal or vertical component of the L-shaped strut of the septum with cartilage grafts.

Overresection of the Alar Base

Overresection of the alar base causes potential problems of inspiratory obstruction and also aesthetic problems. Figure 54-36 shows a patient whose alar base was overresected. The result was vestibular stenosis and a severe aesthetic deformity. Prevention of the problem begins by determining whether the patient has a small external airway. By inserting a small finger into the vestibule, some idea of the size of the airways can be easily appreciated.

If the patient has a small vestibule, the wedge of tissue to be removed should include only the alar skin, not skin from within the vestibule (Fig. 54-37). More often than not, patients do not require an actual reduction of the perimeter of the vestibule. Furthermore, it is seldom necessary to take more than 3 to 4 mm of the ala. By using an Adson-Brown forceps to grasp the wedge of ala to be excised and excising a wedge of tissue that is not much wider than the forceps itself, one can avoid overresection of the ala.

Another way to prevent the problem of stenosis and overresection of the ala is simply not to resect it. The broad nasal base of certain patients is better treated by reducing the in-

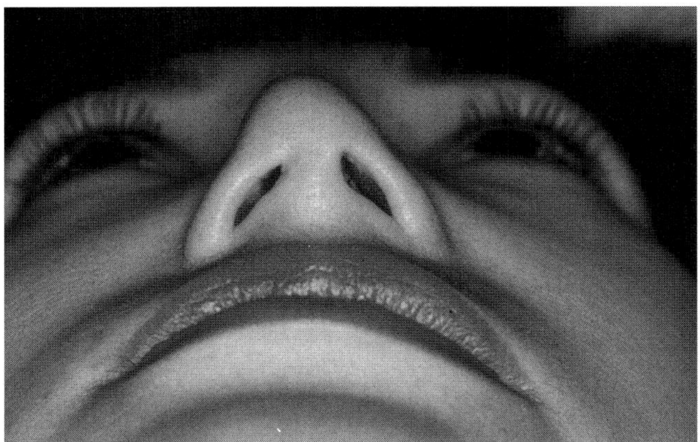

A

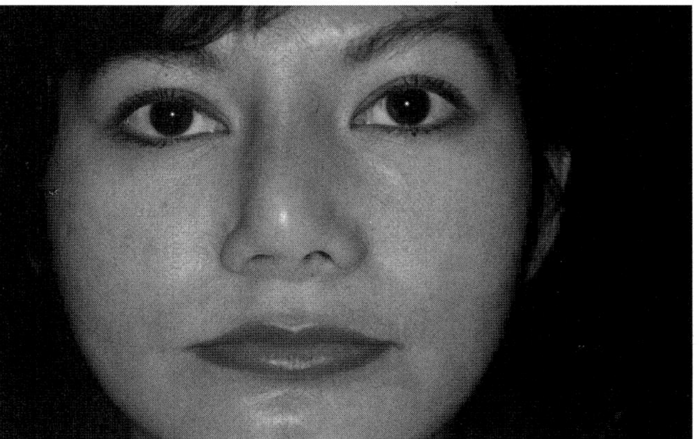

B

FIGURE 54-36. This patient illustrates overresection of the alar base, which created an aesthetic problem in addition to nostril stenosis. **A:** Basal. **B:** Frontal. In general, the width of the excision need not exceed the width of an Adson-Brown forceps.

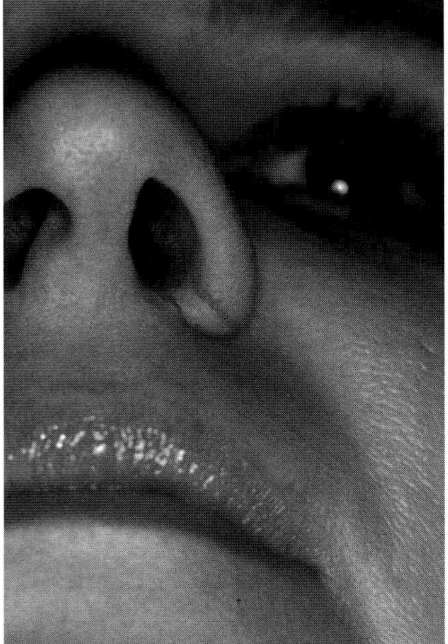
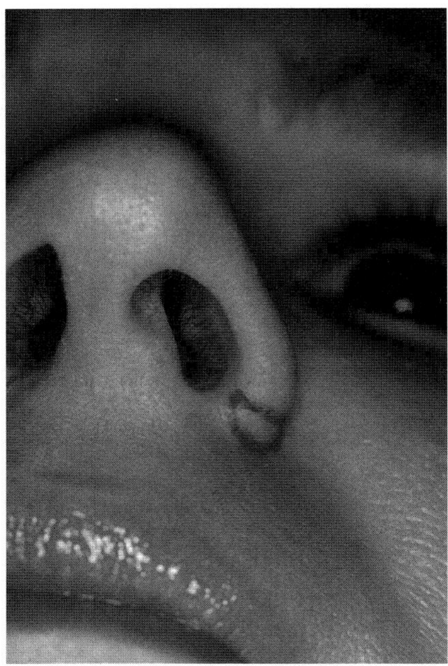

FIGURE 54-37. The alar base excision may extend into the vestibule **(A)**. However, when alar base skin is removed, a decision must be made as to whether the skin within the vestibule should be removed. If not, the excision need not extend into the vestibule **(B)**.

teralar distance. This involves undermining a tunnel between two incisions at the alar base, undermining the tissues, and relying on strong permanent sutures to narrow the interalar distance (23).

Overresection is best managed with an island flap as designed by Constantian (24). In essence, a small island of tissue is developed immediately adjacent to the ala and transferred into a surgically created gap between the ala and the nostril sill. Composite grafts have been used but have a tendency to contract and cause a problem of color mismatch.

RARE COMPLICATIONS

Obstruction of the Lacrimal Duct

Obstruction of the lacrimal duct is usually an early but can be a late complication of nasal surgery. If one looks carefully, many patients exhibit some lacrimal duct obstruction. In most cases, it is temporary and disappears. Occasionally, however, persistent swelling develops in the corner of the eye, sometimes with infection. The origin of the problem is usually the lateral osteotomy, which damages the lacrimal sac and drainage system. In these cases, patients exhibit all the signs and symptoms of a dacryocystitis that requires immediate treatment with antibiotics. Prevention is a matter of careful osteotome positioning. Once the infection is controlled, usually no further treatment is needed, and the lacrimal drainage returns to normal.

Intracranial Complications

Very rarely, intracranial complications develop early after rhinoplasty (25). These include pneumocephalus, cerebrospinal fluid rhinorrhea (26), meningitis, cerebritis, and cavernous sinus thrombosis. Infection can reach the brain through the ophthalmic veins, the bloodstream, or an iatrogenic fracture that extends to the cribriform plate or the anterior cranial fossa. Pneumocephalus (with or without cerebrospinal fluid rhinorrhea) is usually seen in patients with previous nasal trauma. An even rarer problem is penetration by the osteotome. Hematoma or direct injury to the optic chiasm can result in blindness.

Nasal Cysts

Rarely, benign growths in and around the nose may be seen. For example, mucocysts can form either at the dorsum of the nose or in the area along the lateral nasal bone (Fig. 54-38). The cause of this problem is invagination of the mucous membrane, which then forms a cystlike structure. The patient complains of a persistent swelling and sometimes redness. Magnetic resonance imaging helps to make the diagnosis. This problem in the area of dorsal resection is best prevented by resecting the exposed mucoperichondrium carefully so as not to leave a large residual that might fall into the subcutaneous space. The open approach facilitates this type of inspection. In the region of the lateral osteotomy, however,

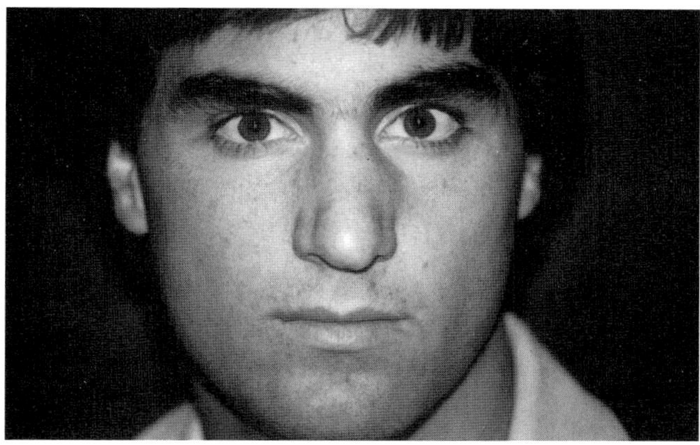

FIGURE 54-38. This patient has a nasal cyst in the lateral aspect of the nose, caused by an invagination of mucous membrane. When persistent isolated swelling is seen in the area of the lateral osteotomy, even along the dorsum, this diagnosis should be suspected.

A

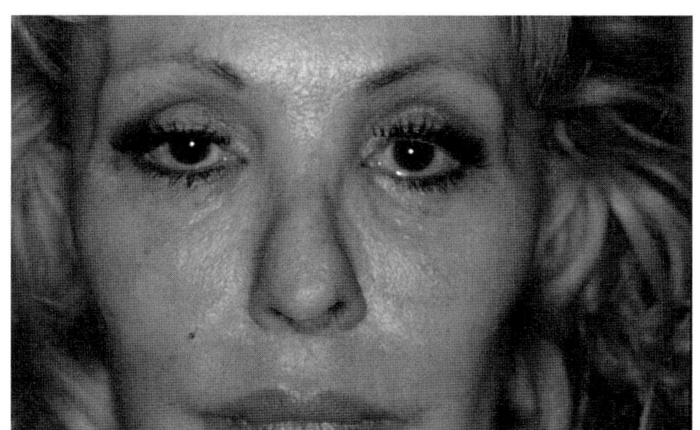

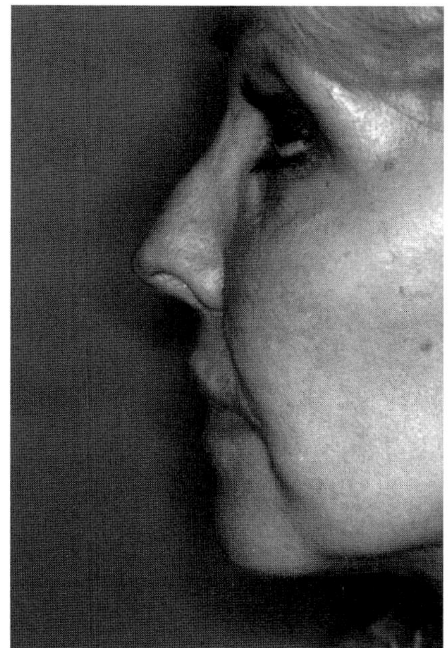

B

C

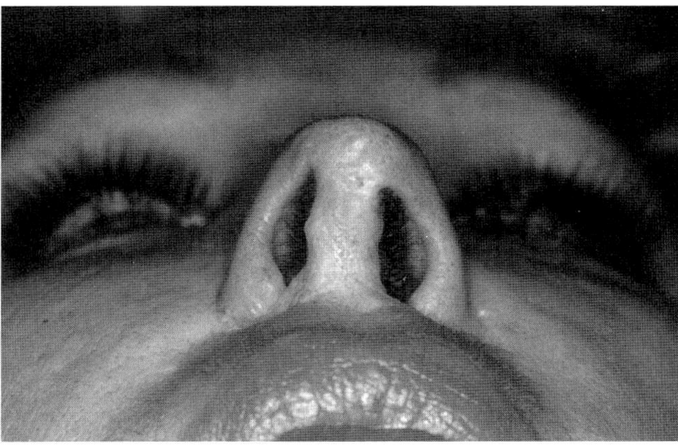

FIGURE 54-39. This patient underwent multiple operations and has a crippled nose. The skin is badly damaged, with irregularities everywhere, including the vestibular rims. **A:** Frontal. **B:** Lateral. **C:** Basal. Further surgery is likely to be futile.

there is not good way to avoid this problem. Treatment involves the use of antibiotics if the cyst is inflamed. Frequently, a surgical resection of the cyst is necessary.

Painful Nose

Although it is infrequent, pain in the nose can be one of the most disabling complications of a rhinoplasty. The mechanism is unclear, but pain is most likely to occur in patients with neurologic or psychological problems and who may also have an altered pain threshold. Physical examination usually reveals nothing wrong, and yet the patient has persistent pain. Prevention is best accomplished by eliciting a history of psychological and neurologic problems, such as trigeminal neuralgia. Treatment is similar to that for other types of pain disorders.

Crippled Nose

Each time the patient is returned to the operating room to improve the nose, the chances for success decrease. The complication rate increases because the skin no longer adapts to the underlying cartilaginous and bony framework and because scar tissue and edema (which may be worse than after the first surgery) mask the underlying anatomical structure. The patient in Fig. 54-39 underwent multiple operations to improve her appearance. Because of her unrealistic expectations and demands, and because multiple surgeons were willing to try to help her, she ended up with a permanently deformed nose. The overlying skin is atrophic and irregular, and the deformities are numerous. At this point, it becomes difficult to do anything for this patient because the skin itself is no longer resilient and will not conform well to further changes in the cartilaginous framework.

Preventing a crippled nose is contingent on the surgeon's refusal to perform further surgery when risk begins to outweigh possible gain. Multiple surgeries performed too close together may also increase the likelihood of a crippled nose. If surgery is undertaken to make some improvement, an open approach should probably not be used in this type of patient because the skin is not adequate for the operation. If anything at all is done, it must be very minor, with the understanding that only minor improvement should be anticipated. Unfortunately, no truly satisfactory surgical treatment is possible for most of these patients.

CONCLUSION

The pertinent complications and unfavorable results following aesthetic rhinoplasty have been reviewed in detail, with special emphasis on the complications germane to the open rhinoplasty technique. The problems associated with the various phases of the rhinoplasty procedure have been considered, including (a) preoperative problems; (b) intraoperative problems, such as hypertension; (c) early postoperative problems, such as hematoma and necrosis; (d) late postoperative problems, such as columellar scarring; (e) architectural and anatomical problems, such as saddle nose deformity, nasal bone collapse, and polly beak deformity; and (f) rare complications, such as intracranial infection and blindness. Ways to prevent and treat these problems have been discussed.

REFERENCES

1. Parks ML, Borowiecki B, Binder W. Functional sequelae of rhinoplasty. *Ann Plast Surg* 1980;4:116–120.
2. Peck GC, ed. *Complications and problems in aesthetic surgery.* New York: Gower, 1992.
3. Teichgraeber JF, Russo RC. *Treatment of nasal surgery complications.* Ann Plast Surg 1993;30:80–88.
4. Marten TJ. Physician-administered office anesthesia. *Clin Plast Surg* 1991;18:877–889.
5. Bryant WM. Ketamine anesthesia and intranasal or intraoral operations. A potentially dangerous combination. *Plast Reconstr Surg* 1973;51:562–564.
6. Goldwyn RM. Unexpected bleeding after elective nasal surgery. *Ann Plast Surg* 1979;2:201–204.
7. Teichgraeber JF, Riley WB, Parks DH. Nasal surgery complications. *Plast Reconstr Surg* 1990;85:527–531.
8. Tobin G, Shaw RC, Goodpasture HZ. Toxic shock syndrome following breast and nasal surgery. *Plast Reconstr Surg* 1987; 80:111–114.
9. Rohrich RJ, Gunter JP, Friedman RM. Nasal tip blood supply: an anatomic study validating the safety of the transcolumellar incision in rhinoplasty. *Plast Reconstr Surg* 1995;95:795–799.
10. Daniel RK. Secondary rhinoplasty following open rhinoplasty. *Plast Reconstr Surg* 1995;96:1539–1546.
11. Shirakabe Y, Shirakabe T, Kishimoto T. The classification of complications after augmentation rhinoplasty. *Aesthetic Plast Surg* 1985;9:185–192.
12. Daniel RK. The Gore-Texed patient. *Plast Reconstr Surg* 1995;95:1336.
13. Sheen, JH. Rhinoplasty complication following the use of banked homologous cartilage. *Perspect Plast Surg* 1990;16:163–166.
14. McKinney P, Cook JQ. A critical evaluation of 200 rhinoplasties. *Ann Plast Surg* 1981;7:357–361.
15. Aiach G. Male aesthetic surgery. In: Marchac D, Granick MS, Solomon MP, eds. *Male aesthetic surgery.* Boston: Butterworth-Heineman, 1996:171–197.
16. Gruber RP. Male rhinoplasty. *Aesthetic Plast Surg* 1994; 18:12–15.
17. Gorney M. Patient selection in rhinoplasty: practical guidelines. In: Daniel RK, ed. *Rhinoplasty.* Boston: Little, Brown and Company, 1993:71–78.
18. Sarwer DB, Wadden TA, Pertshuk MJ, et al. Body image dissatisfaction and body dysmorphic disorder in 100 cosmetic surgery patients. *Plast Reconstr Surg* 1998;101:1644–1649.
19. Sheen JH. *Aesthetic rhinoplasty,* 2nd ed. St. Louis: Mosby, 1987.
20. Gunter JP, Friedman RM. Lateral crural strut graft: technique and clinical applications in rhinoplasty. *Plast Reconstr Surg* 1997;99:943–952.
21. Guyuron B. Nasal osteotomy and airway changes. *Plast Reconstr Surg* 1998;102:856–860.
22. Stuzin JM, Kawamoto HK. Saddle-nose deformity. *Clin Plast Surg* 1988;15:83–94.

23. Gruber RP. Alar base excision. *Aesthetic Video J* 1995;2.
24. Constantian MB. An alar base flap to correct nostril and vestibular stenosis and alar base malposition in rhinoplasty. *Plast Reconstr Surg* 1998;101:1666–1674.
25. Marshall DR, Slattery PG. Intracranial complications of rhinoplasty. *Br J Plast Surg* 1983;36:342–344.
26. Hallock GG, Trier WC. Cerebrospinal fluid rhinorrhea following rhinoplasty. *Plast Reconstr Surg* 1983;71:109–113.

Discussion

OPEN RHINOPLASTY

AMY LAI
MACK L. CHENEY

Drs. Gruber and Aiach have clearly and meticulously elucidated the complications that can be encountered and prevented in open rhinoplasty. There is no question that techniques of open, or external, rhinoplasty are invaluable in certain circumstances and that, in the right hands, they can consistently yield superior results. The indications for open rhinoplasty have been enumerated elsewhere (1,2). In general, open rhinoplasty is preferred over closed approaches in extensive reshaping of the nasal tip (3,4), difficult revision rhinoplasty, insertion of multiple nasal grafts, structural retailoring of support elements such as the columella, and correction of congenital deformities; it is also preferred when direct visualization is required for hemostasis. The open technique avoids trauma to the region of the internal nasal valve, which is often a consequence of intercartilaginous or intracartilaginous incisions. Because of the superior exposure afforded by the open technique, it is the approach we prefer for primary and revision rhinoplasties.

PREOPERATIVE EVALUATION

Drs. Gruber and Aiach astutely point out the importance of patient selection for open rhinoplasty, which should not be performed when a patient does not want an external incision. When the benefits of the open approach are discussed with patients, the great majority of them accept the external incision as a minor consequence. The prepared surgeon should be able to present a surgical plan and discuss with the patient the ideal and realistic achievements of rhinoplasty. Generally, the patient returns for several consultations before surgery is performed. The passage of time eliminates those patients who embark on cosmetic surgery as a whim, and allows the surgeon to determine the patient's motivation and willingness to accept surgery. These preparations are especially important when a patient is undergoing revision rhinoplasty because of a complication or an unfavorable result.

INTRAOPERATIVE TECHNIQUE

In most cases, the senior author performs rhinoplasty under general anesthesia. General anesthesia allows better control of the airway and blood pressure, and the surgeon is free to concentrate on the aesthetic outcome. A solution of 1% lidocaine and epinephrine (1:100,000) is injected into the anterior nasal septal mucoperichondrium, columella, mucosa, periosteum overlying the pyriform apertures bilaterally, and lateral nasal walls. If a concomitant septoplasty is necessary, it is performed through a hemitransfixion incision. An inverted V incision is made in the middle of the columella. Three-point and two-point retraction is used to maximize exposure of the crural cartilage and decrease the risk for injury to the cartilage (1,5). Converse scissors are used to facilitate elevation of the skin-soft tissue envelope (SSTE). When the skin is separated from the medial crura, it is important not to dissect into the intercrural soft tissues or disrupt the interdomal ligament. These structures provide an ideal envelope for a columellar strut. A crucial guideline for a correct plane of dissection in the dome is to elevate the SSTE immediately superficial to the perichondrium of the lower lateral cartilages. Dissection in the subdermal connective tissue leads to excessive bleeding, increased postoperative edema, and an increased risk for fibrosis. Hemostasis is

A. Lai: Department of Otology and Laryngology, Massachusetts Eye and Ear Infirmary, Boston Massachusetts; and Department of Surgery, Winchester Hospital, Winchester, Massachusetts
M. L. Cheney: Department of Otolaryngology, Harvard Medical School; and Department of Otolaryngology, Massachusetts Eye and Ear Infirmary, Boston, Massachusetts

maintained with the bipolar electrocautery. When dissection is in the correct plane, the risk for skin perforation is greatly reduced. We do not advocate "hyperinflating" the SSTE with local anesthesia or saline solution before elevation because this technique distorts the underlying anatomy and causes the soft tissue to become more fragile. Once the anterior septal angle has been identified, dissection proceeds along the nasal dorsum in a subperiosteal plane. The nasal dorsum is directly visualized with an Alfricht retractor. The bands tethering the dorsal SSTE to the lateral nasal walls are divided under direct vision with a knife or scissors. The columellar incision is closed with interrupted 6-0 nylon sutures. Lateral notching at the mucocutaneous junction of the incision is prevented by careful approximation of the corner sutures. If substantial bleeding is encountered, light packing with finger cots is placed for 3 to 24 hours. Early follow-up, between 24 and 48 hours, is recommended to detect early complications. Cast and sutures are removed at 1 week.

EPISTAXIS

Epistaxis is rare in the open technique because bleeding is easily detected and cauterized. However, because of the increased disruption of venous and lymphatic drainage, hematomas in the opened nose can be a devastating complication, potentially leading to scarring, deformity, and skin necrosis. Patients who take aspirin are advised to stop 7 days before surgery. Other nonsteroidal antiinflammatory medications must be discontinued for a period equivalent to at least five half-lives before the time of surgery. Patients are questioned specifically for a personal or family history of excessive bleeding. A history of bleeding is a more reliable indicator of risk than the results of coagulation studies or a determination of the bleeding time. If a submucous resection of the septal cartilage has been performed, the mucoperichondrial layers of the two sides are reapproximated with a horizontal mattress, "quilting" stitch of 4-0 double-armed plain gut suture. Silastic splints may be placed to prevent the formation of synechiae between the septum and the mucosa of the lateral nasal wall, or to stent areas of nasal valve repair. These splints are cut into long ellipses that span the entire nasal septum and affixed with a transseptal 4-0 Prolene suture. As mentioned earlier, packing with finger cots is placed in the anterior nasal cavity for 3 to 24 hours, with ties anterior to the columella to prevent accidental aspiration.

The marginal incision of the open rhinoplasty is closed loosely with 5-0 chromic gut suture to allow blood to leave the ala. This maneuver restores the lower lateral cartilage to its proper anatomical position and prevents its prolapse into the lateral nasal vestibule.

Incisions for the lateral osteotomies overlying the pyriform apertures bilaterally are first injected with lidocaine and epinephrine. Enough time must pass for the vasoconstrictive effects of epinephrine to work. Only a small horizontal incision is made anterior to the inferior turbinate. Subperiosteal dissection in the nasomaxillary suture line is performed over a limited tract of bone with an Anderson dental periosteal elevator. Just enough space is created to pass an osteotome through without tearing the periosteum, which tends to bleed. The osteotomy site is not closed.

IMPLANT COMPLICATIONS

Complications stemming from allograft implants are well-known. Problems with extrusion, infection, hemorrhage, and mobility have been reported with both allografts and irradiated homografts, and they can occur years after graft placement. These complications present a challenge to the rhinoplasty surgeon, who must address both physiologic and aesthetic problems in the patient's nose. After implant removal, a thick fibrous capsule is often present around the graft site that has great potential for contracture. Whatever material is placed into the wound must be strong enough to withstand great forces of distortion.

Secondary augmentation has been described with a variety of allograft materials, the most recent being expanded polytetrafluoroethylene (Gore-Tex). Although complication rates are lower than with silicone implants, the rate of events leading to the removal of Gore-Tex grafts has been reported to be 2% to 4% (6,7). Autogenous grafts such as temporalis fascia, temporoparietal fascia, conchal cartilage, and septal cartilage are suitable for small cartilage defects but may not address a large nasal dorsal defect, such as a saddle deformity. The tendency of rib cartilage to warp with time renders it less than ideal as a graft material. For secondary reconstructions, we prefer to use calvarial bone grafts (8,9). These are strong, reliable grafts that can be obtained from adults and children older than 6 years.

NASAL GRAFTS

An ideal donor tissue for cartilaginous spreader or batten grafts to repair nasal valvular deformities is conchal cartilage. Because of its convexity, it is easily fashioned into an onlay batten graft to repair a collapsed external nasal valve. Such collapse usually results from overly zealous caudal resection of the lower lateral cartilage in the pursuit of a more angular tip. Although cartilage grafts are excellent for correcting functional defects, we avoid using onlay grafts to correct aesthetic deformities. These grafts tend to cause irregularities through the soft tissue envelope of the nose, and are especially noticeable in patients with thin skin. One cannot predict how much of the graft will show through the skin after contracture of the soft tissue envelope with time. In revision rhinoplasty, subtle sculpting of the soft tissues by suturing may achieve as much correction as excision or grafting, and may avoid the excessive overcorrection that results in an unnatural appearance.

SADDLE DEFORMITY

One of the most devastating complications of rhinoplasty, saddle deformity results from overresection of the dorsal and caudal septal cartilage and the consequent loss of tip support. Loss of the dorsal and caudal septum cannot be corrected simply by placing an implant at the anterior septal angle. Over time, the nasal tip will certainly fall. On opening the nose, the surgeon often finds buckled and weak medial crura that have been distorted by scar contracture.

The treatment for saddle deformity is twofold. First, adequate dorsal support must be reestablished. The ideal material to re-create dorsal height is calvarial bone (8). It is easily harvested and firmly incorporated into the nasal complex, and complications at the donor site are few. Rates of infection and migration are significantly lower than when allografts are used. The scalp is prepared with Betadine and draped in sterile fashion at the beginning of the procedure. The hair is not shaved. A horizontal incision is made through all layers of the scalp at the level of the superior temporal line on the nondominant side. A calvarial bone graft measuring 4×1 cm is harvested with a drill and curved osteotomes. The cranial defect is repaired with methylmethacrylate. The graft is fashioned to the right shape with a drill and then placed in a pocket elevated through an external rhinoplasty incision. No screws are used to fix the bone.

Second, caudal support must be reestablished. A columellar strut fashioned from the septal cartilage and placed between the medial crura provides firm tip support. Conchal cartilage lacks sufficient structural integrity to be an effective columellar strut. When the pocket for the columellar strut is created, one is careful to terminate at a point just superior to the nasal spine. If the strut abuts the nasal spine, it may slip to one side of the spine and shift the nasal tip.

SUMMARY

As with closed rhinoplasty, successful avoidance of complications in open rhinoplasty is predicated on careful planning, knowledge of nasal anatomy and physiology, and meticulous surgical technique. Revision rhinoplasty becomes increasingly difficult and the results increasingly less satisfying with each attempt. Open rhinoplasty provides direct visualization and improved exposure of the surgical field. Facility with this technique should be in the armamentarium of the rhinoplasty surgeon.

REFERENCES

1. Johnson CM, Toriumi DM. *Open structure rhinoplasty.* Philadelphia: WB Saunders, 1990:6.
2. Toriumi DM. Open rhinoplasty. In: Bailey BJ, ed. *Atlas of head and neck surgery: otolaryngology.* Philadelphia: JB Lippincott Co, 1993:2128–2140.
3. Goodman WS. Septo-rhinoplasty: surgery of the nasal tip by external rhinoplasty. *J Laryngol Otol* 1980;94:485–494.
4. Tardy ME, Pratt BS, Walter MA. Transdomal suture refinement of the nasal tip. *Facial Plast Surg* 1993;9:275–284.
5. Anderson JR, Johnson CM, Adamson P. Open rhinoplasty: an assessment. *Otolaryngol Head Neck Surg* 1982;90:272–274.
6. Conrad K, Gillman G. A 6-year experience with the use of expanded polytetrafluoroethylene in rhinoplasty. *Plast Reconstr Surg* 1998;101:1675–1683.
7. Godin MS, Waldman SR, Johnson CM. The use of expanded polytetrafluoroethylene (Gore-Tex) in rhinoplasty. A 6-year experience. *Arch Otolaryngol Head Neck Surg* 1995;121:1131–1136.
8. Cheney ML, Gliklich RE. The use of calvarial bone in nasal reconstruction. *Arch Otolaryngol Head Neck Surg* 1995;121:643–648.
9. Hallock GG. Cranial nasal bone grafts. *Aesthetic Plast Surg* 1989;13:285–289.

SUGGESTED READING

Deva AK, Merten S, Chang L. Silicone in nasal augmentation rhinoplasty: a decade of clinical experience. *Plast Reconstr Surg* 1998;102:1230–1237.

55

SEPTAL AND TURBINATE SURGERY

JENNIFER PARKER PORTER
DEAN M. TORIUMI

GENERAL CONSIDERATIONS

Septal and turbinate surgery is difficult to teach and learn because the narrow passages involved frequently can be visualized only by a single surgeon. The complications of septal and turbinate surgery have been reported to decrease as the experience of the operating surgeon increases (1). Endoscopic equipment has facilitated teaching to a certain degree. However, most learning is acquired by observing other surgeons. The key to performing septal surgery without complications is to dissect in the correct plane and preserve mucosal integrity. Dissection should be performed in the space between the mucoperichondrium and the quadrangular cartilage and also between the mucoperiosteum and bony vomer and the perpendicular plate of the ethmoid. Dissection superficial to the perichondrium and periosteum can cause complications that will be discussed in detail.

Turbinate surgery is quite controversial. In dry, cold climates, a minimalistic approach is taken because of potential problems with rhinitis sicca and atrophic rhinitis. However, in areas where warmer, more humid conditions prevail, the turbinates can be operated in conservative fashion to prevent postoperative nasal obstruction. Nonetheless, in all climates, patients are at risk for postoperative complications of turbinate surgery.

Surgical interventions designed to improve respiration through the nasal passages most frequently involve straightening the septum and occasionally debulking the inferior turbinate. However, obstruction can also be caused by an incompetent nasal valve. The nasal valve is defined as the area bounded by the nasal septum medially and the caudal aspect of the upper lateral cartilage laterally (2,3). The nasal valve area encompasses the inferior turbinate and floor of the pyriform aperture, in addition to the caudal septum and caudal edge of the upper lateral cartilage (2). The nasal valve angle should measure approximately 10 to 15 degrees (2,3). Nasal obstruction can therefore have a mechanical cause, such as septal deviation, turbinate hypertrophy, or nasal valve collapse. The causes of an obstruction should be determined carefully so that all aspects of the problem can be addressed at the primary surgery. Failure to diagnose a fixed obstruction with a concomitant nasal valve collapse will inevitably result in failure of the primary surgery. Nasal valve collapse is not discussed further here because it is primarily a complication of rhinoplasty surgery.

A vast array of surgical techniques are available for the treatment of the obstructing nasal septum and turbinate, and the reader is referred to the list of suggested readings. This chapter focuses on the more common unfavorable outcomes of septal or turbinate surgery, including the following: septal perforation, persistent septal deviation, saddle nose deformity, synechiae, septal hematoma, and septal abscess. Complications that may occur secondary to turbinate surgery include atrophic rhinitis, rhinitis sicca, persistent obstruction, and bleeding. Although these lists are not all-inclusive, the scope of this chapter does not permit further discussion of the other, less common reported complications, which include pneumocephalus, cerebrospinal fluid leak, olfactory nerve injury, cavernous sinus thrombosis, toxic shock syndrome, myospherulosis, tooth devitalization, and impaired midfacial growth (4–6).

UNFAVORABLE RESULTS IN SEPTAL SURGERY

Septal Perforation

Septal perforation can be either an acquired or an iatrogenic problem (Table 55-1). The perforation may be caused by the long-term use of intranasal vasoconstrictors, chronic digital trauma, autoimmune disease, carcinoma, or infectious problems. Iatrogenic septal perforation can be caused by septal surgery, tight nasal packing and splints, and nasal cautery. Prior septal surgery is reportedly the most common cause of septal perforation, with studies reporting the inci-

J. P. Porter: Department of Otolaryngology and Communicative Sciences, Baylor College of Medicine; and Department of Otolaryngology, The Methodist Hospital, Houston, Texas

D. M. Toriumi: Department of Otolaryngology—Head and Neck Surgery, University of Illinois at Chicago, Chicago, Illinois

TABLE 55-1. ETIOLOGY OF NASAL SEPTAL PERFORATION

Infectious
Septal abscess
Syphilis
Tuberculosis
Rhinoscleroma
Typhoid
Diphtheria
Autoimmune
Wegener's granulomatosis
Systemic lupus erythematosis
Sarcoidosis
Traumatic
Septal hematoma
Blunt trauma
Digital trauma (nose picking)
Iatrogenic
Septal surgery
Tight nasal packing/splints
Nasal cautery
Nasotracheal intubation
Neoplastic
Carcinoma
Lethal midline granuloma
Irritants
Cocaine
Chromic acid fumes
Toxic fumes
Vasoconstrictors (neosynephrine, oxymetazoline)

dence to range from 1.5% to 6.4% (1,4,7–9). Bilateral mucoperichondrial flap tears that are in direct opposition predispose to the formation of perforations. In addition, tight septal splints or nasal packing may also be a culprit (9).

Septal perforations can cause symptoms of crusting, epistaxis, whistling, and nasal obstruction. On occasion, patients report no symptoms, especially if the perforation is small and posterior in location (10). Obviously, asymptomatic perforations require no treatment, as attempted surgical closure has the potential to worsen the problem. Symptomatic perforations require some form of treatment. This can range from symptomatic medical therapy to closure of the perforation with grafts via the external rhinoplasty approach. Treatment is selected according to the size and location of a perforation.

Supportive medical treatment can be given for a perforation of any size, although most would recommend it particularly for a larger perforation that would be difficult to close surgically (10). In addition, patients who abuse drugs, be it cocaine or over-the-counter intranasal vasoconstrictors, are often best treated with conservative medical therapy because continued abuse inevitably results in a recurrence of the problem. Frequently, the treatment is aimed at decreasing the amount of crusting and minimizing the amount of bleeding. Thus, antibiotic ointment and a nasal spray of saline solution are often recommended for perforations in which surgical repair is precluded. Use of a powered water jet frequently helps to maintain a clean nasal cavity and minimize crusting.

Insertion of a small Silastic button through a perforation may allay symptoms if the perforation is smaller than 3 cm. Although the button may decrease the amount of whistling in small, anterior perforations, it will not eradicate crusting, bleeding, or nasal blockage caused by the perforation. Facer and Kern (7) describe the use of the Silastic button in perforations ranging from 5 mm to 3 cm. Placement of a button through a perforation is similar to placement of a pressure-equalization tube through a myringotomy. The buttons can be fashioned to fit the size of the perforation and can be placed under local anesthesia alone (7). Septal buttons are particularly useful in patients who are not surgical candidates. Some patients continue to have symptoms of crusting and bleeding, even with the button in place. In the study of Kridel et al. (10), improvement was greater when the perforation was closed with local flaps rather than with a septal button, and they recommend flap surgery in all symptomatic patients who have no medical contraindication to surgery (10).

A variety of methods have been described for the surgical closure of septal perforations. A horizontal myomucosal flap has been described by Tardy (11) to be reliable and expedient for the closure of anterior perforations. The tissue is harvested from the undersurface of the upper lip, and a medially based flap is created that begins just lateral to the midline frenulum. A lateral alotomy facilitates exposure of the perforation, and a tunnel is created between the lip and the nasal floor. The flap is passed through this tunnel and secured into position with resorbable sutures, so that the opposite side can reepithelialize.

A more popular method for repair is the external rhinoplasty approach, in which bilateral septal mucoperichondrial flaps are raised in an attempt to close the perforation (10). Closure of the perforation is facilitated through the use of an intraseptal connective tissue graft of periosteum, fascia, perichondrium, or acellular dermis (8,10). After bilateral flap elevation, perforations smaller than 1 cm can be closed primarily with simple interrupted sutures and a connective tissue graft placed between the two sides of the flaps. For perforations larger than 1 cm, lateral relaxing incisions should be made in an anteroposterior direction along the floor of the nose below the inferior turbinates on both sides (Fig. 55-1). In this way, the flap can be mobilized further from below. If additional length is needed, the flap can be elevated from the upper lateral cartilage to facilitate closure. Perforations up to 4 cm in size have been closed with these techniques; the overall success rate has been 77% (9).

Septal Hematoma and Abscess

The development of a septal hematoma after surgery of the nasal septum can have devastating consequences if it is not discovered relatively soon after it forms. The presence of a

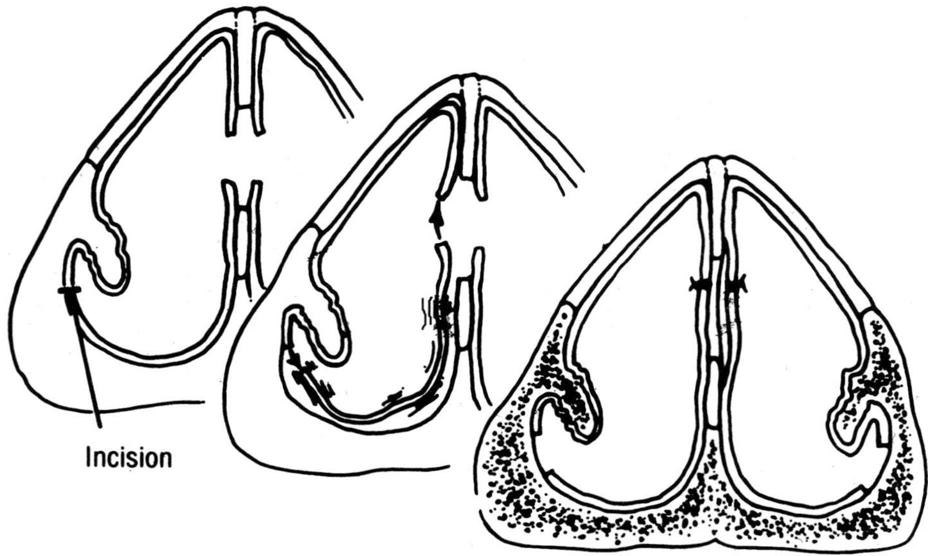

FIGURE 55-1. Repair of a septal perforation requires release of the mucosa underlying the inferior turbinate such that the mucoperichodrial flap can be advanced medially as a bipedicled flap. Final closure is shown with the interposed soft tissue graft. (From Kridel RWH, Foda H, Lunde KC. Septal perforation repair with acellular human dermal allograft. *Arch Otolaryngol Head Neck Surg* 1998;124:78, with permission.)

hematoma between the mucoperichondrial flaps leads to resorption of the septal cartilage, possible abscess formation, and ultimate nasal deformity because of loss of the cartilage. Intracranial extension of the abscess is a far more worrisome complication, and the physician should be on the alert for signs of this during the history and physical examination phase of the evaluation. A loss of the normal blood supply provided by the mucoperichondrium and pressure necrosis from the expanded hematoma result in destruction of the cartilage (12) and create an environment in which bacteria thrive. The time required for cartilage destruction is not well defined. Canty and Berkowitz (13) studied a group of 20 children in whom hematoma or abscess of the nasal septum had been diagnosed. The children in whom cartilage was not resorbed presented for treatment on average 3.6 days after traumatic injury, whereas those with cartilage destruction were seen on average 6.9 days after trauma (13). These data highlight the need to diagnose hematoma early. Bacteria that can thrive in this environment include the usual isolates in the head and neck region, including *Staphylococcus aureus, Streptococcus pneumoniae, Staphylococcus epidermidis,* group A β-hemolytic streptococci, and *Haemophilus influenzae* (13,14).

The prevention of septal hematoma and abscess after septal surgery can be enhanced by using a mattress or quilting suture to reapproximate the cartilage and mucoperichondrial flap, or the mucoperichondrial flaps alone when no intervening cartilage is present. Careful placement of the sutures obliterates the dead space between the flaps such that the amount of fluid collected between the flaps is minimal. The sutures should span the area of flap elevation so that the potential space is nonexistent (Fig. 55-2). When the septum is approached through the external rhinoplasty approach, an incision should be made intranasally through one of the mucoperichondrial flaps to allow for the egress of small amounts of fluid. Studies have not shown that nasal packing decreases the incidence of hematoma formation in the postoperative period (15).

In the event that a hematoma does form, prompt evacuation of the fluid collection is in the best interest of the patient to prevent reabsorption of the septal cartilage. Urgent attention is required. A topical anesthetic can be applied; however, the mucosal edema may prevent penetration of the medications. In the case of previous septoplasty, no further incisions should have to be made to evacuate the hematoma or abscess, as the Killian or hemitransfixion incision sutures can be removed and the clot or pus evacuated. Aerobic and anaerobic cultures should be obtained for microbiology examination. Subsequent to evacuation of the hematoma or pus, the region should be irrigated with saline solution and an antibiotic solution. A quilting suture should be applied to the septum. Intravenous antibiotics should be administered, directed at the most likely pathogens, until a culture-specific antibiotic can be instituted (13). Specific recommendations regarding the duration of intravenous antibiotic therapy are not available; however, studies indicate that it should be continued for approximately 7 days or until clinical improvement (13,14). Subsequent administration of oral antibiotics is recommended. The patient should be observed frequently to detect any reaccumulation of fluid.

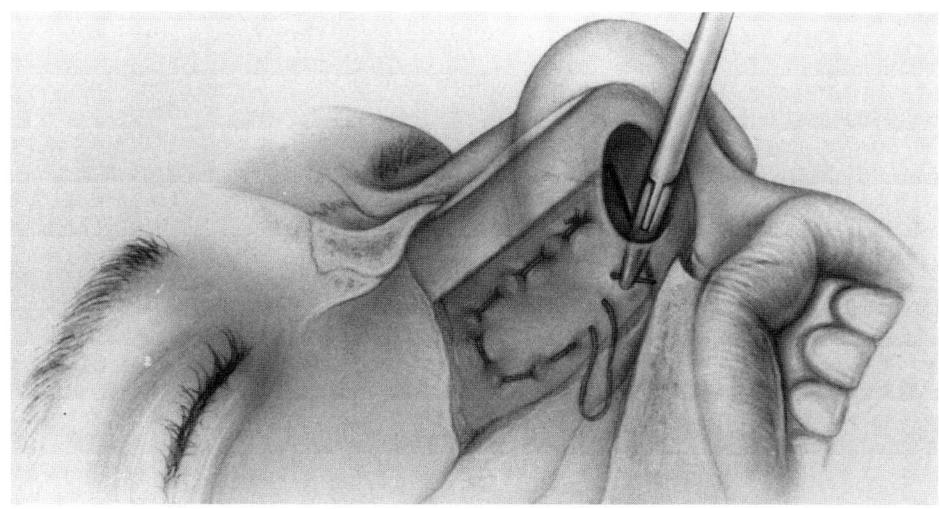

FIGURE 55-2. An absorbable quilting suture is used to reapproximate the mucoperichondrial flaps and prevent an accumulation of fluid during the postoperative period. (From Johnson CM Jr, Toriumi DM. *Open structure rhinoplasty.* Philadelphia: WB Saunders, 1990, with permission.)

Persistent Septal Deviation

Maneuvers to correct a deviated septum sometimes fail. The reasons include inherent memory of the septal cartilage when the cartilage has been scored. Caudal septal deviation may persist because of inadequate attention to the subluxation of cartilage from the bony maxillary crest. Bony deviations of the vomer and perpendicular plate of the ethmoid may persist because they were unrecognized at the time of the first surgery. Our observation has been that failure to examine this area during the initial surgery is often a cause of persistent nasal obstruction.

Preventative measures include accurate assessment at the time of surgery. Aligning the septum at the time of surgery is critical, as no further correction should be expected in the postoperative period despite packing or splinting. The caudal septum must be addressed in a case of deviated or subluxed cartilage. A "swinging door" maneuver may be performed to align the septum in the midline (16,17). The maneuver involves elevation of mucoperichondrial flaps on both sides of the caudal septum with subsequent disarticulation of the quadrangular cartilage from the maxillary crest. Once the caudal septum is mobile, excess cartilage is noted and trimmed so that the cartilage is aligned with the maxillary crest in the vertical plane (Fig. 55-3). Once the cartilage is in place, a permanent monofilament suture (e.g., 4-0 Prolene) is placed through the periosteum on the side opposite the deviation and passed through the caudal end of the cartilage and tied. Suture stabilization of the septum is paramount to prevent postoperative collapse and tip settling.

Bony septal deviations persist primarily because of the previous surgeon's neglect. These areas are corrected with standard septoplasty techniques for the management of

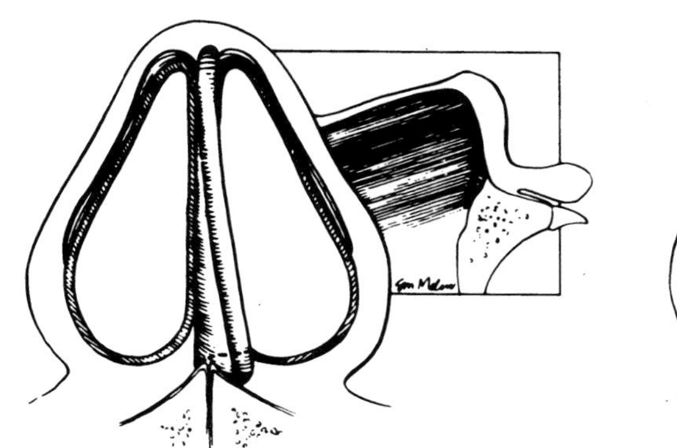

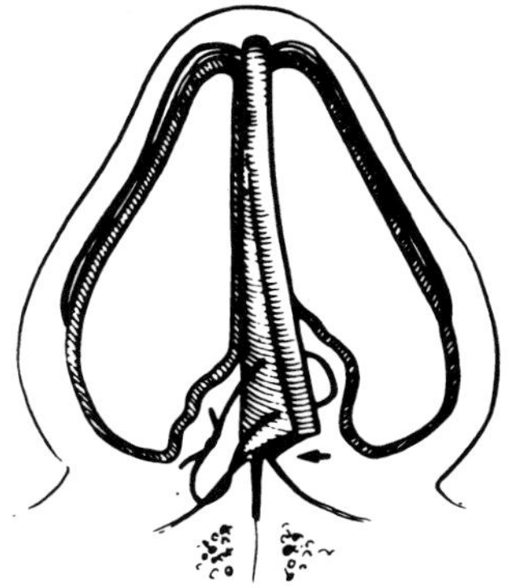

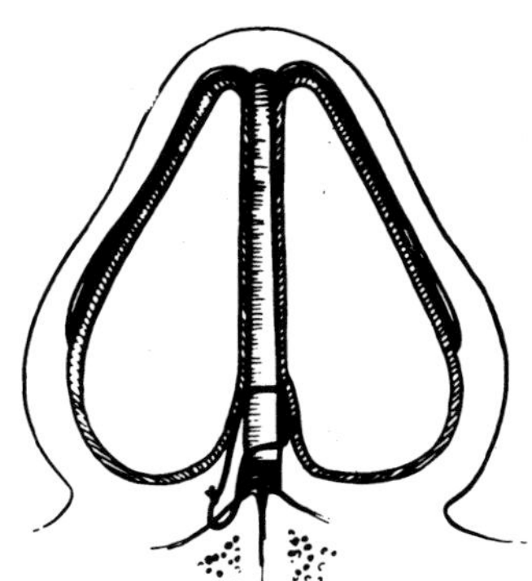

FIGURE 55-3. In the "swinging door" maneuver, the subluxed cartilage is released from the maxillary crest. The cartilage is trimmed to lie in the same vertical plane as the maxillary crest. A 4-0 monofilament nonabsorbable suture is placed through the periosteum on the side opposite the deviation and the caudal aspect of the septum to fix the septum in the midline. (From Toriumi DM, Ries WR. Innovative surgical management of the crooked nose. *Facial Plast Surg Clin N Am* 1993;1:63–78, with permission.)

bony deformities. One of the basic tenets of bony septal surgery is to avoid transmission of forces to the area of the cribriform plate. Small pieces of bone can be removed with the Takahashi forceps to prevent the transmission of significant forces. In addition, scissors can be used to cut the bone above the area of the deviation to eliminate the possibility of disturbing the cribriform plate when the deviated segment is removed.

Saddle Nose Deformity

The causes of saddle nose deformity are numerous, most of them similar to the causes of septal perforation. However, saddle nose deformity in the postoperative state can be caused by overresection of the dorsal quadrangular cartilage or failure to leave an adequate dorsal and caudal L-shaped strut. Likewise, septal hematoma or abscess in the postoper-

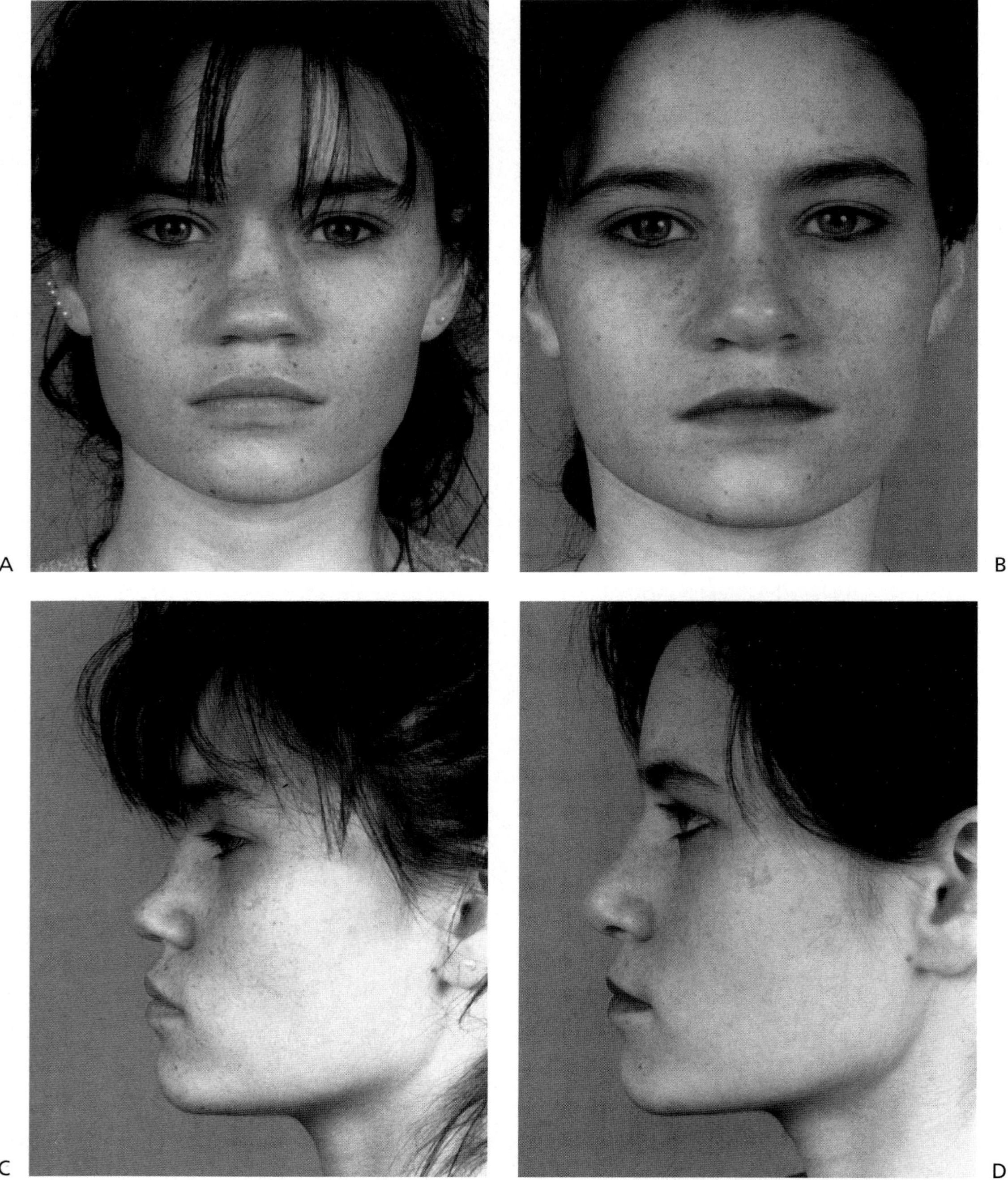

FIGURE 55-4. Patient with saddle nose deformity after blunt nasal trauma. The deformity was corrected by reconstructing the L-shaped strut of the septum with a segment of cartilage harvested from the posteroinferior septum. **A,C:** Preoperative views. **B,D:** Postoperative views.

ative period can lead to cartilage resorption and a dorsal concavity.

Preventative measures include frequent reassessment during rhinoplasty of the dorsal profile relationship. With regard to septal surgery, maintenance of the L-shaped strut, with at least 1.5 cm left dorsally and caudally, will provide adequate support. L-shaped struts that are weakened through cartilage-scoring maneuvers may collapse in the postoperative period if they are not reinforced with cartilage grafts.

Correction of the saddle nose deformity requires augmentation. The extent of augmentation is based on the deformity and the materials available for reconstruction. Most patients with a saddle deformity do not have septal cartilage available for grafting purposes. Thus, autogenous cartilage from the ear or rib are the materials of choice for augmentation. If significant dorsal augmentation is required, autologous rib is preferred. Under certain circumstances, harvesting autologous cartilage is precluded. These include a lack of availability of auricular cartilage and cartilage that is diseased (e.g., relapsing polychondritis). Patients with poor pulmonary reserve or elderly patients are not good candidates for rib cartilage harvest. Therefore, in these cases, the use of irradiated rib cartilage may be indicated. Irradiated rib cartilage is versatile, used for dorsal augmentation and multiple grafting purposes. The risk for disease transmission is minimal, and the cartilage is tolerated well by patients (18,19). Warping has been reported in 2.7% of cases and is minimized by removal of the attached perichondrium before implantation (18). Cartilage resorption has been reported, primarily with grafts in sites other than the nose. Within the nose, few cases of significant resorption have been reported, although long-term follow-up is lacking (18,19). Calvarial bone can also be used for dorsal augmentation. However, calvarial bone is more difficult to shape precisely and also can be resorbed. Numerous alloplastic materials are available for nasal augmentation; however, they are not recommended because of problems of extrusion and infection.

The grafts can be placed through an internal or external approach, although we prefer the external approach. Grafts should be sutured in place unless a precise pocket is present in which the graft can sit. Articulation of the columellar strut further stabilizes the dorsal graft (19). The patient shown in Fig. 55-4 had a saddle nose deformity resulting from previous trauma. The deformity was corrected by using existing posterior septal cartilage to reconstruct the L-shaped dorsal strut.

Synechiae

The formation of synechiae secondary to septal or turbinate surgery results from injury to the mucosal surfaces that are apposed to each other. During the surgical procedure, all incisions should be closed to prevent the coaptation and irregular healing of raw surfaces. In addition, to prevent this unfavorable result, careful attention to cleansing the nose after surgery is required. At follow-up examinations, the nose should be inspected and any early synechiae resolved by breaking up fibrous connections. Nasal irrigation with a spray of saline solution also encourages the healing process.

When well-formed synechiae are noted in the late postoperative period, the adhesions should be lysed and Telfa packing interposed between the raw surfaces for several days. This simple procedure can be performed under local anesthesia in the office. While the packing is in place, the patient should be placed on antibiotics to prevent toxic shock syndrome.

UNFAVORABLE RESULTS IN TURBINATE SURGERY

Persistent Hypertrophy

Turbinate surgery has long been controversial because of the complications that can arise from manipulation. The turbinate can be altered or removed in such a way that the nasal resistance is decreased. Furthermore, partial or total removal of the inferior turbinate decreases the surface area available to humidify the airway and may result in chronic dryness and crusting (16,20).

The causes of turbinate hypertrophy are numerous and include allergic rhinitis, vasomotor rhinitis, rhinitis medicamentosa, rhinitis of pregnancy, hypothyroidism, exogenous hormonal therapy, antihypertensive medications, and antidepressant medications. Compensatory hypertrophy can result from a deviated nasal septum (21). The medical treatment of allergic rhinitis, vasomotor rhinitis, and rhinitis medicamentosa usually reduces the size of the turbinates. Maximal medical therapy should be instituted for an extended period of time before any surgical procedure is undertaken to attempt to reduce the size of the turbinates. Compensatory turbinate hypertrophy may be very subtle and may not be recognized until after surgical correction of a long-standing deviated nasal septum. Recognition of the diagnosis preoperatively will prevent the new onset of nasal obstruction in the contralateral nasal passage during the postoperative period.

The medical treatment of turbinate hypertrophy depends on its cause. Allergic rhinitis is often treated with topical nasal steroids and antihistamines with or without decongestants. This combination therapy helps to diminish the congested nasal tissues. Rhinitis medicamentosa is treated by stopping the offending medicine and applying topical decongestants and topical nasal steroids. A tapered dose of oral steroids is added if the condition is severe. Vasomotor rhinitis can be treated with an anticholinergic medication such as Atrovent nasal spray (ipratropium bromide), which diminishes nasal secretions. Numerous texts describe various other treatments for these conditions. Compensatory hypertrophy is seldom a problem during the preoperative phases of patient evaluation.

Numerous methods have been devised to reduce the size of an enlarged turbinate that does not respond to medical treatment. Once removed, the turbinate cannot be replaced, so that caution is advised. Methods to reduce the turbinate range from conservative to aggressive. Conservative measures include crushing and lateral out-fracture, cauterization of the anterior portion of the inferior turbinate, cryotherapy, and laser vaporization. More aggressive measures include submucous resection of the inferior turbinate, inferior turbinoplasty, and total resection (21). The spectrum of procedures is broad; however, destructive procedures in which the entire turbinate is removed are likely to lead to rhinitis sicca and atrophic rhinitis. In the event of persistent turbinate hypertrophy and obstruction in the postoperative phase, some of the conservative procedures may be utilized to decrease the blockage.

Atrophic Rhinitis and Rhinitis Sicca

Atrophic rhinitis and rhinitis sicca are two conditions that may occur after reductive surgery of the turbinates. Rhinitis sicca is characterized by dry nasal mucosa and mild crusting of the anterior portion of the nose (20). Atrophic rhinitis presents with a triad of symptoms: unusually wide nasal passages; viscous secretions; and greenish yellow, foul-smelling crusting throughout the nasal cavity. Primary atrophic rhinitis occurs without any previous nasal surgery or trauma (22). Secondary atrophic rhinitis develops after surgery or trauma to the nose, and after destructive infectious processes, including tuberculosis and syphilis. Atrophic rhinitis typically heralds an infection with *Klebsiella ozaenae* (22). Of the two conditions, rhinitis sicca is probably the most common sequela of destructive turbinate surgery.

Prevention of these entities requires careful, conservative reduction of the turbinates, especially in arid climates. Turbinate surgery should be performed only when absolutely necessary. Once atrophic rhinitis or rhinitis sicca develops, it is very difficult to relieve the condition surgically. The medical treatment of rhinitis sicca consists mainly of the frequent use of nasal saline spray. Atrophic rhinitis requires more aggressive medical treatment, including culture of the viscous secretions of the nose. Culture-specific antibiotics are instituted. Patients infected with *Klebsiella ozaenae* are treated with tetracycline for 2 to 6 months unless sensitivities indicate otherwise (22). In addition, mechanical cleansing with nasal irrigation is a mainstay of treatment. Numerous surgical options to treat atrophic rhinitis have been reported, including the placement of submucosal implants in the lateral wall or floor of the nose to increase the surface area of the nasal mucosa. Others have recommended intermittent closure of the anterior nasal passage to inhibit air flow through the nasal passage for an extended period of time. Because none of these surgical options is very effective, again, extreme caution is advised before surgery of the turbinates is undertaken.

Hemorrhage

Bleeding is the most common complication following nasal surgery (4,5). In a series of patients undergoing rhinoplasty, bleeding was more common in those who at the same time underwent septoplasty, turbinectomy, or both (4). Bleeding is the most common complication following surgery of the turbinates (21). Bleeding can be caused by a coagulation disorder, excessive activity immediately postoperatively, inadequate cauterization after partial or total turbinate resection, or lack of nasal packing after turbinate resection. The prevention of postoperative hemorrhage actually begins in the preoperative setting with a careful history and physical examination (5). Patients should be questioned about any history of a bleeding disorder, a family history of bleeding disorders, and medications used. All patients should discontinue aspirin and nonsteroidal antiinflammatory medications for 10 days to 2 weeks before surgery.

Postoperative hemorrhage can be prevented by gaining control of bleeding in the operating room. Although endoscopic guidance is not absolutely necessary, it facilitates cauterization by making it possible to target precisely the areas that require attention, particularly in cases concurrently undergoing endoscopic sinus dissection, in which the endoscope is ready and available. Packing is necessary following extensive surgery of the turbinate (23). It is recommended that packing be retained for 48 hours after turbinate surgery.

In the event that hemorrhage does occur in the postoperative period, it may be necessary to repack the nose with a 0.5-in gauze pad impregnated with antibiotic ointment or sponge packs. Should the packing fail to control the bleeding, options include suction cauterization of the site of bleeding under general anesthesia and with endoscopic visualization. If cauterization fails to control the bleeding while the patient is in the operating room, ligation of the sphenopalatine or ethmoid arteries may be necessary. The arterial anatomy of the nose should be borne in mind in any attempt to determine the site of bleeding. If arterial ligation is to be undertaken, then the anatomy will guide the surgeon to the artery that should be ligated first. An alternative to surgical management is angiography with subsequent embolization of the bleeding vessels. Embolization is very successful; however, it cannot be used to control bleeding from the anterior and posterior ethmoid arteries because of the potential risk for causing blindness.

CONCLUSION

Unfavorable results of septal and turbinate surgery occur fairly frequently because of errors in diagnosis and omissions in the preoperative evaluation. Other unfavorable results are caused by failure of the surgical technique employed. Safe septal and turbinate surgery requires an accurate assessment of the problem and implementation of the available techniques, with a good understanding of the possible untoward results and how to manage them effectively. With these tools in hand, it is possible to attain reproducible results.

REFERENCES

1. Tzadik A, Gilbert SE, Sade J. Complications of submucous resections of the nasal septum. *Arch Otorhinolaryngol* 1988; 245:74–76.
2. Kasperbauer JL, Kern EB. Nasal valve physiology: implications in nasal surgery. *Otolaryngol Clin North Am* 1987;20:699–719.
3. Sheen JH. Spreader graft: a method of reconstructing the roof of the middle nasal vault following rhinoplasty. *Plast Reconstr Surg* 1984;73:230–237.
4. Teichgraber JF, Riley WB, Parks DH. Nasal surgery complications. *Plast Reconstr Surg* 1990;85:527–531.
5. Teichgraber JF, Russo RC. Treatment of nasal surgery complications. *Ann Plast Surg* 1993;30:80–88.
6. Wheeler TM, Sessions RB, McGavran MH. Myospherulosis: a preventable iatrogenic nasal and paranasal entity. *Arch Otolaryngol* 1980;106:272–274.
7. Facer GW, Kern EB. Nonsurgical closure of nasal septal perforations. *Arch Otolaryngol Head Neck Surg* 1979;105:6–8.
8. Fairbanks DN, Fairbanks GR. Nasal septal perforation: prevention and management. *Ann Plast Surg* 1980;5:452–459.
9. Schwab J, Pirsig W. Complications of septal surgery. *Facial Plast Surg* 1997;13:3–14.
10. Kridel RWH, Appling WD, Wright WK. Septal perforation closure utilizing the external septorhinoplasty approach. *Arch Otolaryngol Head Neck Surg* 1986;112:168–172.
11. Tardy, Jr ME. *Rhinoplasty: the art and the science.* Philadelphia: WB Saunders, 1997:640–647.
12. Fry HJH. The pathology and treatment of hematoma of the nasal septum. *Br J Plast Surg* 1969;22:331–335.
13. Canty PA, Berkowitz RG. Hematoma and abscess of the nasal septum in children. *Arch Otolaryngol Head Neck Surg* 1996;122: 1373–1376.
14. Ambrus PS, Eavey RD, Sullivan Baker A, et al. Management of nasal septal abscess. *Laryngoscope* 1981;91:575–582.
15. Nunez DA, Martin FW. An evaluation of postoperative packing in nasal septal surgery. *Clin Otolaryngol* 1991;16:549–550.
16. Sulsenti G, Palma P. Tailored nasal surgery for normalization of nasal resistance. *Facial Plast Surg* 1996;12:333–345.
17. Toriumi DM, Ries WR. Innovative surgical management of the crooked nose. *Facial Plast Surg Clin N Am* 1993;1:63–78.
18. Kridel RW, Konior RJ. Irradiated cartilage grafts in the nose. A preliminary report. *Arch Otolaryngol Head Neck Surg* 1993;119: 24–30.
19. Murakami CS, Cook TA, Guida RA. Nasal reconstruction with articulated irradiated rib cartilage. *Arch Otolaryngol Head Neck Surg* 1991;117:327–330.
20. Papay FA, Eliachar I, Risica R. Fibromuscular temporalis graft implantation for rhinitis sicca. *Ear Nose Throat J* 1991;70: 381–384.
21. Mabry RL. Surgery of the inferior turbinates: how much and when? *Otolaryngol Head Neck Surg* 1984;92:571–576.
22. Chand MS, MacArthur CJ. Primary atrophic rhinitis: a summary of four cases and review of the literature. *Otolaryngol Head Neck Surg* 1997;116:554–558.
23. El-Silimy O. Inferior turbinate resection: the need for a nasal pack. *J Laryngol Otol* 1993;107:906–907.

SUGGESTED READING

Johnson CM Jr, Toriumi DM. *Open structure rhinoplasty.* Philadelphia: WB Saunders, 1990.

Ridenour BR. The nasal septum. In: Cummings CW, Fredrickson JM, Harker LA, et al., eds. *Otolaryngology head and neck surgery.* St. Louis: Mosby, 1998:921–948.

Tardy ME. *Rhinoplasty: the art and the science.* Philadelphia: WB Saunders, 1997.

Discussion

SEPTAL AND TURBINATE SURGERY

JENNIFER C. KIM
MACK L. CHENEY

The surgical management of the nasal septum often presents a challenge to even the most skilled nasal surgeon. The authors have clearly and concisely reviewed the unfavorable circumstances that may arise before, during, and after nasal surgery. We elaborate on some of the information presented and discuss several salient points to provide additional perspective regarding this topic.

We begin by stressing the importance of the preoperative

J. C. Kim and M. L. Cheney: Department of Otolaryngology, Harvard Medical School; and Department of Otolaryngology, Massachusetts Eye and Ear Infirmary, Boston, Massachusetts

evaluation. The clinical analysis must consider the complete history, including causes of the problem and any previous nasal surgery, and the results of a physical examination. The patient's nasal anatomy must be analyzed thoroughly before surgery is undertaken so that the surgical indications are appropriately met and the correct surgery performed. The patency of the nasal airway depends on its component structures: the nasal valve, septum, and inferior turbinate. It is important to note that these structures exist in a dynamic state and are continuously reacting and adapting to the environment; the findings of the office nasal examination represent just one point in time.

Preventive measures are as consequential as the treatment. The surgeon can avoid complications by having a thorough knowledge and keen sense of nasal anatomy, physiology, and wound healing combined with good surgical technique and judgment. The list of potential complications is extensive, but the most common ones are perforation, bleeding, hematoma, persistent nasal obstruction, and adhesions.

The authors extensively discuss septal perforations and briefly mention numerous reparative procedures that have been developed for use when supportive medical management has failed. Our approach has been to treat septal perforations only when they are symptomatic. Furthermore, no septal perforation should be repaired until the cause has been determined. If this is not evident from the history and physical examination findings, then blood work, radiographic studies, and biopsy may be indicated.

Most perforations are iatrogenic and result from previous nasal surgery. As the authors state in their introductory paragraph, "The key to performing septal surgery without complications is to dissect in the correct plane and preserve mucosal integrity." This is achieved by taking the time to identify and obtain the submucoperichondrial plane. On inspection, a subtle bluish hue to the cartilage is noted. On palpation, the cartilage feels gritty, not smooth. Once the correct plane has been established, then elevating the perichondrium is effortless. Particular care must be taken during elevation along the maxillary crest. Decussating fibers and numerous bony spurs along the crest make elevation difficult and predispose to tears in the nasal septal mucosa.

Experience indicates that the size and location of a perforation are related to symptoms. We see patients with large iatrogenic septal defects after frontal sinus drill-out surgery who remain asymptomatic, whereas others, with smaller anterior perforations, are incapacitated by excessive crusting and recurrent epistaxis. Perforations located high or posteriorly along the septum are less often symptomatic, even when of considerable size. Because the anterosuperior nasal septal cartilage forms the medial side of the internal nasal valve and is involved in the modulation of air flow, a perforation here causes a disruption of normal laminar air flow, with turbulence and desiccation of the nasal mucosa. The anterior caudal septum is also the region of Kisselbach's plexus, which explains why anterior perforations tend to cause bleeding and crusting.

If supportive medical treatment fails to relieve complaints, many surgical options are cited, ranging from variations of local flap repair (1,2) to the use of temporoparietal fascial flaps (3), turbinate flaps (4), tissue expanders (5), free flaps (6), and acellular grafts (7). Our experience has shown that simplicity is key. Bilateral sliding advancement mucosal flaps are successful for perforations smaller than 1.5 cm. Autogenous or acellular grafts may be interposed. For perforations larger than 2 cm, we recommend partial or complete septectomy. This procedure is easy to perform and relieves whistling, crusting, and bleeding (8).

Postoperative bleeding is rarely a problem, but the potential sequelae of a septal hematoma warrant close attention. It is imperative that the diagnosis be made quickly. On examination, the nasal septum is widened, with notable fluctuance or ballottement of the mucosal flaps. The patient will be more uncomfortable than would be expected. We routinely reapproximate the septal flaps to obliterate the dead space. For this process, we use short, double-armed, straight needles and 4-0 plain gut running horizontal mattress sutures. We also routinely use Silastic splints because they are well tolerated, help stabilize the flaps in the midline, and decrease the chances for adhesion formation, particularly if turbinate work has been performed concurrently. We place finger cots, which are removed before the patient is discharged to home. These ensure postoperative hemostasis as local vasoconstriction wears off.

The paragraph on persistent septal deviation also underscores the importance of preoperative assessment and accurate diagnosis. Surgical failure is often caused by residual, unrecognized deviations or spurs of the bony septum or a dislocated caudal septum. We have obtained excellent results by using a hemitransfixion incision and routinely performing submucous resections. The hemitransfixion incision exposes the entire caudal septum and its insertion into the maxillary crest. Frequently, dislocation or buckling of the caudal septum is found here and can be addressed with the "swinging door" maneuver, as previously mentioned. Once both flaps are elevated through this incision, an excellent view of the entire septum and maxillary crest, starting at the most anterior aspect of the cartilage, is obtained. This exposure also facilitates the harvesting of a large intact segment of septal cartilage for use as graft material in septorhinoplasty. We leave at least a 1.5-cm anterior and dorsal strut and resect the remaining cartilaginous and bony septum. The septal mucosal flaps are reapproximated with a 4-0 chromic quilting stitch, and Silastic stents are placed. We have not had an increased incidence of perforation, bleeding, septal hematoma, adhesions, or persistent nasal obstruction after using this technique.

Saddle nose deformities following septoplasty are caused by overresection and destabilization of the cartilaginous dorsum or septum. Reconstruction of the deformity requires augmentation with a stable, enduring material. Alloplasts, cartilage, and calvarial bone have all been used, and all differ in regard to resorption, warping, extrusion, and availability.

Alloplastic substances resist resorption but, as mentioned, have fallen out of favor because of their tendency to erode underlying bone or extrude through soft tissue. Drs. Porter and Toriumi favor autogenous cartilage from the ear or rib. Costal cartilage has a tendency to warp secondary to internal elastic forces, and both auricular and septal cartilage are relatively fragile and limited in supply (9). Furthermore, the harvesting of rib cartilage is inherently risky, associated with pneumothorax and prolonged pain.

We favor autologous bone over cartilage. Autologous bone, which is available from rib, iliac crest, tibia, and calvarium, provides rigidity and excellent support. Our primary graft choice is calvarial bone. The embryonic origin of calvarium is membranous rather than endochondral (10). Endochondral bone comprises most of the axial skeleton and arises from a cartilaginous precursor, whereas membranous bone in the cranium develops directly from mesenchymal tissue (10). The resorption rates of membranous bone are lower than those of endochondral bone (11). This is possibly a consequence of the earlier revascularization of membranous bone. Others have hypothesized that differences in morphology are responsible, with a thicker cortical plate, a smaller endocortical cancellous region, and stronger intracortical struts found in membranous bone (10).

Calvarial grafts are easily accessible beneath the scalp and lie within the same operative field. The harvest site is relatively pain-free and the scar well hidden. Unlike previous authors, we find less resorption with calvarium, and it is easy to sculpt the graft with an otologic cutting drill.

In our review of 35 consecutive cases, calvarial bone proved to be versatile and reliable, with easy harvesting, excellent contour, and a minimal long-term complication rate (12). A long-term follow-up of 363 cranial bone grafts for nasal reconstruction by Jackson et al. (13) reaffirmed the value of the technique. Graft resorption was absent, the donor site hidden and painless, and the shape excellent (13).

Adhesions, or synechiae, result from the apposition of disrupted mucosal surfaces of the septum and lateral nasal wall. Our routine use of Silastic splints until 1 week postoperatively has minimized this problem. Their function as a barrier is important; postoperative nasal mucosal congestion and edema decrease with time, so that the two sides no longer abut.

Little need be added to the section on turbinate surgery. As the authors point out, the causes of turbinate hypertrophy are numerous, and many treatment strategies are available, all of which share the goal of maximizing the nasal airway and minimizing nasal complaints (e.g., dryness).

Medical management should be optimized before surgery is considered. The many surgical options available vary in regard to associated risks and complications, invasiveness, and duration of symptomatic improvement. In general, one must weigh more aggressive or destructive procedures to optimize the nasal airway (e.g., total turbinate resection) against the risks for complications. The incidence of bleeding and atrophic rhinitis increases with more radical procedures, whereas the likelihood of suboptimal relief of nasal blockage increases with more conservative procedures. We find out-fracture and cautery of hypertrophic turbinates to be a simple and effective procedure associated with minimal morbidity.

Unfavorable outcomes of nasal septal and turbinate surgery are not uncommon, and "avoidance and treatment" are maximized by clinical acumen and good surgical technique. When complications are encountered, strong diagnostic and problem-solving skills are imperative. Always keep in mind that patients differ in regard to protoplasm, lifestyles, and external influences. Addressing the individual patient along with the disease process will optimize appropriate care and a successful outcome.

REFERENCES

1. Jahn AF. How I do it: a simple eversion flap for repair of small septal perforations. *J Otolaryngol* 1994;23:69–70.
2. Yousef M. Repair of nasal septal perforation. *Am J Rhinol* 1997;11:35–40.
3. Delaere PR, Guelinckx PJ, Ostyn F. Vascularized temporoparietal fascial flap for closure of a nasal septal perforation. Report of a case. *Acta Otorhinolaryngol Belg* 1990;44:47–49.
4. Vuyk HD, Versluis RJ. The inferior turbinate flap for closure of septal perforations. *Clin Otolaryngol* 1988;13:53–57.
5. Romo T 3rd, Jablonski RD, Shapiro AL, et al. Long-term nasal mucosal tissue expansion use in repair of large nasoseptal perforations. *Arch Otolaryngol Head Neck Surg* 1995;121:327–331.
6. Murrell GL, Karakla DW, Messa A. Free flap repair of septal perforation. *Plast Reconstr Surg* 1998;102:818–821.
7. Kridel RWH, Foda H, Lunde KC. Septal perforation repair with acellular human dermal allograft. *Arch Otol Head Neck Surg* 1998;124:73–78.
8. Montgomery WW. Surgery of the nose. In: *Surgery of the upper respiratory system.* Baltimore: Williams & Wilkins, 1996: 476–478.
9. Duncan MJ, Thomson HG, Kent-Maneer JF. Free cartilage grafts: the role of perichondrium. *Plast Reconstr Surg* 1984; 73:916–923.
10. Smith TD, Abramson M. Membranous vs. endochondral bone autografts. *Arch Otolaryngol* 1974;99:203–205.
11. Zins JE, Whitaker LA. Membranous vs. endochondral bone: implications for craniofacial reconstruction. *Plast Reconstr Surg* 1983;72:778–784.
12. Cheney ML, Gliklich RE. The use of calvarial bone in nasal reconstruction. *Arch Otol Head Neck Surg* 1995;121:643–647.
13. Jackson IT, Choi HY, Clay R, et al. Long-term follow-up of cranial bone graft in dorsal nasal augmentation. *Plast Reconstr Surg* 1998;102:1869–1873.

SUGGESTED READING

Jackson LE, Koch RJ. Controversies in the management of inferior turbinate hypertrophy: a comprehensive review. *Plast Reconstr Surg* 1998;103:300–312.

Motoki DS, Mulliken JB. The healing of bone and cartilage. *Clin Plast Surg* 1990;17:527–544.

56

LASER FACIAL RESURFACING

THOMAS L. ROBERTS III
JASON N. POZNER

The introduction of lasers to plastic surgery has provided us with another tool to combat aging. Lasers are a two-edged sword; when used properly, they can help produce remarkable results, but when used improperly, like any tool, they can cause problems.

We believe that well-trained plastic surgeons can easily master the technique of laser resurfacing; however, this skill must be combined with a commitment to intensive postoperative care. Unfortunately, the changing face of health care has brought lasers into the hands of physicians not adequately trained in their use and unable to handle the complications that may arise. This situation has delighted the media, giving them graphical material that can be sensationalized, and has resulted in some distrust of lasers by the general public, not unlike the attitude toward silicone breast implants in the early 1990s. Fortunately, the pendulum has now swung back to a more moderate position, and laser resurfacing for the most part is being performed with greater forethought by properly trained persons who are able to manage complications. The technology is such that most problems, unlike those associated with other plastic surgery procedures, do not occur during the actual surgery. Proper patient selection and attention to detail in the postoperative period can avoid most complications. We hope that this chapter will serve as a guide to physicians currently performing or learning laser resurfacing, and that the information presented herein will be used to *prevent* complications or identify and treat them early enough that significant sequelae do not arise.

HISTORY

The era of laser resurfacing began in the United States in 1994 with the introduction of the UltraPulse carbon dioxide (CO_2) laser by the Coherent Medical Group (Palo Alto, California) (1–3). This laser offered high-energy pulses of short duration, which maximized the ablation of unwanted tissue and minimized undesirable thermal effects. In contrast, the older continuous-wave or superpulsed lasers had created uncontrolled thermal damage that often resulted in hypertrophic scarring. The first national plastic surgery presentation on laser resurfacing was by Roberts in 1995 (4). Other companies began producing lasers that similarly minimized the duration of the laser-tissue interaction and the thermal damage to skin (1,5,6). The initial systems used a manual hand piece and had a small spot size (3 mm), an arrangement that proved to be extremely operator-dependent. Occasionally, too much overlap of spots increased thermal damage and resulted in hypertrophic scarring (7). The development of the computer pattern generator made it possible to control spot overlap and minimize the possibility of thermal damage caused by operator error.

The erbium:yttrium-aluminum-garnet (Er:YAG) lasers were introduced as an alternative to CO_2 lasers (8,9). Their affinity for water is much greater than that of the CO_2 lasers, so that skin ablation can be accomplished with much less thermal damage. The Er:YAG lasers were initially promoted for use in younger patients in place of light chemical peels, but they are now used as an alternative to CO_2 lasers in some centers in patients with fine wrinkling because the recovery period is quick and the incidence of hypopigmentation lower.

At present, progress is being made in using CO_2 and Er:YAG lasers together and in developing long-pulse Er:YAG lasers. Investigators hope to combine the ablative technology of the Er:YAG laser with the dermal remodeling and tightening offered by the CO_2 laser. Because long-term clinical use of these lasers is limited, the complication rates have not been fully assessed, although we assume that they will be similar to those for CO_2 and Er:YAG lasers used individually. The goal is to develop a laser that will provide the same dramatic tightening as the CO_2 laser without causing prolonged erythema and delayed hypopigmentation.

TECHNICAL CONSIDERATIONS AND SAFETY

Carbon dioxide and Er:YAG lasers are extremely complex instruments that must be maintained appropriately. If the

T. L. Roberts III: Department of Surgery, Medical University of South Carolina, Spartanburg, South Carolina
J. N. Pozner: Boca Raton Community Hospital, Boca Raton, Florida

laser beam is not aligned properly, inadequate or uneven beam distribution may cause the operator to misjudge the tissue level; in a worst-case scenario, too deep or irregular resurfacing and possibly hypertrophic scarring can result. We know of no cases of problems caused by machine malalignment but surmise that they may arise as the lasers age or change hands. We mention this to remind everyone that lasers are complex instruments that require routine maintenance for safe use. The beam should be checked on a wet wooden tongue blade before each session. The sound and the pattern imprinted will often alert the experienced surgeon to technical problems.

Many reports of safety guidelines for laser use have been published (2,10–13). The two concerns that are most important to plastic surgeons are eye safety and avoiding fires.

Eye protection for the patient and operating room personnel is mandatory (14). Specific lenses for each wavelength are available and should be used for optimal safety. Laser-safe nonreflective metal eye shields should be placed on the patient before periorbital or full facial resurfacing. The sandblasted surface diffuses any laser reflection. Plastic shields should not be used because the laser beam may melt the plastic and cause ocular injury. Patients undergoing only perioral or cheek resurfacing may wear laser-safe goggles. Nonreflective laser-safe instrumentation should also be used to prevent beam reflection.

Fires are possible whenever oxygen is used around the laser. Laser-safe endotracheal tubes or tubes wrapped in crushed (less reflective) aluminum foil should be used to prevent tube injury and combustion. If nasal cannulas are used, it is preferable to wrap them in aluminum foil and place them deep into the pharynx to decrease the oxygen concentration around the nose and mouth. The use of wet drapes and gauze around the face is recommended to prevent accidental fire. Needless to say, operating room explosions or fires can be deadly, and proper prevention is essential.

PATIENT SELECTION

Favorable results in laser surgery stem as much from proper patient selection as from proper technique and aftercare (15–18). A few but important contraindications to laser resurfacing are the following:

1. *Recent or current use of isotretinoin (Accutane).* Laser-resurfaced wounds are reepithelialized by the migration of cells from sebaceous glands, hair follicles, and other skin appendages. Agents that interfere with normal secretory function can impair reepithelialization and possibly lead to scarring. Accutane inhibits secretory function even after the patient has stopped using it. Current recommendations are to discontinue Accutane for 6 to 24 months and then be certain that the skin has clinically recovered. We insist on waiting at least 6 months after skin oiliness and moisture have recovered completely. We feel that this physiologic endpoint is more important than the time that has elapsed since Accutane treatment. We successfully treated several patients off Accutane for less than 1 year previously whose skin oiliness and moisture had recovered immediately; likewise, we have refused to treat patients off Accutane for as long as 3 years because their normal skin oiliness and moisture had not recovered.
2. *Extensive electrolysis or scleroderma.* The wound healing of patients who have undergone extensive facial electrolysis may be impaired because of damaged follicles. Similarly, the appendage function of patients with scleroderma may be impaired.
3. *Active infection.* Patients should not undergo resurfacing if they have active bacterial or viral infections. When resurfaced, the skin temporarily loses its barrier function and can be easily contaminated.
4. *Herpes zoster.* In patients with a history of facial herpes zoster (shingles), an outbreak of infection or post-herpetic neuralgia can result in prolonged severe pain following resurfacing. A history of facial herpes zoster is not a contraindication to resurfacing, but the facial area previously involved should not be resurfaced.
5. *Unrealistic expectations.* Patients who believe that laser resurfacing will substitute for a facelift or who have other unrealistic expectations should be screened carefully.

Relative contraindications to laser resurfacing include red "lipliner" tattoo and "sensitive skin." Laser resurfacing may remove some of the lipliner pigment, and reapplication may be required. Patients with sensitive skin usually cannot tolerate soap and must use hypoallergenic products. Laser resurfacing can result in chronically irritated skin, pain, and intolerance to previously tolerated products.

PITFALLS OF RESURCFACING

The complications of laser resurfacing that stem from the actual procedure can usually be avoided with proper training, conservative surgical judgment, and careful lasering (12). Since the introduction of the computer pattern generator, the evenness of resurfacing has improved dramatically because the problem of excessive or inadequate overlapping of spots, inherent to the use a manual hand piece, has been eliminated. However, excessive treatment can still be applied with the computer pattern generator if the patterns overlap.

It is important to avoid an excessive number of passes with the CO_2 laser. Studies have not shown any benefit to more than three passes with the Coherent laser. Dehydration of tissues and denaturation of surface tissue prevent further ablation and lead to increased thermal damage and the risk for hypertrophic scarring. With the Er:YAG laser, care must be taken to keep a record of the number and depth of passes; otherwise, one can enter the subcutaneous tissues without any warning signs. Similarly, skin thickness, fluence, and the ablative thresholds of the laser must be understood if one is to obtain enough total fluence to ablate to the correct depth.

Careful lasering is important to avoid burning eyelashes. Wet Q-tips are useful to hold eyelashes while the periorbital area is lasered. Lasering 1 to 2 mm into the fine hair of the eyebrows and 3 to 5 mm into the fine hair at the margins of the forehead is advised. The immediate regrowth of these hairs helps blur the demarcation line of the pink lasered skin and the white nonlasered skin and makes camouflage much easier. Some physicians prefer to apply 30% trichloracetic acid into the eyebrows and hairline to blur the demarcation line.

Obvious demarcation lines can turn an otherwise good result in which rhytids are eradicated into a less satisfactory outcome (Fig. 56-1). If a few guidelines are adhered to, obvious demarcation lines can be avoided or at least minimized with the CO_2 laser:

1. *Perform full facial resurfacing whenever possible.* Doing so avoids a change of color or texture in adjacent areas of the face, especially in men, who usually do not like to wear camouflage makeup in the postoperative period. The only regional CO_2 laser resurfacing we perform now is periorbital, which can be easily disguised by glasses or makeup.
2. *Fade (feather) the resurfacing* **over** the jaw line and into the shadow under the jaw to hide any color or texture step-off when full facial resurfacing is performed. The jaw line should be marked preoperatively with the patient in an upright position, and allowances should be made for skin shrinkage. After resurfacing, the previous jaw line mark is often pulled upward as the CO_2 laser tightens the facial skin, and the lower margin of resurfacing must be reassessed after the whole face is treated. The mark may be elevated by 0.5 to 2 cm, depending on the thickness of the skin, number of passes made, and fluence used.
3. *If regional resurfacing is performed, laser only one area.* Do **not** resurface two noncontiguous areas (i.e., periocular **and** perioral) because a "clown"-type mask will be evident for as long as the erythema lasts. To resurface an isolated area, laser one aesthetic unit and fade the resurfacing into the adjacent unit to avoid a sharp demarcation line.

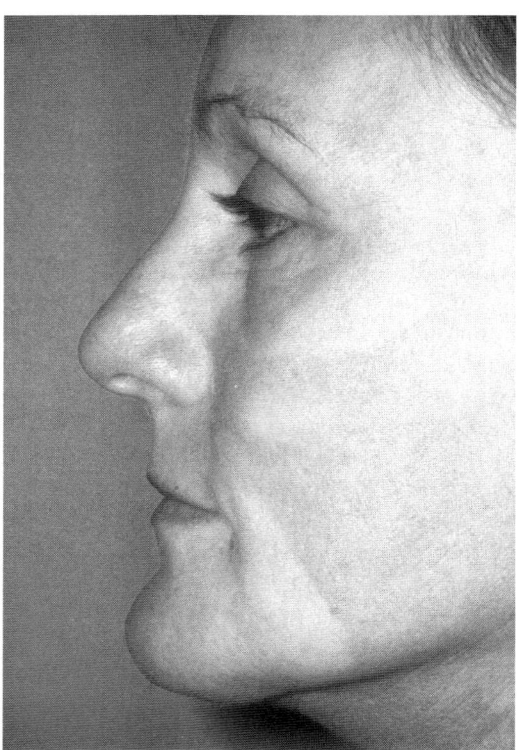

FIGURE 56-1. Demarcation lines from periorbital and perioral regional resurfacing, 1 year postoperatively.

For more superficial resurfacing, the duration of erythema is shorter, fewer textural changes are produced, and the risk for hypopigmentation is less with the Er:YAG laser than with the CO_2 laser. Results of regional resurfacing are much more acceptable with the Er:YAG laser, even when discontinuous areas are lasered. Some textural differences may be apparent between lasered and nonlasered adjacent areas, but they will not be as noticeable as with the CO_2 laser.

POSTOPERATIVE CARE

We believe that proper postoperative care is the key to successful laser resurfacing and therefore to a happy, satisfied patient (19). Problems caught early in the postoperative period can often be minimized, whereas those recognized late are more difficult to resolve. Needless to say, the physician must be involved in the postoperative care, and the task not completely delegated to the nursing staff.

We strongly believe that a "closed" postoperative care regimen (i.e., use of a semipermeable membrane dressing) is preferable to an "open" method (i.e., use of ointments and soaks only); healing is less painful and faster, and the likelihood of patient error is less. Others disagree, arguing that an open approach is associated with a lower infection rate, is cheaper, and requires less nursing care. We refer the readers to our selected references to choose the method that suits their practice best. We suggest that if a "closed" approach is chosen, dressings be kept intact and changed at regular intervals to avoid contamination and possible infection. In any case, the lasered wound must be kept moist until epithelialization is essentially complete (3 to 7 days, depending on the depth of treatment).

Minor Complications

Acne

We try to pretreat all patients who have adult acne with tretinoin (Retin-A) and any other agents necessary to suppress active acne before resurfacing (15–17,19). This helps to minimize postoperative flare-ups, which are a disturbing and dramatic, although temporary, setback (Fig. 56-2). Acne is relatively rare, occurring in up to 3% of patients. Activation of the appendages often causes hypersecretion, which leads to acne in susceptible persons. Avoiding comedogenic products postoperatively is also helpful. Treatment entails discontinuing occlusive agents and using topical Retin-A and glycolic acids with or without tetracycline.

Synechiae

A synechia is an adhesion created when two deepithelialized portions of skin heal together. It occurs most frequently in the lower eyelid and under a dressing and can be avoided by stretching the skin taught as the dressing is applied. We have found synechiae to more common with the Er:YAG laser, although this is purely anecdotal and may be related to the use of thinner dressings following Er:YAG resurfacing. Treatment, which should be initiated as early as possible, consists of pulling the skin bridge apart with cotton-tipped applicators. If the epithelial bridge is allowed to persist, inflammation and possibly even cyst formation can occur. Figure 56-3 shows the typical appearance of a synechia as a crease or white line on the lower lid. The synechia in Fig. 56-4A was not diagnosed until 2 weeks postoperatively, and the adhesion had to be snipped with fine scissors (Fig. 56-4 B–D). Fortunately, the subsequent "tight phase" of skin healing helped remodel the skin to an acceptable appearance.

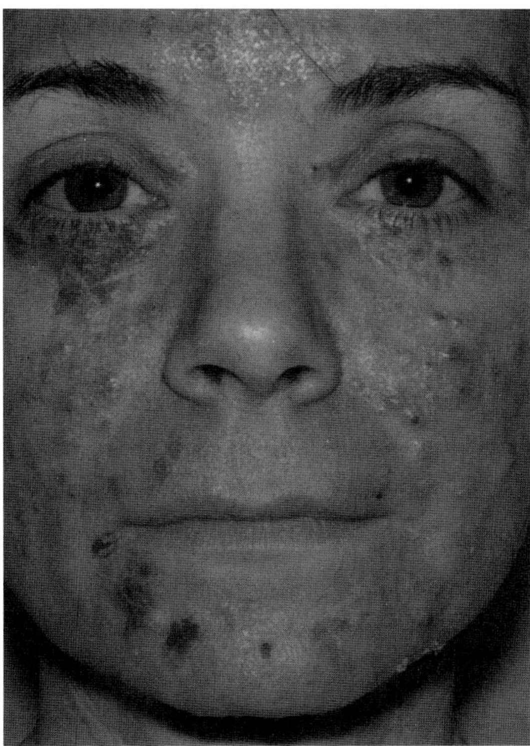

FIGURE 56-2. Acute eruption of acne discovered 7 days postoperatively on removal of opaque, adhesive, semipermeable dressing.

Milia

Milia (tiny white bumps not surrounded by erythema) represent sweat or oil glands whose openings have been sealed over in the reepithelialization process (Fig. 56-5). They are extremely common after resurfacing and should be opened with a fine needle. Patients should be told not to manipulate any acne or milia, either mechanically or with dermatologic products, because the skin is delicate and healing may be delayed.

Transient Hyperpigmentation

Transient hyperpigmentation has been reported in 8% to 30% of patients following CO_2 laser resurfacing, depending primarily on the mixture or skin types in the population. The Fitzpatrick skin types IV and V (which often include the Asiatic, Mediterranean, African-American, and Japanese ethnic groups) are much more likely to become hyperpigmented than the fairer-skinned Fitzpatrick types I through III, although hyperpigmentation can occur in any skin type (Fig. 56-6). Anecdotal evidence suggests that the incidence may be higher following Er:YAG resurfacing, although this may represent earlier exposure to the sun because the shorter healing phase allows a faster return to normal activities. Hyperpigmentation may occur even in the absence of sun exposure. The cause is a migration of metabolically active

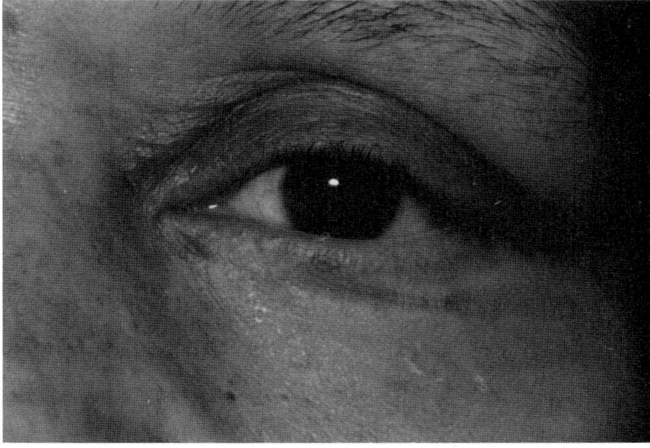

FIGURE 56-3. Typical appearance of a synechia (epidermal adhesion) 1 week following resurfacing.

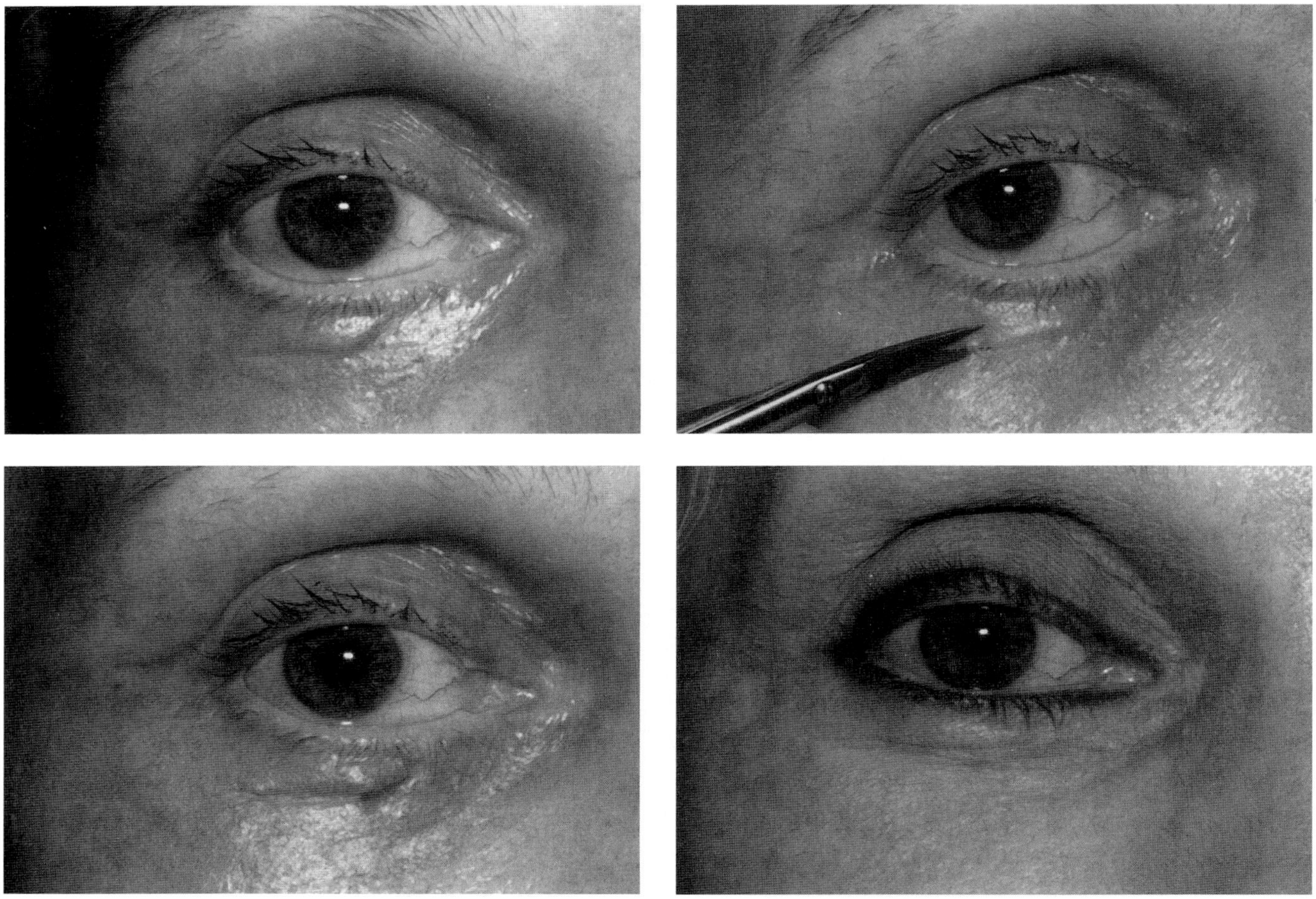

FIGURE 56-4. **A:** Synechia presenting as an unusual crease. It was first noticed 2 weeks following resurfacing. **B:** Same patient. The epidermal bridge is snipped with fine scissors under magnification. **C:** Same patient immediately after release of the synechia. **D:** Same patient 6 months postoperatively.

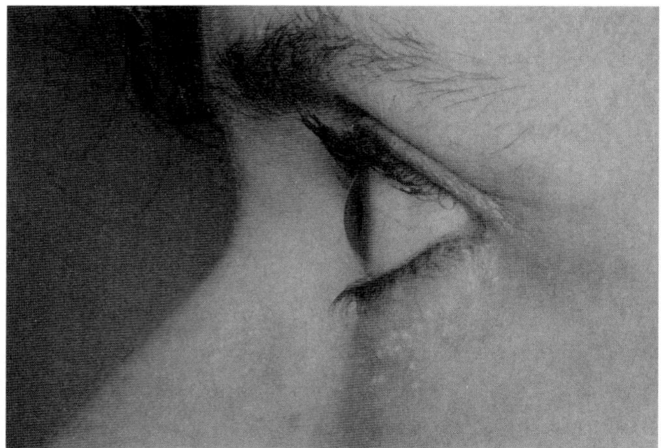

FIGURE 56-5. Multiple milia of lower eyelid 2 months after resurfacing.

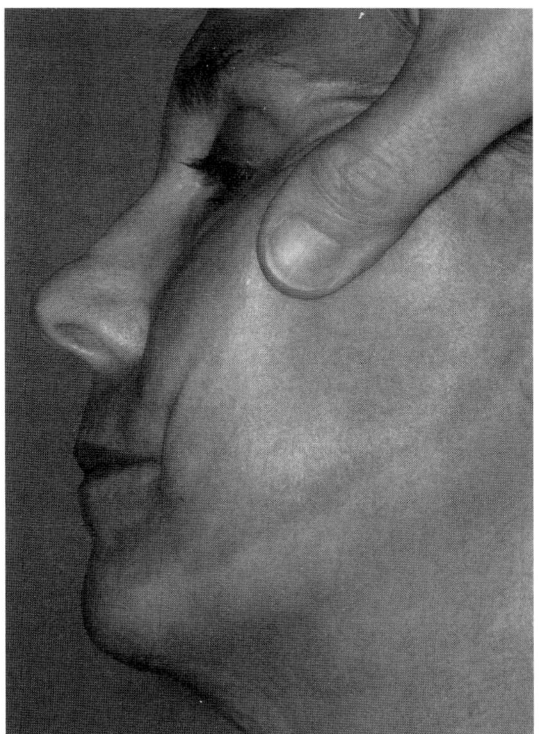

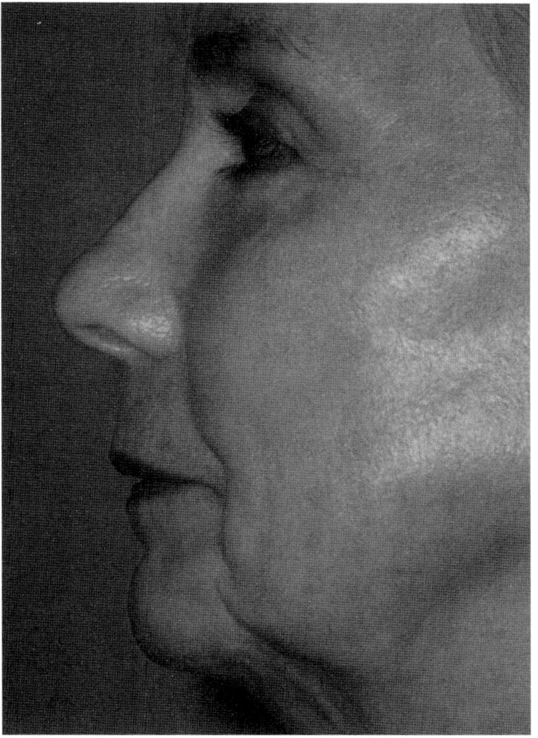

FIGURE 56-6. A: Hyperpigmentation of the entire face 4 weeks after resurfacing. **B:** Complete resolution of hyperpigmentation in same patient after 4 weeks of treatment with retinoic acid and hydroquinone.

melanocytes that are producing new melanin. The process may start as early as 3 weeks following resurfacing and may persist for many months if left untreated.

Whether pretreatment with bleaching agents is necessary before laser resurfacing is controversial. We know of no controlled studies comparing pretreatment with no pretreatment. The argument for pretreatment stems from the chemical peel literature, which is not directly applicable to laser resurfacing. The argument against pretreatment is that the bleaching creams act only on epidermal melanocytes, which are removed on the first laser pass. When practical, the authors prefer to pretreat the Fitzpatrick IV and V skin types with Retin-A and hydroquinone for 6 to 8 weeks if the skin is oily, or for 2 to 3 weeks if the skin is dry.

Although the efficacy of pretreatment in preventing hyperpigmentation is questionable, there is little question that prophylaxis with hydroquinone following epithelialization is effective in reducing the incidence of hyperpigmentation. Our usual treatment regimen is to prescribe glycolic acids and 4% hydroquinone with or without kojic acid twice a day for patients with fairer skin types. Treatment is started 2 weeks following resurfacing and continued for 6 to 8 weeks. If pigmentation persists or is marked, Retin-A can be added at 4 weeks. It is applied every third night and then nightly as tolerance increases. Overly aggressive treatment may lead to irritant dermatitis. Breakthrough pigmentation is treated with increasing concentrations of agents. Patients should be counseled that hyperpigmentation will resolve even without treatment, but that use of the aforementioned regimen will minimize the incidence and degree. We have personally never seen hyperpigmentation persist beyond 8 weeks if treatment is prompt and appropriate.

Patients should apply a hypoallergenic physical sunblock such as titanium dioxide, wear a hat, and avoid both indirect and direct sun exposure, at least until erythema has subsided. Patients often need to be reminded that ultraviolet light penetrates automobile windows and that the sunblock should be applied before travel.

Itching

Itching following laser resurfacing is not an uncommon phenomenon. The key is to avoid subsequent scratching and mechanical trauma. The use of a "closed" postoperative regimen minimizes itching in the epithelialization phase. Topical hydrocortisone or systemic diphenhydramine (Benadryl) or hydroxyzine (Atarax) may be necessary to minimize itching following epithelialization.

Mechanical Trauma

Punctate or linear excoriations or petechial hemorrhages may result from scratching (Fig. 56-7), mechanical trauma (e.g., with a comb) or a Valsalva maneuver (protracted vomiting). We require patients to wear soft cotton gloves at night to minimize manual excoriation during sleep. Scratching areas of itching is the most common cause of petechial hemorrhage, and the resultant red marks may take 3 to 6 weeks to subside.

Irritant Dermatitis

Irritant dermatitis has been reported in up to 7% of patients. In contrast to contact dermatitis, it is not a true allergic reaction, but rather a skin irritation that is usually caused by topical caustic agents. Irritant dermatitis usually occurs following epithelialization because potentially irritating creams are not usually used before this phase. The most common offending agents are Retin-A and bleaching creams, although toners, sunscreens, and glycolic or other alpha-hydroxy acids are also potential irritants. The usual presentation is an increase in redness in the first or second weeks following epithelialization. Treatment is discontinuation of the irritating agent. If there is any question regarding which agent is causing the irritation, discontinue all products and use only a simple cleanser such as Cetaphil.

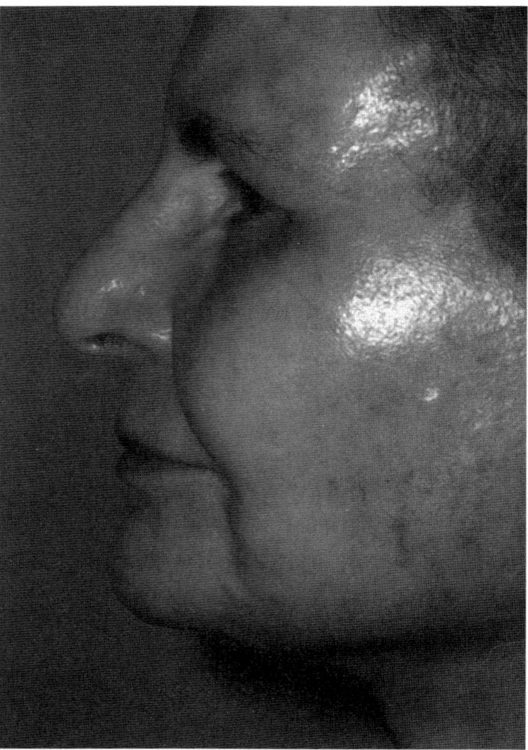

FIGURE 56-7. Petechial hemorrhages as a manifestation of mechanical trauma (scratching) 4 weeks after resurfacing.

Severe irritation may lead to erosions and possible hypertrophic scarring.

Often, irritant dermatitis develops when patients commence their own skin care regimen despite warnings from the plastic surgeon to follow guidelines. Patients have told us of using a certain product for many years without problems but then experiencing severe irritation after using it too soon following epithelialization. Patients need to be made aware of the delicate nature of their new skin. As a general rule, we ask patients not to follow their own regimen for 3 months after resurfacing (with the exception of eyeshadow, eyeliner, and lipstick, which can be worn at 2 to 4 weeks).

Acne Rosacea

Acne rosacea is an incompletely understood inflammatory condition that may be stimulated or triggered by resurfacing. It can lead to sebaceous hypertrophy and prominence of blood vessels, which appear clinically as scattered, red papules or pustules and telangiectasia. Treatment may include topical agents such as metronidazole. Response is variable, and a dermatologic consultation is recommended if the diagnosis is unclear or the condition persists. Severe and chronic forms of acne rosacea can lead to rhinophyma, which is best treated with laser resurfacing.

Telangectasia, Dermal Thinning, and Textural Changes

The quality of the skin is changed following laser resurfacing. Removal of sun-induced pigmentary and dermal changes often produces an initial thinning of the skin and a more translucent quality. This may result in the visible appearance of small veins that previously went unnoticed (Fig. 56-8). Telangiectases present before resurfacing or resulting from capillary fragility may also cause patient dissatisfaction. Telangiectasia is treated with a pulsed dye laser when healing is complete.

Textural changes may become noticeable when regional resurfacing is performed and strikes another argument for full facial resurfacing. Proper blending is important to avoid distinct changes in texture. Treatment entails the use of retinoic acids or even resurfacing the previously unlasered areas.

Major Complications

Skin Eruptions

Bacterial, fungal, and viral infections and contact dermatitis all present with the same clinical picture—new onset of pain and deterioration in the appearance of the skin (7,17,18–21). The symptoms may occur during or after epithelialization. Specimens from any new raw, red, weepy areas with or without exudate should be Gram's-stained and

A 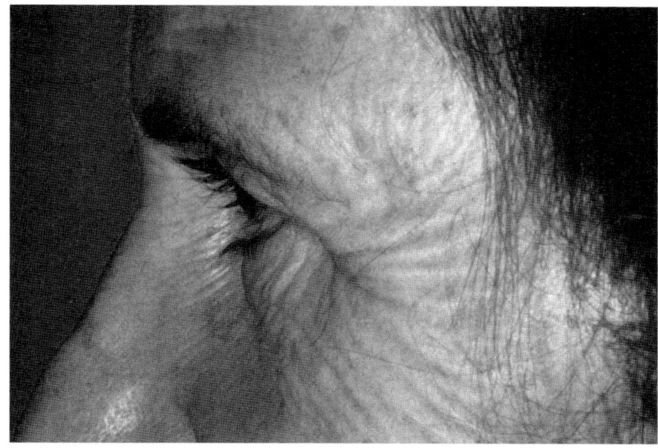

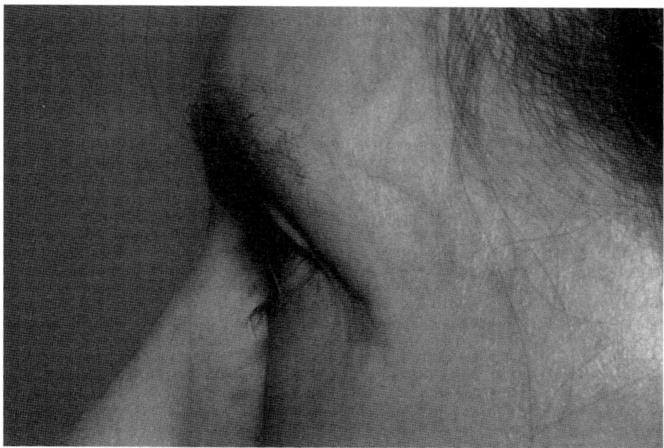 B

FIGURE 56-8. A: Temple area in 65-year-old woman exhibits rhytids and actinic damage. **B:** Same patient, with veins now visible in temple, 6 months after resurfacing, endoscopic browlift, and lower blepharoplasty.

stained for fungi, and cultures should be taken. Appropriate *systemic* (not topical) therapy must be initiated without delay. The patient with these clinical findings plus marked swelling, but with negative Gram's stain and fungal stain results, should be considered to have contact dermatitis. All topical treatments should be stopped and a Medrol Dosepak begun.

Infections are rare following laser resurfacing. Early anecdotal experience has indicated that antibiotic and antiviral prophylaxis decreases the incidence of bacterial and viral infections, respectively. However, we know of no controlled studies specifically aimed at laser resurfacing.

Early detection of infections is the key to successful treatment. Delay may lead to a more severe infection and resultant scarring. Dressings will usually not adhere if an infection is present. If the presence of an infection is questionable, remove the dressings and change to an open technique with warm Pedi-Boro Soak Paks (Pedinol Pharmacal).

Bacterial Infections

The incidence of bacterial infections following CO_2 resurfacing is less than 1% in large series. To the best of our knowledge, no large series have determined the rates after Er:YAG resurfacing, but we suspect they would be similar for resurfacing at the same depth. The offending organism usually cultured is *Staphylococcus aureus.* Methicillin-resistant *S. aureus* infection has been reported in three patients who underwent resurfacing in a hospital setting. *Pseudomanas* infection has also been reported in patients with sinus colonization.

The usual prophylaxis recommended is a first-generation cephalosporin such as cephalexin (Keflex). Antibiotics are usually started the night before surgery and continued until epithelialization is complete. We often also administer intravenous antibiotics just before resurfacing.

Warning signs of bacterial infection include a marked increase in erythema, especially if the erythema was starting to subside. Eruptions are unusual, and the infective process usually resembles a weeping cellulitis (Fig. 56-9). Aerobic and anaerobic cultures should be taken and a broad-spectrum antibiotic started until organisms and sensitivities have been determined. If *Pseudomonas* is suspected, treatment with ciprofloxacin is begun. Severe infections may require hospitalization and treatment with intravenous antibiotics.

Fungal Infections

Fungal infection follows laser resurfacing in fewer than 1% of patients in large series. The most common cultured organism is *Candida albicans.* Suspect signs are similar to those in bacterial infection—a delay or setback in wound healing with new onset of pain (Fig. 56-10). A slimy white exudate may be present and is pathognomonic, but its absence does not rule out infection. Unfortunately, treatment is often begun late because fungal infection is often not considered. Cultures and fungal stains should be obtained and treatment with a systemic oral antifungal agent begun [e.g., 100 mg of fluconazole (Diflucan) daily] if hyphae are seen. Topical agents are not effective.

Viral Infections

The rates of viral infection after laser resurfacing have been reported to be around 3% if prophylaxis is not given and below 1% with prophylaxis. Herpes simplex virus type 1 is usually cultured, although infection with varicella-zoster virus has been described. Current recommendations are to give either 400 mg of acyclovir (Zovirax) four times daily, 500 mg of valacyclovir (Valtrex) twice daily, or 500 mg of famciclovir (Famvir) twice daily. Treatment is begun 1 day before surgery and continued until after reepithelialization is complete (about 10 days). Patients with active herpes infections should not undergo resurfacing until the infection

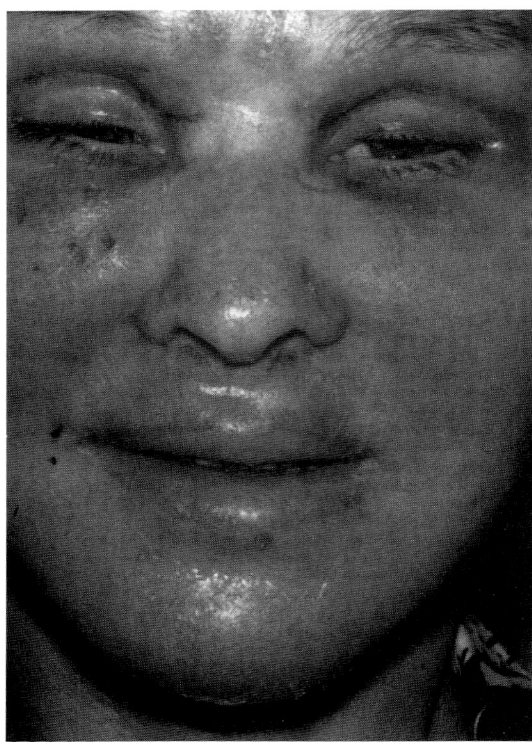

FIGURE 56-9. Bacterial infection (*S. aureus*) on postoperative day 7.

has subsided. Patients with a history of herpes zoster in the treated area may experience a recurrence of neuralgia postoperatively, which may persist for some time. Patients with a history of herpes zoster should undergo resurfacing with caution.

Herpes infections do not usually present with typical vesicles because epithelialization is not complete. The usual presentation is one of discrete, punched-out, punctate ulcerations (Fig. 56-11), but discrete areas of weeping skin

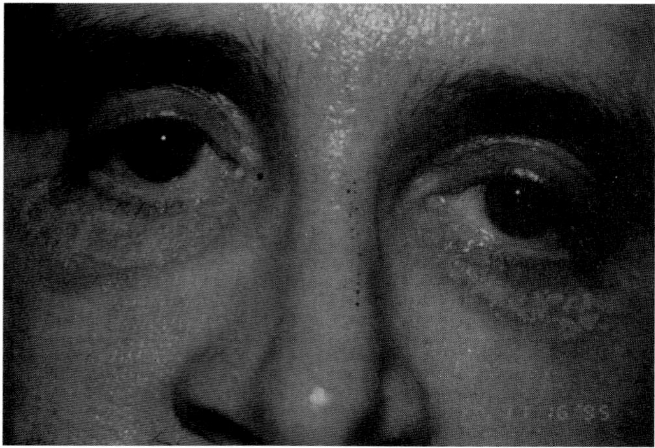

FIGURE 56-10. Fungal infection (*C. albicans*) on postoperative day 5.

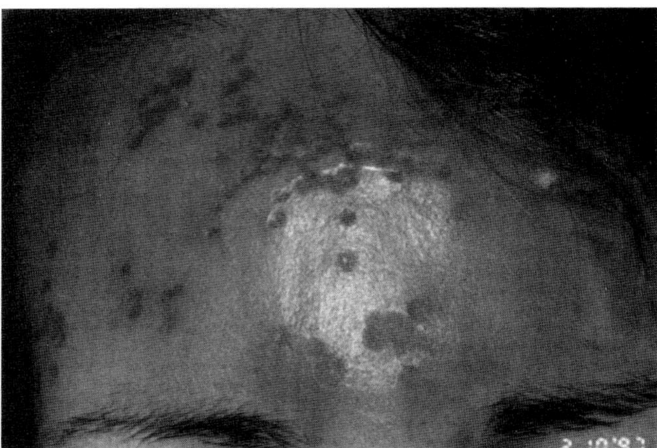

FIGURE 56-11. Typical appearance of viral infection (herpes simplex) 2 1/2 weeks after resurfacing.

that previously were healing well may also develop. If viral infections are not treated promptly, permanent scarring can result. If viral infection is suspected, viral cultures may be taken, but treatment is started empirically by increasing to therapeutic doses of acyclovir (800 mg every 4 hours), valacyclovir (1,000 mg four times daily), or famciclovir (1,000 mg four times daily). Topical acyclovir ointment can be added but should not be the only mode of therapy. More severe infections may require hospitalization and intravenous acyclovir.

Contact Dermatitis

The appearance new pain and a deterioration of skin quality together with marked swelling suggests contact dermatitis (Fig. 56-12). Contact dermatitis is a true allergic reaction caused by the removal of the normal epidermal barrier and exposure of the Langerhans cells to topical antigens. It has been reported in about 1% of cases but was more frequent in the early era of resurfacing, when multiple products were being tried. Most commonly, contact dermatitis develops when topical antibiotic ointment is used, although we have seen it in association with the use of petrolatum jelly, moisturizers, and makeup. It usually appears before epithelialization and presents as a deterioration in wound healing. Contact dermatitis mimics an infectious process, and the diagnosis is often by exclusion. It may develop as late as 4 weeks and present as sudden swelling, weeping, crusting, and discomfort (Fig. 56-13). Treatment is discontinuation of all topical agents except water soaks. Oral and topical steroids may be useful. (We use oral dexamethasone plus a topical high-potency steroid cream.)

Scleral Show and Ectropion

Temporary scleral show following laser treatment has been reported in up to 3% of patients, permanent scleral show in

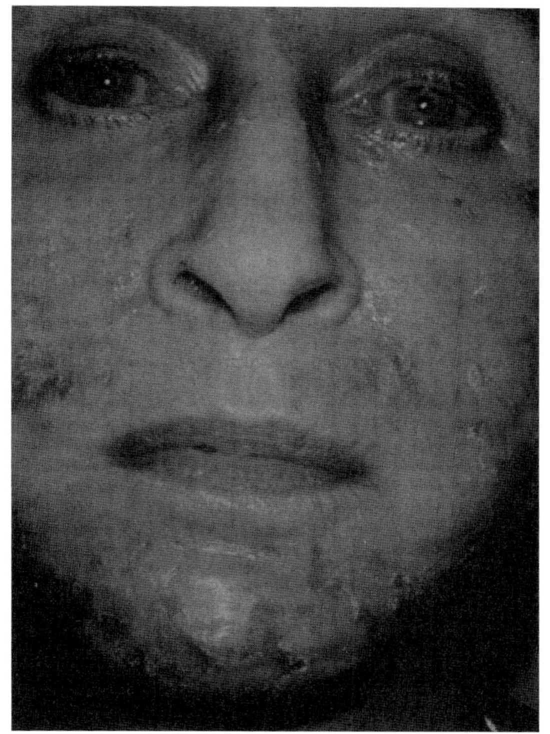

A

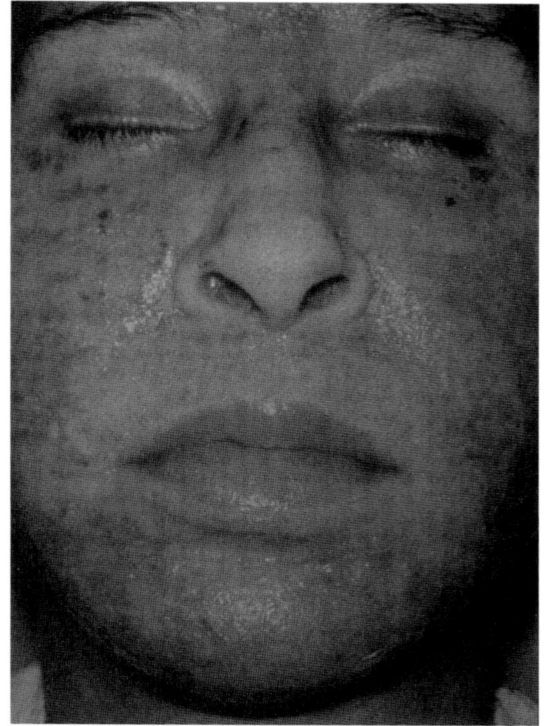

B

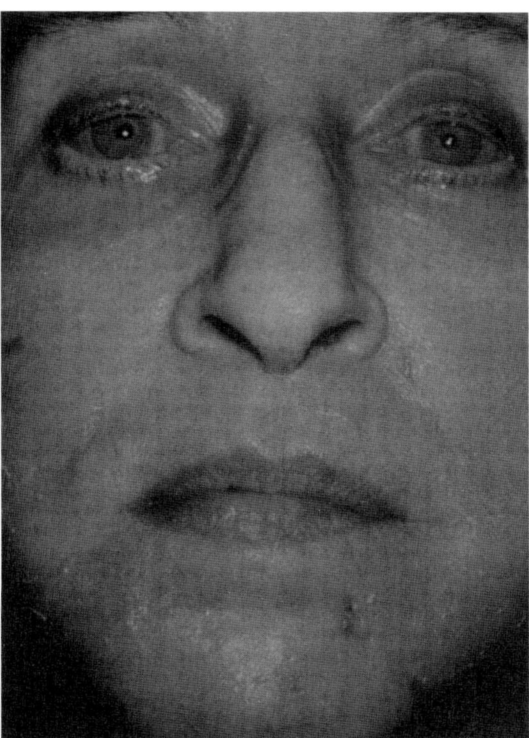

C

FIGURE 56-12. A: Patient 5 days after resurfacing. Note that upper lip is completely healed. **B:** Same patient 3 days later. Contact dermatitis has developed in response to application of ointment. Note deterioration of upper lip and medial cheeks and massive swelling of lips. **C:** Same patient after 5 days of oral and topical steroids, plus withdrawal of all topical treatments except water soaks.

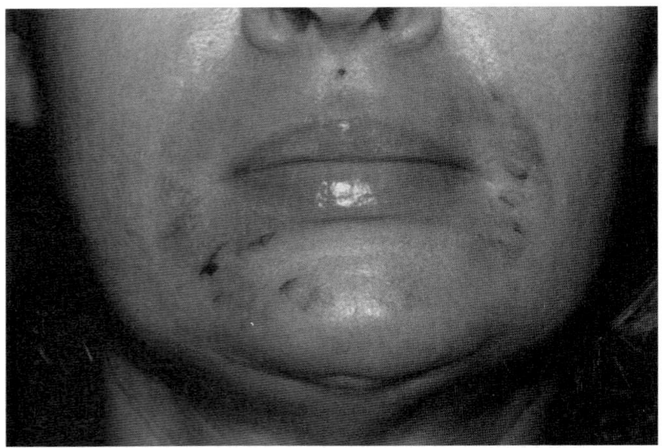

FIGURE 56-13. This patient's face was completely healed at 2 weeks. Contact dermatitis then developed in response to commercial makeup.

up to 2% of patients, and true ectropion in 0.3% of patients in large series (7,14,15,17,21,22). Patients who have previously undergone blepharoplasty (Fig. 56-14) are at risk for scleral show or ectropion, as are patients with shallow orbits or hypoplastic inferior orbital rims, so that on lateral view the inferior orbital rim is several millimeters posterior to the cornea ("negative variance"). Preoperative testing of lid laxity is essential in all patients, regardless of age, to avoid problems in the lower lids. We find the "snap test" to be unreliable (12,14,23). To obtain a quantitative evaluation of lid laxity, we recommend the following: The patient is told to relax the frontalis, levator, and orbicularis muscles. The lower lid is pulled down firmly for 5 to 10 seconds, then gently released. If it takes 5 seconds or more for the lid margin to regain contact with the globe, lid tightening must be performed. The authors' preferred method is lateral canthal suspension. This technique restores about 1 mm of lost canthal elevation, gives excellent support to the lower lid, and has reduced by two-thirds the incidence of minimal scleral show (8%) in comparison with traditional blepharoplasty. No cases of ectropion have occurred since this technique was implemented.

The treatment for mild scleral show is massage and watchful waiting. Most cases resolve without treatment. Mild ectropion can be treated with a temporary tarsorrhaphy suture, but significant ectropion or persistent scleral show greater than 1 to 2 mm should be treated by an appropriate lid shortening or suspension technique.

Hypertrophic Scarring

Hypertrophic scarring is the most dreaded complication of laser resurfacing. Large series report an incidence of approximately 1% (Fig. 56-15). It was more common in the early days of resurfacing, when the use of single-spot hand pieces was associated with excessive overlapping of spots. The introduction of the pattern generator solved many of the problems of overlap. Reports showing that an excessive number of passes caused an increase in thermal deposition without better resurfacing led to a refinement of methods with less scarring. Scarring is caused by a number of factors:

1. *Thin skin.* All skin is not created equally. A failure to detect thin skin preoperatively may lead to excessively deep resurfacing and resultant scarring. Great care should be taken to resurface thin skin conservatively. The skin of elderly patients is often thin, but young people may have genetically thin skin.
2. *Damage or dysfunction of skin appendages.* All healing after resurfacing is a race between the formation of normal epithelium and scar epithelium. Anything that causes a decrease in the quantity or quality of the skin appendages tilts the balance in favor of scar epithelium.

   Oral isotretinoin causes the sebaceous glands, which are necessary for wound healing, to dysfunction. Current

A

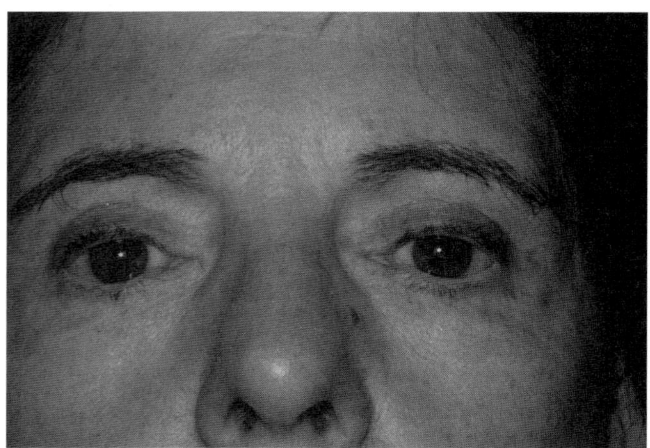

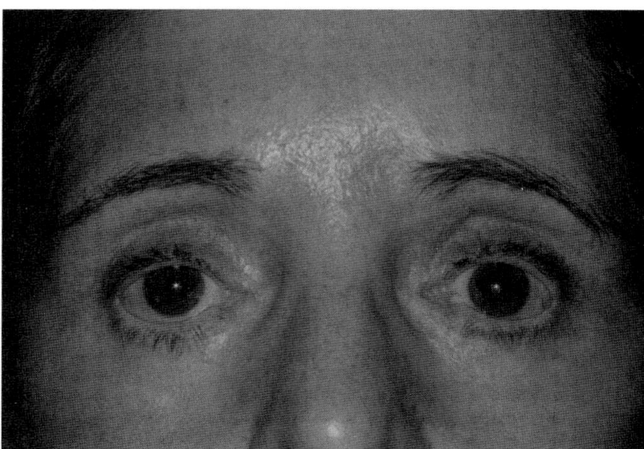

B

FIGURE 56-14. A: Patient with previous blepharoplasty; lid laxity was overlooked before resurfacing was performed. **B:** Same patient 3 weeks after resurfacing; scleral show took 4 months to resolve completely.

A 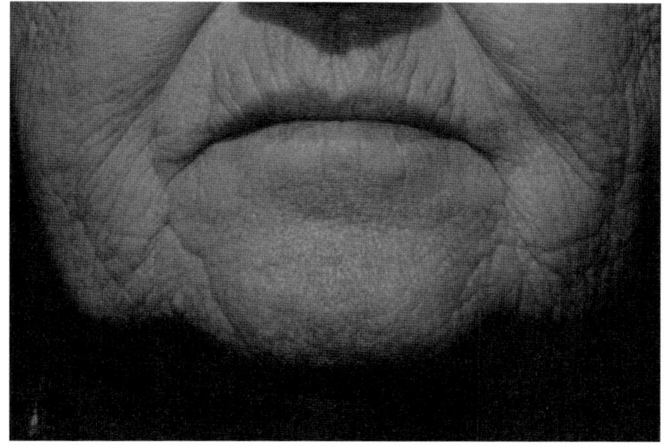

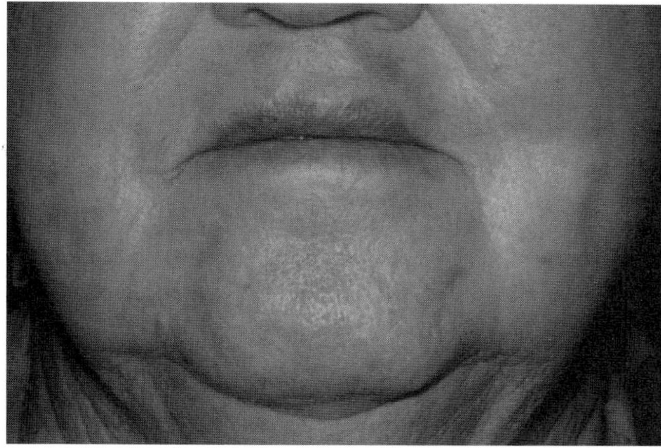 B

C 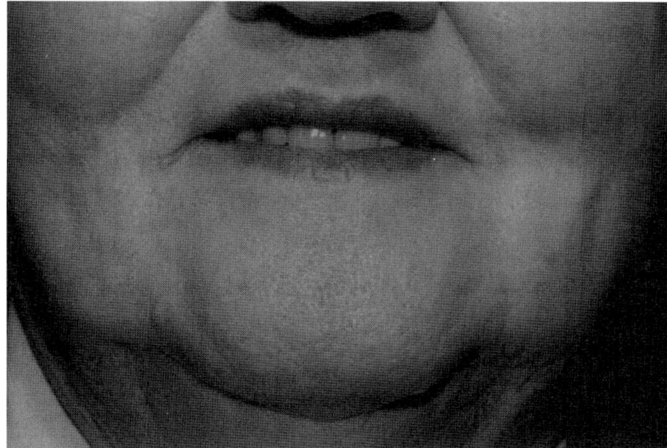

FIGURE 56-15. A: Extremely deep perioral rhytids. **B:** Same patient 4 months following aggressive resurfacing; note flat plaque of hypertrophic scarring on left upper lip and small scar nodule on left midchin. **C:** Same patient with complete resolution of scarring 1 1/2 years postoperatively, after intralesional steroid injections, pulsed dye laser treatments, and application of silicone gel sheeting.

recommendations are to discontinue oral isotretinoin for 6 months to 2 years before resurfacing and then to assess the patient's skin for evidence of sebaceous gland function. (Please see our detailed recommendations in the section on patient selection.)

Extensive electrolysis damages to hair follicles, which also contain accessory glands necessary for proper wound healing following resurfacing. Patients who have had extensive electrolysis should undergo resurfacing with caution.

3. *Infection,* especially if left untreated, can lead to areas of hypertrophic scarring. Treat infections early and aggressively.
4. *Poor technique* results in excessive overlap, too many passes, and thermal damage, all of which increase the risk for scarring. Proper training and careful lasering are essential to good results.
5. *Scratching* can convert a controlled second-degree wound into a third-degree wound with a potential for scarring.
6. *Poor postoperative care* can lead to wound desiccation and a deeper wound, which may lead to scarring.
7. *Neck or hand resurfacing.* The skin of the neck and dorsum of the hands is very thin and has far fewer appendages than are necessary for proper healing following resurfacing. Published reports of neck resurfacing with the CO_2 laser cite an excessively high incidence of hypertrophic scarring (24,25). We do not recommend laser resurfacing of the neck or hands.
8. *Overzealous use of retinoic acid* has been reported to cause erosions, which lead to hypertrophic scarring. Patients should start (or restart) retinoic acid cautiously following epithelialization. We prefer not to begin retinoic acid until 4 weeks postoperatively. It is at first applied every third night until tolerance develops; application is then increased to every other night and finally every night.
9. *Lasering over undermined flaps* may cause devascularization and resultant scarring if not performed cautiously (26–31). Flap vascularity, skin thickness, and thermal effect of the laser chosen should all be considered.

Detection and Treatment of Hypertrophic Scarring

The most important single step to minimize scarring is to feel the entire lasered area gently with the fingertips as soon as epithelialization is complete, and at each subsequent examination. In this way, a small area of induration can be detected 2 months before a scar may be visible. When an induration is detected, we begin careful intralesional injections of dilute (5 mg/mL) triamcinolone acetonide (Kenalog) with a 27- or 30-gauge needle under a magnification of 2.5 to 4. Care is taken not to rupture the epidermis or inject into the subcutaneous tissue. The area is inspected and injected again weekly until the first sign of softening occurs (not disappearance). If the induration does not soften after 4 weekly injections at a concentration of 5 mg/mL, we gradually increase the concentration. Silicone sheeting is used nightly, and difficult lesions are also treated with a pulsed dye laser.

Hypopigmentation

Hypopigmentation is a late phenomenon that occurs in up to 30% of patients following CO_2 resurfacing (Fig. 56-16). Many initial studies reported lower rates of hypopigmentation, but we believe this was because of a short follow-up. The degree of hypopigmentation does not become apparent until after 8 to 10 months and can gradually worsen. True hypopigmentation should be distinguished from the removal of darker, abnormal pigment and sallow color associated with solar damage. We encourage patients to avoid solar exposure following resurfacing, so that their skin color tends to lighten. Some practitioners compare the color of the resurfaced face with the color of the inner upper arm (an area with minimal solar exposure). If the facial color is similar to the arm color, true hypopigmentation does not exist. If the facial color is paler than the arm color, then hypopigmentation is present. This test is useful only as a guide because a great variety of skin colors is found in each person. It is difficult to determine the risk factors, but hypopigmentation is probably related to depth of resurfacing and possibly to the degree of dermal heating. Two theoretical causes of hypopigmentation are melanocyte dysfunction and dermal fibrosis. The melanocyte dysfunction theory suggests that resurfacing irreversibly damages melanocyte function. The dermal fibrosis theory suggests that scar tissue (fibrosis) created in the dermis changes the light reflex of the skin and accounts for the shiny, pale appearance. The fact that hypopigmentation is a late phenomenon somewhat supports the dermal fibrosis theory; the maturation of the collagen during a 1- to 2-year period could change the light reflex and subsequent appearance. At present, the only way to minimize the chance of hypopigmentation is to laser more conservatively. We hope to have enough hard data soon to determine whether the same degree of tightening and improvement in deep wrinkles can be obtained with the newer lasers (Er:YAG, the combined short- and long-pulse Er:YAG, and the combined CO_2 and Er:YAG) as with the CO_2 laser, and if so, whether the same high-quality results can be obtained with a lower incidence of hypopigmentation. A minimum follow-up of 9 months is necessary to obtain these important answers.

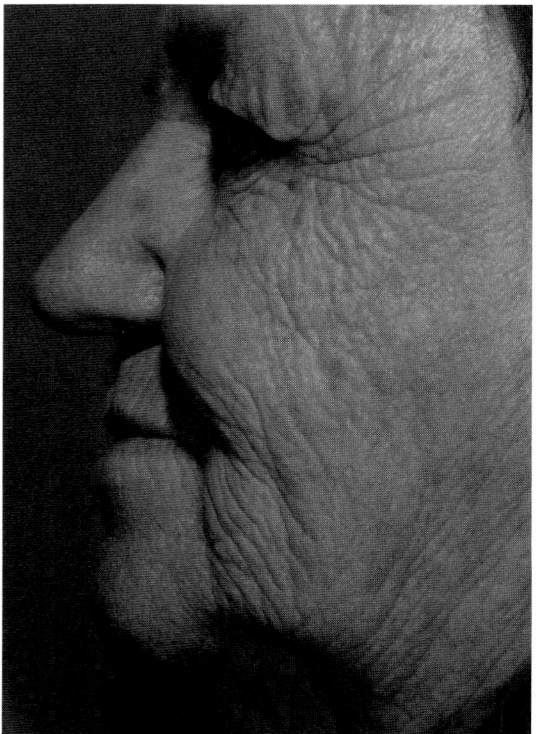
A

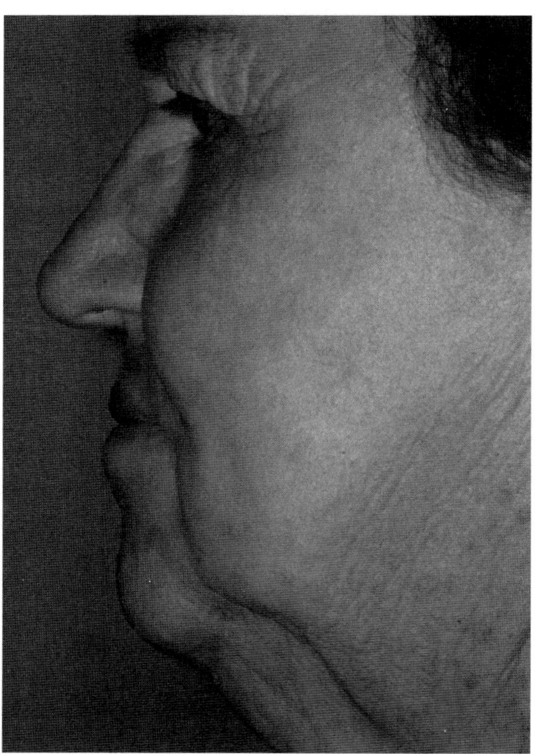
B

FIGURE 56-16. A: Same patient as in Fig. 54-15, with deep facial rhytids preoperatively. **B:** Same patient 1 year after aggressive resurfacing, with smooth skin; however, hypopigmentation and a distinct demarcation line are present.

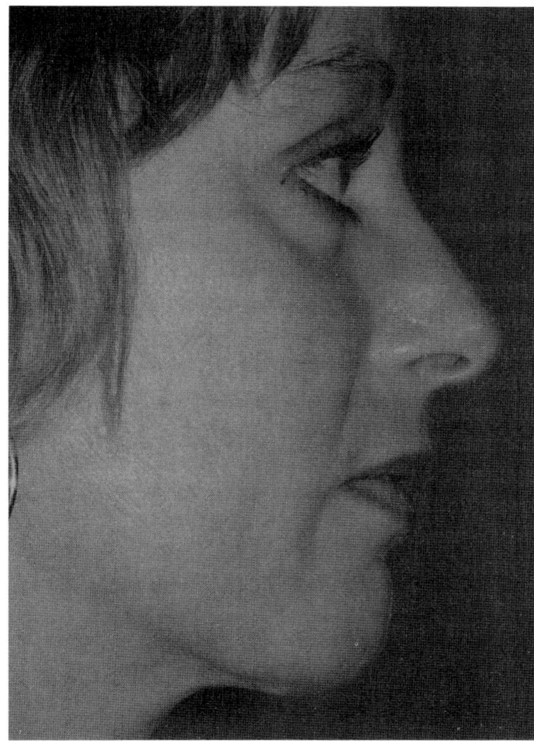

FIGURE 56-17. Visible demarcation line resulting from hypovascularity 10 months after conservative resurfacing of perioral region in a patient with very pink skin of central face.

Hypovascularity

Regional laser resurfacing in patients with pink or ruddy skin may result in a sharp demarcation line that resembles hypopigmentation (Fig. 56-17). On closer evaluation, this demarcation line is not caused by a loss of pigment (a white-brown demarcation line) but by coagulation of the dilated vessels in the uppermost dermis (a white-pink demarcation line).

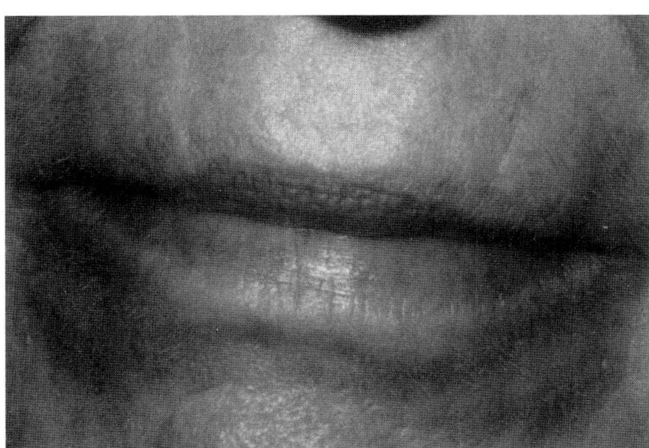

FIGURE 56-18. Loss of vermilion color (hypovascularity) of upper portion of upper lip 1 year following aggressive resurfacing across the vermilion border.

The vermilion of the lip is subject to this phenomenon. Figure 56-18 shows a patient from early in our experience who underwent two to three passes over the vermilion border. The vermilion skin is thin, and only one pass is necessary to improve vermilion wrinkles.

Hypovascularity is generally not evident for at least 6 to 9 months, when all erythema has subsided. The treatment of regional demarcation lines is to resurface the rest of the face with the same parameters. Vermilion color loss can be corrected only by tattooing with red lipliner.

INADEQUATE RESULTS

Inadequate results following laser resurfacing may be caused by poor patient selection, inadequate casing, or unrealistic expectations on the part of both patient and physician. Laser resurfacing is not an alternative to facelifting in the treatment of aging (27–29,31). Plastic surgeons have a significant advantage in comparison with other specialists in that we are able to offer patients a wide variety of procedures. Facelift, blepharoplasty, browlift, fat grafting, Botox, and other procedures may be needed to complete the rejuvenation process. If laser resurfacing is offered as merely another tool in our armamentarium rather than as a miracle treatment, and if patients are informed candidly about how they will look during the healing process and about potential results and limitations, then dissatisfaction is less likely to occur.

Inadequate lasering can be corrected in a subsequent treatment. A certain degree of edema may mask some of the rhytids, so that patients believe their rhytids have recurred when the edema subsides. A second treatment may be initiated at about 3 months, although it is advisable to wait up to a year for final collagen remodeling to occur. Earlier resurfacing does not allow adequate time for final results to become evident.

REFERENCES

1. Anderson RR. Laser-tissue interactions. In: Fitzpatrick RE, Goldman MP, eds. *Cutaneous laser surgery.* St. Louis: Mosby, 1994.
2. Goldman L, Rockwell RJ Jr. *Lasers in Medicine.* New York: Gordon and Breech, 1971.
3. Trost D, Zacherl A, Smith MFW. *Surgical laser properties and their tissue interaction.* St. Louis: Mosby, 1992.
4. Roberts TL. *The ultrapulsed CO_2 laser: an important new tool in the aesthetic plastic surgeon's armamentarium.* Presented at the annual meeting of the American Society for Aesthetic Plastic Surgery, San Francisco, California, March 1995.
5. Roberts TL. Invited discussion of Stuzin JM, Baker TJ, Baker TM, et al. Histologic effects of the high-energy pulsed CO_2 laser on photodamaged facial skin. *Plast Reconstr Surg* 1997;99:2051.
6. Stuzin JM, Baker TJ, Baker TM, et al. Histologic effects of the high-energy pulsed CO_2 laser on photodamaged facial skin. *Plast Reconstr Surg* 1997;99:2036.

7. Weinstein C. Carbon dioxide laser resurfacing: long-term follow-up in 2123 patients. *Clin Plast Surg* 1998;25:109.
8. Bass LS. Erbium:YAG laser skin resurfacing: preliminary clinical evaluation. *Ann Plast Surg* 1998;40:328.
9. Weinstein C. Computerized scanning erbium-YAG laser for skin resurfacing. *Dermatolog Surg*1998;24:83.
10. American National Standards Institute. *American national standards for the safe use of lasers in health care facilities.* Standard Z136.3. New York: ANSI Publications, 1988.
11. Ossoff D, Karlan MS. Safe instrumentation in laser surgery. *Otolaryngol Head Neck Surg* 1984;92:644.
12. Roberts TL, Weinstein C. *Aesthetic laser surgery: blepharoplasty and management of the lax lower lid* [Videotape]. St. Louis: Mosby, 1996.
13. Sliney DH, Wolbarsht ML. *Safety with lasers and other optical sources.* New York: Plenum Publishing, 1980.
14. Roberts TL, Laser blepharoplasty and laser resurfacing of the periorbital area. *Clin Plast Surg* 1998;25:95.
15. Roberts TL, Pozner JN. Aesthetic laser surgery. In: Achauer BM, Eriksson E, Guyuron B, Coleman JJ III, Russell RC, Vander Kolk CA, eds. *Plastic surgery: indications, operations, outcomes.* St. Louis: Mosby, 1999:2457–2486 (*Aesthetic surgery,* vol 4).
16. Roberts TL, Lettieri JT, Ellis LB. CO_2 laser resurfacing: recognizing and minimizing complications. *Aesthetic Surg Q* 1996; 16:142.
17. Weinstein C, Ramirez OM, Pozner JN. Carbon dioxide laser resurfacing complications and their prevention. *Aesthetic Surg J* 1997;17:216.
18. Weinstein C, Roberts TL. Aesthetic skin resurfacing with the high-energy ultrapulsed CO_2 laser. *Clin Plast Surg* 1997;24:379.
19. Weinstein C, Ramirez OM, Pozner JN. Postoperative care following CO_2 resurfacing: avoiding pitfalls. *Plast Reconstr Surg* 1997;100:1855.
20. Fitzpatrick RE, Goldman MP. CO_2 laser surgery. In: Fitzpatrick RE, Goldman MP, eds. *Cutaneous laser surgery.* St. Louis: Mosby, 1994.
21. Roberts TL, Weinstein C, Alexandrides JM, et al. Aesthetic laser surgery: evaluation of 907 patients *Aesthetic Surg J* 1997;17:293.
22. Roberts TL. The emerging role of laser resurfacing in combination with traditional aesthetic plastic surgery. *Aesthetic Plast Surg* 1998;22:75.
23. Roberts TL, Yokoo K. In pursuit of optimal periorbital rejuvenation: laser resurfacing with or without blepharoplasty and browlift. *Aesthetic Surg J* 1998;18:321.
24. Goldberg D. Treatment of neck and hand photoaged skin with the erb:YAG laser. *Lasers Surg Med Suppl* 1998;10:33.
25. Rosenberg G. Full face and neck laser skin resurfacing. *Plast Reconstr Surg* 1997;100:1846.
26. Guyuron B, Michelow B, Schmelzer R, et al. Delayed healing of rhytidectomy flap resurfaced with CO_2 laser. *Plast Reconstr Surg* 1998;101:816.
27. Ramirez OM, Pozner JN. Simultaneous full facial resurfacing at the time of facelifting. *Lasers Surg Med Suppl* 1997;9:60.
28. Ramirez OM, Pozner JN. Laser resurfacing as an adjunct to endoforehead lift, endofacelift, and biplanar facelift. *Ann Plast Surg* 1997;38:315.
29. Ramirez OM, Pozner JN. Subperiosteal minimally invasive laser endoscopic rhytidectomy: the SMILE facelift. *Aesthetic Plast Surg* 1996;20:463.
30. Roberts TL, Ellis C. In pursuit of optimal rejuvenation of the forehead: endoscopic browlift with CO_2 laser resurfacing. *Plast Reconstr Surg* 1998;101:1075.
31. Roberts TL, Ritter EM. *Facelift with simultaneous total facial laser resurfacing: can it be done safely?* Presented at the annual meeting of the European Association of Plastic Surgery, Verona, Italy, May 28–30, 1998.

Discussion

LASER FACIAL RESURFACING

PAUL J. CARNIOL

In a very well-written and informative chapter, Dr. Roberts has described how to avoid and treat the complications of laser resurfacing. Laser resurfacing for the treatment of actinic changes was first reported in 1989 (1). Since then, numerous reports about resurfacing have been presented, both in the literature and at meetings.

Initially, physicians were advised to laser until a chamois appearance of the tissue was achieved. This appearance was the result of thermal injury to the reticular dermis. Significant thermal injury in the reticular dermis can lead to healing problems, hypertrophic scarring (2), and hypopigmentation. In 1995, I presented the first modification of the resurfacing technique, intended to reduce the rate of thermally induced complications (3).

Paul J. Carniol: Department of Surgery, UMDNJ–The New Jersey Medical School, Newark, New Jersey and Overlook Hospital, Summit, New Jersey

LASER SAFETY

Laser safety is important. In 1980, the American National Standards Institute published its first guideline for laser safety. Since then, it has undergone revisions. The latest laser safety standard is Z136.3-1996 (4), which includes a description of laser policies and procedures. Recommendations for updating this standard are currently being drafted by the Laser Institute of America in Orlando, Florida.

The most common injuries related to laser procedures are ocular. Different portions of the eye tend to be injured by lasers of different wavelengths. Certain wavelengths, such as those of the argon, krypton, potassium titanyl phosphate (KTP), copper vapor, helium neon, and neodymium:YAG lasers, pass through the lens and injure the retina (5). These lasers, which are in the visible spectrum, are focused by the lens system on the retina. Focusing magnifies the effect of the laser 100,000 times (6). Use of the carbon dioxide (CO_2) or erbium:yttrium-aluminum-garnet (Er:YAG) laser puts the cornea at risk for injury.

Proper eye protection is important for all medical personnel as well as the patient. The protective eyewear for medical personnel should have an ocular density of at least 4 according to the 1996 ANSI standard. Ocular density is an inverse logarithmic scale. An ocular density of 4 means that at a specific wavelength, the laser light is reduced such that only 1/10,000 of the laser energy passes through the lens (6). Protective eyewear must protect the eyes from both direct and indirect, reflected laser energy. Protective eyewear must be appropriate for the particular wavelength in use. Protective eyewear that is inappropriate for the wavelength in use does not provide protection.

It is important that every facility in which lasers are used have a laser fire protocol (7) (Table 56D-1).

PATIENT SELECTION

Dr. Roberts emphasizes the importance of patient selection and lists five contraindications to resurfacing. A sixth relative contraindication should be added, which is prior radiation therapy. Radiation therapy can have a deleterious effect on both the blood supply and the pilosebaceous units and puts the patient at risk for delayed healing and hypertrophic scarring.

If for any reason a patient's ability to heal after laser resurfacing is in question, a punch biopsy can be taken of the skin. This can be used to evaluate the pilosebaceous units, or a laser test patch can be performed. Both of these techniques are helpful to assess healing, although they are subject to sampling error. Any patient who has a significant deficiency of the pilosebaceous units on biopsy or a significant healing problem on a test patch should not undergo resurfacing.

Other patients in whom healing may be difficult after resurfacing are those with significant rosacea. They are at risk for persistent erythema after resurfacing. Any resurfacing procedure must take this potential problem into consideration.

It is important that patients have appropriate expectations regarding the resurfacing procedure. The preoperative

TABLE 56D-1. LASER FIRE PROTOCOL

In the unlikely event that a laser fire develops, it is critical that the surgeon have a usable management protocol. The authors would recommend the following:

1. Simultaneously stop ventilation, disconnect endotracheal tube from breathing system, and remove endotracheal tube or remove cannula.
2. Mask ventilate with 100% oxygen.
3. Maintain anesthetic to facilitate injury assessment.
4. Apply iced saline-soaked compresses immediately to areas of thermal injury.
5. Use flexible nasal pharyngoscope or bronchoscope to survey upper airway and laryngeal tissues to evaluate injury and remove any large foreign bodies and carbon debris.
6. Use Betadine soap and copious irrigation to remove carbon debris from areas of first- and second-degree burns. Irrigate with copious amounts of water. Be diligent to prevent Betadine from entering orbital tissues.
7. Apply Xeroform gauze or bacitracin ointment to cutaneous areas with first- and second-degree burns.
8. If thermal injury has occurred to nasal airway, consider light packing with Xeroform gauze to stent airway and treat thermally damaged tissues.
9. After stabilizing patient and performing the initial evaluation, consider the following:
   - Administer intravenous steroids—12 mg Decadron (i.v. in adults).
   - Administer antibiotics (consider i.v. cephalosporin in adults if no contraindication exists).
   - Provide high-humidity environment and monitor oxygenation closely. Patient may require ventilator support if laryngeal edema is a potential hazard.
   - Consider chest radiography to assess pulmonary damage to baseline.
   - Consider advisability of ophthalmologic consultation for evaluation of ocular status and baseline.
   - Consider medical consultation to evaluate pulmonary status.
   - Provide for overnight observation regardless of degree of injury.

From Carniol PJ, ed, *Laser skin rejuvenation*. Philadelphia: Lippincott–Raven Publishers, 1998:60.

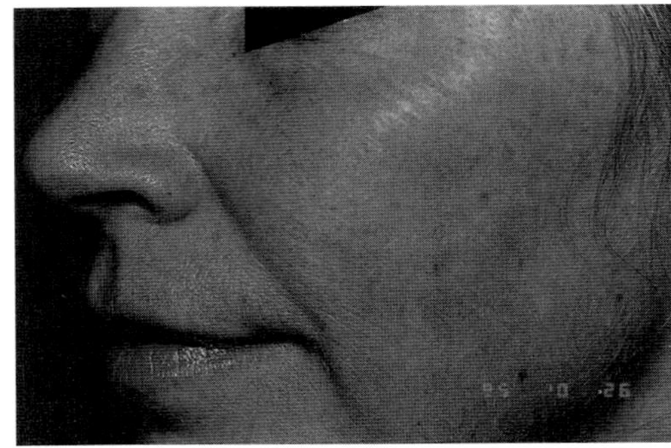

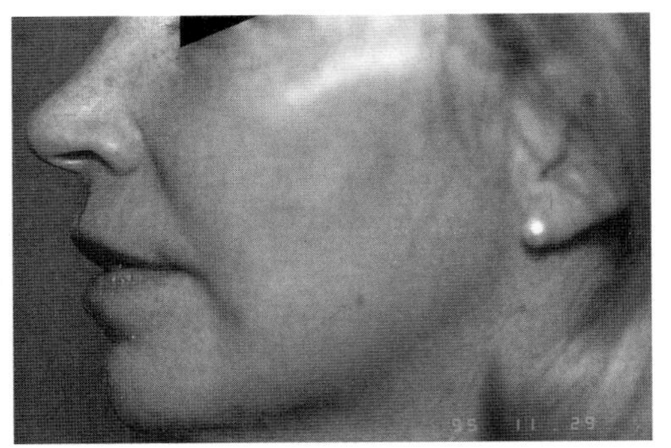

FIGURE 56D-1. A: This patient had significant skin changes of photoaging. **B:** The appearance of the patient's skin improved significantly after resurfacing. (From Carniol PJ, ed. *Laser skin rejuvenation.* Philadelphia: Lippincott–Raven Publishers, 1998:120.)

visit should include a candid discussion of the variability of potential results and the limitations of the procedure. Some deep rhytids extend significantly into the reticular dermis and will at least partially persist after the procedure.

Resurfacing can be used to treat facial photoaging, traumatic scars, and acne scars (Figs. 56D-1 and 56D-2).

PITFALLS IN RESURFACING

The technique for "feathering" the resurfacing margins with the CO_2 laser can be challenging. Each laser has an ablation threshold. If the fluence is set below the ablation threshold to try to "feather," the risk for thermal injury and scarring will be increased (8). It is important that the laser not be set below the ablation threshold to avoid this risk.

Some physicians combine resurfacing with trichloracetic acid peels at the resurfacing margins to blend or feather the laser margins. For those who favor this technique, it is important to mark the laser resurfacing margins and then apply the peel solution before resurfacing. Resurfacing should be performed only after the peel solution has dried and frosted. If the laser resurfacing is performed first, the peel solution may move into the adjacent already resurfaced area and cause an unpredictable degree of injury.

When the Er:YAG laser is used, feathering can be achieved more readily than with the CO_2 laser. This is achieved by performing fewer passes or using less fluence. With the Er:YAG laser, subablative fluence should not be used because it increases thermal injury. A current laser, the Contour (Sciton, Palo Alto, California) uses subablative erbium energy to increase the thermal effect and produce thermal injury in a controlled fashion. The goal of this technique is to stimulate neocollagen formation. Its efficacy in inducing neocollagen deposition is being compared with the efficacy of the more powerful ablative erbium lasers in a current study.

Between passes with the CO_2 laser, it is important to wipe away all desiccated tissue gently to avoid thermal stacking effects and increased thermal injury (9). When ablative fluence is used for the Er:YAG laser, it is not necessary to remove the desiccated tissue between passes. When subablative Er:YAG lasering is performed, as with the Sciton Contour laser, it is important not to overlap scans and to remove all desiccated tissue. Otherwise, thermal injury can be

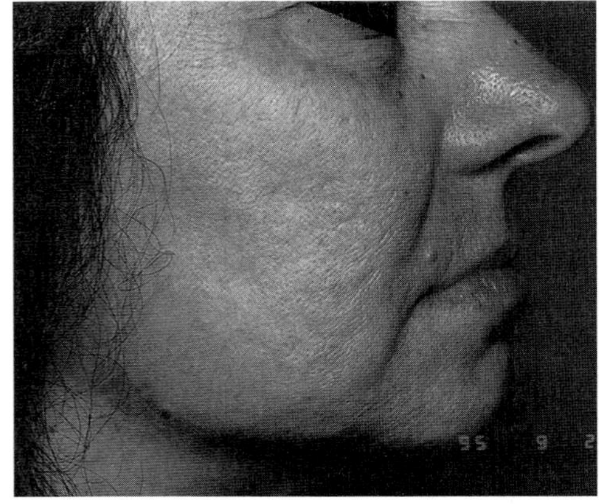

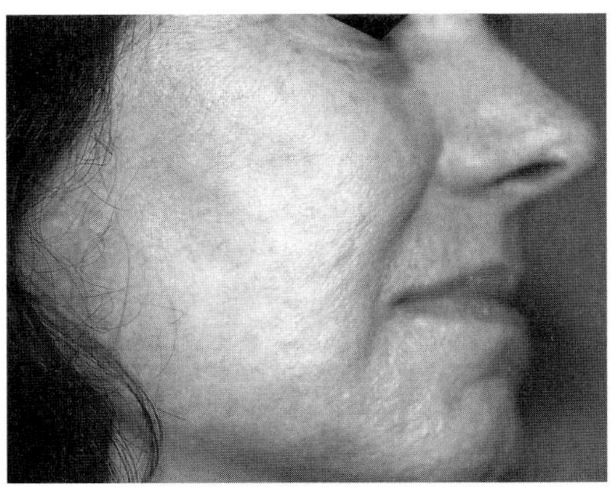

FIGURE 56D-2. A: This patient had significant acne scars, previously treated with dermabrasion. **B:** After two laser resurfacing treatments, her skin showed significant improvement. (From Carniol PJ, ed. *Laser skin rejuvenation.* Philadelphia: Lippincott–Raven Publishers, 1998:121.)

increased and thermal stacking effects produced, as with the CO_2 laser.

Another new technology uses coblation for resurfacing. In this process, a bipolar current is used to create an ionized plasma, which causes an energy-mediated cellular disintegration for resurfacing. This process has been used to treat both rhytids and actinic lesions. Preliminary trials have indicated that this new technology is efficacious, and histologic studies by Dr. Alastair Carruthers (10) have demonstrated that the risk for thermal injury-related complications is smaller than with current lasers.

POSTOPERATIVE CARE

I agree completely with Dr. Roberts about the importance of postoperative care. These patients need to be followed closely. Resurfacing is a process of controlled, partial-thickness injury. In the care of patients after resurfacing, many of the same issues are involved as in in the care of patients with other partial-thickness wounds, such as second-degree burn injuries of varying depth.

The descriptions that have been used by most physicians for wound care after resurfacing are technically inaccurate. "Closed" wound care has been used to describe occlusive dressings, whereas "open" wound care has been used to describe the use of ointments. Ointments actually create an occlusive "closed" environment.

Reepithelialization occurs more rapidly in a moist environment (11–13). Because a closed environment is more likely to become infected, it is important to remove all dressings and clean the wounds before reapplying dressings. I prefer to have the patients change their dressings at home daily. To be sure that the wounds are being properly cleaned along with the daily dressing changes, I have my patients return to the office 2 to 3 days after the procedure. In the office, we change the dressings, clean the wounds, and evaluate early wound healing.

Frequently, I use a hydrogel dressing for the first 3 days after resurfacing. These dressings provide a protective hypoallergenic cover for the wound and a moist environment. Once they are applied, the resurfacing wounds should be only mildy uncomfortable, not really painful. Most patients require only acetaminophen for pain relief. If a semipermeable membrane dressing is used after resurfacing, I recommend changing the dressing 48 hours after resurfacing.

Hyperpigmentation

Hyperpigmentation is common after laser resurfacing. This has been reported to occur as early as postoperative day 15 but usually develops 3 to 4 weeks after resurfacing (14).

To minimize the chance of hyperpigmentation after resurfacing, strict avoidance of the sun both preoperatively and postoperatively is important. I can only reiterate Dr. Robert's recommendation that the patient use a hypoallergenic titanium dioxide sunscreen. Titanium dioxide is a mechanical block for both ultraviolet A and ultraviolet B. The blocking effect on ultraviolet A is important in preventing hyperpigmentation after resurfacing (15). Because hydroquinones are potentially irritating and can prolong erythema after resurfacing, I do not use them routinely after resurfacing in patients with Fitzpatrick skin types I through III. Rather, these patients are followed closely, and if any sign of incipient hyperpigmentation appears, "bleaching agents" are started immediately. In my experience, if patients are followed weekly and treatment is initiated as soon as any minimal hyperpigmentation is noted, the hyperpigmentation responds readily to treatment.

In patients with the Fitzpatrick IV skin type, "bleaching agents" are used routinely before and after resurfacing. These patients are at a significantly greater risk for long-term dyschromia.

Long-term hypopigmentation after resurfacing is a more frequent problem than persistent hyperpigmentation. Hypopigmentation may develop as a result of injury to melanocytes during resurfacing or dermal fibrosis, or it may be caused by "bleaching agents."

Dyschromia is less common when more superficial resurfacing is performed. The actual depth of resurfacing equals the depth of tissue ablation and the depth of adjacent thermal injury.

Another issue is the role of the inflammatory response in delaying healing, prolonging erythema, and causing dyschromia. Some physicians advocate resurfacing down to the desired depth with a CO_2 laser, then using an erbium laser to remove the residual thermally injured tissue. They believe that removing most of the thermally injured tissue with the erbium laser shortens the inflammatory response (16,17).

Infection

The early diagnosis of infections after resurfacing is important. As discussed by Dr. Roberts, infections can present with an increase in erythema. This is most easily diagnosed when the erythema resulting from resurfacing has begun to subside. In some patients, the increased erythema may be difficult to recognize. Infections may also be heralded by the development of pain, burning, or stinging (18). Infection can lead to long-term healing problems and scarring. It is important to obtain cultures before a patient is started on antibiotics for an infection.

Most physicians who perform laser resurfacing use prophylactic antibiotics. The duration of postoperative antibiotic therapy is controversial. For surgical procedures, prophylactic antibiotics are typically started before surgery so that adequate blood levels have been achieved at the start of the procedure. The antibiotics are then discontinued within 48 hours after the procedure.

For laser resurfacing, many physicians advocate using "prophylactic antibiotics" until reepithelialization occurs. As of this writing, no controlled study has demonstrated that a 7- to 10-day course of antibiotics is more effective for "prophylaxis" than the standard regimen used for other surgical procedures. Using antibiotics for a longer period than is customary in prophylaxis may lead to the emergence of resistant organisms and hypersensitivity or increase the chance of a fungal infection.

Fungal infections may present with areas of localized erythema in addition to delayed healing with persistent erythema. The presentation can be subtle; therefore, a high index of suspicion is important in making the diagnosis. Because established fungal infections can be difficult to eradicate, the earlier the diagnosis is made, the easier it is to obtain a clinical response to therapy. Some physicians give prophylactic fluconazole to patients who undergo resurfacing.

Hypertrophic Scarring

The early diagnosis of hypertrophic scarring is important. It presents as areas of residual localized erythema with palpable thickening. Rather than first injecting triamcinolone acetonide (Kenalog) into the scar, I usually treat with a potent topical glucocorticosteroid for 1 week. Silicone paste is applied over the glucocorticosteroid to increase the penetration of the medication. After the week of topical glucocorticosteroid therapy, the topical silicone paste alone is continued for an additional week. Then the involved area is reassessed.

If the hypertrophic scar is resolving, the topical silicone paste alone is continued. If a partial response and some residual scar are noted, the 2-week cycle is repeated. If the area of scarring is continuing to thicken or is unresponsive to topical therapy, then treatment with the 585-nm flashlamp pumped dye laser or injection of corticosteroids is initiated. Any regimen for the treatment of hypertrophic scars must be initiated as soon as any sign of formation is noted. Furthermore, the treatment regimen must be adjusted for each patient.

CONCLUSION

In laser resurfacing, the goals are to minimize complications and optimize results. Patients should be followed closely after resurfacing. Close follow-up facilitates the early diagnosis of postoperative problems. As in other plastic surgical procedures, the early diagnosis and treatment of postoperative problems allow the best possible outcome.

REFERENCES

1. David LM, Lasl GP, Glassberg E, et al. CO_2 laser abrasion for cosmetic and therapeutic treatment of facial actinic damage. *Cutis* 1989;43:583–587.
2. Ohmori S. The problem of keloid formation in burns in Japan. In: Lawless AB, Wilkinson AW, eds. *Transactions of the Second International Congress on Research in Burns.* Edinburgh: Churchill Livingstone, 1966.
3. Carniol PJ. *Laser resurfacing.* Master's seminar, annual meeting of the American Academy of Cosmetic Surgery, September 1995, New Orleans.
4. American National Standards Institute. *American national standards for the safe use of lasers in health care facilities.* Standard Z136.3. New York: ANSI Publications, 1988.
5. Beeson WH. Laser safety. In: Carniol PJ, ed. *Laser skin rejuventation.* Philadelphia: Lippincott–Raven Publishers, 1998:55.
6. Gilmore J, Clark P, Carniol P. Laser safety in facial surgery. In: Carniol PJ, ed. *Facial rejuvenation.* New York: Wiley-Liss, 2001:263–279.
7. Beeson WH. Laser safety. In: Carniol PJ, ed. *Laser skin rejuvenation.* Philadelphia: Lippincott–Raven Publishers, 1998:49–63.
8. Carniol PJ. FeatherTouch, SilkTouch and SureTouch lasers. In: Carniol PJ, ed. *Laser skin rejuvenation.* Philadelphia: Lippincott–Raven Publishers, 1998:120.
9. Carniol PJ. FeatherTouch, SilkTouch and SureTouch lasers. In: Carniol PJ, ed. *Laser skin rejuvenation.* Philadelphia: Lippincott–Raven Publishers, 1998:121.
10. Carruthers A. Coblation: a new method for facial resurfacing in facial rejuvenation. In: Carniol PJ, ed. *Facial rejuvenation.* New York: Wiley-Liss, 2001:413–427.
11. Maibach HF, Rovee DT. *Epidermal wound healing.* St. Louis: Mosby, 1972:132–146.
12. Elson ML. Effect of petroleum jelly on the healing of skin following cosmetic surgery procedures. *Cosmetic Dermatol* 1993;6:18–22.
13. Kannon GA, Garrett AB. Moist wound healing with occlusive dressings. *Dermatol Surg* 1995;21:583–590.
14. Bridenstine JB, Carniol PJ. Managing post resurfacing complications. In: Carniol PJ, ed. Laser skin rejuvenation. Philadelphia: Lippincott–Raven Publishers, 1998:251–254.
15. Weinstein C. Erbium remodeling—long-term wrinkle improvement. In: Carniol PJ, ed. *Facial rejuvenation.* New York: Wiley-Liss, 2001:349–388.
16. Fitzpatrick R, Goldman M. Personal communication, January 1999.
17. Koch JR. Personal communication, April 1999.
18. Bridenstine JB, Carniol PJ. Managing post resurfacing complications. In: Carniol PJ, ed. *Laser skin rejuvenation.* Philadelphia: Lippincott–Raven Publishers, 1998:244.

57

ALLOPLASTIC FACIAL CONTOURING

EDWARD O. TERINO

Surgical procedures to improve the facial appearance have become widely accepted during the 1990s and are now used extensively. The reconstruction of soft tissue and bony defects of the face and torso was first attempted during the First and Second World Wars. Such reconstructive surgery evolved into aesthetic surgical procedures during the 1970s and 1980s. Starting with the superficial soft tissue integument and subcutaneous fat layers, aesthetic surgeons worked their way down through the facial anatomy into the submuscular aponeurotic system (SMAS) and finally the skeleton. Aesthetic skeletal procedures were developed mostly by Dr. Paul Tessier and his disciples, who reconstructed the advanced congenital facial deformities of infants and children.

Lacking extended formal training in the advanced techniques of craniofacial reconstruction, most plastic surgeons practicing in the aesthetic arena are more familiar and comfortable with the use of alloplastic materials to alter the facial skeletal and soft tissue contours. The development of anatomical midface and mandible implants, and of newer, biocompatible alloplastic materials, has made it possible to undertake midface, malar, and premandible facial contouring. Consequently, within the last decade, the public demand for aesthetic facial surgery and facial contouring has exploded and motivated aesthetic plastic surgeons to learn techniques involving the use of alloplastic implants and materials (1,2). These are particularly applicable in the chin, as opposed to the malar and midface regions. Central chin augmentation has been practiced since the 1950s and 1960s (3). The surgical technique is relatively simple and provides a very satisfactory improvement of the facial profile, so that it is now widely accepted and utilized by plastic surgeons.

Midface augmentation and alloplastic enhancement of other areas of the facial skeleton have been less popular among surgeons because the operations require dissections into the midface on a subperiosteal bony plane. Moreover, surgery in this area has been less commonly used because of its potential to produce an artificial appearance (Fig. 57-1).

In the 1990s, all aspects of facial aesthetic surgery were brought together in a new comprehensive, three-dimensional model, so that aesthetic facial surgery is now regarded as a form of living sculpture. Soft tissue plane techniques, both superficial and deep, have been conquered and are being utilized by a growing number of trained aesthetic surgeons. However, these are two-dimensional techniques. The aesthetic surgeon of the future is striving to develop three-dimensional concepts and techniques that can significantly contour the bony architecture of the face in addition to the soft tissues. To achieve these goals, alloplastic techniques are rapidly being developed and are becoming the final frontier in aesthetic facial surgery. The use of midface suspension techniques *combined with midfacial implant augmentation and premandible contouring* is the final phase in the evolution of true three-dimensional artistry in facial aesthetic surgery (4).

Published data on unfavorable results and complications of alloplastic techniques are limited (5,6). To gather accurate, up-to-date data, I conducted a survey among the members of the American Society of Plastic and Reconstructive Surgery (ASPRS) in 1990, more than 10 years ago. Of the 3,200 members, 9% responded. It was felt that these respondents represented surgeons who favored and performed malar and chin augmentations as part of their usual armamentarium. The survey data indicated that approximately 20,000 chin implant procedures and 3,000 malar/chin procedures had been performed by some 300 surgeons. It was obvious from the survey results that the use of alloplastic materials was increasing.

As part of the preparation for this chapter, another survey was performed in 1998 of the current 1,200 members of the American Society for Aesthetic Plastic Surgery (ASAPS). Four hundred members (33%) responded. Again, it appears that the respondents were mainly sur-

Edward O. Terino: Plastic Surgery Institute of Southern California; and Los Robles Regional Medical Center, Thousand Oaks, California

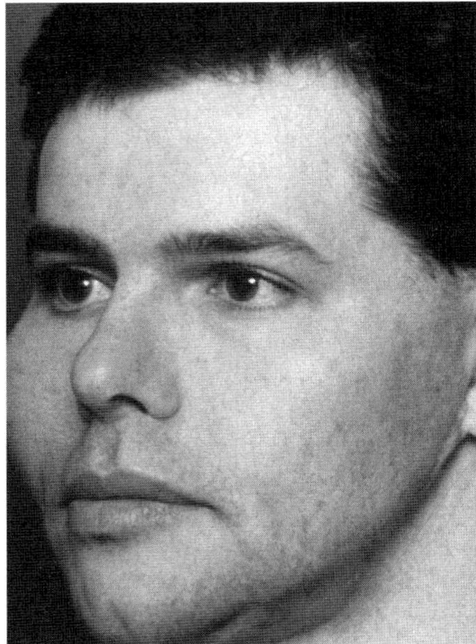

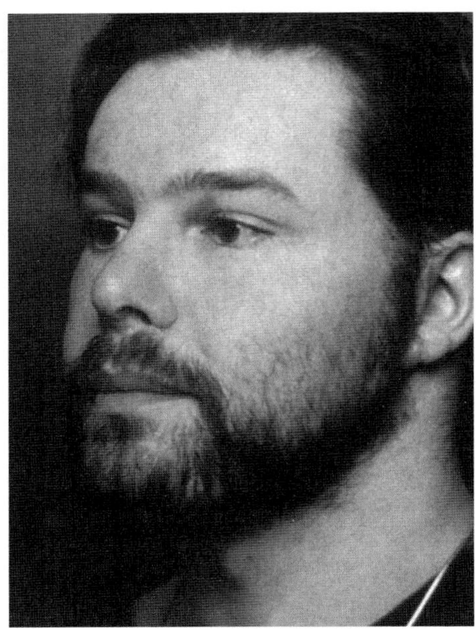

FIGURE 57-1. A chronic right malar infection, abnormal chin contour, and lower eyelid retraction developed in this 30-year-old man after he underwent malar augmentation, placement of a chin implant, and blepharoplasty. **A:** Preoperative. **B:** Postoperative, 8 months after replacement of the malar and chin implants along with upper midface suspension surgery and lateral canthoplasties.

geons who favored these techniques and performed them commonly. Indeed, 95% of the respondents reported using alloplastic materials in their aesthetic facial procedures. The 1998 ASAPS survey showed that more than 80% of surgeons utilize premandible and chin alloplastic procedures, whereas only 65% augment the malar and midface region (Table 57-1). Approximately 25% perform some form of premaxilla augmentation, and only 20% address forehead and temple problems. The suborbital tear trough procedure is performed by 14% of responding members. A corresponding average number of surgeries per location was noted (i.e., 68 for the premandible/chin region, 21 for the malar/midface region, and 4 for the suborbital/tear trough region). Nearly 50% of the surgeons reported using these techniques for the past 10 to 20 years, and an additional 35% had used them for more than 20 years. In other words, more than 80% of the respondents have used alloplastic materials for more than 10 years. Only 3% of the surgeons have used alloplastic techniques for less than 5 years (Table 57-2). Two-thirds of the surgeons who responded categorized alloplastic facial contouring techniques as very useful (50%) and most desirable (12%). An additional 38% considered them occasionally useful. No physicians responded to the description "never useful" (Table 57-3).

TABLE 57-1. 1998 ASAPS SURVEY: USE OF ALLOPLASTIC MATERIALS BY LOCATION

Site	Physician responses (%)
Premandible chin	96
Malar midface	74
Premaxilla	30
Forehead	16
Temple	15
Suborbital tear trough	15

ASAPS, American Society for Aesthetic Plastic Surgery.

TABLE 57-2. 1998 ASAPS SURVEY: DURATION OF USE OF ALLOPLASTIC MATERIALS

Duration (y)	Physician responses (%)	
0–5	3	
6–10	17	
11–20	47	82 (11–20 and 21+)
21+	35	

ASAPS, American Society for Aesthetic Plastic Surgery.

TABLE 57-3. 1998 ASAPS SURVEY: ATTITUDES TOWARD ALLOPLASTIC FACIAL CONTOURING

Attitude	Physician responses (%)	
Very useful	50	62
Most desirable	12	
Occasionally useful	38	
Never useful	0	

ASAPS, American Society for Aesthetic Plastic Surgery.

FACIAL AESTHETICS

Any discussion of unfavorable results and complications with alloplastic materials and implants must include a brief presentation of the relevant aesthetic principles of surgical contouring of the malar/midface and premandible/jaw line regions.

Facial Balance

The first basic consideration in facial aesthetics is balance. Balance is the summation of the size, shape, and form of the soft tissue and skeletal elements and the facial features, all of which are responsible for attractive or unattractive facial architecture and the soft tissue appearance. A face is considered pleasing when the basic relevant anatomical facial structures are similar in size.

Aesthetic Units of the Face

Perhaps most important in establishing an attractive facial balance are the volume-mass relationships of the dominant structural elements of the face. This is particularly true in the midface and jaw line. A strong nose of significant proportions will dominate a face, and so the malar and cheek regions and the chin and jaw line aesthetic unit will appear smaller. Conversely, a larger malar and cheek size will reduce the significance of a large nose in proportion to the rest of the face. Many people born with a prominent midface and nose have a weak aesthetic mandibular unit with microgenia (Fig. 57-2). Augmenting and increasing the volume-mass appearance of the lower third of the face and jaw line can bring about facial balance without a reduction in the size of the nose (Fig. 57-3). Facial balance and aesthetics essentially depend on the relationships between the three major facial promontories (i.e. the nose, the malar/midface cheek region, and the lower mandibular/jaw line segment).

The aesthetic units of the face are three in number: (a) an upper aesthetic facial unit extending from the hairline to the lateral canthi, (b) a midfacial aesthetic unit extending from the lateral canthi to the lateral commissures of the mouth, and (c) the lower third aesthetic facial unit, which extends from the lateral commissures of the mouth to the inferior margin of the central mentum. These three units should be approximately equal, although the lower third unit may be slightly smaller in faces that are nevertheless considered to be optimally attractive. Should one or more of these aes-

A

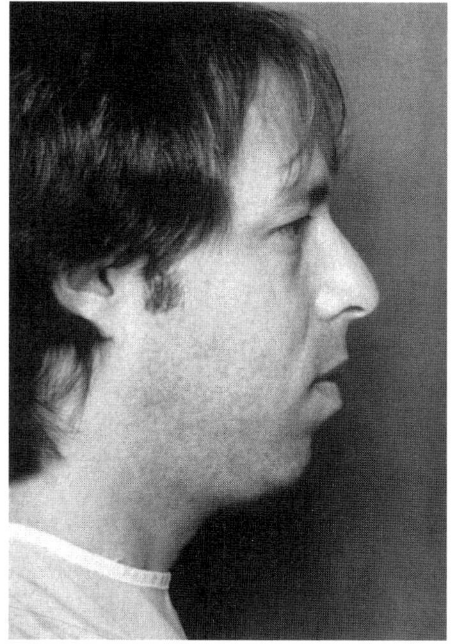

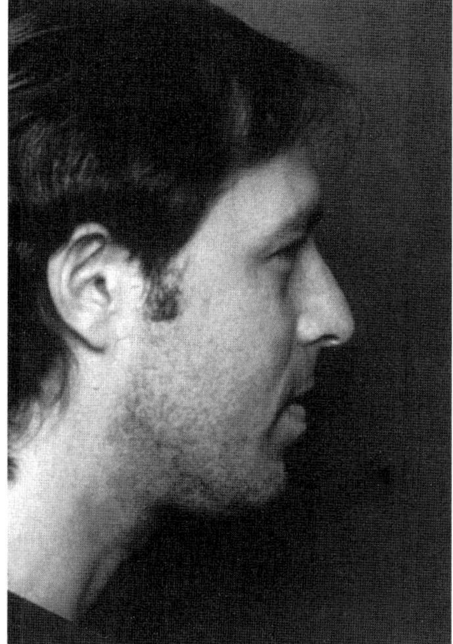

B

FIGURE 57-2. This patient's nose appears prominent because of an aesthetic volume deficiency of the premandible with microgenia. **A:** Preoperative. **B:** Postoperative, 1 year after chin augmentation.

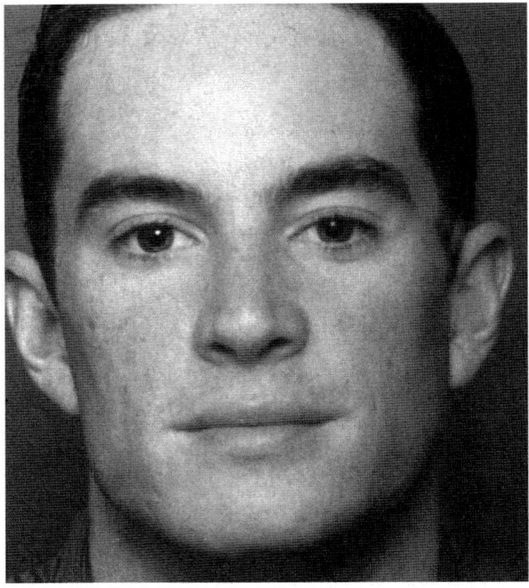

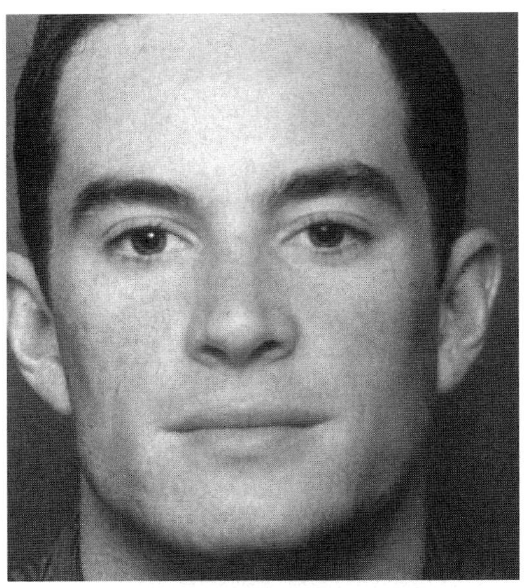

FIGURE 57-3. A 28-year-old man with aesthetic facial imbalance and extreme hereditary volume deficiency of the entire mandible and chin. **A:** Preoperative. **B:** Postoperative, after alloplastic augmentation of the mandibular angle and central mandible.

thetic units have too much mass, volume, or vertical and anteroposterior size, the appearance to most observers will be displeasing.

Gross discrepancies in the size (volume and mass) of the anatomical structures of the midfacial and lower mandibular aesthetic units create unattractive disharmony.

Zonal Anatomy of the Malar/Midface and Premandible/Jaw Line Facial Aesthetic Units

The malar/midface region can be designated as having five aesthetic anatomical zones (Figs. 57-4 and 57-5).

Zone 1, the largest, includes the major body of the malar bone and first third of the zygomatic arch. This zone is the first to be augmented for relative or absolute skeletal deficiencies. Zone 2 comprises the middle third of the zygomatic arch. Augmentation of the malar and zygomatic bones, together with zone 1, produces a significant aesthetic alteration by widening and enhancing the upper midface.

Zone 3 is the paranasal area medial to the infraorbital nerve. The "tear trough sulcus" of aging develops in this zone and may require a volume enhancement through alloplastic techniques. This often includes contouring of the entire suborbital region with implants or with malar soft tissue elevation and suspension techniques.

Zone 4 is the posterior third of the zygomatic arch, an area of lesser significance that never requires augmentation. It is an area to be avoided in dissections because of the dense and adhesive nature of the soft tissues to the bony arch and the proximity of the overlying branches of the facial nerve to the frontalis, orbicularis, and zygomaticus muscles just inferior to the arch.

Zone 5, the submalar zone, consists of the lower half of the midface, or submalar region. The submalar space is the most important zone for improving midface contour with implants, especially in persons with atrophic changes of aging. The submalar zone extends 3 to 4 cm inferiorly over the fibrous tendon of the masseter muscle as it originates from the inferior malar zygomatic arch.

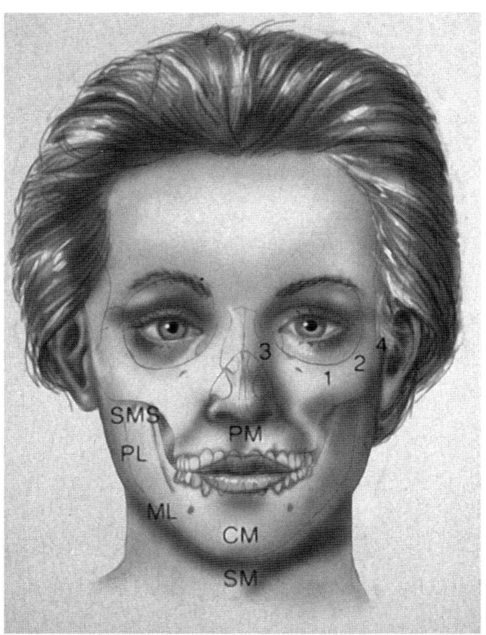

FIGURE 57-4. Five basic malar/midface zones or regions can be augmented and enhanced.

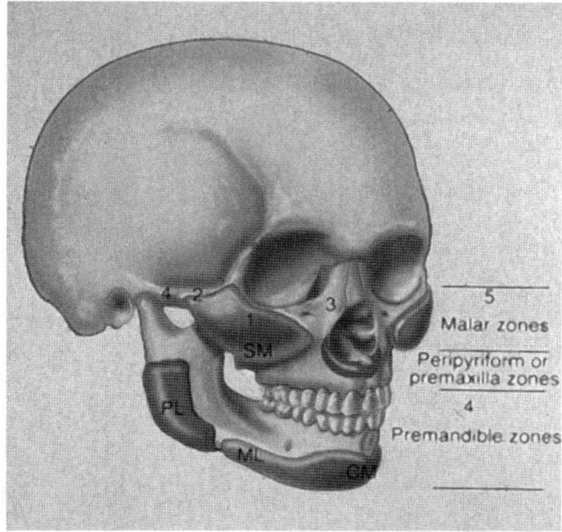

FIGURE 57-5. Implants are commercially available to produce aesthetic improvements in all the anatomical zones of the midface and premandible.

To appear natural and simulate soft tissue augmentation, an alloplastic implant must have a generous surface area (12 to 15 cm^2) with which the malar bone and the submalar zone inferior to the malar bone can be bridged. I have developed a comprehensive malar shell design to provide anatomically natural-looking augmentations that simulate the soft tissues and bone in the midface zones. Similarly, implants have been developed and are commercially available that surgeons can use to create pleasing and relevant contour changes in the mandible/jaw line aesthetic facial unit (Figs. 4 and 5).

The central mentum zone, or zone 1, is located between the two mental foramina. Traditional chin implants used in the 1950s and 1960s were centrally placed and often produced an unattractive central protuberance ("witch's chin"). Recently designed anatomical implants extend from the central mentum laterally onto the middle half of the horizontal ramus to the area of the oblique line. Thus, it is important to augment the midlateral zone of the mandible simultaneously with the central mentum zone to create a natural anterior chin and jaw contour.

The posterolateral mandible zone, or zone 3, includes the mandibular angle and ascending ramus. Augmentation within this zone, with specially designed implants, broadens the posterior jaw line contour. These changes are often desired and sought after by young men who desire a contemporary, strong, masculine image.

Zone 4, the submandibular zone, lies beneath the inferior border of the mandible. A specially shaped commercial implant provides vertical augmentation to lengthen the face from the lower lip to the inferior chin line. This may also help to correct a marionette groove or anterior mandibular prejowl sulcus.

The premaxillary region consists of the peripyriform area, which is most obviously unattractive in persons with genetic midface retrusive deficiencies but is also often subtly apparent in persons with midfacial bony regression associated with aging. Alloplastic implants and materials provide excellent improvement for these deficiencies.

TYPES OF FACIAL IMPLANTS

Optimal Characteristics

Types of implants and materials are of special importance in determining malar, midface, mandible, and jaw line contouring. Undesired complications and unfavorable results may follow the misuse of certain implant shapes and designs or the improper selection of materials.

Ideal alloplastic facial implants should (a) be easy to implant, (b) not be palpable, (c) be easy to replace, (d) conform to and resemble the facial skeleton, (e) be acceptable to the host, (f) withstand infection and inflammation, and (g) be easily modified by the surgeon (Table 57-4). The 1998 ASAPS survey considered the opinions of practicing aesthetic surgeons regarding several alloplastic implant materials for the face, including AlloDerm, even though it is essentially a human tissue derivative.

TABLE 57-4. QUALITIES OF ALLOPLASTIC FACIAL IMPLANT MATERIALS[a]

Quality	Silicone rubber	Gore-Tex	Porex	Hydroxyapatite	AlloDerm	Soft form
Biocompatible	4	3	3	4	4	3
Readily modifiable	3	2	3	3	4	3
Host acceptability	4	3	3	3	4	3
Anatomic contours	4	3	2	2	2	2
Easily exchangeable	4	2	1	1	1	2
Resistant to infection	3	2	2	2	4	3
Visible, palpable	3	2	2	2	4	2

[a] 4, optimal; 1, least optimal.

Implantable Materials

Silicone (Polysiloxane)

Silicone is still the implantable material of choice among plastic surgeons (7–9) (Table 57-5). Indeed, nearly 90% of responding surgeons considered it to be their material of choice for alloplastic implantation. Other materials were used by 8% to 18% of the members surveyed.

A smooth silicone implant placed directly on bone becomes fixed securely and rapidly and resists the biomechanical forces of fibrosis and encapsulation. A most desirable feature of silicone implants is the ease with which they can be removed and exchanged for an implant of another size or shape when necessary.

Medium-grade silicone is easily implantable and conformable. It is flexible enough to be inserted through small tissue apertures and soft enough to mold to the external contour of the bone. When implants made of silicone rubber are finely tapered at the margins, they are not palpable through the soft tissues. Other implant materials, such as Gore-Tex, Medpor, and hydroxyapatite, are either manufactured with less finesse or are of a harder consistency with irregular surface textures that may be both visible and palpable through the skin surface.

Silicone implants also have the favorable feature of being easily shaped, carved, and modified at the operating table or before surgery with scissors, scalpels, or dermabraders. Inflammation surrounding silicone implants can be treated without removing them. Even purulent infection is not an absolute indication for removal. The judicious use of antibiotics, drainage procedures, and perhaps even continuous irrigation can prevent implant loss.

Other Materials

Other commonly used alloplastic materials are porous, such as Gore-Tex (polytetrafluoroethylene) (10–12), polyethylene (Medpor) (13–16), and methylmethacrylate and hydroxyapatite (17,18). According to the ASAPS survey, they are used by plastic surgeons significantly less often than silicone implants, although some surgeons prefer them for chin/jaw line augmentations. Porous materials offer the advantage of immediate implant stability because of rapid stabilization by fibrous tissue ingrowth. In every series reported, however, these substances presented special problems of difficult placement and removal and increased rates of infection because of their matrix characteristics (19,20). Moreover, their hard and sometimes irregular consistency can create problems of external contour shape, size, and palpability.

TABLE 57-5. 1998 ASAPS SURVEY: CHOICE OF IMPLANT MATERIAL

Material	Physician responses (%)
Silicone rubber	88
Gore-Tex	18
Porex	15
Methylmethacrylate	15
Hydroxyapatite	10
Soft form	8

ASAPS, American Society for Aesthetic Plastic Surgery.

Until precise and predictable techniques evolve for the use of the newer implant materials, surgeons would be wise to use nonporous, nonadherent, smooth implants that encapsulate firmly onto bone but can easily be removed and replaced when a correction of size or shape is desired (21).

The most comprehensive review of the world literature regarding the complications and toxicities of implantable materials in facial reconstructive and aesthetic surgery, by Rubin and Yaremchuk, appeared in 1997 in the *Journal of Plastic and Reconstructive Surgery.*

CORRECTION OF THE VARIOUS TYPES OF MIDFACIAL DEFICIENCY

An additional and very useful analysis of facial aesthetics is based on six common facial types with midface volume-mass deficiencies. Knowledge of these facial types enables both surgeons and patients to identify more precisely the size and shape of implants and their proper positioning before surgery is undertaken.

Patients with facial type 1 have insufficient malar and suborbital skeletal mass but good submalar/midface soft tissue fullness. This creates a deficiency in zones 1 and 2 and possibly the paranasal zone 3 tear trough region. Augmentation with malar shell implants and occasionally with tear trough implants in these zones significantly improves facial balance in the upper part of the midface, enhances facial beauty and attractiveness, and helps diminish the "pudgy cheek" appearance.

Patients with a type 2 facial pattern have adequate bony and soft tissue volume and mass in the upper midface zones 1 and 2 but atrophy or soft tissue deficiency in the lower submalar midfacial zone. Youthful fullness can be restored or provided to a face by placing a malar shell into the submalar region on top of the masseter muscle and extending it 3 or 4 cm below the lower margin of the malar bone. This is the most appropriate and commonly performed midfacial augmentation in the aging face. In a young person, augmentation of this facial region can create a round, full, "apple cheek" contour. In an older person, it restores youthful facial fullness.

Type 3 facial deficiency is an exaggerated version of type 2 and is uncommon. It is characterized by dramatically prominent malar eminences and an extremely deficient soft tissue mass in the submalar aspect of the midface. These people often have thin skin, and therefore the transition from the strong malar bone contours to the lower region of extreme soft tissue deficiency is striking. The contrast creates a gaunt, emaciated, hollow appearance. Straightforward traditional and two-dimensional multilayered tissue SMAS tightening or composite deep plane techniques often accentuate this unattractive skeletal appearance.

In type 4 faces, which are rare, severe malar and suborbital hypogenesis is combined with an extreme deficiency of the lower submalar midface soft tissues. This type is more common in men. The totally deficient maxillary/midface region requires considerable augmentation within both the malar and submalar zones (1 and 5). A shell implant with a large surface area (15 to 20 cm) encompasses and augments both the bony malar eminence and the submalar soft tissue triangle sulcus.

In facial type 5, significant suborbital bone deficiency with descent of the suborbital malar/midface soft tissues creates a shadowed infraorbital hollow and the appearance of weariness. Improvement of this type of facial deficiency requires either autologous or alloplastic augmentation in the suborbital region. Alloplastic silicone tear trough implants can be used, or autologous materials such as fascia, fat, galea, and AlloDerm.

Recently developed midfacial suspension techniques elevate the aging and descending soft tissues from the malar and suborbital regions to a higher position adjacent to the inferior orbital rim. These new procedures can be a useful adjunct for correcting types 4 and 5 deficiencies in the suborbital upper maxillary region.

Type 6 facial deficiency is associated with a retrusive central premaxillary appearance. This can be considered a lesser variant of a cleft lip and nose premaxilla deformity or other congenital deformities of midface hypoplasia or retrusion. Recent data confirm that with aging, bony absorption occurs in the central maxilla, a phenomenon that contributes to a retrusive appearance. Premaxillary peripyriform augmentation is extremely useful to improve the appearance in persons with either hereditary or acquired type 6 deficiency. Hydroxyapatite granules, silicone, Gore-Tex, and AlloDerm human tissue implants have all been effective in this region of the face.

TECHNICAL FACTORS CONTRIBUTING TO COMPLICATIONS AND UNFAVORABLE RESULTS

Most complications and unfavorable results in plastic and reconstructive surgery relate to errors in planning and conceptualizing operations more than to technical execution. The plastic surgeon should keep in mind that "an ounce of prevention is worth a pound of cure." Successful alloplastic contouring depends entirely on a specific perception of the aesthetic parameters of the human face, accurate patient-doctor communication regarding what is expected, and an appropriate choice of implant. The size, shape, and positioning of an implant and the type of implantable material must be suitable to establish the image agreed on by both patient and surgeon. This is a tall order. The principles of facial aesthetics, zonal analysis, and facial typing presented in this chapter are not the only tools that surgeons can use to perceive facial aesthetics, understand the facial anatomy pertinent to facial contouring, and improve their technique. Many paths lead to Rome, and surgeons must choose their own methods of studying facial balance that will enable them to achieve the natural appearance that is the desired result.

MALAR/MIDFACE AUGMENTATION

The malar/midface region can be approached from four different routes, all of which can be used successfully. Each one, however, carries its own risks for malposition, nerve damage, and complications.

Subcilial Lower Eyelid Approach

Entrance into the malar space through a subcilial blepharoplasty incision allows accurate visualization, particularly of the upper bony malar/zygomatic region. Visualization of the lower submalar zone with the use of fiberoptic instruments facilitates dissection over the masseter tendon. This approach minimizes contamination and provides a strong inferior base on which implants can rest. This dissection also avoids potential damage to the infraorbital nerve, which does not have to be visualized. Despite these merits, the approach has not been widely utilized because of the potential for morbid distortions of lower eyelid (e.g., ectropion). Should excessive trauma and bleeding into the lid tissues occur, particularly into the middle lamella, fibrosis and contracture can produce severe ectropion (Fig. 57-6). Maneuvers to minimize this outcome are (a) adequate hemostasis, achieved with generous (20 mL) tumescent infiltration of dilute local anesthetic solution; (b) accurate and atraumatic subperiosteal dissection; and (c) implementation of standard, predictable lateral canthopexy or canthoplasty techniques.

The lower eyelid approach to malar/midface augmentation has become more popular with the advent of new midfacial suspension and fat transposition techniques to correct age-related changes. The midface became the focus of facial rejuvenation in the 1990s, and it will remain so. Therefore, aesthetic surgeons must know how to dissect accurately into this region and to use implant contouring precisely.

Once the arcus marginalis is released, the dissection is extended onto the anterior suborbital region of the maxilla and an incision is made down to the subperiosteal level 4 mm below the orbital rim in its lateral aspect. Maintaining a cuff of periosteum, fascia, and fat [suborbicularis oculi fascia (SOOF) layer] along the inferior and lateral orbital rim

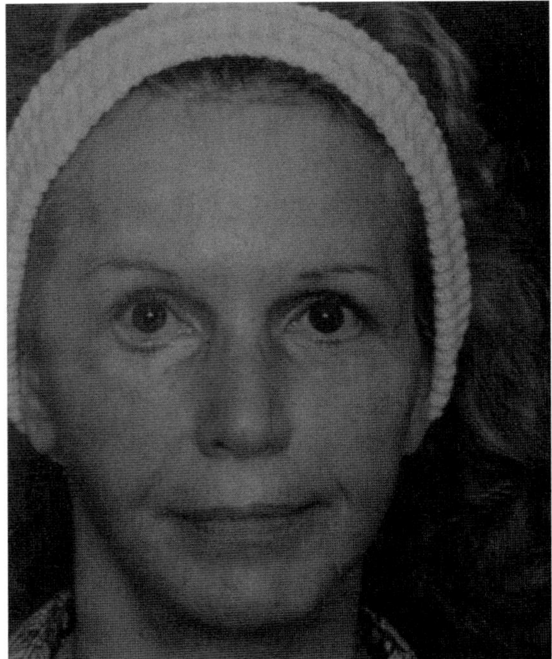
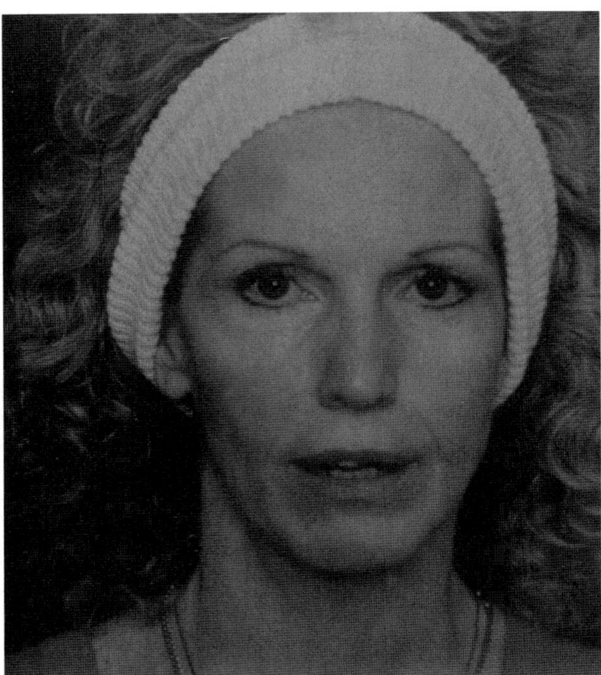

FIGURE 57-6. After this 53-year-old woman underwent malar augmentation through a subciliary blepharoplasty approach, excessive bleeding and trauma to the right lower eyelid produced ectropion. **A:** Preoperative. **B:** Postoperative. Secondary correction of ectropion by canthoplasty techniques.

prevents the development of severe adhesions to structures between the bony rim and the eyelid. These can produce serious retraction. Midfacial/malar suspension techniques can be used to secure this cuff of tissue to the deep temporal fascia above the junction of the lateral orbital rim and zygomatic arch. Canthopexy and midface suspension techniques create an apparent excess of lower eyelid skin and muscle. Resection of these structures should be minimized or avoided, as the normal downward forces of gravity and healing will distribute the tissues in a natural fashion and prevent abnormal retraction. The additional volume expansion produced by an implant under the malar/zygomatic tissues further underscores the need for conservative technique in the resection of lower eyelid tissue.

Intraoral Approach

The traditional and original approach for malar augmentation has been intraoral. Once the anatomy and techniques have been mastered, so that control of bleeding and accurate visualization of the malar and submalar space are consistently reliable for the surgeon, the placement of large shell implants into the malar zones 1 and 2 and into submalar zone 5 is very precise.

Sensory or motor nerve damage can be a disconcerting and serious consequence of this approach. The dissection must be performed directly on bone and in an oblique direction along the maxillary buttress to parallel the infraorbital nerve and not subject it to traumatic dissection. Nonetheless, transection or stretching of small distal branches in the lip and cheek can produce dysesthesias and hypesthesias, which are annoying and upsetting to both patient and surgeon. A mucosa-only oblique incision, 1.5 cm in length, is made above the canine tooth over the anterior maxillary buttress 2.5 cm medial to the orifice of the parotid duct. Blunt muscle penetration is performed directly onto bone at the most inferior aspect of this aperture to minimize damage to branches of the infraorbital nerve and branches of the facial nerve to the orbicularis and zygomaticus muscles. Dissection on the subperiosteal plane is then directed obliquely up onto the malar bone and over to the zygomatic region. The tendinous origins of the masseter muscle must be identified at the leading edge of the malar eminence and the dissection maintained on this plane to elevate the lower midfacial/submalar soft tissues from the masseter. Should dissection into tissue layers above the bony tendinous plane be blunt, forceful, and traumatic, the branches of the facial nerve that enter the zygomaticus and orbicularis muscles from their posterior aspect may be endangered.

The dissection space for midface implants must be adequate to prevent pressure displacement or buckling and yet not so large that an implant can easily rotate or move out of position. The generous surface area of contemporary anatomical midface shell implants minimizes the possibility of significant malposition.

Armed 2-0 Ethibond arthroscopic sutures on 10-in needles are used to pull the implant tail into position and fix it externally to the temporal area posterior to the hairline. This ensures the precise placement and stabilization of midface implants. Further anterior and inferior stabilization of the midface implant is rarely necessary but can be accomplished easily when the surgeon feels that it is required. This choice is made on the basis of direct observation during the surgical procedure. A strong, two-layered closure of the zygomaticus and orbicularis oris muscles and the overlying mucosa creates a strong inferior supporting floor for the malar space that will prevent extrusion or implant descent.

Rhytidectomy Approach

Creating the malar space by penetrating the SMAS lateral or medial to the zygomaticus major muscle over zone 1 prevents complications that can occur when midface implants are placed via other routes. No significant underlying anatomical structures are located over the bone that can be injured when the roof of the malar space is penetrated in this location. The critical maneuver in creating the malar space from a sub-SMAS rhytidectomy approach involves a posterior elevation along the zygomatic arch into zone 2 to allow the implant to be placed without buckling of the tail. This dissection is necessary and not difficult to perform. If the implant space is made over zone 1 directly on the body of the malar bone, damage to the branches of the facial nerve that innervate the orbicularis and frontalis muscles can be avoided.

Implant placement during rhytidectomy offers two advantages: (a) A sterile entry wound is created that is readily accessible during a composite deep plane or SMAS rhytidectomy procedure, and (b) this direct approach permits very accurate placement that can be confirmed by direct observation and palpation.

Midface Surgical Approach

The new midface suspension procedure and the modifications devised by various surgeons (Ramirez, Hester, Little, and Terino) lend themselves readily to midfacial alloplastic contouring. Whether the desired effect is to augment the upper bony zone 1 and 2 regions or the submalar zone 5 of the lower midface, easy visual access to these areas is provided by extensive release of the arcus marginalis and orbicularis oculi structures from the malar bone at their inferior orbital rim location. To provide adequate space for the larger malar shell implants to be placed into the lower submalar midface region, a dissection is performed under direct vision. The fascial tendinous coverings of the masseter muscle are elevated from the inferior aspect of the malar bone into the midface inferiorly for 3 to 4 cm and the buccal fat pad is exposed. Through this approach, the implant position can easily be secured by either of two methods. The implant can be sutured to a previously described cuff of soft tissue and periosteum left attached to the inferior orbital rim when augmentation of the upper zones 1 and 2 is desired, or it implant can be secured to the masseter muscle inferior to the malar bone when submalar/lower midface soft tissue volume contouring is the goal. These fixations are accomplished by means of a large 3-0 Biocyn sutures placed directly through the implant. When the implants are accurately secured with sutures, the overlying midfacial soft tissue envelope can be elevated and suspended over the implants to the deep temporalis fascia by means of a lateral temporal approach.

A midface procedure should be performed under direct visualization, which allows accurate dissection and precise implant positioning and minimizes implant asymmetry and nerve damage. The subcilial suborbicularis approach to the midface facilitates accurate midfacial augmentation and suspension procedures.

PREMANDIBLE/JAW LINE AUGMENTATION

Aesthetic alloplastic augmentation of the central premandible has been performed for 30 years. The techniques for improving profiles ("profileplasty") have been well accepted and utilized by plastic surgeons. New anatomical implants developed in the 1980s provide greatly improved alternatives to effect changes in the lower third aesthetic jaw line segment. Onlay premandible implants that simulate normal anatomy can alter the shape and size of the midlateral and posterior mandible and also the central segment.

The 1991 ASPRS survey revealed that 30% of the respondents used anatomical, extended Silastic chin implants exclusively. They reported considerably greater satisfaction with the chin contour provided by these implants than with the contour provided by the original "central chin"-type implants. Of the members of the ASAPS who responded to the 1998 survey, 95% said they were now using alloplastic materials and implants for facial aesthetic surgery. More than 80% reported using these techniques for more than 10 years, with 95% of the surgeons using alloplastic implantation in the premandible/jaw line (Table 57-1) and 75% in the malar/midface region.

Whether the surgeon approaches the central and midlateral zones of the premandible from the submental or intraoral route, the technical principles for the placement of alloplastic implants are the same: (a) maintain the dissection directly on bone; (b) dissect only along the lower border of the mandible to avoid the mental nerve; (c) ensure accurate placement by appropriate manipulation and fiberoptic visualization; (d) minimize bleeding through the liberal use of local anesthetic infiltration and control blood pressure with general anesthesia; (e) close all layers securely, including muscle and subcuticular (submental) or muscle and mucosa (intraoral).

Surgical Technique

A 2-cm transverse incision is made either intraorally in the mucosa or submentally through the skin. In the submental approach, the muscles are penetrated at the inferior border of the mandible, and a gentle dissection beneath the periosteum is performed from below in an upward direction until the mental nerve and foramen are clearly visualized.

In the intraoral approach, it is important to separate the mentalis muscle pillars vertically through their central fibrous raphe to avoid horizontal transection of the muscle bundles. The customary transverse muscle incisions transect, weaken, and cause laxity of the mentalis muscle, thereby increasing the likelihood of ptosis and the development of a central, drooping chin mound deformity.

To permit the placement of large implants, a tight area of periosteum at the origin of the anterior mandibular ligament and surrounding the mental foramen must be released delicately to free up the soft tissues along the midlateral aspect of the anterior horizontal ramus of the mandible. The mental nerve and foramen are located 2.5 to 3.5 cm from the midline, beneath the first or second premolar, and 8 to 15 mm up from the lower border of the mandible. Anatomical variations at 1.5 to 4.5 cm from the midline have been reported in as many as 20% to 30% of cases. Multiple or double mental nerves and foramina are also possible. Therefore, dissection under direct visualization is important to prevent mental nerve morbidity.

Although the mental nerve is durable and resists avulsion injuries, traction during surgery commonly produces transient postoperative dysesthesia and hypesthesia. Total loss of sensation is rare. When it occurs, it may indicate that implants are misplaced anterior to the mental nerve and are compressing it. This situation requires prompt reexploration within the first 2 weeks after the operation.

POSTEROLATERAL MANDIBULAR AUGMENTATION

The number of patients seeking posterolateral widening and angular definition of the jaw line is increasing. Commercial anatomically designed implants are available for widening a mandibular angle from 6 to 12 mm (12 to 24 mm of total widening bilaterally). A similarly designed implant with dimensions that extend vertically can alter the mandibular-submental angle into a more horizontal direction by 6 to 10 mm. Patients frequently request lateral widening of the face to define the contours in the regions of the inferior and posterior jaw line angles.

The mandibular angle and ascending ramus are accessed through a 2-cm "hockey stick" mucosal incision that extends vertically to parallel the anterior border of the masseter muscle, and horizontally within the posterior buccal sulcus at a distance of 1 cm from the mandible in front of the molar teeth. Direct penetration with an elevator enables an easy subperiosteal dissection to visualize the angle of the posterior horizontal ramus and the ascending ramus. The tendinous attachments of the masseter to the inferior border, ascending ramus, and angle of the mandible, however, must be detached sharply with an Obwegeser mandibular degloving elevator. This permits the commercial angle implant to fit like a glove over the bone. It extends 4 cm up the ascending ramus and 3.5 cm along the horizontal ramus. It is compressed into place by the overlying sturdy masseter muscle. A two-layered closure must be performed. Infection and dehiscence are rare when a secure closure is accomplished. Patient satisfaction is high when mandibular angle augmentation is effective.

AUGMENTATION OF THE SUBMANDIBULAR SPACE

Increasing the vertical height of the lower third aesthetic jaw line segment is possible with a specially designed vertical extension implant. This wraps around the inferior mandibular border to provide 4 mm of anterior projection and 4 mm of height to the central and midlateral mandible. The implant is placed through a submental incision located 1 cm posterior to the natural crease to facilitate expansion of the submental tissue envelope, which occurs because of the unique location of this implant. The inferior border of the mandible is degloved easily under fiberoptic visualization. It is not necessary to observe the mental nerve or dissect above the lower bony margin. The implant fits securely around the inferior border. It is held in place by the mentalis and depressor anguli oris muscle groups. No other premandibular implantation provides such a dramatic improvement in facial balance as submandibular augmentation when the lower third facial aesthetic segment is vertically deficient.

AVOIDING UNFAVORABLE RESULTS AND COMPLICATIONS

The surveys of the ASPRS and the ASAPS, carried out in 1991 and 1998, respectively, revealed the following categories of unfavorable results of facial implantation: patient and doctor dissatisfaction; asymmetries, inappropriate shape, and malposition; hematoma, seroma, inflammation, and infection that necessitate removal; and nerve dysfunction (Table 57-6).

It is interesting to note that in the 1998 survey, more than 90% of the surgeons responding considered the unfavorable results of alloplastic facial augmentation to be relatively insignificant, both emotionally and physically (rating of 1 to 3 on a scale of 1 to 10) (Table 57-7). Perhaps this is because the majority of untoward sequelae were either temporary (asymmetries), partial (nerve dysfunctions), or reversible (removals) (Tables 57-8 through 57-10).

TABLE 57-6. 1998 ASAPS SURVEY: UNFAVORABLE RESULTS

Unfavorable result	Physician responses (%)
Patient dissatisfaction	81
Asymmetries	80
Cellulitis/inflammation	71
Extrusion	70
Nerve damage-motor	67
Wrong contour	64
Purulent infection	57
Nerve damage-sensory	44

ASAPS, American Society for Aesthetic Plastic Surgery.

Nerve dysfunctions can be motor or sensory. Specific nerves damaged in the malar/midface region are those to the frontalis muscle (forehead movement) and the orbicularis oculi muscle (eyelid closure), and motor branches to the zygomaticus muscles (lip elevation and smiling).

In chin and premandible augmentation, the unfavorable results most commonly reported were injuries to the mentalis nerve (sensory). Occasionally, damage to nerves to the lower lip depressor and mentalis muscles produced motor dysfunctions.

The commonly reported problems associated with extended chin/premandible augmentation are similar to those associated with midface augmentation and include (a) surgeon and patient dissatisfaction with implant size, shape, or contour; (b) asymmetries, inappropriate shape, and malposition; (c) hematoma, seroma, inflammation, infection, or extrusion necessitating implant removal; and (d) symptoms related to mental nerve dysfunction. Bone resorption is also reported and is discussed later in this chapter.

Patient Dissatisfaction

Patient dissatisfaction is the most common unfavorable result of facial implant contouring procedures. In both surveys, the rate of disappointment with size, shape, or contour of the cheek or jaw line (81%) was approximately equal to the rate of dissatisfaction regarding asymmetry (80%) (Table 57-6).

TABLE 57-7. 1998 ASAPS SURVEY: SIGNIFICANCE OF UNFAVORABLE RESULTS

Definition: On a scale of 1 to 10 (1 being least and 10 being greatest), how significant – emotionally or physically – do you rate this complication?

Scores	Physician responses (%)
1–3	91
4–6	5
7–10	4

ASAPS, American Society for Aesthetic Plastic Surgery.

TABLE 57-8. 1998 ASAPS SURVEY: SIGNIFICANCE OF UNFAVORABLE RESULTS

	Physician responses (%)		
Unfavorable result	1–3[a]	4–6[a]	7–10[a]
Patient dissatisfaction	53.5	13	4
Asymmetries	53.5	7	5
Cellulitis/inflammation			
Resolved with antibiotics	27	—	—
Removal necessary	24	2	6
Extrusion			
Internal through mucosa	12		
External through skin	9		

[a] Least significant; 10, most significant.
ASAPS American Society for Aesthetic Plastic Surgery.

The best ways to avoid patient dissatisfaction are the following: (a) understand the common facial types and their anatomical zonal deficiencies as they pertain to facial aesthetics; (b) understand and duplicate the patient's expectations regarding shape, size, and specifics of regional facial contours; (c) create surgically the precise subperiosteal spaces required; (d) place implants that achieve the desired contours accurately and appropriately; and (e) choose an implant of the correct size and shape.

Choice of Implant

Detailed discussions with the patient always reveal the subtleties and nuances of the specific contour results they anticipate in facial regions. It remains for the surgeon to evaluate whether their requests can be fulfilled by means of up-to-date implant augmentation techniques.

The following guidelines are based on the author's experience: Implant enhancement of the upper malar/zygomatic bony region (zone 1) produces a sharp, high angular appearance. Placing the implant or choosing one that extends

TABLE 57-9. 1998 ASAPS SURVEY: SIGNIFICANCE OF UNFAVORABLE RESULTS

	Physician responses (%)		
Unfavorable result	1–3[a]	4–6[a]	7–10[a]
Purulent infection			
Resolved antibiotics	16	—	—
Removal necessary	26	—	4
Nerve damage			
Temporary sensory			
Partial	72	—	—
Total	5	—	—
Permanent			
Partial	15	—	—
Total	6	—	—

[a] 1, least significant; 10, most significant.
ASAPS, American Society for Aesthetic Plastic Surgery.

TABLE 57-10. 1998 ASAPS SURVEY: SIGNIFICANCE OF UNFAVORABLE RESULTS

	Physician responses (%)		
Unfavorable result	1–3[a]	4–6[a]	7–10[a]
Nerve damage			
Temporary motor			
Partial	20	—	—
Total	1.5	—	—
Permanent			
Partial	4	—	—
Total	1.5	—	—
Wrong contour			
Patient opinion	39	—	—
Physician opinion	30	—	—

[a] 1, least significant; 10, most significant.
ASAPS, American Society for Aesthetic Plastic Surgery.

laterally into zone 2 widens the upper aspect of the midfacial segment. Augmenting the submalar region to correct a hereditary defect or the appearance of aging (type 2 midface deficiency) produces a fuller midface in the lower aspect of the cheek below the bone. Deciding whether to augment the upper malar bone aspect of the middle third aesthetic facial unit or the lower submalar soft tissue segment is the most important factor in creating specific cheek/midface contours that meet the patient's specifications.

Implant Size

The size of an implant relates to its surface area and thickness. Standard 4-mm commercial shells of large or jumbo sizes are suitable to produce natural and pleasing augmentations in more than 90% of patients. Occasionally, when patients want a more subtle effect, 3-mm medium shells can be used. When a more dramatic effect is desired, 5-mm or 6-mm shells are most advisable. Large shells of 20 cm^2 and jumbo shells of 30 cm^2 are always preferable to small implants of 15 cm^2 or medium implants of 18 cm^2. A broader surface area creates a subtle contour rather than a prominent localized lump.

Implant Positioning

The subperiosteal location has proved to be the most desirable one because of the rapid fixation of implants to the bone or underlying structures, such as the masseter muscle. Subcutaneous placement frequently results in implant mobility because encapsulation occurs within elastic and moveable soft tissues.

Fibrous ingrowth into porous materials or through implant fenestrations is completely unnecessary. When smooth implants are used, the correction of a malposition simply requires that a new, accurately located space be created directly on the bone level and beneath all anatomical tissue planes, including scar tissue and previous capsules. Dissection of a tissue space of slightly larger capacity facilitates placement of the implant without buckling, infolding of the edges, or abnormal bulging.

Facial Asymmetry

Natural facial asymmetry is universal. A form of hemifacial microsomia occurs in more than 90% of patients. On careful examination, the left and right sides of the face are usually quite different in size, shape, or volume. One side is wider and has a greater volume of bone and soft tissue. Also, one orbit, eyebrow, and eye complex is usually lower than the other.

Patients can be very particular and obsessed with asymmetries. Such asymmetries frequently go unnoticed before facial implant contouring. It is imperative, therefore, to evaluate facial asymmetries meticulously, note them in the medical records, and explain them in detail to patients. It is also necessary to warn patients that asymmetries will most likely be present following surgery, even when implants of different sizes are chosen and positioned to compensate for the variations in volume and shape that already exist (Fig. 57-7). Asymmetries can be documented in the patient's chart by computer imaging or photographic modalities. Documentation helps to prevent criticism postoperatively if the asymmetry is still apparent to the patient.

Although Cemax-Icon (Fremont, California) technology can be used to create customized models with asymmetrical skull anatomy, at the present time such advanced methods are usually indicated only for the most complicated problems; they are time-consuming and expensive, and the results at best are only moderately more successful than those obtained with standard, universally designed anatomical implants. Nevertheless, advances in this area of computed technology are rapidly evolving and will soon enable aesthetic plastic surgeons to correlate implant size and shape with desired changes in facial form and contour.

Choosing implants to correct asymmetries is presently more a matter of intuition than of technical precision. Obviously, a thicker implant with a larger surface area is indicated for the side of the face that lacks bone and soft tissue volume. Similarly, for jaw line asymmetries in the posterior mandibular and midlateral zones, implants that provide additional thickness of 1, 2, or 3 mm can be used on the side of the deficient mandible.

Perhaps the most important principle for the surgeon to remember is that minor asymmetries tend to become less noticeable within a 6-month postoperative healing period, during which relaxation of the collagenous capsular matrix around the implants allows the contours to appear softer.

Postoperative Infection and Removal

Complications in the third most frequent category in the two surveys included hematoma, cellulitis, infection, and extrusion requiring implant removal. These problems were

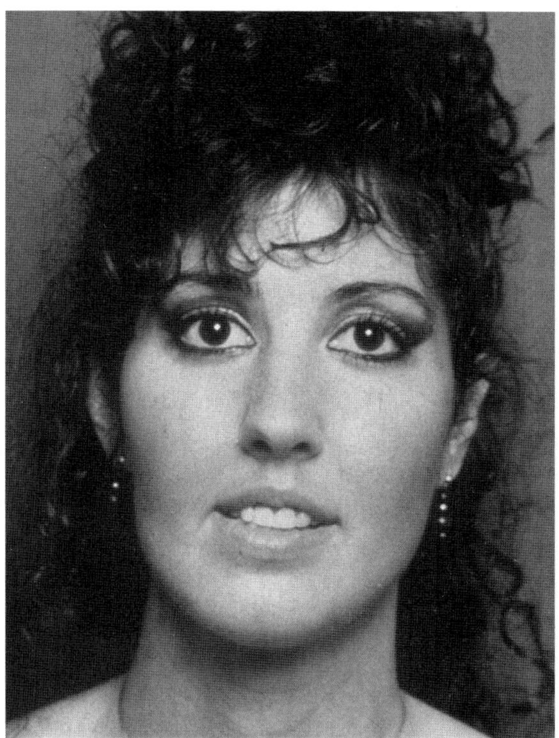
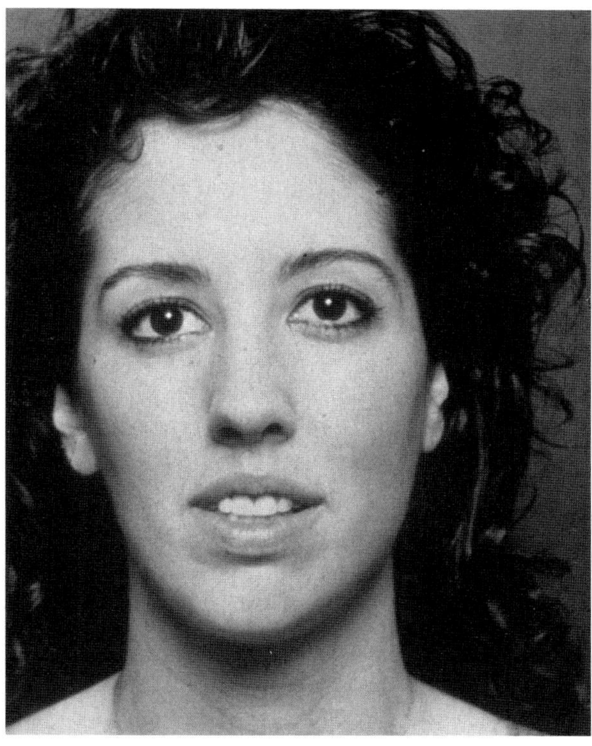

FIGURE 57-7. A 32-year-old woman with significant natural asymmetry of the face. **A:** Preoperative. **B:** Postoperative. The malar and mandibular regions have been augmented with implants of different sizes placed in slightly different positions.

noted by 57% to 70% of the surgeons. In the author's personal experience, the occurrence has been 0.04% in all facial implant procedures performed since 1971.

What are the causative factors? The type of implant material is significant. In all the reported series of intraorally placed implants, the incidence of postoperative infection, extrusion, and necessary removal was highest when an obsolete porous material called Proplast was used. With porous implant substances (e.g., Medpor, hydroxyapatite, and Gore-Tex), tissue, blood, and bacteria can enter the interstices of the implant structure, where a perfect environment for organism proliferation and growth is maintained. With smooth Silastic rubber implants, the infection rate is very low, and the implants can be salvaged even when inflammation, cellulitis, or gross purulence is present. This is a major reason why I prefer to use the latter material.

Infections resolve adequately and promptly when traditional regimens of antibiotics, warm compresses, rest, or even drainage and irrigation are instituted. Sound surgical judgment, combined with courage, close surveillance, and prompt intervention when necessary, are the elements required for the successful management of inflammation surrounding facial implants. Hydroxyapatite and Porex have been reported to resist implant infection as well as Silastic rubber. However, no statistical reports are available to substantiate this claim.

When inflammation, cellulitis, and infection develop in tissues surrounding a Gore-Tex implant, immediate removal is necessary. These problems will not resolve with the traditional treatments mentioned above if a Gore-Tex implant has been used.

Infection of the midface is a significant hazard that surgeons dare not risk. The prognosis for a patient with cellulitis and inflammation surrounding a Silastic facial implant is very favorable. Ultimate control and resolution of such infectious processes have been the norm in the author's extensive experience (Fig. 57-8). Frequent contaminants are skin and intraoral organisms such as *Staphylococcus aureus,* which for the most part are sensitive to penicillin derivatives and the cephalosporins. Acute inflammation, cellulitis, and impending infection are often alleviated with 750 mg of ciprofloxacin taken twice daily for 10 days. An additional 2 or 3 weeks of less potent antibiotic suppression is indicated after the acute process has subsided. When necessary, intravenous antibiotics may be administered for a course of several days. If an acute inflammatory process does not improve rapidly, immediate measures must be taken to drain the area adequately or to remove the prostheses, even when Silastic has been used.

Drainage of a malar or chin implant abscess or seroma by percutaneous needle aspirations, in addition to systemic antibiotic therapy, is indicated when palpable or visible evi-

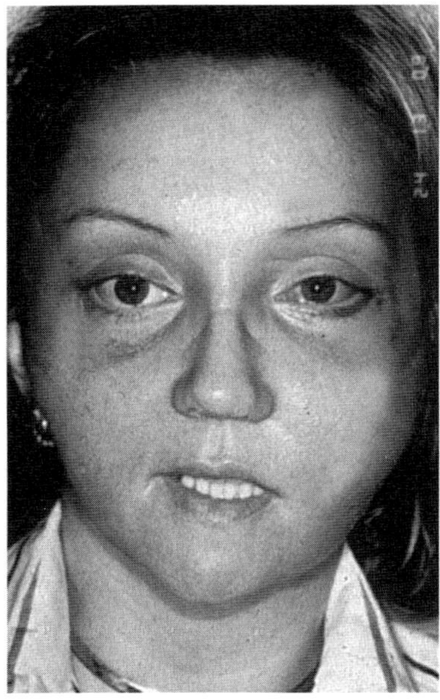
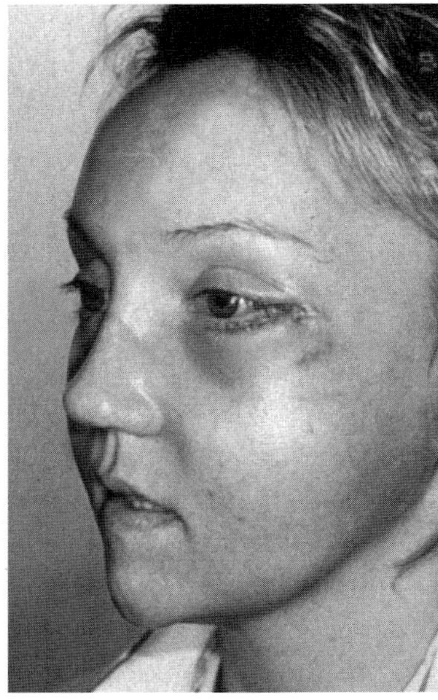
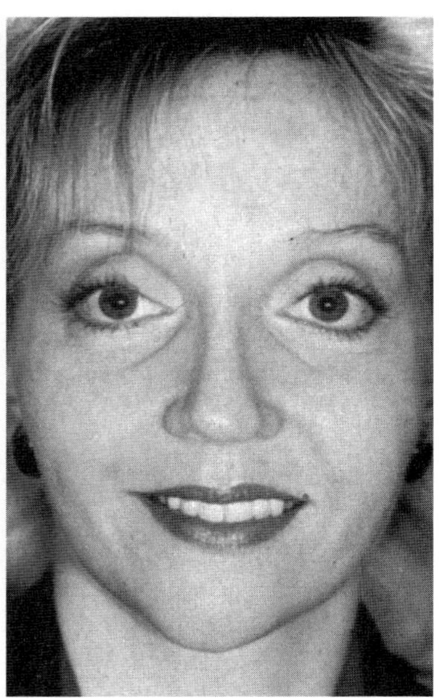

A, B C

FIGURE 57-8. Cellulitis and inflammation developed in this 38-year-old woman after she underwent malar augmentation surgery. **A:** Front view 10 days after surgery. **B:** Oblique view 10 days after surgery. **C:** At 3 weeks after surgery, cellulitis has resolved following treatment with antibiotics and drainage.

dence of a fluid collection around the implant is noted. These may be performed for several consecutive days.

Occasionally, continuous vacuum suction drainage should be instituted. A small percutaneous angiocatheter suction drain can be placed into the implant cavity externally through the submalar cheek region to institute midfacial drainage (Fig. 57-9). An effective means of preventing the accumulation of blood following the primary surgery is the placement of a 7-mm catheter from within the implant space to penetrate the scalp behind the temporal hair line. Thorough and continuous irrigation with antibiotic solution, soaking of implants in Betadine solution, and "no touch" (instruments only) handling of the implant are additional standard measures to prevent contamination and subsequent infection.

Extrusion

Extrusion of facial implants, either in the malar/midface or the premandible regions, should rarely occur. In general, extrusion can be prevented by creating a subperiosteal space that is comfortable for the implant, and by providing adequate, tension-free soft tissue coverage in layers.

Extrusion can follow trauma that has displaced the implant, particularly in the postoperative healing phase. Inadequate healing of the wound following implant placement may be caused by (a) wound tension during insertion and closure, (b) ischemic tissue damage following traumatic dissections, or (c) internal hematoma or seroma, which creates internal pressure and subsequent wound dehiscence.

Even placement of the largest extended anatomical premandible, posterior angle, and malar/midface implants should not result in problematic wound healing or extrusion. These complications are technical and can be avoided by following the technical guidelines described in this chapter.

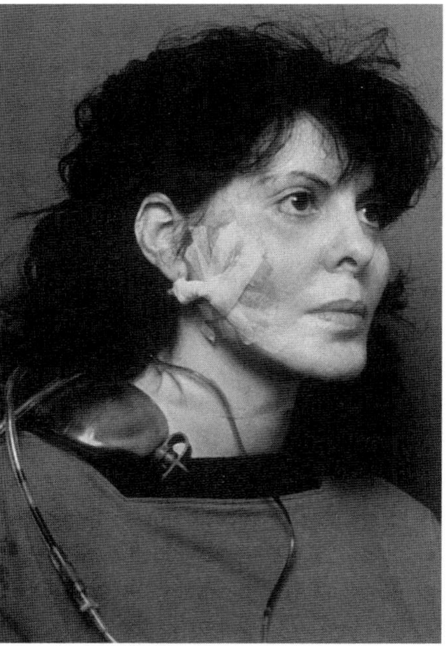

FIGURE 57-9. Percutaneous suction drainage can be combined with intensive antibiotic therapy to manage a midface suppurative infection.

Rarely, some poorly explained internal forces may displace a mandible angle or central chin implant downward, so that pressure necrosis and gradual extrusion through the skin result (Fig. 57-10). Simple removal through the aperture of the extrusion site allows the wound to heal. Secondary insertion in proper fashion may be carried out 6 months later.

Similarly, malar/midface implants can extrude through the upper buccal sulcus (Fig. 57-11). An inferiorly placed submalar implant under pressure from an overlying dental prosthesis can erode the oral buccal mucosa covering the implant.

Poor placement of a malar implant in the upper zone 1 malar bone region can cause extrusion or protrusion above the orbital rim, especially in the lateral aspect. This can result in a visible and palpable deformity and possibly an ectropion. Removal by the subciliary blepharoplasty route is not difficult.

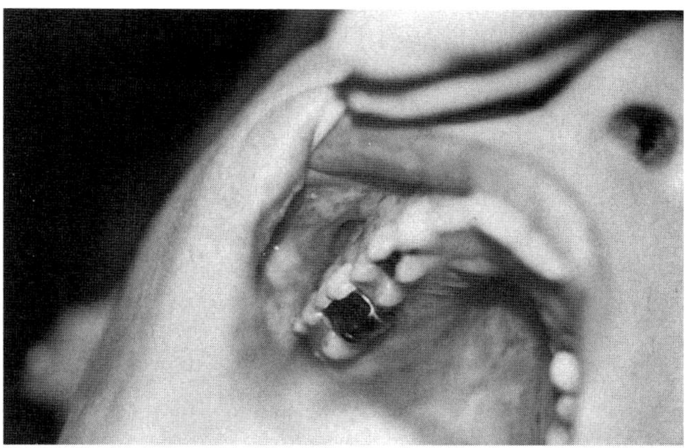

FIGURE 57-11. Intraoral extrusion of a midface implant can follow inferior placement of the implant with overlying pressure erosion caused by a) a dental prosthesis, b) hematoma and infection, or c) inadequate midface anatomical dissection.

Hematoma and Seroma

Hematomas and seromas following malar/midface and chin/jaw line augmentation are so common that they can almost be considered standard. In certain circumstances, fluid and blood collections cause complications:

1. The accumulation of blood and serum products encourages the growth of bacteria and increases the possibility of cellulitis and gross purulent infection.
2. Early postoperative asymmetries result from a distortion of contour caused by fluid collection. Considerable swelling is always present in the first 72 hours following facial implant procedures. Fluid collections and hematomas during that time are difficult to assess. Unusual pain and swelling caused by a hematoma are obvious (Fig. 57-12). Smaller fluid collections may simply appear as excessive postoperative swelling with asymme-

A

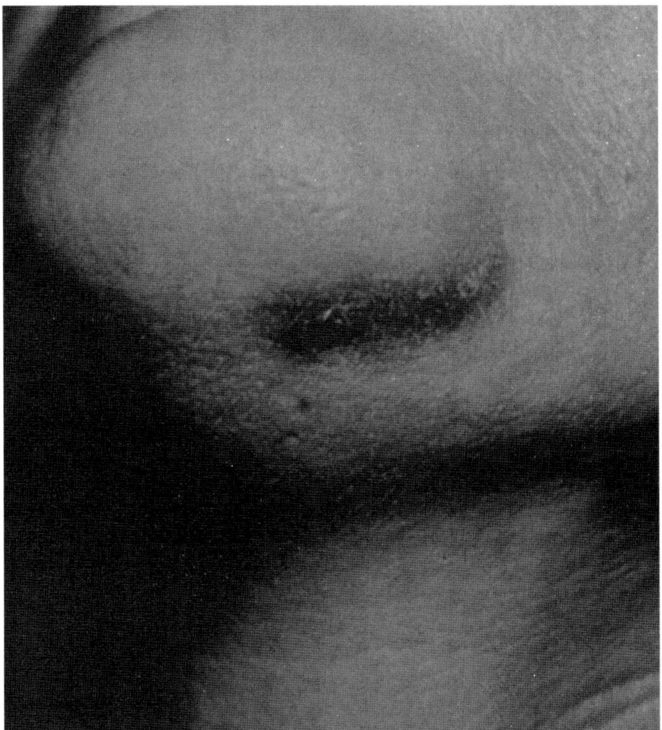

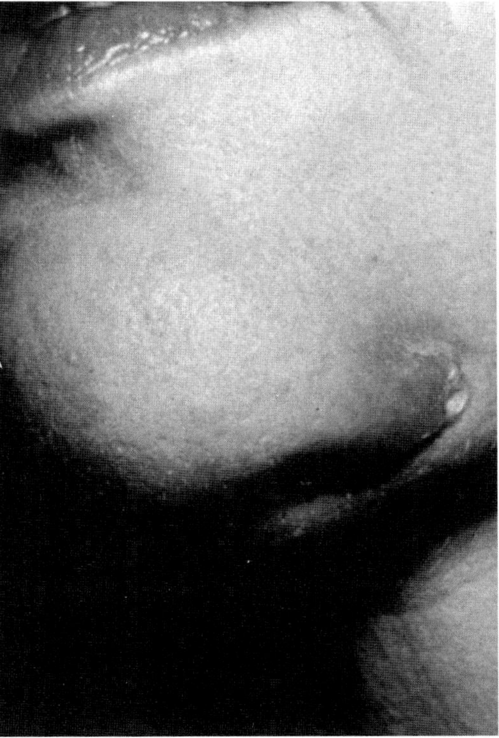

B

FIGURE 57-10. Extrusion of a central mandibular chin implant is rare but can be caused by excessive trauma or internal pressures created by an inadequate space.

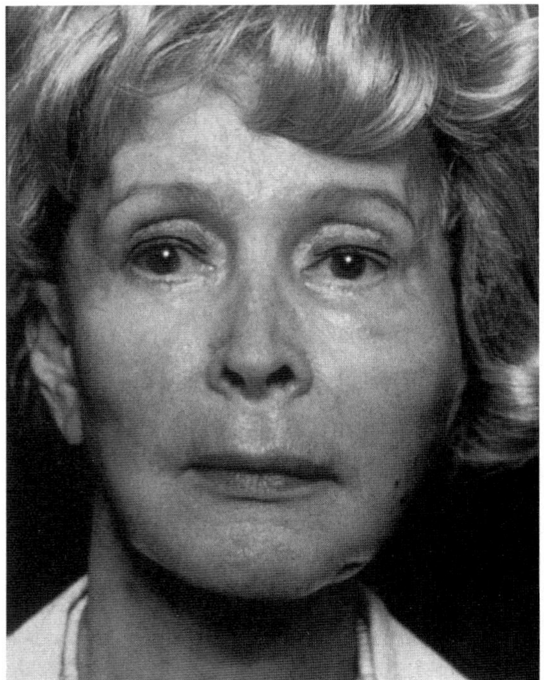

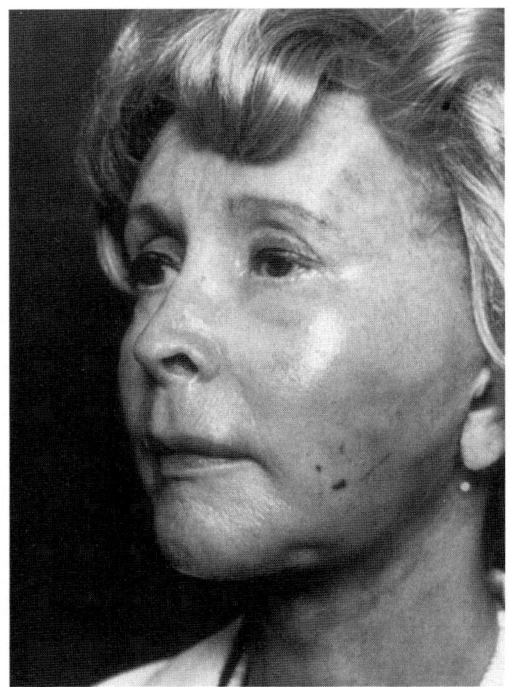

A B

FIGURE 57-12. A hematoma that developed during the first 24 hours after surgery caused pain and swelling in this 61-year-old woman.

try, which resolves adequately without treatment and without sequelae within 10 to 14 days. The implant during the early postoperative period, especially in the presence of surrounding fluid, may be difficult to palpate and can create an asymmetric appearance that alarms the patient.

3. In rare cases, capsular soft tissue contour deformities cause excessive fibrosis after breast augmentation.

Causes

The causes of hematoma and seroma formation are numerous: (a) Traumatic, rough dissection into tissue planes leads to excessive bleeding during and following surgery; (b) because of inadequate anesthesia techniques, both local and systemic, adequate vasoconstriction and control of blood pressure are not obtained; (c) rises in blood pressure occur during recovery, often stimulated by nausea, vomiting, agitation, urinary retention, and pain; (c) trauma to the operative site is caused inadvertently immediately following surgery, possibly by head movement on a pillow or mastication.

Hematoma and seroma are more frequent following secondary procedures because of the need to re-create adequate implant spaces by the surgical lysis of scar tissue. Additionally, the lysis of fibrous adhesions through fenestrations and porous matrices in implants increases trauma and predisposes to bleeding.

Treatment

A great degree of swelling, including hemorrhage into the sclera and other tissues around the orbital region, may indicate significant hematomas of the malar space. Pain elicited by opening or closing the mouth relates to the temporal mandibular joint and may indicate hematomas of the posterior mandible angle space. Large hematomas recognized early should be evacuated. Copious irrigation with antibiotic solution [2 g of cefazolin (Ancef) per liter of saline solution] is also advisable.

The drainage procedures previously mentioned may be used primarily for prophylaxis. Persistent or unrecognized seromas or hematomas may result in excessive capsule formation, malposition of the implant, and infection. To minimize these possibilities, liquefied hematomas or seromas should be aspirated percutaneously within 2 to 3 weeks postoperatively. The need for repeated aspirations can be avoided by effective, continuous drainage, as previously described. Antibiotic coverage is mandatory.

If removal of an implant should be necessary because of gross purulence or cellulitis that is resistant to treatment, secondary implantation can be planned 6 to 12 months later. Another solution, one that should be attempted cautiously, comprises (a) removal of an implant with resterilization and reinsertion, (b) thorough irrigation of the cavity with Betadine solution, and (c) intraoperative drain placement. Leaving the intraoral buccal wound open may also be considered. Removal and reinsertion are probably not indicated unless postoperative infection occurs after the first month or two, when a protective fibrotic capsule has already formed around the implant and acts as a bacterial barrier.

Long-term delayed occurrence of seromas has been observed in rare cases. On three occasions, this was associated with the growth of *Serratia marcescens,* a slowly growing organism that is difficult to eradicate without implant removal. In each instance, the implants were replaced successfully several months later.

Prevention through Anesthesia and Surgical Technique

To facilitate an accurate surgical facial implantation, intraoperative and postoperative control of bleeding is critical. The following routines, adopted by the author, have minimized the incidence of complications to an almost negligible statistic:

1. Maintaining the patient's systolic blood pressure at a level of 90 to 100 mm Hg during the intraoperative and postoperative periods. This is of critical importance and is best accomplished by utilizing general anesthesia.
2. Routine administration of 0.2 to 0.3 mg of clonidine postoperatively on the morning of surgery. This successfully stabilizes the blood pressure and pulse in most patients for a prolonged, 6- to 10-hour period of time.
3. Generous (50 to 75 mL) tumescent infiltration of dilute lidocaine solution (0.2%) with adrenaline (1:800,000) (Table 57-11). This is injected into the midface or premandible dissection zones subperiosteally, and into the tissues surrounding the upper and lower margins of the bony architecture.
4. The use of fiberoptic instruments. This enables the surgeon to perform a gentle and minimally traumatic elevation of soft tissues directly from the bony plane under visualization.
5. Copious irrigation with antibiotic solution during and at the end of the procedure. This eliminates the collection of blood products and minimizes the potential for bacterial contamination.
6. The use of drainage techniques, particularly in secondary procedures. The author does not use compression bandages postoperatively, although it is theoretically sound to consider them initially for 24 to 48 hours.

TABLE 57-11. IDEAL ANESTHESIA FOR ALLOPLASTIC FACIAL CONTOURING

General anesthesia
Maintain systolic blood pressure at 90 to 100 mm Hg
Clonidine 0.1 mg orally preoperatively
Local anesthesia
Lidocaine solution 0.2%
Adrenaline 1:800,000
Generous tissue infiltration into malar and premandibular space (20 to 30 mL each)

The prevention of postoperative bleeding and hematoma formation is worth a pound of cure. This complication can be avoided by the use of proper surgical technique and appropriate hemostatic methods of anesthesia.

Nerve Damage

Damage to the facial nerve branches and sensory nerve branches during malar/midface or chin/jaw line premandible augmentation is the most dreaded complication. Fortunately, such injuries occur in only a small percentage of cases and are usually temporary (Fig. 57-13). According to the 1991 ASPRS survey and 1998 ASAPS survey, 40% to 60% of the surgeons noted nerve complications following midface augmentation and chin/jaw line contouring. However, because of their temporary and partial nature, the surgeons did not consider them significant. The patients are usually the ones who show the greatest concern. For them, disturbances of sensation or motor function constitute the most frightening sequelae of facial surgery. Such occurrences, even when partial or temporary, are worrisome for both surgeons and patients.

In malar/midface augmentation, the infraorbital nerve is the primary sensory nerve of concern. However, its position relative to the dissection and placement of the implant is quite protected. It is necessary to dissect into the region surrounding the infraorbital nerve and foramen only when augmentation of the paranasolabial zone 3 tear trough region or malar/ premaxillary midface suspension is being performed. Nevertheless, disturbances of infraorbital nerve function have been significant according to the surveys. When the necessary precautions are taken and the basic technical guidelines described earlier are followed, such sensory nerve dysfunction should be rare and transient.

Similarly, the mentalis nerve is frequently disturbed during premandible and chin augmentation of the anterior and central zones. The mental nerve, however, appears to recover more quickly, and permanent sensory disturbances are extremely rare.

Disturbances of facial nerve function are even more frightening because motor abnormalities result in animated asymmetries or, even worse, total functional deficits. These complications occur only when dissection instruments penetrate the region of the seventh nerve and its branches. They are more likely to occur when the dissection is not directly on bone, and when excessive traction traumatizes the nerve bundles, especially where they exit from their bony foramina. Posterior dissections along the zygomatic arch that extend superiorly or inferiorly to the middle third of the arch can inadvertently damage the frontal branch to the forehead elevator muscles and branches to the orbicularis oculi muscles simultaneously. The damage is usually transient but can cause lagophthalmos with scleral dryness, tearing, and irritation to the cornea.

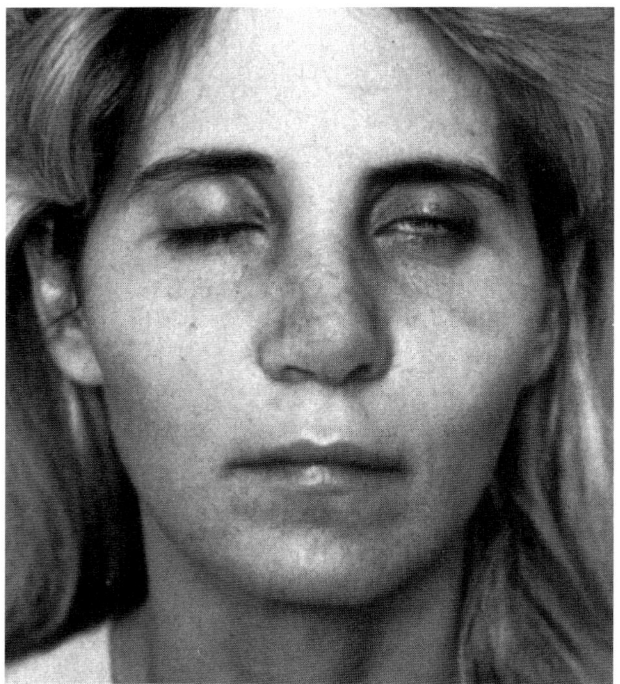
A

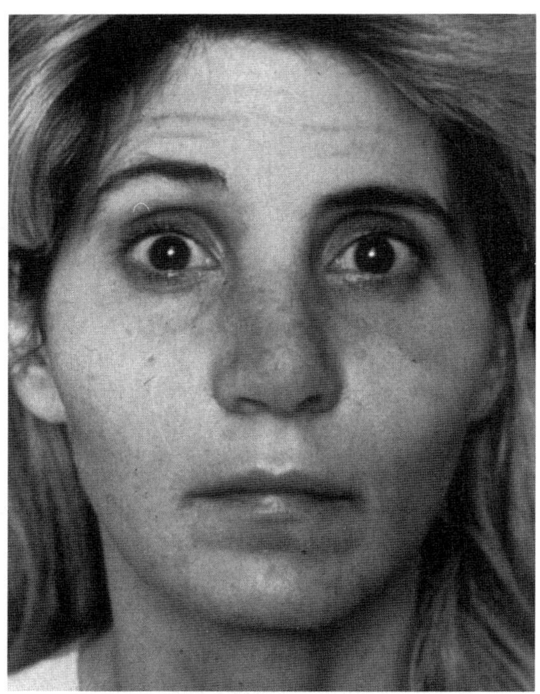
B

FIGURE 57-13. Facial nerve injuries are rare following facial implant surgery and are usually temporary. This is an example of temporary damage to the frontalis and orbicularis branches of the left facial nerve following malar augmentation.

Secondary operations for malar augmentation carry even greater risks for nerve and muscle damage. As many as 30% and perhaps closer to 50% of secondary procedures are associated with some manifestation of nerve and muscle dysfunction. In the author's experience, the actual number of afflicted patients has been few, but the emotional impact of these complications is appreciable.

If porous or fenestrated implants have been used, surgical removal requires tissue dissection techniques that can easily disrupt the surrounding nerve-containing musculature of the midface and premandible. Dissections to expand a previously dissected area and reposition an implant or accommodate one that is larger or differently shaped also predispose to muscle or nerve damage.

The zygomaticus lip elevator muscles and their nerves are another commonly reported area of functional damage, which produces such forms of nasolabial asymmetry as a "crooked" smile or "drooping" lip.

Fortunately, most nerve injuries resolve and function returns completely. Nonetheless, when even a small palsy or diminution of muscle action affects the areas of facial function (i.e., forehead and periorbital, periocular, and perioral regions), it is noticeable and extremely disconcerting to patients. In long-term sensory nerve injuries, the development of crossover sensation is probable and can ultimately resolve the emotional anxieties and preoccupations that result from disturbances of feeling.

Sometimes, when implant removal and accurate replacement are performed, some or all of the morbid signs and symptoms of sensory or motor dysfunction are alleviated.

In the rarest circumstances, operative procedures, such as coronal brow elevation, lateral canthopexy, or midface suspension, are necessary to improve the motor asymmetries that have resulted from midfacial procedures and implant augmentation.

Dissatisfaction with Augmentation of the Premandible/Jaw Line Aesthetic Unit

As has previously been mentioned, no completely accurate scientific method is available to determine the precise size and shape of implants for either the midface or the lower third premandible aesthetic unit. Cephalometrics are used by maxillofacial and craniofacial surgeons. The well-known zero meridian concept popularized by Mario Gonzalez Ulloa provides semiaccurate guidelines for anteroposterior chin augmentation. These methods rely heavily on the surgeon's individual experience and artistic judgment for accurate execution of the parameters that have been measured.

Traditional, centrally placed chin implants are small and nonanatomical in shape. They often create abnormal central chin mounds with visible, unnatural, unattractive lateral prejowl sulcus depressions (Fig. 57-14). Such chin contours are unacceptable to today's surgeons and patients. They are often accentuated by laxity of the lower facial tissues, which develops in an aging jowl just posterior to the anterior

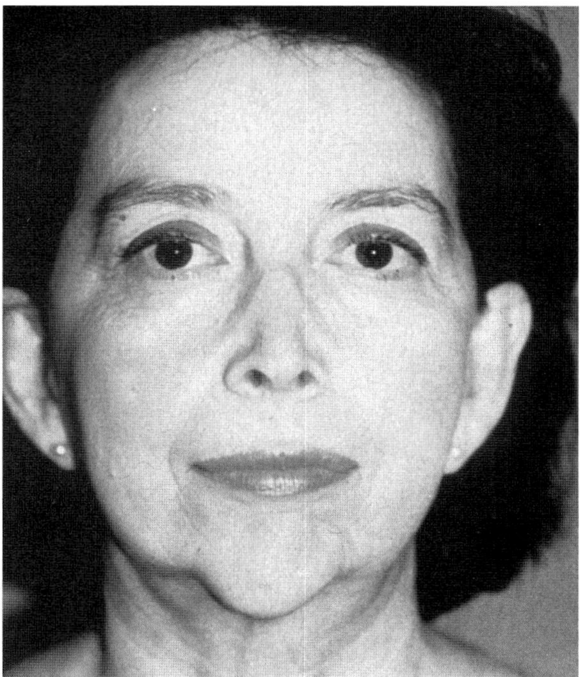

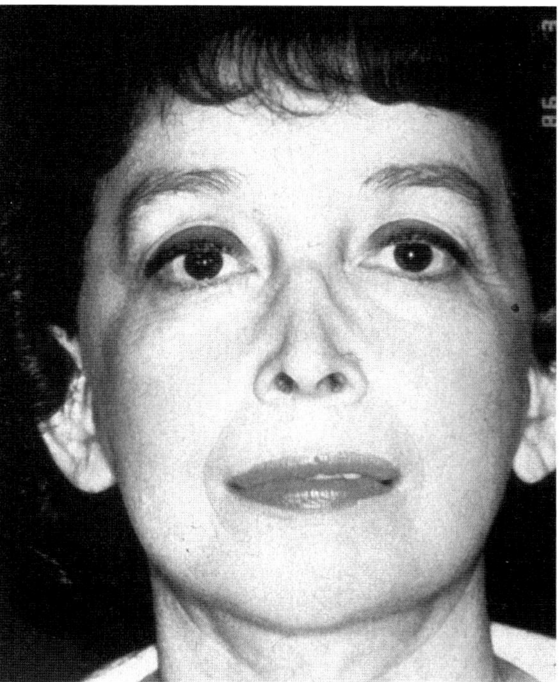

A B

FIGURE 57-14. This 55-year-old women underwent central chin augmentation with a small, centrally placed, nonanatomical implant. **A:** Postoperative. Abnormal, unnatural, unattractive central chin implant deformity. **B:** Secondary postoperative correction with an extended anatomical chin implant.

mandibular ligament. This problem can be corrected only by layered reconstruction (i.e., fat removal, skin tightening, SMAS tightening, and bony augmentation). Mandibular implants inserted at the time of rhytidectomy can minimize this deformity.

Centrally placed implants also tend to rotate. Rotational displacement of even a few millimeters creates noticeable asymmetry. On the other hand, anatomical implants with lateral wings that extend into the midlateral zone beneath the mental nerve and foramen rapidly become stabilized in a horizontal direction, so that the possibility of malrotation is eliminated.

Many young male patients request a bold, square jaw line. This often requires central augmentation of the mandible of 8 to 10 mm and midlateral augmentation of 3 to 5 mm on each side. One implant 12 to 14 cm long can be used to accomplish both these goals. They can be inserted through one central incision, and two lateral intraoral incisions can be used to adjust the tails of the implants.

Mandibular angle implants that create a wider, stronger, and better defined posterior jaw line are becoming more popular. Accurate placement around the inferior and ascending borders of the posterior mandibular angle must be accomplished to avoid asymmetries, possible dislocation of the implant, and intraoral extrusion. Once again, smaller implants predispose to complications more than implants with a larger surface area. As previously discussed, external extrusion through the skin and subcutaneous layer of the posterior jaw line is possible. The author does not use internal fixation, although it has been reported to be useful by other reconstructive aesthetic surgeons. Some easy method of fixation may become available to minimize posterior mandibular angle complications in the future. Nonetheless, the incidence of problems in that region still remains small (1%).

The submandibular vertical wraparound implant, which extends beneath the mandibular border into the submalar zone to enhance vertical length from the lower lip to the submentum by 4 mm, is very useful to augment the volume of the lower third facial segment. A more significant jaw line minimizes the need for extreme dorsal nasal reduction.

Again, the surgeon must have several very specific discussions with the patient to acquire a precise understanding of the visual result that the patient expects. As with all facial contouring, patients tend to be very particular and discerning regarding the details of their jaw line (e.g., pointed, rounded, more square, more defined). Computer imaging technology has greatly advanced and improved communication between aesthetic surgeons and their patients, especially regarding midface, jaw line, and nasal contouring. Although the precise implant size and shape cannot yet be determined by computer, a good visual image of the patient's desired result can be constructed, and the patient's agreement to the computerized images can be obtained.

Available implants can be altered with scalpel, dermabrader, and calipers during surgery to increase the likelihood of a successful outcome.

Bone Erosion and Absorption

No discussion of facial contouring with alloplastic implants would be complete without a discussion of bone erosion. Many investigations of this phenomenon have been reported in the medical literature. It is noteworthy that very few cases of dental damage have been cited (22), and in the ASPRS and ASAPS surveys, bone erosion was not specifically mentioned as a complication in the comments and data provided by the responding surgeons. However, it is certain that for unknown reasons, bone erosion occurs in a significant percentage of patients with implants and may even be a universal phenomenon (23,24). Bone erosion takes place in both the malar/maxillary region and the mandible. Whether erosion occurs more frequently with subperiosteal placement or supraperiosteal dissection has never been established.

Erosion appears to be minimized by the use of extended anatomical implants that have a broader surface area. This is perhaps because the soft tissue pressure forces are more generally dispersed and distributed.

Malar bone erosion does not appear to present a significant problem. Theoretically, if severe enough, it could produce a gross contour deformity or damage the nerve root of a tooth, so that an overlying implant might be required. No statistics in the literature indicate large numbers of dental complications, such as root impingement or abscess. Rather, thousands of successful augmentations have been performed during the past 40 years without such complications having been reported.

Significant bone erosion with small implants is not unusual. It may occur even to a depth of 5 to 8 mm. Overgrowth of bone above the surface onto an implant is more common. This bone is generally very thin, with an egg shell consistency, and can be rongeured easily. It may be necessary to correct surface irregularities resulting from bone erosion with an osteotome or power tool to facilitate the appropriate, stable positioning of a new implant. Another option is to fill the bony excavation with autogenous tissue, such as temporalis fascia or galea. Bone wax or hydroxyapatite may also be used. Bone erosion from alloplastic implants apparently does not cause significant medical problems (25).

When an atrophic mandible is augmented, concern about weakening the structural integrity of the bone by erosion is real (26). This theoretical complication has not actually been reported, but it should always be considered when the patient is older or has frequent dental problems. Mandibular resorption during aging progresses from the tooth socket down toward the mental foramen, whereas implants are located on the bone inferior to the region of resorption. The lower segment of the mandibular architecture remains sturdy throughout life.

Occasional cases of dental infections posing a threat to alloplastic implants have been reported, but in very few of them was removal of the implant necessary. There is always concern when dental infections of the mandible or maxilla arise and when dental procedures, including cleaning, are performed. Dental infections should be treated intensively with antibiotics in the presence of malar or mandible implants. All patients with facial implants should be placed on antibiotic coverage for at least 12 hours before any dental procedure or cleaning. From all reported data, it appears that bone erosion is more of a potential hazard than a real one in facial contouring. However, it should always be acknowledged by the aesthetic surgeon.

CONCLUSION

Remarkable advances have been made in creating three-dimensional changes in facial contours with alloplastic materials since the 1980s. These procedures, in addition to newer midfacial soft tissue suspension techniques, have won acceptance by both physicians and patients. The 1998 ASAPS survey conclusively demonstrates that alloplastic facial augmentation is now a recognized and accepted subspecialty. Premandible chin augmentation was considered to be very successful (52%), a useful adjunct (34%), or occasionally useful (20%) by the responding surgeons. Indeed, 13% of them considered this technique to be indispensable, only 4% felt that it was poor, and only 8% felt that they could do without it (Table 57-12). Malar/midface augmentation was considered to be very successful (28%), occasionally useful (31%), or mediocre (37%) by the responding surgeons. Four percent felt that it was indispensable, only 8% felt that it was poor (8%), and only 16% though they could do without it (Table 57-13). It is evident from the change in attitudes since the 1991 survey that alloplastic facial contouring has achieved a significant place in the armamentarium of aesthetic facial plastic surgeons.

TABLE 57-12. 1998 ASAPS SURVEY: ATTITUDES TOWARD PREMANDIBLE CHIN AUGMENTATION

Attitude	Physician responses (%)
Very successful	52
Useful adjunct	34
Occasionally useful	20
Indispensable	13
Moderately successful	8
Could do without	8
Not bad	4
Poor	4
Mediocre	1

ASAPS, American Society for Aesthetic Plastic Surgery.

TABLE 57-13. 1998 ASAPS SURVEY: ATTITUDES TOWARD MALAR MIDFACE AUGMENTATION

Attitude	Physician responses (%)
Mediocre	37
Occasionally useful	31
Very successful	28
Could do without	16
Useful adjunct	15
Not bad	8
Poor	8
Indispensable	4

ASAPS, American Society for Aesthetic Plastic Surgery.

In the future, computerized technology will allow the aesthetic surgeon to correlate facial images with implant designs and specifications more accurately. The technology to produce precisely customized implants will increase and improve. Postsurgical complications are not rare, but they do not occur in prohibitively high numbers. The newer materials and implant techniques generated from the expanding collective experience of aesthetic surgeons will provide more accurate methods of analysis and the technical finesse with which to reduce complications and patient dissatisfaction dramatically.

REFERENCES

1. Terino EO. *The art of alloplastic facial contouring.* Philadelphia: WB Saunders, 1999.
2. Mladick R. Alloplastic cheek augmentation. *Clin Plast Surg* 1991;18:29–38.
3. Binder WJ, Kamer FM, Parkes ML. Mentoplasty—a clinical analysis of alloplastic implants. *Laryngoscope* 1981;91:383.
4. Terino EO. Facial contouring with alloplastic implants. *Fac Plast Surg Clin North Am* 1999;7:85–103.
5. Wilkinson TS. Complications in aesthetic malar augmentation. *Plast Reconstr Surg* 1983;71:643.
6. Terino EO. Chin and malar augmentation. In: Peck G. *Complications and problems in aesthetic plastic surgery.* New York: Gower Medical Publishers, 1992:6.2–6.30.
7. Zarem HA. Silastic implants in plastic surgery. *Surg Clin North Am* 1968;48:129.
8. McKenzie ML. Mandibular reconstruction using silicone: fifteen-year follow-up. *Plast Reconstr Surg* 1984;74:531.
9. Ivy E, Lorenc Z, Aston S. Malar augmentation with silicone implants. *Plast Reconstr Surg* 1995;96:63–68.
10. Mole B. The use of Gore-Tex in aesthetic surgery of the face. *Plast Reconstr Surg* 1992;90:200–206.
11. Godin M, Waldman R, Johnson C. The use of expanded polytetrafluoroethylene (Gore-Tex) in rhinoplasty. *Arch Otolaryngol Head Neck Surg* 1995;121:1131.
12. Owsley TG, Taylor CO. The use of Gore-Tex for nasal augmentation: a retrospective analysis of 106 patients. *Plast Reconstr Surg* 1994;94:241–248.
13. Rubin L. Polyethylene as a bone and cartilage substitute: a 32-year restrospective. In: Rubin L, ed. *Biomaterials in reconstructive surgery.* St. Louis: Mosby, 1983:474–493.
14. Berghas A. Porous polyethylene in reconstructive head and neck surgery. *Arch Otolaryngol* 1985;111:154–160.
15. Romano J, Iliff N, Manson P. Use of Medpor porous polyethylene implants in 140 patients with facial fractures. *J Craniofac Surg* 1993;4:142–147.
16. Yaremchuk M, Sims D, Casanova R, et al. *Long-term follow-up of expanded polyethylene implants for aesthetic and reconstructive facial skeletal surgery.* Presented at the 6th International Congress of Craniofacial Surgery, Saint Tropez, France, October 21–24, 1995.
17. Wellisz T. Clinical experience with Medpor porous polyethylene implant. *Aesthetic Plast Surg* 1993;17:339–344.
18. Byrd H, Hobar P, Shewmake K. Augmentation of the craniofacial skeleton with porous hydroxyapatite granules. *Plast Reconstr Surg* 1993;91:15–22.
19. Salyer KE, Hall CD. Porous hydroxyapatite as an onlay bone-graft substitute for maxillofacial surgery. *Plast Reconstr Surg* 1989;84:236–244.
20. Merritt K, Shafter J, Brown S. Implant site infection rates with porous and dense materials. *J Biomed Mater Res* 1979;13:101–108.
21. Whear NM, Cousley RRJ, Liew C, et al. Postoperative infection of Proplast facial implants. *Br J Oral Maxillofac Surg* 1993;31:292–295.
22. ASTMF981. Standard practice for the assessment of biocompatibility of biomaterials (nonporous) for surgical implants with respect to effect of materials on muscle and bone. *Annual book of ASTM standards,* vol 13.01, 1994.
23. Hoffman S. Loss of a Silastic chin implant following a dental infection. *Ann Plast Surgery* 1981;7:484.
24. Lilla JA, Vistnes LM, Jobe RP. The long-term effects of hard alloplastic implants when put on bone. *Plast Reconstr Surg* 1976;58:14.
25. Robinson M, Shuken R. Bone resorption under plastic chin implants. *J Oral Surg* 1969;27:116.
26. Friedland JA, Coccaro PJ, Converse JM. Retrospective cephalometric analysis of mandibular bone absorption under silicone rubber chin implants. *Plast Reconstr Surg* 1976;57:144–149.

Discussion

ALLOPLASTIC FACIAL CONTOURING

JOSEPH L. DAW, JR.

The use of alloplastic materials in facial contouring is quite commonplace in the plastic surgeon's armamentarium. Conceptually, it is usually associated with aesthetic procedures of the face, but it can also be a useful adjunct to reconstructive corrections. Dr. Terino has nicely described a systematic method of analysis for determining the needs and requirements of the patient who may benefit from facial augmentation procedures, and he has provided approaches to allow proper execution of the operative plan.

It is of the utmost importance to arrive at a proper diagnosis. This requires an understanding of facial proportions and the changes associated with aging of the facial soft tissues and skeleton (1). The surgeon must know when to augment a particular anatomical location, and must also appreciate the circumstances in which reduction is the indicated procedure, such as when a patient has an excessive transverse dimension at the zygomas or mandibular angles. The initial clinical examination should include an assessment of occlusal and skeletal relations. Augmenting the chin of a patient with mandibular retrognathia and a class II malocclusion without a full understanding of the diagnosis is a disservice to the patient. In this case, orthodontic therapy and orthognathic surgery would be the proper and ideal treatment. Cephalometric analysis is particularly useful to assess patients for whom a change in chin projection is contemplated. In the aged face, repositioning and redistribution of ptotic soft tissue will accomplish the desired aesthetic goals in a purely autologous manner.

Augmentation of the malar region can create or restore a desired facial balance (2). Lower eyelid support is improved by a positive vector orientation. A proper orientation is critical to the correct placement of cheek implants. This must occur in all planes, and when the orientation is incorrect, an unnatural, artificial appearance results. A simple method for determining the position of an implant, in addition to the techniques reported in the literature, which are based on measurements and linear guides, is to place the implant externally on the skin over the malar eminence and orient it to achieve the desired contour. The boundaries are then marked on the skin. This method also provides a guide to accurate dissection of the pocket.

The intraoral approach is the easiest and fastest one to use and is less likely to cause complications than the other techniques. A full-thickness incision through the mucosa, orbicularis oris, and periosteum is preferred to blunt tearing through the muscle; with the former, trauma to the soft tissues is minimized, and so postoperative edema, hemorrhage, and the risk for hematoma formation are reduced. A generous cuff of loose mucosa should be allowed facilitate closure. The intraoral approach provides the best visualization of the infraorbital nerve. When the nerve is identified promptly, it is less likely to be injured. Nevertheless, all patients who are to undergo malar implant augmentation must be informed of the possibility of postoperative numbness. If the patient experiences numbness postoperatively, sensation almost always returns to normal within 2 to 8 weeks because the mechanism of injury is a neurapraxia resulting from either the dissection or retraction. If numbness persists for 6 to 8 weeks or is associated with a dysesthesia, one must consider impingement of the implant on the infraorbital nerve. Exploration and repositioning of the implant will be necessary. As long as the dissection remains in the subperiosteal plane, the risk for injury to branches of the facial nerve should be negligible. Despite attempts at accurate dissection of the subperiosteal pocket, it is often large enough for the implant to move. Movement of the implant leads to asymmetry or an unnatural position of the implant(s). Therefore, stabilization of the implant with one or two titanium screws is advantageous. Porous polyethylene implants are preferred to silicone implants because it is easier to drill the screw holes, and they do seem to provide a more rapid and stable "integration." Although the porosity of the implant is of theoretical concern, infection has not been problematic.

Chin augmentation is a simple way to achieve lower facial balance (3,4). This procedure in and of itself does not necessitate a general anesthetic and can be easily performed under intravenous sedation. Hematoma formation should not be a concern if care is taken to obtain good hemostasis with electrocautery, even directly on the bony sites of bleeding. General anesthesia may result in elevated blood pressure during the emergence, with "bucking" on the endotracheal tube and postoperative emesis. These events are likely to

J. L. Daw, Jr.: Division of Plastic Surgery, The University of Illinois at Chicago, Chicago, Illinois contribute to hematoma formation. Although the infection rates for the intraoral and extraoral approaches are similar, I prefer the submental access because superior malposition or migration of the implant, one of the more common complications after insertion of a chin implant, is less likely to occur. Typically, the mental nerve is located below and between the root apices of the first and second premolars. This guide is more reliable than the measurements reported in the literature. If a careful, deliberate subperiosteal dissection is carried out in a medial to lateral direction, the nerve will be readily identified and protected. Using the position of the teeth can be misleading if either the first or second premolar has been extracted during orthodontic therapy. If any uncertainty exists, a Panorex radiograph will assist in locating the mental foramen preoperatively. Finally, division of the mentalis muscles is an inherent part of the intraoral approach. The muscles must be carefully reapproximated during closure of the incision or else a ptotic lower lip may result. Even with proper repair of the mentalis muscles, reduced animation of the chin may occur postoperatively. This is almost always temporary and resolves within a few months.

Selection of the implant is very important. Use of the longer, anatomical type of implants allows for a gradual taper in the parasymphysis/body region, so that visible areas of demarcation are avoided. Again, stabilization with titanium screws may be useful to avoid postoperative malposition, especially rotational. For younger patients (i.e., in their 20s or even 30s), an osseous genioplasty is a better method for increasing the sagittal projection of the chin. The long-term presence of a chin implant results in gradual erosion of the underlying bone. The gain in projection will eventually be reduced, and the erosion may extend to involve the anterior mandibular teeth (Fig. 57D-1). Such involvement results in pain and sensitivity of the teeth, and root canal therapy may be indicated. This complication has probably been underreported in the literature because it occurs after 20 or 30 years, so that these patients are lost to follow-up with the original surgeon. A vertical deficiency of the chin cannot be corrected by placing an implant. An osteotomy is required, with either a bone graft or hydroxyapatite block placed interpositionally. Postoperatively, the application of light compression to the chin with Microfoam tape or an elastic garment will promote rapid soft tissue adherence and immobilization of the implant and lessen the risk for hematoma formation.

Augmentation of the nasal dorsum with alloplastic implants obviates the need for a donor site, which is required when autologous tissue is used. The avoidance of morbidity at the donor site makes an alloplast an attractive option. Silicone implants and porous polyethylene are well suited to this area. Complications related to the implantation of alloplastic materials in the nose are similar to those occurring when autologous tissue is used and when implants are placed in other regions of the face. These include infection, improper contour, malposition, skin breakdown with exposure, and mobility. Although the use of alloplastic implants in the nose is not as well accepted in the United States, good results, with an acceptable rate of complications, have been reported by Asian surgeons (5).

Augmentation of the posterolateral mandible may be necessary bilaterally for developmental jaw anomalies or unilaterally for cases of hemifacial microsomia or Romberg's disease. The surgical approach utilizes an incision similar to that used for the sagittal ramus osteotomy or intraoral vertical ramus osteotomy. Generally, the superior aspect of the incision should not extend higher than the plane of occlusion of the mandibular teeth. Extending the incision higher will likely lead to exposure of the buccal fat pad, which can herniate into the wound and obscure the view. The incision is placed approximately 1 cm lateral to the external oblique ridge to facilitate wound closure. As described previously,

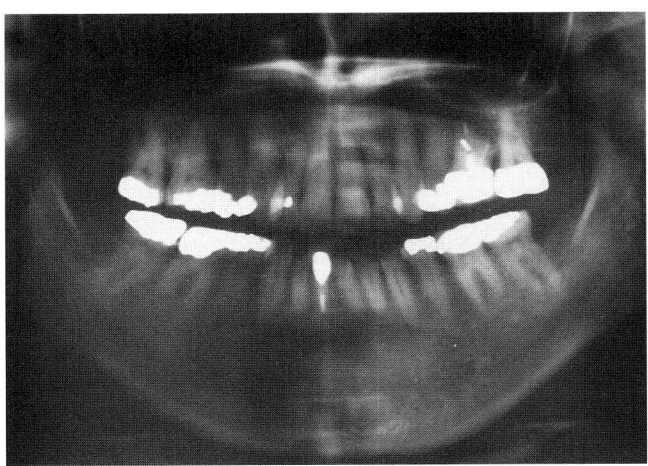

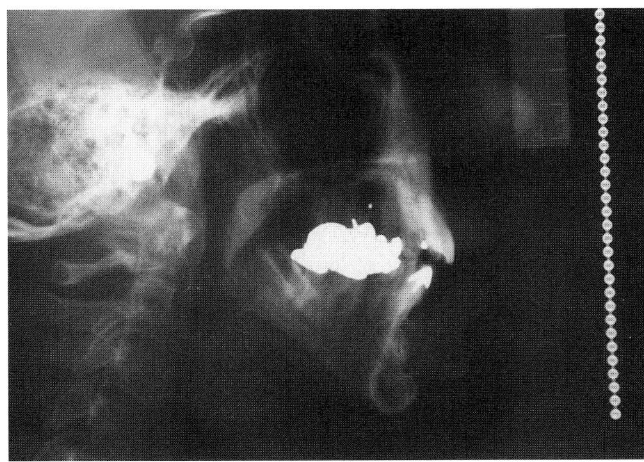

FIGURE 57D-1. Panorex **(left)** and lateral cephalometric radiographs **(right)** of a patient with a Silastic chin implant eroding into the mandibular symphysis and anterior teeth.

the incision is carried sharply through all layers of soft tissue, including periosteum; blunt tearing through the buccinator muscle is to be avoided. Most beneficial is the percutaneous placement of titanium screws through the implant and underlying bone (6) (Fig. 57D-2). This ensures stability of the implant and prevents malposition and asymmetry.

Temporary sensory deficits after the insertion of facial implants, particularly chin and malar implants, should be anticipated and the patient forewarned. As previously mentioned, full recovery generally occurs within 2 to 8 weeks. Persistent numbness or pain may indicate impingement of the implant on the affected nerve. Exploration and repositioning of the implant will be required to resolve the symptoms. Injury to the facial nerve should occur much less frequently than injury to branches of the trigeminal nerve. The likelihood of injury to the facial nerve is greatest during placement of a malar implant via a facelift approach. The temporal branch of the facial nerve can be injured when the subperiosteal pocket is developed along the zygomatic arch; however, one would have to be fairly careless for this to occur.

Implants with a larger surface area allow a more suble tape to their borders and provide an inconspicuous transition from the augmented to the nonaugmented tissue. Smaller implants with an abrupt taper are unnatural and result in a visible contour of the implant. For these reasons, care must be taken when the implant is trimmed and customized for the patient. The implant may move despite being placed in a subperiosteal pocket, usually because the pocket is excessively large. The possibility of fibrous ingrowth into the implant is an advantage of porous polyethylene over silicone. The use of titanium screws can ensure absolute stability.

An infected implant carries a poor prognosis. An attempt at salvage with a 3- to 4-week course of oral antibiotics or even a brief course of intravenous antibiotics is reasonable. However, extending the attempt at salvage beyond this period only prolongs morbidity, and removal of the implant is indicated. Before a new implant is placed, 6 to 12 months should elapse. Mobility, especially in implants placed transorally, may predispose to infection. With the development of chronic infection, a fistulous tract may form (Fig. 57D-3). This clearly necessitates removal of the implant, and the fistula also must be excised. Infection of an implant often follows a dental procedure in which infiltration of local anesthesia in the region of the implant has been required. The implant is then inoculated. Patients should be advised to inform their dentists of the presence of an implant so that this complication can be avoided.

Facial implants may become exposed for a variety of reasons: an inadequate pocket; improper positioning of the implant; excess prominence of the implant, which may cause pressure necrosis of the overlying soft tissue, and hematoma. Implants in the paranasal region seem to be particularly susceptible to exposure, probably because of their proximity to the suture line.

Bone erosion at the undersurface of the implant occurs in every patient with time. This is especially so in areas of relatively high tension, such as the chin. For this reason, I advocate osseous genioplasty rather than alloplastic augmentation for patients in their late teens to 30s. Significant bony erosion over the anterior mandible may extend to involve the anterior mandibular teeth. Such involvement leads to pain or sensitivity of the teeth, so that root canal therapy is sometimes required. This complication is probably underreported in the literature.

One type of alloplastic material available for craniofacial augmentation that has not been mentioned is bone cement (7,8). Several commercially available products are on the market, all of which are a form of calcium phosphate ce-

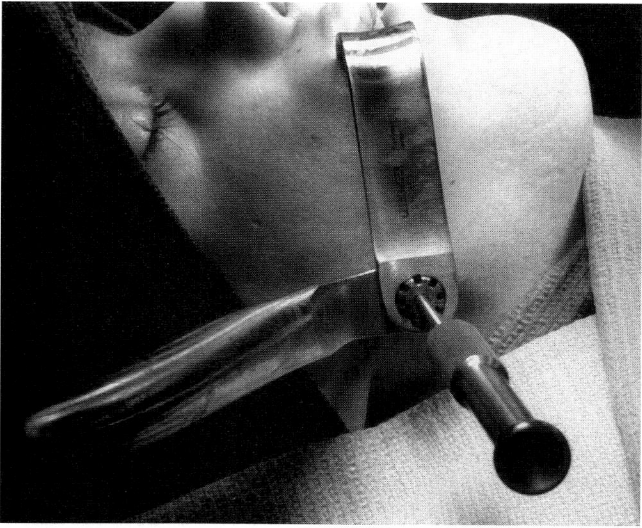

FIGURE 57D-2. Percutaneous placement of a titanium screw to stabilize a lateral mandibular implant.

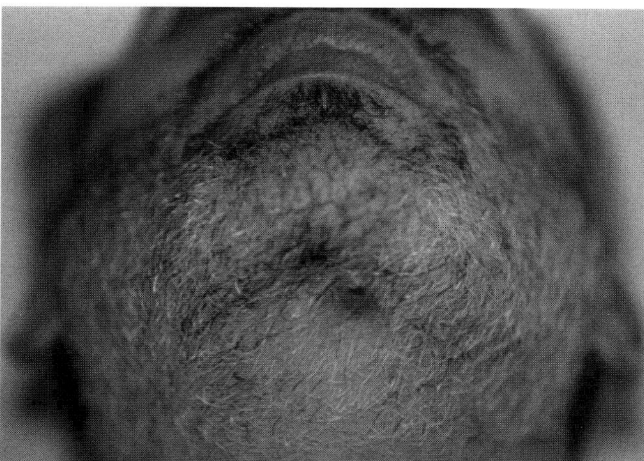

FIGURE 57D-3. Submental cutaneous fistula that developed as the result of a chronically infected Silastic chin implant. This was refractory to long-term antibiotic therapy.

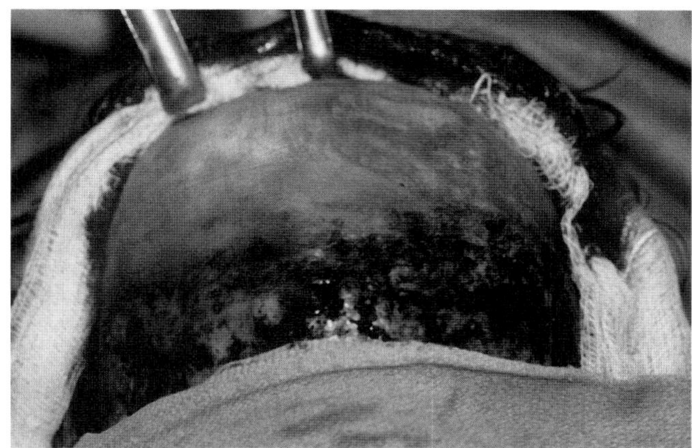

FIGURE 57D-4. Recontouring of the forehead with hydroxyapatite cement.

ment. They typically require a dry field for setting. In addition, deformation may occur before complete setting if significant forces are applied to the material by the soft tissue. For these reasons, the use of bone cement in malar and chin augmentation is not efficacious. Useful applications are in contouring of the forehead (Fig. 57D-4), superciliary ridge, and cranial vault. Surgical approaches for these purposes include a coronal incision, occasionally with endoscopic assistance. It appears that volume maintenance is good and that some degree of replacement with bone or bony ingrowth occurs. Once set, the material is rather brittle and prone to fracture if a strong force is absorbed. Splintering leads to a loss of form and mobility and the formation of seromas. All fractured material must be removed and new or additional bone cement applied.

Although some surgeons have criticized them, alloplastic facial implants have been used with excellent aesthetic results and an acceptable complication rate. However, proper analysis of the patient's aesthetic requirements and precise placement are essential to minimize unfavorable results. Despite the insertion of a facial implant is an operation of small magnitude, it is rather sensitive to technique, and one may expect improved outcomes as experience is gained.

REFERENCES

1. Bartlett SP, Grossman R, Whitaker LA. Age-related changes of the craniofacial skeleton: an anthropometric and histologic analysis. *Plast Reconstr Surg* 1992;90:592–600.
2. Whitaker LA. Temporal and malar-zygomatic reduction and augmentation. *Clin Plast Surg* 1991;18:55–64.
3. Mahler D. Chin augmentation—a retrospective study. *Ann Plast Surg* 1982;8:468–473.
4. Guyuron B, Raszewski RL. A critical comparison of osteoplastic and alloplastic augmentation genioplasty. *Aesthetic Plast Surg* 1990;14:199–206.
5. Deva AK, Merten S, Chang L. Silicone in nasal augmentation rhinoplasty: a decade of clinical experience. *Plast Reconstr Surg* 102;1998:1230–1237.
6. Yaremchuk MJ. Mandibular augmentation. *Plast Reconstr Surg* 2000;106:697–706.
7. Burstein FD, Cohen SR, Hudgins R, et al. The use of hydroxyapatite cement in secondary craniofacial reconstruction. *Plast Reconstr Surg* 1999;104:1270–1275.
8. Jackson IT, Yavuzer R. Hydroxyapatite cement: an alternative for craniofacial skeletal contour refinements. *Br J Plast Surg* 2000;53:24–29.

58

GENIOPLASTY

BAHMAN GUYURON

Because of a growing awareness of the importance of the chin in facial pulchritude, especially in patients who undergo rhinoplasty, genioplasty is becoming an increasingly popular procedure. The high rates of patient satisfaction, ranging from 90% to 95% for osteoplastic genioplasty and from 85% to 90% for alloplastic genioplasty (1), clearly indicate that complications following genioplasty are rare. Genioplasty is a somewhat less exacting procedure than rhinoplasty for two reasons. First, most chins are covered with a significant amount of soft tissue, which mitigates any skeletal imperfections that otherwise would be discernible. Furthermore, the area of the chin is richly supplied with blood vessels, which reduce the potential for infection.

Nevertheless, undesirable results and complications do follow genioplasty, so that a careful analysis of the deformity (2), proper choice of technique and implant material, and meticulous execution of the surgery (3) are essential to minimize complications and inauspicious outcomes. This chapter focuses on the assessment of the patient with undesirable results or complications, and the management of the various categories of complications and poor results.

PATIENT EVALUATION

In all secondary aesthetic procedures, dealing with a patient who is disenchanted with a surgical outcome or who has endured a complication is perplexing and requires experience and special patient management skills. A patient who has undergone genioplasty and experienced a suboptimal result or complication is disappointed, frustrated, and often angered. Trust in surgeons in general, and the former surgeon in particular, has vanished, and restoring some level of comfort and confidence is an important part of the overall patient management.

Many of these patients are searching for facts to justify a potential legal action, and an unfounded or unjustified statement may invoke this process. Impetuous statements, particularly pertaining to the previous surgeon's inadequate knowledge, capability, and experience as the reason for the complication, should be avoided. Generally, such statements are unnecessary and should be eschewed altogether if possible. However, if a statement has to be made in this regard, it should follow a scrupulous analysis of the facts (e.g., a study of the chart notes detailing the surgical technique and postoperative care).

Many of the patients are highly emotional, and it is crucial for the surgeon not to be misled by exaggerated statements. A sagacious analysis of the factors that have led to the complications or dissatisfying results should be conducted to minimize the potential for a similar misfortune following the next surgery. Listening to the patient's version of the events and then comparing it with the facts may enable to surgeon to learn more about the patient and the potential for failure or success of the intended surgery. If a slight imperfection is present, yet the patient perceives it as a significant deformity, such a patient is unlikely to be pleased with any outcome. On the other hand, a patient who has experienced complications and undesirable results and who unjustifiably assumes the blame for a poor surgical outcome, may be an ideal candidate for further surgical correction.

Medical conditions such as diabetes can contribute to complications. They may have been overlooked by the previous surgeon or, more commonly, may not have been known to the patient or the surgeon. Any unexpected and unusual complication should raise suspicions about contributing factors (4,5).

A patient whose devastation over a minimal chin asymmetry has caused her to become a socially inactive hermit is most likely a patient who has an underlying psychological problem that will not be resolved with the most successful surgery. Such a patient should undergo a psychiatric evaluation before undergoing any other surgery, if indeed surgery should be contemplated at all.

A clinical analysis of the entire face must precede the analysis of the lower face and the occlusion. A hasty decision about what needs to be done can result in failure. In many cases of patient dissatisfaction, an underlying mandibular

B. Guyuron: Division of Plastic Surgery, Case Western Reserve University, Cleveland, Ohio

deficiency mistaken for microgenia and an advancement of the chin has been performed, but the entire lower jaw is in an improper position. In such situations, an examination of the oral cavity, occlusion, and inclination of the teeth may aid the surgeon in making a better decision regarding the second operation. If retrognathia or micrognathia is present, the patient is a better candidate for orthognathic surgery than for genioplasty.

The face and neck should be thoroughly examined from the front and in profile. The presence of excess submental fat and redundant skin may prevent an optimal genioplasty result.

The role of cephalometric radiography and life-size photographs cannot be overstressed, particularly when one is dealing with a patient who is not content with the outcome of previous surgery. These studies help to determine what has gone wrong and what may possibly set the stage for a future success.

Genioplasty can be either alloplastic or osteoplastic. These are two totally different procedures, and although they can be cross-utilized in limited situations, by and large the results differ. Although an alloplastic procedure may lead to a reasonably good outcome, generally an osteotomy gives better results, and occasionally, alloplastic materials cannot be used or cannot provide the intended aesthetic result. Often when patients seek a secondary genioplasty, it is necessary to remove the previous implant and convert to an osteotomy, which can cause complications and difficulties. These two categories are considered separately.

COMPLICATIONS AND UNDESIRABLE RESULTS OF OSTEOPLASTIC GENIOPLASTY

In general, autogenous genioplasty is superior to alloplastic genioplasty and leads to fewer complications during long-term follow-up. Potential problems include asymmetry, wound dehiscence, irregularities, step deformity, overadvancement, underadvancement, infection, anesthesia and paresthesia of the lower lip, and chin ptosis ("witch's chin" deformity).

Chin Asymmetry

Chin asymmetry may be observed following genioplasty for a variety of reasons. The most common reason is a preexisting asymmetry of the chin or mandible that was not detected preoperatively. Asymmetry of the mandible is the more common reason for an asymmetric outcome of genioplasty. In this situation, no type of genioplasty will produce a completely symmetrical lower face. Although a genioplasty might camouflage a major mandibular asymmetry to some degree, it would fail to overcome a true mandibular disharmony. With a thorough analysis of the face, including an intraoral examination, such an undesirable result can be avoided. One has to assess the alignment of the maxillary and mandibular midlines. Any misalignment may indicate a mandibular or maxillary discrepancy unless an orthodontic compensation has occurred. When the maxillary mandibular midlines do not correspond but the maxillary midline matches that of the rest of the upper face, then the problem is in the mandible. Given this condition, an optimal result can be achieved only by orthodontic preparation and orthognathic surgery (Fig. 58-1). Patients who decline this approach should be aware that proper harmony of the lower jaw with the rest of the face cannot be achieved.

Asymmetry confined to the chin area can be related to postoperative shift of the caudal segment, absorption of bone, or technical errors. Regardless, if the asymmetry is discernible, surgical correction should be considered. This condition will require an operation through the previous intraoral incision.

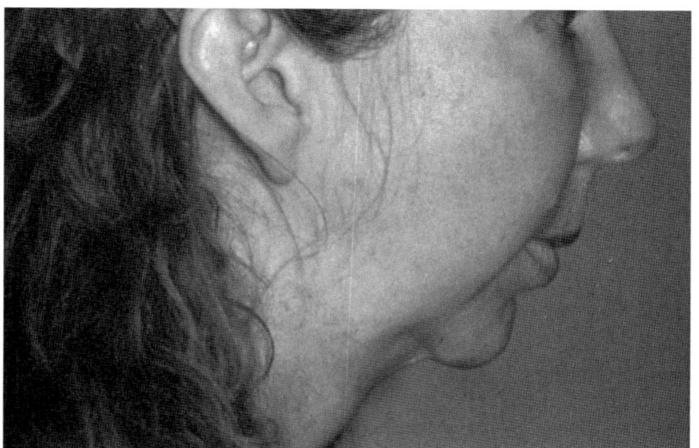
A

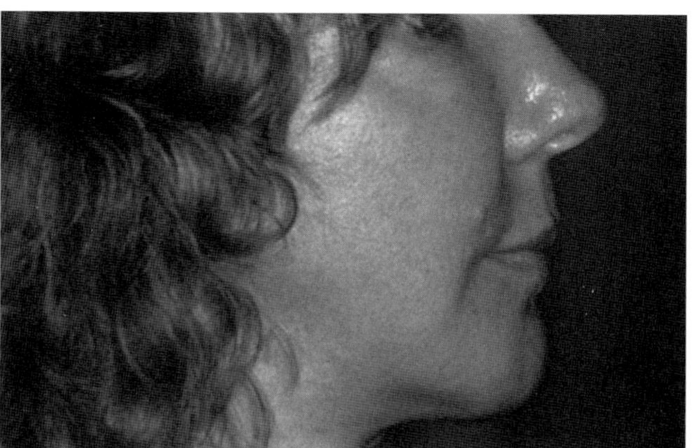
B

FIGURE 58-1. Profile view of a patient who had undergone two previous genioplasties with suboptimal results **(A)** and after orthodontic preparation, mandibular advancement, and osteoplastic genioplasty **(B)**. (From Guyuron B. *Genioplasty.* Boston: Little, Brown and Company, 1993, with permission.)

Secondary osteotomy of the chin is far more difficult than primary osteotomy for three reasons: (a) Scar tissue in the lower labial sulcus makes the incision and dissection difficult; (b) the soft tissue elasticity has been reduced by scar tissue involving the periosteum and the adjacent tissues, so that the exposure is minimized; and (c) removal of hardware implanted in the bone, such as wires or screws and plates, may prove difficult. If bone has deposited on top of the screws or plates, removal is complicated. When the wire loops are buried in the bone and it becomes impossible to remove them, the osteotomy can still be performed by cutting through the wires with a power saw.

The rest of the procedure is similar to what has been described previously (3). Before the osteotomy, the midline of the chin should be marked on the bone with a bone pencil. A horizontal osteotomy is made, and depending on the type of asymmetry, a rotation, lateral transposition, unilateral advancement, or elongation can be accomplished (3). If side-to-side asymmetry is perceived, then a horizontal osteotomy is completed and the caudal segment is moved to the proper position. If one side of the chin is longer but the length of the other side is appropriate, then the long side is shortened by performing a horizontal osteotomy and removing of a segment from the long side. Similarly, the short side is elongated by a horizontal osteotomy with or without bone graft. If the asymmetry is the consequence of a small bone projection, then it can be eliminated by burring the bone. On completion of the osteotomy, the area is irrigated and the incisions repaired in detail; the periosteum and mentalis muscles are approximated to avoid chin ptosis.

Wound Dehiscence

Wound dehiscence following a chin osteotomy is rare. It usually is a consequence of leaving an inadequate amount of soft tissue on the gingival side for a secure repair when the initial incision is made, although a hematoma or infection can also cause wound dehiscence. One undesirable consequence of this complication is chin ptosis resulting from attachment of the mentalis muscle in a more caudal position. For this reason, wound dehiscence has to be treated vigorously.

If the dehiscence is discovered early, an attempt at primary closure can lead to a successful result. However, late discoveries, particularly when no bone is exposed, are best managed with conservative treatment, including frequent mouth irrigation and systemic antibiotics. If the cortical bone is exposed, one has to debride the exposed cortex and the soft tissue and approximate the soft tissues. The advanced soft tissue is then sutured to the remaining gingival tissue. Occasionally, it is necessary to place supporting sutures wrapped around the teeth to avoid early recurrence of the dehiscence. Every effort should be made to repair the wound in anatomical layers. For a delayed repair, monofilament nonabsorbable sutures are preferred over absorbable sutures.

Irregularities and Step Deformities

These are often depressions on either side of the chin. They cause a displeasing outline of the chin and an ungraceful transition of contour from the mandibular body to the chin area. Depending on the cause of the irregularities and depressions, the treatment varies. If the irregularity is the consequence of prominence along the lateral border of the caudal genioplasty segment, it can be easily corrected with an oval bur through an intraoral incision. The excess bone is removed while the soft tissue is protected. Irregularities resulting from a deficiency in the chin area and step deformities can be corrected with either bone graft or hydroxyapatite granules mixed with tribromoethanol (Avertin) and normal saline solution (6). Some step deformities, particularly those that result from a prominent lateral border of the caudal segment, may disappear after 6 months. It is crucial, therefore, not to plan an immediate correction of these imperfections, although the emotional state of the patient may mandate an early correction.

Infection

The incidence of infection following osteotomy is extremely low. In fact, I have never observed this complication. However, when it does occur, it is important to irrigate the oral cavity and infected area copiously. The patient should receive systemic antibiotics and practice vigorous oral care with rinses. Bone debridement is seldom necessary unless the infection has been neglected for a long time.

Overcorrection

Familiarity with the aesthetic proportions of the face can reduce the chances for this complication. Proper knowledge of the soft tissue response to skeletal alteration in this region is also crucial. Generally, an overadvanced chin results in a deep labiomental groove and gives a more aged appearance to the face. (The chin becomes more prominent during the aging process.) The chin may also appear more pointed. This type of result is often dissatisfying for patient and surgeon alike. Excessive vertical elongation or excessive resection of the symphysis may result in soft tissue ptosis, which creates a "witch's chin" deformity.

If the chin has been advanced too much, the appropriate correction is surgical reversal (Fig. 58-2). Sometimes, because of the inclination of the osteotomy plane, the overcorrection may also result in elongation of the lower face. This is specifically undesirable in a patient who has an underlying long face deformity with a receding chin. Even when the chin is advanced to an optimal position, an ostensibly elongated face may result if the patient has a long face deformity. This effect is highly disappointing for both patient and surgeon. In such a case, it is best to correct the maxillary deformity by entering the maxilla.

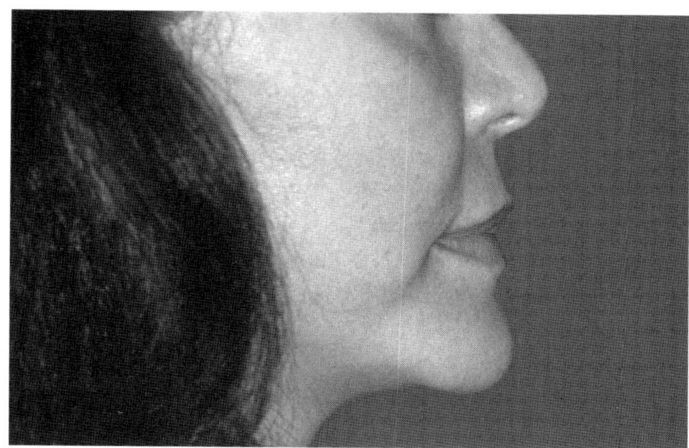
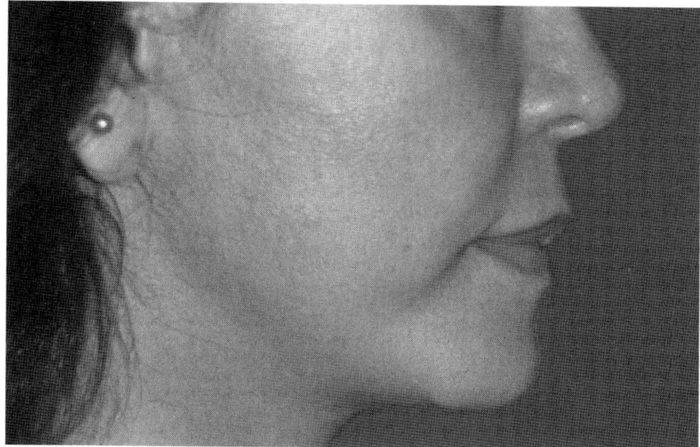

FIGURE 58-2. Profile view of a patient after overadvancement of the chin **(A)** and after osteotomy and setback of the caudal segment **(B)**. (From Guyuron B. *Genioplasty.* Boston: Little, Brown and Company, 1993, with permission.)

An underadvanced chin can readily be advanced further. Through an intraoral incision, an osteotomy is made and the chin is advanced to a new position and fixed in position with screws.

Anesthesia and Paresthesia

Temporary paresthesia and anesthesia are common sequelae of genioplasty. However, the paresthesia is generally minimal and almost always resolves in a matter of weeks to several months, unless the nerve is severed. If the anesthesia persists beyond a year, it is likely that the nerve has been avulsed. Nerve avulsion is generally the consequence of placing an osteotomy too cephalad, either above or at the level of the mental foramen. If the osteotomy is designed approximately 5 to 6 mm caudal to the level of the mental foramen, the chance of permanent numbness is drastically reduced and the nerve cannot possibly be damaged unless vigorous retraction of the soft tissue results in disruption of the mental nerve. Should permanent damage to the nerve follow genioplasty, one may consider exploring the mental nerve and the inferior alveolar nerve canal. If the nerve is not in continuity, it can be approximated with microneurography.

Chin Ptosis

Chin ptosis resulting from overresection of the chin or excessive setback can be corrected by the removal of redundant soft tissue from the submental area (3).

UNDESIRABLE OUTCOMES OF ALLOPLASTIC GENIOPLASTY

Some of the undesirable results of alloplastic genioplasty are related to the limitations of the procedure. Osteoplastic genioplasty is far more versatile than alloplastic genioplasty. In fact, of all the deformities of the chin (2), only horizontal microgenia, and to some degree minimal vertical microgenia, can be corrected with alloplastic chin implants. When the capabilities of alloplastic genioplasty are stretched beyond what it can deliver, the results are suboptimal. The results of an alloplastic genioplasty can also become complicated or the outcomes fail to satisfy the patient for other reasons. These include the use of the wrong size implant, infection, extrusion, malposition, capsular contracture, chin ptosis, and soft tissue chin deformity.

Improper Implant Selection

Choosing a chin implant of the proper size can be difficult. Implant size, which is a major factor in achieving the intended aesthetic goals, is determined by prudent facial evaluation, examination of life-sized photographs, and analysis of soft tissue. One of the most reliable soft tissue criteria for determining the size of a chin implant is Riedel's line (7). This simple line connects the most prominent portion of the upper lip to the lower lip. The chin should be lined up with these two projections; in other words, the most prominent portion of the chin, the upper lip, and the lower lip are ideally in the same plane. Any deficiency reflects microgenia. It is much easier to replace a small implant with a larger implant than vice versa because the excess soft tissue envelope left after removal of a large implant may result in chin ptosis or soft tissue irregularities.

An important factor in selecting the implant size is the soft tissue response to the alloplastic augmentation. In general, the response of the soft tissue to an implant is less than its response to an osteotomy. The soft tissue response to an osteoplastic genioplasty is approximately 1:1 for an advancement, whereas the soft tissue response is 0.8:1 when a implant is used. Another factor in choosing the size of an implant is the depth of the labiomental groove. At no point should the labiomental groove be deeper than 4 mm in a female patient or 6 mm in a male patient.

Implant replacement can be performed as an outpatient procedure with the patient under intravenous sedation. The face is prepared properly and the chin area is infiltrated with lidocaine containing 1:100,000 epinephrine. It is preferable to remove the implant through a submental incision so long as the implant is flexible. An incision is made anterior to the submental incision, even if the previous implantation was performed through an intraoral incision. The incision is deepened to the subcutaneous soft tissue, periosteum, and bone. The symphysis is exposed by elevating the periosteum. Generally, silicone implants will have become encapsulated. The capsule is opened, and the implant is removed and replaced with a larger or smaller implant, depending on the condition. Replacement of a previously placed large implant with a smaller one is not as predictable as replacement of a small implant with a larger one.

Although an intraoral incision can also be used, this is discouraged because it violates the mentalis muscle. However, if this is the only route by which the patient's wishes can be carried out, the oral cavity is irrigated copiously with antibiotic solution and an incision is made in the lower labial sulcus along the previous incisional scar, with adequate soft tissue left on the gingival side for a safe, watertight repair. The incision is then taken down to the capsule of the previous implant, which is opened, and the implant is removed. The cavity is irrigated, and the implant is either replaced with another implant or an osteotomy is performed. If the idea is to replace the implant with an osteotomy, then the intraoral incision is the only proper way of conducting this operation. It is sometimes necessary to remove the capsule to restore the soft tissue elasticity and prevent the collection of fluid in the capsule and ultimate distortion of the chin. Following completion of the implant replacement or the osteotomy, the incision is repaired in two layers.

For the submental incision, 6-0 Vicryl is used. Plain 6-0 catgut is utilized to repair the subcutaneous tissue and skin. For the intraoral incision, a 4-0 chromic is more appropriate. If a porous implant has been previously inserted, the dissection may become more arduous. The larger the pores, the more difficult the removal of the implant. However, every implant can be removed or replaced safely so long as care is taken to perform the dissection right on the implant and not violate the mentalis muscle.

Infection

Infection following augmentation genioplasty remains uncommon. The reported incidence of this complication varies from center to center (3), averaging 5%. Although it is possible to salvage an infected porous implant in an early stage with aggressive antibiotic therapy and oral rinses (8), salvage is seldom successful, particularly if the implant has been placed intraorally; with submental implantation, the chance of success may be greater. Often, it is necessary to remove the implant, irrigate the cavity, and allow the soft tissue to heal. At a later time, the implant is replaced, or, more suitably, an augmentation genioplasty is converted to an osteotomy.

Malpositioned or Displaced Implant

This condition is related either to an initially difficult placement or to rotation of the implant (Fig. 58-3). If the implant is positioned in an appropriately and symmetrically dissected pocket, rotation is unlikely, particularly if the implant is porous. However, silicone implants placed in a larger pocket may shift and cause asymmetry. Another possibility is cephalic migration of the implant (Fig. 58-4). This is a fairly common problem if the implant has been placed through an intraoral incision. Another common reason for asymmetry is preexisting asymmetry on the underlying bone that has gone undetected and shifts the implant in an undesirable direction. Should the implant malposition be discernible at an early stage, the implant is repositioned surgi-

A

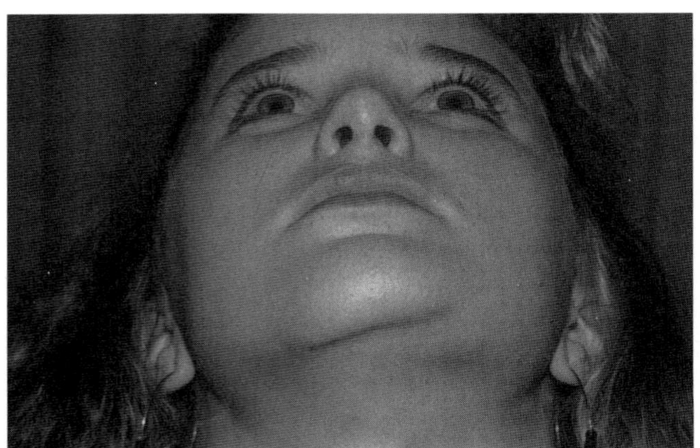

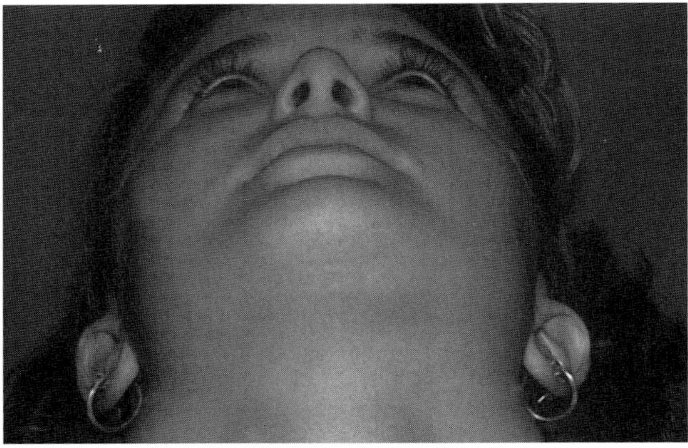

B

FIGURE 58-3. Basilar view of a patient with a malpositioned chin implant **(A)** and after removal of the implant and osseous genioplasty **(B)**. (From Guyuron B. *Genioplasty.* Boston: Little, Brown and Company, 1993, with permission.)

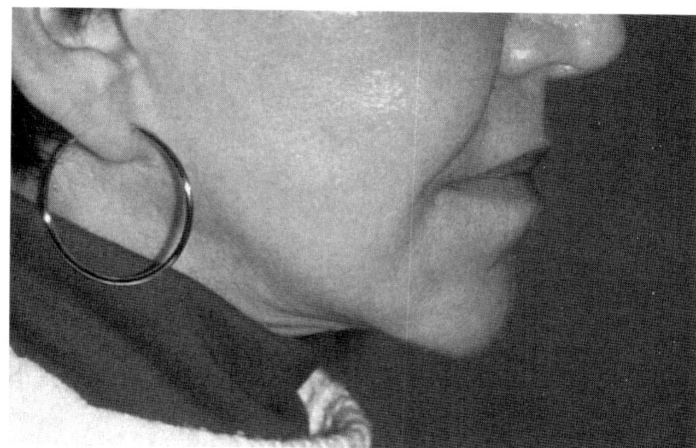
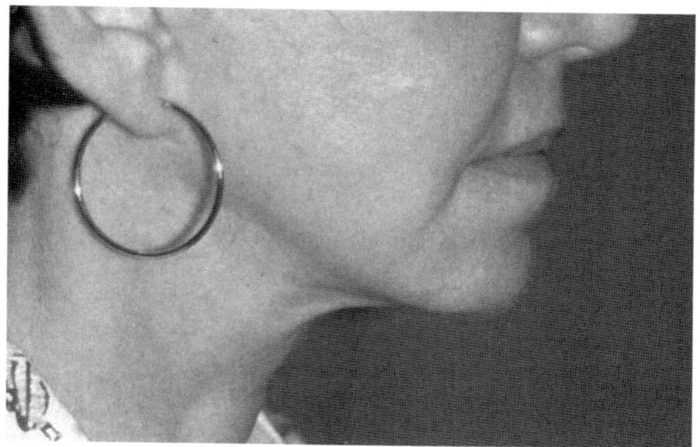

FIGURE 58-4. A: Caudal migration of this implant has resulted in loss of projection and elongation of the lower face. **B:** After replacement of the implant through a submental incision.

cally. However, if the rotation or asymmetry is noted at a later time, then, depending on the degree of asymmetry, one may choose to leave it alone or replace it. Once more, in this situation, conversion of an implant to an osteotomy may produce more desirable results (Fig. 58-3).

Capsular Contraction

In general, a capsule does not form around a porous implant, whereas a thick capsule may form around a smooth implant, specifically one of silicone. As long as the implant is placed in the subperiosteal plane, the formation of a capsule may not be consequential, although positioning the implant in this anatomical plane increases the likelihood of bone erosion. On the other hand, when capsular contraction takes place in the subcutaneous plane, it often results in an unnatural appearance, implant palpability, and skin irregularity. This is a more difficult problem to correct, and often violation of the mentalis muscle causes skin dimpling. Whenever capsular contraction produces a visible deformity, one has no choice but to correct the contraction. It is often necessary to resect the capsule carefully and either convert the alloplastic genioplasty to an osteoplastic genioplasty or replace the silicone implant with one of a porous material, such as HTR.

Chin Ptosis

Chin ptosis is often the consequence of detachment of the mentalis muscle from the anterior mandible, although elongation of the muscle and a deficiency in muscle bulk can also cause chin ptosis (9). This problem is rarely iatrogenic, a consequence of placement of the implant in an improper position, in which it extends the length of the anterior chin (Fig. 58-4). In patients with chin ptosis, excessive exposure of the lower incisors often develops because of lip ptosis, and in a profile view, the soft tissue is seen to extend beyond the horizontal plane of the submental area. This arrangement is aesthetically displeasing, and the problem must be corrected. Surgical correction, however, produces unpredictable results. Even with dissection and reattachment of the soft tissue at a higher level, one may not be able to secure a lip position and chin form that are aesthetically optimal.

The surgical correction can be performed under intravenous sedation. The anterior mandible and the submental area are degloved to slide the soft tissue cephalad, and with the technique of bone tunneling, the periosteum is reattached in a higher level. Initial overcorrection is required because some degree of ptosis may recur. The suspension can be carried out with PDS sutures and bone tunneling; the techniques are similar to those used in endoscopic forehead rejuvenation (10). With the application of external supportive dressing following redraping of the skin in a cephalic position, better results can be achieved.

Bunching and Dimpling of the Skin

One of the most difficult problems to correct is bunching and dimpling of the skin as a consequence of violation and dysfunction of the mentalis muscle. For this reason, it is best to make incisions in the submental area, or if an intraoral incision is used, then the mentalis muscle must be reattached. Should this problem arise, the best solution is to place a layer of dermis or fascia graft between the subcutaneous tissue and the mentalis muscle through a submental incision. The chin is dissected and a sheath of thin dermis graft or fascia graft is placed in the subcutaneous plane. This procedure generally eliminates the dimpling.

TIMING OF SURGERY

Many of the undesirable outcomes of genioplasty may become less visible as time elapses. Dehiscence should be repaired immediately, particularly if the cortical bone is exposed. However, if the bone is not exposed and some time has elapsed, one can allow healing to take place spontaneously. Some irregularities may disappear within a year, so that undertaking corrective surgery before a year has passed may not be justifiable.

REFERENCES

1. Guyuron B, Kadi J. Problems following genioplasty. *Clin Plast Surg* 1997;24:507–514.
2. Guyuron B, Michelow BJ, Willis L. Practical classification of chin deformities. *Aesthetic Plast Surg* 1995;19:257–264.
3. Guyuron B. *Genioplasty.* Boston: Little, Brown and Company, 1992.
4. Guyuron B, Raszewski R. Undetected diabetes and the plastic surgeon. *Aesthetic Plast Surg* 1990;86:471–474.
5. Guyuron B, Zarandy S, Tirgan A. Von Willebrand's disease and plastic surgery. *Ann Plast Surg* 1994;32:351–355.
6. Byrd HS, Hobar PC, Shewmake K. Augmentation of the craniofacial skeleton with porous hydroxyapatite granules. *Plast Reconstr Surg* 1993:91:15–22.
7. Riedel RA. An analysis of dentofacial relationships. *Am J Orthod* 1957;43:103.
8. Rosen HM. The response of porous hydroxyapatite to contiguous tissue infection. *Plast Reconstr Surg* 1991;88:1076–1080.
9. Zide BM, McCarthy J. The mentalis muscle: an essential component of chin and lower lip position. *Plast Reconstr Surg* 1989;83:413–420.
10. Guyuron B, Michelow BJ. Refinements in endoscopic forehead rejuvenation. *Plast Reconstr Surg* 1997;100:154–160.

Discussion

GENIOPLASTY

S. ANTHONY WOLFE

It has always been curious to me that so few aesthetic surgeons of the highest caliber have become truly comfortable with the osseous genioplasty. Bahman Guyuron is one of the few, and he has had considerable experience with the procedure, as evidenced by the wisdom and experience he presents in his chapter.

I would differ with him in his choice of terms. To me, the term *genioplasty* is reserved for a direct osseous procedure involving an osteotomy of some sort, with movement of the basilar segment in a variety of directions, with or without an interpositional bone graft. It is because of the many possible movements that the osseous genioplasty is such a versatile procedure, suitable for managing with vertical abnormalities (chin too short or too long) in addition to laterogenias. For the experienced maxillofacial or craniofacial surgeon, an osseous genioplasty is often a complementary procedure, performed after some other, more complex intervention on the facial skeleton, and it may do *more* to improve the patient's facial appearance than the orthognathic or orbitocranial procedure that preceded it.

For an alloplastic material used to augment the chin, I would use the term *chin implant.* The main advantage of alloplastic chin implantation is that it is easy, and no facility in performing facial osteotomies is required of the surgeon, which is certainly why it is performed so much more frequently than osseous genioplasty.

Although I have not performed an alloplastic chin implantation in more than 25 years, because I feel I can obtain a similar result in all cases with an osseous genioplasty, I am by no means opposed to the use of chin implants. They should be used in appropriate cases: mild retrogenia, without vertical or lateral discrepancies. My only other comment regarding chin implants is to suggest that they be placed through a submental incision, which limits their tendency to ride upward. If they are placed over the thick, hard bone of the basilar segment (and I do not think it makes any difference whether they are above or below the periosteum), they may sink into the underlying bone a bit, but this shift will serve to anchor them. Occasionally, they will sink all the way into the underlying bone, but this is rare. If they are displaced superiorly, they will be over thinner, alveolar bone, and in this situation, significant resorption can threaten underlying dental roots.

Dr. Guyuron's chapter deals with unfavorable results after genioplasty, and because the osseous procedure, as mentioned, is performed so much less frequently, it is relatively rare to see a complication after an osseous intervention. The complications of the osseous genioplasty that I discuss

S. A. Wolf: Department of Plastic and Reconstructive Surgery, University of Miami School of Medicine; and Department of Reconstructive Surgery, Miami Children's Hospital and Victoria Hospital, Miami, Florida

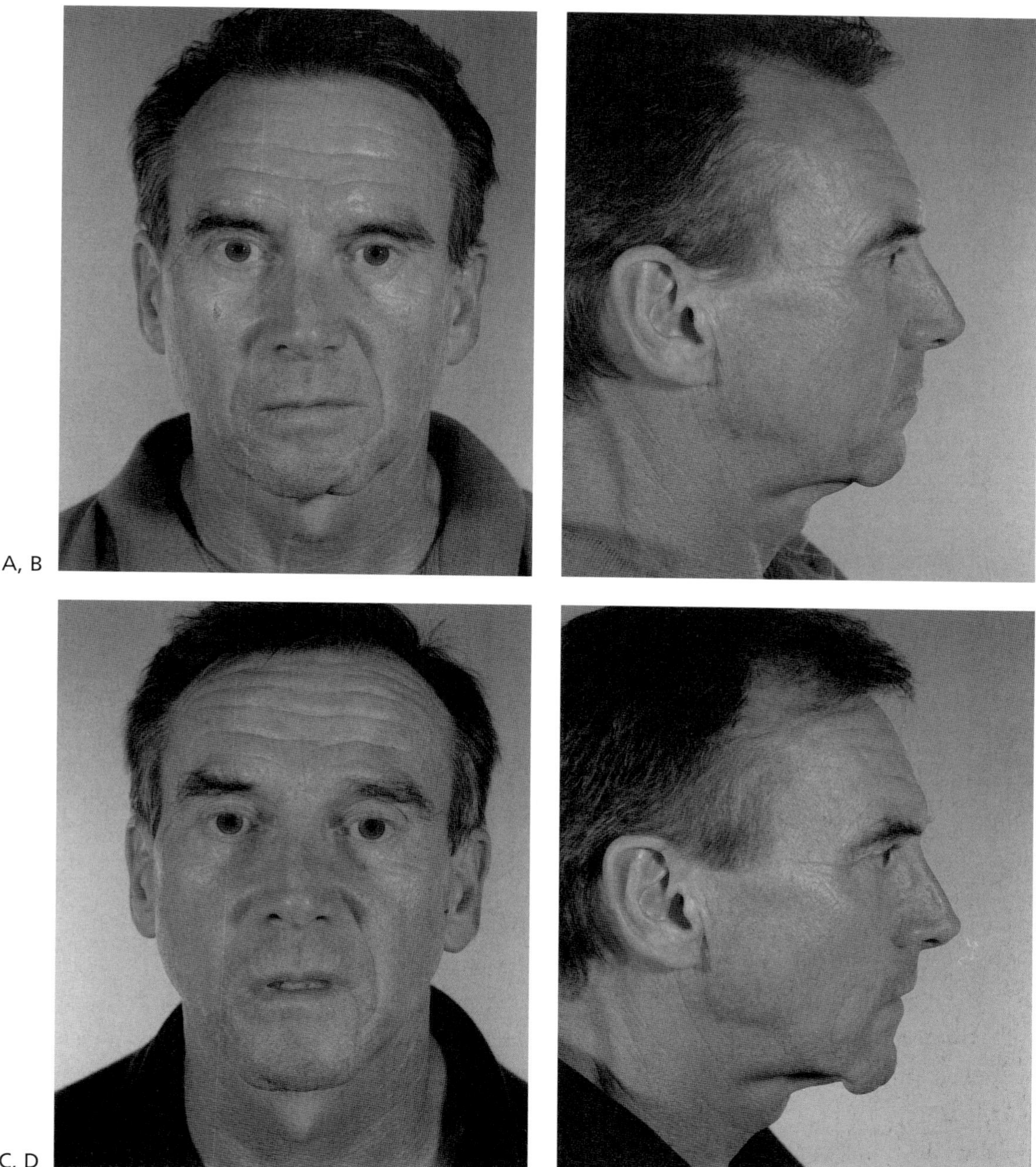

FIGURE 58D-1. A–J: A 58-year-old man who had previously undergone three chin implants, all removed because of infection and displacement, presented with some irregularities in the chin pad, most noticeable on smiling, and a mild "witch's chin" deformity. First, an osseous genioplasty was performed through an intraoral approach. All capsular material encountered from the previous operations was removed. In a second procedure, performed several months later under local anesthesia, some of the redundant skin was removed, the chin pad was suspended to the upper portion of the genioplasty segment, and the submental muscles were sutured to the mentalis muscle over the lower border of the symphysis. No other work was performed on the neck.

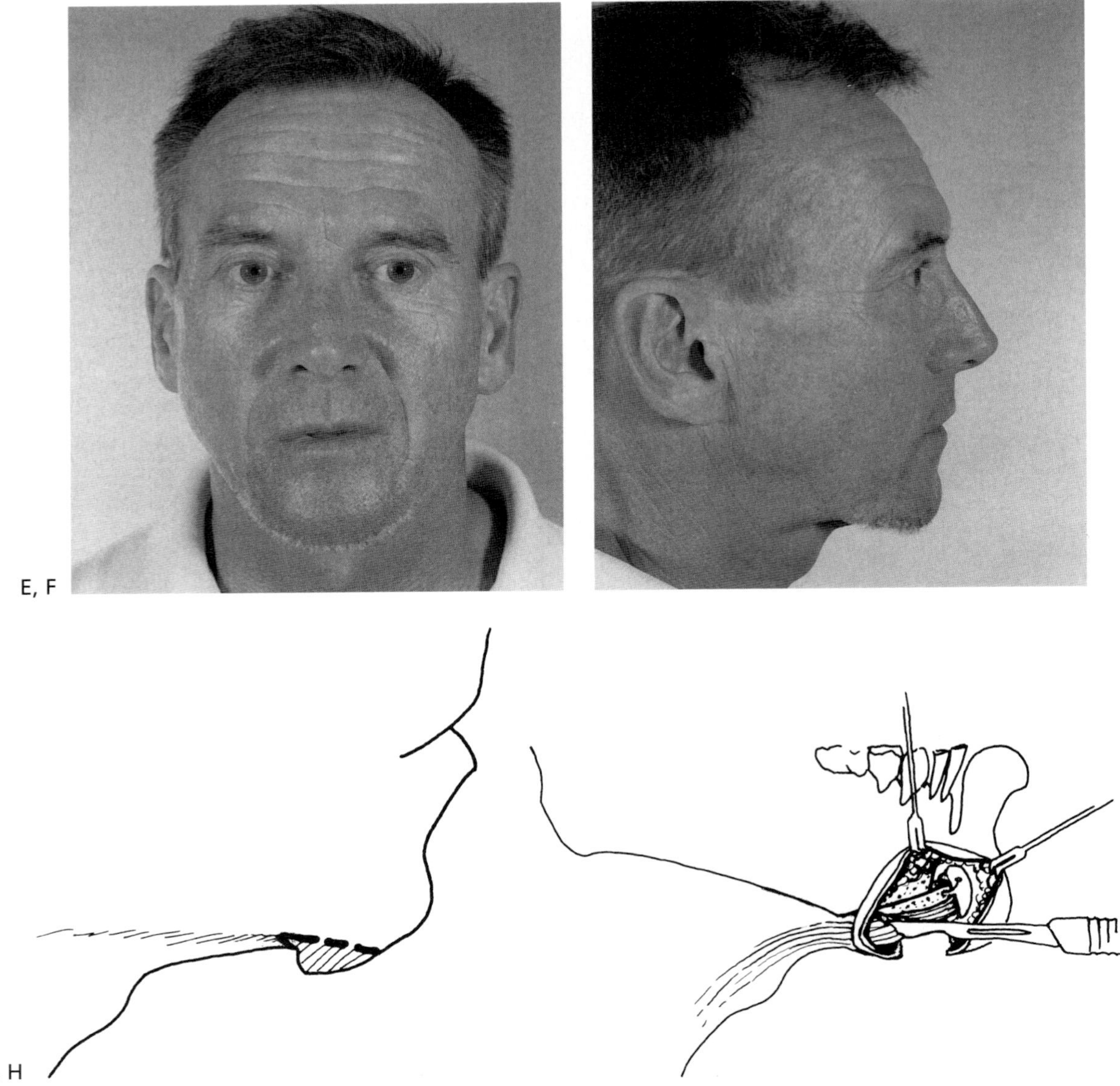

FIGURE 58D-1. (Continued)

herein are therefore largely ones that I have encountered in the approximately 500 cases that I have performed myself. Before I begin this discussion, I would like comment on a few other points that Dr. Guyuron brings up in his chapter.

1. *The patient with a major reaction to an ostensibly minor deformity.* In this situation, I have not found that a psychiatrist is of much help, unless one is blessed with having in one's community a psychiatrist with a particular interest in the sometimes unusual reactions of patients seeking plastic surgery. Generally, the plastic surgeon must be the one to recognize and deal with this type of aberration.

2. *The versatility of osseous genioplasty.* Patients who have mild occlusal abnormalities, such as hemifacial microsomia with a mild cant of the occlusal plane, or who have a mandibular midline that is several millimeters off in relation to the maxillary midline and a chin point that is modestly deviated to one side, can be dealt with satisfactorily with a "centering" genioplasty. One often also sees patients who have an underlying class II malocclusion that has been "corrected" by the orthodontist, often with dental extractions, lingual tilting of the maxillary incisors, and labial tilting of the mandibular incisors. These patients, if they have retrogenia, are not often willing to undergo orthodontics in the reverse direction so that a proper orthognathic correction can be carried out, and they are better camouflaged with an osseous genioplasty.

3. *Dehiscence of the intraoral incision.* This would be a disaster with an alloplastic chin implant; with a simple sliding genioplasty, the basilar segment has an excellent blood

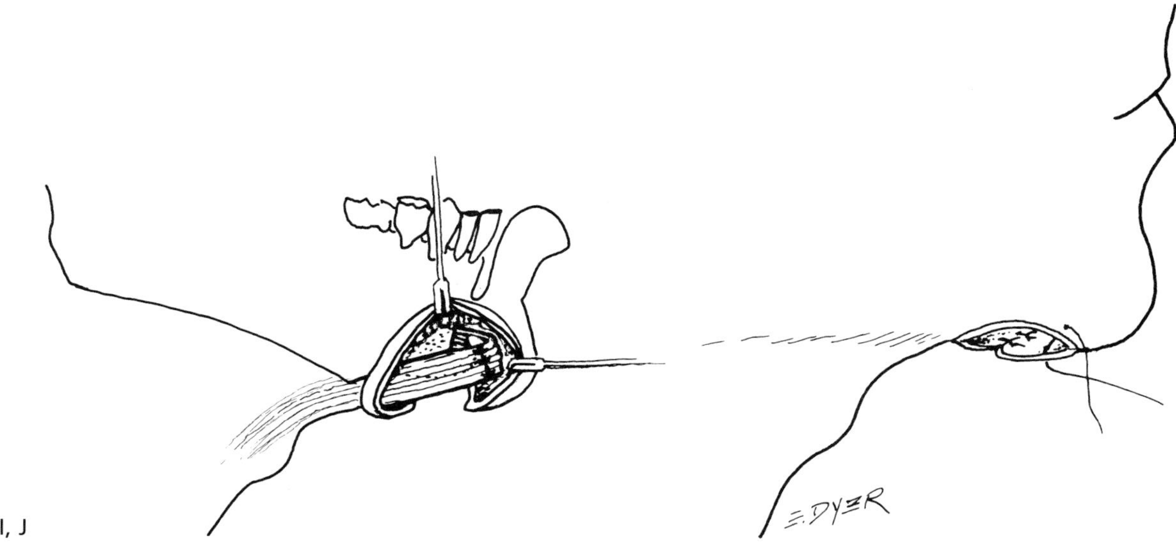

FIGURE 58D-1. (Continued)

supply, and with simple wound care, a healed wound and a good result can be obtained.

4. *Step deformity at the lateral extent of the osteotomy.* This can occur and, as Dr. Guyuron points out, usually smooths out with time. It is not such an easy matter as he suggests simply to bur down the offending bone through the intraoral incision because the mental nerves are often directly in the way. If this problem persists after 6 months, the addition of hydroxyapatite in any of its various forms through an intraoral approach would be appropriate.

5. *Infection.* Like Dr. Guyuron, I have never seen infection after a simple sliding genioplasty. Several decades ago, I had a number of patients in whom a lengthening genioplasty had been performed with an interpositional bone graft, and wire osteosyntheses had been used. Wound infections developed in several of these patients at about 1 month, and debridement and removal of the wires became necessary. Since I have been using rigid fixation with plates and screws, I have had no further infections in this type of case.

6. *Overcorrection.* In my experience, this is the most common "complication," or source of patient discontent, after an osseous genioplasty. The osseous genioplasty is a powerful tool, and when one is using a wire osteosynthesis between the posterior border of the lower segment and the anterior border of the remaining symphysis, it is easy to overcorrect. When one wishes only 2 to 4 mm of correction, it is better to use lag screw fixation. The best way of avoiding this problem is *never* to bring the basilar segment out in front of the lower lip. This may mean in some cases, as Harvey Rosen has pointed out (1), that one lengthens more than one advances.

7. *Numbness.* It is best to tell all patients to expect some. I like to identify the mental nerves, so that they can be protected, and do not extend the cut laterally higher than 5 mm below the mental foramina. In two of my cases, the nerve was either cut or avulsed. This was recognized; the nerve was repaired (a time-consuming process), and sensation returned after about 6 months.

8. *Show of the lower incisors.* This is a disaster that I think may be caused by a lower labial sulcus incision cutting through—and denervating—a good bit of the mentalis muscle. I do not know of a reliable and reproducible way to correct this problem.

The results of the genioplasties that I have performed have been studied by several of my fellows. In one series, 50 patients who had had genioplasties along with facelifts were scrutinized (2), and the main cause for discontent was overcorrection, which could be easily corrected by simply burring down the basilar segment a bit, a procedure amenable to local anesthesia.

The results of a review of all my genioplasty patients (now around 500) were presented to the American Association of Plastic Surgeons a few years ago (3), and they have been submitted for publication. In short, the complications were somewhat less than those reported for similar series of patients with chin implants.

Two of my patients demonstrate several of the points that Dr. Guyuron and I have mentioned:

Patient 1 (Fig. 58D-1). This 58-year-old man had previously undergone three chin implants, all removed because of infection and displacement. He presented with some irregularities in the chin pad, most noticeable on smiling, and a mild "witch's chin" deformity. He was told that cor-

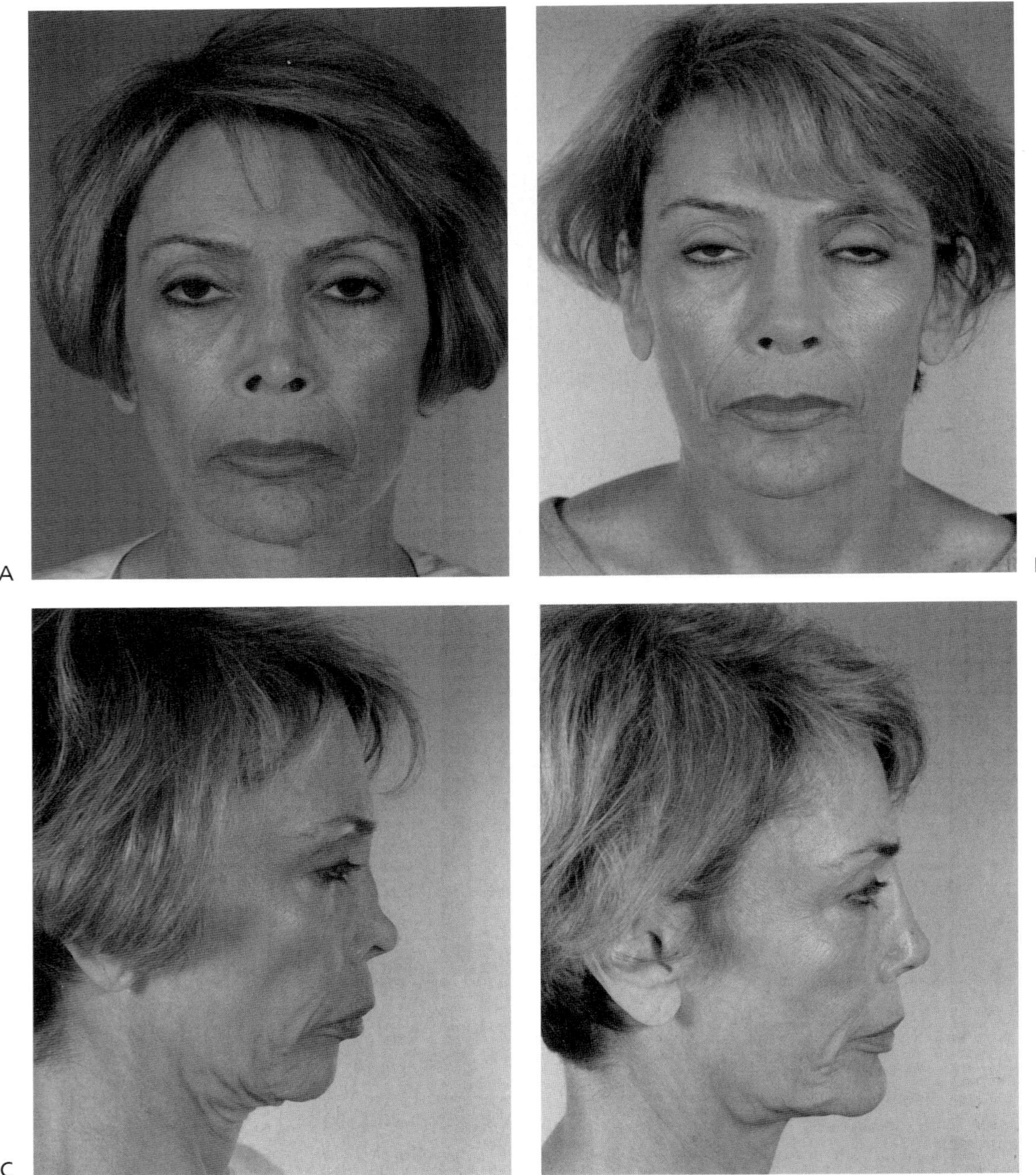

FIGURE 58D-2. A–F: A 64-year-old woman who had undergone multiple operations on her nose, including several extrusions of alloplastic materials, presented with mentalis strain and difficulty obtaining lip seal. She had a class II malocclusion before surgery. Her nose was improved with a calvarial bone graft to the dorsum and conchal cartilage grafts to the tip, and a *limited* osseous genioplasty was performed (5 mm of advancement and fixation with lag screws).

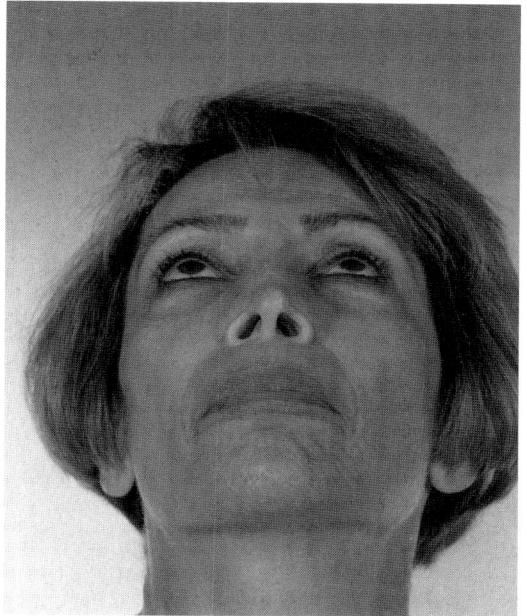

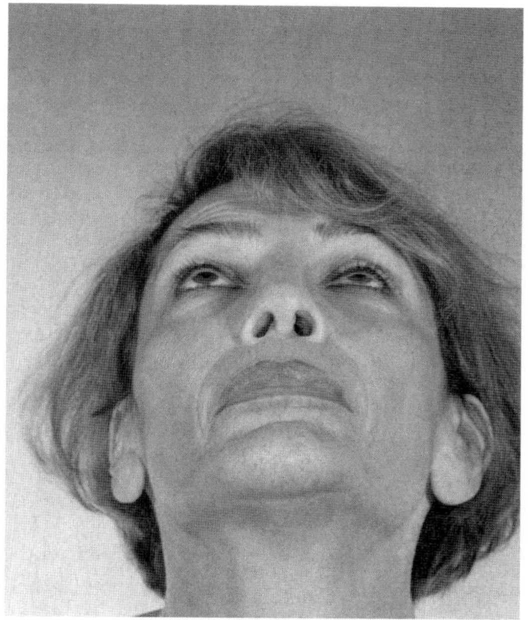

FIGURE 58D-2. (Continued)

rection would require two procedures. First, an osseous genioplasty was performed through an intraoral approach. All capsular material encountered from the previous operations was removed. This reduced the surface irregularities and gave him a somewhat longer chin. It also accentuated the hang of the submental chin pad and the show of the lower incisors. In a second procedure, performed several months later under local anesthesia, some of the redundant skin was removed, the chin pad was suspended to the upper portion of the genioplasty segment, and the submental muscles were sutured to the mentalis muscle over the lower border of the symphysis.

No other work was performed on the neck. The point to be made by this case is that when a problem has developed with a chin implant or implants, one should proceed to an osseous genioplasty and be prepared to perform a subsequent procedure for residual soft tissue problems. The drawings attempt to show the soft tissue portion of the procedure.

Patient 2 (Fig. 58D-2). This 64-year-old woman had undergone multiple operations on her nose, including several extrusions of alloplastic materials. Preoperatively, she showed mentalis strain and difficulty obtaining lip seal, and she had a class II malocclusion. Her nose was improved with a calvarial bone graft to the dorsum and conchal cartilage grafts to the tip, and a *limited* osseous genioplasty was performed (5 mm of advancement and fixation with lag screws). She was extremely happy with the result of her nasal surgery, and almost as unhappy with the results of her genioplasty, which she felt made her chin look too large. With time, she came to accept it, but if it had been moved in front of her lower lip by even the slightest amount, it is unlikely that she would have done so. She is currently thinking about a facelift, and possibly later some fat injections to her quite thin lower facial third. The lesson to be learned from this case is not to overadvance, particularly in patients whose faces are already quite thin.

REFERENCES

1. Rosen HM. Aesthetic guidelines in genioplasty: the role of facial disproportion. *Plast Reconstr Surg* 1995;95:3.
2. Wider TM, Spiro SA, Wolfe SA. Simultaneous osseous genioplasty and meloplasty. *Plast Reconstr Surg* 1997;99:1273–1281.
3. Fenner G, Wolfe SA. *An analysis of 478 genioplasties over a 21-year period.* Presented to the American Association of Plastic Surgeons, May 1997.

59

HAIR REPLACEMENT

WALTER P. UNGER

Patients may be dissatisfied with the results of hair transplantation for reasons that any objective observer would agree ought to cause dissatisfaction. Alternatively, patients may be dissatisfied because the results fall short of their idea of what could reasonably be expected from the treatment. Most of this chapter deals with the former situation, but the importance of a thorough and frank preoperative consultation cannot be overstated. One should be particularly careful not to design hairlines that will look unnatural to most observers, especially as the patient ages; one should also not promise patients more density or coverage than can reasonably be expected, or create hair density or coverage that is far less than the patient can reasonably expect. If the surgeon has any reason to suspect that a patient's expectations are beyond what can be safely promised, it is always better to walk away rather than try to satisfy unrealistic expectations. In addition, any patient who appears to have significant emotional problems should be referred to a psychiatrist or psychologist before the surgeon agrees to proceed.

Unfavorable results can occur in either the recipient or the donor area. In the recipient area, they include the following: (a) poor hairline design; (b) attempting to cover a recipient area that is too large or, at the other extreme, limiting the transplant to an area far smaller than the patient could reasonably hope to have covered; (c) extension of male pattern baldness beyond what was originally predicted; (d) inadequate density in the transplanted sites or poor hair survival; (e) plugginess; (f) incorrect hair direction or angle; (g) depressed or elevated grafts; and (h) mistakes related to alopecia reduction. Unfavorable results in the donor area include (a) wide scars, (b) overharvesting, and (c) severe temporary hair loss. Usually, a combination of a variable number of the previously noted errors is seen in one patient; however, for purposes of clarity, each is discussed separately.

RECIPIENT AREA

The terminology used in this chapter is summarized in Table 59-1.

W. P. Unger: Department of Dermatology, Mt. Sinai Medical School, New York, New York

Poor Hairline Design

The most frequent error made in designing a male hairline is to fill the frontotemporal triangles with grafting. Alopecic frontotemporal triangles develop in the vast majority of men as they age (Fig. 59-1A), and transplanting these triangles draws attention to the hairline. A hairline ideally should begin at the most anterior and superior temporal points and extend toward the midline of the forehead, so that it runs more or less horizontally when viewed laterally. Natural hairlines also usually have a slight bell shape (1). Thus, if one of the objectives is to fill the frontotemporal triangles, the patient should be made fully aware that this hairline will probably be noticed often by casual observers, and the patient must be comfortable with that idea. In addition, the surgeon must be very skilled, so that when others are looking at the hairline, they will not appreciate the fact that it has been transplanted. If you or the patient is not entirely confident about both of the above, then the frontotemporal triangle should be left untransplanted. The patient should also be aware that additional donor tissue will be used in the anterior third of the area of male pattern baldness if these triangles are treated, and therefore in the long run it may not be possible to transplant as large a proportion of the rest of the area of male pattern baldness as he would like.

Should a male patient want transplanted frontotemporal triangles eliminated, one is left with the following four options:

1. Electrolysis or laser therapy to remove the hair
2. Punching out the grafts and either suturing the sites or filling them with alopecic plugs taken from elsewhere in the area of male pattern baldness (Fig. 59-1B,C)

Either of these methods may still leave noticeable scars that may or may not be made less conspicuous with subsequent dermabrasion or resurfacing.

3. An alopecia reduction posterior to the hairline zone—with or without prior tissue expansion of the forehead skin—with the goal of pulling up its lateral borders to create a frontotemporal triangle.
4. A V-shaped excision of tissue to produce a more normal-looking frontotemporal area. If this route is chosen, any

TABLE 59-1. GRAFT TERMINOLOGY

	No. hairs	Type of recipient site	No. follicular units	Tissue removed
Micrograft (always a single follicular unit)	1–3	Puncture hole	1	No
Beaver graft	2–4	Beaver mini-ES blade slit	2	No
Minigraft "small"	3–5	Hole or slot	2–3	Yes
Minigraft "large"	5–7	Hole or slot	2–4	Yes
Slit graft "small"	3–5	Blade slit	2–3	No
Slit graft "large"	5–7	Blade slit	2–4	No
Standard graft	8–30	3.0+ mm hole	6–22	Yes

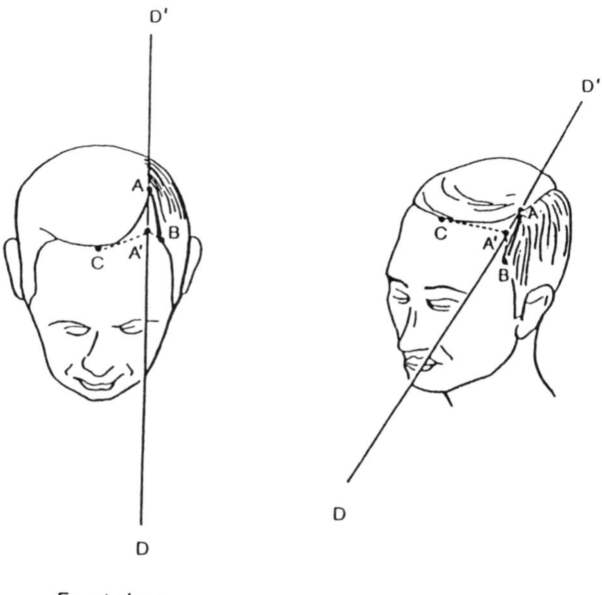

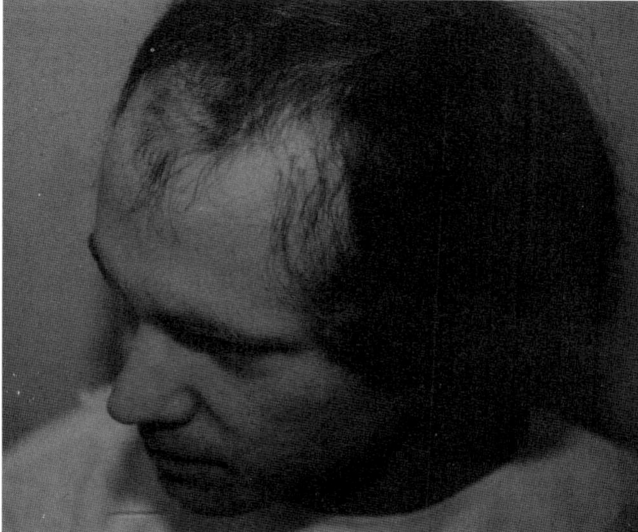

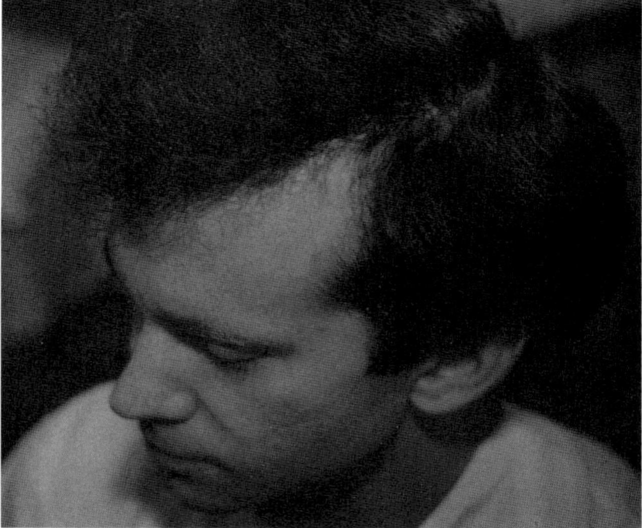

FIGURE 59-1. A: *Dotted line A[1]* represents minimal temporal recession. *Solid line A,B* represents more advanced temporal recession. *Dotted line C,A[1]*,B represents minimal frontal recession. *Solid line C,A,B* represents more extensive frontal recession. Although *apex A* obviously represents more extensive alopecia than *apex A[1]*, the hair when parted at A still appears natural and balanced relative to the other facial features because it falls on the *line D,D[1]*. **B:** Before corrective transplanting, the results of poorly placed grafts performed elsewhere are obvious just anterior to the temporal hair. The frontotemporal area, into which these grafts were placed, should rarely be transplanted because persisting hair in this triangle beyond the age of 30 years is very uncommon. **C:** Grafts that were improperly placed in the frontotemporal triangle were excised and sutured. Further grafting was carried out concomitantly. The patient was being seen for further grafting at the hairline and part at the time this photograph was taken.

noticeable postoperative scar will require subsequent micrografting.

On the other hand, women normally do not have alopecic frontotemporal triangles and should therefore have such areas transplanted (2) (Fig. 59-2). If they have not been treated, it is relatively simple to correct the problem with additional grafting.

The other major problem that can occur with conventionally transplanted hairlines is that they are too abruptly dense. Normal hairlines are not lines at all but rather irregular zones with irregular densities. The hair is also usually fine in texture and less dense anteriorly; it gradually becomes coarser and denser as one moves posteriorly. Thus, one should utilize fine-textured single-hair grafts most anteriorly, then follicular units with two hairs posterior to those, and three-hair, single- or double-follicular units grafts posterior to the latter. Three- to four-hair slit grafts or round minigrafts with slightly coarser hair are used to complete the more posterior portion of the hairline zone.

If the hairline is too abrupt or dense, the best treatment is usually to create a new hairline zone slightly anterior to the original one with micrografts and minigrafts containing appropriately textured hair (Fig. 59-3). Alternately, if the hairline is already low or if adding a new hairline zone will make it too low, electrolysis can be used to destroy some of the previously transplanted hair to create a less dense and softer zone. The treatment of plugginess in the hairline is discussed later in this chapter.

Treatment of an Inappropriate Proportion of the Area of Male Pattern Baldness

This problem may be the result of an extension of male pattern baldness beyond what was originally predicted. It may also by caused by failure to connect transplanted areas to each other during initial treatments carried out while the patient still had some of his original, persisting hair. In the latter case, further hair loss reveals "islands" of unnaturally disconnected transplanted hair. Objectives of minimal coverage may also result in patient dissatisfaction.

Most frequently, treatment of an inappropriate proportion of the area of male pattern baldness means treatment of an area that is too large relative to the available donor reserves. New donor harvesting techniques, combined with minigrafting and micrografting, have greatly increased the proportion of an area of male pattern baldness that can be treated to produce natural-looking results. However, the younger the patient, the more difficult it is to predict accurately the eventual extent of his male pattern baldness and the required size of his donor area. If one limits oneself to micrografting and minigrafting, most patients can have at least the anterior two-thirds of the eventual area of male pattern baldness treated and obtain a natural-looking coverage of hair. Trying to treat a larger area than that requires (a) a particularly favorable family history, (b) a patient ideally in his 40s or older, and most importantly (c) a willingness to consider alopecia reduction at some point during the course of treatment (3). Without the latter, it is unwise to treat the entire developing area of male pattern baldness in patients under the age of 40 years, and in many cases even in those older than 40 years.

Should the patient present with patchy areas of grafting separated by untransplanted areas or new areas of alopecia that were not anticipated, the best course is to perform alopecia reduction to remove as much bald tissue as possible (without utilizing limited donor reserves) and micrografting/minigrafting to join the previously transplanted areas to each other and the temporoparietal rim hair (Fig. 59-4). As

A

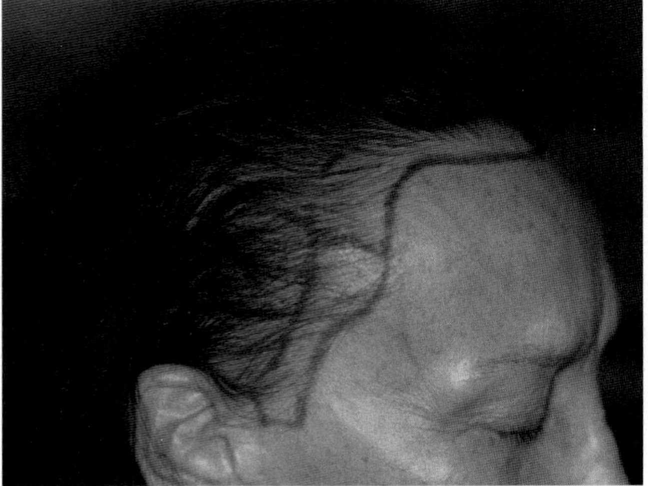

B

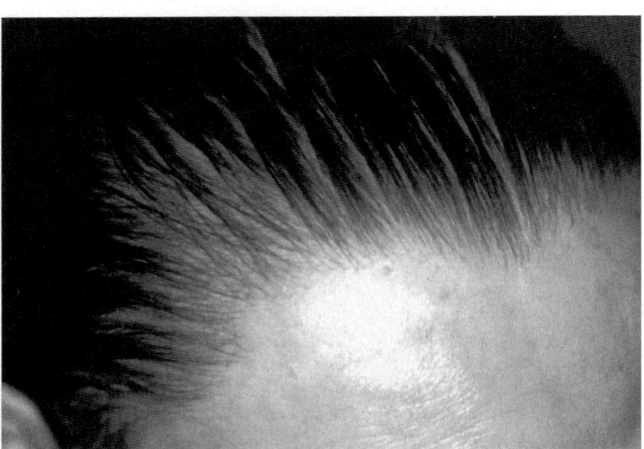

FIGURE 59-2. A: Patient before her first hair transplant. The areas outlined in *black crayon* were to be thickened. Note that the frontotemporal triangles are minimal to nonexistent. **B:** Five months after the second transplant.

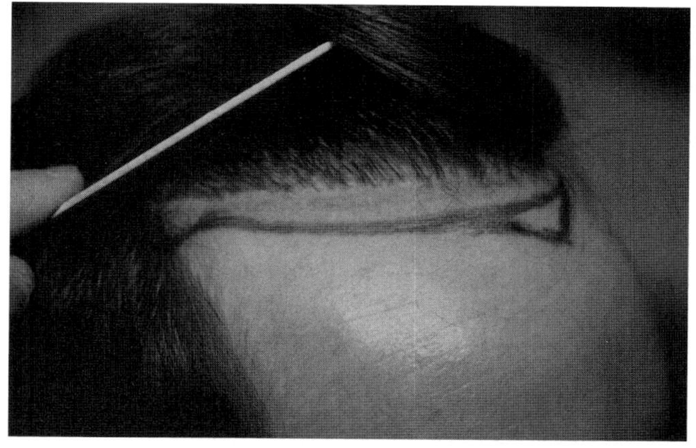
A

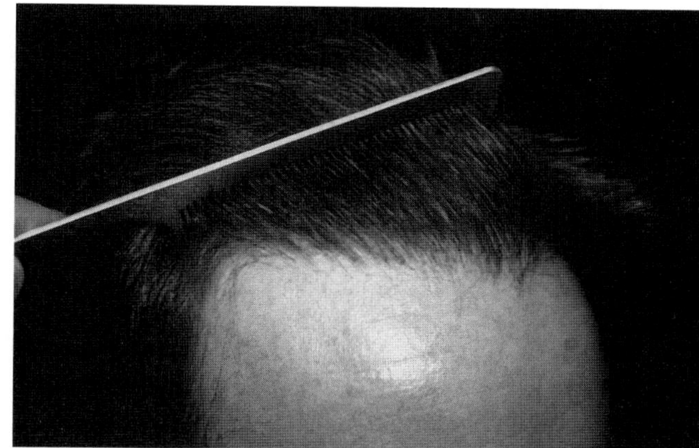
B

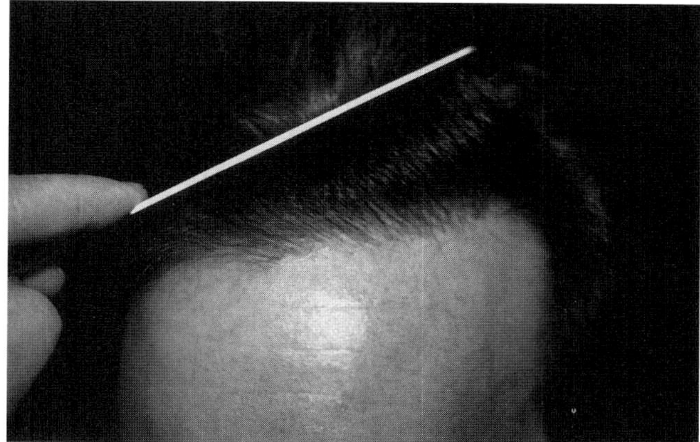
C

FIGURE 59-3. A: This patient demonstrates not only an abrupt hairline that is too dense but also a pluggy appearance. The *black grease pencil* outlines a new hairline that is to be constructed with micrografts and minigrafts. **B:** After three repair sessions. Note the density of the area that was treated previously with large grafts. Spaces between larger grafts were completely filled with new and appropriately sized grafts at the same time that the new hairline was constructed (see also Figs. 59-11 and 59-13). The result is a "silver lining" of great hair density. **C:** Contralateral hairline after three repair sessions.

an alternative to the latter, frontal transplanting can be converted into a larger-than-usual isolated frontal forelock (discussed in more detail below) by "finishing" the lateral and posterior borders with one to three sessions of micrografting and minigrafting (4).

In contrast to the patients in whom too large an area is treated are the young patients who are treated only with an isolated frontal forelock (Fig. 59-5). This pattern of hair transplantation has become quite popular within the last 5 to 10 years and is unsatisfactory for many young persons. Virtually all patients with male pattern baldness types 1 to 5 (Fig. 59-6) can have a much larger area covered than can be accomplished with an isolated frontal forelock. Approximately 80% of patients 80 years old or younger are included in this group (5); however, because one can never be 100% certain that a particular young man is not one of the approximately 20% who will progress to type 6 or 7 male pattern baldness, some practitioners have advocated an isolated frontal forelock for *all* patients (6). These surgeons are obviously well-meaning, but their approach has resulted in *most* patients being undertreated. A more reasonable approach is to treat patients who have a family history of type 6 or 7 male pattern baldness with an isolated frontal forelock and to formulate a more ambitious objective, described below, for the others.

To establish the borders of an eventual area of male pattern baldness, wet the hair and try to discern the true extent of the thinning hair (Fig. 59-7). Then transplant into those areas that still have hair but can reasonably be expected to lose it with the passage of time. This approach avoids a never-ending chase of an expanding area of alopecia. Taking the patient's age into consideration and obtaining a careful family history will aid the surgeon in estimating accurately how far the male pattern baldness will progress in the long run. The lateral borders of any area treated should always be finished with micrografts and minigrafts (Fig. 59-8), so that if the male pattern baldness progresses beyond what is expected some years later, the patient will be left with a large isolated frontal forelock that will look natural despite the development of alopecic "alleys" lateral to the transplanted area. The surgeon should also always try to leave a reserve of donor hair so that in case such alleys develop, and the patient is dissatisfied with his appearance, donor tissue will be available for transplanting them.

Of course, it is *not* necessary to wait until such alleys are totally alopecic before treatment is started. As soon as it is obvious that thinning is affecting areas that were untreated previously, and if the patient states that he is unhappy with the development of these alleys, they can be treated with a combination of micrografts and minigrafts as the hair is lost.

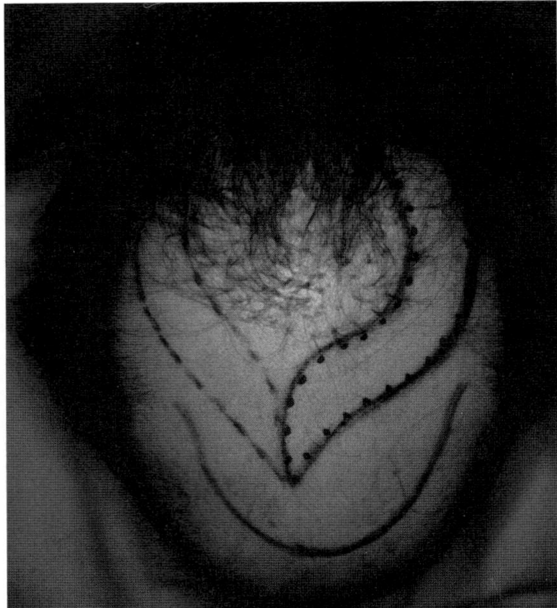

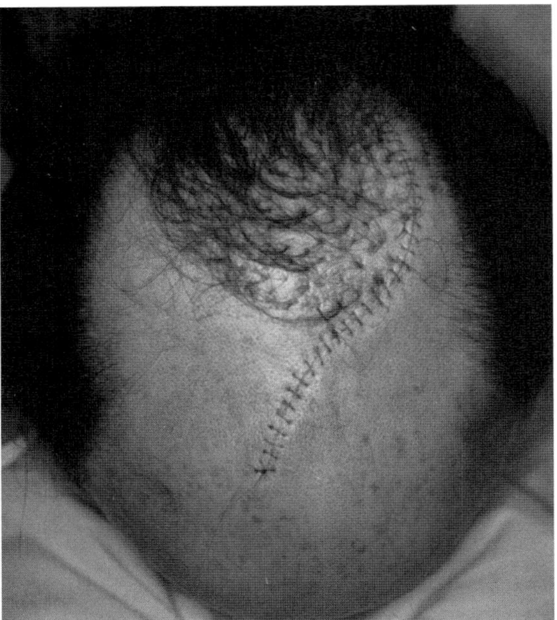

FIGURE 59-4. A: Before repair sessions. This 56-year-old man had undergone transplanting in the vertex area many years earlier. His male pattern baldness had progressed to leave an "island" of pluggy-looking grafts in the central vertex. The photograph shows the pattern of proposed alopecia reduction to the left and right of the island of grafts, and the proposed new hairline. By removing as much alopecic tissue as possible with alopecia reduction, one can utilize grafts that would have been needed to fill these areas to improve previously transplanted areas or treat new ones. **B:** Immediately after the second alopecia reduction on the left side, showing essentially complete removal of the alopecic "alley" on that side. Two alopecia reductions were also performed on the right side. **C:** After four alopecia reductions, three minigraft/micrograft sessions for the anterior male pattern baldness and one minigraft/micrograft session for the vertex were performed. (The alopecia reductions were carried out by Dr. Martin Unger; grafting was done by the author.)

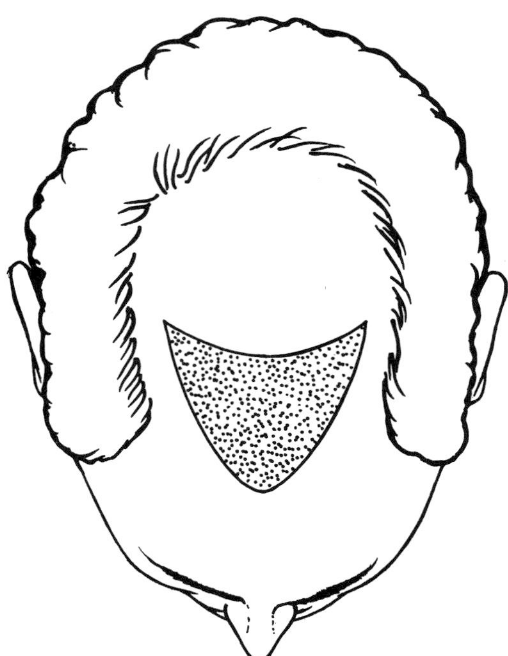

FIGURE 59-5. Pattern of an isolated frontal forelock. Grafts at the periphery of the forelock are generally micrografts and become progressively larger as one moves toward the center of the area.

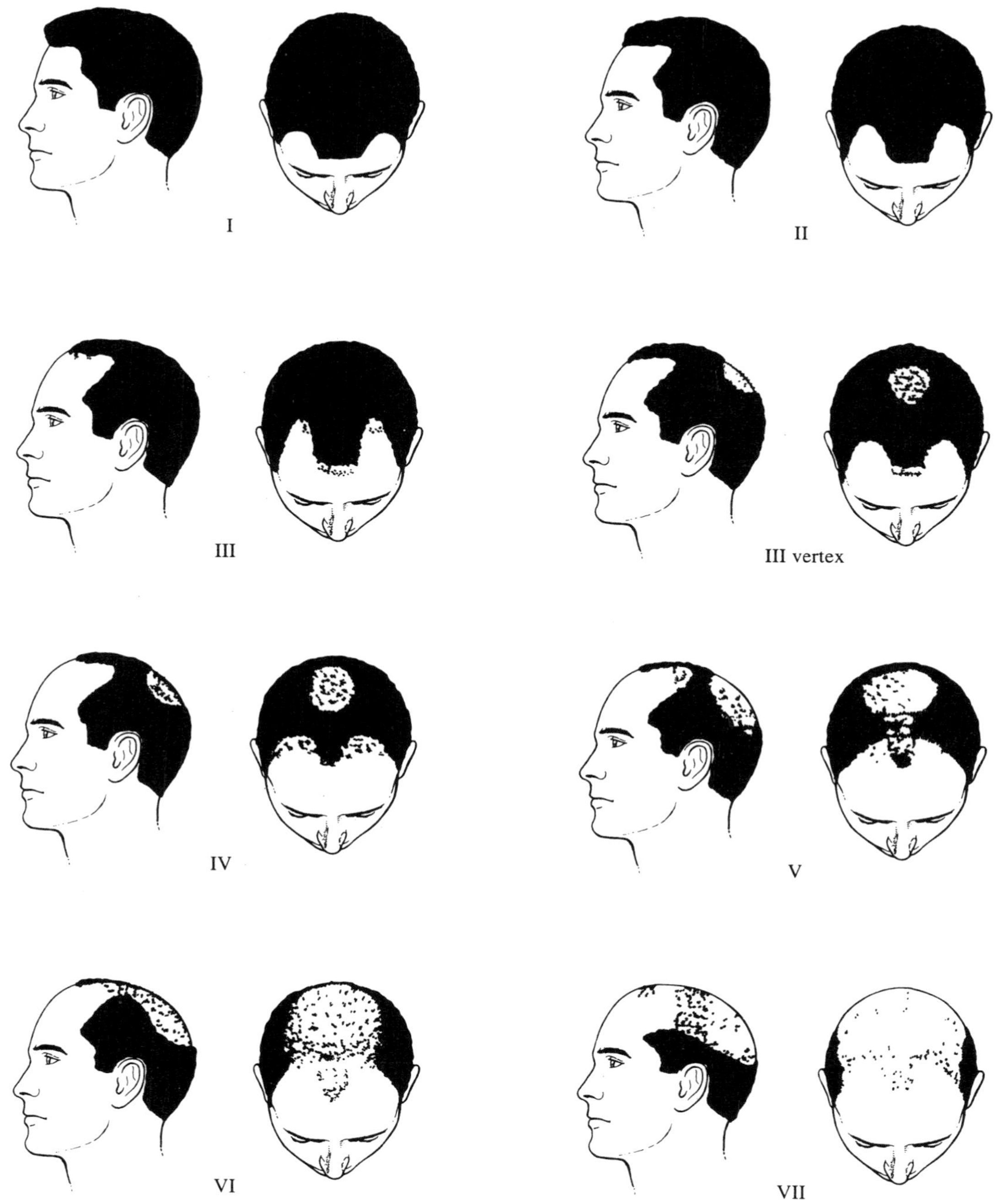

FIGURE 59-6. A: The Norwood classification of the most common types of male pattern baldness. (*continued*)

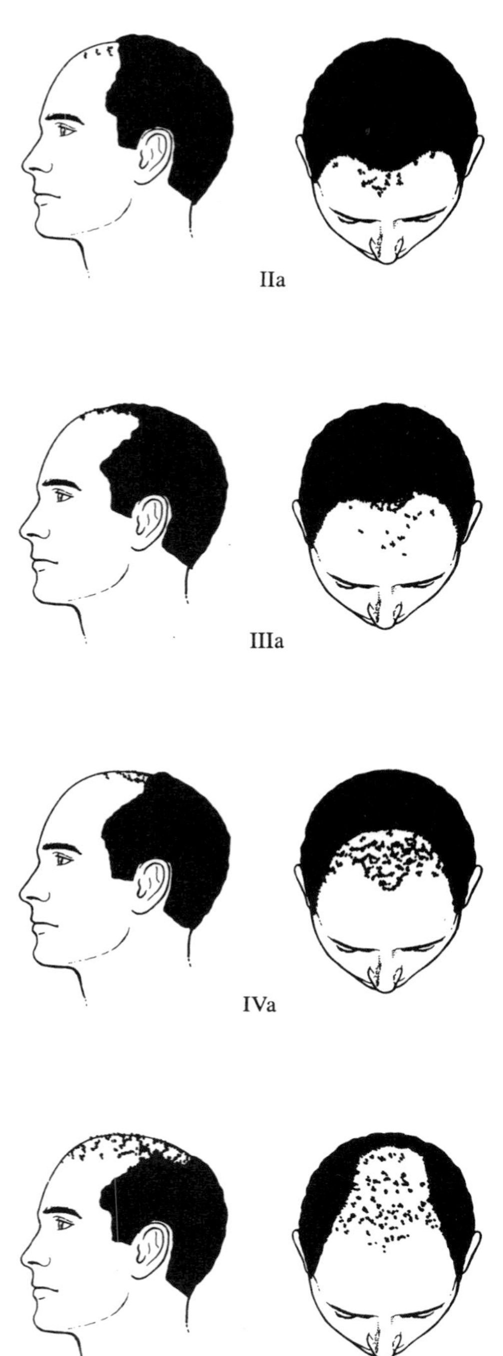

FIGURE 59-6. (*Continued*) **B:** Classification of type A variant male pattern baldness. (From Norwood O'T, Shiell R, eds. *Hair transplant surgery,* 2nd ed. Springfield, Illinois: Charles C Thomas, 1984:5–10, with permission.)

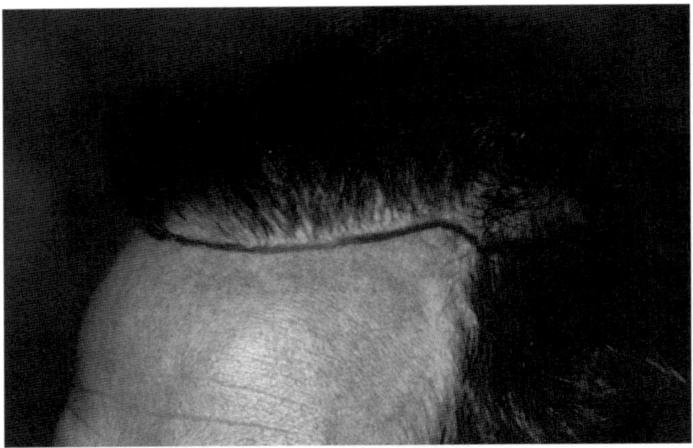

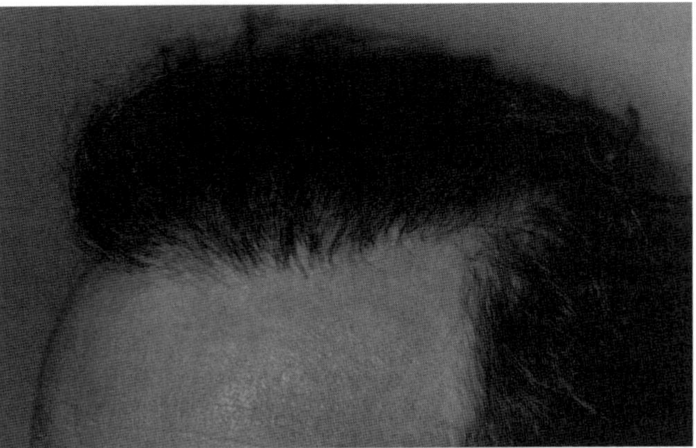

FIGURE 59-7. A: The *black crayon mark* delineates the new hairline for this patient, seen for repair. The patient has a pluggy and overly irregular hairline, and the transplanting did not extend into zones of thinning hair superior to the left and right temporal areas. The area of thinning is clarified by wetting the hair and is demarcated in the photograph by the *black crayon line* extending posteriorly from the most anterior and superior point of the temporal area. Transplanting should ideally extend into those areas that still have hair but can reasonably be expected to lose it with the passage of time. **B:** Same patient after a single repair session. Micrografts were added anteriorly and between previously transplanted grafts, and grafting was extended into the areas superior to the left and right temporal hair. The latter will have to be transplanted at least two more times during the lifetime of this patient, as hair originally present at this location is lost.

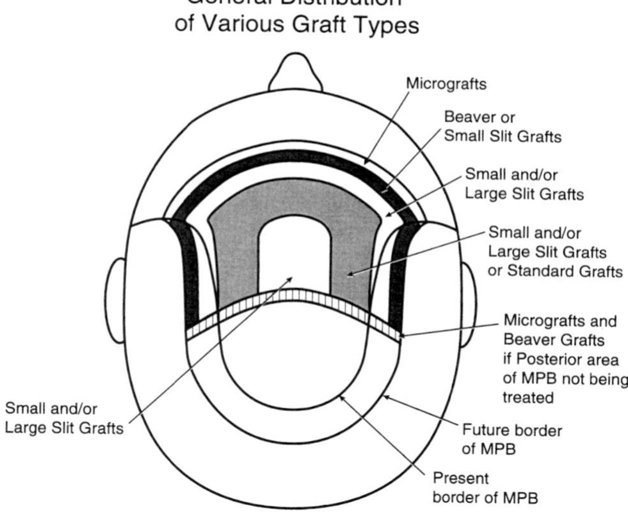

FIGURE 59-8. Schematic drawing of the general distribution of various graft types in a typical hair transplant session to the anterior third to half of an area of male pattern baldness. Note that the periphery of the treated area is transplanted with "beaver grafts" or small slit grafts (in addition to micrografts along the hairline and posterior border). If some years later the male pattern baldness progresses beyond what was originally anticipated, the patient will be left with a large isolated frontal forelock, which will look natural despite the development of alopecic "alleys" lateral to the transplanted area.

As noted earlier, the surgeon can also excise the new alopecic areas, then micrograft and minigraft the scars.

Patients who have had an isolated frontal forelock intentionally created and who want fuller coverage are easily treated with the addition of micrografts and minigrafts to join the forelock to the temporoparietal fringes. Usually, an alopecic alley can be satisfactorily transplanted with two or three sessions of micrografting and minigrafting.

Inadequate Hair Density

Hair density in the recipient area can appear inadequate to the patient, or it may actually be inadequate as the result of objectively poor graft hair survival. It bears repeating that during the initial consultation, it is important to establish with the patient what hair density he expects and to make it clear to him whether you in fact feel that you can produce that density. Most patients are not candidates for dense hair transplantation because they lack adequate donor reserves, unless they are prepared to treat only the anterior third to half of the developing area of male pattern baldness. It is also wise to remember that dense frontal transplanting is appropriate only if the patient can be reasonably expected to maintain dense temporal hair over his lifetime. One does not want to create very dense frontal hair adjacent to what eventually will become an area of sparse temporal hair; in this situation, the patient looks as if he is wearing a hairpiece. Only approximately 10% to 15% of my patients are candidates for dense transplanting of the frontal third to half of their area of male pattern baldness (7). For such persons, a combination of micrografts, minigrafts, and standard grafts is recommended. The standard grafts are used in a zone approximately 2 to 2.5 cm wide and are sandwiched between a hairline zone, lateral zones, and areas posterior to the standard grafts—all of which are treated with micrografts and minigrafts (Fig. 59-8). Although "dense" hair transplanting is limited to a relatively narrow zone in which densities of 160 to more than 200 hairs per square centimeter can be achieved, one can still produce an *appearance* of remarkable overall density (7) (Fig. 59-9).

The most common causes of inadequate density despite good hair survival are (a) the use of micrografts or slit grafts only, and (b) the employment of too few grafts per session. The smaller the number of hairs per graft, the greater the number of grafts that must be used per session to produce a satisfactory density per session, and the greater the number of sessions that will be required to create dense hair. Furthermore, preparing the recipient sites for micrografts/follicular units and slit grafts does not involve the removal of any alopecic skin. Thus, one is just adding hair (and also some skin), and not concomitantly removing alopecic skin, as one does with round grafts and slot grafts (8). Transplanting the same number of hairs but utilizing round grafts and slot grafts therefore tends to produce more density per session than does using micrografts and slit grafts. I routinely use round minigrafts and slot grafts in second, third, or later sessions in the same areas to maximize density per session (8). Nevertheless, cosmetically excellent results are possible in many cases with the use of only micrografts or micrografts and slit grafts if the practitioner and staff are sufficiently skilled, and particularly if the patient has good donor hair density or if the contrast between the color of the patient's hair and skin is minimal (Fig. 59-10).

The second reason for inadequate hair density is poor graft hair survival. Two common causes of poor hair yield are (a) placing the recipient sites too close together and (b) performing too many grafts in a single session. Although "megasessions" of 1,500 to 3,000 grafts and "dense packing" (in which the grafts are placed very close to each other) are popular with some hair transplant surgeons, reports of poor growth in portions of the area transplanted are not uncommon (9–11). Patients generally want to be "done in one session," and surgeons are naturally anxious to satisfy them. Sessions of more than 1,500 micrografts or minigrafts, however, increase the risk for poor hair yield. Most surgeons consequently limit the number of grafts per session to 500 to 1,200. The size of the graft is an important factor. The larger the graft, the fewer number of grafts that should be utilized per session and the farther apart they should be because the interruption of the blood supply will be greater

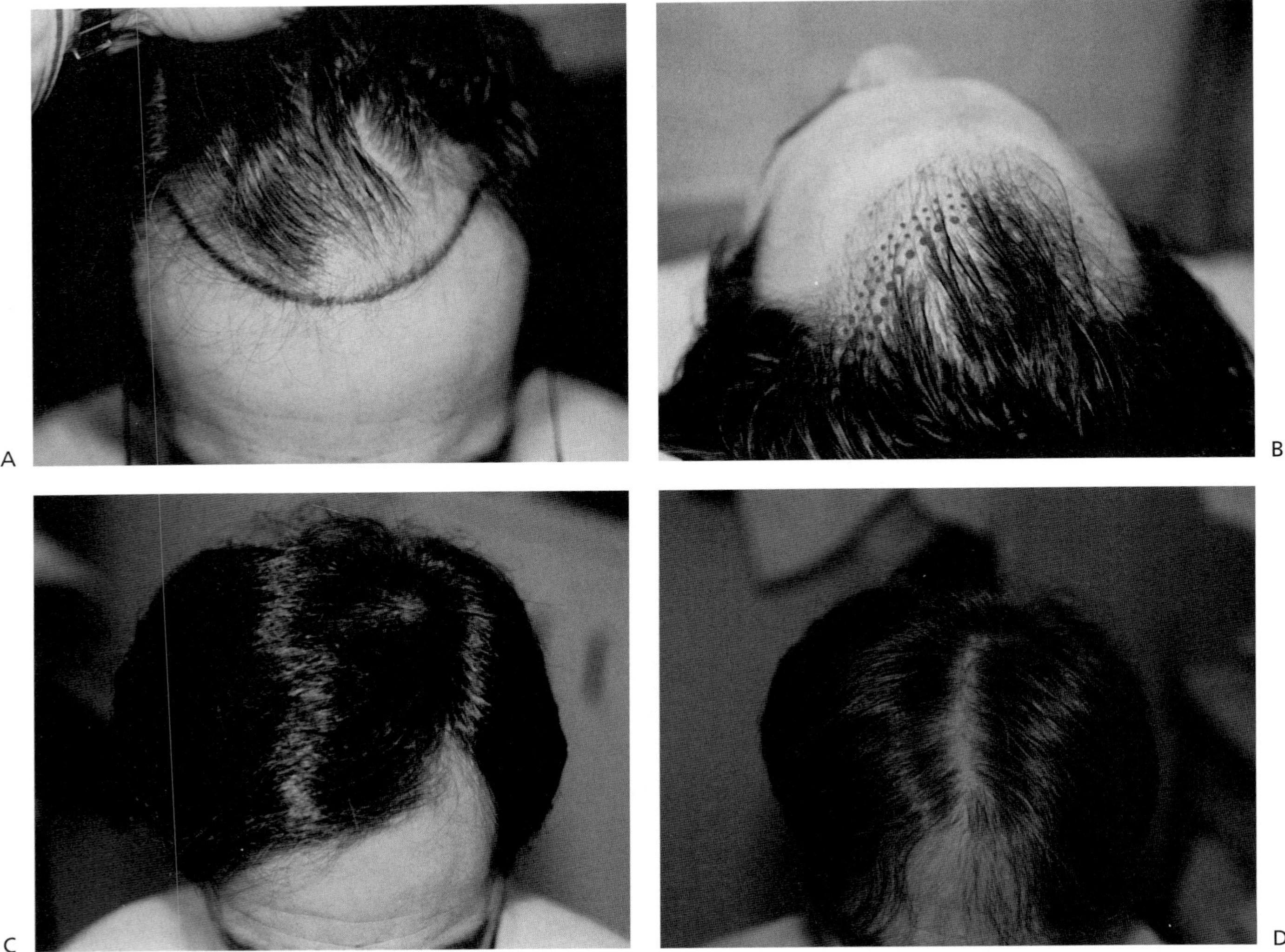

FIGURE 59-9. A: The patient before his first session. **B:** The pattern of grafting used in this patient. It consisted of micrografts and minigrafts to create a hairline zone, followed by two rows of 2-mm grafts and a row of grafts of standard size. The rest of the frontal area was treated with minigrafts. **C:** One year after the third transplant. **D:** One year after the third transplant, with the hair parted for critical evaluation. An appearance of remarkable density can be created with a mixture of micrografts, minigrafts of various types, and standard grafts.

when larger recipient sites are prepared. Although the space between micrografts or follicular units may be 1 mm or less, slit and minigrafts are best spaced approximately 2 to 3 mm apart, and standard grafts should be 3 to 3.5 mm apart. In a typical session of only micrografts or micrografts and minigrafts, approximately 1,500 to 2,750 hairs are transplanted as 800 to 1,200 micrografts or as 250 micrografts and 350 to 450 slit and minigrafts. A typical session that includes standard grafts can reasonably total 2,500 to 2,750 hairs and may include, for example, 250 micrografts, 300 to 350 slit and minigrafts, and 50 to 55 standard grafts (7).

The third major cause of poor hair yield is poor graft preparation. It is essential that grafts be kept moist at all times. Dehydration probably is responsible for more follicular death than poor handling of the donor tissue. In addition, one should utilize whatever magnification is required to prepare grafts with minimal injury to the hair follicles. Most experienced technicians are able to produce excellent grafts with a magnification of 1 to 3×. However, some technicians do far better with stereoscopic microscopes (magnification of 7 to 10×), especially if the hair is light-colored. Proper lighting and background lighting are also important components of good graft preparation (12).

Lastly, poor hair yield may result from rough handling of the grafts as they are inserted into the recipient sites. Grafts should be grasped by their subcutaneous tissue "tails" rather than around the hair matrix and should be eased gently into recipient sites, with care taken that the forceps approaches the recipient site at an angle or direction similar to that of the site itself.

A

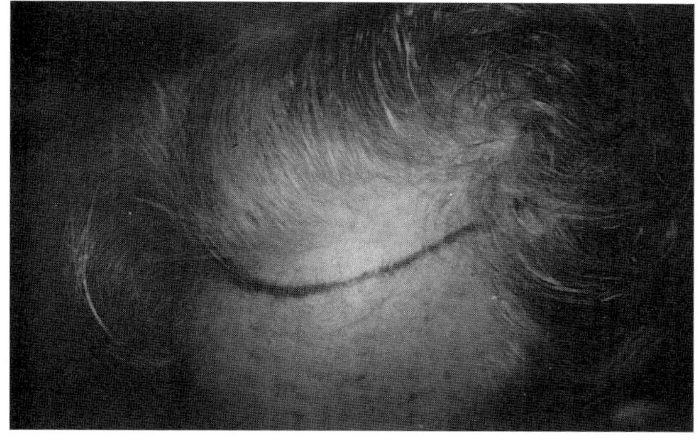

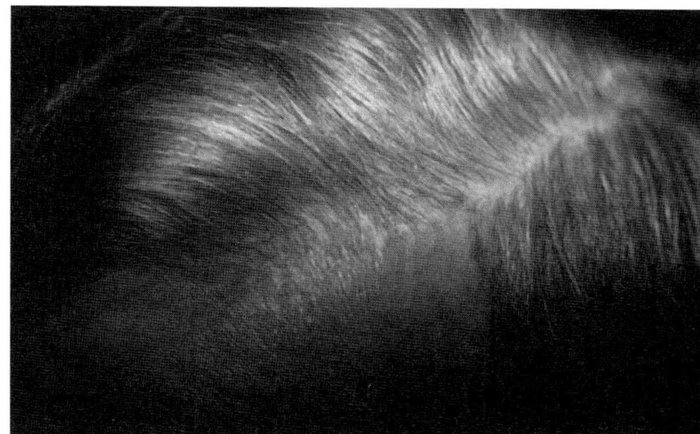

B

C

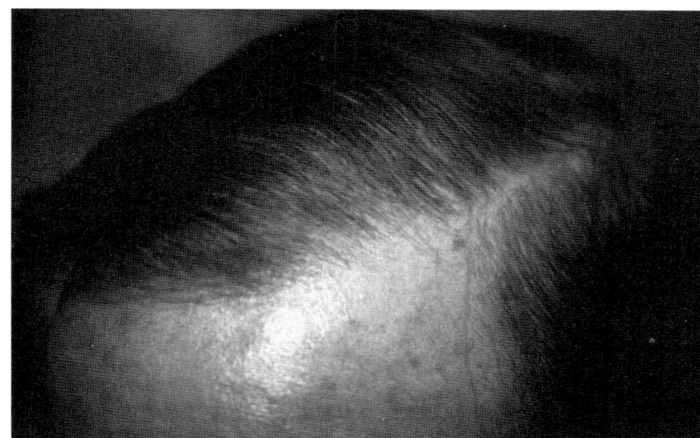

FIGURE 59-10. A: The patient before treatment. He had fine, dense, white hair and was therefore an excellent candidate for the procedure. **B:** The same patient 14 months after his first hair transplant, which consisted of 150 micrografts and 364 small slit grafts. It is possible to obtain cosmetically excellent results in many patients with only micrografts and slit grafts, particularly if the patient has good hair density in the donor area or if the contrast between the hair and skin color is minimal. **C:** The same patient 12 months after a second transplant, which consisted of 50 micrografts, 675 small slit grafts, and 11 standard round grafts. The patient has now dyed his hair red, and the results are cosmetically similar to those seen after a single session when his hair was white. The less the contrast between the hair and skin color, the more natural and thicker the hair appears.

If a patient is dissatisfied with the density of previously otherwise satisfactory treatments, one can increase the density by additional transplanting with micrografts, slit grafts, or ideally small round grafts or slot grafts placed between the previously transplanted hair.

Plugginess

Plugginess in a recipient area in a new patient can be avoided by choosing grafts with fine hair for the hairline, and by minimizing the use of grafts containing more than three to six hairs in a hairline zone, especially if the contrast between the color of the hair and that of the skin is significant. Grafts containing more than three to six hairs can be used in areas posterior to the hairline zone if the hair texture is fine or if the color contrast is minimal (8).

For patients who have been unsatisfactorily treated previously with round grafts, and especially those who have undergone transplantation with standard grafts, repair is best carried out by using a combination of grafts of different sizes within the area previously treated and, if possible, creating a new hairline zone anterior to that area. The spaces between existing round grafts containing relatively dense hair should be totally excised with appropriately sized punches.

The density of hair obtained with micrografts and minigrafts can never equal that obtained with round grafts that have good hair survival. For example, it is not possible using only micrografts to produce more than 20 hairs in a round area with a diameter of only 3.25 mm (7). Thus, if a hairless space is present between two round grafts containing relatively dense hair, the best way to eliminate the space is to excise it completely with a round trephine of appropriate size and replace it with another round graft with hair density and texture similar to that of its neighbors (Figs. 59-11, 59-12). An alternate approach is to punch out a portion of the dense larger grafts and reuse the tissue to create small round grafts or slit grafts elsewhere. This latter approach in combination with micrografting and minigrafting is useful as an adjunct to adding standard grafts to areas previously treated with standard grafts, but it is not satisfactory in its stead. The only exception to this general rule can be made when the spaces between previously transplanted larger grafts are very small. In such cases, micrografting and minigrafting (without standard grafts) can produce acceptable results (Fig. 59-13).

If one has utilized micrografts and slit grafts to create a new hairline zone anterior to an area treated with standard grafts and the spaces between the standard grafts have been

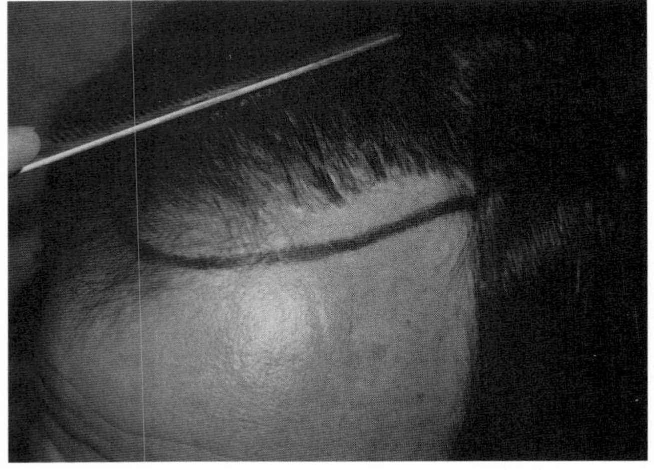

A

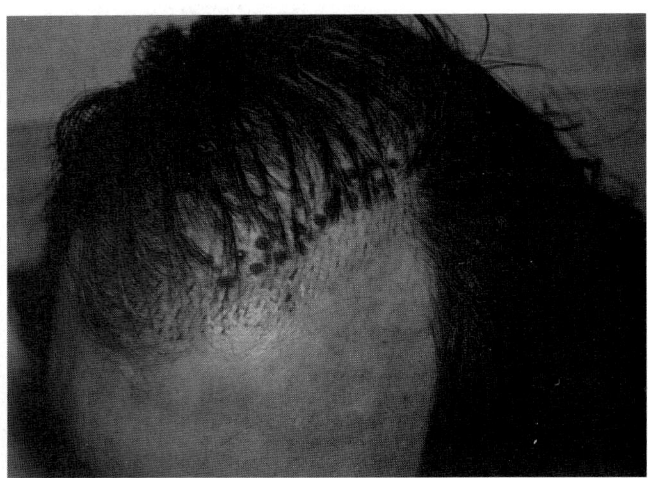

B

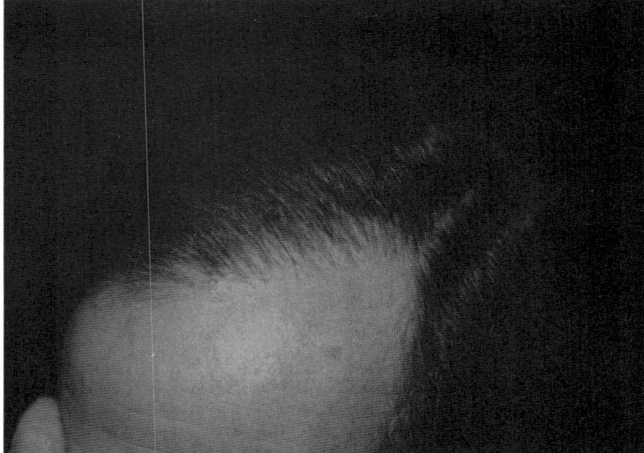

C

FIGURE 59-11. A: Patient before corrective procedure. The *black crayon line* denotes the limits of the new hairline to be constructed anterior to the previous transplant. **B:** A new hairline was constructed with micrografts and slit grafts. The empty spaces between the standard grafts were punched out with a punch large enough to remove the alopecic spaces between the grafts entirely. These were filled with standard grafts. In subsequent sessions, some of the grafts with coarser, denser hair were also punched out and moved more posteriorly, to be replaced with grafts having a hair texture and density more consistent with that of the adjacent grafts. **C:** Same patient after three corrective transplants.

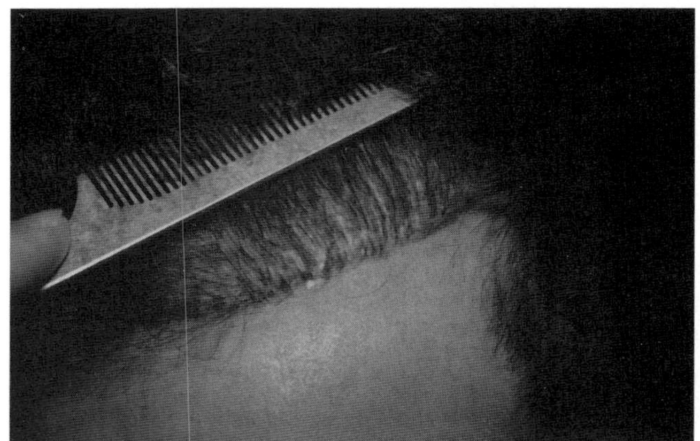

A

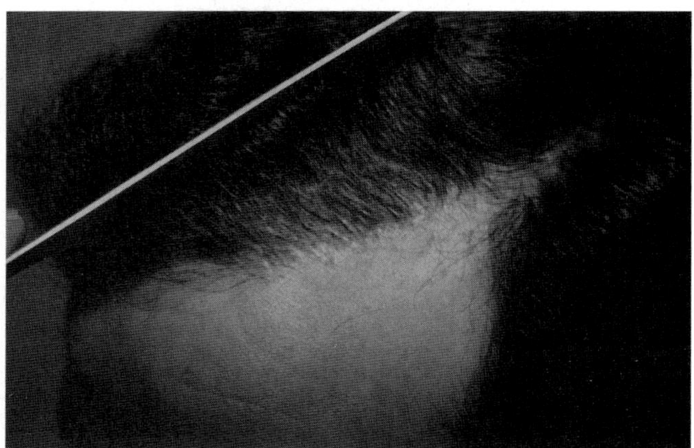

B

FIGURE 59-12. A: Another patient seen for corrective hair transplanting. Once again, trephines of various sizes have been used to punch out alopecic spaces. Small round grafts are sprinkled throughout the hairline zone at the same time that micrografts and minigrafts are added to this area to minimize the change of density between the hairline zone and standard grafted areas more posteriorly, where the density is greater. **B:** Same patient after two repair sessions.

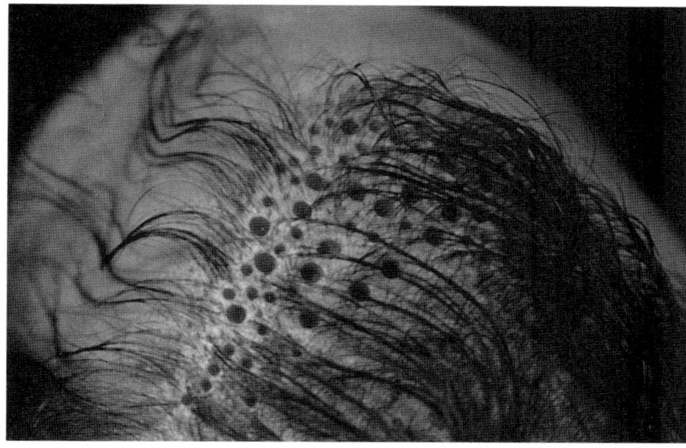
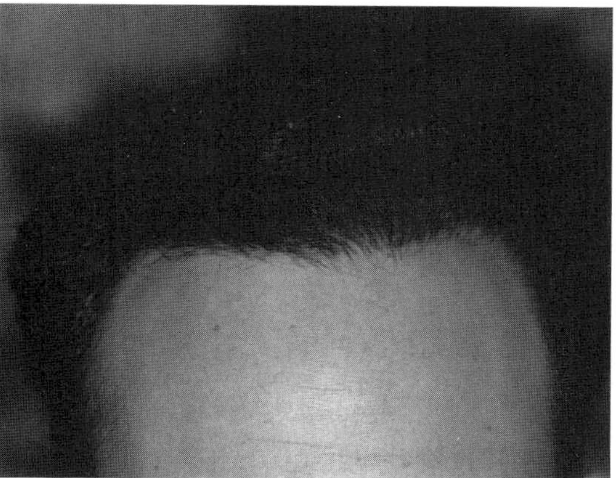

FIGURE 59-13. A: Before corrective transplanting, this patient had a hairline constructed primarily with small grafts of various sizes. The spaces left between the grafts were relatively small and were treated with small round grafts, slit grafts, and micrografts. **B:** Six months after a single corrective session. When spaces between previously transplanted grafts are very small, micrografting, slit and minigrafting alone are often sufficient to produce good results.

filled with other standard grafts, one generally will have produced a fairly sharp demarcation between a hairline zone of relatively low density and a dense area treated with larger grafts. Small round grafts should therefore always be used throughout the hairline zone to blur and minimize changes in density (Fig. 59-12).

Lastly, any grafts containing particularly coarse or numerous hairs near the anterior border of the hairline zone should be punched out and moved in whole or part more posteriorly. A pluggy appearance is frequently caused not only by too many hairs per graft and alopecic spaces between grafts—especially standard grafts—but also by inconsistent hair density and texture in adjacent grafts (Figs. 59-11, 59-14). This problem can be avoided by carefully selecting and using in the same area, from the first session onward, grafts of consistent hair density and texture. Micrografts with hair that is too coarse or dense also occasionally turn up in otherwise good transplanting and should be punched out and retransplanted (Fig. 59-15). One of the advantages of waiting 5 months or longer between sessions is that such grafts are easily recognized and corrected during the next session. The site of the inappropriate graft should be sutured or filled with a graft containing hair of more suitable hair density and texture.

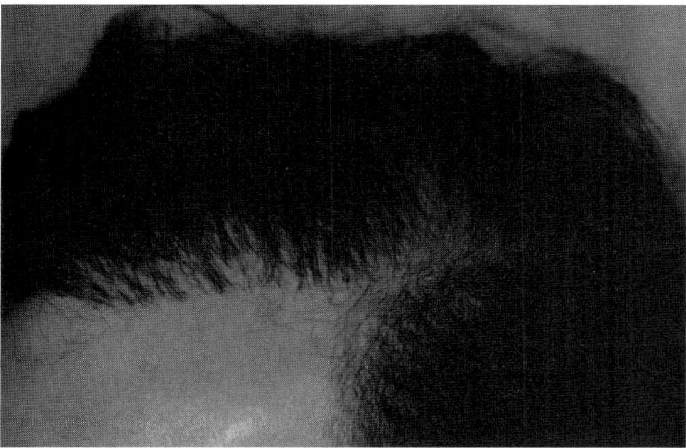
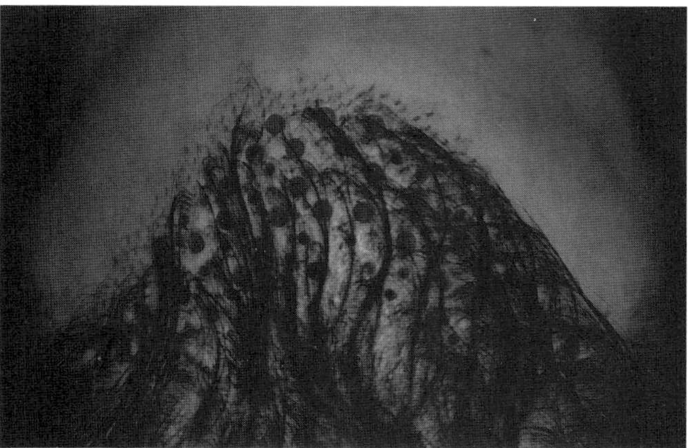

FIGURE 59-14. A: A pluggy appearance is frequently caused not only by too many hairs per graft and alopecic spaces between the grafts, especially standard grafts, but also by inconsistencies in hair density and texture, as shown above. Grafts with hair that differs in texture or density from the hair of neighboring grafts are punched out and utilized elsewhere. They are replaced with grafts of appropriate density and texture. **B:** An intraoperative picture showing the type and sizes of grafts used in this patient. Note the sites for micrografts anterior to the previous grafting. These will soften an otherwise too abruptly dense hairline.

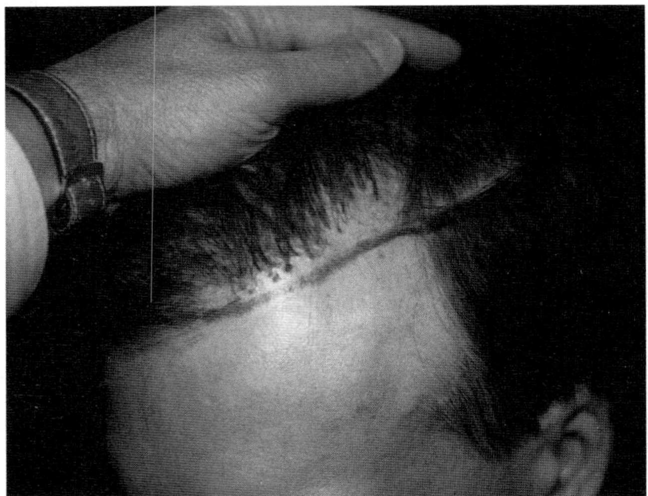

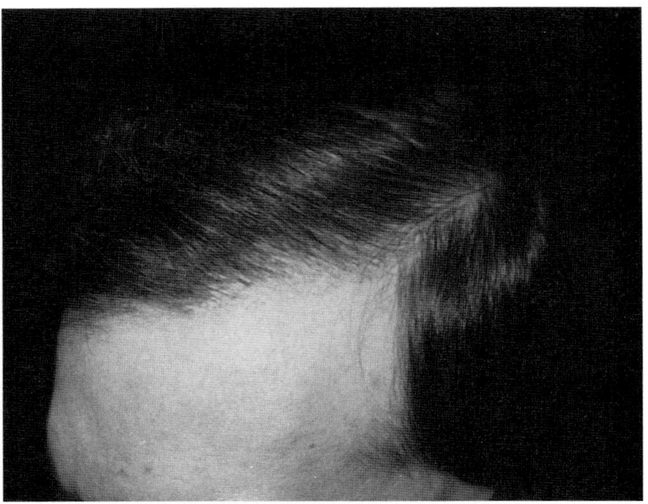

FIGURE 59-15. A: A patient before his first repair session. **B:** The same patient 6 months after his second repair session. Generally, this is an acceptable result except for a single minigraft, seen on the left side of the hairline near the midpoint, containing hair that is too dense. This small graft should be punched out and replaced with a graft containing finer-textured and slightly less dense hair. The inappropriate graft should be retransplanted more posteriorly.

Incorrect Hair Direction

Figure 59-16 provides a general idea of the usual hair directions in various areas of the recipient site. However, the normal direction and angle of hair for any area varies from person to person. It can virtually always be discerned by looking for persisting terminal or vellus hairs in the recipient area and attempting to mimic them. When preparing a recipient site, I constantly comb these hairs in various directions to see which way they want to fall. My assistants try to hold the hair at the apparent angle and direction once these parameters have been chosen. It is difficult to describe in writing how this is accomplished except to say that the hair is kept moist, that combing is continued virtually every minute if any significant amount of hair is present in the recipient area, and that the assistants use gauze to grip the ends of the hairs and push them forward slightly in such a way as to reveal their angle and direction.

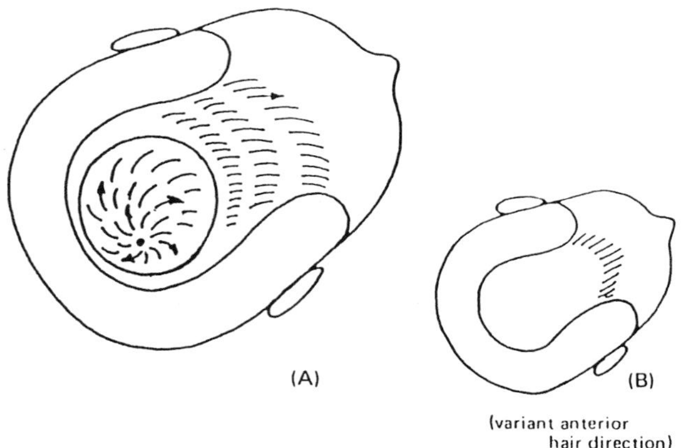

FIGURE 59-16. This schematic drawing provides a general idea of the usual hair directions in various areas of the recipient site.

The angle or direction of hair in poorly executed hair transplants can be only slightly or grossly incorrect (Fig. 59-17). If the discrepancy is slight and located in an inconspicuous area, it can frequently be ignored. If it is pronounced or situated in a cosmetically more important area, such as the anterior border of the hairline zone, the grafts should be punched out with a punch of appropriate size and the site sutured or left to heal by secondary intention if it is small enough (e.g., ≤ 2 mm in diameter). If the misdirected grafts are numerous, it is often wise to excise them in one or more separate sessions devoted entirely to this purpose. Frequently, however, they can be removed in stages as part of the repair procedures. All such excised hair should, of course, be reused at once in other areas.

Depressed or Elevated Grafts

One should be careful to place grafts in the recipient site flush with the surrounding skin. Prolonged pressure is in some cases necessary to prevent graft elevation and "cobblestoning," whereas in others the graft tends to sink below the surrounding skin. If an even surface cannot be achieved with pressure and repositioning, the use of a drop of cyanoacry-

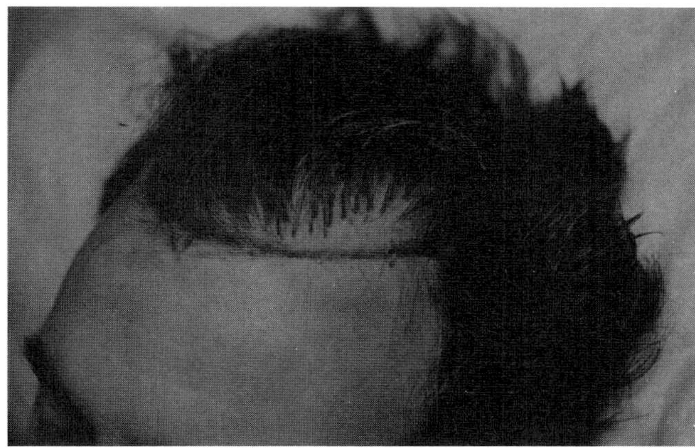

A

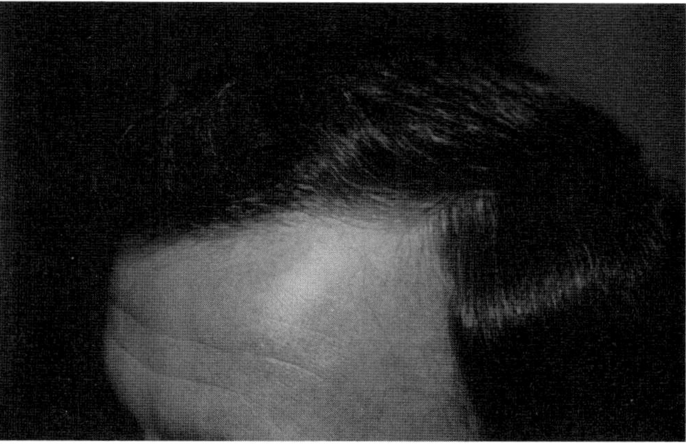

B

FIGURE 59-17. A: A patient before corrective surgery. The direction of grafts in some areas is satisfactory, but in other areas (e.g., at the depth of the frontotemporal recession), the hair is grossly misdirected posteriorly and laterally instead of anteriorly. Such grafts often must be punched out and the sites sutured in a separate session before grafts are added to the same area. If the direction or angle of transplanted hair is less unnatural, or if the graft is in a less cosmetically important area, it frequently can be ignored or at least excised at the same time that additional grafts are transplanted. **B:** The same patient 8 months after the first corrective session.

late glue at the edge of each graft is recommended (12). Slight elevation of grafts is preferable to depression or "dimpling." The former is easily corrected with light electrodessication at a later date; depressed grafts are best punched out and replaced with new and properly positioned ones. (The old grafts are reused elsewhere.) The easiest way to avoid depressed grafts is to use instruments that limit the depth of the recipient site. Minde knives (A to Z Surgical, 2021 The Alameda No. 385, San Jose, California 95126; (408) 243-3006), which are used for micrograft sites, have short blades that are designed to penetrate no deeper than deep dermis or superficial subcutaneous tissue. Beaver blades (Robbins Instruments, 2 North Passaic, Box 441, Chatham, New Jersey; (201) 635-8972) can be mounted on a needle driver with the length of the exposed blade limited to the depth suitable for the "beaver grafts" that will be placed into the sites.

Errors in Alopecia Reduction

When alopecia reduction is used, it is important to use a two-layered closure and avoid excess tension on the suture line. One should also generally not remove so much of the bald area that the remaining hair lateral to the excision site takes on an abnormal direction (13). [Scalp extension as described by Frechet is sometimes the exception to this rule (14).] In addition, alopecia reduction scars should not extend into areas that will not be treated with grafts at some point in the future, and the alopecia reductions should not overly stretch the donor area such that hair density in that area becomes unsatisfactory. With regard to the latter, it is important to realize that hair in the "permanent rim" will gradually become more sparse with advancing age, so that the density in the rim should not be reduced to what is minimally acceptable at the patient's current age. Allowance must be made for future thinning of the rim hair.

Wide scars can be corrected by reexcision and closure under proper tension. Misdirected hair is more difficult to correct but can usually be improved with Frechet three-flap or two-flap procedures (14) (Fig. 59-18). In general, it is best not to reduce the alopecic area to a width of less than 4 to 6 cm, and to use grafts directed and angled properly to eliminate the rest of it.

DONOR AREA

Wide Scars

Wide scars in the donor area are most commonly caused by excision of a donor strip that is too wide and closure of the donor wound with too much tension. Be careful not to be too ambitious when deciding on the width of the strip to be excised. Excessive closing tension is most likely to occur post-auricularly or in the midline of the occipital area. We record the width of the strip that is excised during each procedure, and note on the operative report the amount of closing tension on a scale of 1 to 10. This provides guidance for subsequent sessions. If any tension is present on closure, the edges of the wound should be undermined, and both galeal and superficial sutures should be utilized. It is best, however,

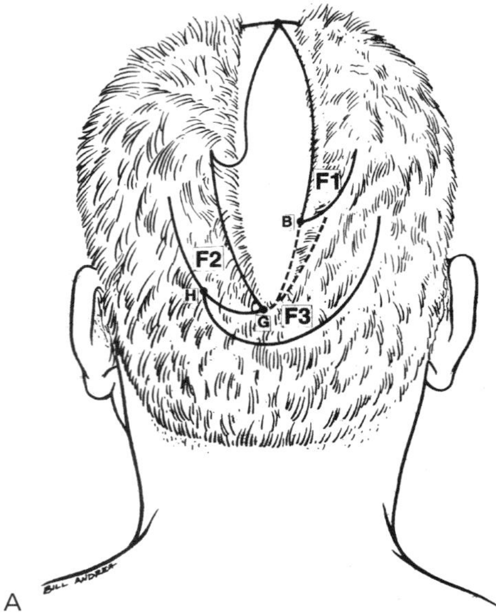

A

FIGURE 59-18. A: A schematic drawing of incision lines of the three hair-bearing scalp flaps before transposition. Points *B* and *H* are the distal ends of the superior and inferior flaps, respectively. They will be rotated to the left. Point *G* is the distal end of the intermediate flap, to be rotated to the right. Although the alopecia reductions in the particular patient shown in **B** were carried out with a view to creating a slot defect before correcting it with a Frechet three-flap procedure, similar defects that are unintentionally created can also be treated in this fashion. (From Frechet P, Scalp Extension. In: Unger W, ed. *Hair transplantation*, 3rd ed. New York: Marcel Dekker Inc., 1995:625–657, with permission. Drawing courtesy of Patrick Frechet.) **B:** Patient before slot correction. **C:** Patient immediately after the three hair-bearing scalp flap procedure. (Photographs courtesy of Patrick Frechet.)

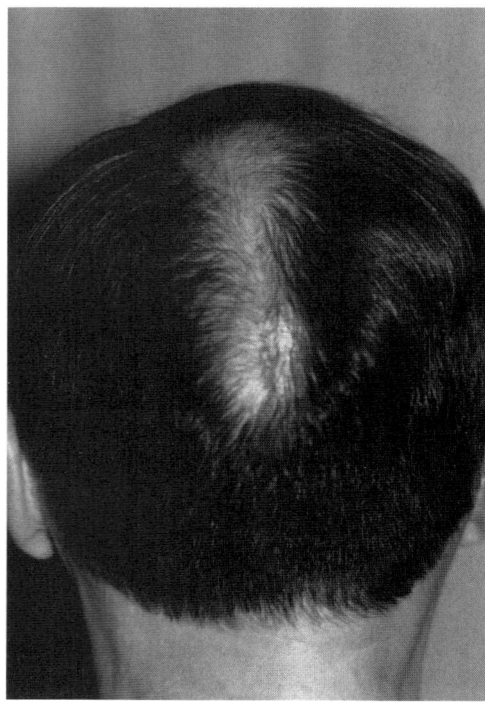

B

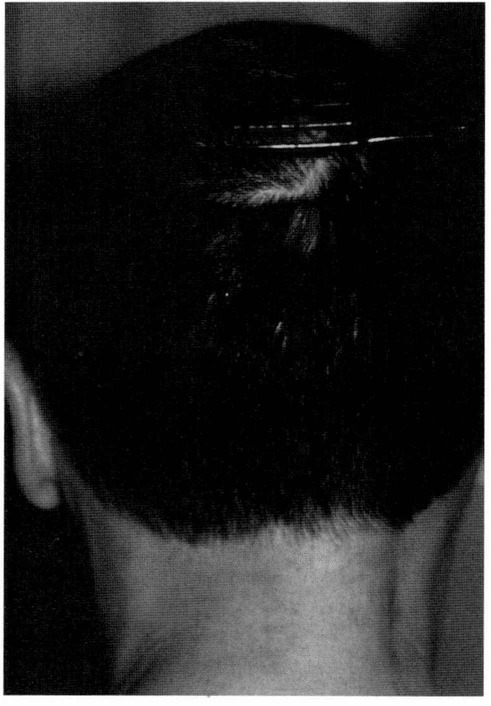

C

not to excise a strip so wide that galeal sutures and undermining are necessary rather than optional.

The best treatment of a scar that is too wide is reexcision of the site and appropriate undermining with or without the use of galeal sutures. In a few isolated cases, if the scar is very wide, some tissue expansion before the excision may be necessary.

The second most frequent cause of wide scars in the donor area is compromise of the blood supply to the donor site by scar tissue resulting from previous donor area harvesting. One can minimize this problem by excising tissue for new donor areas immediately adjacent to the scar(s) from the previous ones and including the scars in the new donor strip(s). This practice is referred to as a *total excision technique* (5). With this approach, only one or occasionally two scars are ever produced in the donor area, so that inter-

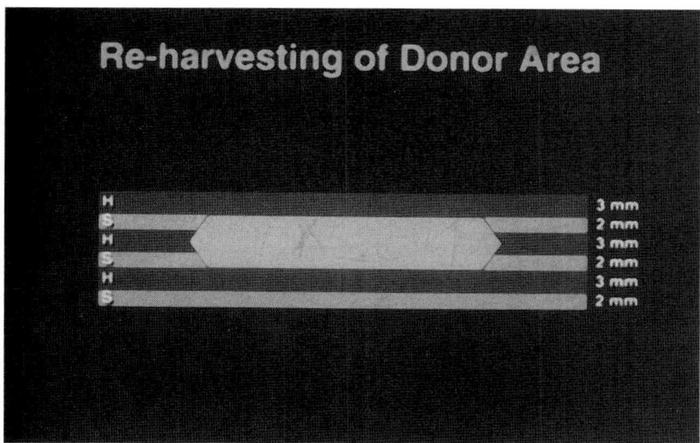

FIGURE 59-19. A schematic drawing of alternating rows of hair *(H)* and scar *(S)* indicates the donor area excision pattern, which includes two rows of scar and one row of hair. Once this area has been excised and the defect sutured, a single scar will replace two wider scars. Also, two rows of hair will now be adjacent to each other. Thus, the overall density of the donor area will be increased rather than decreased despite the removal of more hair from this area.

ruption of its blood supply is minimal. Should one be working in an area that has previously been harvested by another physician and in which many scars are present, it is best to take strips sufficiently narrow that essentially no tension is created on closure.

Overharvesting

If too many grafts have been taken from a donor area, scars may become noticeable either immediately or with advancing age as the hair in the donor "rim" gradually thins. The best way to avoid this problem is to utilize a total excision technique and close with minimal tension to obtain optimal scars. If the area has been overharvested, especially with standard grafts, it is usually possible to excise a strip in such a way that hair-bearing tissue will be supplied and the amount of scar will be reduced to improve the appearance of the donor area. *This approach must nearly always be used to obtain the grafts required to correct virtually all the problems noted in the first section of this chapter.* In a well-organized, previously harvested donor area, for example, one can often excise two rows of scars with a row of hair between them. In this way, hair is obtained for transplanting and a single narrow scar is created from two usually wider scars, while two hair-bearing rows are left adjacent to each other (Fig. 59-19).

Severe Temporary Hair Loss

Severe hair loss may occur in the donor area in cases with a bad combination of closing tension and substantial preoperative scarring in the donor area from previous surgeries. This happens most often in patients undergoing repair whose donor areas are heavily scarred and have a poor blood supply (Fig. 59-20). Once again, taking a narrow enough donor strip to allow for closure under minimal tension and without undermining will help to prevent this problem, as will the use of a solution of 3% minoxidil applied twice daily for the first 5 weeks postoperatively. Fortunately, this effluvium is usually temporary, and the patient requires only reassurance.

A
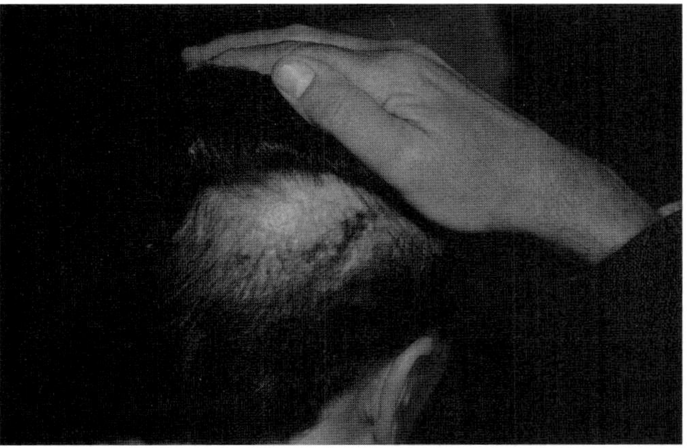

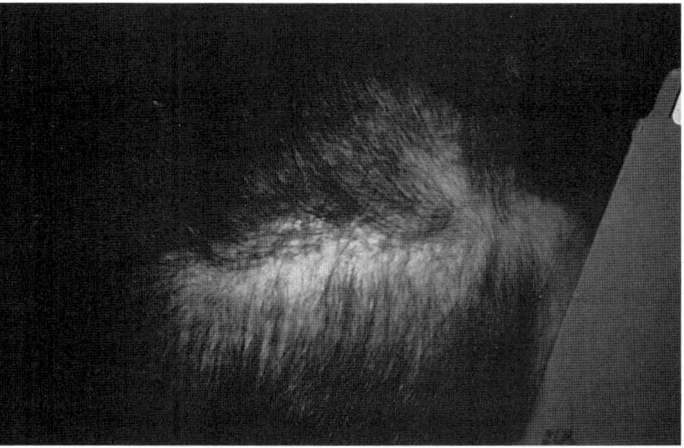
B

FIGURE 59-20. A: Severe alopecia developed in this patient superior and inferior to a donor area closed with minimal tension. A combination of even minimal closing tension but substantial donor area scarring after previous surgeries led to this hair loss. Virtually all this hair will begin regrowing within 3 months of the surgery. **B:** Same patient 5 months later. Lost telogen hair has regrown. A donor area scar that was slightly wider than usual was excised 10 days before this photograph was taken.

REFERENCES

1. Unger WP, Knudsen R. General principles of recipient site organization and planning. In: Unger WP, ed. *Hair transplantation.* New York: Marcel Dekker Inc, 1995:105–158.
2. Cotterill PC. Hair transplantation in females. In: Unger WP, ed. *Hair transplantation.* New York: Marcel Dekker Inc, 1995: 287–292.
3. Unger M. Alopecia reductions. In: Unger WP, ed. *Hair transplantation.* New York: Marcel Dekker Inc, 1995:509–624.
4. Beehner M. The frontal forelock. *Hair Transplant Forum* 1995;5:1–5.
5. Unger WP. The donor site. In: Unger WP, ed. *Hair transplantation.* New York: Marcel Dekker Inc, 1995:183–187.
6. Marritt E, Dzubow LM. Reassessment of male pattern baldness: a reevaluation of the treatment. In: Stough DB, Haber RS, eds. *Hair replacement.* New York: McGraw-Hill, 1995:30–41.
7. Unger WP. Different grafts for different purposes. *Am J Cosmetic Surg* 1997;14:177–183.
8. Unger WP. Recipient area. In: Unger WP, ed. *Hair transplantation.* New York: Marcel Dekker Inc, 1995:215–321.
9. Pomerantz M. More problems with megasessions. *Hair Transplant Forum* 1995;5:4–5.
10. Arnold J, Marzola M, *Barcelona report—part III.* Hair Transplant Forum International, 1998, 8:1, 1.
11. Arnold J. On Marzola, Barcelona report part II. *Hair Transplant Forum Int* 1998;8:1.
12. McKeown M, Preparation and insertion of grafts. In: Unger WP, ed. *Hair transplantation.* New York: Marcel Dekker Inc, 1995:331–348.
13. Unger M. Scalp reduction. In: Unger WP, ed. *Hair transplantation.* New York: Marcel Dekker Inc, 1995:509–570.
14. Frechet P. Scalp extension. In: Unger WP, ed. *Hair transplantation.* New York: Marcel Dekker Inc, 1995:625–642.

SUGGESTED READING

Anderson R. New expanded scalp flap techniques for elimination of male pattern baldness. In: Unger WP, ed. *Hair transplantation.* New York: Marcel Dekker Inc, 1995:673–691.

Brandy DA. The bilateral occipito-parietal flap. *J Dermatol Surg Oncol* 1986;12:1062–1066.

Limmer BL. Elliptical donor stereoscopically assisted micrografting as an approach to further refinement in hair transplantation. *J Dermatol Surg Oncol* 1994;20:79–93.

Nordstrom REA. Micrografts for improvement of the frontal hairline after transplantation. *Aesthetic Plast Surg* 1981;5:97–101.

Stough DB, Haber RS. *Hair replacement.* New York: McGraw-Hill, 1995.

Unger M. The Unger-modified major reduction. In: Unger WP, ed. *Hair transplantation.* New York: Marcel Dekker Inc, 1995:564–567.

Unger WP, Solish B, Giguerre D. Delineating the "safe" donor area for hair transplanting. *Am J Cosmetic Surg* 1994;11:239–243.

Unger WP, Stough DB, Jimenez FJ, et al. Alopecia reduction. In: Ratz JL, ed. *Textbook of dermatologic surgery.* Philadelphia: Lippincott–Raven Publishers, 1998:501–504.

Weidig JC. An approach to the younger patient. In: Stough DB, Haber RS, eds. *Hair replacement.* New York: McGraw-Hill, 1995:62–67.

Discussion

HAIR REPLACEMENT

JAMES E. VOGEL

For plastic surgeons who routinely perform a myriad of cosmetic and reconstructive procedures, hair restoration surgery in general, and hair transplantation in particular, should be among the procedures with the fewest complications. When successful, the restoration of hair to a bald pate can be received with the same or greater enthusiasm than that seen after other well-planned and well-executed cosmetic surgical operations. As in all cosmetic procedures, it is essential to select patients carefully and establish the surgeon's ability to achieve the patient's anticipated goals preoperatively. Thus, I would point out and echo the first paragraph of Dr. Unger's chapter, in which he emphasizes the importance of frank and thorough discussion with the patient before surgery is undertaken.

When technical complications follow hair restoration procedures today, they are usually the consequence of neglect of some basic principles of hair restoration surgery. These principles have been outlined in the preceding chapter, and in numerous journals (1,2) and texts, including the one edited by Dr. Unger (3,4).

In clinical practice, however, most of the truly unfavorable results seen are the result of hair restoration procedures performed according to techniques or philosophies that are

James E. Vogel: Division of Plastic Surgery, The Johns Hopkins University School of Medicine, Baltimore, Maryland 21208 now outdated. This is true of alopecia reductions, hair flap surgery, and hair grafting. Most of these complications of previous hair restoration surgery can generally be attributed to previous hair grafting or the unanticipated progression of baldness.

Dr. Unger's classification of unfavorable results in hair restoration surgery as occurring in the recipient or donor area is logical, and this discussion is organized accordingly.

UNFAVORABLE RESULTS IN THE RECIPIENT AREA

All the entities listed in the preceding chapter are potential complications, but those most frequently seen are an inappropriately placed hairline and a pluggy appearance. A pluggy hairline is the unattractive and unnatural result of hair grafting with large plugs of hair. A pluggy look can be best be avoided by using small grafts at the anterior hairline and larger grafts posteriorly. The best method for correcting a pluggy appearance of grafts was first described by Lucas (5). The technique described by Dr. Unger is a variation of this original description. The following technique for correcting pluggy grafts represents our current modification of the Lucas operation, which we have termed *plug reduction and recycling* (1) (Fig. 59D-1). To correct the anterior hairline, the technique of plug reduction is aggressively applied to the anterior two rows of plugs. In general, during the first corrective session, every other plug in a row can be selected for plug reduction and recycling. The plugs to be reduced are selected and trimmed to a length of approximately 3 mm. A punch biopsy tool that is the same size as the plug or slightly smaller is selected. For example, the size of a traditional plug is typically 4 mm, and so we would select a 3.5-mm punch

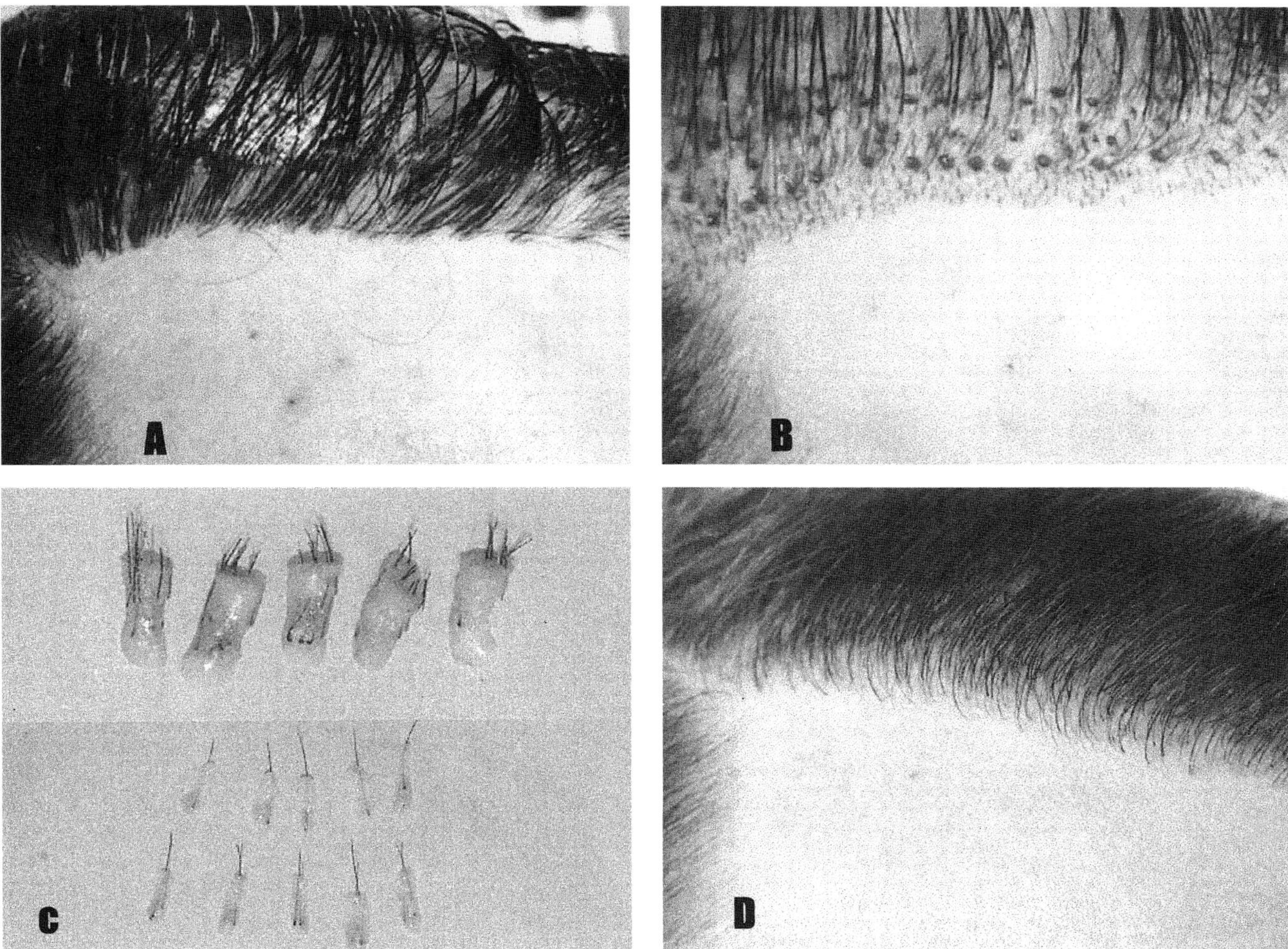

FIGURE 59D-1. Technique of plug reduction and recycling. **A,B:** Straight, pluggy hairline, two anterior rows of plugs, and intervening areas of alopecia. **C,D:** Every other plug is cut to a length of 3 mm, and a punch excision is eccentrically performed to leave behind a linear graft with three to four hairs. The plug excisions are closed, and recycled grafts and newly harvested grafts are transplanted anteriorly and placed to create an irregular hairline.

biopsy for the plug reduction. Using a smaller punch size would leave too much residual plug and incompletely treat the clumped and often compressed appearance of the plug. The punch is positioned eccentrically to leave a crescent shape of the remaining original plug. This effectively leaves behind a linear graft of approximately three to four hairs.

The circular punch sites can be left open to heal by secondary intention or closed primarily. When we first started with this technique, the wounds were uniformly left open. However, because of annoying serous seepage from these sites and the delay in separation of the plug reduction site eschar, we began closing the wounds primarily. A 3-0 chromic suture is used for to close the plug reduction site.

The recycled hair and additional hair harvested from the occipital region are densely transplanted anterior and posterior to the plug reduction sites. Usually, several wide tracks of alopecia are present between the linear rows of plugs, and these need to be transplanted densely. Plugs that are more than 2.5 to 3 cm posterior to the anterior hairline can generally be left intact. Aggressive management of the first two or three rows of plugs as described is usually all that is needed to soften and camouflage the corn row appearance. In this way, the density of the plugs posteriorly, the only redeeming quality of large circular grafts, can be combined with the soft look of the anterior hairline zone. Most pluggy hairlines can be significantly improved after one session; however, it is not unusual for two or more corrective sessions to be needed.

The correct design of an anterior hairline just as important as the use of hair grafts that are natural and undetectable. The principles of hairline design have been reviewed elsewhere (3–5). Briefly, the hairline must be symmetrical and exhibit bilateral temporal recessions. In men, the distance from the glabella to the most anterior point of the hairline is usually not less than 8.0 to 8.5 cm. The most common problems associated with hairline design are blunted temporal angles or placement of the hairline too low on the forehead. Dr. Unger's methods for correcting a low hairline are appropriate and useful. In addition, the combined use of modified forehead lifting, scalp reduction with use of an M-shaped pattern, and plug reductions can result in a very satisfactory improvement in patients with problems of hairline design (6).

Alopecia reductions are a source of debate among hair restoration surgeons. Most would agree that a visible scar on the bald head is to be avoided. However, the debate is primarily focused on whether it is possible to hide a scalp reduction scar completely with hair grafting. Those who feel it is not possible to hide a scar on the scalp predictably argue that scalp reduction has no role. Those who favor scalp reduction feel the scars are either acceptable or easily camouflaged. The obvious reason for performing a scalp reduction at all is to reduce the area that must be grafted. Dr. Unger states that when wide scars result from scalp reduction, reexcision and closure under proper tension can correct them. This same advice applied to the treatment of wide scars in the donor area. It would have been impressive to see a surgical photograph exemplifying this type of scar management in either of the two settings described. My experience is that wide scars in these areas exist because of tension on the wound. Even with undermining and multilayered closure, further excision and reapproximation are not successful because a tension-free closure cannot be obtained. In these cases, traditional, prolonged tissue expansion is the only reliable method to revise already tight wounds that have resulted in a wide scar.

Hair-bearing flap surgery is mentioned only briefly in the chapter, in a description of the Frechet triple flap. When a hair flap dies or is malpositioned, the result can be disastrous. A flap that is too short to cover the anterior hairline, maldirection of the hair, and progressive alopecia that causes a flap to appear as an isolated strip of hair are other complications of flap surgery. Furthermore, flap donor scars are often wide and occasionally impossible to hide with surrounding hair. Repair of these problems ranges from difficult to impossible. The approach includes the use of a myriad of techniques included in the chapter and this discussion. Avoidance is based on very careful patient selection and familiarity with the hair flap of choice.

Finally, it is worth commenting on hair restoration surgery in women. Unlike men, most women are not good candidates for hair restoration surgery because their donor hair is too sparse. In general, only about 30% of women are satisfactory candidates for hair transplantation. When women are deemed candidates for a transplant, they need to know that temporary telogen effluvium or anagen effluvium (i.e., hair loss) can occur. They can be reassured that in 3 to 5 months, most of the shed hair will return. In addition, the transplanted hair will appear thicker and stronger.

In conclusion, Dr. Unger's years of experience with hair transplantation have resulted in many "pearls" that can help the plastic surgeon avoid an unfavorable result with these procedures. Stated several times in his chapter is the importance of a thorough preoperative consultation with the patient regarding the goals and limitations of hair restoration surgery. Issues of obtainable density and the extent of possible coverage must be completely understood and documented preoperatively. The limitations and goals of surgical hair restoration must take into consideration the patient's age, hair loss classification, donor density, and willingness to complete the necessary number of procedures.

When patients do present with problems caused by hair restoration surgery, it is not at all uncommon to hear them lament that their entire lifestyle revolves around the concealment of plugs, a low hairline, or some other unnatural appearance of their hair. Often, patients rise early to devote extra time to hair grooming and concealment, plan social engagements in areas with dim lighting, and avoid swimming or getting caught in the rain all to avoid the obvious display of their hair plugs. In addition, patients who bear this burden of surgical misadventure are often constant wearers of hats or hairpieces, or they resort to the perpetual use of scalp-coloring creams or sprays. Finally, the unfortunate patients with unsightly plugs on their head often carry with them an emotional burden of anger and distrust derived from past experiences with hair restoration procedures. Thus, it is easy to understand how grateful patients are when the corrective techniques described in the preceding chapter successfully reverse the unfavorable result of their hair restoration surgery.

REFERENCES

1. Vogel JE. Correction of the corn row transplant and other common problems in surgical hair restoration. *Plast Reconstr Surg* 1999;105:1529–1536.
2. Vogel JE. Advances in hair restoration surgery. *Plast Reconstr Surg* 1997;100:7.
3. Stough DB, ed. *Hair replacement,* 1st ed. St. Louis: Mosby, 1996:306.
4. Unger WP, ed. *Hair transplantation,* 3rd ed. New York: Marcel Dekker Inc, 1995:375.
5. Lucas MWG. Partial retransplantation. A new approach in hair transplantation. *J Dermatol Surg Oncol* 1994;20:511.
6. Marzola M. A new slopecia reduction design: no visible scars, no slots, no frechet flaps. *Am J Cosmetic Surg* 1997;2:167.

60

MASTOPEXY

SCOTT L. SPEAR
MICHAEL S. BECKENSTEIN

A mastopexy may be performed to correct ptotic changes in the breast by any one or all of the following methods: elevating the nipple-areolar complex, increasing projection, or creating a more aesthetic shape (1–10). When properly executed, a mastopexy nearly always produces improvement, but disappointment to both patient and surgeon may occasionally arise from bad luck or a procedure that is poorly planned or executed. A basic approach to mastopexy should include an accurate assessment of the degree and nature of the ptosis, the selection of an appropriate procedure, obtaining informed consent, adequate preoperative planning, and, finally, sound execution. The surgeon should do everything possible to minimize unfavorable results and the need for revisional procedures. In addition, the surgeon should become familiar and comfortable with at least one periareolar procedure, one short scar mastopexy, and some type of inverted-T procedure. By mastering these techniques, the surgeon will acquire the versatility needed to achieve success in aesthetic breast surgery. Mastopexy typifies the trade-offs involved in plastic surgery. The breast is nearly always improved in shape, but at the cost of scars around the areola and perhaps the breast itself. Although poor scars are one type of unfavorable result of this operation, they may be unavoidable. Poor results caused by errors in planning or execution are another matter. In these cases, careful planning and surgical technique can be highly effective in avoiding or correcting problems.

ASSESSMENT

The first step toward attaining a favorable result with a mastopexy is to assess the status of the breasts accurately. During careful inspection, the surgeon must note the position of the nipple in relation to the inframammary fold. It is important also to measure the extent to which the breast overhangs the inframammary fold. With these findings, the degree of breast ptosis can be determined, and this information aids in the selection of appropriate corrective methods. In the youthful breast, the nipple ideally lies above the level of the inframammary fold. *Pseudoptosis* is characterized by a lax, often "inelastic" breast; the breast overhangs the fold but the nipple is positioned above the fold. In *first-degree ptosis,* the nipple lies at the inframammary fold. In *second-degree ptosis,* the nipple lies between the inframammary fold and the lowest contour of the breast. In *third-degree ptosis,* the nipple is located at the lowest contour of the breast (1). It is also important to note the longitudinal position of the nipple-areolar complex on the breast mound. A complex located away from the breast meridian can be repositioned centrally during the procedure. A careful assessment of the breast volume and distribution must also be made; this will help the surgeon choose an appropriate procedure and decide if an augmentation or a reduction might be in order.

Any asymmetry must be noted and demonstrated to the patient preoperatively, including discrepancies in nipple location, contour, and volume. It is important to determine whether asymmetry is the result of an irregularity of volume, of contour, or both because the treatment varies accordingly. Contour irregularities are usually disguised when the patient is wearing a brassiere, whereas volume differences persist in a brassiere (2). The operative plan must address any asymmetries, and it must be decided whether or not an attempt should be made to rectify them. If asymmetries are not addressed, they can be magnified in the final result.

CHOOSING AN APPROPRIATE PROCEDURE

After the breasts have been thoroughly assessed, a method must be chosen that will address all contributing factors and, it is hoped, produce an aesthetically pleasing result. The patient should be included in this decision. A number

Scott L. Spear: Division of Plastic Surgery, Georgetown University Hospital, Washington, DC
Michael S. Beckenstein: Department of Breast and Aesthetic Surgery, Georgetown University Hospital, Washington, DC

of mastopexy procedures are available that are suitable for the various types of ptosis, which implies that no single method is best to correct each type of ptosis. With this fact in mind, the surgeon must become proficient in at least one method to address each level of ptosis and the contributing factors.

Guidelines for which methods to use for the various types of ptosis have been described by others. In patients with *pseudoptosis* or *first-degree ptosis,* an augmentation mammoplasty may produce a good aesthetic result (3,4). Smaller volumes may be sufficient to restore the desired breast contour; however, larger volumes can certainly be utilized if the patient wants larger breasts, particularly because excess skin and a large volume capacity are typical of the ptotic breast. When the nipple is slightly lower than the inframammary fold, a small hemiareolar or periareolar mastopexy may be sufficient to relocate the nipple. Augmentation alone will not correct greater degrees of ptosis, particularly because with time, the breast tissue will migrate caudally. If an implant is placed totally submuscularly, the combination of a high implant and a ptotic breast will exaggerate the problem and create the appearance of a "double bubble." On the other hand, the use of a subglandular implant in the ptotic breast risks magnifying the ptosis.

Second-degree ptosis cannot be satisfactorily rectified with a breast implant alone, regardless of how large. If correction with an implant alone is attempted, even though the breast will be larger, the nipple will remain at the same level and the result will be unattractive. To correct the problem, the nipple must be elevated to the desired position. A periareolar mastopexy is appropriate when this distance is only a few centimeters. Periareolar mastopexy is limited, however, because as the amount of skin that must be excised increases, the resulting breast projection decreases, and the potential for poor scars and inadequate correction increases. This trade-off must be acknowledged by both surgeon and patient (5). For patients with a greater degree of ptosis, procedures that transpose the nipple farther are required. Usually, a short vertical scar or inverted-T method is suitable. An augmentation, reduction, or plication of the tissue of the lower pole may also help to obtain the desired aesthetic result. If the breast volume is limited or the patient wants a larger volume, then a supplemental augmentation may be performed. Sufficient skin must be excised in these cases to prevent the nipple from drifting inferiorly below the implant. With lower pole fullness, a tight closure over the existing breast tissue may help to elevate the breast, but such cases may also benefit from a small, lower pole reduction to prevent flap necrosis and widened scars that result from an excessively tight closure. If the patient does not want any alteration of breast volume, superior repositioning with or without plication of the central lower pole is another option to produce the desired contour.

Cases of *third-degree ptosis* are similar to the more severe second-degree cases. A skin excision with a short vertical scar or an inverted-T procedure combined with an augmentation, reduction, or plication is warranted. Occasionally, along with a reduction or plication, an augmentation is paradoxically helpful to provide upper pole fullness at the same time that the lower pole is being reduced. It is important to realize that with ptosis, upper pole volume is often lacking, even when a lower pole reduction is necessary and the breast tissue is elevated. The upper pole paucity will become more apparent as the tissues descend late in the postoperative period.

OBTAINING INFORMED CONSENT

Patients may be unhappy despite an excellent technical result. This situation often arises when something was not fully understood by the patient preoperatively. Informed consent is a helpful way to minimize such misunderstandings. As with all surgical procedures, a vigorous effort at educating the patient about all the associated risks and benefits of a procedure and available alternatives ultimately helps to reduce patient dissatisfaction.

With regard to mastopexy, the patient must be made aware of the scars that will result and their often unpredictable potential to become hypertrophic. The location of the scars must also be explained to the patient, especially with the inverted-T methods. Patients should be made aware that the benefits of a mastopexy may be to some extent temporary. Within a year or two, ptosis may recur, although typically not to the degree that was present preoperatively. Patients who elect to undergo a supplemental breast augmentation should be informed about the associated risks of implants and the issues associated with the various locations where they may be placed—subglandular, subpectoral, or totally submuscular. The effects of subsequent pregnancies should be presented to women of childbearing age, as postpartum changes may affect the outcome of a mastopexy. Asymmetries should be pointed out to the patient preoperatively, and the patient should be told that, depending on the methods used, they may persist or become more pronounced postoperatively. If an attempt is to be made to achieve symmetry, the patient should not be promised that this will be possible. The possible effects a mastopexy might have on subsequent mammography should also ideally be discussed with the patient, especially those undergoing augmentation, reduction, or plication procedures. Women who have reached the age at which screening mammography is recommended should have a mammogram before their surgery. Finally, the major complications associated with mastopexy should be explained, including, but not limited to, unsightly scarring, skin loss, distortion or misplacement of the areolae, sensory changes, misshapen breasts, asymmetries, and persistent ptosis.

PREOPERATIVE PLANNING AND PREPARATION

Preoperative planning and marking are helpful to verify that the method chosen is in fact appropriate and also provide the template for the actual surgery. Preoperative marking should be performed with the patient standing or sitting with her arms at her sides. The suprasternal notch reference point, midline, breast meridians, and inframammary folds should be marked. The new nipple position should be selected and marked on each breast, and any preexisting asymmetries addressed. In second- and third-degree ptosis, the

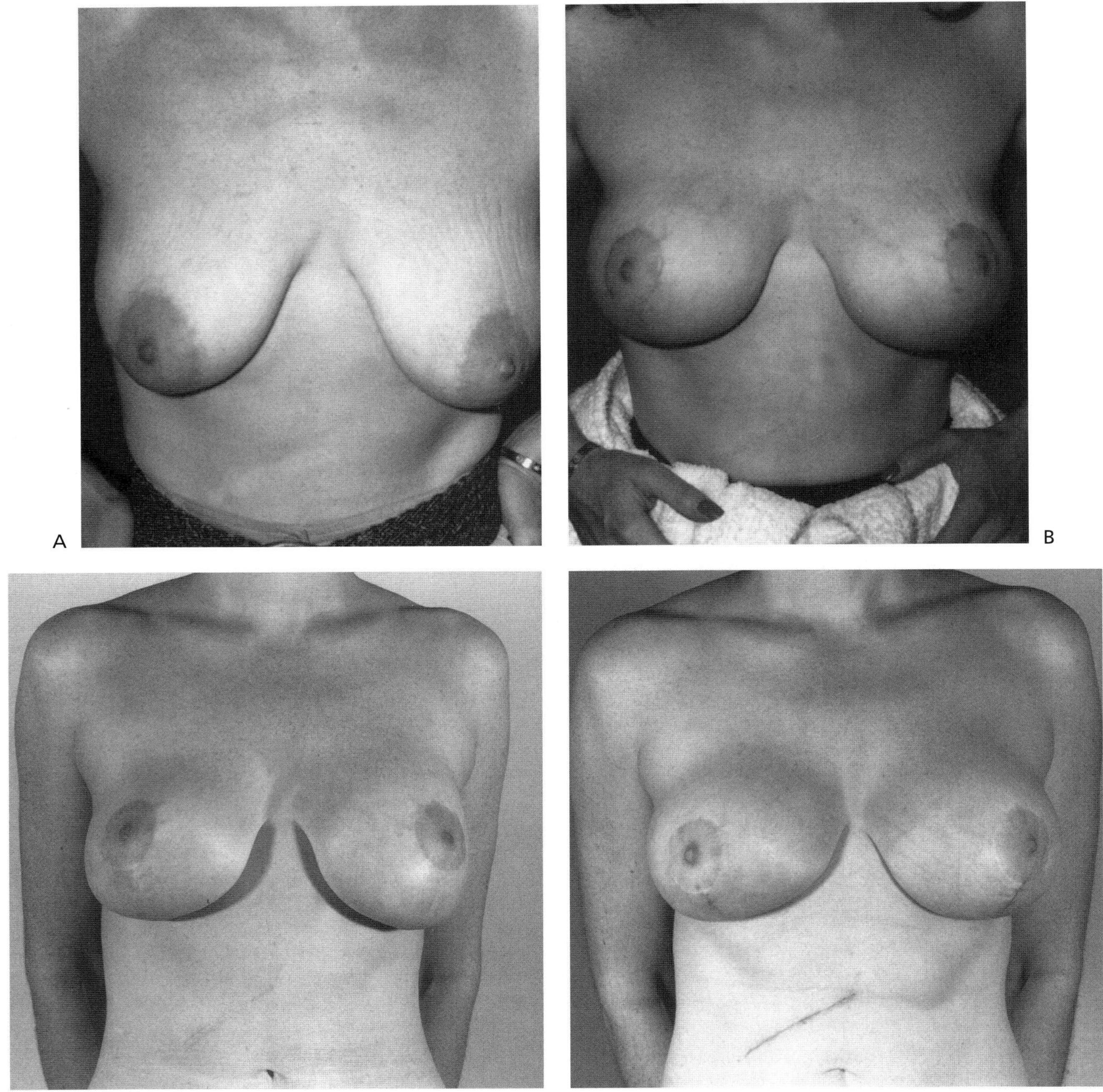

FIGURE 60-1. This 36-year-old woman had undergone a mastopexy and subglandular augmentation with textured, saline solution-filled implants 2 years earlier. She noticed progressive postoperative distortion of her breasts. Note the initially favorable result, followed by gradual bottoming out of the breast and superior migration of the nipples, particularly the left one. The problem was corrected by repeating the mastopexy and removing excess skin inferiorly. **A:** before the mastopexy. **B:** After initial mastopexy. **C:** Late bottoming out and nipple migration. **D:** After revision mastopexy.

nipple position must be set at a higher level. An aesthetically pleasing nipple should be located at or a few centimeters above the inframammary fold and near the anticipated apex of the newly reshaped breast. In the average patient, this position may be 22 to 23 cm from the sternal notch (7). The decision of how far to relocate the nipple will be influenced by the type of method used. Because some degree of nipple or gland ptosis may return, overcorrection of the nipple position should be cautiously considered. If an inverted-T technique is used without internal breast glandular remodeling, the distance from the inframammary fold to the areola may increase with time, and the nipple will be further elevated relative to the breast gland (Fig. 60-1). This distance can increase by 1 to 2 cm or even more in subpectoral or subglandular augmentations, in which caudal implant migration may also appear to increase nipple elevation (2). In these circumstances, the tendency toward overcorrection of the nipple location should be restrained. Nipple longitudinal "centricity" should be noted, and correction should be incorporated in the operative plan (9,10).

When planning to use a periareolar method, the surgeon must be careful not to compromise breast projection to restore nipple position (Fig. 60-2). Mathematical formulas based on the diameters of the proposed skin excision along with the current and desired areolae can serve as guidelines to prevent excessive distortion of the breast and areolae (5). If these guidelines indicate that projection will be lost, then a short vertical scar or inverted-T method may be a better

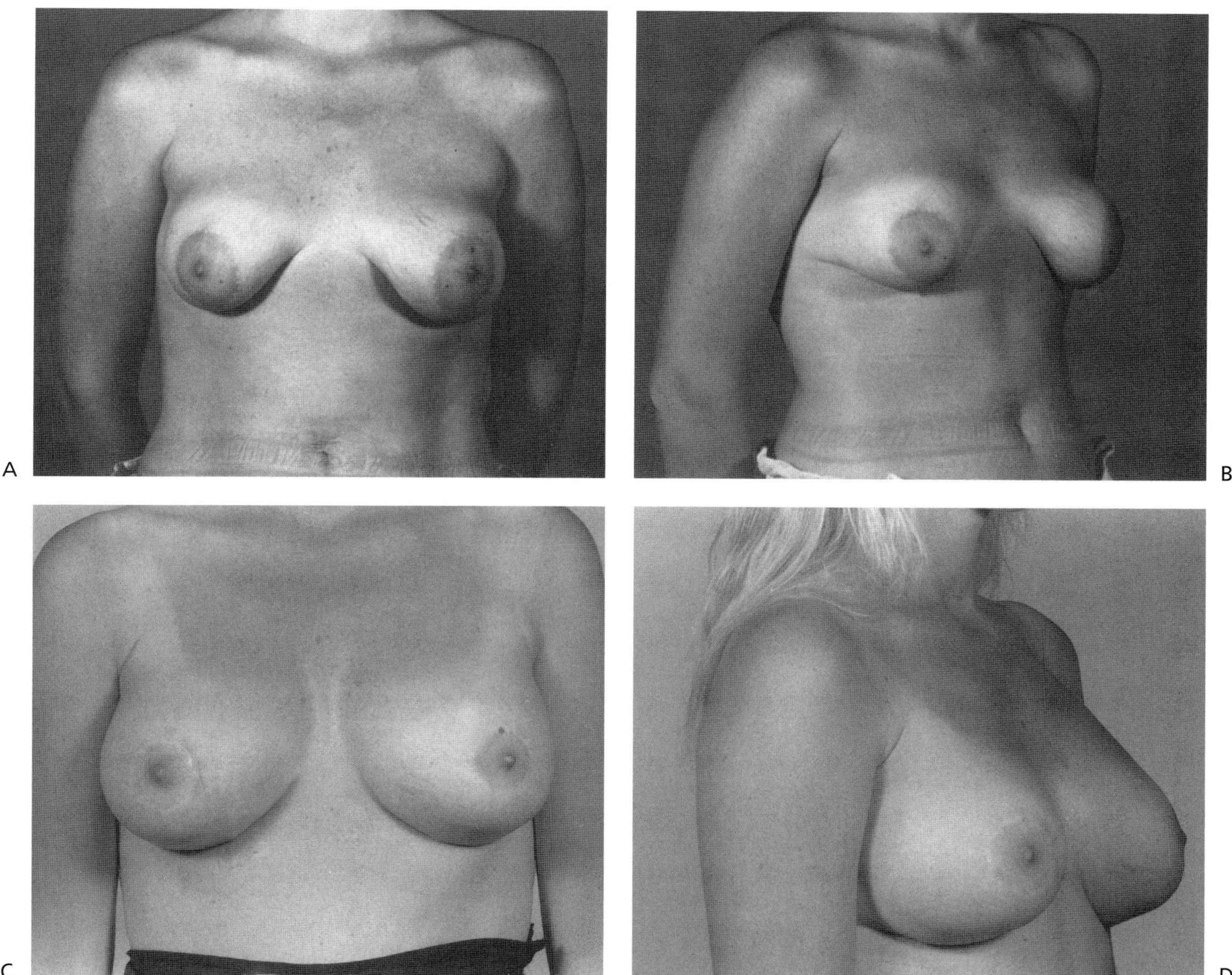

FIGURE 60-2. A,B: This 29-year-old woman had previously undergone a breast augmentation in an unsuccessful effort to camouflage her ptotic, tuberous breasts. **C,D:** After correction with circumareolar mastopexy and reaugmentation with larger silicone gel implants.

choice. Adding an implant or aggressive internal gland remodeling can help reduce the flattening effects of periareolar mastopexy.

If a short scar method is chosen, the skin should be pinched along the limb to determine if the excision is adequate. An L-shaped extension or inverted-T procedure may be required if a dog-ear develops along the lower aspect of the vertical limb with this maneuver. If tension is noted or the skin cannot be approximated, a reduction by means of sharp excision or liposuction may be necessary to prevent excess tension on the closure. A similar maneuver should be performed for an inverted-T technique to ensure a tension-free closure.

When an augmentation/mastopexy is planned and it is not certain which mastopexy method will be used, a periareolar approach should be used for the augmentation. The augmentation may achieve most of the desired goals, so that a lesser mastopexy may suffice. Use of the periareolar approach avoids the possibility of unnecessary scars, particularly an unnecessary inframammary incision.

OPERATIVE EXECUTION

Once all the preoperative planning and preparation have been completed, execution of the surgical technique commences. The patient should be positioned on the middle of the operating table, with the shoulders square and arms abducted 90 degrees or tucked "akimbo" along her sides. The hips should be located at the break in the table so that the patient can be placed in the sitting position during the procedure. Careful preparation and draping should be performed to preserve the markings. It is often useful to employ triangulation sutures, placed at the sternal notch and xiphoid, to help verify symmetry between the various points.

When an augmentation is to be performed, it should precede any mastopexy because the presence of the implant will alter the dynamics of the breast. Once the implants are correctly positioned, the patient should be placed in the sitting position, and the mastopexy can be simulated by tacking the skin previously marked for excision. Any adjustments can then be made. In our experience, this intraoperative simulation does tend to underestimate the actual degree of ptosis that the patient will experience postoperatively and thus may lead to some degree of undercorrection of the ptosis.

In any periareolar technique, care must be taken when the lower pole tissue and subglandular or subpectoral spaces are accessed. Elevating a skin flap in the lower periareolar area can lead to flap necrosis or contour deformities if the flap is too thin or tension is excessive on closure. Depending on the plan, access to these areas is sometimes best gained through direct parenchymal transection, which preserves perfusion to the lower mammary skin. Closure of the periareolar wound must be devoid of excess tension; a deep dermal purse-string suture performed with a straight needle helps to prevent this problem. If a nonabsorbable suture is used, it should be placed particularly deeply in the dermis to avoid visibility and decrease the incidence of erosion. The knot should be inverted and again placed in the deep dermis. To prevent puckering of the periareolar scar, meticulous suturing is essential. The careful placement of interrupted mattress sutures along the circumference in quadrants, halved each time, is one way to avoid this unsightly result. If a dog-ear is noted at the 6-o'clock position, it can be rectified with a short vertical skin excision.

When short scar or inverted-T techniques are performed, it is imperative that the vertical limbs be closed without excessive tension. If closure is difficult, a small reduction of lower pole tissue may be appropriate; forcing the skin edges together can lead to an unattractive shape or skin necrosis. Closure in layers helps reduce tension along the vertical and horizontal limbs. If the vertical limbs appear too long, an elliptical excision along the central portion of the inframammary fold can be used to shorten them. If the nipples appear too low when the patient is in the sitting position, the surgeon should measure the distance from the fold to the areola. The nipples will rise when the breast tissue settles, and if the distance measures 4 to 6 cm, no adjustment should be made.

Postoperative care should consist of long-term support with a surgical brassiere. If an augmentation/mastopexy was performed, an adhesive dressing such as Tegaderm may help the skin "redrape" over the implant. This can be worn for up to 3 weeks. For early signs of hypertrophied scarring, topical silicone sheet therapy is available and may be helpful.

SCARRING AND OTHER UNFAVORABLE RESULTS

Scarring

Unattractive scars are usually related to the skin type of the patient or the location of the incisions. The best way to avoid this problem is to choose patients carefully. Patients of Asian or African descent are at higher risk. Of course, this is the argument for keeping the scars as short as possible.

Any unsightly scars that persist beyond 1 year can be excised. For wider scars, some mobilization of flaps and a layered closure are required to alleviate tension. Widened periareolar scars can be excised circumferentially with an additional mastopexy effect. It is important to realize that circumferential excision may diminish breast projection. If this is the case, a vertical extension may be used to alleviate tension, but at the expense of an additional scar (3).

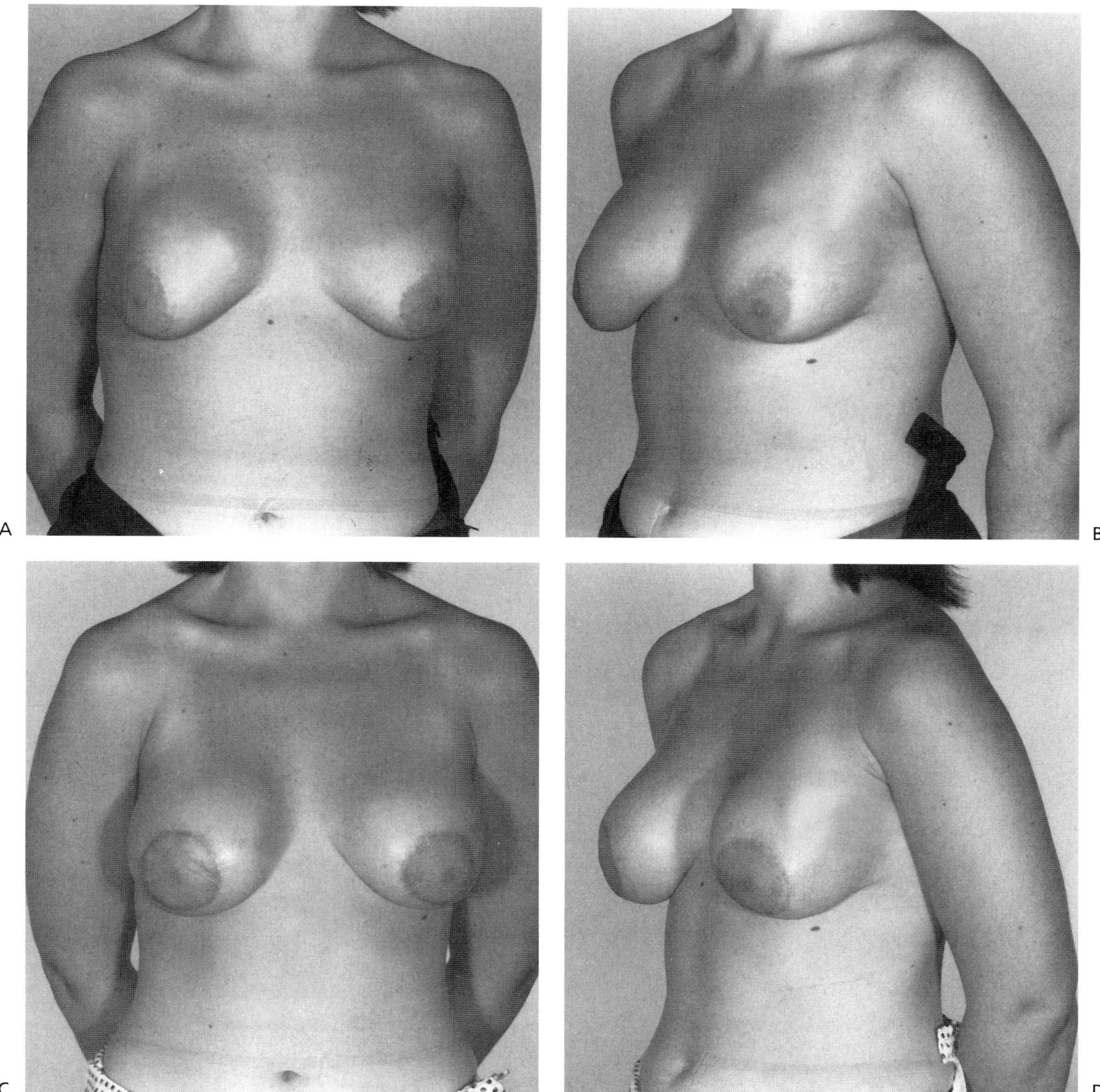

FIGURE 60-3. A,B: A 30-year-old woman 10 years previously had undergone a subglandular breast augmentation with silicone gel implants and simultaneous circumareolar mastopexy. Her result 10 years postoperatively was unsatisfactory, with capsular contracture, superior migration of the implants, and a disproportionately large and ptotic areola. **C,D:** After replacement of her subglandular gel-filled implants with subglandular round, textured, saline solution-filled implants and repeated periareolar mastopexy. Although the breast shape is improved, the nipple remains too low and the areola too wide. A repeated circumareolar mastopexy, perhaps with a short vertical excision inferiorly, will be necessary to elevate the nipple and reduce the areola.

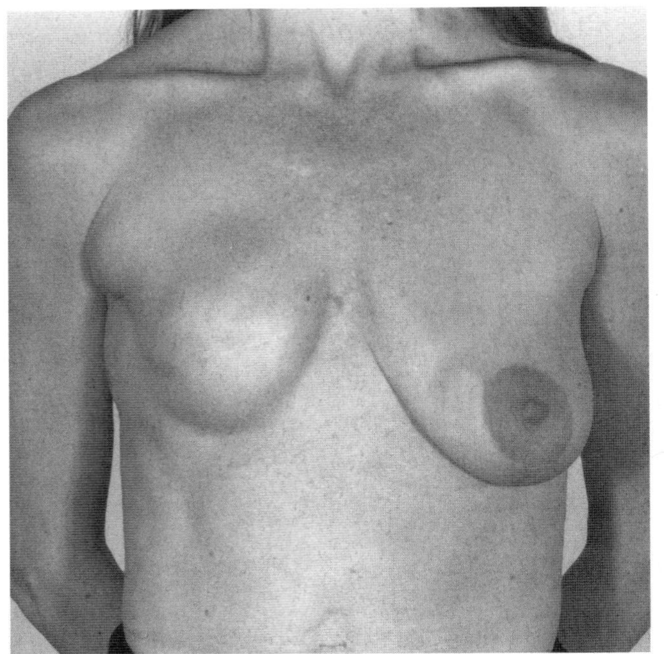
A

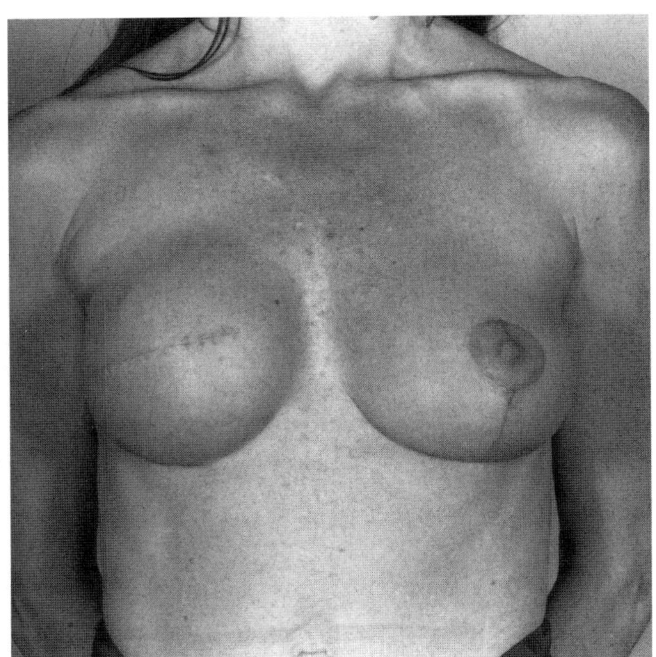
B

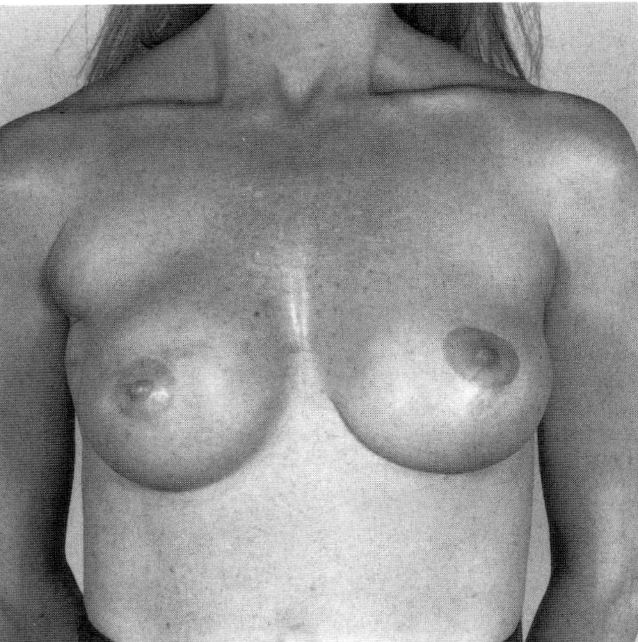
C

FIGURE 60-4. A: A 40-year-old woman had previously undergone a two-staged reconstruction of the right breast with a tissue expander and implant and a mastopexy of the left breast. **B:** Her initial left mastopexy revision with simultaneous augmentation set the nipple slightly high. **C:** A few months later, the left breast had bottomed out even more and the nipple had migrated even further superiorly. The left nipple was lowered by removing an ellipse of breast skin at the level of the inframammary fold. The right breast was ultimately reconstructed with an adjustable silicone gel-saline implant.

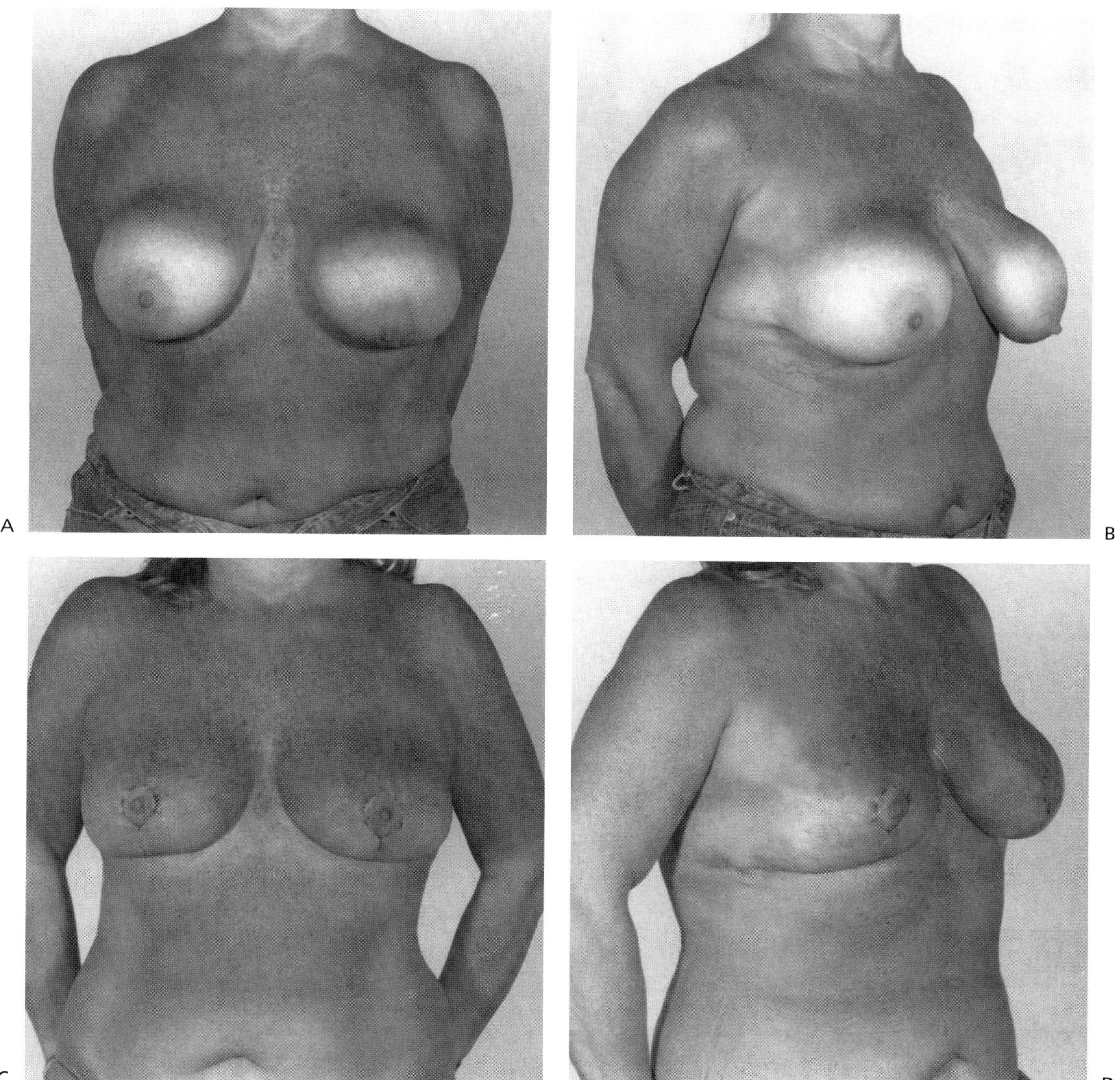

FIGURE 60-5. A,B: The previously placed implants of this 43-year-old woman from outside the United States were unsuccessful in camouflaging her ptotic breasts. **C,D:** After removal of her implants and successful correction of her ptosis with bilateral mastopexies.

Nipple Deformities/Malposition

Areolar distortion resulting from uneven tension can be corrected simply with skin excision around the distorted section and closure. Occasionally, circumferential excision is required to attain a circular areola. Nipples may be too high because of subsequent sagging of the breast or overaggressive elevation of the nipple (3). Small relocations can be accomplished with crescent excisions (2). Correction may require relocating the nipple-areolar complex as a free nipple graft or a dumbbell graft, or excising an ellipse of inframammary skin (2,6). Removing an ellipse of inframammary skin shortens the vertical limb and so lowers the nipple. In patients who have already had an inverted-T reduction, this method is preferable because it does not produce new scars. Nipple-areolar complexes that are too low can be elevated with a hemiareolar, periareolar, or complete mastopexy.

Asymmetries/Contour Deformities

Gross asymmetry in areolar diameter can be corrected by circumferential excision. Contour asymmetries may have existed preoperatively or be the result of improper planning and execution. If the discrepancy is caused by volume differences, a reduction of the larger breast is easier than augmentation of the smaller breast (2). Contour asymmetries may be caused by differences in the skin envelope, even if the volumes are similar. A skin excision on one or both sides with use of the original technique if possible may suffice and avoid additional scarring (2).

Periareolar or short scar techniques that incorporate lower pole wedge excisions or plication may create a tubular deformity as the lower pole and fold are narrowed. An inverted-T method is one way to reshape this breast (2).

Recurrent Ptosis

Adequate correction of recurrent ptosis depends on addressing the causative factors. A careful assessment must be made to determine whether the recurrence is caused by skin excess, parenchymal sagging, loss of upper pole volume, or any combination of these. When a correction is planned, knowledge of the previous procedure is helpful. If another surgeon performed the original procedure, the operative report is an important source of information. This will help the surgeon determine where additional skin excision is needed, where parenchymal alteration is required, and whether an implant is required or an existing one needs to be altered. If a recurrence following a periareolar mastopexy is caused by skin excess, a more substantial skin excision will usually be required to elevate the breast (Fig. 60-3). Rarely, an inframammary component may be necessary. Unfortunately, this requires new scars. Any parenchymal component can be addressed with a vertical plication or reduction. An upper pole volume deficit can be rectified with a small implant. Careful planning of the skin excisions in these cases is essential because the dynamics of the breast are altered with augmentation or plication. Ptosis following short scar or inverted-T techniques can be revised by means of the same technique, with the addition of parenchymal alterations or augmentation (1–3) (Fig. 60-4).

A recurrence of ptosis following an augmentation may be caused by capsular contracture suspending the implant above the breast tissue. It can be corrected with a revision of the augmentation, preferably with capsulectomy. If the contracture alone is responsible for the recurrence, then the revision will suffice to solve the problem. A formal mastopexy may also be required to address any skin or parenchymal component (Fig. 60-5).

REFERENCES

1. Regnault P. Breast ptosis. *Clin Plast Surg* 1976;3:193.
2. Grotting JC. Reoperative surgery of the breast after reduction mammoplasty and mastopexy. In: Grotting JC, ed. *Reoperative surgery,* 1st ed. Baltimore: William & Wilkins, 1995:914–962.
3. Regnault P. Unfavorable result after mastopexy. In: Goldwyn R. *The unfavorable result in plastic surgery: avoidance and treatment,* 2nd ed. Philadelphia: JB Lippincott Co, 1984:703–714.
4. Spear SL, Majidian A. Mastopexy. In: Spear SL, ed. *Breast surgery: principles and art.* Philadelphia: Lippincott–Raven Publishers, 1998:673–684.
5. Spear SL, Little JW. Guidelines for concentric mastopexy. *Plast Reconstr Surg* 1990;85:961.
6. Spear SL, Beckenstein MS. Secondary prosthetic cases. Ch29 p443. In: Spear SL, ed. *Breast surgery: principles and art.* Philadelphia: Lippincott–Raven Publishers, 1998:443–462.
7. Penn J. Breast reduction. *Br J Plast Surg* 1954;7:357.
8. Kroll SS, Doores S. Nipple centralization for the correction of breast deformity from segmental mastectomy. *Ann Plast Surg* 1990;24:271–275.
9. Smith JW, Gillen FJ. Repairing errors of nipple-areolar placement following reduction mammoplasty. *Aesthetic Plast Surg* 1981;4:179–187.
10. Millard DR, Mullin WR, Lesavoy MA. Secondary correction of the too high areola and nipple after a mammaplasty. *Plast Reconstr Surg* 1976;58:568.

Discussion

MASTOPEXY

JAMES C. GROTTING
ELIZABETH FOX

Despite technologic advances in plastic surgery of the breast, the aesthetic result of a mastopexy procedure can be disappointing to both patient and surgeon. Part of the reason for this is that the breast is not a static organ. Because the breast changes according to the influences of hormones, weight changes, pregnancy, and gravitational effects on tissue, plastic surgeons are often defeated in their attempts to achieve a long-lasting aesthetic shape. This excellent chapter by Drs. Spear and Beckenstein focuses on a number of important problems that develop following mastopexy, including scars, poor contour, recurrence of ptosis, and mammographic alterations. Many of these problems lead to a repeated operation or an unhappy patient who seeks the services of another plastic surgeon.

Because so many factors influence outcome in mastopexy, the thorough evaluation will include an assessment of the degree of ptosis, parenchymal distribution, quality of the skin, and, perhaps most importantly, the expectations of the patient. Because mastopexy remains an imperfect and nonpermanent procedure, patients must be made aware that some recurrence of ptosis is the rule rather than the exception. The well-educated patient will understand the relationship between parenchymal volume and skin relaxation, the limitations of implant use, and the location and extent of permanent scars.

The addition of scars dissuades many patients from choosing to undergo mastopexy. However, in most cases, patients will accept scars of good quality if a beautiful shape can be produced. Clearly, poor-quality scars do seriously compromise the aesthetic advantage of mastopexy, and hypertrophic scars may be difficult to manage postoperatively. Fortunately, we are beginning to see some progress in scar amelioration with new developments that appear to provide measurable benefit. The time-honored steroid injections can now be supplemented with the use of silicone sheeting or gel. Several other modalities are effective in scar modulation; these are listed in Table 60D-1. The future of scar modulation may involve the manipulation of antibodies to growth factors such as transforming growth factor-β_1 and -β_2. The fact that scarring is reduced in elderly persons, in whom levels of growth factors are decreased, indicates that they may be significant.

The choice of technique in mastopexy must also take into account skin quality. Because short scar techniques rely on some skin retraction to achieve the final result, patients with breast striae are poor candidates for short scar procedures, especially those with significant ptosis. Patients with normal skin elasticity and lesser degrees of ptosis may be candidates for the newer periareolar techniques. Traditionally, "doughnut mastopexy" has deserved its reputation for flattening and widening of the breast without providing a permanent lift. Periareolar skin excision techniques yield acceptable results if only minimal correction is needed. However, recently improved periareolar methods, which separate the breast into its skin and parenchymal components, appear to yield vastly superior and permanent correction (1,2). Goes (1) has popularized the use of an internal mesh support to maintain optimal shape during the phase of scar maturation. External taping of the skin also helps counteract gravitational descent as the skin contracts. One might deduce that postoperative external support for all patients after breast surgery is crucial in preventing the early recurrence of ptosis. Does brassiere or external garment support during breast growth and development counteract the eventual descent of the breast by preventing the stretching of Cooper's ligaments? No scientific study to date has proved the validity of this concept; however, the theoretical advantage of continued external support is widely held.

TABLE 60D-1. METHODS FOR SCAR IMPROVEMENT

Topical and intralesional steroids
Retinoic acid
Vitamin E
Topical zinc
Intralesional hyaluronidase
Topical putrescine
Pressure therapy
Cryotherapy
Laser treatment
Radiation treatment
Surgical revision
Silicone gel
Antihistamines
Lathyrogens

J. C. Grotting: Division of Plastic Surgery, University of Alabama, Birmingham, Alabama
E. Fox: Miami, Florida

Until mastopexy can be accomplished without objectionable scars, it will continue pose a maximal challenge to the aesthetic breast surgeon. Could skin-shrinking modalities such as ultrasound or laser be utilized to this end? Until such time as these technologic improvements can be made, we will all have to deal with unfavorable results from time to time in treating the ptotic breast.

REFERENCES

1. Goes JCS. Periareolar mastopexy and reduction with mesh support: double skin technique. In: Spear SL, ed. *Surgery of the breast: principles and art.* Philadelphia: Lippincott–Raven Publishers, 1998:697–708.
2. Benelli L. A new periareolar mammaplasty: round block technique. *Aesthetic Plast Surg* 1990;14:99.

61

BREAST AUGMENTATION

JOHN B. TEBBETTS

Augmentation mammaplasty is not a simple operation if the goal is a predictable, long-term result without complications and with minimal trade-offs. Breast augmentation, like all surgical procedures, involves inevitable risks and trade-offs. Inevitable risks result in a low rate of complications and unfavorable results that are largely *unpredictable* and *unavoidable.* However, many complications and unfavorable results that occur in augmentation *are avoidable.* This chapter focuses on *avoidable* problems in breast augmentation. Avoidable problems are caused by omissions or errors in

1. Diagnosis,
2. Decision making and alternative selection,
3. Technical execution, or
4. Postoperative care and treatment.

Avoiding any surgical problem is easier than correcting it. To avoid a problem, a surgeon must understand why a problem is likely to occur and *choose alternatives* (sometimes difficult alternatives for the patient and surgeon) that *reduce the risks* of that problem occurring. Some of the most severe (and sometimes uncorrectable) complications and untoward results occur in reoperation cases, often after multiple previous procedures. Complications and compromises increase at a nonlinear rate with the number of reoperations. In augmentation, as in most surgical procedures, the first operation, optimally performed, has less risk of a complication or untoward result than any subsequent operation. Decisions made and alternatives chosen at the *primary* operation often determine the necessity of a reoperation, even decades later. In residency and continuing education, too much emphasis is placed on the treatment of complications rather than analyzing and understanding the circumstances and the method of decision making that allowed the problem to occur. If surgeons make better decisions at the *primary* operation and educate their patients about the consequences of their choice(s) of alternatives, fewer patients will need reoperations to correct complications or unfavorable results.

J. B. Tebbetts: Private Practice, Dallas, Texas

One chapter cannot adequately and comprehensively cover all of the treatments for complications that can occur in augmentation. Instead, this chapter focuses on *avoiding* problems and unfavorable results in augmentation by addressing the decision-making process at the primary operation and at reoperations.

AUGMENTATION PRINCIPLES TO AVOID UNFAVORABLE RESULTS

Adhering to specific principles during each of the four stages of treatment (diagnosis, decision making and technique selection, surgery, and postoperative care) can reduce risks of unfavorable results. In a retrospective analysis of most unfavorable results, failure to recognize and follow basic principles often contributes to an unfavorable outcome. Focusing on principles can dramatically reduce *unavoidable* complications and compromised results and virtually eliminate the avoidable ones.

The Surgeon and the Patient

The surgeon's role should be more than addressing a patient's request. The surgeon should know more about the many factors involved in achieving an optimal *short-term and long-term* outcome. The following principles are important during the consultation process:

1. *Listen carefully to the patient.* Preconsultation with a well-trained patient educator often provides valuable information that the patient is often more likely to communicate to a female patient educator than to the surgeon.

2. *List the patient's objectives in the presence of the patient.* Ask pointed questions to clarify any areas of a patient's requests that are unclear and document the answers in the patient's presence.

3. *Discuss your role with the patient.* "I want to clearly understand your desires and objectives. I cannot produce what you want if we do not communicate well and if we are not honest with each other. When I understand your objectives, I will help you understand our choices to achieve your de-

sires. Most importantly, no surgical procedure is without risks and trade-offs. One of my jobs is to educate you about the limitations, risks, and trade-offs of any choice that you make or that we make together, and be sure that you understand and accept those risks and trade-offs. It also is important that I help you understand the possible long-term consequences of any choice that we make."

4. *Force the patient to make specific decisions and accept specific trade-offs, and document the process.* For any decision that can potentially affect the result or cause a misunderstanding, clearly state and list the alternatives and force the patient to make the decision and accept the risks and trade-offs. Document the choice or decision and the patient's acceptance of risks, trade-offs, and limitations in the patient's presence. This process does not need to be unnecessarily burdensome. A well-structured checklist of alternatives and trade-offs checked by the surgeon and initialed by the patient can be very effective. Table 61-1 is excerpted from my clinical evaluation sheet and lists basic risks and trade-offs I discuss with every patient. Specific circumstances are listed under "Other." Specific examples are detailed later in this chapter.

5. *Educate the patient and obtain detailed informed consent.* Preoperative patient education by the patient educator and surgeon is infinitely preferable to postoperative education by someone else, often in an adversarial atmosphere. Personalized (nongeneric) information written by the surgeon, consultations with a well-trained patient educator and the surgeon, and complete documentation are key components of an efficient and thorough system of patient education. Video and multimedia information systems can be effective *adjuncts*, but nothing replaces thorough discussion and documentation by qualified personnel and the surgeon.

TABLE 61-1. BASIC RISKS AND TRADE-OFFS FROM THE CLINICAL EVALUATION SHEET THAT ARE DISCUSSED WITH THE PATIENT DURING THE PHYSICAL EXAMINATION

- My breasts will definitely not match following my augmentation.
- Sensory loss can occur, the degree is not predictable, and it can be complete and permanent.
- Infection can occur, and, if it occurs, will require implant removal without replacement.
- I may require additional operations in the future to replace my implant(s) or correct other problems. Increased costs are possible.
- I may be able to feel or see edges or portions of my implant, depending on my tissue characteristics.
- The position of my implants will change over time, depending on my tissue characteristics. Dr. Tebbetts cannot control these changes, and additional surgery may be necessary.
- If I request a different size implant following my augmentation, I will assume all of the costs and risks of exchange.

Patient's initials: __________
Surgeon's initials: __________

Additional informed consent documents reinforce each of these issues in greater detail.

Diagnosis

Errors in diagnosis, especially errors of omission, are one of the most common causes of adverse outcomes. Failure to recognize and acknowledge clinical information and tissue characteristics that determine long-term chances of success or failure risks unfavorable consequences. The result of a breast augmentation is more than the volume of the breast implant, and thoroughly planning each component of the augmented breast increases the predictability of the result. Clinically *recognizing what is achievable* from each patient's tissues and *acknowledging tissue limitations* in the decision-making process avoid postoperative misunderstandings and untoward results.

Assessing the Tissues

Specifically characterize each patient's skin, subcutaneous tissue, and breast parenchyma. Are the tissues excessively thin? Excessively tight? How much parenchyma is present? Is it soft and malleable over an implant, or firm and tightly concentrated, unlikely to drape well over an implant? Is the parenchyma–muscle interface tight or mobile?

Implant–soft tissue dynamics (discussed in detail later in this chapter) determine long-term outcomes in every augmentation patient. Every surgeon should specifically characterize each patient's tissues during the clinical examination and integrate those tissue characteristics into the decision-making process preoperatively. Unfortunately, tissue characteristics are often a minor consideration compared to defining desired implant volume or incision location, risking significant long-term consequences. In reoperations, tissue characteristics can preclude a successful long-term outcome, regardless implant or surgical technique. Recognizing two distinct categories of breast tissues can help the surgeon avoid many potential complications: (i) excessively *thin* tissues and (ii) excessively *tight* tissues.

Inadequate soft tissue coverage (parenchyma, subcutaneous tissue, skin) over any breast implant is a major cause of complications and compromised long-term results in both primary and reoperation breast surgery. In today's society, minimizing body fat is a goal of many patients. If patients with minimal subcutaneous tissue have minimal breast parenchyma (a common characteristic of patients who seek augmentation), soft tissue coverage is minimal, even at the primary operation. In many reoperation cases, parenchyma is minimal *and* the skin envelope may have been stretched and thinned by a large implant or a prolonged capsular contracture. Any implant placed under thin soft tissue cover (anything less than 1 cm of measured thickness) introduces inevitable trade-offs and risks. Specific considerations for clinical situations involving thin soft tissue cover in primary and reoperation cases are discussed in detail later in this chapter.

Excessively *tight* soft tissue envelopes inherently risk untoward results that often require reoperation. Two categories of patients often have tight envelopes: (i) nulliparous patients with minimal breast parenchyma, and (ii) patients who have an excellent (genetic) quality breast envelope that is already filled by substantial parenchyma (even if the patient wants more). In each of these tight envelope patients, the key to an optimal long-term result is an *accurate estimate of the degree of stretch achievable to achieve optimal aesthetics without compromising the patient's tissues* (stretching, thinning of skin, atrophy of parenchyma) *long term.* Excessively large implants in thin tissue envelopes almost guarantees a compromised short-term result (high-riding implant, excessive upper pole bulge that does not resolve) and introduces significant long-term adverse consequences (parenchymal atrophy, excessive stretching of the envelope with or without pregnancy, implant lateralization, traction rippling, and less predictable aesthetic result long term). Conservatism in implant size or volume is key to avoiding problems in the tight envelope breast, even if it means the patient accepting some aesthetic compromises and focusing on improvement instead of a preconceived "ideal" result.

Clearly explain to the patient how her specific tissue characteristics could affect her potential results, both short and long term. Document any compromises in aesthetics or patient desires that are needed to achieve a more risk-free long-term result, and document the patient's acceptance of all trade-offs and risks. For example, a patient with a wide base width breast on a wide torso with a very tight envelope may request a very large implant and a very narrow intermammary distance (cleavage) with a full but natural slope to the upper breast. With a tight envelope, the base width of the implant required to adequately narrow the intermammary distance might contain excessive volume for the patient's envelope, producing excessive upper pole bulging, possible long-term parenchymal atrophy, excessive stretching of the lower envelope (bottoming), and/or thinning of the soft tissue envelope. A reasonable trade-off might be to accept a slightly wider intermammary distance, selecting a smaller base dimension (and hence smaller volume) implant to avoid most of the potential problems. Regardless of the choices, clear documentation in the presence of the patient during preoperative consultation is invaluable when the patient comes in postoperatively complaining that the intermammary distance is not narrow enough. The preoperative discussion gives the surgeon an opportunity to assess the patient's listening and comprehension skills and the appropriateness of her choices. Poor communication and inappropriate choices often guarantee poor outcomes.

Specific breast measurements provide objective, quantifiable data that can affect patient decisions, surgeon decisions, potential results, and complications in augmentation mammaplasty. Defining a patient's desires by measurements is objective and quantifiable, and helps the patient understand the dimensions of her existing breast and how the dimensions of the implant selected may affect the dimensions and appearance of the result. Examples of quantifiable dimensions that affect breast appearance are (a) *base width of the breast* (affects medial fullness, intermammary distance or cleavage, and lateral fullness); (b) *intermammary distance* (the distance between the breast mounds, affects patient's perception of cleavage); and (c) *areola or nipple-to-inframammary fold distance* (affects the position of the inframammary fold, lower breast fullness, and nipple–areola tilt or position). *The base width of the implant* selected is also an important dimension in discussions with the patient. If the implant base width exceeds the base width of the patient's existing breast parenchyma, implant edges are covered by skin and subcutaneous tissue only, and the patient must accept a greater risk of implant edge palpability and visibility or select a narrower base dimension (smaller) implant. *Caliper-measured pinch thickness of the skin and subcutaneous tissue,* especially superior to the existing parenchyma, is an excellent method of determining when soft tissue cover is adequate to offer a patient a retromammary versus a partial retropectoral pocket location for the implant. If pinch thickness is less than 2 cm superior to the parenchyma (Fig. 61-1), risks of edge visibility or palpability and visible wrinkling increase, especially with noncohesive filler implants; hence, a partial retropectoral implant pocket location is a better alternative.

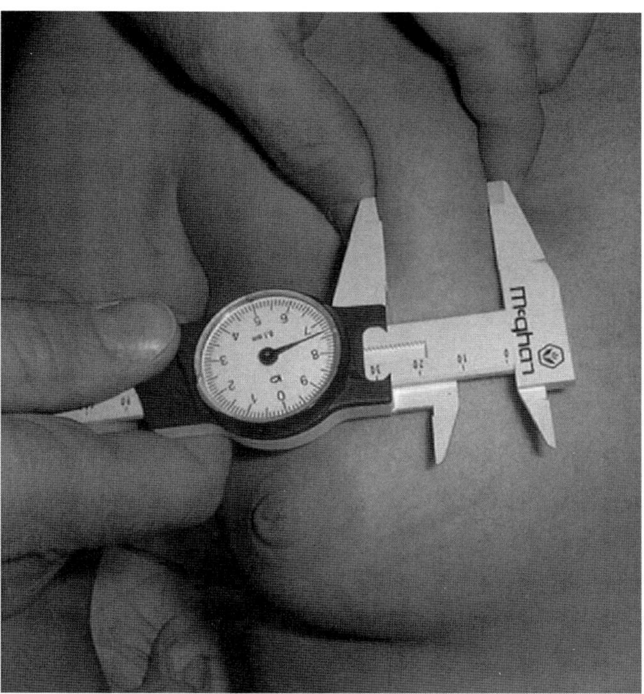

FIGURE 61-1. Pinch test to quantify thickness of soft tissues superior to the breast parenchyma. If pinch thickness is less than 2 cm to firm pinch, a partial retropectoral implant placement usually is optimal to ensure adequate soft tissue cover superiorly and avoid implant edge visibility.

Document clinical findings in the breast with high-quality photographs. High-quality photographic documentation provides another perspective that yields essential, invaluable information during operative planning, intraoperative decision making, and postoperative discussion results. Photographs in the operating room are as helpful and meaningful in breast augmentation as they are in rhinoplasty, yet many surgeons still do not use quality photographs in the operating room.

Avoid augmentation in patients that are high risk for any breast disease based on family history, past medical history, or clinical evidence, and rule out breast masses in every patient by clinical examination and/or mammography.

Each surgeon must establish individual criteria that preclude a patient having breast augmentation and interpret those criteria with respect to clinical factors and the patient's understanding and acceptance of risks. An aggressive position toward *not* operating patients that are at risk for breast disease limits risks, complications, and unfavorable outcomes for both the patient and the surgeon.

Consultation, Decision Making, and Selection of Alternatives

Figure 61-2 is a flowchart that summarizes a basic systematic approach to the augmentation patient, beginning with the patient's requests during consultation, determining what is achievable, defining the range of available alternatives, and completing the decision-making process. A systematic approach to every augmentation patient, adhering to specific principles at each step, minimizes unfavorable results and complications. Figure 61-3 is a decision support algorithm for defining the desired breast and selecting alternatives.

Components of the Result

The result in a breast augmentation is produced by the patient's envelope, the parenchyma, and the implant, or stated as a formula: Result = Envelope + Parenchyma + Implant. Failure to consider all three components during operative planning and implant selection risks unfavorable results. Implant selection should not be based entirely on volume of the implant or on base dimension of the implant without considering the characteristics of the patient's envelope and the amount of parenchyma already present. *A specific volume implant does not produce a specific cup size breast in a range of patients.* Consider the following comparison. A 300-mL implant placed in a tight envelope patient with a minimal amount of firm parenchyma and an areola-to-inframammary fold distance of 3.5 cm will produce a certain result. The same implant will produce a totally different result in a

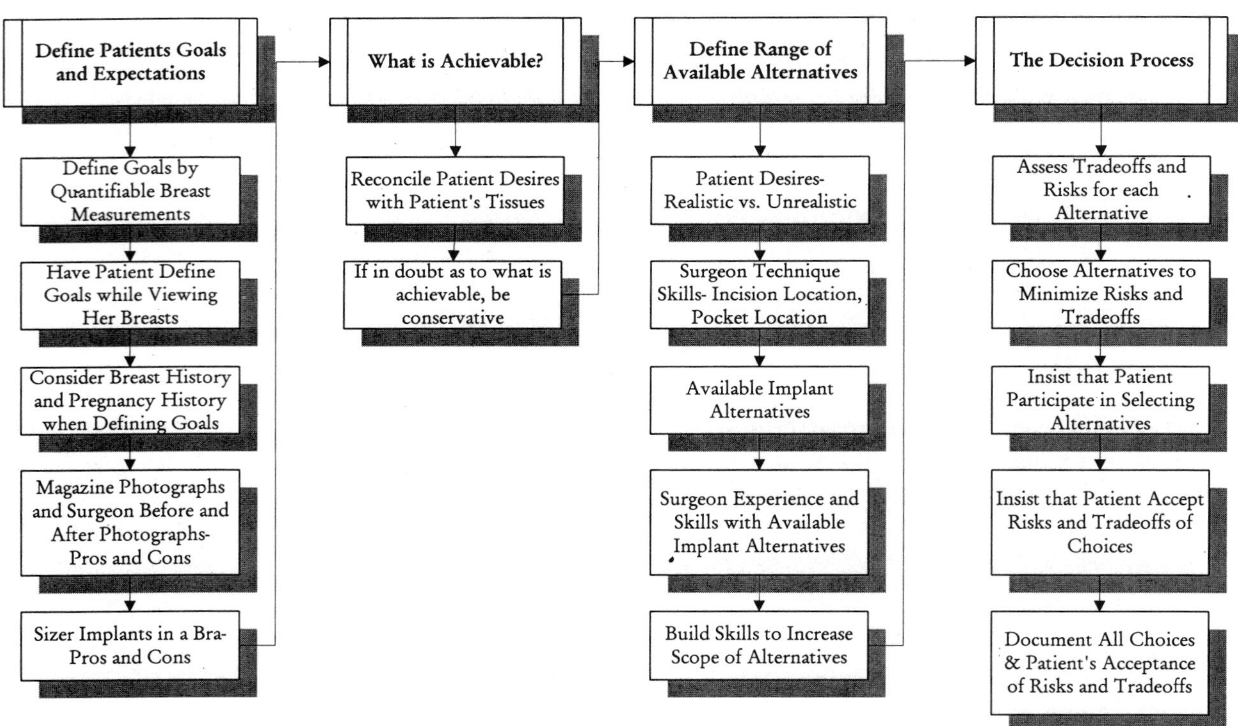

FIGURE 61-2. Systematic approach to the augmentation patient, beginning with the patient's requests during consultation, determining what is achievable, defining the range of available alternatives, and completing the decision making process. (© 1998 John B. Tebbetts. Used with permission.)

patient with a thin stretched envelope with glandular ptosis, a substantial amount of very soft, pliable parenchyma situated only in the lower envelope, and an areola-to-inframammary fold distance of 7.0 cm. To predict implant–soft tissue dynamics and avoid long-term compromises and complications, a surgeon must understand the interaction of envelope and parenchyma with the implant. Consider another comparison. A round, smooth shell, 250mL high-profile (narrower base dimension, more projection) implant placed in a breast with a wide base dimension, thin envelope, and minimal parenchyma, risks traction rippling in the lower breast, even if placed retropectoral. This same implant could be an excellent choice for an optimal result in a constricted lower pole breast with a narrow base dimension on a narrow torso with a normal skin envelope and narrow base width parenchyma that has been expanded by scoring.

What the Patient Wants: Defining the Goals

The surgeon must clearly understand what the patient wants and help the patient define any areas that are not absolutely clear. Some patients have very specific ideas of the result they desire. Other patients do not. Rarely does any patient consider the individual characteristics of her tissues and the limitations or implications of her tissue characteristics on her desired result. Even more rarely does the average patient consider the long-term implications of her desires in augmentation. The surgeon must clearly understand what the patient has in mind in order to discuss limitations, trade-offs, and the range of alternatives. Regardless of implant and surgical techniques chosen, the surgeon should initially document what the patient wants and clearly document any deviations from that request that occur during the consultation process. If the patient does not know what she wants, the surgeon must assist the patient in defining the desired result and document the patient's acceptance of the goals, risks, and limitations of the augmentation.

Define goals by quantifiable measurements to the extent possible. During diagnosis, show the patient the existing width of the breast mound. Emphasize that the wider the breast mound, the narrower the distance between the breasts (the intermammary distance). If one of the patient's goals is to narrow the distance between the breasts, ask her to push the breasts inward to demonstrate the desired intermammary distance and measure the desired distance with a caliper. If achieving the desired narrowing of the intermammary distance will require an implant with a base dimension greater than the base dimension of the patient's existing parenchyma, the surgeon must discuss the trade-offs of an implant that is wider than the existing parenchyma (edge visibility, palpability, possible rippling). Using measurements during discussions is much better than simply agreeing with the patient that "we want more cleavage" and then postoperatively having the patient complain, "Well, the distance between my breasts may be narrower, but it's not narrow enough." When the desired measurement is not achievable given the trade-offs, the surgeon must counsel the patient to accept a trade-off of a slightly wider intermammary distance with less risk of visible implant edges, or accept a much higher risk of visible implant edges.

When possible, define the patient's desires while looking at the patient's breasts. Ask the patient to demonstrate desired medial fullness, upper fullness, intermammary distance, and projection by displacing her breast tissue in different directions or pointing with a finger while the surgeon measures the desired breast dimensions. When the patient demonstrates her desires while looking down at her breasts, the surgeon and patient develop a more realistic and quantifiable image of what the patient wants.

The patient's pregnancy history (or lack thereof) and breast history provide key information preoperatively. In parous patients, the pregnancy history and patient's perspective of her bra cup size before, during, and after pregnancy provide important information. If the envelope has been stretched during pregnancy, the envelope must be adequately filled during augmentation to produce an optimal result. Although patients' perception of bra cup size often is inaccurate, it nevertheless gives the surgeon some idea of how much the breast enlarged during pregnancy and nursing. An important question to ask every parous patient is, "Did you like the fullness or size of your breasts (not how they felt) when they were the fullest during your pregnancy or nursing?" If the answer is, "Yes," the surgeon usually can fill the stretched envelope without the patient complaining of an excessively large breast postoperatively. If the patient was a D cup during pregnancy and requests a full B or small C cup with augmentation, the surgeon must point out to the patient that her request may produce inadequate fullness in the upper breast because of inadequate fill of her stretched envelope.

Photographs of another woman's breasts (from a magazine or other source) to define a desired result in augmentation can be helpful or disastrous. If used realistically and productively, images can indicate a patient's general preferences or desires and assist in the communication process. In every instance, however, the surgeon must point out that the woman in the picture has tissues that are different than that of the patient, and that what was achievable in the picture may not be achievable in the patient. Discuss specific differences in the pictured breast and the patient's breasts. The surgeon should point out the effects of any bra or clothing that is shaping the breast in the picture and the effects of any specific posing position on the visual appearance of the breast. When defining the goal of any breast augmentation, focus the patient on the appearance of the breast with her standing without any type of clothing. Never define goals in any type of clothing. Before and after results of a surgeon's own patients can be very helpful in pointing out to a patient another patient with similar tissue characteristics versus patients with different breast

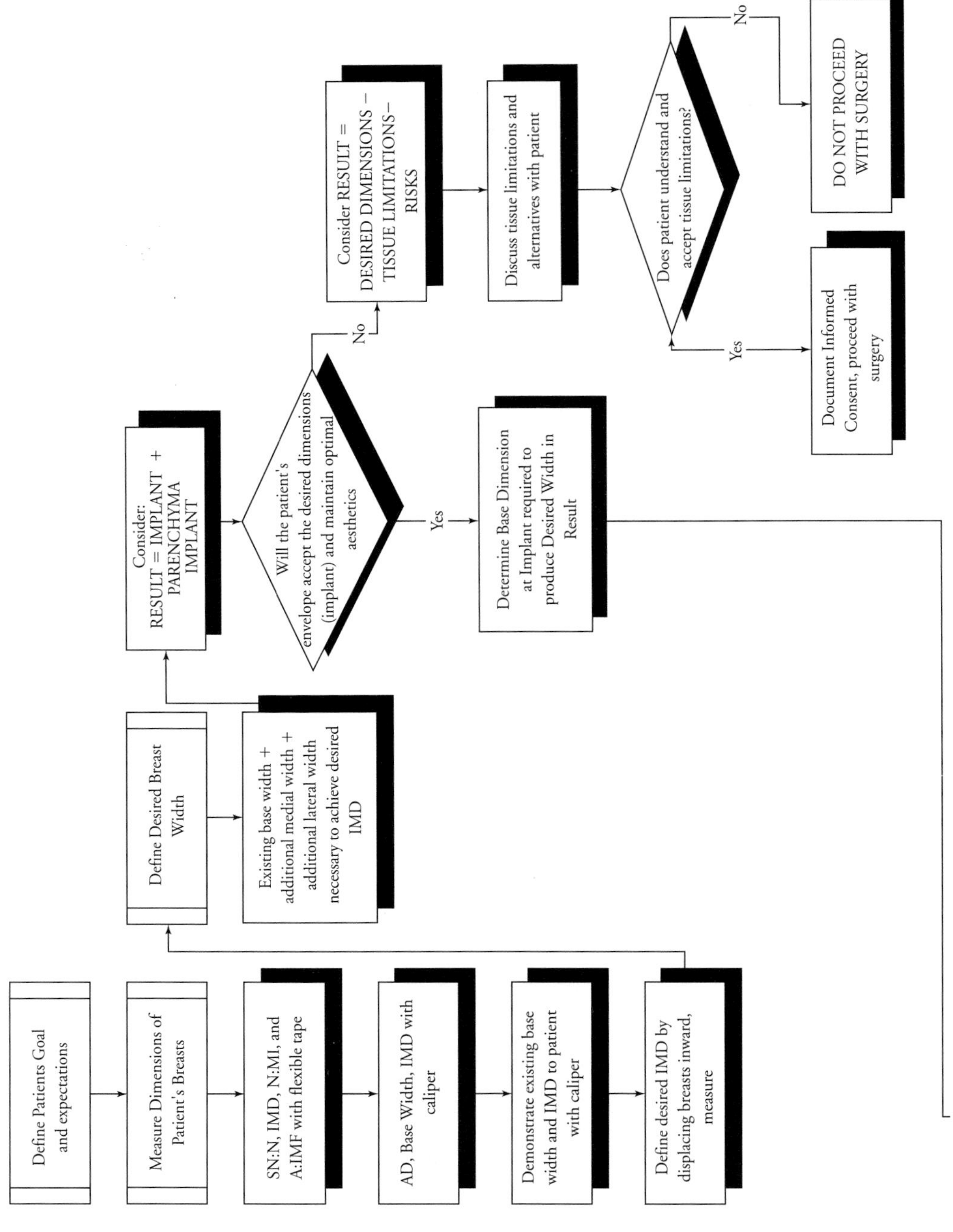
Define Patients Goal and expectations
Measure Dimensions of Patient's Breasts
SN:N, IMD, N:MI, and A:IMF with flexible tape
AD, Base Width, IMD with caliper
Demonstrate existing base width and IMD to patient with caliper
Define desired IMD by displacing breasts inward, measure
Define Desired Breast Width
Existing base width + additional medial width + additional lateral width necessary to achieve desired IMD
Consider: RESULT = IMPLANT + PARENCHYMA IMPLANT
Will the patient's envelope accept the desired dimensions (implant) and maintain optimal aesthetics
Yes
Determine Base Dimension at Implant required to produce Desired Width in Result
No
Consider RESULT = DESIRED DIMENSIONS – TISSUE LIMITATIONS – RISKS
Discuss tissue limitations and alternatives with patient
Does patient understand and accept tissue limitations?
Yes
Document Informed Consent, proceed with surgery
No
DO NOT PROCEED WITH SURGERY

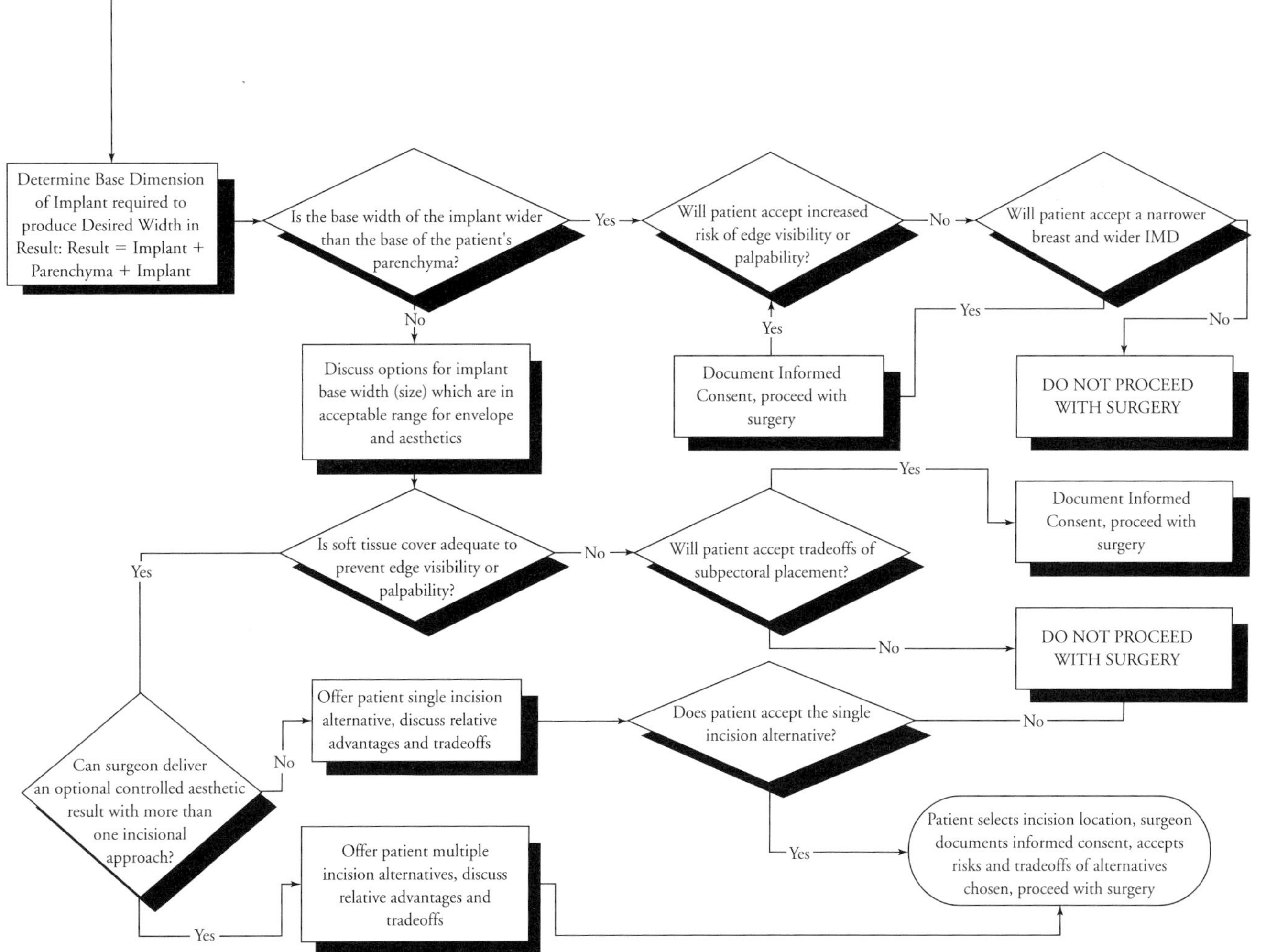

FIGURE 61-3. Decision support algorithm for defining the desired breast and selecting alternatives. (© 1998 John B. Tebbetts. Used with permission.)

characteristics, carefully emphasizing that no photographic result can be duplicated surgically because no photograph can accurately reflect the stretch characteristics of the tissues.

If sizer implants in a bra are used to define desired cup size, the surgeon must be extremely careful to explain to the patient that a bra is not the same as her soft tissue envelope. Although this method may give the surgeon an idea of what the patient wants, if the surgeon then honors the patient's specific request for implant size, the surgeon is failing to consider tissue limitations and long-term implications. Remember, Result = Envelope + Parenchyma + Implant. A bra is not the patient's envelope. An implant placed into a bra ignores implant–soft tissue dynamics and the long-term implications of those dynamics. When a patient chooses an implant using this method, the surgeon must reconcile her request with (i) tissue characteristics, (ii) implant–soft tissue dynamics, and (iii) long-term implications of the choice, then document the discussion and patient's acceptance of the final choice.

What is Achievable? Reconciling Patient Desires with Reality

Any planned result in a breast augmentation should be based on the patient's desires, any tissue limitations that are present, and the patient and surgeon's acceptance of trade-offs and risks that are present in each clinical situation. Stated as a formula: *Result = Desired Result − Tissue Limitations − Trade-offs/Risks.* During the consultation, this formula is invaluable to remind the surgeon to discuss the inevitable tissue limitations, risks, or trade-offs that relate to the patient's tissue characteristics and her specific desires. This formula applies to every patient. No clinical setting or choice of alternatives exists in breast augmentation that does not involve trade-offs that should be discussed and documented preoperatively.

One of the most important questions a surgeon must answer preoperatively is, "What is achievable, given the patient's tissue characteristics, pregnancy history, and available implant and technique alternatives?" Early in a surgeon's career, this can be a very difficult question to answer. For the long-term welfare of the patient, if in doubt, every surgeon should plan the augmentation based on a conservative estimate of what is achievable. Pushing the envelope risks complications and unfavorable results. Tissue limitations are present in a large percentage of augmentation patients, including (i) an extremely tight envelope in a nulliparous patient; (ii) a thin, stretched envelope in a parous patient; genetically thin, delicate tissues that are prone to stretch; (iii) thin tissues that have already proved they will stretch in a patient with ptosis; and (iv) thin, often compromised tissues in many reoperations. All are examples of tissue limitations that the surgeon must recognize and acknowledge preoperatively. Each of these tissue limitations carries trade-offs for the patient. If "Result = Desired Result − Tissue Limitations − Trade-offs," the surgeon must preoperatively reconcile the inherent trade-offs of any tissue limitations with the patient and with the operative plan.

A common example of a situation that risks unfavorable results is the nulliparous, tight envelope and thin envelope patient who requests a very large breast. Although it is technically possible to place a large (more than 350 mL) implant in this patient, short-term risks include excessive upper pole bulging that may not resolve, increased postoperative morbidity with pain, increased sensory loss in the short or long term, and increased risk of palpable or visible implant edges. Potential long-term trade-offs include excessive "bottoming" of the breast, excessive ptosis, parenchymal atrophy, thinning of the subcutaneous tissue and skin, visible implant edges, traction rippling, and increased need for reoperations, such as mastopexy. All of these potential risks are discussed in detail later in this chapter when discussing the trade-offs of larger implants.

If in doubt about what is achievable, conservatism with implant size and operative techniques can avoid unfavorable results. If a patient asks for a result that exceeds what is achievable given the patient's tissues and the surgeon's range of alternatives and skills, the surgeon should not perform an augmentation. If the surgeon is not confident of what is achievable, a second opinion from a more experienced colleague is imperative. The surgeon should clearly point out to the patient and document any tissue limitations that are present preoperatively. The patient should clearly acknowledge the limitations, and the surgeon and patient together must adjust the range of alternatives and make appropriate choices. Any choice that involves a compromise in the aesthetic outcome compared to the patient's request and the patient's acceptance of the compromise both must be clearly documented. In reoperation cases, conservatism is even more important. If the soft tissues are severely compromised (thinned and/or scarred), implant removal without replacement, regardless of the aesthetic trade-offs, may be better for many patients in the long term.

Define the Range of Alternatives

The range of alternatives in any breast augmentation case that will produce a predictable, optimal result depends on (a) the patients desires, (b) the patient's tissues, (c) the surgeon's skills with a range of alternative surgical techniques, and (d) available implant alternatives and the surgeon's experience with various implant alternatives. When a surgeon and patient select alternatives that (a) exceed what is achievable due to tissue limitations or (b) exceed the surgeon's skills and experience with surgical techniques or implants, an unfavorable result or complication is more likely.

Every surgeon must recognize and acknowledge the range of skills and experience that the surgeon has acquired in training and in practice, and avoid choosing alternatives of implant or technique that are not within that range. When learning to use new techniques or implant technology, the surgeon should develop experience in *routine* cases, not in more difficult cases that introduce more surgical variables and unpredictability. Implant technology virtually never solves clinical problems, but can certainly add to clinical problems. For example, if a surgeon has minimal or no experience using anatomical implants, this implant should not be an alternative the surgeon considers when presented with a patient with capsular contractures who has developed recurrent contractures after two previous capsulectomies and implant replacements. In this type of case, controlling the pocket precisely is difficult for the most experienced surgeon, and using an anatomical implant without optimal pocket control risks implant malposition or rotation. For the less experienced surgeon, a round implant is more controllable.

Every surgeon can operate a wider range of patients without incurring unfavorable results and complications by building surgical skills with a range of alternative techniques and implants. Unfortunately, many plastic surgeons select one incision approach, one pocket location, and one type of implant, and apply these choices to virtually every augmentation patient, often in primary and reoperation cases. A "one solution for every clinical problem" approach often results from familiarity with only one technique or implant. Patients differ, and optimal results (short and long term) in augmentation require individualizing the operation and the implant to the patient. Skill development should be a never-ending process for every surgeon, with an inviolate time commitment and plan for expanding the range of skills throughout the surgeon's career.

If a surgeon has a limited range of skills and alternatives from which the patient can choose, the surgeon will often "talk the patient into" the set of alternatives the surgeon prefers. Postoperatively, if the result is anything less than spectacular, patients frequently look for something to explain the unfavorable result, and one area of blame can be a surgeon's failure to allow adequate patient input or offer the patient viable choices. Offering patients a wider range of choices (implying building a wider range of surgical skills) and insisting that the patient make the choices and accept trade-offs and risks avoids potential problems postoperatively.

The Decision-making Process

The decision process is a major determinant of potential success or compromise in the augmentation patient's result. This process must involve the patient and the surgeon, with each assuming specific roles described earlier in this chapter.

The surgeon and the patient must assess each realistic alternative with respect to relative risks and trade-offs, choosing the alternative that minimizes risks and trade-offs, address the patient's goals, and provide acceptable risks and trade-offs to both the patient and the surgeon. The surgeon presents the patient with realistic alternatives tempered by the patient's tissue limitations and the surgeon's range of skill and experience. When choosing alternatives, the surgeon must ensure that the patient understands the relative trade-offs or risks of choosing that alternative, and that *the patient makes the ultimate choice and accepts the responsibility for that choice, documented in the medical record.* This principle applies to each of the following areas: (a) an aesthetic characteristic of the result; (b) incision location; (c) pocket location; and (d) implant shape, shell type, and size.

Insist that the patient participate in the decision-making process. After educating the patient, the surgeon should insist that the patient participate in selecting alternatives. More importantly, the surgeon must insist that the patient *accept* the inevitable trade-offs and risks that accompany any alternative and *document* the patient's understanding and acceptance of the choice, trade-offs, and risks.

Never let economic considerations overrule good judgment. No surgeon can charge a surgery fee adequate to compensate for bad choices by the patient or the surgeon. When a patient's requests impose inherent risk of an unfavorable outcome, either short or long term, the situation becomes "no-win" for both the patient and the surgeon. Because the surgeon is the one who should recognize this type of situation, it is the surgeon's responsibility to try to help the patient modify requests or to decline the operation. If more surgeons declined "no-win" requests, fewer unfavorable outcomes would occur.

The surgeon should think long term by assuming that the patient will return for routine follow-up for the next 50 years. When considering alternatives, the surgeon must think long term as well as short term. Meeting a patient's requests short term may make the patient happy and yield economic return, but may risk long-term unfavorable consequences. An example is the patient who presents with thin, delicate soft tissues, deep stretch marks following a pregnancy, and minimal breast parenchyma desiring a DD cup breast, specifically requesting a 450-mL implant. Although any surgeon probably could satisfy this patient's request, if that same surgeon acknowledged that the patient might present 15 or 20 years later with marked ptosis and impending implant extrusion, needing a mastopexy, the surgeon might be more prone to discuss long-term consequences and alter implant and technique choices.

The Operation: Technical Execution

Precise preoperative marking with the patient standing or sitting upright are critically important to avoid unfavorable results. A detailed description of techniques of preoperative marking is beyond the scope of this chapter, but preoperative markings should include the following: existing inframammary fold; desired new inframammary fold; medial and lateral pocket borders; existing and desired intermammary distance; and precise incision location and length.

Optimal Instrumentation

Optimal instrumentation avoids complications by increasing exposure, increasing accuracy and control of dissection, reducing operative trauma, reducing bleeding, increasing accuracy of pocket borders, and reducing operative times. Bleeding and tissue staining obscure anatomical detail and increase postoperative inflammation in the pocket, decreasing control at the implant–soft tissue interface, increasing postoperative discomfort and morbidity (even in small amounts), and probably increasing the incidence of capsular contracture and pocket border irregularities. For optimal control, the surgeon must control vessels *before* cutting them. Electrocautery pocket dissection allows dissection of a retromammary or partial retropectoral pocket with less than 2 mL of blood loss using refined techniques, controlling all larger vessels *before* they are cut and simultaneously coagulating smaller vessels *as* they are cut. Reduction of intraoperative bleeding requires (i) optimal retraction and exposure to see the vessel, and (ii) prospective control of vessels, avoiding tissue staining that obscures subsequent vessels. Fiberoptic retractors with smoke evacuation capabilities (if electrocautery dissection is used) and optimal electrodissection instruments provide optimal control, reducing bleeding during dissection of the pocket. Two types of electrodissection instruments are invaluable: (i) a handswitching electrocautery pencil with short and extended needlepoint tips, and (ii) long, unipolar handswitching electrocautery forceps with very sharp, fine tips that can be used simultaneously for both dissection and hemostasis. A fiberoptic headlight and spatula or malleable retractors are invaluable to protect the implant while allowing visualization and minor pocket adjustments after the implant is in place.

Choice of pocket location should be determined primarily by adequacy of soft tissue coverage, determined by the pinch test and caliper measurement described earlier in this chapter. If soft tissue pinch thickness superior to the parenchyma is less than 2 cm to firm pinch, a partial retropectoral pocket location provides more soft tissue coverage superiorly and reduces risks of a visible or palpable implant edge. Soft tissue pinch thickness should always be reassessed intraoperatively before beginning pocket dissection to ensure optimal soft tissue coverage and avoid undesirable problems postoperatively.

Dissection Techniques and Trauma

Blunt dissection of either a retromammary or partial retropectoral pocket, although expedient, is rapidly becoming obsolete. Controlled dissection under direct vision is possible through every incision approach except the periumbilical approach. Blind blunt dissection can never be as accurate as dissection under direct vision, regardless of the incision approach. Tearing or separating tissues with a blunt instrument invariably causes more tissue trauma and morbidity compared to precise electrocautery dissection under direct vision. With blunt dissection, tissues are mechanically torn, and bleeding invariably occurs to a greater degree compared to electrocautery dissection under direct vision. Once the tissues are stained, identification of smaller bleeders is more difficult, and more blood remains in the tissues or in the pocket. This increases the inflammatory process postoperatively and potentially increases the risks of capsular contracture or fibrous tissue replacement that can compromise results.

Precise electrocautery dissection techniques (using newer electrocautery generators set at optimal settings with blended cut and coagulation currents) under direct vision are available through all incisional approaches. Combined with optimal instrumentation, electrocautery dissection is much more precise, more controlled, and less traumatic compared to blind blunt dissection techniques. After an initial learning curve, electrocautery pocket dissection times can be substantially less than blunt pocket dissection times when hemostasis time is considered, currently less than 5 minutes per side. Precise electrocautery dissection eliminates the necessity of drains in primary augmentation cases. Patients uniformly dislike drains, and drains can potentially allow contamination of the periprosthetic pocket, so any technique that reduces the necessity of drains potentially reduces morbidity.

Optimal Hemostasis

Hemostasis during pocket dissection is a major factor affecting postoperative morbidity and unfavorable results. Bleeding can be virtually nonexistent using today's state-of-the-art techniques. The percentage risk of a hematoma that requires evacuation is relatively small compared to excessive inflammation and fibrous tissue replacement that can occur with smaller amounts of bleeding. Even small amounts of blood in the pocket or tissues increases the inflammatory response. Blood in the periprosthetic pocket (i) interferes with optimal action of a textured surface implant with the soft tissue interface; (ii) can collect in pocket borders inferiorly and laterally, subsequently undergoing fibrous replacement and causing pocket border distortions and/or implant displacement; and (iii) can increase risks of infection and/or capsular contracture.

The less bleeding *during* and *after* pocket dissection, the less risk of morbidity, complications, or unfavorable results. Prospectively establishing hemostasis as dissection proceeds is far preferable to creating bleeding and then trying to achieve hemostasis. In the latter case, more blood is deposited in the tissues, tissue staining obscures smaller vessels that may bleed postoperatively, pocket dissection is less accurate, and the surgeon has less control of the inflammatory process postoperatively.

Accurate Pocket Borders

Accuracy of pocket borders is critical to avoid implant displacement, asymmetries, and other visible irregularities. With smooth and textured shell implants, pocket borders determine the range of implant position in a mediolateral direction, depending on the patient's body position. With textured surface implants, pocket borders largely determine whether the textured surface is in contact with adjacent soft tissues, allowing it to exert control at the implant–soft tissue interface to affect capsule characteristics.

Dissection under direct vision is much more accurate than blind blunt dissection in creating accurate pocket borders. During dissection, small needles passed percutaneously through skin markings at the desired pocket borders are visible inside the pocket and can precisely define the desired pocket borders for the surgeon. Retraction forces sometimes can open a pocket past the desired borders; hence, the surgeon should limit retraction forces to amounts necessary for exposure and anticipate this problem in patients with thin or delicate tissues.

After pocket dissection is complete, the surgeon can insert one or two fingers and lift the soft tissues, allow the pocket to fill with air, then insert the fingers further to occlude the incision. This traps air in the pocket to define pocket borders and ensure accuracy.

Implant Sizers

Implant sizers are unnecessary and undesirable in primary augmentation cases. With proper preoperative evaluation and planning, implant selection is straightforward. Sizer implants have many potential risks and trade-offs. Characteristics of the sizer implant shell or filler often differ from the permanently implanted device. Every device inserted through an incision into the pocket increases potential bacterial contamination of the pocket and increases tissue trauma. Sizer implants are reused frequently and often are reused many, many times, further increasing possible contamination risks. Operative times are increased, often unnecessarily, when intraoperative decision making using sizer implants replaces optimal preoperative planning. Implant sizers for primary augmentation are unnecessary and should rapidly become obsolete.

Implant Positioning

With smooth shell implants, the borders of the pocket and the patient's body position largely determine implant position. With textured implants, especially textured, anatomically shaped implants, the surgeon must accurately position the implant within a pocket carefully created to fit the implant. Implant positioning is facilitated by maintaining optimal implant position *as the implant is inserted into the pocket,* reducing the necessity of implant repositioning or removal and reinsertion that can increase the risks of contamination and increase tissue trauma.

The most common error in positioning textured anatomical implants is failing to accurately position the inferior border of the implant at the desired, new inframammary fold. In the retropectoral plane, if the origins of the pectoralis are left intact along the inframammary fold, the pressure of the muscle on the lower pole of the implant prevents the implant from resting at the inferior most extent of the pocket. In this instance, the pocket must be dissected slightly lower and the implant positioned slightly lower to avoid an excessively upwardly displaced implant and bulging upper breast. The same situation exists with a retromammary pocket placement in a nulliparous patient with a tight lower pole envelope.

When placing inflatable implants, as the implant fills and the anterior shell moves away from the posterior shell, the inferior edge of the implant moves superiorly. To avoid an excessively high implant position, the surgeon should reposition the implant back down to the desired, new inframammary fold level when the implant is approximately two-thirds full, or after the implant is completely filled.

Every augmentation patient should be elevated to a sitting or near-sitting position intraoperatively to check implant position and symmetry. It is categorically impossible to comprehensively assess implant position as accurately with the patient supine as with the patient sitting. Upper pole fullness and contour are impossible to assess with the patient supine. Other deformities, such as parenchyma sliding off the front of an implant, producing a "double-bubble" deformity, are virtually impossible to assess or predict in the supine position. Regardless of the nuisance of dealing with intravenous lines, anesthesia tubing, and monitoring leads, every patient should be assessed in the sitting position intraoperatively to avoid preventable implant malposition postoperatively. Hypostatic effects on the patient can be minimized by providing adequate fluids intraoperatively and avoiding excessively long periods with the patient sitting.

Parenchyma–Implant Relationships

The relationship of the patient's parenchyma to the underlying implant has a significant effect on the aesthetic result. If the parenchyma is visibly distinct from the implant postoperatively, a visible step-off or "double-bubble" deformity results. If the parenchyma is very firm and has a much narrower base width than the implant (e.g., in a tubular or constricted lower pole breast), the surgeon may need to consider redistributing the parenchyma over the implant by scoring to avoid visible deformities. In the glandular ptotic breast, the parenchyma "slides off" the anterior surface of the pectoralis. If an implant is placed beneath the pectoralis without carefully repositioning the inferior border of the pectoralis upward, disrupting the sliding interface and allowing the implant to project and contact the parenchyma, a "double-bubble" deformity often results.

Photographs in the Operating Room

Preoperative photographs in the operating room can help the surgeon avoid unfavorable results. A surgeon cannot substantially change the quality or quantity of tissues in a routine primary breast augmentation. Following placement of implants intraoperatively, if residual visible asymmetries are present, they often are due to differences in the tissues of the breasts that existed *preoperatively*. Without preoperative photographs in the operating room, accurate assessment and optimal decision making are virtually impossible.

Postoperative Care

Most unfavorable results and complications are prevented by thorough preoperative planning and precise intraoperative execution. There are few, if any, postoperative devices, drugs, or regimens that can *produce* a good augmentation result or prevent a complication, but less than optimal postoperative management can contribute to morbidity. The more thorough and precise the planning and surgery, the simpler the postoperative regimen required.

Activity and Bleeding

Limitation of normal motion and activities following augmentation is unnecessary after augmentation mammaplasty if optimal, state-of-the-art dissection techniques described earlier in this chapter are used. Aerobic activity, or any activity that has the potential to substantially increase pulse and/or blood pressure, increases risks of postoperative bleeding and probably should be restricted for 2 weeks. In more than 1,000 patients in my own practice, I encouraged immediate return to full normal activity and had two hematomas that required evacuation in 20 years.

Devices for Positioning

Devices or taping to attempt control or maintain implant position are largely unnecessary in primary augmentation if optimal intraoperative techniques are used. Support beneath the breast is unnecessary if (i) pocket dissection is accurate, and (ii) accurate preoperative planning of the desired position of the inframammary fold based on the existing nipple-to-inframammary fold distance and the base dimension of the implant selected is performed. Pressure on the upper breast by tape or other device is unnecessary if (i) an excessively large implant is not used, (ii) the lower pocket is dissected accurately, and (iii) the implant is positioned adequately inferiorly at surgery. Pressure on the soft tissue envelope to achieve contact with a textured implant shell is unnecessary if (i) pocket dissection is accurate, and (ii) no excess fluid is present in the pocket. If any of these criteria are not met, then the devices may be helpful. I have used no bandages, bras, binders, or other pressure devices in primary breast augmentations for the past 15 years. Several other potential problems can occur from the use of postoperative devices. Devices complicate postoperative care, increase costs, and often irritate patients. Patient compliance is unpredictable at best. Any device that can position an implant has the ability to malposition the implant if improperly applied or if the patient can manipulate the device.

Drugs

No postoperative drug or combination of drugs has been proved to prevent postoperative complications or unfavorable results. However, excessive analgesics can reduce patient mobility and compliance, and can create drug dependence. Many surgeons use preoperative and/or postoperative antibiotics. Although this use seems logical when placing a large foreign body in or near tissues that normally harbor bacterial organisms, conclusive scientific evidence that the drugs prevent postoperative complications is lacking. Levels of postoperative pain medications required are extremely variable, depending on the degree of surgical trauma and the patient's pain tolerance. No drugs conclusively reduce the incidence of capsular contracture. Precise intraoperative dissection techniques can substantially reduce postoperative pain and the need for analgesics. Avoiding blunt dissection, avoiding bleeding and cauterization on rib perichondrium, and using muscle relaxants to avoid excessive retraction forces on the pectoralis muscle allowed more than 95% of my retropectoral augmentation patients to raise their arms above their heads, drive their cars, and lift normal weight objects within 24 hours. In this group of patients, ibuprofen (Motrin) was the only pain medication used postoperatively.

Drains

Drains are totally unnecessary in primary augmentation if the surgeon uses optimal electrocautery dissection technique and avoids blunt dissection. If the surgeon uses blunt dissection, drains may reduce fluid accumulation in the pocket. Closed drainage systems are preferable to open systems to reduce risks of pocket contamination.

IMPLANT–SOFT TISSUE DYNAMICS

Implant–soft tissue dynamics can significantly affect short- and long-term results in breast augmentation. The breast soft tissue envelope and parenchyma have individual unique characteristics in each patient. Tissue characteristics in the breast change as a patient ages. The skin frequently becomes thinner and loses support for the weight of normal breast tissue. The skin stretches in the lower pole and allows redistribution of parenchymal fill to the lower pole, decreasing upper pole fill.

In addition to normal changes with aging, a breast implant exerts forces on adjacent tissues, can stretch tissues, pull the breast inferiorly (due to gravitational forces), cause formation of a capsule that can exert forces on the tissues, and potentially cause pressure atrophy of adjacent tissues. Many of these factors potentially can cause unfavorable results or complications, but most can be avoided by understanding and respecting implant–soft tissue dynamics.

Implant Size: Long-term Effects

The larger the breast implant, all other factors being equal, the greater the chance of an unfavorable result or complication in the long term. Based on my 21-year clinical experience, I consider any implant over 350 mL, regardless of the filler material, a large implant. The larger the implant, the greater the weight of the implant, regardless of implant type or filler material. A heavier implant exerts greater forces on the soft tissues, stretching and thinning the soft tissue envelope over time. Because the patient's tissue quality declines with increasing age, a larger implant may appear ideal for a short period of follow-up but will adversely affect the tissues in the long term.

When the soft tissue envelope and parenchyma of the breast are subjected to the pressures and weight of excessively large implants, soft tissue dynamics and changes are predictable. The pressure of the implant on the parenchyma usually produces some degree of parenchymal atrophy. The lower pole envelope stretches, allowing the implant to move inferiorly, often increasing the degree of ptosis. The breast loses upper pole fill. As the implant pulls inferiorly, traction on the upper envelope may produce visible traction rippling. The skin and subcutaneous tissue usually thin over time, with the degree of thinning directly related to the size of the implant and the patient's tissue characteristics.

Placement of excessively large implants unquestionably increases the risk of potential complications and reoperations in the long term. Patients should be given informed consent preoperatively regarding increased long-term risks and complications if they request large implants. Later, if reoperation surgery is necessary for ptosis, traction rippling, or excessive tissue thinning with visible irregularities, the surgeon is forced to operate on compromised tissues. Soft tissue coverage is compromised, healing may be compromised, and risks of unfavorable results or complications increase. In extreme cases, excessively large implants can exert forces that are clearly destructive to soft tissues.

Characterizing the Soft Tissues

When evaluating a patient for augmentation, the surgeon should carefully consider the individual tissue characteristics of the patient's breasts. These characteristics are unchangeable. If tissue limitations are ignored or not respected in selecting the implant and pocket location, the tissues or tissue quality can be irreversibly compromised. If the tissues are delicate, thin, or "stretchy," the surgeon should make the patient aware of these tissue limitations and advise the patient toward conservatism with regard to implant size, regardless of other aesthetic compromises.

In reoperation cases, adequacy of soft tissue coverage often is the single most important factor affecting outcome. Whenever an implant is placed under inadequate soft tissue coverage, risks of an unfavorable result or complication increase exponentially. Problems that can occur as the result of inadequate soft tissue coverage include visible and palpable implant edges; visible traction and/or underfill rippling; ptosis; asymmetry; implant displacement or malposition; incision line dehiscence; infection; implant exposure; and implant extrusion.

REOPERATION FOLLOWING AUGMENTATION

The primary surgical procedure offers the best chance of achieving a good result with minimal complications. With every reoperation procedure following breast augmentation, the surgeon must address more variables, has less control over these variables, and both surgeon and patient must accept a greater risk of unfavorable results and/or complications. Because these facts are inescapable, the decision process for reoperations is different compared to primary operations. To prevent outcomes that will require additional surgeries (with even greater risks and trade-offs), the surgeon must (a) recognize and acknowledge tissue limitations that are present; (b) narrow the range of alternatives for technique and implant to minimize unfavorable outcomes, regardless of the patient's desires; and (c) remember in cases with significant tissue limitations that implant removal without replacement sometimes is the best option. In any case where a patient refuses to acknowledge and accept the limitations that are present, the surgeon should decline the reoperation.

Some of the more common reasons for reoperation following augmentation include capsular contracture, size exchange, visible rippling or wrinkling, asymmetry, implant malposition, or an unsatisfactory cosmetic result. Earlier in this chapter, we emphasized principles and techniques to avoid these problems. When a surgeon is confronted with a reoperation problem, the surgeon should follow the same principles for *avoidance*, but additionally recognize existing compromises and limitations, and formulate a *treatment plan that narrows alternatives* to those that have the most reasonable and predictable chance of success.

Decision Support Flowchart

Figure 61-4 shows a decision support flowchart that addresses some common reoperation problems following aug-

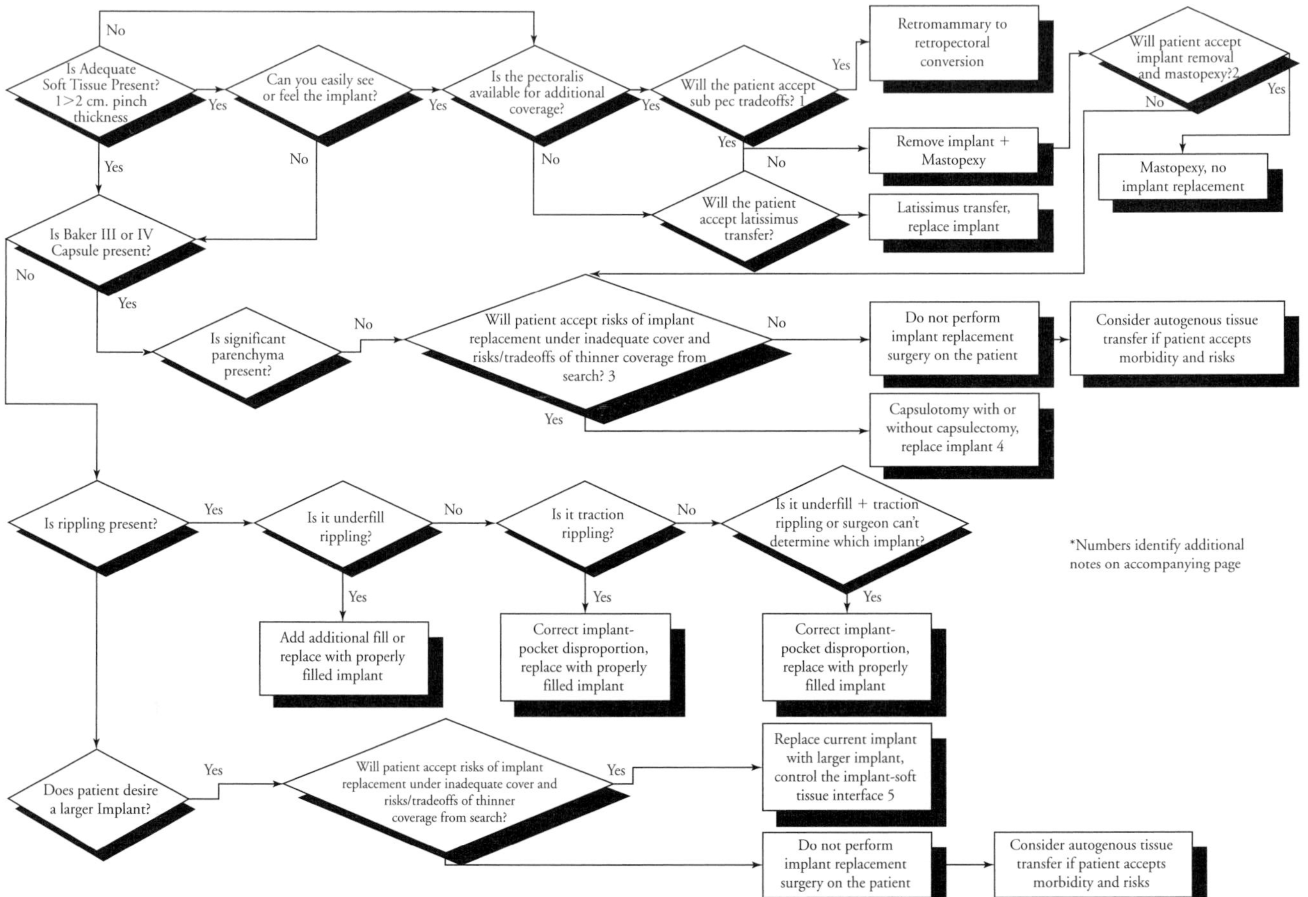

FIGURE 61-4. Decision support flowchart that addresses common reoperation problems following augmentation. (© 1998 John B. Tebbetts. Used with permission.)

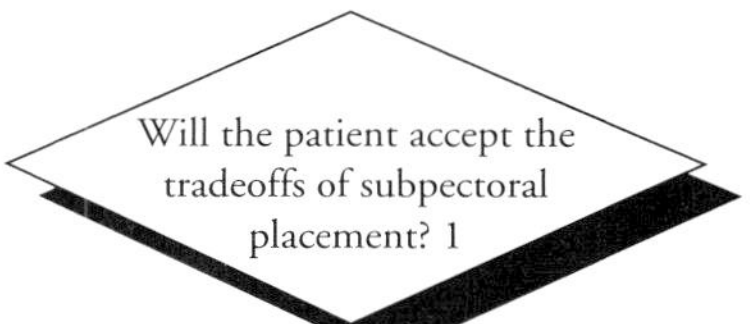

Tradeoffs of subpectoral or partial subpectoral placement:
1. Wider intermammary distance
2. More lateral implant displacement
3. More lateral fullness
4. Less medial fullness
5. Breast distortion with pectoralis contraction
6. Less overall control of breast shape
7. Less control of upper pole fullness and shape
**If caliper measured pinch thickness of tissues superior to parenchyma is less than 2 cm., partial retropectoral coverage or additional soft tissue coverage (latissimus) is mandatory.

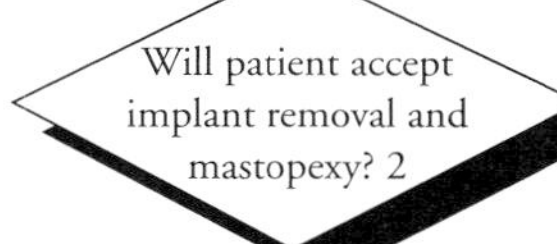

1. Whenever future soft tissue thinning is inevitable, the patient should first be offered the option of removing the implant and having mastopexy as necessary without implant replacement
2. Capsulectomy and/or placement of a larger saline implant inevitably results in future stretch and thinning of the envelope

---

Will patient accept risks of implant replacement under inadequate cover and risks/tradeoffs of thinner coverage from scratch? 3

Risks of Implant Replacement Under Inadequate Soft Tissue Cover
(Any cover less than 1 cm thick or less than 2 cm to pinch thickness)
1. Unsatisfactory breast appearance
2. Increased risk of extrusion with:
Possible additional surgery, time off work, costs
3. Possible increased risk of infection if thin tissue healing is compromised
4. Implant edge visibility and/or palpability
5. Visible rippling or wrinkling in the breast
6. Increased likelihood of needing implant removal all in the future

Tradeoffs of thinner coverage occurring from stretch whenever a larger implant is placed:
1. Inevitable further thinning of overlying soft tissue and/or parenchyma
2. Inevitable increase in breast sagging
3. High-likelihood of requiring mastopexy and exchange to smaller implant or no implant in the future

Capsulotomy with or without capsulectomy, replace implant 4

1. Capsulectomy or site change minimizes risks of recurrent capsular contracture
2. The surgeon must weigh recurrence risk against the need for additional coverage by leaving capsule

---

Replace current implant with larger implant, control the implant-soft tissue interface. 5

To optimally control the implant-soft tissue interfaces
1. Create a "virgin" soft tissue interface to the extent possible
2. Consider capsulectomy or site exchange (RM to PRP or the reverse)
3. May be forced to compromise recurrence risk to maintain adequate coverage by preserving portions of capsule
4. Assure adequate fill of the soft tissue envelope for an optimal aesthetic result
5. Assure adequate implant base width to prevent implant-pocket disproportion that risks traction rippling
6. Adjust the pocket to "fit" the implant if using an anatomic implant
7. If you cannot control the pocket, do not use an anatomic implant
8. Adjust the envelop (mastopexy) to correct excessive laxity (much more control if implant placement is staged 3-6 months after mastopexy)
9. Use closed drainage to minimize fluid in the periprosthetic pocket

FIGURE 61-4. *(Continued)*

mentation mammaplasty. This flowchart reflects my personal approach to reoperations, but it does not address every reoperation problem or factor that is present in each individual case. Surgeon's decisions must involve many factors that are not addressed here. The intent of this flowchart is to emphasize the importance of adequate soft tissue coverage in reoperations and to outline common problems and decisions that are present in reoperations. Numbered annotations are listed in some of the decision diamonds to expand on specific topics.

RIPPLING AND WRINKLING

Visible rippling and wrinkling of the breast soft tissue envelope following augmentation mammaplasty has become a more common problem as the use of inflatable implants with noncohesive filler materials (e.g., saline, peanut oil, soy oil) has increased, but this problem is not limited to saline or other noncohesive filler implants. It can occur (i) with any *underfilled* implant (due to the manufacturer defining and recommending inadequate fill or the surgeon inadequately filling the implant); and (ii) when any type of implant causes significant traction on a thin overlying soft tissue envelope.

To correct visible wrinkling or rippling, the surgeon must understand the causes of the problem and select alternatives for correction that address (a) potential problems with the implant; (b) soft tissue problems and limitations; and (c) long-term implant–soft tissue dynamics.

Types of Rippling and Wrinkling

Two basic types of rippling and wrinkling occur: *underfill rippling* and *traction rippling.* When wrinkling or rippling is visible on the breast when the patient is upright, one or both of these problems may be present.

Underfill rippling occurs when the amount of filler material in the implant shell is inadequate to adequately expand the implant shell, which allows the shell to partially collapse or fold (Fig. 61-5). Under thin soft tissues or minimal parenchyma, the implant shell collapse can be visible. The thinner the skin and subcutaneous tissue and the less parenchyma overlying the implant, the more likely that underfill rippling will be visible. Underfill rippling can occur with *any type of implant* and *any type of filler,* but it usually is more visible with noncohesive filler implants such as saline or oil. Underfill rippling often is visible in the upper pole of the breast, but it also can be visible in the medial and lateral areas of the breast if the soft tissue envelope is thin or the implant has been placed under inadequate soft tissue cover. Underfill rippling can occur as early as 3 to 4 months following augmentation, but it usually is not apparent until

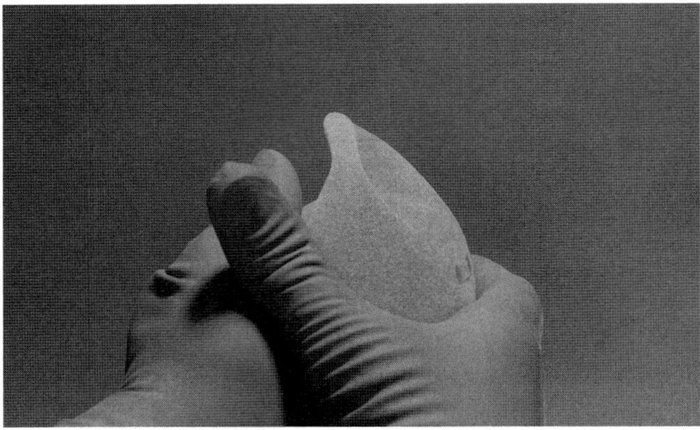

FIGURE 61-5. When any implant, regardless of filler material, is inadequately filled to maintain expansion of the upper implant shell, shell collapse or folding can occur.

the lower pole envelope stretches enough to decrease pressure on the implant. Following primary augmentation, the earlier that visible wrinkling or rippling occurs, the more likely implant underfill is a factor. Underfill rippling is almost totally preventable by the surgeon selecting and using only adequately filled implants, or filling inflatable implants adequately by the tilt test described later in this chapter.

Traction rippling occurs when an implant falls to the inferior-most portion of the breast soft tissue envelope and applies traction to the capsule and overlying soft tissue envelope (Fig. 61-6). Traction rippling can be visible superiorly, medially, or laterally, depending on the soft tissue characteristics of the envelope and capsule, adherence of the capsule to the soft tissues, the type and size of the implant, and implant–soft tissue dynamics. Traction rippling can occur with any type of implant and any type of filler material, but it usually is more common with larger implants (smooth or textured shell) that are placed under thin or "stretchy" soft tissue envelopes. Traction rippling is uncommon in the first 6 months following augmentation and usually becomes apparent over time as a larger implant stretches and thins the soft tissues, or as the patient ages.

On clinical examination, it may be impossible to distinguish underfill rippling from traction rippling. The distinction is made at surgery when implant fill can be definitively measured. Underfilled implants do not always produce visible underfill rippling. In many cases, underfilled, smooth shell implants fall to the bottom of the pocket where the wrinkled or collapsed implant shell is covered by breast parenchyma and is not visible. In other cases, underfilled implants placed subpectorally are wrinkled and the shell is collapsed and folded, but the additional thickness of the pectoralis superiorly obscures the shell collapse.

Textured surface implants are *not* more likely to cause visible wrinkling or rippling compared to smooth shell implants. Both textured and smooth shell implants experience shell collapse when inadequate filler is placed in the implant. The major difference is that smooth shell implants tend to fall to the bottom of the periprosthetic pocket where the rippling is more likely camouflaged by overlying parenchyma. Shell collapse and wrinkling, risking shell folding and fatigue, are present, but may not be visible. With textured implants, when visible wrinkling is present, the surgeon has an opportunity to correct the problem *before* shell failure occurs. With smooth shell implants that fall to the bottom of the pocket where shell folding is camouflaged by overlying parenchyma, the surgeon may not have the opportunity until shell integrity is lost and other clinical manifestations occur.

Determining Adequate Implant Fill

What is adequate implant fill? This is a difficult question that brings a variety of answers. Based on my personal clinical experience, an implant is adequately filled when the upper pole of the implant shell does not collapse or fold when the implant is help upright with the implant supported evenly across the entire lower pole without applying additional pressure to the lower pole. If the upper shell of an implant collapses and folds when upright, regardless of the implant type, shell type, or filler material, the implant shell will be subjected to fold and abrasion stresses that could shorten shell life. Implant shell life is a major factor that affects the rates of reoperation in large numbers of patients over time. Shell folding is not the only factor affecting shell life, but it is one factor that surgeons and manufacturers can easily address prospectively.

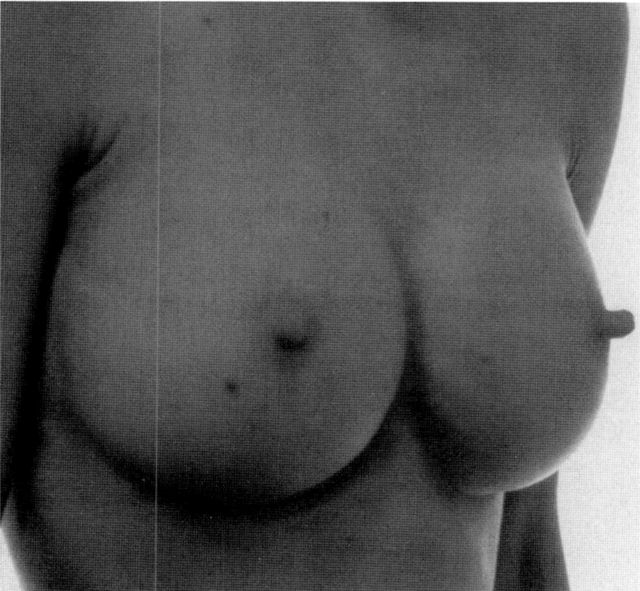

FIGURE 61-6. Traction rippling occurs when an implant falls to the inferior-most portion of the breast soft tissue envelope and applies traction to the capsule and overlying soft tissue envelope. Traction rippling can occur with smooth or textured implants, round or anatomical. Traction rippling is most common when soft tissue cover is thin and implant size is excessive for the degree of support provided by the soft tissue envelope.

With currently available biomaterials, the more filler that is placed in any implant shell, the firmer the implant feels, regardless of the type of filler material or type of shell. The additional firmness of any adequately filled implant has been a major factor in determining manufacturer's recommended fill volumes for implants. During implant design and testing, surgeons consulted by the manufacturer frequently examine and feel implants lying flat on a table and held in the hand. Surgeons frequently complain that implants filled adequately to prevent shell folding feel excessively firm. Manufacturers in the past have responded by defining fill volumes that are based more on palpable firmness than on the volume required to prevent shell collapse. In clinical use, however, patients virtually never complain about excessive implant firmness from adequate fill, especially if preoperatively the surgeon has given them a choice between a softer, underfilled implant that might rupture sooner and a slightly firmer, adequately filled implant with potentially longer shell life. In my personal series of more than 1,000 patients who chose adequately filled implants by the tilt test, no patient with up to 5-year follow-up requested an implant exchange to a softer implant.

With any type of implant and any type of filler, a simple tilt test that any surgeon can use preoperatively or intraoperatively provides an excellent indication of adequacy of implant fill to prevent shell folding (Fig. 61-7A–C). With the implant lying flat in the hand, evenly support (but do not apply pressure) the lower pole of the implant across the entire lower pole, then tilt the implant vertically. If the upper shell collapses and/or folds, the implant is underfilled, regardless of the manufacturer's recommended fill volume. *All currently manufactured round implants (both silicone and saline filled) are underfilled by the tilt test.* With an underfilled implant, the surgeon is in a difficult situation. If the surgeon fills the implant *above* the manufacturer's recommended volume, the surgeon voids the manufacturer's warranty. If the surgeon fills *to* the manufacturer's recommended volume, the surgeon risks underfill rippling, shell folding, and possible premature shell fold fatigue and shell failure. Manufacturers should define recommended fill volumes of round implants to prevent upper shell folding with the implant upright for optimal shell longevity and lowest possible reoperation rates. Anatomically shaped implants that have a higher recommended fill pass the tilt test, so the surgeon need not fill above the recommended level to prevent shell collapse and folding.

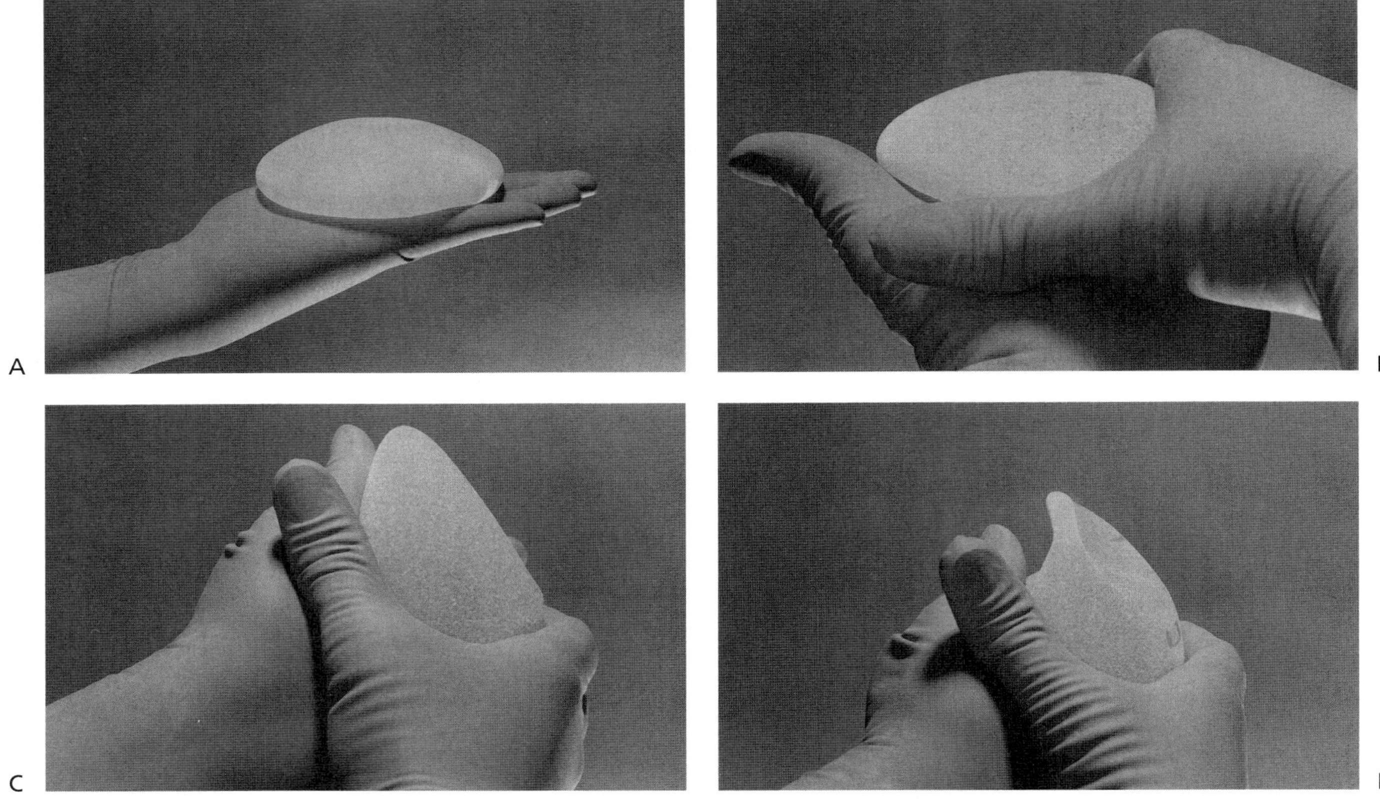

FIGURE 61-7. A–D: With any type of implant and filler, a simple tilt test that any surgeon can use preoperatively or intraoperatively provides an excellent indication of adequacy of implant fill to prevent shell folding. This test simulates the worst-case clinical scenario of an implant in a loose or lax soft tissue envelope. **A:** Place implant flat in palm. **B:** Support, but do not compress the lower pole, and tilt the implant vertically. **C:** The upper pole of an adequately filled implant does not collapse or fold. **D:** Under-filled implants experience upper shell collapse and/or folding.

Diagnosis and Correction: An Algorithm

Figure 61-8A shows a flowchart that addresses diagnosis and correction of visible rippling or wrinkling following primary augmentation. Figure 61-8B addresses diagnosis of rippling following reoperations, and Fig. 61-8C addresses prevention of rippling or wrinkling at the primary operation and treatment at reoperations.

INFECTION

Infection following breast augmentation is one of the most challenging problems a surgeon faces. Although many techniques have been promoted to salvage an infected implant, my personal clinical experience in treating periprosthetic space infections has led me to the following conclusions.

1. A substantial percentage of infected implants remain infected despite all drainage, medication, and topical treatment measures.
2. Every infected implant should be removed; the sooner the better.
3. Removing one implant and leaving the other in place is not an optimal solution clinically. The presence of the remaining implant and the inconveniences to the patient of the asymmetry exert influence on the surgeon to replace the infected implant, sometimes sooner than ideal.
4. At the time of removal of an infected implant, removal of virtually all of the capsule and contents of the capsule does not predictably create a satisfactory environment for replacement of an implant. Any lesser technique risks a higher reinfection rate if the implant is replaced.
5. No waiting interval following removal of an infected implant is long enough to ensure against recurrent infection if the implant is replaced.
6. A substantial reinfection risk is present despite all measures when placing an implant in a previously infected breast.
7. Even if reinfection does not occur, the incidence of capsular contracture is extremely high when replacing an implant in a previously infected breast.
8. Reinfection and/or capsular contracture require additional reoperations and risk additional complications and possible permanent tissue damage or uncorrectable deformities.

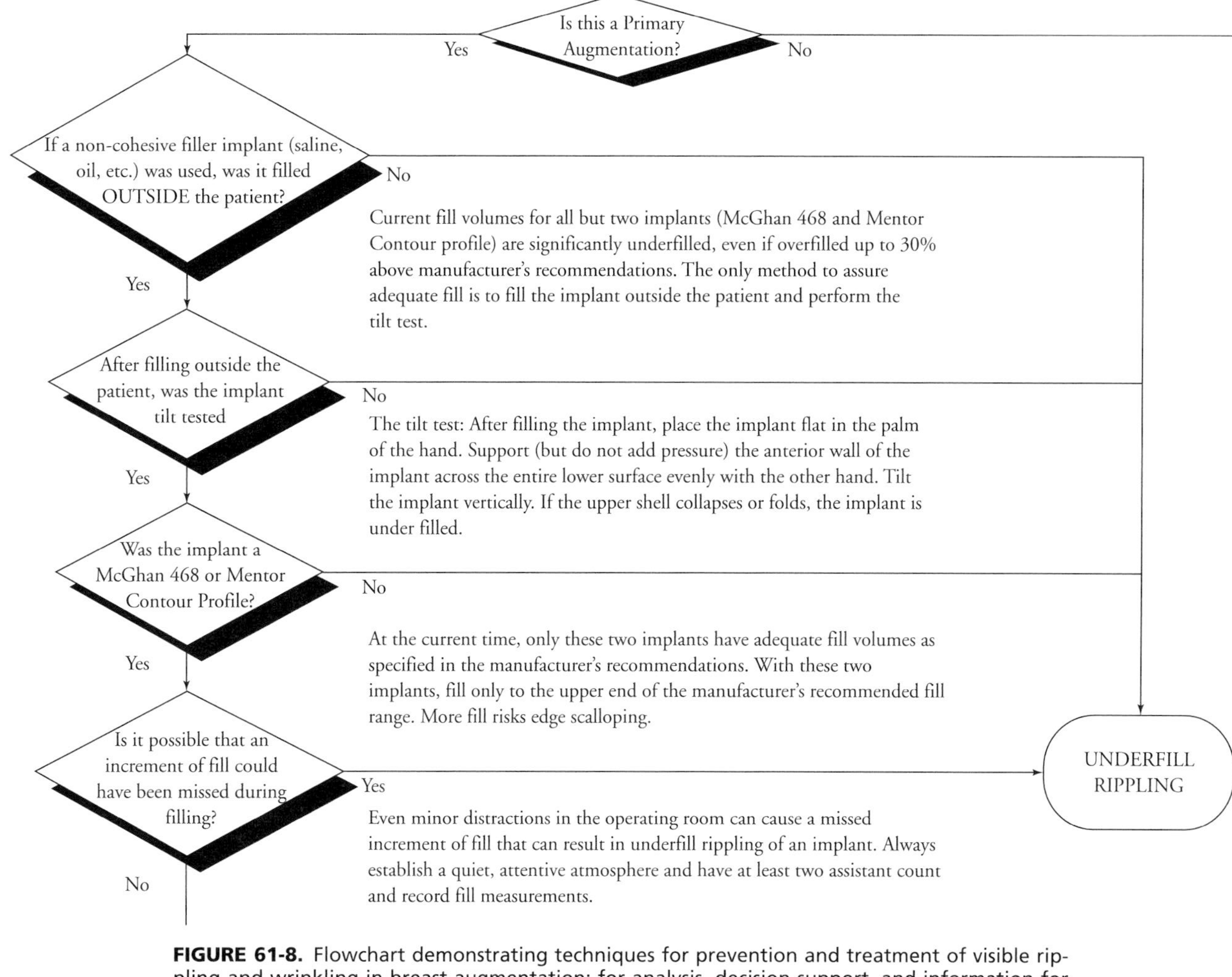

FIGURE 61-8. Flowchart demonstrating techniques for prevention and treatment of visible rippling and wrinkling in breast augmentation; for analysis, decision support, and information for rippling following primary breast augmentation; and for analysis, decision support, and information for visible rippling following breast augmentation reoperations. (© 1998 John B. Tebbetts. Used with permission.) (*continued*)

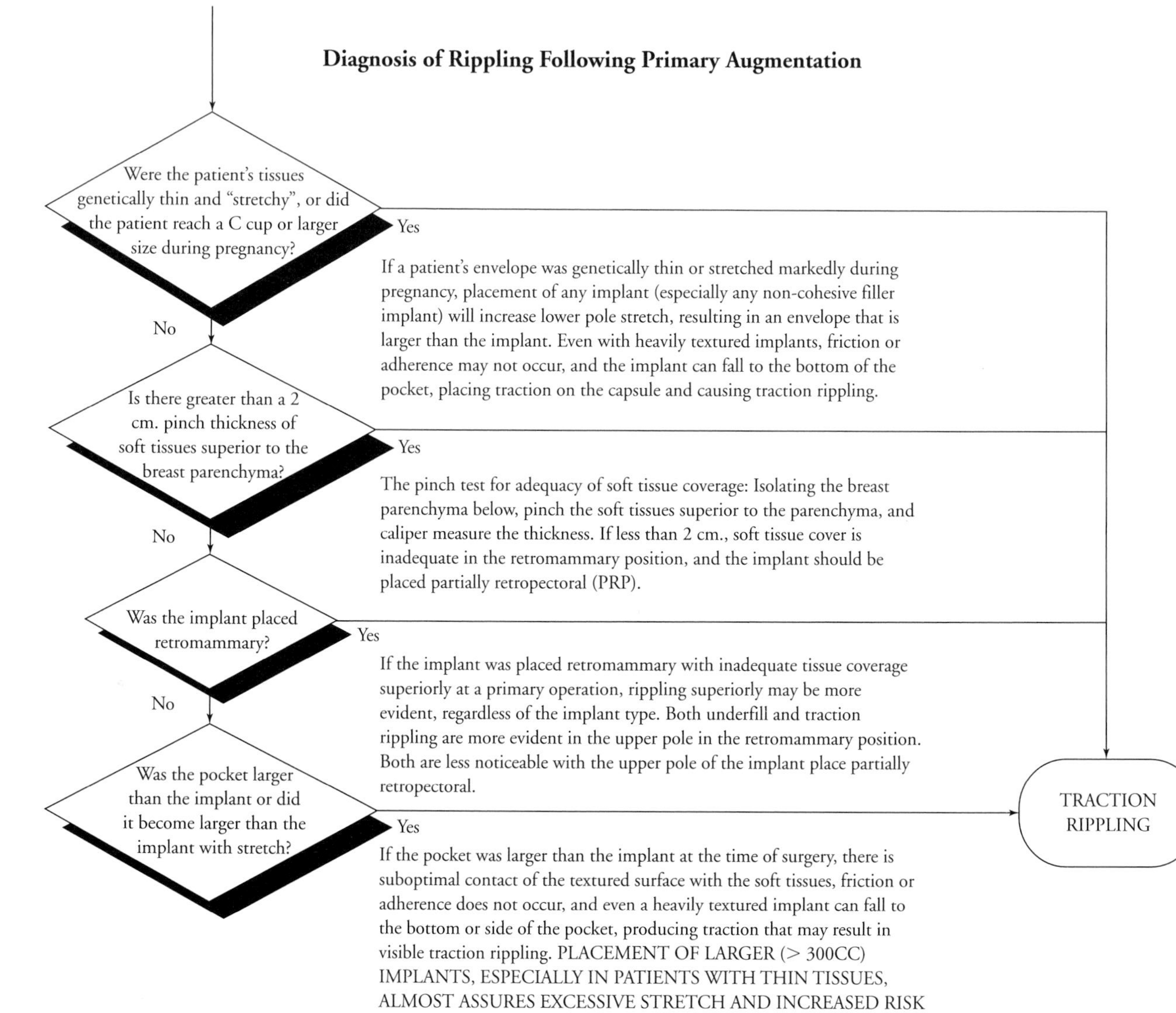

FIGURE 61-8. *(Continued)*

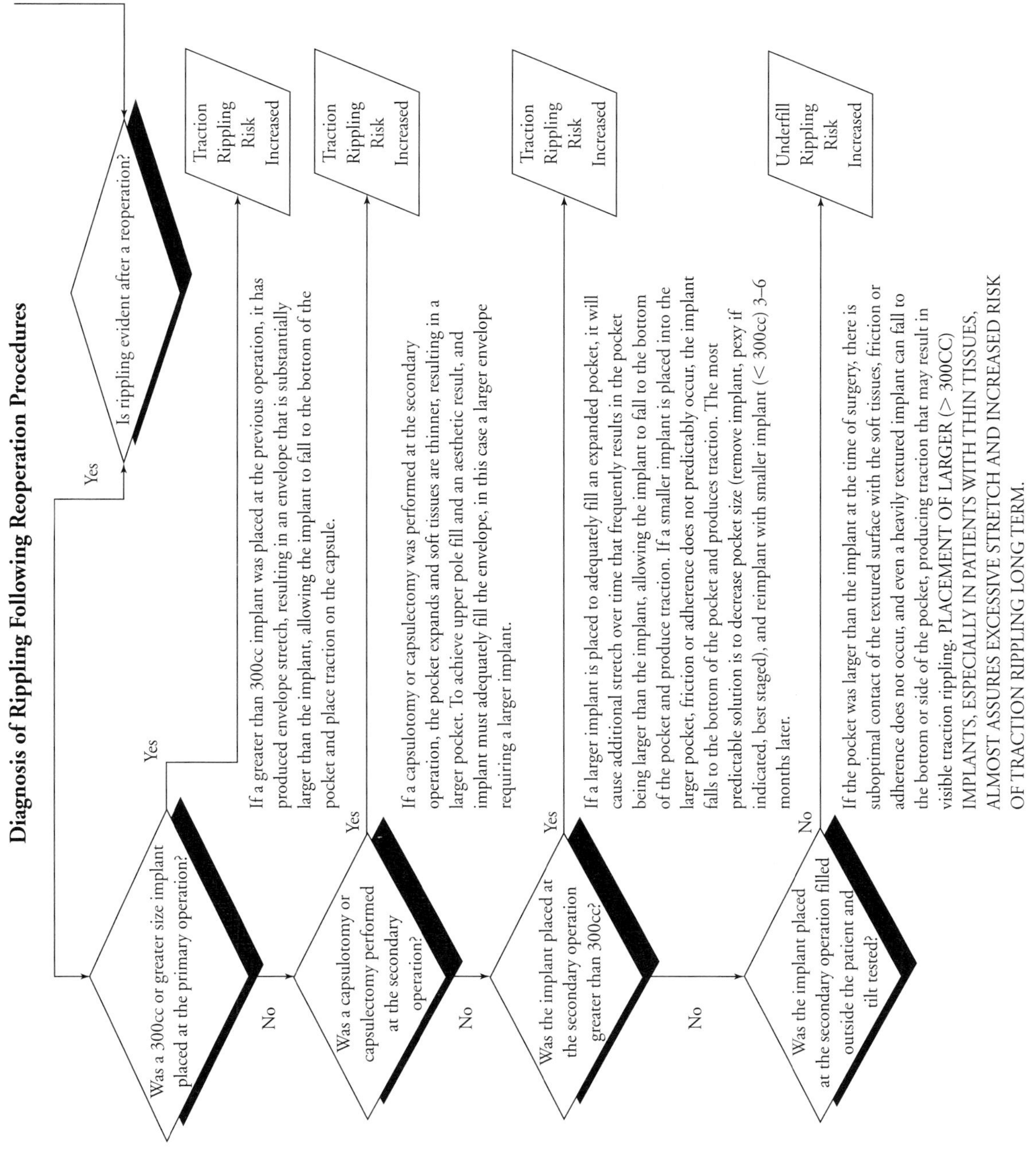

FIGURE 61-8. *(Continued)*

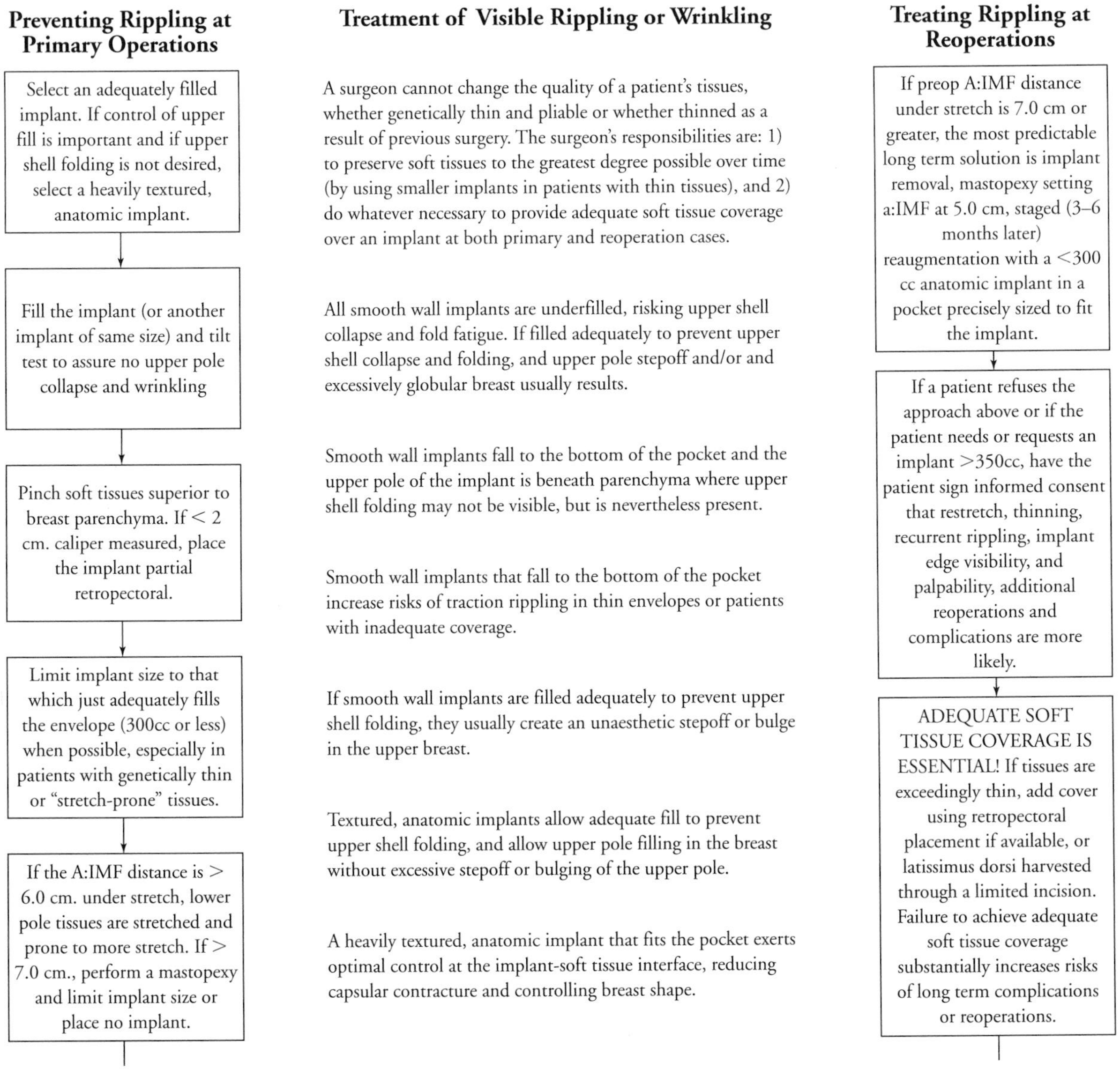

Preventing Rippling at Primary Operations

Select an adequately filled implant. If control of upper fill is important and if upper shell folding is not desired, select a heavily textured, anatomic implant.

↓

Fill the implant (or another implant of same size) and tilt test to assure no upper pole collapse and wrinkling

↓

Pinch soft tissues superior to breast parenchyma. If < 2 cm. caliper measured, place the implant partial retropectoral.

↓

Limit implant size to that which just adequately fills the envelope (300cc or less) when possible, especially in patients with genetically thin or "stretch-prone" tissues.

↓

If the A:IMF distance is > 6.0 cm. under stretch, lower pole tissues are stretched and prone to more stretch. If > 7.0 cm., perform a mastopexy and limit implant size or place no implant.

Treatment of Visible Rippling or Wrinkling

A surgeon cannot change the quality of a patient's tissues, whether genetically thin and pliable or whether thinned as a result of previous surgery. The surgeon's responsibilities are: 1) to preserve soft tissues to the greatest degree possible over time (by using smaller implants in patients with thin tissues), and 2) do whatever necessary to provide adequate soft tissue coverage over an implant at both primary and reoperation cases.

All smooth wall implants are underfilled, risking upper shell collapse and fold fatigue. If filled adequately to prevent upper shell collapse and folding, and upper pole stepoff and/or and excessively globular breast usually results.

Smooth wall implants fall to the bottom of the pocket and the upper pole of the implant is beneath parenchyma where upper shell folding may not be visible, but is nevertheless present.

Smooth wall implants that fall to the bottom of the pocket increase risks of traction rippling in thin envelopes or patients with inadequate coverage.

If smooth wall implants are filled adequately to prevent upper shell folding, they usually create an unaesthetic stepoff or bulge in the upper breast.

Textured, anatomic implants allow adequate fill to prevent upper shell folding, and allow upper pole filling in the breast without excessive stepoff or bulging of the upper pole.

A heavily textured, anatomic implant that fits the pocket exerts optimal control at the implant-soft tissue interface, reducing capsular contracture and controlling breast shape.

Treating Rippling at Reoperations

If preop A:IMF distance under stretch is 7.0 cm or greater, the most predictable long term solution is implant removal, mastopexy setting a:IMF at 5.0 cm, staged (3–6 months later) reaugmentation with a <300 cc anatomic implant in a pocket precisely sized to fit the implant.

↓

If a patient refuses the approach above or if the patient needs or requests an implant >350cc, have the patient sign informed consent that restretch, thinning, recurrent rippling, implant edge visibility, and palpability, additional reoperations and complications are more likely.

↓

ADEQUATE SOFT TISSUE COVERAGE IS ESSENTIAL! If tissues are exceedingly thin, add cover using retropectoral placement if available, or latissimus dorsi harvested through a limited incision. Failure to achieve adequate soft tissue coverage substantially increases risks of long term complications or reoperations.

FIGURE 61-8. *(Continued)*

Preventing Rippling at Primary Operations

Make the pocket fit the implant medially, laterally and inferiorly (and superiorly if using a reduced height anatomic implant). An excessively large pocket allows the implant to fall to the bottom of the pocket, risking traction rippling.

↓

Perform adequate superior mobilization (RM or PRP) to allow proper draping, and decrease pressure of upper pole tissues on the implant, causing increased lower pole stretch.

↓

Try to avoid augmentation in combination with mastopexy with any non-cohesive filler implant (e.g., saline, oil, etc.). The tissues have already shown that they are prone to stretch or the patient would not need mastopexy.

↓

If performing mastopexy augmentation (in patients with A:IMF >7.0 cm under stretch), stage the augmentation 3–6 months later. Use smaller implants, and develop the pocket to precisely fit the implant when the tissues are no longer surgically mobile.

Treatment of Visible Rippling or Wrinkling, con'd

In primary operations, making the pocket fit the implant with textured anatomic implants means developing the pocket to fit the base dimension of the implant. An additional superior mobilization for redraping and to avoid excessive pressure on the implant upper pole is also important. If the pocket fits the implant, the implant surface can exert maximal control of the implant-soft tissue interface. SMOOTH WALL IMPLANTS EXERT TO CONTROLS OF THE IMPLANT SOFT TISSUE INTERFACE, with increased risks of capsular contracture and less control of breast shape, fill, and breast border definition.

If the pocket does not fit the implant, there is less or no control of the implant-soft tissue interface, the implant can displace unpredictably, and anatomic implants can more easily rotate or malposition.

Despite making the pocket fit the implant at the primary operation, an excessively large implant or excessively thin, stretch-prone tissues, or a combination of both can produce envelope stretch and thinning, increasing risks of traction rippling and implant edge or shell visibility. Avoid these problems by recognizing this type of tissue preoperatively and limiting implant size and weight regardless of the aesthetic tradeoffs. Long term preservation of the soft tissues is much more important.

Each reoperation on the breast usually leaves the envelope larger and the tissues thinner and more stretched. Achieving an aesthetic result requires filling the existing envelope, but in a thinned, stretched envelope that requires reoperation, larger implants inevitably produce more stretch, loss of upper pole fill, and increased risk of traction rippling. With thin tissues in a patient requiring a >300cc implant to fill the envelope, the better long term decision is often implant removal, mastopexy if A:IMF is >7.0 under stretch, and staged reaugmentation if the patient insists 3–6 months later with a <300 cc implant in a precisely controlled pocket when the tissues are not as surgically mobile as at the time of mastopexy.

FIGURE 61-8. *(Continued)*

Based on these observations over the past 20 years, I currently advise every primary augmentation patient of the following and obtain informed consent of their understanding and agreement:

1. If infection occurs in either breast, both implants will be removed.
2. For optimal safety, the least risk of reoperations, and the least risk of tissue damage or uncorrectable deformities, for the long-term welfare of the patient, no implants will be replaced.

Although this approach may seem unduly harsh to some surgeons, it is, quite possibly, the safest and best solution for the patient. In my opinion, most "disasters" that occur following augmentation are not caused by a device, but more likely occur when well-meaning perseverance cannot overcome inevitable tissue compromises and the limits of biologic systems. Removal of a breast implant without replacement is emotionally trying for both patient and surgeon, but not as emotionally trying as a permanent deformity or significant medical complication. Preoperative discussion of these issues is critically important to help a patient deal with the consequences if this rare but potentially devastating complication occurs.

CAPSULAR CONTRACTURE

Capsular contracture is not a complication. It is a normal, predictable biologic response to the presence of an implanted prosthetic device. When the capsule surrounding a breast implant contracts excessively, excessive firmness, distortion of shape, implant displacement, and discomfort can occur and require correction. Arguably the most common clinical situation that requires reoperation following augmentation, capsular contracture is a problem that every surgeon who performs augmentation will experience clinically. Rates of capsular contracture vary widely with implant type, filler material type, shell surface characteristics, pocket location, and operative techniques. A detailed discussion of these factors is beyond the scope of this chapter.

Having used virtually every implant type through every incision location, retromammary, and retropectoral over the past 20 years, I have experienced an overall long-term capsular contracture rate of 7% to 10% in patients whom I have been able to follow. In a series of patients operated on using smooth shell gel implants via an axillary approach with blunt dissection with up to 9-year follow-up, an initial capsule rate of approximately 6% overall gradually increased with another 10 years of follow-up to a rate of nearly 11%. My experience with polyurethane-covered implants over a 7-year period produced a capsular contracture rate of less than 1% in primary cases followed up to 7 years. This rate over an ensuing 7-year period increased to approximately 2%. With current, textured, anatomical saline devices, my capsular contracture rate in more than 1,000 patients followed up to 7 years is less than 1%. Whether this rate will rise with time remains a question.

Based on clinical experience treating my own capsular contractures and more than 300 cases in which I was not the primary surgeon, I currently believe the following:

1. Closed capsulotomy is not an effective, predictable method of treating clinically significant capsular contractures.
2. Recurrent contracture following closed capsulotomy in my experience approaches 75%.
3. Closed capsulotomy rarely provides optimal correction, even when it is successful.
4. Closed capsulotomy risks bleeding, implant rupture, and surgeon injury, and is painful to the patient. Complication rates can be substantial.
5. Any procedure that is, at best, 50% successful and carries a substantial complication rate is, in my opinion, not an optimal treatment alternative for capsular contracture compared to other treatment modalities.
6. Complete capsulectomy is more effective at preventing recurrent contracture than partial capsulectomy or capsulotomy. The only clinical situations in which I leave capsule are (a) exceedingly thin soft tissue envelopes, and (b) on the posterior surface of the pectoralis major following retropectoral capsular contracture. In all other cases, I remove all capsule possible using needlepoint electrocautery dissection.
7. Closed drainage is helpful following capsulectomy to reduce fluid accumulation, which prevents a textured implant from controlling the implant–soft tissue interface.
8. Textured surface implants are more effective at preventing recurrent contracture than smooth shell implants.
9. Following capsulectomy, the pocket expands. Adequate fill of the soft tissue envelope for optimal aesthetics and optimal contact of a textured shell with the soft tissues to control the implant–soft tissue interface usually requires a larger implant than was removed.
10. The more aggressive the texturing on a silicone shell surface implant, the more effectively the surface can reduce capsular contracture.
11. An aggressively textured surface implant is more effective at preventing capsular contracture than a smooth shell implant in a large pocket combined with implant displacement exercises.
12. Capsulectomy is optimally performed using a handswitching electrocautery pencil with short and long needle tips for the most precise, complete removal with minimal bleeding.

THE UPWARDLY DISPLACED IMPLANT

Figure 61-9 shows a flowchart that addresses the causes and treatment of the upwardly displaced breast implant.

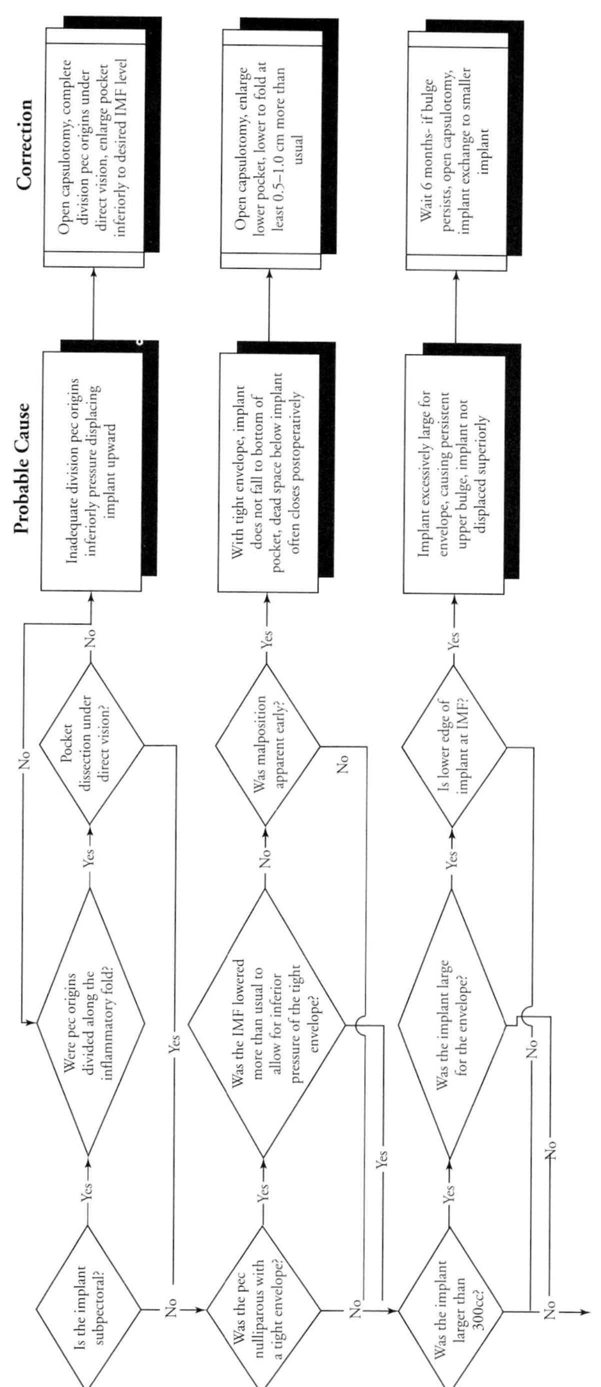

FIGURE 61-9. The upwardly displaced implant: diagnosis and correction. (© 1998 John B. Tebbetts. Used with permission.) (continued)

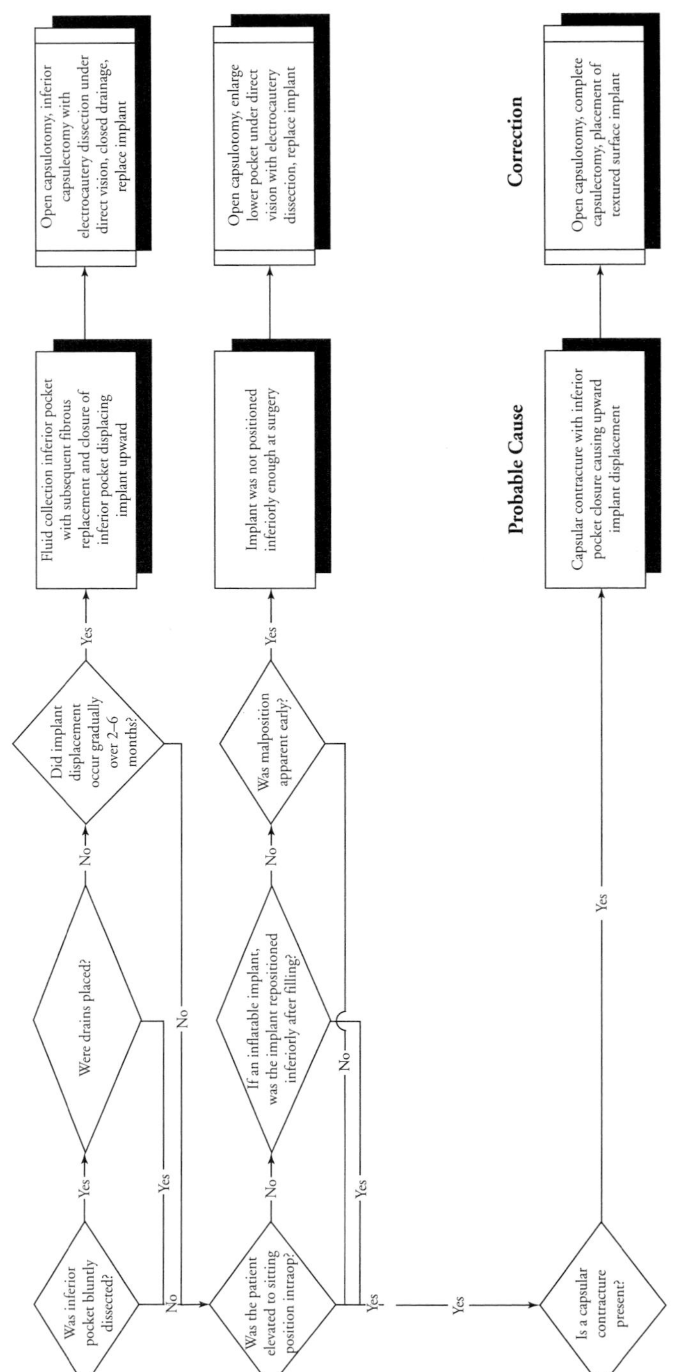

FIGURE 61-9. *(Continued)*

THE "DOUBLE-BUBBLE" DEFORMITY IN THE LOWER BREAST

Figure 61-10 shows a flowchart that addresses correction of a "double-bubble" deformity of the lower breast.

SUMMARY AND CONCLUSION

Based on my personal 20-year experience using every type of implant available through every incision approach and pocket location, I believe that the following are the primary causes of complications in breast augmentation:

1. Underfilled implants that cause visible shell rippling and/or premature shell failure
2. Excessively large implants
3. Placing implants under inadequate soft tissue coverage
4. Hesitancy to remove implants, regardless of the cosmetic consequences, to limit reoperations to a maximum of two
5. Attempting to fulfill the patient's requests without fully understanding and informing the patient of the consequences of her requests.

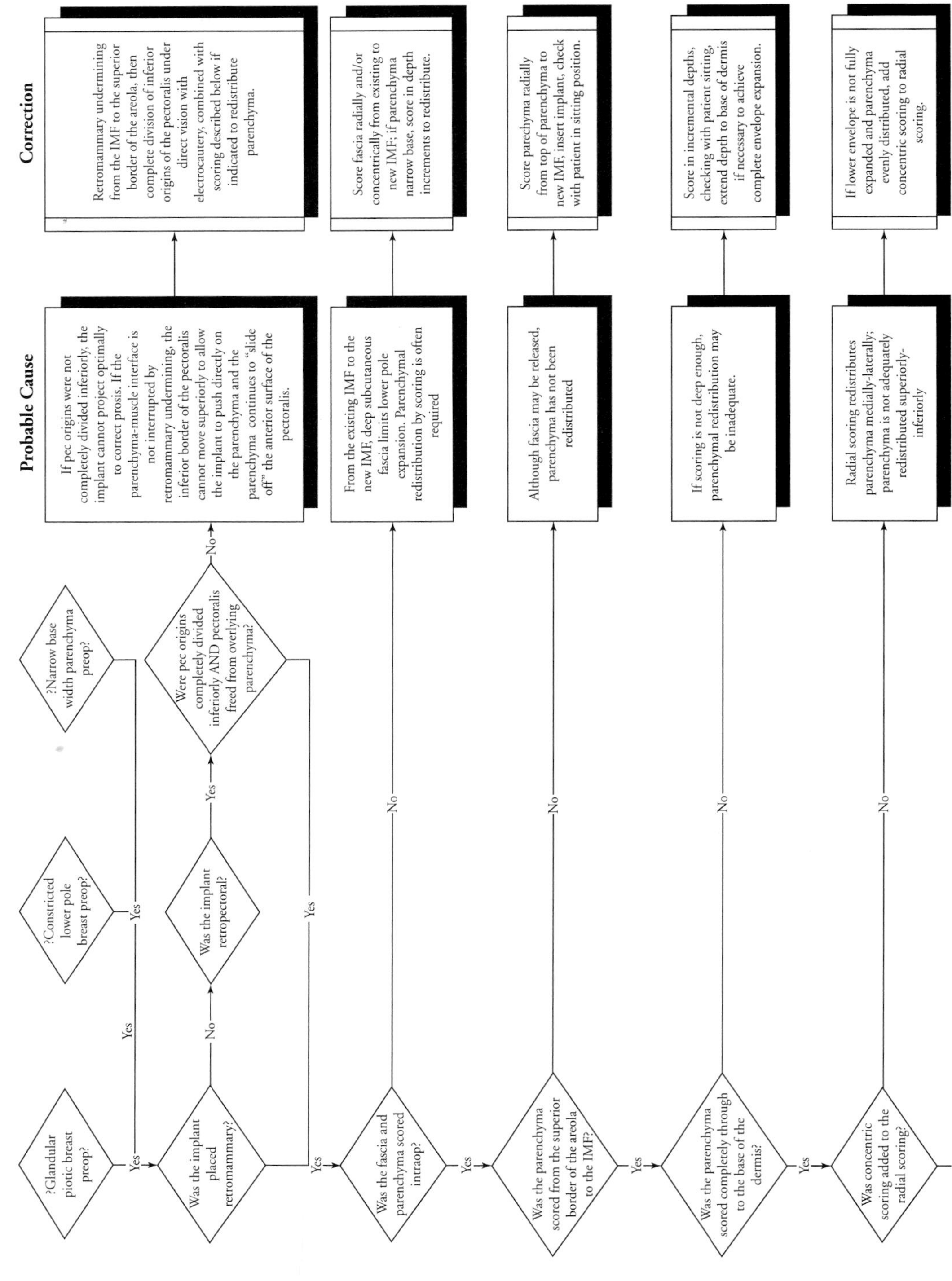
Probable Cause
Correction
?Glandular ptotic breast preop?
?Constricted lower pole breast preop?
?Narrow base width parenchyma preop?
Yes
Yes
Yes
Was the implant placed retromammary?
No
Was the implant retropectoral?
Yes
Were pec origins completely divided inferiorly AND pectoralis freed from overlying parenchyma?
No
Yes
Yes
If pec origins were not completely divided inferiorly, the implant cannot project optimally to correct ptosis. If the parenchyma-muscle interface is not interrupted by retromammary undermining, the inferior border of the pectoralis cannot move superiorly to allow the implant to push directly on the parenchyma and the parenchyma continues to "slide off" the anterior surface of the pectoralis.
Retromammary undermining from the IMF to the superior border of the areola, then complete division of inferior origins of the pectoralis under direct vision with electrocautery, combined with scoring described below if indicated to redistribute parenchyma.
Was the fascia and parenchyma scored intraop?
No
From the existing IMF to the new IMF; deep subcutaneous fascia limits lower pole expansion. Parenchymal redistribution by scoring is often required
Score fascia radially and/or concentrically from existing to new IMF; if parenchyma narrow base, score in depth increments to redistribute.
Yes
Was the parenchyma scored from the superior border of the areola to the IMF?
No
Although fascia may be released, parenchyma has not been redistributed
Score parenchyma radially from top of parenchyma to new IMF, insert implant, check with patient in sitting position.
Yes
Was the parenchyma scored completely through to the base of the dermis?
No
If scoring is not deep enough, parenchymal redistribution may be inadequate.
Score in incremental depths, checking with patient sitting, extend depth to base of dermis if necessary to achieve complete envelope expansion.
Yes
Was concentric scoring added to the radial scoring?
No
Radial scoring redistributes parenchyma medially-laterally; parenchyma is not adequately redistributed superiorly-inferiorly
If lower envelope is not fully expanded and parenchyma evenly distributed, add concentric scoring to radial scoring.

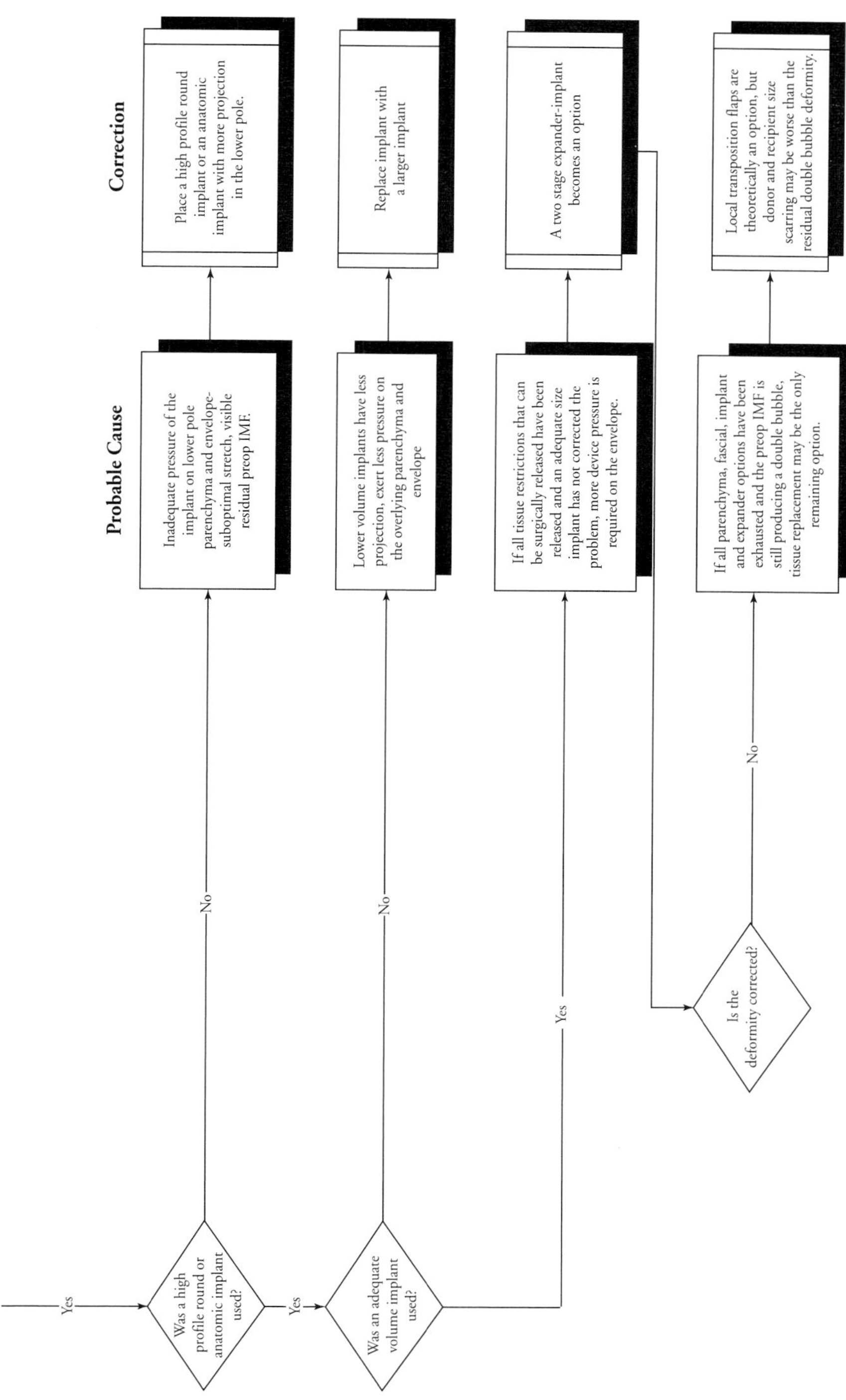

FIGURE 61-10. The "double bubble" deformity of the lower breast: diagnosis and correction. (© 1998 John B. Tebbetts. Used with permission.) *(continued)*

Discussion

BREAST AUGMENTATION

SUMNER A. SLAVIN

Achieving a successful long-term result in breast augmentation is a complex task, according to one of the masters of the field, Dr. John Tebbetts. It requires more than technical expertise because the physical characteristics of the patient's breast anatomy predicts, to a large extent, the stability and predictability of the result. In his chapter, Dr. Tebbetts reviews both the basic ingredients of a favorable result and the pitfalls that lead elsewhere. He provides numerous specific clinical algorithms for treating every potential mishap—from capsular contracture to rippling to double-bubble deformity. The approach is rigorously scientific, emphasizing preoperative analysis of the patient and identification of quantifiable anatomical characteristics.

Any plastic surgeon performing breast augmentation with saline implants needs to learn how to conduct a comprehensive preoperative consultation and physical examination. Dr. Tebbetts' chapter emphasizes communication of potential risks and complications by categorizing them as either avoidable or inevitable. Like most experienced plastic surgeons, he prefers to focus on the avoidable in order to produce the favorable. There are overriding principles that are repeatedly stressed: choose an implant that is appropriate for that specific patient; maximize the opportunity for a favorable primary operation, because successive reoperations introduce more complexity and hazard. This chapter preaches what every student of plastic surgery has heard throughout his or her training—a need to "get it right the first time" and customize the procedure to the patient.

Recognizing the surgical implications of breast measurements is a basic principle. Patients with certain physical characteristics—ptosis, a nipple–areolar complex with a large diameter, a short distance from the inferior border of the areola to inframammary crease, or a wide intermammary distance—pose formidable challenges for the plastic surgeon. These findings should be explained carefully during the preoperative consultation so that the patient appreciates the technical implications of unfavorable breast anatomy. Although quantifiable data can be obtained from meticulous preoperative measurements, as this chapter demonstrates, Dr. Tebbetts' dictum to "define goals by quantifiable measurements" may at times be more theoretical than practical.

Most plastic surgeons will agree that a patient will be pleased postoperatively if the breast is larger and shapely. Certain limitations imposed by surface and interior characteristics of the breast are acceptable if a reasonably aesthetic result has been achieved. Those patients requesting an appearance of improved cleavage, for example, can still be satisfied by augmentation once they realize that their preoperative intermammary distance precludes a result in which the breasts appear pressed closer together. In general, the action of the pectoralis major muscle when a submuscular technique has been chosen is to push the implant inferiorly and laterally over time, making a generously cleaved breast unlikely, if not impossible. Failure to explain this inevitable result leads to disappointment. It is, as Dr. Tebbetts says, a matter of avoidable risks, trade-offs, and choosing the right alternatives.

Unfortunately, many risks and complications of breast augmentation cannot be eliminated by either meticulous preoperative measurement or the collection of quantifiable data. Rippling and wrinkling of saline implants continue to predominate as causes of an unfavorable result, along with deflation and encapsulation. Although there may be agreement that underfilling of saline implants and traction on adjacent soft tissues are common causes of deformity, a precise solution to this problem has not been identified. Surface characteristics of the implant—both smooth and textured—have been associated with both rippling and capsular contracture. Overfilling of a saline prosthesis produces a firm breast, whereas underfilling predisposes to rippling and ultimate collapse of the device. In addition, overfilling may expose the plastic surgeon to legal problems because the fill volume selected in the operating room to eliminate wrinkling may exceed the manufacturer's guidelines. For most patients, underfilling represents more of an aesthetic hazard than overfilling. This may be most evident along the lower pole of the augmented breast where an absence of the pectoral musculature makes wrinkles more easily palpable. Informing a patient in advance of the "unavoidable" risk improves patient acceptance immeasurably.

If rippling cannot be definitively eliminated as an inevitable risk of breast augmentation, providing adequate

S. A. Slavin: Department of Surgery, Beth Israel-Deaconess Hospital, Brookline, Massachusetts

soft tissue cover treats this problem in most patients. Subglandular saline implants are associated with both common complications—rippling and capsular contracture. In my opinion, saline implants do poorly in this location, except when correction of moderate ptosis is one of the preoperative goals. Even then, the amount of correction is modest, not usually exceeding 1 cm. Despite the lack of muscular cover along the inferior pole of the breast, subpectoral placement should be considered as the site of first choice for saline implants. The benefit of this approach is most appreciated when the patient leans forward and is not embarrassed by the bizarre appearance of upper pole surface undulations.

Over the past several years, this author has observed an increasing number of young women seeking augmentation mammoplasty who are bodybuilders or trainers or who are remarkably physically fit. Societal trends support this finding on an empirical basis, and no doubt published statistics will confirm it. As a hallmark of their commitment, they have a significantly developed pectoral musculature that presents the plastic surgeon with concomitant opportunity and danger. Their enhanced pectoral muscles, by virtue of sheer thickness, lend an extremely dense layer of soft tissue over saline implants. These patients almost never reveal the tell-tale upper pole waves and ripples of augmentation mammoplasty using saline implants placed in a subglandular position. Leaning forward, there is no retraction or distortion of the upper pole surface. However, such advanced muscular development often is associated with low levels of body fat, a measurable quantity that the physically fit seek to eliminate altogether! For the plastic surgeon, diminished amounts of body fat, or subcutaneous fat as we know it, contribute to a loss of breast contour and, more importantly, softness. These types of patients in particular make poor candidates for subglandular breast augmentation and should be informed of this concern preoperatively. With the exception of the lower pole of the breast, exaggerated muscular development will conceal the implant's surface characteristics. As a result, any debate over the putative benefits of textured versus smooth implants is moot.

Bodybuilders create an additional challenge: their pectoral muscles are not only thick but taut. The unyielding tension in the pectoralis major muscle is evident even under general anesthesia, restricting placement to a smaller size device. Otherwise, the implant's shape is flattened and any desired projection will be limited. This type of patient is one of the most difficult to assess preoperatively, with or without breast measurements and other "quantifiable data." Exceptionally strong muscles deform the surface of a saline implant by exerting high levels of pressure directly on the device during contraction. Consequently, the prosthesis will be flattened *in vivo,* defying all attempts at preoperative quantification. Breast base width and other measurable components lose their meaning when subjected to strong deforming forces in an awake patient. For this reason alone, anatomically shaped implants may be aesthetically ineffective. Instead of enhancing lower pole contour and providing upper pole fullness, anatomical implants assume the contour of a round implant. This simple clinical observation is more evident postoperatively, but also can be ascertained when neuromuscular blockade is avoided or reduced intraoperatively. Another factor that reduces the advantage of an anatomically shaped implant is the common occurrence of postoperative periprosthetic seroma. Sometimes a boon to both patient and plastic surgeon because it provides a softer result, ultimately, a seroma may contribute to malrotation of an anatomical implant and loss of its cosmetically pleasing shape.

Along with consideration of breast shape, scarring of the breast surface preoccupies many patients seeking augmentation. The advent of endoscopic instruments with improved magnification and visualization have made it possible to reintroduce transaxillary subpectoral placement as a highly desirable technique for breast enlargement. Through incisions as small as 2.5 cm tucked into an axillary fold, excellent access to the subpectoral pocket can be obtained. Transaxillary subpectoral endoscopic breast augmentation delivers on its promise—a scarless breast—and is rapidly becoming the preferred access site among those who are comfortable with all of the commonly used incisions. In addition to elimination of incisions on the surface of the breast, the transaxillary approach does not violate the integrity of the breast parenchyma, nor does it disrupt ductal integrity. The subpectoral space is approached easily along the lateral border of the pectoralis major muscle, eliminating muscle splitting in the central portion of the muscle. Placement of anatomical implants through an axillary incision, however, should be avoided in most instances because the device is inserted in a collapsed state, and if it is not precisely situated and oriented at the lower pole of the breast, some rotation is possible. Malpositioning may not be evident intraoperatively or may become more manifest postoperatively. As mentioned, postoperative seroma formation contributes to malrotation and a distorted cosmetic result. Based on my personal experience, round smooth saline implants are excellent choices for transaxillary subpectoral endoscopic placement. Removing a prosthesis for a size change or deflation is not technically difficult because the plane of dissection can be identified on successive procedures. However, it is necessary to deflate intentionally an intact prosthesis or it will not fit through the small axillary incision.

Another important advantage of the endoscopic transaxillary approach has been a decrease in sensory loss following augmentation. In addition to unsightly scarring, diminution of feeling on the surface of the breast, and especially the nipple–areolar complex, is an extremely disturbing complication for any patient. The exact incidence of this problem is difficult to determine, because many patients manifest variable degrees of numbness, often in a patchy distribution, over the breast surface. Numbness also can be an early postoperative finding that improves or completely disappears over weeks to months. When it is permanent, however, it constitutes an extremely unfavorable result for the patient, who may suffer chronic pain and dysesthesias of the breast. For some patients, loss of sensation over the breast surface can mean a severe disturbance in the quality of their sexual function.

Because the endoscope visualizes all areas of the subpectoral space with the exception of the most lateral and superolateral aspects, injury to the fourth intercostal nerve and other associated sensory branches as they enter laterally is most uncommon, and direct severance of the main sensory fibers is, fortunately, technically difficult to do. More likely, decreased sensory function postoperatively reflects a neuropraxic type of injury caused by stretching during implant placement. Whether sensory injuries can be related quantitatively to increasing amounts of stretch is not known and would pose a challenge for a study of this problem Most patients note a return to approximately the same level of sensation as was present preoperatively.

As more patients with ever increasing pectoral dimensions seek breast enlargement, achieving a cosmetically satisfying result in this particular group has stimulated interest in a variety of intraoperative maneuvers directed at improving muscular compliance. Those patients with extremely low percentages of total body fat have a greater reliance on the saline implant for both breast contour and consistency. Conversely, creating a natural convexity of the implant beneath the pectoralis major muscles was not forthcoming by simple placement of the device. The resulting flattening of the prosthesis yielded an exaggeration of the muscular contour of the upper chest rather than improved breast aesthetics. This conflict has been resolved to a considerable extent by the intraoperative placement of implant sizers that serve the dual role of tissue expander and size selector. Inexpensive and never reused, the sizers provide intraoperative expansion of the pectoralis major muscle by inflating to approximately twice the desire end volume. Improved muscle compliance is observed intraoperatively, followed by better projection of the breast. In addition, there is relaxation of the tense cutaneous envelope that often mirrors the underlying musculature.

Sizers have proved useful in other patients who are neither bodybuilders nor well developed. The sizer aids in expanding the lower pole skin when the areola-to-inframammary crease distance is shortened, sometimes to 2 or 3 cm. In patients with this configuration, lower pole projection is absent and the breast appears as truncated and masculine. Stretching of the skin is most effective when the transaxillary incision has been selected, allowing direct pressure against the lower pole without intervening incisions. The extent of the improvement in contour is remarkable if one side is not expanded with the sizer before implant placement. Intraoperative expansion times of 15 to 30 minutes appear to be adequate. Some patients with mild ptosis may benefit as the sizer fills the lower pole glandular tissues and mimics the improved breast appearance and elevation of a completely subglandular prosthesis. Even patients with less severe forms of tuberous breast deformity are improved by the intraoperative use of implant sizers, as the skin deficiency of a tuberous breast is expanded and the base diameter of the breast becomes widened. For some patients, it has been possible to achieve a one-stage reconstruction of this notoriously difficult problem.

There are few risks associated with the intraoperative use of a sizer. Infection rates in augmentation mammoplasty are extremely low, less than 1% in my experience. Since we began to use sizers in 1995, no patient has developed a wound infection following transaxillary subpectoral breast augmentation. Sizers do not traumatize tissues because the dissection is completed before their introduction. Filling of the sizer through its attached tubing does not appear to increase the risk of infection. Rather than becoming obsolete, implant sizers continue to confer enormous benefits intraoperatively in a wide variety of patients with unfavorable breast configurations.

Poor results following breast augmentation will not be eliminated by the use of sizers, despite the benefits described. Encapsulation following augmentation, for example, is another unresolved problem that has not been eliminated completely by recent technical advances and appears unrelated to the process of selecting appropriate candidates for the procedure. Similarly, excessively large implants lead inevitably to overstretched skin and disfigurement. Skin stigmatized by striae and nipple–areolar complexes with oversized diameters remain refractory to correction. Avoidance, as Dr. Tebbetts emphasizes, is truly the best treatment and, for some problems, the only one.

62

REDUCTION MAMMAPLASTY

ROBERT M. GOLDWYN

Although reduction mammaplasty usually has a high rate of patient satisfaction (1–7), many things can go wrong (8–11). The fact that the breast has sexual significance makes misfortune especially difficult for the patient and for the surgeon. Problems may be relatively minor, such as a stitch reaction, or distinctly major, such as nipple loss.

Some complications that can occur after any operation may happen after reduction mammaplasty and are the most serious: cardiac arrest and death. They will not be discussed in this chapter, but every plastic surgeon must be alert to their possibility and hopefully to their prevention.

PREOPERATIVE CONCERNS

The Wrong Patient

Operating on a patient who is physically or emotionally ill suited can be catastrophic (8). Proper patient selection is mandatory in every elective procedure. The patient to avoid is the one with unrealistic expectations, particularly about scarring. She may not truly comprehend emotionally, not just intellectually, that she could have hypertrophic scars or keloids. Telling a prospective patient that scars "tend to fade" may mistakenly convey the idea that the scars will disappear and not merely lessen. I have found a good way to get the patient to be realistic is to show her postoperative photographs of someone with very bad scars. If this is done, it should be noted in the record, because it could be useful later in discussions with her or an attorney. I usually have slides of patients with a range of results: from poor to excellent. I want to be sure that when I show a patient a photograph of someone whom I believe has a very good result, the patient agrees and does not expect an outcome beyond my power to effect.

The patient with an emotional illness or systemic disease may be unfit for reduction mammaplasty at the time of initial consultation. A careful history, physical examination, and laboratory investigation, to detect coagulopathy, for example, should be done. One should communicate with her primary physician and, if indicated, with those whom she is consulting for other problems.

The patient with a disorder of body image, who may have anorexia nervosa or bulimia, may still be a good candidate for reduction mammaplasty, but only if her psychotherapist concurs (12). Frequently, it is the therapist who has suggested the operation. Part of the medical history should include whether the patient is a smoker. If she is and has not stopped and cannot do so within 4 months of the operation, her procedure should be canceled because the likelihood of necrosis of the skin and nipple–areola is greater.

Inadequately Examined Breasts

It is surprisingly easy to examine a patient for reduction mammaplasty without actually thinking about each breast, both breasts, and those areas of the breast that would require modification to produce an excellent result, including the axillary tail. Seeing without observing and examining without thinking characterize medicine by rote or routine, an unfortunately easy pattern to lapse into when one is fatigued. To prevent this from happening, one should think carefully about the procedure when the patient is in the office and not think about it for the first time when you are both in the operating room. One should study the patient's photographs the day before operation and thoughtfully examine her again before the procedure commences, even if the method to be used does not necessitate preoperative marking.

In no patient for reduction should one forget that the breast potentially harbors a malignancy (13–15). For those with a relevant family history, such as a mother or sister with breast cancer, especially if premenopausal, and in a patient 35 years or older, I routinely obtain preoperative mammograms.

Incorrect Size

The surgeon should never guarantee the patient a specific cup size; yet, one must be aware of the size the patient wants

R. M. Goldwyn: Division of Plastic Surgery, Beth Israel Deaconess Medical Center, Harvard Medical School, Boston, Massachusetts

to be. If, for example, someone who is a DDD and weighs 185 lb and is 5 feet 7 inches tall desires a small B, her eventual appearance may not be satisfactory and trying to achieve this technically could result in necrosis of the nipple. The patient must understand these considerations before, not after, operation.

Poor Rapport

If the surgeon and the patient have good rapport, the course of treatment will be much easier and more satisfying to each. This is not just a matter of good public relations; it is the essence of medicine and surgery: truly caring about the patient. If the patient rightfully perceives her surgeon to be uncaring, she will not do well emotionally, especially should a complication arise.

Preoperatively the patient should not feel inhibited about calling and asking more questions. Failure to return a call or respond to a letter is a serious mistake and one that is easily avoidable. If the surgeon senses that the patient wants another appointment, she should receive it speedily and, I suggest, without charge. It is better to facilitate communication before operation than afterward. Having said all this, however, I, like others, have patients who are unrealistic in their expectations or unstable in their emotions. It is better to sever the relationship before one gets involved its booking the operation.

The Improperly Informed Patient

Not only should patients have realistic expectations about scars and breast size, but they should understand the possibility of complications, including death; infection; bleeding; asymmetry; decreased, altered, or absent sensation of the nipple–areola or skin of the breast (16,17); dehiscence (disruption of the wound); and loss of the nipple–areola on one or both sides. One should not only give the patient these possibilities in writing, but should dictate them in the record with a note that they have been thoroughly discussed, the assumption being that that is true. The informed consent that I use (Table 62-1) is helpful but is not offered as the only one to use. Each surgeon must decide what is best for his or her needs in accordance with the advice of the malpractice carrier.

Failure to Cancel or Postpone an Operation

Any patient who develops a significant medical or emotional problem near the time of or even on the day of operation should not have the procedure. The anesthesiologist usually examines the patient and screens her, but this no reason for the surgeon to abrogate responsibility about deciding whether and when to operate. If, for example, the patient has an acute infection, such as conjunctivitis, bronchitis, or cystitis, her surgery should be canceled.

Faulty Preoperative Marking

Proper marking of the patient is best done with the patient in the upright position before the administration of medication. The most common error is to place the site of the new nipple too high.

INTRAOPERATIVE CONCERNS

Improper Positioning of the Patient

Improper positioning of the patient on the operating table can result in pressure sores, musculoskeletal strains, and cervical and brachioplexus injuries. If the cautery is used, it must be working safely with the patient appropriately grounded.

Failure to Try to Prevent Pulmonary Embolism

Hospitals and surgeons vary with regard to measures taken to prevent pulmonary embolism. For me, the use of leg tourniquets is easy and helps prevent pulmonary embolism, although no method can eliminate that possibility. If tourniquets are to be used, the surgeon should be sure that they are functioning before induction of anesthesia.

Errors of Anesthesia

Every surgeon should be aware of what is happening to the patient from the point of view of the anesthesia she is receiving. Has she been properly intubated? One can observe the movement of her chest with ventilation. One should also check oxygen saturation and the electrocardiogram, and pay attention to readings of blood pressure and pulse. This does not mean that the surgeon should neglect what he or she is doing on the field, but it does mean that the surgeon should not isolate the anesthetist or the course of anesthesia from his or her ken.

Technical Errors

Cutting the wrong thing because of inattention, carelessness, fatigue, or ignorance obviously can cause a poor surgical result. When an operation becomes "routine," the patient is more at risk.

Faulty Incision

Even though the incisions may have been marked preoperatively, it is advisable to check their location during operation, especially with regard to the medial extension of the inframammary incision to avoid going outside the fold. Care

TABLE 62-1. ROBERT M. GOLDWYN, M.D., INC.-AUTHORIZATION-REDUCTION MAMMAPLASTY

Patient's Name____

1. I authorize Robert M. Goldwyn, M.D. (the "Doctor") and his assistants to perform upon me (or my ______________________________) the operation known as reduction mammaplasty (breast reduction).
2. The nature and effects of the operation, the risks and complications involved, as well as alternative methods of treatment, have been fully explained to me by the Doctor and I understand them.

   The following points, among others, have been specifically made clear:
   a. The scars are permanent.
   b. Although having the breasts match is the surgical objective, perfect symmetry of nipples, areolae, and breasts cannot be achieved.
   c. Complications after reduction mammaplasty can be those after any surgical procedure.
   d. Bleeding and infection following reduction may occur and may require an additional procedure(s) for treatment.
   e. There is a possibility that the blood supply to one or both nipples and areolae and skin of the breasts may become impaired and necrosis (death of tissue) may result. This complication may require later reconstruction.
   f. There is a decreased likelihood of breast nursing after reduction mammaplasty.
   g. As far as now known, this operation does not influence the later development of breast cancer.
   h. Swelling and ecchymosis (black-and-blue marks) takes several weeks to disappear; several months are necessary for the breasts to assume their final shape.
   i. While every attempt will be made to make each breast, including nipple and areola, as normal and pleasing in appearance as possible, the objective cannot always be attained.
   j. Sensation to the breast, including nipple and areola, usually is altered and may be decreased permanently.
3. I authorize the Doctor to perform any other procedure which he may deem desirable in attempting to improve the condition stated in Paragraph 1, or any unhealthy or unforeseen condition that may be encountered during the operation.
4. I consent to the administration of anesthetics by the Doctor or under the direction of the physician responsible for this service.
5. I understand that the practice of medicine and surgery is not an exact science and that reputable practitioners cannot guarantee results. No guarantee or assurance has been given by the Doctor or anyone else as to the results that may be obtained.
6. I understand that the two sides of the human body are not the same and can never be made the same.
7. For the purpose of advancing medical education, I consent to the admittance of authorized observers to the operating room.
8. I give permission to Robert M. Goldwyn, M.D., Inc. to take still or motion clinical photographs with the understanding that such photographs remain the property of the corporation.
9. I am not known to be allergic to anything except: (list)

   ____

I certify that I have read the above authorization, that the explanations referred to therein were made to my satisfaction, and that I fully understand such explanations and the above authorization.

Signed ____

Patient or person authorized to consent for patient

Witness ______________________________ Date ____________________

taken at this stage will eliminate a problem that might require revision.

Asymmetry

In teaching centers, one cause of asymmetry can be asymmetry of the breasts before operation or the same surgeon not operating on both breasts. This is not the place to argue how to train residents or how to use assistants. The patient should be informed that another surgeon, under the careful supervision of the primary surgeon, will be doing part of the operation.

Throughout the procedure, the surgeon must know not only the amount but also the location of tissue removed. Periodically weighing it and having the patient sit are helpful in attaining symmetry.

The surgeon should judge the breast from the foot of the table. Enlisting the opinion of others also is helpful, although the surgeon is ultimately responsible.

Faulty Placement and Asymmetry of the Nipples

No matter what the preoperative markings or how they were done, either before or during operation, the location of the nipple must be checked to be certain that it is correct and that both nipple–areola complexes are symmetrical and of equal diameter and shape. A few minutes spent in assessing the position of the nipple can avoid later anguish for the patient and the surgeon, including the need for another operation (18). It is critical to measure the distance of each nipple from the midline and/or the sternal notch and from the submammary sulcus.

Impending Nipple and Areola Necrosis

The nipple–areola must be inspected during operation to determine its apparent viability by noting its color and by testing its capillary filling. If the nipple–areola does not appear healthy, it is necessary to open the incision to rule out torsion or bleeding. The wound may have to be closed differently or more tissue might have to be resected to decrease tension. Occasionally, it is necessary to close the wound only partially around the nipple–areola and/or along the vertical incision. Leaving sutures in place for delayed closure is helpful. Secondary healing, if required, proceeds with surprising rapidity. To delay suturing is a much better alternative than to confront nipple necrosis.

If one has doubt abort the viability of the nipple or areola after these maneuvers, intravenous fluorescein in conjunction with a Wood lamp can furnish some guidance. In a black patient, a small piece of epidermis should be removed by abrasion or as a split graft to see the uptake of the fluorescein. I have found this test to be right more often than wrong. If the nipple–areola and part of its pedicle have poor blood flow, the nipple–areola should be removed as a graft and the avascular segment of the pedicle amputated. The nipple–areola then must be placed on a dermal bed, where it usually survives (19). In grafting the nipple–areola, it is necessary for the nipple to be in contact with the substrate by stitching it down and using a pressure dressing to get maximum attachment. Even then, a portion of the nipple, especially if hypertrophic, may not survive.

With regard to nipple necrosis, the chief error is undercutting the pedicle laterally or medially, or trimming it excessively at its base or behind the nipple–areola.

Improper handling is another factor contributing to necrosis of the nipple–areola. Carelessly allowing the flap to fold on itself during the operation will compromise vascularity.

Dog-ears

At the end of the procedure, most surgeons become slightly fatigued, and it is easy not to take special care to eliminate dog-ears. One commonly used method is to close the wound from the ends toward the midline. This maneuver has additional advantages of decreasing tension centrally so that there is less chance for necrosis at the junction of the inverted T. The other advantage is that it decreases the length of the inframammary incision if it has not already been fully made. However, one disadvantage is that as more tissue is brought centrally, the nipple–areola distance to the inframammary fold can lengthen, which is another reason to check the distance to be sure that it does not exceed 6.5 to 7.0 cm to the point of the nipple.

From a technical point of view, it is easier to eliminate dog-ears by turning the patient slightly to the opposite side and by sitting down when suturing. One must be sure that the extension of the incision, if necessary, to eliminate the dog-ear does not rise too high or extend too far and that it matches as much as possible that of the opposite side. Going too far laterally or medially can produce hypertrophy of the scar.

Excessive Blood Loss

Careful dissection and the punctilious use of electrocautery will decrease blood loss. In the last 37 years, I have never needed to transfuse a patient having a reduction mammaplasty.

Infiltration with epinephrine, in low concentrations, is effective in minimizing blood loss. Although this technique has the theoretical disadvantages of interfering with pedicle vascularity and causing rebound bleeding after the epinephrine effect has passed, these usually do not happen (20).

Some patients will want to donate blood because they fear the possibility of transfusion and wish to avoid the acquired immunodeficiency syndrome. They should be allowed to do so even if the blood is not to be used.

Nipple and Areola Inversion and Distortion

The surgeon is wise not to attempt to correct preexisting nipple inversion at operation for reduction, as the blood supply to the nipple–areola may be compromised.

IMMEDIATELY POSTOPERATIVE CONCERNS

Errors of General Management

Many things can go wrong postoperatively. The first is incomplete or faulty orders. The surgeon should write orders or check those written by someone else. For example, one must be certain that the patient in the recovery room has received her antibiotics, if ordered; her proper diabetic regimen, if required; or cortisone, if needed. If the patient is to continue pneumatic boots, they not only should be ordered, but also used. Writing an order is not synonymous with having it carried out. Orders must include instructions for examining the nipple–areola to detect necrosis. Dressings should be loose and permit easy access for that purpose. Tight wraps around the chest restrict respiration and can increase venous congestion of the nipple–areola.

Instructions concerning voiding should be explicit. At the request of the anesthesiologist, I generally use an indwelling catheter if the procedure is to last more than 4 hours. The catheter can be removed at the end of the operation or left until midnight if the patient stays overnight.

How long the patient is hospitalized varies, depending on the health of the patient, the nature of the operation, and the stipulations of the insurance company. The surgeon, however, is ultimately responsible for the well-being of the patient, and no insurance company or financial considerations should overrule good judgment. The criterion of what is best for the patient should never be abandoned.

If the patient has nausea or vomiting or feels weak, discharge the day of operation is not in that patient's best interests.

Impending Nipple Necrosis

Impending nipple necrosis is the dread of every surgeon. If the nipple–areola appears to be extremely blue and engorged postoperatively, one should remove a few stitches. If this produces no change in color, the patient may have to return to the operating room to rule out torsion of the pedicle or underlying hematoma. If, despite these measures, the nipple–areola complex still shows marked venous obstruction, then it should be removed and grafted.

Sometimes venous obstruction is mild and can be reversed with medicinal leeches (21). Because the leech *(Hirudo medicinalis)* carries *Aeromonas hydrophila,* the patient can develop an infection and should prophylactically receive tetracycline or another antibiotic to which the leech is sensitive. *Aeromonas* is resistant to penicillin and ampicillin. Hyperbaric oxygen also has proven helpful. Several patients I have seen in consultation have benefitted remarkably from it. I admit that I was skeptical initially, but I believe it is worth trying because it is safe.

Infection

Wound infection in the immediate postoperative period is unusual but can occur. In most instances, the cause of organisms is *Streptococcus.*

Although prophylactic antibiotics may not be necessary, I administer them and continue their use orally for 5 days. Some might argue with that regimen, but few would dispute that when a patient becomes febrile and the wound looks erythematous, she should be given an antibiotic.

Ransjo et al. (22) showed that cultures taken during reduction mammaplasty grew predominantly *Staphylococcus epidermidis* and anaerobic *Propionibacterium acnes.* It is assumed that these bacteria are normal inhabitants of the mammary ducts of most women.

Rand and Bostwick (23) reported pyoderma gangrenosum in a 19-year-old patient 4 days after reduction mammaplasty. She had received oral cephalosporin but developed a fever with negative cultures results, perhaps because she had received antibiotics. Subsequently, she needed debridement and the tissue showed only nonspecific inflammation. She was managed successfully with intravenous globulin (because of her hypogammaglobulinemia) and with prednisone.

In a prospective study of approximately 22,500 wounds, Cruse and Foord (24) determined that the electrocautery doubled the incidence of infection in four varieties of wounds: clean, clean-contaminated, contaminated, and dirty.

Drains, especially the nonsuction type such as a Penrose drain, increase infection, although they decrease the likelihood of seromas. I now use no drains, a change due less to medical reasoning than to socioeconomic changes leading to decreased hospitalization.

Hemorrhage and Hematoma

Hemorrhage is always possible after any operation, but fortunately it is uncommon after reduction mammaplasty. One should be quick to evacuate an expanding hematoma before it leads to pressure necrosis of the skin or the nipple–areola.

Although most hematomas occur in the first 24 hours, McKissock (11) noted that infrequently hemorrhage can happen up to 9 days following operation and even consecutively in the same patient. Possible factors for late bleeding are extreme physical exertion, aspirin ingestion, and unrecognized coagulopathy.

The presence of a hematoma, even if evacuated, may predispose the patient to infection. The patient should be given antibiotics if she is not already receiving them.

EARLY POSTOPERATIVE COMPLICATIONS AND UNFAVORABLE RESULTS

Wound Dehiscence

Frequently, a suture line will disrupt, most likely at the junction of the inverted T if closure was too much tight or if the stitches were removed too early. A small skin flap based on the inframammary fold in the midline decreases tension on the closure and helps avoid this problem.

The use of 4-0 Monocryl intradermally provides additional support and has the added advantage of eliminating the tedium and the pain of removal of sutures.

Occult Cancer

On rare occasions, a patient without a worrisome family history or suspicious mammograms and physical examination has an unsuspected malignancy detected microscopically during or soon after operation (13,15). The patient should be referred to an appropriate surgeon and oncologist. It is possible that she will require mastectomy. This happened in two of my patients and was devastating. Both women required psychotherapy before undergoing modified radical mastectomy (in each instance no nodes were involved).

If a malignancy is recognized at the time of operation, the procedure must be terminated. No attempt should be made to reduce the opposite breast or perform a mastectomy without informing the patient. The decision of how to treat this cancer usually is not in the province of the plastic surgeon.

In a recent study, 27,527 women who had breast reduction in Ontario, Canada, 18 were found to have breast cancer at the time of operation (25). Sixty-seven percent underwent total mastectomy: 33% partial mastectomy, 46% irradiation, and 23% chemotherapy. Their survival at 5 years of about 80% was the same as for patients from the general population treated for breast cancer.

Mondor's Disease

Mondor's disease is benign, self-limiting, superficial thrombophlebitis of a vein or veins of the anterolateral wall that can occur spontaneously or 3 to 7 weeks after trauma, such as reduction mammaplasty (26). A visible, palpable, vertical cord is present, generally but not always in the submammary area. It becomes noticeable when the patient raises her arms, which puts the skin under tension. Because Mondor's disease disappears by recannulization and remodeling of collagen, no treatment is indicated. Only rarely, however, because of pain or cosmesis, is it necessary to divide or remove the thrombosed vein.

Systemic Problems

Space does not allow detailing the many possible problems, medical and surgical, the patient might develop postoperatively. It is important, however, to be alert for atelectasis and pneumonia, urinary infection, cardiac arrhythmia or ischemia, deep phlebitis, and pulmonary embolism.

LATE COMPLICATIONS AND UNFAVORABLE RESULTS

Bad Scarring

Although scars are inevitable, some are worse than others; those especially prone to becoming hypertrophic are the ends of the inframammary incision, particularly lateral, and the circumareolar incision. The last is more likely to occur if there has been partial loss of the areola in a young patient, who is more prone to develop hypertrophic, thick, red scars.

The secondary healing that commonly occurs at the junction of the inverted T does not usually produce a thick scar. If it does occur, it is in a hidden location. It might require steroid injection or revision.

The use of silicone sheeting beginning 1 or 2 weeks after operation and extending for 3 to 6 months supposedly is helpful in reducing unwanted scarring. I usually have patients order the product themselves; they are eager to comply in order to have a better outcome.

Surgical revision of scars is disappointing in young patients who have healed primarily without infection. Patients must be informed about the possible futility of scar revision, which should not be attempted until 9 to 12 months have elapsed and only after the patient has received steroid injections or has used silicone sheeting or steroid creams.

The popularized techniques that use only circumareolar incisions with possibly an additional vertical and/or a short inframammary incision obviously decrease the development of objectionable scarring (27–36). These procedures are difficult, at least in my hands, for patients who are *extremely* large breasted.

With the round block method of reduction mammaplasty, as popularized by Benelli (27,37), the periareolar scar may show pleating, which a revision under local anesthesia can ameliorate but not always eliminate. Patients, nevertheless, are willing to accept the secondary procedure in order to avoid the anchor (inverted T) scar with the more traditional methods.

Tear-drop Nipple and Areola

Hallock and Altobelli (38) reported on this problem and recommended that if it is perceived at operation, it can be avoided by releasing the areola, usually at the 6 o'clock position.

If the tear-drop configuration is a problem postoperatively, it can be handled similarly in one's office with just local anesthesia.

Asymmetry and Undesirable Shape or Size

Unfavorable results in terms of contour and shape can be judged only after sufficient time has passed—at least 6 months or even longer. Occasionally, it may be necessary to remove more tissue. This usually can be done under local anesthesia, very often with liposuction because what remains is more likely to be fat rather than breast tissue. When it is both, sharp dissection may be necessary.

A patient may complain that her breasts are still too large. Although this is not an outcome that the patient or the surgeon wants, it is better than having removed too much tissue and resorting to an implant in the future.

Despite what is shown at meetings and in the literature, the reality is that only rarely are both breasts *absolutely* symmetrical before or after reduction (5). Whether or not the patient is satisfied depends not just on how much difference but also how much discrepancy the patient (and the surgeon) can tolerate (Fig. 62-1). Symmetry is in the eye of the beholder.

For secondary procedures performed to achieve a desired shape or size, I do not charge patients, but they must pay hospital costs. Prior to operation, they sign a form stipulating their obligation (Table 62-2), but it is never easy to have the patient accept that financial burden. Surgeons with their own operating rooms have a great advantage under these circumstances.

TABLE 62-2. STIPULATION OF OBLIGATION TO PAY HOSPITAL COSTS FOR SECONDARY PROCEDURES

ROBERT M. GOLDWYN, M.D.

Because insurance coverage varies with different companies, I understand that I may be responsible for the hospital costs associated with any surgery undertaken to improve a result or to treat a complication. While I understand that Dr. Goldwyn would be willing to forego his fee for additional work if it is not covered by insurance, I understand that he cannot assume responsibility for the hospital charges.

I understand also that it is not his policy to return the original surgical fee in the event that I am displeased with the result and wish to consult another physician/surgeon for evaluation, treatment, or reoperation.

____
Date

____
Signature

____
Witness

Fat Necrosis

If fat has been left attached but lying beyond the pedicle, it may later necrose because of its insufficient blood supply. Drainage, a sterile abscess, or even a hard mass may result. A lump that persists a few months despite a normal pathology

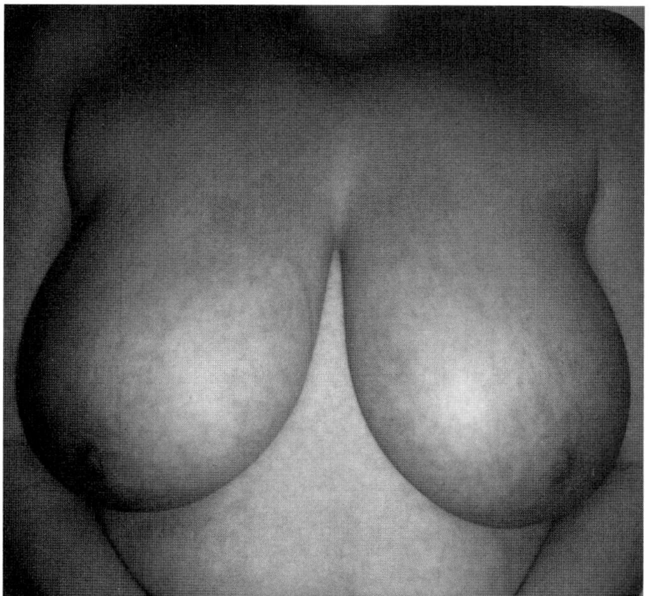
A

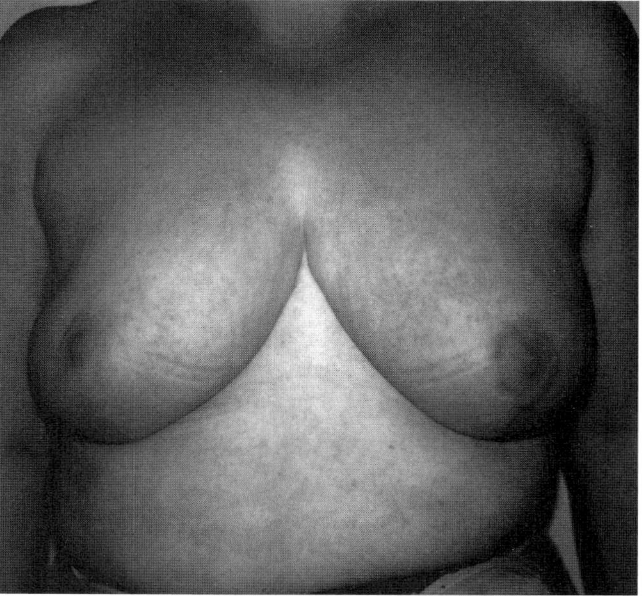
B

FIGURE 62-1. A: Preoperative view in a 51-year-old woman. **B:** Postoperative view 13 months after the patient had 630 g removed from the right breast and 620 g from the left breast. The patient is bothered by the greater concavity in the upper outer quadrant of the right breast compared to the left breast. She realizes rationally that the asymmetry is moderate, but she is still concerned. She wants no other procedure to help correct the difference.

report of the tissue previously removed must be biopsied to be certain of the diagnosis.

There is a possibility of a malignancy in any breast at any time, and not only in patients with a history of breast cancer (39), because most women who develop this malignancy have a negative family history.

Strombeck (14) reported, as have others,an increased incidence of fat necrosis in obese patients having a resection greater than 1,000 g. In my experience, with the inferior pedicle technique, necrotic fat is rare unless nipple–areola necrosis occurred or too much breast tissue was left beyond the pedicle. Prompt attention with aggressive debridement will shorten recovery time considerably.

Nipple and Areola Necrosis

This dreaded event usually can be noticed impending intraoperatively or certainly within 48 hours postoperatively. Sometimes, however, necrosis occurs 7 to 10 days later, particularly in patients who may have never stopped smoking or secretly resumed it. We all can remember anxiously seeing patients in the office and hoping that the bluish nipple–areola will reverse itself. Many times it does, but sometimes it does not. At this stage, leeches and hyperbaric oxygen usually are unsuccessful. Debridement may be necessary, but, if one is in doubt, waiting a few days may yield an unexpected good outcome.

If there is debridement and the wound is now open, the patient must be taught to care for it. This decreases her dependency and will help her physically and emotionally. Visiting nurses may be necessary, but the surgeon still is responsible for the patient and must see her frequently to offer support and to debride the wound if required. I usually have the patient use saline dressings three to four times a day. I believe strongly in having patients shower and cleaning the wound with soap and water.

If the nipple or areola or both have undergone significant loss, reconstruction and replacement will be necessary if the patient desires. The sane kinds of techniques used in nipple–areola reconstruction and breast reconstruction are applicable here. For a minimal loss of the areola, tattooing may be the answer.

Total loss of the nipple–areola usually is accompanied by some loss of the pedicle. If severe, additional tissue may be necessary for symmetry. The latissimus dorsi is excellent for this purpose.

Inversion of the Nipples

Inversion of the nipples cannot always be avoided at operation and should not be corrected if the patient already has this condition, a fact that should be explained to her. Some techniques, such as that of Strombeck, are associated with this problem more than other methods of reduction mammaplasty. McKissock (11) noted that with his vertical bipedicle flap technique, areolar retraction usually results from an excessively broad-based superior flap. Correction is possible by narrowing the attachment with incisions around the areola made from 11 o'clock to l o'clock.

Every surgeon has his or her own technique for correcting nipple inversion, which attests to the difficulty of the problem. I have found buried flaps of dermis, slid under the nipple and joined together, to be helpful (40,41). I also have used various techniques of purse-string suturing (42). With no method can one guarantee a patient long-term success.

The use of external suction may work in a small percentage of patients, but I have not found it to be effective when the inversion was secondary to operation.

Residual Areola

Patients with very large areolae should be told preoperatively that it may be impossible to remove as much of the areola as aesthetically desirable, because it would compromise closure and create unsafe tension. Excising the remaining areola as a secondary procedure usually is not difficult, because in most cases it lies adjacent to the vertical incision–from areola to inframammary fold.

Pouting Nipple and Areola

Occasionally the nipple–areola complex will look redundant and pouting. If one notes this phenomenon at operation, trimming more tissue from its underside may be the solution. Often this fails, and it is better to accept the problem and not whittle away to the point of jeopardizing vascularity.

If this pouting persists in the areola that is smaller, one can increase the diameter of the keyhole but one should wait at least 6 to 8 months. Tacking the undersurface to the deeper tissue with nonabsorbable sutures of nylon also is helpful, but I have had a couple of patients in whom nothing was effective. The cause was likely too much tension in approximating the vertical incision.

Convergent Areolae

Areolae that are too medial and point inward toward each other can be difficult to correct. Sometimes a simple semicircular excision of skin may be all that is necessary, but only if the nipple–areola is not too far medial.

Nipple Too High

Nipple placement that is too high is one of the most challenging and exasperating problems. Its prevention, as mentioned, is being careful to place the new nipple site low. With the inferior pedicle technique, this is usually 23 to

24.5 cm from the sternal notch on the midclavicular line.

For the nipple–areola that is too high, resecting an inferior segment of tissue above the inframammary sulcus may lower it. For a nipple that is extremely high, it is not possible to lower it without leaving a scar above it, unless an expander is used, as described by Raffel (43). The expander can be placed superiorly to create more tissue with subsequent relocation of the nipple–areola. This involves another operation but not another new scar, as would result from closure of the old nipple–areola site after bringing it down to where it belongs.

Nipple Too Low

The unfavorable result of a nipple that is too low is less disturbing to the patient because a lien nipple stays in the brassiere. Yet, it is not an outcome that pleases either the patient or the surgeon. Unless the nipple is excessively low, a simple crescent excision of skin immediately superior to the areola is sufficient to raise it. If more length is required in the vertical closure, a Z-plasty of the vertical scar can be effective.

Although I have not used an expander in this situation, it might be useful. Another solution, but one I would assiduously avoid, is to use a skin graft or a flap from below the inframammary fold to raise the nipple–areola.

Inability to Lactate

Despite the large numbers of women who had reduction mammaplasty, only a few studies about lactation have been reported. These indicate a 50% to 70% chance of nursing in patients who had breast reduction by transposition techniques. Many patients who would be able to nurse do not because of their fear of resulting ptosis and hypertrophy.

Galactorrhea

Galactorrhea immediately after reduction mammaplasty has been reported. It may occur because of a combination of several factors: (i) prolactin, which is a stress hormone, and its increased secretion after operation; (ii) a rebound phenomenon following discontinuance of birth control pills, if the patient was taking them, which results in decreased progesterone that might increase prolactin-releasing factors; (iii) stimulation of prolactin production by a sucking reflex that is well known and can be mimicked by transposing the mammilla on its pedicle; (iv) elevation of steroid concentration as a result of surgical stress that may stimulate prolactin receptors; and (v) hypersensitivity to prolactin receptors (44). This sequence is still conjectural.

Galactorrhea usually can be managed successfully by giving the patient bromocriptine, a prolactin inhibitor, which induces cessation of galactorrhea.

Recurrent Hypertrophy

The recurrence of hypertrophy after reduction mammaplasty is extremely rare, except in very young patients, ages 12 to 14 years, whose breasts are massive and whose operations had to be performed because of enormous rapid growth. Sometimes a patient in that age group may have to undergo subcutaneous mastectomy with implants to provide a solution, which is a drastic measure that one would try to avoid. The administration of hormones under these circumstances may be indicated, but the long-term effect of such treatment is unknown.

Late Changes of Shape and Volume

Vilain and Mitz (45) reported that patients followed for more than 20 years after reduction mammaplasty by the Biesenberger method showed little change in the appearance of the breast despite weight fluctuation, pregnancy, and aging. If changes occurred, they did so within 2 years of the procedure. Hoffman (46), however, found that asymmetry and ptosis made their appearance after 5 years and were partially due to failure at operation to resect enough breast tissue inferiorly and by placing the nipple too high.

In my experience, it is a rare patient who returns years after her reduction to have a repeat reduction. This does not necessarily mean that the appearance of the breasts would not be helped by an additional operation or revision. What it does indicate is that patients adapt well to mild or moderate changes in their breasts if they happen slowly.

Damage to the Long Thoracic Nerve

Rarely a patient may develop a winged scapula as a result of damage to the long thoracic nerve at operation. Prevention by adequate visualization, careful dissection, and nontraumatic traction are preferable to what could be an extensive and futile procedure of reopening the wound and performing a neurorrhaphy.

Paul (*personal communication,* April 9, 1998) reported the complication of damage to the long thoracic nerve in a patient seen in consultation, but fortunately it resolved completely. Its cause was most likely traction and electric cauterization.

Impaired Sensation

As mentioned, every patient for reduction mammaplasty must be warned about the possibility of impaired sensation to their nipples. Courtiss and Goldwyn (47) found that after reduction mammaplasty by dermal pedicle transposition (inferior pedicle technique), almost all breasts had decreased sensibility to pain (measured by a dental pulp voltimeter), crude touch, and light pressure for about 6 months. After 1 year, the skin of the breast in most patients regained its sensibility, but the nipple had decreased sensation in 35% of patients, even at 2 years. These changes related more to the amount of tissue removed rather than the type of technique used. Even though the nipple objectively had some degree of numbness, women subjectively reported a higher degree of sensitivity in their breasts, a finding that suggests their better body image permitted them to enjoy more physical intimacy. Craig and Sykes (48) found that 80% of patients had normal sensation following reduction with the use of a pedicle, but only 50% had adequate sensation when the technique used grafting of the nipple–areola.

Sarhadi and Souter (17) found in female cadaver breasts that in all instances nerve branches other than those from the fourth intercostal nerve alone gave additional nerve supply to the nipple.

As a practical matter, sensation to the breast is more likely to be preserved by leaving tissue on the pectoral fascia and not exposing the nerves at the time of operation. One can contour the breast nicely without excising the small amount of additional tissue that gives protection to the sensation of the breast.

For the woman in whom reduction mammaplasty has caused persistent numbness that still is present at 2 years, nothing now known can be done to improve sensation with predictability.

In my experience with women who had their reductions done elsewhere and complained of their persistent numbness, what seems to have bothered them equally is their allegation that the surgeon had not warned them of that possibility. This postoperative problem should be part of the informed consent (Table 62-1).

Cysts

This problem, which should be avoidable, is more common than is recognized and admitted. If a procedure involved a dermal pedicle, the surgeon should have inspected it carefully with magnification lenses if necessary, to be sure that all the epidermis had been removed, whether by knife, cautery, dermatome, or laser. Many of these remnants will disappear, but some can produce exasperating cysts and recurrent infection that necessitate exploration of the area with full-thickness excision. Primary closure without additional tissue in the form of a flap almost always is possible.

Patient Dissatisfaction

Although most patients are satisfied with the result, not all are or should be. Some patients are unhappy when they should not be, and some are happy when the surgeon, if honest, will consider the result below par. Strombeck (14) found that satisfaction was related to age: the older the patient, the happier she was with the result. As a general rule, the more the patient considers her reduction mammaplasty to be reconstructive and not cosmetic, the greater the likelihood that she will be satisfied with her result. It also is true, however, that what begins as reconstructive becomes cosmetic.

When a complication or an unfavorable result produces noticeable asymmetry of breast size, women have problems in adaptation because of difficulties with buying clothes or interpersonal relations. In this regard, what that "important other" says or how he or she reacts becomes the determining factor in persistent dissatisfaction.

Sometimes patients who are dissatisfied with a result that is not easy to improve or may, in fact, be impossible to ameliorate develop persistent *pain.* This may have an anatomical base, but generally its cause is unknown or ambiguous, and its correction is difficult or impossible. The patient may be depressed, but it is hard to separate the soma from the psyche. If one has access to a pain clinic, the patient may receive the treatment and support that she needs. The surgeon, however, should continue to see the patient on a regular basis.

REFERENCES

1. Aboudib JH Jr, de Castro CC, Coehlo RS, et al. Analysis of late results in postpregnancy mammoplasty. *Ann Plast Surg* 1991;20:111–116.
2. Berg A, Palmer B. Quality assurance in plastic surgery: reduction mammaplasty. *Scand J Plast Reconstr Hand Surg* 1997;31: 327–331.
3. Brown DM, Young VL. Reduction mammaplasty for macromastia. *Aesthetic Plast Surg* 1993;17:211–223.
4. Kinell I, Beausang-Linder M, Ohlsen L. The effect on the preoperative symptoms and the late results of Skoog's reduction mammoplasty. *Scand J Plast Reconstr Hand Surg* 1990;24:61–65.
5. Lieberman C. Corrective surgery for mammary hypertrophy on ambulant patients. *Am J Cosmetic Surg* 1996;13:25–29.
6. Tobin HA, Houting TV. Breast reduction—an analysis of 105 cases comparing the superior–and inferior–pedicle techniques. *Am J Cosmetic Surg* 1996;13:31–46.
7. Wallace WH, Thompson WOB, Smith RA, et al. Reduction mammaplasty using the inferior pedicle technique. *Ann Plast Surg* 1998;40:235–240.
8. Goldwyn RM. Complications and unfavorable results of reduction mammaplasty. In: Goldwyn RM, ed. *Reduction mammaplasty.* Boston: Little, Brown and Company, 1990: 561–577.
9. Mandrekas AD, Zambacos GJ, Anastasopoulos A, et al. Reduction mammaplasty with the inferior pedicle technique: early and late complications in 371 patients. *Br J Plast Surg* 1996;49:442–446.
10. McKissock PK. Reduction mammaplasty. In: Courtiss EH, ed. *Aesthetic surgery. Trouble: how to avoid it and how to treat it.* St. Louis: Mosby, 1978:189–203.
11. McKissock PK. Complications and undesirable results with reduction mammaplasty. In: Goldwyn RM, ed. *The unfavorable result in plastic surgery: avoidance and treatment,* 2nd ed. Boston: Little, Brown and Company, 1984:739–752.
12. Losee JE, Serletti JM, Kreipe RE, et al. Mammaplasty in patients with bulimia nervosa. *Ann Plast Surg* 1997;39:443–446.
13. Sgouras N, Porfyris E, Harkiolakis J, et al. Incidental histopathological findings in patients with reduction mammaplasty. In:

Hinderer UT, Vilar-Sancho B, Moll JQ, eds. *Proceedings of the X Congress of the International Confederation for Plastic and Reconstructive Surgery, Madrid, 28 June–3 July 1992.* Amsterdam: Excerpta Medica, 1992:653–654.

14. Strombeck JL. The Strombeck procedure for reduction mammaplasty. In: Goldwyn RM, ed. *Reduction mammaplasty.* Boston: Little, Brown and Company, 1990:131–146.
15. Titley OG, Armstrong AP, Christie JL, et al. Pathological findings in breast surgery. *Br J Plast Surg* 1996;49:447–451.
16. Jaspars JJP, Posma AN, van Immerseel AH, et al. The cutaneous innervation of the female breast and nipple-areola complex: indications for surgery. *Br J Plast Surg* 1997;50:249–259.
17. Sarhadi NS, Soutar DS. Nerve supply of the nipple: only from the fourth or from several intercostal nerves? A clinical experiment and an anatomical investigation. *Eur J Plast Surg* 1997;20: 209–211.
18. Spear SL, Hoffman S. Relocation of the displaced nipple-areola by reciprocal skin grafts. *Plast Reconstr Surg* 1998;101:1355–1358.
19. O'neal RM Goldstein JA, Roluich R, et al. Reduction mammaplasty with free-nipple transplantation: indications and technical refinements. *Ann Plast Surg* 1991;26:117–121.
20. DeBono R, Rao GS. Vasoconstrictor infiltration in breast reduction surgery: is it harmful? *Br J Plast Surg* 1997;50:260–262.
21. Gross MP, Apesos J. The use of leeches for treatment of venous congestion of the ripple following breast surgery. *Aesthetic Plast Surg* 1992;16:343–348.
22. Ransjo U, Asplund OA, Gylbert L, et al. Bacteria in the female breast. *Scand J Plast Reconstr Surg* 1985;19:87–89.
23. Rand RP, Bostwick J III. Pyoderma gangrenosum. *Perspect Surg* 1988;2:176–180.
24. Cruse PJE, Foord R. A five-year prospective study of 23,649 wounds. *Arch Surg* 1973;107:206–210.
25. Tang CL, Brown MH, Levine R, et al. Breast cancer found at the time of reduction mammaplasty. *Can J Plast Surg* 1998;6:52.
26. Green RA, Dowden RV. Mondor's disease in plastic surgery patients. *Ann Plast Surg* 1988;20:231–235.
27. Benelli L. Technique de plastic mammarie le "round block." *Rev Fr Chir Esth* 1988;13:7–11.
28. Chen TH, Wei F-C. The evolution of the vertical reduction mammaplasty: the s approach. *Aesthetic Plast Surg* 1997;21:97-104.
29. Gray LN. Liposuction breast reduction. *Aesthetic Plast Surg* 1998;22:159–162.
30. Lassus CL. Breast reduction: evolution of a technique–a single vertical scar. *Aesthetic Plast Surg* 1987;11:107–112.
31. Lejour M, Abboud M. Vertical mammaplasty without inframammary scar and with breast liposuction. *Perspect Plast Surg* 1990;4:67–90.
32. Lejour M. Vertical mammaplasty as secondary surgery after other techniques. *Aesthetic Plast Surg* 1997;21:403–407.
33. Marchac. D. Reduction mammaplasty with a short horizontal scar In: Goldwyn RM, ed. *Reduction mammaplasty.* Boston: Little, Brown and Company, 1990:317–335.
34. Shin KS. Reduction mammaplasty with the short submammary scar (s-s) technique In: Hinderer UT, Vilar-Sancho B, Moll JQ, eds. *Proceedings of the X Congress of the International Confederation for Plastic and Reconstructive Surgery, Madrid, 28 June–3 July 1992.* Amsterdam: Excerpta Medica, 1992:595–596.
35. Thomas WO, Moline S, Harris CN. Design-enhanced breast reduction: an approach for very large, very ptotic breasts without a vertical incision. *Ann Plast Surg* 1998;40:229–234.
36. Toledo LS. Mammaplasty using liposuction and the periareolar incision. *Aesthetic Plast Surg* 1989;13:9–13.
37. Benelli L. A new periareolar mammaplasty: round block technique. *Aesthetic Plast Surg* 1990;14:99
38. Hallock GG, Altobelli JA. Prevention of the teardrop areola following the inferior pedicle technique in breast reduction. *Plast Reconstr Surg* 1988;82:531–534.
39. Isaacs G, Romer L, Tudball C. Breast lumps after reduction mammaplasty. *Ann Plast Surg*1985;15:394–399.
40. Haseker B. The application of de-epithelialised "turn-over" flaps to the treatment of inverted nipples. *Br J Plast Surg* 1984;37: 253–255.
41. Hinderer UT, Del Rio JL. Treatment of the postoperative inverted nipple with or without asymmetry of the areola. *Aesthetic Plast Surg* 1983;7:139–144.
42. Crestinu JM. Inverted nipple: the new method of correction. *Aesthetic Plast Surg* 1989;13:189–197.
43. Raffel B. Technique for correction of areola misplacement with no new scars. *Plast Reconstr Surg*1991;88:895–897.
44. Menendez-Graino F, Fernandez CP, Burrieza PI. Galactorrhea after reduction mammaplasty. *Plast Reconstr Surg* 1990;85: 645–646.
45. Vilain R, Mitz V. The Biesenberger technique in mammary ptosis and hypertrophy. In: Goldwyn RM, ed. *Long-term results in plastic and reconstructive surgery.* Boston: Little, Brown and Company, 1980:708–734.
46. Hoffman S. Medicalegal aspects of reduction mammaplasty. In: Goldwyn RM. ed. *Reduction Mammaplasty.* Boston: Little, Brown and Company, 1989:59.
47. Courtiss EH, Goldwyn RM. Breast sensation before and after plastic surgery. *Plast Reconstr Surg* 1976;58:1–13.
48. Craig RDP, Sykes PA. Nipple sensitivity following reduction mammaplasty. *Br J Plast Surg* 1970;23:165–172.

SUGGESTED READING

Hinderer U. Plastia mamaria modelante de dermoplexia superficial y retromamaria. *Rev Esp Cir Plast* 1972;5:65–86.

Discussion

REDUCTION MAMMAPLASTY

SAUL HOFFMAN

Reduction mammaplasty is one of the most common operations done by plastic surgeons. There were approximately 48,000 breast reduction procedures performed in 1997, and 90,000 were performed 3 years later, an increase of 88%. Although most of these women were satisfied with their results, not all were, and some dissatisfied patients were unhappy enough to begin a malpractice action against their plastic surgeons. In the words of Dr. Paul McKissock, "The nature of surgery for breast reduction, with all its attendant risks, makes it a fertile field for complications, beyond which, moreover, there lies a vast minefield of potential errors that are hazard to the unwary surgeon."

Dr. Goldwyn's chapter should be read and re-read by all plastic surgeons who do this operation. In it, he gives the reader the benefit of his vast experience. By following his advice, many of the complications and poor results can be prevented.

In 1989, a questionnaire was sent to the members of The American Society of Plastic and Reconstructive Surgery in a sort of outcome study, in an effort to determine the degree of patient satisfaction, the complication rate, and the incidence of malpractice actions. Eleven percent of the responding surgeons stated that a malpractice suit had been precipitated by a dissatisfied reduction mammaplasty patient.

The majority of the unhappy patients complained about the appearance of their scars. This led to a proliferation of techniques to reduce the amount of scarring. Other areas of dissatisfaction were asymmetry, loss of sensation, and nipple position.

Dr. Goldwyn stresses several important principles, including proper selection of patients and a detailed informed consent. A careful discussion with the patient is mandatory in order to determine what she expects and to inform her about the limitations as well as the possible complications. It may be helpful to show photographs to help the patient understand what to expect. The tendency to show only good results should be avoided. The possible need for future revision should be part of the discussion. This should include a discussion of payment policies for revisional surgery, because patients who require revision may be upset by the additional unexpected charges.

Dr. Goldwyn's chapter covers this subject in great detail. Nothing is left out. Once again, I urge everyone to study this chapter carefully.

SUGGESTED READING

Hoffman S. Medicolegal aspects of reduction mammaplasty. In: Goldwyn RM, ed. *Reduction mammaplasty.* Boston: Little, Brown and Company, 1989:59.

S. Hoffman: Department of Surgery, Mount Sinai School of Medicine, New York, New York

63

BODY CONTOURING BY LIPOPLASTY

PETER B. FODOR

Lipoplasty rapidly gained popularity after the early 1980s and remained the most commonly performed aesthetic procedure. In the great majority of patients, the recovery is uneventful, scarring is minimal, if not negligible, and the results are predictable. The satisfaction rate is high, and the reoccurrence of localized fat deposits is unusual. Abuse and misuse of the procedure results in unfavorable outcomes, which range from minor sequelae to serious complications. In addition to insufficient training, a casual or cavalierish attitude toward this seemingly simple operation is the most common cause for unsatisfactory results. There also has been a trend for wide-scale introduction of technical and technologic changes in advance of appropriate laboratory and clinical research backing these "innovations."

The routine procedure consisting of proper patient selection, judicious uses of wetting solutions, blunt-tipped cannulas, preservation of the superficial layer of subcutaneous fat, moderate-pressure postoperative garments, and a healthy postoperative lifestyle will produce a satisfactory result in most instances (Fig. 63-1)

As with most surgical procedures, prevention of unfavorable results is far simpler than their subsequent management. A comprehensive discussion of all aspects of liposuction is beyond the scope of this chapter; therefore, the "tips, tricks, and traps" I have helpful in carrying out the procedure will be emphasized. Specific treatments for various body regions will not be described.

PATIENT SELECTION

Wrong choices in psychological, medical, physical, and aesthetic evaluation lead to unsatisfactory results, nagging patients, more difficult repeat surgical interventions, and lawsuits.

The psychologically unfit patient or an individual with low self-esteem, marked anxiety, fear, paranoia, or unrealistic expectations can be difficult to diagnose preoperatively. Time spent with patients showing them representative photographs, encouraging patients to provide magazines or other pictures illustrating their expectations, and using computer imaging (not used in the author's practice) can go a long way in detecting a lurking psychological problem. First impressions, input from the office staff, and the prospective patient's attitudes toward previous aesthetic surgical outcomes and surgeons are all important. When in question, it is best to avoid surgery. The impression of needing an extensive psychological evaluation or a psychometric analysis in order to accept a patient for surgery is a warning sign by itself.

A comprehensive medical evaluation is in order for the lipoplasty patient as it is for other aesthetic procedures. Specifically, it should rule out a history of chronic lung disease, bleeding disorders, thromboembolic disease, and acute or chronic systemic diseases. For example, use of oral contraceptives places the patient at higher risk for pulmonary embolus. Lifestyle and dietary habits can lead to protein deficiency and fluid or electrolyte imbalance. In addition to bulimia, many people have bizarre dietary habits; others exercise excessively without adequate nutritional support and are chronically malnourished, with low iron source, low albumin levels, low potassium levels, or all three. Others may have taken medications such as fenfluramine-phentermine (Fen-Phen), dexfenfluramine (Redux), steroids, diuretics, cathartics, and other potentially hazardous medications in order to influence some aspect of their physiology. In addition to alcohol and recreational drug dependence, taking megadoses of certain vitamins and other over-the-counter remedies is common, for example, consumption of vitamin E, which can influence clotting.

Large-volume lipoplasty, defined arbitrarily by the author as removal in excess of 4,000 cc of supernatant fat in one operative session, should be considered only in patients of low anesthetic risk: American Society of Anesthesiologists class I patients who are at least in average aerobic shape and have preoperative hemoglobin and hematocrit measurements of above 11 g and 30%, respectively. A bleeding time to detect coagulopathy and an erythrocyte sedimentation rate, although nonspecific, detect cryptic disease processes and are informative. Testing for hepatitis B or C, or the human immunodeficiency virus, although prudent, does not remove all risks.

Complete physical examination should evaluate patients for preexisting orthopedic and neurologic conditions that may be aggravated when the patient is put under anesthesia on the operating table.

P. B. Fodor: Department of Plastic Surgery, University of California Los Angeles Medical Center, Los Angeles, California

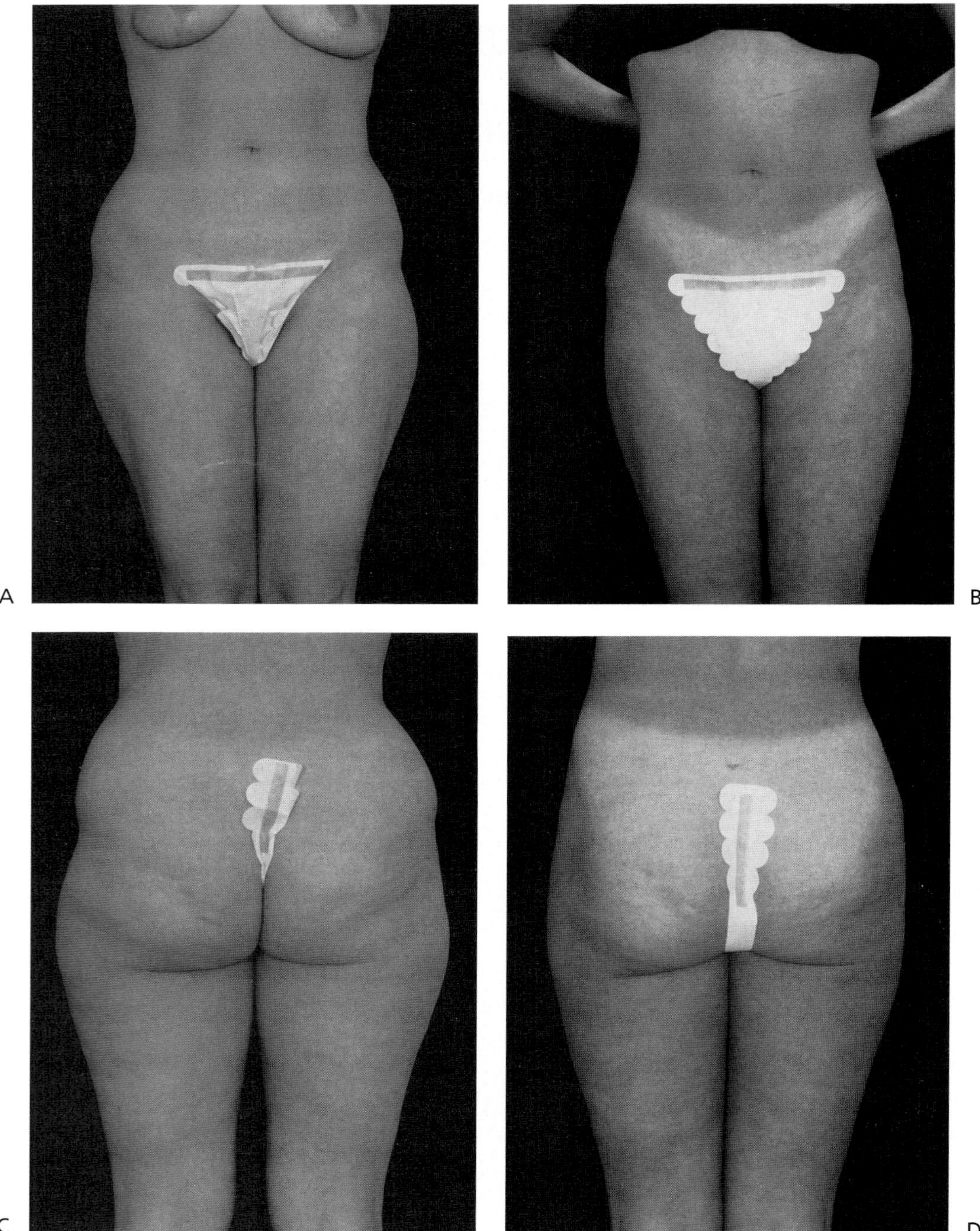

FIGURE 63-1. A 31-year-old patient before **(A,C,E)** and after **(B,D,F)** liposuction of the abdomen, inner knees, inner and outer thighs, and hip rolls. The volume removed was 3,560 cc.

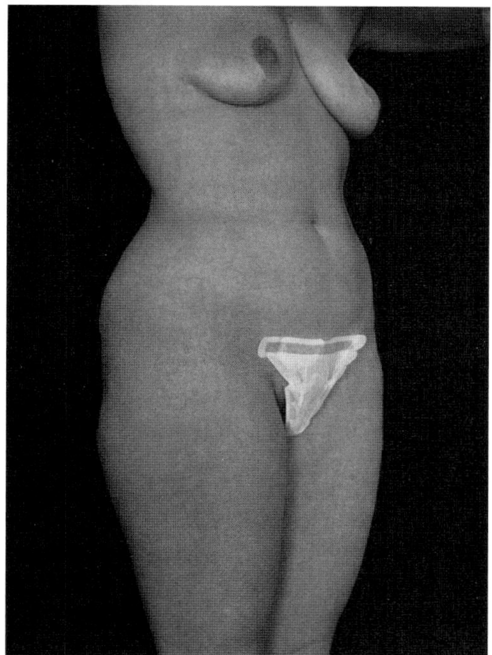

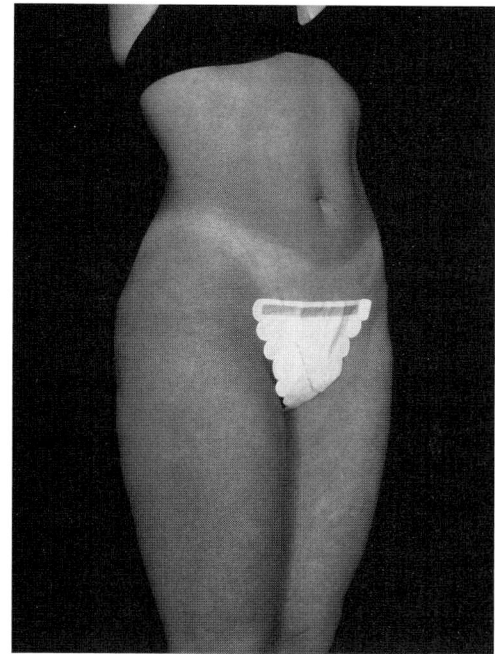

FIGURE 63-1. (*Continued*)

From an aesthetic standpoint, the ideal patient for lipoplasty is a relatively healthy thin young person with highly localized fatty excess: "figure faults" with taut skin.

The *average candidate* is over 40 years of age, weighs 15 to 20 pounds over ideal, has a history of weight fluctuations, and has some degree of skin relaxation and/or striae. Although such a patient will experience some improvement from lipoplasty, which may incorporate superficial suction, autologous fat transfer (AFT), and intraoperative and postoperative Endermologie, he or she should be informed that subsequent suctioning and dermolipectomy may be necessary for the most optimal result.

The *less than ideal patient* is older, is more than 20 pounds overweight or generally obese, has a history of weight fluctuations, and has clearly loose skin. Striae, soft tissue ptosis with cascading folds of redundant skin, the beginning of abdominal ptosis, banana rolls (sometimes multiple), inner thigh ptosis, or a combination of these features are present on physical examination. In this group, patients older than 55 years seem more readily satisfied with the results of the procedure than their younger counterparts. The patient should repeatedly be informed before surgery of the limitations imposed by their anatomy. A more conservative approach followed by secondary suctioning, after interim skin contraction, and eventual dermolipectomy may be required.

Visual inspection is not sufficient for adequate preoperative evaluation. Palpation for skin turgor, elasticity, and strength is important. If pinched skin does not return instantly to normal position, lipoplasty by itself is a poor choice. The pinch test demonstrates the difference between body regions with excess localized fat deposits and the surrounding areas. For example, pinching the hypogastric area should demonstrate thickness several folds over fat lateral to it. Patients readily relate to this demonstration. It helps them to understand that not all fat is to be removed, that what remains will be in better proportion to the rest of the body, and that what is left is more important than what is removed. In men with large "beer bellies," the pinch test often demonstrates that the epigastric area has an amount of fat similar to the area lateral to it, which renders this type of patient a poor candidate for liposuction. In these individuals, most of the fat is intra-abdominal (greater omentum) and retroperitoneal.

Showing Polaroid photographs, especially from the posterior view, to patients during consultation is an important tool to demonstrate what can and, as importantly, what cannot be done about their concerns.

PREOPERATIVE MARKINGS

Patient markings are carried out with the patient in a standing position and usually are done in a topographic manner. Sights of maximum removal and dells or valleys are appropriately noted. In addition to the localized fat deposits to be suctioned, the areas to be augmented with AFT, undesirable skin adhesions to underlying tissue (such as the folds between back rolls), and location of folds to be created (such as better definition of the gluteal folds or design of abdominal etching) are marked. Excess incisions needed to reach the areas to be suctioned are placed as close as possible. Shorter cannulas provide better control. Using indelible marking pens of different colors is useful. When cannula (without suctioning) discontinuous undermining is planned to facilitate skin contraction beyond the borders of suctioning (as in larger cases of gynecomastia), this is also drawn. Polaroid photographs taken with the markings in place are used to confirm the surgical plans with the patient and serve as documentation of what was treated. Standardized multiple-view preoperative and postoperative photographs are taken.

SURGICAL INTERVENTION

Postoperative garment size is determined before surgery. Prepping, whether circumferential (in the standing position) or sequential (on the operating table), is a function of the body areas to be treated and the surgeon's preference. Surgeon's preference also dictates optimal patient positioning. Before induction of anesthesia, the different patient positions on the operating table required for a given procedure and the placement of access incisions is checked and adjusted as necessary. Attention is given to padding pressure points (by protecting bony prominences), and care is taken in turning and in preventing injury to the extremities, brachial plexus, face, chest, and genitalia. The neck should be placed in the normal postural position to avoid pinching of the cervical roots.

WETTING SOLUTIONS, ANESTHESIA, AND LARGE-VOLUME REMOVALS

Wetting solutions have played a pivotal role in lipoplasty. Schrudde first reported on "lipexeresis" (lipexhairesis), which is the removal of subcutaneous fat through small incisions, using blind small scissors undermining and a sharp curette-like instrument. No wetting solution, i.e., "the dry technique," was used (1). Complications were many.

Yves-Gerard Illouz (2), the forerunner of modern lipoplasty in the early 1980s, reported on the blunt-tip cannula technique. No undermining, no sharp instruments, and very high vacuum were used to extract fat. The complications, such as prolonged drainage, lymphorrhea, hematoma, and skin necrosis, seen with sharp instrumentation were reduced by sparing most of the structures intervening between skin and muscle fascia. Illouz also infused a hypotonic hyaluronidase-containing fluid to liquefy the fat before aspiration, i.e., "the wet technique," and termed the procedure lipolysis. He initially used 200 to 300 mL of infusate, regardless of the amount of estimated aspirate. Blood loss in the aspirate diminished by about half from the 25% to 40% seen with the dry technique. In 1984, Hetter (3) added epinephrine in low concentrations to the infusate. Blood in the aspirate decreased further to about 4% to 8%.

Blood loss in the aspirate can be assessed by a hematocrit measurement, known as the lipocrit, in a sample obtained from either the centrifuged undecanted aspirate or from the infranatant portion of the decanted specimen.

In 1986, the "superwet" concept of infusing approximately 1 mL of epinephrine-containing isotonic solution for each milliliter of estimated aspirate was introduced by Fodor (4). This resulted is further reduction of blood in the aspirate to a lipocrit of less than 1% (5).

With any technique there is additional blood in the tissues, acute and delayed, which is not assessed by lipocrit measurements in the aspirate. The patient's hemoglobin level will fall substantially (1 to 3 g/L) when measured 5 days postoperatively (5). Therefore, a yellow aspirate in itself is not indicative of total blood loss. With all lipoplasty operations, blood and/or serum is lost into a third space.

Table 63-1 lists the lipocrit values reported for different lipoplasty approaches.

Until the early 1990s, lipoplasty was the most commonly performed aesthetic surgical procedure and had the lowest rate of complications. At this time, the "tumescent technique," which consists of infusing massive amounts of wetting solutions, using tissue turgor as an endpoint, was popularized. These solutions contain large amounts of lidocaine (Xylocaine), and the goal was to provide anesthesia for the procedure. Proponents of this technique consider the need for an intravenous line and the presence of an anesthesiologist during the procedure unnecessary. The tumescent technique, as popularized primarily by dermatologists (6,7), is the very gradual (up to 3 hours) installation of wetting solution until there is tissue turgor, the body area is white, and the skin has a *peau d'orange* appearance. Advocates of this technique state that they inject between 3 and 6 mL of wetting solution per milliliter of estimated aspirate. Thus, many liters of lidocaine-containing fluid may be injected, which amounts to a highly variable clysis. The volumes removed as reported by the advocates of the technique often are much larger than with other methods. However, the aspirate contains much more of the instilled wetting solutions and cannot be compared with volumes removed when smaller amounts of wetting solutions are used. With the superwet

TABLE 63-1. EVOLUTION OF WETTING SOLUTIONS USED IN LIPOPLASTY

Technique	Year	Author	Lipocrit
Dry	1983	Fournier	20–40%
	1992	Courtiss	
Wet	1980	Illouz	8–10%
Wet + Epinephrine	1984	Hetter	4–8%
Superwet	1986	Fodor	
	1990	Samdal	1%
Tumescent	1993	Klein	1%

method, for example, the supernatant fat routinely comprises as much as 75% to 80% of the aspirate.

For small to moderate volumes of removal, any technique is comparatively safe when performed in a healthy, young, aerobically fit patient. The potentially hazardous nature of massive wetting solution infusion techniques applied to large-volume lipoplasty can result in fluid and lidocaine overload. This scenario was readily predictable (8) as the trend using the tumescent technique for large-volume removals was adopted around 1994. Unfortunately, the incidence of major complications and fatalities associated with lipoplasty rose rapidly after 1995 (Table 63-2). Consequently, the public's perception of the procedure changed from a safe to a hazardous one.

Detailed analysis of fluid overload and lidocaine toxicity issues will not be presented in this chapter. These topics are well described elsewhere (4,8–13) and will be mentioned here only in general terms. Patient tolerance to initial fluid load and the ability to maintain postoperative fluid and electrolyte balance are determined by many factors, such as general health, age, obesity, aerobic condition, volume of aspirate, and size of the surface area suctioned. All of these factors should be considered when determining the safe volume of infusate and aspirate. Flow sheets documenting input and removal volumes are recommended. Lipocrit measurements and the percentage of supernatant fat in the aspirate also are informative.

It is generally accepted that lidocaine up to 35 mg/kg, injected in the subcutaneous fat in solutions containing epinephrine, is safe. It is notable, however, that this dose is in direct contrast with the recommendation of less than 7 mg/kg published in the *Physicians' Desk Reference* (14). Absorption rates vary significantly, and measurements of peak plasma lidocaine levels are more meaningful than absolute amounts of injected lidocaine in assessing potential toxicity. The danger is amplified by the fact that lidocaine absorption from the subcutaneous fat can peak as late as 10 to 12 hours after injection (6,13,15), by which time the patient usually has been discharged from the surgical facility. Other factors can affect lidocaine toxicity, such as the amount of unbound versus protein-bound lidocaine. In turn, protein binding is influenced by several factors, such as stress, chronic disease, cigarette smoking, oral contraceptives, and anorexiants. Therefore, the correlation between total plasma lidocaine concentration and the predictability of specific toxicity occurring in a given patient is weak at best.

TABLE 63-2. LIPOPLASTY FATALITIES IN THE UNITED STATES

- 1982–1995: ~12 deaths
  Primarily from sepsis, pulmonary embolus

Widespread adaption of tumescent technique

- 1995–1997: ~100 deaths
  Primarily from fluid overload and lidocaine toxicity

TABLE 63-3. COMPARISON OF SUPERWET AND TUMESCENT TECHNIQUES

	Superwet (~1 cc/cc aspirate)	Tumescent (~3 cc/cc aspirate)
Volume removal	+ + +	+ + +
Blood loss	− − −	− − −
Ecchymosis	− − −	− − −
Time to inject	+	+ + +
Fluid load	+	+ + +
Tissue turgor	+	+ + +
Ease to sculpt	+	? ?
Lidocaine load	0 → +	+ + +

In summary, the benefits of the tumescent technique, e.g., low blood loss and decreased need for colloid and crystalloid replacement, are realized with the "superwet technique," but without the hazards of delayed fluid uptake by large clysis, need for drainage, risk of pulmonary edema (9), and potential for lidocaine toxicity. Table 63-3 compares the tumescent and superwet techniques.

Several different formulations of wetting solutions have been recommended (4,7,16). These formulations do not differ significantly from each other. For most part, they are isotonic in nature and contain low concentrations of epinephrine and lidocaine. The formulation I currently favor is listed in Table 63-4.

As a general rule, the volume of wetting solutions administered to a patient undergoing a lipoplasty procedure should not be more than 5,000 mL. The lidocaine load should not exceed 35 mg/kg of body weight.

Bupivacaine (Marcaine) or lidocaine is mixed in the solution to provide preemptive and some postoperative analgesia. Which local agent is used from the standpoint of toxicity is a mute point. An extensive review of the literature failed to disclose any evidence of cardiac toxicity associated with bupivacaine when infused in low concentration into subcutaneous fat. This use of local anesthetics in the wetting solutions is notably different from the use of lidocaine as proposed with the tumescent technique. Although small-volume removals can be performed safely with the analgesia provided by the lidocaine contained in the wetting solutions, this author is of the definite opinion that wetting solutions are not a practical or safe anesthesia delivery system for major-volume lipoplasty. General or epidural anesthesia is recommended.

TABLE 63-4. INFUSION FORMULATION FOR SUPERWET TECHNIQUE

- Sequential/segmental infusion
- 1–1.5 mL infusate/mL of estimated aspirate
- 1,000 mL Ringer Lactate + 0.5–1 cc epinephrine 1/1,000
  + 25 mL 0.25% bupivacaine
  + 1 mL (40 mg) gentamicin
  +/– Hyaluronidase

TABLE 63-5. LIPOPLASTY CLASSIFICATION BY VOLUME OF ADIPO-ASPIRATE

• Small	<1,500 mL	40%
• Moderate	1,500–4,000 mL	40%
• Large	>4,000 mL	20%

Supranatant fat commonly ~75% of aspirate.

An arbitrary classification of lipoplasty patients according to the volume of aspirate currently used by the author is listed in Table 63-5. Large-volume lipoplasty carries a significantly higher risk. Patient tolerance for this procedure is a function of several different factors, and as such, safety considerations need to be accordingly observed. In addition to age and general health, the percentage of body surface area to be treated is important. The fluid shifts that occur after lipoplasty are not unlike those that occur after a second-degree burn. If the area of injury exceeds 15% of body surface area, morbidity rises disproportionately. The palmar surface of the patient's own hand and fingers represents 1% of the body surface.

The need to monitor fluid shifts and hemodynamic changes requires close intraoperative and postoperative monitoring, which is best provided by an accredited surgical facility. Injudicious ambulatory discharge of large-volume lipoplasty patients may lead to many potentially dire consequences, such as hypovolemia, oliguria, fat embolism syndrome, shock, renal shutdown, pulmonary embolism, and myocardial infarction.

Large volumes can be removed safely in properly selected patients. Our general guidelines for the preoperative, intraoperative, and postoperative care of lipoplasty patients are listed in Tables 63-6 through 63-8. It should be stressed that the amount of wetting solutions (crystalloids) delivered alters the amounts of intravenous fluids required over time. Close communication with the anesthesiologist and careful patient monitoring are essential. Sequential infusion, as opposed to infusing all areas to be suctioned at once, lessens acute fluid load by clysis and variability of tissue distortion by the wetting solutions. Uniform layering of infusion facilitates sculpting. For small volumes, such as treatment of necks or inner knees, 60-mL syringes with infusion cannulas are used. Infusion pumps are better suited for removal of larger volumes.

TABLE 63-6. SAFETY ISSUES IN LARGE-VOLUME LIPOPLASTY: PREOPERATIVE CONSIDERATIONS

- Low anesthetic risk: ASA class I
- Erythropoietin + RE for hematocrit <35%
- Discontinue Fen-Phen and other potentially hazardous prescription drugs
- Rule out past medical history of deep vain thrombosis
- Rule out lifestyle and dietary habits leading to protein deficiency and fluid and electrolyte imbalance
- Should be in at least average aerobic shape

TABLE 63-7. SAFETY ISSUES IN LARGE-VOLUME LIPOPLASTY: INTRAOPERATIVE CONSIDERATIONS

- Body heat preservation; silver cap, Bair Hugger, warm infusion fluids
- Anesthesia: general or epidural (not local)
- Superwet technique (not tumescent!!!)
- Low or only keep, open volumes of intravenous fluids
- Foley catheter
- Sequential pneumonic leg compression

SUBCUTANEOUS ANATOMY AND SURGICAL TECHNIQUE

The superficial fascia, an important membrane in some areas of the body and less well developed in others, divides the subcutaneous fat into a superficial areolar and a deeper laminar fat. Localized fat deposits are defined by the superficial fascia enveloping the deposit and fusing with the muscle fascia at the perimeter of the deposit. This fusion is strong and is readily felt when a cannula pierces through it. When a surgeon transgresses this resistance and inadvertently enters with suction the subcutaneous layer of fat, depressions, divots, or dimples can result. In body regions such as the neck, lower abdomen, and outer thighs, this deep fascial layer is well defined. In the epigastrium, hip rolls, knees, calves, and ankle, the superficial fascia is less well defined and is more like a fibrous structure resembling a honeycomb. The superficial fascia is anchored to the undersurface of the dermis by vertical arches of connective tissue, the retinacula cutis. When these are stretched beyond their limits of elasticity, dimples or *peau d'orange* as seen in cellulite occur.

The author believes that this entire superficial fibrous fascial system, which extends between the superficial muscular fascia and the undersurface of the dermis, is the human derivative of the panniculus carnosus (17). The vertical fibrous attachments play an essential role in skin contracture after liposuction. In conventional lipoplasty, suction of the deep fat compartment is common. This is the workhorse area, where the most improvement is seen in the majority of cases. The beginner should concentrate on these areas. Suction of the superficial layer as well as cannula "discontinuous undermining" over and adjacent to the area suctioned promotes postoperative skin contracture. Therefore, with the superficial technique, the procedure can be used for larger removals and can be offered to older patients and to

TABLE 63-8. SAFETY ISSUES IN LARGE-VOLUME LIPOPLASTY: POSTOPERATIVE CONSIDERATIONS

- Overnight observation
- Early ambulation
- Sequential pneumonic leg compression
- Patient able to void before discharge
- Hematocrit at 24 hours (of questionable value)

patients with more flaccid skin. Superficial suction does not eliminate skin excisional body sculpting procedures. Properly performed superficial suction reduces the need for dermolipectomies. Creative combination of these different techniques allows a customized approach for each patient. With experience, the conventional and superficial suction techniques can be combined skillfully. For example, when suctioning the abdomen, superficial and deep suction are used in the epigastrium. In the hypogastric area, the deep fat under the Scarpa fascia is suctioned primarily. Most suction in the neck is superficial to the platysma and hence is in the superficial layer.

Errors in fat removal from the superficial layer are highly visible. Fat removal from this layer should be as even as possible; otherwise, grooves and irregularities may result. Avoidance is far simpler than subsequent treatment. If a problem caused by excessive extraction is recognized at the time of the initial procedure, whether in standard or superficial suction, fat reinjected at that time seems to survive better than when done as part of a later procedure. Many patients consult for correction of surface irregularities associated with various degrees of skin laxity. In many instances, the degree of preoperative skin redundancy was not fully appreciated, and superficial liposuction was carried out instead of dermolipectomy (Fig. 63-2). In other instances, these unfavorable results follow improper use of the superficial technique in a patient who was a good candidate for this approach. In most of these patients, the success rate of secondary surgery is modest at best. It is tedious to perform and consists of suction of the residual fat around the low points combined with AFT into the depressed areas (Figs. 63-3, 63-4). In other instances, additional suction and AFT are combined with skin resection procedures, such as an inner thigh-plasty (Fig. 63-5), or other dermolipectomies. These procedures are described elsewhere in this book.

Too superficial a level of suction using sharp cannulas that penetrate just subjacent to the dermis places the deep dermal plexus in jeopardy. This technique has the potential not only for creating surface irregularities, but also for chronic pigmentary, sensory changes, and even skin sloughs. These outcomes usually are permanent and not correctable (Fig. 63-6).

Briefly, cannulas should be blunt at the tip, with the opening(s) located sufficiently proximal from the tip to avoid inadvertent removal of subdermal fat. With smaller-lumen cannulas, the suction power and, therefore, the rate of removal are exponentially reduced. The finer the tunnels, the fewer waves and surface irregularities occur. Cannula diameter is reduced as the procedure progresses from initial debulking to fine sculpting and from a deeper to a more superficial level. Multihole cannulas extract fat quickly and therefore require greater attention. Cobra cannulas, which have their openings at the tip, and other combinations of cutting tip designs are useful in fibrous areas (for treatment of gynecomastia), the epigastrium, or the periumbilical area. Their use requires diligence.

For the vacuum source, the suction machine or the syringe aspiration technique can be used equally well. Familiarity with both is recommended. Personally, I favor pumps for speed, and use syringes only for small removals,

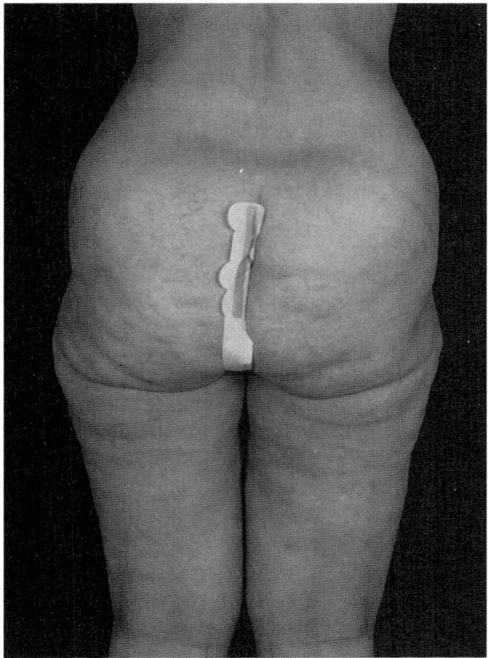
A

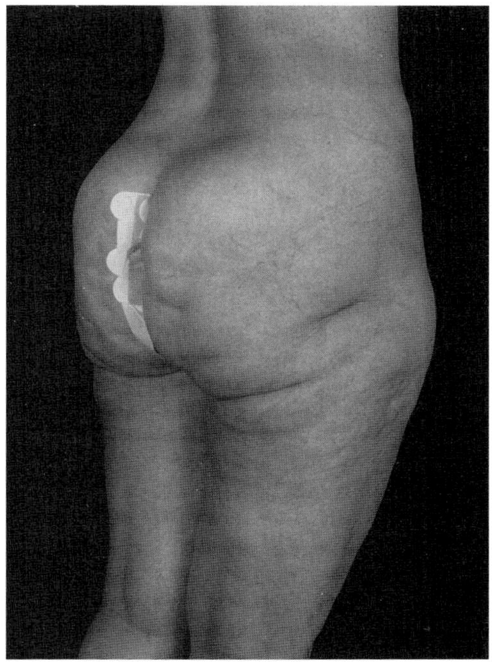
B

FIGURE 63-2. A,B: A 47-year-old patient 6 months after liposuction performed by another surgeon.

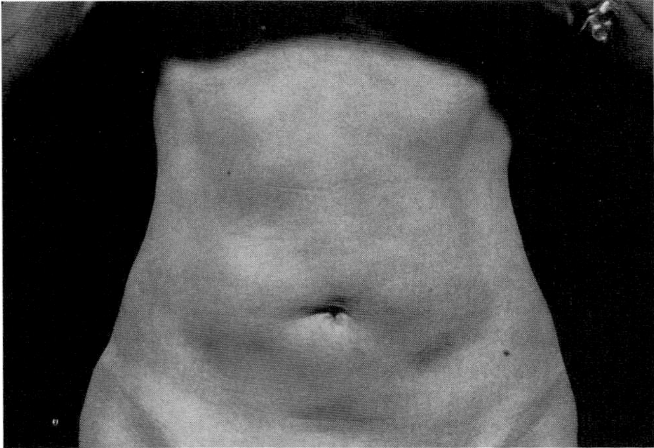

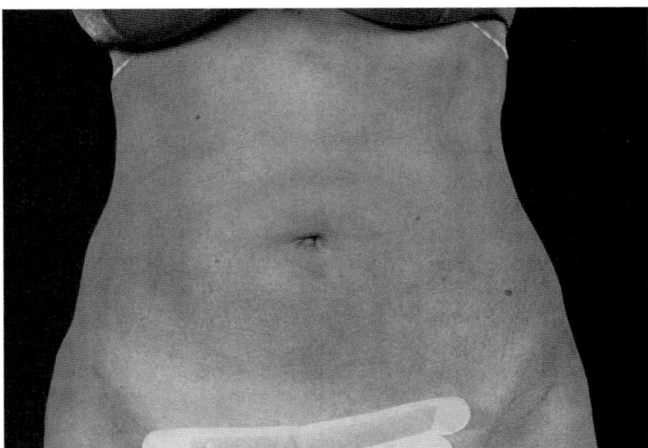

FIGURE 63-3. A 41-year-old patient before **(A)** and 2 years after **(B)** revision lipoplasty of the abdomen, including autologous fat transfer.

some touchup procedures, and to harvest fat for AFT. The skill of the surgeon is far more important than the type and size of the cannula or the suction source.

Pretunneling, i.e., passing the cannula when no suction is attached, helps to define the proper plane. The feel in the superficial layer is "gritty," whereas the feel in the deep fat is smoother. A cannula that is too pointed or has a sharp tip does not as readily provide this important tactile feedback. Suction, once applied, detracts from the tactile sense. By passing the cannula in regular radiating thrusts, a pseudoplane that better defines the fat to suction is developed. The easy movement of the cannula stops where the superficial fascia fuses at the limits of the localized fat deposits. When no suction is attached, a puncture wound into the superficial fat causes no lasting effect. Pretunneling is helpful to define the depth and extent of suction. The extraction should be in radial, not coalescing, tunnels, with long even strokes and additional passes where "plus" signs indicate more fat. The edges of the deposits are feathered, and "mesh undermining" without suction is extended laterally as needed. Cross tunneling at right angles to the first tunnels can result in additional fat extraction. Beware of overresection, and

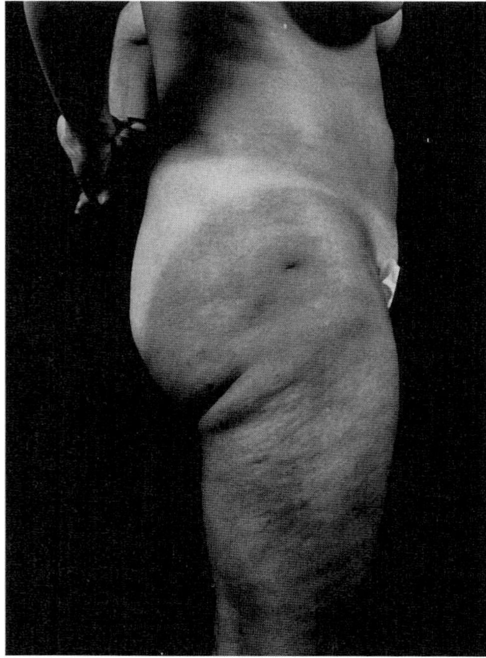

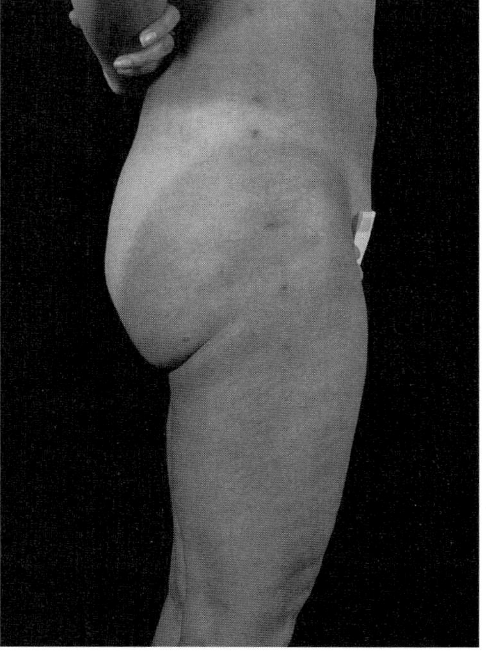

FIGURE 63-4. A 45-year-old patient before **(A)** and 3.5 years after **(B)** revision lipoplasty of the lateral thighs, including autologous fat transfer.

A 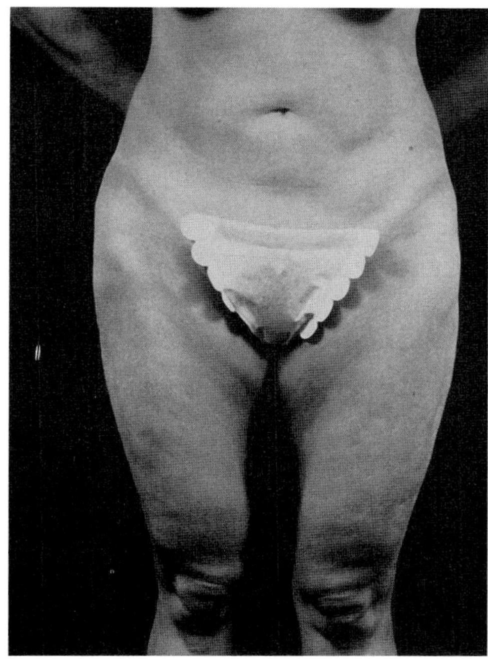 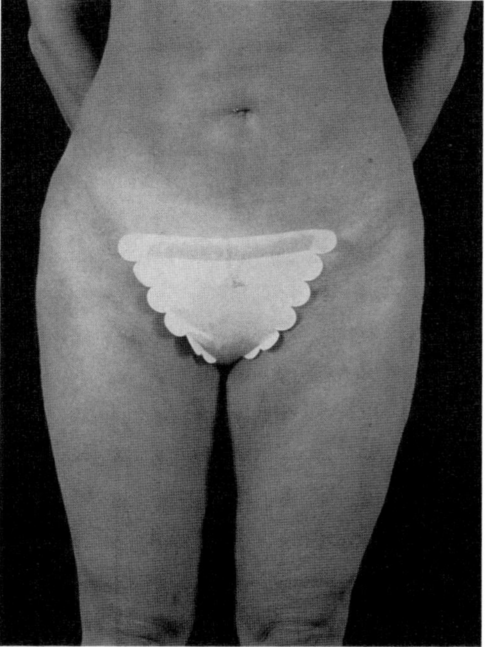 B

FIGURE 63-5. A 41-year-old patient before **(A)** and 2 years after **(B)** revision inner thigh surgery consisting of secondary lipoplasty, Colles fascia anchor medial thigh-plasty, and inner thigh autologous fat transfer.

avoid an unpleasant surprise by inspecting from different angles and performing the pinch and roll tests often. Avoid a side-to-side windshield wiper motion, which promotes seroma and pseudobursa formation. The cannula lumen is not turned against the deep dermal surface (unless an indentation is being created on purpose), and persistent overworking of a bloody area is avoided.

Knowing when to stop is the hardest part of all endeavors. What is left behind, not how much is extracted, determines the quality of the result. When the aspirate turns

A 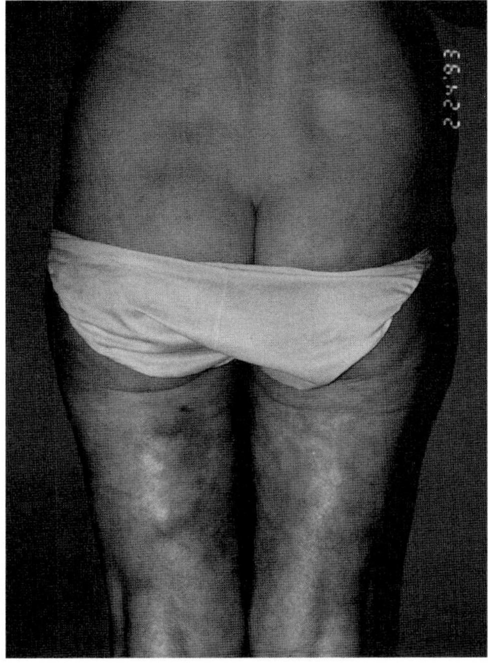 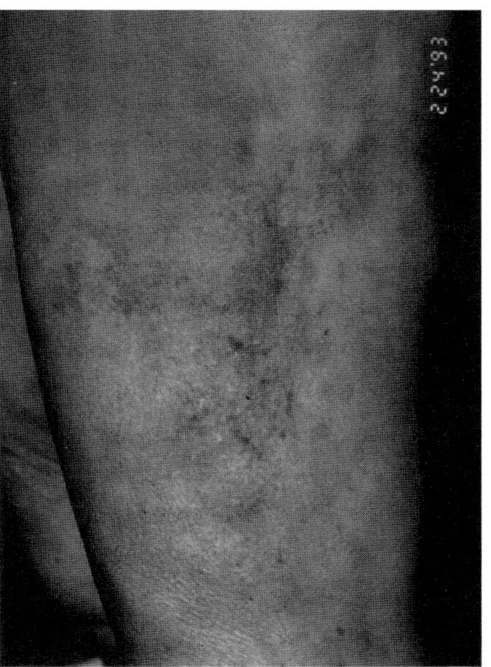 B

FIGURE 63-6. A,B: A 60-year-old woman 9 months after "superficial lipoplasty."

bloody, it is time to move to the next tunnel. If the skin appears lax, especially over the abdomen and inner or outer thighs, it is reasonable to stop or, based on the surgeon's skill and experience, to proceed with the superficial technique. Be careful and remember that secondary suction after initial skin contracture, performed some months later, is an option.

It is important to compare the extracted area for evenness, within itself and to the surrounding untreated areas, visually and by palpation. Aesthetic sense is hard to describe and is more innate than learned. Overresections performed in an attempt to comply with a patient's preoperative wishes for a "flat stomach" or "skinny straight thighs" may not in proportion with aesthetically natural curves of the body, which should be known and respected. For example, when less fat than ideal is left over the trochanter in a female patient with residual hip rolls, she will appear masculinized in the posterior view. Similarly, a scaphoid abdomen void of any periumbilical fullness is not feminine in appearance.

Small refinements can be made with fine cannulas attached to low suction or to syringes. Autologous fat after anaerobic washing and decanting can be transferred to fill areas of preexisting depressions or overresection. Selective division of retinacula cutis combined with rolling massage and injection of a thin layer of autologous fat following superficial suction has resulted in limited improvement in the appearance of cellulite.

Since late 1996 in the author's practice, Endermologie has been added intraoperatively to lipoplasty in two phases: just after infusion of wetting solutions for their better dispersion and after fat extraction to assist with even distribution of the remaining fat. Postoperative edema and ecchymosis have been reduced dramatically by this maneuver. Long-term smoother postoperative skin surfaces have been noted. These subjective observations have been partially substantiated in laboratory and clinical studies (18–20).

Application of focused energy to lipoplasty has excited interest. A laser-tipped unit was subjected to a multicenter study (21), but the project was abandoned.

The benefits of applying ultrasound energy after infusion of wetting solutions and before fat extraction, such as external ultrasound-assisted lipoplasty (EUAL), has not yet been clearly defined. It appears that it may assist with dispersion of wetting solutions. Contralateral or other forms of controlled studies are lacking. The concept of using external ultrasound for body sculpting without fat extraction, known by some as external hydrolipoclasia, although attractive to patients, has not proved to be of any benefit. The hazardous effects of high-frequency ultrasound energy on biologic structures are unknown at best. Internal ultrasound-assisted lipoplasty (UAL) also has been advocated as a technologic advance in lipoplasty. The fat is emulsified concurrently (hollow cannula technology) or before (solid probe technology) its extraction. To date, the process of emulsification is not fully understood. Although cavitation has been proposed as the principal mechanism, the micro "sledge hammer" effect, imparted by the application of the ultrasound energy to the adipose tissue, also may play an important role. In addition to thermal effects, concerns regarding sonoluminescence and sonochemistry have been raised. Studies supporting the safety of UAL have been reported (22–25). Additional experience and research combined with evolving technology will define the proper place for UAL in body sculpting surgery. At this point in its evolution, when safety precautions are taken, it can be of benefit in the treatment of fibrous areas, such as gynecomastia, back rolls, hip rolls, and the epigastrium, and in secondary suction by diminishing tissue resistance encountered by the advancing cannula.

Larger removals, lower blood loss, better skin contraction/retraction, faster recovery, and smoother postoperative skin surfaces have not been demonstrated convincingly enough to justify replacement of traditional lipoplasty with UAL. Currently, it is best used in combination with the traditional technique (22,25). In addition to expense, there is a tedious learning curve for the surgeon, imposition on the staff, and side effects particular to UAL, including larger access incisions, longer surgical times, and higher seroma and dysesthesia rates. The extracted fat is unsuitable for transfer. Thermal damage can occur at the access incisions and at distant sites, but appropriate training can minimize most of these. In UAL, the following measures are recommended: skin protectors at incision sites, a wet surgical towel between the shaft of the cannula and the subjacent skin in contact with it, constant cannula movement while ultrasound energy is being delivered, avoiding extensive ultrasound times in one location (less than 10 minutes), avoiding "end hits," and keeping the cannula at least 1 cm below the deep surface of the dermis. These general recommendations apply to all UAL devices currently available in the United States. The more powerful the unit is, the steeper the learning curve and the lower the relative safety of the device. The relative power and safety ratings of these machines based on the author's personal opinion and experience in over 200 cases are listed in Table 63-9. These relative power ratings represent the maximum output these units are capable of delivering. The

TABLE 63-9. POWER AND SAFETY RATINGS OF ULTRASOUND-ASSISTED LIPOPLASTY MACHINES[a]

Equipment	Manufacturer	Power	Safety
First-generation solid (probe) technology	SMEI	+++++	+
Second-generation hollow (cannula) technology	Medicamat	+	++++
	Surgitron	+++	+++
	Sebbin	++	++++
	MDA	++	+
	Mentor	+++	++
	Morwel	+	+++

[a]Arbitrary subjective ratings.

novice UAL surgeon is advised to begin with a lower setting, especially if using one of the more powerful devices. The SMEI machine, which has a long probe with less than 30 W of output and a short probe with less than 15 W of output, falls into this category. Technical improvements in UAL machines are constantly being made. The names of the machines change as some companies enter and others abandon their manufacturing. A wet environment is mandatory for fat emulsification. The superwet technique used in combination with UAL adequately satisfies this requirement without the hazards imposed by the tumescent approach. As long as the superficial layer of fat is not exposed to ultrasound energy, the more severe complications, such as permanent pigmentary and prolonged, if not permanent, sensory changes, fibrosis, and extensive skin sloughs, can be mostly avoided. The solid probe approach, unlike the hollow cannula method, does not provide the surgeon with continuous visual feedback of the emulsified fatty material. Still, the solid probe technique may prove to be safer because the subcutaneous structures (nerves, lymphatics, blood vessels, and deep dermis) are not suctioned up against the tip of the cannula, where most of the ultrasound energy is being delivered. When first beginning UAL, the value of attending properly selected teaching courses, cautious graduated experience, and solid surgical judgment cannot be overemphasized.

Another focused-energy cannula approach on the horizon is a reciprocating device marketed by Microaire. This device currently is powered by pressurized nitrogen readily available in most operating rooms. Early trials in several centers are in progress. To date, the best application is similar to UAL, but at a fraction of the cost. It lessens resistance to cannula passage in body regions where the fat is fibrous. Preliminary observations show that the aspirate, while bloodless, remains suitable for AFT.

More than any other aesthetic procedure, lipoplasty has witnessed the wide-scale clinical introduction of new modalities without adequate research preceding their popularization. Although patients are quick to request these "innovations," surgeons need to proceed with caution.

POSTOPERATIVE MANAGEMENT

The postoperative care of lipoplasty patients is straightforward. For treatment of discomfort, analgesics and muscle relaxants often suffice. Attention is paid to prevent thromboembolic phenomena and urinary retention and to ensure fluid and electrolyte balance.

A pressure garment is applied to provide even tension; a localized tourniquet effect is to be avoided. Padding with a sponge-like material can assist in accomplishing this. Tension should be relieved periodically, for example, by temporarily undoing the hook-and-loop closure of an abdominal binder.

Orthostatic hypotension is not uncommon, especially in patients who underwent large-volume removals. It almost invariably is transient in nature and responds to simple measures. If not, the patient should be evaluated immediately for the need for intravascular volume expansion to prevent oliguria, hypoxia, hemoconcentration, and embolic phenomena. Prompt treatment with oral fluids or, if necessary, crystalloids and/or hetastarch (Hespan) administration is imperative. Blood transfusion is used only as a last resort. It seldom, if ever, is necessary, as long as the safety guidelines for large-volume removals outlined earlier in this chapter are followed. In the author's lipoplasty practice expanding over 15 years, not a single patient received heterologous blood transfusion. Autologous transfusions also have been eliminated by the superwet technique and by pretreatment with erythropoietin in estimated removals exceeding 4,000 cc of supernatant fat.

The first dressing change is at 3 to 5 days, at which time access incision sutures are removed.

Perioperative antibiotics, postoperative Endermologie, or massage and ultrasound treatments can be used in accordance with the surgeon's preference and what is practical for a given patient. Although ultimately the results are indistinguishable at 1 year, physical therapy modalities are comforting during convalescence. The worried or anxious patient is especially well served by these measures.

Adipocyte regrowth is limited to nonexistent following lipoplasty. Some patients eat with abandon and gain weight primarily in body areas not suctioned. However, most patients experience a renewed enthusiasm for a lifestyle that incorporates a healthy diet and a moderate exercise program. These patients experience additional weight loss often far in excess of what was suctioned.

Gradual resumption of exercise or beginning exercise can begin safely 3 to 4 weeks after the procedure.

CONCLUSIONS

Nutritional counseling often is greatly appreciated by the post-lipoplasty patient. The suggestions made in this chapter will assist surgeons to avoid unfavorable results in lipoplasty. Experience with less complex procedures, combined with judicious application of new technology, is strongly recommended before advancing to more complex procedures and approaches.

REFERENCES

1. Rogers BD. The father of lipoplasty. *Lipoplasty Newsletter* 1991;8:6.
2. Illouz YG. Body contouring by lipolysis: a 5 year experience with over 3000 cases. *Plast Reconstr Surg* 1983;72:591.
3. Hetter GP. The effect of low dose epinephrine on the hematocrit drop following lipolysis. *Aesthetic Plast Surg* 1984;8:19.

4. Rohrich RJ, Beran SJ, Fodor PB. The role of subcutaneous infiltration in suction-assisted lipoplasty: a review. *Plast Reconstr Surg* 1992;99:514.
5. Samdal F, Amland PF, Bugge JF. Blood loss during suction-assisted lipectomy with large volumes of dilute adrenaline. *Scand J Plast Reconstr Hand Surg* 1995;29:161.
6. Klein JA. Tumescent technique for regional anesthesia permits lidocaine dose of 35 mg/kg for liposuction. *J Dermatol Surg Oncol* 1990;16:248.
7. Klein JA. The tumescent technique. *Dermatol Clin* 1994;8:425.
8. Fodor PB. Wetting solutions in aspirative lipoplasty: a plea for safety in liposuction. *Aesthetic Plast Surg* 1995;19:379.
9. Gilliland MD, Coates N. Tumescent liposuction complicated by pulmonary edema. *Plast Reconstr Surg* 1997;99:215.
10. Grazer FM, Meister FL. Factors contributing to adverse effects of the tumescent technique. *Aesthetic Surg J* 1997;17:411.
11. Grazer FM, Meister FL. Complications of the tumescent formula for liposuction. *Plast Reconstr Surg* 1997;100:1893.
12. Meister FL. Possible association between tumescent technique and life-threatening pulmonary complications. *Clin Plast Surg* 1996;23:642.
13. Mottura AA. Tumescent technique for liposuction. *Plast Reconstr Surg* 1994;94:1096.
14. *Physicians' desk reference.* Mountvale, NJ: Medical Economics Data Production Company, 1995:571.
15. Samdal F, Amland PF, Bugge JF. Plasma lidocaine levels during suction assisted lipectomy using large doses of dilute lidocaine with epinephrine. *Plast Reconstr Surg* 1994; 93:1217.
16. Hunstad JP. Tumescent and syringe liposculpture: a logical partnership. *Aesthetic Plast Surg* 1995;19:32.
17. Fodor PB. From the panniculus carnosus (PC) to the superficial fascia system (SFS). *Aesthetic Plast Surg* 1993;17:179.
18. Fodor PB, Watson J. Endermologie and Endermologie-assisted lipoplasty update. *Aesthetic Surg J* 1998;18:302.
19. Shack RB. Personal communication analysis of the cutaneous, subcutaneous and systemic effects of an Endermologie device in the porcine model. ASAPS Global Summit on Aesthetic Surgery, Los Angeles, California, May 3, 1998.
20. Watson J, Fodor PB. Personal communication physiologic effects of Endermologie: a preliminary report. *Aesthetic Surg J* 1998; 18:4.
21. Apfelberg DB, Rosenthal S, Hunstad JP, et al. Progress report on multicenter study of laser-assisted liposuction. *Aesthetic Plast Surg* 1994;18:3:259.
22. Fodor PB, Watson J. Personal experience with ultrasound-assisted lipoplasty: a pilot study comparing ultrasound assisted lipoplasty with traditional lipoplasty. *Plast Reconstr Surg* 1998; 101:1103.
23. Kenkel JM, Robinson JB Jr, Beran SJ, et al. The tissue effects of ultrasound-assisted lipoplasty. *Plast Reconstr Surg* 1998; 102:213.
24. Kloehn RA. Liposuction with "sonic sculpture": six years experience with more than 600 patients. *Aesthetic Surg Q* 1996;16:123.
25. Rohrich RJ, Beran SJ, Kenkel JM, et al. Extending the role of liposuction in body contouring with ultrasound-assisted liposuction. *Plast Reconstr Surg* 1998;101:1090.

Discussion

BODY CONTOURING BY LIPOPLASTY

YVES GERARD ILLOUZ

I would like to congratulate Dr. Fodor for his work and I agree with almost all of what he said. My discussion will be short, almost an outline. The main points of this book and this chapter are unfavorable results, how to avoid complications, and obviously how to treat them.

From 1982, when my technique started to be performed after the blue ribbon committee favorable report, to 1995 (over 13 years), there were only three deaths and very little morbidity. During these 13 years, only my traditional technique was performed. From 1995 to 1998, which is only 3 years, there were almost 100 deaths, frequent morbidity, many bad results, many lawsuits, and significant loss of prestige of the technique.

Y. G. Illouz: Department of Aesthetic Surgery, Saint Louis Hospital, Paris, France

Why? During those 3 years, many so-called "new" techniques came onto the market. We will discuss the complications and unfavorable results of the "traditional" technique, the complications and unfavorable results of the "new" techniques, the problems of postoperative care, and the treatment of these unfavorable results

THE TRADITIONAL ILLOUZ TECHNIQUE

When I first presented lipoplasty in Hawaii in October 1982 after 5 years of experience (I innovated lipoplasty in 1977), I warned surgeons about the complications and unfavorable results. In general, systemic complications can occur after 3,000 mL is removed. Burn syndrome, like a "crush syndrome," can occur after a procedure involving more than one-third of body surface. Unfavorable results (Fig. 63D-1) include dimples, depressions, or furrows, separate or together, which can occur after suction that is too superficial (Fig. 63D-2). Adhesions can occur after suction that is too deep (Fig. 63D-3). A moon-surface appearance can occur after an "anarchic suction," which is too superficial in some places and too deep in others (Fig. 63D-4). Excess skin can occur when the indication for surgery was poor, e.g., skin that was already present in excess or skin that was not elastic enough.

At the time, my technique was simple, safe, reliable, and capable of providing dramatic results (Figs. 63D-5 through 63D-9). However, the technique must be performed very precisely, because each step has potential traps. With regard to patient selection, before performing lipoplasty, we must answer three main questions to avoid pitfalls: Is there enough fat? Is the skin tonic enough, or is there an excess of skin? What will be the aspect of the skin after surgery? Marking must be carried out with the patient in the standing position, but it must be corrected when the patient is in the operative position, because some fatty masses "move" to different areas. I do not advocate hetching, because if patients gain or lose weight or develop excess skin (with age), the placement of the hetching changes and gives a poor appearance to the abdomen. Thus, the surgical technique must achieve fat-to-fat healing to avoid an unattractive appearance, subdermal healing that results in dimpling, and aponeurosis healing that results in adhesions.

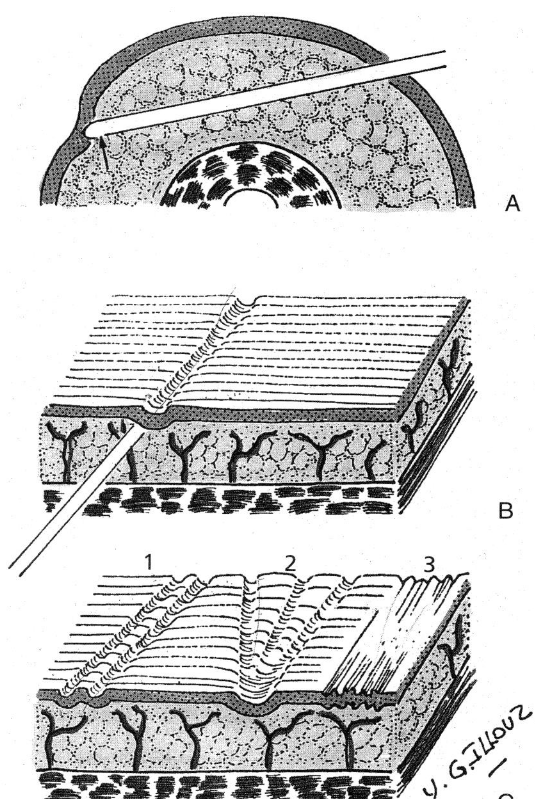

FIGURE 63D-2. Causes of complications. **A:** Dimple caused by cannula colliding with the surface. **B:** Furrow caused by stroke that was too superficial. **C1:** Waves caused by parallel furrows. **C2:** Fan-shaped furrows. **C3:** Wrinkling due to subdermal technique.

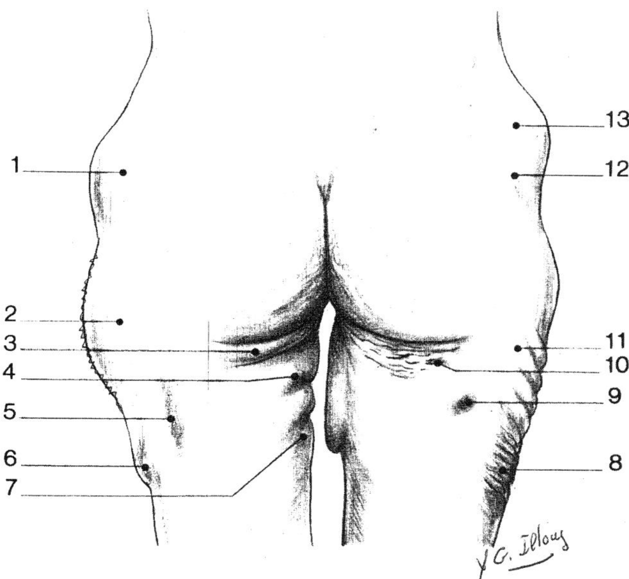

FIGURE 63D-1. Complications that can occur after lipoplasty include remaining bumps; postoperative false bumps by "accordionization of the skin"; double folds and postoperative banana; adhesions due to suction that was too deep, with musculoaponeurotic trauma; furrows; step deformities; adjacent adhesions giving a wavy aspect; wrinkles; dimples; slight excess of skin; waves caused by irregular suction; cavities; and bumps due to seroma.

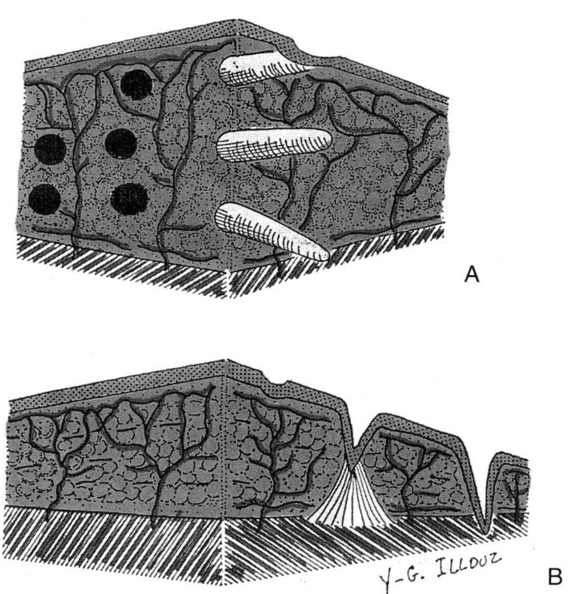

FIGURE 63D-3. Causes of defects. **A:** In the middle, normal way to do a lipoplasty in plain fat (to the skin induces a dimple) to the muscle induces a trauma of the musculoaponeurotic plane. **B:** Trauma to the muscle induces a fibrotic reaction that results in an adhesion.

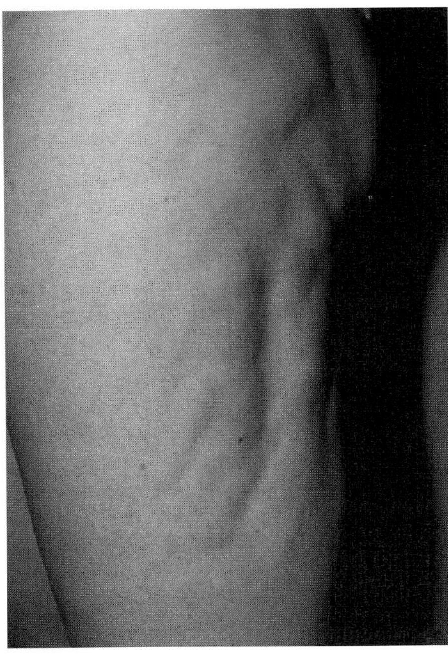

FIGURE 63D-4. Sample of complications, such as irregularities, adhesions, dimples, and waviness.

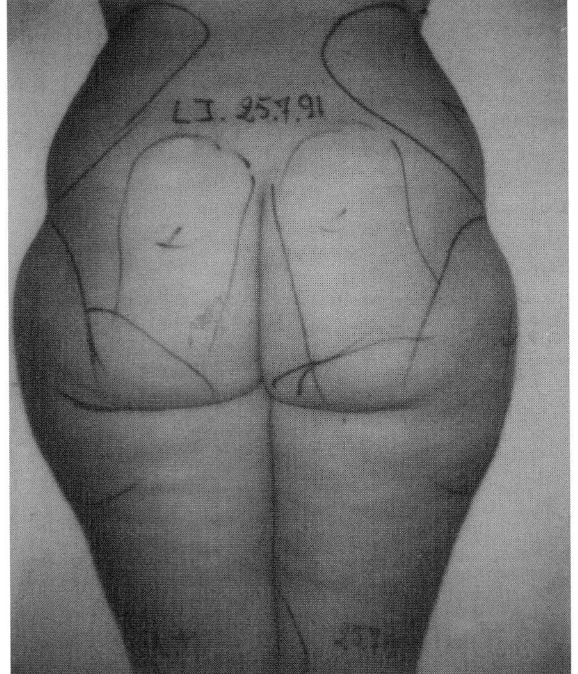

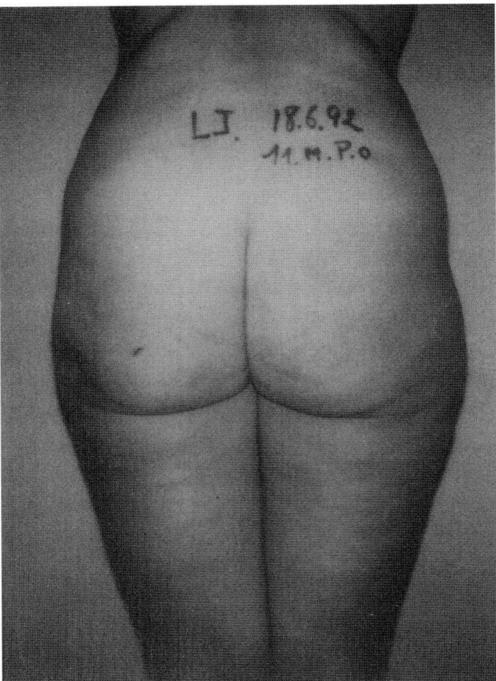

FIGURE 63D-5. Spectacular result 11 months after lipoplasty of the entire basin: riding breeches, hips, and buttocks.

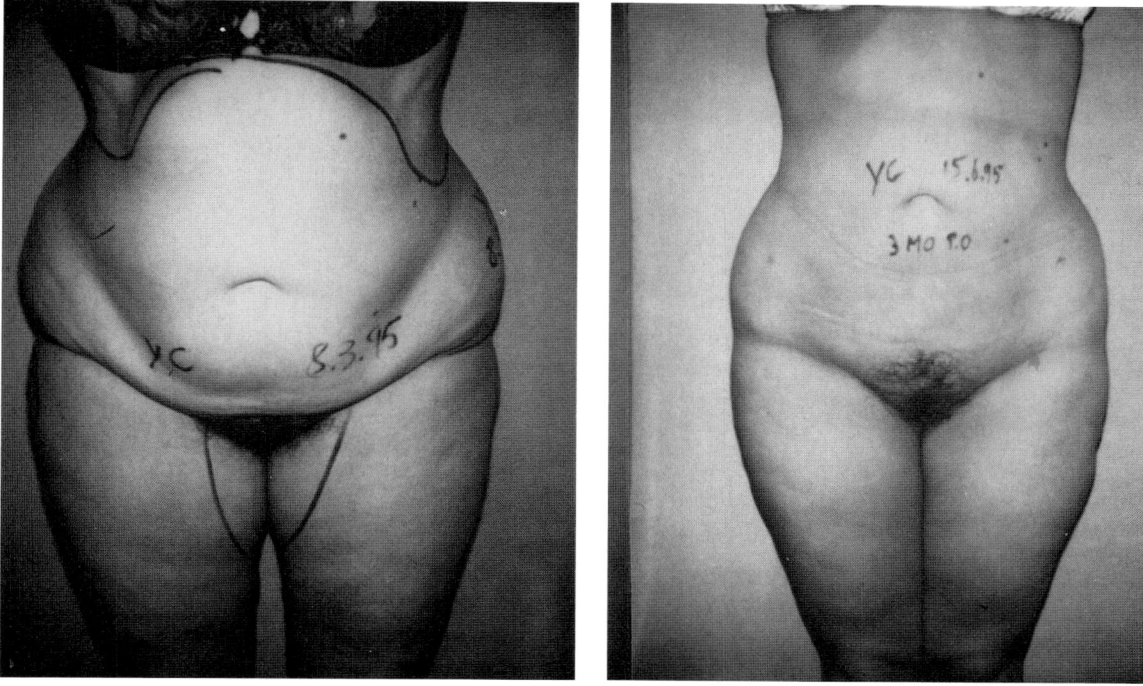

FIGURE 63D-6. Spectacular result 3 months after lipoplasty of the abdomen and inner thighs.

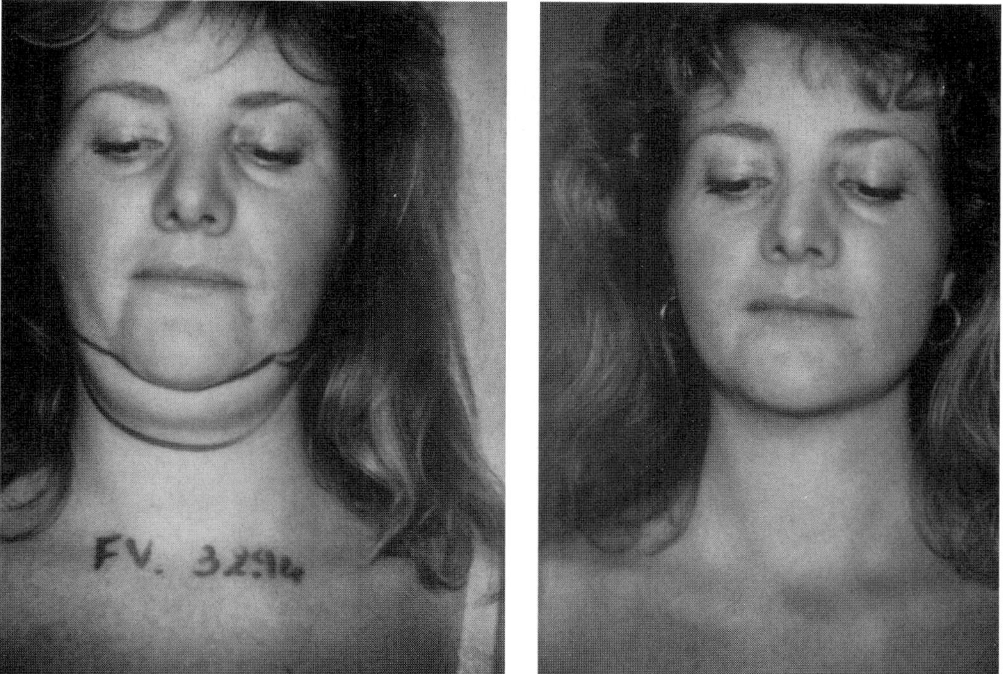

FIGURE 63D-7. Dramatic result of face suction.

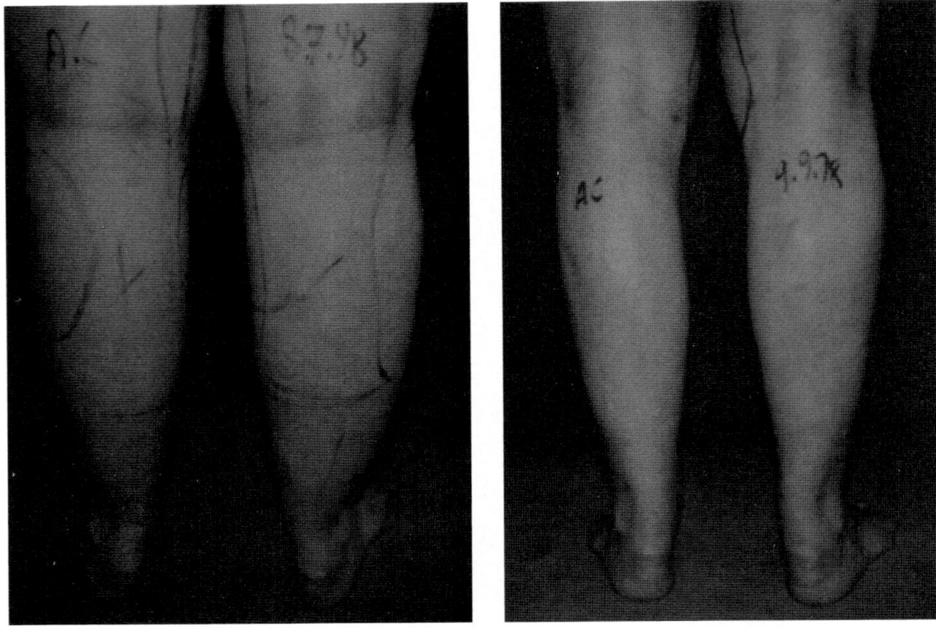

FIGURE 63D-8. Very good result of circumferential suction performed on the legs.

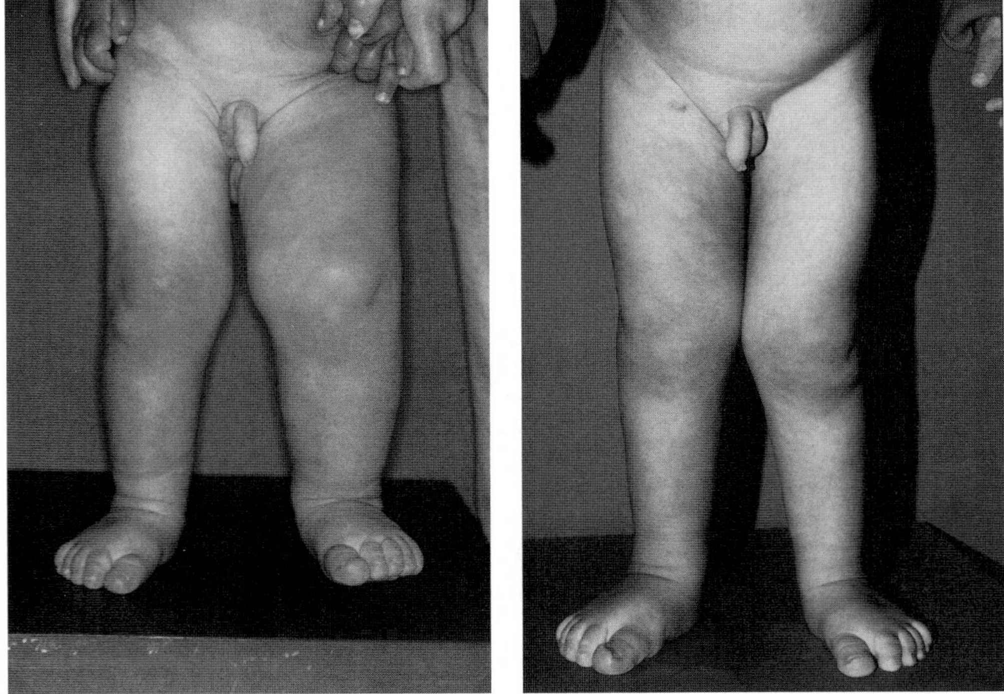

FIGURE 63D-9. Suction for congenital hypertrophy of the thigh and leg after 1 year.

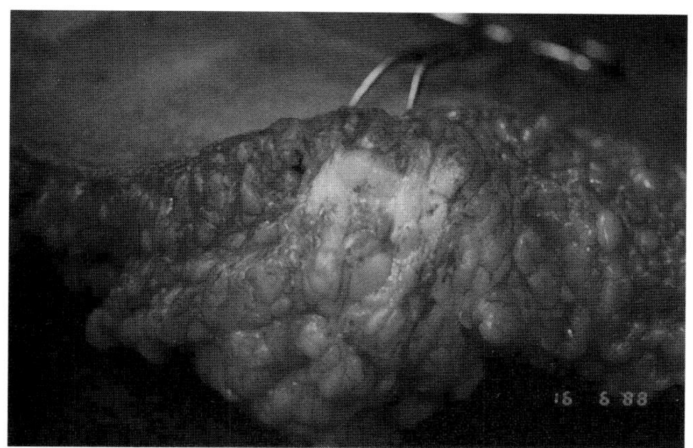

FIGURE 63D-10. Subcutaneous fat anatomy. Superficial layer (skin to fascia superficialis) divided vertically. Deep layer (fascia superficialis to fascia muscle) divided horizontally.

THE NEW TECHNIQUES AND THEIR PROBLEMS

Injection

Since the beginning, I have advocated a wet technique, with an infiltration of 1:1. At the beginning, my formula for 1,000 mL of normal saline was 200 mL of distilled water, 1,000 IU of Wydase, or Hyaluronidase, to diffuse the solution, 1 mg of epinephrine in local anesthesia to avoid problems in general anesthesia with cyclopropane, and 500 mg of lidocaine (Xylocaine) in case local anesthesia was needed. We quickly stopped using cyclopropane for general anesthesia and began to use epinephrine in all cases.

In the meantime, Hetter (1) advocated epinephrine in any kind of anesthesia, and other surgeons were advocating different injections: the dry technique (2), which now is almost never used; the tumescent technique (3:1) (3), which has already resulted in more than ten deaths as a result of pulmonary edema and still others as a result of toxicity of the solution; and the superwet technique, for which Fodor in 1988 reported an excellent study on infiltration. He showed that a ratio of less that 1:1 is not efficient and that a ratio of more than 1.5:1 is not useful and can even be dangerous (he called this ratio the *superwet technique*). It is largely agreed that the best infiltration ranges from 1:1 to a maximum of 1.5:1.

Superficial Technique

The anatomy shows two layers of fat (Fig. 63D-10). The first is the deep layer, which is divided horizontally into genetic and reserve fat. This layer creates the bump. The second layer is the superficial, current fat. This layer is divided vertically and produces cellulite or the "mattress phenomenon." It is estrogen dependent, and the vertical septi produce retraction (Fig. 63D-11). Histology shows the vertical septi and how the orange skin phenomenon occurs (Fig. 63D-11). Endoscopy shows that when the cannula has a diameter larger than 2 mm, the suction destroys almost everything in the superficial layer, which is dangerous (Fig. 63D-12). Unfavorable results are produced by suction that is too superficial (subdermal) and an irregular technique (Figs. 63D-13, 63D-14).

We can conclude the following. (i) Too superficial of an approach (subdermal) is dangerous in all cases. (ii) Suction

1

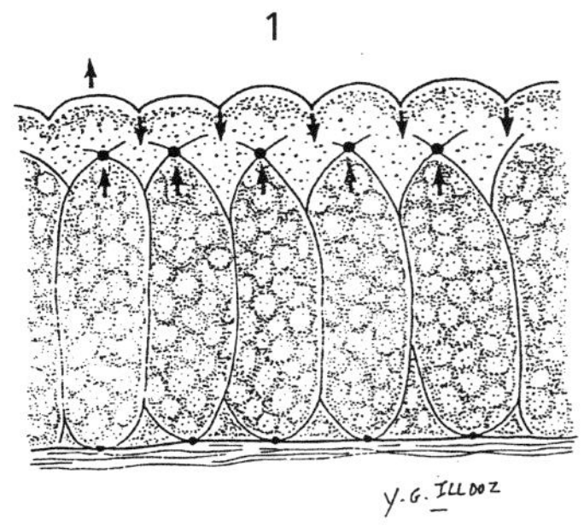

2

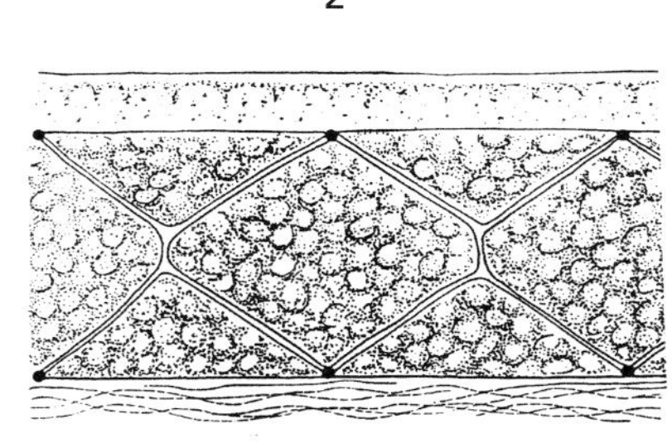

3

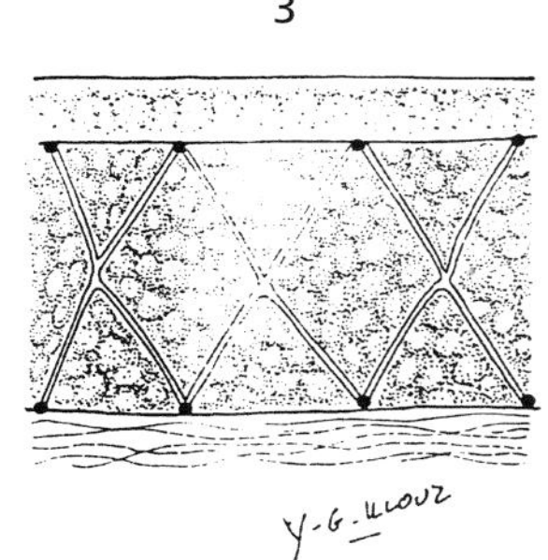

4

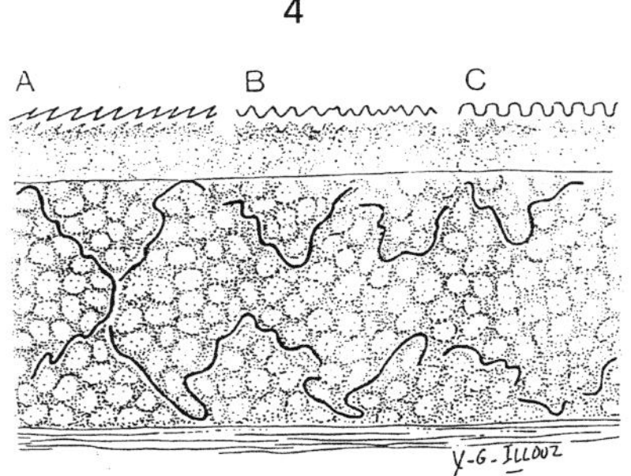

FIGURE 63D-11. (1) How the "cellulite aspect" occurs by fat hypertrophy of the chambers. The pressure goes "up" and induces a dimpling aspect (orange skin phenomenon). (2) The "septa" are horizontally elastic and seem to be responsible for skin retraction (3). (4) If the subdermal accordion is destroyed by suction that is too superficial, the skin can no longer retract normally and it wrinkles (Fig. 63D-13 through 63D-14).

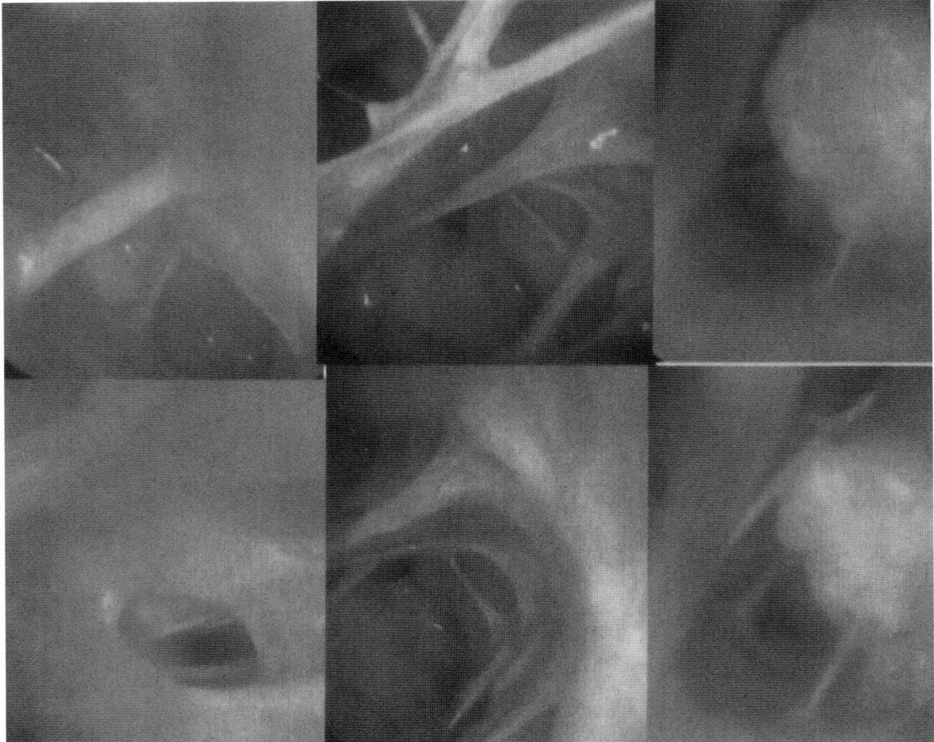

FIGURE 63D-12. Endoscopy shows that a cannula with diameter larger than 2 mm can destroy the subdermal conjunctive tissue; thus, superficial suction must not use a cannula with diameter larger than 2 mm.

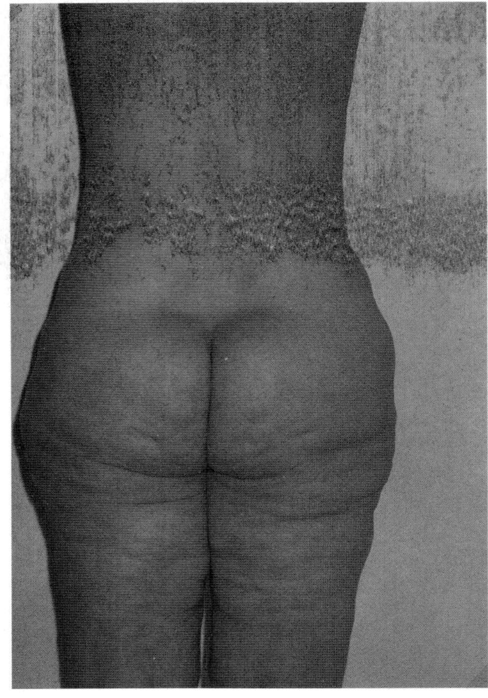

FIGURE 63D-13. Waviness and irregularities after superficial suction.

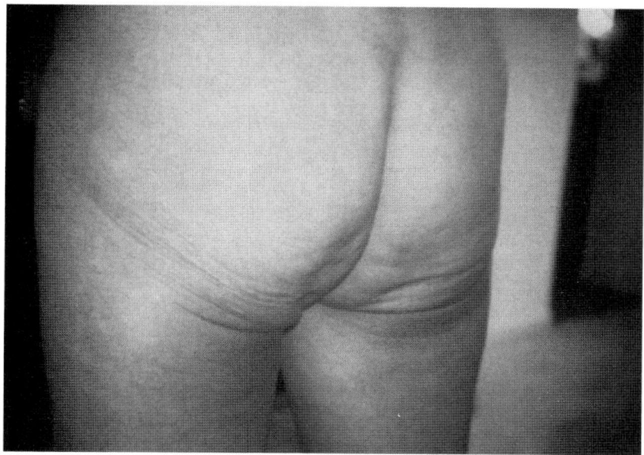

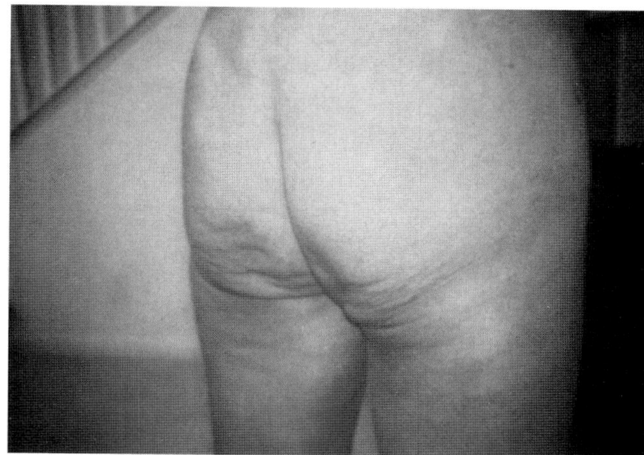

FIGURE 63D-14. Wrinkles and skin excess after superficial suction.

within in the first 5 mm can destroy everything in the superficial layer and thus is dangerous, inappropriate, or both. (iii) Suction within the first 5 mm is acceptable because it respects the vessels, nerves, and conjunctive tissues, which are responsible for skin retraction. (iv) Superficial lipoplasty that respects the first 5 mm results in good skin retraction without posing danger to the first 5 mm.

INSTRUMENTATION

Normal Cannulas

Endoscopy shows that a cannula diameter larger than 2 mm risks damage to vessels and nerves, and that the tip of the cannula and the edges of the hole must be blunt, which I have always advocated. The safer cannula is one that respects these principles (Fig. 63D-15). Some cannulas are sharper or do not have blunt tips. They are more efficient but also are more dangerous. They can be useful for some sclerous tissues, such as those encountered in gynecomastia, or for performing touchups.

Mechanical Cannulas

Rotative cannulas are dangerous and now are almost never used. Back-and-forth vibrating cannulas may provide easier penetration but require further testing.

MEGALIPOPLASTIES

Early in 1982, I advocated a limit of 3,000 mL, after which general or systemic problems can occur, especially shock, crush syndrome, or burn syndrome, which results from the creation of a very important "third space" by the tunneling technique. Do we have the same limits today? Theoretically, we could say that we have no more limits, because of refinements in the technique and the progress made in resuscitation and anesthesiology. However, there are always limits to avoid any risk, and a lethal risk in aesthetic surgery is not acceptable. Thus, the limits I advocate are 10% of body weight, 40% of body surface, and no more than one unit of blood in the aspirate. Almost all the lethal "accidents" reported in lipoplasties occur beyond these limits. Patients who require procedures exceeding these limits must undergo two or more stages, which most patients can tolerate well.

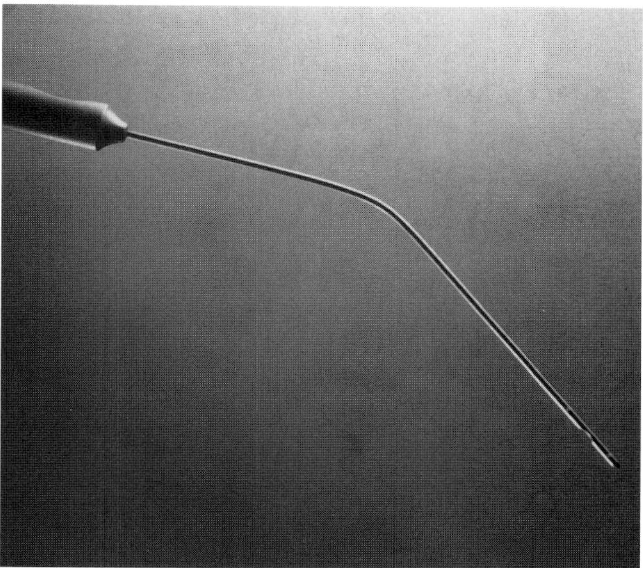

FIGURE 63D-15. Titane cannula, designed by the author, with one ventral hole and two lateral holes less than 2 mm on each side. This cannula can perform deep suction by the ventral orifice and more superficial suction by the lateral holes. The cannula is malleable and easily bent, and the design avoids criss-cross of the tunnels.

ULTRASOUND

Ultrasound-assisted Lipectomy

In 1988, I tried using an ultrasonically powered machine, and in 1989, I published a report regarding use of such a machine (Fig. 63D-16). Ultrasound is a wonderful idea because it is absolutely selective for the fat calls that "explode" and lose their lipids. In addition, they theoretically respect the vessels, nerves, and conjunctive tissues. Unfortunately, they have two negative side effects. First, the mechanical energy of the ultrasound can be transformed into thermal energy that can reach 150°C and result in burns; some biopsies show vessel coagulation resulting from the ultrasound beam. Second, the same mechanical energy can, mainly with a hollow cannula, work like a jackhammer or an electrical knife, cutting vessels and inducing necrosis (Fig. 63D-17). These complications are rare but can occur, even with skilled surgeons. I hope that these side effects will dissipate with better machines. The machines we have today are not appropriate because they are not safe, are too slow, do not produce better results, and do not allow for larger quantities. At this time, ultrasound-assisted lipectomy has no obvious advantages over traditional lipoplasty. The small advantages (better performance with sclerous or dense tissues) are not enough to compensate for the huge disadvantages and risks they can induce.

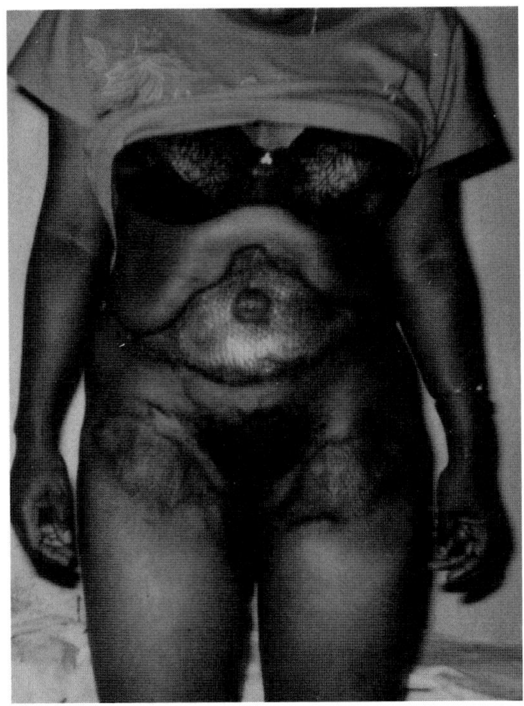

FIGURE 63D-17. Large amount of skin necrosis after ultrasound lipoplasty.

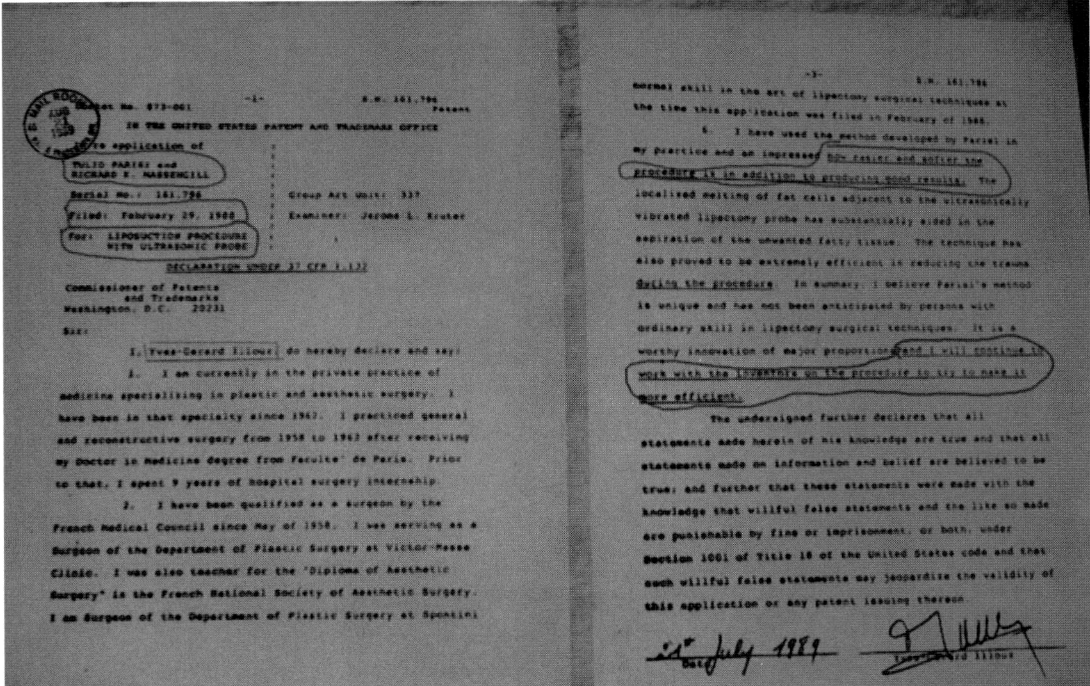

-1-

Docket No. 873-061 S.N. 161,796
Patent

IN THE UNITED STATES PATENT AND TRADEMARK OFFICE

In re application of

TULIO PARISI and
RICHARD F. MASSENGILL

Serial No.: 161,796 Group Art Unit: 337

Filed: February 29, 1988 Examiner: Jerome L. Kruter

For: LIPOSUCTION PROCEDURE
WITH ULTRASONIC PROBE

DECLARATION UNDER 37 CFR 1.132

Commissioner of Patents
and Trademarks
Washington, D.C. 20231

Sir:

I, Yves-Gerard Illouz, do hereby declare and say:

1. I am currently in the private practice of medicine specializing in plastic and aesthetic surgery. I have been in that specialty since 1962. I practiced general and reconstructive surgery from 1958 to 1962 after receiving my Doctor in Medicine degree from Faculte' de Paris. Prior to that, I spent 9 years of hospital surgery internship.

2. I have been qualified as a surgeon by the French Medical Council since May of 1958. I was serving as a Surgeon of the Department of Plastic Surgery at Victor-Masse Clinic. I was also teacher for the "Diploma of Aesthetic Surgery" in the French National Society of Aesthetic Surgery. I am Surgeon of the Department of Plastic Surgery at Spontini

-3- S.N. 161,796

normal skill in the art of lipectomy surgical techniques at the time this application was filed in February of 1988.

5. I have used the method developed by Parisi in my practice and am impressed how easier and softer the procedure is in addition to producing good results. The localized melting of fat cells adjacent to the ultrasonically vibrated lipectomy probe has substantially aided in the aspiration of the unwanted fatty tissue. The technique has also proved to be extremely efficient in reducing the trauma during the procedure. In summary, I believe Parisi's method is unique and has not been anticipated by persons with ordinary skill in lipectomy surgical techniques. It is a worthy innovation of major proportions and I will continue to work with the inventors on the procedure to try to make it more efficient.

The undersigned further declares that all statements made herein of his knowledge are true and that all statements made on information and belief are believed to be true; and further that these statements were made with the knowledge that willful false statements and the like so made are punishable by fine or imprisonment, or both, under Section 1001 of Title 18 of the United States code and that such willful false statements may jeopardize the validity of this application or any patent issuing thereon.

21st July 1989 — Date

Yves-Gerard Illouz

FIGURE 63D-16. Evaluation of ultrasonic power for lipoplasty used by Illouz in 1989 before the introduction by the media of ultrasound-assisted lipectomy in 1992.

External Ultrasound

We have long been aware of the use of external ultrasound, which was advocated by Illouz and De Villers (4) for postoperative care to reduce edema, pain, and sclerous tissue. Can its use be extended? The main effect of external ultrasound is heat, which can be directed to a certain depth. Controlled by endoscopy, we can see that the ultrasound beams do not destroy the adipocytes or any cell types. In fact, they simply heat an injected solution for better melting. If the beam is too superficial, it can burn; if the beam is too deep, it can reach the muscles or the bones. Perhaps in the future we can completely master these effects and use them more efficiently.

POSTOPERATIVE CARE

Dressing

Early in my practice, I used elastic semicircular bandages. They were efficient and not dangerous, but they were difficult to apply and very painful to remove. "It is the most painful part of the procedure," a patient once told me. "Ready-made" dressings then became available. They are circular, compressive garments that are easy to apply and to remove, but difficult to apply when the patient is sedated.

As soon as these bandages are applied, thrombophlebitis and emboli can occur. Because the bandages are circular, they can become too tight and induce stasis. Stasis can result in thrombosis, which in turn can induce emboli. To avoid such a complication, the compression of the garment must be less than 24 mm Hg (venous pressure) but more than 18 mm Hg to be efficient. Not many bandages have such parameters. To avoid stasis or compression, I recommend the following. Never apply the bandages when the patient is sedated and on the operating table. Instead, apply the bandages only when the patient is awake and able to stand up, so that he or she can report whether the garment is too tight. If so, put on a larger garment. Ask the patient to check his or her feet to see if there is any abnormal edema or purple color. If so, remove the garments immediately.

Physiotherapy

I have recommended postoperative physiotherapy (massages, alternative compression, lymphatic drainage, external ultrasound, and ionization) from the early days of my practice. However, I believe that the effects are more psychological than of any actual physical benefit. Some patients do not undergo any postoperative care and have the same results as those who do, although the postoperative time may have been somewhat shorter: 12 weeks without physiotherapy versus 10 weeks with physiotherapy. Regardless of the type of physiotherapy (manual or mechanical massages, ultrasound), there may be no scientific advantage. Nevertheless, we must continue to refine our technique and find efficient postoperative physiotherapy.

TREATMENT

Skin Excess

Abdominoplasty

Abdominoplasties are now very rare (Fig. 63D-18). A good lipoplasty often is sufficient even for an huge abdomen with significant ptosis (Fig. 63D-6). However, when the results are not favorable or after an unsuccessful lipoplasty, abdominoplasty may be required. Unhappily, a classic abdominoplasty associated with aspiration may result in severe shock or significant necrosis.

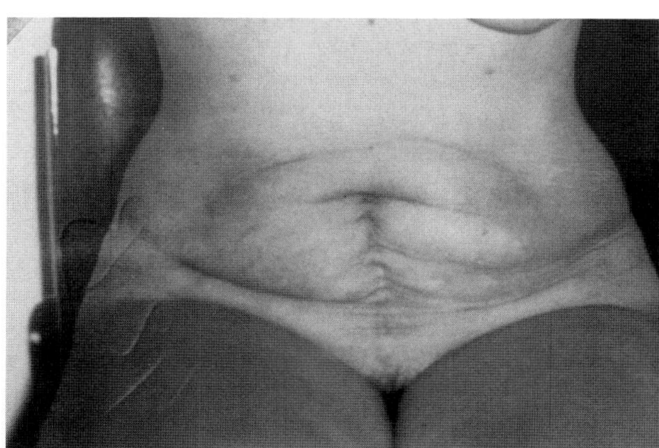

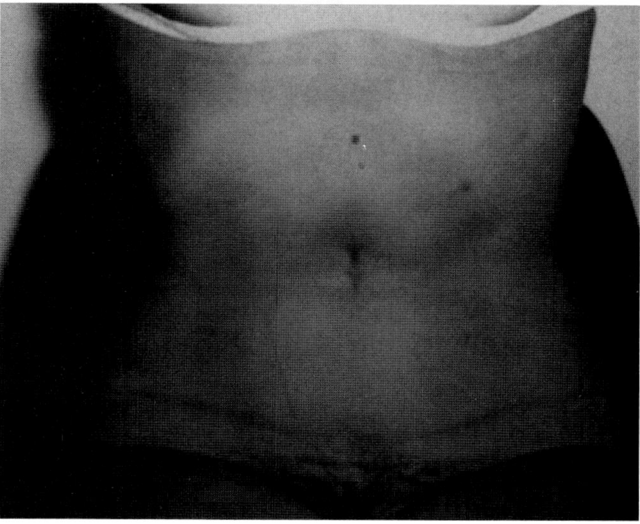

FIGURE 63D-18. Result of Illouz *en bloc* abdominoplasty performed on a slim patient with a vertical neoumbilicoplasty.

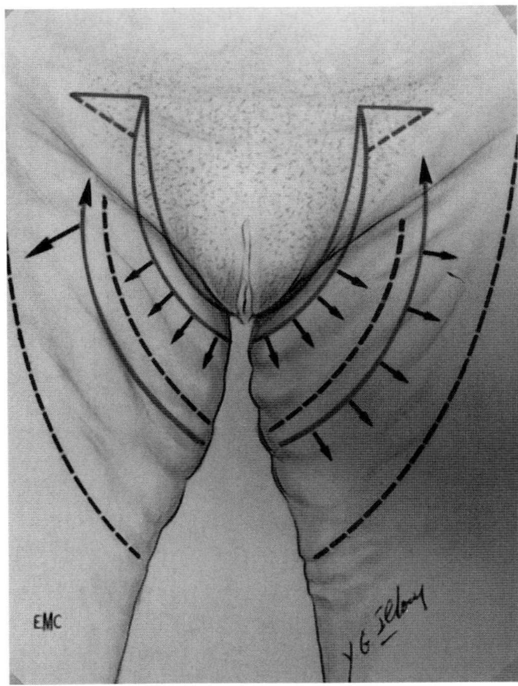

FIGURE 63D-19. Illouz inner thigh-plasty.

For this reason, in 1984 I innovated a safe *en bloc* abdominoplasty with an immediate neoumbilicoplasty that consists of the following: suction in the upper abdomen; *en bloc* resection of the excess of skin with the navel; no undermining of the upper abdomen (the absence of undermining explains the absence of general complications); and vertical neoumbilicoplasty (Illouz type) a good distance from the pubic hair (minimum 10 cm; maximum 13 cm).

Inner Thigh-plasty

To avoid descent of the scar and deformation of the vulva, Ted Lockwood described how to fix the inferior flap to Colles ligament (4). It was a great improvement, but the scar was too long. This is why in 1988 I innovated a new technique that results in a very short scar that is almost hidden in the pubic hair (Fig. 63D-19). For the inner and anterior thighs, the inferior flap is fixed to the Colles ligament in the inner part and to the crural arcade in the anterior part (Illouz 1990). Complete bodylift requires a circular incision.

Depression

Good results are permanent, but so are bad results. When a depression occurs, it is permanent. The problem is how to fill a depression. At this time, fat injection seems to be the best solution (no cost and no allergic reaction) (Fig. 63D-20). I innovated fat injection in 1983 and published widely on this technique. In the last report from 1989, I reviewed 100 cases after 4 years of experience and concluded that 40% to 60% of fat "remains" and the rest is resorbed. More recently, other authors such as Fournier and Coleman reported less resorption.

Another way to fill a depression permanently is to use alloplastic material. Gore-Tex can be useful, but very often is too visible and leaves nonaesthetic results. Artecoll and Arteplast also can leave nonaesthetic results and induce granuloma. Silicone can induce catastrophic results (Fig. 63D-21).There currently is no completely reliable material

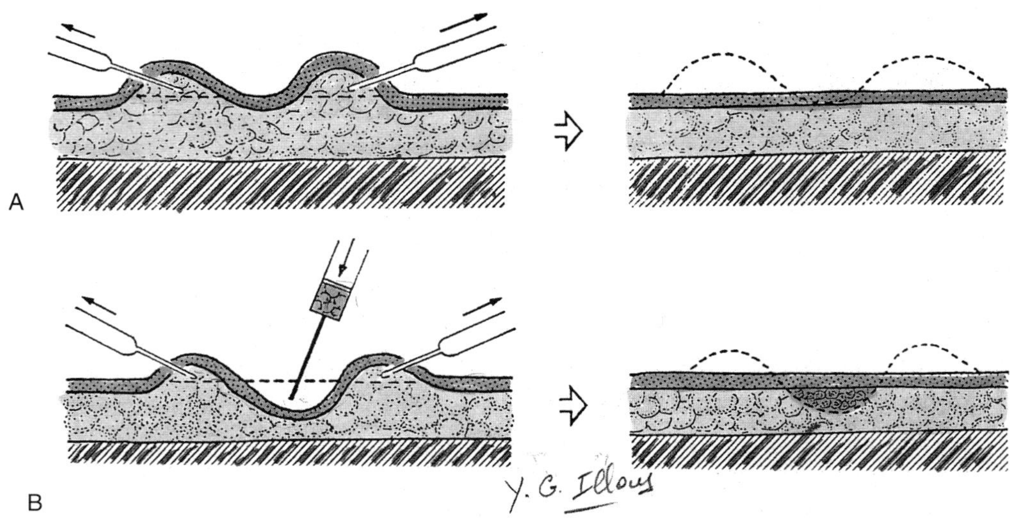

FIGURE 63D-20. Method to correct a depression. **A:** When the depression is *above the ideal line* between two bumps, we need only to "suck" the two bumps. **B:** When the depression is *under the ideal line*, we must suck the bumps *above* the ideal line and fill the depression with fat.

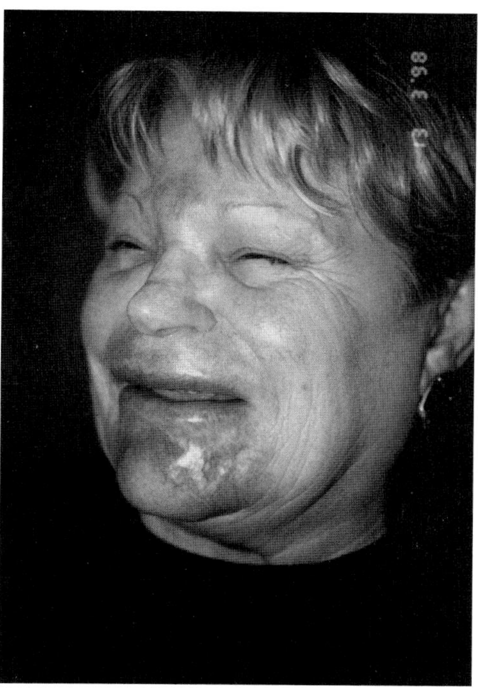

FIGURE 63D-21. Catastrophic sequelae 5 years after injection of "silicone" in the face.

to fill a depression or to augment soft tissue. We must work to find a technique that is 100% reliable.

Cellulite

Lipoplasty removes excess fat but does not remove cellulite. Cellulite (Fig. 63D-11) is skin characterized by orange skin peel aspect, a mattress phenomenon, or Chesterfield canapé that sometimes is very visible or sometimes is visible only with a "pinch test." It is the result of hypertrophy of the superficial layer of fat, which in women is divided vertically. Because of this division in women, any hypertrophy results in turgescence, or cellulite, which is not pathologic but normal and dependent on estrogen. Fat cells in culture grow faster and larger with β-estradiol. Cellulite is a normal aspect of skin.

Surgical Treatment

Some surgeons tried to remove cellulite by cutting the vertical divisions using a superficial technique or a special instrument designed like a tiny fork. Does it work? To study it, I performed a deep suction and a superficial suction and cut the septa. After a few months I performed a biopsy, which showed that the septa reappeared and the cellulite returned. Because cellulite is dependent on estrogen, it (re)appears with a certain level of female hormones.

Physiotherapeutic Treatment

Physiotherapy cannot remove cellulite. Manual or mechanical massages and external ultrasound can help temporarily, but they cannot produce a cure. At this time, nothing can make cellulite disappear without taking femininity with it. Many "sophisticated" devices have appeared on the market, but their effects are more psychological than physical.

Medical Treatment

Perhaps in the future, an antagonistic characteristic female hormone that induces hypertrophy of fat cells will be identified. This antagonist must be very selective to avoid any diminution of femininity.

CONCLUSIONS

Although lipoplasty appears to be simple, it is one of the most difficult procedures in aesthetic surgery. It is easy to remove fat with this technique and it is very easy to remove a large volume of fat, but it is very difficult to remove exactly what must be in an even, harmonious, and aesthetic manner. The surgeon must be an "*in vivo* sculptor" but not make a mistake, particularly removing too much fat. A reliable and ideal "filling" procedure is still to be discovered. No machine can replace the hands of the surgeon. The skill of the surgeon prevails over any material. For the patient, it is better to have a good surgeon with only skilled hands than a poor practitioner with very sophisticated machines.

REFERENCES

1. Hetter GP. The effect of low dose epinephrine on the hematocrit drop following lipolysis. *Aesthetic Plast Surg* 1984;8:19.
2. Fournier PE, Otteni FM. Lipodissection in body sculpturing: the dry procedure. *Plast Reconstr Surg* 1983;72:598.
3. Klein JA. Tumescent technique for regional anesthesia permits lidocaine dose of 35 mg/kg for liposuction. *J Dermatol Surg Oncol* 1990;16:248.
4. Illouz YG, De Villers YT. *Body sculpturing by lipoplasty.* London: Churchill Livingstone, 1989.

SUGGESTED READING

Illouz YG. Body contouring by lipolysis: a 5 year experience with over 3000 cases. *Plast Reconstr Surg* 1983;72:591

Illouz YG. The utilization of fat after liposuction. *Rev Chir Esthet Lang Fran* 1984;IX(36):13–14, X(38):19–22.

Illouz YG. The fat cells "graft," a new technique to fill depressions [Letter]. *Am Soc Plast Reconstr Surg J* 1986;78:122.

64

BODY CONTOURING WITH EXCISIONS

TED LOCKWOOD

Excisional body contour surgery may be one of the most challenging areas in aesthetic surgery in which to obtain consistently favorable results. The aesthetic deformities of the body and extremities are extremely varied, the surface areas to be contoured are great, and the lifting distances are long. Long incisional scars are required, and wound repair is under high tension. The need for symmetry of scars and contours is essential. The resultant body contours will be viewed circumferentially from all angles and positions, often in a skimpy bikini. Contours should be natural and appropriate in repose and with physical activities.

The challenges of excisional surgery are daunting. Long labor-intensive surgeries, complex preoperative planning and postoperative care, and the risk of potential complications and other unfavorable results limit the popularity of body lifts. Obtaining consistently superior results in excisional body lift surgery may be one of the last frontiers in aesthetic surgery. In the past decade, there have been significant advances in excisional body lifting based on an improved understanding of both youthful and aged soft tissue anatomy (1–6). Using current anatomical and design concepts is the first step in reducing potential unfavorable results with excisional body contour surgery.

Modern body contour surgery began 40 to 45 years ago with the development of various excisional designs for the arms, abdomen, thighs, and buttocks (7–16). These surgical lifts were designed in a practical fashion to remove hanging skin and fat with incisions hidden in swimwear patterns of the day. Although technical modifications and improvements were reported over the decades, the anatomical principles upon which these lifts were founded have not changed. Classic body lift techniques, based on original but dated anatomical precepts, often have lacked consistency and predictability and, except for abdominoplasty, have failed to gain widespread acceptance.

The introduction of liposuction in the early 1980s revolutionized body contour surgery, making classic body lifts even less popular (17). However, liposuction deals only with fat excess, not with skin quality problems (to any significant degree or with any long-lasting effect). Proper skin tone adds immeasurably to the body aesthetic in both static and dynamic activities. There is a need for excisional lifting for optimal aesthetic results in selected individuals.

Body lifts are designed to treat skin quality problems of the aesthetic body contour deformity. Laxity and sagging of the skin will occur in everyone with the normal aging process. As our population ages, there may be increased demand for safe and effective body lifts. Body lifts are a useful adjunct to liposuction and should be considered when developing an overall surgical plan for an individual patient.

Lifts may be used at the time of initial liposuction or may be required to treat skin laxity and contour irregularities that appear after liposuction. Patients should be aware of the limitations of liposuction and that subsequent body lifting may be required to gain optimal body contours. This discussion before initial liposuction helps the patient understand that their *skin tone is the primary determinant of the aesthetic success or failure of liposuction,* even with the best liposuction technique. Patients who understand this principle rarely have unrealistic expectations about the results of liposuction and are reasonably prepared to consider body lifts in the future, if needed.

ALL BODY LIFTS

Avoidance of Unfavorable Results

Patient Selection

Appropriate patient selection is essential to limiting unfavorable results. Although liposuction and body lifts both are useful in body contour surgery, the indications for surgery are not the same. Liposuction treats localized fat deposits; lifts treat skin quality problems. It is important to dispel the myth that "liposuction tightens skin." Liposuction does not tighten or lift *relaxed skin and fat,* but it does allow *youthful and elastic* skin to retract and conform to smaller contours. This is true for both traditional small-cannula liposuction and ultrasonically assisted liposuction. In patients with flaccid skin, attempts to use liposuction to gain maximum skin

T. Lockwood: Private Practice, Overland Park, Kansas

retraction often results in significant and permanent skin contour irregularities.

Likewise, excisional lifts should not be used as the primary treatment for localized fat deposits. Because many patients have both fat deposit and actual or potential skin laxity problems, body lifts and liposuction can be combined in one or multiple surgical procedures. Clear indications for body lifts include skin laxity without significant fat deposits, excessive skin laxity and cellulite, patients in whom skin tightening is their primary goal, aged medial thigh deformities, and buttock ptosis.

Because surgical complication rates for body lifts are higher than for moderate-volume liposuction, patients selected for excisional surgery should have moderate-to-severe laxity problems and should be well informed of the potential risk of complications and unfavorable results. To reduce the risk of unfavorable results, avoid patients consuming any form of nicotine and patients with generalized obesity or other medical problems (cardiovascular, respiratory, history of deep vein thrombosis).

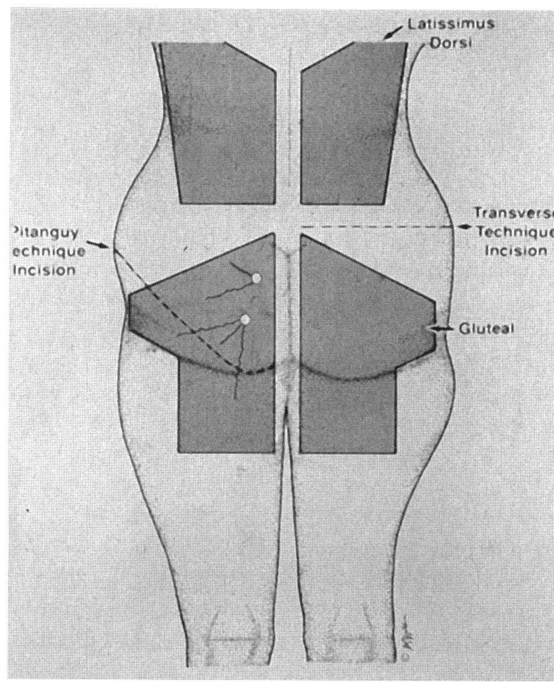

FIGURE 64-1. Placing the thigh/buttock lift incision in a transverse direction between the major vascular territories established in the 1970s yields improved vascularity. The Pitanguy thigh/buttock lift design (1964) transects the dominant gluteal vascular territory.

Surgical Design

After proper patient selection, the next step in reducing potential unfavorable results with excisional body contour surgery is the utilization of current anatomical and design concepts. Classic dermolipectomies were based on anatomical concepts that are no longer valid. These include misunderstanding the support structure of the skin/subcutaneous fat unit, the vascular anatomy of skin, and the mechanisms resulting in the aged (relaxed) aesthetic body deformity.

Anatomists and surgeons have always believed that the major structural support for the skin/subcutaneous fat unit was the skin, specifically the dermis (18,19). Plastic surgeons have used dermis or deepithelialized dermal flaps to anchor high-tension wound repair. This basic concept was challenged in an article on the superficial fascial system (SFS) reported in 1991 (2). Functionally, the SFS of the subcutaneous tissue is primarily responsible for supporting the weight of the soft tissues of the body over many decades of rather constant vertical gravitational force. In addition, the SFS holds the skin onto the body, so that the position, contour, and tone of the skin are determined by the position and tone of the SFS and its fibrous attachments to the underlying musculoskeletal tissues. SFS suspension with nonabsorbable sutures should be used for all high-tension wound repairs to reduce the risk of widened and hypertrophic scars and to provide a more secure and long-lasting lift of the tissues.

Skin vascular territories established in the 1970s should be respected to reduce the risk of ischemic necrosis, delayed wound healing, and poor scarring (Fig. 64-1). The Pitanguy thigh/buttock lift design (1964) transects the dominant gluteal vascular territory (11). Placing the thigh/buttock lift incision within high-cut bikini lines yields improved vascularity to both wound edges, because the incision lies between the major vascular territories of the trunk and thighs.

A better understanding of the mechanisms of aging in producing the typical aged body appearance allows improved surgical design. For example, the lower body lift design (1993) to simultaneously tighten the relaxed tissues of the trunk and thighs recognized that the maximum relaxation of the body generally occurs along the lateral body contour (4). Resecting maximally along the lateral contour shifts lax tissues of the trunk and thighs toward their youthful position, reducing unfavorable aesthetic results often seen with classic techniques. The high-lateral-tension abdominoplasty design (1995) also uses this concept to produce natural aesthetic contours with a body lift effect via an abdominoplasty incision (5).

The medial thigh aesthetic deformity is another area that often is misunderstood by the patient and surgeon. In many patients, anterior medial thigh laxity is due, in large part, to a descent of relaxed abdominal, pubic, and inguinal tissues after pregnancy or weight loss. Attempting a medial thigh lift before the support tissues of the lower trunk are lifted often leads to unfavorable aesthetic results. In addition, trying to lift the distal thigh via a medial thigh lift incision usually is unsuccessful. Relaxation of the anterior and medial distal thighs primarily results from a "down and in" rotational descent away from the point of maximal relaxation along the lateral body. Therefore, a strong thigh lift laterally is most effective in rejuvenating the distal thigh.

Technique

Markings should be symmetrical and the incisional scar should hide within bikini outlines for trunk/thigh contouring. Patients are positioned to allow initial overcorrection of the lift with hip flexion of 30 degrees for both abdominoplasty and thigh lifting and thigh abduction of 30 to 40 degrees for thigh lifting. The flap to be resected is undermined. Further undermining is limited. In abdominoplasty, central undermining is limited to the rectus diastasis, extending onto the medial edge of the rectus muscle. Because vascular perforators move laterally as the rectus muscle diastasis widens, such limited undermining preserves maximal vascularity to the abdominal flap. In a minority of patients, there is flaccid skin in the epigastrium without a familial fat deposit. Undermining must be extended in this small group of patients if dimpling or bunching of the abdominal flap occurs after rectus plication. In patients with an epigastric fat deposit (even a small one), liposuction after the abdominoplasty wound repair will eliminate any bulging or dimpling of the abdominal contour.

In thigh/buttock lifting, direct undermining of the lateral thigh is limited to the trochanteric area, preserving the anterior and posterior (gluteal) blood supply. Discontinuous cannula undermining into the distal thigh can be used, if needed. Also, do not infuse dilute epinephrine solutions into the wound edges of directly undermined flaps. Although epinephrine may or may not affect the viability of an undermined flap in the trunk or thighs, avoiding epinephrine allows monitoring of the flap color during the procedure.

Resection is performed using a D'Assumpcão marking clamp, leaving more skin than SFS. A *two-layer SFS repair using nonabsorbable sutures* should result in a minimal-tension skin repair, reducing the risk of wound and scar complications. In the high-lateral-tension abdominoplasty design, the highest wound tension is placed laterally, reducing the tension on the undermined central flap and producing a body lift effect on adjacent tissue (waist, groin, upper thigh) for a natural, balanced rejuvenation.

Several fluted Blake drains are left in place for 7 to 14 days to minimize the risk of seroma formation. Light gauze dressings are applied. Compression garments or binders are unnecessary and may compromise the vascularity of undermined flaps.

Postoperative Management

In addition to appropriate patient selection, procedure design, and surgical technique, thoughtful postoperative care is required to limit unfavorable results after major body lifting. A hospital setting is appropriate for postoperative care after surgical trauma to large body surface areas. Prophylactic antibiotics are used on all body lift patients and are continued for 7 to 10 days or until after the last drain is removed (7 to 14 days).

The initial 24-hour period is critical to skin flap viability. To ensure adequate cardiac output and tissue perfusion, vigorous intravenous lactated Ringer (nondextrose) fluid resuscitation and frequent urinary output monitoring is performed in the early postoperative period. In addition, a slow intravenous (piggyback) drip of 500 mL of hetastarch (Hespan) is started at the end of the procedure and continues over 5 hours to help stabilize intravascular blood volume. In addition to adequate fluid resuscitation, proper patient positioning reduces postoperative wound tension, enhancing tissue perfusion of the wound edges.

Prophylaxis for deep vein thrombosis in patients without prior pathology includes leg elevation, support hose, pulsatile stockings, anemia (hemodilution), bed exercises and ambulation, and, in the absence of a significant blood loss problem, enteric-coated aspirin started on the first postoperative day.

Performing major body lifts in a hospital setting ensures appropriate nursing care and monitoring. Should the need arise, pulmonary x-rays or scans, pulse oximetry, intensive care unit availability, and specialty medical consultants will be available in a timely manner.

Treatment

The risk of life-threatening complications, such as pulmonary embolus or massive infection, is rare (less than 0.25%). Medical consultation, diagnostic scans, anticoagulation, and intensive care monitoring can successfully treat many pulmonary emboli. Massive infection also will require infectious disease consultation, diagnostic wound cultures, antibiotics, surgical drainage as needed, and in-hospital monitoring.

The risk of major skin necrosis is unusual (less than 3%) with new body lift designs and appropriate postoperative care. The risk of lesser complications is more significant, occurring in 10% to 20% of body lift patients. These complications include wound infection; delayed healing including wound dehiscence; minor degrees of necrosis; poor scarring; suture reactions and infection; seromas or hematomas; anemia; nonautologous blood transfusion; dog-ears; significant areas of anesthesia or paresthesia; inadequate lifting of tissues; and prolonged hospitalization or recovery.

Until ample experience is gained with body lift procedures, perform surgical rejuvenation of the entire circumferential trunk/thigh aesthetic unit in appropriate stages. This also allows one to "touch up" the results of the previous surgery with the next stage.

Wound Complications

If skin ischemia is noted after body lifting, treat initially with either 2% nitroglycerin ointment applied to the ischemic area every 4 to 6 hours or silver sulfadiazine cream applied twice daily. Either technique is useful in reducing the risk and extent of full-thickness skin loss. If marginal skin necrosis is minimal, delayed wound healing should occur uneventfully. Continue the silver sulfadiazine cream until healing is complete. If skin necrosis is more significant, conservative debridement is performed once wound healing is stable (3 to 5 weeks). After wound debridement is completed and granulations have appeared, secondary wound repair with antibiotic prophylaxis frequently is successful in treating areas of skin loss or of wound dehiscence. For larger wounds, secondary healing over weeks or months will allow wound contraction to reduce the size of the scar for future scar revision (Fig. 64-2A,B). Skin grafting may be necessary for patients who desire rapid wound closure.

Hypertrophic scars are less common with strong two-layer SFS repair, but still may occur in a small minority of patients. Excessive scars generally require many months or years to improve. Silicone elastomer sheeting may speed scar maturation. Scar revision after 1 year may be indicated.

Suture Complications

Suture reaction or infection is somewhat more common when using nonabsorbable sutures in the subcutaneous tissues. Braided nylon SFS sutures are dipped in povidone-iodine or antibiotic solution before use to help reduce suture complications. Suture granulomas or sinus tracts or exposed sutures will require suture removal for healing to progress.

Hematomas/Seromas

Hematomas are uncommon after body lifts. Significant hematomas will require surgical drainage. Seromas occur in 3% to 5 % of body lift patients. Prevention of seromas begins with surgical technique. Minimizing direct undermining in both abdominoplasty and thigh lifts will decrease the seroma rate. If wider undermining techniques are used, tacking the undermined flap to muscle fascia with multiple absorbable sutures is recommended. In addition, strong suturing of the SFS with nonabsorbable sutures avoids the subincisional dead space that can occur if the SFS repair separates in the first weeks after surgery. Using ample drains with slits rather than holes allows the drains to function longer without becoming plugged, even with minimal amounts of drainage. In general, long 15- or 19-French drains are used.

In abdominoplasty, two or three drains are brought out through the pubic area and remain in place for 7 to 8 days, regardless of the amount of drainage. The drains are removed when the drainage is minimal. In procedures involving thigh lifting, two large drains are placed into each thigh as far distal as the tissues have been raised. The drains exit the body through separate ports, in the pubic area and near the incision posteriorly. Drains should not exit through the incision. Because thigh drains must drain against gravity, two drains are used in case one fails early on. One of the drains is left in place for a minimum of 12 to 14 days.

If the diagnosis of seroma is in doubt, ultrasound can be effective in confirming the diagnosis (20). Once diagnosed, seromas must be treated early with frequent, repetitive external drainage and compression dressing or by the placement of a percutaneous drainage system (Seroma-Cath,

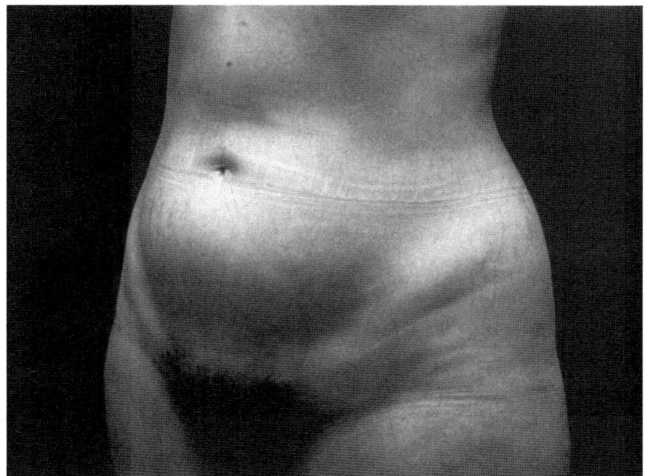
A

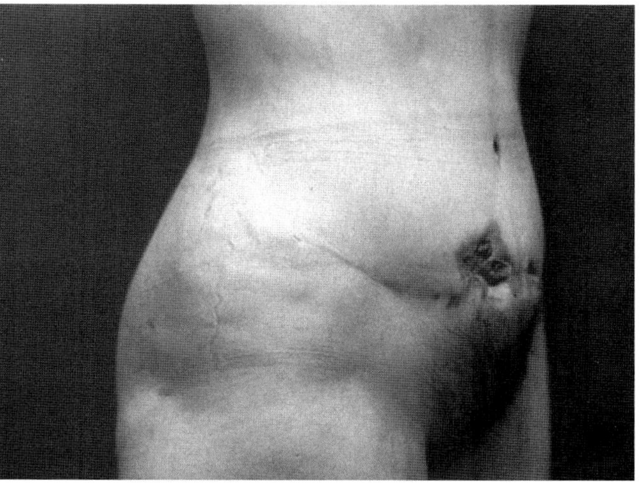
B

FIGURE 64-2. Preoperative **(A)** and postoperative **(B)** views after abdominoplasty, complicated by major skin necrosis due to a tight tape dressing. Conservative debridement and wound care over several months allowed maximal wound contraction without further surgery. Complications are better tolerated by the patient if the aesthetic contour results are significant and dramatic.

Greer Medical, Santa Barbara, CA, USA). Sclerosing agents, such as tetracycline, have been recommended for treatment of seromas, although the success rate varies and the treatment often is painful (21). Animal studies using tissue adhesives, such as fibrin glue or polyethylene oxide hydrogel, intraoperatively to help prevent seromas have been reported, although clinical human trials are lacking (22). Neglected seromas can evolve into a pseudobursa that requires surgical treatment (23).

ABDOMINOPLASTY

Modern abdominoplasty techniques were developed in the 1960s. Although many modifications were presented during the past 30 years, the surgical principles for standard abdominoplasty have remained largely the same. These principles include a transverse lower abdominal incision, wide undermining to the costal margins, tightening of the abdominal musculature, resection of the redundant abdominal flap with the maximum resection centrally, umbilical transposition, and skin closure with hips flexed.

Although the operation has been standardized, the long-term aesthetic results of standard abdominoplasty often have been inconsistent and disappointing. Common unfavorable features following standard abdominoplasty include initial overtightening of the central abdomen; residual laxity of the inguinal and lateral abdominal regions; late suprapubic scar depression with soft tissue bulges above and below the incisional scar; superior displacement of the pubic hair; poor waist definition; and asymmetrical, irregular, and hypertrophic scars (Fig. 64-3A, B) (24).

Avoidance of Unfavorable Results

All standard abdominoplasty techniques are based on faulty principles. Maximal truncal laxity occurs laterally in most patients, not centrally as assumed by standard abdominoplasty designs. The strong midline adherence of the epigastrium to the linea alba limits true vertical descent above the umbilicus. A more effective abdominoplasty design would tighten the lateral abdomen, waist, groin, and upper thighs more than the central abdomen, as well as allow circumferential liposculpturing of the trunk and thighs in a single stage. The high-lateral-tension abdominoplasty addresses the practical and theoretic faults of standard abdominoplasty design (5). Key features include limited direct undermining, increased lateral skin resection with highest-tension wound closure along lateral limbs, two-layer SFS repair, and significant truncal liposuction when needed (Fig. 64-4). The high-lateral-tension design limits the unfavorable features of standard abdominoplasty noted earlier and produces balanced, natural aesthetic contours (Fig. 64-5A,B).

Indications

The high-lateral-tension abdominoplasty is indicated for moderate-to-severe actual or potential skin laxity of the anterolateral trunk and upper thighs.

Design

Resection maximally along the lateral limbs of the abdominoplasty more accurately reverses truncal aging; provides lifting of the waist, inguinal area, and upper thighs; and decreases the tension on the suprapubic wound repair.

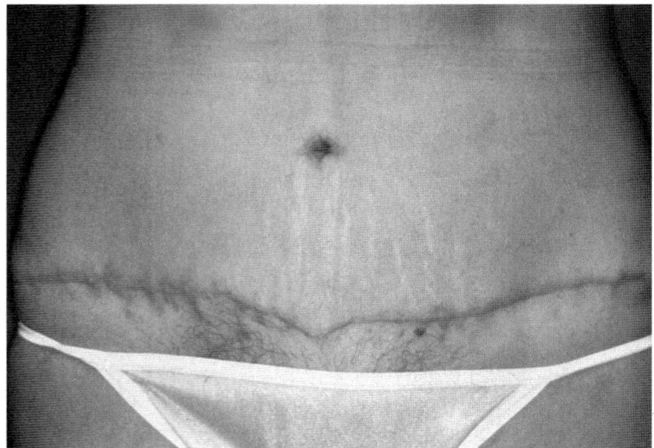
A

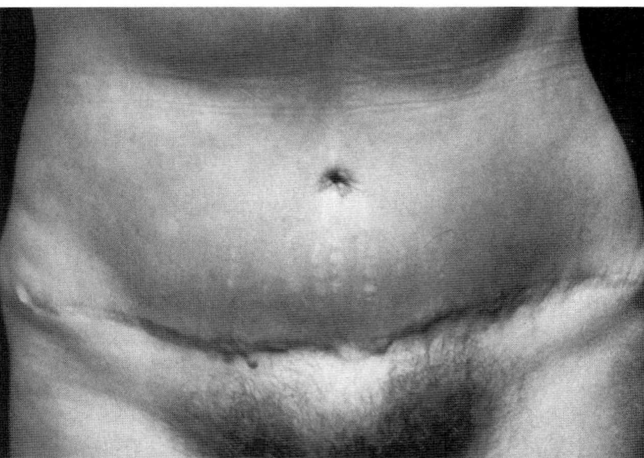
B

FIGURE 64-3. Postoperative views 3 months **(A)** and 15 months **(B)** after standard abdominoplasty demonstrate common delayed unfavorable results, which include late suprapubic scar depression with soft tissue bulges above and below the scar; superior displacement of the pubic hair; residual laxity of the inguinal and lateral abdominal regions; poor waist definition; and asymmetrical, irregular, and hypertrophic scars.

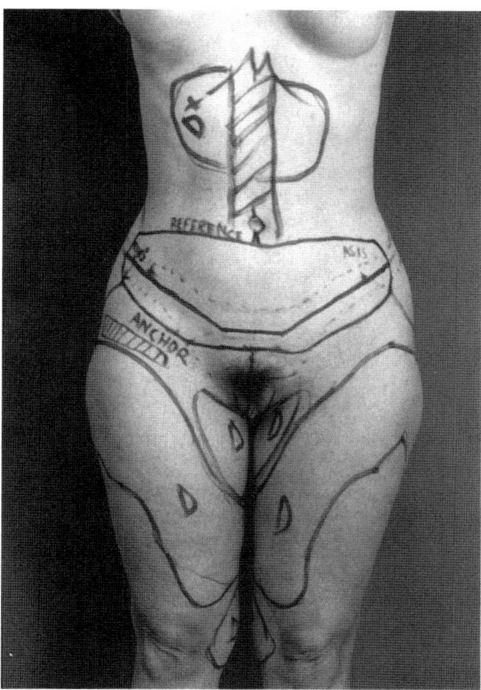

FIGURE 64-4. Design of the high-lateral-tension abdominoplasty places the highest wound tension in the lateral thirds of the incision and limits the direct undermining to just beyond the rectus diastasis. The superior blue line of the abdominoplasty pattern is for reference only; the actual resection is less than the pattern.

Less tension centrally reduces the risk of skin necrosis and superior migration of the pubic hair. SFS repair reduces tensions on the skin repair, resulting in improved scars with less late scar depression. Limiting direct undermining to the diastasis centrally and to the tissues to be resected laterally will reduce the risk of seromas and hematomas and will allow circumferential truncal liposuction in all areas except the new hypogastrium.

Treatment of Unfavorable Results

Delayed wound healing, suture reactions, seromas, and dog-ears are the most common unfavorable results following abdominoplasty. Dog-ears should be treated at the time of abdominoplasty. Dog-ears are produced by a folding of the entire skin/SFS/subcutaneous fat unit. Treatment begins with liposuctioning the fat within the SFS meshwork as well as the subdermal fat. Next, the skin of the dog-ear is sharply detached from the subcutaneous tissue (SFS complex) at the subdermal level. This dissociates the skin from the SFS, minimizing the dog-ear and allowing final trimming of the redundant skin. This technique successfully treats dog-ears even with a lateral resection angle of 90 to 100 degrees.

BRACHIOPLASTY

In the 1970s, significant innovations in brachioplasty techniques included careful preoperative planning and marking; incisional scar placement along the medial bicipital sulcus;

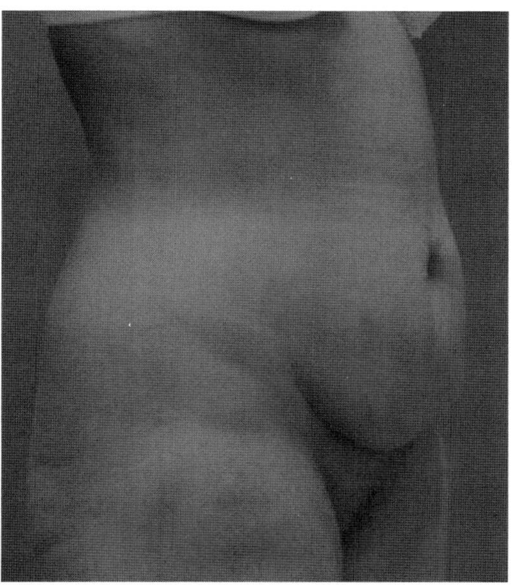

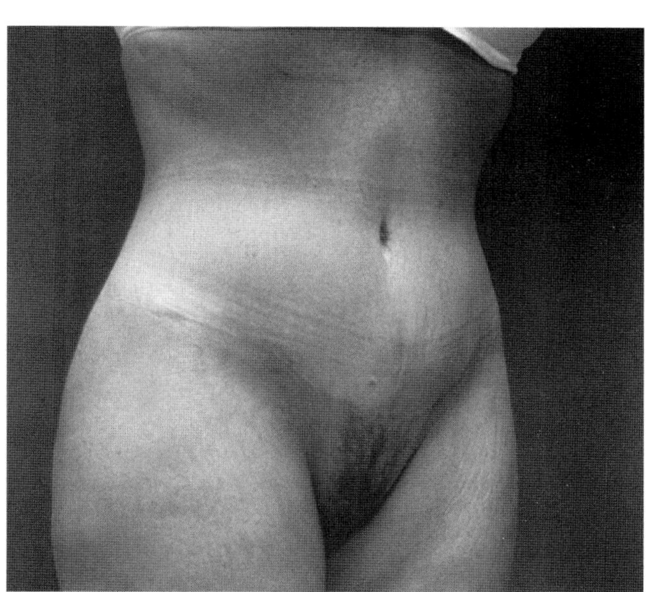

FIGURE 64-5. Preoperative **(A)** and 1-year postoperative **(B)** views after high-lateral-tension abdominoplasty and circumferential liposuction in a 34-year-old woman. The entire lower trunk and upper thighs are rejuvenated, producing balanced, natural contours.

cross-reference lines; axillary Z-plasties; straight, sinuous, or W-plasty incisions; and flap advancement techniques.

Despite these improvements, brachioplasty remains an unpopular procedure today for two reasons. First, liposuction has greatly reduced the number of patients requiring excisional surgery. Second, current brachioplasty techniques are somewhat unpredictable and are commonly associated with significant unfavorable results. Frequent problems include misplaced, widened, or hypertrophic scars; contour deformities due to overresection centrally and underresection proximally and distally; transverse cutaneous folds; and delayed wound healing due to marginal skin necrosis and suture dehiscence. (Fig. 64-6).

Avoidance of Unfavorable Results

All previous brachioplasty techniques are based on the assumption that relaxation of arm soft tissues is primarily responsible for the aesthetic deformity of the aging arm. A second, and perhaps more important, etiologic mechanism of the aesthetic arm deformity is relaxation of a longitudinal fascial system sling that extends from the clavicle to the posteromedial arm soft tissues via the clavipectoral and axillary fasciae (6). Re-anchoring of the posteromedial arm soft tissues to the axillary fascia with nonabsorbable sutures addresses the relaxation of this axillary fascial sling and forms the basis for the anchor brachioplasty. Similar to anchoring the medial thigh soft tissues to Colles fascia (perineum) in medial thigh lifts, fascial anchoring of brachioplasties provides more predictable results while reducing complications.

Indications

The primary indication for anchor brachioplasty is moderate-to-severe skin laxity of the arms with or without associated arm fat deposits. Patients with significant arm fat deposits with limited skin laxity should be treated with liposuction with postoperative compression for 3 to 4 months. Patients with lesser degrees of arm/axillary laxity can be treated with an axillary anchor brachioplasty without an arm incision.

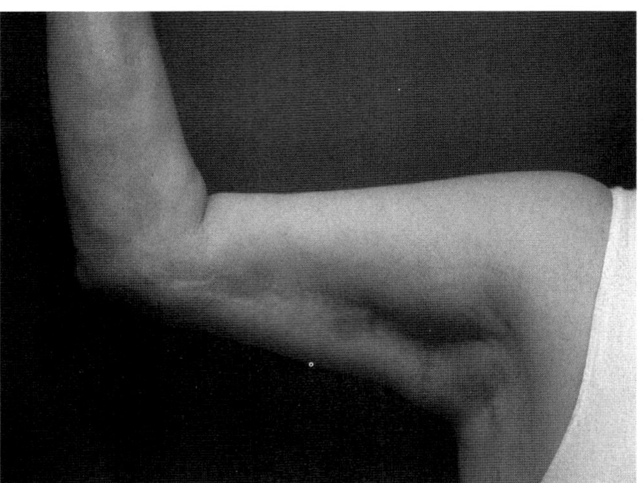

FIGURE 64-6. Common unfavorable results after standard brachioplasty include overresection centrally, with widened, misplaced scars, and underresection proximally and distally.

Design

Loosening of the connections of the arm SFS to the axillary fascia as well as relaxation of the axillary fascia itself with age, weight fluctuations, and gravitational pull yields a "loose hammock" effect, resulting in significant ptosis of the posteromedial arm. The degree of ptosis caused by loosening of the fascial support mechanism can be assessed in the preoperative patient by digitally forcing the lax upper medial arm soft tissues high into the axillary dome. In addition, as noted in high-tension closures in other excisional lifts of the body, repairing the SFS of all incisions with nonabsorbable sutures will provide a more secure wound closure and reduce the risk of hypertrophic scarring and scar widening.

The axillary incision is used to recreate an axillary hollow both to hide the incision and to provide support to the arm soft tissues. The longitudinal arm incision should fall in the medial bicipital sulcus after closure. This incision design avoids the central overresection ("dumbbell" deformity) that can occur with an elliptical resection of the medial arm.

Treatment of Unfavorable Results

Misplaced, Widened, or Hypertrophic Scars

Although scar revision may be useful in some cases, it often is limited due to scar malposition and overresection of the central arm tissues.

Contour Deformity

The dumbbell contour deformity is produced by central overresection and underresection proximally and distally. Liposuction of proximal and distal arm bulges along with adding an axillary resection and anchoring to axillary fascia may improve contours to some degree.

MEDIAL THIGH LIFT

Skin laxity in the medial thigh is frequently the earliest sign of aging in the thighs and is one of the first signs of significant ptosis in the body. The skin of the medial thigh is quite thin and inelastic, resulting in early relaxation with age and poor retraction after liposuction even by the age of 35 years. Laxity of the medial thighs may occur at even earlier ages when there is a history of obesity or a familial trait of early skin relaxation.

Avoidance of Unfavorable Results

The classic medial thigh lift has been plagued with persistent problems, such as inferior migration and widening of scars, lateral traction deformity of the vulva (Fig. 64-7), and early recurrence of ptosis. In an attempt to limit unfavorable results, the medial thigh lift was modified to allow anchoring the inferior skin flap to the tough, inelastic deep layer of the superficial fascia of the perineum (1). Using Colles fascia as the central anchor for the medial thigh lift has produced more consistent, long-lasting results and decreased the risk of problems commonly associated with the classic skin suspension medial thigh lift.

Indications

Significant actual or potential laxity of the medial thigh tissues remains the standard indication for medial thigh lifting. As noted earlier, the "medial thigh lift" effect of the high-lateral-tension abdominoplasty has reduced the need for medial thigh lifting in many patients. Also, tightening the medial thigh without first tightening lax tissues of the lower abdomen, pubis, and groin will create an unaesthetic appearance of this region.

Design

Since originally describing the fascial anchoring technique for medial thigh lifts in 1987 (1), numerous technical refinements have been developed to provide enhanced predictability and aesthetics. The *design* of the lift has changed due to a better understanding of thigh aesthetic deformities. Because the majority of skin laxity occurs at the juncture of the anterior and medial thighs, the resectional pattern has rotated anteriorly, allowing the entire procedure to be performed with the patient in the supine position (Fig. 64-8). In contrast to previous descriptions, the incision should not extend into the buttock fold posteriorly. The resectional ellipse can be extended to the anterior superior iliac spine for more extensive problems in the anterior thigh and inguinal areas.

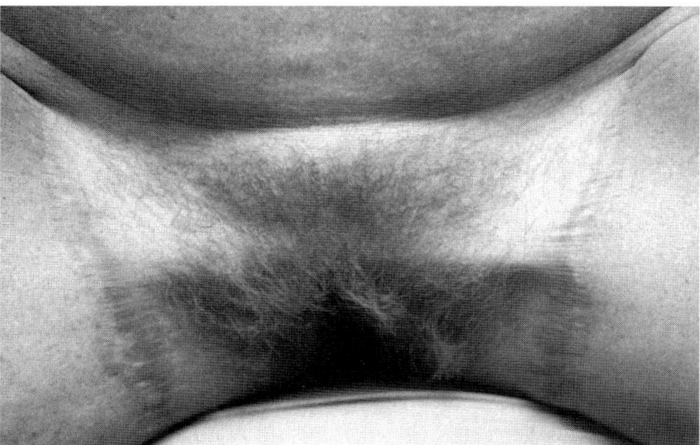

FIGURE 64-7. Lateral traction deformity of the vulva and inferior displacement of the scars are common unfavorable results after standard skin suspension medial thigh lifting.

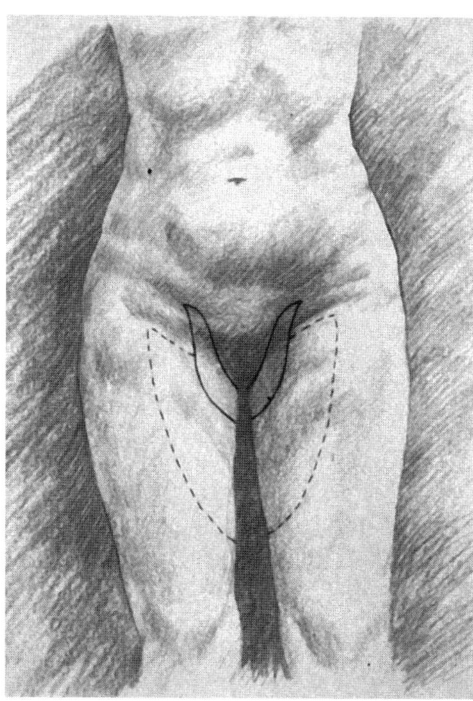

FIGURE 64-8. The medial thigh lift resectional pattern has rotated anteriorly, because most laxity occurs in the anteromedial area of the upper thigh. Do not extend the incision into the buttock fold posteriorly.

Technique

To reduce scar widening and migration, the actual skin resection has become more conservative over the years, averaging 5 to 7 cm of stretched skin at the anteromedial corner of the thigh. Anchoring the perineal thigh crease into Colles fascia provides an additional 3 to 5 cm of lift. The excision of redundant tissue and subsequent repair are performed with the knees shoulder-width apart (rather than frog-leg) to avoid undercorrection. Superficial (8 to 10 mm) undermining lateral to the mons pubis preserves the external pudendal blood and lymphatic vessels, reducing the risk of lymphatic complications.

Anchoring the inferior skin flap to Colles fascia of the perineum with nonabsorbable sutures reduces the risk of scar widening, scar migration, and lateral traction deformity of the vulva. When identifying Colles fascial roll, it is important not to overdissect this fascia. Digital dissection using a dry gauze sponge over the adductor muscles most reliably preserves Colles fascial anatomy. Retracting the skin and superficial fat of the vulva medially will expose the Colles fascial roll at the deepest and most lateral aspect of the vulvar soft tissues. Nonabsorbable anchoring sutures into Colles fascia are used (0 braided nylon, dipped in povidone-iodine solution). In addition, Scarpa fascia is used as the anchor anteriorly and the buttock fold SFS posteriorly. Next, the 0 braided nylon sutures are placed into the thigh flap SFS. Dermal repair is completed with 3-0 absorbable sutures followed by interrupted 3-0 nylon sutures. Light dressings are applied. Drains generally are not used.

Treatment of Unfavorable Results

Scar Widening/Migration and Vulvar Deformity

This is the most common long-term unfavorable result of medial thigh lifting. This usually can be prevented by avoiding overresection and by strong anchoring to Colles fascia with nonabsorbable sutures. Once established, treatment is primarily a resuspension of the anteromedial thigh tissues. For moderate problems, anchoring to Colles fascia may suffice. For more severe problems, perform an extended medial thigh lift by essentially combining the medial thigh lift with a high-lateral-tension abdominoplasty. This provides a much stronger anchor than perineal thigh crease anchoring alone.

Delayed Wound Healing

Medial thigh lifts have a higher risk of delayed healing than other body lifts (30% to 35%), especially in patients with heavier thighs (who require much liposuction and have minimal space between the thighs). In patients undergoing multiple body contouring procedures, performing the medial thigh lift at a second stage is advisable. Delayed wound healing should be treated conservatively with frequent wound cleansing, air drying, light gauze dressings, and antibiotics as indicated. Exposed permanent anchoring sutures are removed. Resultant scar widening can be treated in 6 to 12 months as noted earlier.

Inadequate Thigh Lifting

The most common causes of residual medial thigh relaxed deformity are poor surgical design and failure to accurately anchor to Colles fascia with nonabsorbable sutures (see earlier). Poor anchoring rather than underresection is usually the problem. The lower abdominal, inguinal, and pubic tissues are the foundation for the anteromedial thigh. Any significant laxity of these tissues must be treated (high-lateral-tension abdominoplasty) before or at the time of medial thigh lifting.

Major Skin Necrosis

Major skin necrosis with medial thigh lifting is rare. Significant thigh flap undermining with or without hematoma and superficial liposuction at the time of the medial thigh lift may result in major necrosis. This can largely be prevented by not undermining the thigh flap and by only performing deep liposuction during medial thigh lifting. Long-term wound care, which includes silver sulfadiazine cream, antibiotics, and conservative debridement, is indicated. Skin grafting may be required.

THIGH/BUTTOCK LIFT

The thigh/buttock lift of Pitanguy (11) originally was designed in 1964 to allow direct excision of trochanteric fat deposits. For 30 years, the Pitanguy lift also was used as the standard surgery for laxity and cellulite of the lateral thigh and buttock region.

Avoidance of Unfavorable Results

Pitanguy's thigh lift has been performed infrequently due to problems such as noticeable scars, early recurrence of deformities, unnatural contours, significant wound complications, long operative times, and prolonged postoperative disability (Fig. 64-9) (25). With the advent of liposuction and better knowledge of the vascular anatomy of skin and the anatomy of the SFS (2), a new thigh/buttock lift procedure was designed (3). The flank/thigh/buttock lift design uses a transverse resection of redundant tissue of the body (between major vascular territories of the trunk and thighs) with an incisional scar within high-cut bikini lines (Fig. 64-1).

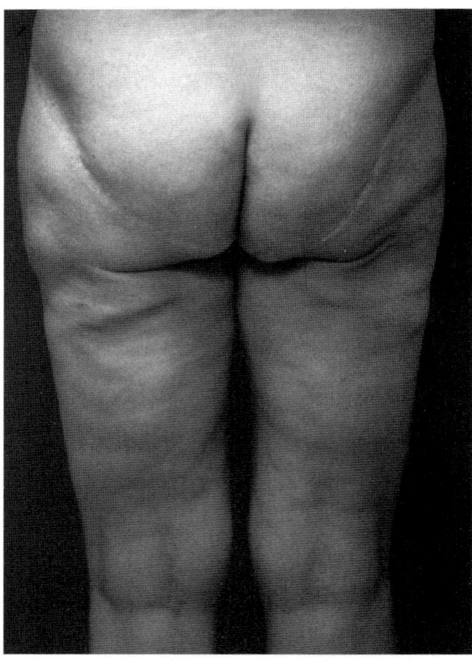

FIGURE 64-9. Common unfavorable results after the Pitanguy thigh/buttock lift include scars outside of current bikini lines, unnatural contours, supratrochanteric depression, inadequate lifting, significant wound complications, and long postoperative disability.

Indications

The transverse flank/thigh/buttock lift is indicated for moderate-to-severe laxity and cellulite of the trunk and thighs and/or buttock ptosis.

Design

The transverse thigh/buttock lift provides numerous advantages over the Pitanguy lift. There is improved skin flap vascularity; strong yet dynamic fascial support; simultaneous lifting of the trunk, buttock, thigh tissues; natural youthful contours; and a stable scar that remains hidden in bikini lines. Patients presenting with laxity and cellulite of the flank/lateral thigh/buttock region usually have associated relaxation of the abdomen and medial thighs. Strong lifting of the posterolateral trunk and thighs without concomitant abdominoplasty increases the degree of abdominal relaxation, resulting in marked disharmony of the body aesthetic unit. The transverse thigh/buttock lift alone is used infrequently, except as a staged procedure after previous abdominoplasty. Even then, a modified secondary abdominoplasty often is required.

The thigh/buttock lift most commonly is combined with the high-lateral-tension abdominoplasty (lower body lift, version 2) (Fig. 64-10A,B). As noted earlier, this combination will produce a moderate lift of the medial thighs. A more significant medial thigh problem will require a staged medial thigh lift. The medial thigh lift is combined with the thigh/buttock lift (lower body lift, version 1) as a primary procedure in patients with minimal abdominal problems (or previous abdominoplasty) and significant medial thigh relaxation.

Technique

The amount of soft tissue laxity superior to the planned line of closure is estimated (4 to 5 cm). The lax tissue inferior to the line of closure generally ranges from 10 to 18 cm, producing a total vertical resection of 14 to 23 cm. In the lateral decubitus position, the hip is flexed anteriorly 30 to 45 degrees, and the thighs are abducted with foam blocks to keep the knees 15 inches apart. The superior resection line is incised. Direct undermining should extend beneath the flap to be resected and into the trochanteric region. No undermining is performed over the buttocks. Discontinuous cannula undermining is performed more distally if the aesthetic deformity extends into the lower half of the thigh.

The redundant soft tissue is resected, being careful to leave more skin than underlying SFS. This allows a minimal-tension skin repair after SFS anchoring sutures are placed (two-layer, No. 1 and 2-0 braided nylon). The anterior incisions meet across the suprapubic area to resect skin excess and repair muscle laxity of the lower abdomen. Two 19-French fluted (Blake) silicone drains are inserted into

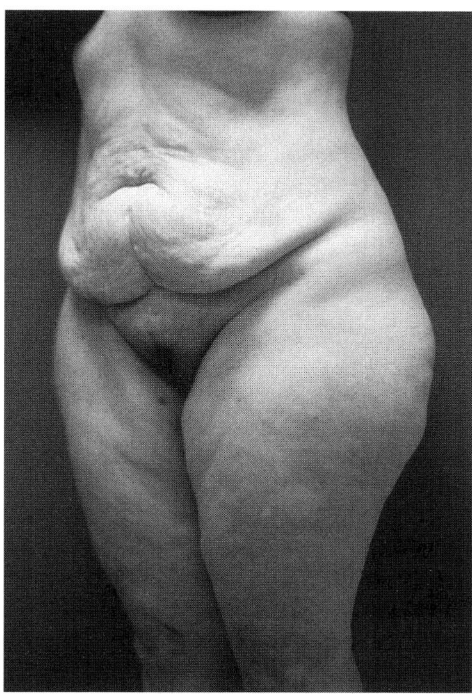
A

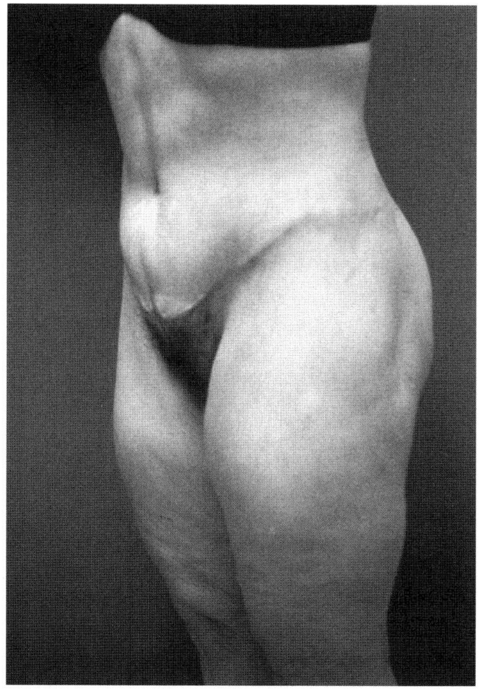
B

FIGURE 64-10. Preoperative **(A)** and 4-month postoperative **(B)** views after lower body lift (version 2) in a 52-year-old woman. The suture line ridge created at surgery with all superficial fascial system repairs usually takes 5 to 8 months to totally flatten. This reduces the risk of hypertrophic or widened scars.

each thigh as far distally as possible, exiting in the mons pubis anteriorly and near the incision posteriorly. The procedure is performed on the opposite side in similar fashion. Light dressings are applied and no compression garment is used.

Lower Body Lift, Version 1 (Combined with Medial Thigh Lift)

After completion of the thigh/buttock lift, the patient is placed supine with knees shoulder-width apart and the hips flexed 30 degrees. Follow the described medial thigh lift technique. No undermining is performed over the femoral triangle lymphatics.

Lower Body Lift, Version 2 (Combined with High-lateral-tension Abdominoplasty)

The high-lateral-tension abdominoplasty is performed first, closing the incisions to the anterior superior iliac spine region. The thigh/buttock lift is completed in the lateral decubitus position.

Treatment of Unfavorable Results

Scarring

Widened, asymmetrical, misplaced, or hypertrophic scars may occur after thigh lifting. Careful preoperative planning and avoiding excessive wound repair tensions reduce scar complications. Treatment of scar complications generally should be delayed for 8 to 12 months. Widened or hypertrophic scars may be improved with simple scar revision. Misplaced scars often require further body lifting.

Inadequate Lifting

Long incisions around the body are well tolerated if incisions are hidden in bikinis and the aesthetic results are dramatic. Select patients with significant laxity and cellulite problems for body lifting. Photographic documentation of the laxity problem is essential. Appropriate lift design with overcorrection is important. Unfortunately, a second body lift is required to correct inadequate lifts or asymmetrical or misplaced scars.

In conclusion, modern body lifting is an exciting frontier for plastic surgeons. Although the results can be dramatic and fulfilling, the surgeries are labor intensive and challenging. Life-threatening complications are rare, but there is a significant risk of unfavorable results that can be minimized with proper patient selection, careful surgical design, planning, and execution, and appropriate postoperative care.

A final caveat: Complications are reasonably well tolerated if the aesthetic results are dramatic and significant (Figs. 64-2, 64-11). Likewise, if the aesthetic results are mediocre or poorly documented, even very minor complications may seem quite troublesome to the patient.

A

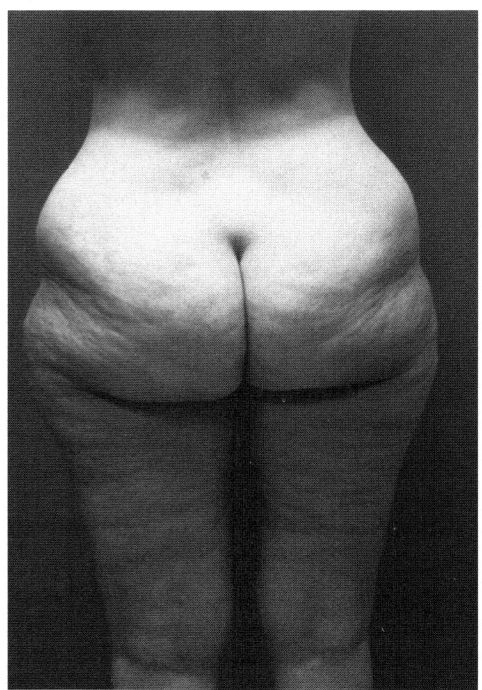

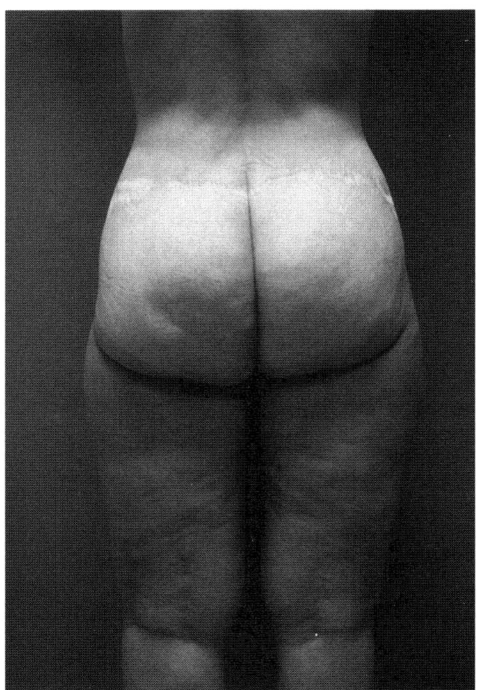

B

FIGURE 64-11. A,B: Lower body lift complicated by bilateral areas of skin necrosis and scarring laterally. Conservative debridement and care for several months resulted in healing without further surgery. Significant complications are reasonably well tolerated by the patient if the aesthetic results are significant and dramatic.

REFERENCES

1. Lockwood T. Fascial anchoring in medial thigh lifts. *Plast Reconstr Surg.* 1988;82:299–304.
2. Lockwood T. Superficial fascial system (SFS) of the trunk and extremities: a new concept. *Plast Reconstr Surg.* 1991;87: 1009–1018.
3. Lockwood T. Transverse flank-thigh-buttock lift with superficial fascial suspension. *Plast Reconstr Surg.*1991;87:1019–1027.
4. Lockwood T. Lower body lift with superficial fascial system suspension. *Plast Reconstr Surg.*1993;92:1112–1122.
5. Lockwood T. High-lateral-tension abdominoplasty with superficial fascial system suspension. *Plast Reconstr Surg* 1995; 96:603–615.
6. Lockwood T. Brachioplasty with superficial fascial system suspension. *Plast Reconstr Surg* 1995;96:912–920.
7. Callia W. *Dermolipectomia abdominal.* Sao Paulo, Brazil: Centro de cinematografia Carlo Erba, 1965.
8. Correa-Iturraspe M, Fernandez, JC. Dermolipectomia braquial. *Prensa Med Argent.* 1954;34:24–32.
9. Gonzalez-Ulloa M. Belt lipectomy. *Br J Plast Surg* 1961; 13:179–184.
10. Lewis J. The thigh lift. *J Int Coll Surg* 1957;27:330–334.
11. Pitanguy I. Trochanteric lipodystrophy. *Plast Reconstr Surg* 1964;34:280–286.
12. Pitanguy I. Abdominal lipectomy: an approach to it through an analysis of 300 consecutive cases. *Plast Reconstr Surg* 1967; 40:384–391.
13. Pitanguy I. Correction of lipodystrophy of the lateral thoracic aspect and inner side of the arm and elbow dermosenescence. *Clin Plast Surg* 1975;2:477–483.
14. Somalo M. Dermolipectomia circular del tronco. *Semana Med* 1940;47:1435–1441.
15. Spadafora A. Abdomen pendulo: dermolipectomia anterolateral baja (technica persona). *Prensa Med Argent* 1962;49:494–503.
16. Vilain R, Dubousset J. Techniques et indications de la lipectomie circulaire: a propos de 150 interventions. *Ann Chir* 1964; 18:289–294.
17. Illouz YG. Body contouring by lipolysis: a 5-year experience with over 3000 cases. *Plast Reconstr Surg* 1983;72:591–597.
18. Hardy J, ed. *Hardy's textbook of surgery,* 2nd ed. Philadelphia: JB Lippincott, 1988.
19. Peacock E. Wound healing and wound care. In: Schwartz S, Shires GT, Spencer F, eds. *Principles in surgery,* 5th ed. New York: McGraw-Hill, 1989:307–330.
20. Mohammad JA, Warnke PH, Stavraky W. Ultrasound in the diagnosis and management of fluid collection complications following abdominoplasty. *Ann Plast Surg* 1998;41:498–502.
21. McCarthy PM, Martin JK, Wells DC, et al. An aborted, prospective, randomized trial of sclerotherapy for prolonged drainage after mastectomy. *Surg Gynecol Obstet* 1986;162:418–420.
22. Silverman RP, Elisseeff J, Passaretti D, et al. Transdermal photopolymerized adhesive for seroma prevention. *Plast Reconstr Surg* 1999;103:531–535.
23. Ersek RA, Schade K. Subcutaneous pseudobursa secondary to suction and surgery. *Plast Reconstr Surg* 1990;85:442–445.
24. Guerrerosantos J, Spaillat L, Morales F. Some problems and solutions in abdominoplasty. *Aesthetic Plast Surg* 1980;4:227–237.
25. Regnault P, Daniel RK. Secondary thigh-buttock deformities after classical techniques: prevention and treatment. *Clin Plast Surg* 1984;11:505–513.

SUGGESTED READING

1. Baroudi R, Keppke EM, Tozzi Neto F. Abdominoplasty. *Plast Reconstr Surg* 1974;54:161–167.
2. Baroudi R. Dermatolipectomy of the upper arm. *Clin Plast Surg*1975;2:485–494.
3. Baroudi R, Moraes M. Philosophy, technical principles, selection, and indications in body contouring surgery. *Aesthetic Plast Surg* 1991;15:1–18.
4. Grazer FM. Abdominoplasty. *Plast Reconstr Surg* 1973;51: 617–623.
5. Grazer FM, ed. *Atlas of suction assisted lipectomy in body contouring.* New York: Churchill Livingstone, 1992.
6. Guerrerosantos J. Brachioplasty. *Aesthetic Plast Surg* 1979;3: 1–14.
7. Illouz YG, De Villers Y. *Body sculpturing by lipoplasty.* New York: Churchill Livingstone, 1989.
8. Juri J, Juri C, Elias JC. Arm dermolipectomy with a quadrangular flap and "T" closure. *Plast Reconstr Surg* 1979;64:521–525.
9. Pitman GH. *Liposuction and aesthetic surgery.* St. Louis: Quality Medical Publishing, 1993.
10. Planas J. The "crural meloplasty" for lifting of the thighs. *Clin Plast Surg* 1975;2:495–503.
11. Regnault P. Abdominoplasty by the W technique. *Plast Reconstr Surg* 1975;55:265–274.
12. Regnault P. Brachioplasty, axilloplasty, and preaxilloplasty. *Aesthetic Plast Surg.* 1983;7:31–36.
13. Regnault P, Daniel RK. *Aesthetic plastic surgery: principles and treatment.* Boston: Little, Brown and Company, 1984.

Discussion

BODY CONTOURING WITH EXCISIONS

IVO PITANGUY

Body contouring surgery is a field where surgical creativity meets anatomical limitations and at the same time where the highly motivated patient frequently encounters the surgeon's reluctance to perform surgery. Dissatisfaction may begin well before surgery, and proper indication is perhaps the most important step to avoid the unhappy patient. The experienced surgeon should be able to perceive the patient's hidden desires and weigh the factors that may or may not be within a realistic goal. The unfavorable results in body contouring surgery are always a source of frustration for the surgeon, yet revisions and touchups are fallbacks that, in this area of plastic surgery, are commonly performed with greater acceptance.

Over the past decades, we have witnessed the constant evolution of body contouring. With the advent of suction-assisted lipectomy, surgeons finally gained the capacity to "sculpt" the patient's body with greater finesse and minimal incisions, relegating the large removal of excess fat, by means of extensive scars, to selected cases. Nevertheless, basic precepts of excisional body contouring procedures have continued to expand, for example, with better understanding of functional anatomy. The ultimate goal of these procedures remains a challenge to this day: the removal of excess cutaneous and fatty tissue, while maintaining a natural contour and leaving the patient with socially acceptable scars.

One of the many contributors to this field has been Dr. Lockwood, who is well known for his dedication to body contouring. His descriptions of the superficial fascial system, whose function is to encase, support, and shape the fat of the body, together with techniques based on this structure, have been valuable additions to our understanding of body contouring (1–5). In this splendid chapter, Dr. Lockwood presents an overall view regarding excisional lipectomy in a clear and didactic manner, pointing out, by different anatomical regions, the many pitfalls of which the younger surgeons should constantly be aware. The avoidance of each potential problem is covered extensively and needs no further comment.

Body contouring presents the plastic surgeon with many conflicting issues (6–9). In today's aesthetically aware society, patients are almost impelled to correct even the smallest deformity. Furthermore, the dichotomy between ideal form and opposing factors, such as weight gain, skin flaccidity, and the inevitable aging process, becomes the source of personal frustration. On the other hand, increasing leisure time and sports activities result in constant exposure of the body. Body contour deformities may involve aspects regarding the patient's psychosocial status and overall health, and so the surgeon must always consider the possible benefit of including the participation of a multidisciplinary team approach.

It should be remembered that, although these deformities may be treated by a single operation, they may demand more complex, combined procedures. Multiple or severe deformities, such as in patients who have undergone dramatic weight loss, will require a multistage plan. Body contouring in these cases should be considered a surgical program; consequently, a second and even a third stage will be seen as part of a continuum (10–12). Above all, the full participation of the patient is to be encouraged. This is especially true in cases where more than one operation is indicated, the order of which is an important aspect to be decided. It is a good strategy to begin the surgical program addressing those areas that present with the greatest possibility of patient satisfaction, thus encouraging the patient to continue with subsequent operations. Each patient should have his or her intimate desires evaluated and, wherever possible, the surgeon should be supportive of these motivations.

These preliminary considerations serve to underscore the obligation that every plastic surgeon has to measure patient expectations and to be very honest regarding the limitations of the different surgical techniques. A deep understanding of the person as a lucid body, one that is constantly interacting with his or her social and emotional environment, allows the surgeon to capture the true nature of these procedures. Furthermore, possible revisions are foreseen and discussed, thus maintaining patient credibility (13,14). Dr. Lockwood has very adequately covered these points, stressing the importance of a frank discussion beforehand to avoid frustration with the results obtained.

As the author mentioned, core concepts in body contouring surgery have remained basically unchanged, and in our hands they have given consistent and predictable results. They will be reviewed briefly. Adequate planning begins before the patient is examined, by discouraging those who are

I. Pitanguy: Clinica Ivo Pitanguy, Rio de Janeiro, Brazil

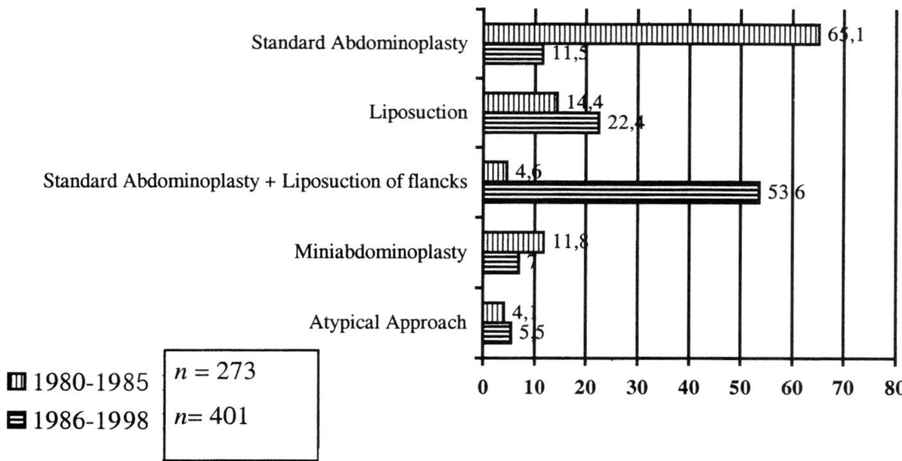

FIGURE 64D-1. Body contour surgery of the abdomen. Comparison of two periods: 1980 to 1985 and 1986 to 1998. Cases are grouped by procedures.

grossly overweight, who have unrealistic results in mind, or whose motivations are centered on the will of others. Although liposuction has greatly decreased the indications for dermolipectomies, excess skin requires skin removal with the necessary implication of permanent scars, and this should be explained to the patient (Figs. 64D-1, 64D-2).

In preparation for surgery, our routine includes complete clinical and laboratory examinations. When two or more simultaneous procedures are planned and a large blood loss is expected, autologous blood transfusion may be indicated. This is begun at least 2 weeks before surgery. A well-coordinated surgical team is essential to optimize operative time (11). The anesthesiologists should be familiar with the long duration of the operation and the different stages of surgery, as some procedures require that the patient be placed in different positions.

Excisional techniques that were in use more than 40 years ago commonly resulted in large scars that widened and displaced with time, and whose final position was aesthetically unacceptable in many cases. Contouring of the abdomen was restricted to large deformities, with simple resection of excess tissues and limited concern for function. Together with other colleagues who shared our interest in excisional techniques, personal contributions were reported that emphasized respect for anatomy and the dynamics of areas presenting with contour deformities, with the aim to correctly position scars.

These precepts, applied to *trochanteric lipodystrophy* and the "riding breeches" deformity, included limiting dissection to those tissues to be resected, curving incisions to better camouflage scars, and rotating flaps rather than simply pulling on them (7,15–17). It was understood that direct traction leads to high tension, and when this is applied to the skin/dermis unit, will cause the drawbacks mentioned by Dr. Lockwood. Rotation, on the other hand, implies a repositioning of the tissues. When this is done together with meticulous suturing in layers, which includes the superficial fascial system, tension is removed from the skin.

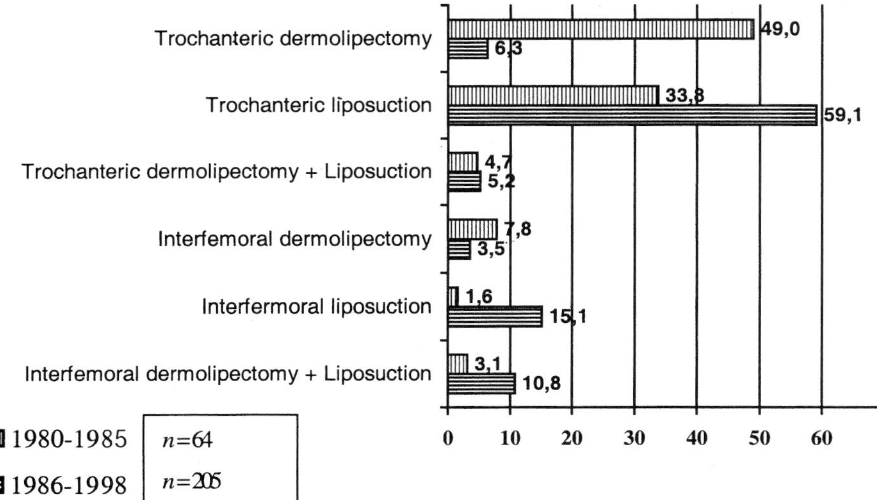

FIGURE 64D-2. Procedures in trochanteric and interfemoral regions. Comparison of two periods: 1980 to 1985 and 1986 to 1998. Cases are grouped by procedures.

Excision of *upper limb flaccidity accompanied by lateral thoracic lipodystrophy* has been described as a single procedure (16,18,19). A sinuous, curving incision demarcates excess tissue of the inner aspect of the arm, continues along the axilla taking care to "break" the incision to avoid a cicatricial band, and finishes at the submammary fold to better camouflage scars. This procedure currently is reserved for patients who present with gross weight loss.

The approach to *abdominal lipodystrophy and flaccidity*, as first described in 1967 (20), includes a lower positioning of the final scars so that they are hidden under bathing trunks. Incision positioning should respect the patient's preferences, and social and sports activities. We tend to place the incision lower due to greater body exposure in our country, yet the higher positioning of scars, as seen in Dr. Lockwood's cases, is acceptable if this is planned with the participation of the patient.

Dissection of the abdominal wall is restricted to the central portion, leaving the flanks to be treated with liposuction. Plication of the rectus abdominis aponeurosis is done with inverted nonabsorbable suture, without opening of the aponeurosis, from the xiphoid process down to the pubis. This causes tension toward the midline, resulting in reinforcement of the abdominal wall. The umbilicus is repositioned through a transverse incision that, following tension on the flaps, is transformed into a smooth ring. The abdominal flaps, once ready for final positioning, are rotated towards the midline, causing the lateral abdomen to be further shaped and avoiding dog-ears to decrease the extension of the scar.

Finally, it has been our observation that placing a plaster mold over a thick, soft dressing over the flap has significantly decreased our rate of serosanguinous collection. In the first 48 hours, a small weight is positioned on this shield, so that constant and even pressure is exerted over dissected tissues.

We believe that these contributions have established a methodology that has allowed for consistent and aesthetically pleasing results, with a very low rate of unfavorable results (Table 64D-1) (21,22).

TABLE 64D-1. COMPARISON OF COMPLICATIONS OF ABDOMINOPLASTY IN DIFFERENT TIME PERIODS

Complication	1955–1960 (n = 32)	1961–1979 (n = 637)	1980–1998 (n = 631)
Dehiscence	6.2	2.8	1.0
Serosanguinous collection	15.6	4.2	0.3
Infection	3.1	0.6	0.1
Hypertrophic scar	3.1	2.9	1.3
Residual fat	3.1	0.9	0.5
Wide umbilical scar	2.0	1.0	0.3

Values are given on percentages.

TABLE 64-2. ASSOCIATED PROCEDURES IN AESTHETIC PLASTIC SURGERY PERFORMED IN 1967–1979

Associated Procedures	Percentage
Face lift + rhinoplasty	28.3
Rhinoplasty + mentoplasty	14.5
Face lift + mammaplasty	12.3
Mammaplasty + abdominoplasty	9.0
Face lift + mentoplasty	8.6
Face lift + abdominoplasty	7.9

n = 3,342.

FINAL COMMENTS

With experience, the surgeon who follows these principles of excisional surgery should obtain natural contour, with infrequent complications and acceptable final scars. Solid knowledge and respect for anatomy and a keen aesthetic sense cannot be overstressed. We have been rewarded in these contributions by the high degree of patient satisfaction and by the results reported by colleagues who comprehended these principles. Body contouring often is performed in association with other aesthetic procedures. The preparation of an expert surgical team is essential. Tables 64D-2, 64D-3 list our experience with combined surgery in all areas and show the importance of body contouring in our practice.

A few selected cases illustrate the principal contributions to body contouring.

Patient 1: Correction of the "Riding Breeches" Deformity

This 45-year-old woman presented with excess skin and fat in the lateral aspects of the thighs. Although performed many years ago, excisional removal for similar cases remains the correct indication if the patient requests complete correction of the trochanteric lipodystrophy and agrees with final scars. An alternative approach is to plan serial liposuctions to allow the skin to gradually adapt to the new contour. Preoperative views of the patient are shown in Fig. 64D-3A–C). Postoperative views at 1 year shows a satisfactory final contour and acceptable scars (Fig. 64D-3D–F).

TABLE 64-3. ASSOCIATED PROCEDURES IN AESTHETIC PLASTIC SURGERY PERFORMED IN 1980–1998

Associated Procedures	Percentage
Face lift + rhinoplasty	13.1
Face lift + abdominoplasty	11.7
Face lift + mammaplasty	10.4
Face lift + lipo suction (body contouring)	9.7
Mammaplasty + abdominoplasty	7.6
Rhinoplasty + mentoplasty	4.5

n = 2,427.

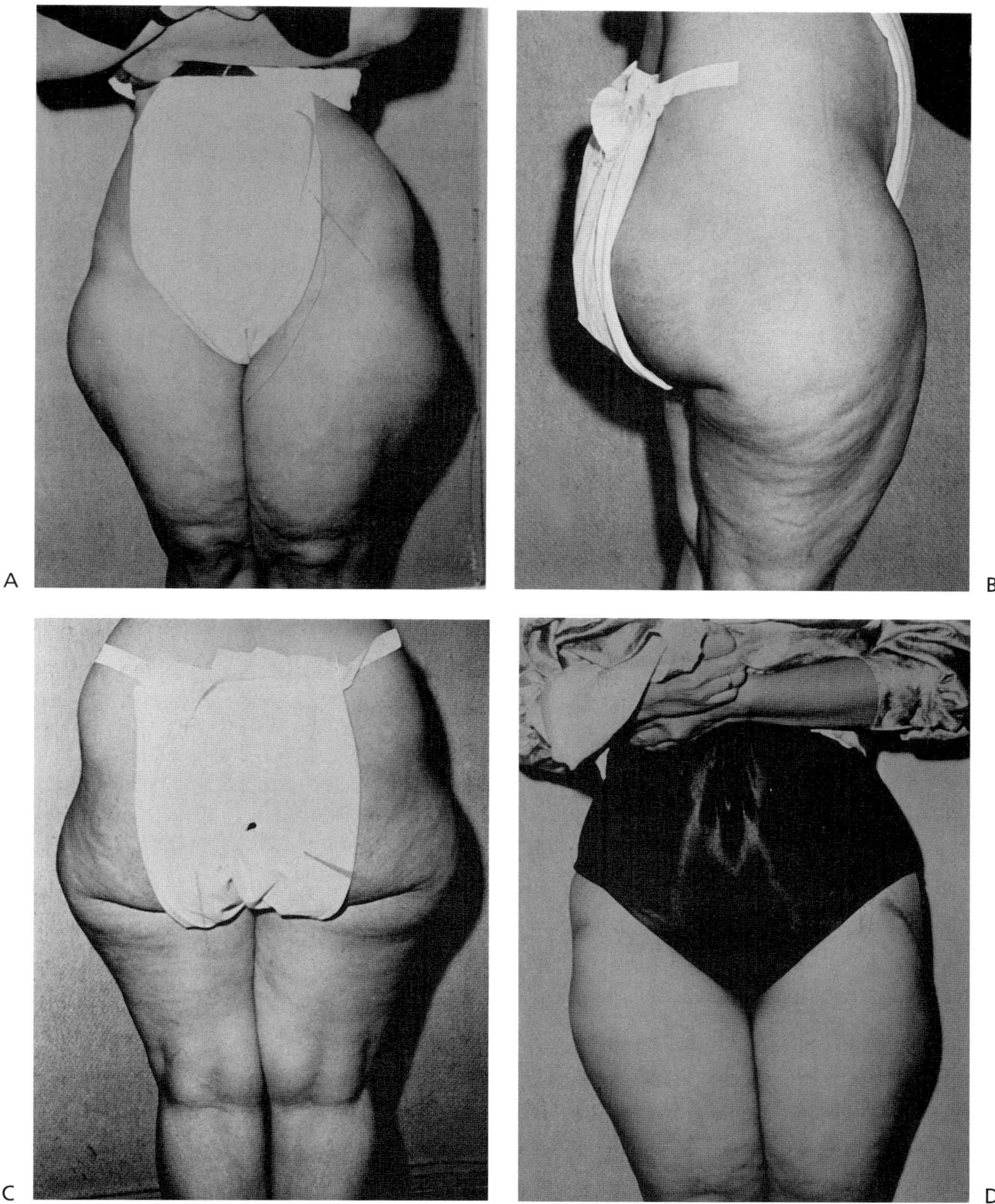

FIGURE 64D-3. Correction of the "riding breeches" deformity. A 45-year-old woman presented with excess skin and fat in the lateral aspects of the thighs. Although performed many years ago, excisional removal remains the correct indication if the patient requests complete correction of the trochanteric lipodystrophy and agrees with final scars. An alternative approach is to plan serial liposuctions to allow the skin to gradually adapt to the new contour. **A–C:** Preoperative views. **D–F:** One-year postoperative views show a satisfactory final contour and acceptable scars. (*continued*)

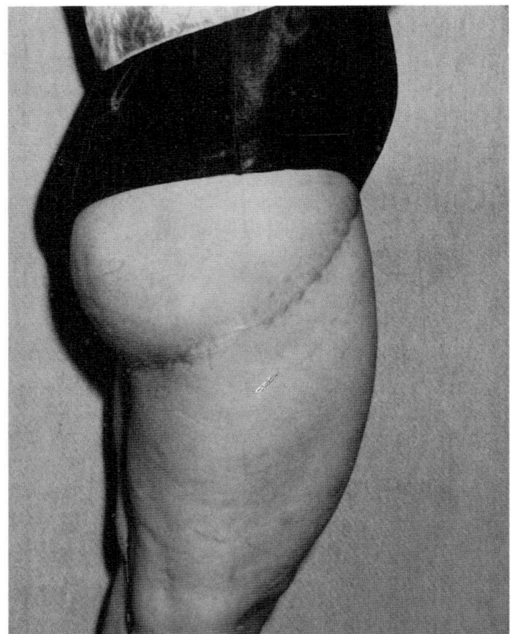

E

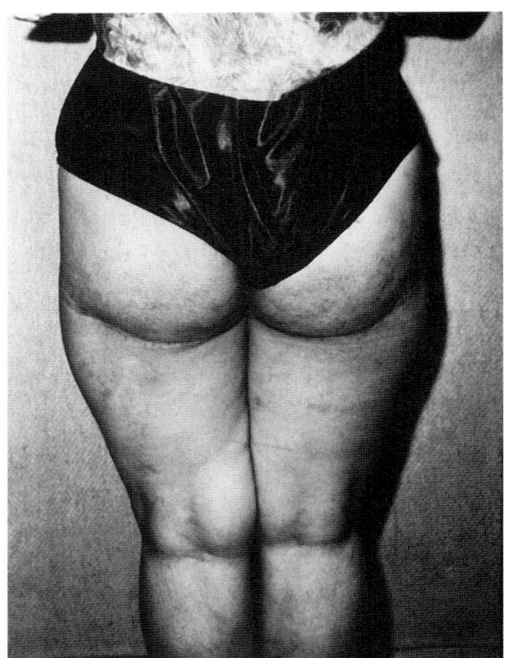

F

FIGURE 64D-3. (*Continued*)

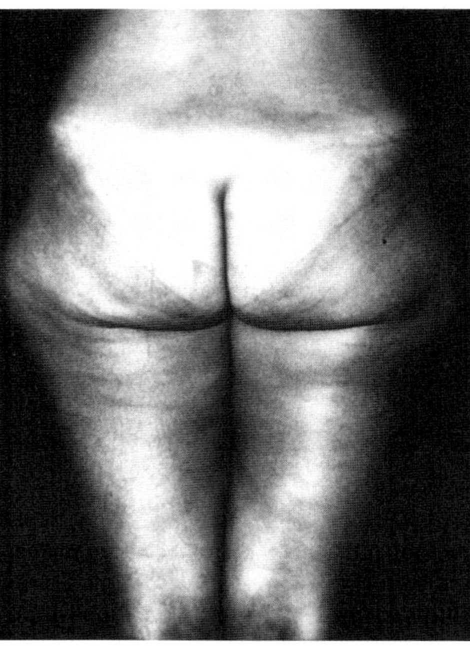

A

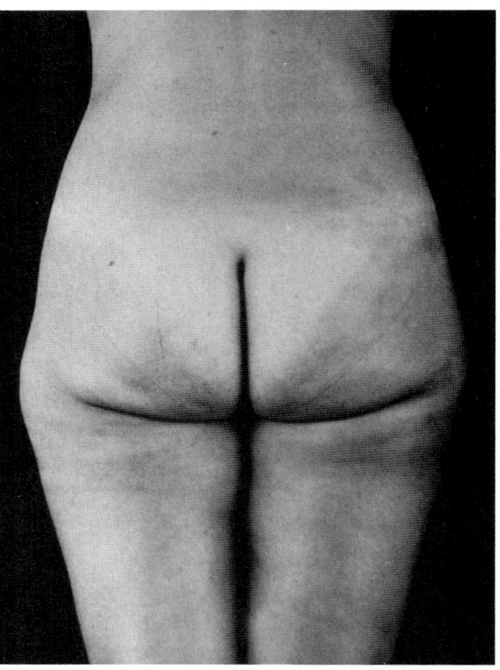

B

FIGURE 64D-4. Simple suction-assisted liposuction. A 33-year-old patient was treated with one liposuction. It is interesting to observe that the area demarcated for excision in the classic trochanteric dermolipectomy, as see in patient 1, matches the exact pattern that today is treated by suction-assisted lipectomy. **A:** Preoperative view. **B:** One-year postoperative view shows satisfactory final contour.

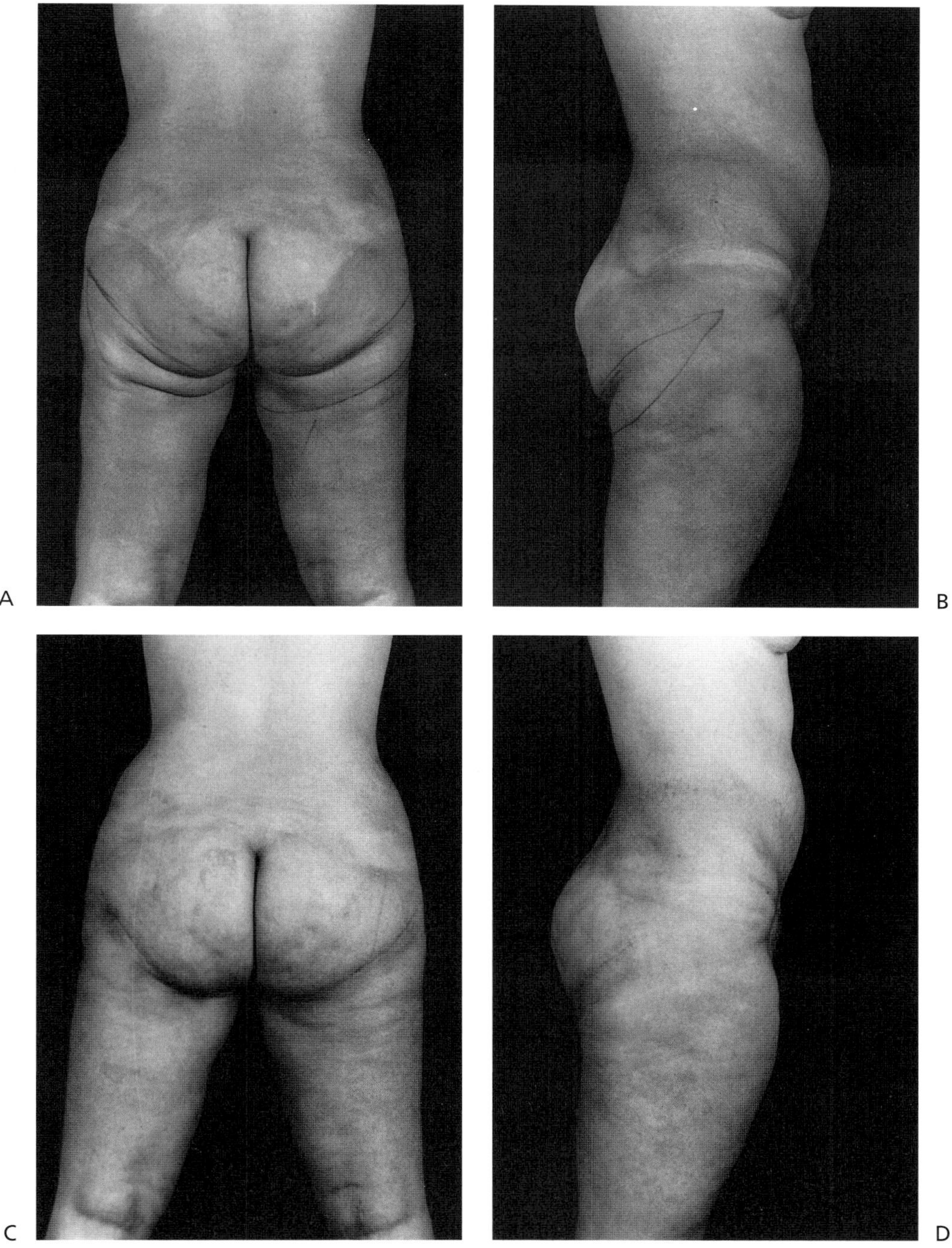

FIGURE 64D-5. Excisional surgery after suction-assisted lipectomy. A 22-year-old patient had undergone liposuction elsewhere and subsequently developed a gross irregularity. A classic dermolipectomy was indicated. **A–B:** Preoperative views. **C–D:** One-year postoperative views show a satisfactory final contour and acceptable scars.

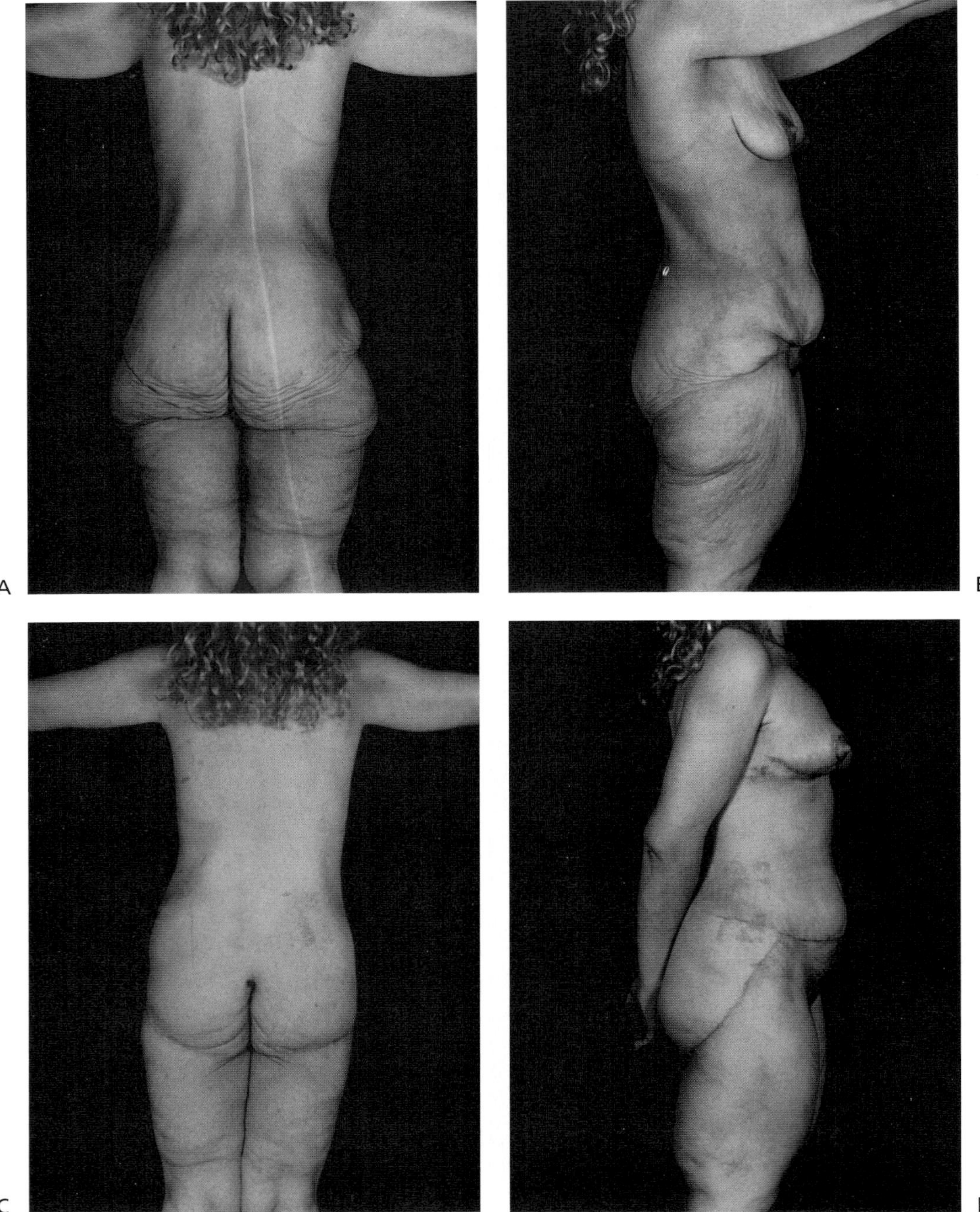

FIGURE 64D-6. Combined body contour surgery after large weight loss. This 30-year-old woman had a weight loss of approximately 40 kg over a 2-year period. She was highly motivated for multiple contour procedures, and a surgical program was planned. The first operation consisted of dermolipectomy of excess tissue of the thighs. One month later, she underwent brachioplasty associated with abdominoplasty. A third stage was performed after 1 month, with breast reduction by the rhomboid technique. **A–B:** Preoperative views. **C–D:** Postoperative views 1 month after the last procedure.

Patient 2: Simple Suction-assisted Liposuction

As mentioned throughout the text, suction-assisted lipectomy has considerably decreased the indications for dermolipectomy of the thighs. Cases that present with a large volume of adipose tissue and firm skin tone, as seen this 33-year-old patient, can be treated with one liposuction. It is interesting to observe that the area demarcated for excision in the classic trochanteric dermolipectomy, as presented in case 1, matches the exact pattern that today is treated by suction-assisted lipectomy. The preoperative view of the patient is shown in Fig. 64D-4A. The postoperative view at 1 year shows satisfactory final contour (Fig. 64D-4B).

Patient 3: Excisional Surgery Following Suction-assisted Lipectomy

Trochanteric dermolipectomy is still a very attractive procedure in selected patients who present with an unfavorable result following liposuction. This 22-year-old patient had undergone liposuction elsewhere and subsequently developed gross irregularity. A classic dermolipectomy was indicated. Preoperative views of the patient are shown in Fig. 64D-5A–B. Postoperative views at 1 year show a satisfactory final contour and acceptable scars (Fig. 64D-5C–D).

Patient 4: Combined Body Contour Surgery Following Large Weight Loss

This 30-year-old woman had weight loss of approximately 40 kg over a 2-year period. She was highly motivated for multiple contour procedures, and a surgical program was planned. The first operation consisted of dermolipectomy of excess tissue of the thighs. One month later, she underwent brachioplasty associated with abdominoplasty. A third stage was performed after 1 month, with breast reduction by the rhomboid technique. The patient was seen 2 months after this last stage. Preoperative views of the patient are shown in Fig. 64D-6A–B. Postoperative views 1 month after the last procedure are shown in Fig. 64D-6C–D.

ACKNOWLEDGMENTS

The author is grateful to Drs. Francisco Salgado and Henrique N. Radwanski for their collaboration in preparing this discussion.

REFERENCES

1. Lockwood T. Superficial fascial suspension (SFS) of the trunk and extremities: a new concept. *Plast Reconstr Surg* 1991;87:1009–1015.
2. Lockwood T. Transverse flank-thigh-buttock lift with superficial fascial suspension. *Plast Reconstr Surg* 1991;87:1019–1027.
3. Lockwood T. High-lateral-tension abdominoplasty with superficial fascial system suspension. *Plast Reconstr Surg* 1995;96:603–615.
4. Lockwood T. Brachioplasty with superficial fascial system suspension. *Plast Reconstr Surg* 1995;96:912–920.
5. Lockwood T. Lower body lift with superficial fascial system suspension. *Plast Reconstr Surg* 1995;92:1112–1122.
6. Baroudi R. Thigh and buttock lift. In: Courtiss EH, ed. *Aesthetic surgery: trouble and how to avoid it.* St. Louis: Mosby, 1978:227–255.
7. Pitanguy I. Thigh lift and abdominal lipectomy. In: Goldwyn RM, ed. *Unfavorable results in plastic surgery.* Boston: Little, Brown and Company, 1972:387.
8. Pitanguy I. Body contour. *Am J Cosmetic Surg* 1987;4:283–293.
9. Pitanguy I. Complications in aesthetic surgery: what experience has taught us over the years. Lecture at the 2nd International Symposium, Eilat, Israel, 1996
10. Pitanguy I, Cavalcanti MA. Methodology in combined aesthetic surgeries. *Aesthetic Plast Surg* 1978;2:331–340.
11. Pitanguy I. Combined aesthetic procedures. *Aesthetic plastic surgery of head and body.* Berlin: Springer-Verlag, 1981:353–359.
12. Pitanguy I, Ceravolo M. Our experience with combined procedures in aesthetic plastic surgery. *Plast Reconstr Surg* 1983;71:56–63.
13. Baroudi R. Discussion: lower body lift with superficial fascial system suspension. *Plast Reconstr Surg* 1995;92:1123–1125.
14. Pitanguy I. Evaluation of body contouring and facial cosmetic surgery today: a 30 year perspective. *Plast Reconstr Surg* 2000;105:1499–1514.
15. Pitanguy I. Trochanteric lipodystrophy. *Plast Reconstr Surg* 1964;34:280–286.
16. Pitanguy I. Dermolipectomy of the abdominal wall, thighs, buttocks and upper extremity. In: Converse JM, ed. *Reconstructive plastic surgery, vol. 7,* 2nd ed. Philadelphia: WB Saunders, 1977:3800–3823.
17. Pitanguy I. Thigh and buttock lift. In: Lewis JR, ed. *The art of aesthetic surgery, vol. 2.* Boston: Little, Brown and Company, 1989:1060–1067.
18. Pitanguy I. Lipectomy, abdominoplasty and lipodystrophy of the inner side of the arm. In: Grabb W, Smith J, eds. *Plastic surgery: a concise guide to clinical practice,* 2nd ed. Boston: Little, Brown and Company, 1973:1005–1013.
19. Pitanguy I. Correction of lipodystrophy of the lateral thoracic aspect and inner side of the arm and elbow dermosenescence. *Clin Plast Surg* 1975;2:477–483.
20. Pitanguy I. Abdominal lipectomy: an approach to it through an analysis of 300 consecutive cases. *Plast Reconstr Surg* 1967;40:384–391.
21. Pitanguy I. Abdominal lipectomy. *Clin Plast Surg* 1975;2:401–410.
22. Pitanguy I. Abdominoplasty: classification and surgical techniques. *Rev Bras Cir* 1995;85:23–44.

65

COSMETIC PROCEDURES OF THE LOWER EXTREMITY

ADRIEN E. AIACHE

IMPLANTATION

Calf Implant-related Complications

Due to the particular problems related to leg circulation gravity and constant leg use, implantation of prostheses is problematic in those cases most requiring implantation.

After poliomyelitis, the leg can be devastated, devoid of muscle, and consequently present with an anatomical situation different from the usual healthy one. The deep fascia is nonexistent, and because there are no muscular elements, the vascular supply is drastically reduced (1–4).

This anatomical situation causes immense postoperative difficulties when a large implant is introduced. These complications, which are more severe in females than in males, probably are related to the difference in musculature and physical activity between men and women.

In contrast to the difficulties encountered in legs that are underdeveloped because of specific conditions, results can be gratifying in underdeveloped healthy legs if the size of the implant is not disproportionate with the tissue (5,6).

The author has seen half a dozen cases of poliomyelitis and clubfoot reject implants where thin but otherwise healthy legs can be corrected if one is reasonable and provides a modest-size increase.

Extremely large implants in thin legs are a recipe for disaster and should be avoided (Fig. 65-1).

Expander-related Complications

Use of tissue expanders for calf implantation is reserved for cases where the desired volume cannot be achieved in one surgical procedure because of the paucity of leg tissue. Patients with poliomyelitis, clubfoot, or Charcot-Marie-Tooth disease have a very small amount of leg tissue, scant muscle development, if any, and poor blood supply to the tissues. It is erroneous to expect these tissues to be able to accept and tolerate very large implants. In males, the ratio of implant to leg tissue is larger than in females, and this can lead to difficulties. Expanders are used in these cases to expand the soft tissue envelope and allow for placement of a longer implant. Complications from these procedures include poor tissue healing, pain, swelling, inflammation, and inability to use the leg, with claudication and contracture of the ankle posteriorly. Some implants must be removed almost immediately, while others last for a few months before they need to be removed (Figs. 65-2, 65-3).

Late Complications

Capsular Contracture

Capsular contracture was a common occurrence in the early cases of implantation using cigar-shaped soft silicone gel implants. The capsule distorts the shape of the calf and forces the implants in many directions. At times, it creates a round mass that seems unnatural and firm, with eventual displacement of the implant either posteriorly or inferiorly. Treatment consists of removal of the soft implants or replacement with firm implants (Figs. 65-4, 65-5).

Nerve Injury

The sciatic nerve divides into the tibial and common peroneal nerve above the popliteal fold. The common peroneal nerve passes laterally and posteriorly above the bony peroneal head and subdivides into the peroneal anastomotic, which joins the sural nerve, and the deep peroneal nerve. Injuries at this level can result in footdrop and sensory loss over the lateral aspect of the leg and the lateral plantar aspect of the foot by injury to the lateral plantar nerve. Injuries to the tibial nerve, which lies deep under the soleus muscle, can occur rarely. Injuries at the lower level can result in numbness to the calcaneal skin and paralysis to the gastrocnemius muscle, soleus, and plantaris muscle. The junction of the peroneal anastomotic nerve (branch of the common peroneal nerve) and the medial sural cutaneous nerve (branch of the tibial nerve) gives rise to the sural nerve. This junction

A. E. Aiache: Department of Plastic Surgery, Cedars-Sinai Medical Center, Beverly Hills, California

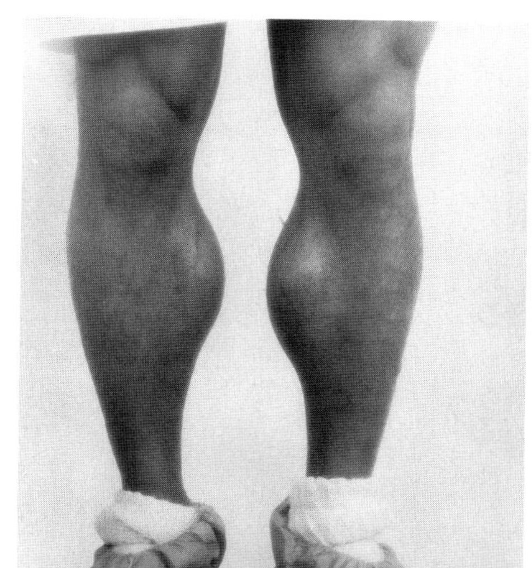

A

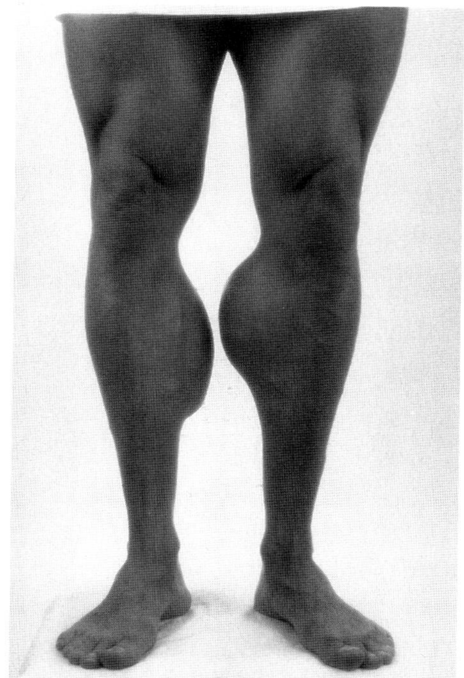

B

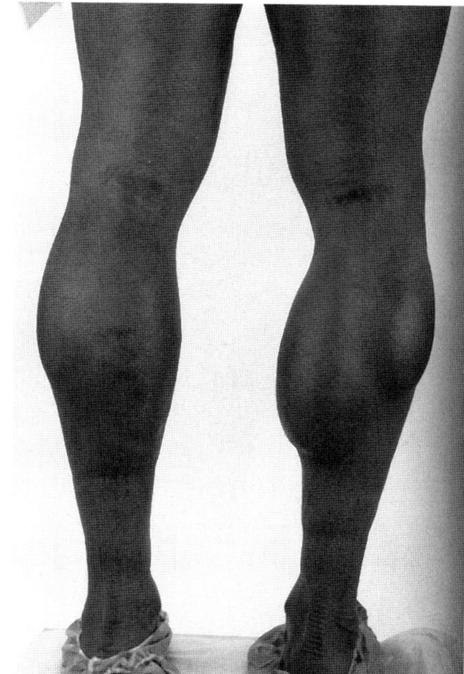

C

FIGURE 65-1. A: A 43-year-old man who underwent an uneventful calf implantation with soft silicone gel implants. **B:** Eighteen months after the operation, the patient developed severe capsular contracture with secondary distortion of the leg contour. **C:** The implants in the right leg were removed and replaced with a hard silicone implant. The patient developed seroma and hematomas, and removal of the implant was eventually necessary.

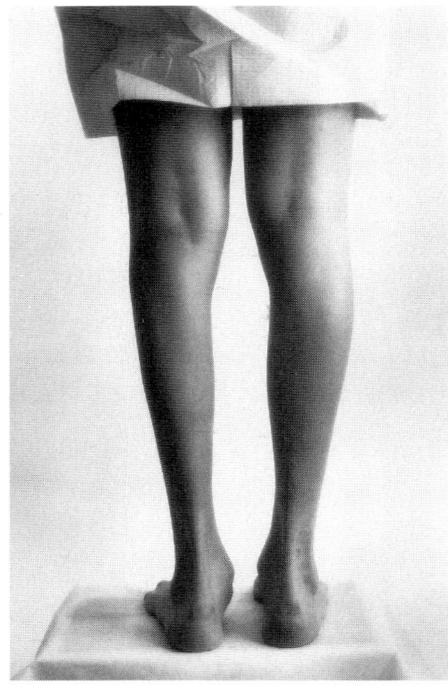

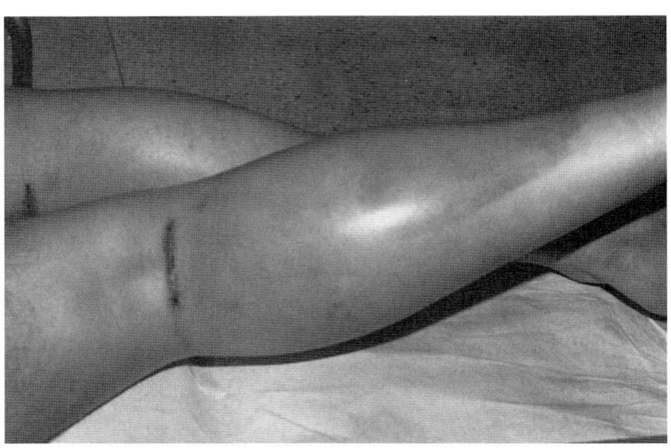

FIGURE 65-2. A: An 18-year-old man with left leg underdevelopment secondary to poliomyelitis. **B:** Red, swollen, tender leg with high fever in the days immediately after implantation. This was treated successfully with drainage and antibiotics.

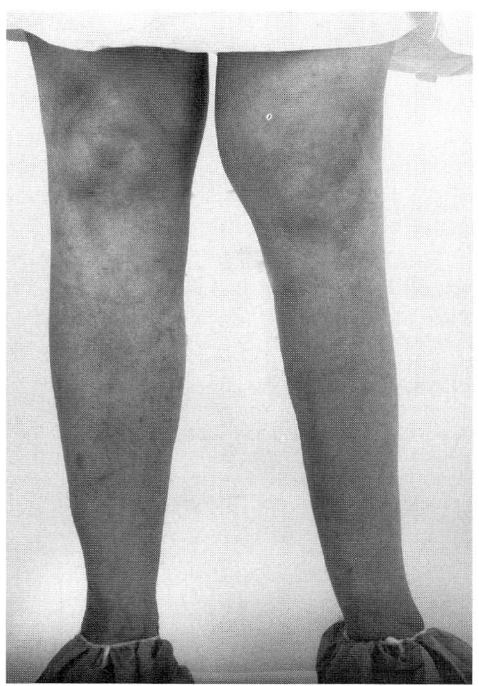

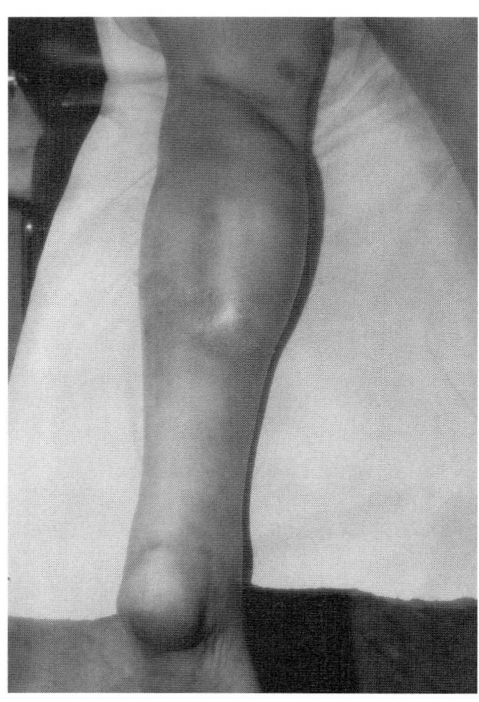

FIGURE 65-3. A: A 45-year-old woman with right leg underdevelopment secondary to poliomyelitis with relatively good amount of fat in the leg. **B:** Red, swollen, tender left leg with high temperature in the days after an implant exchange, which was performed because the patient wanted a better leg shape after the first calf implant. This implant eventually had to be removed.

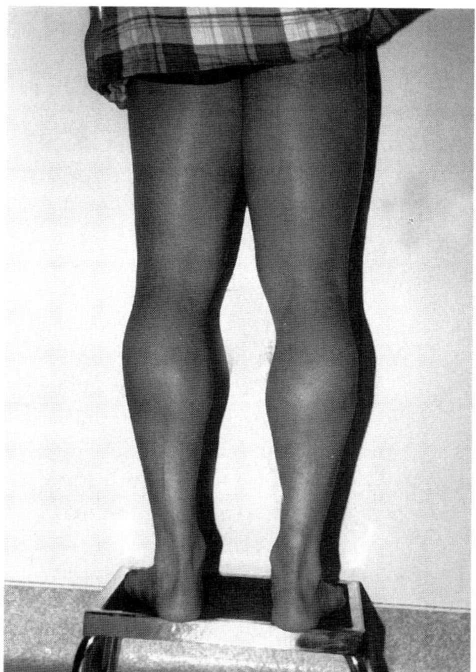
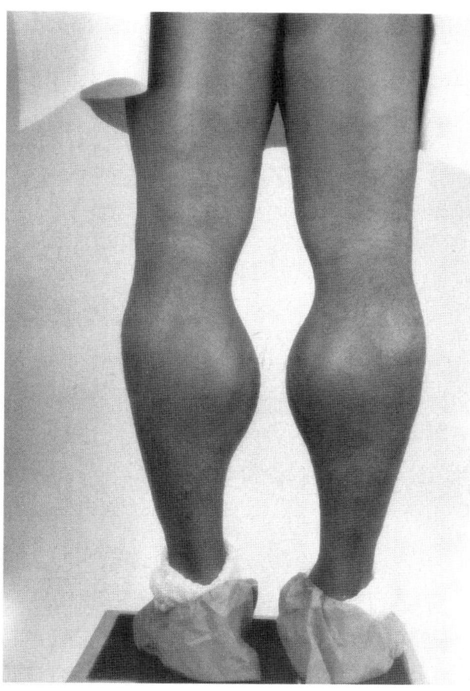

A B

FIGURE 65-4. A: A 32-year-old bodybuilder who desired to increase the size of his calves. **B:** After 2 years, capsular contracture developed around his soft silicone gel implants.

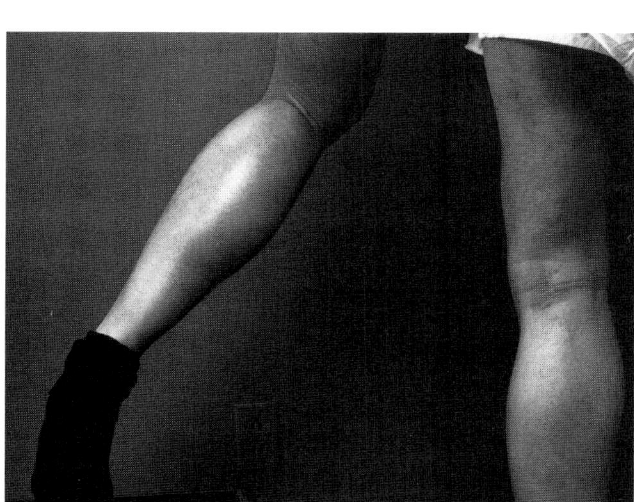
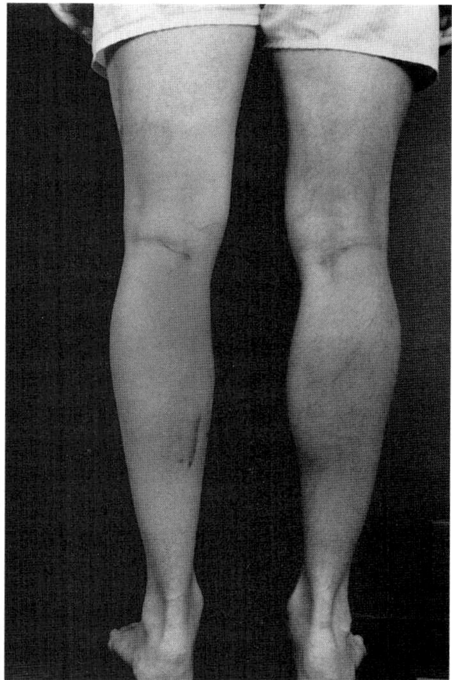

A B

FIGURE 65-5. A: A 28-year-old man who underwent bilateral calf augmentation with implants. He experienced pain, swelling, redness, and infection around the implants. **B:** The right leg infection was eventually drained by a general surgeon while the patient was in another city. The surgery left him with a visible scar in the lower leg.

appears more superficial between the two heads of the gastrocnemius muscles at the mid-third of the leg. Injury to the sural nerve can cause numbness of the posterior aspect of the leg laterally and posteriorly, the lateral aspect of the dorsum of the foot, and the most lateral aspect of the plantar area of the foot. This injury can occur when the implant is placed too medial because it is too wide or when an implant is made to occupy the full posterior aspect of the leg, without regard to the fact that the gastrocnemius has two heads.

Injuries to the very medial aspect of the leg can result in numbness of the inner aspect of the calf caused by injury to the saphenous nerve, which wraps around the knee medially and courses anteriorly to supply the anterior and medial skin of the calf. Such injury results in numbness to the medial and anterior calf area.

Discussion

The tibial nerve, which is the larger of the two terminal divisions of the sciatic nerve, travels between and under the two heads of the gastrocnemius muscle and under the soleus muscle. It gives rise to two terminal branches, the medial plantar and the lateral plantar nerve, which supply the plantar aspect of the foot from the proximal third to the toes. The tibial nerve itself supplies the posterior part of the plantar aspect of the foot. The tibial nerve rarely is injured because it lies so deep and divides so low. At the upper third of the leg, the tibial nerve gives rise to the medial sural cutaneous nerve, which is a sensory nerve that anastomoses with the peroneal anastomotic nerve from the common peroneal nerve and provides sensation to the posterior aspect of the leg. This nerve is one of the most commonly injured in calf implantation. When injured, the common peroneal nerve will cause loss of sensation to the outer aspect of the leg as well as footdrop, because the nerve is motor to the anterior compartment of the leg. The muscular branches of the deep peroneal nerve go to the extensor digitorum brevis and other extensors, such as the tibialis anterior, extensor digitorum longus, peroneus tertius, and extensor hallucis longus. Injury to this nerve is more prone to cause motor impairment. Only in cases of compartment syndrome can the tibial nerve be injured by a combination of devascularization of the nerve associated with myonecrosis of the posterior muscles of the calf.

Hematoma/Seroma

Early hematomas usually are not seen, but if the muscle is injured during implantation, bleeding can become troublesome and difficult to control, even with endoscopic assistance.

Bleeding during and immediately after surgery occurs more commonly in secondary cases of implant replacement with pocket enlargement or displacement, or implant introduction after expanders are placed in preparation for the implants.

If bleeding is more severe than usual, drainage is mandatory after exhaustive attempts at hemostasis. Seromas are rarer and usually follow hematomas that were not been drained fully. Conservative drainage is necessary but may not be sufficient, leading to eventual implant removal.

Compression syndromes are seen after injury to muscle causes bleeding and secondary compression of the tissues, leading to muscle necrosis, nerve damage, and vascular insufficiency. Acute leg pains should not always be attributed to nerve compression or compression syndromes, because it can be secondary to a simple large implant with tissue compression that, in many cases, will improve in a few days. In some cases where there is no improvement, decompression surgery with a long open incision along the fascia of the gastrocnemius muscle belly is necessary. Fasciotomies are the eventual final treatment for compression syndromes. Pressure gradients can be measured at the muscle level to determine the proper diagnosis and assess the treatment to be given.

Cases of total compartment syndrome of the extensors eventually leading to muscle necrosis and complete loss of the anterior lateral leg soft tissue have been reported.

In compartment syndrome, the skin usually shows some degree of distress, such as a shiny pinkish discoloration, blood formation, extreme pain, tenderness, and swelling, sometimes followed by frank skin slough. Early intervention with fasciotomy usually is the treatment of choice. The early signs of compartment syndrome sometimes are limited, and surgery might be avoided using elevation and a conservative approach. However, the surgeon should always be suspicious, and assessment with careful frequent follow-up can be helpful in the eventual diagnosis and treatment.

Early Infections

Early infections often occur after a large hematoma develops immediately after surgery. Often it is difficult to assess the condition of the leg, because hematoma with tissue compression results in skin distress, characterized by redness, shininess of the skin, and blebs formation. Occasionally the pustules become purulent, making the diagnosis of deep infection more difficult.

Fluid evacuation or hematoma drainage should be performed, with culture and sensitivity tests to determine proper antibiotic coverage.

Antibiotics can be given on an outpatient basis or, in more acute cases, intravenously while the patient is in the hospital. If the response is not rapid enough, it would be wise to remove the implants, drain the leg through an inferior stab wound, and treat the leg with saline soaks and antibiotics and dependent drainage.

Infection

Given this relatively new type of procedure, calf implantation, and especially due to the lower extremity location of surgery, some complications naturally have arisen.

Some of the complications are similar to those of silicone implantation, such as infection, displacement, and capsule formation; others are especially related to the procedure itself, such as irregular protruding areas of compression and ankle edema.

The most common serous complication is infection that occurs either during the immediate postoperative period or afterward. The typical symptoms of infection—pain, redness, tenderness, swelling, and temperature—may develop.

The pain consists of a constant ache that is exacerbated by walking or increased activity. The pain eventually becomes severe and requires immediate attention.

Redness is present over the entire area of the infected implant and can expand above the incision line. It is either a mild redness that may be difficult to distinguish from ordinary postoperative redness, or a frank, reddish, shiny discoloration of the skin indicating underlying pus formation.

Swelling is present and consists of a hard, painful, swollen area situated over the gastrocnemius muscle belly. The skin becomes tense and shiny, and the swollen area is extremely tender to palpation if infection has developed into pus formation.

The infected area is hot to the touch, as opposed to the opposite leg. The patient often presents with a fever of 101 to 103°. Formation of blebs and pustules indicates a combination of skin distress and circulatory problems.

Comments

The pain present is distinguishable from postoperative pain by its excessiveness and by the fact that this deep, dull ache is more marked than that in the opposite noninfected leg. The pain apparently increases daily and can become unbearable.

At times, the skin is barely touchable and the patient feels extra discomfort only in the infected area. The swelling may be difficult to distinguish from the simple presence of fluid or blood. Sometimes it is helpful to have the associated signs of pain, redness, and temperature, without which the diagnosis of infection is difficult to make.

Redness often is present in the early postoperative stages and improves in a few days. It can be troublesome, and its persistence and localization to only one area can be significant, indicating the presence of fluid with or without infection

The diagnosis is easier to make if the symptoms are new and appear after an asymptomatic period.

At an advanced and acute stage of the infection, the redness is frank and associated with other signs of infection, such as discoloration and skin turgor.

In short, the four cardinal signs of infection are present most of the time and will help make the diagnosis.

Once the diagnosis of infection is made, the choice of treatment is important. In mild or early cases, a combination of higher doses of antibiotics, rest, elevation, and saline soaks seems to be helpful.

In cases where the response to treatment is slow and there does not appear to be frank abscess formation, careful introduction of a plastic drain has been useful.

A plastic catheter is introduced into the lower part of the pocket while the opposite hand holds the implant above it, and then the catheter is advanced slowly until fluid becomes apparent. This fluid can be turbid, but it is often relatively clear, negating the presence of infection. The drain is maintained in place for a few days, which allows complete drainage of fluid from the leg. Improvement using this technique has been remarkable, reducing fluid formation.

In the very advanced stages of infection where neither antibiotics alone nor antibiotics plus drainage is sufficient, one must completely reopen the popliteal wound, irrigate copiously with Betadine and antibiotic solutions, remove the implant, and introduce a drain into the lower portion of the cavity. This drain will remain in place for approximately 2 to 4 days, which allows complete drying of infected material from the pocket. Once the drain is removed, antibiotic treatment is continued until the infection is completely eliminated. Reinsertion of the implant usually is postponed for 3 to 6 months to ensure that no further infection supervenes. The author has seen reinfections in a case where the drain was removed using this technique and the implant was reintroduced 3 months after infection. Thus, it is better to wait for a longer period of time to be absolutely sure all sources of infection have been eradicated from the area of the wound. Broad-spectrum antibiotics are given according to the type of bacteria identified from cultures. Most often the infection is due to either *Staphylococcus alba* or *Staphylococcus aureus,* but mixed flora have been seen in some cases.

Myonecrosis Secondary to Implantation

In rare cases, postoperative immediate acute pain can indicate an acute compartmental syndrome secondary to either too large a volume of implant in a tight subfascial space or increased bleeding and hemorrhage within the space containing the implants. Muscle fiber necrosis results from increased counterpressure. The time interval from introduction of the implant to release of tension is important. This problem has been described in the acute crush syndrome of the extremities. Symptoms in these cases are very similar to the process of acute crush syndrome. The synergistic forces of obliteration of endomysial capillaries with ischemia or direct pressure from acute bleeding on the muscle compressed under the deep fascia can cause this problem. The consequence of these severe problems is muscle necrosis necessitating wide debridement and general support measures to prevent possible systemic effects. Treatment is implant removal as soon as it is diagnosed.

Late Seroma/Hematoma Formation

A complication related to implants is sudden swelling around the implant area. This problem can be seen imme-

TABLE 65-1. LOWER EXTREMITY AESTHETIC SURGERY COMPLICATIONS

Early Complication	Method to Avoid Complication
Bleeding	
At surgery	Careful hemostasis
Immediate postoperative	Pain control (to avoid hypertension)
	Proper plane of dissection
Infection	
Immediate postoperative	Proper operative technique
	Proper Preparation
	Atraumatic surgery
Nerve Injury	
At surgery	Proper plane of dissection
	Careful dissection
	Anatomy knowledge
Seroma	
Unknown reasons	Immediate postoperative
Constant drainage and secondary infection	Aseptic techniques
	Antibiotics wash

diately, or it may occur 1 or 2 to 10 years after initial implantation. Tissue distortion is due to the tension and is similar to the phenomenon of capsular contracture, except that the process consists of increased fluid distension of the leg. Pain is mild and constant and sometimes has a burning characteristic. Some patients have this swelling for a few weeks before they seek help. In some patients, the swelling can be bilateral, with one side always larger than the other. There is no redness, lymph node enlargement, or fever. The only symptoms are extreme swelling of the leg zone over the calf implants and mild pain. Treatment consists of relieving the discomfort by aspirating the collected fluid. The fluid usually consists of a bloody dark-red fluid. In most cases, the results of culture and sensitivity tests for these specimens are negative. In many cases, the liquid will reaccumulate and require multiple sessions of aspiration, which can lead to secondary infection. The ultimate treatment for this condition is complete removal of the implant.

After implant removal, complications still can occur, such as recurrence of fluid accumulation even in the absence of implants and secondary infection of the pocket that was drained, because it is laid by an inner capsule that is not very responsive to possible secondary infection. In some cases, the leg must be drained inferiorly with long-term drainage and debridement, even after the implants have been removed for a couple of weeks (Table 1).

SUCTION LIPECTOMY COMPLICATIONS

Suction lipectomy of the lower extremities can present complications related to the general technique of liposuction and problems specific to the lower extremity, such as edema, skin conditions secondary to reduced blood supply with arterial insufficiency, venous congestion, or areas of cellulite that can be troublesome (Figs. 65-6, 65-7).

Avoidance of these problems consists of strict triage of the patient. A history of leg swelling and claudication, as well as persistent edema, vein congestion, and ankle deformities, suggests a contraindication to surgery. It is interesting that patients who present with chronic leg edema and congestion are the first to request liposuction because they desire a reduction in leg circumference.

The older age of the patient is often a good reason for contraindication. Even if the medical history does not appear highly positive, it should be researched in depth to avoid unexpected problems. One may find chronic edema that is unappreciated by the patient or the internist but could be a telltale sign of incipient problems in the legs.

Complications consist of chronic pain, swelling, induration of the ankle, and skin difficulties leading to frank skin slough.

Prolonged pain often is secondary to scarring and nerve entrapment in the scar. Elevation of the leg, rest, and support can be helpful.

Specific liposuction complications related to the lower extremities include irregularities, scarring, and depression. One must be aware of the potential for depressions when the cannula travels too far superficially and its trajectory is not monitored constantly.

Long grooves of depression can result from accidental traveling of the tip in a more superficial area. Scar adhesion

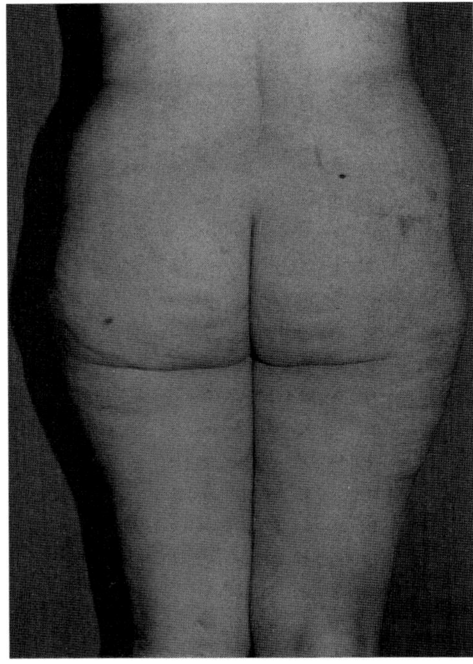

FIGURE 65-6. Early postoperative results showing the lack of symmetry after saddlebag liposuction in a very large woman. Dents irregularities and extreme lengthening of the gluteal fold on the left are seen.

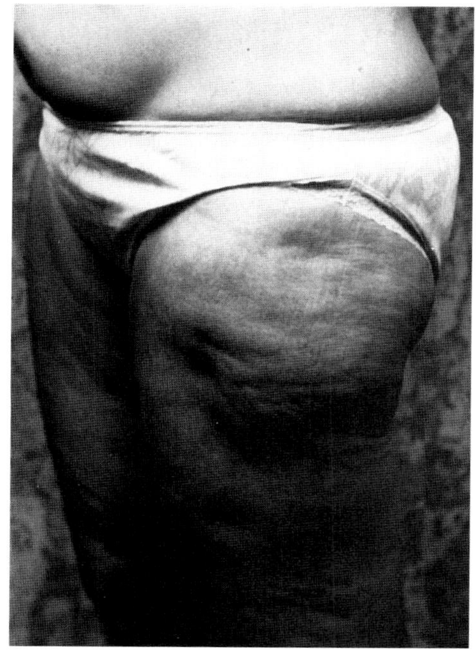

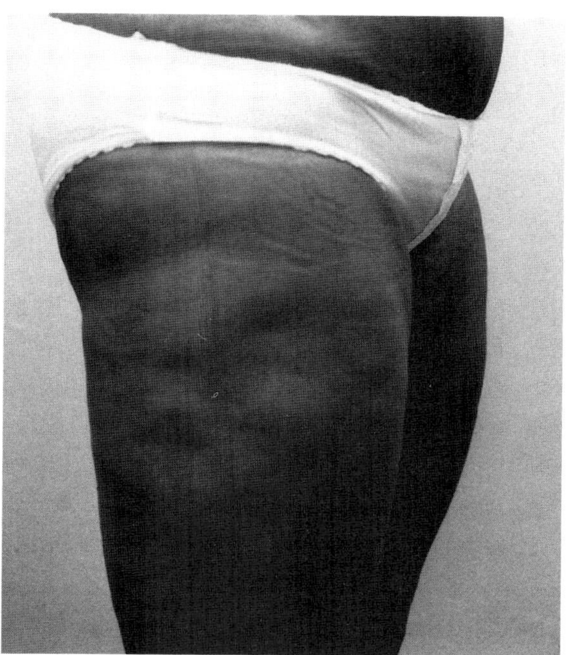

FIGURE 65-7. A: Skin dimples, waviness, and an irregular skin surface can result from poorly performed liposuction surgery. **B:** Uneven work can result in a deformed skin surface. Notice the checkerboard-type deformity of this hip.

and skin discoloration can result. The liposuction cannula should remain under the deep fascia of the legs. Accidental traveling of the tip toward the surface can result in a zone of depression.

Induration, edema, and pain of the ankle can last up to 6 months after liposuction. Treatment consists of pain medication, elevation, and rest.

Liposuction Complications

Thigh liposuction is especially delicate. Areas of irregularities, dents, depressions, and deformity can result. Avoidance consists of painstaking care during application of suction, with an attempt at evenness by keeping the cannula deep and controlling the traveling of the cannula tip at all times. When correcting the inner thigh, the suction can be superficial as long as it is even. The complications of unevenness are secondary to lack of experience or carelessness during liposuction. In the anterior thigh, a certain depth of suction should be maintained because the subcutaneous tissue is dense and interspersed with many connective septa that prevent evenness of the area if suction is not performed carefully. The recommendation is to stay deep, use only very fine suction cannulas in the subcutaneous tissue, use multiple strokes, and maintain evenness (Figs. 8 and 9).

Laterally, saddlebags and lateral thigh can be corrected by multiple-layer liposuction in a multiple layer of depth of the

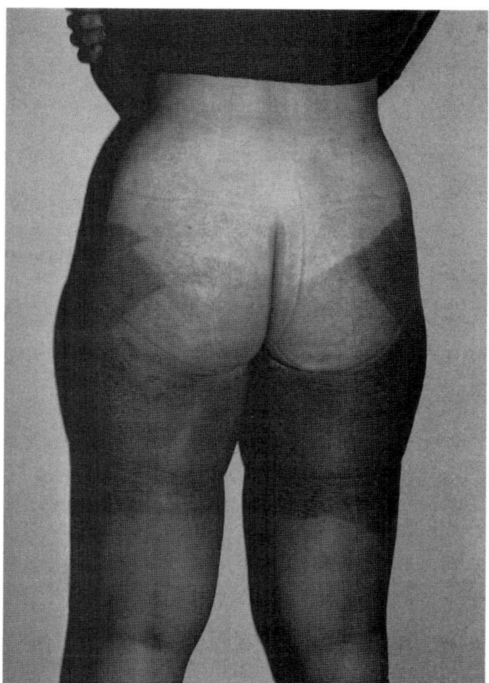

FIGURE 65-8. An allergic reaction seen after management of liposuction areas with elastic tape. Elastic tape no longer is advised, and only garments are necessary.

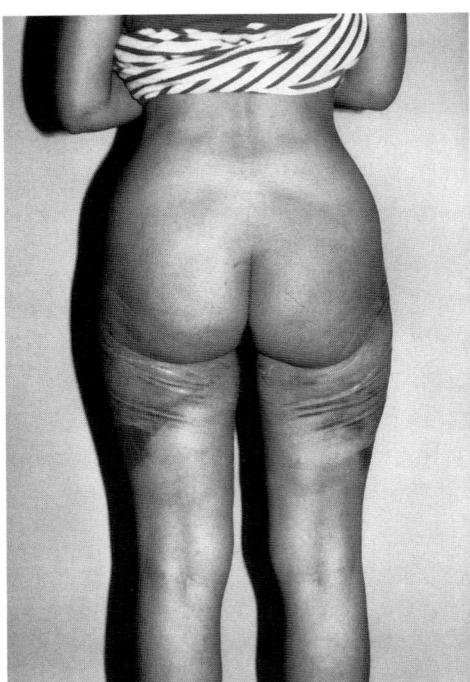

FIGURE 65-9. Bilateral bruising after saddlebag liposuction often can lead to skin discoloration and permanent pigmentation.

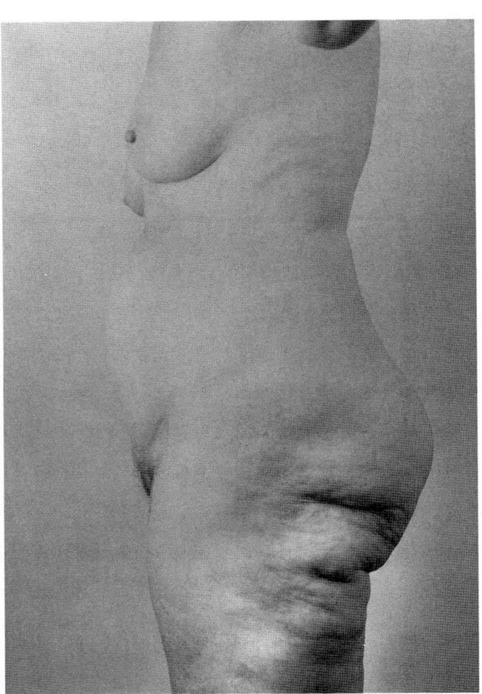

FIGURE 65-10. A very-large-volume liposuction should be performed in a superficial plane in addition to the deep plane to avoid such postoperative waviness and irregularities.

cannila if going too superficial with control of the evenness. Entry into the field should be done through a minimum of two approaches, which allows criss-crossing of suction and ensures more evenness; otherwise complications can result in complete unevenness, dents, depressions, bumps, long lines of depressed areas due to the traveling of the cannula, and poor matching with the surrounding tissues. To avoid these problems, evenness of suction, feathering the edges, and careful monitoring of the cannula tip to prevent its traveling in a too superficial plane as opposed to the remaining strokes will ensure success (Figs. 65-10 through 65-12).

The posterior thighs can be suctioned with a deep and superficial suction mechanism to correct cellulite, which is very common in that area. Correction of cellulite consists of releasing the fibers that attach the skin to the superficial fascia system while expanded fat cells bloat the areas between. Release of these septa and filling with fat will help prevent secondary depressions and dents. Deep liposuction will help to reduce overall excess.

Patient Dissatisfaction

Although not a complication *per se,* patient dissatisfaction can create severe problems for the plastic surgeon unless he or she is prepared with the eventuality, preoperatively and postoperatively.

One of the most common causes of dissatisfaction is the patient's judgment of insufficient removal of fat. Surgeons know too well the patient whose result is excellent by all

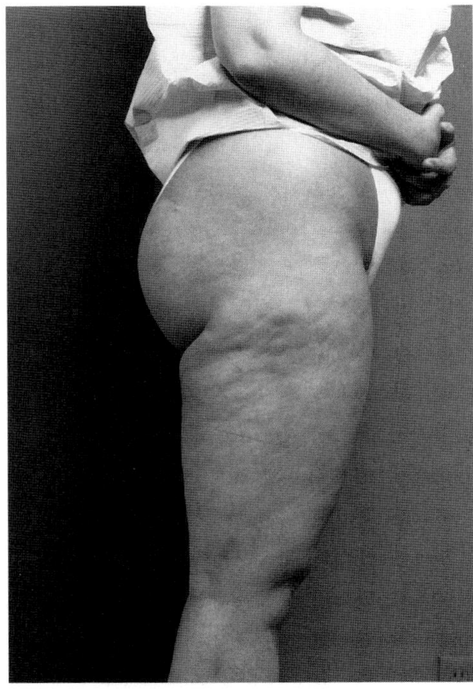

FIGURE 65-11. Dents are present and cellulite sometimes worsens after liposuction if the cellulite is not treated by superficial suction and cellulite release.

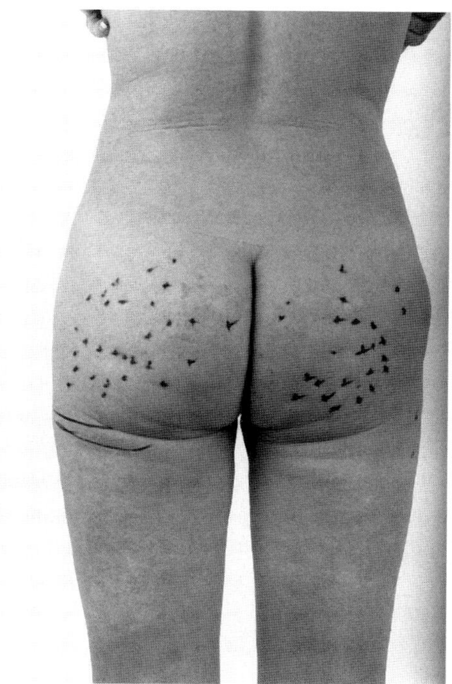

FIGURE 65-12. Cellulite and poor gluteal folds are often the results of liposuction.

clinical standards but who, nevertheless, for unrealistic expectations or unobtainable goals, complains of a poor result.

Preoperative evaluation and patient counseling can help. Postoperative patience and support also can be helpful, although patient dissatisfaction, justified or not, often is more intense in the early postoperative period. The dissatisfaction improves gradually with time and, in most cases, patients adjust to their new body image.

Liposuction Scars

Although minimal, liposuction scars can annoy patients, who then express their dissatisfaction. The scars can be inverted, discolored, and relatively conspicuous. Ultrasound suction scars can be even more objectionable, because the scars usually are larger and often exhibit burned areas around them.

Scar revision can help in the hip, anterior thigh, and waist. Steroid injection helps hypertrophic scars when given at 3-week intervals two or three times. Taping and silicone sheeting also are useful.

There is no way to avoid these scars, which are a minimal way to obtain the desired surgical results. Good placement in Langer's line and in areas that are inconspicuous is advised.

Sensory Disturbances

Although not a complication *per se,* sensory disturbances often are noted. There is no real cure; time will help these problems. These disturbances seem more prominent with the new ultrasound liposuction, and patients should be warned about them.

Long-term Discoloration

No specific treatment is known. The discoloration is due to increased bruising in a tight area of the body. The skin may be discolored permanently. The posterior thighs, ankles, and lower part of the arms can exhibit this problem (Fig. 65-13).

Skin Slough

Although skin slough is uncommon, when it occurs it is located in zones of reduced circulation or excess venous congestion. Usually it is treated conservatively. The eschar is allowed to separate spontaneously. Often the resulting defect beneath the eschar reepithelializes or heals by contraction of the surrounding tissues.

Scar debridement may prevent infection if it is suspected, but it will result in a larger scar than conservative treatment.

Postoperative Distortion

In cases of where excess suction is performed in the inner thighs or hips, ptosis of the tissue may develop. This is rare and is limited to much older patients over 60 years of age with poor skin tone. Conservative compression garments may help. Secondary liposuction also may help the tissue contract further.

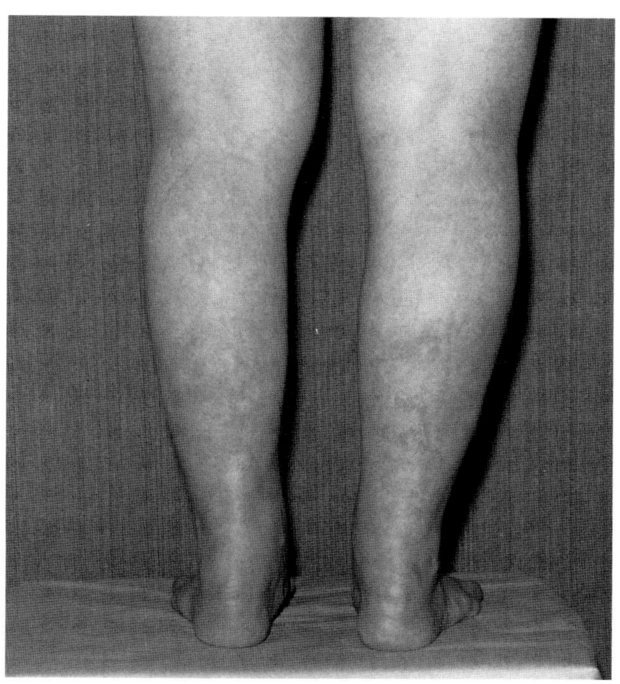

FIGURE 65-13. Ankle suction complications other than frank slough in the Achilles tendon area can result in swelling, discoloration, and poor circulation of the foot.

Asymmetry

Asymmetry can exist preoperatively and often is difficult to improve to the patient's satisfaction. It can result postoperatively when a larger amount of fat excess is removed from one area than is removed from the opposite side. This is a common problem, and patients should be warned about its possible occurrence and advised that a secondary suction can help if they are not fully satisfied. Although the surgeon tries to prevent this occurence as much as possible during surgery, immediate postoperative swelling and distortion may hide the actual asymmetry, which only becomes apparent in the long-term postoperative period (Fig. 65-14).

Postoperative Edema and Induration

Excessive postoperative edema and induration may be caused by interruption of the lymphatic pathways located in the lower leg anteriorly and posteriorly. This occurrence is unavoidable if one wants to achieve a satisfactory liposuction. Although conservative liposuction may prevent this problem, it will not satisfy the patient fully in all cases; only more aggressive liposuction may help. In older patients, lymphatic problems can lead to edema, induration, and constant pain and soreness in the area. Treatment consists of systematic steroids followed by long-term doses of naproxen (Aleve), which causes the swelling to disappear gradually.

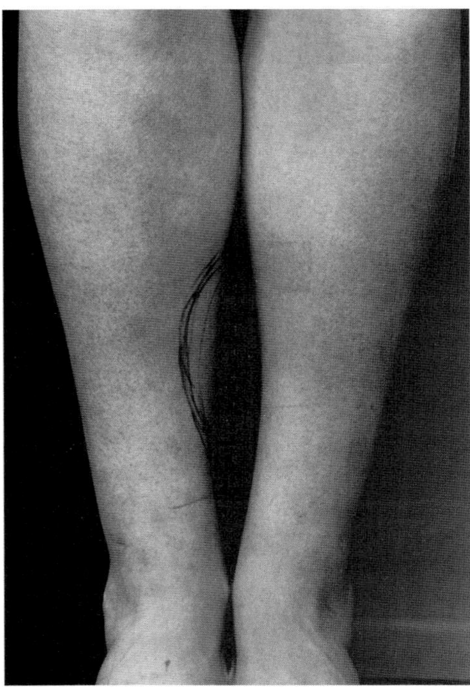

FIGURE 65-14. A straight ruler between the legs shows the uneven result after ankle liposuction. A more careful procedure could have prevented these problems.

Constant massage and exercises may help the problem, but there is no specific way to avoid this condition.

Dermatologic Complications

Increased telangiectasia can be seen after liposuction in the lower leg area or ankle. It usually is present to some degree preoperatively and should be called to the patient's attention. Increased pigmentation usually is seen in patients who have excessive bruising, hematomas, or slough caused by hemosiderin deposition. Sun exposure should be avoided postoperatively until all evidence of bruising has resolved. The use of sunscreens is recommended when the possibility of prolonged sun exposure exists. The use of sun-sensitizing antibiotics, such as minocycline or tetracycline, should be avoided. Resolution of hyperpigmentation occurs slowly; it may take more than 1 year to resolve, or it may be permanent. Hyperpigmentation might be improved slightly by the use of cutaneous bleaching creams, such as hydroquinone or kojic acid.

Skin Distortion

Skin distortion can occur after liposuction. It may be secondary to the deep ligaments holding the skin to the deep fascia while the liposuction freed the tissues or a hematoma distending the skin, which prevents it from adhering in the right area. Secondary freeing of these distortions can be accomplished by lysis of the adhesions similar to cellulite treatment using a butterfly cannula.

VEIN LIGATION AND SCLEROTHERAPY COMPLICATIONS

These procedures, reserved for use in the lower extremity, can present their own complications.

Hemorrhage can result from poorly ligated vessels; a vein retraction can make its ligation impossible because it retracts.

Infection and hematoma leading to infections are relatively uncommon. Avoidance of these problems involves strict asepsis and careful venous ligation.

Accidental peripheral nerve injuries lead to pain and neuroma formation. Knowledge of the anatomy is a good base for prevention of these problems.

Sclerotherapy complications are common; ecchymosis, skin slough, and pigmented areas can result from this procedure. A strict technique with careful injection to avoid extravasation can prevent this problem. Some sclerotherapy agents are more noxious than others and should be chosen carefully. Even hypertonic saline injections, which supposedly are less dangerous than the other sclerotic agents, can present problems, such as superficial extravasation with skin necrosis and permanent discoloration.

REFERENCES

1. Aiache A. Calf contour correction with implants. *Clin Plast Surg* 1991;18:857–862.
2. Hallock JJ. Myonecrosis as a sequela of calf implants. *Ann Plast Surg* 1993;30:456–458.
3. Howard P. Calf augmentation and correction of contour deformities. Clinical correlation is suggested. *Plast Surg* 1991;18:601–613.
4. Lemperle G, Kostka K. Calf augmentation with new solid silicone implants. *Aesthetic Plast Surg* 1993;17:233–237.
5. Morillas C, et al. Contour treatment through silicone prosthesis implants. *Am J Cosmetic Surg* 1989;6:4 254–255.
6. Novack PH, Alloplastic implants for men. *Clin Plast Surg* 1991;18:828.

Discussion

COSMETIC PROCEDURES OF THE LOWER EXTREMITY

LLOYD N. CARLSEN

Dr. Adrian Aiache has covered a wide range of complications in cosmetic plastic surgery of the lower extremities.

The neuroanatomical description, although not an untoward result, will enhance the surgeon's knowledge of the area and thereby help prevent complications.

Our experience from 1971, when we did the first calf implantation, is of 338 patients, 212 bilateral and 126 unilateral, for a total of 550 legs.

During the early 1970s, I observed some skin circulatory problems and immediately removed the implants. In 1980, I realized the importance of staying below the deep investing fascia and consequently never had a skin slough. In essence, one is elevating a large fascia–cutaneous flap of the leg. We believe it is of paramount importance to place the implant below the deep investing fascia to preserve the integrity of the skin housing. This will prevent skin sloughs.

Dr. Aiache discussed implant complications together with skin housing problems. Care must be taken with the hypoplastic leg, whether congenital or acquired. I believe the deep investing fascia exists in most of these hypoplastic legs, but is of poorer quality or, more commonly, disrupted by previous orthopaedic procedures. Blunt dissection in these patients is very important. Endoscopic dissection may be of value. Expansion is required in almost all hypoplastic legs. It may require weekly injections for 2 to 5 months. Implantation can be carried out to balance the leg discrepancy to a large degree (Fig. 65D-1A,B).

L. N. Carlsen: Department of Plastic Surgery, Scarborough Hospital General Division, Scarborough, Toronto, Ontario and Department of Surgery, McMaster University, Hamilton, Ontario, Canada

NERVE AND MUSCLE COMPRESSION

Overimplantation can lead to a compression syndrome or myonecrosis.

In our series, one patient developed anterior compartment syndrome with footdrop. The implant was removed and the fascia and skin split the full length of the leg. She regained total function, but is left with a scar the full length of her leg. This complication occurred because the external dressing became too tight. The night of surgery, the dressing on the other leg was released and that leg had no sequela.

A bodybuilder who had undergone four-quadrant augmentation developed severe pain and edema in one leg 36 hours postoperatively. Compartment pressure recordings did not indicate a compression syndrome, but the implants still were removed and the deep fascia split internally. The patient developed some muscle necrosis and the leg drained for 3 weeks. To my knowledge, he has regained full function.

I believe that if a patient has severe pain within 24 hours with the leg at rest, then removal of the implant should be contemplated. Do not wait 4 days. Expansion can be carried out with a later implantation.

In the cases I was consulted about or that I reviewed because of disputes, the most common offense was insertion of

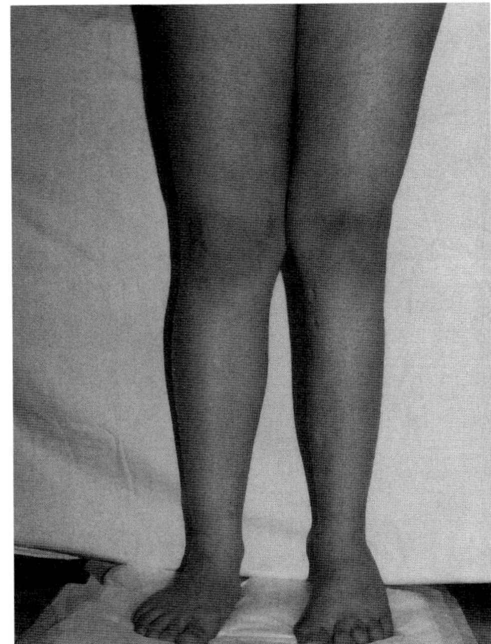

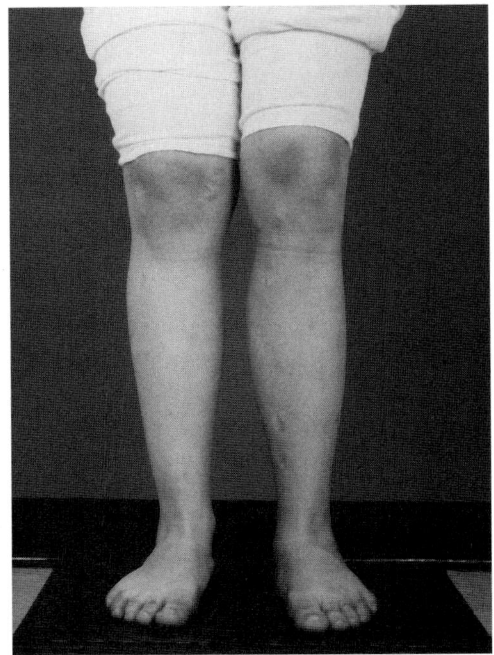

FIGURE 65D-1. A,B: Implantation carried out to balance the large degree of leg discrepancy.

too large an implant leading to pressure problems. If in doubt, take it out.

IMPLANT PROBLEMS

The first six implants I inserted were carved from a block of Silastic foam (Fig. 65D-2), as silicone rubber and gel implants were not available at that time. Contraction of these implants was observed, and one that was removed 26 years later had shrunk to one-third its original size (Fig. 65D-3). In the mid-1970s and again in 1983 and 1984, we used gel implants that were manufactured by Dow Corning, McGahn, Heyer Schulte, and Surgitec. The manufacturers had problems with polymerization of the gel in these implants. Some of them broke down and had to be removed and replaced with silicone rubber implants. One silicone rubber implant disintegrated and had to be removed 12 years after insertion (Fig. 65D-4).

I prefer soft silicone rubber implants. The edges of the extra soft implants are difficult to insert flush and tend to curl under, thereby creating a space that leads to seroma formation. The hard silicone implants do not feel natural, but they are requested by some bodybuilders.

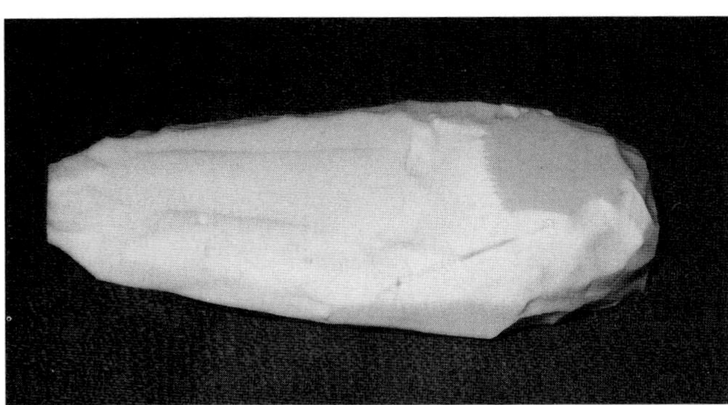

FIGURE 65D-2. An implant carved from a block of Silastic foam.

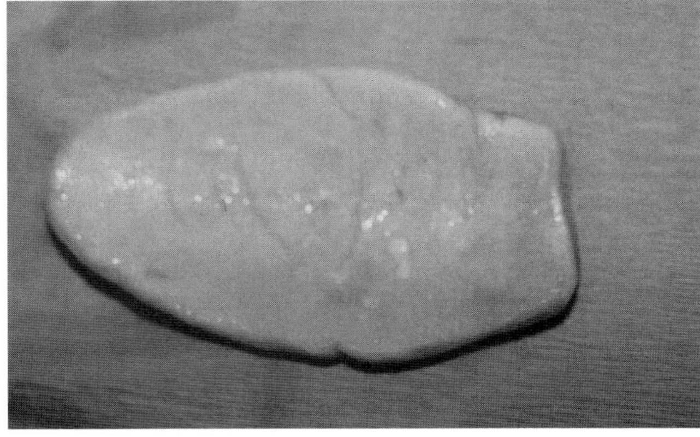

FIGURE 65D-3. Contraction of a Silastic foam implant, removed 26 years after implantation, that had shrunk to one-third its original size.

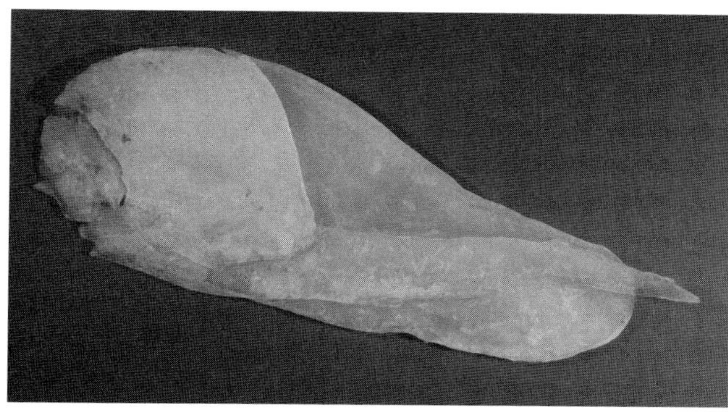

FIGURE 65D-4. Silicone rubber implant that had disintegrated and had to be removed 12 years after insertion.

BLEEDING AND HEMATOMA

Bleeding and subsequent hematoma formation has not been a problem in our bilateral cosmetic cases. The subfascial space is highly avascular. It is important not to violate the muscle. If the surgeon stays in the subfascial plane and uses blunt dissection, bleeding should not be a problem. I do not advocate putting the implant behind the muscle, as some surgeons do.

SEROMA

Seroma is the main complication caused by the implant moving away from the muscle; this creates a space that then fills with fluid. We believe it is important that the patient wear firm support hose for 4 weeks to prevent the implant separating from the muscle until the capsule forms to hold it in place. As Dr. Aiache pointed out, repeated aspiration is required until the space is closed.

Late seroma is an enigma. I had one patient develop seroma 18 years after implantation. I suspect it was probably on a traumatic basis. Computed tomographic scan showed buckling of the implant, with changes of implant shape.

One patient who had bilateral calf augmentation performed in 1976 developed a seroma in one leg that required nine aspirations. Twenty-two years later, she developed extensive calcification of the capsule on that side but not the contralateral side. She had bilateral implant and calcification debris removal.

Infection has not been a problem in our series, but it has been covered extensively by Dr. Aiache.

SUCTION-ASSISTED LIPECTOMY

The author has addressed the problem from his experience in fat removal of the thigh and lower leg. The lower leg is unforgiving in terms of contour deformities. The fat for removal is between the skin and the deep investing fascia, so this is the area that needs to be addressed.

Dr. Aiache does not address the problems that occur following medial thigh-plasty. The most common problem is drifting of the groin scar. To prevent this occurrence, the skin flap should be attached as securely as possible to the adduction tendon insertion and to the deep perineal fascia. The tension must be taken by these deep structures rather than the skin. This will prevent drifting of the scar but also distortion of the labia majora.

Troublesome posterior dog-ears can be avoided by gathering the skin upward toward the adductor tendon area. The wrinkling of skin will smoothen out with time. The scars that drift downward can be repositioned using the aforementioned technique 1 year after primary surgery.

SUGGESTED READINGS

Carlsen LN. Calf augmentation: a preliminary report. *Ann Plast Surg* 1979;2:508–510.

Aiache AE. Calf implantation. *Plast Reconstr Surg* 1989;89:488–493.

Montellano L. Calf augmentation. *Ann Plast Surg* 1991;27:429–438.

von Szalay L. Calf augmentation: a new calf prosthesis. *Plast Reconstr Surg* 1985;75:83–87.

Serra JM, Mesa F, Paloma V, Ballesteros A. Use of calf prosthesis and tissue expansion in aesthetic reconstruction of the leg. *Plast Reconstr Surg* 1992;89:684–688.

Kon M, Baert CM, de Lange MY. Thigh augmentation. *Ann Plast Surg* 1995;35:519–521.

Cocke WM, Ricketson G. Gluteal augmentation. *Plast Reconstr Surg* 1973;52:93.

Vergara R, Marcos M. Intramuscular gluteal implants. *Aesthetic Plast Surg* 1996;20:259–262.

Hallock GG. Myonecrosis as a sequela of calf implants. *Ann Plast Surg* 1993;30:456–458.

SUBJECT INDEX

Page numbers followed by *f* indicate figures; page numbers followed by *t* indicate tables

B

C

F

G

H

J

M

N

Q

R

S

U

V

W

X

Z